DESIGNED FOR THE MAINTENANCE OF GOOD NUTRITION OF PRACTICALLY ALL HEALTHY PEOPLE IN THE UNITED STATES

Water-Soluble Vitamins							Minerals						
Vitamin C (mg)	Thiamin (mg)	Riboflavin (mg)	Niacin (mg NE)	Vitamin B_6 (mg)	Folate (μg)	Vitamin B_{12} (μg)	Calcium (mg)	Phosphorus (mg)	Magnesium (mg)	Iron (mg)	Zinc (mg)	Iodine (μg)	Selenium (μg)
30	0.3	0.4	5	0.3	25	0.3	400	300	40	6	5	40	10
35	0.4	0.5	6	0.6	35	0.5	600	500	60	10	5	50	15
40	0.7	0.8	9	1.0	50	0.7	800	800	80	10	10	70	20
45	0.9	1.1	12	1.1	75	1.0	800	800	120	10	10	90	20
45	1.0	1.2	13	1.4	100	1.4	800	800	170	10	10	120	30
50	1.3	1.5	17	1.7	150	2.0	1,200	1,200	270	12	15	150	40
60	1.5	1.8	20	2.0	200	2.0	1,200	1,200	400	12	15	150	50
60	1.5	1.7	19	2.0	200	2.0	1,200	1,200	350	10	15	150	70
60	1.5	1.7	19	2.0	200	2.0	800	800	350	10	15	150	70
60	1.2	1.4	15	2.0	200	2.0	800	800	350	10	15	150	70
50	1.1	1.3	15	1.4	150	2.0	1,200	1,200	280	15	12	150	45
60	1.1	1.3	15	1.5	180	2.0	1,200	1,200	300	15	12	150	50
60	1.1	1.3	15	1.6	180	2.0	1,200	1,200	280	15	12	150	55
60	1.1	1.3	15	1.6	180	2.0	800	800	280	15	12	150	55
60	1.0	1.2	13	1.6	180	2.0	800	800	280	10	12	150	55
70	1.5	1.6	17	2.2	400	2.2	1,200	1,200	320	30	15	175	65
95	1.6	1.8	20	2.1	280	2.6	1,200	1,200	355	15	19	200	75
90	1.6	1.7	20	2.1	260	2.6	1,200	1,200	340	15	16	200	75

Retinol equivalents. 1 retinol equivalent = 1 μg retinol or 6 μg β-carotene.

[d]As cholecalciferol. 10 μg cholecalciferol = 400 IU of vitamin D.

[c]α-Tocopherol equivalents. 1 mg d-α tocopherol = 1 α-TE.

[f]1 NE (niacin equivalent) is equal to 1 mg of niacin or 60 mg of dietary tryptophan.

ESTIMATED SAFE AND ADEQUATE DAILY DIETARY INTAKES OF SELECTED VITAMINS AND MINERALS[a]

		Vitamins	
Category	Age (years)	Biotin (μg)	Pantothenic Acid (mg)
Infants	0-0.5	10	2
	0.5-1	15	3
Children and adolescents	1-3	20	3
	4-6	25	3-1
	7-10	30	4-5
	11+	30-100	4-7
Adults		30-100	4-7

		Trace Elements[b]				
Category	Age (years)	Copper (mg)	Manganese (mg)	Fluoride (μg)	Chromium (μg)	Molybdenum (mg)
Infants	0-0.5	0.4-0.6	0.3-0.6	0.1-0.5	10-40	15-30
	0.5-1	0.6-0.7	0.6-1.0	0.2-1.0	20-60	20-40
Children and adolescents	1-3	0.7-1.0	1.0-1.5	0.5-1.5	20-80	25-50
	4-6	1.0-1.5	1.5-2.0	1.0-2.5	30-120	30-75
	7-10	1.0-2.0	2.0-3.0	1.5-2.5	50-200	50-150
	11+	1.5-2.5	2.0-5.0	1.5-2.5	50-200	75-250
Adults		1.5-3.0	2.0-5.0	1.5-4.0	50-200	75-250

*Because there is less information on which to base allowances, these figures are not given in the main table of RDA and are provided here in the form of ranges of recommended intakes.

*Since the toxic levels for many trace elements may be only several times usual intakes, the upper levels for the trace elements given in this table should not be habitually exceeded.

PERSPECTIVES IN NUTRITION

GORDON M. WARDLAW, Ph.D., R.D., L.D.
The Ohio State University

PAUL M. INSEL, Ph.D.
Stanford University School of Medicine

SECOND EDITION

with 305 illustrations created by Medical and Scientific Illustration:

WILLIAM C. OBER, M.D.
CLAIRE GARRISON, R.N., B.A.

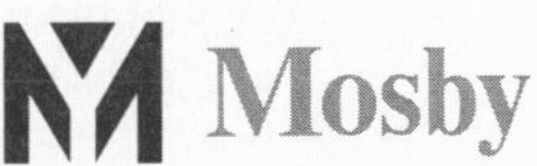

St. Louis Baltimore Boston Chicago London Philadelphia Sydney Toronto

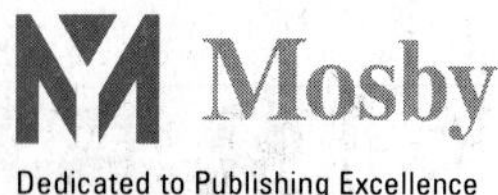

Dedicated to Publishing Excellence

Editor-in-Chief: James M. Smith
Acquisitions Editor: Vicki Malinee
Developmental Editor: Loren M. Stevenson
Project Manager: Karen Edwards
Production Editor: Cindy Miller
Designer: Liz Fett

SECOND EDITION

Printed in the United States of America

Mosby–Year Book, Inc.
11830 Westline Industrial Drive
St. Louis, Missouri 63146

Library of Congress Cataloging-in-Publication Data
Wardlaw, Gordon M.
Perspectives in nutrition / Gordon M. Wardlaw, Paul M. Insel ; illustrations by William C. Ober, Claire Garrison.—2nd ed.
p. cm
Previously published: 1990.
Includes bibliographical references and index.
ISBN 0-8016-6570-1
1. Nutrition. I. Insel, Paul M. II. Title.
QP141.W38 1992
613.2—dc20 92-30682
CIP

93 94 95 96 97 GW/CD/VH 9 8 7 6 5 4 3 2 1

CONTENTS

PART ONE
Nutrition Basics

PART TWO
The Energy-Yielding Nutrients

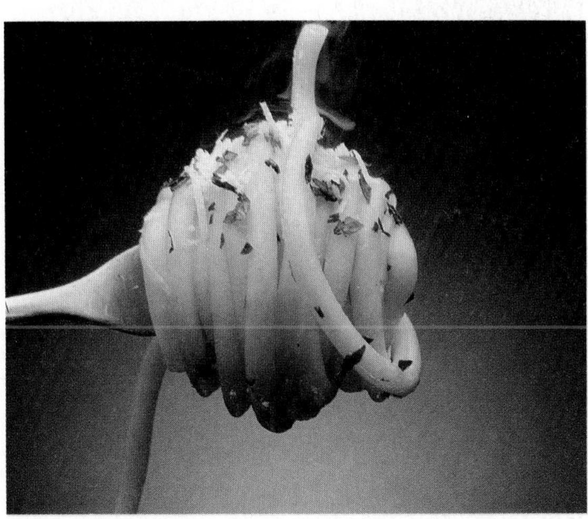

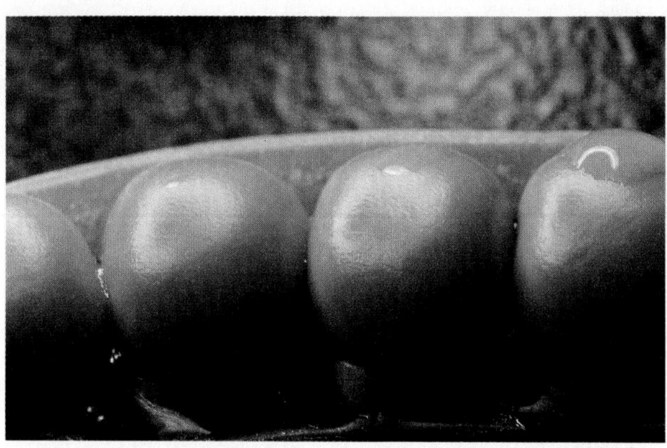

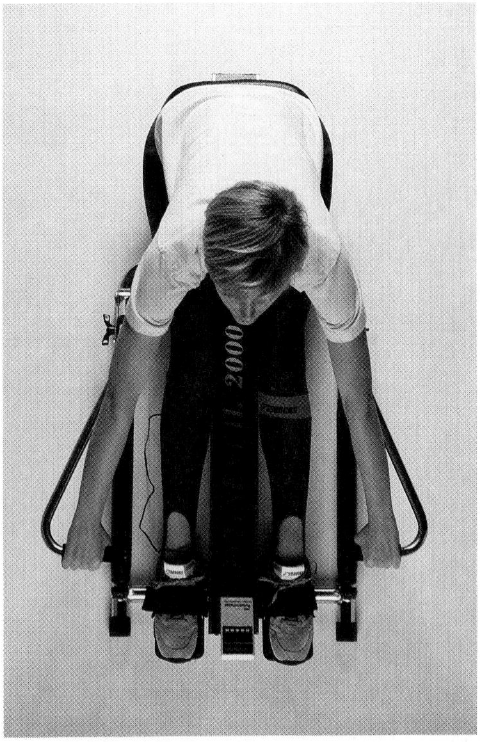

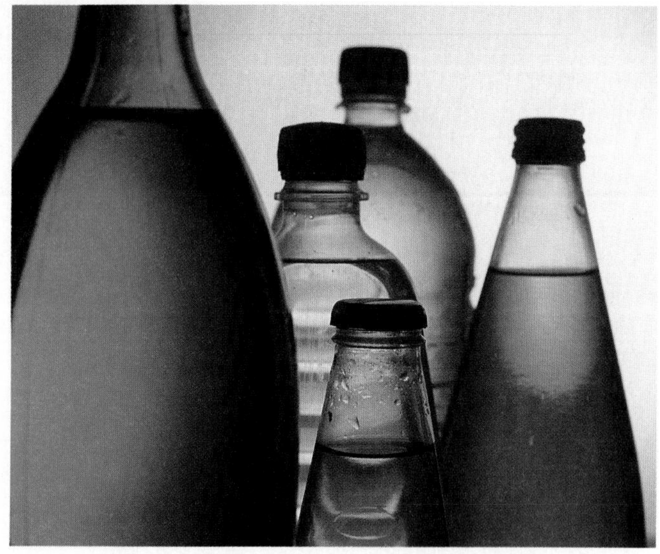

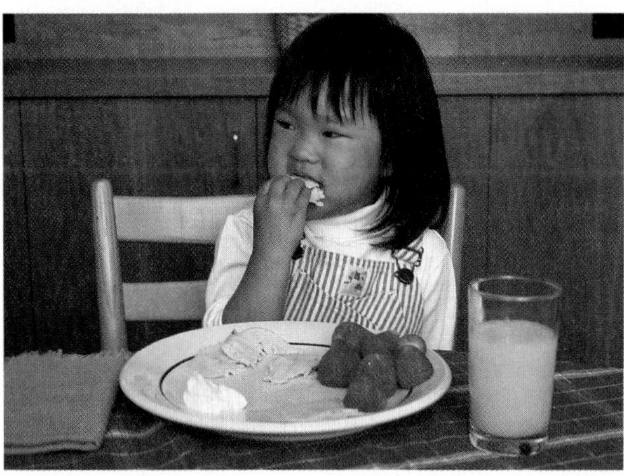

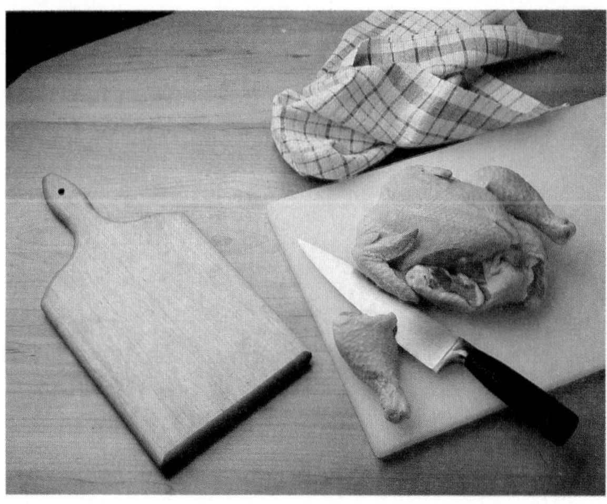

ABOUT THE AUTHORS

GORDON M. WARDLAW, Ph.D., R.D., L.D., teaches nutrition to a variety of students at The Ohio State University. Dr. Wardlaw is the author of numerous articles in prominent nutrition, biology, physiology, and biochemistry journals and was the 1985 recipient of the Mary P. Huddleson Award from the American Dietetic Association. Dr. Wardlaw is a full member of the prestigious American Institute of Nutrition and is certified as a specialist in Human Nutrition by the American Board of Nutrition.

PAUL M. INSEL, Ph.D., is currently Clinical Associate Professor of Psychiatry and Behavioral Sciences at Stanford University. He has been the principal investigator of numerous NIH studies, is the senior author of the leading introductory health text, and is Editor-in-Chief of *Healthline* magazine.

PREFACE TO THE INSTRUCTOR

As a professor, you undoubtedly already find nutrition a fascinating topic. However, it can also be quite frustrating to teach. Claims and counterclaims abound about the need for certain constituents in our diet, such as sodium. One group of researchers promotes a low sodium diet as an effective preventive measure for hypertension, while other groups state normal blood pressure values can be maintained in many of us even on our typical excess intakes.

We, too, are aware of conflicting opinions in our field, and so have continued to draw on as many sources as possible in the revision of this textbook. We have incorporated much new material, especially from the numerous supplements to the American Journal of Clinical Nutrition published in the last year. We also have consulted with a number of experts and continue to provide their insights on the current state of nutrition research.

We feel this textbook continues to make a break from all others in the field. Like other textbooks, it focuses on the latest research in nutrition but goes further to document important research studies throughout the chapters, list those references at the back of the chapters, and provide Expert Opinions in each chapter to reexamine the most controversial issues in the chapter. In all, we strive to provide you with many perspectives of current nutrition research so that you and your students can more clearly understand and take part in the debate of current nutrition issues.

Personalizing Nutrition

One overriding theme in nutrition research today is *individuality*. Not all of us find that saturated fat in our diets raises our blood cholesterol levels over recommended standards. We often respond in an idiosyncratic manner to nutrients, and that is something we constantly point out in this textbook.

Even at this basic level we do not try to put every nutrition student through the same square hole. We constantly ask students to learn more about themselves and their health status and apply the information in a manner appropriate to improving their own health. After reading this textbook, students will have a much clearer understanding of how the nutrition information given on the evening news, on cereal box labels, in popular magazines, and by government agencies applies to them. They will become learned consumers of nutrients and nutrition information, realizing that nutrition knowledge allows them to personalize the information rather than follow every guideline issued to a population—which by definition actually consists of separate individuals with separate genetic backgrounds and responses to diet.

In addition, we cover important questions that students often raise concerning vegetarianism, diets for athletes, the safety of our food supply, and fad diets. We emphasize the importance of behavior in terms of understanding one's food choices and changing one's diet. We discuss food behaviors in Chapter 1 and focus on behaviors that lead to obesity in Chapter 9.

Audience

This book has been designed for a diverse audience. It is most useful for students majoring in nutrition, the health sciences, home economics, nursing, physical education and other health-related areas, and premedical and predental students. However, due to the flexibility of chapter organization and content and outstanding student appeal, it can be adapted to students of diverse backgrounds. While not absolutely necessary, most students will find that having studied a course in biology, whether at the high school or college level, or having an understanding of basic biological concepts will provide a helpful background for taking the introductory nutrition course.

While the book is most suitable for a semester-length course, it can also be used in a quarter-length course by omitting chapters or skimming various sections. An important feature of this text is that it is presented in six segments:

PART ONE:	Nutrition Basics
PART TWO:	The Energy-Yielding Nutrients
PART THREE:	Energy Production and Energy Balance
PART FOUR:	The Vitamins and Minerals
PART FIVE:	Nutrition Applications in the Life Cycle
PART SIX:	Putting Nutrition Knowledge into Practice

This organization facilitates the ease of tailoring the text to your specific course needs.

New to the Edition

The second edition of *Perspectives in Nutrition* incorporates several new features to enhance student learning:

Two new chapters. Chapter 10, Nutrition for Fitness, exposes students to information on a key issue for the 1990s. In it, students will find a detailed discussion of energy metabolism and nutritional needs of athletes and active people. Chapter 20, Undernutrition Throughout the World, focuses on the seriousness of undernutrition in the United States and in other countries, and the conditions that create it. This chapter will provide students with the information they need to examine possible solutions and visualize hope for the future.

Minimal use of chemistry. An explanation of chemistry principles is presented in the appendix to help students with weak chemistry backgrounds. We use some chemistry concepts to help students more fully comprehend the nature of nutrient metabolism. Overall, this is kept to a minimum, and chemical structures are found primarily in the margins to be used at your option.

Later introduction of digestion and absorption. These topics are discussed after the energy-yielding nutrients. This enables students to obtain a good background in the basic concepts surrounding key nutrients before they learn how nutrients are digested and absorbed in the body.

Emphasis on behavior change strategies. Behavior change strategies have been integrated into Chapter 9, Weight Control, to encourage students to plan their own diets to enhance health maintenance. The strategies allow students to take the foundations of the course and apply them to daily life. Once students are able to put all the concepts into perspective, they can then set nutritional goals and change their diets accordingly.

Additional Features

We have organized this text in response to the needs of current instructors and students:

Content and controversial topics are well referenced. Approximately 80% of the referenced material is from sources published since the last edition in 1990. As instructors, we demand the latest information to present to our students. Providing this up-to-date research will not only give students the most accurate picture of nutrition today but will also point them to current materials for further study.

Separate chapters on energy balance, weight control, and anorexia nervosa and bulimia. The student receives a thorough discussion on these very controversial and current topics.

Emphasis on nutrient density. Discussions of nutrients are based on the most nutrient-dense sources of foods. Leading food sources in the U.S. diet are identified for each nutrient when those data are available.

Emphasis on the exchange system. An outline of the exchange system is presented in Chapter 2 and can be used or not used at your option. The use of the exchange system is reinforced in Chapters 3 through 5 and in the Student Study Guide and Nutrient Analysis Software that accompany the book.

Summary tables. Some chapters contain large detailed summary tables that include the major points made in the chapter. These tables provide convenient capsules for reference.

Design

Organizing the illustration program for this textbook has been quite exciting. We have drawn heavily from the biology and physiology expertise of Mosby–Year Book, Inc., and especially the illustrators, under the direction of William Ober, M.D. This textbook is far ahead of any in the field in depicting important biological and physiological phenomenon, such as cell membranes, emulsification, glucose regulation, digestion and absorption, the progression of cancer, and fetal development. The extensive, three-dimensional graphic presentations in this book will make nutrition and relevant physiological principles come alive for students.

In addition, we have drawn on many sources to provide what we consider the best photographic program in any nutrition text. The numerous four-color photos for this text were researched and selected to reflect a modern view of food presentation and food consumption. This provides the student with the most outstanding and timely view of the nutrition arena today.

Humor has been sprinkled throughout the text to aid the learning process. We have combed recent newspapers for the best work of our nation's leading cartoonists. The cartoons make important nutrition points in a way students will remember.

Pedagogy

The following extensive pedagogical features were designed not only to interest the student but also to constantly reinforce the learning process:

Nutrition Awareness Inventory. This set of 15 true/false questions serves to heighten awareness of chapter content. This feature also provides students with a gauge of how much they learned by repeating the quiz and comparing their scores. The answers are listed by chapter at the end of the book.

Margin notes. A liberal number of margin notes appear throughout the book. These notes provide clinical examples, references to other chapters, clarification of ideas, and further details for important concepts.

Margin definitions. Important key terms are boldfaced at first mention. More difficult terms include a definition in the text's margin. All boldfaced terms are included in the glossary at the back of the text.

Concept Check boxes. This material summarizes recent chapter content every few pages, providing the student with the opportunity to monitor his or her understanding of the material presented.

Nutrition Focus boxes. Each chapter contains one to two short boxed essays on often controversial topics in nutrition, such as bottled water and fat replacements.

Take Action boxes. This activity at the end of each chapter provides the student with an opportunity to put theory into practice. The suggested assignments are usually proactive and at times involve the student in an activity in which a registered dietitian or nutritionist may perform.

Summary points. Chapter content is summarized by highlighting seven to ten major points. This feature, together with the Concept Checks, should help students to study for examinations.

Suggested Readings. This feature helps students find interesting and timely articles.

Study Questions. Five questions at the end of each chapter encourage the student to probe deeper into the chapter content, making connections and experiencing new insights.

Up-do-date references. Each chapter contains approximately 30 current references, most published since 1988.

Nutrition Perspective boxes. This essay at the end of each chapter extends the chapter content by adding more detailed and controversial material.

Expert Opinion boxes. Each chapter contains an "Expert Opinion" written by a noted researcher. In most cases, the expert has received recognition from the American Dietetic Association or the American Institute of Nutrition.

Glossary. A comprehensive glossary of more than 500 words is included for the student's reference. The glossary also contains pronunciation inclusions for many unfamiliar terms.

Supplementary Materials

Both the student and the instructor are provided with the latest materials to make better use of the text and the concepts of the course:

Instructor's manual and test bank. Prepared by Margaret Kessel, Ph.D., R.D., L.D., this comprehensive teaching aid includes chapter summaries with suggestions for teaching difficult material; activities; suggested readings; nutrition assessments; conversion notes; source lists of supplementary materials; and a unique "Survival" chapter, addressed to the novice instructor, that discusses class organization, scheduling, and problem areas such as cheating.

Extensively reviewed for clarity and accuracy, the test bank features approximately 2000 test items (multiple-choice, short-answer, and matching) coded for level of difficulty, the kind of knowledge being tested, topic, and text page reference. Test items in each chapter follow the sequence of chapter discussions to make selection easy. The resource manual also includes 75 transparency masters of key illustrations from the text and other sources.

Computerized test bank. Qualified adopters of the text receive a computerized test bank package compatible with the IBM, Macintosh, Apple IIc, or Apple IIe microcomputers. This software provides a unique combination of user-friendly aids and enables the instructor to select, edit, delete, or add questions, and construct and print tests and answer keys. The Gradebook segment features computerized record-keeping, and class, test, or individual grade analysis displayed as bar charts. The Proctor segment allows instructors to set up student tutorials, using items from the test bank or specially written tests.

Study guide. Prepared by Gordon M. Wardlaw, this student aid has been thoroughly reviewed by experienced instructors and developed in consultation with a learning theory expert. This comprehensive guide reinforces concepts presented in the text and integrates them with study activities, such as the use of flash cards to reinforce key concepts. It features vocabulary review and sample examinations structured to reflect the actual examinations students will face in the classroom. An ongoing dietary analysis highlights the content of each chapter.

Nutrient analysis software. This interactive software includes a unique food list with more than 2250 items, selected activities, and food exchange lists. The disk allows students to input food intake and physical activities to determine total kcalories consumed and expended in a 24-hour period.

Transparency acetates. Seventy-two full-color transparency acetates feature key illustrations from the text with large, easy-to-read labels.

Acknowledgments

TEXT DEVELOPMENT

The authors wish to thank Ann Voss, Ph.D., R.D., Diane Cicenas, M.S., R.D., Jeffrey Harris, D.H.Sc., R.D., Margaret Kessel, Ph.D., R.D., Robert DiSilvestro, Ph.D., and Scott Madwar, B.S., for help in various stages of chapter revisions. We also thank Dr. Allan Burkett for his revisions to the chemistry review, Appendix B. Their insights contributed greatly to the final product, and we are greatly indebted to them.

REVIEWERS

As with the first edition, our goal is to provide the most accurate, up-to-date, and useful introductory nutrition text available. We would like to recognize and thank those people whose direction and insight guided us in the first and second editions.

For the second edition:

Paul Abernathy, Ph.D.
Purdue University

Ellen Brennan, M.S.
San Antonio College

Charlotte Britto, M.S.
San Joaquin Delta College

Thomas Castonguay, Ph.D.
University of Maryland
(Chapter 8)

Veryan Cumberbatch, M.S., R.D.
University of Kentucky

Robert DiSilvestro, Ph.D.
The Ohio State University

Hazel Forsythe, Ph.D.
University of Kentucky

Art Gilbert, Ph.D.
University of California-Santa Barbara

Jeffrey Harris, D.H.Sc., M.P.H., R.D.
West Chester University

Susan Houston, M.S.
City College of San Francisco

Carol Johnston, Ph.D.
Arizona State University

Murray Kaplan, Ph.D.
Iowa State University
(Chapter 7)

Robert Lee, D.H.Sc., M.P.H., R.D.
Central Michigan University

Lisa McKee, Ph.D.
New Mexico State University

Christopher Melby, D.H.Sc., M.P.H.
Colorado State University

Nina Mercer, Ph.D.
University of Guelph

Carol Mitchell, Ph.D., R.D.
Memphis State University

Cathy Rozmus, D.S.N., R.N.
Columbia State Community College

Anne Shaw
United States Department of Agriculture
(Chapter 2)

LuAnn Soliah, Ph.D.
Baylor University

Carol L. Thomas, M.A.
San Joaquin Delta College

Adrienne White, Ph.D.
University of Maine

Gregory Williams, Ph.D.
California State University—Fullerton

For the first edition:

Richard Ahrens, Ph.D., R.D.
University of Maryland

Kathy Beerman, Ph.D.
Washington State University

Wen Chiu, Ph.D.
Shoreline Community College

Sylvia Gartung, B.S.
Michigan State University

Catherine Justice, Ph.D., R.D.
Purdue University

Michael Keenan, Ph.D.
Louisiana State University

RoseAnn Kutschke, Ph.D.
University of Texas—Austin

Joseph Leichter, Ph.D.
University of British Columbia

Ricki Lewis, Ph.D.
State University of New York—Albany

Sandra Mitchell, Ph.D., R.D.
California State University—Chico

Jean Peters, M.S.
Oregon State University

Harry Sitren, Ph.D.
University of Florida

Joanne Slavin, Ph.D., R.D.
University of Minnesota

Anne Smith, Ph.D., R.D.
The Ohio State University

Linda Vaughan, Ph.D., R.D.
Arizona State University

A unique feature of this book is the "Expert Opinion" boxes. We would like to thank the following experts whose outstanding and insightful articles highlight this text:

Paul Addis, Ph.D.
University of Minnesota

Stephen Barrett, M.D.
Psychiatrist and Consumer Advocate
Allentown, PA

Robert DiSilvestro, Ph.D.
The Ohio State University

James Ferguson, M.D.
University of Utah

Constance Geiger, Ph.D., R.D.
University of Utah

Helen Guthrie, Ph.D., R.D.
The Pennsylvania State University

Al Harper, Ph.D.
University of Wisconsin (Emeritus)

John Hathcock, Ph.D.
Food and Drug Administration

Jeffrey Harris, D.H.Sc., R.D.
West Chester University

Jules Hirsch, M.D.
Rockefeller University

Murray Kaplan, Ph.D.
Iowa State University

Ann Kittlaus
Food Research and Action Center

David Klurfeld, Ph.D.
Wistar Institute of Anatomy and Biology

David Kritchevsky, Ph.D.
Wistar Institute of Anatomy and Biology

David Lamb, Ph.D.
The Ohio State University

James Leklem, Ph.D.
Oregon State University

Judy Loper, Ph.D.
Weight Loss Counselor
Columbus, OH

Donald McCormick, Ph.D.
Emory University

Gerald Reaven, M.D.
Stanford University

Ellyn Satter, M.S., R.D.
Family Therapy Center
Madison, WI

Bonnie Worthington-Roberts, Ph.D., R.D.
University of Washington

Special Acknowledgments

We would like to thank our developmental editor, Loren Stevenson, who nurtured and assisted us through every step of the revision. Vicki Malinee, Acquisitions Editor, and Jim Smith, Editor-in-Chief, facilitated the difficult decisions that frequently arose. Kathy Sedovic researched most of the oustanding photographs, and Cindy Miller provided excellent and careful copyediting and production work.

While this book was taking every free minute for the last two years, our children William and Elizabeth Wardlaw and Claire and Philip Insel had to sometimes wait for their fathers to finish the book in order to have their bedtime stories, go to the swimming pool, or walk the dog. The book originally began with a dream. The revision was fostered by the excitement that each improvement brought and has ended in the reestablishment of an innovative and exciting textbook that we feel continues to set a standard for introductory nutrition textbooks.

GORDON M. WARDLAW
PAUL M. INSEL

STUDENT PREFACE

Cholesterol, sports drinks, food labeling, bulimia, artificial sweeteners, vegetarianism, and *Salmonella* food-borne illness—we suspect you have heard these terms. Which of them are important enough to be a consideration in your life or the life of someone you know?

Americans pride themselves on being individuals. Nutritional advice should be given in that manner. Not all of us have high cholesterol levels, and so don't face the risk of heart disease. The need to tailor dietary advice to our individual nature is the basic philosophy behind this book. First, we give you a brief introduction to the study of nutrition and give you information on how to be a good consumer. With so much information floating around—both accurate and inaccurate—you will need to know how to make informed decisions about your nutritional well-being. Then, we encourage you to discover the basics of nutrition and how to apply the concepts in this book that specifically pertain to you.

We think you will find the study of nutrition fascinating. The text discusses some of the most interesting and important elements of nutrition and food consumption to help you understand both how your body works and how what you eat affects your health.

FEATURES

We have included some features in this book that you should find especially interesting and valuable:

Planning a new way of eating. Early in the text, we present many of the basic guidelines of planning a healthy diet, including a description of the USDA's new Food Guide Pyramid in Chapter 2. Later, in Chapter 9, we give you the steps involved in setting nutritional goals and designing a diet plan to attain these goals.

Understanding the world around us. In a college environment, it is often difficult to envision how real the problem of world hunger is. Chapter 20 examines the problem of undernutrition and the conditions that create it. The chapter allows you to examine possible solutions and visualize hope for the future of our world.

Chemistry review. In Appendix B, we discuss in detail the critical chemistry concepts you need to know for an introductory study of nutrition. Written by an expert, this information will give you a better understanding of how nutrients work and how nutrition information applies to you.

PEDAGOGY

Perspectives in Nutrition, second edition, incorporates some important tools (called pedagogy) to help you learn nutrition. The next few pages show how to use these to aid in your study of the material.

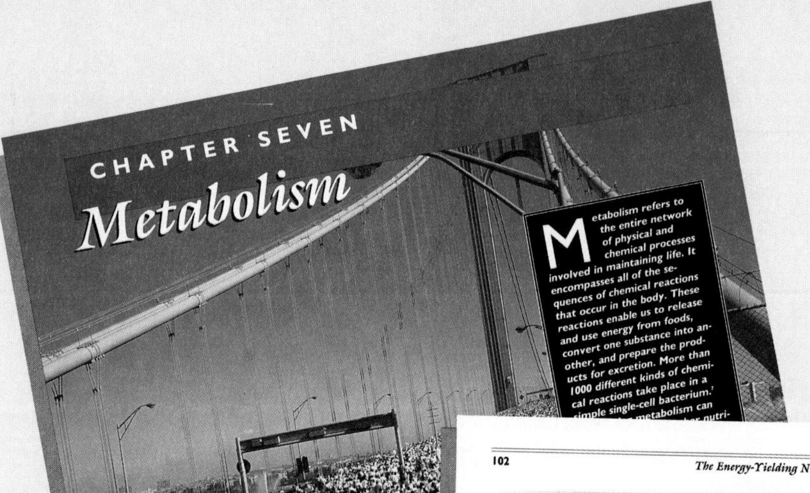

CHAPTER SEVEN
Metabolism
Metabolism refers to the entire network of physical and chemical processes involved in maintaining life. It encompasses all of the sequences of chemical reactions that occur in the body. These reactions enable us to release and use energy from foods, convert one substance into another, and prepare the products for excretion. More than 1000 different kinds of chemical reactions take place in a simple single-cell bacterium.

Each chapter begins with a Nutrition Awareness Inventory. This group of fifteen true/false questions helps you determine how much you already know about the chapter content. Take this examination again when you finish the chapter and you will see how much you have learned.

102 *The Energy-Yielding Nutrients*

NUTRITION AWARENESS INVENTORY

Here are 15 statements about lipids. Answer them to test your current knowledge. If you think a statement is true or mostly true, circle T. If you think the statement is false or mostly false, circle F. Use the scoring key at the end of the book to compute your total score. Take this test again after you have read the chapter. Compare the results.

1. T F Lipids composed of polyunsaturated fatty acids are liquid at room temperature.
2. T F A lipid has more kcalories per gram than carbohydrate or protein.
3. T F One's total serum cholesterol level is the most important blood test in assessing risk for heart attack and stroke.
4. T F Cholesterol is found only in the purely animal-derived foods we eat.
5. T F Animal fat is the major dietary factor that raises serum cholesterol levels.
6. T F Triglycerides are the main form of fat found in foods.
7. T F Fat is not absolutely necessary in our diet.
8. T F Hydrogenation makes vegetable oils more solid at room temperature.
9. T F Fruits and vegetables are essentially fat free.
10. T F Antioxidants provide protection from foods turning rancid.
11. T F The small intestine absorbs some vitamins better when dietary fat is present.
12. T F A blood cholesterol test is not necessary if you are age 40 years or less.
13. T F Butter and margarine contain about the same amount of fat.
14. T F Some of the fat present in fish is especially healthy.
15. T F Nondairy creamers are healthier for you than low-fat milk.

Structures and Forms of Lipids

You probably know lipids as fats and oils. At room temperature, fats are solid and oils are liquid. Referring to them both as lipids simplifies the terminology and makes considering a food's temperature irrelevant. Otherwise, butter can be an oil on a hot day and a fat on a cold day.

Lipids are a diverse group, but they share two main characteristics: (1) they all dissolve in chloroform, benzene, and ether, and (2) they are not soluble in water. Think of an oil and vinegar salad dressing; the oil is not soluble in the water-based vinegar. Lipids also contain fewer oxygen atoms per carbon atom than do carbohydrates, protein, or alcohol. There are few other characteristics that are common to all lipids. For example, compare the structures of lecithin and cholesterol as these are discussed in the following pages.

When we discuss lipid chemistry or metabolism, we will use the term lipid or the actual name of the compound, such as serum **triglycerides.** When we discuss lipids in foods, we will use the terms fats, or fats and oils. This usage is common today in health care settings.

FATTY ACIDS

The **fatty acid** is common to most of the lipids in the body and in foods. Its basic structure is a long chain of carbons bonded to hydrogen atoms. At one end of the molecule, called the alpha end, is an acid (specifically carboxyl) group (—C(=O)—OH). At the other end is a methyl group ($-CH_3$) (Figure 4-1). This is called the omega end. In the Greek alphabet, alpha means beginning and omega means end.

If all bonds between the carbons are single bonds, a fatty acid is called **saturated.** In other words all the carbons are saturated with hydrogens, like a sponge saturated with water. Animal fats are often high in saturated fatty acids. If a fatty acid has one carbon-carbon double bond, it is **monounsaturated.** Olive and canola oils have

saturated fatty acid A fatty acid with no carbon-carbon double bonds.

monounsaturated fatty A fatty acid containing one carbon-carbon double bond.

Throughout each chapter are boldfaced key terms. The more difficult terms will include a definition in the text's margins. All boldfaced terms will appear with their definitions and pronunciations in the glossary at the end of the text.

184 *The Energy-Yielding Nutrients*

Table 6-2 Summary of digestive enzymes

Secretion origin	Enzyme	Substrate	Major end products
Salivary glands	Salivary amylase	Starch, glycogen	Maltose and dextrins
Lingual glands	Lingual lipase	Short-chain triglycerides, medium-chain triglycerides	Fatty acids, monoglycerides
Stomach glands	Pepsin	Protein	Peptides, peptones
	Gastric lipase	Short-chain triglycerides, medium-chain triglycerides	Fatty acids, monoglycerides
Pancreas	Trypsin	Protein, peptides	Polypeptides, smaller peptides
	Chymotrypsin	Protein, peptides	Same as trypsin, more coagulating power for milk
	Carboxypeptidase	Polypeptides	Smaller peptides, free amino acids
	Pancreatic amylase	Starch, glycogen, dextrins	Maltose
	Lipase	Triglycerides	Monoglycerides, free fatty acids
Intestinal wall	Aminopeptidase	Peptides	Amino acids, smaller peptides
	Maltase	Maltose	Glucose
	Sucrase	Sucrose	Glucose, fructose
	Lactase	Lactose	Glucose, galactose
	Enterokinase	Trypsinogen	Trypsin

CARBOHYDRATE DIGESTION

Digestion of the large carbohydrates—starches—coming mostly from the flour in the banana bread begins as these mix with saliva during the chewing of food. Saliva contains an enzyme called salivary **amylase.** This enzyme breaks down starch (a chain of thousands of glucose units) into many small sugar units called maltose (merely two glucose units bonded together). You can observe this conversion by chewing a saltine cracker. Prolonged chewing of the cracker ... become more sweet as some starch is broken down ...

Salivary amylase ...

amylase Starch-digesting enzymes from the salivary glands or pancreas.

The numerous tables throughout the text provide convenient capsules of information for reference.

At the end of each chapter is a Take Action box that will help put major concepts in each chapter into focus for your own life. The activity may include looking more carefully at your diet, examining your family history, or applying information you've learned to others.

376 *The Vitamins and Minerals*

TAKE ACTION

Measuring your vitamin intake against the RDAs

This activity requires you to reexamine the nutritional assessment you did for Chapters 1 and 2. You recorded all the foods and drinks you consumed for 1 day and their quantities. Then you assessed your intake by recording the total amounts of nutrients you consumed. You were then asked to compare your nutrient intake to certain standards. Many of the standards you used were the 1989 RDAs found on the inside front cover of this book. Take your completed assessment and look at your intakes of vitamins A, E, C, B-6, B-12, and thiamin, riboflavin, niacin, and folate. Record these numbers in the table below. Next, record the RDAs for each of these nutrients off your assessment. Then, record the percentage of the RDA you consumed for each vitamin. Lastly, place a +, −, or = in the space provided reflecting an intake higher than, lower than, or equal to the RDA.

VITAMIN	INTAKE	RDA	% OF RDA	+, −, =
A				
E				
C				
THIAMIN				
RIBOFLAVIN				
NIACIN				
B-6				
FOLATE				
B-12				

ANALYSIS

1. Which of your vitamin intakes equaled or exceeded the RDA?

2. Which if your vitamin intakes were below the RDA?

3. What foods could you eat to improve your dietary intake of vitamins in low amounts in your diet? (Review sources of certain vitamins in this chapter and the next.)

222 *Energy Balance*

CONCEPT CHECK

In the process of losing an amino group, individual amino acids form carbon skeletons. Many carbon skeletons can be further metabolized so that they enter either the citric acid cycle or glycolysis pathway. If so, the carbons can be pushed through gluconeogenesis to ultimately form new glucose molecules. If the carbon skeleton enters metabolism as acetyl-CoA, glucose production is not possible. The amino groups go on to form part of urea. This is excreted from the body via urine.

The Concept Checks list the major points made in a chapter section. If you don't understand the Concept Check, you should go back and reread the preceding section to get a clearer understanding.

NUTRITION FOCUS

Alcohol Metabolism

Alcohol is still another substance that can supply energy for the body: 7 kcalories per gram. The liver metabolizes most of the alcohol consumed. A social drinker who weighs 150 pounds and has normal liver function metabolizes about 7 to 14 grams of alcohol per hour (100 to 200 milligrams per kilogram of body weight per hour).[6] This is about 8 to 12 ounces of beer or half an ordinary-sized drink. When the rate of alcohol consumption exceeds the liver's metabolic capacity, the blood alcohol content rises and symptoms of intoxication appear.

Pathways for alcohol metabolism

Alcohol at low doses first reacts with NAD to form the compound acetaldehyde. The enzyme used is alcohol dehydrogenase (Figure 7-10).[2] This enzyme requires the mineral zinc for activity. Acetaldehyde is then converted into acetyl-CoA. Both reactions yield an NADH molecule. The acetyl-CoA enters the citric acid cycle, and the NADH, $FADH_2$, and GTP molecules produced in the citric acid cycle can then be used to generate ATP.

In structure, the end of ethanol with the hydroxyl group (−OH) resembles a carbohydrate. But since it breaks down directly into acetyl-CoA, alcohol carbons cannot support glucose production. So alcohol is metabolized more like a fat than like a carbohydrate, and thus is considered a fat in metabolic terms.

When a person drinks a lot of alcohol, the enzyme alcohol dehydrogenase cannot keep up with the demand to metabolize all of it into acetaldehyde. For this and other reasons, another enzyme system in the liver begins metabolizing alcohol. This system is called the microsomal ethanol oxidizing system (MEOS).[2] The MEOS is usually used by the liver to metabolize drugs and other "foreign" compounds. The liver registers excessive molecules of alcohol as foreign compounds, and thus the MEOS kicks in. Once the MEOS is active, alcohol tolerance increases because the rate of alcohol metabolism increases.

There are two interesting aspects about this use of the MEOS. First, instead of forming NADH as does alcohol dehydrogenase, the MEOS uses NADPH, a compound analogous to NADH. Now, instead of yielding "potential" ATP molecules from the first step in alcohol metabolism, the MEOS uses "potential" ATP molecules. This helps explain why people with alcoholism do not gain as much weight as expected from the amount of kcalories they consume via alcohol. High doses of alcohol are inefficiently used by the liver because they require energy for the first metabolic step. The person with alcoholism basically wastes some alcohol kcalories by inducing this alternate metabolic pathway.[2] Liver damage from alcohol, such that other metabolic pathways are hampered, also is implicated in the loss of kcalories associated with high alcohol use.[1,2]

The use of the MEOS also increases the potential for an overdose of alcohol. While the MEOS system is metabolizing alcohol, it has a reduced capacity to metabolize drugs, such as many sedatives. If high amounts of alcohol and these sedatives are mixed, the user may lapse into coma and die. The liver is not able to break down the sedatives in the body fast enough. Alcohol itself is toxic in high quantities. Mix it with sedatives and an extremely toxic combination results. Nutrient deficiencies associated with excess alcohol intake also are likely. We discuss these possible negative health implications in detail in Chapter 18.

Alcohol is metabolized most like a fat as compared to carbohydrate or protein.

Nutrition Focus boxes allow you to explore timely topics that your instructor may not have time to cover, but that may be of interest to you.

Each chapter ends with Summary points. These points convey the major ideas in the chapter. We also include five Study Questions per chapter. Both of these elements provide an excellent review for studying for examinations.

We provide you with detailed References to back up material presented in the chapter. The research cited is from the most current publications—approximately 70% are from 1990 to present. If you are preparing a research paper for your class or would just like more information on specific topics, consult the Suggested Readings section at the end of each chapter for interesting and informative articles.

Summary

1. Some trace mineral deficiencies are difficult to detect in humans and were first observed in small geographically isolated groups or in patients on total parenteral nutrition. Eating a variety of foods maximizes your chances of consuming adequate amounts of trace minerals. Supplementing with trace minerals is potentially harmful, since so many questions remain regarding daily needs and interactions.
2. Iron is the only nutrient for which the RDA is greater in adult women than men because of women's iron losses that occur during menstruation. Iron absorption depends mainly on the form of iron present and the body's need for it. Heme iron from animal sources is better absorbed than the nonheme iron obtained primarily from plant sources. Consuming vitamin C simultaneously with iron will increase nonheme absorption.
3. The main function of iron is for synthesizing hemoglobin and myoglobin. It is also important in the synthesis of some enzymes, cytochromes, and in the action of the immune system. A prolonged low iron intake can lead to decreased production of red blood cells, and in turn reduced ability of the blood to carry sufficient oxygen. Such a condition is called iron-deficiency anemia and may result in fatigue, apathy, and decreased learning ability.
4. Foods rich in iron include beef, oysters, broccoli, and liver. Other sources are spinach and enriched breads and cereals. However, iron from plant sources is not well absorbed. Iron toxicity usually results from a genetic disorder called hemochromatosis. This disease causes overabsorption and accumulation of iron, which can result in severe liver and heart damage.

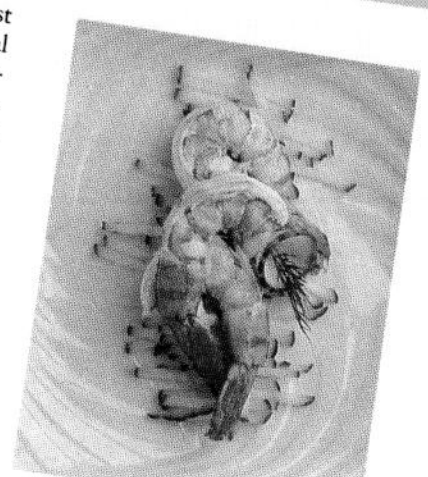

Study Questions

1. Minerals in the diet are likely to interact with each other. Provide two examples of this for trace minerals.
2. Describe how a "mucosal block" lessens the risk of developing an iron or zinc toxicity state.
3. Outline the histories of iodide and fluoride in human nutrition—from epidemiological observations to dietary intervention.
4. Relate the role of two nutrients to immune function, including at least one trace mineral.
5. Describe what is meant by a marginal deficiency state with respect to trace minerals. What two factors make studying this state of health difficult?

REFERENCES

1. Anderson RA and others: Supplemental-chromium effects on glucose, insulin, glucagon, and urinary chromium losses in subjects consuming controlled low-chromium diets, *American Journal of Clinical Nutrition* 54:909, 1991.
2. Anonymous: Manganese deficien... mans: fact or fiction? N... 46:348, 1988.
3. Black MR an... serum...
4. Castillo-Duran C, Uauy R: Copper deficiency impairs growth in infants recovering from malnutrition, *American Journal of Clinical Nutrition* 47:710, 1988.
5. Chandra RK: 1990 McCollum Award Lecture. Nutrition and immunity: lessons from the past and new insights into the future, *American Journal of Clinical Nutrition* 53:1087, 1991.
6. Clydesdale FM: The relevance of mineral chemistry to bioavailability, *Nutrition Today,* March/April 1989, p 23.
7. Cook JD and others: Calcium supplementation: effect on iron absorption, *American Journal of Clinical Nutrition* 53:106, 1991.

Continued on next page

EXPERT OPINION

Ergogenic Aids: Some Substances can Enhance Athletic Performance

DR. DAVID LAMB

Manipulating one's diet for better performance has a long history. As long as 80 years ago, American football players were encouraged on hot practice days to "toughen up" for competition by liberally consuming salt tablets before and during practice and by not drinking water. Now it is widely recognized that this practice can be fatal. Today's athletes are as likely as their predecessors to experiment—artichoke hearts, bee pollen, dried adrenal glands from cattle, seaweed, freeze-dried liver flakes, gelatin, and ginseng are just some of the worthless substances now used by athletes in hopes of gaining an "ergogenic" (work-producing) edge.

Still, modern-day athletes can benefit from recently-documented scientific evidence that a few dietary substances do have ergogenic properties. These ergogenic aids include sufficient water, lots of carbohydrate, and a balanced and varied diet that follows suggestions in the Guide to Daily Food Choices. Protein and amino acid supplements are presently not on the list. The average American apparently eats plenty of protein, athletes included.

Clearly, it is not possible to change average athletes into champions simply by altering diets. This means nutrient supplements require careful evaluation. Use should be designed to meet a specific dietary weakness, such as a poor iron intake. These and other aids whose benefit is often dubious and which nonetheless can pose health risks must be given close scrutiny before use. The risk-benefit ratio of these ergogenic aids especially needs to be examined. Athletes must stay on guard against false promises.

Carbohydrate loading

For athletes who compete in events lasting 90 to 120 minutes or longer or in shorter events repeated in a 24-hour period, it is often advantageous to undertake a **"carbohydrate-loading"** regimen to maximize muscle glycogen stores. One possible regimen includes a gradual reduction or "tapering" of exercise intensity and duration, coupled with a gradual increase in dietary carbohydrate as a percentage of energy intake. The procedure can begin 6 days before competition, with the athlete completing a hard workout lasting about 60 minutes. Workouts for the next 4 days then last about 40, 40, 20, and 20 minutes, respectively, with exercise intensities being progressively reduced each day. On the final day before competition, the athlete rests.

The dietary carbohydrate on the first 3 days of this regimen (about 450 grams) contributes 45% to 50% of energy intake. This rises to 65% to 75% carbohydrate (about 600 grams per day) for the last 3 days leading up to competition. This carbohydrate-loading technique usually increases muscle glycogen storage by 50% to 85% over usual conditions (i.e., when a typical amount of carbohydrate is consumed [46% of kcalories]). The greater carbohydrate stores then often result in improved athletic endurance.

A potential disadvantage to carbohydrate loading is that along with the glycogen, some water is also stored in the muscles. The water adds body weight and may cause muscle stiffness. For some people, this makes carbohydrate loading an unfeasible practice. Athletes considering carbohydrate loading should try it during training (and well before an important event) to experience its effects on performance. They can then determine if it is worth the effort.

Carnitine supplementation

The majority of the energy stored in the body for muscle use is found in fat. During physical activity, fatty acids are released from the fat depots into the bloodstream and travel to the muscles, where they are taken into each cell and "aerobically" broken down to carbon dioxide and water. These fatty acids must enter the cell's mitochondria before they can be broken down. The fatty acids are mostly transported from the fluid portion of the cell into the mitochondria using a transport system that contains a compound called carnitine. Athletes sometimes take carnitine supplements hoping carnitine will help them burn fat faster in exercise. But since our cells can make carnitine quite easily, carnitine supplements provide no reliable benefit.

Bicarbonate loading

We have noted that muscles that contract vigorously during athletic performance produce lactic acid. Lactic acid buildup inhibits the activity of enzymes involved in energy metabolism, and may lead to early fatigue. In the 1930s, athletes' attempts to counter this lactic acid accumulation by ingesting small doses of **sodium bicarbonate** (a base) failed to improve their athletic performances. On the other hand, more recent experiments using large doses of bicarbonate (300 milligrams per kilogram body weight) that were consumed 1 or 2 hours before exercise generally showed improved strenuous performance lasting 2 to 10 minutes. About 20 minutes of warm-up has typically preceded the exercise performance in these experiments. The bicarbonate loading apparently speeds the removal of lactic acid from contracting muscle cells and increases sodium levels in body fluids to help reduce acidity. Unfortunate side effects of large doses of sodium bicarbonate are nausea and diarrhea, often at unpredictable times. For this reason, bicarbonate loading has so far not become popular with athletes.

Caffeine supplementation

Drinking 2 to 4 cups of coffee (4 to 9 milligrams of caffeine per kilogram body weight) or using caffeine suppositories about 1 hour before an endurance competition (lasting more than 2 hours) enhances performance in some, but not all, athletes. The effect is less apparent in athletes who have ample stores of glycogen or are highly trained. The reason for the overall effect is not well established; sparing of muscle glycogen by increasing the use of fatty acids for muscle fuel, psychological effects, or enhancement of glycolysis in muscle all deserve consideration. However, some athletes experience changes in heart rhythm, nausea, or lightheadedness that can actually impair performance. Olympic officials view caffeine as a drug and do not condone its use. They consider a body level of caffeine exceeding the equivalent of 5 to 6 cups of coffee illegal.

In the Expert Opinion boxes, an expert in the field of nutrition and health outlines information you need to understand nutrition issues of our day. Consider these boxed discussions like "visiting speakers" coming into your classroom to inform you of the latest research findings.

Nutrition Perspectives are essays at the end of chapters that develop current topics in nutrition in greater detail than the chapter can. Topics include nutrition labeling, the effects of alcohol, nutrition and cancer, and heart disease.

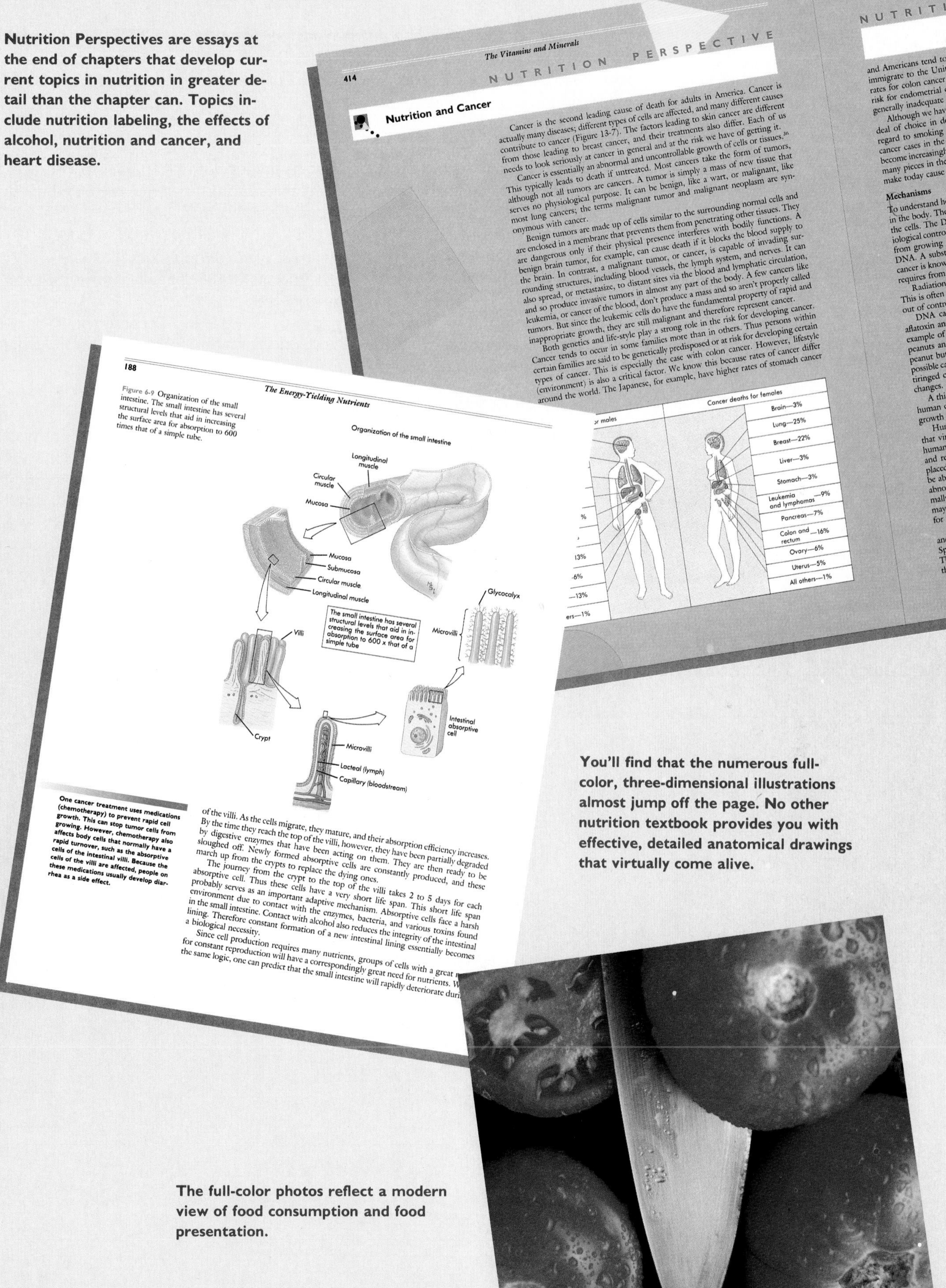

414 *The Vitamins and Minerals*

NUTRITION PERSPECTIVE

Nutrition and Cancer

Cancer is the second leading cause of death for adults in America. Cancer is actually many diseases; different types of cells are affected, and many different causes contribute to cancer (Figure 13-7). The factors leading to skin cancer are different from those leading to breast cancer, and their treatments also differ. Each of us needs to look seriously at cancer in general and at the risk we have of getting it.

Cancer is essentially an abnormal and uncontrollable growth of cells or tissues.[36] This typically leads to death if untreated. Most cancers take the form of tumors, although not all tumors are cancers. A tumor is simply a mass of new tissue that serves no physiological purpose. It can be benign, like a wart, or malignant, like most lung cancers; the terms malignant tumor and malignant neoplasm are synonymous with cancer.

Benign tumors are made up of cells similar to the surrounding normal cells and are enclosed in a membrane that prevents them from penetrating other tissues. They are dangerous only if their physical presence interferes with bodily functions. A benign brain tumor, for example, can cause death if it blocks the blood supply to the brain. In contrast, a malignant tumor, or cancer, is capable of invading surrounding structures, including blood vessels, the lymph system, and nerves. It can also spread, or metastasize, to distant sites via the blood and lymphatic circulation, and so produce invasive tumors in almost any part of the body. A few cancers like leukemia, or cancer of the blood, don't produce a mass and so aren't properly called tumors. But since the leukemic cells do have the fundamental property of rapid and inappropriate growth, they are still malignant and therefore represent cancer.

Both genetics and life-style play a strong role in the risk for developing cancer. Cancer tends to occur in some families more than in others. Thus persons within certain families are said to be genetically predisposed or at risk for developing certain types of cancer. This is especially the case with colon cancer. However, lifestyle (environment) is also a critical factor. We know this because rates of cancer differ around the world. The Japanese, for example, have higher rates of stomach cancer

188 *The Energy-Yielding Nutrients*

Figure 6-9 Organization of the small intestine. The small intestine has several structural levels that aid in increasing the surface area for absorption to 600 times that of a simple tube.

One cancer treatment uses medications (chemotherapy) to prevent rapid cell growth. This can stop tumor cells from growing. However, chemotherapy also affects body cells that normally have a rapid turnover, such as the absorptive cells of the intestinal villi. Because the cells of the villi are affected, people on these medications usually develop diarrhea as a side effect.

of the villi. As the cells migrate, they mature, and their absorption efficiency increases. By the time they reach the top of the villi, however, they have been partially degraded by digestive enzymes that have been acting on them. They are then ready to be sloughed off. Newly formed absorptive cells are constantly produced, and these march up from the crypts to replace the dying ones.

The journey from the crypt to the top of the villi takes 2 to 5 days for each absorptive cell. Thus these cells have a very short life span. This short life span probably serves as an important adaptive mechanism. Absorptive cells face a harsh environment due to contact with the enzymes, bacteria, and various toxins found in the small intestine. Contact with alcohol also reduces the integrity of the intestinal lining. Therefore constant formation of a new intestinal lining essentially becomes a biological necessity.

Since cell production requires many nutrients, groups of cells with a great n... for constant reproduction will have a correspondingly great need for nutrients. W... the same logic, one can predict that the small intestine will rapidly deteriorate duri...

You'll find that the numerous full-color, three-dimensional illustrations almost jump off the page. No other nutrition textbook provides you with effective, detailed anatomical drawings that virtually come alive.

The full-color photos reflect a modern view of food consumption and food presentation.

A Student Study Guide and nutrient analysis software are available to you with *Perspectives in Nutrition,* second edition. These instructional aids are designed to help you practice the major concepts developed in each chapter and prepare for classroom examinations.

STUDENT STUDY GUIDE

Reviewed by instructors and developed in consultation with a learning theory expert, this valuable Study Guide by Gordon Wardlaw reinforces concepts presented in the text and integrates them with activities to facilitate learning.

- Sample examinations reflect the actual tests you will face in the classroom.
- Vocabulary reviews increase your knowledge of the terminology.
- Flash cards help you review the major concepts in the chapter, and in turn test your understanding of these important concepts.
- Activities include fill-in tables, labeling, and matching terms. These activities follow the text discussion and are anchored with quotations and page citations from the text. An ongoing dietary analysis highlights the content of many chapters.

NUTRIENT ANALYSIS SOFTWARE

Created by N-Squared Computing, the nutrient analysis software is designed to help you quickly calculate the nutrient content of your diet, learn more about the exchange system, and calculate how many kcalories you use each day. You will find that learning to use this software will help you analyze your diet more efficiently.

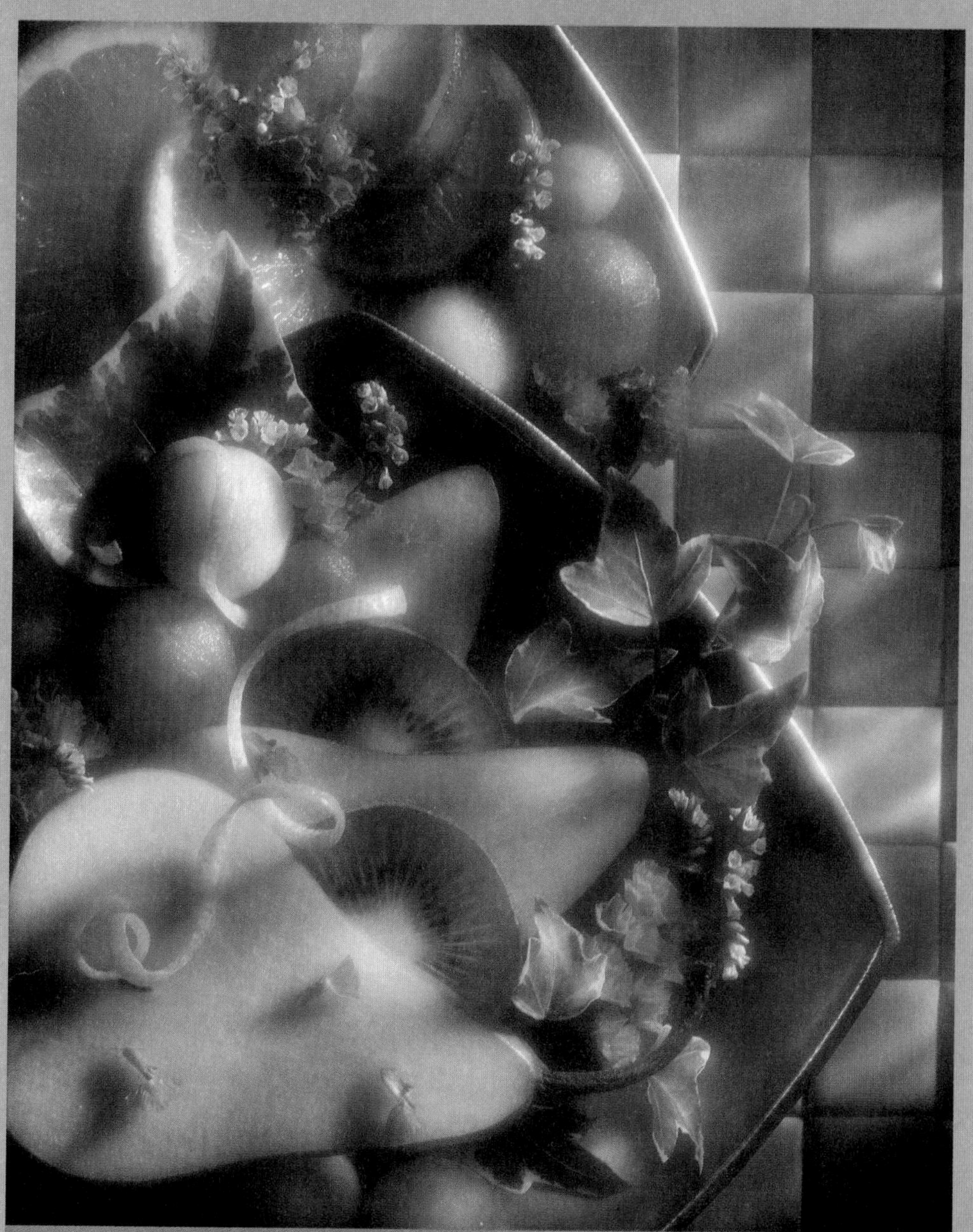

PART ONE
Nutrition Basics

CHAPTER ONE

What Nourishes You?

We are continually bombarded with information about nutrition and health. Almost daily, the news media report new studies showing how diet affects our well-being. The best-seller list usually contains at least one book about diet and health. Bookstores display rows and rows of books telling us what to eat and what to avoid. We're constantly getting mixed messages, which are confusing. Worse, some diet "experts" encourage us to follow unbalanced and gimmicky diets. They try to exploit a concerned public seeking information on diet that gives shortcuts to health and beauty.

Turning to a more knowledgeable source, the 1988 Surgeon General's Report on Nutrition and Health *reminds us that "for the two out of three adult Americans who do not smoke and do not drink excessively, one personal choice seems to influence long-term health prospects more than any other: what we eat."[19] Some of us have nutritional lifestyles that are out of balance with our physiology. And since we live longer than our ancestors did, we have to focus more on preventing nutrition-related diseases.[6]*

By changing our "problem" food habits, we can strive to bring the goal of optimum health within reach. This is a theme, not only for this chapter, but for this book as well.

NUTRITION AWARENESS INVENTORY

Here are 15 statements about nutrition and food habits. Answer them to test your current knowledge. If you think the answer is true or mostly true, circle T. If you think the answer is false or mostly false, circle F. Use the scoring key at the end of the book to compute your total score. Take this test again after you have read this chapter. Compare the results.

1. T F Many foods are mostly water.
2. T F Minerals can be broken down into vitamins in the body.
3. T F The terms kcalories and calories can be used interchangeably; both are correct.
4. T F Fats yield more energy per gram than do carbohydrates.
5. T F Vitamins directly provide energy to the body.
6. T F Nutritional stores refer to nutrients your body can call upon when needed.
7. T F The body generally requires greater daily amounts of vitamins than minerals.
8. T F One gram of water can provide 1 kcalorie of energy when metabolized by the body.
9. T F The term organic is similar to the term organic gardening.
10. T F When referring to nutritional states of health, the terms undernutrition and malnutrition can be used interchangeably.
11. T F Fatigue and poor body temperature control can be signs of an advanced iron deficiency.
12. T F Problems of overnutrition are more common than those associated with undernutrition in our society.
13. T F Vitamin and mineral supplements in any dose are safe to use.
14. T F Alcoholic beverages provide a large source of energy for some people.
15. T F Food choices are most often determined by nutrition knowledge.

The Importance of Exploring Your Own Food Habits

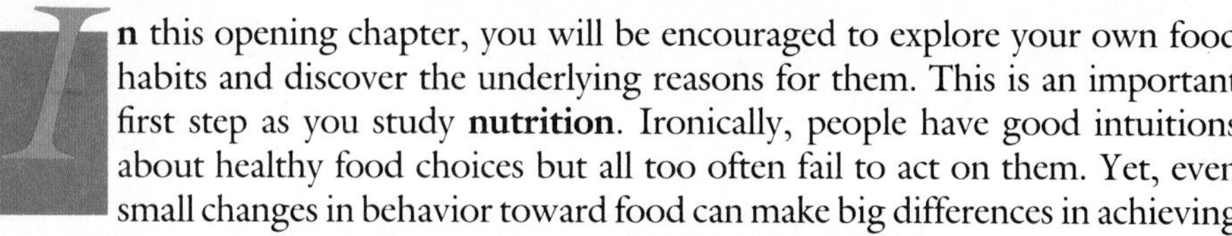

In this opening chapter, you will be encouraged to explore your own food habits and discover the underlying reasons for them. This is an important first step as you study **nutrition**. Ironically, people have good intuitions about healthy food choices but all too often fail to act on them. Yet, even small changes in behavior toward food can make big differences in achieving a long and vigorous life. The more you know about both nutrition and your health risks, the better you can plan a diet to meet your nutritional needs.

Recent evidence suggests that a poor diet is a **risk factor** for the major **chronic** diseases that are the leading causes of adult death: **heart disease, stroke, hypertension, diabetes mellitus**, and some types of **cancer**. Together, these disorders account for two thirds of all deaths in America. In addition, **cirrhosis** of the liver, accidents, and suicides are associated with excessive alcohol consumption as shown in Table 1-1. All of these consequences of modern living are partly an "affliction of affluence."[16] The great tragedy here is that much of this illness is preventable. An understanding of nutrition and the role it plays in your short-term and long-term health can significantly minimize your risks for these diseases.

nutrition The Council on Food and Nutrition of the American Medical Association defines nutrition as "the science of food; the nutrients and the substances therein; their action, interaction, and balance in relation to health and disease; and the process by which the organism (i.e., body) ingests, digests, absorbs, transports, utilizes, and excretes food substances."

heart disease A disease characterized by the deposition of fatty material in the blood vessels in the heart. This restricts blood flow through the heart and can in turn lead to heart damage and death.

diabetes mellitus Diabetes mellitus is a disease characterized by high blood sugar levels due to poor insulin (a hormone) action. It is commonly referred to as just diabetes in typical usage.

nutrients Chemical substances in food that nourish the body by providing energy, building materials, and factors to regulate needed chemical reactions.

WHAT ACTUALLY DOES NUTRITION REPRESENT?

The Council on Food and Nutrition of the American Medical Association defines nutrition as "the science of food, the nutrients and the substances therein, their action, interaction, and balance in relation to health and disease, and the process by which the organism ingests, digests, absorbs, transports, utilizes, and excretes food substances."

To begin your study of this process we call nutrition, we must start at the foundation—the **nutrients** themselves. We will first examine the nutrients and their function in the body. This especially sets the stage for understanding the basis behind the food plans discussed in Chapter 2. Then we will discuss how to assess a person's nutritional health and introduce the four chief components used in evaluating a

Table 1-1 Ten leading causes of death in the United States (1990)

Rank order	Cause of death	Percent of total deaths
...	All causes	100.0
1	Diseases of heart*	34
2	Malignant neoplasms, including neoplasms of lymphatic and hematopoietic tissues (cancer)*	23
3	Cerebrovascular diseases (stroke)*	7
4	Accidents and adverse effects†	4
...	Motor vehicle accidents	2
...	All other accidents and adverse effects	2
5	Chronic obstructive pulmonary diseases and allied conditions (lung diseases)	4
6	Pneumonia and influenza	4
7	Diabetes mellitus*	2
8	Suicide†	1
9	Homicide and legal intervention†	1
10	Chronic liver disease and cirrhosis†	1

NOTE: Acquired immune deficiency syndrome (AIDS) is ranked no. 11.
Modified from National Center for Health Statistics: Annual Summary 39(13), 1990.
*Causes of death in which diet plays a part.
†Causes of death in which excessive alcohol consumption plays a part.

person's nutritional status. The "health" status of the American diet will be described. Finally, we will discuss the factors that influence our food habits.

Nutrients Come from Food

Food, water, and oxygen are the life-giving and life-sustaining substances we need. Food provides you with both the energy and materials needed to build and maintain all your body cells.

It is important to distinguish between food and nutrients. Food is the source of nutrients. Nutrients are the nourishing substances in food that are **essential** for the growth of the infant, the development that leads to adulthood, and the maintenance of body functions throughout life. In this context, the term *essential* means that if a nutrient is left out of a diet, aspects of human health decline. If the nutrient is later added back to the diet before permanant damage occurs, those aspects of human health hampered by lack of the nutrient return to normal function. In other words, the lost aspects of health are restored when the essential nutrient is now consumed.

essential nutrient In nutritional terms, this represents a substance which, when left out of a diet, leads to signs of poor health. The body either can't make these nutrients or can't make them fast enough for its needs.

CLASSES OF NUTRIENTS

The nutrients in food can be organized into six classes (Table 1-2). First there are the energy-yielding nutrients, which, excluding water, constitute the major portion of most foods:

1. **Carbohydrates** are composed of mainly carbon, hydrogen, and oxygen. Carbohydrates provide a major source of fuel for the body. Small carbohydrate forms are called sugars or simple sugars. Table sugar is an example. Simple sugars, such as **glucose**, can chemically link together to form large storage carbohydrates called complex carbohydrates. An example is the **starch** in potatoes.

   Sugars impart sweetness to many foods we eat. Aside from enjoying this taste, we need sugars and other carbohydrates in our diets primarily to satisfy the

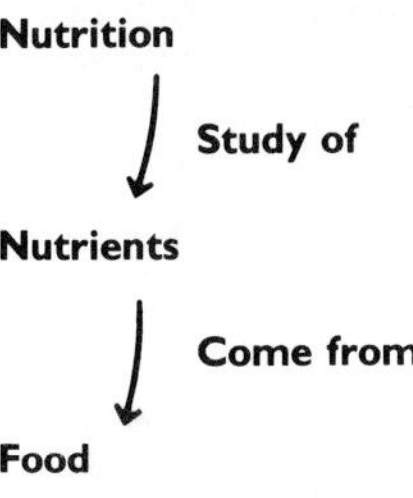

Table 1-2 Essential nutrients* in the human diet and their categories

Energy nutrients			
Carbohydrate	**Fat (lipid)†**	**Protein (amino acid)**	**Vitamins Fat-soluble**
Glucose‡ (or a carbohydrate that yields glucose)	Linoleic acid (omega-6)	Histidine	A
	α-Linolenic acid (omega-3)	Isoleucine	D§
		Leucine	E
		Lysine	K
		Methionine	
		Phenylalanine	
		Threonine	
		Tryptophan	
		Valine	

	Minerals			
Vitamins water-soluble	**Major**	**Trace**	**Questionable**	**Water**
Thiamin	Calcium	Chrominum	Arsenic	Water
Riboflavin	Chloride	Copper	Boron	
Niacin	Magnesium	Cobolt	Nickel	
Pantothenic acid	Phosphorus	Fluoride ‖	Silicon	
Biotin	Potassium	Iodide		
B-6	Sodium	Iron		
B-12	Sulfur	Manganese		
Folate		Molybdenum		
C		Selenium		
		Zinc		

This table includes nutrients that the current RDA publication lists for humans. Some debate over the questionable and other minerals not listed exists.
*Dietary fiber could be added to the list of essential substances, but it is not a nutrient (see Chapter 3).
†The lipids listed are needed in only slight amounts, about 2% of total energy needs (see Chapter 4).
‡In order to prevent ketosis and thus the muscle loss that would occur as protein was used to synthesize carbohydrate (see Chapter 3).
§Sunshine on the skin also allows the body to make vitamin D for itself (see Chapter 12).
‖Primarily for dental health.

energy needs of certain body cells, such as red blood cells. When you do not eat enough carbohydrates to supply one particular sugar (glucose) to cells, your body is forced to make this sugar from proteins. However, a typical diet contains more than enough carbohydrate to prevent this from happening.

We begin digesting some of the starches in our diets as soon as we put them into our mouths. The process continues until starches and large sugars break down into single sugar molecules (such as glucose) to be absorbed into the bloodstream. The links between the sugar molecules in certain complex carbohydrates cannot be broken down by human digestive processes. These carbohydrates are part of what is called **dietary fiber**. These fibers then pass down the intestinal tract to provide bulk for the stool (feces) that is formed in the large intestine (colon). Chapter 3 focuses on carbohydrates.

dietary fiber Substances in food (essentially all from plants) that are not digested by the processes present in the stomach and small intestine.

2. **Lipids (mostly fats and oils)** are composed of mainly carbon and hydrogen whose structures can't dissolve (in other words, are not **soluble** in water). These can dissolve in certain organic solvents, such as ether and benzene. Note that

there are fewer oxygen atoms in lipids than in carbohydrates. This allows lipids to yield more energy per gram than carbohydrates, namely nine versus four. The main form of lipid in food is called a **triglyceride**. This is a key fuel for the body. Triglycerides also are the major form for energy storage in the body.

In most cases we will use the more familiar terms fats and oils, rather than lipids, in this book. But by definition, fats are solid at room temperature and oils are liquid. There are two basic types of fat found in food: saturated and unsaturated.

Certain unsaturated fats are essential parts of the diet. Their components help regulate some important body functions, such as blood pressure. They are also needed for synthesizing and repairing vital cell parts. You need only about 1 tablespoon of a common vegetable oil (such as that found in supermarkets) each day to supply the essential fats. The average American diet supplies about three times this amount.

Fats in food are a combination of both saturated and unsaturated fatty acids.The dominant type of fat present determines the fat's characteristics; for example, whether it is solid or liquid at room temperature. Plant oils tend to be unsaturated. This makes them liquid. Animal fats are often quite saturated, which makes them solid. Chapter 7 focuses on fats.

3. **Proteins** are composed of mostly carbon, nitrogen, oxygen, and hydrogen. The presence of nitrogen in the structure is a distinguishing feature of proteins. Proteins form a major part of the body structure. Muscles contain much protein. A major part of bone is protein. Important parts of blood, cell membranes, and components of the immune system come from proteins.

   The basic unit of protein structure is the **amino acid**; these join together to form proteins. Twenty common amino acids are found in food; nine of these are essential parts of an adult's diet. Chapter 5 focuses on proteins.

Appendix B reviews many basic chemistry concepts. If you are unfamiliar with chemistry terms, you will find that review quite helpful.

• • •

Two other classes of nutrients are vitamins and minerals. Again, aside from water, food is mostly a mixture of carbohydrates, fat, and proteins. While vitamins and minerals are vital to good health, they are needed only in small amounts in our diet and provide no direct source of energy for the body.

vitamins Compounds needed in very small amounts in the diet to help regulate and support chemical reactions in the body.

4. **Vitamins** exhibit a wide variety of structures and can contain carbon, hydrogen, nitrogen, oxygen, phosphorus, sulfur, and other atoms. The main role of vitamins is to enable many chemical reactions in the body to occur. Some of these reactions help release the energy trapped in carbohydrates, fats, and proteins. Remember, however, vitamins themselves provide no energy for us to use.

   Vitamins are divided into two groups: those that are fat soluble (vitamins A, D, E, and K) and those that are water soluble (vitamin C and the B vitamins). The individual vitamins found in each group often act quite differently. Under cooking conditions, water-soluble vitamins break down much more readily than fat-soluble vitamins. Water-soluble vitamins also are stored in the body to a lesser extent than fat-soluble vitamins. This in turn makes the fat-soluble vitamins much more likely to build up in excessive amounts in the body. This can cause illness. The vitamins are the focus of Chapters 12 and 13.

Although many of these nutrients perform life-sustaining functions, the essential nature of each one in terms of a diet is sometimes not that clear cut. Need is sometimes offset by the body's ability to compensate for a missing nutrient. This can be done in some cases by the body synthesizing its own supply. For example, the body requires a daily source of vitamin D, but the skin is capable of synthesizing its own vitamin D upon receiving sunlight. This reduces the daily need from dietary sources.

5. **Minerals** are structurally very simple, existing as groups of one or more of the same atoms. Although not clearly as complex as the vitamins, minerals nevertheless are critical players in nervous system function, metabolic processes, water balance, and structural (e.g., skeletal) systems. And again, minerals themselves yield no energy as such for our use. The degree to which the body requires certain amounts of the 20 or so essential minerals varies enormously. Thus they are divided into two groups: major minerals and trace minerals. The actual need for some trace minerals in the human body has yet to be determined. Minerals are the focus of Chapters 14 and 15.

minerals Elements used in the body to promote chemical reactions and form body structures.

Provide Energy	Promote Growth and Maintenance
carbohydrate	protein
protein	fat
lipids (fats and oils)	minerals
	water

Regulate Body Processes
vitamins
minerals

6. **Water,** chemically H_2O, nourishes in many ways. It is vital in the body as a **solvent** and lubricant, as a medium for transporting nutrients and waste, and as a medium for maintaining body temperature regulation. It is for these reasons, and the fact that the human body is approximately 60% water, that we require great amounts of it—about 2 liters (2000 grams or 8 cups) of fluid every day. Compare this to our daily need of less than 60 grams of protein (about 2 ounces) and less than 30 grams for the total of all vitamins and minerals.

   Water is not merely available from the most obvious sources; it is often the major component in foods, such as many fruits and vegetables (e.g., lettuce, grapes, and melons). The body even makes some water as a by-product of **metabolism.** Water is examined in detail in Chapter 14.

Because minerals and water do not contain carbon atoms bonded to hydrogen atoms, they are called **inorganic** compounds. The other nutrients contain carbon atoms bonded to hydrogen atoms and so are called **organic** compounds. These terms have nothing to do with organic gardening, but instead are based on simple chemistry concepts that we describe in Appendix B.

metabolism Chemical reactions in the body that allow for life.

inorganic Free of carbon atoms bonded to hydrogen atoms.

organic Contains carbon atoms bonded to hydrogen atoms.

alcohol Ethyl alcohol or ethanol (CH_3CH_2OH).

kcalorie The heat needed to raise the temperature of 1000 grams (1 liter) of water 1 degree Celsius.

Nutrients—Further Perspectives

Nutrients have three functions in the body: (1) they provide the many substances essential for life, including materials for building and maintaining the body; (2) they act as regulators for key metabolic reactions; and (3) they participate in reactions in a cell that ultimately provide the energy that is necessary to sustain life.

ENERGY SUPPLIES FOR BODY FUNCTIONS

We get the energy necessary to perform body functions and to do work from carbohydrates, fats, and proteins (and **alcohol** for some of us). Energy is held in the chemical bonds of these compounds. In Chapter 7 we discuss how that energy is released and used by cells.

The energy in food is often measured in terms of calories. A calorie is the amount of heat it takes to raise the temperature of 1 gram of water 1 degree **Celsius** (1° C, centigrade scale). Because a calorie is such as tiny unit of heat measurement—like a penny in relation to a $10 bill—we can more efficiently express food energy in terms of kilocalories, which are 1000-calorie units. A kilocalorie (**kcalorie** or kcal) is the amount of heat it takes to raise the temperature of 1000 grams (1 liter) of water 1° C. The abbreviation kcalorie (or kcal) is used throughout this book, although note the term *calorie* is commonly used in everyday life.

Today scientific journals often require the use of the term kilojoule (kjoule) instead of kcalorie to express the energy content of a food. One kcalorie equals 4.8 kjoules. A kjoule is a measure of work, not heat. It is the amount of work involved in moving 1 kilogram for 1 meter with the foce of 1 newton. Heat and work are just two forms of energy. Energy expressions in the form of either heat or work can be exchanged for each other. In kjoule units, 1 gram of carbohydrate equals 17 kjoules, 1 gram of protein equals 17 kjoules, 1 gram of fat equals 38 kjoules, and 1 gram of alcohol equals 29 kjoules.

DETERMINING THE KCALORIE CONTENT OF A FOOD

A bomb calorimeter is used to determine the number of kcalories in a food portion (Figure 1-1). The food is burned inside a chamber that is surrounded by water. As the food burns, it gives off heat. This raises the temperature of the water surrounding the chamber. The increase in water temperature seen after the food has burned indicates the number of kcalories the food contained. Any food can be burned in the calorimeter, but some foods must be dried first.

The bomb calorimeter provides values for the amount of energy that can be derived from carbohydrates, fat, protein, and alcohol. Specifically, carbohydrates yield 4 kcalories per gram, proteins yield 4 kcalories per gram, fats yield 9 kcalories per gram, and alcohol yields 7 kcalories per gram. These kcalorie figures have been adjusted for (1) **digestibility** and (2) those substances in food that will burn in the bomb calorimeter but that the human body cannot use for energy needs, such as waxes and some fiberous parts of plants.

digestibility The proportion of food substances eaten that can be broken down in the intestinal tract and absorbed into the bloodstream.

Once you know the gram quantities of these substances in a food, you can estimate the total kcalories in that food using the kcalorie values. For example, if a banana milk shake has 45 grams of carbohydrate, 7 grams of protein, and 10 grams

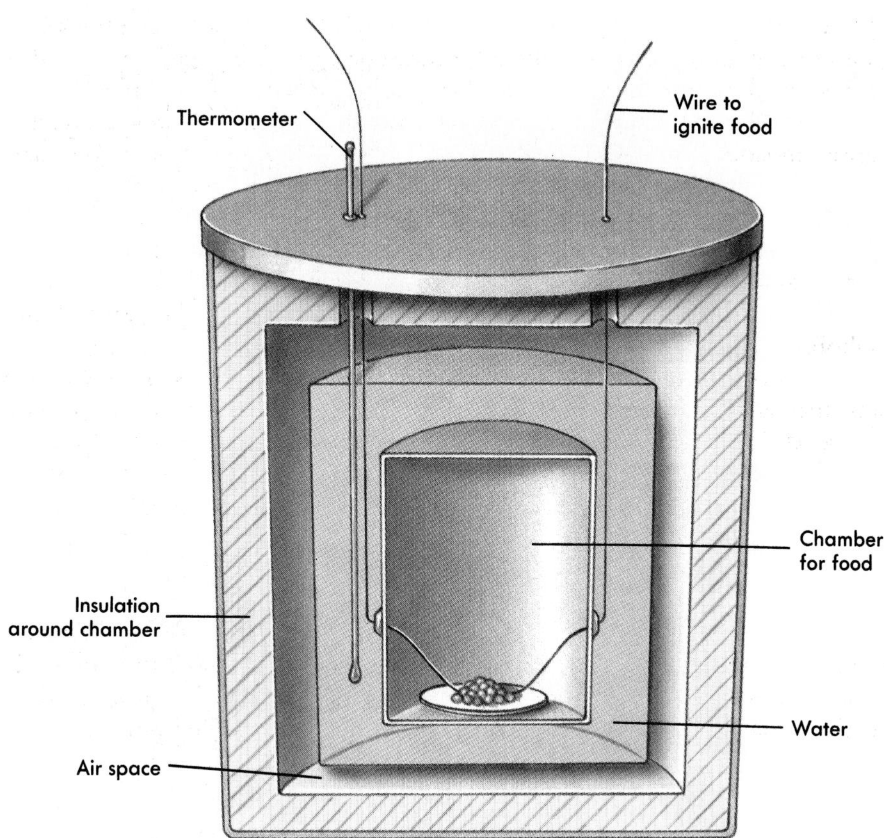

Figure 1-1 Cross-section of a bomb calorimeter. First, a dried portion of food is burned inside a chamber charged with oxygen that is surrounded by water. Then as the food is burned, it gives off heat. This raises the temperature of the water surrounding the chamber. The increase in water temperature indicates the number of kcalories the food contains.

of fat, it would contain 298 kcalories ($45 \times 4 + 7 \times 4 + 10 \times 9 = 298$). If a banana-flavored rum drink has 10 grams of carbohydrate, 1 gram of protein, 1 gram of fat, and 15 grams of alcohol, it would contain 158 kcalories ($10 \times 4 + 1 \times 4 + 1 \times 9 + 15 \times 7 = 158$).

Chapter 2 reviews the metric system. If you are not familiar with the metric system, you will find that review quite helpful.

ARE YOU WHAT YOU EAT?

The quantities of nutrients that a human consumes vary widely from one nutrient to another. Nutrient quantities found in food also vary a great deal. Together, daily protein, fat, and carbohydrate intakes amount to about 500 grams. Contrast that to typical daily mineral intake of about 20 grams and daily vitamin intakes of less than 300 milligrams. Although each day we require nearly a gram of some minerals like calcium and phosphorus, many minerals are also needed in quantitites of only milligrams or less. For example, you need about 15 milligrams of zinc per day, which is just a few specks of the mineral. Figure 1-2 contrasts the relative concentration of all of the major classes of nutrients in a human body with the composition of both a cooked steak and a cooked stalk of broccoli. Note how your nutrient composition differs from the nutritional profiles of foods you eat.

CONCEPT CHECK

Food contains vital nutrients that are essential for good health: carbohydrates, lipids (fats and oils), proteins, vitamins, minerals, and water. The chemical elements (atoms) that make up these life-sustaining nutrients include nearly half of those found in nature. Carbohydrates, lipids, and proteins yield energy for the body. The unit for this energy is the kcalorie. Vitamins and minerals aid in energy production, among other functions. Water is the solvent of life—the medium for transport of the body's substances.

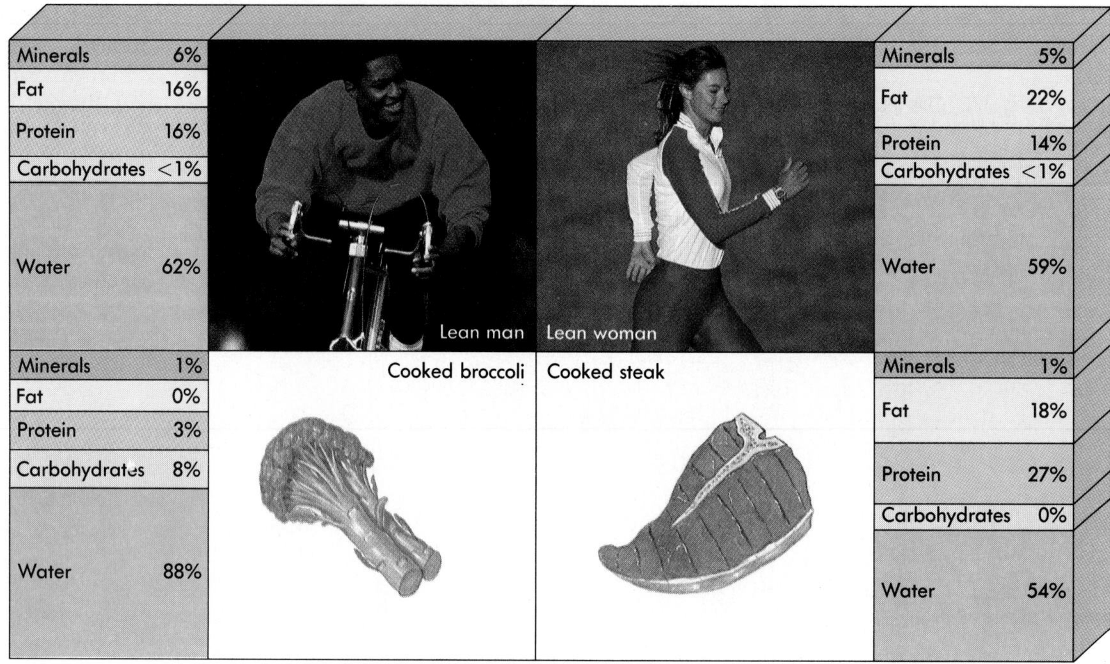

Figure 1-2 You aren't what you eat! The proportions of nutrients in the human body do not match those found in typical foods—animal or vegetable.

nutritional status The nutritional health of a person as determined by anthropometric measures (height, weight, circumferences, and so on), biochemical measures of nutrients or their by-products in blood and urine, a clinical (physical) examination, and a dietary analysis.

States of Nutritional Health

DESIRABLE NUTRITIONAL STATUS

Theoretically, the body's nutritional status varies for each individual nutrient it needs (Table 1-3). Desirable **nutritional status** for a nutrient is achieved when body tissues have enough of a nutrient for both (1) metabolic functions and (2) surplus stores of it, which can be mobilized in times of increased need.[3]

UNDERNUTRITION

When nutrient intake does not regularly meet the nutrient needs dictated by cell activities and body maintenance, stores of nutrients soon become depleted, some sooner than others. Although body stores may be sufficient to compensate for an inadequate diet for a brief period of time, in the long run serious problems can arise from an inadequate diet. Some women in the United States, for example, do not consume sufficient iron and eventually deplete their iron stores.

biochemical lesion Nutritional deficiency symptoms observed in the blood or urine, such as low levels of nutrient by-products or low enzyme activities, indicating reduced biochemical function.

Reduced Biochemical Functions

Once nutrient stores are depleted, a continuing nutrition deficit drains body tissues further. The body will try to compensate but can only do so to a point (see the discussion on homeostasis in Chapter 7). When tissue levels fall far enough, the body's metabolic processes eventually slow down, or even stop. Poor enzyme function can be at the heart of the problem. A **biochemical lesion** then develops. This deficiency is termed subclinical because there are no outward signs or symptoms. At the **subclinical** stage for poor iron status, low levels of hemoglobin (a red blood cell protein) are found in the bloodstream. Synthesizing hemoglobin requires iron.

clinical lesion Nutritional deficiency sign seen on physical examination.

Clinical Signs and Symptoms

If a biochemical deficit becomes very severe, clinical signs and symptoms eventually develop and become outwardly apparent. It is now possible to actually note **clinical lesions** in the body, perhaps in the skin, hair, nails, tongue, and eyes (see Appendix

Table 1-3 Levels of nutritional status with respect to iron†

General conditions:	Condition with respect to iron:
Overnutrition: nutrients consumed in excess of body needs (degree of toxicity varies for each nutrient).	Results in toxic damage to liver cells.
Desirable nutritional status: nutrients consumed to support body functions and stores of nutrients for times of increased need.	Adequate liver stores of iron, adequate blood values for iron-related compounds.
Undernutrition: nutrient intake does not meet nutrient needs:	Many changes in body functions are associated with a decline in iron status:
Stores depleted: tissue levels fall.	Serum* ferritin, and iron-containing protein in the blood, drops below 12 nanograms per 100 milliliters.
Reduced biochemical function (biochemical lesion).	Hemoglobin, an iron-containing pigment in the red blood cell, drops below 11 grams per 100 milliliters of blood.
Clinical signs and symptoms (clinical lesion).	Pale complexion, greatly increased heart rate during activity, "spooning" of the nails in a severe deficiency, poor body temperature regulation.

*Serum is the liquid portion of blood present after blood clots.
†This general scheme can apply to all nutrients. We have chosen iron because you are likely to be familiar with this nutrient.

A sign is visible on examination, such as flaky skin on a child. A symptom is a change in body function that is not necessarily apparent to an examiner, such as the stomach pains a child experiences.

C for common clinical signs and symptoms of nutritional deficiencies). The person also lacks that vigorous glow that good health conveys. In the case of an iron deficiency, the person may become very pale, and his or her heart rate can increase greatly during even moderate activity.

OVERNUTRITION

One nutritional state that is reaching epidemic proportions in our society today is **overnutrition**, especially from overloading the body with too many kcalories.[19]

overnutrition A state where nutritional intake exceeds the body's needs.

At the beginning of the twentieth century undernutrition was the battle cry for nutrition science. Today attention needs to be directed to both undernutrition and overnutrition. In fact, the major nutritional problems we face today are the result of overnutrition, principally caused by excess intakes of energy compared with energy needs and overconsumption of sodium and fat. Some of us are especially susceptible to ill health when we consume too many of these nutrients.

In the short run, for instance a week or two, overnutrition may cause no sign or symptom. But keep it up and eventually body weight, as well as blood levels of some nutrients, will increase. In the long run, this overnutrition can then lead to serious diseases, such as **obesity**, and its often related diseases diabetes and hypertension. Vitamin A toxicity also can result. The first form of overnutrition noted, excessive energy intake, has been possible for many people for centuries. With the recent and popular introduction of vitamin and mineral supplements, many forms of vitamin and mineral overnutrition have now become a concern.[14]

obesity A condition characterized by excess body fat, usually defined as 20% above desirable body weight.

For most nutrients, the gap between an optimal intake and overnutrition is wide. Therefore, even if people take a typical multiple vitamin and mineral supplement daily, they probably won't receive a harmful amount of any nutrient. Some possible

For vitamins A and D, a potentially harmful dose is only 5 to 10 times greater than the amount recommended to meet health needs.

exceptions are vitamin A, vitamin D, and iron toxicities. Recent studies indicate that very high doses of the vitamins B-6 and niacin can also cause health problems. Usually supplements need to be taken in large amounts on a regular basis to build up toxic levels in the body. Still, it is important to remember that for some vitamins and minerals, high doses are toxic to the body.

In the United States more than 40% of adults take vitamin and mineral supplements.[14] Although this practice usually causes no harm, some people have overdone it and have become sick and even hospitalized. If you take nutrient supplements, keep a close eye on your total vitamin and mineral intake both from food and from supplements (see Chapter 12 for further advice on use of nutrient supplements).

Nutritional Assessment

How nutritionally-fit are you? How can you find out? A nutrition assessment protocol—either in total or in part—needs to be performed. First, family history plays an important role in determining nutritional and health status and therefore must be analyzed as a preliminary measure of nutritional assessment. Other related factors to consider include: (1) your medical history, especially for any disease states or treatments that could impede nutrient absorptive processes; and (2) your socioeconomic history to determine the ability to purchase and prepare appropriate foods needed to maintain health (Table 1-4).

EVALUATING YOUR ABCDs

A thorough assessment of nutritional status then requires further examination. There are four components that in combination add to the complete nutritional picture. Due to ease and generally good reliability, **anthropometric** measurements of height, weight, body skinfolds, and body circumferences are an excellent first line of attack. However, an in-depth examination of nutritional health is impossible without the rather expensive process of biochemical assessment. This involves the analysis of specific blood **enzyme** activities and measurement of blood-nutrient and nutrient–by-product levels.

anthropometric The measurement of weight, lengths, circumferences, and thicknesses of the body.

enzyme A compound that speeds the rate of a chemical reaction but is not altered by the chemical reaction. Almost all enzymes are proteins.

Table 1-4 Components of a nutritional assessment

Component	Example
Background histories	Medical history including current diseases and past surgeries Medications history Social history; married, cooking facilities Family history Economic status
Nutrition parameters	**A**nthropometric assessment; height, weight, skinfold thickness, arm muscle circumference, and other parameters **B**iochemical (laboratory) assessment of blood and urine; enzyme activities, levels of nutrients or their by-products **C**linical assessment (physical examination); general appearance of skin, eyes, and tongue, rapid hair loss, sense of touch, ability to walk **D**iet history; usual intake or record of previous days' meals

NUTRITION FOCUS

Genetics and Nutrition

The genetic code in cells directs cell growth and development. The genes that form this code establish your individual traits, such as height and eye color. Most chronic diseases in which nutrition plays a role also are influenced by genetic background. The risk for developing heart disease, high blood pressure (hypertension), obesity, diabetes mellitus, cancer, and osteoporosis is influenced by interactions between genetic and nutritional factors. Studies of families, including those with twins and adoptees, provide strong support for the effect of genetic background in the above disorders.[16] In fact, family history is considered to be one of the greatest risk factors for many key diseases that influence human health (Figure 1-3).

Heart disease

Present in about one of every 500 persons in the general North American population is a gene defect that results in greatly slowing cholesterol removal from the bloodstream. As you will learn in Chapter 5, this leads to a high risk for developing heart disease at a young age. Diet changes can help these people, but medications and possibly surgery often are also needed to address this problem.

Hypertension

An estimated 10% to 15% of individuals are very sensitive to salt intake. When these salt-sensitive people consume too much salt, their blood pressure values tend to climb out of the desirable range. The fact that more of these people are African-Americans than Caucasian suggests a genetic link to the problem. At present, there is no certain method for identifying which persons with hypertension are salt-sensitive. A salt-restricted diet needs to be followed to see what effect it has on an individual's blood pressure.

Obesity

Most obese individuals have at least one parent who is obese. Findings from many human studies suggest that a variety of genes are involved in the regulation of body weight. Little is known, however, about the specific nature of these genes or how the actual changes in body metabolism, such as a lower kcalorie use at rest, are produced. Some individuals may be genetically predisposed to store body fat, but whether or not they actually do depends on how much excess energy—above energy needs—they ultimately consume.

A common thread in nutrition is the concept of nurture—how one conducts his or her life—allowing nature—genetic background—to be expressed. Not every person with a genetic tendency toward obesity develops the problem, but a lifetime risk most likely exists for some individuals.

Diabetes

Both of the two common types of diabetes have genetic links, as shown by studies of families and twins. Only sensitive and expensive testing can determine who is at risk. The major form of diabetes that leads to 80% to 90% of all cases has a strong link, however, to obesity. Again, we see nurture affecting nature. A genetic tendency for the major form of diabetes will be expressed once the person becomes obese, but often not before.

Cancer

A few cancers have a strong genetic link, such as some forms of colon cancer. Still, cancer provides another example of the interaction of genetic tendency with environmental factors, such as diets high in kcalories and fat. Obesity raises the risk for many forms of cancer. One third of all cancers result from smoking. Again, often a genetic tendency is not enough—environment must also contribute to the risk profile.

Osteoporosis

Twins and mother-daughter pairs show similarities for bone mineral density, and so bone strength. The relative importance of genetic versus dietary factors is unknown, but scientists strongly support the need to consume enough calcium in childhood and adolescence to build a strong bone structure. Still, genetic background does influence the overall risk for developing osteoporosis in later life. Note in Chapter 14 we cover the good news—this disease can be virtually prevented by a combination of medical and nutritional means if therapy is started at least by mid-life.

Implications

The fact that genetic background influences disease risk means that not all people will necessarily benefit equally from the same dietary advice.[12] Recommendations to eat more calcium or less salt are more important for individuals who have a genetic risk profile and so especially require this advice. It is not presently possible, given the resources allocated to medical care in America, to identify all people at genetic risk for the major chronic "killer" diseases. Thus many health authorities feel it is reasonable to give a general nutrition message to everyone, noting that some people will benefit from the advice much more than others.[19] In an ideal world, dietary advice would be tailored to one's unique health-risk profile—pointing out how to avoid the "controllable" risk factor(s) that make genetically-linked diseases more likely to appear in one's life.

Throughout this book we will try to point out how you can personalize nutriton advice based on your genetic background. Overall, keep in mind that a family history for certain diseases should raise your awareness for the potential of you developing that disease and desire to prevent this from happening. Consider discovering what your family history is for the diseases listed in Table 1-1 (consider siblings, parents, and grandparents for a start).

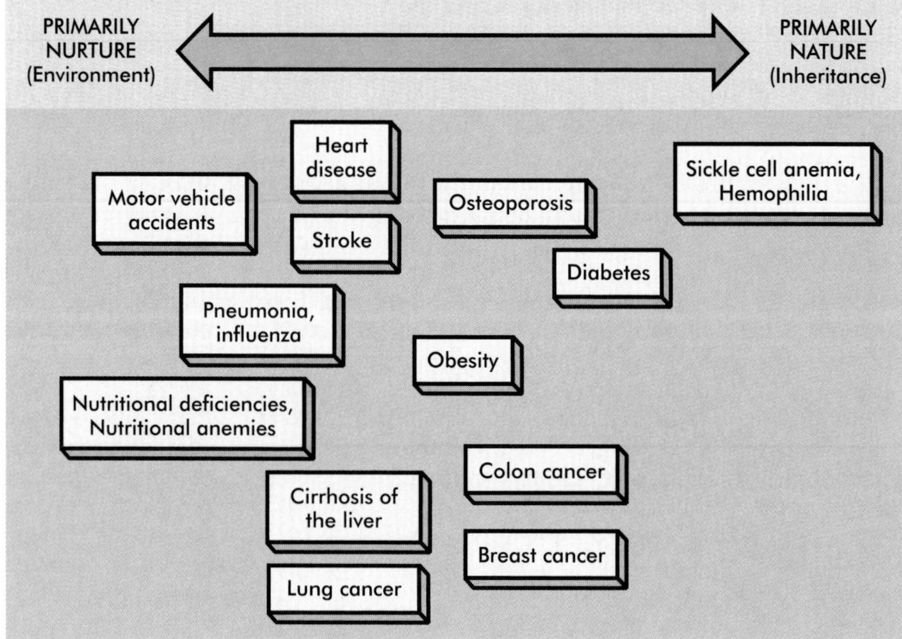

Figure 1-3 Common causes of death and illness in our population vary in their links to genetic background versus environmental influences. We must consider both influences as we study each disease.

A clinical examination would follow, wherein a health professional could detect the presence of any diet-related physical signs of diseases. Last, but certainly not least, a diet history, documenting at least the previous few days' intake, is an invaluable tool for insight into possible problem areas.[2] Together these activities form the **ABCDs** of nutritional assessment.

A WARNING

cholesterol A waxy lipid; it has a structure containing multiple chemical rings.

Often a long time elapses between the initial development of poor nutritional health and the first clinical evidence of a problem. For example, a diet high in animal fat often increases one's blood **cholesterol** level without showing any clinical signs or symptoms for years. But when the blood vessels become sufficiently blocked by cholesterol and other materials, chest pain during physical activity may develop. This buildup of fatty substances also may eventually provoke a heart attack. Thus a person may be on the road to developing a serious disease but because it progresses slowly, the effects won't be obvious until quite late—perhaps too late.

An example of this gray area that should be of specific interest to adolescent females relates to calcium intake. A goal should be to build dense bones during the years of growth and development by consuming adequate calcium. Still, young women who consume well below the recommended amount of calcium often suffer no ill effects in their younger years. However, these women whose bone densities do not reach full potential during the years of growth are likely to face significant risk for osteoporosis later in life.[16] This is why it is important for us to try to meet our nutrient needs each day. Prolonged inadequate nutrient intake, such as for calcium, can result in a subtle decline in health and performance that will initially go unnoticed.

Furthermore, clinical signs and symptoms of nutritional deficiencies are often not very specific. Typical signs to look for—diarrhea, an irregular walk, facial sores—can be caused by many different problems. It is often hard to decide if the problem is caused by faulty nutrition or by some other medical disorder. Long lag times and vague signs and symptoms often make it difficult to establish a link between an individual's current diet and nutritional state.

As you study nutrition and learn the importance of nutrients in foods, you may notice people who, in spite of very poor diets, show no outward clinical signs or symptoms of poor health. Such cases primarily reflect the need for more research in nutrition. Better methods for early detection of nutritional disease are needed. Often it is not possible to separate the best nutritional state from one that is slightly jeopardized. We can usually distinguish between **overt malnutrition** and good nutrition, but the gray area—the gradual slide from a "good" to a poor nutritional state—is hard to detect.

malnutrition Failing health that results from a long-standing dietary intake that fails to match nutritional needs.

CONCEPT CHECK

A desirable nutritional state results when the body has enough nutrients to function fully and contains stores to use in times of increased needs. When nutrient intake fails to meet body needs, undernutrition develops. Poor body functioning and physical signs and symptoms of a nutrient deficiency eventually can develop. Overnutrition is another potential problem to avoid, with excessive intake of kcalories being the biggest risk. Eating a wisely planned diet can help you avoid both poor states of nutritional health.

The American Diet: How Good Is It?

As we said, the major energy sources in our diets are carbohydrates, fats, and proteins. Alcoholic beverages provide a large source of energy for some people; in fact, alcoholic beverages—generally rich sources of carbohydrate as well—are the third leading contributor to kcalorie intakes and supply about 11% of all kcalories consumed in the United States.[5] Outside of kcalories from alcohol, adults in the United States currently consume about 14% to 16% of kcalories as proteins, 44% to 48% of kcalories as carbohydrates, and 35% to 38% of kcalories as fats.[22] These percentages change slightly from year to year.

Most of our protein intake comes from animal sources; vegetable sources supply only about one third of our protein. In many other parts of the world, it is just the opposite: vegetable proteins—those found in rice, beans, corn, and other vegetables—dominate protein intake. About half of carbohydrates in our diets come from simple sugars; the other half come from starches (such as in pastas, bread, and potatoes). About 60% of fats come from animal sources and 40% from vegetable sources.

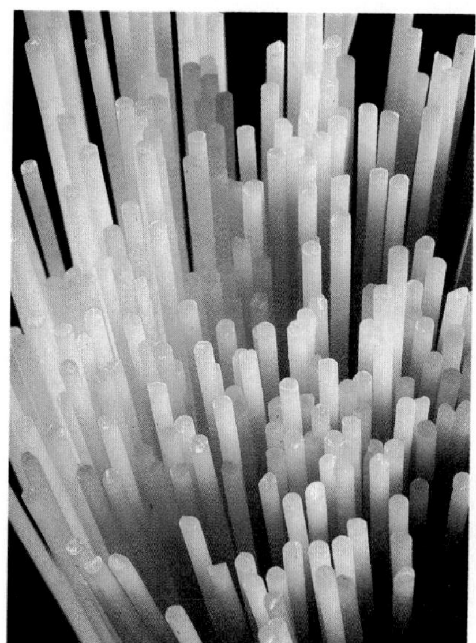

Carbohydrate is the nutrient most promoted for the American diet in the last 20 years.

SURVEYS IN THE UNITED STATES AND CANADA ASSESS NUTRITIONAL HEALTH

Federal governments perform large surveys to estimate the actual levels of nutrients in our food supply, as well as our nutrient intakes. The first such survey in the United States was the *Ten State Survey* done in the late 1960s. In Canada the first survey, called *Nutrition Canada,* began in the early 1970s. Because the *Ten State Survey* focused on mostly low-income people in the participating ten states, it did not accurately assess the average nutrient intake of people in the United States. Therefore another study—the first National Health and Nutritional Examination Survey (NHANES I 1971-74)—was conducted in the United States, followed by NHANES II (1976-80). The NHANES surveys included a cross section of about 20,000 Americans. This survey collected data about food intakes; assessed heights, weights, and blood pressures; measured vitamin and mineral levels in the blood; and examined other health parameters. Each time the NHANES survey is performed more and more parameters are added. NHANES III, already in process, will include

The current fruit and vegetable top 20 in the U.S. *FRUITS:* banana, apple, watermelon, orange, cantaloupe, grape, grapefruit, strawberry, peach, pear, nectarine, honeydew melon, plum, avocado, lemon, pineapple, tangerine, sweet cherries, kiwi fruit, and limes. *VEGETABLES:* potato, head lettuce, tomato, onion, carrot, celery, sweet corn, broccoli, green cabbage, cucumber, bell pepper, cauliflower, leaf lettuce, sweet potato, mushroom, green onion, green (snap) bean, radish, summer squash, and asparagus.

40,000 people.[21] Results should be available between 1992 and 1995. The U.S. Department of Agriculture (USDA) also conducts, as it has since the beginning of this century, various other types of surveys that document the types of foods people eat.[22] Agriculture Canada performs the same type of food-consumption surveys.

AN AMERICAN NUTRITION PROFILE

Results from the NHANES, Nutrition Canada, and various other food-consumption surveys show quite a diversity in our diets. Many people are meeting their nutrient needs; others are not. The studies suggest that some of us need to consume more foods that are rich in iron, calcium, vitamin A, vitamin C, magnesium, zinc, and dietary fiber.[13,16,19,22] This in part stems from the fact that a high proportion of the population does not eat from all the major food groups each day: dairy, meats, grains, fruits, and vegetables. Only about 33% of us consume foods from all five nutrient sources each day, and only 2.9% consume the desired number of servings from each food group.[13] Foods from the fruit and dairy groups are the most likely to be omitted on any given day. In addition, we must consider the possibility that, often linked to cultural influences, individual lifestyles may provide a diet excessive in kcalories, alcohol, and sodium.

HOW DO WE RATE OUR DIETS?

salt Generally refers to a compound of sodium and chloride in a 40:60 ratio.

Judging from the responses given by people in several recent surveys, most of us are extremely concerned about good nutrition and are well aware of possible health hazards from excessive intakes of fat, **salt,** and sugar.[15] Ninety percent of participants in one survey said that they chose foods for health reasons and 81% claimed that they would like to eat healthier foods more often. Fifty-six percent of adults "try a lot" to avoid consuming too much fat, 33% "try a little," and only 10% "don't try at all." Two-thirds of the shoppers interviewed said that they were eating healthier foods than one year ago.[9] These shoppers ranked nutrition second only to taste as the most important factor they consider when purchasing food—97% thought nutrition was a somewhat or very important factor in grocery-shopping decisions. Most shoppers (95%) were at least somewhat concerned about the nutritional content of foods; 56% of shoppers were very concerned about nutrition.

A telephone survey of the dietary habits and attitudes of 1000 adult Americans representative of the U.S. population showed that 26% of the respondents felt that nutrition was important, that they were careful about what they ate and that they were doing things right. Another 36% knew they were not doing much to manage their diets, but were not interested in changing, since it would mean giving up their favorite foods and would take too much time. The remaining 38% thought that diet was fairly important, but only about half of them were doing as much as they thought they should do because most did not want to give up the foods they like and they thought that it would take too much time. Thus the unwillingness of some people to significantly change many of their nutritional practices is probably the major impediment to improving their diet—concern does not necessarily translate into change.

In the survey of shoppers mentioned earlier, more than two thirds thought their diets could be more healthful.[9] Only 10% considered their diets already as healthful as possible. Still, people in a recent USDA survey were not convinced they needed to know more about nutrition, in spite of scoring low on nutrition-knowledge questions. Only 7% of people surveyed said they were not very well informed on the subject. Most viewed food and cooking as a pleasure, not as a science. We hope you will think of it as both. One third agreed that "nobody really knows the answers on the best foods to eat for a balanced diet." Almost one half agreed that "learning the basic ideas in nutrition will probably alter my personal eating habits very little." We hope we can convince you to do otherwise.

EXPERT OPINION

Junk Foods—or Junk Diets

HELEN A. GUTHRIE, PH.D., R.D.

Over the past few decades, the phrase "junk food" has invaded our vocabulary. To nutritionists, this term is meaningless, it should be banned. There is no totally worthless food, any more than there is a perfect food that meets all our nutritional needs.

Obviously, some foods contribute more nutrients than do others. But almost any food has some redeeming value under the right circumstances. The problem arises when foods that contribute more calories than nutrients become so important in our diet that foods of higher nutritional value are excluded. It is equally possible to make an unbalanced selection from among our most sacred nutritious foods, for instance milk and apples, and wind up with a diet overabundant in some nutrients yet deficient in others. In both cases, the result can be labeled a "junk diet."

Some foods go hand-in-hand

In terms of nutrient density—roughly defined as the nutrients delivered per kcalorie—food with low values seldom carry much nutritional weight. For example, in some cakes and cookies, most of the kcalories come from fat and sugar, and relatively few from nutrient-rich milk, flour, and eggs. However, if eating a cookie means that a child also drinks milk or fruit juice, we should look at cookie-and-milk or cookie-and-beverage as a unit and judge them together rather than condemn one and applaud the other. For an 8-year old, milk and one or two cookies makes a nutritious combination. Milk and five cookies, though, may create an imbalance between kcalories and nutrients—and thus must be considered lower in nutrition.

Potato chips are another example of a food that can be valuable in the right context. Eaten alone, potato chips have sufficient vitamin C, vitamin B-6, and copper to make them a meaningful source. Eaten with sandwich, potato chips become part of a balanced meal. But if we eat so many potato chips that we're too full to eat dinner, we are misusing them. What about the salt, you ask? One ounce of potato chips provides about ⅛ gram of sodium—less than the amount in the bread in a sandwich and considerably less than the amount in two slices of bread with salted butter. Just because we see and taste the salt on potato chips doesn't mean they have more than those foods in which it is hidden.

For another example, consider pizza. All too frequently people see it as a junk food high in kcalories, cholesterol, and fat. But with essentially the same ingredients, pizza has nutritional merits comparable to a meat-and-cheese sandwich served with tomato, providing valuable amounts of protein, calcium, iron, and many vitamins.

Too much of a good thing?

How about the classically "healthful" foods like milk, chicken, orange juice, and oatmeal? Are they always desirable? Surprisingly, no. Milk, especially nonfat milk, has one of the most impressive nutrient profiles of any food. But it isn't perfect. Although high in calcium, protein, and riboflavin, it is low in iron and vitamin C. In contrast, oranges are high in iron and vitamin C, but low in calcium, protein, and riboflavin.

What does all this have to do with junk food? When a food doesn't meet an immediate nutritional need, its nutritional value is limited. After an adult has had two or three glasses of milk (which would meet many nutritional needs), additional milk becomes less and less useful. If the additional milk (which does not provide vitamin C) displaces a fruit juice that does have vitamin C, that milk becomes of limited nutrition value, or even worthless, except as a source of kcalories. In this context, the extra milk would be a "junk" food. So foods should not be judged in isolation, but in relation to the total diet and the individual's needs.

If all our daily nutrient needs are met except for kcalories, technically we can obtain the rest of our kcalorie requirements from any food. In reality we recommend that the extra kcalories come from a food with a reasonable amount of other nutrients. In selecting food, moderation is a virtue. And so is avoidance of excess amounts of fat, sodium, and kcalories, all of which are essential in controlled amounts. Getting a maximum of 10% to 15% of our total daily kcalories from foods of limited nutritional value is reasonable—more than this can lead to nutritional problems.

Cost per nutrient

In choosing nutritious foods, cost per nutrient is also important. Many parents feel good about giving their children toast with margarine and honey for breakfast but feel guilty if they serve a doughnut. Since both bread and doughnuts are made with enriched flour—where by definition certain vitamins and minerals have been added—there is no appreciable difference in their overall nutrient content. There is also no big advantage of honey over jam nor margarine over oil. Costwise, however, the doughnut is not as good a buy. Similar considerations hold for french-fried and baked potatoes. Nutritionally, a serving of french fries cooked in oil compares favorably with a baked potato served with a fat such as sour cream or butter. However, the cost per nutrient of commercially prepared French fries can be considerably higher than that of home-prepared baked potatoes. Nutritionists want people to eat the right amount and combinations of nutrients to promote health, but they also want everyone to eat in a rational way, without feeling guilty about including a favorite food merely for pleasure. Special medical considerations aside, a healthful diet can include at least small amounts of any food you enjoy as long as your overall diet is moderate in kcalories and balanced to provide essential nutrients.

Dr. Guthrie is Professor of Nutrition at The Pennsylvania State University.

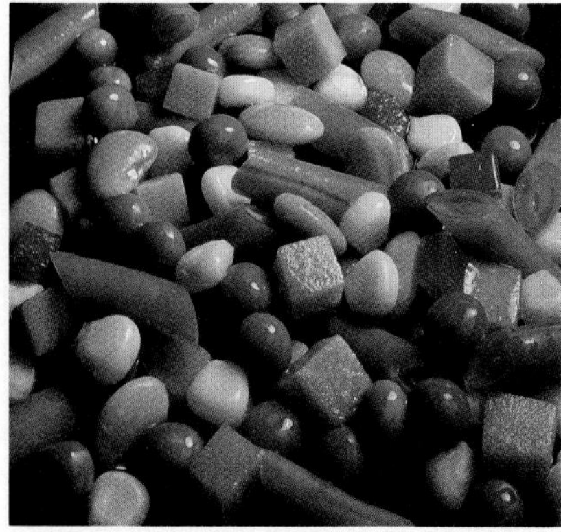

Vegetables are a good source of dietary fiber—eat them every day.

Currently the aspects of our diets that concern us the most are fat, cholesterol, and salt.[9] Kcalories, sugar, and additives are of less concern. On a per person basis, Americans consumed roughly 18 pounds of butter and 270 pounds of whole milk in the 1920s and 1930s, compared with less than 5 pounds of butter and 111 pounds of whole milk in the late 1980s. Therefore progress is being made in reducing key sources of fat and cholesterol in our diets. But for many of us more work needs to be done, as we discuss in Chapter 2.

CONCEPT CHECK

Surveys show that we have plenty of food available to us in the United States. However, some of us could improve our diets by focusing on good food sources of iron, calcium, vitamin A, vitamin C, magnesium, zinc, and dietary fiber. In addition, some of us should use more moderation when consuming kcalories, fat, sodium, and alcoholic beverages. Often we don't realize these diet changes are needed.

What Shapes Our Food Tastes?

The basic purpose of food is nourishment, but to us it means far more than that, and that is fine. Food symbolizes much of what we think about ourselves.[1] We bond relationships and express friendships around the dinner table. We enhance and maintain our social status by entertaining creatively or lavishly. We cope with stress and tension by eating or not eating. We influence other's behaviors through our food practices. Some of us express religious beliefs and display our creative talents through food preparation and ceremonies. Since people eat 80,000 to 100,000 times in a lifetime (which takes 13 to 15 years of our waking hours), eating becomes an important key to the way we define ourselves politically, religiously, and socially (Figure 1-4).

Food likes and dislikes are probably the most important determinants of what we eat. Respondents to a USDA survey rated taste as the chief consideration in selecting foods to serve their families; budget came in second. Respondents were

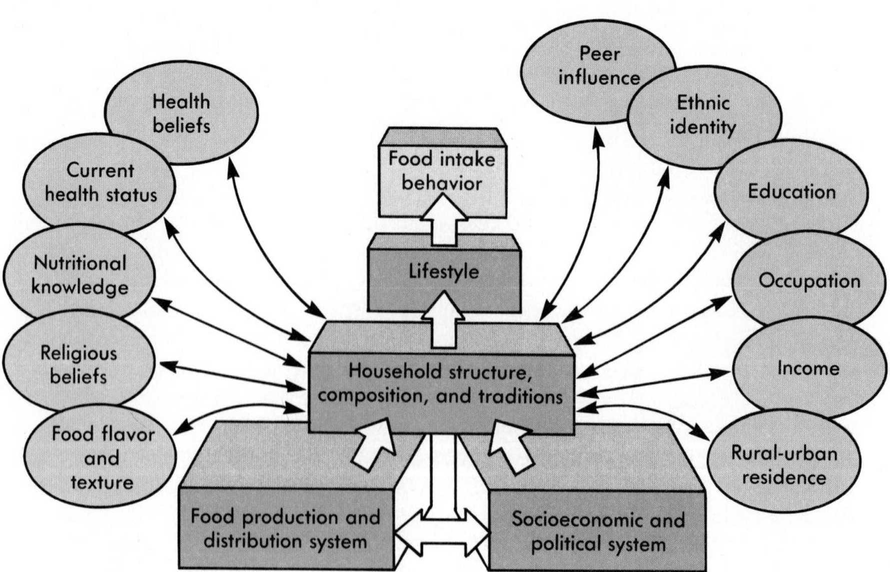

Figure 1-4 Food behavior can be influenced by many sources. Which are important in your life?

much more likely to serve a meal based on taste, compared with one they knew would be more nutritious.

EARLY EXPERIENCES

Food preferences are learned early as social and cultural preferences (Figure 1-5). They are refined through interactions with parents and friends, social class, and the need for status.[4] Unfortunately for young children, adult caregivers may severely limit the child's experience with food. Adults may purchase only a small subset of foods available and may even consider many of these foods inappropriate for children. For example, at what age were you first introduced to okra, kiwis, lentils, spinach salad, or salmon?

Mere exposure to a variety of foods can help reduce the resistance to trying new foods. Young children tend to prefer foods that are sweet or familiar, but preschoolers are often quite willing to try new things. Caregivers need to provide that opportunity. It may take as many as fifteen introductions, but the odds are in favor of final acceptance.

Our built-in preferences are important, including universal enjoyment of sweet foods and dislike of bitter and sometimes spicy, burning ones. Bitter tastes often signal poisonous substances. However, built-in responses can be modified through exposure and conditioning (i.e., learning).[18] This allows some people—even entire cultures—to learn to enjoy very sour or hot, spicy foods, such as jalapeño peppers and fiery curries.

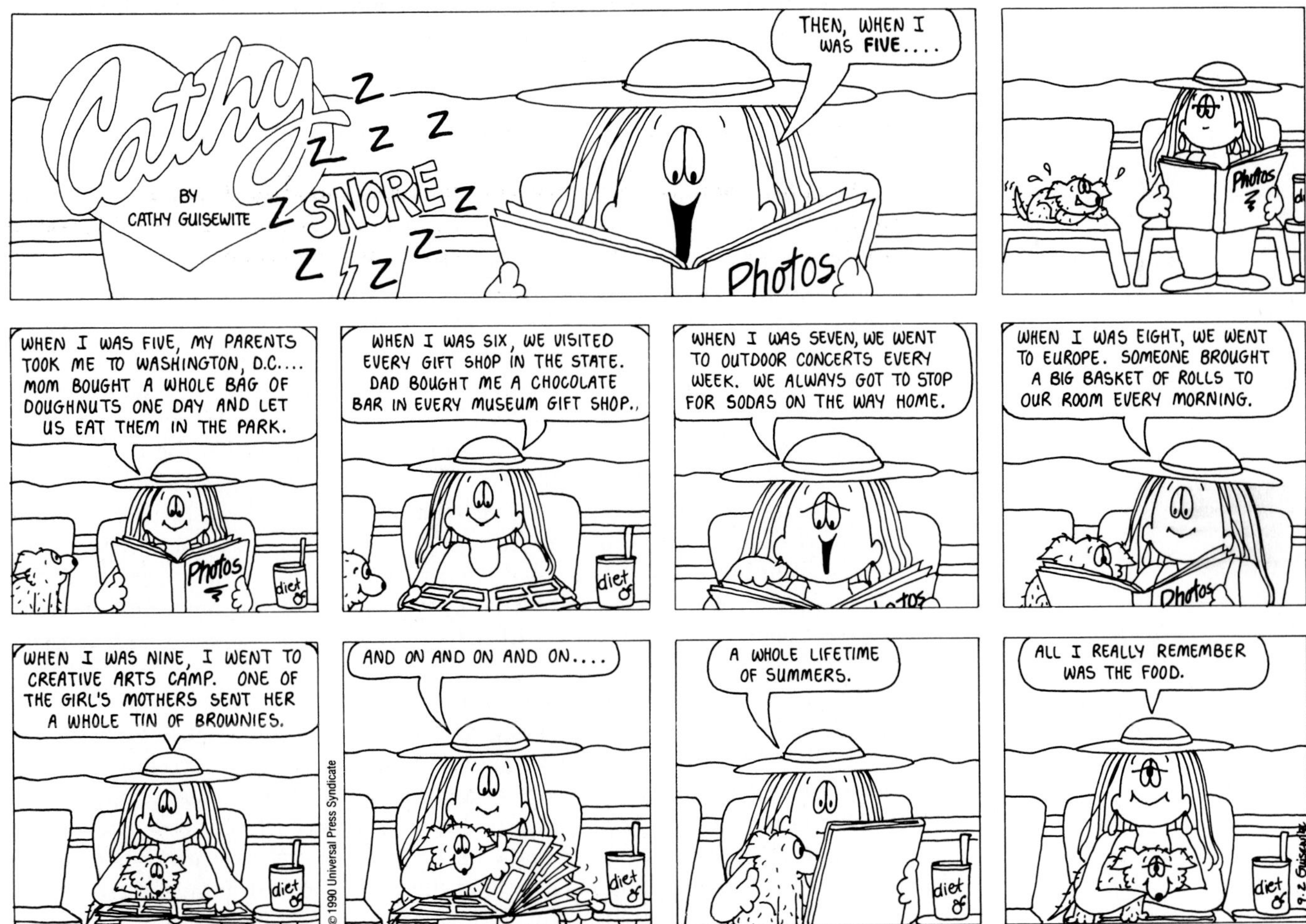
Cathy
BY CATHY GUISEWITE
Z Z Z Z SNORE Z Z Z Z
THEN, WHEN I WAS FIVE....
Photos
WHEN I WAS FIVE, MY PARENTS TOOK ME TO WASHINGTON, D.C.... MOM BOUGHT A WHOLE BAG OF DOUGHNUTS ONE DAY AND LET US EAT THEM IN THE PARK.
WHEN I WAS SIX, WE VISITED EVERY GIFT SHOP IN THE STATE. DAD BOUGHT ME A CHOCOLATE BAR IN EVERY MUSEUM GIFT SHOP..
WHEN I WAS SEVEN, WE WENT TO OUTDOOR CONCERTS EVERY WEEK. WE ALWAYS GOT TO STOP FOR SODAS ON THE WAY HOME.
WHEN I WAS EIGHT, WE WENT TO EUROPE. SOMEONE BROUGHT A BIG BASKET OF ROLLS TO OUR ROOM EVERY MORNING.
WHEN I WAS NINE, I WENT TO CREATIVE ARTS CAMP. ONE OF THE GIRL'S MOTHERS SENT HER A WHOLE TIN OF BROWNIES.
AND ON AND ON AND ON....
A WHOLE LIFETIME OF SUMMERS.
ALL I REALLY REMEMBER WAS THE FOOD.
diet
© 1990 Universal Press Syndicate

Figure 1-5 Cathy.

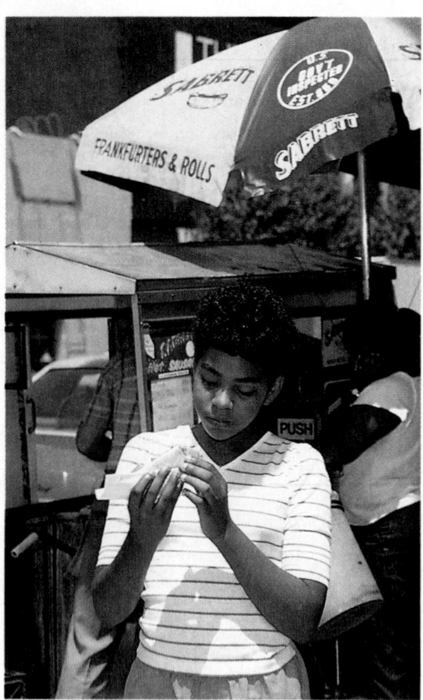

Food preferences often are rooted in childhood experiences.

HABIT

Most of us eat only from a core group of foods. Only about 100 basic items account for 75% of the total amount of food we consume. We may think we buy foods mainly based on their sensory appearance, freshness, safety, nutritional quality, healthfulness, convenience, and price. Those factors do figure in, but we still work within very narrow constraints, primarily dictated by the routines and habits surrounding the selection of foods. Many of us could use cooking classes to expand our nutritional horizons. Of the respondents in a USDA survey of women, 51% agreed that their cooking habits were very similar to those of their mothers. Did your mother teach you healthy food habits?

Taboos further limit cuisine: Hindus would no more eat beef than we would eat a dog. And Swedish people, who regard corn in general as food for hogs, do not enjoy a good ear of sweet corn. Adults even limit the time of day foods can be eaten. When did you last have nourishing vegetable noodle soup for breakfast, even though it can be highly comforting on a cold morning? Many Asian people prefer it at that time of day.

HEALTH

As we have noted, several surveys have revealed that most of our population considers nutrition, or what they think is good nutrition, an important factor in influencing their food purchases.[8,9] Only about one fourth of people report that price is more important than nutrition. The people in this country who focus on better nutrition are mainly the well-educated professionals of the middle-class, the health-oriented and active lifestyle segment of the population whose tastes can set a trend. Still, all of us should pay attention to nutritional health. In fact, increased health awareness among minority people is a major goal of the current U.S. federal government health strategies.

In the past sugar was the main diet monster; today fat and cholesterol have the limelight.[20] As a result, manufacturers are racing to the market with reduced-fat or nonfat items. According to a 1991 national consumer survey conducted by the Calorie Control Council, about two thirds of the adult population reported consuming low-fat or reduced-fat foods and beverages on the day of the survey. Low-kcalorie sweeteners accounted for about 13% of overall sweetener consumption in 1988, compared with 6% in 1980 and 5% in 1970.

Some of the most successful products introduced in recent years to the U.S. markets are those with a healthy image, whether or not they actually contain healthful ingredients. Popular products of the 1980s have included fruit rolls and bars, bottled mineral water, granola bars, fruit juices, bulk frozen vegetables without sauce, and oriental meals. What will the 1990s hold? Food scientists suggest that the demand for quick, easy, and nutritious meals will continue to grow as we spend less time in the kitchen. Some 75% to 80% of American households now have microwave ovens. Current estimates show that women want to spend a half hour or less each day selecting and cooking foods, and men only want to spend 15 minutes. Overall, we like to eat on the run; note that 8% of all food purchased at restaurants is consumed in the car.

The recent movement toward better nutritional health was sparked in the 1960s when the American Heart Association labeled the fat-rich and cholesterol-rich diets in the United States a major contributor to heart disease. More recently, research shows diet may be linked to 10% to 35% of all cancers.[7] Some of us are responding to these health risks by attempting to change our diets. Nevertheless, as we said earlier, taste and habit still profoundly dictate food choice. Recently, when people were asked why they did not include foods they knew were healthy in their diets—for instance, yellow vegetables, low-fat milk, margarine, and whole-wheat bread—they said they didn't like them. The response to why they didn't give up foods they thought they should decrease—such as whole milk, cheese, and fatty meat—was that they liked them too much.

The food industry is responding to our health concerns. A modern supermarket provides extensive choices among fresh, frozen, international, gourmet, ethnic, vegetarian, and even not-so-healthy foods. Salad bars in supermarkets are a big hit, especially where single people shop. Stores are moving toward foods lower in fat, salt, and sugar. They are carrying unsalted nuts, pure fruit juices, high-fiber cereals, whole-grain breads, fruits canned in natural juices, low-sodium soups and sauces, low-fat turkey and chicken franks, and many kinds of fish. Bulk foods sold in bins now include beans, rice, flours, dried fruits, nuts, and grains.

Some shelf tags in markets provide information on the nutritional content of foods, such as kcalories, vitamins and minerals, sodium, and cholesterol. The road to good nutrition is paved with the ready availability of appropriate sign posts and choices.

ADVERTISING

To capture consumers' interest, the food industry spends annually well over $6 billion on advertising and another $26 billion on packaging (another form of advertising)—a total of more than $32 billion (Table 1-5). Some of this advertising is helpful—when it promotes the importance of calcium and dietary fiber in our diets and encourages us to consume more low-fat and nonfat milk products, fruits, vegetables, and lean meats. The food industry, however, does not promote all foods equally: sellers tend to emphasize brand-name foods because they bring higher profits, especially highly sweetened cereals, cookies, cakes, and pastries. Food manufacturers often pay for the best place in the supermarkets: at the end of the aisle and, depending on the product, at the child's or adult's eye level.

Today, foods are also often unfairly promoted. Fat content may be expressed on a label in terms of product weight rather than in terms of total product kcalorie content. Sausages with 50% of their kcalories as fat may be labeled as 90% fat-free (by weight). The water in the sausage is the reason for the discrepancy. Keep in mind that meats are usually greater than 50% water by weight—which yields no

Table 1-5 On a typical day in the United States. . .

* 34 new restaurants open and 8 fold.
* 134 million people eat out, of which 16 million eat at McDonald's. Note that McDonald's spends $500 thousand in advertising per day to encourage this.
* Each person spends about 1 hour and 20 minutes at meals, in turn eating about 4 pounds of food. This includes 16 teaspoons of fat and 32 teaspoons of sugar.
* 11,000 girls ages 12-19 go on a diet, joining the 101 million people already on diets.
* 100 million M&Ms are sold. 2 million Hershey's Kisses and 17 million Tootsie Rolls are produced.
* 25 million hot dogs are eaten.
* 524 million Cokes are consumed. To encourage this, Coca-Cola spends $500 thousand per day on advertising.
* $3.5 million are spent on vitamin supplements, while $10.4 million are spent on potato chips and $3.5 million on tortilla chips.
* In total, $22 million are spent on snack foods, while $203 million are spent on low-calorie foods. $1.4 million are spent on laxatives.
* Children see five beer and wine commercials on television as part of the $3 million spent to advertise beer, wine, and liquor.
* $2 million are spent on baby food.

The United States has about 250 million people.

Adapted from Heyman T: *On An Average Day*, New York, 1989, Fawcett Columbia.

kcalories. Currently, basing nutrient content on weight is legal advertising, but quite misleading to the weight conscious public. Fortunately, new labeling laws that will be in effect by mid 1993 will put a stop to most of the fraudulent food advertising we see today (see Chapter 2).

RESTAURANTS AND EATING OUT

Restaurants have been a big growth industry in America. About 45% of all food dollars are spent on meals outside the home. On weekdays lunch is eaten out by 30% of all adults and dinner by 24%. Restaurant excursions are no longer a splurge. For some people, such as traveling sales representatives, students, and truck drivers, it is convenient to stop at a quick-service (also called "fast-food") restaurant on a regular basis. Drive-through restaurants are now especially a part of our culture, whereas 40 years ago they were much less common. Today people drive through, wolf down 1200 kcalories (about half their daily needs) via the burger, fries, and shake, and they are on their way.

Many restaurants do offer healthy alternatives to their high-kcalorie and salty foods. This includes quick service restaurants. They in fact have led the way in publishing consumer nutrition information, have begun to use yogurt instead of ice cream in their shakes; switched from beef fat to vegetable oil for frying; and now have low-fat hamburgers. Carrots go on their salads, along with cheese. Salad bars are everywhere. Grilled chicken, fresh fruit, whole grain muffins, and low-fat milk are widely available.

Still, the temptation to consume foods rich in fat and salt is often too hard to resist when we eat out. The reality is that a hamburger, french fries, and a milk shake often have a greater appeal than a well-stocked salad bar. Thus food chosen in a restaurant is generally poorer in nutritional quality than food eaten at or taken from home. For regular visitors to quick service restaurants, what they choose to eat is crucial if they want to have a nutritious diet.[17]

SOCIAL FACTORS

Many social changes in recent years have strongly affected the food marketplace. The increase in the number of working women and single parents, both young and old, means that less time is available for preparing meals. In the last 20 years, the number of families headed by women doubled from 5.5 million in 1970 to 10.9 million today. Three out of four women 35 to 44 years old are now in the labor force. Even for married women with a child less than 6 years old the participation rate reached about 60% in 1989. A general "time-famine" is emerging. Most people turn to quick service restaurants for meals on the run, but supermarket food counters are stealing some of these restaurant customers. The appeal of microwave ovens and frozen foods is especially strong. Quick to meet the need, food producers have increased the number of foods that require little or no preparation. Almost 1000 new microwave products were introduced in 1989. Surveys show one third to one half of people state that to save time, those are the type of foods they eat consistently. Ready-to-eat or microwaveable products marketed directly to children and the calorie-conscious are especially on the rise.

The advent of the ever-present shopping mall has created a new generation of "mall munchers," eating everything from ethnic foods to high-priced cookies.

As the age of our population has increased, so has the consumption of certain foods: for example, shellfish, fresh vegetables, and alcoholic beverages. For the elderly, new health and nutrition problems often arise and compel changes in food habits (see Chapter 18).

Overall, in today's fast-paced world, many people are looking for ways to make time. One area they seem perfectly willing to cut is in meal planning. Today, it's relatively common to eat away from home and to skip meals. In one study, over one half of college students reported that they ate only two meals a day, eating many snacks to make up the difference. For families, approximately 30% of adults skip breakfast. Ironically, breakfast is the time to replace carbohydrate stores used during the night's sleep. Skipping it will give you more time, but you may end up less alert and less efficient. You will most likely get much more accomplished during the day if you just take the 20 minutes to relax and enjoy a morning meal.

It also is desirable to try to eat with others often. Meal time is a key social time of the day. The Japanese are ahead of us in recognizing that food's powers go beyond the realm of nutrition. Their national dietary guidelines, which like ours stress the importance of eating a variety of foods, maintaining healthy weight, and limiting fat in the diet, also advise people to make all activities pertaining to food and eating pleasurable.

ECONOMICS

The amount of money available for food influences eating habits. As income increases, so do meals eaten away from home. More affluent people also tend to consume more vegetables, fruits, cheeses, meats, fish, poultry, and fat, but they eat less dried beans, and rice. However, the relationship between income and overall food consumption is not as strong as you might expect, probably because food is relatively inexpensive in America. An average of only 11.8% of after-tax income was spent for food in 1990; 7.3% for food at home and 4.5% for food away from home. Compare this to about 50% of income spent on food in China or India. Nevertheless, high meat prices have led to the use of beef as an ingredient rather than as a centerpiece in some households; chicken, turkey, and fish are used as alternatives.

Given Our Food Choices, We Can Do Better

In the United States our cultural diversity, varied cuisines, and generally high nutritional status should be points of pride for us. In 1993, we have available a tremendous variety of food choices. Some 9200 new food products were introduced last year. We are eating more breakfast cereals, pizza, pasta entrees, stir-fried meat

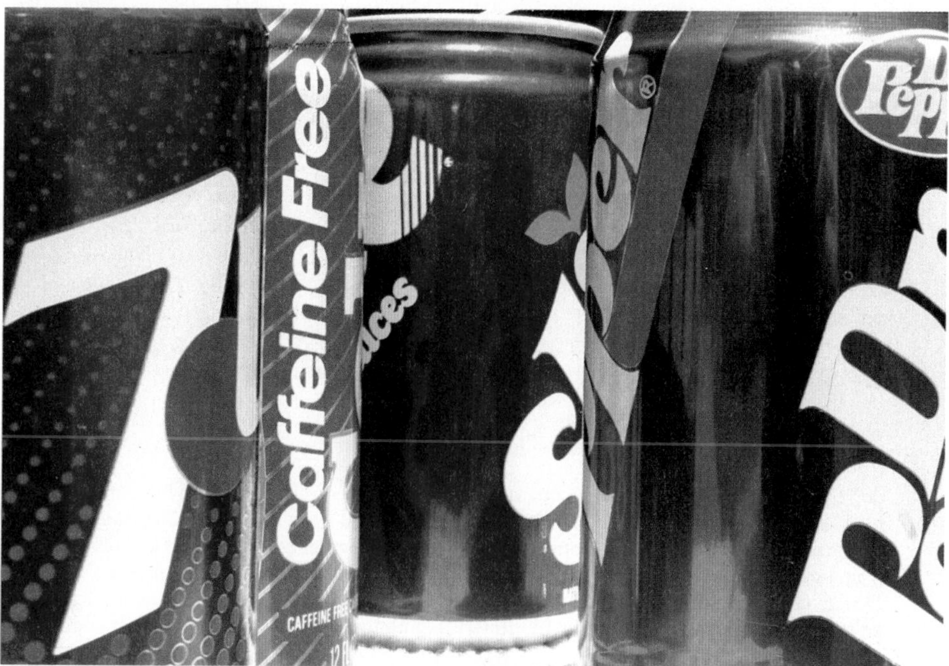

Soft drinks are today more popular than milk, although not as beneficial to a diet.

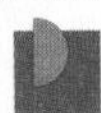

How to Spot Front-Page Fallacies

BY ANTHONY SCHMITZ

YOUR NEWSPAPER probably prints some type of food news every day. It may be important, it may be meaningless. Don't count on the paper's editors knowing the difference. You can defend yourself against half-baked findings and wild advice—if you read carefully. Here's how to pick apart a food news piece, one that hit the pages of the *Minneapolis Star Tribune* on April 26, 1991.

1. Study: Eating citrus can help against cholesterol

Associated Press

MIAMI—Eating citrus can reduce cholesterol plaque in clogged arteries and help reverse atherosclerosis, a leading cause of heart attacks and strokes, researchers said Wednesday.

2. A two-year experiment with pigs found that citrus pectin—the sticky substance that's used to make jelly—reduces the formation of fatty plaque in coronary arteries, said D. Sigurd Normann of the University of Florida.

3. "The practical impact of our investigation is that we can tell a patient with severe atherosclerosis all is not lost," said fellow researcher Dr. James Cerda. "Based on this research, I would advise my patients with high cholesterol levels to eat a low-fat diet, get some exercise, and eat at least one grapfruit or several fresh oranges every day."

4. The researchers emphasized that citrus juice doesn't have the same beneficial effects because pectin is found only in the rind and in the pulp.

5. Normann, chief of cardiac pathology at the university's college of medicine, presented the study Thursday to the Federation of American societies of Experimental Biology in Atlanta.

6. The primary grant for the research came from the Florida Citrus Commission, a state-appointed, industry-funded panel, but the commission played no role in reviewing the results, university officials said.

Norman said the study used pigs because their arteries and susceptibility to atherosclerosis are similar to humans'.

7. Dr. Margo Denke, a specialist with the Center for Human Nutrition at the University of Texas's Southwestern Medical Center in Dallas, said she was impressed with the research. The findings fit in with previous studies showing pectin, a type of soluble fiber, can reduce cholesterol levels.

"They saw the change in a very short period of time, which is quite dramatic," she said. "But I think that more research is going to need to be done, and we might not expect such a dramatic effect in humans."

The study indicated as little as one grapefruit a day was enough to show results, but Denke said some other research has suggested that higher amounts might be necessary.

Dr. George Lumb, a scholar in residence at Duke Medical School who has conducted research on heart disease for 30 years, questioned whether people would be willing to eat that much fresh citrus fruit every day. He said his research team is conducting studies on 24 volunteers with high cholesterol levels to test the effects of pectin-enriched fruit punch.

1. The bold, beckoning words at a newspaper story's top are usually cranked out by a special headline writer whose familiarity with the subject can be measured in minutes. If eating citrus can help against cholesterol, your first questions should be: How much citrus? Whom does it help?

2. Now you know they're talking about pigs. Even if you have four legs and a snout, you shouldn't go for the pectin quite yet. The writer left out the study size—seven control pigs, seven pigs on pectin—which is too small to make the results widely applicable *even for pigs*. For humans, the conclusions are shakier still. That's not to say the research is irrelevant. Human arteries harden about the same way pigs' do. But the story doesn't say what else the pigs ate. Pigs are more sensitive to food's cholesterol; we're more sensitive to fat. Animal studies alone can't prove anything about human nutrition and health.

3. Did the pigs eat an amount of pectin that a reasonable pig, or a reasonable person, might eat? The answer (not that it's here) is no. Researchers fed 60-pound Yucatan micropigs half an ounce of pure pectin a day. Chances are you weigh two or three times more than a micropig. To have any hope of a cholestrol drop like that of the pigs you'd have to eat at least *two dozen* grapefruit a day.

4. Great news if you eat grapefruit *rind*. Most people don't.

5. There's a big difference between papers delivered at a conference, such as this one, and papers published in the *Journal of the American Medical Association*, the *New England Journal of Medicine, Science, Nature,* and the like. Journal articles are usually reviewed by experts who help editors toss out the scientific chaff. Presentations at conferences aren't as carefully winnowed and shouldn't be taken as seriously.

6. If the bills are paid by the citrus industry, wouldn't the researchers inevitably find *something* good to say about grapefruits and oranges? Maybe; maybe not. You can't jump to conclusions about bias, warns *Washington Post* science writer Victor Cohn. Some crooked researchers *do* get money from corporations, he notes. "But the peddler of a biased point of view is as likely to be an anti-establishment crusader or an academic ladder-climber as a corporate darling." You have to judge each study on its own merits.

7. The last paragraphs are often more helpful than the first. This is usually where outside experts comment, putting the finding in perspective. In this case Margo Denke, a member of the American Heart Association's nutrition committee, makes three good points: This study confirms others showing that soluble fiber lowers cholesterol. Humans, however, aren't the same as pigs. And there ought to be more research done before anyone warms up the citrus bandwagon.

Anthony Schmitz is a contributing editor to Health magazine.

and vegetables served on rice, salads, tacos, burritos, and fajitas. Sales of whole milk dropped 7% in 1989 compared with the previous year. Over the same time period, sales of 1% low-fat milk increased almost 13% and skim milk sales increased by 25%. More than half the shoppers in a recent survey (57%) said they are eating more fruits and vegetables to ensure healthful diets. Shoppers said they are also eating less meat (34%), fats and oils (25%), and sugar (19%). About one sixth reported eating more chicken (16%) or dietary fiber (16%), and 14% said they are eating more fish.[9] Soft drinks now are more popular than milk, although not as beneficial to the diet, but frozen as opposed to canned vegetable consumption is also on the rise. Many of these recent diet changes are advantageous; some are not.

Today, we live longer than ever before and enjoy better general health.[6] Some of us also have more money, more overwhelming food and lifestyle choices to consider, and more time to relax and enjoy life. The end results of these trends are not fully known, but deaths from heart disease and strokes have dropped dramatically since the late 1960s. Better medical care and diets deserve some of the credit. Still, affluence, when it leads to sedentary lifestyles and high intakes of fat and alcohol, can be a villain.[19] Because of better technology and greater choices, we can have a much better diet today than ever before—if we know what to do with the choices. Overall, we are doing well, but many of us can do better. The goal here is to help you find your best path to good nutrition. Chapter 2 contains key information to aid you in that goal.

CONCEPT CHECK

Our food choices are influenced mainly by taste and habit. Of late, factors such as health, economics, convenience, and social structure also are becoming important dietary determinants. Good food habits developed and strengthened now will benefit you in years to come.

Summary

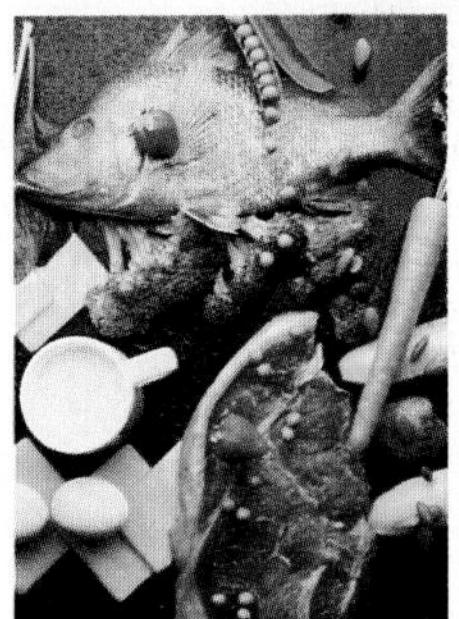

1. Nutrition is the study of the food substances vital for health and how the body uses these substances to promote and support growth, maintenance, and reproduction of cells.
2. Nutrients in foods fall into six classes: carbohydrates, lipids (mostly fats and oils), proteins, vitamins, minerals, and water. The first three, along with alcohol, provide energy for the body to use.
3. As nutritional health diminishes, nutrient stores in the body are depleted first. The body will try to compensate, but eventually biochemical reactions in the body slow down. Finally, clinical evidence (signs and symptoms) can be seen.
4. Overnutrition is a focus today in America. This condition includes overconsumption of energy and certain vitamins and minerals.
5. The focus for nutrition planning should be food, not supplements. Using foods to supply nutrient needs essentially eliminates the possibility of severe nutrient imbalances.
6. Genetic background influences a person's risk for developing many chronic diseases, such as obesity, heart disease, cancer, and diabetes. Evidence of these diseases in one's family should make a person more attentive to avoiding "controllable" risk factors for these diseases. We will cover these risk factors throughout this book.
7. Results from large nutrition surveys in the United States suggest that some of us need to concentrate on consuming foods that supply more vitamin A, calcium, magnesium, iron, zinc, and dietary fiber.
8. Our food choices are greatly affected by our culture, our family, our upbringing, our self-image, and the image we want to present to others.

Study Questions

1. Describe how genetic tendencies and other risk factors interrelate in terms of contracting a nutrition-related chronic disease. Name some of the chronic diseases associated with nutrition and a few corresponding risk factors.
2. Outline the concept behind measurement of kcalories in foods and how these values are determined.
3. Describe the states of nutritional health from overnutrition to undernutrition.
4. Outline the "ABCD" activities often performed to assess nutritional status.
5. List some changes brought on in your nutritional intake by the recent changes seen in our "modern-age" society (within the past 20 years).

REFERENCES

1. Axelson ML: The impact of culture on food-related behavior, *Annual Review of Nutrition* 6:345, 1986.
2. Basiotis PP and others: Number of days of food intake records required to estimate individual and group nutrient intakes with defined confidence, *Journal of Nutrition* 117:1638, 1987.
3. Beaton GH: Towards harmonization of dietary, biochemical, and clinical assessments: the meaning of nutritional status and requirements, *Nutrition Reviews* 44:349, 1986.
4. Birch LL: The acquisition of food acceptance patterns in children. In Boakes RA and others, editors: *Eating habits: food, physiology, and learned behavior,* London, 1987, John Wiley & Sons.
5. Block G and others: Nutrient sources in the American diet, *American Journal of Epidemiology* 122:13, 1985.
6. Burkitt DP, Eaton SB: Putting the wrong fuel in the tank, *Nutrition* 5:189, 1989.
7. Butrum RR and others: NCI dietary guidelines: rationale, *American Journal of Clinical Nutrition* 48:88, 1988.
8. Cassell JA: Commentary: American food habits in the 1980s, *Topics in Clinical Nutrition* 4:47, 1989.
9. Checking out the supermarket shopper, *Journal of the American Dietetic Association* 91:1511, 1991.
10. Garn SM, Leonard WR: What did our ancestors eat? *Nutrition Reviews* 47:337, 1989.
11. Harper AE: Nutrition: from myth and magic to science, *Nutrition Today*, Jan/Feb 1988, p 8.
12. Harper AE: The 1990 Atwater lecture: the science and the practice of nutrition: reflections and directions, *American Journal of Clinical Nutrition* 53:413, 1991.
13. Kant AK and others: Dietary diversity in the U.S. population NHANES II, 1976-1980, *Journal of the American Dietetic Association* 91:526, 1991.
14. Koplan JP and others: Nutrient intake and supplementation in the United States (NHANES II), *American Journal of Public Health* 76:287, 1986.
15. McBean LD: Consumer knowledge and attitudes about diet and nutrition, *Diary Council Digest* 62:19, 1991.
16. National Research Council—National Academy of Sciences: *Diet and health,* Washington DC, 1989, National Academy Press.
17. Reese CP and others: Impact of commercial eating on nutrient adequacy, *Journal of the American Dietetic Association* 87:463, 1987.
18. Rozin P: Acquisition of stable food preferences, *Nutrition Reviews* 48:106, 1990.
19. Surgeon General's report on nutrition and health, *Nutrition Today,* Sept/Oct 1988, p 22.
20. Webb L: Changing dietary habits of consumers, *Topics in Clinical Nutrition* 5:34, 1990.
21. Woteki CE and others: National Health and Nutrition Examination Survey—NHANES, *Nutrition Today,* Jan/Feb 1988, p 25.
22. Wright HS and others: The 1987-88 Nationwide Food Consumption Survey, *Nutrition Today,* May/June 1991, p 21.

SUGGESTED READINGS

We want to call your particular attention to the article by Beaton that describes the many theoretical problems surrounding the establishment of nutrient needs. This article reminds us that we should not attribute extravagant values to nutrients, but instead have foods as our major focus. Axelson looks in detail at various social influences on our food behavior, including income, education, gender, race, and attitude. Articles like this one published in *Annual Review of Nutrition* are generally quite detailed and provide numerous references. Finally, the articles by Harper provide interesting looks at the science of nutrition and emphasize the importance of maintaining a skeptical mind when evaluating nutritional claims. He reminds us that nutrition-related diseases, such as diabetes mellitus and heart disease, are common not only because of our food habits, but also because of genetic background and the long life that all of us have the potential to enjoy. As we age, these diseases have a longer time to develop.

TAKE ACTION

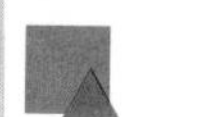

Examine the factors affecting your eating habits

Choose 1 day of the week that is typical of your eating pattern. In the table below, list all foods and drinks you consumed for 1 day. In addition, write down the approximate amounts you ate in units like CUPS, OUNCES, TEASPOONS, and TABLESPOONS. Check the food composition table in Appendix A for examples of appropriate serving units for different types of foods, such as meat, vegetables, etc. After completing this activity you will use this list of foods for future activities.

After you record each food, drink, and serving size, indicate in the table why you choose to consume each item. Use the following symbols to indicate your reasons. Place the corresponding letter in the space provided, indicating why you picked that particular food or drink.

TAST	Taste/Texture	**HUNG**	Hunger
CONV	Convenience	**FAM**	Family/Cultural
EMO	Emotions	**PEER**	Peers
AVA	Availability	**NUTR**	Nutritive value
ADV	Advertisement	**$**	Cost
WTCL	Weight Control	**HLTH**	Health

There can be more than one reason for choosing a particular food or drink.

Time	Minutes spent eating	M or S	H*	Activity while eating	Place of eating	Food and quantity	Others present	Reason for food choice

M or S: Meal or snack
H: Degree of hunger (*0 = none; 3 = maximum)

Application

Now ask your self what is your most frequent reason for eating or drinking. To what degree is health a reason for your food choices? Should it be made a greater priority? ▲

NUTRITION PERSPECTIVE

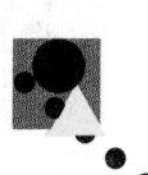

Establishing Nutrient Needs by Scientific Research

The study of nutrient needs and nutrient metabolism relies on information obtained by use of the scientific method, a method designed to detect and eliminate error. Scientists begin by observing physical phenomena. They conjecture and speculate about the causes of the phenomena, and then suggest possible explanations or **hypotheses** about them. They critically examine these possibilities using rigorous experimental tests to either support or refute them. If many lines of evidence support hypothesis, it gains the status of a **theory.**

hypothesis An "educated guess" by a scientist to explain a phenomenon.

theory An explanation for a phenomenon that has numerous lines of evidence to support it.

Science obliges us to view hypotheses and theories skeptically, avoiding hasty acceptance of them based on meager evidence and discarding those that fail to pass critical analyses (see Figure 1-6).[11] Nutrition science requires skeptical minds that impose a critical evaluation of all current ideas. In other words, don't react to one research study by radically changing your life. Looking for consistency of results in science, coupled with critical evaluation, are important tools for you to use when evaluating nutrition research.

Generating Hypotheses

Historical events often give us clues to important relationships in nutrition science. For example, in the fifteenth and sixteenth centuries, when European explorers left Europe to come to the Americas, the disease **scurvy** developed during long voyages. This deficiency disease developed because the sailors ate few fruits and vegetables, and thus consumed very little vitamin C. Eventually British scientists discovered that lime juice cured the scurvy. About 300 years later vitamin C was discovered. Meanwhile the British Navy, run by "Limeys," had a healthy work force, and in turn dominated the seas worldwide.

scurvy The deficiency disease that results after a few months of consuming a diet free of vitamin C.

During World War II, the German army blockaded the Russian city of Leningrad, causing widespread semistarvation there. Noting that this lack of food was associated with increased infant **mortality,** scientists in North America reevaluated the finding and eventually showed that food supplements given to poor women improved their chances of delivering a healthy baby.

mortality This represents a population's death rate. The term morbidity refers to the number of sick persons in a population.

Still, viewed from a historical perspective, man appears capable of surviving on a diet consisting either mainly of meat or almost entirely of vegetables and fruit. The human species is known to have subsisted for many thousands of years on a diet high in vegetable content and low in animal products. Early diets were about one third from animal sources and two thirds from plant sources and were generally higher in protein, lower in fat, and higher in dietary fiber than ours. This was not for any nutritional reason, but because that was what was available. We examine the diet of early humans further in Chapter 18. For now, note that history can give us clues to the path to a healthy diet, but any "answers" deserve close scrutiny. Just because early humans ate differently than we do, diet superiority is not necessarily indicated.[10] Only closer scientific scrutiny can provide that assessment.

Epidemiology

Another approach scientists pursue to establish nutritional hypotheses is to study the different dietary and disease patterns among various populations in the world. If one group tends to develop a certain disease while another group does not, speculation can occur about the role diet plays in this difference. The study of diseases in populations is called **epidemiology.**

epidemiology The study of how disease rates vary between different population groups, such as the rate of stomach cancer in Japan compared with that in Germany.

pellagra A disease characterized by inflammation of the skin, diarrhea, and eventual mental incapacity due to lack of the vitamin niacin in the diet.

In the 1920s, epidemiological studies helped Dr. Joseph Goldberger determine that the disease **pellagra** was a dietary deficiency disease, rather than an infectious disease. He noticed that prisoners in jail—but not their jailers—suffered from

NUTRITION PERSPECTIVE

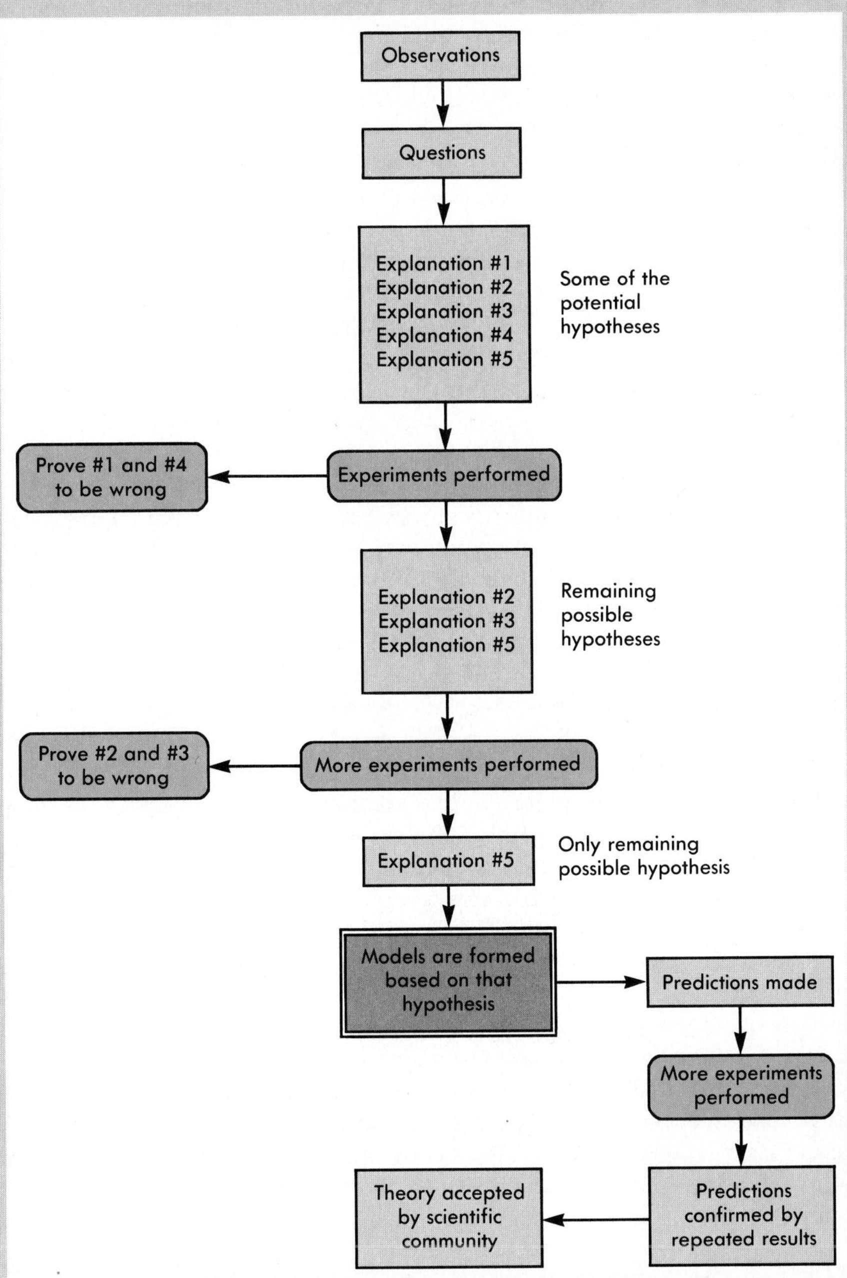

Figure 1-6 From question to theory—the process of science applied to nutrition. Only after careful and thorough analysis does a research finding deserve to have influence over our food choices.

NUTRITION PERSPECTIVE

Establishing Nutrient Needs by Scientific Research—cont'd

infectious disease Any disease caused by an invasion of the body by microorganisms, such as bacteria, fungi, or viruses.

experiment A test made to examine the validity of a hypothesis.

animal model A disease in animals that duplicates human disease and thus can be used to understand more about the human disease.

pellagra. If pellagra was an **infectious disease,** both populations would be expected to suffer from it.

In the 1970s, Dr. Denis Burkitt noted the low rate of intestinal problems in Africans compared with Americans. Burkitt speculated that the large amount of dietary fiber that Africans eat leads to greater intestinal health, and that the low dietary fiber intakes seen in the United States cause problems.

Confirming Epidemiological Impressions

Epidemiological evidence, however, was still not enough for either Goldberger or Burkitt to establish that a dietary problem caused the diseases they studied. Getting better evidence required **experimental** testing. In the 1920s, various foods were fed to people in mental asylums who suffered from pellagra. The experiment showed that yeast and high-protein foods could cure pellagra. Similarly, when typical Americans' diets were improved to contain more dietary fiber in the 1970s, intestinal health often improved. The research on pellagra is largely complete, but research on the importance of dietary fiber to health still continues.

Using Animals to Explore Epidemiological Associations

When scientists cannot test their hypotheses on humans, they often use animals. Much of what we know about human nutritional needs and functions has been generated from animal experiments. Still, human experiments are the most convincing for scientists. In the 1930s, scientists showed that a pellagra-like disease seen in dogs, called blacktongue, was cured by nicotinic acid. But only when nicotinic acid actually cured the disease in humans were scientists convinced that nicotinic acid, later called niacin, was the critical dietary factor.

Today we know that low doses of the mineral fluoride can stimulate growth in rats. However, we still do not know whether that is true for humans because no human experiment can be conducted. It is just not practical to control the fluoride intake of humans accurately enough. Thus there is speculation that fluoride might stimulate growth in humans, but real proof is lacking.

In addition, some human experiments would not be ethical, and so are impossible. Careful, humane use of animals is then the typical option used. You may think it is reasonable to feed rats a low-copper diet to study copper's importance in the formation of blood vessels. (Some people argue that performing animal experiments is unethical.) Almost universally, however, people would find it unethical to study how copper affects the formation of blood vessels in infants.

Unfortunately, this means scientists often cannot advance their findings in humans beyond the point of epidemiology. In addition, perhaps no disease exists in animals that is comparable with a particular human disease, so no **animal model** can be used to further pursue the question. Adding a further roadblock is perhaps insufficient funds for experimentation in humans.

Using Human Subjects to Answer Research Questions

The Case-Control Study. A case-control study can almost be considered a microscopic epidemiological study. It is a study wherein one looks at individuals with the condition in question, and compares them to a group without the condition but matched subject by subject in other major characteristics not under study, such as age and gender. This comparison may point out factors, other than the condition in question, that differ between the two groups. Such knowledge may equip the researchers with a clue towards the possible cause of the condition.

NUTRITION PERSPECTIVE

The Double-Blind Study. An important approach used to test hypotheses is the double-blind study. By definition, this requires that a group of subjects follow a specific protocol, such as eating a certain food. A corresponding control group then must follow the normal pattern of living. People are randomly assigned to each group, such as by a flip of a coin. Scientists then observe the experimental group over time to see if there is any effect that is not found in the control group. Sometimes subjects are used as their own control: first, they are observed for a period of time, and then they are treated and their responses noted.

double-blind study An experimental design where neither the subjects nor the researchers are aware of the subject's assignment (test or placebo) nor the outcome of the study until it is completed. An independent third party holds the code and the data until the study is completed.

Bias (prejudice) can easily affect the outcome of an experiment. Researchers need to limit the amount of bias they and the subjects contribute in the experiment. The best way to do that is to make sure the subjects and researchers are "blind," in that neither knows which subjects are in the experimental group and which are in the **control group.** In addition, the effects of the experimental protocol are not disclosed until after the entire study is completed. This approach avoids the possibility that researchers may see the change they want to see in the subjects in order to prove a certain hypotheses, even though the change did not actually occur. This approach also avoids the chance that the subjects may begin to feel better, for example, simply because they are part of the experimental group.

control group Participants in an experiment whose habits are not altered.

The effect of mere suggestion is referred to as the placebo effect. The Latin word placebo means I shall please. The placebo effect cannot be accounted for on the basis of pharmacological or other direct physical action. Feeling better when the physician walks into the room is a common example of the placebo effect.

placebo A fake medicine used to disguise the roles of participants in an experiment; if fake surgery is performed, that is called a sham operation.

In a double-blind experiment a **placebo** (fake medicine), such as a sugar pill, is often given to the control group in order to camouflage who is in what group and so defeat the bias introduced by the placebo effect. Until the experiment is complete, an independent third party holds the code that identifies each participant and his or her treatment. Sometimes only a single-blind protocol is possible, in which either the subjects or the researchers are kept in the dark.

Drug studies lend themselves to a double-blind protocol because it is often easy to disguise the drug with a placebo. However, food studies often cannot be placebo controlled. It is hard to disguise a diet high in fruits and vegetables from one devoid of them. However, in that case, the experimenters should try to ensure that the results from the blood assays or other samples are not revealed until the end of the study. In addition, the results should be kept from the subjects until the end of the study. In that way much potential bias can be eliminated. The more bias is controlled in the experiment, the more confidence we can have in the results.

When you read accounts of scientific experiments, ask yourself: "Was a double-blind study protocol used? If the use of a placebo was possible, was it used? During the progress of the experiment, were the researchers 'blinded' as much as possible to who received the experimental treatment and to the effects of that treatment?"

Peer-Review of Experimental Results

Once an experiment is complete, scientists summarize the findings and publish the results in a scientific journal. At the ends of the chapters in this book, we list many citations for important experiments that have been published in scientific journals. Most of these journals are peer-reviewed. This means other scientists have judged the quality of the research, striving to allow only the highest quality research findings to be published. Research results published in the *American Journal of Clinical Nutrition,* the *New England Journal of Medicine,* or the *Journal of The American Dietetic Association* are much more reliable than those found in popular magazines or promoted on television talk shows. A major difference is that scientific journals are closely scrutinized by the scientific community to make sure the research results are of sufficient quality to deserve your attention.

The American Dietetic Association has established a toll-free hotline, staffed by registered dietitians, to answer consumers' food-related questions. Call (800) 366-1655, weekdays from 10 a.m. until 5 p.m. EST.

NUTRITION PERSPECTIVE

Establishing Nutrient Needs by Scientific Research—cont'd

The Need for Follow-Up Studies

Finally, even if the study contains all the right factors and is accepted by the scientific community, one examination is not enough. Results from one laboratory must be confirmed by other laboratories. Only then can we really trust and use the results. We don't advise accepting new ideas as fact or incorporating them into your health habits until they are proven by several lines of evidence. Until then, the best goal is variety in the diet and moderation with any food.[11]

CONCEPT CHECK

Nutrition knowledge often proceeds from epidemiological findings through laboratory animal studies to the human study. Throughout this book we will point out areas where more research is needed to answer important nutritional questions. Many of these questions will have been raised by epidemiological studies or by other observations of scientists; they now await support from experiments done in the animal and, especially, the clinical laboratory. Until overwhelming evidence supports the hypothesis, ideally from more than one blinded study, it should not be considered a nutrition "fact."

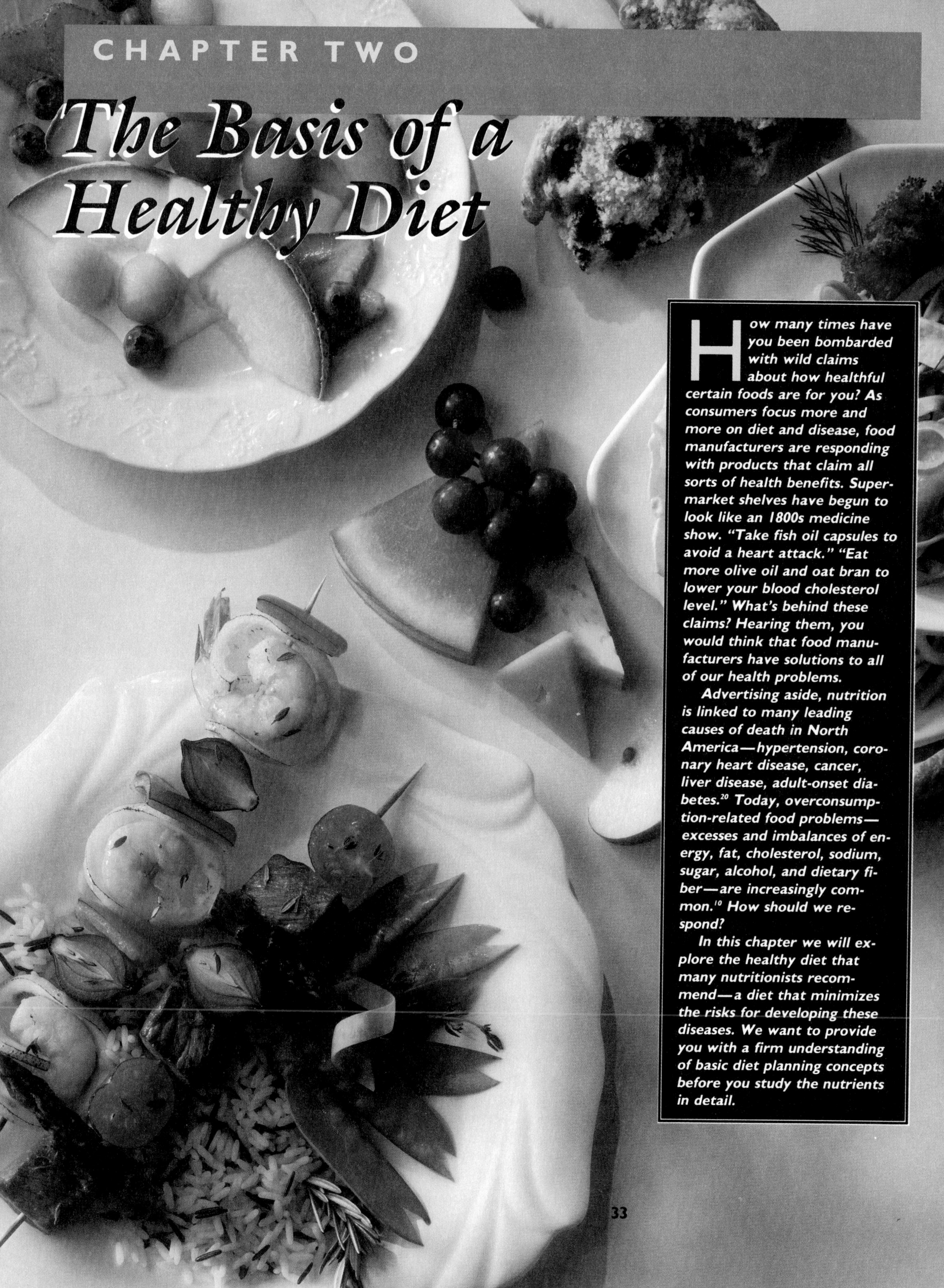

CHAPTER TWO

The Basis of a Healthy Diet

How many times have you been bombarded with wild claims about how healthful certain foods are for you? As consumers focus more and more on diet and disease, food manufacturers are responding with products that claim all sorts of health benefits. Supermarket shelves have begun to look like an 1800s medicine show. "Take fish oil capsules to avoid a heart attack." "Eat more olive oil and oat bran to lower your blood cholesterol level." What's behind these claims? Hearing them, you would think that food manufacturers have solutions to all of our health problems.

Advertising aside, nutrition is linked to many leading causes of death in North America—hypertension, coronary heart disease, cancer, liver disease, adult-onset diabetes.[20] Today, overconsumption-related food problems—excesses and imbalances of energy, fat, cholesterol, sodium, sugar, alcohol, and dietary fiber—are increasingly common.[10] How should we respond?

In this chapter we will explore the healthy diet that many nutritionists recommend—a diet that minimizes the risks for developing these diseases. We want to provide you with a firm understanding of basic diet planning concepts before you study the nutrients in detail.

NUTRITION AWARENESS INVENTORY

Here are 15 statements about the tools for studying nutrition. Answer them to test your current knowledge. If you think the statement is true or mostly true, circle T; if you think the statement is false or mostly false, circle F. Use the scoring key at the end of the book to compute your total score. Take this test again after you have read this chapter. Compare the results. Make sure to correct answers as needed.

1. T F The basic nutrients are carbohydrates, fats, proteins, vitamins, minerals, and water.
2. T F It is sufficient for children to just have protein intake to meet daily losses.
3. T F In addition to eating a balanced diet, it is important for most adults to take vitamin supplements to be certain they are getting enough nutrients.
4. T F A cup of water equals a milliliter (ml) of water.
5. T F 100 grams equals about 1 pound.
6. T F RDA is the abbreviation for recommended daily allowance.
7. T F Most vitamins are needed daily to maintain good health.
8. T F Recommended nutrient intakes differ from country to country.
9. T F Establishing personal nutritional needs is the main purpose of the RDAs.
10. T F An intake of 1500 kcalories per day is considered adequate for most people.
11. T F Although potatoes are vegetables, their nutrient content more closely resembles that of bread than that of broccoli.
12. T F The exchange system works on the premise that foods with similar fat, protein, and carbohydrate composition can be substituted for each other.
13. T F Nutrient density is based on the nutrient to kcalorie ratio in a food.
14. T F A kcalorie is the amount of heat required to raise the temperature of 1 liter of water 1° C.
15. T F There is no perfect food.

What Should I Eat?

You may be surprised to learn that what you should eat is exactly what you've heard many times before—a great variety of foods balanced by moderation with each food. A variety of foods is best because no natural food meets all your nutrient needs. Human milk comes close for the infant, except it provides only low amounts of iron and vitamin D. Cow's milk also contains very little iron and no dietary fiber. Meat provides protein but little calcium. Eggs have no vitamin C, and the calcium is mostly in the shell. This is why you need a variety of foods—the nutrients you need are scattered among many foods.

Many people would like to live on pizza alone. What are pizza's nutrient strengths and inadequacies? Check the food composition table, Appendix A, for the vitamin C content of cheese pizza. How many slices would you need to eat to yield the RDA of 60 milligrams? (Answer: 25 slices)

A FOOD PLAN THAT WORKS

One way to balance your diet as you consume a variety of foods is to select foods from the five major food groups everyday. These groups are (1) vegetables; (2) fruits; (3) breads, cereals, and other grain-based foods; (4) milk, cheese, and other dairy products, such as yogurt; and (5) meats, fish, poultry, eggs, dry beans and peas, and nuts. The foods are grouped based on similar nutrient contents. A bean burrito with tomatoes accompanied by a glass of milk and an apple takes care of all groups. Fats, oils, and sweets also can be added to one's diet to increase its desirability. An easy way to further "balance" your total diet is to vary the foods within each group so you don't eat only a small group of foods.

Eating **moderately** requires planning: by reviewing your entire day's diet, you can plan ahead on how to juggle nutrient sources. For example, when you plan to eat something relatively high in fat, sugars, salt, or kcalories, such as a bacon cheeseburger at a quick-service restaurant, you should eat other foods that are lower in the same nutrients, like fruits and salad greens, the same day. If you choose salty ham for dinner, opt for fresh or frozen vegetables prepared without salt to accompany it. If you prefer whole milk to low-fat or skim milk, cut the fat elsewhere in your meals. Try low-fat salad dressings or use jam instead of butter or margarine on toast.

NUTRITION FOCUS

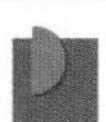

Mathematical Tools in Nutrition

The mathematical concepts you need for studying nutrition are few. Besides performing addition, subtraction, multiplication, and division, you need to calculate simple ratios and proportions (expressed as percentages) and convert English units of measurement to metric units. Note that Chapter 1 covered the conversion of kcalories to kjoules. This is important to know since many scientific journals today will only accept energy units in kjoules.

Percentages

The term percent (%) refers to a part of the total when the total represents 100 parts. For example, if you earn 80% on your first nutrition examination, you will have answered the equivalent of 80 out of 100 questions correctly, and the other 20 questions incorrectly. We have already discussed percentages when describing the American diet in Chapter 1. The best way to master this concept is to calculate some percentages. We have included some problems below.

Question	Answer
What is 6% of 45?	0.06 × 45 = 2.7
What is 32% of 8?	0.32 × 8 = 2.6
What percent of 16 is 6?	6/16 = .375 or 37.5%
What percent of 99 is 3?	3/99 = 0.03 or 3%

Joe ate 15% of the adult RDA for vitamin C at lunch. How many milligrams did he eat? (RDA = 60 milligrams)

0.15 × 60 milligrams = 9 milligrams

Joe ate 200 grams of carbohydrate, 100 grams of fat, and 70 grams of protein yesterday. Turn those values into percentages of total kcalories:

total kcalories = (200 × 4) + (100 × 9) + (70 × 4) = 1980

% of kcalories as carbohydrate = (200 × 4)/1980 = .404 or 40.4%

% of kcalories as fat = (100 × 9)/1980 = .455 or 45.5%

% of kcalories as protein = (70 × 4)/1980 = .141 or 14.1%

It is difficult to succeed in a nutrition course unless you know what a percentage means and how to calculate one. We use the concept of percentages frequently in referring to diets and nutrient composition.

The metric system

The basic units of the metric system are the meter for length, the gram for weight, and the liter for volume. The inside cover of this book contains conversion factors for the English system units of pounds, feet, and cups to metric units. Here is a brief summary.

A meter is 39.4 inches long, or about 3 inches longer than 1 yard (3 feet). A meter is divided into 100 units called centimeters. A meter divided into 1000 units yields millimeters. There are 2.54 centimeters in 1 inch, and about 30 centimeters in 1 foot. A 6-foot tall person is 183 centimeters tall.

A gram is about 1/28 of an ounce (1/28.3 to be exact). Thus an ounce equals 28 grams. Five grams of sugar or salt is about 1 teaspoon. A kilogram is 1000 grams, a kilogram is equivalent to 2.2 pounds. A 156-pound man weighs 71 kilograms. A milligram breaks a gram into 1000 parts; a microgram breaks 1 gram into 1,000,000 parts.

Liters are divided into 1000 units called milliliters. One teaspoon equals about 5 milliliters, 1 cup is about 240 milliliters, and 1 quart (4 cups) equals almost 1 liter (0.946 liters to be exact).

If you plan to work in any realm of science, you should study the metric system until you become quite comfortable with it. For now, remember that a kilogram equals 2.2 pounds, 2.54 centimeters equals 1 inch, and a liter is almost the same as a quart. In addition, know what the prefixes micro-, milli-, centi-, and kilo- represent. With that knowledge you can get an approximation of any metric quantity into English units and approximate English units into the metric system.

Overall we should strive to moderate—as opposed to feeling we must eliminate—intake of some foods.[20]

Most important, eat foods that appeal to you. There are no “good” or “bad” foods. Focus on your total day’s intake when you make a “health” evaluation. Fortunately we live in a time when the food supply is abundant and safe. For most of us a good diet is affordable, and we have a huge variety of food choices. A well-balanced and healthful diet can be planned to match your family and cultural traditions, lifestyle, and budget. Even so, white bread, whole milk, doughnuts, cookies, French fries, hot dogs, hamburgers, and meat loaf—all high in fat—along with sugared soft drinks make up a major part of the American diet.[6] Many of us have our work cut out for us to improve our nutrition and health habits.[15]

Health professionals have recommended the same basic diet plan for the last 10 years: watch how much you eat, focus on the major food groups, and stay physically active.[9] Whole grains, fruits, and vegetables have always been among the "good guys" in our diet. Let's now fine-tune this advice.

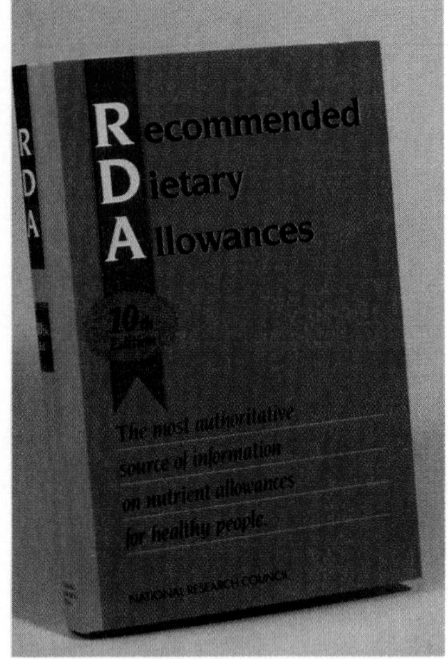

Figure 2-1 The 1989 RDAs are contained in a publication, which incorporates much supporting evidence and discussion of the various nutrient recommendations made by the Food and Nutrition Board of the National Academy of Sciences.

Recommended Dietary Allowances (RDAs)

Before designing a diet, we need to know how frequently we need to consume each nutrient and how much is enough (or too much). People have puzzled over these questions for centuries. In fact a major nutrition controversy arose when many men were rejected from military service during World War II because of the effects of poor nutrition on their health. In response, a group of 25 scientists met in the early 1940s and formed the first Food and Nutrition Board. They were given the responsibility to establish dietary standards that could be used to both evaluate the nutritional intakes of large population groups as well as provide a guide for planning agriculture production. This board developed the first RDAs, issued in May 1941.[11] Because their standards had to be based on insufficient scientific information, they realized the RDAs would need alterations as new information became available. This is still true today—RDAs change as new knowledge necessitates.[16]

Subsequently, the RDAs were revised every 4 to 5 years (Figure 2-1). To set new RDA levels or reevaluate existing values the Food and Nutrition Board does the following:[12]

1. Estimates the average **requirement** of a population for a given nutrient and the **variability** for that requirement in a population. In other words, the board estimates how much of a nutrient each person requires to be healthy and how much those requirements vary among people.
2. Increases that average requirement by amounts sufficient to meet the needs of nearly all members of the population. This usually means increasing the average requirement by about 30% to 50%. Thus if the average requirement for a vitamin is 20 milligrams per day, the RDA may be approximately 28 milligrams per day, or 40% higher than the average figure.
3. Increases the RDAs to account for inefficient use by the body of the nutrients once consumed. This inefficiency could be caused by poor absorption, poor conversion of an inactive form to an active form, or other causes.
4. Uses scientific judgment to interpret and establish allowances when information about requirements is limited. In other words the members of the Food and Nutrition Board need to use their scientific judgment in lieu of specific scientific data in certain cases.

Recommended Dietary Allowances (RDAs) Recommended intakes of nutrients that meet the needs of almost all healthy people of similar age and gender. These are established by the Food and Nutrition Board of the National Academy of Sciences.

Using this process, the board sets the RDAs for males and females according to various age groups (see the inside cover of this textbook for the specific recommendations).

One important fact to note is the RDAs serve as a guide to help you meet your nutritional needs with food, rather than relying on vitamin and mineral supplements. The RDAs are based on the assumption that we eat a wide variety of foods (in other words follow a mixed diet). This aim is important because only 19 of approximately 40 necessary nutrients—not counting essential amino acids—have an RDA. Not enough is known about many nutrients for the Food and Nutrition Board to establish an RDA. However, all essential nutrients should be part of your diet.

THE RDA ARE NOT FOR AMATEURS

One common misconception about the term RDA is that the "D" stands for "daily." It does not; it stands for "dietary." It is not necessary to consume the RDA for each nutrient every day. Think instead of averaging the RDA for vitamins and minerals over a week's time. No nutrient (even water) need absolutely be consumed every day. A typical adult can survive for a few days on a diet without water, months without an intake of vitamin A, and about 1 to 3 years on a diet without vitamin B-12. Notice also that the "R" stands for recommended, not required.

requirement The amount of a nutrient required by one person to maintain health. This varies between individuals. No one knows his or her true requirements for various nutrients.

variability The variation one would expect to see in nutrient requirements within a group of individuals.

Because the RDAs are based on our average needs and increased to account for variability in the population, it is by definition a generous allowance. The Food and Nutrition Board expects that the allowances are high enough so that healthy people will demonstrate no improvement in health from consuming more than RDA levels.[12] The board believes the RDA generally covers any possible benefit that may be achieved from the nutrients obtainable in a typical diet. A key goal of the RDA is to protect Americans from receiving either too much or too little of the needed nutrients; the RDA guidelines provide good protection against both possibilities. Too often people think that if a little of something is good, a lot must be better. This can lead to trouble with some nutrients, as you will see in Chapter 12.

Thus the RDAs are estimates of the amount of each nutrient that should be consumed by healthy people to meet their nutritional needs. The word healthy needs emphasis. The RDA guideline also assumes that people are not taking medications or suffer from diseases that increase nutrient needs, are not experiencing temperature extremes, and do not participate in long, strenuous physical activity.[12]

Correct uses of the RDAs include:

- Planning and obtaining food supplies for groups, such as schools, hospitals, and health care facilities.
- Designing sample diet plans for food assistance programs, such as the USDA Thrifty Food Plan.
- Evaluating dietary survey data, such as NHANES, and other scientific research.
- Developing food and nutrition information and education, such as given in federal food assistance programs.
- Establishing food labeling standards, such as U.S. RDA and RDI.
- Regulating food fortification, such as setting standard fortification policies for enriched bread, milk, and infant formulas.
- Developing new or modified food products, such as for use in military combat and space rations.

A CLOSE LOOK AT ONE RDA: PROTEIN

The RDA of 0.8 grams of protein per kilogram of body weight per day for an adult aims for a state of protein **equilibrium:** where protein intake balances daily losses.[12] This ends up to be about 50 to 60 grams (0.8×70 kg $= 56$). Balance studies also are used to set RDAs for many nutrients; other methods are used for various other nutrients. One alternate approach is eating a diet that causes depletion of stores of a specific nutrient in a person and then seeing how much of that nutrient it takes to regain adequate status for that nutrient. For the balance method the nutrient allotment includes the amount needed to meet body losses and to keep stores full in the body (Figure 2-2).[18] Thus the overall economy of the nutrient in the body, in this case protein, should remain stable.

equilibrium A state where nutrient intake equals nutrient losses. Thus the body maintains a stable condition.

In setting the RDAs for children, scientists include enough protein to meet daily losses and maintain stores, plus some extra to accommodate growth and storage in new tissue that is built each day. The RDAs for children then must attempt to promote a positive protein balance. Equilibrium is not good enough because children need to gain new protein tissue. Children, then, should regularly consume a greater amount of protein than they lose. The same is true for pregnant women and people recovering from significant injuries and weight loss caused by disease.

positive balance A state where a nutrient intake exceeds losses. This causes a net gain of the nutrient in the body, such as when tissue protein is gained during growth. The opposite of this would be negative balance, where losses exceed intake, as in cases of starvation.

Whether we need to be in equilibrium or **positive balance,** none of us knows exactly how much protein we need each day. Based on the adult RDA for protein, if we each consume 0.8 grams of protein per kilogram of body weight per day (again, 56 grams for a 70 kilogram—154 pound—person), probably all of us will meet our needs. However, the RDA does not indicate that if you eat only 0.6 grams per kilogram instead, you will necessarily not get enough protein. Because allowances are generous, many of us get enough protein when we eat less than the RDA. This is an example of why the RDAs do not actually apply to individuals.

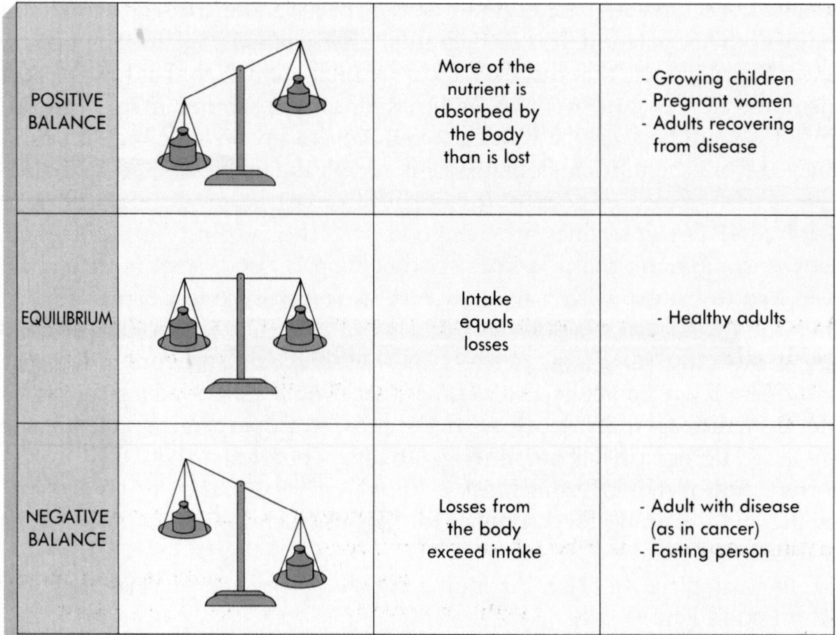

Figure 2-2 Nutrient balance using protein as an example. The concept of positive balance, equilibrium, and negative balance applies to the health status of a person with respect to all nutrients.

If you calculate the amount of protein you eat in a week, divide by 7, compare it with the RDA, and find that your intake is close to the RDA, fine. You are most likely consuming enough protein. However, if you take in less protein than the RDA suggests, you do not know whether you are eating enough protein. You could need less than the RDA. Overall, the further you stray from an RDA, the greater your risk of a nutritional deficiency. Based on statistical theory, when you are eating less than half of an RDA, it is likely that you are not eating enough of that nutrient.

Signs and symptoms of nutritional deficiencies may be subtle and develop slowly. Decreased effectiveness of the immune system, reduced enzyme functions, or an impaired ability to carry oxygen in the bloodstream may not become apparent for a long period of time. You may become ill more often and not know the cause. Though your diet may be inadequate, you still may show no telltale signs. No "smoke detector" will sound the alarm. Thus it is best to eat a diet that meets the RDAs for your age and gender, rather than run the risk of developing health problems from poor nutrition. This recommendation forms the basis for the dietary advice in this book.

CORRECTLY APPLYING THE RDAs TO GROUPS

From this discussion it should be clear RDAs are not meant as requirements for individuals. These are set for the nutrient needs of groups and should be used primarily to plan and evaluate what groups eat.[12] Recall one original purpose of the RDAs when established in the 1940s: to plan and evaluate soldiers' diets. That is still the basic function of the RDAs, except its scope now includes all healthy groups of Americans, such as college students eating on campus.

ESTIMATED SAFE AND ADEQUATE DAILY DIETARY INTAKES

Estimated Safe and Adequate Daily Dietary Intake (ESADDI) Nutrient intake recommendations first made in 1980 by the Food and Nutrition Board, where a range for intake of some nutrients was given because not enough information was available to set an RDA.

As noted above, the Food and Nutrition Board revises the RDAs every 4 to 6 years in response to new scientific information. In 1980, **estimated safe and adequate daily dietary intakes (ESADDI)** were listed for several nutrients that previously had no RDA, including copper, biotin, and chromium (see inside cover). The Food and Nutrition Board felt that there were insufficient data on these nutrients to set an RDA, but enough data existed to suggest a range for a reasonable intake for groups. In 1989, the tenth edition of the RDAs included a category called minimum requirements for sodium, potassium, and chloride, rather than ESADDIs, which were in the ninth edition.[16] Even with the estimated safe and adequate daily dietary intakes and minimum requirements included with the RDAs, some nutrients—like carbohydrates, fats, boron, and nickel—still are not covered by specific numerical amounts. They have no set number. Meeting all nutrient needs stated by the Food and Nutrition Board through diet, not with supplements, should account for these other nutrients.

RDA FOR ENERGY NEEDS

RDAs for nutrients are set high enough to meet the needs of almost all healthy people. In comparison, The Food and Nutrition Board sets the RDA for energy at the average energy needs for various age groups, and also provides a wide range for the allowance (see inside cover of this textbook for recommendations). Note that no extra amount is added for human variabilities, as is done for nutrient RDAs. Excess kcalories consumed (above energy needs) are not easily excreted, as is the case with most vitamins and minerals. Thus to promote weight maintenance a more conservative standard must be set for energy needs. The board also warns that the energy RDA is only a rough estimate.[12] Energy intake should depend more on energy use. For most adults, weight maintenance is the best yardstick of energy balance—kcalorie intake that matches kcalorie output.

WORLD NUTRIENT GUIDES

Canada has its own version of RDAs, called Recommended Nutrient Intakes (RNIs), set by the Department of National Health and Welfare (Appendix D).[8] Great Britain also has its own guideline, as do other countries. The World Health Organization, together with the Food and Agriculture Organization (FAO/WHO) of the United Nations publishes a counterpart to the RDAs to apply worldwide. All these nutrient recommendations are set by separate groups of scientists. The groups do not always agree, so the recommended nutrient levels may differ from country to country, although they are usually close (see Table 2-1). If they are not close, a good expla-

Table 2-1 Comparison of United States (1989), United Kingdom (1985), Canadian (1990), and WHO (1974) dietary standards for the adult male and adult female

Classification	Kcal	Protein (grams)	Calcium (mg)	Iron (mg)	Vitamin A (RE)	Thiamin (mg)	Riboflavin (mg)	Vitamin C (mg)
United States								
Female (63 kg, 1.63 m)	2200	50	800	15	800	1.1	1.3	60
Male (79 kg, 1.76 m)	2900	63	800	10	1000	1.5	1.7	60
United Kingdom								
Female	2150-2500	54-62	500	12	750	0.9-1.0	1.3	30
Male	2150-3350	63-84	500	10	750	1.0-1.3	1.6	30
Canada								
Female (59 kg)	1900	51	700	13	800	0.8	1.0	30
Male (74 kg)	2700	64	800	9	1000	1.1	1.4	40
FAO/WHO								
Female	2200	29	400-500	14-28	750	0.9	1.3	30
Male	3000	37	400-500	5-9	750	1.2	1.8	30

Modified from Shils ME, Young UR: *Modern nutrition in health and disease,* ed 7, Philadelphia, 1988, Lea & Febiger.

nation for the difference often exists. For example, different populations worldwide consume different amounts of protein. This can lead to varying vitamin and mineral needs. Philosophies also vary on the role of the dietary allowances, which can alter the amount set.

CONCEPT CHECK

Recommended Dietary Allowances represent the nutrient needs of groups, not of individuals. RDAs are established for specific age and gender categories. No one knows his or her own personal nutritional requirements. The best general rule is that the further you stray from the RDAs for your age and gender, the greater the chance of experiencing a nutritional deficiency.

U.S. Recommended Daily Allowances (U.S. RDA) Standards established by the FDA for use on nutrition labels. Generally the four existing versions use the highest nutrient recommendation in the appropriate age and gender category from the 1968 publication of the RDA. The version that includes children over 4 years of age and adults is most commonly seen on nutrition labels.

U.S. RDA AND RDIs

One practical application of the RDAs is the **U.S. Recommended Daily Allowances (U.S. RDA).** Note that the "D" stands for Daily. The U.S. RDA, set in 1974 by the FDA, is used on nutrition labels on foods. It replaced the minimum daily requirements (MDR). The U.S. RDA for adults basically represents a compilation from the 1968 publication of the RDAs and primarily uses the highest RDA values within specific age categories. For example, consider iron: In 1968 the RDA for adult men was 10 milligrams per day; for adult women and adolescents it was 18 milligrams per day. The U.S. RDA for adults used the higher value of 18 milligrams per day. Table 2-2 lists U.S. RDA values for the category that refers to children

Table 2-2 U.S. Recommended Daily Allowances (U.S. RDA) and provisional Reference Daily Intakes (RDI) compared to values from the 1989 RDA publication

Vitamins and minerals	Units of measurement	U.S. RDA for adults and children 4 or more years of age*	RDI‡	RDA (or ESADDI) Males 19 years old	RDA (or ESADDI) Females 19 years old
Protein	Grams	65†	50	58	46
Vitamin A	Retinol Equivalents	1000	875	1000	800
Vitamin D	"	400	260	400	400
Vitamin E	"	30	9	10	8
Vitamin C	Milligrams	60	60	60	60
Folate	"	0.4	0.180	0.200	0.180
Thiamin	"	1.5	1.2	1.5	1.1
Riboflavin	"	1.7	1.4	1.7	1.3
Niacin	"	20	16	19	15
Vitamin B-6	"	2.0	1.5	2.0	1.6
Vitamin B-12	Micrograms	6.0	2.0	2.0	2.0
Biotin	Milligrams	0.3	0.06	0.03-0.1	0.03-0.1
Pantothenic Acid	"	10	5.5	4-7	4-7
Calcium	Grams	1.0	0.9	1.2	1.2
Phosphorus	"	1.0	0.9	1.2	1.2
Iodine	Micrograms	150	150	150	150
Iron	Milligrams	18	12	10	15
Magnesium	"	400	300	350	280
Copper	"	2.0	2.0	1.5-3.0	1.5-3.0
Zinc	"	15	13	15	12

*These U.S. RDA values are on most nutrition labels.
†If protein efficiency ratio of protein is equal to or better than that of casein. RDA is 45 g for adults, 20 g for children under 4 yrs, and 18 g for infants (see Chapter 6).
‡Note the RDI will soon replace U.S. RDA (by 1993), but also might undergo some fine tuning beforehand.

over 4 years of age through adults. Note also that certain nutrients do not quite follow the rule. The highest adult and adolescent RDA in 1968 was 1200 milligrams for calcium, but the U.S. RDA is 1000 milligrams. FDA believed that 1000 milligrams was high enough.

Four versions of the U.S. RDA exist: (1) children over 4 years and adults, (2) infants less than 1 year, (3) toddlers 1 to 4 years, and (4) pregnant and lactating (breast-feeding) women. Most nutrition labels that list the U.S. RDA use the "adult" version. Infant formulas will use the infant U.S. RDA, "junior" baby foods use the "toddler" U.S. RDA, and vitamin supplements designed for pregnant women use the U.S. RDA designed for pregnant and lactating women.

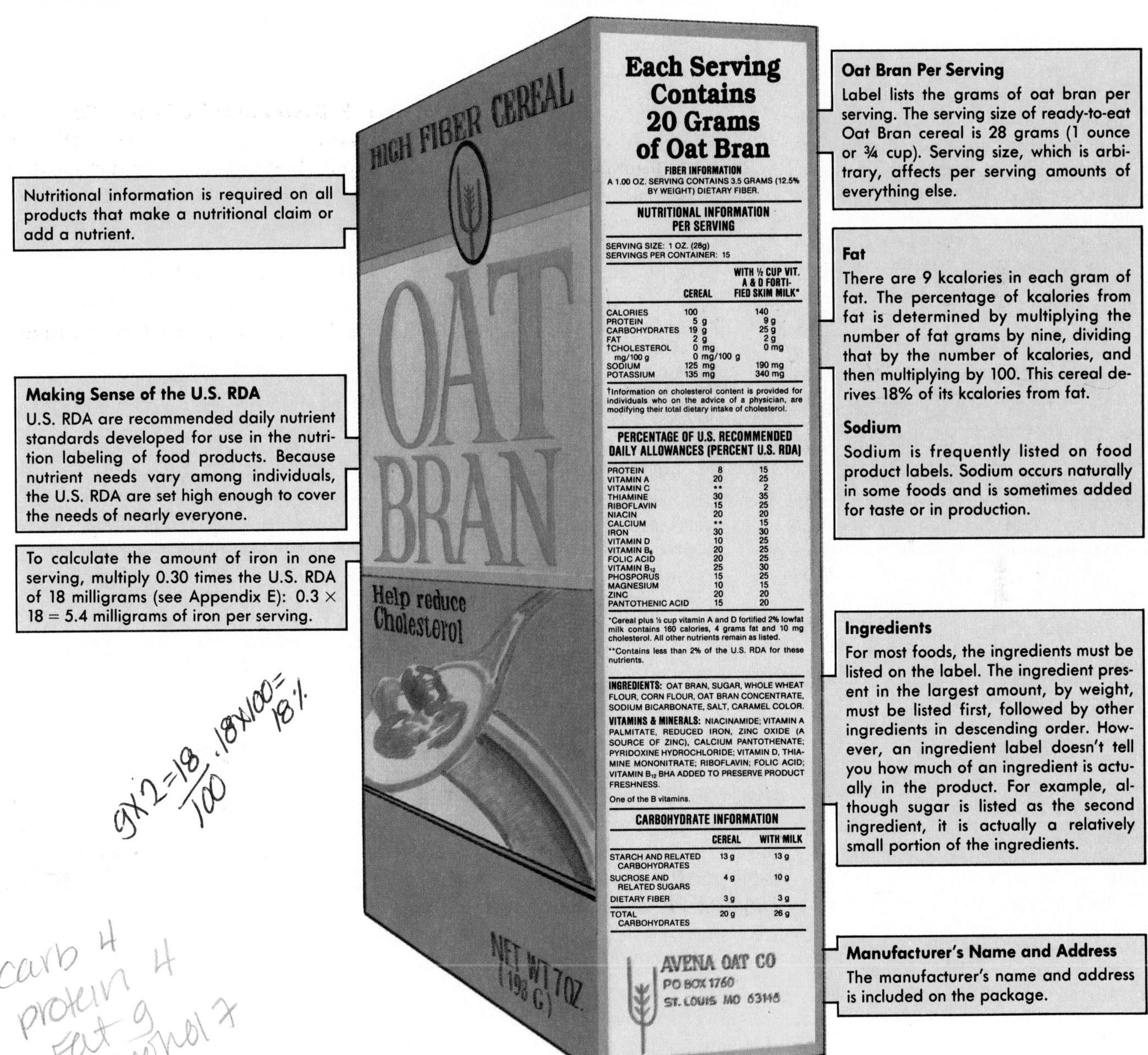

Figure 2-3 A nutrition label. This label is a source of much important nutrition information, such as the kcalorie and fat content of a food. The Nutrition Perspective reviews the parts of this label in detail. The format of this label will likely change by May 1993, but what changes will take place are still under study. Overall, nutritionists recommend that all of us read these labels in order to understand more about our current nutrient intakes.

EXPERT OPINION

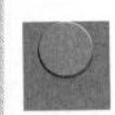

What's on the Label?

CONSTANCE GEIGER, PH.D. R.D.

Today, people are very interested in nutrition and health. A recent Louis Harris survey found that the percentage of Americans buying low-fat, low-cholesterol foods went from 36% in 1986 to 61% in 1989, which indicates that health is increasingly important in consumer food selection. Increased consumer interest in health has resulted in greater availability of decreased-kcalorie, decreased-sodium, decreased-fat, and increased-fiber products in the supermarket. Consumers have more nutrition information than ever before. However, they do not always interpret it correctly. So what can you do as a consumer to learn more about nutrition? What can a food label tell you or how can it help you learn about nutrition?

In 1990 FDA began a three-step approach to update the nutrition label, and in November 1990 the Nutrition Labeling and Education Act (NLEA) became law. This act affects the entire nutrition label. The following are some important highlights that you can look for as a consumer to help you make more informed food choices:

1. Before the NLEA, nutrition labeling was required only for fortified foods and those for which nutrition claims were made. The NLEA now makes nutrition labeling information mandatory on virtually all packaged foods.
2. USDA and FDA regulations will be synchronized, and so nutrition labeling also will be mandatory for all processed meat and poultry products.
3. Nutrients that must be listed on a label will change to keep pace with the nation's changing health concerns. We are now concerned more with chronic disease prevention than with deficiency diseases. The proposed mandatory nutrients reflect this concern and include kcalories from fat, saturated fat, complex carbohydrates, sugars, and dietary fiber. Other familiar nutrients that will continue to stay on the label include total kcalories, total fat, cholesterol, total carbohydrates, protein, sodium, vitamin A, vitamin C, calcium, and iron.

   Thiamin, niacin, riboflavin, and other nutrients would become optional in listings as the concern about deficiencies for these nutrients no longer exists. Polyunsaturated and monounsaturated fats and soluble and insoluble fibers will be required on the label if a health claim is made for the product, such as high in fiber.
4. The names of nutrient allowances will be changed to percent of Daily Value (DV). The Recommended Dietary Intakes (RDIs) and Daily Recommended Values (DRVs), as mentioned in the chapter, are meant to serve as reference values to help you compare how nutrient levels in foods contribute toward general recommendations for a total diet. For the first time ever, standards for labeling are being proposed for such nutrients as total fat, saturated fatty acids, unsaturated fatty acids, cholesterol, total carbohydrate, fiber, sodium, and potassium.

   A nutrition profile is proposed for the bottom portion of the nutrition label for those nutrients that have established DRVs. The nutrients would appear with the absolute amount along with percent of DRV. These standards

Reference Daily Intakes (RDI) Standards for expressing nutrient content on nutrition labels. RDI are based on average 1989 RDA values set for a nutrient that span a particular age range, such as children over 4 years through adults. RDI will replace the U.S. RDA by May 1993. FDA wants to use the RDI and Daily Reference Values (DRV) as a single list of reference values known as "Daily Values" (or some other variant) in showing nutrition information on food labels.

Mainly for economic reasons, the U.S. RDA have not been updated since 1968, but new food labeling laws will soon lead to changes. The new name for U.S. RDA will be **Reference Daily Intakes (RDIs).**[3] Values will be based on the 1989 RDAs and represent an average value of the RDA for that nutrient over the age range that the RDIs is applied to (Table 2-2 and Appendix F). In addition, **daily reference values (DRVs)** will also be set by FDA for certain parts of a diet that have no true 1989 RDA, such as carbohydrate, fat, sodium, potassium, and dietary fiber. The DRVs are intended to help us further evaluate food choices as we compare food values of these substances to desirable (or maximum) intakes (Appendix F).

Figure 2-3 shows a current **nutrition label** and how the U.S. RDA for children over 4 years of age and adults are depicted as percentages. The label we show states that one serving of this breakfast cereal contains 30% of the U.S. RDA for iron. Since the U.S. RDA for iron is 18 milligrams and 0.3 × 18 is 5.4 milligrams, this product contains about 5.4 milligrams of iron per serving. For the vitamin niacin, the label states a content of 20% of the U.S. RDA. With a U.S. RDA of 20 milligrams, the niacin content is 0.2 × 20, or about 4 milligrams.

Note that the U.S. RDA values (currently still in use) are in general slightly higher than 1989 RDAs. An example is the abovementioned U.S. RDA for iron for adults. Even though the highest RDA value for iron for adult women was 15

EXPERT OPINION

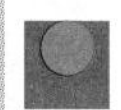

What's on the Label?—cont'd

CONSTANCE GEIGER, PH.D. R.D.

have created some controversy, as could be expected, in the scientific community. Overall, however, they can help you interpret how much you need (or should limit) per day.

5. An exciting development is a "dictionary of terms" for consistent and uniform definitions with regard to nutrient content claims. You have probably seen these claims on labels but not realized that they have had no legal definition. For example, the term light, lite, etc. can mean light in color, weight, or kcalories. Now, there will be uniform definition. Nutrient content claims will include two types of claims: (1) content claims and (2) comparative claims. The new regulation will establish criteria for use and allowed terms. The content claims include *free, low, source of, and high*. The comparative claims include the terms *reduced, light or lite, less, fewer, more, and fresh*.
6. Definitions will also be specific for the fatty acid and cholesterol content of food. Many of you have seen products that say "95% fat free." The product is 5% fat by weight, not 5% of kcal from fat. The new proposed regulations indicate "percent fat free" can be used only on low-fat foods; in other words, those with less than or equal to 3 grams of fat per serving. Another important term is "reduced fat," which can be used only if it has less than or equal to 50% fat of the typical food and if the reduction is greater than 3 grams of fat per serving. A "cholesterol free" claim can be made if the food contains less than 2 grams of saturated fat per serving and less than 2 milligrams of cholesterol per serving.
7. Guidelines for voluntary labeling of raw fruits and vegetables and fish have also been recommended. So you will be seeing nutrition labeling on produce, most likely as placards above the products.
8. A new format for nutrition labeling is being proposed. No one is sure what this format will be; however, there has been a push for the use of graphics in nutrition labeling. Some studies have indicated that consumers prefer this format and comprehend it better than a numerical format. Several food manufacturers are already using pie charts and bar graphs on food labels with great success.

In summary, the new regulations will be helpful to you because nutrition labeling will be required on almost all processed food products and voluntary food labeling will be seen on many fresh items. You will be able to know the nutrient content of your candy bar or cookie or other foods that have not been required to be labeled prior to this time. Standardized terminology will be used for nutrient content claims and there will be strict definitions for those claims. Nutrition profiles will provide you with reference amounts so you can gauge about how much you should consume in a day. This is indeed an exciting time for nutrition labeling and for consumers. The Nutrition Perspective at the end of this chapter further discusses some of the concepts examined here.

Dr. Geiger is currently Assistant Professor and Director, Division of Foods and Nutrition, University of Utah. Her research involves nutrition labeling, with a special focus on meeting consumer needs.

milligrams per day in 1989, the U.S. RDA still uses an earlier estimate of 18 milligrams of iron per day for adults. Therefore when you read a cereal label that claims a serving provides 25% of the U.S. RDA for a nutrient, you can be sure that it will provide at least 25% of the RDA for your age and gender. This is especially true for vitamin E, vitamin B-12, and folate. Your need, if it is different from the U.S. RDA, will probably be lower. An exception is calcium for the age group 11 to 24 years; the U.S. RDA is 200 milligrams lower than the RDA. The proposed RDI values follow the adult RDAs much more closely (Table 2-2). See the Nutrition Perspective to learn more about regulations that apply to nutrition labels on foods.

NUTRIENT DENSITY

The RDAs are used to evaluate the diets of groups, but what is used to evaluate the nutritional quality of an individual food? **Nutrient density** is a concept that has gained acceptance in recent years. To estimate nutrient density, simply compare the vitamin or mineral content of the food with the number of kcalories it provides. For any nutrient, the higher the nutrient density in the food the more nutrient—say vitamin C—there is per kcalorie, and so the better the food source is for that particular nutrient. Still, the focus on menu planning is the total diet, not whether

nutrient density The ratio formed by dividing a food's contribution to nutrient needs by its contribution to kcalorie needs. When the contribution to nutrient needs exceeds that of its kcalorie contribution, the food is considered to have a favorable nutrient density.

one food is the key to an adequate diet. Nonetheless, nutrient-dense foods like skim and low-fat milk, lean meats, beans, nuts, oranges, carrots, broccoli, whole-wheat bread, and whole-grain breakfast cereals do help balance less nutrient-dense choices we often make, like cookies and chips. The latter are often called empty-calorie foods because they tend to supply energy as sugar and fat, but little else.

CONCEPT CHECK

The U.S. RDA, designed in 1974 by the FDA, is currently used as a benchmark for representing the nutrient content of foods on nutrition labels. Nutrient content is expressed as a percentage of the U.S. RDA. The values used to set the U.S. RDA were taken primarily from the 1968 publication of the RDA. This standard will soon be updated to reflect 1989 RDA values and be renamed reference daily intakes (RDIs). The concept of nutrient density evaluates the nutrient contributions made by each food in a diet in comparison with its contribution to total kcalorie needs. Nutrient-dense foods supply much of one or many nutrients for a modest amount of kcalories.

Meal Planning Tools

In the 1940s nutritionists began translating the RDA into more practical terms so that people with no special training could estimate whether their nutritional needs were being met. A seven-food-group plan was one of many early formats. Daily food choices had to include food from each group. This plan later was simplified to five food groups. By the mid-1950s a four-food-group plan was established that included a milk group, a meat group, a fruit and vegetable group, and a breads and cereals group. In 1979 the names of the groups were revised, and a fifth group containing fats, sweets, and alcoholic beverages was added as part of the "Hassle-Free Daily Food Guide." Caution was urged in consuming this last group, though some foods in it can supply needed vitamin E and essential fatty acids. The entire plan was designed to provide a minimum foundation for a complete diet and represents about 1200 to 1400 kcalories.

In 1985 the USDA revised the Hassle-Free Daily Food Guide to represent a total diet, rather than simply a foundation for a diet. This latest plan is called USDA's Food Guide Pyramid—A Guide to Daily Food Choices (Figure 2-4). The major changes are an increase in fruit and vegetable servings from four per day to five to nine per day, and an increase in bread and cereal servings from four per day to six to eleven per day. One goal of these changes is to provide the bulk of dietary energy intake from carbohydrate while limiting fat intake.

From this point on we will refer to USDA's Food Guide Pyramid as The Guide to Daily Food Choices. This emphasizes the content rather than the shape of the plan.

USING THE GUIDE TO DAILY FOOD CHOICES TO BUILD A BETTER DIET

The number of servings to eat from each food group in the current Guide to Daily Food Choices depends on a person's age and kcalorie needs. Serving size is also adjusted for young children. Table 2-3 lists serving sizes and amounts for various ages. The traditional plan for an adult over age 24 basically consists of two servings from the milk, yogurt, and cheese group; two to three servings from the meat, poultry, fish, dry beans, eggs, and nuts group (5 to 7 ounces total); three to five servings from the vegetable group; two to four servings from the fruit group; and six to eleven servings from the bread, cereals, rice, and pasta group. A final group that requires cautious use includes fats, oils, and sweets. Some population groups—children, teenagers, adults under age 25, and pregnant or lactating women—need three servings of the milk, yogurt, and cheese group. Table 2-3 lists the major nutrients each food group supplies. Note the similarities and differences between the groups. Table 2-4 uses the plan to construct a 1-day meal plan.

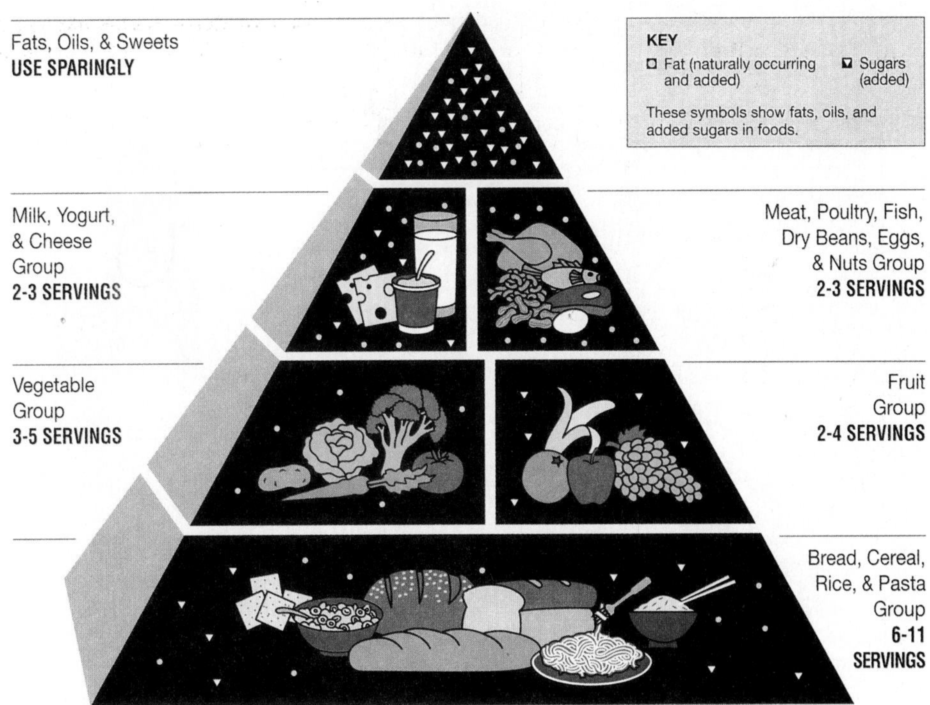

Figure 2-4 USDA's Food Guide Pyramid—A Guide to Daily Food Choices. This guide lists the food groups and number of servings to consume of each. Note for children, teenagers, and adults under age 25, three servings should be chosen from the milk, yogurt, and cheese group.

Here are several important points to keep in mind when you use The Guide to Daily Food Choices:

1. The guide does not deal with infant feeding.
2. No one food is absolutely essential to good nutrition. Each food is low in at least one essential nutrient.
3. No one food group alone provides all essential nutrients in adequate amounts. Each food group makes an important, distinct contribution to nutritional intake.
4. Variety is the key to the guide and is first guaranteed by using all the groups. Furthermore, one should consume a variety of foods within each group.
5. The foods within a group can still vary widely with respect to nutrient and kcalorie content. Comparing the kcalories in 3 ounces of baked potato (98) to that in 3 ounces of potato chips (470) helps to make this point. Do the same comparison for an orange and apple with respect to vitamin C using Appendix A.

Again, the foundations of balanced nutrition are variety and moderation. The Guide to Daily Food Choices specifically speaks to all of these parameters. Choosing from every group and varying choices within groups allows for a healthy variety of foods. The nutritional adequacy of the guide is compromised unless variety of choices is practiced. In addition, to ensure enough vitamin E, vitamin B-6, magnesium, iron, and zinc—nutrients sometimes low in diets based on this plan—we recommend the following advice:

1. Choose low-fat and nonfat items from the milk, yogurt, and cheese group. This saves kcalories to allow for more of other food group choices.
2. Make sure to regularly include servings of vegetable protein sources, at least several times a week.
3. For vegetables and fruits, try to include a dark green vegetable each day. In the NHANES II survey, only 25% of those interviewed had eaten such a vegetable that day. Efforts to increase use of these foods are needed.[5]
4. Choose whole-grain varieties of breads, cereals, rice, and pasta often.
5. Moderate use of foods rich in fats and sugars. This again saves kcalories to allow for more of other food group choices.

Table 2-3 The Guide to Daily Food Choices—a summary

Food group	Serving	Major contributions	Foods and serving sizes*
Milk, yogurt, and cheese	2 (adult‖) 3 (children, teens, young adults, and pregnant or lactating women)	Calcium Riboflavin Protein Potassium Zinc	1 cup milk 1½ oz cheese 2 oz processed cheese 1 cup yogurt 2 cups cottage cheese 1 cup custard/pudding 1½ cups ice cream
Meat, poultry, fish, dry beans, eggs, and nuts	2-3	Protein Niacin Iron Vitamin B-6 Zinc Thiamin Vitamin B-12†	2-3 oz cooked meat, poultry, fish 1-1½ cups cooked dry beans 4 T peanut butter 2 eggs ½-1 cup nuts
Fruits	2-4	Vitamin C Fiber	¼ cup dried fruit ½ cup cooked fruit ¾ cup juice 1 whole piece of fruit 1 melon wedge
Vegetables	3-5	Vitamin A Vitamin C Folate Magnesium Fiber	½ cup raw or cooked vegetables 1 cup raw leafy vegetables
Bread, cereals, rice, and pasta	6-11	Starch Thiamin Riboflavin§ Iron Niacin Folate Magnesium‡ Fiber‡ Zinc‡	1 slice of bread 1 oz ready-to-eat cereal ½-¾ cup cooked cereal, rice, or pasta
Fats, oils, and sweets		Foods from this group should not replace any from the other groups. Amounts comsumed should be determined by individual energy needs.	

This is a practical way to turn the RDA into food choices. You can get all essential nutrients by eating a balanced variety of foods each day from the food groups listed here. Eat a variety of foods in each food group and adjust serving sizes appropriately to reach and maintain desirable weight.

*May be reduced for child servings.
†Only in animal food choices.
‡Whole grains especially.
§If enriched.
‖≥ 25 years of age.

Table 2-4 Putting the Guide to Daily Food Choices into practice

Breakfast

1 peeled orange
1½ cup Cheerios with ½ cup 1% milk
1 slice raisin toast, 1 teaspoon margarine
Optional: coffee or tea

Lunch

Ham sandwich
  2 slices whole wheat bread
  2 ounces ham
  2 teaspoons mayonnaise
Banana
4 oatmeal raisin cookies (small)
Optional: diet soda

3 PM Study Break

1 whole bagel
2 tablespoons peanut butter
½ cup 1% milk

Dinner

Lettuce salad
  1 cup romaine lettuce
  ½ cup sliced tomatoes
  2 tablespoons 1000 Island dressing
  1 grated carrot
4 ounces broiled salmon
½ cup rice
¾ cup green beans with teaspoon margarine
Optional: coffee or tea

Late night snack

1 cup fruited low-fat yogurt

Nutrient breakdown:

2100 kcalories

carbohydrate	52% of kcalories
protein	18% of kcalories
fat	30% of kcalories

Meets RDA/ESADDI values for all vitamins and minerals for adult age 25. For adolescents and adults under age 25, add 1 additional serving of milk, yogurt, and cheese group.

Overall, excessive consumption of any single food is risky. Our diets must continue to be balanced, though with less of a bias towards meat and dairy products in order to moderate fat intake.[4]

By following the Guide to Daily Food Choices it is easy to create daily diets that contain as little as 1600 kcalories. This level of kcalories does not meet the needs of an active adult, but it will probably meet the needs of a sedentary adult or an elderly person. If 1600 kcalories are too many kcalories for you, first try to become more active. It is very difficult to obtain enough nutrients from a food plan that supplies less than about 1600 kcalories total. You probably don't need to meet the RDA for all nutrients, but you may never know for which ones those are. If you can't increase your energy output, you may need to include some nutrient-fortified foods, like ready-to-eat breakfast cereals. Chapter 12 discusses whether nutrient supplements are a wise choice; they are usually not needed. In addition, if your diet does not include meat or other animal products, see the Nutrition Perspective on vegetarianism in Chapter 5.

CONCEPT CHECK

The Guide to Daily Food Choices translates nutrient needs into a food plan. This guide recommends that adults over age 24 consume:

1. Two servings from the milk, yogurt, and cheese group (three if age 24 or younger, pregnant, or lactating).
2. Two to three servings from the meat, poultry, fish, dry beans, eggs, and nuts group for a total equivalent of 5 to 7 ounces of lean meat per day.
3. Three to five servings from the vegetable group.
4. Two to four servings from the fruit group.
5. Six to eleven servings from the bread, cereals, rice, and pasta group.
6. Cautious use of fats, oils, and sweets.

THE DIETARY GUIDELINES

The Guide to Daily Food Choices was designed to help meet nutritional needs for protein, vitamins, and minerals. However, most of the major chronic "killer" diseases in America, such as heart disease, cancer, and diabetes, are not associated with deficiencies in protein, vitamins, or minerals. Deficiency diseases such as rickets (vitamin D deficiency) and pellagra (niacin deficiency) are no longer common. It appears the real problems in the American diet for many of us are excess kcalories, saturated fat, cholesterol, alcohol, and sodium (salt) (Figure 2-5).[20] You can also add insufficient calcium, iron, zinc, and dietary fiber in the diets of some people to that list.[15]

Dietary Goals Specific goals for nutrient intakes set in 1977 by a Committee of the U.S. Senate.

Dietary Guidelines General goals for nutrient intake and diet composition now set by the USDA and DHHS.

In response to concerns regarding disease patterns in the United States, a Senate Select Committee developed **dietary goals** for the United States. The first dietary goals were published and then quickly revised in 1977 (Appendix I). In response to criticisms that the dietary goals lacked sufficient scientific data to support the strict recommendations listed, the USDA and Department of Health and Human Services (DHHS) published more general **Dietary Guidelines** in 1980, with slight revisions in 1985 and 1990.[19] The latest version is as follows:

1. Eat a variety of foods. Following the Guide to Daily Food Choices is advised.
2. Maintain healthy weight.

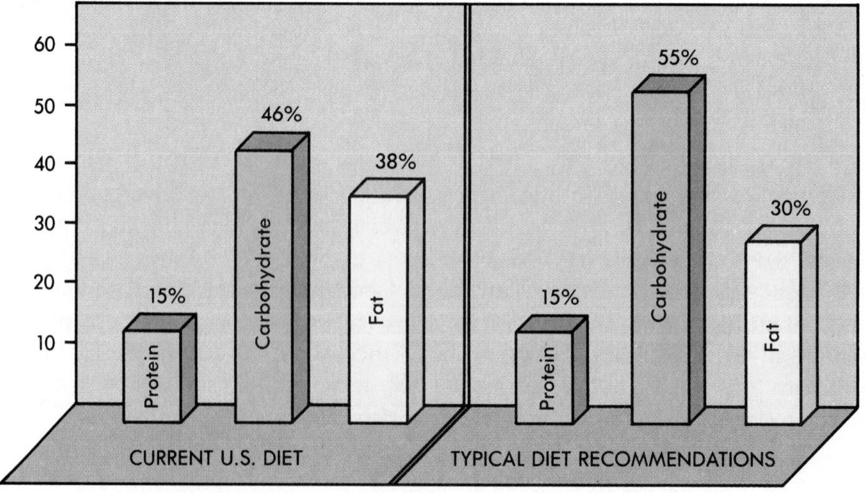

Figure 2-5 Is our current diet in our best interests? Many nutrition scientists, after evaluating the relationship between diet and health, have concluded that we should eat more carbohydrate-rich foods and less fat-rich foods. For carbohydrate-rich foods, choices should be often high in dietary fiber and ideally low in simple sugars.

3. Choose a diet low in fat, saturated fat, and cholesterol. Reducing fat to 30% of kcalories and saturated fat specifically to 10% of kcalories is recommended.
4. Choose a diet with plenty of vegetables, fruits, and grain products.
5. Use sugars only in moderation.
6. Use salt and sodium only in moderation.
7. If you drink alcoholic beverages, do so in moderation. A moderate alcohol intake consists of 2 or fewer servings of: 12 ounces of beer, 5 ounces of wine, or 1½ ounces of distilled spirits (80 proof).

Note that no change in current protein intakes is suggested in this plan.

This plan, published in a pamphlet called *Nutrition and Your Health—Dietary Guidelines for Americans,* tries to ensure adequate vitamin and mineral intake with the first guideline: eat a variety of foods. Then the guidelines try to create changes that will reduce risk for obesity, hypertension, heart disease, diabetes, and alcoholism. We will discuss diet recommendations for adults issued by other scientific groups in Chapter 18. In essence, the current recommendations of the American Heart Association, U.S. Surgeon General,[20] National Academy of Sciences,[17] American Cancer Society, Canadian Ministries of Health, and World Health Organization are consistent with the spirit of these guidelines. These groups do not wish to have people focus on health alone in deciding what to eat but, rather, to encourage them to modify their eating behaviors in ways that are both healthful and pleasurable.[21]

A shortcut method for healthy weight gives 100 pounds for the first 60 inches for women and an extra 5 pounds for every inch thereafter. The corresponding values for males are 105 pounds to start and 6 additional pounds per inch over 60 inches (see Chapter 8).

COMBINING THE MAJOR FOOD PLANS

Ideally, we should combine concepts from the Guide to Daily Food Choices and the Dietary Guidelines as just indicated. Good eating habits can yield life-long dividends.

PUTTING DIETARY GUIDELINES INTO PRACTICE

Some nutritionists are uneasy about the Dietary Guidelines. They think the plan is too general because it does not acknowledge that individual people may need to follow different dietary objectives. As we show in later chapters, some people's health is greatly affected by saturated fat in foods, while the health of others is not; one person's health may be affected by sodium in foods, while another's may not. As individuals, we vary in our tendencies toward developing high blood cholesterol levels, hypertension, obesity, cancer, and other health problems that the guidelines are designed to help prevent.[14] Genetic background is one key reason for the variation, as we covered in Chapter 1. In addition, controversy exists over the harmfulness of sugar. For now, keep in mind these two plans—the Guide to Daily Food Choices and the Dietary Guidelines. If what you are currently eating is far from what these plans recommend, try to make some appropriate changes (Table 2-5).

In your study of the next few chapters, you may find it exciting to design a more personal set of plans for yourself. This is the power of studying nutrition: You no longer must follow general recommendations. You can learn more about your body and find ways to stay healthy, even from plans that vary from those we have just reviewed.

CONCEPT CHECK

Dietary guidelines have been set by a variety of private and government organizations. These guidelines are designed to reduce the risk of developing obesity, hypertension, heart disease, and alcoholism. To do so, they first encourage us to eat a variety of foods, ideally, by following the Guide to Daily Food Choices. Then they encourage us to limit consumption of kcalories to match energy output and to limit total fat, saturated fat, salt, sugar, and alcohol intake while focusing more on fruits, vegetables, and grain products. No alteration in protein intake—another kcalorie contributor—is suggested.

Table 2-5 Advice for applying the Dietary Guidelines to practical situations

You usually eat this:	Reconsider and eat this:
white bread	whole-wheat bread (less nutrients lost in refinement/processing)
sugared breakfast cereal	low sugar cereal (use the kcalories you save for a side dish of fruit)
cheeseburger and french fries	hamburger (hold the mayonnaise) and baked beans (for less fat and the benefits of plant proteins)
potato salad at the salad bar	three-bean salad
doughnut, chips, salty snack foods	bran muffin or bagel (no cream cheese)
soft drinks	diet soft drinks (save the kcalories for more nutritious foods)
boiled vegetables	steamed vegetables (for more nutrient retention)
canned vegetables	frozen vegetables (less nutrients lost in processing)
fried meats	broiled meats (watch the fat drain away)
fatty meats, like ribs	lean meats, like ground round; also, eat chicken and fish often
whole milk and ice cream	1% or skim milk and sherbet or frozen yogurt (to reduce saturated fat intake)
mayonnaise or sour cream salad dressing	oil and vinegar dressings, or diet varieties (to save kcalories)
cookies for a snack	popcorn (air popped with minimal margarine)
heavily salted foods	foods flavored primarily with herbs, spices, and lemon juice

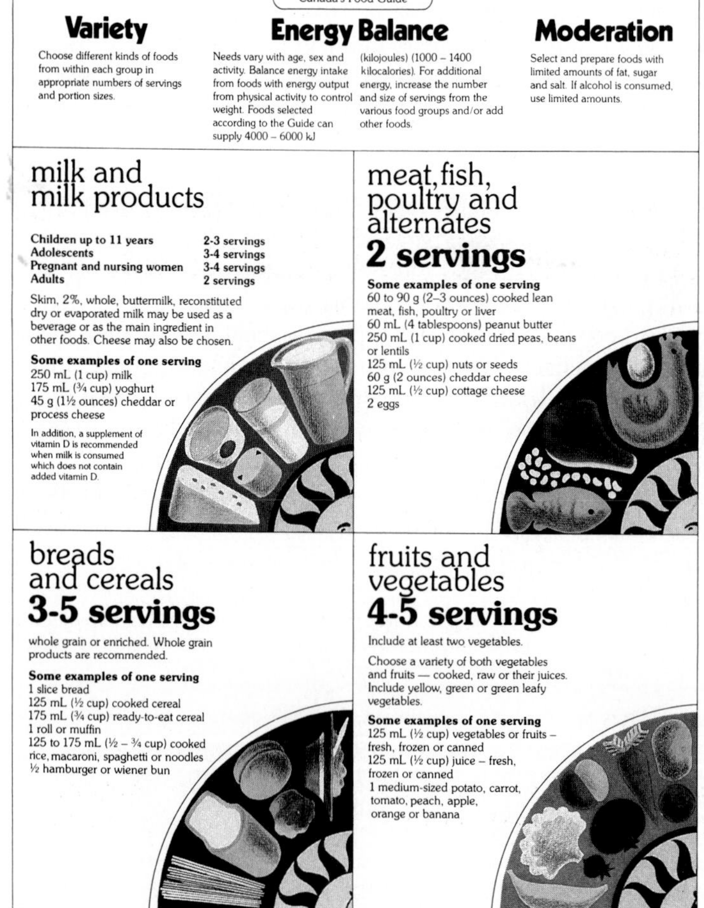

Figure 2-6 The Canadian food guide.

NUTRITION FOCUS

Dietary Advice for Canadians

Canada has its own version of RDA, called Recommended Nutrient Intakes (RNIs), published by the Minister of National Health and Welfare.[8] These are listed in Appendix D. A separate Canadian food guide provides a plan to meet these nutrient needs (Figure 2-6).

A summary of the desired characteristics of a diet for Canadians includes:[8]

1. **The Canadian diet should provide energy consistent with the maintenance of body weight within the recommended range.**
   Physical activity should be appropriate to circumstances and capabilities. While the importance of maintaining some activity throughout life can be stressed, it is not possible to specify a level of physical activity appropriate for the whole population. As a general guideline it is desirable that adults, for as long as possible, maintain an activity level that permits an energy intake of at least 1800 kcalories while keeping weight within the recommended range.
2. **The Canadian diet should include essential nutrients in amounts recommended in this report.**
   While it is important that the diet provide the recommended amounts of nutrients, it should be understood that no evidence suggests that intakes in excess of the RNIs confer any health benefit. There is no general need for supplements except for vitamin D for infants and folate for women during pregnancy. Vitamin D supplementation might be required for elderly persons not exposed to the sun, and iron for pregnant women with low iron stores.
3. **The Canadian diet should include no more than 30% of energy as fat (33 g/1000 kcalories) and no more than 10% as saturated fat (11 g/1000 kcalories).**
   Dietary cholesterol, though not as influential in affecting levels of blood cholesterol, is not without importance. A reduction in cholesterol intake normally will accompany a reduction in total fat and saturated fat intakes. The recommendation to reduce total fat intake does not apply to children under the age of 2 years.
4. **The Canadian diet should provide 55% of energy as carbohydrate (138 g/1000 kcalories) from a variety of sources.**
   Food sources should be selected that provide complex carbohydrates, a variety of dietary fiber, and beta-carotene.
5. **The sodium content of the Canadian diet should be reduced.**
   The present food supply provides sodium in an amount greatly exceeding requirements. While there is insufficient evidence to support a precise recommendation, potential benefit would be expected from a reduction in current sodium intake.
6. **The Canadian diet should include no more than 5% of total energy as alcohol, or two drinks daily, whichever is less.**
   The deleterious influence of alcohol on blood pressure provides a more urgent reason for moderation. During pregnancy it is prudent to abstain from alcoholic beverages because a safe intake is not known with certainty.
7. **The Canadian diet should contain no more caffeine than the equivalent of four regular cups of coffee per day.**
   This is a prudent measure in view of the increased risk for cardiovascular disease associated with high intakes of caffeine.
8. **Community water supplies containing less than 1 mg/liter should be fluoridated to that level.**
   Fluoridation of community water supplies has proven to be a safe, effective, and economical method of improving dental health.

More details are available on RNIs and diet recommendations in the 1990 publication entitled *Nutrition Recommendations: The Report of the Scientific Review Committee.*

In essence, suggested actions toward healthy eating as listed in Canada's Guidelines for Healthy Eating include:

- Enjoy a variety of foods.
- Emphasize cereals, breads, other grain products, vegetables, and fruits.
- Choose low-fat dairy products, lean meats, and foods prepared with little or no fat.
- Achieve and maintain a healthy body weight by enjoying regular physical activity and healthy eating.
- Limit salt, alcohol, and caffeine.

The Exchange System

The **exchange system** is a valuable tool for quickly estimating the energy, protein, carbohydrate, and fat content of a food or meal. Using it also creates greater understanding about what one eats. Rather than memorizing the tables of composition of all foods, your work is greatly simplified by using the exchange system because it generalizes those details into a manageable framework.

exchange system A grouping of foods in six lists. When the serving size for any food in a list is consumed, all foods within the list yield a similar amount of carbohydrate, fat, protein, and energy.

The exchange system arranges foods based on nutrient composition not origin.

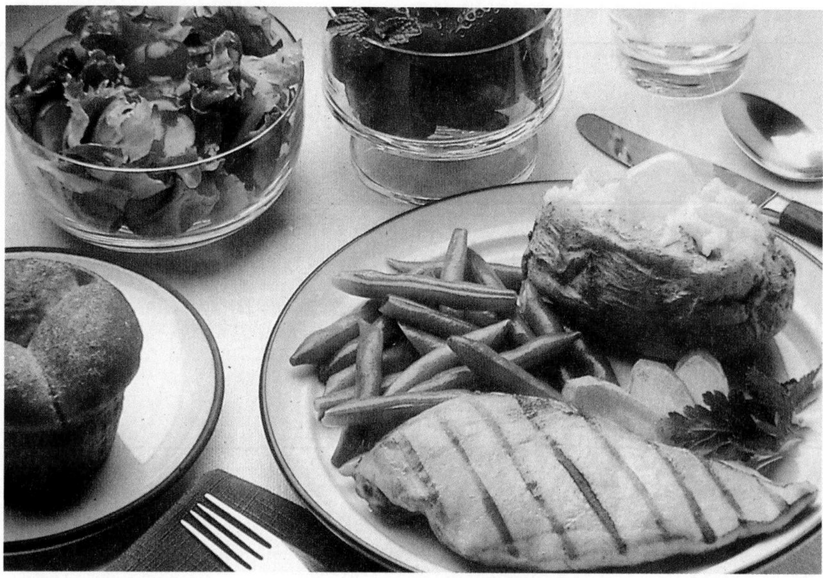

The exchange system arranges food into six different categories: milk, fruit, vegetables, starch/bread, meat, and fat.[1] These categories are designed so that after noting the proper serving size, each food within a category provides about the same amount of carbohydrate, protein, fat, and kcalories. This equality allows the exchange of foods within a category. Hence the term exchange system.

The exchange system was developed in the 1950s for planning diabetic diets. Diabetes is easier to control if the person's diet has about the same composition day after day. If a certain number of **"exchanges"** from each of the six categories is eaten each day, that regularity is easier to achieve. However, the utility of this system goes beyond that, since it yields a quick way to estimate energy, carbohydrate, protein, and fat content in a food or meal. Learning it is a bit tedious. As in learning a foreign language, you will need some practice before you feel comfortable with the exchange system.

exchange The serving size of a food within a specific exchange group.

USING THE EXCHANGE SYSTEM

The exchange system was revised in 1976 and again in 1986. Each time it has changed slightly. When using the exchange system listed in any book, it is important to note which version you are consulting.

To use the exchange system you must know which foods are in each group and the serving sizes for each food. We have listed the entire U.S. exchange system in Appendix G. You will need to consult this appendix many times before you can apply the system.

Table 2-6 shows the carbohydrate, protein, fat, and energy composition of each of the six exchange groups. The starch/bread group has 15 grams of carbohydrate, 3 grams of protein, and a trace of fat per exchange. The trace of fat is calculated as 1 gram of fat when the total energy contribution of a starch/bread exchange is determined. The meat group is divided into three subclasses: lean, medium fat, and high fat. Each exchange has 7 grams of protein. Lean meats contain 3 grams of fat per exchange, medium-fat meats have 5 grams of fat per exchange, and high-fat meats have 8 grams of fat per exchange. Meats have essentially no carbohydrate. The vegetable group contains 5 grams of carbohydrate, 2 grams of protein, and no fat per exchange. The fruit group has 15 grams of carbohydrate per exchange. Fruit has no appreciable fat or protein.

The milk group is divided into three subclasses: nonfat, low-fat, and whole. Each exchange has 12 grams of carbohydrate and 8 grams of protein. Nonfat milk has a trace of fat (calculated as 1 gram when energy content is expressed) per exchange.

Table 2-6 The exchange lists composition (1986 edition)

Exchange list	Household measures*	Carbohydrate (grams)	Protein (grams)	Fat (grams)	Kcalories
Starch/Bread	1 slice, ¾ cup raw, or ½ cup cooked	15	3	trace†	80
Meat	1 ounce				
Lean		—	7	3	55
Medium-Fat		—	7	5	75
High-Fat		—	7	8	100
Vegetable	½ cup cooked	5	2	—	25
Fruit	1 small piece	15	—	—	60
Milk	1 cup				
Skim		12	8	trace†	90
Low-fat		12	8	5	120
Whole		12	8	8	150
Fat	1 teaspoon	—	—	5	45

The American Diabetes Association and American Dietetic Association: *Exchange lists for meal planning,* 1986.
*Just an estimate. See exchange lists for actual amounts.
†Calculated as 1 gram for purposes of energy contribution.

Low-fat milk has 5 grams of fat per exchange, and whole milk has 8 grams of fat per exchange. Finally, the fat group contains 5 grams of fat per exchange. Fats contain no appreciable amount of carbohydrate or protein.

An exchange from the starch/bread group contains 80 kcalories. Lean meats have 55 kcalories per exchange, medium-fat meats have 75 kcalories per exchange, and high-fat meats have 100 kcalories per exchange. Vegetables have 25 kcalories per exchange. Fruits have 60 kcalories per exchange. Skim milk has 90 kcalories per exchange; low-fat milk has 120 kcalories per exchange; and whole milk has 150 kcalories per exchange. Finally fat has 45 kcalories per exchange.

TAKING A CLOSER LOOK AT THE EXCHANGE GROUPS

Before you can turn a group of exchanges into a meal plan for one day, you first have to see what each exchange group contains (see Appendix G). The starch/bread group contains dry cereal, cooked cereal, rice, pasta, baked beans, corn on the cob, potatoes, bread, and tortillas. This list is not the same as that used for the groups in the Guide to Daily Food Choices. The exchange system is not concerned about the origin of the food, whether animal or vegetable. It is primarily concerned with the nutrient composition in terms of carbohydrate, protein, and fat of each food in a group. For example, the carbohydrate composition of potatoes resembles that of bread more than of broccoli, although potatoes are vegetables.

The lean meat list contains round steak, lean ham, veal, chicken (without skin), fish, cottage cheese, and 95% fat-free luncheon meat. The medium-fat meat list contains T-bone steak, pork roast, lamb chops, well-drained duck and goose, salmon, mozzarella cheese, and eggs. The high-fat meat list contains prime cuts of beef (marbled), ribs, sausage, fried fish, cheddar cheese, salami, and peanut butter (Figure 2-7).

The vegetable list contains most vegetables. Some starchy vegetables were listed above in the starch/bread group. Some vegetables, such as cabbage, celery, mushrooms, lettuce, and zucchini, are "free foods"; their minimal energy contribution does not count in the calculations when eaten in moderation (2 to 3 servings per day). The fruit list contains fruits and fruit juices.

The milk exchange list contains milk, plain yogurt, and buttermilk. The amount

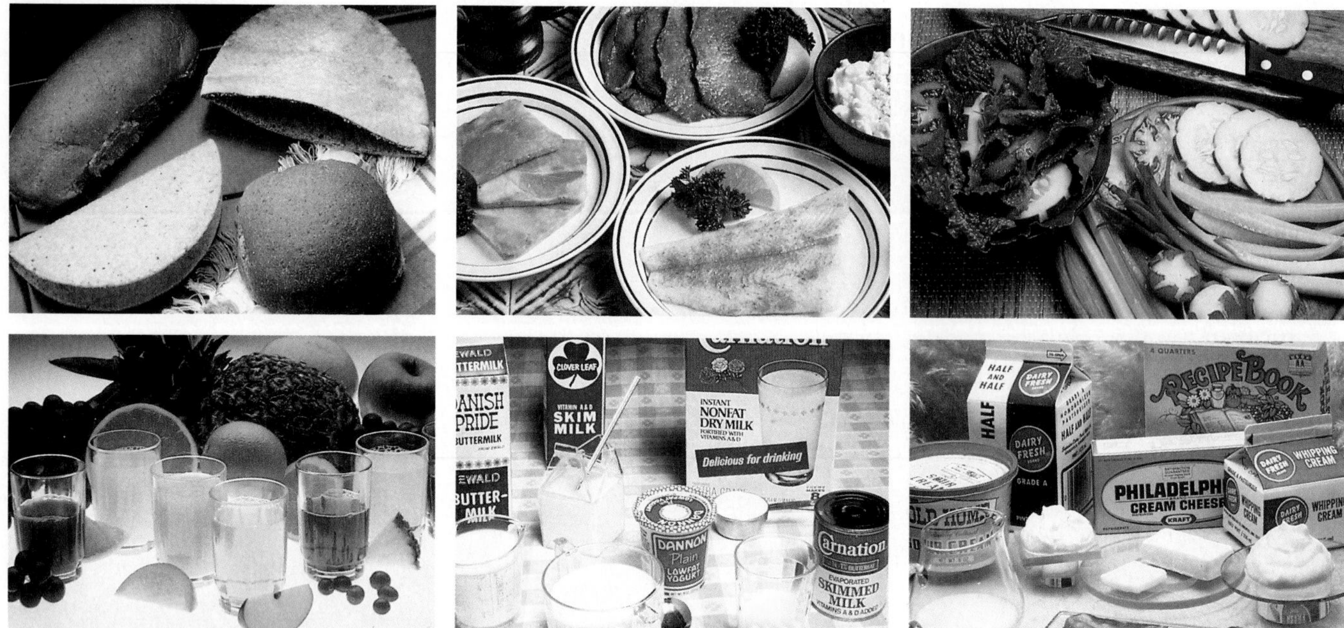

Figure 2-7 The exchange system groups. *Above left,* the starch/bread exchange group; *above center,* the meat exchange group; *above right,* the vegetable exchange group; *below left,* the fruit exchange group; *below center,* the milk exchange group; *below right,* the fat exchange group.

Table 2-7 Exchange patterns to get you started

kcalories/day	1200	1600	2000	2400	2800	3200	3600
Exchange group							
Milk (low fat)	2	2	2	2	2	2	2
Vegetables	2	2	3	3	3	3	3
Fruit	5	4	5	8	8	10	10
Bread	4	8	11	11	15	17	20
Meat (medium fat)	2	2	3	5	5	7	8
Fat	4	7	8	9	12	12	14

These are just one set of options. More meat could be included if less milk is used, for example. The breakdown is: 55% kcalories as carbohydrate, 30% kcalories as fat, 15% kcalories as protein.

of fat in a product determines whether the serving is nonfat, low-fat, or whole.

The fat list contains margarine, mayonnaise, nuts and seeds, salad oils, olives, sour cream, and cream cheese. Bacon is considered a fat, rather than a high-fat meat.

Free foods, other than the vegetables already mentioned, include bouillon, diet soda, coffee, tea, dill pickles, and vinegar, as well as herbs and spices.

Let's now turn an exchange food plan into 1 day's menu. We want 2000 kcalories, consisting of 55% energy from carbohydrates (1100 kcalories), 15% energy from protein (300 kcalories), and 30% energy from fat (600 kcalories). This can be translated into 2 low-fat milk exchanges, 3 vegetable exchanges, 5 fruit exchanges, 11 bread exchanges, 3 medium-fat meat exchanges, and 8 fat exchanges (Table 2-7). Note this is only one of many possible combinations; the exchange system offers great flexibility.

Table 2-8 arbitrarily separates these exchanges into breakfast, lunch, dinner, and a snack. Breakfast includes 1 low-fat milk exchange, 2 fruit exchanges, 3 starch/bread exchanges, and 2 fat exchanges. This total corresponds to ¾ cup cold cereal eaten with 1 cup of 1% milk, 2 slices of bread with 2 teaspoons margarine, and 1 cup of orange juice.

Table 2-8 Turning an exchange system plan into a menu for one day

Breakfast	
1 low-fat milk exchange	1 cup 1% milk (put some on cereal)
2 fruit exchanges	1 cup orange juice
3 bread exchanges	¾ cup cold cereal, 2 pieces whole-wheat toast
2 fat exchanges	2 teaspoons margarine on toast
Lunch	
4 bread exchanges	2 slices whole-wheat bread, 16 animal cookies
3 fat exchanges	2 slices bacon, 1 teaspoon mayonnaise
1 vegetable exchange	1 sliced tomato
2 fruit exchanges	1 banana (9 inches)
1 low-fat milk exchange	1 cup 1% milk
Dinner	
3 medium-fat meat exchanges	3 ounces broiled T-bone steak
2 bread exchanges	1 large baked potato
1 fat exchange	1 teaspoon margarine
2 vegetable exchanges	1 cup broccoli
1 fruit exchange	1 kiwi fruit
	coffee (if desired)
Snack	
2 bread exchanges	1 bagel
2 fat exchanges	2 tablespoons cream cheese

Values calculated using a computer and nutrient analysis software		Prescription
kcalories	2037	2000
Carbohydrate	55%	55%
Protein	16%	15%
Fat	29%	30%

Lunch consists of 3 fat exchanges, 4 starch/bread exchanges, 1 vegetable exchange, 1 low-fat milk exchange, and 2 fruit exchanges. This translates into 2 slices of bacon with 1 teaspoon mayonnaise, two slices of bread, and tomato. In other words, a bacon and tomato sandwich. Add to this a 9-inch banana (1 exchange = ½ banana), 1 cup of 1% milk, and 16 animal crackers.

Dinner consists of 3 medium-fat meat exchanges, 1 fruit exchange, 2 vegetable exchanges, 1 fat exchange, and 2 starch/bread exchanges. This total corresponds to a 3-ounce broiled t-bone steak (meat only, no bone), 1 large baked potato (1 exchange equals 1 small baked potato) with 1 teaspoon of margarine, 1 cup broccoli, and 1 kiwi fruit. Coffee (if desired) is not counted, as it contains no appreciable kcalories.

Finally, we have a snack containing two starch/bread exchanges and two fat exchanges. This translates into 1 bagel with 2 tablespoons of cream cheese.

We have listed only one of many possibilities for a day's food plan. Orange juice could replace apple juice. The banana could be two apples. The T-bone steak could be 3 ounces of chicken breast with the skin. The choices are endless. Notice that an exchange diet is much easier to plan if you use individual foods, as we have; however, the exchange system tables list some combination foods to help you (see

Appendix G).[1] Using combination foods, such as pizza or lasagna, however, makes it more difficult to calculate the number of exchanges in a serving. For instance, lasagna has meat exchanges, vegetable exchanges, and starch/bread exchanges.

With experience, you will be able to tackle such complex foods. For now, using individual foods makes learning the exchange system much easier. Finally, you might want to prove to yourself that our food choices really meet the exchange plan. This demonstration will give you practice turning exchanges into actual food servings.

Note that the exchange system values closely match the computer analysis shown in Table 2-8. The exchange system is a very useful tool for diet planning. If used correctly, there is no easier way to plan a precise menu pattern.

CONCEPT CHECK

The exchange system enables us to design and follow a precise diet that yields desired ratios of carbohydrate, fat, and protein, while accounting for total energy intake. Within each of the six exchange lists, when serving sizes are considered, all foods yield similar contributions of carbohydrate, fat, protein, and kcalories. Their similar nutrient profiles allow the foods in each group to be "exchanged" for each other.

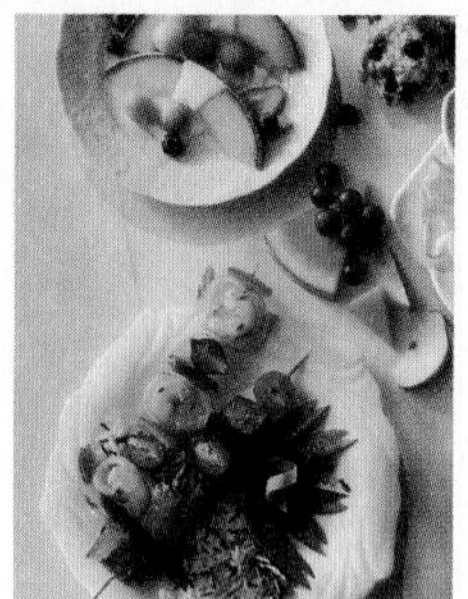

Summary

1. The metric system is used throughout science. Lengths are expressed in meters, weights are expressed in grams, and volumes are expressed in liters. A meter equals about 39 inches, a kilogram is about 2.2 pounds, and a liter is about 1 quart.
2. Recommended Dietary Allowances (RDAs) are set for many nutrients. These levels represent the amount of each nutrient that meets the needs for essentially all healthy people for that nutrient. Different RDA guidelines have been set for different genders and ages.
3. The four versions of the U.S. RDA are based primarily on the highest RDA levels found in the 1968 RDA publication. The U.S. RDA is used as a basis for expressing the nutrient levels in foods on nutrition labels. Soon Reference Daily Intakes (RDIs) will replace U.S. RDA. These standards are based on values from the 1989 RDA publication.
4. The Guide to Daily Food Choices is designed to convert nutrient recommendations from the RDAs into a food plan. The guide is best implemented by focusing on low-fat (or nonfat) dairy products, some vegetable proteins in addition to animal protein foods, citrus fruits, and dark green vegetables, and emphasizing liberal breads and cereals.
5. Dietary Guidelines have been issued to help reduce the amount of chronic "killer" diseases. The guidelines emphasize eating a variety of foods; maintaining healthy body weight; and limiting consumption of fats, cholesterol, sugar, salt, and alcohol, while emphasizing fruits, vegetables, and grain products.
6. The exchange system provides a powerful tool for estimating the carbohydrate, fat, protein, and kcalorie content of a food or meal and for planning a diet to correspond to specific goals for carbohydrate, fat, protein, and kcalorie consumption.

Study Questions

1. What three key points would you want to make as you explained to a friend what the RDAs represent?
2. How do the RDAs differ from U.S. RDA (and RDI) in intention and application? Which standard more accurately reflects the needs of people your age and gender?
3. Put the term nutrient density into common language. For instance, how would you explain the concept to a fourth grade class?
4. Describe how use of the exchange system would aid the control of a disease process, based on what the system can predict and monitor.
5. Nutritionists encourage all people to read nutrition labels to learn more about what they eat. What four nutrients could easily be tracked in your diet if you regularly read nutrition labels?

REFERENCES

1. American Dietetic Association and the American Diabetes Association: *Exchange lists for weight management,* 1989.
2. American Dietetic Association: Nutrition information on food labels, *Journal of the American Dietetic Association* 90:583, 1990.
3. Anonymous: United States nutrition labeling and education act of 1990, *Nutrition Reviews* 49:273, 1991.
4. Anonymous: Diet, nutrition and the prevention of chronic diseases—a report of the WHO study group on diet, nutrition and prevention of noncommunicable diseases, *Nutrition Reviews* 49:291, 1991.
5. Block G: Dietary guidelines and the results of food consumption surveys, *American Journal of Clinical Nutrition* 53:356S, 1991.
6. Block G and others: Nutrient sources in the American diet, *American Journal of Epidemiology* 122:13, 1985.
7. Blumenthal D: A new look at food labeling, *FDA Consumer* Nov 1989, p 15.
8. Canadian nutrient and dietary recommendations, *Nutrition Today,* Nov/Dec 1990, p 4.
9. Cronin FJ and others: Developing a food guidance system to implement the dietary guidelines, *Journal of Nutrition Education* 19:281, 1987.
10. Dwyer JT: Dietary change: convergence of prevention and treatment measures, *Topics in Clinical Nutrition* 6:42, 1991.
11. Filer LJ: Recommended dietary allowances: how did we get where we are? *Nutrition Today* Sept/Oct 1991, p 25.
12. Food and Nutrition Board, National Academy of Sciences—National Research Council: *Recommended dietary allowances, revised 1989,* Washington, DC, 1989.
13. Goldberg JP: Nutrition and health communication: the message and the media over half a century, *Nutrition Reviews* 50:71, 1992.
14. Harper AE: Scientific substantiation of health claims: how much is enough, *Nutrition Today* March/April 1989, p 17.
15. Harris SH and Welch S: How well are our food choices meeting our nutrition needs? *Nutrition Today* Nov/Dec 1989, p 20.
16. Monsen ER: The 10th edition of the recommended dietary allowances: what's new in the 1989 RDAs, *Journal of the American Dietetic Association* 89:1748, 1989.
17. National Research Council: *Diet and health,* Washington, DC, 1989, National Academy Press.
18. Olson JA: Should RDA values be tailored to meed the needs of their users? *Journal of Nutrition* 117:220, 1987.
19. Perkin BB: Dietary guidelines for Americans, 1990 edition, *Journal of the American Dietetic Association* 90:1725, 1990.
20. Surgeon General's report on Nutrition and Health: *Nutrition Today,* Sept/Oct 1988, p 22.
21. Wotek CE, Thomas PR: Eat for life, Washington, DC, 1991, National Academy Press.

SUGGESTED READINGS

The articles by the American Dietetic Association and Harper provide an excellent background for understanding the issues surrounding health claims on food labels. The articles by Monsen and Filer will help you understand how the Food and Nutrition Board thinks about the RDA and how, as scientists, they must work together to form a consensus using the information available at one time. Finally, the article by Olson will add further insights to setting the RDA. Reading these articles, along with the RDA book itself, will help you develop a deep understanding of this concept and the ramifications inherent in setting a specific RDA.

TAKE ACTION

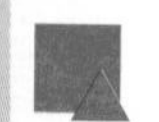

Does your diet meet the RDAs and Guide to Daily Food Choices?

Perform either part I or part II. Then perform parts III, IV and V. (For assistance in following the instructions for this activity, see the sample Assessment in Appendix E.)

Part I

A. Take the information from the 1-day food intake record you completed in Chapter 1 and record it on the blank form provided in Appendix E or by your instructor. Make sure to record the food or drink ingested and the amount (e.g., weight) consumed. NOTE: Your instructor may require keeping the food record for more than 1 day.

B. Review the 1989 RDAs on the inside cover of the book and choose the appropriate recommendations for your gender and age. Write the appropriate value for each nutrient on the line on the form labeled "Your RDA." NOTE: The values for sodium and potassium from the table on the inside cover of the book are labeled, "Estimated Sodium, Chloride, and Potassium Minimum Requirements of Healthy Persons."

C. Look up the foods and drinks that you listed on the form in the food composition table, Appendix A. Record on the form the amounts of each nutrient and kcalories present in them. If the food is not listed choose a substitute.

D. For each food and drink, add the amounts in each column and record the results on the line labeled "Totals."

E. Compare the totals to your RDAs. Divide the total for each nutrient by the specific RDA or minimum requirement and multiply that by 100. Record the result on the line labeled, "% of Your RDA."

F. Keep this assessment for use in subsequent activities for other chapters.

Part II

A. Obtain copies of the computer software from your instructor. Load the software into the computer.

B. Choose RDAs for you based on your age and gender.

C. Enter the information from the 1-day food intake record you kept in Chapter 1. Make sure to enter each food and drink, and the appropriate serving size.

D. This software program will give you the following results:
   a. the appropriate 1989 RDA value for each nutrient.
   b. the total amount of each nutrient and kcalories consumed for the day.
   c. the percentage of the RDA 1989 values you consumed for each nutrient.

E. Keep this assessment for use in subsequent activities for other chapters.

Part III

Evaluation

Remember that you don't necessarily need to consume 100% of the 1989 RDA values. A safe standard is at least a 70% average over 5 to 8 days. It would be best not to exceed 500% to avoid potential toxic effects. There is no proven advantage for a healthy person to exceed 100%.

A. For which nutrients do you fall below 70%?

B. Did you exceed the minimum requirements for sodium? To what degree?

C. For which nutrients did you exceed the RDA by greater than 500% (5 times greater)?

D. What dietary changes could you make to correct or improve your dietary profile? If unsure, future chapters will help guide your decisions. ▲

TAKE ACTION

Does your diet meet the RDAs and Guide to Daily Food Choices?—cont'd

Perform either part I or part II. Then perform parts III, IV and V. (For assistance in following the instructions for this activity, see the sample Assessment in Appendix E.)

Part IV
Guide to daily food choices

Use the following table to again record your food intake. Now place each food item in the correct categories of the Guide to Daily Food Choices. Note that a food like toast with margarine would contribute to two catagories, namely to bread, cereals, rice, and pasta group, but also to fats, oils, and sweets group. You can expect that many food choices contribute to more than one group.

Indicate number of servings that each food represents							
Food or beverage	**Amount eaten**	**Milk, yogurt, and cheese**	**Meat, poultry, fish, beans, nuts, and seeds**	**Fruits**	**Vegetables**	**Bread, cereals, rice, and pasta**	**Fats, oils, and sweets**

Part V
Evaluation

Do the weaknesses suggested in your nutrient analysis, if any, correspond to missing servings in the Guide to Daily Food Choices? Consider improving the latter to aid improving the former. ▲

NUTRITION PERSPECTIVE

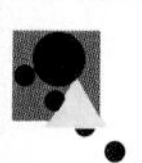

What's on the Label?

In the United States FDA is responsible for most food labeling, except for meat and poultry products, which are regulated by the USDA, and alcoholic beverages, which are regulated by the Bureau of Alcohol, Tobacco and Firearms. The Federal Trade Commission (FTC) regulates the advertising of food products and has authority to take action against unsubstantiated claims. In doing so, it uses FDA as the leading agency.

Foods packaged and sold in any United States supermarket usually are labeled with the product name, the name and address of the manufacturer, the amount of product in the package, and the ingredients, which are listed in descending order of weight. With the exceptions of fresh fruits, vegetables, and meats, almost all other foods are so labeled.[7]

Another exception to this labeling system is given to foods with a **standard of identity.** Products under FDA jurisdiction with a standard of identity must follow a certain recipe on file with FDA. In those cases, the manufacturer does not have to list ingredients, unless optimal ingredients are included, such as extra spices or flavors. These foods include catsup, ice cream, mustard, and mayonnaise. Notice, however, that many manufacturers now list the ingredients on labels for these foods, though they do not have to by current law. This trend is caused by consumer demand. Most of us want to see what ingredients are in our foods, now more than ever. New labeling laws to be inacted are likely to eliminate this labeling exception.

Since 1973 if a manufacturer (1) adds a nutrient to the food product or (2) makes a nutritional claim about the product, a "nutrition label" must also be provided. The next time you see a food package that announces the product is "low in sodium" or "high in fiber" check the nutrition label for more specific information. Today 60% of the foods under FDA control carry a nutrition label. Of those, about half are voluntary—no nutrition label is legally required. Many foods, however, give us no nutrient information, aside from contents. This will change soon because of a new law passed in 1990 that requires most foods to be labeled.

An example of the current "nutrition label" is shown in Figure 2-3. The label lists the serving size of the product; servings per package; and kcalorie, protein, carbohydrate, fat, and sodium amounts per serving. If the product contains more than 2% of the U.S. RDA for certain vitamins and minerals, these percentages must be listed. These nutrients include protein, vitamin A, vitamin C, thiamin, riboflavin, niacin, calcium, and iron.

Additional information may be provided on dietary fiber, the amount of sugars and cholesterol, and other information the manufacturer believes the consumer wants. The Surgeon General of the United States has encouraged manufacturers to make full use of this opportunity to educate the public.[20]

Always check serving sizes when comparing nutrition labels because under current law manufacturers determine their own serving sizes, and these vary from product to product. A product may be lower in kcalories than another similar one because the manufacturer simply listed a small serving size. Don't be fooled.

FDA is in the midst of changing labeling regulations. Proposed regulations will lead to changes in the nutrition label. The new nutrition labels also generally will have more information, with a mandatory listing of:[7]

- saturated fat content
- cholesterol content
- total dietary fiber content
- total kcalories from fat in the product

The U.S. RDA will be updated to more closely conform to the current RDA and undergo a name change to Reference Daily Intakes (RDIs), as we noted earlier. Serving size will follow more uniform patterns. As well, Daily Reference Values (DRVs) will also be set by FDA for certain parts of a diet not covered by the 1989 RDA, such as carbohydrate, fat, and dietary fiber. The DRVs are intended to help us further evaluate food choices as we compare food values of these substances to desirable (or maximum) intakes. The bulk of final changes in food labeling regulations will be in place by May 1993.

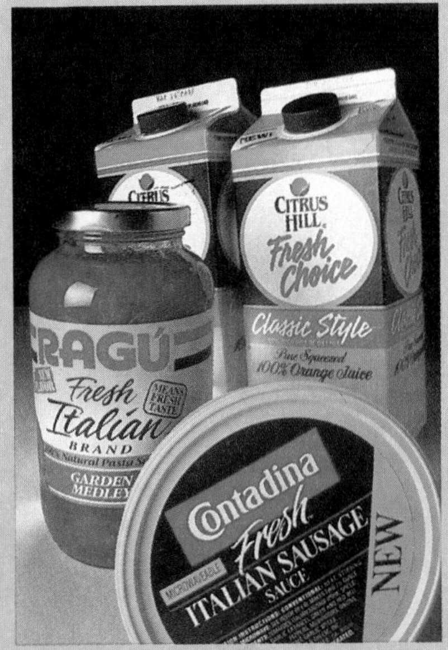

FDA currently is enforcing labeling regulations more strictly. This includes foods that use the term "fresh" but are obviously not since they are packaged.

LABELING PITFALLS

Some pitfalls accompany label reading. The meanings of terms on labels are not always apparent. Food marketers are happy to satisfy our cravings for "healthy" foods with healthy-sounding choices labeled "no cholesterol," "low-fat," "organic," and "sugar free." How trustworthy are these claims? Though technically true, many of the claims are irrelevant; others are misleading or only paint part of the picture. Consider the recent controversy over the labeling of jars of heat-processed spaghetti sauce as "fresh." Table 2-9 lists some legal definitions for terms you are likely to see on food labels. Note that these definitions may change in the future as food labeling laws change, especially for specific terms—light (lite), free, low, reduced, less, more, high, fresh, and source of—as they relate to nutrient content.

HEALTH CLAIMS ON LABELS

A debate exists concerning the extent to which a manufacturer can make health claims on a food product label. It is permissible to state that a food contains certain nutrients: This simply requires a nutrition label to back up the claim. The debate concerns whether a manufacturer can state that these nutrients will provide specific health benefits, such as the claim that dietary fiber in food helps prevent some types of cancer. The current trend is for manufacturers to make health claims. Since 1984 the Kellogg Company has marketed its high-fiber cereals as a possible preventive measure against certain forms of cancer. Whether this should be allowed is far from settled. After relaxing laws to allow this to happen in 1987, government agencies are not sure how far they should let manufacturers go. Many nutritionists think this particular claim lacks scientific merit and that claims in general are a bad idea.[14]

As we noted, labeling regulations currently under development will set standards for some of the more common claims, such as "light" ("lite"), "no cholesterol," and "high fiber." Currently, FDA proposes to limit the use of health messages to six areas in which there is general scientific agreement of a relationship between a nutrient and a chronic disease. These may include: fiber and cancer, fiber and heart disease, fat and cancer, fat and heart disease, sodium and hypertension, and calcium and osteoporosis.

Some groups oppose the use of health messages on food labels. A major problem is that a "good food/bad food" comparison is promoted by many claims on labels, and the emphasis on total diet is ignored. As we have discussed, one's total meal plan and nutrient intake should be the focus because nutrients work together to maintain health—not as separate entities existing in a vacuum. Protein metabolism uses vitamin B-6, iron metabolism uses vitamin C, and folate metabolism uses vitamin B-12.

Again, health claims for specific foods or food supplements ignore the importance on the entire diet and may be irresponsible because they do not warn of the dangers of excess intakes of the specific foods or supplements. Thus the idea of having health claims on labels may not be a particularly good one.

NUTRITION PERSPECTIVE

What's on the Label?—cont'd

Table 2-9 Definitions for terms on food labels

Free and Low:

- ***Free:*** an amount that is "nutritionally trivial" and unlikely to have a physiological consequence.
- ***Calorie Free:*** fewer than 5 kcalories per serving.
- ***Sugar Free:*** less than 0.5 grams per serving.
- ***Sodium Free*** and ***Salt Free:*** less than 5 milligrams of sodium per serving.
- ***Low:*** would allow frequent consumption of a food "low" in a nutrient without exceeding the dietary guidelines. Per serving and per 100 grams (a little less than half a cup) of food, these amounts would be defined as:
  - ***Low Sodium:*** less than 140 milligrams per serving and per 100 grams of food.
  - ***Very Low Sodium:*** less than 35 milligrams per serving and per 100 grams of food.
  - ***Low Calorie:*** less than 40 per serving and per 100 grams of food.

A food that is *normally* free of or low in a nutrient may make such a claim, but the claim must indicate that the condition exists for all similar foods—for example, "Fresh spinach, a low-sodium food."

High and Source of:

- ***High*** and ***Source of:*** terms intended to emphasize the beneficial presence of certain nutrients, not to characterize levels of nutrients that increase the risk for chronic diseases. "High" is 20% or more of the dietary reference values. "Source of" is 10% to 19% of these values. Any high-fiber claim for a food containing more than 3 grams of fat per serving and per 100 grams of the food must be accompanied by a declaration of total fat.

Relative Terms:

- ***Reduced, Light, Less,*** and ***More:*** Use of these terms must be accompanied by information about the food that is the basis for comparison—the identity of the comparable food, the percentage (or fraction) by which the referenced food has been modified, and the amount of the nutrient that is the subject of the claim.
- ***Reduced:*** may be used for sodium only if the food contains no more than half the sodium of the comparison food. *Reduced* may be used for kcalories, however, if the referenced food has been reduced by one third.
- ***Less:*** may be used to describe nutrients if the reduction is at least 25%.

Light: may be used on foods that contain one-third fewer calories than a comparable product. Any other use of the term *light* must specify if it refers to the look, taste, or smell; for example, "Light in color."

- ***More:*** could be used to show that a food contains more of a desirable nutrient, such as fiber or potassium, than does a comparable food. To use the term *more,* a food must contain at least 10% more of the given nutrient than the comparable food.

Definitions related to fat and cholesterol:

- ***Fat Free:*** less than 0.5 grams of fat per serving, providing that it has no added fat or oil ingredient.
- ***Low Fat:*** 3 grams or less of fat per serving and per 100 grams of the food.
- ***(Percent) Fat Free:*** may only describe foods that meet FDA's definition of "low fat."
- ***Reduced Fat:*** no more than half the fat of an identified comparison. To avoid trivial claims, the reduction must exceed 3 grams of fat per serving.
- ***Low in Saturated Fat:*** may be used to describe a food that contains 1 gram or less of saturated fat per serving, and not more than 15 percent of kcalories from saturated fat.

NUTRITION PERSPECTIVE

Table 2-9 Definitions for terms on food labels—cont'd

- ***Reduced Saturated Fat:*** no more than 50% of the saturated fat than the food with which it's compared. Foods with a reduction of 25% or greater may have a comparative claim using the term "less." If "reduced saturated fat" or a comparative claim is used, it must indicate the percent reduction and the amount of saturated fat in the food with which it's compared. The reduction of saturated fat must exceed 1 gram.
- ***Cholesterol Free:*** less than 2 milligrams of cholesterol per serving and 2 grams or less saturated fat per serving.
- ***Low in Cholesterol:*** 20 milligrams or less per serving and per 100 grams of food, and 2 grams or less of saturated fat per serving.
- ***Reduced Cholesterol:*** 50% or less of cholesterol per serving than its comparison food. Foods with reductions in cholesterol of 25% or more may bear comparative claims using the term "less," but both "reduced cholesterol" and comparative claims must be fully explained, and the reduction in cholesterol must exceed 20 milligrams per serving.

All claims of cholesterol content are prohibited when a food contains more than 2 grams of saturated fat per serving. The label of a food containing more than 11.5 grams of total fat per serving or per 100 grams of the food must disclose those levels immediately after any cholesterol claim.

Fresh:

- ***Fresh:*** can only be linked to raw food, food that has not been frozen, processed, or preserved.
- ***Freshly:*** with a verb such as "prepared," "baked," or "roasted" this term may be used if the food is recently made and has not been frozen, heat processed, or preserved.

Adding approved waxes or coatings, using approved pesticides after harvest, or applying a mild chlorine wash or mild acid to raw produce would not prohibit the use of the term "fresh."

Terms such as "fresh frozen" and "quickly frozen" are also defined.

Other terms:

- ***Diet or dietetic:*** Usually the product contains no more than 40 kcalories per serving (also called low-calorie), or has at least one-third fewer kcalories than the regular product (also called reduced-calorie). NOTE: this does not mean *diabetic;* foods for persons with diabetes mellitus need not be dietetic to be appropriate for use.
- ***Imitation:*** The product does not follow the usual recipe for that type of product. For instance, more water may have been added to margarine to make it lower in kcalories. Note that such products may also be lower in nutrients, such as protein, vitamins, or minerals. The "cheese" used on frozen pizza is sometimes imitation cheese.
- ***Natural:*** This term is usually meaningless. It simply states that the product occurs in nature. When applied to meats, it means the meat contains no added artificial flavors, colors, preservatives, or synthetic ingredients and was minimally processed—just enough to make it safe or edible.
- ***Organic:*** This term has no legal meaning as far as the U.S. federal law is concerned.
- ***Wheat:*** The product contains wheat but not necessarily whole wheat. The label will say whole wheat if the product uses only whole-wheat flour.
- ***Enriched:*** The vitamins thiamin, riboflavin, and niacin and the mineral iron have been added to the product to replace (and in some cases augment) what is lost in processing.
- ***Fortified:*** Vitamins and/or minerals have been added to the product in amounts in excess of those originally present in the product.

NUTRITION PERSPECTIVE

What's on the Label?—cont'd

The American Dietetic Association feels health claims are permissible as part of a labeling or marketing system as long as they are presented in the context of a total diet and are generally supported by the scientific community.[2] Those claims supporting the messages given in *Dietary Guidelines for Americans* are deemed especially appropriate. The association supports both positive and negative health claims on food labels to prevent the public from being misled. For example, a high-fiber claim on a food product should also state if the food is high in fat. Such an approach would protect the consumer against deception by omission.

The danger with health claims is that not all the facts may be presented. For example, with dietary fibers, some adverse facts are omitted: No studies clearly show that Americans who eat wheat bran cereals develop less cancer than Americans who do not; many kinds of dietary fiber exist; too much bran can lead to poor absorption of iron, zinc, and calcium, as well as intestinal problems such as gas. The warning should be that too much—as well as too little—dietary fiber can be harmful (see Chapters 3 and 6 for more details).

The bottom line for health claims on food packages is honesty (Figure 2-8).[2,13] The whole story needs to be told. How federal agencies in the United States will ensure that honesty prevails remains unanswered. For you the best tactic will continue to be defensive shopping: Read the small print and be skeptical.

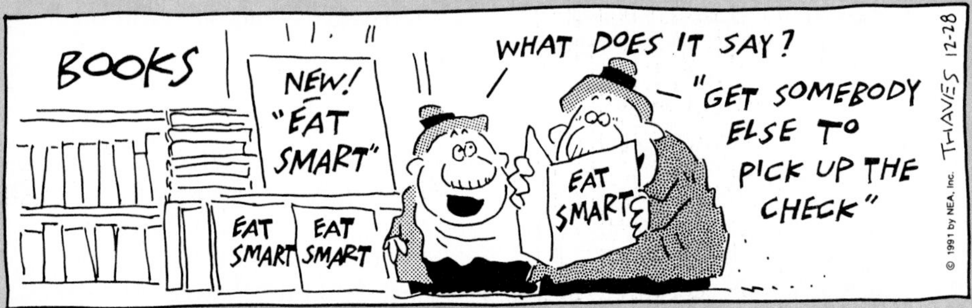
FRANK & ERNEST ® by Bob Thaves
BOOKS
NEW! "EAT SMART"
EAT SMART
EAT SMART
WHAT DOES IT SAY?
EAT SMART
"GET SOMEBODY ELSE TO PICK UP THE CHECK"
THAVES 12-28
© 1991 by NEA, Inc.

Figure 2-8 Frank and Ernest.
Reprinted by permission of NEA, Inc.

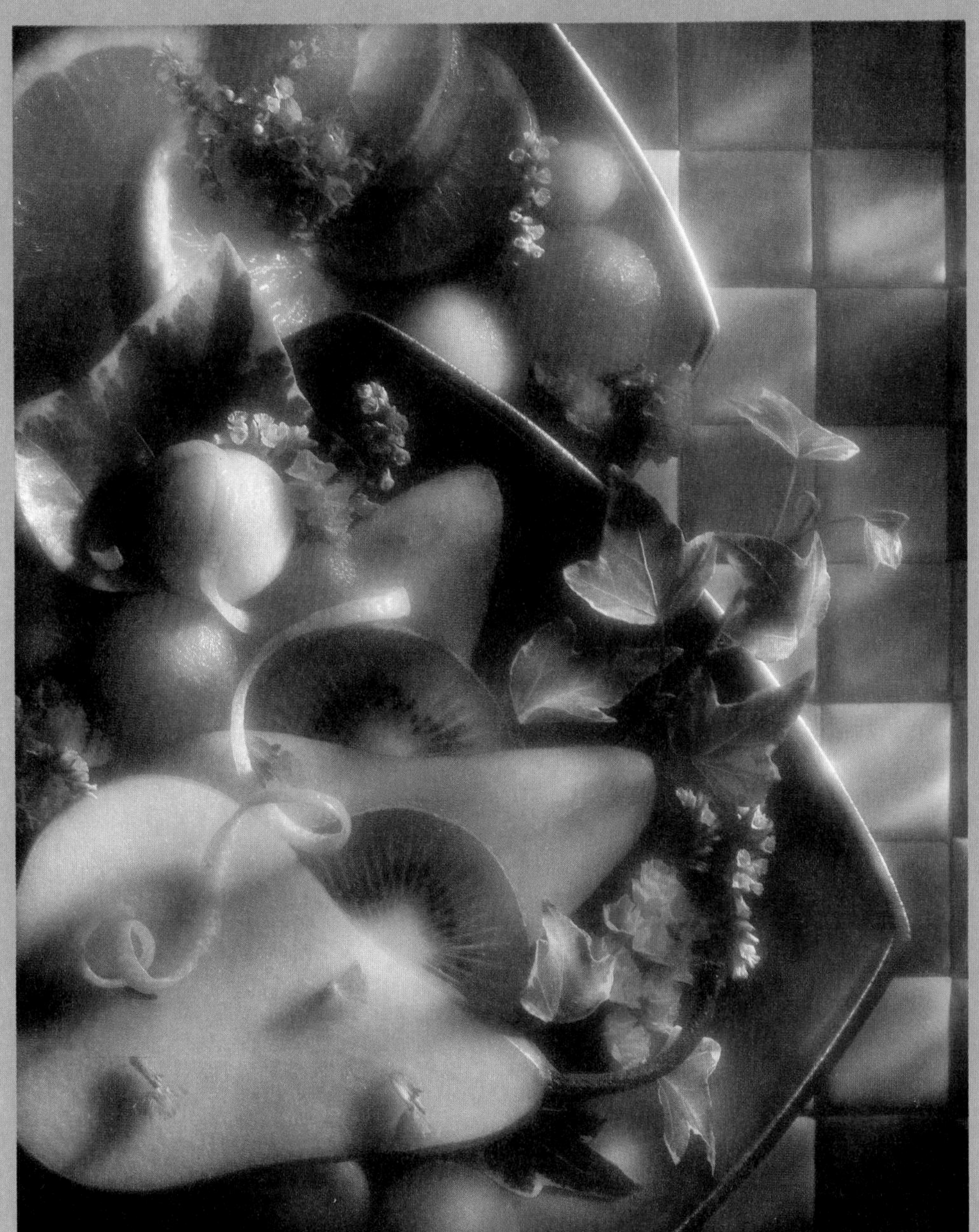

PART TWO

The Energy-Yielding Nutrients

CHAPTER THREE

Carbohydrates

You have now studied what we eat, why we eat those foods, and basic tools used to plan diets. The next three chapters examine the energy-yielding nutrients—carbohydrates, proteins, and fats. Knowing about them will give you an advantage over the average consumer. Most people know that potatoes have carbohydrates and steak has fat and protein, but few people know what those terms actually mean. These chapters give you the opportunity to learn that, and much more.

The largest amount of any single biochemical compound on earth is the carbohydrate cellulose. This forms part of the structure of many plants. Another carbohydrate, chitin, forms part of the structure of many insects and crustaceans. Carbohydrates also should be the major source of energy for the human diet. Overall, this makes carbohydrates the ideal place to begin our detailed nutrient discussions.

It is important to study carbohydrates in detail because these compounds are often misunderstood. People may think carbohydrates cause diabetes—they do not. Some people think carbohydrates can make them hyperactive—again, this is unlikely. In fact, carbohydrates, especially complex varieties, have been the nutrient most promoted by nutritionists in the last 10 years.[10] The link between fat—especially animal fat—and heart disease should prompt us to switch our focus away from so many high-fat food choices to more high-carbohydrate food choices.

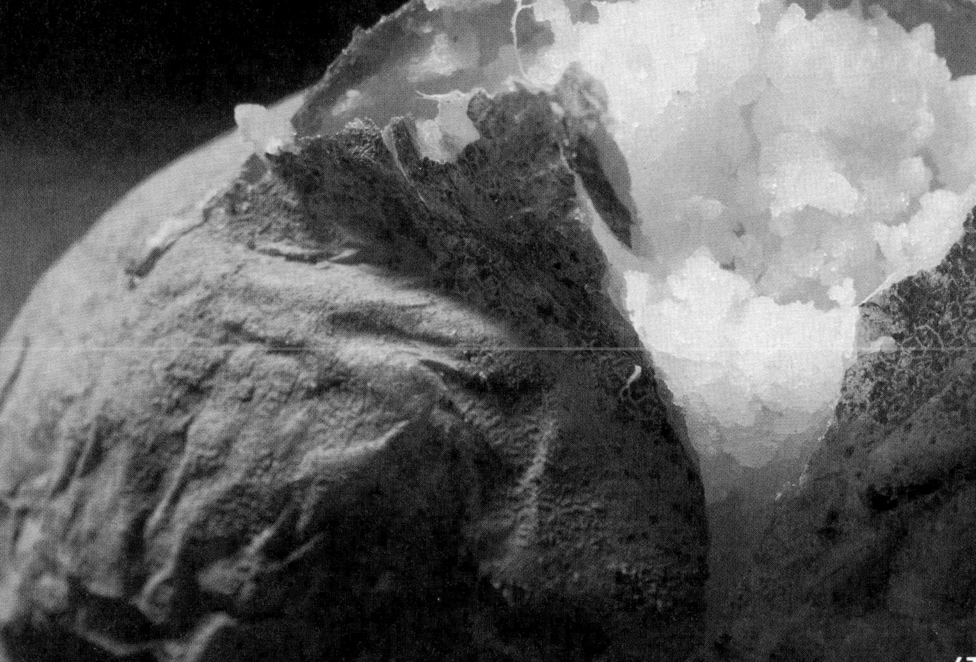

NUTRITION AWARENESS INVENTORY

Here are 15 statements about carbohydrates. Answer them to test your current knowledge of carbohydrates. If you think the statement is true or mostly true, circle T. If you think the statement is false or mostly false, circle F. Use the scoring key at the end of the book to compute your total score. Take this test again after you have read this chapter. Compare the results.

1. T F Common table sugar is called sucrose.
2. T F Starch is a storage form of carbohydrates in plants.
3. T F Carbohydrates are necessarily fattening.
4. T F The primary role of carbohydrates is to supply energy.
5. T F Fiber and "roughage" are the same thing.
6. T F There is an RDA for carbohydrates.
7. T F The human body uses dietary fiber mainly for energy.
8. T F Sugar plays a role in the production of dental caries.
9. T F Excess dietary carbohydrates are converted into fat in the body.
10. T F Wheat bread is a good source of dietary fiber.
11. T F No desirable level of sugar intake has been established, but current intakes may be too high.
12. T F Honey is not safe to feed to infants.
13. T F Diabetes is a disorder of low blood glucose levels.
14. T F Sugar causes hyperactivity and juvenile delinquency.
15. T F Africans show fewer intestinal disorders than Americans.

Structures and Forms of Simple Carbohydrates

Most forms of carbohydrates are composed of carbon, hydrogen, and oxygen in the ratio of 1:2:1, respectively. The general formula is $(CH_2O)n$, where *n* stands for the number of times the ratio is repeated. Glucose, being $C_6H_{12}O_6$, is $(CH_2O)_6$. The simpler forms of carbohydrates are called **sugars** and often take the form of single or double sugars. The more complex forms are typically either starches or dietary fibers. Plants use carbon dioxide, water, and energy (from the sun) to produce the carbohydrates we eat:

6 carbon dioxides (CO_2) + 6 waters (H_2O) →
the carbohydrate glucose ($C_6H_{12}O_6$) + 6 oxygens (O_2).

MONOSACCHARIDES

Monosaccharides are simple sugars (*mono* meaning one and *saccharide* meaning sugar). Glucose, fructose, and galactose are monosaccharides.

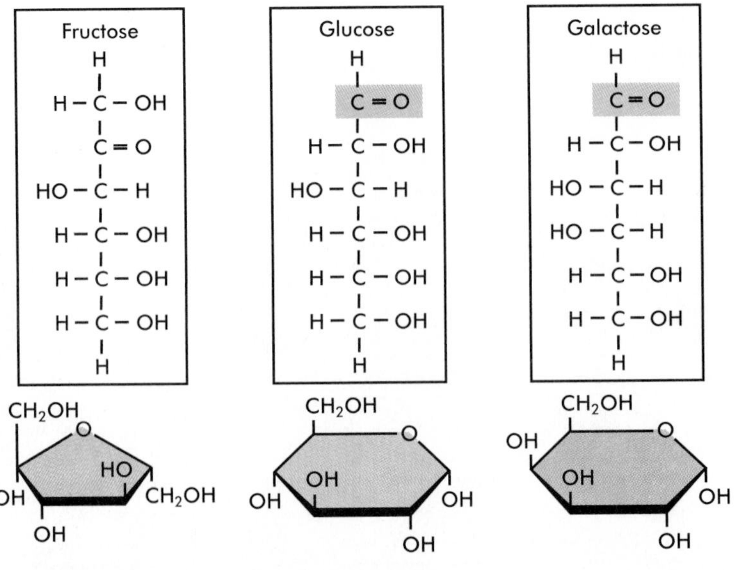

Figure 3-1 Structure of three monosaccharides—fructose, glucose, and galactose—shown in six-carbon linear form (when solid) and ring form (when in solution). Note the similarities in the structures.

Glucose is the major monosaccharide in the body. Other names for glucose are dextrose and blood sugar. In Figure 3-1 the D isomer of glucose is drawn in both linear and ring forms. The ring form is how glucose exists in the body. Your body can metabolize only the D isomer of glucose. This makes the possibility of developing the L isomer into an alternative sweetener very enticing. (Appendix B reviews the concept of isomers.)

For a learning technique study the structure of glucose. Then only learn the difference between glucose and the other two monosaccharides, fructose and galactose.

Glucose is a six-carbon monosaccharide and so is called a **hexose** (*hex* meaning six; *ose* is the standard ending for carbohydrates). Note the six-membered ring formed includes oxygen.

Fructose is a structural isomer of glucose and although it is a hexose, it can form either a five- or six-membered ring, which includes oxygen (Figure 3-1). Fructose is also called levulose and is found in:

- fruit
- honey (about half fructose, half glucose)
- **high fructose corn syrup,** which is found in soft drinks, frozen desserts, and confections. The presence of fructose in these products is quickly making it a major simple sugar in our diets.

Fructose, after absorption by the small intestine and transport to the liver, is quickly metabolized, mainly into glucose (Figure 3-2). Some fructose is converted into **glycogen, lactic acid,** or fat, depending on the metabolic state of the individual.[14]

glycogen A carbohydrate made of multiple units of glucose containing a highly branched structure; sometimes known as animal starch. It is the storage form of glucose and is synthesized (and stored) in the liver and muscles.

Galactose is the last major monosaccharide of nutritional importance. Compare

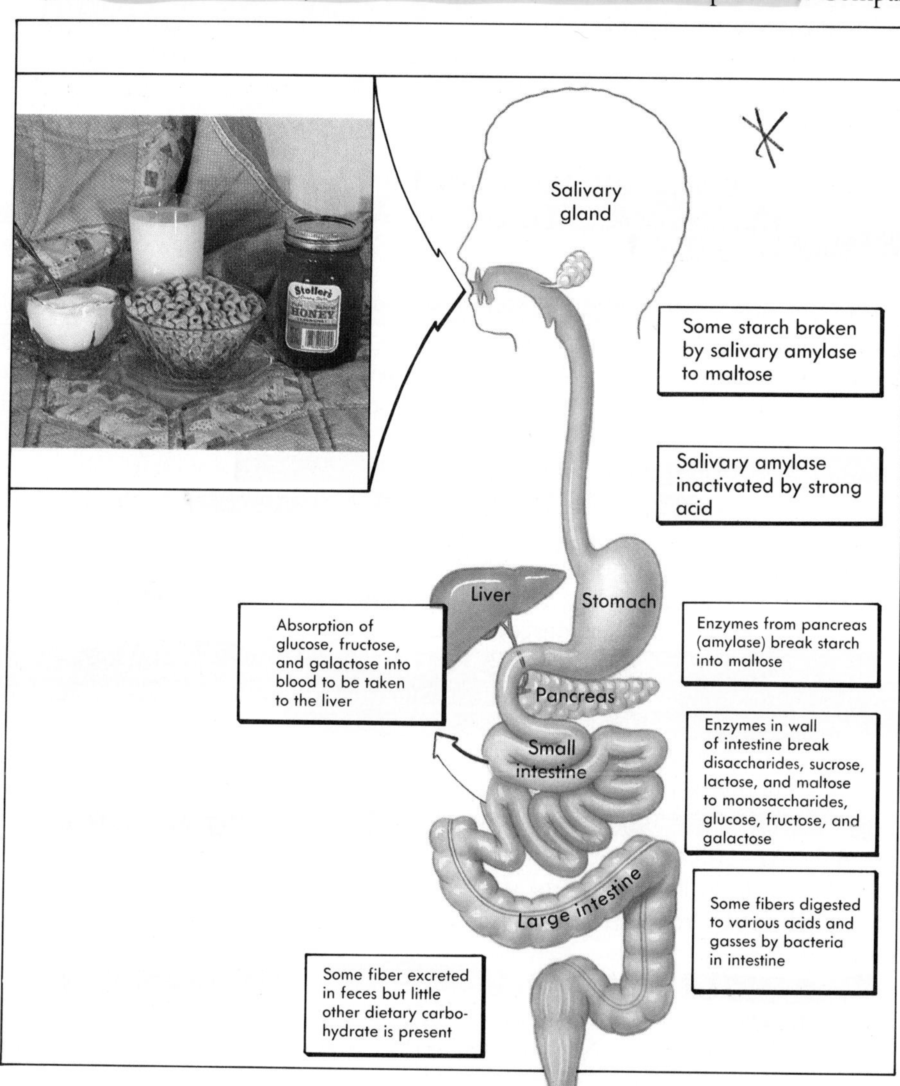

Figure 3-2 For your information. A brief summary of carbohydrate digestion and absorption. Chapter 6 covers this in detail.

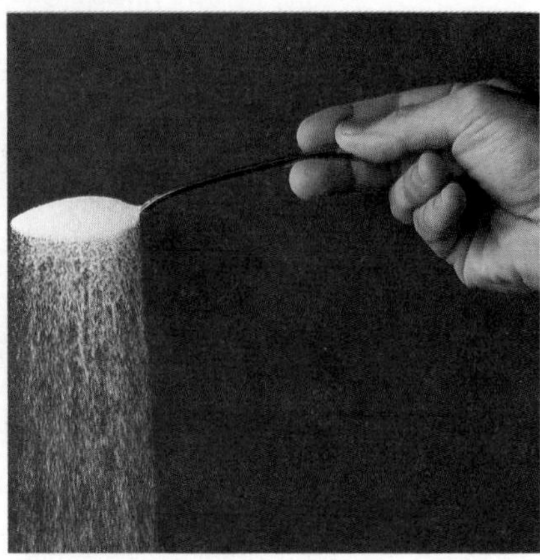

Use sugars only in moderation.

the structure of this simple sugar to glucose in Figure 3-1. The two structures are identical except the hydrogen (−H) and the hydroxyl group (−OH) are reversed on carbon no. 4. Galactose is not usually found free in nature in large quantities, but rather combines with glucose to form a double sugar called **lactose.** This is present in milk and other dairy products. Once absorbed into the body, galactose is transformed into either glucose or built into a storage form of glucose in the liver and muscle, called glycogen.

Now is a good time to begin to emphasize a key concept in nutrition—the difference between eating a compound or substance and using that same compound. In many instances, when a substance is not an essential nutrient (recall the definition of an essential nutrient in Chapter 1), the body does not always use that substance when it is presented. The substance instead may be stored or broken down and later reassembled into the same or different compound when and where necessary. In the case of galactose, it is metabolized to glucose or glycogen. When later required, as in the mammary gland of the lactating female, galactose is resynthesized at the appropriate time and place.

The other monosaccharides found in nature, such as **ribose** (a five-carbon sugar present in a cell's genetic material), are not so plentiful in our diets. In addition, this is a compound made from other things that we eat. A few single-sugar alcohols appear in foods and will be discussed in the section on nutritive sweeteners. Currently, the major ones used in the manufacture of edible products are **sorbitol** and **mannitol.**

Once you are familiar with the chemical forms of the simple sugars, it is much easier to understand how they are interrelated, combined, broken apart (digested), broken down (metabolized), and reassembled (synthesized).

ribose A five-carbon sugar found in genetic material, specifically RNA.

disaccharides Class of sugars formed by the chemical bonding of two monosaccharides.

glycosidic bond The covalent bond formed between two monosaccharides when a water molecule is lost.

alpha bond A type of glycosidic bond that can be digested by human intestinal enzymes.

beta bond A type of carbohydrate bond that is not digested by human intestinal enzymes when it is part of a long chain of monosaccharides.

DISACCHARIDES

There are three double sugars **(disaccharides)** that are common in the diet. Disaccharides are formed when two monosaccharides combine (*di* means two). A condensation reaction occurs: the two monosaccharides are joined, and a water molecule is released (Figure 3-3).

This reaction forms a **glycosidic bond** (C—O—C). Two forms of this bond exist and are labeled alpha (α) and beta (β). An **alpha bond** is drawn as └O┘, and a **beta bond** looks like ┌O┘. When glucose molecules bond together, we can digest the compound if it has alpha—but not beta—bonds. This will be discussed in detail later.

Maltose is formed when two glucose molecules combine using an alpha bond (Figure 3-3). Our major source of maltose is germinating grains. As the starch in grains breaks down during germination, maltose is formed. This occurs before grains are used to make beer. In the process of beer making, yeast changes the maltose into "malt," which is easier for the yeast to metabolize than the original starch in the grain. We have few other sources of maltose in our diets.

Sucrose, the most familiar of the disaccharides, is glucose and fructose joined together to form table sugar (Figure 3-3). Sucrose comes only from plants and is found in sugar cane, sugar beets, honey, and maple syrup. The sucrose from these sources may be purified in various degrees to yield the brown, white, or powdered sugars commonly seen in grocery stores.

A common misconception is that honey contains vitamins and minerals. You can prove to yourself that honey is also no more nutritious than sucrose by using Appendix A. Only the sweetener molasses, a by-product of sugar production, contains any appreciable amount of minerals. However, our consumption of molasses in foods is very low.

Lactose is glucose joined to galactose to form the sugar found in dairy products (Fig. 3-2). As we discuss later in the chapter, many people are unable to digest large amounts of lactose. This can cause intestinal gas, bloating, cramping, and discomfort as any unabsorbed lactose is metabolized by bacteria in the large intestine into acids and gases.[17]

Monosaccharides and disaccharides are often referred to as "simple" sugars. Food labels sometimes lump all these sugars under that one category, listing them as "sucrose and other sugars." Note the way sugar often is listed on the label of cereal

Condensation reactions

Glucose + Glucose → Maltose + H_2O

Glucose + Fructose → Sucrose + H_2O

Galactose + Glucose → Lactose + H_2O

Figure 3-3 Condensation between two monosaccharides forms, a disaccharide. **A,** Maltose is made of two glucose molecules and is found in germinating grains. **B,** Sucrose, or common table sugar, is made of glucose and fructose. **C,** Lactose, or milk sugar, is made of glucose and galactose. Note that lactose contains a different type of bond than maltose and sucrose, a property that can make lactose difficult to digest for individuals who show a relative or total lack of a specific enzyme (lactase).

boxes in Figure 3-4. Then note how much sugar is in the cereal that you usually eat (see Table 3-1 and Appendix A).

Although the amount of sucrose eaten by Americans has declined over time, the total amount of sugars eaten has increased. There are many "smoke screen" words for sugar, including the words found in Table 3-2.

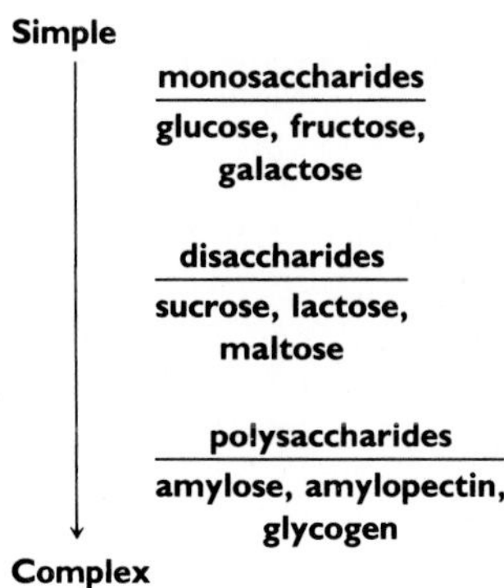

CONCEPT CHECK

Monosaccharides are single sugars. Important monosaccharides in the diet are glucose, fructose, and galactose. Disaccharides are double sugars. The major disaccharides in the diet are sucrose (glucose bonded to fructose), maltose (glucose bonded to glucose), and lactose (glucose bonded to galactose). Once absorbed into the body, the majority of these carbohydrates are ultimately transformed into glucose by the liver.

Structures and Forms of Complex Carbohydrates

If a carbohydrate contains more than two monosaccharide units, it is no longer a simple sugar.

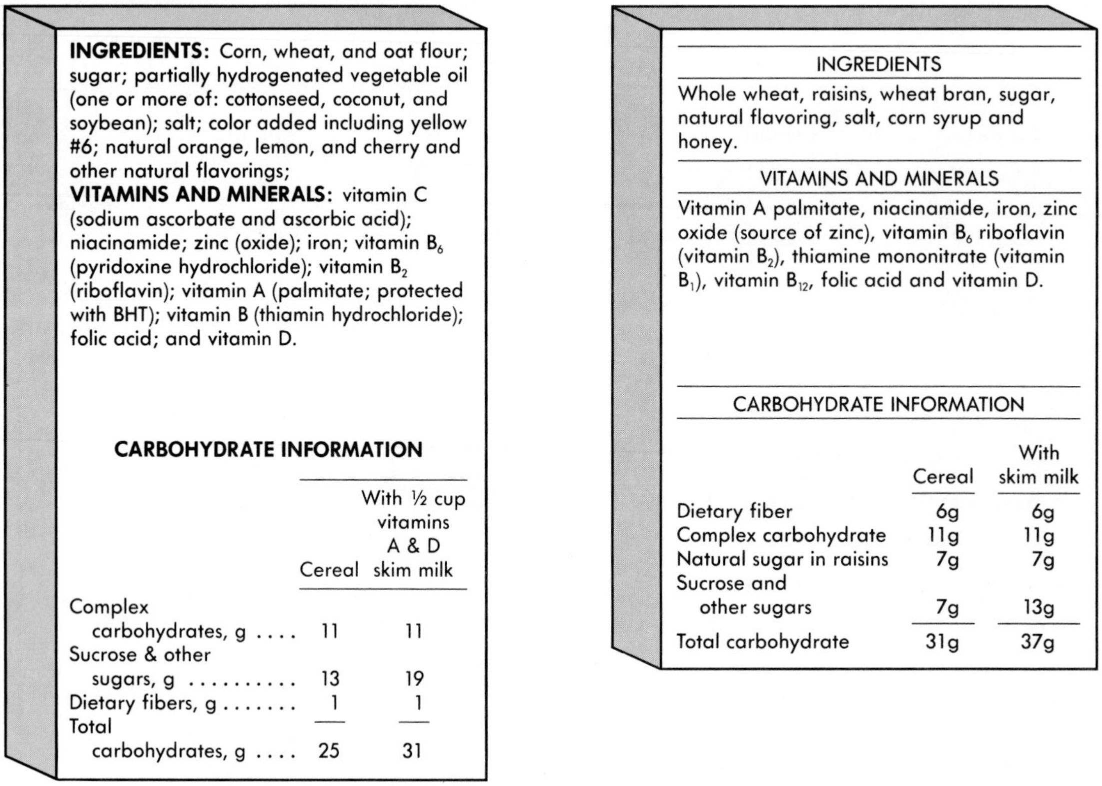

INGREDIENTS: Corn, wheat, and oat flour; sugar; partially hydrogenated vegetable oil (one or more of: cottonseed, coconut, and soybean); salt; color added including yellow #6; natural orange, lemon, and cherry and other natural flavorings;
VITAMINS AND MINERALS: vitamin C (sodium ascorbate and ascorbic acid); niacinamide; zinc (oxide); iron; vitamin B_6 (pyridoxine hydrochloride); vitamin B_2 (riboflavin); vitamin A (palmitate; protected with BHT); vitamin B (thiamin hydrochloride); folic acid; and vitamin D.

CARBOHYDRATE INFORMATION

	Cereal	With ½ cup vitamins A & D skim milk
Complex carbohydrates, g	11	11
Sucrose & other sugars, g	13	19
Dietary fibers, g	1	1
Total carbohydrates, g	25	31

INGREDIENTS

Whole wheat, raisins, wheat bran, sugar, natural flavoring, salt, corn syrup and honey.

VITAMINS AND MINERALS

Vitamin A palmitate, niacinamide, iron, zinc oxide (source of zinc), vitamin B_6 riboflavin (vitamin B_2), thiamine mononitrate (vitamin B_1), vitamin B_{12}, folic acid and vitamin D.

CARBOHYDRATE INFORMATION

	Cereal	With skim milk
Dietary fiber	6g	6g
Complex carbohydrate	11g	11g
Natural sugar in raisins	7g	7g
Sucrose and other sugars	7g	13g
Total carbohydrate	31g	37g

Figure 3-4 Reading labels helps us choose more nutritious foods. Based on the information from their nutrition labels, which cereal is the better choice for breakfast? Consider the amount of dietary fiber and sugars in each cereal. Did the ingredient lists give you any clues (NOTE: Ingredients are always listed in descending order by weight on a label)?

OLIGOSACCHARIDES

Oligosaccharides contain three to ten single sugar units (*oligo* means scant). Two oligosaccharides of nutritional importance are **raffinose** and **stachyose.** These are constructed of typical monosaccharides but bonded together in such a way that the digestive enzymes our bodies make cannot break them down. Thus when we eat these carbohydrates in beans and other legumes, the raffinose and stachyose molecules remain undigested upon reaching the large intestine. Bacteria in the large intestine then metabolize them, producing gas and other by-products. Plant breeders have been trying to produce "gasless" beans—those without a great amount of oligosaccharides.

raffinose An indigestible oligosaccharide with three monosaccharide units (galactose-glucose-fructose).

stachyose An indigestible oligosaccharide with four monosaccharide units (galactose-galactose-glucose-fructose).

Recently available in stores is an enzyme preparation (Beano) that prevents the unpleasant side effects of intestinal gas if consumed right before a meal. The enzyme preparation, once consumed, breaks down much of the undigestible oligosaccharides in legumes and other vegetables in a meal before they reach the large intestine. This allows for their absorption in the small intestine, as is the case for digestible carbohydrates.

POLYSACCHARIDES

Polysaccharides contain many monosaccharide units, and for the most part these are glucose. Some have 3000 or more units. You may have heard the terms starch and complex carbohydrates. These are the main terms used for the major digestible polysaccharides in our diet. In general, starches are the storage form of carbohydrates and are a source of energy for plants and animals. These forms include **amylose** and

amylose A straight-chain digestible polysaccharide made of glucose units; part of starch.

Table 3-1 Some sources of sugars

Food	Serving	Teaspoons of Sugar
BEVERAGES		
Cola drinks	1 (12 oz bottle or glass)	7
Ginger ale	12 oz	10
Orange-ade	1 (8 oz glass)	5
Root beer	1 (10 oz bottle)	4½
Seven-up	1 (12 oz bottle)	7½
CAKES AND COOKIES		
Angel food cake	1 (4 oz piece)	7
Applesauce cake	1 (4 oz piece)	5½
Banana bread	1 (2 oz piece)	2
Cheesecake	1 (4 oz piece)	2
Chocolate cake (plain)	1 (4 oz piece)	6
Chocolate cake (iced)	1 (4 oz piece)	10
Coffee cake	1 (4 oz piece)	4½
Cupcake (iced)	1	6
Fruit cake	1 (4 oz piece)	5
Jelly-roll	1 (2 oz piece)	2½
Orange cake	1 (4 oz piece)	4
Pound cake	1 (4 oz piece)	5
Sponge cake	1 (1 oz piece)	2
Strawberry shortcake	1 serving	4
Brownies unfrosted	1 (¾ oz)	3
Chocolate cookies	1	1½
Fig newtons	1	5
DAIRY PRODUCTS		
Ice cream	⅓ pt (3½ oz)	3½
Ice cream bar	1	1-7 accord. to size
Ice cream cone	1	3½
Ice cream soda	1	5
Ice cream sundae	1	7
Malted milk shake	1 (10 oz glass)	5
Frozen yogurt	3 oz	3
JELLIES AND JAMS		
Apple butter	1 T	1
Jelly	1 T	4-6
Orange marmalade	1 T	4-6
Peach butter	1 T	1
Strawberry jam	1 T	4
CANDIES		
Av. chocolate milk bar (ex. Hershey)	1 (1½ oz)	2½
Chewing gum	1 stick	½
Fudge	1 oz square	4½
Gum drop	1	2
Hard candy	4 oz	20
Lifesavers	1	½
Peanut brittle	1	3½
CANNED FRUITS AND JUICES		
Canned apricots	4 halv./1 T syr.	3½
Canned fruit juices sweetened	½ cup	2
Canned peaches	2 halv. & 1 T syr.	3½
Fruit salad	½ cup	3½
Fruit syrup	2 T	2½
Stewed fruits	½ cup	2
BREAKFAST CEREALS*		
Cheerios	1 oz	⅕
Special K	1 oz	⅔
Total	1 oz	⅔
Quaker 100% Natural	1 oz	2
Sugar Frosted Flakes	1 oz	2
Sugar Smacks	1 oz	3
Raisin Bran*	1 oz	1½
Cracklin' Oat Bran	1 oz	1½
Fruit Loops	1 oz	2½
Cap'n Krunch	1 oz	2½
Rice Krispies	1 oz	⅔

*As served; no sugar added by the consumer.

amylopectin in plants and glycogen in animal tissues. Most vegetables turn glucose into starch as they age, so peas and corn are sweetest when they are young. On the other hand, fruits, such as bananas and peaches, turn starches into sugars as they age.

amylopectin A branched-chain digestibel polysaccharide made of glucose units; part of starch.

Amylose is a long chain of many glucose molecules linked together with alpha bonds. For comparison, maltose is just two glucose units linked with an alpha bond. Recall that these alpha bonds can be broken during digestion, especially if the starch-containing food has been cooked. Cooking makes the starch more available for attack by digestive enzymes.

Amylopectin starts out the same as amylose (a long chain of glucoses with alpha bonds), but has some branches off of the straight chain that also use alpha bonds.

Table 3-2 Names of sugars used in foods

Sugar	Invert sugar	Lactose	Maple syrup
Sucrose	Glucose	Mannitol	Dextrin
Brown sugar	Sorbitol	Honey	Dextrose
Confectioner's sugar (powdered sugar)	Levulose	Corn syrup or sweeteners	Fructose
Turbinado sugar	Polydextrose	High-fructose corn syrup	Maltose
		Molasses	Caramel
		Date sugar	Fruit sugar

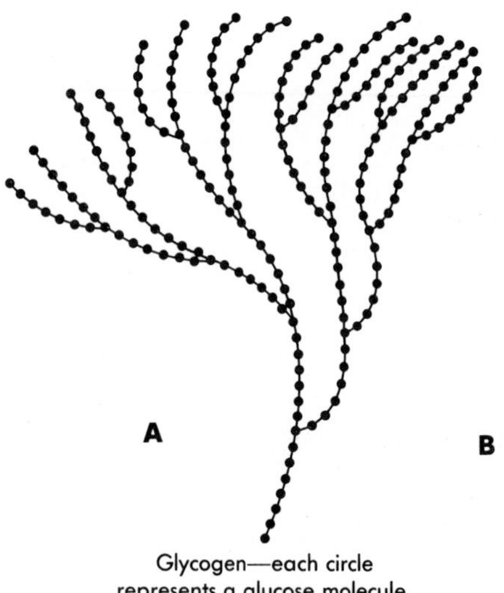

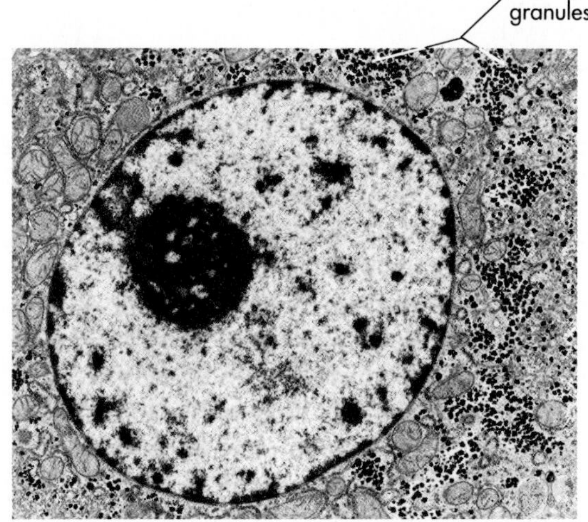

Figure 3-5 A, Glycogen structure. **B,** Glycogen stores as found in the cell.

The only difference in the alpha bonds at the branch points is that they occur on the sixth carbon atom of the molecule rather than the fourth carbon as in the main chain formation. Either way, the body can digest these links in starches.

Amylose and amylopectin can be found in potatoes, beans, breads, pasta, rice, and other food products, typically in a ratio of about 1:3. The branches in amylopectin allow it to form a very stable starch gel, enabling it to retain water and resist water seepage. Food manufacturers commonly use starches rich in amylopectin (like waxy cornstarch) in sauces and gravies for frozen foods for this reason. Manufacturers may also use processes to bond the starch molecules to each other, further increasing their stability. These products are listed as **modified food starch** on food labels of baby foods, salad dressings, and instant puddings.

Glycogen is the storage form of carbohydrate in animals and is made of glucose molecules with alpha bonds and many, many branches. Overall, the structure of glycogen is similar to amylopectin, but the branching patterns are more complicated (Figure 3-5).

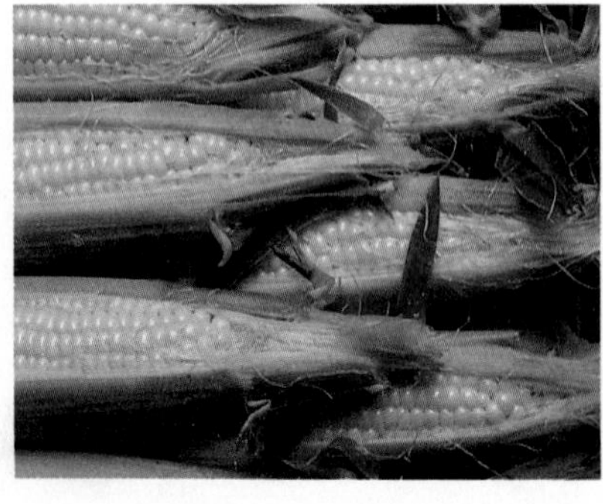

As the corn plant ages sugars are turned into starches, making young corn the sweetest kind.

Enzymes that digest starches can start digestion only at the ends of the glucose chains. The more numerous the branches of a molecule, the more sites (ends) available for enzyme action. Because it is highly branched, glycogen is quickly broken down. Therefore it is an ideal form for carbohydrate storage in the body. In other words, when the body needs an immediate source of blood glucose, the many branches of glycogen provide many points at which a glucose molecule can be broken off rather than waiting for each glucose molecule in a single chain to be removed sequentially.

The liver and muscles are the major storage sites for glycogen.[18] Liver glycogen can be turned into blood glucose but muscle glycogen cannot. Chapter 7 discusses why this is the case. Still, the glycogen in muscles can supply glucose for muscle use, especially during high-intensity and endurance exercise. (See Chapter 10 for a discussion of carbohydrate use in exercise.)

DIETARY FIBER

Dietary fibers are primarily polysaccharides in terms of chemical composition, but these cannot be digested by the human stomach or small intestine. Dietary fiber consists of the carbohydrates **cellulose, hemicelluloses, pectins, gums,** and **mucilages,** as well as the only noncarbohydrate fiber, **lignins** (an alcohol derivative).[16] All the forms of dietary fiber come from plants (Table 3-3).

Cellulose is a polysaccharide with a structure very similar to amylose. However, instead of alpha bonds, which link the glucose units in amylose, cellulose has beta bonds. As we noted earlier, beta bonds are not digestible by humans. Thus cellulose is a part of dietary fiber and not a starch. The glucose chains of cellulose are linear and form many attractions to adjacent cellulose molecules, producing fibrous structures of great strength. Overall, cellulose, hemicelluloses, and lignins form the structural part of the plant. A cotton ball is pure cellulose. Bran fiber is rich in hemicelluloses. The woody fibers in broccoli are partly lignins. These compounds generally will not dissolve in water and so are called **insoluble fibers.**

Pectins, gums, and mucilages are found inside and around plant cells. They help "glue" plant cells together. These compounds either dissolve or swell when put into water and so are called **soluble fibers.** They exist as gum arabic, guar gum, locust bean gum, and various pectin forms in foods, especially in salad dressings, inexpensive ice creams, jams, and jellies.

One workable definition of dietary fiber is: the foodstuffs that remain undigested as they enter the human large intestine.[23] Since some dietary fibers—especially the soluble fibers—are digested by bacteria in the large intestine, it is not accurate to say that dietary fiber is the carbohydrate found in the feces.

Bacteria in the large intestine metabolize soluble dietary fibers into products such as acids (e.g., acetic acid and propionic acid) and gases.[24] Both can then be absorbed, in turn yielding about 3 kcalories per gram. The actual value is still in question. Some gases produced by the bacteria, such as methane (CH_4) and hydrogen (H_2) gas, increase in the breath when dietary fiber intake increases, but this is not harmful.

Another term used for dietary fiber is **crude fiber.** This term arose in the early 1900s to reflect the amount of indigestible foodstuff present in animal feed. The animal feed was boiled for 1 hour in acid, then for another hour in an alkaline solution. The remains of that chemical digestion was called crude fiber; it consisted mostly of cellulose and lignins. All other types of fibers were destroyed by the chemical action. Food composition tables may still report dietary fiber values in terms of crude fiber. These values often bear little resemblance to dietary fiber values because crude fiber no longer contains many fiber components. This point is important. When nutrition scientists talk about fiber, they refer to dietary fiber. Other outmoded terms for dietary fiber include roughage and bulk.

cellulose A straight-chain polysaccharide of glucose molecules that is undigestible due to the presence of beta glycosidic bonds; part of insoluble fiber.

hemicelluloses A group of insoluble fibers containing the monosaccharides xylose, galactose, glucose, and other monosaccharides bonded together.

pectins A group of soluble fibers containing chains of galacturonic acid and other monosaccharides; characteristically found between plant cell walls.

insoluble fibers Fibers that mostly do not dissolve in water and are not digested by bacteria in the large intestine. These include cellulose, some hemicelluloses, and lignins.

soluble fibers Fibers that either dissolve or swell in water or are metabolized (fermented) by bacteria in the large intestine. These include mostly pectins, gums, and mucilages.

The term fiber almost defies definition. Fiber differs from other nutrients, such as the B vitamins, because there is really no common thread that characterizes fibers. Rather, fibers are a group of diverse and complex compounds whose single common property is their ability to resist digestion in the human stomach and small intestine. Note insoluble fibers are also defined as those that are not metabolized (nonfermentable) in the large intestine, while soluble fibers are those that are metabolized (fermentable) in the large intestine.

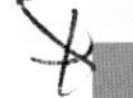

CONCEPT CHECK

Amylose, amylopectin, and glycogen are all storage forms of glucose, called polysaccharides. Amylose and amylopectin combine in varying proportions to form the starch in foods like potatoes and bread. Glycogen is a storage form of glucose in animals, and liver glycogen yields a ready source of blood glucose.

Dietary fiber is essentially the portion of ingested food that remains undigested as it enters the large intestine. Components include cellulose, hemicelluloses, lignins, pectins, gums, and mucilages. There are two types of dietary fiber: insoluble and soluble. Insoluble fibers are made up mostly of cellulose, hemicelluloses, and lignins. Soluble fibers are made up of mostly pectins, gums, and mucilages.

Table 3-3 Classification of dietary fibers

Type	Component	Examples	Physiological Effects	Major Food Sources
Insoluble				
Noncarbohydrate	Lignins	Wheat bran	Uncertain	All plants
Carbohydrate	Cellulose	Wheat products	Increases fecal bulk	All plants
	Hemicelluloses	Brown rice	Decreases transit time	Wheat, rye, vegetables
Soluble				
Carbohydrate	Pectins, gums, mucilages	Apples Bananas Citrus fruits Carrots Barley Oats Kidney beans	Delays gastric emptying; slows glucose absorption; can lower blood cholesterol level	Citrus fruits, oat products, beans

Putting Carbohydrates to Work in the Body

Functions of carbohydrates in the body start with energy production, but that is only the beginning.

ENERGY PRODUCTION

The main function of the simple sugar glucose (and so carbohydrates in general, since most sugars can eventually yield glucose) is to supply energy for the body. Certain tissues in the body derive energy only from glucose, such as the red blood cells and most parts of the brain. In fact, except when the diet contains almost no carbohydrates, the brain and nervous system use mostly carbohydrates for fuel. Carbohydrates can also fuel muscle cells and other body cells, but many of these cells can usually use fats for energy needs.[18]

FLAVORING AND SWEETENING FOODS

From birth humans respond to sugars with a smile. On the tip of the tongue are receptors for tasting sweetness. These recognize a variety of sugars, and even some noncarbohydrate substances. The sugars are not equally sweet; on a per gram basis fructose is almost twice as sweet as sucrose under either acid or cold conditions; sucrose is 30% sweeter than glucose; lactose is less than half as sweet as sucrose (Table 3-4).

SPARING PROTEIN

The sugars and starches (as they break down into sugars) we eat are protein sparing. This term means that dietary protein can be used to make body tissues and perform other vital processes only when carbohydrate intake is sufficient. As mentioned before, red blood cells and the brain require glucose for fuel under normal circumstances. Therefore if you do not eat enough carbohydrates to yield that glucose, your body is forced to make it from other nutrients, such as proteins. This process is termed **gluconeogenesis,** which means "production of new glucose." The hormone cortisol stimulates this process, and the liver and kidney perform most of the gluconeogenesis in the body.

gluconeogenesis The production of new glucose molecules by metabolic pathways in the cell. Amino acids usually provide the carbons for these new glucose molecules.

The source of most of this new glucose must be protein because fats generally cannot be synthesized into glucose. Amino acids from the proteins in muscles, heart, liver, kidneys, and other vital organs supply the carbons needed to make this glucose. If the process occurs over weeks at a time, these organs can become partially weakened. Generally, Americans have more than adequate sources of protein, so sparing

Table 3-4 The sweetness of sugars and alternative sweeteners[4]

Type of sweetner	Relative sweetness* (sucrose = 1.0)	Typical sources
Sugars		
Lactose	0.2	Dairy products
Maltose	0.4	Sprouted seeds
Glucose	0.7	Corn syrup
Sucrose	1.0	Table sugar, most sweets
Invert sugar†	1.3	Some candies, honey
Fructose	1.7	Fruit, honey, some soft drinks
Sugar alcohols		
Sorbitol	0.6	Dietetic candies, sugarless gum
Mannitol	0.7	Dietetic candies
Xylitol	0.9	Sugarless gum
Alternate sweetners		
Aspartame	200	Diet soft drinks, diet fruit drinks, sugarless gum, powdered diet sweetener
Acesulfame-K	200	Sugarless gum, diet drink mixes, powdered diet sweetner, puddings, gelatin desserts
Saccharin (sodium salt)	500	Diet soft drinks

*On a per gram basis.
†Sucrose broken down into glucose and fructose.

protein is not an essential function of carbohydrate under such conditions. It does become important in some low-kcalorie, low-carbohydrate diets, and in semi-starvation. (See Chapters 5 and 20 for a discussion of the specific effects of semi-starvation.)

PREVENTING KETOSIS

Sugars and starches (as these form sugars) are necessary for complete fat metabolism. Insufficient carbohydrate intake (intake not meeting glucose needs) leads to an incomplete breakdown of fats in the metabolic pathways. Without sufficient dietary carbohydrates, carbon dioxide (CO_2) and water (H_2O) molecules are not readily formed during fat metabolism. Instead, fats mostly are turned into **ketones**—acetoacetic acid and its derivatives. The liver is the major organ that produces these ketones.[18] We discuss ketone metabolism and situations that lead to extensive production in detail in Chapter 7.

ketone Incomplete breakdown products of fat containing three or four carbons. These contain a ketone chemical group, hence, the name. An example is acetoacetic acid.

For now, remember that you need to eat at least 50 to 100 grams of carbohydrates per day to ensure complete fat metabolism and to avoid ketosis. This prevents the body weakness that usually results from an insufficient carbohydrate intake. Note that normally we eat at least twice that much carbohydrate each day (about 200+ grams per day).

In starvation conditions, people do not eat enough carbohydrates and so ketones soon appear in their bloodstreams. Again, this is the normal metabolic response. Part of the brain and other tissues can use these ketones for fuel. In fact, the use of ketones by the brain and other organs, such as the heart, is an important adaptation measure for survival during starvation; it reduces protein breakdown by about one third. If part of the brain could not use ketones, the body would be forced to produce much more glucose from protein to support the brain's extra needs. The resulting self-cannibalization would rapidly break down muscle, heart, and other organs, severely limiting the body's ability to tolerate starvation. Thus a person could not exist nearly as long in starvation if the brain could not use ketones for energy.

insulin A hormone produced by the beta cells of the pancreas. Insulin increases the synthesis of glycogen in the liver and the movement of glucose from the bloodstream into muscle and adipose cells, among other processes.

In untreated **insulin-dependent diabetes,** ketones also can be formed, partly because there is not enough **insulin** to allow for normal glucose metabolism.[13] For more information on ketone production in diabetes, see the Nutrition Perspective.

CONCEPT CHECK

The major reason for consuming carbohydrates is to provide glucose for the energy needs of red blood cells and parts of the brain and nervous system. Eating less than 50 to 100 grams of carbohydrates per day forces the liver and kidneys to make glucose (via gluconeogenesis), primarily using carbons from amino acids. These amino acids come from proteins in vital organs. A poor carbohydrate intake also inhibits efficient fat metabolism by the liver and in turn can lead to ketosis.

HEALTH OF THE LARGE INTESTINE

Why do we need dietary fiber? Dietary fiber supplies mass to the feces, making elimination much easier. When enough fiber is consumed, the stool will be large and soft because many types of plant fibers can attract water. The larger size stimulates the intestinal muscles, which aids elimination (see Chapter 6). Consequently, less pressure is necessary to expel the larger stool. This link between dietary fiber and the large intestine's function has interested people for hundreds of years.

When eating too little dietary fiber, the opposite can occur: the stool may be small and hard. Constipation may result, which can force one to exert pressure in the large intestine during defecation. These high pressures can force parts of the large intestine wall to pop out from between the surrounding bands of muscle, forming small pouches. A person can have many of these pouches, called **diverticula.** About 50% of elderly people have diverticula (Figure 3-6). **Hemorrhoids** may also result from excessive straining during defecation (see Chapter 6).

diverticula Pouches that protrude through the outside wall of the large intestine.

hemorrhoid A pronounced swelling in a large vein, particularly those found in the anal region.

diverticulosis The condition of having many diverticula in the large intestine.

Diverticula are normally asymptomatic; that is, they are not noticeable. The asymptomatic form of this disease is called **diverticulosis.** If the diverticula become filled with food particles, such as hulls or seeds, bacteria can metabolize these food particles into acids and gases. The acids and gases irritate the diverticula and may eventually cause them to become inflamed. This condition is known as **diverticulitis.** Antibiotics then may be needed to lessen the bacterial action, and dietary fiber intake may be reduced to also limit further bacterial activity. Once the inflammation subsides, a high dietary fiber intake (but free of seeds and hulls) is begun to ease stool elimination and reduce the risk of a future attack.

As noted above, diverticula commonly occur in the lower large intestine (colon) of elderly people in Western countries. These rarely occur in people in Third World countries.[7] The low dietary fiber intake in Western countries, in contrast to that of the Third World, is probably the major reason for the difference.

The Nutrition Focus on page 80 mentioned dietary fiber may also play a key role in the prevention of colon cancer. Among the deadly cancers, colon cancer ranks in the top three in the U.S. About half the studies on the subject—epidemiological and case-control—have been able to link colon cancer to lack of fiber in the diet. Still researchers know little about how dietary fiber might affect cancer development. There is good reason for suggesting that potential carcinogens in the intestinal contents are (1) being diluted by fluid attracted to the fibers, (2) bound

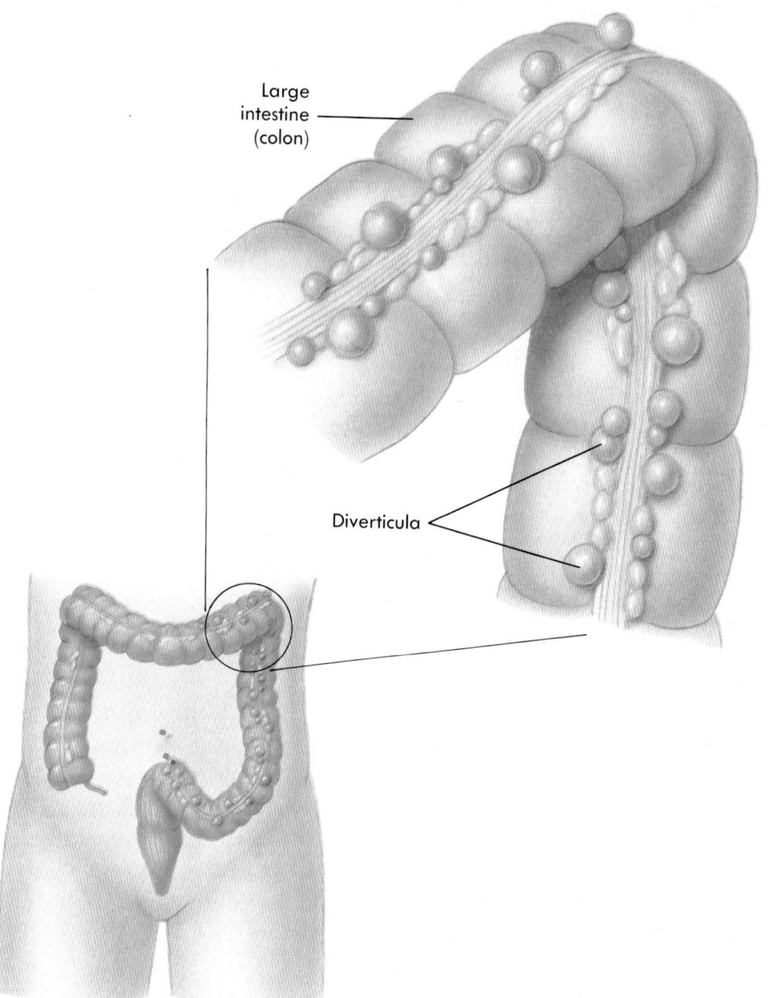

Figure 3-6 Diverticula in the colon. A low-fiber diet increases the risk for their development.

to the fibers, and (3) more rapidly excreted as fibers speed passage of feces through the intestinal tract.

Colon cancers have been prevented in laboratory animals by adding dietary fiber to the diet. Cellulose, hemicelluloses, and lignins have the major protective role. In human studies fiber from fruit and vegetable sources have tended to be most protective.[1] Overall, accumulating evidence suggests that too much fat and total energy content of the diet, as well as too little dietary fiber, may be important causal factors in colon cancer. Inactivity is also implicated; regular physical activity aids bowel regularity.

More About Soluble and Insoluble Fibers

All dietary fibers do not have the same effect on the body (Table 3-3). Insoluble fibers, particularly certain types of hemicelluloses, are the best fiber source for increasing stool size. Bran, the fibrous covering of grain kernels, is rich in hemicelluloses. Bran adds mass to stool most effectively if it is coarsely ground. Finely ground bran does not significantly increase stool size or frequency. Since bran layers form the outer covering of all grains, **whole grains** are good sources of insoluble fiber.

Soluble fibers are the best fiber source for inhibiting cholesterol absorption from the small intestine and for slowing down glucose absorption from the small intestine.[2] Rich sources of soluble fibers include fruits, vegetables, legumes (dry beans), soybean fiber, **psyllium** seeds (found in many commercial fiber laxatives and some breakfast

psyllium A mostly soluble type of dietary fiber found in the seeds of the plantain plant.

NUTRITION FOCUS

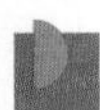

History of Fiber in America

Folklore surrounding dietary fiber has been a part of American culture since the 1800s. Sylvester Graham, a minister, traveled up and down the East Coast extolling the virtues of fiber in the 1820s and 1830s. He left us a legacy—the Graham cracker. However, today's graham cracker bears little resemblance to the whole-grain product he promoted.

The next wave of fiber frenzy crested in the mid-1870s. Dr. John Harvey Kellogg was hired by the Seventh Day Adventist Church to manage their health sanitarium in Battle Creek, Michigan. He believed fiber would cure many of the ills that existed in his time. People came from throughout the United States, including many famous people, to "take the cure" at the sanitarium. Fiber was an important part of that cure. Dr. Kellogg became the first person to earn a million dollars from "health foods."

One gentlemen who came for a cure in 1891 was Charles W. Post. Post saw what Dr. Kellogg was doing and decided he could do the same. He created the Post Toasted Cornflakes Company and started producing Postum Cereal Food Coffee and Grape Nuts Cereal. Not to be outdone, William Kellogg, John Harvey Kellogg's brother, revived the Kellogg Toasted Corn Flake Company in 1906. Today both companies are active in the breakfast cereal market. True to form, the Kellogg Company is still "promoting" fiber to Americans.

Fiber finally received its scientific letters in the early 1970s. Dr. Denis Burkitt, a noted British physician, observed that in Africa many "western" diseases did not exist. These included diverticulosis, colon cancer, appendicitis, hemorrhoids, constipation, and other intestinal disorders. He also noted that heart disease was rare in Africa. Burkitt surmised that the high-fiber intake of Africans was an important reason that these diseases did not occur.[7] He noticed that Africans had very large stools, almost twice the weight of stools from Westerners.

Many researchers followed Burkitt's lead. Soon studies showed that high-fiber intakes decreased transit time. That is, by eating more fiber less time is needed for the undigested part to pass through the intestinal tract and be eliminated. Researchers suggested that if stool stayed in the large intestine for only a short time, less bacterial metabolism of the stool would occur, thus probably fewer toxins and perhaps fewer carcinogens would form. This faster transit time is especially true for insoluble fibers. Researchers also found that soluble fibers can bind cholesterol-containing substances in the intestine. This finding strengthened the link between a high-fiber diet and low levels of coronary heart disease.

An argument arose in the mid-1980s when the Kellogg Company began promoting high-fiber cereals in the war against colon cancer. Actually, the company was following the lead of the National Cancer Institute. Scientists at the National Cancer Institute believed that a verifiable link existed between low-fiber diets and colon cancer and thought the public needed to be alerted. But the bold move by the Kellogg Company to promote fiber to Americans was and still is criticized as premature by some scientists. Fiber is important for regular bowel habits, and it can help control hyperglycemia in diabetes and lower blood cholesterol levels.[3] However, scientific research does not support the promotion of fiber much beyond that. In other words, the jury is still out on the extent to which dietary fiber can reduce colon cancer risk. Clinical studies are ongoing.

cereals), and oat bran. Still, intake must be considerable to have an effect on serum cholesterol levels (60 to 100 grams/day of oat bran, which is about ½ to ¾ cup).

CONCEPT CHECK

Dietary fiber has been the focus of human attention for centuries. Dietary fiber forms a vital part of the diet by providing mass to the stool, which helps ease elimination. Certain forms are also useful for controlling blood glucose levels in people with diabetes and in lowering blood cholesterol levels. Some types of fibers yield energy after they are metabolized by bacteria in the large intestine. Whole grains, vegetables, legumes, and fruits are excellent sources of dietary fiber.

Regulating Energy Sources in the Bloodstream

Now you understand the structure, form, and function of simple and complex carbohydrates. One of the most important functions of carbohydrates is supplying a source of energy. The next question then becomes, how is this essential energy source regulated in the bloodstream?

Under normal circumstances, blood glucose usually varies between about 70 and 115 milligrams per 100 milliliters of blood. If blood glucose rises above 170 milligrams per 100 milliliters of blood, it begins to spill over into the urine. If blood glucose falls below 40 to 50 milligrams per 100 milliliters of blood, a person begins to feel nervous, irritable, and hungry, and may develop a headache. Having high levels of blood glucose is called **hyperglycemia.** Having low levels of blood glucose is called **hypoglycemia.**

As carbohydrates are digested and absorbed in the small intestine, the resulting monosaccharides—glucose, fructose, and galactose—go directly to the liver.[18] Here much of the galactose and fructose is turned into glucose. The liver is a main organ for controlling the amount of glucose that eventually is found in the bloodstream. Since it is the first organ to screen the absorbed sugars, the liver appropriately serves as guard, helping to control the amount of glucose that enters the bloodstream after a meal (Figure 3-7).

Small amounts of the hormone insulin are released by the pancreas as soon as a person begins eating. Once glucose has entered the bloodstream, the pancreas releases large amounts of insulin. Insulin affects the body in a variety of ways. It promotes increased glycogen synthesis in the liver to stimulate glucose storage, as well as increased glucose uptake by the muscle cells, **adipose (fat) cells,** and many other cells. By this means, insulin triggers both glucose storage in the liver and glucose movement out of the bloodstream into cells. This dual action of insulin is one key to maintaining blood glucose levels within a narrow, normal range.

adipose (fat) cells Fat storing cells.

Other hormones counteract the effects of insulin. Now when a person has not eaten carbohydrates for a few hours, and the blood glucose level begins to fall, it

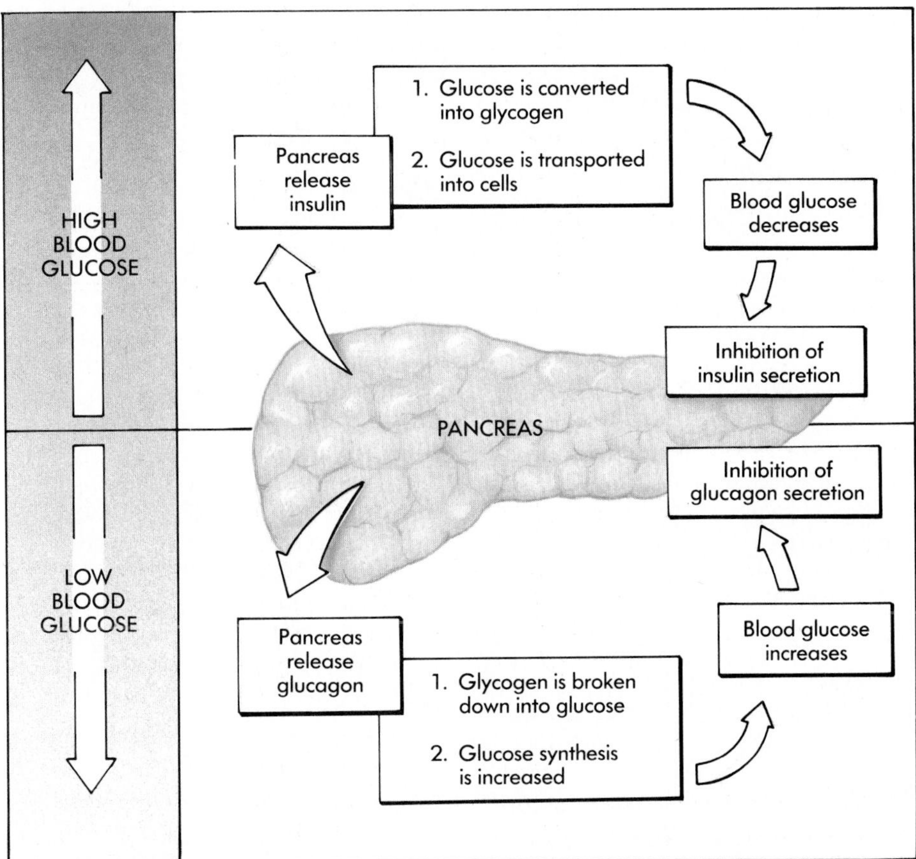

Figure 3-7 The regulation of blood glucose. Insulin and glucagon levels for key control points with regards to blood glucose levels.

EXPERT OPINION

Dietary Fiber: Different Types, Different Effects

DAVID KRITCHEVSKY, PH.D.

One of the most enduring dietary interests of the 1980s worldwide has been dietary fiber. One probable reason is that, for once, physicians and other health professionals have been asking us to add something to the diet instead of declaring another taboo. Another reason may be that any substance that is touted to help prevent or cure a large number of maladies—from obesity, constipation, and ulcers to cancer, diabetes, and heart disease—is bound to garner considerable attention.

What is fiber? Grandmother called it "roughage" and it is presently defined as a plant substance that resists breakdown by the body's digestive processes in the stomach and small intestine. Whenever we eat vegetables, fruits, legumes, grains, or seeds, we're ingesting fiber.

There is no universally accepted method for analyzing dietary fiber. The method used to provide data found in older tables was inadequate: it crudely measured what was called "crude fiber" (a meaningless term still found on some labels)—completely missing the soluble fibers—while also giving poor recovery of the insoluble ones. Most modern methods are based on enzymatic breakdown of the carbohydrate materials followed by analysis of individual sugars. Protein, mineral ash, and lignins are determined separately. Although the variations in methodology are complex, all are coming up with similar answers. Accurate tables of fiber content of various foodstuffs are now becoming available. A simple (possibly oversimple) classification of fibers is into insoluble (the brans) and soluble (pectin, various gums). Most foods contain both.

Whereas people generally think of wheat bran as pure fiber, as you have seen in the chapter discussion, it is actually a mixture of a number of types of fiber. It also contains some protein, fat, and trace minerals. Soy and rice brans differ from wheat bran in their makeup of nutrients. The age of a vegetable may also influence its fiber composition; thus young carrots contain very little lignin, whereas old carrots may contain 10% to 20% of this material. And the form in which fruit is eaten affects the fiber content. For example, an apple (with skin) has far more fiber than applesauce, and apple juice has virtually no fiber at all.

Not all soluble fibers are alike, either. Pectin, for example, consists of a uronic acid (a carbohydrate) backbone with natural carbohydrate side chains. Oat gum, on the other hand, is primarily a beta glucan, which is a mixture of three or four linked glucose units. Whether one type of structure is more effective than others, regarding physical or metabolic properties, remains to be seen.

In almost every case, insoluble fibers, such as wheat bran and corn bran, have no effect on serum cholesterol levels. Doses of wheat bran as high as 60 grams per day have been ineffective in lowering these levels. On the other hand, 60 grams of oat bran per day does have a cholesterol-lowering action, probably because it contains a soluble fiber, oat gum. Likewise, when 6 grams to 36 grams per day (an average of 19 grams) of pectin is ingested for 2 to 12 weeks (an average of 7 weeks), cholesterol levels decrease by 5% to 18% (an average of 8%). Guar gum has similar effects at similar dosages. Another fiber that has been shown to be effective in lowering cholesterol is psyllium.

Why do fibers, such as pectin and oat gum, have cholesterol-lowering effects? The existence of several competing hypotheses suggests that none is totally satisfactory. According to one hypothesis, some fibers tend to link bile acids, which are needed for the absorption of cholesterol. But scientific data are not consistent enough to validate this idea. Another hypothesis involves the roles of volatile fatty acids. The intestinal bacteria degrade soluble fibers to a greater extent than they do insoluble fibers. The acids produced (acetic, propionic, butyric) are absorbed from the colon and enter the circulation. The result is an increase in serum concentrations of acetate and propionate, which have been shown to inhibit cholesterol synthesis by some workers but not by others. One hypothesis is that the effect of soluble fibers is due to their physical, rather than chemical, properties. The fibers, when they reach the intestine, form a gel-like aggregate from which nutrients are absorbed with difficulty.

Are there risks from eating too much fiber? In countries whose populations ingest low-kcalorie, high-fiber diets, there is evidence of growth retardation primarily due to negative zinc balance—since virtually all fibers bind positive ions, such as zinc, calcium, and magnesium. There is always the danger that a diet too high in fiber will lead to a mineral imbalance and, indeed, such cases have been reported. It is easy to overshoot fiber in the diets of certain groups such as elderly people, whose energy intake is normally low. In addition, some people can tolerate more fiber than others. In any case, if you want to increase fiber consumption, do so gradually because your body needs time to learn to deal with the added bulk and to let you know when enough's enough; if the change is made too fast, your body will complain by producing gas and bloating.

Expert panels convened in Canada and the United States have arrived independently at similar suggestions for fiber intake. They propose that it be geared to energy intake and recommend 10 grams to 13 grams of fiber per 1000 kcalories. This amount would provide 20 grams to 35 grams of dietary fiber for the average healthy adult. The ratio of insoluble to soluble fiber should be about 3 : 1, as it is in nature. The same panels suggest that the fiber we do eat comes from the grocery store and not the pharmacy.

Dr. Kritchevsky is Associate Director and Institute Professor at the Wistar Institute of Anatomy and Biology in Philadelphia.

can be restored. As the level of blood glucose falls, the pancreas releases the hormone **glucagon.** This prompts the breakdown of glycogen in the liver, and the resulting glucose is released into the bloodstream. In this way glucagon helps restore blood glucose levels to a normal level.[18]

At the same time, the hormone **epinephrine** (adrenaline) triggers a breakdown of glycogen in the liver and so a release of glucose into the bloodstream. Other hormones, such as **cortisol,** growth hormone, and thyroid hormone also help regulate the blood glucose level.

In essence, the actions of insulin on blood sugar regulation in the body are counterbalanced by the actions of glucagon, epinephrine, cortisol, and other hormones. If hormonal balance is not maintained, such as when insulin or glucagon are either overproduced or underproduced, major changes in blood glucose levels occur. See the Nutrition Perspective for examples of this phenomenon.

Before we move on, let's take a step back and look at one of the intricacies of our body metabolism. Blood glucose is such a key source of energy for so much of the body that it makes sense we have evolved with a system that calls on many factors for its regulation. Imagine the consequence if only one system, such as using a nerve connection between the brain and pancreas, controlled blood glucose levels. If this nerve was severed, dire consequences would result. As it is, a perturbation in one body system—like that in the pancreas—can greatly influence blood glucose levels, but it doesn't knock out the entire regulatory system. The liver and adrenal glands still can contribute to blood glucose regulation. This example of checks and balances is typical of how the body controls levels of its key constituents (see the discussion of homeostasis in Chapter 7).

glucagon A hormone made by the alpha cells of the pancreas that stimulates the breakdown of glycogen in the liver into glucose; this raises the blood glucose level. It also performs other functions.

epinephrine A hormone also known as adrenaline; it is released by the adrenal gland and various nerve endings in the body and acts to increase glycogen breakdown in the liver, among other functions.

cortisol A hormone made by the adrenal gland that stimulates production of glucose from amino acids, among other functions.

Epinephrine is responsible for the "flight or fight" reaction. This is how the body responds to a threat, such as suddenly seeing a car approaching head-on. Epinephrine is released in large amounts from the adrenal gland and various nerve endings. The resulting rapid flood of glucose into the bloodstream helps promote a quick reaction.

CONCEPT CHECK

Blood glucose levels are maintained within a very narrow range, between about 70 and 115 milligrams per 100 milliliters of blood. When blood glucose rises after a meal, the hormone insulin attempts to restore normal levels, partly by increasing glucose uptake by muscles and adipose tissues. If blood glucose levels fall during fasting, then glucagon, epinephrine, and other hormones increase the liver's release of glucose into the bloodstream to restore normal levels. Whether a person has just eaten or fasted overnight, hormone activity and the action of the liver together attempt to maintain blood glucose levels within a very narrow range.

Can We Eat too Much of Certain Types of Carbohydrates?

Can one get too much of a good thing? In a word—yes. Moderation, balance, and variety are the important watchwords of nutrition.

SUGARS

Many people think it is not healthy to consume simple sugars. True, simple sugars by themselves have very low nutrient densities. In other words, sugary foods may supply few, if any, vitamins, minerals, or proteins compared with the number of kcalories they supply. However, if one can afford to consume some extra kcalories, there is nothing wrong with eating sugar. Scientists believe that simple sugars become a problem when substituted for more nutritious foods. In that case, a person could become deficient in vitamins and other important nutrients.

Some people claim simple sugars cause heart disease, diabetes, hyperactivity, juvenile delinquency, obesity, and other problems. Little or no credible research supports these allegations. A systematic, cause and effect relationship between these conditions and the eating of sugar either has not been established or has eluded

cariogenic Literally "caries producing"; a substance, often carbohydrate-rich (such as caramels), that promotes dental caries.

careful testing. Many major scientific groups have examined the current research surrounding the typical sugars in our diet and basically given them a clean bill of health, except for the tendency for many to cause **dental caries.**[4,11] (See Chapter 17 for a full discussion of whether diet causes hyperactivity in children.)

Dental caries are formed when sugars and other carbohydrates are metabolized to acids by bacteria that live in the mouth (Figure 3-8). The acid then dissolves the tooth enamel and underlying structure. Sticky or gummy foods high in sugars, such as caramels, are the worst types as these stick to the teeth and supply the bacteria with a long-lived carbohydrate source. These foods are **cariogenic;** *cario* means cavity. Liquid sugar sources—for example, fruit juices—are not as potent at causing dental caries but still warrant consideration. Snacking regularly on sugary foods is also likely to cause caries since it allows the bacteria on the teeth a source of carbohydrate from which to continually make acids. Sugar-containing foods are not the only foods that may be turned to acid by the bacteria in the mouth. Starch containing foods, such as saltines and bread, if held in the mouth a long time, may be acted on by enzymes in the mouth that break down the starch to sugar. (More about this in Chapter 6.) Overall the frequency and retentive nature of sugar and starch consumption plays the greatest role in the cariogenicity of a food.

It is important to begin to understand the benefits and risks of certain recommendations made by those giving nutrition advice. There are few black and white answers. For example, raisins are a fruit containing vitamins and minerals and are recommended as a good snack for the preschool age child. What about the cariogenic nature of raisins? Does that make it a "bad" snack? The answer is yes only for those particularly susceptible to dental caries, especially poor dental hygiene.

In the final analysis, use of sugars should be guided by the same advice given for many other food products—moderation. By regularly visiting the dentist and keeping blood sugar levels and weight under control, sugar can be enjoyed in "moderation," meaning a limit of about 10% of total kcalorie intake, or about 10

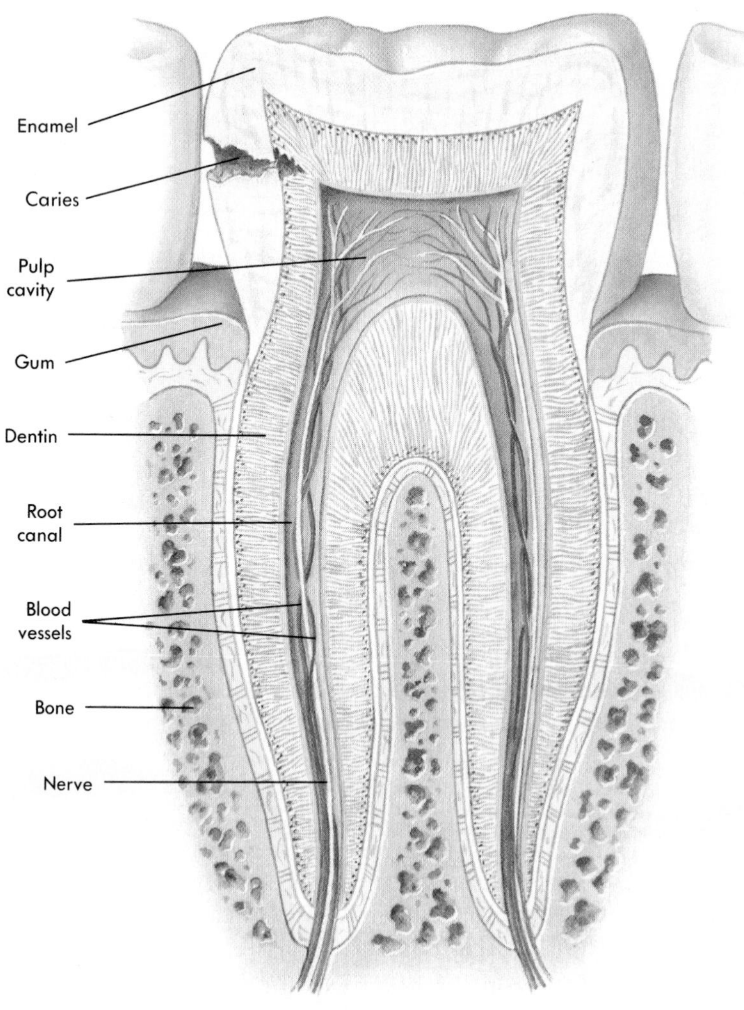

Figure 3-8 Dental decay. Bacteria can collect in various areas on a tooth. Using simple sugars, bacteria create acids that can dissolve tooth enamel, leading to cavities. If the caries process progresses and enters the pulp cavity, damage to the nerve may occur. The bacteria also produce plaque to adhere themselves to the tooth surface.

total teaspoons in a day's diet (one teaspoon contains 15 kcalories). In the last 15 years, simple-sugar consumption has remained about constant in the United States, but dental-caries rates have decreased by 30%. This decline is primarily due to the addition of fluoride to water. When teeth develop in the presence of the mineral fluoride, they become much more resistant to acid (see Chapter 15). Fluoride in

NUTRITION FOCUS

Lactose Intolerance

The inability to digest lactose is the result of a reduction in activity of the enzyme lactase, the function of which is to split the disaccharide lactose into glucose and galactose. Lactase, embedded within the surface of the intestinal cells, ensures that lactose is divided into glucose and galactose so these can be absorbed via the small intestine. If instead the lactose travels as such unaltered into the large intestine, bacteria there will metabolize the lactose to acids and gases. This often causes intestinal gas, bloating, cramping and discomfort (see Chapter 6 for more details on carbohydrate digestion).

Primary lactose intolerance is common in Asians, Hispanics, Native Americans, people of Mediterranean descent, African-Americans, and other dark-skinned races. Some individuals may be born with little or no lactase, but more commonly the lactase levels decline with age. Even though lactose intolerance is more prevalent in some ethnic groups than others, as many as 70% of adults worldwide experience a large decrease in their ability to synthesize lactase. Although when younger they could digest lactose, as they age lactose from milk products tends to remain undigested. This loss of lactase activity is not due to disease; it happens naturally, hence the designation primary.

Secondary lactose intolerance by definition develops as a result of another disease, such as an intestinal bacterial infection. The inability to digest lactose may occur during use of certain medications or cancer chemotherapy. Both processes can inhibit the growth of the rapidly reproducing cells that line the gastronintestinal tract and produce lactase.

Clinically, lactose intolerance can be diagnosed from a history of gas and bloating after milk consumption. This history can then be confirmed by having the person consume 50 grams of lactose, which is equal to 1 liter (4 cups) of milk. If the blood glucose level does not rise much after consuming the lactose, poor digestion is the likely cause. Some clinicians prefer using 12.5 grams of lactose, a more realistic amount for the test dose. Other more technical procedures are available to confirm the diagnosis of lactose intolerance.

Most people quickly learn how much lactose they can tolerate and easily adjust the amount of dairy products in their diet. Few people need to avoid all lactose, but the person who is sensitive to even small amounts of lactose must become an avid lable reader and avoid products with ingredients such as milk, milk solids, casein, and whey. Some medications contain lactose as binders or fillers.

If one is only moderately intolerant to lactose, it is not a good idea to avoid all milk and milk products because these are very good sources of calcium, riboflavin, potassium, and magnesium. All four of these nutrients are present in other foods in our diets, but there are groups of people who don't consume enough of them. Planning a diet for these nutrients is much easier if one uses milk and milk products.

Several options are available then to moderately lactose-intolerant people who prefer to continue using milk products. First, they could consume smaller serving sizes of milk products and take them with other foods; this often works because they are able to digest some lactose, but not large amounts at one time. Secondly, they can eat cheese. Much lactose is lost when milk is made into cheese. Finally, they can consume yogurt. The bacteria that make yogurt can provide their own lactase activity so the lactose in yogurt essentially digests itself.[17] However, typical sweetened yogurt may have as many as 240 kcalories per serving, approximately three times more kcalories than a glass of skim milk, making it a high-kcalorie option. Available now in groceries are low-fat, aspartame-sweetened, fruit-flavored yogurts with as few as 60 kcalories per 4-ounce serving.

In the last few years, manufacturers have been producing low-lactose milk. This type of milk greatly reduces symptoms. Regular milk is treated with lactase that has been isolated from yeast. After a day of treatment, 70% of the lactose is digested into glucose and galactose. This milk tastes a bit sweeter, since glucose is much sweeter than lactose.

One can also reduce the lactose content of milk at home by putting drops of a commerical enzyme preparation into a gallon of milk and waiting 24 hours before consuming it. Lactase can be bought at drug or grocery stores; it works at refrigerator temperatures. Lactase pills can also be purchased for consumption with milk products. These procedures inhibit the unpleasant symptoms associated with lactose intolerance,[6] and although they do increase the cost of using dairy products, the nutritional benefits can be worth it.

Thus several options are available to lactose-intolerant people, only one of which is abandoning milk products. People with severe lactase deficiency who avoid all dairy products should seek other sources of calcium (see Chapter 14).

toothpaste also contributes to dental health as it promotes mineralization of the teeth. Certainly, good nutrition and routine visits to the dentist also have contributed to the improved dental health we enjoy today.

PROBLEMS WITH HIGH-FIBER DIETS

Very high dietary fiber intakes—for example, 60 grams per day—can pose some health risks. A high dietary fiber intake requires a high water intake. Not consuming enough water with the dietary fiber can leave the stool very hard and make it difficult and painful to eliminate. Large amounts of dietary fiber may also bind important minerals, such as calcium, zinc, and iron.

phytobezoars Pellets of dietary fiber, characteristically found in the stomach.

High-fiber diets also often contribute to intestinal gas. In addition, high dietary fiber intakes may lead to the production of fiber balls, called **phytobezoars,** in the stomach.[9] These have been found in diabetic people who consume large amounts of dietary fiber and can lead to blockage of intestinal flow. Finally, great amounts of dietary fiber may add such an excess of bulk to a child's diet that energy consumption would suffer; dietary fiber would fill the child before food intake could meet kcalorie needs.

Recommendations for Carbohydrate Intake

No RDA for carbohydrates has been established. As discussed before, it is important to consume at least 50 to 100 grams of carbohydrates per day to prevent ketosis. Remember, this is just the minimum; much more carbohydrate continues to spare protein and helps meet energy needs (Figure 3-9).

It is easy to consume 50 grams of carbohydrates. Just three pieces of fruit or three slices of bread or a little more than three cups of milk will suffice. In fact, it is difficult to follow a diet that will produce ketosis. The average American eats more than 200 grams of carbohydrates per day. The top five contributors of carbohydrates to the U.S. diet are white breads, sugared soft drinks, baked goods, sugar itself, and milk.

We have mentioned several times that milk and some dairy products contain the milk sugar lactose. This should in no way be construed to mean that this is a food to avoid in order to limit simple carbohydrate consumption. In fact, low-fat and skim dairy products have an overall high nutrient density and would be one of the last sources of sugars to eliminate.

On a percentage of energy basis, carbohydrates supply about 48% of dietary energy needs of adults in the United States. About half of that comes from sugars both naturally occurring and added to foods, and half is from starches. Worldwide, however, carbohydrates account for about 70% of all kcalories consumed. In some countries, carbohydrates account for up to 80% of kcalories consumed. In America

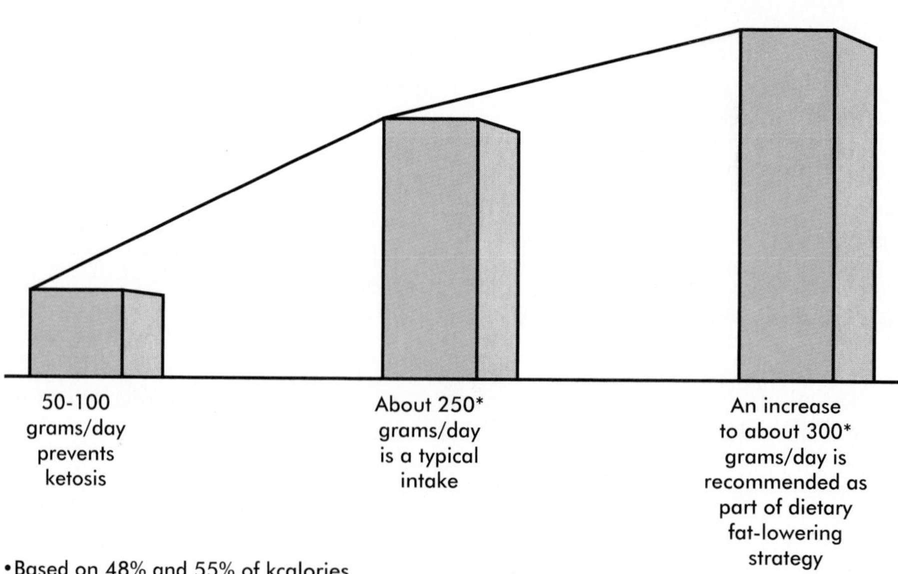

Figure 3-9 The dietary carbohydrate continuum. Relatively little dietary carbohydrate is needed to prevent ketosis. Much more is advised, especially complex varieties, as we reduce our fat intake and search for kcalories to replace those fat kcalories.

and in many other industrialized areas where fat intake is high, carbohydrates supply a lower percentage of total kcalories.

Nutrition experts in the United States and Canada are recommending we place a greater emphasis on starch and fiber in the diet (Figure 3-10).[10] A reasonable goal is to aim for about 45% of kcalorie intake as starches, with a total carbohydrate intake of about 55% of total kcalories. As carbohydrate intake increases, dietary fiber intake should naturally increase and fat intake should decrease.

The American diet supplies about 135 pounds of simple sugars per year for each citizen. About half of this comes from sucrose and half comes from corn sweeteners. Most of these sugars are added to foods and beverages in manufacturing. During processing of food, the sugar content often is increased. The more processed the food is, the higher the sugar content often is. An apple has 0 grams of added sugar, canned apples in heavy syrup have 10 to 15 grams (2 to 3 teaspoons), and ⅙ of a 9-inch apple pie has 30 grams (6 teaspoons) of added sugar.

The rest of the sugars in our diets are present naturally in foods and come from the sugar bowl. Overall consumption of sucrose has dropped in the last 10 years, but consumption of corn sweeteners has increased.[4] Corn sweeteners are cheaper and easier to transport than other forms of sugar used by food manufacturers.

Not only do nutrition experts suggest we increase complex carbohydrates (starches) in the diet, but we should also avoid too much sugar. Although "use

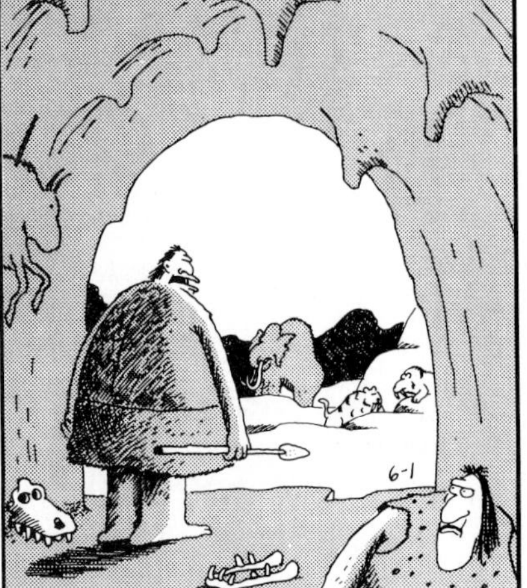

"Once in a while couldn't we just have some pasta?"

Figure 3-10 The Far Side.

The Far Side copyright 1986 Universal Press Syndicate. Reprinted with permission. All rights reserved.

Table 3-5 Suggestions for reducing sugar intake

At the supermarket

- Read ingredient lables. Identify all the added sugars in a product. Select items lower in total sugar when possible.
- Buy fresh fruits or fruits packed in water, juice, or light syrup rather than those in heavy syrup.
- Buy fewer foods that are high in sugar such as prepared baked goods, candies, sugared cereals, sweet desserts, soft drinks, and fruit-flavored punches and soft drinks. Substitute vanilla wafers, graham crackers, bagels, English muffins, and diet soft drinks, for example.
- Buy nuts (dry roasted), sunflower seeds, and popcorn (use hot-air popper) to replace candy for snacks.

In the kitchen

- Reduce the sugar in foods prepared at home. Try new recipes or adjust your own. Start by reducing the sugar gradually until you've decreased it by one third or more.
- Experiment with spices such as cinnamon, cardamom, coriander, nutmeg, ginger, and mace to enhance the flavor of foods.
- Use home-prepared items (with less sugar) instead of commerically prepared ones that are higher in sugar, when possible.

At the table

- Use less of all sugars. This includes white and brown sugar, honey, molasses, and syrups.
- Choose fewer foods high in sugar such as prepared baked goods, candies, and sweet desserts.
- Reach for fresh fruit instead of a sweet for dessert or when you want a snack.
- Add less sugar to foods—coffee, tea, cereal, or fruit. Get used to using half as much; then see if you can cut back even more.
- Cut back on the number of sugared soft drinks and punches you drink. Substitute water, fruit juice, or diet soft drinks.

Modified from USDA Home and Garden Bulletin No. 232-5, 1986.

sugars only in moderation" is a little vague, this has been interpreted to mean less than 10% of total kcalorie intake should come from sugar, as we noted earlier. This corresponds to about 44 pounds of simple sugars per year, or about a one-third decrease from the current amount. Table 3-5 provides ideas to help us reduce our intake of simple sugars.

CONCEPT CHECK

The American diet supplies about 135 pounds of simple sugars a year for each citizen. About two thirds of these sugars are added to foods and beverages in manufacturing. The rest occurs naturally in foods or is added from the sugar bowl. To reduce simple sugar consumption one must reduce consumption of items that have had much sugar added, such as some baked goods, sweet beverages, and presweetened breakfast cereals.

HOW MUCH DIETARY FIBER DO WE NEED?

In his Expert Opinion Dr. Kritchevsky noted that a reasonable goal for dietary fiber intake is 20 to 35 grams per day (10 to 13 grams per 1000 kcalories). Our average intake is closer to 10 to 13 grams per day. Thus most of us should probably increase our dietary fiber intake. A goal of 20 to 35 grams should prevent much of the diverticulosis that typically develops in western countries and is not hard to attain, as we will show later.

To help control blood glucose levels in persons with diabetes, some researchers recommend consuming up to 60 grams of dietary fiber per day, emphasizing soluble fibers.[2] A carefully planned diet is necessary to meet this fiber recommendation. This also carries the risk of producing a stool too large for comfortable elimination and other problems that we discussed earlier.

Before embarking on increasing your dietary fiber intake, first calculate the amount of fiber you are already eating. If it is less than 20 to 35 grams per day, find some higher-fiber foods to substitute for foods you already eat, or add some new ones (Table 3-6).

Eating a high-fiber cereal for breakfast is one possible step. We suggest whole food sources over bran supplement sources because foods can provide a broader variety of nutrients. This is especially true for many natural high-fiber foods.

Table 3-7 lists a diet containing about 25 grams of dietary fiber but only 1500 kcalories. We think you will agree this would be an easy diet to follow if you like fruits and beans. By eating whole-grain breads, legumes, high-fiber cereals, and fruits and vegetables, it is easy to eat enough dietary fiber. However, some people may need to minimize their intake of foods made with refined flour, such as doughnuts, sweet rolls, coffee cakes, and white bread, to control kcalorie intake. Table 3-8 lists tips on increasing dietary fiber intake.

Note that manufacturers are now listing enriched white flour as wheat flour on food labels. Most people think that if "wheat bread" is on the label, they are getting a whole-wheat product. Not so. The label must say "whole-wheat flour" in the ingredient list. If it does not say whole-wheat flour, it is not whole-wheat bread, and so probably will not contain as much dietary fiber as it could. Careful reading of labels is important as you search for more dietary fiber—look especially for whole grains.

Carbohydrates in Foods

In the exchange system the milk group yields 12 grams of carbohydrates per exchange. The starch/bread group and the fruit group both yield 15 grams of carbohydrates per exchange, and the vegetable group yields 5 grams of carbohydrates per exchange (Table 2-6).

Table 3-6 Dietary fiber values for fiber-containing foods

Food group	Serving	kcalories	Grams of dietary fiber*
Breads and cereals			
Air-popped popcorn	1 cup	25	2.5
All Bran	½ cup	100	12
Bran Buds	½ cup	110	7.9
Bran Chex	1 cup	150	4.6
Cracklin' Oat Bran	½ cup	110	4.3
Grapenuts	¼ cup	100	1.4
Oatmeal (cooked)	1 cup	144	4.0
Raisin Bran	1 cup	150	4.0
Whole-wheat bread	1 slice	60	1.9
Legumes, cooked			
Kidney beans	½ cup	110	5.2
Lima beans	½ cup	95	4.5
Navy Beans	½ cup	115	9.3
Vegetables, cooked			
Beans, green	½ cup	15	1.0
Broccoli	½ cup	20	3.0
Brussels sprouts	½ cup	30	3.2
Cabbage, red & white	½ cup	15	0.6
Carrots	½ cup	25	1.9
Cauliflower	½ cup	15	2.0
Corn	½ cup	70	2.0
Green pepper	½ cup	12	1.3
Green peas	½ cup	55	3.3
Lettuce	1 cup	7	0.8
Potato, with skin	1 small	110	2.5
Tomato, chopped	½ cup	17	0.7
Fruits			
Apple	1 medium	80	3.0
Apricot, fresh	3 medium	50	1.8
Apricot, dried	½ cup	100	1.4
Banana	1 medium	105	2.0
Blueberries	½ cup	40	2.0
Cantaloupe	1 cup	50	1.0
Cherries	10	50	1.2
Dates, dried	½ cup	240	1.9
Grapefruit	½ cup	40	1.6
Grapes	10	35	0.5
Orange	1 medium	60	2.2
Peach	1 medium	35	1.9
Pineapple	½ cup	40	0.5
Prunes, dried	½ cup	190	3.0
Raisins	¼ cup	110	2.1
Strawberries	1 cup	45	3.0

*Most values taken from ref no. 16.

Table 3-7 A 25-gram fiber diet for 1500 kcalories

	Carbohydrate Protein Fat		61% of kcalories 19% of kcalories 20% of kcalories
Menu	**Fiber**	**Exchanges**	**Carbohydrate content based on the exchange system**
Breakfast			
1 cup orange juice	—	2 fruit	30
¾ cup Wheaties	3.0	1 starch/bread	15
½ cup 1% milk	—	½ low-fat milk	6
1 slice whole-wheat toast	1.9	1 starch/bread	15
1 t margarine	—	1 fat	0
coffee	—	free	0
Lunch			
2 oz lean ham	—	2 lean meat	0
2 slices whole-wheat bread	3.8	2 starch/bread	30
⅓ cup cooked white beans	3.5	1 starch/bread	15
2 t mayonnaise	—	2 fat	0
¼ cup lettuce	.2	free	0
1 pear (with skin)	4.3	1 fruit	15
Dinner			
3 oz broiled chicken (no skin)	—	3 lean meat	0
1 baked potato (large)	3.6	2 starch/bread	30
1-½ t margarine	—	1-½ fat	0
1 cup green beans	2.0	2 vegetable	10
½ t margarine	—	½ fat	0
1 cup 1% milk	—	1 low-fat milk	12
1 apple (with peel)	3.0	1 fruit	15
TOTAL:	25 grams	TOTAL:	172

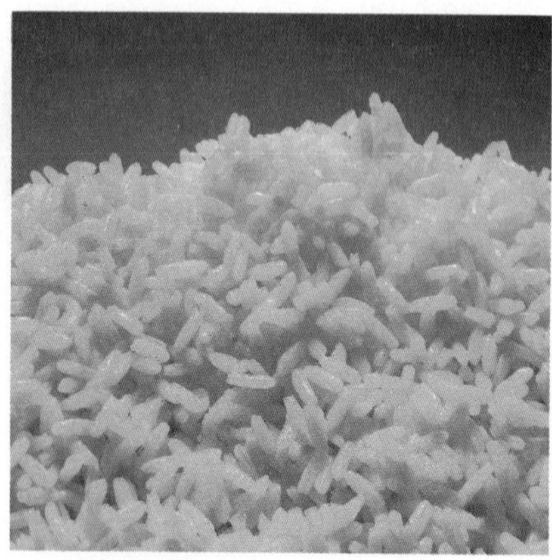

The carbohydrates in rice supply much of the fuel in the Asian diet.

For foods in general, the greatest nutrient densities for carbohydrates (greatest percentage of kcalories from carbohydrates) are found in sugar, honey, jams, jellies, fruit, and plain baked potatoes. They contain essentially all food energy as carbohydrate (Figure 3-11). Corn flakes, rice, bread, and noodles all contain at least 75% of kcalories as carbohydrates. Foods with moderate amounts of carbohydrate energy are peas, broccoli, oatmeal, dry beans and other legumes, cream pies, French fries, and skim milk. In these foods the carbohydrate content is diluted either by protein, as in the case of skim milk, or by fat, as in the case of a cream pie.

Chocolate, potato chips, and whole milk contain 30% to 40% of kcalories as carbohydrates. Again, the energy supplied from carbohydrate content of these foods is overwhelmed by either their fat or protein content. Foods with essentially no carbohydrates include beef, chicken, fish, vegetable oils, butter, and margarine.

Recall that the recommendation for a high-carbohydrate diet primarily means one high in energy from complex carbohydrates. Figure 3-11 shows that the emphasis for a high-carbohydrate diet needs to be on potatoes, grains, pasta, and vegetables. A person cannot form a diet high in carbohydrate energy from chocolate, potato chips, and French fries because these foods contain too much fat. The per-

Table 3-8 Increasing dietary fiber intake is not that hard to do

Try this:	Instead of this:
Whole-wheat bread	White bread
Brown rice	White rice
Baked potato in the skin	Mashed potatoes
Unpeeled apple (or applesauce made with unpeeled apples)	Regular applesauce
Orange segments	Orange juice
Whole-grain cereals (hot or ready-to-eat)	Sweetened cereals
Popcorn (lightly seasoned with margarine or salt, if at all)	Potato chips
Bean dip	Sour cream dip
Kidney beans or garbonzo beans on salad	Bacon bits on salad
Fruit juice	Coffee or tea
Salad bar	French fries

centage of kcalories from carbohydrate is more important than the total grams of carbohydrate in a food choice.

Sweeteners in Foods

Do you want the kcalories along with the sweetness? The choice is yours.

NUTRITIVE SWEETENERS

All of the monosaccharides (glucose, fructose, and galactose) and disaccharides (sucrose, lactose, and maltose) that we discussed earlier are nutritive sweeteners. In other words, they contain nutritive value in the form of energy. The taste and sweetness of sucrose makes it the tried-and-true sweetener. Sucrose comes from sugar cane and sugar beets. It is the benchmark against which all other sweeteners are measured. A relatively new sweetener in food is high-fructose corn syrup, which contains 40% to 90% fructose. To make this, cornstarch is first treated with acid and enzymes. Much of the starch is broken down into glucose, then some to almost all of the glucose is changed by enzymes into fructose. The syrup is usually as sweet as sugar. Its major advantage is that it is cheaper than sugar. Also, it doesn't form crystals and it has better freezing properties. High-fructose corn syrups are used in soft drinks, candies, jams, jellies, other fruit products, and desserts.[4]

In addition to sucrose and high-fructose corn syrup, brown sugar, turbinado sugar, honey, maple syrup, and other sugars are also added to foods (refer to Table 3-2). No raw (unrefined) sugar can be sold in the United States because the U.S. Food and Drug Administration (FDA) considers raw sugar unfit for human consumption. Turbinado sugar, a partially refined version of raw sugar, can be sold and has a slight molasses flavor. Brown sugar is basically white sugar containing some molasses; either the molasses is not totally removed from the sugar during processing or it is added back to the sucrose crystals.

Maple syrup is made by boiling down and concentrating the sap that runs in the spring and autumn from sugar maple trees. Most pancake syrup sold in supermarkets is not maple syrup. Pure maple syrup is available in specialty food shops and from catalogs.

Honey is a product of plant nectar that has been altered by bee enzymes. The enzymes break down much of the nectar's sucrose into fructose and glucose. As we noted earlier, honey basically offers the same nutritional value as other simple sugar sources—a source of energy and little else. However, honey is not safe to use with infants because it can contain spores of the bacterium *Clostridium botulinum*.[4] These

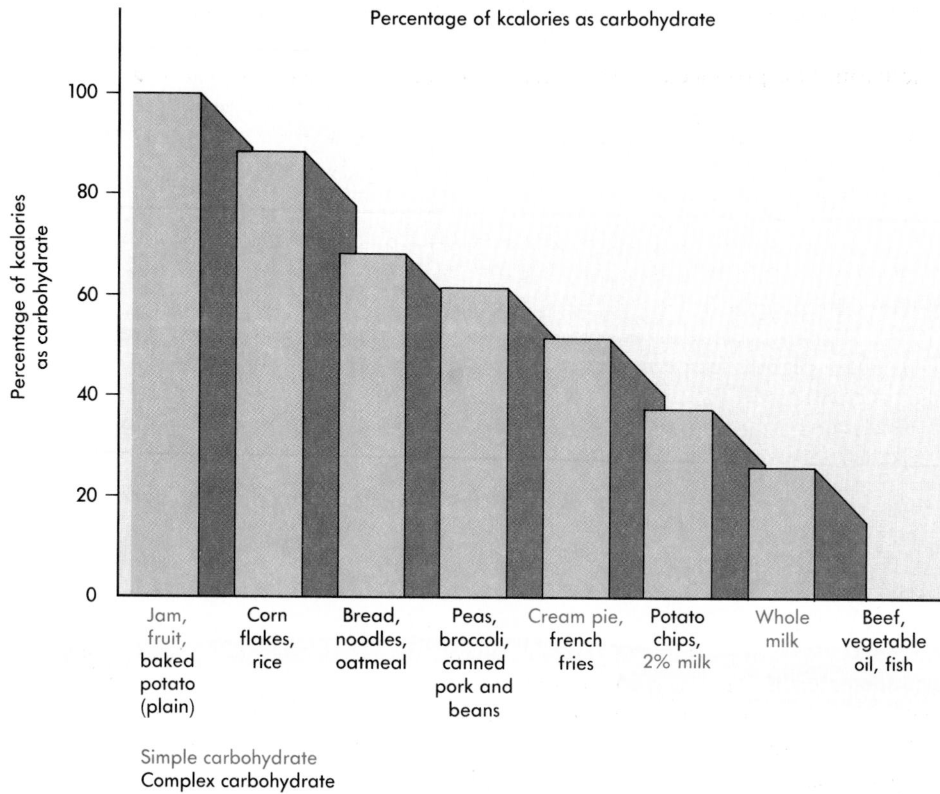

Figure 3-11 Percent of kcalories as carbohydrates in foods. Jams, fruits, rice, and many breakfast cereals provide almost all kcalories as carbohydrates.

spores can become the bacteria that cause fatal food-borne illness. Honey does not pose a problem for adults because the acidic environment of an adult's stomach inhibits the growth of the bacteria. An infant's stomach, however, does not have a very acidic environment, making infants susceptible to the risks that this bacterium poses.

SUGAR ALCOHOLS

Also in the category of nutritive sweeteners are the sugar alcohols: sorbitol, mannitol, and **xylitol.**[4] They are absorbed or metabolized to glucose more slowly than other sugars. Because they do contribute energy and may effect blood glucose levels, they are of little or no advantage in planning diabetic diets. This is a source of confusion to many people with diabetes, because products containing these sugar alcohols are marketed to them.

Sorbitol is used in sugarless gum, breath mints, and candy. It yields kcalories but is not readily metabolized by the bacteria in the mouth. Thus sorbitol does not promote dental caries nearly so readily as other simple sugars, like sucrose. Another sugar alcohol, xylitol, is no longer used widely in the United States, partly because of past safety concerns, although its use is still legal in the United States. It is used widely in Canada and Scandinavia. Any of these sugar alcohols consumed in excess have a tendency to remain in the intestine unabsorbed, and so can cause diarrhea.[11] Refer to Table 3-4 for the relative sweetness of both nutritive and non-nutritive sweeteners.

aspartame An alternate sweetener made of two amino acids and methanol; it is 200 times sweeter than sucrose.

acesulfame An alternate sweetener that yields no energy to the body; it is 200 times sweeter than sucrose.

ALTERNATE SWEETENERS

Often called artificial sweeteners, alternate sweeteners are **saccharin,** cyclamate, **aspartame,** and **acesulfame.** These yield little or no energy at amounts typically used in food products. Only three are available in the United States today—saccharin, aspartame, and acesulfame (see Appendix J for their structures). Cyclamate was banned for use in the United States in 1970, although it was never conclusively proven to cause cancer in human beings. Cyclamate is used in Canada as a sweetener in medicine and as a table-top sweetener.

Saccharin, first produced in 1879, has been recently linked with cancer. Laboratory animals suffer from bladder cancer when given high doses of saccharin, especially animals in the second generation after exposure. Arguments continue concerning the amount of cancer actually resulting from saccharin use. We will discuss this issue further in Chapter 19.

In 1977 FDA attempted to ban saccharin because of this link to cancer. Many users protested because it left them with no low-kcalorie sweetener. The others mentioned above were either not yet available or, as in the case of cyclamate, had also been banned. Although knowing of the association between saccharin and cancer, some people still wanted to use saccharin. Due to this public pressure, Congress prevented FDA from banning saccharin. Until the current moratorium set by Congress expires, FDA cannot act with regards to the future of saccharin.

Some officials at FDA now believe, after considering new research, that the ban on cyclamates in the U.S. may be unwarranted. Thus Americans could see it back on grocery store shelves soon.

Aspartame

In 1981 a new alternate sweetener, aspartame, became available. Its trade name is NutraSweet when added to foods and Equal when sold as powder. Aspartame is composed of the amino acids phenylalanine and aspartic acid, with the addition of methanol. Recall that amino acids are the building blocks of proteins. Thus aspartame belongs more in the protein class than in the carbohydrate class. Aspartame yields energy—4 kcalories per gram—but is 180 to 200 times sweeter than sucrose. Such a small amount is needed to obtain the desired sweetening potency that the energy added is considered to be insignificant unless abused. Today aspartame is used in beverages, gelatin desserts, chewing gum, and other food items that are not heated. Aspartame, like other proteins, is damaged when heated.

CALCIUM AND IRON.
CONTAINS: CARBONATED WATER, ORANGE JUICE, CITRIC ACID, NUTRASWEET* BRAND OF ASPARTAME**, POTASSIUM BENZOATE (A PRESERVATIVE), CITRUS PECTIN, POTASSIUM CITRATE, CAFFEINE, MALTODEXTRIN, GUM ARABIC, NATURAL FLAVORS, BROMINATED VEGETABLE OIL, YELLOW #5 AND ERYTHORBIC ACID (TO PROTECT FLAVOR).
*NUTRASWEET® AND THE NUTRASWEET SYMBOL ARE REGISTERED TRADEMARKS OF THE NUTRASWEET COMPANY.
PHENYLKETONURICS: CONTAINS PHENYLALANINE.

Note the warning for people with PKU to not consume aspartame.

Aspartame never has been linked with cancer, but some complaints have been filed with FDA by individuals claiming adverse reactions to aspartame. These individuals complain of headaches, dizziness, seizures, nausea, allergic reactions, and other side effects.

It is important for people who are sensitive to aspartame to avoid it. But the percentage of sensitive people is likely to be extremely small. Considering its wide use in food products, the relatively small number of complaints made against aspartame means that most people can use it. In addition, careful double-blind research casts doubt on whether it causes headaches,[22] and suggests it does not stimulate subsequent food intake either.[8,20,21]

Aspartame's phenylalanine content has concerned some people. The blood levels of this amino acid may increase too much if aspartame is not consumed with the other amino acids normally found in protein foods. This problem can be easily avoided by consuming aspartame with protein foods. Some people also are concerned about aspartame's methanol content. However, the amount of methanol in a soft drink sweetened with aspartame is not more than is found in a cup of fruit or vegetable juice.

Overall, the scientific community does not agree that aspartame itself is harmful. In fact numerous scientific and medical groups support its use. The acceptable daily intake set by FDA is 50 milligrams per kilogram of body weight per day. This is equivalent to about 14 cans of diet soft drinks a day for an adult. Aspartame appears to be safe for pregnant women[15] and children, but some scientists suggest cautious use by these groups. As more and more foods incorporate aspartame, there is a possibility that more adverse reactions may occur. For now its use is quite limited, and therefore so is our consumption of it.

One final note about aspartame. A rare disease called **phenylketonuria (PKU)** limits a person's ability for metabolizing phenylalanine. (We discuss PKU further in Chapter 5.) Labels on products containing aspartame warn people with PKU to not use the product.

phenylketonuria (PKU) A disease in which the liver has a limited ability to metabolize the amino acid phenylalanine into the amino acid tyrosine.

Acesulfame

The newest alternate sweetener in the United States, acesulfame (Sunette), was approved by the FDA in July 1988. Acesulfame is 200 times sweeter than sucrose. For the present it can be used in chewing gum, powdered drink mixes, gelatins, puddings, and nondairy creamers. It contributes no kcalories to the diet because it is not broken down by the body.[11]

Some studies show that laboratory animals develop cancer after exposure to acesulfame. However, FDA analysis of these studies suggests that the tumors were not due to acesulfame consumption because they could be routinely expected in the animal species studied. Therefore acesulfame has FDA approval. It is already used as a sweetener in foods and beverages in at least 20 countries. Acesulfame can be used in baking, whereas aspartame cannot because current forms break down when heated. So acesulfame may soon see wider uses. Some nutrition professionals think the approval of acesulfame occurred very rapidly in comparison to other non-nutritive sweeteners, and so still view use of this substance with caution. Acesulfame is currently used in many European countries.

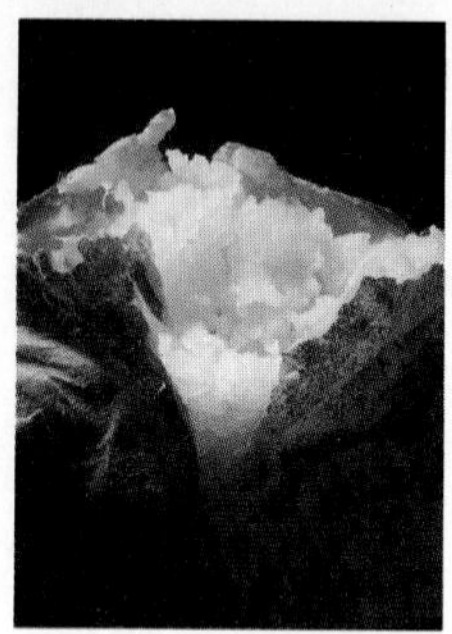

Summary

1. The monosaccharides in our diet include glucose, fructose, and galactose. Once these are absorbed via the small intestine and enter the liver, much of the fructose and galactose is turned into glucose.
2. The major disaccharides are sucrose (glucose plus fructose), maltose (glucose plus glucose), and lactose (glucose plus galactose). When digested, these yield the monosaccharide forms. The ability to digest lactose often diminishes with age. Some ethnic groups show a lower amount of lactose digestion from birth.
3. One major group of polysaccharides contains multiple glucose units linked together with alpha bonds. These bonds allow for the digestion of the straight-chained amylose and the branched-chained amylopectin starches, primarily in the small intestine. Glycogen is the storage form of carbohydrate in animals and is stored in the liver and muscle. Muscle glycogen is a ready source of energy for the muscle but is not released to the bloodstream; glucose from liver glycogen can enter the bloodstream.
4. Carbohydrates provide energy, protect against wasteful breakdown of body protein to supply a constant source of glucose for brain and other tissues, prevent ketosis, and provide flavor and sweetness to foods.
5. Dietary fibers include the carbohydrates cellulose, hemicelluloses, pectins, gums, and mucilages, as well as the noncarbohydrate lignins. Dietary fiber provides mass to the stool, thus easing elimination. In high doses certain forms can help control blood glucose levels in diabetic people and lower high blood cholesterol levels.
6. There is no RDA for carbohydrates. An intake of at least 50 to 100 grams should be consumed to prevent ketosis. If carbohydrate consumption is inadequate, the body can make what it needs to support energy production. However, the price is loss of body protein and ketosis. This in turn can lead to a general weakening of the body if a low-carbohydrate diet is continued for weeks at a time.
7. Diets high in complex carbohydrates are encouraged as a replacement for high-fat diets. A goal of at least 45% of kcalories as complex carbohydrates is a good one, with about 55% of total kcalories coming from carbohydrates in general. Foods to emphasize are potatoes, whole grains, pastas, legumes, fruits, and vegetables.

Study Questions

1. What are the three major disaccharides? Describe how each plays a part in the human diet.

2. How do amylose, amylopectin, and glycogen differ from each other? Why is this important in a metabolic sense and in food preparation?

3. What are the important roles that dietary fiber plays in the diet?

4. What, if any, are the ill effects of sugars in the diet?

5. After reading the Nutrition Perspective, comment on how insulin-dependent diabetes differs from noninsulin-dependent diabetes in cause and treatment?

REFERENCES

1. Alcorn JM: Colorectal cancer prevention: a primary care approach, *Geriatrics* 47(2):24, 1992.
2. Anderson JW and others: Metabolic effects of high-carbohydrate, high-fiber diets on insulin-dependent diabetic individuals, *American Journal of Clinical Nutrition* 54:936, 1991.
3. Anderson JW and others: Lipid responses of hypercholesterolemic men to oat-bran and wheat bran intakes, *American Journal of Clinical Nutrition* 54:678, 1991.
4. American Dietetic Association Reports: Position of The American Dietetic Association: appropriate use of nutritive and non-nutritive sweeteners, *Journal of The American Dietetic Association* 87:1689, 1987.
5. Beebe CA and others: Nutrition management for individuals with noninsulin-dependent diabetes mellitus in the late 1990s, *Journal of The American Dietetic Association* 91:196, 1991.
6. Brand JC, Holt S: Relative effectiveness of milks with reduced amounts of lactose in alleviating lactose intolerance, *American Journal of Clinical Nutrition* 54:148, 1991.
7. Burkitt DP: Dietary fiber and cancer, *Journal of Nutrition* 118:531, 1988.
8. Canty DJ, Chan MM: Effects of consumption of caloric vs noncaloric sweet drinks on indices of hunger and food consumption in normal adults, *American Journal of Clinical Nutrition* 53:1159, 1991.
9. Cooper SG and others: Small-bowel obstruction caused by oat-bran bezoar, *New England Journal of Medicine* 320:1148, 1989.
10. Cronin FJ and Shaw AM: Summary of dietary recommendations for healthy Americans, *Nutrition Today*, Nov/Dec 1988.
11. Greeley A: Not only sugar is sweet, *FDA Consumer*, April 1991, p 17.
12. Grundy SM: Diet therapy for diabetes mellitus, *Diabetes Care* 14:796, 1991.
13. Guthrie RA: New approaches to improve diabetes control, *American Family Physician* 43(2):570, 1991.
14. Henry RR and others: Current issues in fructose metabolism, *Annual Review of Nutrition* 11:21, 1991.
15. London RS: Saccharin and aspartame: are they safe to consume during pregnancy, *Journal of Reproductive Medicine* 33:17, 1988.
16. Marlett JA: Content and composition of dietary fiber in 117 frequently consumed foods, *Journal of The American Dietetic Association* 92:175, 1992.
17. Martini MC and others: Lactose digestion from yogurt: influence of a meal and additional lactose, *American Journal of Clinical Nutrition* 53:1253, 1991.
18. Mayes PA: Regulation of carbohydrate metabolism. In Murray RK and others, editors: *Harper's biochemistry*, East Norwalk, Conn, 1988, Appleton & Lange.
19. Nelson RL: Hypoglycemia: fact or fiction, *Mayo Clinic Proceedings* 60:844, 1985.
20. Rodin J: Comparative effects of fructose, aspartame, glucose, and water preloads on calorie and macronutrient intake, *American Journal of Clinical Nutrition* 51:428, 1990.
21. Rolls BJ: Effects of intense sweeteners on hunger, food intake, and body weight: a review, *American Journal of Clinical Nutrition* 53:872, 1991.
22. Schiffman SS and others: Aspartame and susceptibility to headache, *New England Journal of Medicine* 317:1181, 1987.
23. Slavin JL: Dietary fiber: mechanism or magic on disease prevention, *Nutrition Today*, Nov/Dec 1990, p 6.
24. Topping DL: Soluble fiber polysaccharides: effects on plasma cholesterol and colonic fermentation, *Nutrition Reviews* 49:195, 1991.
25. Yost DA: Clinical safety of aspartame, *American Family Physician* 39(Nov):201, 1989.

SUGGESTED READINGS

To learn more about aspartame read the article by Yost, which provides a summary of the major research surrounding this popular alternate sweetener. For more information about dietary fiber, study the article by Slavin. Although quite detailed, it is in a very readable and understandable format. We recommend that you read the journal it is published in, *Nutrition Today*, regularly if you want to learn more about nutrition. Cronin and Shaw chronicle the various recommendations for carbohydrate intake given by scientific bodies of the last 20 years. This review points out the consistency of our promotion of complex carbohydrates in the diet, especially as a replacement for fats.

TAKE ACTION

How does your diet rate for carbohydrate and dietary fiber?

Let's reevaluate the nutritional assessment you completed at the end of Chapter 2. Here are your tasks:

1. Look at your analysis and find the total number of grams of carbohydrate you ate.
   TOTAL GRAMS OF CARBOHYDRATE ____________
   A. Did you consume more than the minimum amount to avoid ketosis, 50 to 100 grams?
   B. Now calculate the percentage of kcalories in your diet from carbohydrate. You will need the total grams of carbohydrate from your assessment as well as the total kcalories you ate. Use this formula to calculate it:
   TOTAL GRAMS OF CARBOHYDRATE × 4
   ____________ × 100 = % OF KCALS FROM CARBOHYDRATE TOTAL KCALORIES

   Did you eat 55% of kcalories from carbohydrate or greater as suggested?
   If you did not, what could you do to increase your carbohydrate intake?

   ____

   ____

   ____

2. Look again at the list of foods you ate, including the amounts. Refer to the software printout for your dietary fiber intake. Or using the food composition table in Appendix A, look up the dietary fiber content of each food you ate, taking the amount of that food you ate into account. Total the amount of dietary fiber you ate for that day and record it in the blank provided below.
   TOTAL AMOUNT OF DIETARY FIBER CONSUMED ____________ grams.
   A. Did you eat the 20 to 35 grams suggested in this chapter?
   B. If not, what could you do to increase your dietary fiber intake? What foods could you substitute for some of the foods you ate?

   ____

   ____

   ____

3. Finally, use Table 3-5 to see if you can reduce your intake of sugars, especially if you find you need to watch your total kcalorie intake to maintain an appropriate weight. ▲

NUTRITION PERSPECTIVE

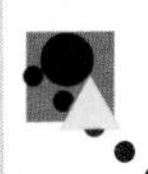

When Blood Glucose Regulation Fails

Two problems arise with blood glucose regulation; the major one is blood glucose that is too high, a disease called diabetes mellitus. About ten million Americans have this disease. The other problem, much rarer, is low blood glucose or hypoglycemia.

Diabetes Mellitus

There are two forms of diabetes—insulin dependent (also called Type I or juvenile-onset diabetes) and **noninsulin dependent** (also called Type II or adult onset). The insulin-dependent form often begins in late childhood, around the age of 8 to 12 years, but can strike at any age. A genetic link is clear—the disease runs in certain families. The hallmarks of the disease are high blood glucose levels after eating and the tendency to develop ketosis.[13] An exciting new finding on the cause of this form of diabetes may help treat and even prevent its occurrence in the future. An immunological disorder causes the destruction of beta cells of the pancreas. Most likely a virus or protein foreign to the body sets off the destruction. In turn, the attacked beta cells release proteins that stimulate a more furious attack. The pancreas then gradually loses its ability to make insulin. For this reason early treatment to stop the immune-linked destruction may be an important therapy. Research on this is ongoing.

As insulin levels decline, blood glucose rises, especially after eating. Excess glucose spills over into the urine. Hence the term diabetes mellitus, which means flow of much urine (diabetes) that is sweet (mellitus). Figure 3-12 shows a typical glucose tolerance curve seen in diabetes after a person eats 50 grams (10 teaspoons) of glucose.

Diabetes is treated by having the person eat three regular meals and one or more snacks (including one at bedtime) of a precise carbohydrate:protein:fat ratio to maximize insulin action and minimize swings in blood sugar levels.[5] A diet high in complex carbohydrates is emphasized, along with ample dietary fiber. Replacing the missing insulin, either with injections one to six times a day or with an insulin pump is also important. The pump dispenses insulin on a regular basis into the body and higher amounts after each meal. Regular meals are especially important for people with diabetes who use insulin because insulin requires a continuing source of glucose in the bloodstream on which to act. This adds much regulation and possible inconvenience to a person's life. Note also a person with diabetes must work with a physician to make the correct alterations in diet and medications to perform exercise safely. This is because physical activity can enhance glucose uptake by muscles, in turn inducing lower blood sugar. This outcome of exercise is beneficial, but people with diabetes need to be aware of their blood glucose response to exercise and compensate appropriately.

If the person with diabetes does not eat, the injected insulin can cause severe hypoglycemia as it acts on whatever little glucose is available. Not taking enough insulin to cover needs also poses problems. The resulting hormone imbalance in the body causes fat to flood into the liver cells. Ketosis is the end result as the fat is converted mostly into ketones. The ketone level can then rise excessively in the bloodstream, eventually spilling ketones into the urine. These pull sodium and potassium ions with them. This series of events can contribute to a chain reaction that can eventually lead to dehydration, ion imbalance, coma, and even death in people with poorly controlled insulin-dependent diabetes.

The noninsulin-dependent form of diabetes usually begins in adulthood. Ketosis is not usually seen in this group.[13] This is the most common type of diabetes,

NUTRITION PERSPECTIVE

When Blood Glucose Regulation Fails—cont'd

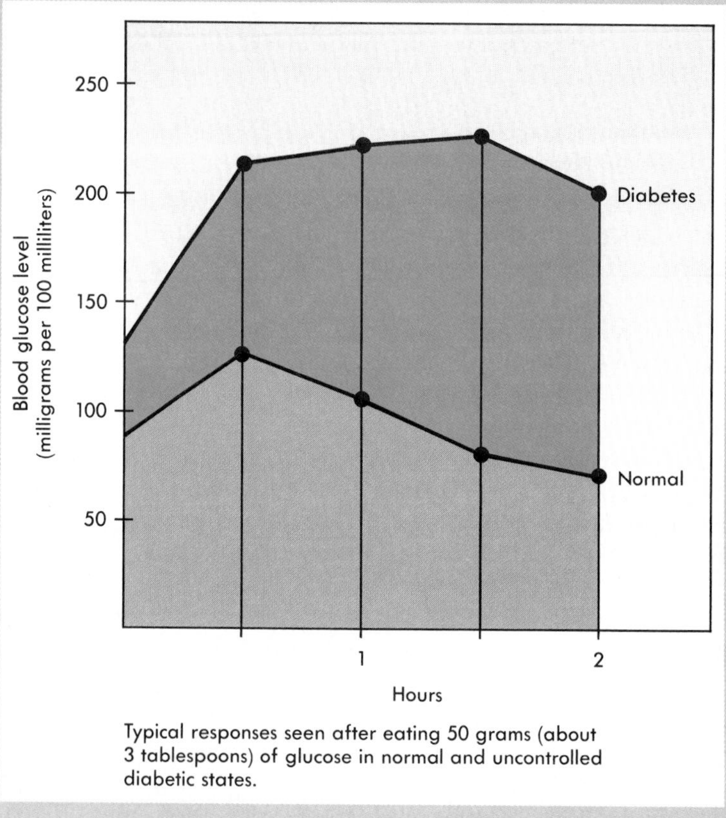

Figure 3-12 Glucose tolerance test. These are typical responses seen after eating 50 grams (10 teaspoons) of glucose in a healthy person and in a person with uncontrolled diabetes mellitus. Blood glucose levels are determined at fasting and then at regular intervals after the person consumes the glucose load.

accounting for about 80% of the cases seen in the United States. The number of people affected is on the rise, linked to widespread inactivity and obesity in our population. This type of diabetes is also genetically linked, but the problem is not only with the beta cells of the pancreas, but also with the insulin receptor on the cell surface of peripheral tissues, especially muscles. Instead of insufficient insulin, there is an abundance of insulin in early stages of the disease, but poor use of it. As the disease develops, pancreas function can later fail, leading to poor insulin output.

Many of the cases of the noninsulin-dependent form of diabetes are associated with obesity, but the hyperglycemia is not necessarily caused by obesity. In fact there is a growing population of lean people with this type of diabetes. Obesity, with its large fat cells, simply increases the risk for a state of insulin resistance in the body. In this case blood glucose is not readily transferred into cells, and so the person develops hyperglycemia as glucose remains in the bloodstream. The pancreas tries to increase insulin output to compensate, but there is a limit to its ability to do this.

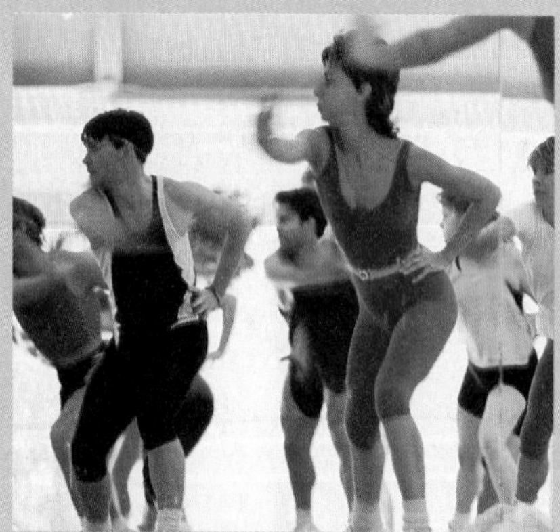

Regular exercise is an important part of the therapy for people who have diabetes.

The noninsulin-dependent form of diabetes often disappears if the obesity is corrected, so achieving a desirable weight should be a primary goal of treatment.[5] Oral medications, which increase the ability of the pancreas to produce insulin, are often prescribed. Sometimes even insulin injections are used. Regular exercise also helps because the muscles will take up more glucose. And regular meal patterns, again with an emphasis on complex carbohydrate and ample dietary fiber, help.

NUTRITION PERSPECTIVE

Eating carbohydrates throughout the day's diet is also important, as this helps minimize the high and low swings in blood glucose levels.[5] If this diet therapy is not sufficiently effective, the diet can be switched to one high in monounsaturated fats with smaller amounts of carbohydrates.[12] The approach to diet is up to the person and his or her medical advisors.

There is one more diet tool a person with diabetes can use. Research concerning the body's response to various carbohydrates has led to the development of a clinical tool known as the glycemic index. This index compares the total amount of glucose appearing in the bloodstream after eating a food with the total amount of glucose appearing in the bloodstream after eating the same amount of carbohydrate in the form of white bread or glucose.

The glycemic index for common foods

100	**white bread**
90	**whole-wheat bread, shredded wheat cereal, raisins**
80	**rice, oatmeal, potatoes**
70	**bananas, All-Bran cereal**
60	**orange, baked beans, spaghetti**
50	**yogurt, apple**
40	**skim milk, peach**

Several factors must be considered when predicting the glycemic index of a food, including the food's amount of dietary fiber, the food's digestion rate, and its total fat content. Some foods, such as oatmeal, contain much soluble fiber. Soluble fibers yield a slow increase in blood glucose after eating.[2] In contrast, foods such as potatoes are quickly digested, in turn producing a rapid increase in blood glucose after eating. If a diabetic person eats many foods having low glycemic indexes, then each meal in the entire diet will encourage normal glucose levels.

Although many cases of the noninsulin-dependent form of diabetes can be relieved by losing excess fat stores, many people are not able to lose weight. They remain affected with diabetes and suffer the complications that are seen in both forms of this disease—blindness, loss of fingers and toes, kidney failure, and heart disease. These problems are linked to microscopic changes in the small blood vessels, called capillaries. There is also nerve deterioration, resulting in many changes where proper nerve stimulation is lacking. Examples include the GI tract where intermittent diarrhea and constipation occur, and the extremities as people with diabetes lose feeling of the pain of injuries or infections. The combination of delay in treatment and a rich environment for bacterial growth (bacteria love the high glucose content) set the stage for problems.

High blood glucose levels also contribute to a rapid progression of fatty buildup in blood vessels, which eventually chokes off the blood supply to nearby organs. See Chapter 4 for details on this latter process called **atherosclerosis.** Many specialists in diabetes now believe that the blood vessel and nerve complications of the disease can be prevented with aggressive treatment directed at keeping blood glucose levels within the normal range.

atherosclerosis A buildup of mostly fatty material (plaque) in the arteries, including those surrounding the heart.

Hypoglycemia

The second carbohydrate disorder is hypoglycemia. This problem comes in two forms—reactive and fasting.[19] **Reactive hypoglycemia** is characterized by irritability, nervousness, headache, sweating, and confusion 2 or 4 hours after eating a meal, especially one high in simple sugars. It is not clear what causes reactive hypoglycemia. It may be due to an over production of insulin by the pancreas in response to rising blood glucose levels.

The second type, **fasting hypoglycemia,** is usually caused by cancer in the pancreas, which may lead to excessive insulin secretion. Blood glucose levels fall to low levels after fasting for about 8 hours to 1 day. This form of hypoglycemia is rare.

reactive hypoglycemia Low blood sugar that follows a meal high in simple sugars, with corresponding symptoms of irritability, headache, nervousness, sweating, and confusion.

fasting hypoglycemia Low blood sugar that follows about a day of fasting.

To diagnose hypoglycemia a physician needs to observe the usual symptoms and a low blood glucose level at the same time. This level of blood glucose is about 40 to 50 milligrams per 100 milliliters of blood. Some of us have bouts of hypoglycemia

NUTRITION PERSPECTIVE

When Blood Glucose Regulation Fails—cont'd

and never know it. Just having a low blood glucose level after eating, however, is not enough evidence to make the diagnosis of hypoglycemia. Both a low blood glucose level and the typical symptoms must appear together to make up the whole pattern.

Many people think they have hypoglycemia but few actually do. Hypoglycemia has been popularized by the popular press and television talk shows and related to symptoms that most all people experience occasionally. There is no clear evidence that the catalog of difficulties attributed to hypoglycemia—depression, chronic fatigue, allergies, nervous breakdowns, alcoholism, juvenile delinquency, childhood behavior problems, drug addiction, or inadequate sexual performance—are actually linked to the disorder. Nevertheless, if you sometimes feel you do develop hypoglycemia, the nutrition therapy is one we all could follow. You need to eat regular meals, make sure you have some protein and fat in each meal, and eat complex carbohydrates with ample soluble fiber. Avoid meals or snacks that contain little more than simple carbohydrates. If symptoms continue, try small, protein-containing snacks between meals. Fat, protein, and soluble fiber in the diet tend to moderate swings in blood glucose.

CHAPTER FOUR

Lipids

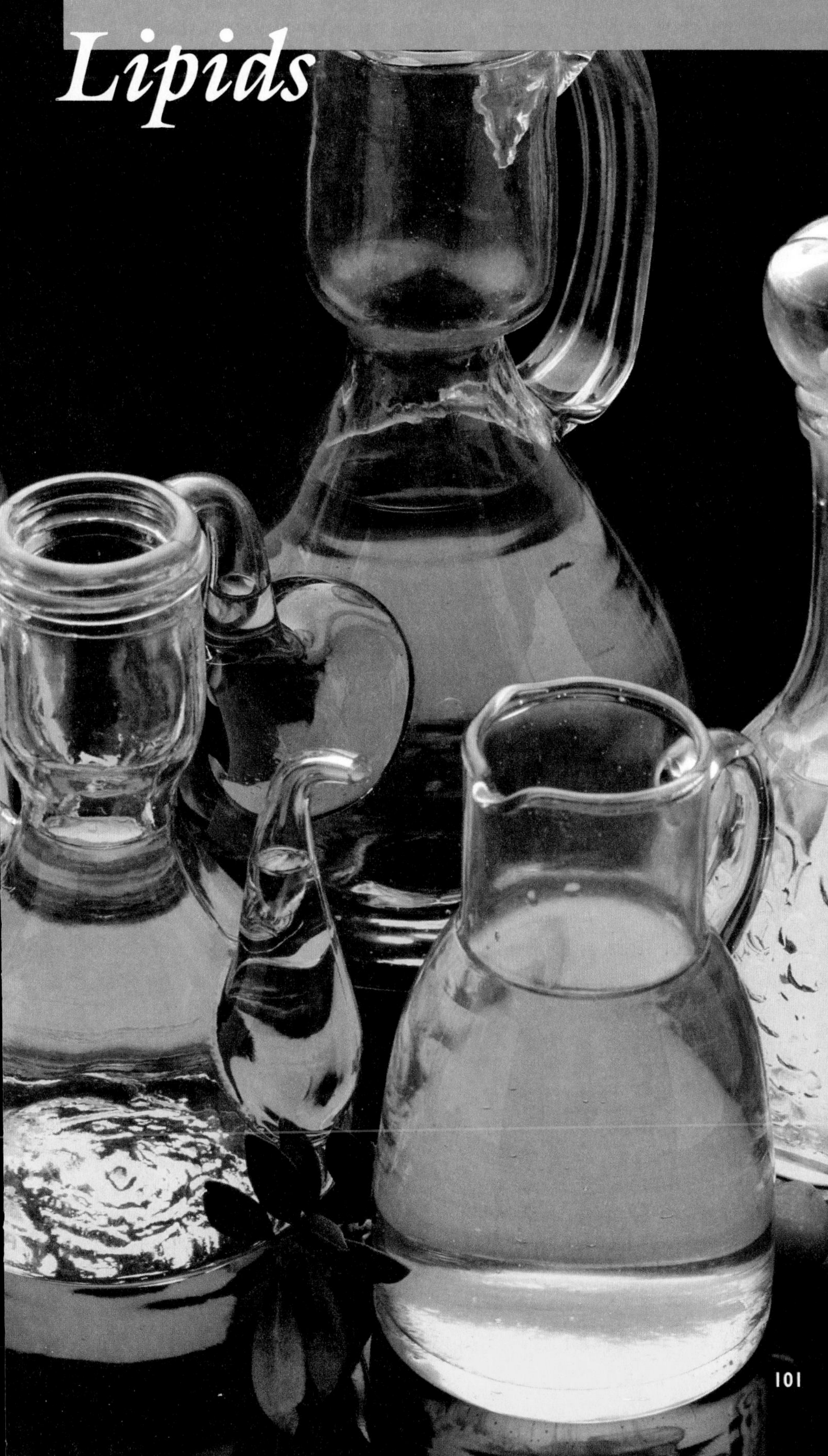

Your doctor informs you that your "triglycerides are up." Your bill from a medical laboratory reads, "Blood lipid profile—$35." A health-food store advertisement suggests using omega-3 fatty acids from fish oils to lower your blood cholesterol level. Advertisers plug "lowest in saturated fat." We often hear these terms: triglycerides, blood lipids, omega-3 fatty acids, and cholesterol. What do they mean?

Lipids, a word that encompasses the fats and oils we just mentioned, also are the nutrients that probably concern us most. Lipids contain more than twice the kcalories per gram (9 instead of just 4) compared with proteins and carbohydrates. Certain types of dietary saturated fats are closely linked to high serum cholesterol levels and consequently to the risk of rapidly developing heart disease. Some concern about lipids is warranted, but lipids also play several very important roles in the body and in foods. Their presence in the diet is vital to health. Let's look at the lipids in detail as we just did for carbohydrates—their forms, functions, metabolism, and food sources. We then will finish with a look at their link to the major "killer" disease in the United States, heart disease.

NUTRITION AWARENESS INVENTORY

Here are 15 statements about lipids. Answer them to test your current knowledge. If you think a statement is true or mostly true, circle T. If you think the statement is false or mostly false, circle F. Use the scoring key at the end of the book to compute your total score. Take this test again after you have read the chapter. Compare the results.

1. T F Lipids composed of polyunsaturated fatty acids are liquid at room temperature.
2. T F A lipid has more kcalories per gram than carbohydrate or protein.
3. T F One's total serum cholesterol level is the most important blood test in assessing risk for heart attack and stroke.
4. T F Cholesterol is found only in the purely animal-derived foods we eat.
5. T F Animal fat is the major dietary factor that raises serum cholesterol levels.
6. T F Triglycerides are the main form of fat found in foods.
7. T F Fat is not absolutely necessary in our diet.
8. T F Hydrogenation makes vegetable oils more solid at room temperature.
9. T F Fruits and vegetables are essentially fat free.
10. T F Antioxidants provide protection from foods turning rancid.
11. T F The small intestine absorbs some vitamins better when dietary fat is present.
12. T F A blood cholesterol test is not necessary if you are age 40 years or less.
13. T F Butter and margarine contain about the same amount of fat.
14. T F Some of the fat present in fish is especially healthy.
15. T F Nondairy creamers are healthier for you than low-fat milk.

Structures and Forms of Lipids

You probably know lipids as fats and oils. At room temperature, fats are solid and oils are liquid. Referring to them both as lipids simplifies the terminology and makes considering a food's temperature irrelevant. Otherwise, butter can be an oil on a hot day and a fat on a cold day.

Lipids are a diverse group, but they share two main characteristics: (1) they all dissolve in chloroform, benzene, and ether, and (2) they are not soluble in water. Think of an oil and vinegar salad dressing; the oil is not soluble in the water-based vinegar. Lipids also contain fewer oxygen atoms per carbon atom than do carbohydrates, protein, or alcohol. There are few other characteristics that are common to all lipids. For example, compare the structures of lecithin and cholesterol as these are discussed in the following pages.

When we discuss lipid chemistry or metabolism, we will use the term lipid or the actual name of the compound, such as serum **triglycerides.** When we discuss lipids in foods, we will use the terms fats, or fats and oils. This usage is common today in health care settings.

FATTY ACIDS

The **fatty acid** is common to most of the lipids in the body and in foods. Its basic structure is a long chain of carbons bonded to hydrogen atoms. At one end of the molecule, called the alpha end, is an acid (specifically carboxyl) group ($-\overset{\overset{\displaystyle O}{\|}}{C}-OH$). At the other end is a methyl group ($-CH_3$) (Figure 4-1). This is called the omega end. In the Greek alphabet, alpha means beginning and omega means end.

saturated fatty acid A fatty acid with no carbon-carbon double bonds.

monounsaturated fatty A fatty acid containing one carbon-carbon double bond.

If all bonds between the carbons are single bonds, a fatty acid is called **saturated.** In other words all the carbons are saturated with hydrogens, like a sponge saturated with water. Animal fats are often high in saturated fatty acids. If a fatty acid has one carbon-carbon double bond, it is **monounsaturated.** Olive and canola oils have

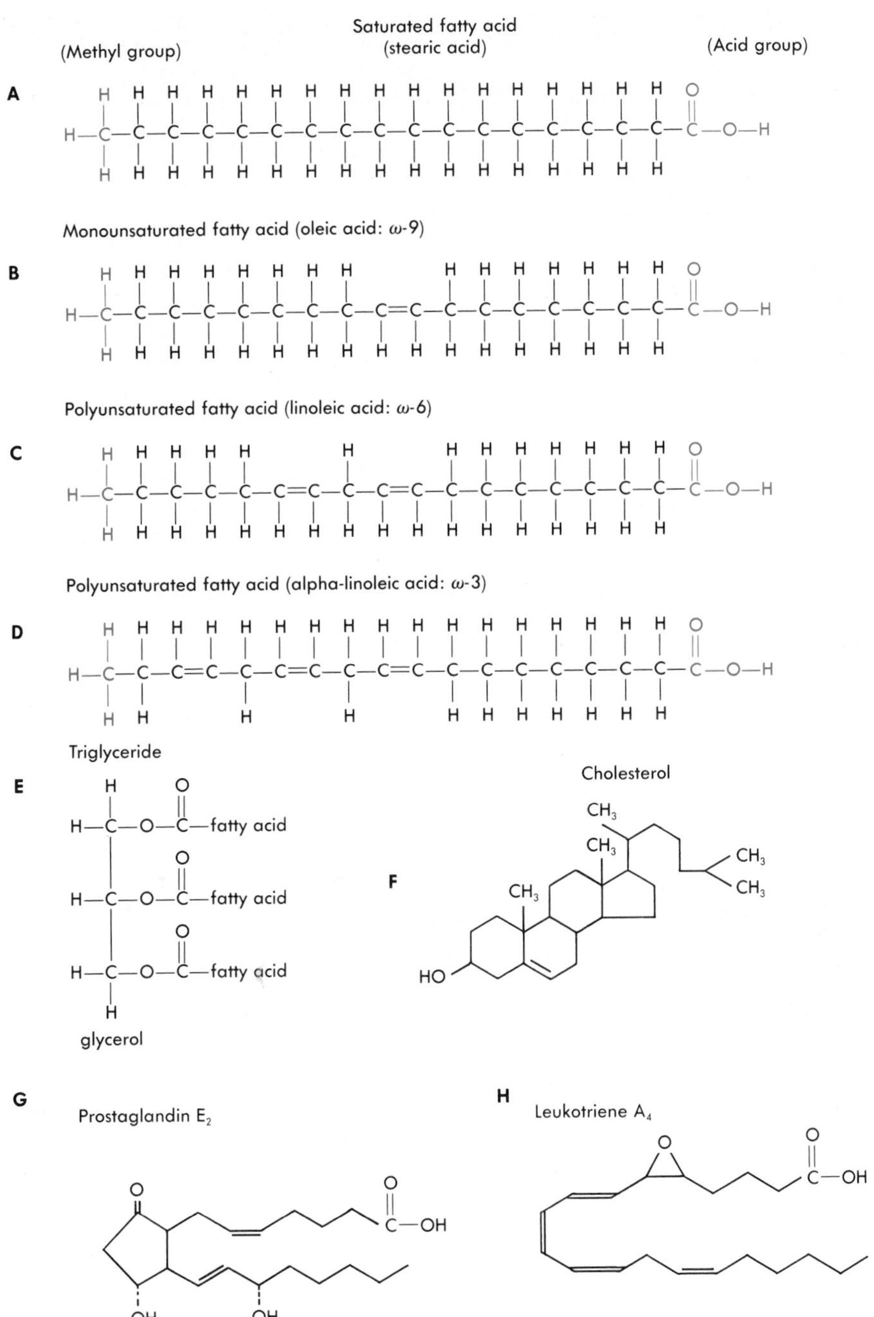

Figure 4-1 The families of fatty acids and some key metabolic products—eicosanoids. Note that the last three structures have most of the carbons and hydrogens deleted for simplicity's sake. Wherever there is a corner in the structure a carbon resides, and it will have up to two hydrogens added to follow the rule that a carbon must have four bonds to form a stable structure.

a high percentage of fatty acids with only one carbon-carbon double bond, and so are often called monounsaturated oils. If two or more bonds between the carbons are double bonds, the fatty acid is **polyunsaturated.** Corn, soybean, and safflower oils are good sources of polyunsaturated fatty acids and so are often called polyunsaturated oils (Figure 4-2). Note, however, that all fats contain a mixture of saturated and unsaturated fatty acids. The fatty acids in greatest concentration are just what we typically focus on.

polyunsaturated fatty acid acid containing two or more carbon-carbon double bonds.

The actual placement of the carbon-carbon double bonds—where they begin—in the fatty acid can make a big difference in how the body metabolizes it. If the double bonds located near the methyl end (-CH3) first appear at the third carbon, it is an **omega-3 (ω-3) fatty acid.** If the double bonds near the methyl end first appear at the sixth carbon, it is an **omega-6 (ω-6) fatty acid** (Figure 4-1). **Alpha-**

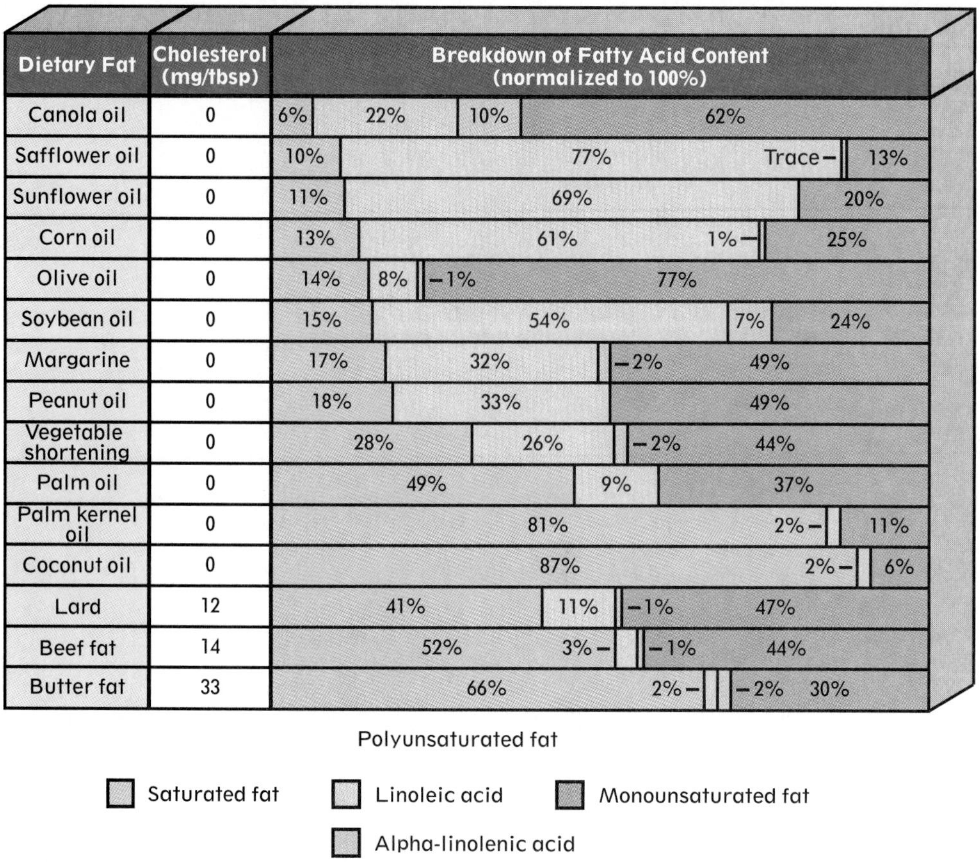

Dietary Fat	Cholesterol (mg/tbsp)	Breakdown of Fatty Acid Content (normalized to 100%)
Canola oil	0	6% 22% 10% 62%
Safflower oil	0	10% 77% Trace– 13%
Sunflower oil	0	11% 69% 20%
Corn oil	0	13% 61% 1%– 25%
Olive oil	0	14% 8% –1% 77%
Soybean oil	0	15% 54% 7% 24%
Margarine	0	17% 32% –2% 49%
Peanut oil	0	18% 33% 49%
Vegetable shortening	0	28% 26% –2% 44%
Palm oil	0	49% 9% 37%
Palm kernel oil	0	81% 2%– 11%
Coconut oil	0	87% 2%– 6%
Lard	12	41% 11% –1% 47%
Beef fat	14	52% 3%– –1% 44%
Butter fat	33	66% 2%– –2% 30%

Polyunsaturated fat

Saturated fat · Linoleic acid · Monounsaturated fat · Alpha-linolenic acid

Figure 4-2 Comparison of dietary fats in terms of saturated fat, the most common unsaturated fats, and cholesterol content.

linolenic acid is the major omega-3 fatty acid in food; **linoleic acid** is the major omega-6 fatty acid; **oleic acid** is the major omega-9 fatty acid.

Humans can obtain omega-3 and omega-6 fatty acids only by ingesting them.[6] A human cell can only produce carbon-carbon double bonds after the ninth or later carbons (numbered from the methyl end). In other words, humans do not have the capacity to place double bonds between the ninth carbon and the methyl end. Any fatty acids with carbon-carbon double bonds in that location were not made by a human cell. Nevertheless, omega-3 and omega-6 fatty acids not only form parts of vital structures in the body, they perform roles in immune system activity and vision, help form cell membranes, and produce hormonelike compounds called **eicosanoids.**[17] So we must eat these fatty acids to maintain good health.

Aspirin has such diverse effects on the body—from lowering body temperature to easing muscle pain—because it blocks the synthesis of certain eicosanoids.

ESSENTIAL FATTY ACIDS

Some polyunsaturated fatty acids—linoleic acid and alpha-linolenic acid—are called **essential fatty acids** because (1) they cannot be made by humans, (2) they are required for important functions, and (3) they are available to us only by ingestion.[6] The 1989 RDA publication states that adults need to consume about 1% to 2% of their total kcalories from linoleic acid; current consumption is about 7%. Up to 10% of kcalories from polyunsaturated fatty acids is generally recommended as a safe upper level of intake.[5] Since common plant oils—corn, soybean, cottonseed,

NUTRITION FOCUS

Cis and Trans Fatty Acids

Monounsaturated and polyunsaturated fatty acids can exist in two isomeric forms—**cis** and **trans**. Isomers share the same chemical formula but have different chemical structures. The cis form has the hydrogen atoms on the same side of the carbon-carbon double bond. The trans form has the hydrogen atoms on opposite sides of the carbon-carbon double bond (Figure 4-3). Plant fatty acids are in the cis form. A few trans fatty acids are in milk because the bacteria in a cow's multiple stomachs (rumen) rearrange the fatty acids from the cis form into the trans form. However, margarine and shortenings, the latter used commonly in food products and deep fat fryers, have the highest concentrations of trans fatty acids.[14]

As you can see in Figure 4-3, the cis bond causes the fatty acid to bend while the trans bond allows the fatty acid to remain straight. Increasing the number of cis double bonds allows the fatty acid to take on a variety of shapes that require more space in a membrane. For example, arachidonic acid with four cis carbon-carbon double bonds takes on a "U" shape. This may have significance for the position occupied by fatty acids in the cell membrane. The presence of fatty acids with trans carbon-carbon double bonds, as they will be straighter, will in turn alter the space requirements in the cell membrane.

Presently many studies show that trans fatty acids are not linked to significantly increased risk for any disease, notably heart disease and cancer, probably because we eat so little of these.[14] Margarine—a major source of trans fatty acids in our food—has been used increasingly for the last 30 years while blood cholesterol levels and heart disease rates have declined,[3] and cancer rates, except for lung cancer, have remained steady. Trans fatty acids are metabolized like saturated fatty acids in that some forms of trans fatty acids raise blood cholesterol levels when fed in amounts about four times our average intake.[19] For those people who eat a large number of commercially prepared foods and fast food, this is of concern. Trans fatty acids also provide no essential fatty acid activity.

Although the research on the effects of trans fatty acids in the amount present in our diet is still controversial, the main concerns are twofold. First, their status on the food label. Presently trans fats are "hidden" on the food label in the United States as monounsaturated fats. Because they are not identified, the consumer is left unaware of their presence. Since trans fatty acids tend to behave as saturated fats, labeling trans fatty acids as monounsaturated fats leaves consumers unaware of the true contribution of trans fatty acids to the diet. Second, there is a potential for a high intake by some of us. As quick-service restaurants have switched from beef fat (tallow) to vegetable shortenings, the trans fatty acid content of some of their various food products has risen.

Still, it is easy to avoid a high intake of trans fatty acids: (1) use little or no stick margarine or shortening; substitute with softer, tub margarine and vegetable oils; and (2) minimize consumption of deep fat fried food in restaurants, including French fries, fried pies, potato skins, and any deep fat fried meat, fish, or poultry at quick-service restaurants. For instance, a typical hamburger sandwich, bowl of chili, and soft drink or milk contain few trans fatty acids. At this time we feel this approach is a prudent one to take.

sunflower, and safflower oils—generally contain over 50% of fatty acids as linoleic acid, they should supply about 4% of our total kcalorie intake. On a 2500 kcalorie diet, this corresponds to 1 tablespoon of highly polyunsaturated vegetable oil per day.

The 1989 RDA publication also states that in the future an allowance for omega-3 fatty acids should be considered. Leading researchers support that statement.[25] Currently Canada is the only national government to establish dietary guidelines for omega-3 fatty acids. The Canadian recommendations suggest about a 4:1 ratio of omega-6 to omega-3 fatty acids. The current ratio in diets in the United States is about 10:1. Many scientists today think diet planning should include a regular supply of alpha-linolenic acid[4,15] or one of its related omega-3 fatty acids, **eicosapentaenoic acid (EPA)** and **docosahexaenoic acid (DHA).** This would essentially require weekly consumption of fatty fish, such as salmon, tuna, and sardines, or regular intake of canola or soybean oil. All are good sources of omega-3 fatty acids. Omega-3 fatty acids are a vital research area today that we will explore further in the next few pages.

eicosapentaenoic acid (EPA) An omega-3 fatty acid with 20 carbons and five carbon-carbon double bonds that is present in fish oils. EPA may also be synthesized from linolenic acid.

docosahexaenoic acid (DHA) An omega-3 fatty acid with 22 carbons and six carbon-carbon double bonds. DHA is also present in fish oils and may be synthesized from alpha-linolenic acid.

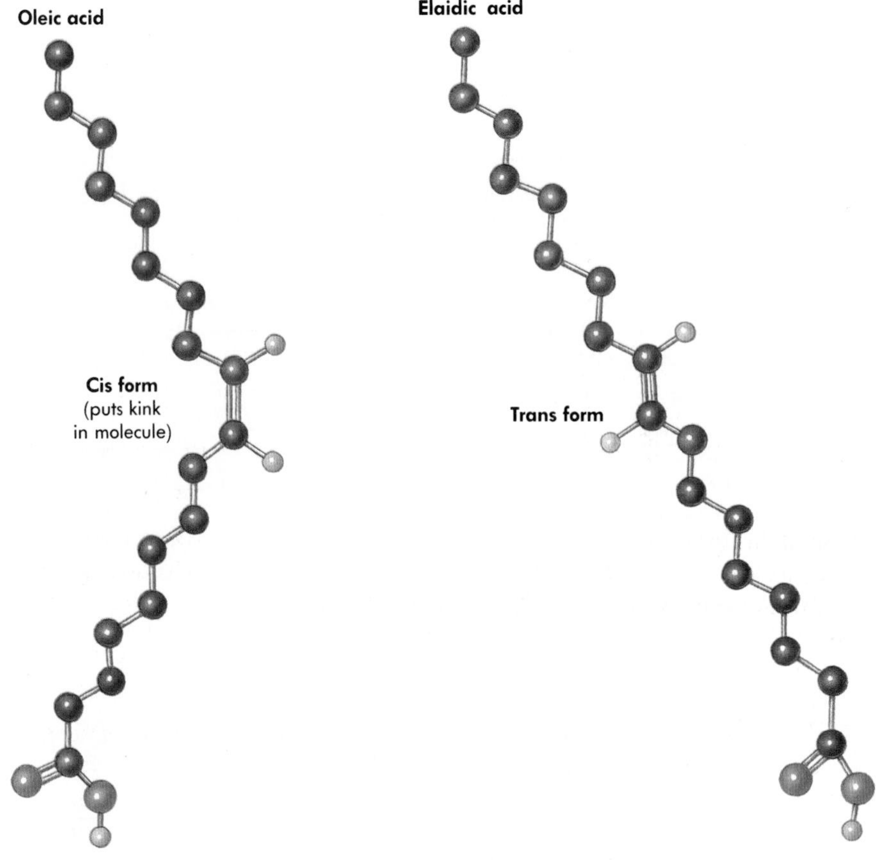

Figure 4-3 Cis and trans isomers of fatty acids. Cis forms are the most common forms in foods.

ESSENTIAL FATTY ACID DEFICIENCY

Unless enough essential fatty acids are consumed, the skin becomes flaky and itchy, sores may develop on the scalp, diarrhea and other symptoms often develop, and growth may be retarded.[6] Today these signs of deficiency appear in people fed **intravenous** solutions that contain no lipid for long periods or infants receiving formulas low in fat. However, since we need only about 1 tablespoon of polyunsaturated plant oil a day to meet essential fatty acid needs, even a low-fat diet, if it follows the Guide to Daily Food Choices, is likely to provide enough.

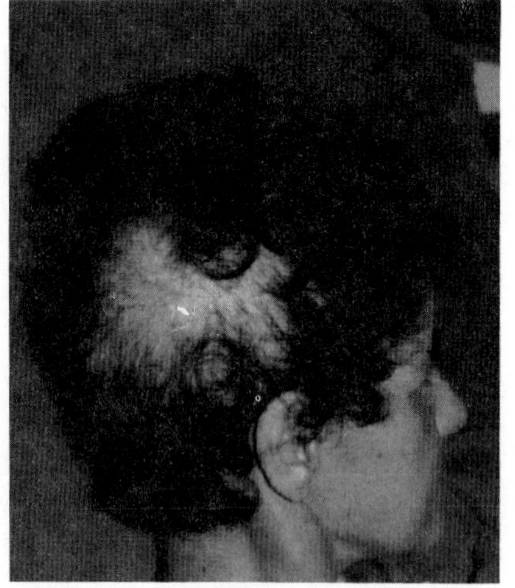

Essential fatty acid deficiency produces changes in the skin, resulting in hair loss.

CONCEPT CHECK

Lipids are a group of compounds that have few oxygen atoms in their structures and dissolve in chloroform, benzene, or ether. Fatty acids form one class of lipids. Saturated fatty acids contain no carbon-carbon double bonds, monounsaturated fatty acids contain one carbon-carbon double bond, and polyunsaturated fatty acids contain two or more carbon-carbon double bonds. If the carbon-carbon double bonds near the methyl end ($—CH_3$) first involve the third carbon, the fatty acid is an omega-3 fatty acid. If the carbon-carbon double bonds near the methyl end first involve the sixth carbon, it is an omega-6 fatty acid. Both omega-3 and omega-6 fatty acids are essential parts of a diet since they cannot be made within the body and are required for health.

TRIGLYCERIDES

Fatty acids usually do not exist in a free form in the body. Some free fatty acids are bound to the protein, albumin, in the bloodstream while they are transferred from

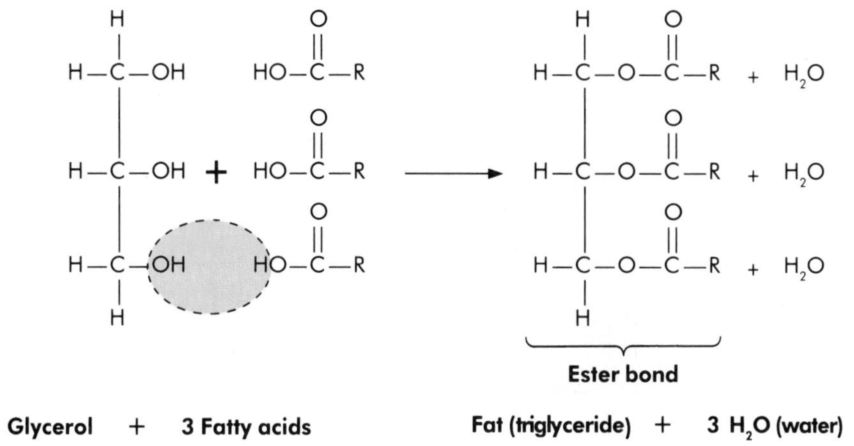

Glycerol + 3 Fatty acids → Fat (triglyceride) + 3 H_2O (water)

Ester bond

Figure 4-4 Forming a triglyceride. This yields water as a by-product while creating ester bonds. The R stands for a long chain of carbons bonded together, with hydrogens attached.

storage in the adipose cells to the liver, muscles, and other sites. However, about 95% of all fat, both in the body and in food, is in the form of triglycerides.

Triglyceride molecules contain a backbone of a three-carbon alcohol, called **glycerol.** On the three hydroxyl groups (-OH) of the glycerol are attached three fatty acids. Three water molecules are released in the process. The net result is that glycerol and three fatty acids form a triglyceride and three water molecules. Note that triacylglyceride is a more formal name of the molecule (Figure 4-4).

glycerol A 3-carbon atom alcohol-containing three hydroxyl groups (-OH); used to form triglycerides.

Most triglycerides are in mixed forms, meaning they contain different types of fatty acids on each glycerol molecule. These fatty acids can be of differing chain lengths and varying degrees of saturation.

The bonds formed in a triglyceride between glycerol and fatty acid are called ester bonds. So the process of putting fatty acids on the glycerol molecule is called **esterification.** Taking the fatty acids off the glycerol molecule is called deesterification. Removing the fatty acids from the glycerol molecule and then putting them back on is called reesterification. Surprisingly, the body reesterifies triglycerides over and over again. Every time a triglyceride crosses a cell membrane it must be broken down, or deesterified. Then, when the fatty acids enter the cell, they often must be reesterified into a triglyceride.

esterification The process of attaching fatty acids to a glycerol molecule, creating an ester bond. Removing a fatty acid is called deesterification; reattaching a fatty acid is called reesterification.

A glycerol containing only one fatty acid forms a monoglyceride. A glycerol that contains two fatty acids forms a diglyceride. During digestion most fatty acids must be removed from the triglyceride molecules. This aids fat absorption because triglycerides are so large they cannot easily cross the intestinal wall and eventually reach the bloodstream. What occurs is that many triglycerides are turned into monoglycerides. When the free fatty acids, monoglycerides, and any free glycerol molecules are absorbed into the intestinal cells, the majority of these parts are rebuilt into triglycerides (Figure 4-5).

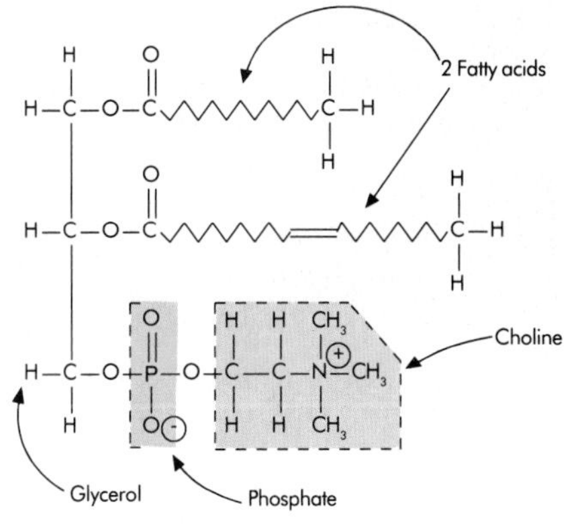

2 Fatty acids

Choline

Glycerol

Phosphate

Lecithin

PHOSPHOLIPIDS

Some lipids look like triglycerides at first glance but contain only one or two fatty acids. Structures other than fatty acids bond to other sites on the glycerol backbone. For example, **lecithin,** also called a phospholipid, is an important component of all cell membranes and a participant in fat digestion in the intestine. Egg yolks contain lecithin in abundance. On the bottom carbon of the glycerol molecule in lecithin is a phosphate group bonded to a choline molecule. This phosphate group is what makes lecithin a phospholipid. You can see from the diagram in the margin that lecithin not only looks like a triglyceride but likely originates from a triglyceride. This is correct.

Many other types of phospholipids exist in the body, such as sphingomyelins and cerebrosides, both found in the brain. However, even though lecithin and other

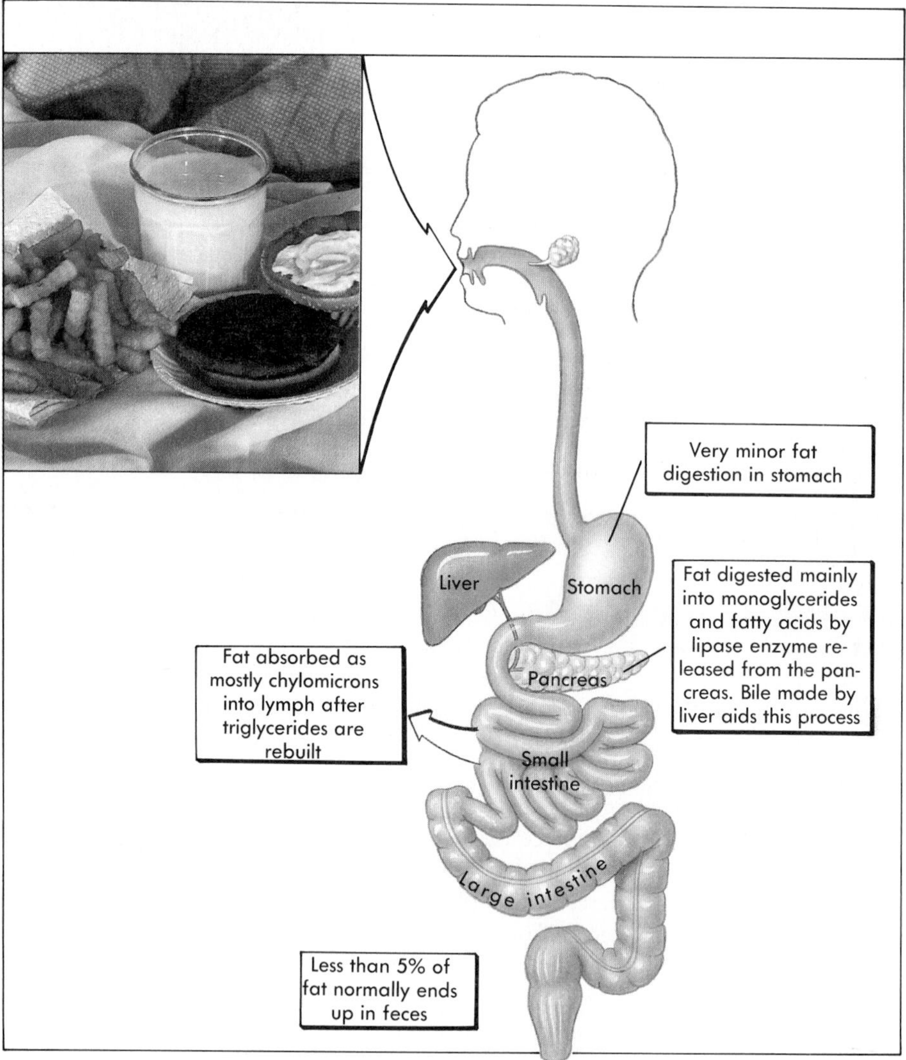

Figure 4-5 For your information—a summary of fat digestion and absorption. Chapter 6 covers this in detail.

phospholipids are found in food, it is not necessary to eat these. The body makes lecithin and other phospholipids when and where it is necessary.

Healthfood literature promotes one component of lecithin, choline, as a vitamin. However, because the human body readily makes choline from the amino acid methionine, choline is not a vitamin for humans (see Chapter 13).

STEROLS

Sterols show how diverse lipids can be. These compounds have a multiringed (steroid) structure. An important sterol is the waxy substance, cholesterol. The hydroxyl group (-OH) on the cholesterol molecule makes it a sterol (Figure 4-1). Cholesterol does not look like a triglyceride, but since it dissolves in ether, it is a lipid. It shares another characteristic with fatty acids, triglycerides, and phospholipids—synthesis of most parts of these molecules uses a derivative of the smallest fatty acid, acetic acid ($CH_3\overset{O}{\overset{\|}{C}}—OH$).

Cholesterol is found only in the animal-derived foods we eat (Table 4-1). Each day your liver makes about 800 milligrams of cholesterol, which circulates through the bloodstream to function as the body needs it. Every type of human cell studied to date makes cholesterol; it is an essential part of a cell. Some hormones also are made from cholesterol. We eat about 300 to 500 milligrams of cholesterol per day.[5] We make cholesterol whether we eat it or not, and when following diets very low in cholesterol, we make even more. Some plants have related sterols, such as er-

Table 4-1 Cholesterol content of common measures of selected foods (in ascending order)

Food	Amount	Cholesterol in milligrams	Food	Amount	Cholesterol in milligrams
Milk, skim	1 cup	4	Clams, halibut, tuna	3 oz	55
Mayonnaise	1 T	10	Chicken, turkey, light meat	3 oz	70
Butter	1 pat	11			
Lard	1 T	12	Beef*, pork*	3 oz	75
Cottage cheese	½ cup	15	Lamb, crab	3 oz	85
Milk, low fat, 2%	1 cup	22	Shrimp, lobster	3 oz	90-110
Half and half	¼ cup	23	Heart, beef	3 oz	164
Hot dog*	1	29	Egg (egg yolk)*	1 each	213
Ice cream, ≈ 10% fat	½ cup	30	Liver, beef	3 oz	410
Cheese, cheddar	1 oz	30	Kidney	3 oz	587
Milk, whole*	1 cup	34	Brains	3 oz	2637
Oysters, salmon	3 oz	40			

*Leading contributors of cholesterol to the U.S. diet.

gosterol, that can form a type of vitamin D. However, the plants we typically eat do not contain cholesterol.

Manufacturers who advertise peanut butter, vegetable shortening, margarines, and vegetable oils as containing no cholesterol are taking advantage of consumer naivete. Of course peanut butter and margarine have no cholesterol—no purely plant food we eat has it. However, some plant-based foods do have a high saturated fat content, and that can make them important in affecting serum cholesterol levels; much more so than the actual cholesterol content of a food. More on this in the Nutrition Perspective.

CONCEPT CHECK

Triglycerides are the main form of fat found in the body and in food. A triglyceride has three fatty acids attached onto a molecule of glycerol. The fatty acids can be of any length and either saturated or unsaturated. Triglycerides must be made smaller to be absorbed and so are disassembled in digestion and then rebuilt for transport in the blood. Phospholipids are derivatives of triglycerides. They form important parts of cell membranes and other body molecules. Cholesterol forms compounds vital to the body, such as hormones and parts of cell membranes. Cholesterol is essential to the body. The body synthesizes cholesterol for its needs, but some may also be consumed in food.

Putting Lipids to Work in the Body

We have touched on some of the roles of lipids in the body. Lets now look at these in detail.

FATTY ACIDS

Forming eicosanoids is a key function of various fatty acids. Once linoleic acid is in a cell, it can be lengthened to 20 carbons and have two more carbon-carbon double bonds added (in other words undergo desaturation) to yield arachidonic acid. Alpha-linolenic acid can be elongated to 20 carbons and have two carbon-carbon double bonds added to form EPA.[4] In some instances, arachidonic acid and EPA are made even longer by having more carbons added. The rate at which this happens and the significance depends on the type of human cell.

arachiodonic acid A fatty acid with 20 carbons and four carbon-carbon double bonds; an omega-6 fatty acid.

The long chain, highly polyunsaturated fatty acids, which include arachidonic acid and EPA, form a group of biologically active compounds called eicosanoids:

prostacyclin A potent inhibitor of blood clotting made by the blood vessel walls.

thromboxane A stimulant of blood clotting made by particles in the bloodstream.

leukotriene An important regulator of many diseases involving inflammatory or hypersensitivity reactions, such as asthma.

prostaglandins, **prostacyclins, thromboxanes,** and **leukotrienes** (Figure 4-1).[17] As mentioned, these eicosanoids are important and potent regulators of vital body functions. These include blood pressure, childbirth, blood clotting, immune responses, inflammatory responses, and stomach secretions. In essence the eicosanoids act as hormonelike compounds.

The ω-3 fatty acids, EPA and DHA, can be made from alpha-linolenic acid or are ingested via fish intake, with the latter being a much more reliable source. EPA and DHA are especially concentrated in marine mammals and cold water fishes. Research has shown that Greenland Eskimos have one tenth the risk of heart attacks compared with Danish people.[18] These Eskimos eat fat primarily from marine sources (fish, whale, seal and walrus)—about 40% of their kcalories comes from fish oils. Studies have also shown that people with very high serum lipid levels markedly reduce those levels (primarily the level of serum triglycerides) by consuming about 20% to 25% of their daily kcalories from fish oils (about 50 grams).[13] Scientists now wonder whether the wide variety of effects of the eicosanoids made from fish oils (EPA and DHA) suggests that they should also be considered essential to the diet, particularly since converting alpha-linolenic acid—another omega-3 fatty acid—to EPA appears to be inefficient.[25] To increase the EPA and DHA content in cells we essentially need to eat fish regularly.

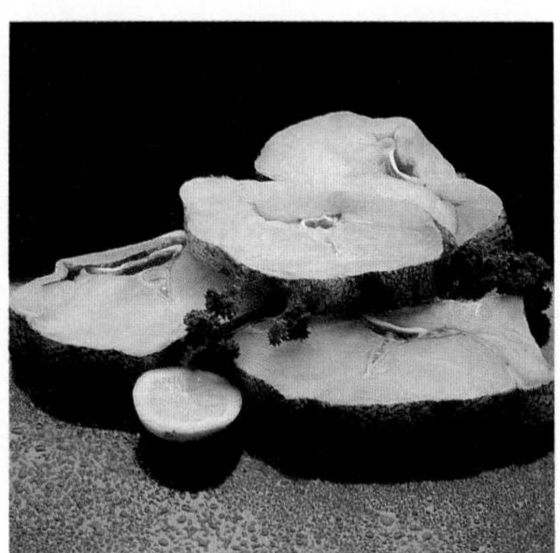

Fish twice a week makes a healthy contribution to a diet.

As we noted above, the ω-3 fatty acids in our diets tend to reduce blood clotting. This line of evidence also supports the recommendation to regularly eat fish. Some studies show that people who eat fish about 2 times a week (240 grams or 8 ounces of total weekly intake) run lower risks for heart disease than people who rarely eat fish. In these cases the fish oil is most likely affecting blood clotting. We will soon discuss how blood clots are linked to heart attacks. Decreasing the tendency for blood to clot reduces the risk of heart attack, especially for people at high risk.

Fish oils reduce the tendency for blood to clot by changing the nature of eicosanoid synthesis in the body. An important class of prostaglandins and thromboxanes are usually made from arachidonic acid, an omega-6 fatty acid. Since fish oils contain a lot of the omega-3 fatty acids (EPA and DHA), cells of people who eat a lot of fish have a greater tendency to synthesize eicosanoids with EPA and DHA. In effect, EPA and DHA compete with arachidonic acid for the same metabolic pathways. When they are highly concentrated in a cell, EPA and DHA win more often.

Now when cells use these different starting compounds, they synthesize different types of eicosanoids. Arachidonic acid yields one type of prostaglandin and thromboxane, while EPA and DHA makes another type of prostaglandin and thromboxane. The subtle differences in eicosanoid structure between the two forms of the compounds yield key differences in function, an important example of which concerns blood clotting. Overall, many of the eicosanoids made from arachidonic acid (omega-6) increase blood clotting, while those made from EPA and DHA (omega-3) primarily decrease it.[18] The net effect is that diets high in arachidonic acid increase the tendency for blood to clot, while diets high in EPA and DHA do not.

Does This Mean We Should Eat "Eskimo" Diets?

Blood clotting is a normal physiological process. Eskimos who eat a lot of fish have a higher risk for strokes than Danish people, maybe because their blood does not readily clot. This is not the case in some parts of Japan, however, where fish consumption is also high. Still, significantly altering blood clotting may be a two-edged sword. Because of this possibility we recommend eating fish about twice a week. Atlantic and Pacific Herring, sardines, Atlantic halibut and salmon, lake trout, coho, pink and king salmon, blue fish, albacore tuna, and Atlantic mackerel are among those fish with the greatest omega-3 fatty acid contents (see Appendix K). New research may soon add more types of fish to this list.

We do not recommend consuming fish oil capsules without a physician's advice.

The potential for seriously altering the effects of the type of eicosanoids formed is only one possible result of fish oil capsules. As we previously discussed, eicosanoids have significant and wide-ranging effects, so altering their production can have profound consequences on your health. The treatment of any condition with fish oil capsules should be considered experimental.[31] The caution regarding fish oil capsules should not be confused, however, with the suggestion that we increase the amount of fish in our diets. There are a number of good reasons to eat more fish than we presently do. It is very difficult to create nutrient toxicities with foods. However, using concentrates of anything, including vitamins, minerals, or fish oils, can be dangerous.

The fish oil story unfolds daily. We mentioned increasing fish oil in the diet can reduce blood pressure as well as inflammation in certain diseases, such as psoriasis and asthma. It will be exciting to follow this new area of research.

CONCEPT CHECK

When cells use omega-3 fatty acids to synthesize hormonelike compounds called eicosanoids, the synthesized products differ markedly from those using omega-6 fatty acids. In general, products made from omega-3 fatty acids tend to lower blood clotting, blood pressure, and inflammatory responses in the body. In the future, there may be more specific recommendations in the United States for the deliberate inclusion of omega-3 fatty acids in diet planning, as is seen in Canada. Presently the recommendation to eat fish about twice a week is a good guide. Other functions of the essential fatty acids are separate from those of the eicosanoids formed from those same essential fatty acids, such as forming a key part of cell membranes.

TRIGLYCERIDES

Energy Storage and Use

Triglycerides are the main form of energy storage in the body. The ability to store lipid is essentially unlimited. The storage sites, adipose cells, can increase about 50 times in weight. If the amount of lipid to be stored exceeds the ability of the cells to expand, the body can form new adipose cells.

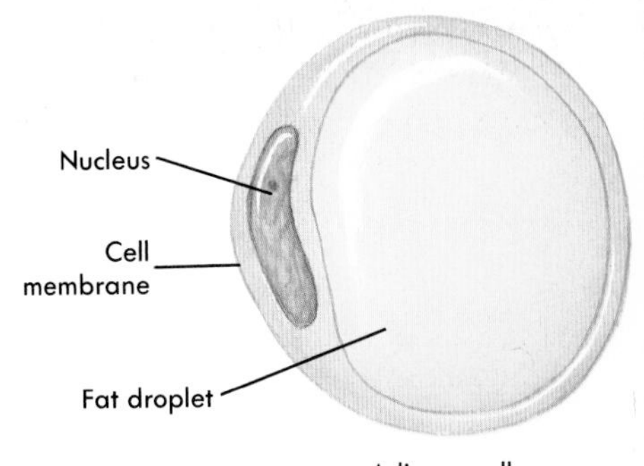

Adipose cell

When we store lipids in adipose cells, we store little else. Adipose cells are about 80% lipid and only 20% water and protein. In contrast, if we stored energy as muscle tissue, we would need to store much water, since muscle is about 73% water. The same is true for energy stored as glycogen. About 2.6 grams of water are stored along with every gram of glycogen. A 3-day supply of energy as glycogen would weigh about 14 pounds (6 kilograms). Think of the consequences if we stored energy as muscle tissue or glycogen—for most of us, body weight would greatly increase due to the excess water we would need to carry. Another advantage to storing triglycerides for energy is that they are energy dense. Recall that triglycerides yield over twice the kcalories per gram as proteins and carbohydrates do.

The free fatty acids on triglycerides go on to make up the main fuel for muscles at rest and during light activity. In endurance exercise the muscles burn a lot of carbohydrate in addition to fatty acids. (See Chapter 10 for a detailed account.) Mostly, however, muscles derive energy from fatty acids. Other body tissues also use fatty acids for energy—about 40% of the energy used by the entire body at rest and during light activity comes from fatty acids. This amount, perhaps coincidentally, is about the same as the percentage of total kcalories in our food that comes from fat.

Insulating and Protecting the Body

A layer of adipose tissue made mostly of triglycerides insulates and protects the body, especially the breasts and kidneys. Women, typically have more adipose tissue in the hips, buttocks, and lower abdomen than men. The preservation of the species depends on the protection of the organs of reproduction. The ovaries and uterus are protected in women, and a testicular fat pad protects the testes in men. We usually don't notice the important insulating function of adipose tissue because we wear clothes, but it is quite apparent in animals. Polar bears, whales, and other animals that live in cold climates build a thick layer of adipose tissue around themselves to insulate against their cold-weather environment. It also represents stored energy for winter.

anorexia nervosa An eating disorder involving a psychological loss of appetite and self-starvation, due in part to a distorted body image and various social pressures associated with puberty (see Chapter 11).

lanugo Downlike hair that appears after much body fat is lost due to semistarvation. As the hair stands erect and traps air, it acts as insulation to the body, replacing that usually supplied by body fat.

fetus A developing infant in utero from 8 weeks until birth.

People with the disease **anorexia nervosa** often lose 25% or more of body weight, resulting in a body-fat percentage that is much too low. We can never be totally fat free, because fat is an essential part of all cells. A level of fat below 5% of body weight can lead to harmful side effects, especially in women (see Chapter 11). However with anorexia nervosa, a person may get as lean as it's biologically possible. The person then often develops downy hair all over the body, called **lanugo.** These hairs stand up, trapping air around them. The air acts as insulation and represents an attempt to substitute for the missing layer of adipose tissue usually present under the skin. Lanugo also insulates a growing **fetus** before its layer of adipose tissue is produced late in pregnancy.

Transporting Fat-Soluble Vitamins

Triglycerides and other lipids carry fat-soluble vitamins to the small intestine and aid their absorption. If the small intestine is diseased, dietary fat may not be properly digested and absorbed. Rather, the fat passes through the small intestine and ends up in the colon. When this happens, the fat-soluble vitamins are bound by the unabsorbed fat and carried into the colon, bypassing their absorption sites in the small intestine. People who absorb fat poorly, such as those with cystic fibrosis, are at risk for deficiencies of fat-soluble vitamins, especially vitamin K. People who use mineral oil as a laxative close to mealtimes are also at risk, since we cannot digest or absorb mineral oil. The undigested mineral oil, which itself is a mixture of liquid petroleum hydrocarbons, carries fat-soluble vitamins into the colon where they are eliminated in the stool. This can make mineral oil a poor choice for a laxative, especially near mealtimes.

Unabsorbed fatty acids can also bind minerals, such as calcium and magnesium, and pull them into the stool for elimination. This can harm mineral status (see Chapter 14).

PHOSPHOLIPIDS

Phospholipids form important parts of cell membranes. A cell membrane looks much like a sea of phospholipids with protein islands (Figure 4-6). The protein islands

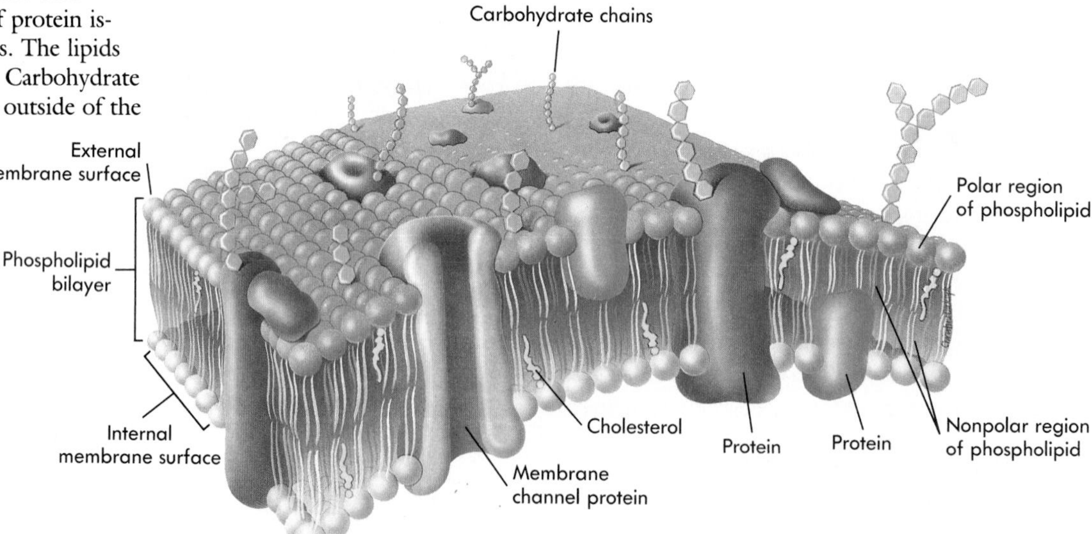

Figure 4-6 A cell membrane. This membrane is composed of protein islands within a sea of lipids. The lipids are mostly phospholipids. Carbohydrate chains are attached to the outside of the cell membrane.

form receptors for hormones, function as enzymes, and act as transporters, among other functions. Notice also the carbohydrates on the surface of the receptor proteins. We mention this here rather than in Chapter 3 so you will first have a better understanding of the cell membrane. A function of this carbohydrate is to help an incoming molecule identify the protein receptor on the cell surface.

Phospholipids also function as emulsifiers, compounds that allow fat globules to break into small droplets. In doing so emulsifiers have the ability to suspend fat in water. Look at Figure 4-7. The charged end of a lecithin molecule attracts water while the other end attracts lipids. The lipid-attracting end is made of fatty acids. These long chains of carbons and attached hydrogens show no positive or negative charges, so they have no polarity. They are **nonpolar.** Triglycerides are also nonpolar and so are attracted to fatty acids.

nonpolar A compound with no charges present.

Water, in contrast, is **polar.** The slightly negative-charged oxygen and the two slightly positive-charged hydrogens create poles similar to magnetic poles. The phosphate group and nitrogen at the bottom of the lecithin molecule are charged—so this area is also polar. The polar water is attracted to the charges on lecithin. This part of lecithin is called **hydrophilic,** which means "liking water." In contrast, the parts with fatty acids are **hydrophobic,** since they don't attract (they fear) water.

polar A compound with distinct positive and negative charges on it. These act like poles on a magnet.

hydrophilic Attracts water (literally means "water loving").

hydrophobic Repels water (literally means "water fearing").

When many emulsifier molecules are mixed together with oil and water, the emulsifiers organize into **micelles** by orienting their hydrophobic parts to the inside and their hydrophilic parts to the outside. Oil is attracted to the hydrophobic core of the micelles, and water is attracted to the hydrophilic shells. The mixture produced then has tiny oil droplets surrounded by thin shells of water. In an emulsified solution there are millions of these tiny oil droplets, all separated from each other by shells of water (Figure 4-7).

micelles An emulsification product in which individual emulsifiers organize with their hydrophobic parts to the center of the micelle and their hydrophilic parts to the outside.

Complete digestion and absorption of fat requires emulsification of dietary fats in the small intestine. Breaking the fats in foods into tiny oil droplets by emulsification, intestinal mixing, and the warming action of the body greatly increases their surface areas and so improves the process of digestion. (Chapter 6 provides a full account of this process.)

Lecithin and **bile acids** are produced by the liver and secreted into the small intestine via the gallbladder to emulsify dietary fats. These two substances—one a phospholipid and the other a sterol—are the body's main emulsifiers.

bile acids Emulsifiers synthesized by the liver and released by the gallbladder during digestion to aid in fat digestion.

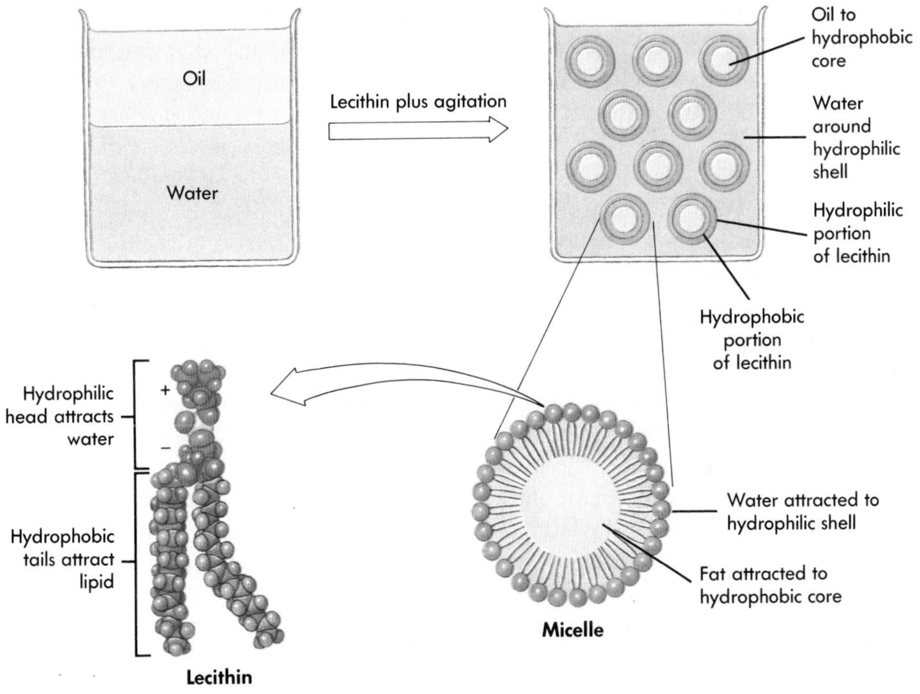

Oil
Water
Lecithin plus agitation
Oil to hydrophobic core
Water around hydrophilic shell
Hydrophilic portion of lecithin
Hydrophobic portion of lecithin
Hydrophilic head attracts water
Hydrophobic tails attract lipid
Lecithin
Micelle
Water attracted to hydrophilic shell
Fat attracted to hydrophobic core

Figure 4-7 Emulsification and emulsifiers. Emulsifiers can organize oil and water into micelles—droplets of oil surrounded by shells of water. Forming micelles is a key step in fat digestion.

calcitriol The active hormone form of vitamin D; it contains a derivative of cholesterol as part of its structure.

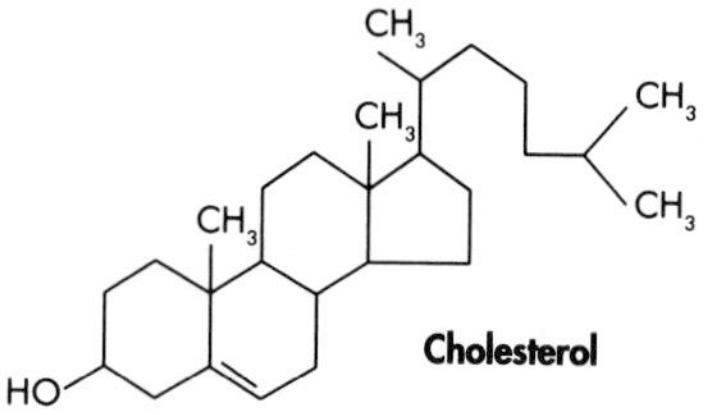

STEROLS

Cholesterol forms part of some important hormones, such as corticosteroids, the estrogens, testosterone, and the active vitamin D hormone, **calcitriol.** Cholesterol also forms the bile acids needed for fat digestion, as we just mentioned. Cholesterol is an essential structural component of membranes and of the outer layer of the particles that transport lipids in the blood (Figure 4-6). (We cover this in a later section entitled "Carrying Lipids in the Bloodstream.") Table 4-1 should help you understand the critical nature of cholesterol in certain organs. The cholesterol content of heart, egg (embryonic stage of life), liver, kidney, and brain is quite high. Because infants and toddlers are forming new tissue, especially brain, this is no time to greatly restrict lipids in the diet!

Cholesterol

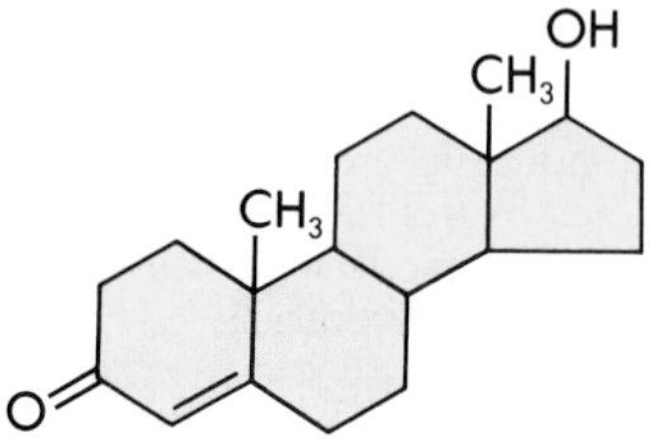

Testosterone

CONCEPT CHECK

Triglyceride is the major form of fat in food and in the body. Triglycerides in the body provide energy, as well as insulate and protect it. Triglycerides are the form in which energy is stored. Phospholipids are important components of cell membranes. If polarities are present, these make the phospholipids effective emulsifiers—compounds that can suspend fat in water. Emulsification of fat improves digestion and helps carry lipid particles in the bloodstream. Cholesterol is a building block for hormones and bile acids and is incorporated into cell membranes and particles that transport lipids in the bloodstream.

Carrying Lipids in the Bloodstream

By their natures, lipids and water don't mix. Overcoming this incompatibility challenges the ingenuity of the body.

CARRYING LIPIDS FROM DIETARY SOURCES

lipoprotein A compound found in the bloodstream containing a core of lipids with a shell of protein, phospholipid, and cholesterol.

apolipoproteins Proteins that are in each lipoprotein. Some are attached to the surface of the lipoprotein while others are imbedded in the outer shell of lipoproteins. Apolipoproteins can help another enzyme function, act as a lipid transfer protein, or help bind to a receptor.

lipoprotein lipase An enzyme that breaks down triglycerides into free fatty acids and glycerol from lipoproteins (especially chylomicrons) for the uptake into extra hepatic cells.

Once dietary fat is digested and absorbed into the cells of the small intestine, triglycerides are reformed. They combine with phospholipids and cholesterol and are packaged into a chylomicron, which is a large droplet of lipid surrounded by a thin shell of protein, cholesterol, and phospholipid. This combination of lipid and protein is called a **lipoprotein** (Figure 4-8). The shell around the chylomicron allows the lipid inside to float freely in the water-based bloodstream. Some of the proteins, **apolipoproteins,** also help other cells identify this particle as a chylomicron.

The chylomicron structure, in essence, emulsifies dietary fats before they enter the bloodstream. This process resembles the action of lecithin and bile acids in the small intestine when they emulsify dietary fats during digestion. The difference is that in digestion a layer of bile acids—rather than of protein, cholesterol, and phospholipid—surrounds the droplets.

Chylomicrons enter the lymphatic system and travel to the thoracic duct, which is located along the spinal column. This duct opens into a large vein in the neck called the subclavian vein. Chylomicrons enter the bloodstream at this point.

Chylomicrons in the bloodstream are acted on by **lipoprotein lipase.** This enzyme is attached to the outside surface of adipose (fat) cells, muscle cells, and blood vessel cells. Action of this enzyme is needed to get fats inside cells. Lipoprotein lipase deesterifies (breaks down) the triglycerides in the chylomicrons into free fatty acids and glycerol.[5] Much of the glycerol travels via the blood to cells in the liver or kidney. There it can be made into glucose. Muscle, adipose, and other cells in the vicinity absorb most of the fatty acids. The absorbed fatty acids can immediately be used for fuel or reesterified (reformed) into triglycerides. The source of the new glycerol molecule is a metabolite of glucose. Muscle cells tend to deesterify and then metabolize the fatty acids, while adipose cells tend to reesterify and store the fatty acids as triglycerides. Once lipoprotein lipase has removed most of the triglycerides

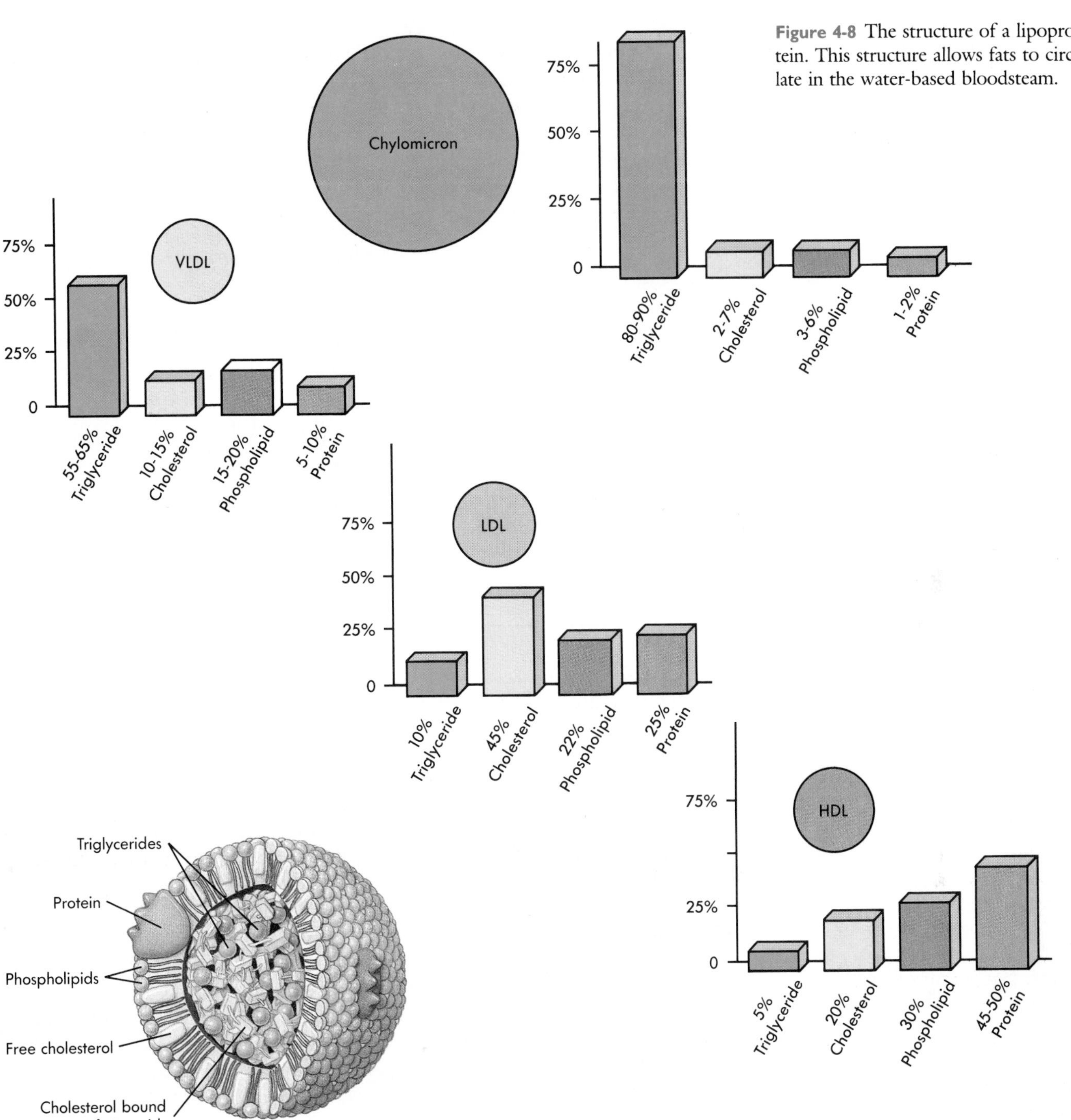

Figure 4-8 The structure of a lipoprotein. This structure allows fats to circulate in the water-based bloodsteam.

from a chylomicron, the remnant, which contains mostly cholesterol and protein, is taken up by the liver and metabolized (Figure 4-9).

The whole process of clearing chylomicrons from the bloodstream after eating takes about 2 hours or more. After 14 hours of fasting, they should be absent from the bloodstream. This is why people should fast for 14 hours before certain blood tests—then there is little chance the presence of chylomicrons will affect the results.

CARRYING LIPIDS FROM NONDIETARY SOURCES

The liver supplies the body with triglycerides and cholesterol. When you eat more kcalories than you need, some of the proteins and carbohydrates are degraded by

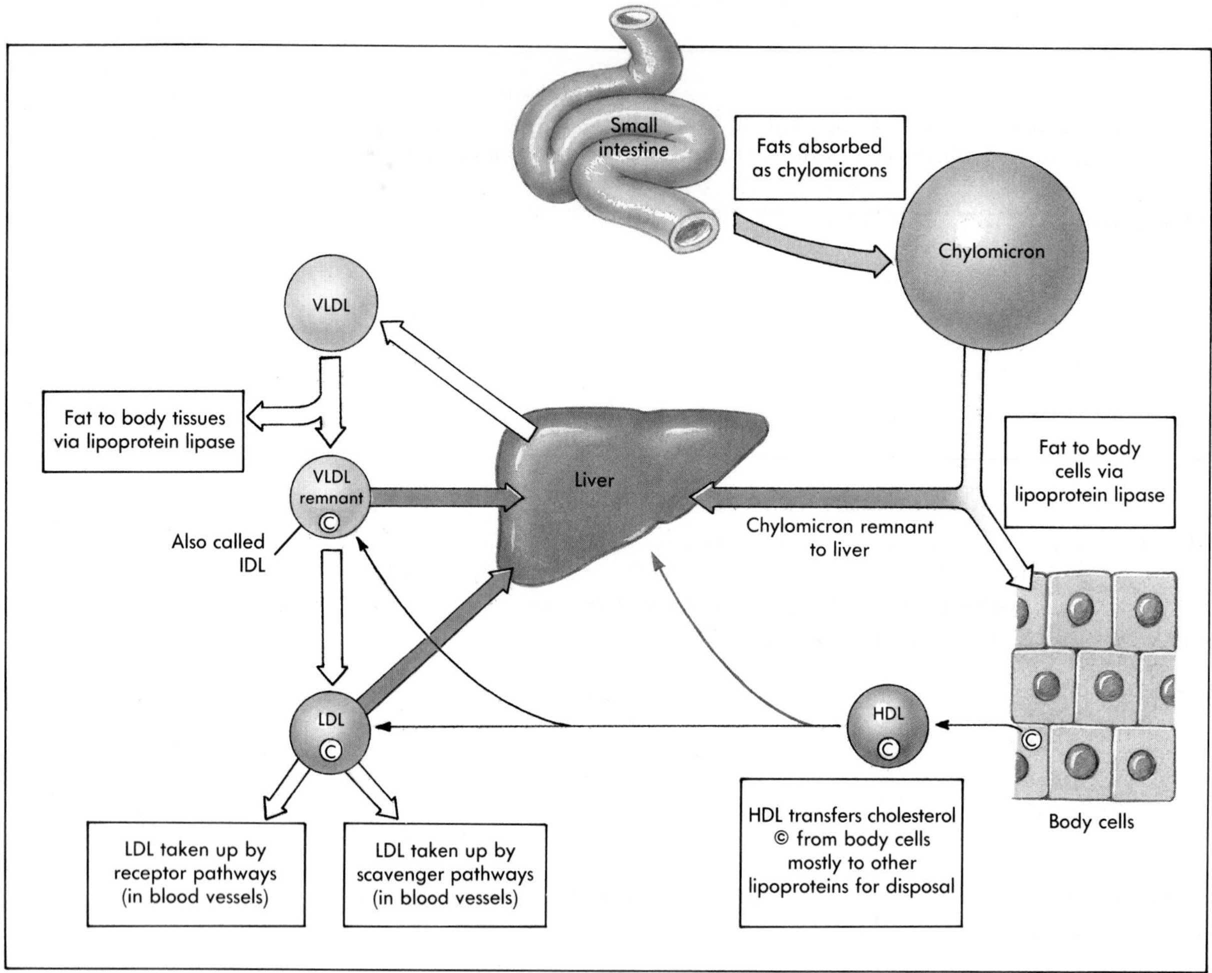

Figure 4-9 Lipoprotein interactions. Chylomicrons carry absorbed fat to body cells. VLDLs carry fat synthesized in the liver to body cells. LDLs arise from VLDLs and carry mostly cholesterol to cells. HDLs carry cholesterol from cells to other lipoproteins and the liver for excretion.

lipogenic Means "creating lipid"; the liver is the major lipogenic organ in the human body.

very low density lipoprotein (VLDL) The lipoprotein created in the liver that carries cholesterol and lipids newly synthesized by the liver.

intermediate-density lipoprotein (IDL) The product formed after a very low density lipoprotein (VLDL) has most of its triglyceride removed.

the liver and the resulting carbons and hydrogens are used to make triglycerides and cholesterol. The liver is the major lipid-producing **(lipogenic)** organ in the body. Adipose tissue primarily stores rather than makes lipid. This is why it is important to not only moderate fat in the diet but also to make sure the total kcalories consumed do not exceed those expended. Otherwise, the liver may turn the extra proteins and carbohydrates (and alcohol as well) into fat.

The liver must resolve the same problem with which the small intestine is faced—equip newly synthesized lipids so they can float in the water base of the bloodstream. So when the liver synthesizes cholesterol or triglycerides, it, too, coats the lipid with a protein, cholesterol, and phospholipid shell, just as the small intestine does for chylomicrons. The liver's version of a chylomicron is a **very low density lipoprotein (VLDL).**[5]

As with chylomicrons, when the VLDLs leave the liver, lipoprotein lipase again deesterifies the triglyceride in the VLDLs. With less triglyceride in the VLDL, it becomes more dense (i.e. no longer a *very low* density lipoprotein), because lipids are less dense than water. The remnant of the VLDL then becomes an **intermediate-density lipoprotein (IDL)**—called intermediate density because of the lipid it has lost. About two thirds of the IDLs are taken up by the liver and the rest are converted to **low-density lipoproteins (LDLs).** An LDL is composed primarily of cholesterol because most triglyceride was removed from the original VLDL. It is even lower in lipid than an IDL and so even more dense. For a cell to absorb an LDL, it needs a receptor to bind it.

To review, VLDL has most of its triglyceride removed on leaving the liver. This process changes it to an IDL, then to an LDL. The LDL particle in the bloodstream still contains cholesterol that originally left the liver. Cells with LDL receptors pick up the LDL particles in a process called the **receptor pathway.**[27] When the LDL particles are received by a cell, they are broken down and parts of the LDL—the cholesterol and protein—are transported throughout the cell. In this way the cell absorbs the building blocks it can use to support the growth and development of the cell.

Research has demonstrated the importance of the LDL receptor. About 1 in 500 people have a genetic defect; they make only about half the LDL receptors needed to latch onto and remove circulating LDLs from the bloodstream.[5] Recall that LDLs are high in cholesterol.

With regard to the development of heart disease, certain scavenger white blood cells tend to leave the bloodstream and end up buried in the blood vessels. When these cells detect circulating LDL particles, they engulf and digest them. This process is called the **scavenger pathway** for LDL uptake and proceeds more rapidly as a person's LDL cholesterol level increases. A key part of this process appears to be alteration of the LDL molecule (more specifically oxidation) by the scavenger cells so that it cannot reenter the bloodstream. Cholesterol then inundates the scavenger cells.[27]

Note that some nutrients have antioxidant properties, as we cover in detail in Chapters 12 and 13. Fruits and vegetables are rich in many of these, such as β-carotene and vitamins C and E.[8] Eating fruits and vegetables regularly is likely one positive step we can take to try to slow the progression of heart disease.[12,16]

When this scavenger process recurs over many years, cholesterol builds up on the vessel wall, and **plaque** develops (see Figure 4-13 in the Nutrition Perspective for an illustration of this process). This plaque, which is probably first deposited to repair injuries in a vessel lining, is eventually mixed with protein and then covered with a cap of muscle cells and calcium.[10] The injuries are likely caused by smoking, high blood pressure, and elevated serum levels of LDL cholesterol. Viral infections also are implicated.

One important key to this process of fat and cholesterol deposition in the arteries—called atherosclerosis—lies in the liver. Because it contains about 50% to 75% of the LDL receptors in the body, the liver is the main regulator of blood cholesterol levels. To illustrate this point, consider the case of a child born essentially without LDL receptors in her liver who received a liver transplant. Before the operation the patient's cholesterol level was 1100 milligrams per 100 milliliters of serum. After the operation her serum cholesterol level dropped to 270 milligrams per 100 milliliters. A desirable serum cholesterol level is below 200 milligrams per 100 milliliters. This demonstrates the importance of the liver in controlling serum cholesterol levels.

A final critical participant in this whole process of lipid transport is the **high-density lipoprotein (HDL).** The liver and intestine produce HDLs that roam the bloodstream, picking up cholesterol from dying cells and other sources. HDLs donate the cholesterol primarily to other lipoproteins for transport back to the liver for excretion (Figure 4-9). Some HDLs may interact directly with the liver as well. This process is called **reverse transport of cholesterol.**[5]

Large-scale studies clearly show that a person's HDL cholesterol level is a good way to predict the risk for heart disease. If the serum HDL level is greater than 60 milligrams per 100 milliliters, the risk of heart disease is likely to be low. If the HDL cholesterol level is less than 35 milligrams per 100 milliliters, the risk of

low-density lipoprotein (LDL) The product of the intermediate density lipoprotein (IDL) containing primarily cholesterol; an elevated level is strongly linked to heart disease.

receptor pathway for cholesterol uptake A process by which LDL molecules (cholesterol-containing) are bound by cell receptors and incorporated into the cell.

scavenger pathway for cholesterol uptake A process by which LDL molecules (cholesterol-containing) are taken up by scavenger cells imbedded in the blood vessels.

plaque A cholesterol-rich substance deposited in the blood vessels; it contains various white blood cells, cholesterol and other lipids, and eventually calcium.

Rates of heart disease in many countries are higher in subpopulations who consume relatively few fruits and vegetables in their diets.[15]

high-density lipoprotein (HDL) Lipoprotein synthesized by the liver and small intestine that picks up cholesterol from dying cells and other sources and transfers it to the other lipoproteins in the bloodstream. A low HDL level increases the risk for heart disease.

reverse transport of cholesterol The process by which cholesterol is picked up by HDL molecules and transferred to other lipoproteins that can dispose of it.

EXPERT OPINION

Beyond Cholesterol: What Other Metabolic Abnormalities are Associated with Coronary Heart Disease?

GERALD M. REAVEN, M.D.

Considerable evidence has accumulated demonstrating that patients with high plasma total and LDL cholesterol concentrations are at increased risk of developing coronary heart disease. Studies also show that the risk of coronary heart disease is decreased following the lowering of serum LDL cholesterol. In response, the National Cholesterol Education Program (NCEP) has published specific guidelines regarding how to lower serum LDL cholesterol concentrations.

The general approach suggested by the NCEP is to screen individuals by measurement of plasma cholesterol concentration and to recommend that dietary intake of saturated fat be decreased. These suggestions are only a start, however, as having a high blood cholesterol level (hypercholesterolemia) is only one metabolic abnormality that increases risk of heart disease. It is now clear that significant risk exists in populations and individuals without elevated serum LDL cholesterol concentrations. Studies of Asian Indians in London have shown that these populations have a death rate from coronary heart disease approximately 50% higher than the British national average, which is already one of the higher rates in the world. This was true despite the fact that plasma total cholesterol levels were actually lower in Asian Indians. In addition, Indians in northwest London were found to have lower dietary intake of saturated fat and a higher intake of polyunsaturated fat than the British average. Even the most enthusiastic proponent of hypercholesterolemia in the genesis of heart disease would have difficulty in ascribing the increased risk in the Indian population to elevated serum cholesterol levels.

Fortunately, there is an explanation to account for the high rates of heart disease in Asian Indians. This population has been shown to have higher blood insulin levels (hyperinsulinemia), higher blood triglyceride levels (hypertriglyceridemia), and lower blood HDL cholesterol levels than British men and women. All these metabolic abnormalities—hyperinsulinemia, hypertriglyceridemia, and a low HDL cholesterol concentration—have been identified as risk factors for coronary heart disease. There seems little reason to doubt that their presence in Asian Indians is strongly related to the high prevalence of heart disease in this ethnic group.

Furthermore, it appears that these same risk factors apply to individuals of European descent. For example, data from Framingham, Mass. show that if the total cholesterol level is low (<200 mg/dl), but the HDL cholesterol concentration is also low (<40 mg/dl), the risk of a heart attack within the next 4 years is as great as if the total cholesterol level were >260 mg/dl. These high-risk individuals with low HDL cholesterol levels would be missed by screening and treatment programs that focus only on total and LDL cholesterol levels.

In addition, data from at least two prospective studies document hypertriglyceridemia as a primary risk factor for heart disease in women. The results of the Paris Prospective Study have shown triglyceride levels to be a significant, independent predictor of death from coronary heart disease in subjects with total cholesterol <220 mg/dl, as well as in subjects with impaired glucose tolerance or diabetes.

It has recently been suggested that a cluster of risk factors tends to occur in

---

developing heart disease is increased,[2] especially if the total cholesterol to HDL cholesterol ratio exceeds 4.5 to 1. Men often have HDL cholesterol levels in the high 30s to low 40s. Overall, however, the ratio of total cholesterol to HDL cholesterol is more important in predicting heart disease risk than considering either of them alone. Still, either way men are often more at risk.

menopause The cessation of menses in women, usually beginning at about 50 years of age.

Women on the other hand often have HDL cholesterol levels in the low 50s to low 60s and favorable total cholesterol to HDL cholesterol ratios. This is one reason why women, at least before **menopause,** have a lower risk for atherosclerosis, and therefore for heart attacks, than men. The estrogen produced by women in their childbearing years appears to help keep serum HDL cholesterol levels high. Estrogen replacement after menopause acts in the same way to keep heart disease risk low (see Chapter 14). Scientists believe that raising HDL levels may be just as important as lowering total cholesterol. Regular exercise, smoking cessation, and restricting kcalories to achieve a desirable weight all tend to raise HDL cholesterol levels.[12] Special attention should be focused on increasing exercise if one is sedentary.[29]

Since a high HDL cholesterol level is associated with a lower chance of developing heart disease, the HDL form of cholesterol has been considered "good" cholesterol. If so, the LDL form would be the "bad" cholesterol because a high

EXPERT OPINION

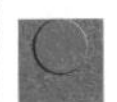

Beyond Cholesterol: What Other Metabolic Abnormalities are Associated with Coronary Heart Disease?—cont'd

individuals, and the underlying defect may be resistance to insulin-stimulated glucose uptake. Overall, hyperinsulinemic individuals (who are by implication insulin resistant) with either normal or impaired glucose tolerance, will tend to have high triglyceride levels and blood pressure and lower HDL cholesterol levels. This cluster of risk factors has been referred to as Syndrome X, in an effort to emphasize the existence of an entity that may have an important role in the etiology of coronary heart disease.

On the basis of the above discussion, it seems not unreasonable to suggest that a substantial proportion of risk is not just linked to high LDL cholesterol levels, but is also related to a series of associated abnormalities of carbohydrate and lipoprotein metabolism and blood pressure regulation. Indeed, this symptom complex may play a major role in the increasing frequency with which heart disease is observed in individuals and/or societies as they become "Westernized."

The implications of these findings are potentially of great significance. For example, knowledge of one's "cholesterol count" will not necessarily serve to identify all subjects at increased risk for development of heart disease, and heart attacks do occur in individuals with cholesterol concentrations less than 200 mg/dl—a value that would not be considered to be high by NCEP guidelines in an otherwise healthy individual. In addition, as we change our view of the proper screening approach to decreasing risk of heart disease, it also seems apparent that public health measures to reduce the risk through dietary changes—aimed at lowering serum LDL cholesterol levels—should be reconsidered for people whose metabolic abnormalities require another intervention. For example, all Americans are urged to follow a "prudent" diet, in which saturated fat is replaced by carbohydrate. Although this advice, if followed, should lead to a fall in LDL cholesterol concentration, it also tends to be associated with increases in serum glucose, insulin, and triglyceride concentrations and a fall in HDL cholesterol concentration. Obviously, it is necessary to question the advocacy of this "prudent" diet in individuals who already are insulin resistant and glucose intolerant as well as have high triglyceride and insulin and low HDL cholesterol levels. Indeed, in this situation, replacing saturated fat with monounsaturated and polyunsaturated fat would seem to represent more useful dietary advice.

In conclusion, there is little reason to doubt that increases in serum total and LDL cholesterol level play an important role in the etiology of coronary heart disease. At the same time, there is increasing evidence that a cluster of associated changes in carbohydrate and lipoprotein metabolism and blood pressure regulation are also of great importance in the genesis of heart disease. Until now, efforts to reduce morbidity and mortality from coronary heart disease have focused on hypercholesterolemia at the expense of these other processes. It seems reasonable to suggest that this narrow approach may no longer be appropriate for all people at risk.

Dr Reaven, a nationally recognized expert in both diabetes and heart disease, practices medicine in Palo Alto, California.

serum LDL cholesterol level increases the risk for heart disease. However, LDLs are not all bad; they carry needed cholesterol to cells and take cholesterol from the HDLs back to the liver for excretion. Probably only when serum LDL cholesterol level is high—greater than 130 to 160 milligrams per 100 milliliters—are LDLs really "bad" for the body.

CONCEPT CHECK

The bloodstream carries absorbed dietary fat as chylomicrons. Lipid synthesized by the liver is carried in the bloodstream as very low density lipoproteins (VLDLs). Once VLDL has most of its triglycerides removed, it eventually turns into a low-density lipoprotein (LDL). This lipoprotein is high in cholesterol. The LDLs are picked up by body cells, especially liver cells. A final lipoprotein is the high-density form, HDL. It picks up cholesterol from cells and transports it primarily to other lipoproteins for eventual transport back to the liver. An elevated serum LDL cholesterol level or total cholesterol to HDL cholesterol ratio above 4.5 to 1 is associated with high risk for heart disease, as is a low serum HDL cholesterol level.

Putting Lipids to Work in Food

While there is some overlap, the functions of fat in foods are often distinct from those in the body.

FATTY ACIDS

long-chain fatty acids Fatty acids that contain more than 12 carbons.

A factor that provides certain characteristics to food is the chain length of the fatty acids on the triglycerides present. Fats in foods that contain primarily saturated fatty acids are solid at room temperature, especially if the fatty acids have a **long chain** (12 carbons or longer). **Medium-chain** saturated **fatty acids** (6 to 10 carbons), such as those found in coconut oil, can produce liquid oils at room temperature. The shorter chain length overrides the effect of saturation. **Short-chain fatty acids** (two to four carbons) also form liquid oils at room temperature. Food sources of short-chain fatty acids include dairy fats (see Appendix H). Fats containing primarily polyunsaturated or monounsaturated fatty acids are usually liquid at room temperature. Chain length is not an issue.

The capability of some saturated fatty acids of short- or medium-chain lengths to form oils at room temperature is significant. Nondairy creamers initially appear to be a healthful substitute for cream because of cream's high content of saturated fats. However, many dry coffee creamers contain coconut oil, which is also high in saturated fatty acids. Manufacturers use coconut oil or **hydrogenated** vegetable oils partly because this allows the product a long shelf life without turning rancid. You will see why in the following section. Low-fat or skim milk is a healthier choice than either liquid or dry nondairy creamers.

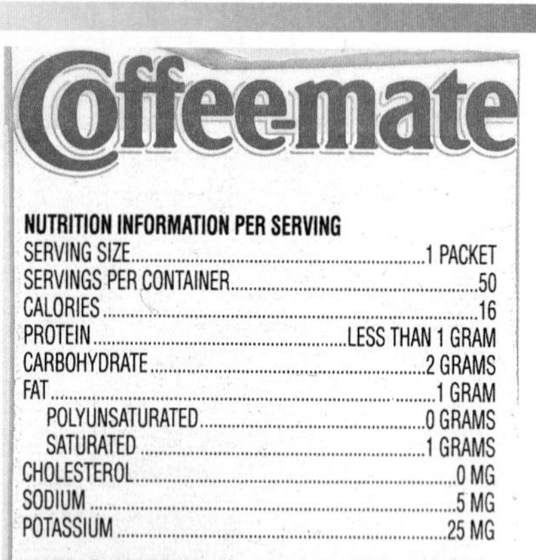

Hydrogenation of Fatty Acids

To solidify vegetable oils into margarines and shortenings the polyunsaturated fatty acids in plant oils must become more saturated. Hydrogens are added across the carbon-carbon double bonds in the fatty acids. This process, called hydrogenation, turns many of the carbon-carbon double bonds into single bonds (Figure 4-10). It

Hydrogen source

Unsaturated vegetable oil (liquid)

Adding hydrogen under pressure

Hydrogenated fat (solid or semisolid)

Figure 4-10 How liquid fatty acids become solid fat. **A,** Unsaturated fatty acids are present in liquid form. **B,** Hydrogens are added (hydrogenation), changing double bonds to single bonds and producing trans fatty acids. This structural change also causes the fats to raise serum cholesterol levels (like many saturated fats), providing another reason for us to limit intake of hydrogenated fat. **C,** The hydrogenated product, likely to be used in margarine, shortenings, or deep fat frying applications.

also produces some trans fatty acids, as we discussed in the earlier Nutrition Focus. Both changes increase hardness. Generally, the harder the product—stick margarine compared with tub margarine—the more hydrogenation has occurred.

Hydrogenated fats are easier to use in some techniques of food production, such as in making pastries and cakes. Manufacturers also prefer to use solid shortening for the production of many crackers and snack products. As public pressure has persuaded manufacturers to remove the tropical oils (palm and coconut) from foods, partially hydrogenated soybean oil has become the major replacement. Notice how many chips, snack products, and crackers contain "partially hydrogenated vegetable oil (soybean oil)" on the label.

Rancidity

Another reason manufacturers hydrogenate plant oils is to reduce their deterioration. The carbon-carbon double bonds in polyunsaturated fatty acids easily break down and form **rancid** products. Ultraviolet light, air, heat, and various chemicals attack the carbon-carbon double bonds and break them, destroying the structure of the polyunsaturated fatty acids. You may have recognized the disagreeable odor and sour, stale taste of decomposing oils. Even though rancid oils are potentially toxic, their unappealing taste and odor most likely discourage people from eating enough to pose a threat. However, rancidity reduces a product's shelf life and is therefore costly to the manufacturer.

Nature provides polyunsaturated fatty acids some natural protection against rancidity. Vitamin E is an **antioxidant** found in plant oils. Other naturally occurring antioxidants include vitamin C and beta-carotene. Antioxidants stop **oxidizing agents** from breaking the carbon-carbon double bonds in fatty acids. Oxidizing agents usually seek electrons to capture. Vitamin E and antioxidants donate electrons to oxidizing agents. This keeps the electrons in the carbon-carbon double bonds of fatty acids, and the bonds they form, safe from attack (see Chapter 12).

When food manufacturers want to prevent rancidity in polyunsaturated fats, they often add the antioxidants **BHA** and **BHT.** Look for these food additives in salad dressings, breakfast cereals, cake mixes, and other products that contain fat. Manufacturers also tightly seal their products from the atmosphere and use other methods to reduce the presence of oxygen inside packages.

rancid Containing products of decomposed fatty acids; they yield unpleasant flavors and odors.

antioxidant A compound that prevents the oxidation of substances in food or the body, particularly lipids. Antioxidants are especially important in preventing the oxidation of polyunsaturated lipids in the membranes of cells. An antioxidant is able to donate electrons to electron-seeking compounds in turn reducing electron capture and thus breakdown of unsaturated fatty acids and other cell components.

oxidizing agents Compounds that seek electrons. A compound is "oxidized" when, among other possible changes, it loses an electron.

BHA and BHT Butylated hydroxyanisol and butylated hydroxytoluene—two common synthetic antioxidants added to foods.

CONCEPT CHECK

At room temperature saturated fatty acids tend to form solid fats, and polyunsaturated and monounsaturated fatty acids tend to form liquid oils. Hydrogenation is the process of turning carbon-carbon double bonds of fatty acids into single bonds by adding hydrogen atoms. As this occurs, some trans fatty acids are created. Hydrogenation solidifies the fat and reduces the breakdown of fatty acids commonly found in polyunsaturated varieties, in turn reducing rancidity. The presence of antioxidants in oils, such as vitamin E, naturally protects unsaturated fatty acids against rancidity.

TRIGLYCERIDES

Triglycerides in foods are very important for **satiety,** that is, feeling satisfied after eating. The composition of what is eaten helps determine the rate of stomach clearance, due to a hormonal response (see Chapter 6). Slower emptying allows food to remain in the stomach longer while acidic secretions complete this important phase of digestion. Since eating fat in our diets causes the stomach to empty slower than eating carbohydrate or protein, a high-fat meal makes us feel full longer.

Many people who want to reduce weight know that fats are high in kcalories. They find it easiest to cut kcalories by cutting out much of the fat they eat. However, if dieters lower fat intake too much, they lose its satiety value and get hungry quicker.

satiety A state in which there is no desire to eat, a feeling of satisfaction.

Thus lowering fat intake too much when dieting can actually be self-defeating. (See Chapter 9 for further discussion.)

Triglycerides and other fats in foods also provide important texture and carry flavors. The most tender cuts of meat are high in fat. This fat can be seen in the marbling of meat. Low-fat meats such as flank steak or brisket require special preparation techniques, such as marinating or slow, moist cooking, to ensure tenderness. Many flavors are fat soluble; their essences dissolve in fat, and the fat carries them to the sensory cells in the mouth that discriminate taste and smell. Perhaps you have used an oil flavoring in baking or to make candy. Heating spices in oil intensifies the flavors of an Indian curry or Mexican dish far more than simply adding them at the table. We thus associate flavorful foods with fatty foods for good reason.

If you have ever eaten a high-fat cheese or cream cheese, you will probably agree that fat melting on the tongue feels good. This love of fat is universal. Western diets, Eskimo diets, and Mediterranean diets are all high in fat. Immigrants to Western cultures quickly embrace the high-fat diet found here.

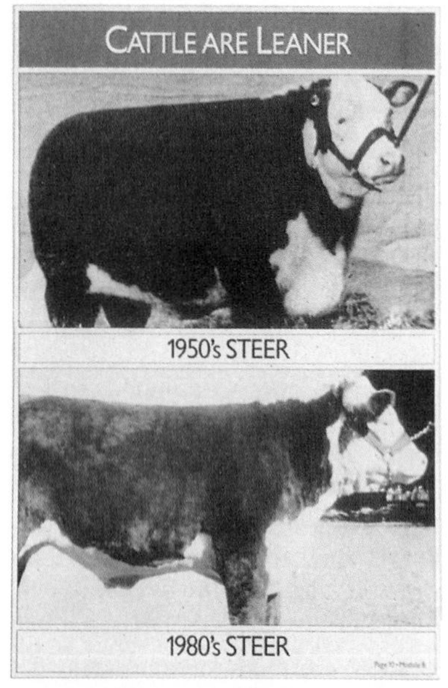

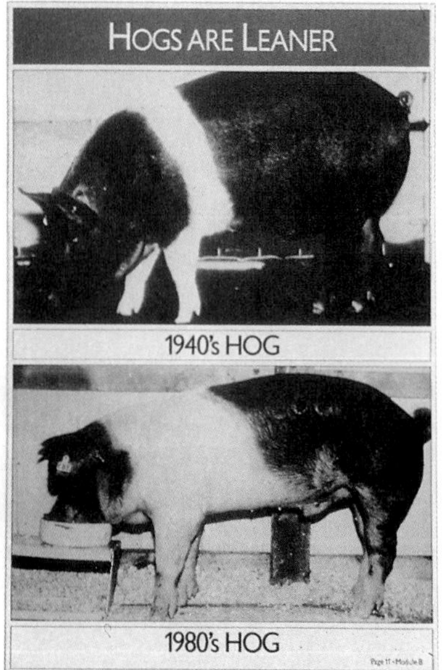

Today's leaner animals make it easier for us to reduce saturated fat intake.

PHOSPHOLIPIDS AND CHOLESTEROL

Phospholipids act as emulsifiers not only in the process of digestion, but they also play a role in the emulsification of fats and oils in foods. Commercial salad dressings are examples of emulsification put to practical use—emulsifiers, such as Polysorbate 60 and lecithin, are added to salad dressings to keep the vegetable oil suspended in the water. Eggs used in cake recipes likewise emulsify the fat with the water in the milk used. Notice the label on salad dressings or cake mixes and examine the ingredients listed. See if emulsifiers are listed. The breakdown products that arise during fat digestion, monoglycerides and diglycerides, are also good emulsifiers, and are sometimes used in cake mixes and salad dressings for that reason.

Cholesterol does not have a particular role in food, as is seen for some of the other fats. It should be remembered, however, that cholesterol intake arises from the animal-based products we eat.

CONCEPT CHECK

Via foods, triglycerides provide satiety after eating. Fats also provide flavor and texture. Phospholipids serve as emulsifiers in foods.

Recommendations for Fat Intake

There is no RDA for fat. A good goal, as suggested earlier, is to consume about 4% of energy from plant oils incorporated into foods to get the essential fatty acids. Recall that this percentage amounts to only about 1 tablespoon of oil per day, so generally all of us easily do that. Currently our diet contains about 7% of energy from polyunsaturated fat. A limit to 10% of kcalories is often recommended,[5] in part because fat breakdown—when part of lipoproteins—is linked to increased cholesterol deposition in the arteries, as we just covered.[12]

The U.S. diet contains about 38% of total kcalories as fat. Vegetable sources supply about half this fat and animal sources supply the other half. Major sources of fat in the U.S. diet include animal flesh, whole milk, pastries, eggs, cheese, margarine, and mayonnaise.

The American Heart Association (AHA) and many other health agencies recommend a fat intake of up to 30% of total kcalories, with a ratio of about 10:10:10 for saturated to monounsaturated to polyunsaturated fatty acids (Table 4-2). Table 4-3 shows a diet that follows this basic recommendation. One added bonus is that the missing fat kcalories in these diets allows additions of more healthful foods, like fruits, vegetables, and whole grains.[22] A good start on this type of diet is a low-fat breakfast—a high-fiber cereal, low-fat or nonfat milk, and fruit juice are options.

Table 4-2 Dietary guidelines for healthy American adults* A statement for physicians and health professionals by the Nutrition Committee, American Heart Association (AHA)

1. Total fat intake should be less than 30% of kcalories.
2. Saturated fat intake should be less than 10% of kcalories.
3. Polyunsaturated fat intake should not exceed 300 mg/day.
4. Cholesterol intake should not exceed 300 mg/day.
5. Carbohydrate intake should constitute 50% or more of kcalories, with emphasis on complex carbohydrates.
6. Protein intake should provide the remainder of the kcalories.
7. Sodium intake should not exceed 3 g/day.
8. Alcholic consumption should not exceed 1 to 2 oz of ethanol per day. Two ounces of 100 proof whiskey, 8 oz of wine, or 24 oz of beer, all of which contain 1 oz of ethanol.
9. Total kcalories should be sufficient to maintain the individual's recommended body weight.
10. A wide variety of foods should be consumed.

*Chapter 2 listed the Dietary Guidelines for both Americans and Canadians. Chapter 18 reviews all these guidelines in the context of adult health. "Eat less fat" is a common general health message given to adults of North America, not withstanding who issues the report.

The AHA further recommends lowering fat intake to no more than 20% of total kcalories in cases where elevated serum cholesterol level does not respond to this moderate recommendation. This is a difficult diet to plan. Advice and counsel of a registered dietitian would be helpful.[26]

The National Cholesterol Education Program, established in 1985 in the United States, recommends reducing saturated fatty acids to 7% of total kcalories if a high serum cholesterol level does not respond to reducing it to 10%.[5] In other words, the lower the better. By encouraging a reduction in total fat and saturated fat intake, all these suggestions are in line with the dietary guidelines issued for Americans.

Fats in Foods

Table 4-3 provides an example of the amount of fat in foods in a day's menu. In the exchange system, foods from both the vegetable and fruit groups are essentially fat free. In the milk group the amount of fat varies with food choice—skim milk has a trace (sometimes calculated as 1 gram), low-fat has 5 grams, and whole has 8 grams per cup. Whole milk was the major source of fat in dairy products until low-fat varieties gained in popularity. Now cheese is the primary source of fat from dairy products. Most foods from the grain group contain small amounts of fat, so this is ignored in the exchange system. However, read the label carefully as some gourmet breads, snack crackers, and cereals can surprise you! In the meat group, fat values vary with food choice—lean has 3 grams, medium-fat has 5 grams, and high-fat has 8 grams per ounce. The fat group has 5 grams of fat per serving.

For foods in general the highest nutrient density for fat is found in salad oils, butter, margarine, and mayonnaise. All contain about 100% of kcalories as fat (Figure 4-11). Walnuts, bologna, avocados, and bacon have about 80%. Peanut butter and cheddar cheese have about 75%. Steak and hamburgers have about 60%, and chocolate bars, ice cream, doughnuts, and whole milk have about 50% of kcalories as fat. Pumpkin pie and cupcakes have 35%. Bread contains about 15% of its kcalories as fat. Corn flakes, sugar, and skim milk have essentially no fat.

Careful label reading is necessary to determine the true fat content of a food. Lets say you read on the package sticker that a certain brand of hot dog is only 27% fat, or 73% fat-free. This might initially impress you. However, it currently means that the hot dog is 27% fat by weight, not in terms of kcalories. Remember

Table 4-3 Menus containing 2000 kcalories and various percentages of fat

30% of Kcalories as Fat		20% of Kcalories as Fat	
Breakfast	Teaspoons of fat		Teaspoons of fat
1 cup orange juice	0	same	0
¾ cup shredded wheat	⅕	same	⅕
1 toasted bagel	⅕	same	⅕
2 t margarine	1¾	same	1¾
1 cup 1% milk	½	1 cup nonfat milk	⅒
Lunch			
2 slices whole-wheat bread	½	same	½
2 oz lean roast beef	1	2 oz boiled ham	½
2 t mayonnaise	1½	same	1½
lettuce	0	same	0
1 sliced tomato	0	same	0
8 animal crackers	⅕	same	⅕
Snack			
1 apple	⅙	same	⅙
Dinner			
3 oz broiled lamb chop	2⅓	3 oz broiled halibut	⅔
1½ pasta	⅔	same	⅔
2 t margarine	1¾	1 t margarine	⅞
½ cup broccoli	0	same	0
1 cup 1% milk	½	1 cup nonfat milk	⅒
		1 banana	⅒
Snack			
2 T raisins	0	¼ cup	0
6 cups air-popped popcorn	½	same	½
		with 1 t margarine	⅞
with 2 t margarine	1¾		
TOTALS	14		8½

that water makes up a significant part of the weight of many foods, including a hot dog. Actually, 83% of the kcalories in this product come from fat (Figure 4-12). So until the new labeling laws that we talked about in Chapter 2 are in place to stop this practice, take care not to be deceived by these kinds of statements.

Animal fats contain about 40% to 60% of total fat as saturated fatty acids and are the chief contributor of saturated fatty acids to the U.S. diet. Saturated fatty acids with 12 to 16 carbons are the primary contributors to high serum cholesterol levels.[5] These problem saturated fatty acids constitute about 25% to 50% of the total fat in animal fats. So despite the fact that some saturated fatty acids in meats are not linked to high blood cholesterol levels (the 18 carbon stearic acid),[7] meat

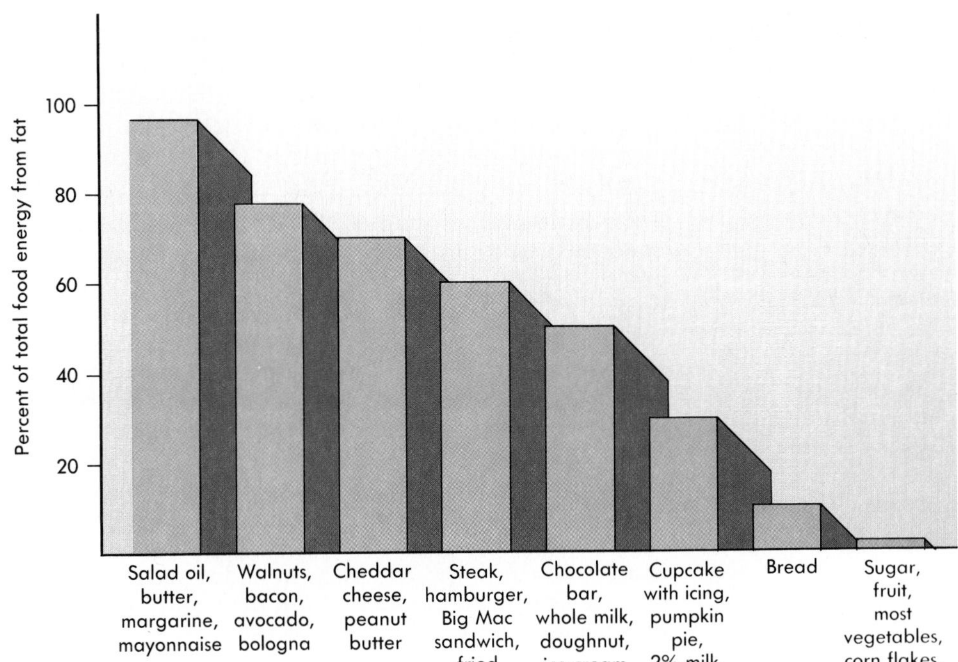

Figure 4-11 Percentage of kcalories as fats in foods. Vegetable oils, butter, margarine, and mayonnaise provide almost all kcalories as fats.

BEEF FRANKS

73% Fat Free

Ingredients: Beef, Water, Corn Syrup, Salt, Dextrose, Flavorings, Sodium Ascorbate (Vitamin C), Sodium Nitrate, Extract of Paprika.

Nutrition Information Per Serving
Seving Size - 1 link, 1.6 ounces (45 grams)

Servings Per Package - 10

Calories	130	Fat	12 Grams
Protein	5 Grams	Sodium	450 mg (0.45 Grams)
Carbohydrates	1 Gram		

On a weight basis: $\frac{\text{fat weight (12 grams)} \times 100}{\text{total weight (45 grams)}}$ = 27% weight is fat

On a kcalorie basis: $\frac{\text{fat kcalories } (12 \times 9) \times 100}{\text{total kcalories (130)}}$ = 83% kcalories from fat

Figure 4-12 Is this hot dog 27% or 83% fat?

Fat Replacements

For years manufacturers have used starch-derivatives and other carbohydrates to bind water in foods in an attempt to find a substitute that captures the flavor and feeling of fat in the mouth and provides satiety following meals. These include cellulose, plant gums, N-Oil, Paselli SA2, Sta-Slim 143, and Maltrin.[28] The goal is to have products that feel like ice cream melting on the tongue but contain few fat kcalories. In the past it has been difficult for individuals to change food choices, to use different preparation techniques, and to limit intake of many culturally based or favorite foods that are high in fat. Recently, public and scientific interests have focused on two newer fat replacements—Olestra and Simplesse. Still other products are in development and could be in use as you read this chapter.[23]

Olestra

Olestra is a sucrose polyester made by adding fatty acids to the hydroxyl groups (—OH) on a sucrose (table sugar) molecule. Ester bonds are formed, so it is called a sucrose polyester. Usually eight fatty acids are added to each sucrose molecule. The manufacturer can change the characteristics of the product by adding greater or fewer numbers of fatty acids. Sucrose polyester with many fatty acids attached cannot be digested by either human digestive enzymes or bacteria that live in the intestine; therefore, it yields no kcalories to the body. As it leaves the body, it can even pull cholesterol-containing substances found in the intestine with it, thereby eventually lowering the person's blood cholesterol level. The product is quite versatile as an ingredient. The manufacturer feels it can replace up to 35% of the fat in oils and shortenings in the home, and 75% of the fats used for deep-fat frying in restaurants and food manufacturing.[1] Presently, however, the manufacturer's petition to the FDA for approval is limited to replacing 100% of the fat used in the preparation of "savory snacks."

There are still some problems with sucrose polyester. It tends to bind the fat-soluble vitamin E, reducing its absorption. The manufacturer has proposed adding enough vitamin E to compensate for the amount bound and excreted from use of sucrose polyester. Some years ago the FDA would not permit the use of mineral oil in foods as a no-kcalorie fat because it bound fat-soluble vitamins. Because of that and other questions, it is unclear when this product will be available.

Sucrose polyester (with the maximum number of fatty acids attached)

Simplesse

The manufacturer of Simplesse has developed a technique in which egg and milk proteins are mixed together with heat in such a way that microscopic, mistlike protein globules are produced. The globules feel like fat in the mouth. While it yields energy, Simplesse has only about 1.3 kcalories per gram, which is much less than regular fat's 9 kcalories per gram.[28] Protein usually has 4 kcalories per gram; however, much water is incorporated into this product, diluting the caloric density.

Simplesse is most useful for replacing fat in mayonnaise, salad dressings, sour cream, yogurt, frozen or refrigerated desserts, and cheese. Because high heat alters Simplesse's structure so much that it no longer resembles fat, it cannot be used for frying, but various forms can be used in many high temperature situations, such as pie crusts, soups, and sauces. Since cheese has become primary source of fat from dairy products, pizza, lasagna, and other main dishes prepared from cheeses, that made with Simplesse could be a healthful method of decreasing the fat content in the diet while still providing a good source of calcium. When Simplesse is used in frozen desserts, it reduces kcalories by about one-half and fat content to a negligible amount.

Fat replacements in perspective

If you look at the 15 major contributors of total fat in the U.S. diet listed in Table 4-4, you will understand why the beneficial effects of fat replacements are uncertain, and may not be very substantial. Overall, many major contributors to fat in the diet will remain so. The main benefit from using fat replacements will be cutting some fat in the diet, most importantly saturated fat and cholesterol. Several estimates suggest foods that are realistic candidates for fat modification could produce the reduction in fat necessary to bring the average diet within the 30% of kcalories from fat, the goal set by many health-related agencies.[5] The actual kcalorie reduction will probably be less impressive because people tend to make up the lost energy by eating more.

We will always need balanced eating habits and moderation in food choices. A diet rich in fruits, vegetables, whole grains, and lean animal products still deserves the most attention. Lowering the amount of fat in recipes we make at home is also important, such as using low-fat or nonfat milk instead of whole milk. Fat replacements can reduce intake of saturated fat and cholesterol in popular foods many of us are unwilling to give up, such as ice cream. But we won't know the true impact of fat replacements on our diets until they are approved for more general use. For now, note that there is much scientific and economic interest in producing flavorful snack and dessert foods that yield less fat

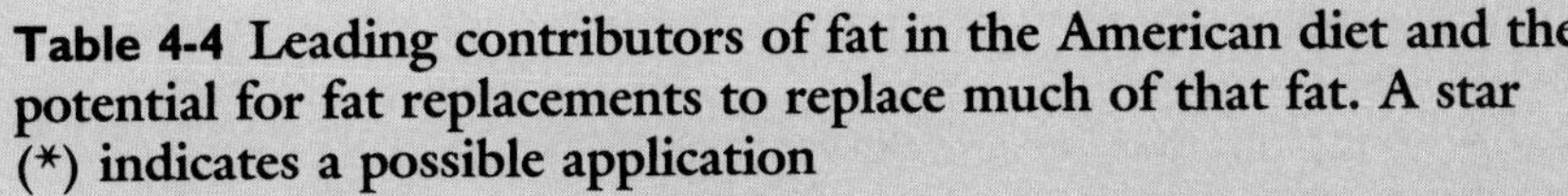

Table 4-4 Leading contributors of fat in the American diet and the potential for fat replacements to replace much of that fat. A star (*) indicates a possible application

Food source of fat &	% of total fat in diet†	Applications for Olestra	Applications for Simplesse
hamburgers, cheese-burger, meatloaf	7.0	—	—
hot dogs, lunch meat	6.4	—	sausage, pate*
whole milk	6.0	—	—
doughnuts, cakes, cookies	6.0	shortenings, frying*	—
beef steaks, roasts	5.5	—	—
white bread, rolls, crackers	4.9	shortenings*	—
eggs	4.6	—	—
cheese	4.5	—	spreads*
margarine	4.5	—	spreads; not for frying
mayonnaise	4.3	—	*
pork	4.0	—	—
French fries, fried potatoes	2.7	frying*	—
salad and cooking oils	2.6	(?)*	—
butter	2.4	—	—
ice cream, frozen desserts	2.1	—	*!

†Based on NHANES II.
—no application as of yet.
NOTE: The use of Simplesse is limited mostly because it cannot be heated to frying temperatures without losing its desirable properties.

is still rich in those fatty acids that are linked to high blood cholesterol levels. Some plant products also contain significant amounts of problem saturated fatty acids in comparison to total fat; for example, cottonseed oil (27%), palm oil (46%), palm kernel oil (79%), and coconut oil (89%).

Plant fats contain mostly unsaturated fatty acids, ranging from 73% to 94% of total fat, excluding palm and coconut oils. Plant oils supply the majority of the linoleic and alpha-linolenic acid in the U.S. food supply. Olive oil, canola oil, and peanut oil contain a moderate to high amount of total fat as monounsaturated fatty acids (49% to 77%). Some animal fats are also good sources (30% to 47%; Figure 4-2). Corn, cottonseed, sunflower, soybean, and safflower oils contain mostly polyunsaturated fat (54% to 77%) in terms of total fat. Note that plant oils vary in their amounts of polyunsaturated fat. While many oils are similar in composition, significant variations are common. "Vegetable oil" is too general a term to list on a label. The specific oil used, for example, corn or palm oil, should be known. Unfortunately, the label may list a variety of oils, and any one could have been used. That makes it difficult for people trying to limit their intake of saturated fat.

Note that some fat in food is obvious: butter on bread, mayonnaise in potato salad, and marbling in raw meat. Fat is less obvious in other foods. Still these foods contribute much fat to our diets. Fat is hidden in whole milk, pastries, cookies, cake, cheese, hot dogs, crackers, French fries, and ice cream. When you can't find a nutrition label, remember that moderating portion size is a good way to keep fat intake down. Overall, as we try to cut fat from our diets, these hidden fats need to be exposed and controlled, along with the more obvious sources. Chapter 17 reviews how to reduce fat intake when eating at quick-service restaurants.

The latest fat research points to the 14-carbon myristic acid as the main blood cholesterol-raising fatty acid. This is especially high in dairy fats and helps explain why palm oil is not as cholesterol raising as butter. Palm oil is low in myristic acid (see Appendix H).

CONCEPT CHECK

There is no recommended dietary allowance for fat. We need about 4% of total energy intake from plant oils to get the needed essential fatty acids. Many health-related agencies recommend a diet containing no more than 30% of energy as fat, and no more than one third of that as saturated fat. The current American diet contains about 38% of energy as fat, with two fifths of that from saturated fat. Foods high in fat (over 60% of total kcalories) include plant oils, butter, margarine, mayonnaise, walnuts, bacon, avocados, peanut butter, cheddar cheese, steak, and hamburger.

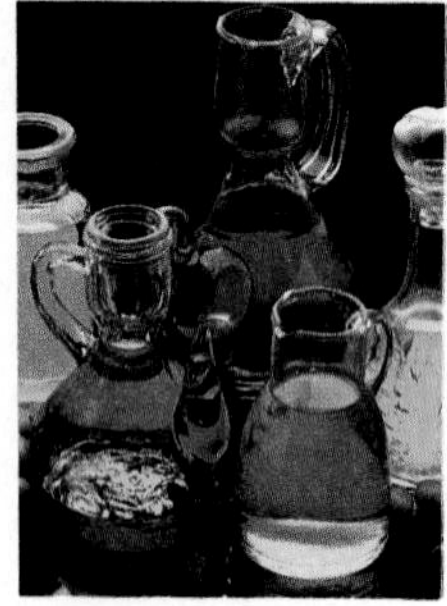

Summary

1. Lipids are a group of relatively oxygen-poor compounds that dissolve in chloroform, benzene, or ether. Saturated fatty acids contain no carbon-carbon double bonds, monounsaturated fatty acids contain one carbon-carbon double bond, and polyunsaturated fatty acids contain two or more carbon-carbon double bonds.
2. If the carbon-carbon double bonds starting from the methyl end ($-CH_3$) in the fatty acid first appear at the third carbon atom, then the fatty acid is an omega-3 fatty acid. If the carbon-carbon double bonds starting from the methyl end first appear at the sixth carbon atom, it is an omega-6 fatty acid. Both omega-3 and omega-6 fatty acids are essential parts of a diet.
3. When cells use omega-3 fatty acids rather than omega-6 fatty acids to synthesize hormonelike compounds called eicosanoids, the products tend to reduce blood clotting, blood pressure, and inflammatory responses in the body.
4. The triglyceride is the major form of fat in food and in the body. Phospholipids are derivatives of the triglycerides. Phospholipids are important parts of cell membranes, and some act as efficient emulsifiers.
5. Cholesterol forms vital compounds, such as hormones, parts of cell membranes, and bile acids. Cells in the body make cholesterol whether we eat it or not.
6. Lipids are carried in the bloodstream by various lipoproteins: chylomicrons, very low density lipoproteins (VLDLs), low-density lipoproteins (LDLs), and high-density lipoproteins (HDLs).
7. The ratio of total cholesterol to HDL cholesterol is a better predictor of cardiovascular disease than total cholesterol, although an elevated serum LDL cholesterol level and a low serum HDL cholesterol level also are risk factors.
8. Lipids composed of saturated fatty acids tend to be solid at room temperature and those with polyunsaturated fatty acids are usually liquid at room temperature. Hydrogenation is the process of turning carbon-carbon double bonds in fatty acids into single bonds by adding hydrogens. This solidifies vegetable oils and reduces the rancid breakdown of fatty acids, but increases trans fatty acid levels.
9. There is no RDA for fat. We need about 4% of total energy intake from plant oils to get the needed essential fatty acids.
10. The typical American diet contains about 38% of the kcalories from fat. Many health agencies and scientific groups suggest reducing fat intake to no more than 30% of kcalories consumed.

Study Questions

1. Describe the difference between a saturated and polyunsaturated fatty acid in both food and their effects on the human body. Be sure to consider the structure of these two types of fatty acids.
2. Describe the structures and roles of the four major blood lipoproteins.
3. What are the recommendations of health care professionals regarding fat intake? What does this mean in terms of actual food choices?
4. What are 3 functions of fat in food? How are these different than the functions of lipids in the human body?
5. What are the significance and three possible usages of the new fat replacements?

REFERENCES

1. Position of the American Dietetic Association: Fat replacements, *Journal of The American Dietetic Association* 91:1285, 1991.
2. Buring JE and others: Decreased HDL_2 and HDL_3 cholesterol, Apo A-I and Apo A-II, and increased risk of myocardial infarction, *Circulation* 85:22, 1992.
3. Burke GL and others: Trends in serum cholesterol levels from 1980 to 1987, *New England Journal of Medicine* 324:941, 1991.
4. Cunnane SC and others: a-Linolenic acid in humans: direct functional role or dietary precursor? *Nutrition* 7:437, 1991.
5. Dalen JE: National Cholesterol Education Program, *Archives of Internal Medicine* 151:1071, 1991.
6. Das UN and others: Clinical significance of essential fatty acids, *Nutrition* 4:337, 1988.
7. Denke MA, Grundy SM: Effects of fats high in stearic acid on lipid and lipoprotein concentrations in men, *American Journal of Clinical Nutrition* 54:1036, 1991.
8. Frei B: Ascorbic acid protects lipids in human plasma and low-density lipoprotein against oxidative damage, *American Journal of Clinical Nutrition* 54:1113S, 1991.
9. Fried RE and others: The effect of filtered-coffee consumption on plasma lipid levels, *Journal of the American Medical Association* 267:811, 1992.
10. Epstein FH: The pathogenesis of coronary artery disease and the acute coronary syndromes, *New England Journal of Medicine,* 326:242, 1992.
11. Grover SA and others: The benefits of treating hyperlipidemia to prevent coronary heart disease, *Journal of the American Medical Association* 267:816, 1992.
12. Grundy SM: Cholesterol and coronary heart disease: future directions, *Journal of the American Medical Association* 264:3053, 1990.
13. Harris WS: Fish oils and plasma lipid and lipoprotein metabolism in humans: a critical review, *Journal of Lipid Research* 30:785, 1989.
14. Hunter JE, Applewhite TH: Reassessment of fatty acid availability in the U.S. diet, *American Journal of Clinical Nutrition* 54:363, 1991.
15. James P and others: Meeting summary, *Nutrition Reviews* 50:68, 1992.
16. Kritchevsky D: Antioxidant vitamins in the prevention of cardiovascular disease, *Nutrition Today,* Jan/Feb 1992, p 30.
17. Lands WEM: Biosynthesis of prostaglandins, *Annual Review of Nutrition* 11:41, 1991.
18. Leaf A, Weber PC: Cardiovascular effects of n-3 fatty acid, *New England Journal of Medicine* 318:549, 1988.
19. Mensink PR, Katan MB: Effect of dietary trans fatty acids on high-density and low-density lipoprotein cholesterol levels in healthy subjects, *New England Journal Of Medicine* 323:439, 1991.
20. Ornish D and others: Can lifestyle changes reverse coronary heart disease? *Lancet* 336:129, 1990.
21. Otani H and others: Long-term effects of a cholesterol-free diet on serum cholesterol levels in zen monks, *New England Journal of Medicine* 326:416, 1992.
22. Retzlaff BM and others: Changes in vitamin and mineral intakes and serum concentrations among free-living men on cholesterol-lowering diets: the dietary alternatives study, *American Journal of Clinical Nutrition* 53:890, 1991.
23. Segal M: Fat substitutes: a taste for the future? *FDA Consumer,* Dec 25, 1990.
24. Seppa K and others: Moderate and heavy alcohol consumption have no favorable effect on lipid values, *Archives of Internal Medicine* 152:297, 1992.
25. Simopoulos AP: Omega-3 fatty acids in health and disease and in growth and development, *American Journal of Clinical Nutrition* 54:438, 1991.
26. Smith-Schneider LM and others: Dietary fat reduction strategies, *Journal of The American Dietetic Association* 92:34, 1992.
27. Steinberg D, Witztum JL: Lipoproteins and atherogenesis, *Journal of the American Medical Association* 264:3047, 1990.
28. Stern JS, Hermann-Zaidins MG: Fat replacements: A new strategy for dietary change, *Journal of The American Dietetic Association* 92:91, 1992.
29. Thompson PD and others: Modest changes in high-density lipoprotein concentration and metabolism with prolonged exercise training, *Circulation* 78:25, 1988.
30. Whyte JL: Oat bran lowers plasma cholesterol levels in mildly hypercholesterolemic men, *Journal of The American Dietetic Association* 92:446, 1992.

SUGGESTED READINGS

To learn more about interactions between diet and lipoproteins see the articles by Grundy and Steinberg. Both focus strongly on the effects of diet. For a detailed discussion of omega-3 fatty acids see the article by Simopoulos. After reading this article consider reading the more technical reports by Leaf and Yetiv. These three articles will give you a strong background in this developing area of nutrition research. Finally, see the article by the ADA on fat replacements for a detailed look at this topic for the 1990s.

TAKE ACTION

Are you at risk for heart disease?

In the 1980s, a flood of products touting oat bran hit grocery shelves. But that was a mere trickle compared to the number of products bearing "reduced-fat" and "fat-free" labels. From cakes and condiments to meats and snacks, it's become a $6 billion industry. Fat-free and low-fat have become the buzzwords of the 1990s.

How do your food practices today reflect these dietary trends and stack up against guidelines that have been suggested in this chapter for fat, saturated fat, and cholesterol intake? Compare the dietary evaluation you completed at the end of Chapter 2 with the guidelines issued by the American Heart Association and the National Cholesterol Education Program. These suggest the following practices for heart health:

- limit or reduce total fat intake to less than 30% of total kcalories.
- reduce saturated fat intake to 7% to 10% of kcalories or less.
- limit cholesterol to less than 200 to 300 milligrams/day.

To see whether the diet you wrote down for your nutritional assessment at the end of Chapter 2 met these guidelines, the following pieces of information are needed from your assessment (write the numbers in the blanks given):

TOTAL KCALORIE INTAKE ______________
TOTAL GRAMS OF FAT ______________
GRAMS OF SATURATED FAT ______________
MILLIGRAMS OF CHOLESTEROL ______________

Now complete the following steps:

1. Multiply your total grams of fat by 9 (kcalories/gram of fat). Then divide the result by your total kcalorie intake. Next multiply this number by 100. THIS WILL GIVE YOU THE % OF KCALORIES YOU CONSUMED FROM FAT.
   % OF KALORIES FROM FAT ______________
   IS IT LESS THAN 30% OF YOUR TOTAL KCALS?
   YES __________ NO __________
2. Multiply the grams of saturated fat you ate by 9 (kcals/gram of fat). Divide the result by your total kcalorie intake. Now multiply this number by 100. THIS WILL GIVE YOU THE % OF KCALORIES YOU CONSUMED FROM SATURATED FAT.
   % OF KCALORIES FROM SATURATED FAT ______________
   IS IT 10% OF YOUR KCALORIES OR LESS? YES __________ NO __________
3. Look at your milligrams of cholesterol.
   IS IT LESS THAN 300 MILLIGRAMS? YES __________ NO __________
4. Look back at the foods you ate and notice the foods that contributed the most fat, saturated fat, and cholesterol. If you didn't meet one or more of the guidelines, how could you change what you ate that day to improve your diet.?
5. Now take the next step. Do you know your HDL and LDL cholesterol levels and your total cholesterol to HDL cholesterol ratio? If not, try to have them checked soon.
6. Finally, fill in the following assessment of your risk for developing premature cardiovascular disease. Then describe how you could modify your diet and lifestyle, if necessary, to reduce your risk. You may not prevent the disease by controlling the factors, but you can most likely slow its development.

Do you have . . .	Yes	No
• a history of smoking?	______	______
• high blood pressure?	______	______
• a high LDL cholesterol level?	______	______
• a low HDL cholesterol level?	______	______
• a high total cholesterol to HDL cholesterol ratio?	______	______
• diabetes mellitus?	______	______
• a history of inactivity?	______	______
• a family history of premature cardiovascular disease?	______	______
• a history of obesity?	______	______
• male gender?	______	______

Other factors also could be considered, as discussed in the Nutrition Perspective, but this provides a good start for assessing your risk. ▲

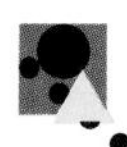

Cardiovascular Disease

Cardiovascular disease is the major killer of Americans. About 600,000 people die of heart disease each year in the United States. The figure rises to almost 1 million if we include strokes and other circulatory diseases in this more global term—cardiovascular disease. These are chronic diseases—they take years to show symptoms. There is no single cause of cardiovascular disease, but many factors increase the risk for its development.

Heart disease and strokes are associated with poor blood circulation. When the flow of blood through arteries supplying the heart muscle with oxygen and nutrients is interrupted, part of the heart muscle can be affected. A heart attack, or myocardial infarction, may ensue (Figure 4-13).[10] This may cause the heart to beat irregularly or not at all, leading to little or no heart function. If blood flow to part of the brain stops, that part of the brain may die. This event is called a cerebrovascular accident (CVA), or stroke. When it causes loss of muscle control, death may result.

Blood clots are the agents that stop the blood flow to the heart or brain. These clots have a greater tendency to form when cholesterol plaque has built up in the arteries that lead to the heart or brain. As we noted earlier, the plaque is probably first deposited to repair injuries in the vessel lining. This is called the "initiation phase."

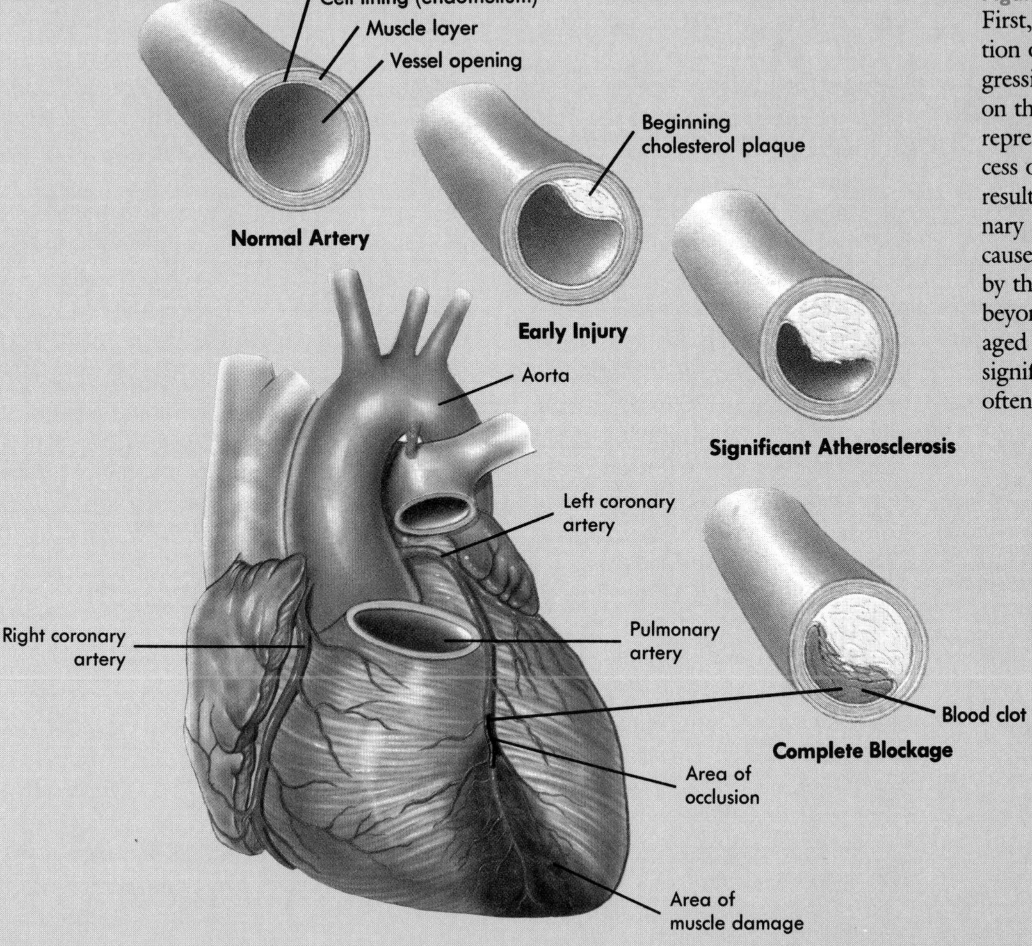

Figure 4-13 The road to a heart attack. First, an injury most likely causes initiation of the process. Then there is progression caused by buildup of plaque on the artery walls. The heart attack represents the termination of the process of atherosclerosis—in this case it resulted from blockage of the left coronary artery by a blood clot, the typical cause. The heart muscle that is serviced by the portion of the coronary artery beyond the point of blockage is damaged and may die. This can lead to a significant drop in heart function and often total heart failure.

NUTRITION PERSPECTIVE

Cardiovascular Disease—cont'd

The rate of further plaque deposition—called the "progression phase"—then partly depends on the amount of LDL cholesterol in the bloodstream. Eventually, arteries harden and narrow as plaque builds up, making them less elastic, and so unable to expand to accommodate various blood pressures. Arteries become damaged even further as blood pumps through and the pressure changes. Finally, in the "termination phase," a clot or spasm in the plaque-clogged artery leads to the myocardial infarction.[10]

What is your Risk for Cardiovascular Disease?

The three most important risk factors for cardiovascular disease are smoking, hypertension (high blood pressure), and high serum LDL cholesterol levels.[5] Family history is also important, particularly if a parent suffers a heart attack or stroke before age 60. Also of importance is a low serum HDL cholesterol level, especially if the total cholesterol to HDL cholesterol ratio exceeds 4.5 to 1. In addition, a serum triglyceride level over 200 to 250 milligrams per 100 milliliters should be cause for concern, mostly because it can lead to deleterious changes in other lipoproteins.

These factors should signal us to take aggressive early steps for prevention. Still significant but less important risk factors are stress, inactivity, diabetes, and obesity. All of these factors can contribute to the problem, as well as some rare lipoprotein metabolism disorders and other factors under study but still poorly understood. However, the most important contributors—smoking, hypertension, high serum LDL cholesterol levels, and total cholesterol to HDL cholesterol ratios—are the ones we should focus on first to prevent early cardiovascular disease. These still account for much of the overall risk for cardiovascular disease. The others can be added to our effort when the first four risk factors are eliminated. Then, at least, if we develop cardiovascular disease, all that was reasonably possible was done to postpone the problem in order to live as disease-free a life as possible.

systolic blood pressure The pressure in the bloodstream associated with the pumping of blood from the heart.

diastolic blood pressure The pressure in the bloodstream found when the heart is between beats.

Do you smoke? Do you have hypertension? Specifically, is your **systolic blood pressure** above 140 millimeters of mercury or your **diastolic blood pressure** above 90 millimeters of mercury? Is your serum LDL cholesterol level over 130 milligrams per 100 milliliters? In addition, what is your serum HDL-cholesterol level and total cholesterol to HDL cholesterol ratio? If the level is below 35 milligrams per 100 milliliters or the ratio is above 4.5 to 1, you have an increased risk for coronary heart disease. Finally, what is your total cholesterol level? If it is greater than 200 milligrams per 100 milliliters of serum, you could have a greater risk of cardiovascular disease. (Have yourself tested at least two more times if you show unhealthy values the first time because all the levels can vary from day to day.) If you add your family history to the other risk factors we mentioned, you can put cardiovascular disease risk into perspective for yourself.

Serum LDL and HDL cholesterol levels and the total cholesterol to HDL cholesterol ratio—rather than the total cholesterol level alone—are really the most important levels to consider. If a total serum cholesterol level greater than 200 milligrams per 100 milliliters is primarily due to a high HDL cholesterol level such that the total cholesterol to HDL cholesterol ratio is low, the risk of cardiovascular disease is still low. This is sometimes the case for women. Unfortunately, when men have elevated total cholesterol levels, it is usually due to an elevated LDL cholesterol level.

The National Institutes of Health in the United States encourage all people over age 20 to have their total serum cholesterol level checked.[5] We recommend having your serum HDL cholesterol and triglyceride levels checked also. That is necessary for the serum LDL cholesterol to be calculated. If you don't know your cholesterol

NUTRITION PERSPECTIVE

levels, you don't know key pieces of information that help predict your risk of developing premature cardiovascular disease.

Preventing early cardiovascular disease, before age 70, should be the focus. Eventually we all die. The key is to prevent premature death. Cardiovascular diseases at age 40 through 60 are closely linked to these risk factors. Preventing this at these ages is an important goal. See Chapter 18 for a further discussion of this concept of premature disease and how to prevent it.

Lowering an Elevated Serum LDL Cholesterol Level

If a high serum LDL cholesterol level and/or other undesirable lipoprotein levels are discovered, one should first consult a physician. Some diseases raise serum LDL cholesterol levels. By treating the disease, the levels will naturally fall. If disease isn't present, diet change should be addressed.[5]

To lower an elevated serum LDL cholesterol level through diet modification, one should first reduce the amount of saturated fat eaten.[5] This diet change can also reduce the fat levels in the bloodstream that appear after eating. Lowering dietary saturated fat intake is more important for most people than reducing dietary cholesterol. Only about 10% to 25% of people find that they lower their fasting serum LDL cholesterol level when they eat less cholesterol. Most people show only a minimal effect or no effect. Still, the recommendation to reduce dietary cholesterol intake can still be justified when one considers that this can lessen the cholesterol content of the chylomicrons produced after food consumption. There is concern that remnants of chylomicron metabolism contribute dietary cholesterol to growing atherosclerosis sites in the bloodstream.

Many people who lower saturated fat intake can lower an elevated serum LDL cholesterol level, often about 10% to 20%, especially if he or she is already eating many foods high in saturated fats. Levels also appear to stay down as long as the diet is followed.[21] Table 4-5 contains tips for lowering saturated fat intake. Saturated fats in the diet probably affect serum LDL cholesterol levels by changing the number of receptors for LDL cholesterol in the liver. When saturated fat intake is low, the number of LDL receptors in the liver increases.[12] Recall that the liver is the major organ for clearing LDL cholesterol from the bloodstream. Serum LDL cholesterol levels fall as more cholesterol is cleared from the bloodstream and pulled into the liver for excretion as bile acids into the small intestine. This uptake of cholesterol by the liver likely also leads to less cholesterol synthesis by the liver itself. Both actions help account for why the blood cholesterol level falls after changing one's diet.

A reasonable goal is to eat no more than 10% of kcalories as saturated fats. A reduction to only 7% is better. To do this one must watch the intake of fatty animal products, butter, coconut oil, palm oil, shortening, and other hydrogenated (solid) fats. Reading labels is important. Saturated fats are often hidden in foods. In addition, broil, bake, or boil meats; don't fry them. Limit use of gravies and fatty desserts. Use only low-fat—and preferably nonfat—dairy products. Thus important foods to avoid should be processed meats (like sausage), butter, ice cream, cheese (except maybe mozzarella and other low-fat cheeses), whole milk, stick margarine, sour cream, nondairy coffee creamers, many granola bars (read the label), most crackers, biscuits, and all visible animal fat (Table 4-5).

To lower dietary cholesterol intake, start by eating fewer egg yolks; egg whites have no cholesterol. The American Heart Association recommends no more than 3 egg yolks per week. If you cook for yourself, it is easy to avoid egg yolks. In making many recipes, such as those for pancakes, French toast, cookies, and cakes, you can substitute egg whites as an economical option. Cholesterol-free commercial egg alternatives are also available in the grocery store. These are usually egg whites colored yellow, to which a small amount of oil has been added to improve their flavor and performance. Table 4-1 lists the amount of cholesterol in some foods.

NUTRITION PERSPECTIVE

Cardiovascular Disease—cont'd

Table 4-5 Tips for avoiding too much fat and saturated fat

1. Steam, boil, or bake vegetables. For a change, stirfry in a small amount of vegetable oil. Consider buying an insert for a pot so you can easily steam your vegetables.
2. Season vegetables with herbs and spices rather than with sauces, butter, or margarine.
3. Try lemon juice on salad or use limited amounts of oil-based salad dressing.
4. To reduce saturated fat, use tub margarine instead of butter or stick margarine in baked products. When possible, use vegetable oil instead of either of these solid fats or hydrogenated shortenings.
5. Limit baked goods made with large amounts of fat, especially saturated fats: croissants, doughnuts, muffins, biscuits, and butter rolls.
6. Try whole-grain flours to enhance flavors when baking goods with less fat and cholesterol-containing ingredients.
7. Replace whole milk with skim or low-fat milk in puddings, soups, and baked products.
8. Substitute plain low-fat yogurt, blender-whipped low-fat cottage cheese, or buttermilk in recipes that call for sour cream or mayonnaise.
9. Choose lean cuts of meat. Limit bacon, ribs, and meat loaf.
10. Trim fat from meat before and after cooking.
11. Roast, bake, or broil meat, poultry, and fish so fat drains away as the food cooks.
12. Remove skin from poultry before cooking. This eliminates the temptation to eat it along with the meat.
13. Use a nonstick pan for cooking so added fat will be unnecessary; use a vegetable spray for frying.
14. Chill meat or poultry broth until the fat solidifies. Spoon off the fat before using the broth.
15. Eat a vegetarian main dish at least once a week. Include fish (cooked without much added fat) in the diet about two times a week.
16. Choose ice milk, low-fat frozen yogurt, sorbets, and popsicles as substitutes for ice cream.
17. Try angel food cake, fig bars, and ginger snaps as substitutes for commercial baked goods high in saturated fat.
18. Limit high-fat cheese intake.
19. Read lables of commerically prepared foods to find out what type of fat or how much saturated fat they contain.
20. Think about the balance of fats in your menu. If your meal contains whole milk, cheese, ice cream, a higher fat meat, or poultry with skin, use margarine and unsaturated vegetable oils for your spreads and dressings. Small amounts of butter, sour cream, or cream cheese can be included if other menu items are low in saturated fat.
21. Use jam, jelly, or marmalade on bread and toast instead of butter or margarine.
22. Buy whole-grain breads and rolls. They have more flavor and do not need butter or margarine to taste good. The dietary fiber present is an added bonus.

NUTRITION PERSPECTIVE

If the fat is trimmed before and after cooking, a 3 ounce serving of chicken, beef, and pork meats has surprisingly little cholesterol, roughly a third to half of that in an egg. It is generally the portion size that causes us trouble with meat and cholesterol intake. A 10 ounce serving of meat can contain 260 milligrams of cholesterol, more than is in one egg. Meats have a reputation for being high in cholesterol. However, this mainly is due to the amount of meat we eat.

Monounsaturated Versus Polyunsaturated Fats

There are some encouraging new observations on the ability of monounsaturated fatty acids in the diet to lower serum LDL cholesterol levels. Recall that these have only one carbon-carbon double bond. In the past saturated fatty acids were thought to contribute to high serum LDL cholesterol levels, and polyunsaturated fatty acids were believed to lower serum LDL cholesterol levels. Polyunsaturated fatty acids were then recommended to replace saturated fatty acids. However, studies show that when foods high in monounsaturated fatty acids replace those high in saturated fatty acids, serum LDL cholesterol levels also fall.[12] So both are now considered good replacements for saturated fatty acids. In fact, monounsaturated fatty acids may be more beneficial since these do not readily lead to oxidation of LDL.[27] Recall oxidized LDL is taken up preferably by plaque in the arteries. To put this recommendation into practical use, reaching for canola oil and olive oil in the grocery store is one possibility, as opposed to choosing only polyunsaturated oils.

Fiber and Reduced Cardiovascular Disease

A recent development in lowering serum LDL cholesterol levels is increasing the intake of soluble fiber, which is found in oatmeal, oat bran, beans, vegetables, and fruits. Some laxatives—those with psyllium fiber—are also sources of soluble fiber. Manufacturers were very quick to realize the marketing potential of a product that might lower serum LDL cholesterol levels. But oat bran isn't the "magic bullet" manufacturers would have us believe (Figure 4-14). You would need to eat about a cup of oat bran a day to reap the desired effect; an oat bran muffin alone won't do it. Diets very high in overall fiber (50 to 60 grams per day), especially those that emphasize soluble fibers, can lower serum LDL cholesterol levels. The fiber probably binds cholesterol and bile acids in the small intestine and carries them into the colon for elimination.[30] This action resembles that of some medications in lowering serum LDL cholesterol levels; removing bile acids from the body forces the liver to pull more cholesterol out of the bloodstream to make new bile acids. Additionally, high-fiber foods tend to replace foods high in saturated fat, which is desirable. Other

FRANK & ERNEST® by Bob Thaves

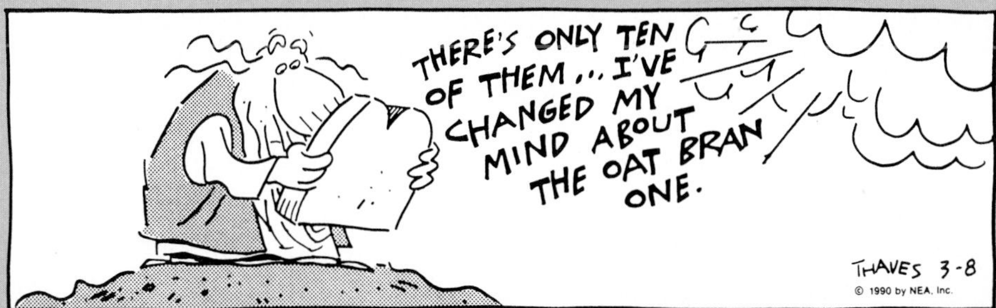
THERE'S ONLY TEN OF THEM... I'VE CHANGED MY MIND ABOUT THE OAT BRAN ONE.
THAVES 3-8
© 1990 by NEA, Inc.

Figure 4-14 Frank and Ernest.
Reprinted by permission of NEA, Inc.

NUTRITION PERSPECTIVE

Cardiovascular Disease—cont'd

mechanisms to account for the effects of soluble fibers have also been suggested (see Chapter 3).

One may have to considerably change eating habits in order to follow a diet high in soluble fiber, but the change is possible. Currently researchers caution against eating more than 35 grams of dietary fiber a day, so it is best to consult a physician before embarking on a very high-fiber diet. We think that eating a diet low in saturated fats may be an easier and safer alternative to raising fiber intake so dramatically.

Raising the Serum HDL Cholesterol Level

An important step in lowering a serum LDL cholesterol level is to keep the HDL cholesterol level in a healthy range at the same time. If levels fall too far, emphasizing monounsaturated fatty acids in a diet at the expense of both saturated and polyunsaturated fatty acids is one strategy.[12] Regular eating habits (three balanced meals per day), an energy intake matched to energy output, and a lower total fat intake often help to lower serum triglyceride levels, which in turn typically results in increased serum HDL cholesterol levels. Why this is so is not clear. In this regard the goal is to have fasting serum triglyceride levels below 150 to 200 milligrams per 100 milliliters. Certain medications also act to lower serum triglyceride levels. When this happens, serum HDL cholesterol levels also often increase.

Exercise often provides a moderate, but beneficial effect on the serum HDL cholesterol level.[29] In men, adding exercise to the regimen increases HDL, and in women exercise blunts the reduction in HDL that often occurs with weight loss without exercise. Exercise is also good for the general condition of the heart and so should be part of any plan to reduce cardiovascular risk. Finally, losing excess weight and avoiding smoking also help to maintain or raise HDL cholesterol levels.

Raising HDL cholesterol levels is usually much more difficult than lowering LDL cholesterol levels. Although drinking alcohol can raise HDL cholesterol, too many other risks—such as liver and heart damage and accidents—are associated with the heavy drinking needed to justify using it for this purpose.[24] Moderation or avoidance is still the overriding recommendation for consumption of alcohol.

Treating high blood pressure is covered in Chapter 14.

What Should One Do?

To lower a high serum LDL cholesterol level:

- Reduce saturated fatty acid and cholesterol intake. Consume more foods low in fat instead. This is the best method and should be the major focus.
- Perform regular exercise. This helps protect serum HDL cholesterol levels.
- Lose weight to attain a desirable body weight. This helps reduce serum triglyceride levels—primarily VLDLs and chylomicrons. This is important since the longer chylomicrons and VLDLs stay in the bloodstream, the greater their tendency to be metabolized to forms of LDLs and other lipoproteins that especially contribute to atherosclerosis.
- Increase intake of soluble fiber. This binds cholesterol and bile acids in the small intestine to encourage their elimination via the colon rather than absorption into the bloodstream; there also may be other causes for the drop.
- Eat fish on a regular basis. This tends to reduce blood clotting and so lessens the risk of developing a myocardial infarction. Regular use of aspirin for people at high risk of a myocardial infarction (under a physician's scrutiny) is promoted for the same reason.

NUTRITION PERSPECTIVE

- Keep all types of coffee consumption to prudent levels—about 2 to 3 cups a day. Studies show moderate increases in LDL cholesterol level with heavy consumption of many types of coffee, including decaffeinated brands.[9]

Everyone needs to find what works best in his or her particular situation. The plan should be to make some changes and recheck the various serum cholesterol levels and total cholesterol to HDL cholesterol ratio in a couple of weeks to compare results. Steady progress toward these goals often reaps the benefit of a lower risk for developing cardiovascular disease. Eating right doesn't mean completely giving up favorite foods, even if they do contain higher-than-desirable levels of saturated fats. If you eat carefully most of the time, you can allow yourself latitude for occasional treats. If you indulge in a meal high in saturated fat, it should be part of the larger picture that includes meals of lower-than-usual amounts of saturated fats in order to balance your diet. Excessive restriction sets one up for failure and guilt.

For children age 2 years or older, a diet with up to 30% of total kcalories as fat is an appropriate goal, with no more than 10% of kcalories from saturated fat. Parents should not go overboard with fat restrictions because children need about 30% fat in their diets to grow properly. We do not advise parents to feed fat-restricted diets to children under age 2 years (see Chapter 17).

Medications to Lower Serum Cholesterol Levels

Medications are a last resort for treating high serum LDL cholesterol levels because of their expense and side effects. Nevertheless, the effects of diet changes are sometimes insufficient to control high serum LDL cholesterol levels, especially in people with strong genetic tendencies toward that problem. Current medications work in one of two ways. One group decreases lipoprotein synthesis by the liver and includes nicotinic acid, lovastatin, probucol, and gemfibrozil. Nicotinic acid and gemfibrozil are also notable for raising HDL cholesterol levels. The side effects of these medications require a physician's careful evaluation. The other group—which includes cholestyramine and colestipol—binds bile acids in the small intestine and prevents their reabsorption. This forces the liver to synthesize new bile acids. The liver pulls cholesterol out of the bloodstream to do this, which lowers the serum LDL cholesterol level.

All of these medications work better when a proper diet is followed—they do not substitute for diet changes.

A controversy currently rages about using medications to combat cardiovascular disease. The question is not whether a link exists between a high LDL cholesterol level or a high total cholesterol to HDL cholesterol ratio and an increased risk of a heart attack. This link is clear in large population studies; most people with high levels of either develop cardiovascular disease in their lifetime. Furthermore, countries worldwide where smoking and diets high in animal fat and other significant sources of saturated fat still predominate lead the world in heart disease risk. The question concerns the point at which a person's risk is sufficient to warrant medical treatment.[11] The need for diet changes are also questioned for the same reason. We feel changes in the diet and the use of medications (if needed) to lower elevated LDL cholesterol levels are a good idea. This is especially important in light of new research showing that (1) plaque regresses in arteries supplying the heart when LDL cholesterol levels are aggressively lowered with either diet,[20] medications, or with surgery on the small intestine to decrease bile acid reabsorption; and (2) both cardiovascular-related mortality and total mortality are reduced when treatment is followed for a long enough period of time, approximately 10 years or more.

National Cholesterol Education Program for Adults—Dietary Advice

GOAL: Total blood cholesterol <200 mg/dl*
LDL cholesterol <160 mg/dl or <130 mg/dl with 2 or more risk factors

If total blood cholesterol is >200 mg/dl and an individual has two or more of the following risk factors:

- **Family history of coronary heart disease**
- **Smokes cigarettes**
- **Diabetes**
- **Obesity**
- **Hypertension**
- **Low HDL cholesterol**
- **Male**

Test for LDL cholesterol

If LDL cholesterol >130 mg/dl:

- **Reduce saturated fat intake to 10% of total kcalories**
- **Reduce total fat intake to 30% of total kcalories**
- **Reduce cholesterol intake to 300 mg/day**

Do this for 6 months

If unsuccessful (that is, LDL cholesterol >130 mg/dl)

- **Reduce saturated fat intake to 7% of total kcalories**
- **Reduce cholesterol intake to 200 mg/day**

Do this for 6 months

If still unsuccessful, a physician may prescribe a cholesterol-lowering medication.

*mg/dl represents milligrams per 100 milliliters of serum.

CHAPTER FIVE

Proteins

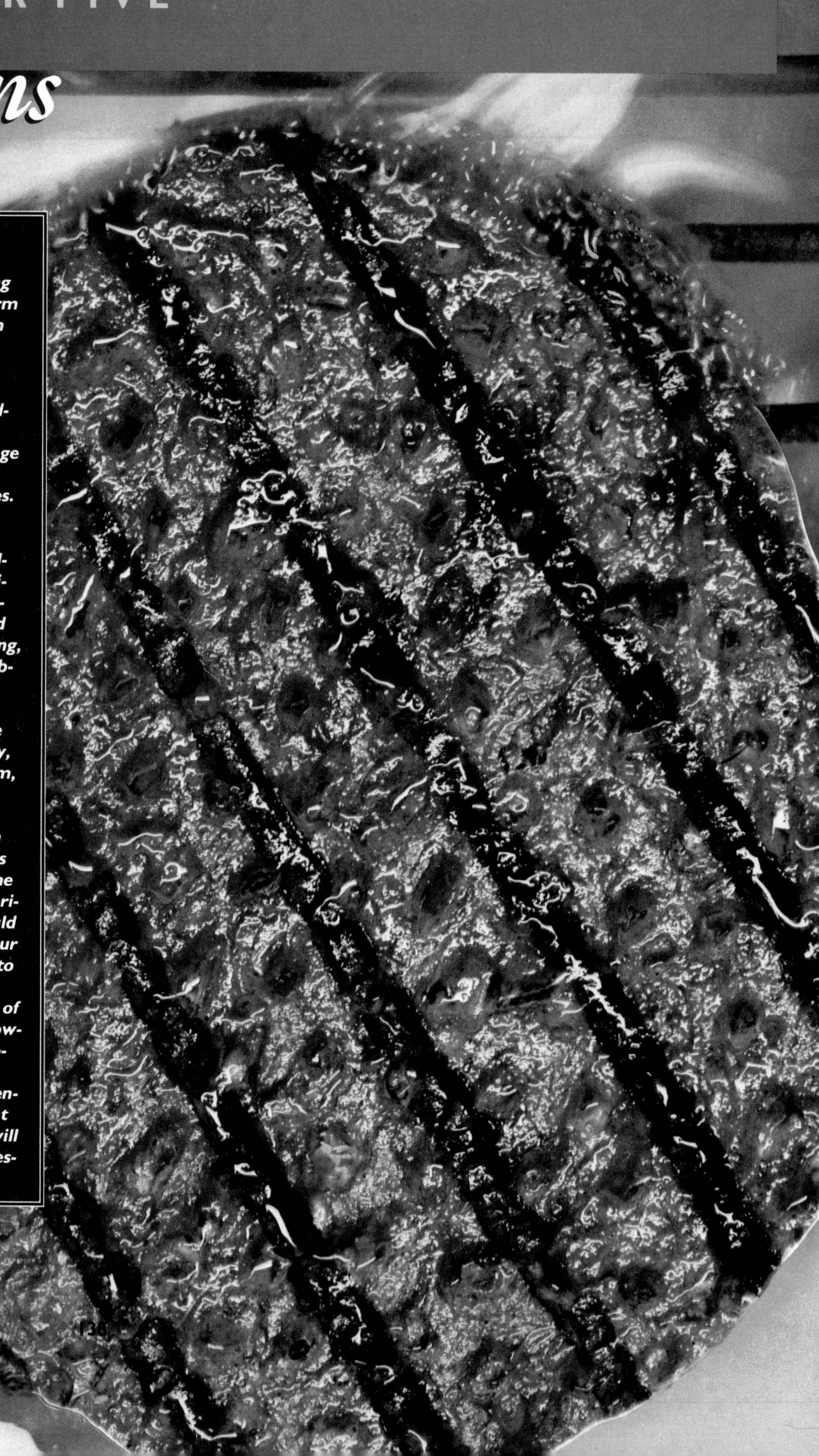

A regular dietary intake of protein is vital for maintaining health. Proteins form important structural parts in body, make up much of the blood, help regulate many body functions, and can fuel body cells. According to studies by anthropologists using fossilized teeth, our Stone Age ancestors obtained most of their protein from vegetables. Not until the emergence of our immediate ancestors, Homo erectus, about 1.5 million years ago, was there evidence of much meat in a primarily vegetarian diet.[6] Food gathering, rather than hunting, was the primary means of obtaining dietary protein.

Today, animal products hold a central position in the American diet—roast turkey, grilled hamburgers, ice cream, and T-bone steak are just a few of the animal protein foods that most of us hold in high regard. Animal products contribute considerably to the total nutrient intake of Americans, but plant proteins should also play a valuable role in our diets. Few of us would wish to exchange our comfortable modern lifestyles with those of our Stone Age ancestors. However, it is possible to incorporate the best of both worlds nutritionally, enjoying the benefits of both animal and plant protein. In this chapter we will discuss why this nutrition message is important.

NUTRITION AWARENESS INVENTORY

Here are 15 statements about proteins. Answer them to test your current knowledge. If you think a statement is true or mostly true, circle T; if you think the statement is false or mostly false, circle F. Use the scoring key at the end of the book to compute your total score. Compare the results.

1. T F Most people have trouble eating a diet containing all the essential amino acids.
2. T F Not enough protein in the diet can stunt a child's growth.
3. T F Most enzymes are proteins.
4. T F Many hormones, including insulin, are proteins.
5. T F The quality of protein can be measured by its biological value—nitrogen retention divided by nitrogen absorption.
6. T F Milk provides higher quality proteins than most other foods.
7. T F In the life span, protein needs are the greatest in the older years.
8. T F Athletes usually need at least double the protein intake of nonathletes. Supplements are the preferred source.
9. T F Animal protein sources often contain high amounts of saturated fat.
10. T F Lack of energy can be a symptom of severe protein deficiency.
11. T F Gelatin supplements can strengthen the protein in fingernails.
12. T F Marasmus is a disease caused by starvation and can be seen in large cities of impoverished countries.
13. T F The nonprotein nutrient content of animal and vegetable protein is about the same.
14. T F Most of the energy in water-packed tuna is in the form of protein.
15. T F Fruits generally contain very little protein.

Proteins—Vital to Life

P**roteins** compose about 16% of body weight in a lean individual. Virtually all the building blocks for these proteins—amino acids—were originally made by plants. Plants combine nitrogen from the soil and air with carbon and other chemical substances to form amino acids. Plants then convert these into proteins. Humans ordinarily consume nitrogen in the form of amino acids via proteins (Figure 5-1). Directly using simpler forms of nitrogen is, for the most part, impossible for humans.

The day-to-day and minute-to-minute regulation and maintenance of the body requires a variety of proteins. As we noted in the chapter overview, proteins contribute to key body functions, including blood clotting, fluid balance, production of hormones and enzymes, vision, and cell repair. Many of these proteins are very large: their molecular weights can exceed 1 million. In contrast, glucose has a molecular weight of only 180. Furthermore, the thousands of different varieties of proteins made by the body greatly exceed the variety found among either carbohydrates or lipids. Thus proteins deserve their name, which means "to come first."

If a person regularly fails to eat enough protein, major metabolic changes occur. An important change is a decrease in immune function. Whether this is a child suffering in a famine or an adult hospitalized with a severe body burn, a poor protein intake can increase the risk of infections, disease, and possibly death.[16]

Amino Acids

Amino acids contain carbon, hydrogen, oxygen, nitrogen, and sometimes sulfur. All 20 types of the amino acids that are found in our diets and used to make protein have similar backbones. Each is composed of a carbon bonded to a nitrogen group (—NH_2). This form is called an amine "amino" group. An acid group

$$(\text{—}\overset{\text{O}}{\overset{\|}{\text{C}}}\text{—O—OH})$$

, a hydrogen (—H), and another group, often signified by R,

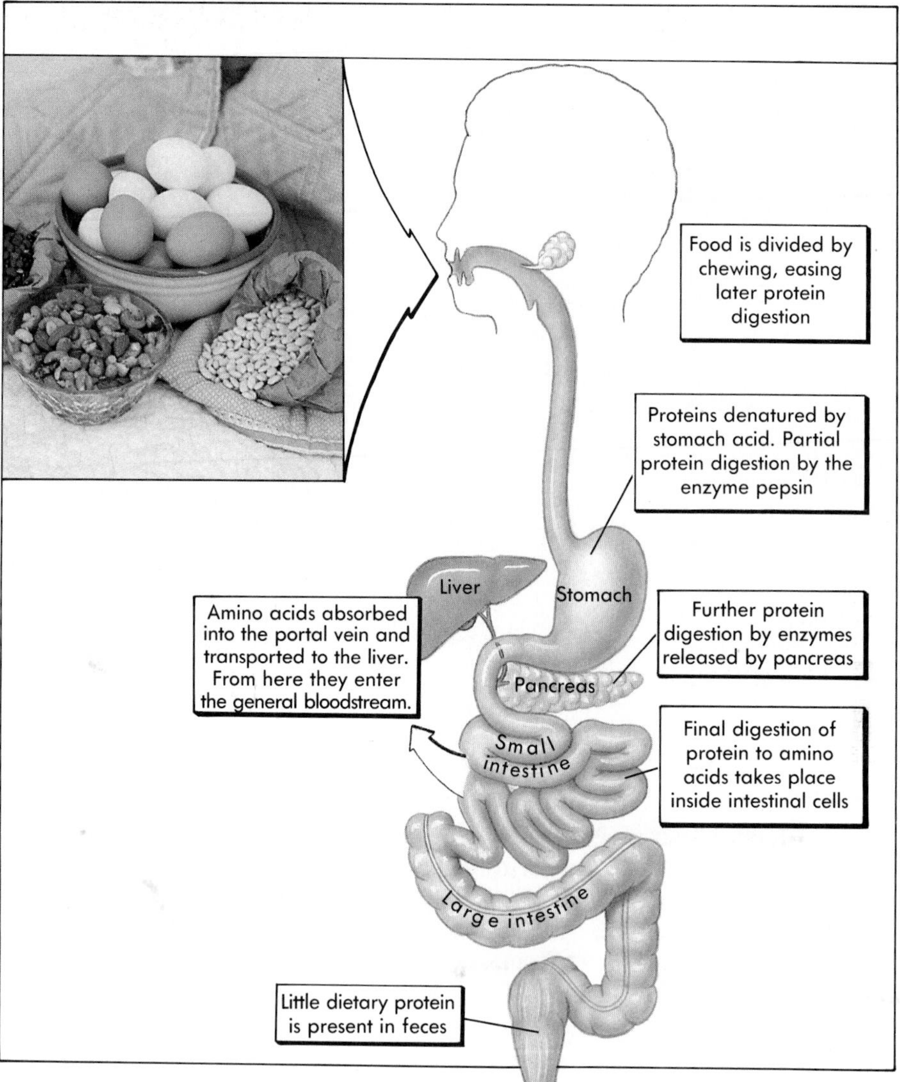

Figure 5-1 A summary of protein digestion and absorption. Chapter 6 covers these concepts in detail.

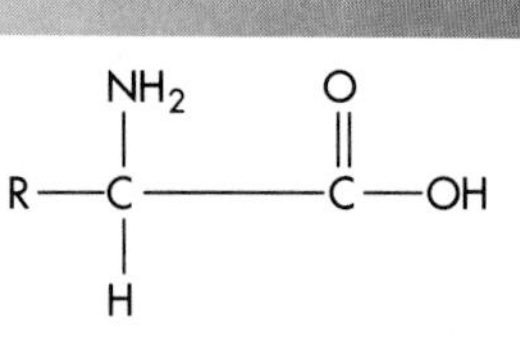

"Generic" amino acid

NH_2 O

H—C—C—OH

H

Glycine

NH_2 O

CH_3—C—C—OH

H

L-alanine

complete the amino acid. In the margin we show a basic model of an amino acid and the actual structures of glycine and alanine.

AMINO ACID FORM DETERMINES FUNCTION

The form that the R portion in the amino acid assumes determines the type and name of the amino acid. If the R is a hydrogen, the amino acid is glycine. If the R is a methyl group (—CH_3), the amino acid is alanine, and so on (see Appendix B). Some amino acids have chemically similar R portions. These related amino acids form special classes, such as acidic amino acids, basic amino acids, or branched-chain amino acids.

The key part of the amino acid is the amino group. This is the distinguishing feature of amino acids.

Cells can produce carbon skeletons and then add amino groups from other amino acids to synthesize 11 of the 20 different types of amino acids the body needs. In the case of the other nine amino acids the body needs, body cells either cannot make the needed carbon skeleton, cannot put an amino group on the carbon skeleton, or just cannot do the whole process fast enough to meet body needs. The amino acids that body cells cannot make are called **essential (indispensable) amino acids** and must be consumed (Table 5-1). The 11 amino acids the body can make are then

essential (indespensible) amino acids The amino acids that cannot be synthesized in sufficient amounts by humans and must therefore be included in the diet; there are nine essential amino acids.

Table 5-1 Classification of amino acids

Essential amino acids	Nonessential amino acids
Histidine	Alanine
Isoleucine	Arginine§
Leucine	Asparagine
Lysine‡	Aspartic acid
Methionine†	Cysteine (Cystine)*
Phenylalanine	Glutamic acid
Threonine	Glutamine‖
Tryptophan	Glycine
Valine	Proline
	Serine
	Tyrosine*

*These amino acids are also classed as semiessential.
†The limiting amino acid in legumes and vegetables. You can consume legumes with grains, nuts, and seeds to supply complete protein at a meal if no animal protein is eaten.
‡A limiting amino acid in grains, nuts, and seeds. You can consume grains with legumes to supply complete protein at a meal if no animal protein is eaten.
§Synthesized at rates inadequate to support growth of children and so is considered essential during growth.
‖Currently considered essential to the diet in some states of traumatic injury and so is often supplemented in specialized formulas used with hospitalized patients.

If the R portion on the amino acid is anything other than a hydrogen, the amino acid will have four different groups attached to it. You may recall from basic chemistry that a carbon with four different groups attached to it can exist as two isomer forms, in this case D and L. In nature almost all amino acids are the L form. However, we can metabolize some D isomer forms (see Appendix B for a review of the concept of isomers).

called **nonessential (dispensable) amino acids.** Note that both essential and nonessential amino acids are present in foods that contain protein.

All amino acids are necessary, considering how imperative they are for proper body function. However, only the essential amino acids must be derived from the diet.[21] If we don't eat enough essential amino acids, the rate of protein synthesis slows progressively until protein breakdown exceeds protein synthesis. A state of poor health can then result.

nonessential (dispensible) amino acids Amino acids that can be readily synthesized by the body; there are 11 nonessential amino acids in the diet.

Two amino acids—cysteine and tyrosine—are in a special category as they can be considered semiessential (conditionally indispensable). They can spare the need for two essential amino acids. For example, cysteine and methionine are just such a pair of nonessential and essential amino acids, as are tyrosine and phenylalanine. Both methionine and phenylalanine are essential amino acids. Cysteine and tyrosine are amino acids that must be made from their essential amino acid counterparts (methionine and phenylalanine) unless they are consumed in the diet. If cysteine and tyrosine are consumed, the body uses them—instead of their essential amino acid partners—to synthesize protein. Thus cysteine and tyrosine spare methionine and phenylalanine from being transformed into cysteine and tyrosine, leaving more methionine and phenylalanine to be used for protein synthesis. About 50% of dietary methionine need is spared if ample cysteine is consumed.

When health is compromised, such as when a child is born prematurely, some amino acids normally nonessential in the adult diet may become an essential part of the diet of the compromised person—an example would be the amino acid arginine. This also appears to be the case for glutamine in adults experiencing traumatic injury.

TRANSAMINATION AND DEAMINATION

A common metabolic process for synthesizing nonessential amino acids is called **transamination**. This requires the participation of vitamin B-6. Figure 5-2 illustrates transamination: pyruvic acid accepts the nitrogen group (—NH2) from the amino acid glutamic acid and becomes the amino acid alanine. In the process, by losing its nitrogen group, glutamic acid turns into a carbon skeleton, called alpha-ketoglutaric acid.

Some amino acids, such as glutamic acid, can simply lose their nitrogen group without transferring it to another carbon skeleton. This process is called **deamination.** The nitrogen group is incorporated into urea in the liver, transferred through the blood to the kidneys, and excreted in the urine (Figure 5-3). Once an amino acid breaks down to its carbon skeleton, the carbon skeleton can be burned for fuel

transamination The transfer of an amine group from an amino acid to a carbon skeleton to form a new amino acid.

deamination The removal of an amine group from an amino acid.

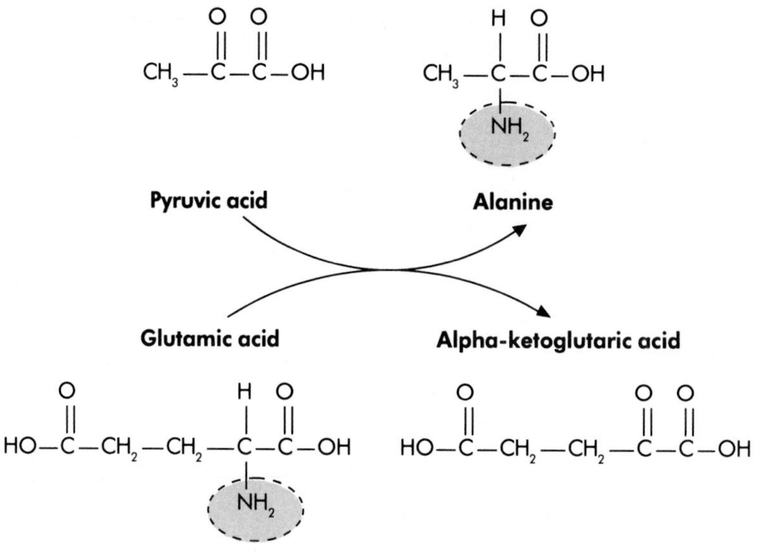

Figure 5-2 Transamination. This pathway allows cells to synthesize nonessential amino acids. In this example, pyruvic acid gains a nitrogen group to form the amino acid alanine.

$$CH_3-\overset{O}{\overset{\|}{C}}-\overset{O}{\overset{\|}{C}}-OH \qquad CH_3-\underset{NH_2}{\underset{|}{\overset{H}{\overset{|}{C}}}}-\overset{O}{\overset{\|}{C}}-OH$$

Pyruvic acid → **Alanine**

Glutamic acid → **Alpha-ketoglutaric acid**

$$HO-\overset{O}{\overset{\|}{C}}-CH_2-CH_2-\underset{NH_2}{\underset{|}{\overset{H}{\overset{|}{C}}}}-\overset{O}{\overset{\|}{C}}-OH \qquad HO-\overset{O}{\overset{\|}{C}}-CH_2-CH_2-\overset{O}{\overset{\|}{C}}-\overset{O}{\overset{\|}{C}}-OH$$

or synthesized into other compounds, such as fatty acids (see Chapter 7).

The amino acids provided by cell breakdown combine with amino acids from protein in the diet to allow the body to build new protein. Each cell contains amino acids that should be thought of as available for a limited time, and in limited quantity. If the pool of amino acids becomes too large, the amino acids are used for energy, glucose, or fat production. From Figure 5-3 you can imagine the amino acid pool would diminish if there was inadequate protein intake, and so additional amino acids would need to come from cell breakdown. This could lead to the breakdown of essential body tissue. Thus eventually essential amino acids need to be replaced by the diet.

PUTTING ESSENTIAL AMINO ACIDS INTO PERSPECTIVE

Physiological Aspects

The disease phenylketonuria (PKU) illustrates the concept of essential and nonessential amino acids. Again, phenylalanine is an essential amino acid. Tyrosine is a nonessential amino acid because phenylalanine can be converted into tyrosine. However, the liver of a person with PKU can lack sufficient enzyme activity to efficiently convert phenylalanine to tyrosine. This defect can vary from a mild to severe impairment of enzyme activity. Two problems result from the lack of this enzyme. Phenylalanine no longer can be broken down when present in excess, and tyrosine is not made from phenylalanine. Tyrosine then becomes an essential amino acid because it now must come from food.

The diet of a person with PKU often must be carefully designed to contain enough phenylalanine for protein synthesis—because it is an essential amino acid—but no more than that. Foods like milk then have to be limited in the diet as this is just one of the many protein foods that is rich in phenylalanine. The inability to readily metabolize excess phenylalanine to tyrosine can lead to a buildup of abnormal products from alternate routes of phenylalanine metabolism. These products are thought to cause the severe mental retardation seen in untreated PKU cases.

Dietary Considerations

Animal proteins and plant proteins can differ greatly in composition of essential and nonessential amino acids. Animal proteins, except gelatin, contain ample amounts of all essential amino acids. With regards to gelatin, not only does it not contain all of the essential amino acids (it lacks the sulfur-containing amino acids), heat and acid processing destroys the tryptophan present. Plant proteins, when compared with human needs, are always relatively low in one or more of the essential amino acids (Table 5-2).[11]

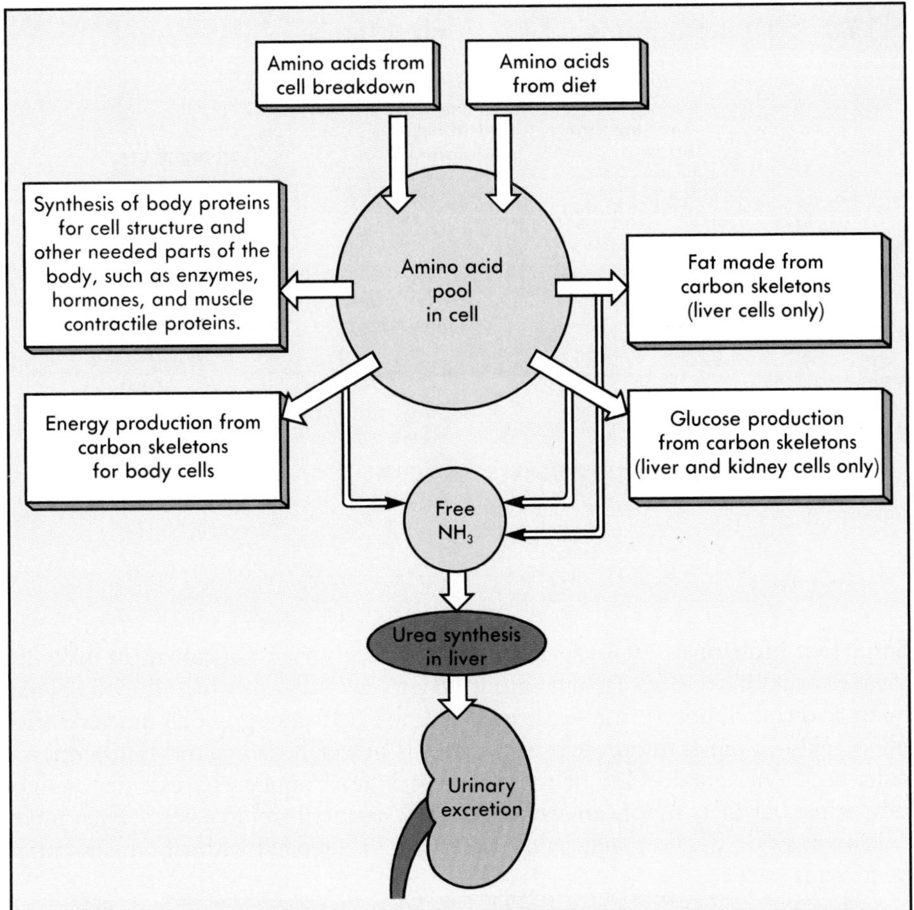

Figure 5-3 Amino acid metabolism. The amino acid pool shown is supplied both by the release of amino acids from the breakdown of old cells and by amino acids from protein in the foods we eat. Each cell builds new protein from amino acids that are available from this pool. Should the pool become too large, the amino acids become a source of energy, or the amino acids are converted to either glucose or body fat.

In essence, human tissue composition resembles that of animal tissue far more than it does plant tissue. As a result of the similarities, proteins from animal sources are used more efficiently to support human growth and maintenance because they are closely matched to the human pattern of essential amino acids. Thus animal proteins, except gelatin, are considered **high-quality proteins** (often called complete proteins). They can support body growth and maintenance because they contain all of the essential amino acids in sufficient amounts.[9] Plant proteins are usually considered **low-quality proteins** (often called incomplete proteins). This means single plant proteins cannot easily support body growth and maintenance because each protein lacks adequate amounts of one or more essential amino acid.[7] An exception exists only if very large amounts are consumed.

High-quality proteins Dietary proteins that contain ample amounts of all nine essential amino acids.

Low-quality proteins Dietary proteins that lack an ample amount of one or more amino acids essential for human protein needs.

If you eat foods that contain low-quality protein—that is foods that do not provide an appropriate balance of all nine essential amino acids—you will also need to eat some high-quality protein to obtain enough of the essential amino acids needed for protein synthesis. Otherwise protein synthesis would soon stop when the supply of any one essential amino acid was depleted. Considering body needs, the amino acid in shortest supply in a food or diet is called the **limiting amino acid.** When protein synthesis stops because one type of essential amino acid is used up, the "all-or-none law" is said to apply: If all nine essential amino acids are not available to synthesize needed protein, the ones present cannot be used at that time, and protein synthesis stops.

limiting amino acid The essential amino acid in lowest concentration in a food in proportion to body needs.

Both the "all-or-none law" and the concept of the limiting amino acid are interesting but can be overemphasized when typical American eating patterns are

Table 5-2 Limiting amino acids in plant foods

Food	Limiting amino acids	Good plant source of limiting amino acids	Traditional uses
Soybeans and other legumes	Methionine	Grains; nuts and seeds	Tofu (soybean curd) and rice
Grains	Lysine, threonine	Legumes	Lentil curry and rice
Nuts and seeds	Lysine	Legumes	Soybeans and ground sesame seeds (miso)
Vegetables	Methionine	Grains; nuts and seeds	Green beans and almonds
Corn	Tryptophan, lysine	Legumes	Corn tortillas and pinto beans

considered. Most of us eat large amounts of such a varied assortment of proteins that we would have to go far out of our way to eat a diet in which the combined amino acid contributions from each food did not yield enough of all nine essential amino acids—even if the protein in the diet is not of high quality. Furthermore, adults need only about 11% of their protein intake supplied by essential amino acids, while our diets supply an average of 50% essential amino acids.[21] Even most adults worldwide who eat sufficient protein will be supplied with all nine essential amino acids.

So there is little reason for the average adult to worry about balancing proteins that specifically complement the deficiencies of amino acids in other proteins consumed. However, vegetarians and populations with access to little or no animal protein, are exceptions to this concept. In these cases two low-quality protein foods can be combined in a meal; the lack of particular essential amino acids in one protein food is complemented by another that contains those amino acids.[11] (See Table 5-2 and the Nutrition Perspective. The latter provides more details on protein complementarity as it examines vegetarianism.)

Infants and preschool children, on the other hand, require that approximately 32% to 43% of their protein come from essential amino acids.[21] So food for young children must be more carefully planned to include enough of all nine essential amino acids. If an infant consumes enough breast milk or commercial formula to meet its protein needs, essential amino acid needs will be automatically met. A major health risk for children occurs in famine situations where only one type of grain is available, increasing the probability that all nine essential amino acids may be lacking in the total diet.[16]

CONCEPT CHECK

Twenty amino acids useful to the body exist in food. A healthy body synthesizes 11 of these—nonessential (dispensable) amino acids. The other nine must be consumed—essential (indispensable) amino acids. Foods that contain all nine essential amino acids in about the proportion needed provide high-quality protein, while proteins that provide a low-quantity of one or more essential amino acids are lower in quality. When different low-quality protein foods are eaten together in a meal, their amino acids often complement each other, providing a high quality protein meal.

Proteins—Amino Acids Joined Together

One way of classifying proteins is based on their number of amino acids. Two amino acids bonded together form a dipeptide, and three amino acids bonded together form a tripeptide. An oligopeptide has more than three amino acids but less than 50. A **polypeptide** has 50 to 100 amino acids, and a protein has at least 100 amino acids. Most foods contain just the large protein form. However, specialized feeding supplements used in hospitals often contain various sizes of peptides.

Amino acids are joined together by a **peptide bond.** A nitrogen group (—NH2) reacts with a carboxyl group (—C(=O)—OH)) and a water molecule is split off. The process requires an enzyme to catalyze the reaction. In this peptide bond, electrons are shared (covalent), and so it is a difficult bond to break apart. The body can synthesize many different proteins by joining together the 20 different types of amino acids with peptide bonds. Imagine the number of combinations that can be made using multiple amounts of the 20 amino acids, especially considering the great lengths of many proteins.

A peptide bond can be broken—water is added back to the molecule. In this fashion, acids, enzymes, or other agents can lead to the breakdown of a peptide bond.

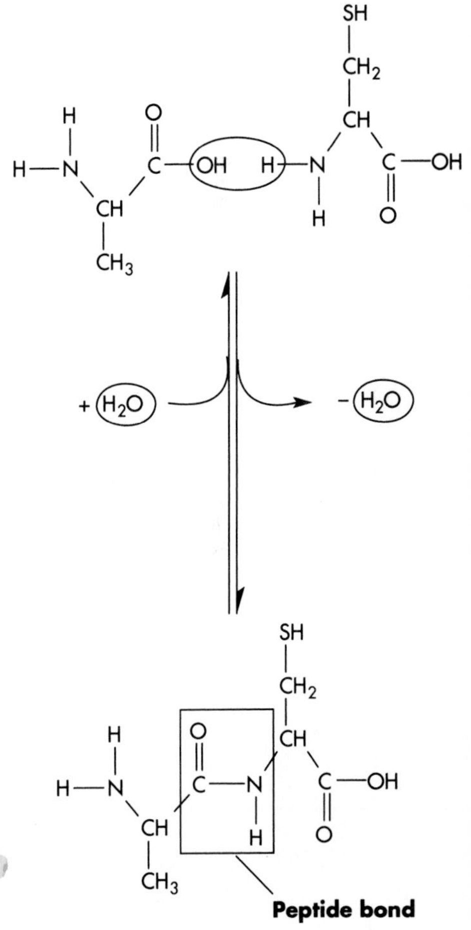

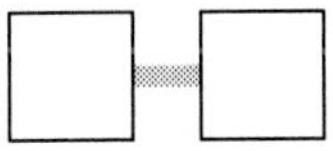

polypeptide Fifty to 100 amino acids bonded together.

peptide bond A chemical bond formed by the reaction of an amino group from one amino acid with an acid group from another amino acid, while splitting off a water molecule; the main bond that links amino acids in a protein.

LEVELS OF PROTEIN ORGANIZATION

Sequence

The order of amino acids in a protein—in other words the sequence created by amino acids bonded to each other—dictates the structure of the protein. This is often called a protein's primary structure. The sequence of the amino acids eventually yields a specific three-dimensional shape to the protein. This shape in turn determines the function that protein will have.

Shape

As we have just alluded to, the chain of amino acids in a protein does not remain as a long, straight string, but rather becomes a three-dimensional structure. The three-dimensional shape begins by the folding, twisting, and turning of the amino acids linked in the sequence. The particular location of an amino acid may allow for a fold or twist to occur at a certain spot. For example, a very small amino acid like glycine or alanine permits a fold to occur at a certain location. It is easy to understand that a fold is unlikely to occur in a location where there is a very large amino acid.

The R groups (side chains) on the amino acids each have special characteristics that may attract or repel other amino acids in the chain. Some amino acids may be hydrophilic or hydrophobic (remember those definitions from the chapter on lipids). The hydrophilic amino acids will remain on the outside of a large protein molecule, while hydrophobic molecules will be hidden on the inside. Again, this is why amino acid sequence determines the shape that the protein assumes. The shape is then stabilized by hydrogen bonds and disulfide bonds (S—S), as well as by other forces.

Configuration

The final configuration the protein assumes is globular (spherical) or coiled (fiber-like). This is often called tertiary structure, to reflect the three-dimensional nature of the protein. Occasionally two or more separate protein units interact to form an even larger new protein form. This organization becomes significant when it is important to have a protein active only at certain times. A protein may be active when the units are joined but inactive when the units are separate (Figure 5-4).

Sickle-cell disease (also called sickle-cell anemia) illustrates the importance of having a protein with the correct sequence of amino acids. African-Americans are

Peptide bond

dipeptide

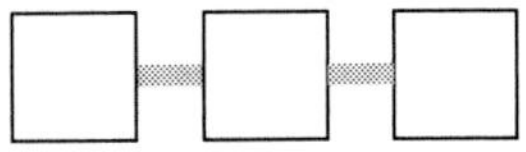

tripeptide

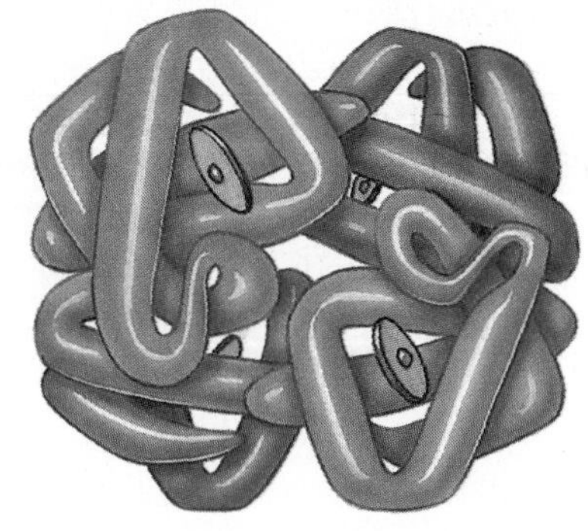

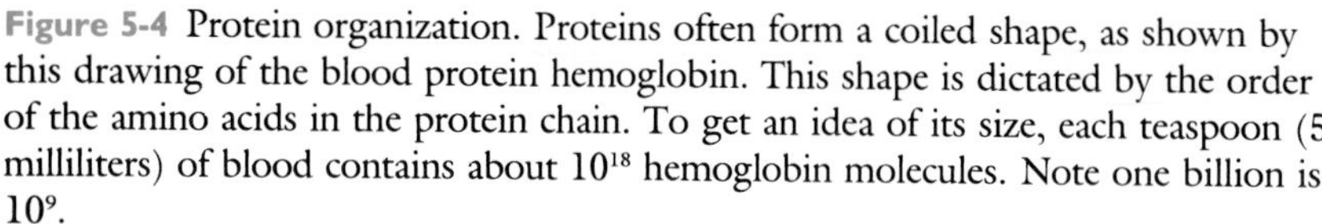

Figure 5-4 Protein organization. Proteins often form a coiled shape, as shown by this drawing of the blood protein hemoglobin. This shape is dictated by the order of the amino acids in the protein chain. To get an idea of its size, each teaspoon (5 milliliters) of blood contains about 10^{18} hemoglobin molecules. Note one billion is 10^9.

especially prone to this genetic disease. The major problem is an altered formation of the protein chains in the red blood cell protein, hemoglobin. Only one incorrect amino acid is present in each of two of the four protein chains. However, this small error produces a profound change in the structure of hemoglobin: it can no longer form the proper shape needed to carry oxygen efficiently inside the red blood cell. The red blood cells then form crescents rather than circles (Figure 5-5). Sickness results, which can lead to episodes of severe bone and joint pain, abdominal pain, headache, convulsions, and paralysis. This demonstrates how critical even a minor error in the primary structure can be. The template containing directions for this proper primary structure lies in the genetic material (the DNA, which forms genes on chromosomes) found in the nucleus of almost every cell in the body (see Chapter 6 for a brief review of this concept).

DENATURATION OF PROTEINS

denature Alteration of a protein's three dimensional form, usually due to treatment by heat, acid or alkaline solutions, or agitation.

Treatment with acid or alkaline substances, heat, or agitation can severely alter the three-dimensional shape of a protein, leaving the protein in an unfolded, or **denatured,** state. Now the protein can no longer function as originally intended. For example, once an egg is cracked into a hot frying pan and solidifies, it can no longer produce a chicken. (The same is true for whipped egg whites.) Once the bacteria

A

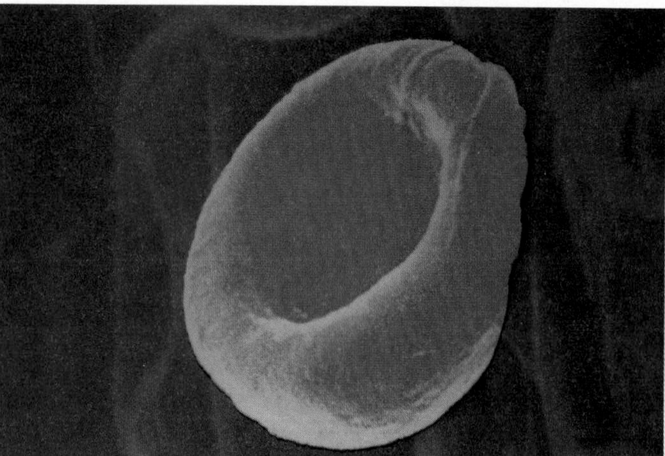

B

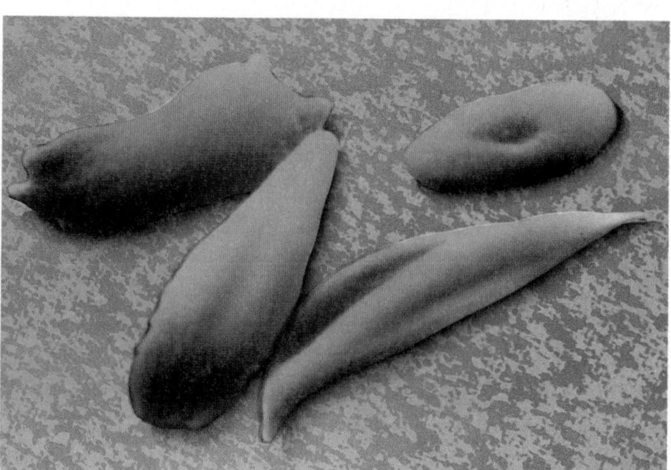

Figure 5-5 Sickle-cell disease from the perspective of the red blood cell. **A,** Normal red blood cell. **B,** Blood from a patient with sickle-cell disease. Note the abnormal, sicklelike shape of the red blood cell near the center.

in yogurt have synthesized enough acid and enzymes to precipitate the milk protein casein, the protein can never be resuspended in the water base.

Destroying a protein's three-dimensional shape often effectively destroys its normal physiological function. The body uses this characteristic of protein to its advantage. When foods reach the stomach, stomach acid denatures some bacteria, plant hormones, many active enzymes, and other forms of proteins in the food. These processes render foods safer to eat and contribute to the digestive process. Denaturing proteins in some foods can also reduce their tendencies to cause allergic reactions. Recall that we need proteins in the diet to supply essential amino acids—we do not need the active proteins themselves. We can build all the proteins we need for amino acids.

CONCEPT CHECK

The proper sequence of amino acids that form the makeup of a protein ensures that each amino acid in the protein will end up in the right position in relationship to the other amino acids when the folds and twists form. It may help to view the protein structure as first being stabilized by attractions formed between amino acids located close together. A more complex structure later may be created by attractions among amino acids located far apart in the sequence of amino acids. Only appropriately positioned amino acids can bond properly so that the correct folded shape—whether coiled or globular—forms. Destruction of the structure or shape of protein by acid or alkaline conditions, heat, or other factors unfolds—denatures—the protein, yielding an inactive form.

Functions of Proteins

Proteins play a myriad of key roles in body metabolism and the formation of body structures. As discussed above, we rely on diet to supply this protein. However, to use dietary protein efficiently, we must also consume enough total kcalories to meet energy needs. Otherwise, the amino acids in proteins will be broken down and used for energy production, rather than for synthetic purposes. In other words, protein can be used for energy, but it is not its most effective use.

PRODUCING VITAL BODY CONSTITUENTS

Proteins form muscle contractile tissue, connective tissue, blood-clotting factors, blood transport proteins, lipoproteins, visual pigments, and the support structure (protein matrix) inside bones. Measurements of the amount of certain structural proteins in the body, such as the circumference of the upper arm muscle, can be used to estimate body protein levels in health and disease.

Each cell membrane contains protein. In fact, as discussed in Chapter 4, a cell membrane is essentially composed of islands of protein in a sea of lipids. Some cell membrane proteins act as receptors for absorption of nutrients into the cell. Others act as receptor sites for some hormones or as pumps to help maintain ion balance in a cell.

Most of these vital body proteins are in a constant state of breakdown, rebuilding, and repair, especially in the intestine and bone marrow. Most of the protein breakdown products, namely amino acids, can be reused, and so add to the pool of amino acids available for future protein synthesis (Figure 5-2). However, other protein breakdown products end up being lost to reuse. When a person continually does not eat enough protein to replace lost protein, the rebuilding and repairing process slows. Then the skeletal muscles, heart, liver, blood proteins, and other organs all decrease in size or amount. The exception is the brain. It is quite resistant to breakdown in this case. For health's sake, a person must eat enough protein to ensure growth and maintenance of the body's structures.

MAINTAINING FLUID BALANCE

The blood proteins—albumin and globulin—help maintain fluid balance in the body. Blood pressure in the arteries acts to force the blood fluid (serum) out of the blood vessels into the capillary beds. The fluid then spills out into the **extracellular spaces** to provide nutrients to cells (Figure 5-6). Proteins in the bloodstream can counteract this effect of blood pressure because they are too large to move out of the capillary beds into the tissues. Their presence in the blood vessels attracts fluid to them, counteracting the force of the blood pressure. This causes most of the fluid to remain in the blood vessels.

extracellular space The space between cells.

The ability of blood proteins, simply by their presence, to attract and retain fluid in the bloodstream is due to their **osmotic potential** (see Chapter 14 for a full discussion of osmosis). In essence, the blood proteins exert an attraction—also called **oncotic** force—on the fluid in the bloodstream that counters the force of blood pressure.

osmotic potential The tendency to attract water across a semipermeable membrane, usually to dilute some constituent in a fluid.

oncotic force The osmotic potential exerted by blood proteins in the bloodstream.

If a person doesn't eat enough protein, eventually the amount of protein in the bloodstream decreases. Blood pressure then can force excessive fluid out of the blood vessels and into the extracellular spaces because there is no strong counteracting force to oppose it. As more and more fluid pools in the extracellular spaces, clinical **edema** results.[16] Other conditions, such as heart failure, kidney disease, liver disease, and pregnancy can also lead to edema. Because edema sometimes leads to serious medical problems, the cause needs to be investigated. A first step is to measure the blood protein concentration to see if it is adequate.

edema The buildup of excess fluid in extracellular spaces.

Children with protein malnutrition often show severe edema.[16] If they are fed

Arterial end of capillary bed

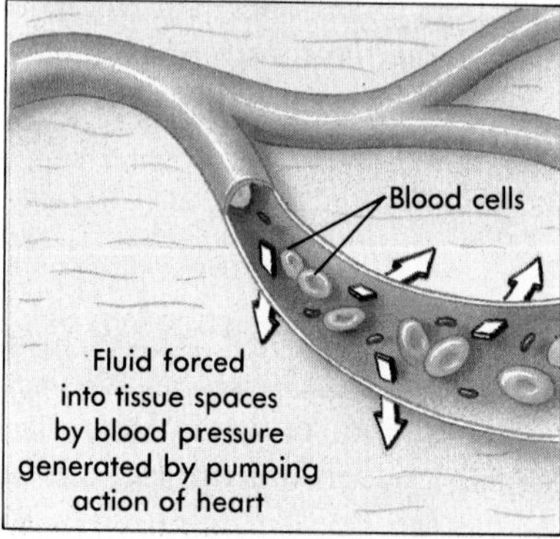

Blood pressure exceeds counteracting force of protein

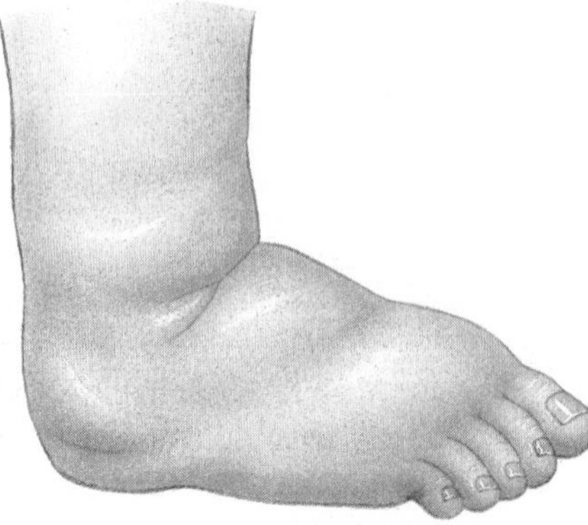

Swollen tissue (edema)

Venous end of capillary bed

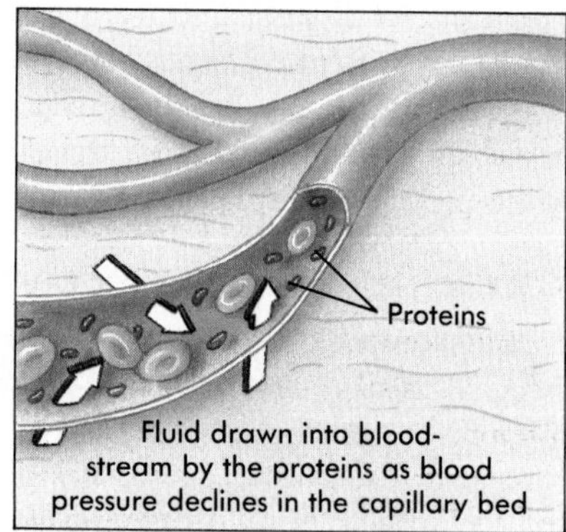

Blood pressure balanced by counteracting force of protein

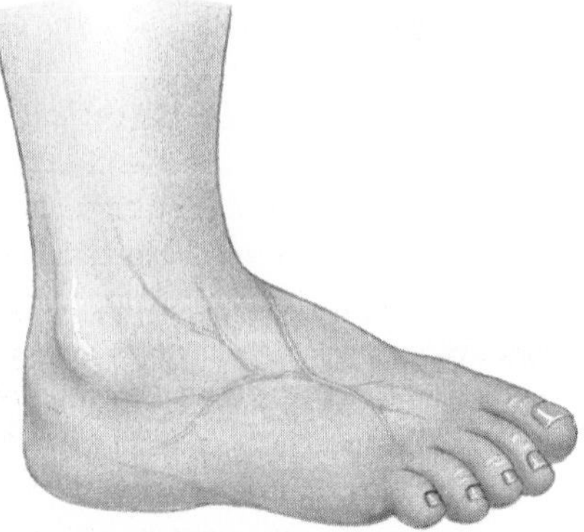

Normal tissue

Figure 5-6 Blood proteins are important for maintaining the body's fluid balance. Without sufficient protein in the bloodstream, edema develops.

protein along with the other nutrients needed for optimal health, their bodies can make more blood proteins. The fluid is then attracted back into bloodstream, and the edema disappears. We will discuss this in detail along with other effects of a protein deficiency later in this chapter.

CONTRIBUTING TO ACID-BASE BALANCE

The concentration of hydrogen ions in the bloodstream determines the acid-base balance (pH) of the blood. Proteins help regulate the amount of free hydrogen ions by readily accepting or donating hydrogen ions. This regulation helps to keep the blood pH fairly constant and slightly alkaline (pH 7.35 to 7.45). Compounds that act to keep pH within a narrow range are called **buffers.** Blood proteins are especially important buffers in the body.

buffer Compounds that can take up or release hydrogen ions to maintain a certain range of pH values in a solution.

FORMING HORMONES AND ENZYMES

Many hormones, such as the thyroid hormones T_3 and T_4, are derivatives of amino acids, while insulin is a polypeptide. These and other hormones that belong within the protein classification perform many important regulatory functions in the body, such as increasing glucose uptake from the bloodstream and controlling metabolic rate.

Neurotransmitter compounds, those made by nerve endings, are often derivatives of amino acids. This is true for dopamine, epinephrine, and serotonin. A current area of research is the study of how diet influences the synthesis of some of these neurotransmitters.

Many hormone medicines from the protein class, such as insulin, must be injected. If taken orally, insulin would be destroyed: the stomach and small intestine would digest the hormone, dismantling it into amino acids, as they do with foods. The digestive tract is unable to distinguish between a protein like insulin, which is being taken for medication, and a protein like hamburger, which is being consumed for nutrients.

Almost all enzymes are proteins (a few are composed of nucleic acids). Enzymes are organic compounds that catalyze (speed) chemical reactions. Occasionally a cell lacks the correct DNA structure for instructions on how to make needed enzymes. An infant, for example, suffering from the disease **galactosemia** cannot make the enzyme needed to metabolize the single sugar galactose. If the infant is not put on a galactose-free diet soon after birth, its growth and mental development will be depressed. This case demonstrates the crucial roles that enzymes, and thus proteins, play in cell function.

galactosemia A rare, genetic disease characterized by the buildup of the monosaccharide galactose in the bloodstream due to the inability of the liver to metabolize it. If present at birth and left untreated, it results in severe growth and mental retardation.

CONTRIBUTING TO THE IMMUNE FUNCTION

Proteins compose key parts of the cells used by the immune system (Figure 5-7). Also, the **antibodies** produced by one type of immune cell (β-lymphocytes) are proteins. These antibodies can bind to foreign proteins in the body, an important step in ridding invaders from the body (see Chapter 15 for a description of how the immune system works). Without enough protein in the diet, the immune system will lack the cells and other tools needed to function properly.[16] Thus immune incompetence—**anergy**—and a protein deficient diet often appear together. Anergy can turn measles into a fatal disease for a malnourished child. It also can encourage unusual infections, such as widespread yeast *(Candida)* growth in the mouth and throat of hospitalized adults. This yeast can more easily reproduce and spread when an immune system functions poorly.

antibody A protein that inactivates foreign proteins found in the body to prevent infections.

anergy Lack of an immune response to foreign compounds entering the body.

FORMING GLUCOSE

In Chapter 3 we noted that the body must maintain a fairly constant level of glucose in the bloodstream to supply energy for red blood cells and nerve tissue. The brain uses about 35% of the body's energy needs at rest, and it gets most of that energy from glucose. If a diet does not contain enough carbohydrate to supply the glucose, the liver and to a lesser extent the kidneys will be forced to metabolize amino acids to make the glucose (Figure 5-3). Many types of amino acids can be used for this purpose. Recall the metabolic process of turning amino acids into glucose is called gluconeogenesis.

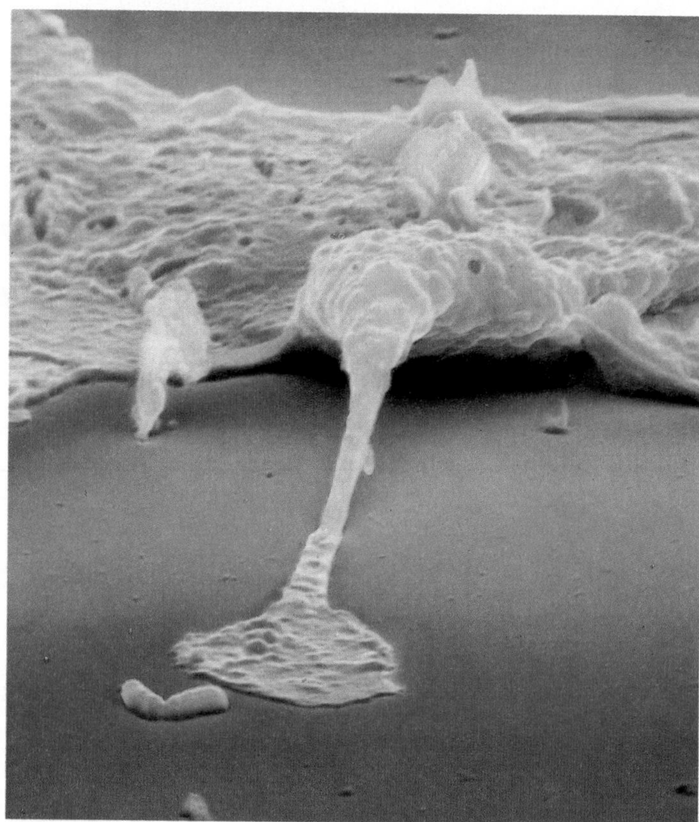

Figure 5-7 Going in for the kill. Ever vigilant, a patrolling white blood cell (macrophage) attacks a bacterium. Adequate protein in the diet aids immune system responses like this one.

Some gluconeogenesis is normal, for example, it occurs after skipping breakfast when you haven't eaten since 7 PM the night before. Taken to the extreme, however, a constant need for gluconeogenesis causes much of the muscle wasting that occurs in starvation.

PROVIDING ENERGY

We have discussed how proteins can be used for energy. About 10% of body energy comes from this source. Still, most cells more readily use carbohydrates and fatty acids for energy. Proteins and carbohydrates contain the same amount of usable energy, 4 kcalories per gram. However, proteins are a very costly source of energy, in terms of both the amount of metabolism and handling required by the liver and kidneys and the original cost of protein foods.

CONCEPT CHECK

Proteins form vital body constituents, such as muscles, connective tissues, blood transport proteins, enzymes, hormones, and immune bodies. Proteins can also provide fuel for the body and carbons for the synthesis of glucose. Through the formation of important body proteins, many key body processes are affected by proteins, such as acid-base balance, fluid balance, and immune function.

Evaluation of Protein Quality

Protein quality refers to the ability of a food protein to support body growth and maintenance. Methods exist to both measure and estimate protein quality. We will discuss the more important approaches.

BIOLOGICAL VALUE

The **biological value (BV) of a protein** is a measure of how efficiently food protein can be turned into body tissues. If a food possesses enough of all essential amino acids, it should allow a person to efficiently incorporate the food protein into body proteins. The biological value of a food then depends on how closely its amino acid pattern reflects the amino acid pattern in body tissues. The better the match, the more completely food protein turns into body protein.

biological value (BV) of a protein A measurement of the body's ability to retain protein absorbed from a food.

$$\text{BV} = \frac{\text{nitrogen retained}}{\text{nitrogen absorbed}} = \frac{\text{dietary nitrogen} - (\text{urinary nitrogen} + \text{fecal nitrogen})}{\text{dietary nitrogen} - \text{fecal nitrogen}}$$

We actually measure protein retention by measuring nitrogen retention. Nitrogen itself is easier to measure than protein, and all amino acids contain nitrogen. Both humans and laboratory animals are used to generate data for biological value determinations (Table 5-3).

If the amino acid pattern in a food is quite unlike human tissue amino acid patterns, many amino acids in the food will not become body protein. They simply end up leftovers. Their nitrogen groups are removed and excreted in the urine as urea. The carbon skeleton that remains is turned into either glucose or fat, or is burned for energy needs (Figure 5-2). Since the nitrogen is not retained, the ratio of retained nitrogen to absorbed nitrogen, and consequent biological value, is small.

Egg white protein has the highest biological value of any single protein source. Milk and meat proteins also have high biological values. This makes sense because humans and other animals have similar amino acid compositions. Because plant amino acid patterns differ greatly from those of humans, corn has only a moderate biological value: It is high enough to support body maintenance, but not growth. Peanuts eaten alone have a poor biological value.

As with essential amino acids, the importance of the biological value of a single food can be overemphasized. It is the biological value of an entire meal that must be considered. Rarely will a meal yield an overall low biological value, even if only plant foods are eaten. The amino acids in peanuts and bread of a peanut butter and jelly sandwich combine to yield complete protein. In other words the two proteins complement one another. Given a variety of foods in a meal, different amino acids usually combine to yield complete protein.[7] This then gives a good overall amino acid pattern, hence a high biological value for the meal.

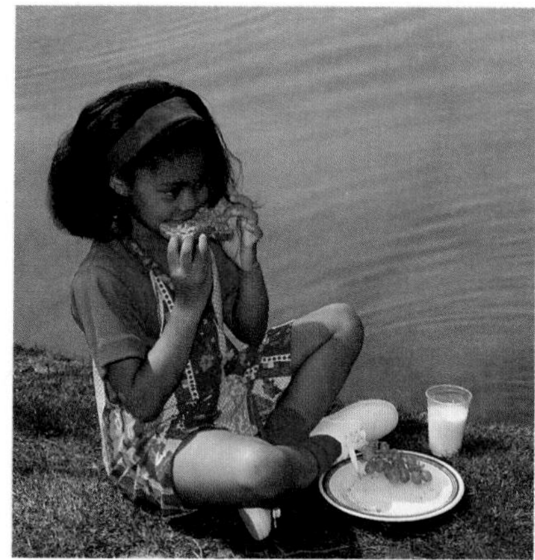

Plant proteins in a peanut butter sandwich combine to yield high quality (complete) protein in the meal.

Table 5-3 Comparative protein quality of selected foods

Food	Chemical (amino acid) score	BV*	PER†
Egg	100	100	3.92
Cow's milk	95	93	3.09
Fish	71	76	3.55
Beef	69	74	2.30
Unpolished rice	67	86	—
Peanuts	65	55	1.65
Oats	57	65	2.19
Polished rice	57	64	2.18
Whole wheat	53	65	1.53
Corn	49	72	—
Soybeans	47	73	2.32
Sesame seeds	42	62	1.77
Peas	37	64	1.57

* Biological value
† Protein efficiency ratio

The concept of biological value is very important in treating some kidney and liver diseases. These organs must help metabolize and dispose of extra amino acids, especially the nitrogen groups. In treating these diseases it is desirable to have as much protein as possible synthesized into body tissues, with as few amino acids as possible left over to burden the already elevated blood urea ($H_2N{-}\overset{\overset{\displaystyle O}{\|}}{C}{-}NH_2$) or ammonia ($NH_3$) levels. Egg or milk proteins are then the sources of choice. These provide the highest biological value possible from foods, in turn allowing protein synthesis to occur without generating large amounts of unneeded amino acids.

PROTEIN EFFICIENCY RATIO

protein efficiency ratio (PER) A measure of protein quality in a food determined by the ability of the protein to support growth in a young rat.

The **protein efficiency ratio (PER)** provides another means for measuring a food's protein quality. FDA uses this method to set standards for food labeling. The PER compares the amount of weight gained by a growing rat after 10 or more days of eating a set amount of protein (9.09% of its kcalorie intake) from one food source to the total grams of protein eaten, given a constant amount of energy in the diet.

$$\text{PER} = \frac{\text{weight gained in a time period (grams)}}{\text{protein intake in that time period (grams)}}$$

The PER of a food reflects its biological value, since both basically measure protein retention by body tissues (Table 5-3). Plant proteins, due to their incomplete nature, yield low PER values. However, as with biological value, the low PER values for individual plant proteins are often of little consequence. Usually we eat many foods—not just one—at a meal. The PER of a peanut butter sandwich will be higher than that of either the bread or peanut butter alone. Why?

The PER also has a practical side. By definition, the PER of the milk protein casein is 2.5. If the PER of a protein is less than 2.5, the U.S. RDA currently used on nutrition labels increases from the standard value of 45 grams to 65 grams to compensate for the amount that food protein is to be compared to. In essence, the label penalizes the food for its lower quality of protein by indicating more of it must be eaten to meet typical protein needs.

CHEMICAL SCORE OF PROTEINS

chemical score A ratio comparing the essential amino acid content of the protein in a food with the essential amino acid content in a reference protein, such as one established by the Food and Agriculture Organization of the United Nations; the lowest ratio for any essential amino acid becomes the chemical score.

Protein quality of a food can be estimated by its **chemical score.** To calculate a food's chemical score, the amount of each essential amino acid provided by a gram of protein in the food is divided by an "ideal" amount for that essential amino acid per gram of food protein. The "ideal" protein pattern is based on the minimal amount (in milligrams) of each essential amino acid that is needed per gram of the food protein to provide all nine essential amino acids.

$$\text{chemical score} = \frac{\text{milligrams of essential amino acid per gram of test protein} \times 100}{\text{milligrams of essential amino acid per gram of the "ideal" protein}}$$

The lowest amino acid ratio calculated for any essential amino acid is the chemical score. Various "ideal" patterns are available. The pattern set by the Food and Agriculture Organization (FAO) of the United Nations for preschool children is often used. It is designed to represent the amino acid levels in human tissue proteins. Note that because children need a greater percentage of protein as essential amino acids than do adults, applying the children's standard to adults underestimates the chemical score value for adults.

For an example of a chemical score calculation, assume the "ideal" lysine level in a diet is 5.5% or 5.5 milligrams per 100 milligrams of total protein. Wheat protein is most deficient in lysine, with a concentration of 2.4% of total protein. The chemical score for wheat would be:

$$\frac{2.4}{5.5} \times 100 = 44$$

The chemical score is quite similar in concept to biological value since both are based on meeting the body's need for the right balance of essential amino acids. The main advantage of the chemical score method is that it can easily be determined because of the availability of instruments that can measure the amino acid content of a food. Two disadvantages for using the chemical score for protein evaluation are (1) it does not consider digestibility, and (2) it does not account for whether toxic substances, such as present in some root crops and tubers, are also present in the food source of the protein. Feeding the protein to animals, as is done for a biological value or PER determination, would indicate both.

Again, keep in mind that we usually eat meals, not single foods, as protein sources. The concepts of biological value, PER, and chemical score have important uses, such as in designing diets for sick people, evaluating individual proteins for famine relief, and determining the effects of food processing on food proteins. However, if you eat enough protein from a variety of foods, you will meet your essential amino acid needs. Remember also that protein quality is an issue only if the food you eat provides adequate kcalories. Otherwise, high quality or not, protein will be used for energy needs first, not protein needs.

CONCEPT CHECK

Protein quality can be measured by determining a food's biological value. This essentially represents the body's ability to retain the food protein absorbed. Protein quality can also be measured by a food's capability to support weight gain in a young growing rat: this measurement is the protein efficiency ratio. To simply estimate protein quality, the essential amino acid composition of the protein can be compared with a reference protein. A chemical score can then be calculated that indicates how well the food protein matches body tissue needs. The protein quality values of individual foods are important, but the protein quality of a total meal is primarily what counts.

The Recommended Dietary Allowance For Protein

How much protein (actually, how many of each essential amino acid) do we need to eat each day? If a person is not growing, he or she simply needs to eat enough protein to match daily losses from the urine, feces, skin, hair, nails, and so on. In short, the person needs to balance protein intake with losses.[8] This maintains the body in a steady state of protein equilibrium.

When either growing or recovering from an illness, the body needs to achieve a positive balance to supply the resources needed for producing new tissues. Consequently protein intake must exceed daily losses. This positive balance requires an appropriate hormonal state. The hormones insulin, growth hormone, and testosterone all stimulate positive protein balance. Merely eating protein does not guarantee a positive balance; the body also needs the right hormonal condition to build extra tissues.

During starvation or illness, protein losses from the body often exceed intake, and the body falls into a negative balance.[12] Hormones that encourage this state are cortisol and thyroid hormone (Table 5-4). They both can stimulate muscle tissue breakdown.

To measure the balance between protein gain and loss by the body, we actually calculate nitrogen balance; only the nitrogen from proteins is excreted to any degree by the body. Nitrogen makes up about 16% of the weight of a protein. So nitrogen intake or output divided by 0.16 yields a rough estimate of protein intake or output. We can also multiply by the reciprocal of 0.16, which is 6.25:

$$\textbf{nitrogen (grams)} \times \textbf{6.25} = \textbf{protein (grams)}$$

The nitrogen excreted in a variety of forms by the body is derived from proteins,

Table 5-4 Protein balance in practical terms

Protein equilibrium: body protein constant
Protein intake = Protein excretion
Positive protein balance: Increase in body protein
Protein intake > Protein excretion
Negative protein balance: decrease in body protein
Protein excretion > Protein intake

Positive protein balance	*Negative protein balance*
Growth	Inadequate intake of protein (fasting, intestinal tract diseases)
Pregnancy	Inadequate energy intake
Recovery stage after illness	Illnesses, such as fevers, burns, and infections
Athletic training*	Bed rest (days)
Increased secretion of hormones, such as insulin, growth hormone, and testosterone	Deficiency of essential amino acids
	Increased protein loss (as in some kidney diseases)
	Increased secretion of certain hormones, such as thyroid hormone and cortisol

*Only when additional lean body mass is being gained. Nevertheless, the athlete is probably already eating enough protein to support this extra protein synthesis: protein supplements are not needed.

so this calculation also gives a measure of the protein lost from the body.

In a healthy person the amount of dietary protein needed to maintain protein (nitrogen) balance can be determined by increasing protein intake until protein intake just equals protein losses. Energy needs must be met so that amino acids are not diverted for energy use. Any protein intake above that needed for protein equilibrium also will lead to an equal intake and output. However, in order to estimate the requirement we actually need to determine the least amount of protein intake that still allows for intake to equal output. An optimal protein intake should yield a balance in the rate of protein synthesis and breakdown. Too little protein in the diet will slow protein synthesis and may not allow synthesis to keep up with breakdown.

Desirable body weight is based on height (see Chapter 8). Desirable body weight is preferred to actual body weight because extra fat storage does not increase protein needs. You may also see the terms ideal or healthy body weight. Both terms—ideal and healthy—represent about the same thing as desirable.

The best estimate for the amount of protein required to meet the needs of nearly all adults—where intake equals output—is 0.8 grams of protein per kilogram of desirable body weight. (We will discuss values for infants and children in future chapters.) This works out to about 56 grams of protein per day for a 70-kilogram (154-pound) man, and about 44 grams of protein per day for a 55-kilogram (120-pound) woman.

Recall that an RDA is an allowance, not a requirement. Some people require less protein than this RDA amount. Even so, the average man and woman in the United States consumes about 90 to 70 grams of protein, respectively, per day, a level in excess of the RDA. Canadian values are similar. People just happen to eat many high-protein foods in North America and can afford them. The excess protein cannot be stored as such. As noted before, the nitrogen group is removed and the carbon skeleton is turned into glucose or fat and then either stored or burned for energy needs (Figure 5-2).

RDA calculations

$$\frac{\textit{154 pounds}}{\textit{2.2 kilograms/pound}} = \textit{70 kilograms}$$

$$\textit{70 kilograms} \times \frac{\textit{0.8 grams protein}}{\textit{kilograms body weight}}$$

$$= \textit{56 grams protein}$$

Mental stress, physical labor, and routine, weekend sports activities do not require an increase in the RDA for protein. Elderly people might need 1 gram of protein per kilogram of body weight. In addition, to support either training needs of endurance athletes, substantial gains in muscle tissue in highly trained athletes, or a large muscle mass formerly acquired, increasing the allowance up to 1.5 times the RDA might be considered. But keep in mind that many of us eat that much protein already. Protein intakes above usual adult intakes are rarely needed for athletes. In addition, there is usually no reason for athletes to take either protein or individual amino acid supplements. All of us—athletes included—can meet our protein needs using basic foods.

Canadians estimate protein needs using 0.82 grams of protein per kilogram of body weight for adult men and 0.74 grams of protein per kilogram of body weight for adult women.

ARE THE HIGH-PROTEIN INTAKES OF AMERICANS HARMFUL?

It is unclear whether or not our high intake of protein is harmful. The extra vitamin B-6, iron, and zinc provided by high-protein foods is often a welcome addition. But research in the 1970s suggested that a high-protein diet might cause greater calcium loss in the urine. This worried researchers because they thought that protein caused calcium to leach out of the bones. In the long run this depletion can demineralize bones and lead to **osteoporosis**, a severe bone disease. However, follow-up studies show that if extra phosphorus is also consumed, urine calcium does not increase so much. Animal foods are excellent sources of both protein and phosphorus. Thus typical American intakes probably don't threaten calcium balance as long as the RDA for calcium is met[20] (see Chapter 14 for further discussion).

osteoporosis A bone disease characterized by decreased bone density that develops primarily after menopause in women.

There is some concern that high-protein intakes may unduly burden the kidneys to excrete the resulting excess nitrogen (mostly as urea) into the urine.[3] Animal studies show that protein intakes that just meet nutritional needs preserve kidney function over time better than high-protein diets. However, the same can be said for low-kcalorie diets.[19] Thus the animal research has yet to determine which is more important for preserving kidney function—a conservative protein intake or a conservative energy intake.

Preserving kidney function is especially important for people with diabetes mellitus and for people who have only one functioning kidney. Thus high-protein diets are discouraged in these cases. For people without diabetes the risk of suffering kidney failure is very low and so the risk of a high-protein diet contributing to kidney disease in later life is probably also low.

Infants' diets must not contain excess protein since their kidneys have difficulty excreting the excess urea and minerals leftover after protein metabolism. Thus regular cow milk must not be used by itself for feeding young infants—it is too high in protein and other nutrients (see Chapter 17 for details).

Overall, the caution against high-protein intakes issued by the National Academy of Sciences in their 1989 *Diet and Health Report* deserves consideration. The panel recommended we not consume more than twice the RDA for protein on a regular basis.

THE IMPORTANCE OF PLANT PROTEINS

Vegetable proteins deserve more attention. These proteins, in proportion to the amount of energy they supply, provide much magnesium, soluble fiber, and other important benefits. Whenever the U.S. Department of Agriculture has rated foods according to the best protein buy for your dollar, dry beans have always been at or near the top of the list. Furthermore, vegetable proteins contain no cholesterol and are low in saturated fat, unless saturated fat is added during commercial processing or home preparation.

As we discovered in Chapter 2, one to two servings of plant proteins per day are consistent with the recommendations of the Guide to Daily Food Choices. Presently plant proteins are not very popular in America, except for maybe peanut butter, baked beans, and refried beans. Should you give them a second look?

CONCEPT CHECK

The Recommended Dietary Allowance of protein for adults is 0.8 grams of protein per kilogram of desirable body weight. For a 70-kilogram (156-pound) person, this means 56 grams of protein per day. The average American man consumes about 90 grams of protein per day, and the average woman consumes about 70 grams of protein per day. Thus our typical protein intakes are more than ample to meet protein needs.

EXPERT OPINION

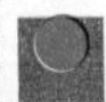

How Much Protein Do We Really Need?

A.E. HARPER, Ph.D.

In 1862, Dr. Edward Smith, a British physician who had studied energy and protein metabolism, concluded that to ensure the working capacity of the labor force during periods of food shortage, a physically active man would need 80 grams of protein daily. During the next 40 years, other estimates of protein needs, which were based on records of the amounts of protein consumed by healthy working men, ranged up to 150 grams per day. But a controversy developed in the early 1900s after Russell Chittenden, an American chemist, concluded from the results of studies on himself, his colleagues, and his students at Yale that 35 to 45 grams of protein per day was sufficient for healthy adults. This controversy has not been entirely resolved but the gap between the lower and higher estimates of protein needs of adults has narrowed.

Problems in establishing protein needs

Researchers face five problems in determining how much protein we need. First, there's the matter of measurement. Until the early 1900s, a measurement of the nitrogen content of a food was accepted as a reliable estimate of its value as a protein source ($N \times 6.25$ = protein). About that time, however, the amount of dietary protein required to prevent loss of body nitrogen was found to differ from one food source to another. The differences were explained when some amino acids in proteins were discovered to be essential nutrients and proteins were shown to differ in their content of these amino acids. This meant that the protein requirement was a dual one and that the ability of foods to supply certain indispensable amino acids could not be estimated from their nitrogen content alone. Some measure of this ability was also needed. How this should be measured is still being debated.

Second, clear signs of protein deficiency don't develop until protein depletion is severe. So it is not possible to reduce the protein intake of human subjects to the point where signs of severe depletion appear and then establish the requirement by determining how much is needed to just prevent their appearance. The initial effect of consuming a protein-deficient diet is loss of body protein. To gauge this loss requires accurate measurements of the amount of nitrogen consumed and the amounts lost in urine and feces. By feeding subjects a series of diets in which the protein content has been increased incrementally and determining the amount required to achieve nitrogen equilibrium, we can estimate the requirement. It tends to be an underestimate, however, because nitrogen lost in sweat, hair, and minor body secretions is rarely measured. An element of judgment is therefore involved in appropriately correcting for the loss.

Third, if protein intake is reduced, adaptation occurs and nitrogen equilibrium is achieved at the lower intake.

Fourth, amino acids, besides being essential nutrients, can also serve as sources of energy. If energy intake is low, a portion of the amino acids from dietary protein will be burned for fuel and additional protein will be required to compensate for this; hence protein requirements will be overestimated. If energy intake is high, amino acids are used more efficiently than usual so protein requirements may be underestimated.

Protein in Foods

The exchange system provides an easy means of estimating the protein content of a food. The fruit and fat groups contain no protein; the vegetable group yields 2 grams of protein; the starch/bread group yields 3 grams of protein; the meat group yields 7 grams of protein; and the milk group yields 8 grams of protein per exchange.

Note that Table 5-5 also shows that it is quite easy to obtain the RDA for protein by following the Guide to Daily Food Choices, even when consuming only 1200 kcalories a day.

The most nutrient-dense source of protein is water-packed tuna, which has over 80% of kcalories as protein (Figure 5-9). Notice that all the foods with more than 20% of kcalories as proteins are animal foods. They are also the major sources of protein in the American diet; over two thirds of our protein comes from animal sources. Worldwide, 54% of protein comes from animal sources. In Africa and East Asia less than 25% of the protein eaten comes from animals.

In the United States in 1990, red meat and poultry consumption (on a boneless basis) was 175 pounds per person per year. Beef and chicken tied with an annual per person consumption of 64 pounds each. Fish consumption averaged 15 pounds per person.

EXPERT OPINION

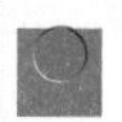

How Much Protein Do We Really Need?—cont'd

A.E. HARPER, Ph.D.

Fifth, if one or more of the indispensable amino acids is present in disproportionately low amounts in relation to the requirements, the protein will be used inefficiently for synthesis of body proteins. That's true of cereal grain proteins, which are low in lysine. In many poor countries where diets are composed largely of plant products, mixtures of cereal grains and legumes are traditionally used. The amino acid patterns of the two complement each other. Thus the mixture is used more efficiently than either source alone.

Quantifying protein needs—the modern view

The FAO/WHO/UNU committee has estimated from the results of the best nitrogen-balance studies that the average need of adults for high-quality proteins is 0.6 grams per kilogram of body weight per day. As half the population should have protein requirements below the average (and half above) public health recommendations for meeting protein needs must be high enough to cover the needs of those with the highest requirements. The FAO/WHO "safe" intake was therefore set at 0.75 grams of high-quality protein per kilogram of body weight per day. The RDA for adults in the United States is 0.8 grams per kilogram of body weight. Men and women don't differ in their protein requirements per unit of body weight but women, because they generally weigh less, need less total protein than men.

If you're doing heavy work in a hot, humid environment, the amount of nitrogen lost in sweat can increase substantially. Under most conditions, the loss appears to be small and transitory so no extra allowance for protein is recommended for physically active people. They usually eat enough extra food to meet their increased energy needs and ensure that their protein intake will also meet any increased needs.

Appropriate intakes of protein

Recommended intakes of protein for different age groups are listed on the inside cover of this textbook. These are sufficient to meet protein needs if there's adequate consumption of all other essential nutrients and energy. That these amounts of protein are a lot less than most people desire is evident from the average U.S. intake of nearly 100 grams per day. So perhaps the question we should ask is "What is an appropriate dietary guideline for protein?" rather than "How much protein do we really need?"

The committee that established the Recommended Intakes of Nutrients for the United Kingdom proposed a guideline for protein of not less than 10% of kcalories. We might well recommend from 10% to 15% of kcalories as protein—not on the basis of meeting protein needs as such but rather on the basis of evidence that diets rich in protein are ordinarily highly nutritious. There is no evidence of risk to health from such intakes. As caloric expenditure declines during aging, the appropriate guideline for the elderly should probably be toward the upper end of the range but, as kidney function also tends to decline with increasing age, it should probably not exceed 15% of total kcalories.

Dr. Harper is Professor Emeritus of Nutritional Sciences at the University of Wisconsin at Madison.

Table 5-5 The protein content of a 1200- and a 2400-kcalorie diet

This table illustrates how few kcalories can be consumed while still meeting the RDA for protein. It also shows how much protein we eat when we consume typical kcalorie intakes.

1200 Kcalories	Grams of protein	2400 Kcalories	Grams of protein
Breakfast			
1 cup skim milk	8	1 cup 2% milk	8
¾ cup Cheerios	3	¾ cup Cheerios	3
1 orange	—	2 soft-cooked eggs	12
		1 orange	—
Lunch			
2 slices whole-wheat bread	7	2 slices whole-wheat bread	7
2 oz chicken breast	18	2 oz chicken breast	18

Continued.

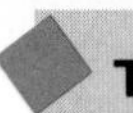

Table 5-5 The protein content of a 1200- and a 2400-kcalorie diet—cont'd

1200 Kcalories	Grams of protein	2400 Kcalories	Grams of protein
Lunch—cont'd			
1 cup carrot sticks	1	1 T mayonnaise	—
1 fig	0.5	2 oatmeal raisin cookies	2
diet soda	—	2 figs	1
		diet soda	—
Dinner			
2 oz beef tenderloin	18	4 oz beef tenderloin	36
1 cup spinach pasta with 1 t garlic butter	7	1 cup spinach pasta with 1 t garlic butter	7
½ cup zucchini sautéed in 1 t oil	0.5	½ cup zucchini sauteed in 1 t oil	0.5
1 cup skim milk	8	1 cup 2% milk	8
Snack			
½ bagel	4	1 bagel	7
	75 grams		122 grams

NUTRITION FOCUS

Do You Need to Rediscover Legumes?

Legumes are the plant family with seed pods that contain one row of seeds: garden peas, green beans, lima beans, pinto beans, black-eyed peas, garbanzo beans, lentils, and soybeans. Dried varieties of the seeds—what we know as beans—yield an impressive contribution to the protein, vitamin, mineral, and dietary fiber content of a meal (Figure 5-8).

Many people dismiss beans from their diets. This unfortunate oversight may be rooted in the Depression of the 1930s when people could afford little else. Beans are such a versatile food: They can anchor or blend into soups, salads, casseroles, sandwich spreads, and cracker dips; they can be added in small quantities wherever extra body, texture, and/or nutritional value is desired. Incorporating them into your week's menu can add variety and new flavors (Table 5-6).

Most legumes except lentils need to be softened before cooking. Soak them overnight. Or, boil for two minutes, uncovered; then remove from heat, cover, and let stand one hour. Dried beans double or triple in volume as they cook. Once cooked, discard any liquid as this is loaded with undigestible carbohydrates (see page 159). Because legumes tend to soak up flavors during the cooking process, it is possible to incorporate delicate flavors from combinations of herbs, spices, and broths.

When you initially add legumes to your diet, they may cause intestinal gas. Split peas, limas, and lentils are less likely to do so than the others, so start with them. Take small servings at first and give your GI tract a few weeks to adjust. Many people have no trouble with legumes, but it's best to be cautious. An enzyme preparation called Beano is also available to ease gas symptoms. Taken right before a meal, it helps digest the undigestible carbohydrates in beans that contribute to intestinal gas (see Chapter 3).

Like all foods, though, legumes do not offer every nutrient, and so they do not make a complete diet by themselves. They contain no vitamin A, vitamin C, or vitamin B-12. The protein in beans is somewhat deficient in methionine, one of the essential amino acids, and therefore is considered an incomplete protein source. This lack is easily made up by serving beans with a food high in methionine, such as meat, eggs, or cheese in typical diets, or with rice, corn, or other grains in vegetarian diets (see the Nutrition Perspective). Many traditional ethnic dishes combine legumes with grains and vegetables to yield a high-quality protein balance: lentil curry on rice; pinto beans and corn tortillas; tofu (soybean curd) and rice; and corn and lima beans (succotash). Try these combinations or create your own.

As you prepare foods or order them in a restaurant, look for beans—salad bars usually provide a few choices. Black bean and other bean soups, baked beans, chili, red beans and rice, and soy burgers are other possibilities. Regularly consuming vegetable proteins, as noted in Chapter 2, can add substantial amounts of nutrients to a diet. And as discussed in Chapter 3, the soluble fiber in them can help lower your blood cholesterol level as well and moderate the swings in blood glucose seen after eating a meal.

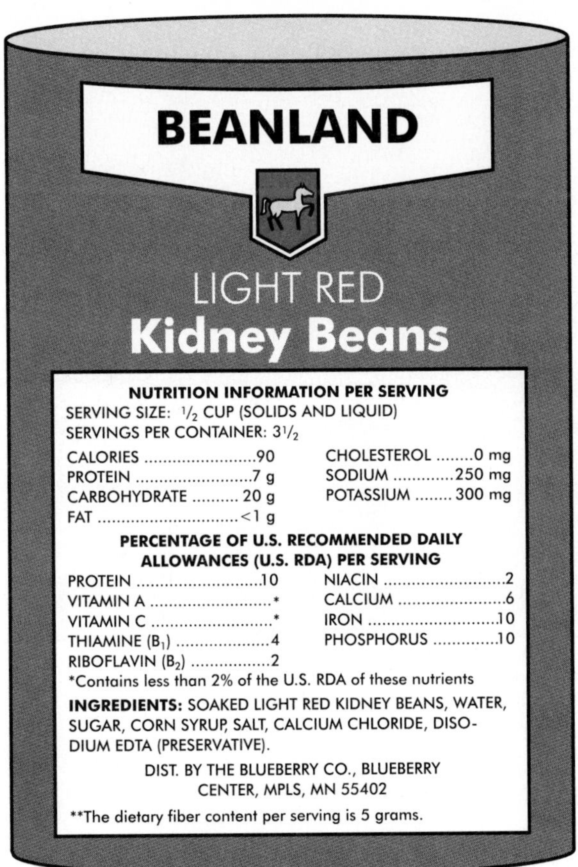

Figure 5-8 Legumes are rich sources of protein. One-half cup meets about 10% of protein needs, and at a "cost" of only about 5% of energy needs. The addition of dietary fiber to one's diet is an added bonus.

Table 5-6 Get to know the legumes

Type	Color	Use
Black beans	Black	Baked, soups, stews
Black-eyed peas	White with a black spot	Casseroles
Garbanzo beans (chickpeas)	Brown	Dips, casseroles, salads, soups, stews
Great northern beans	White	Baked, casseroles, chowder, soups, stews
Kidney beans	Red	Casseroles, chili, salads, soups
Lentils	Brown or green	Casseroles, salads, soups
Lima beans	White	Casseroles, soups
Navy beans	White	Baked, soups
Pinto beans	Pink	Baked, casseroles, soups
Red beans	Red	Casseroles, chili
Soybeans	Tan	Casseroles, salads
Split peas	Green or yellow	Soups

Adapted from Neiman, Butterworth, Neiman: *Nutrition,* 1990, William C Brown.

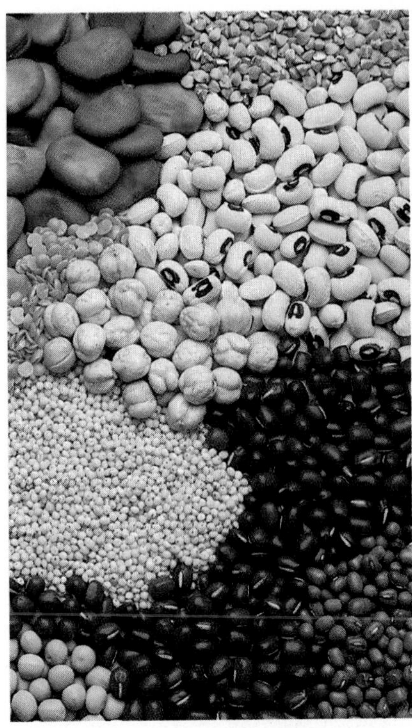

Legumes—another protein source that can meet a body's protein needs. An added bonus is the many other nutrients also present in legumes.

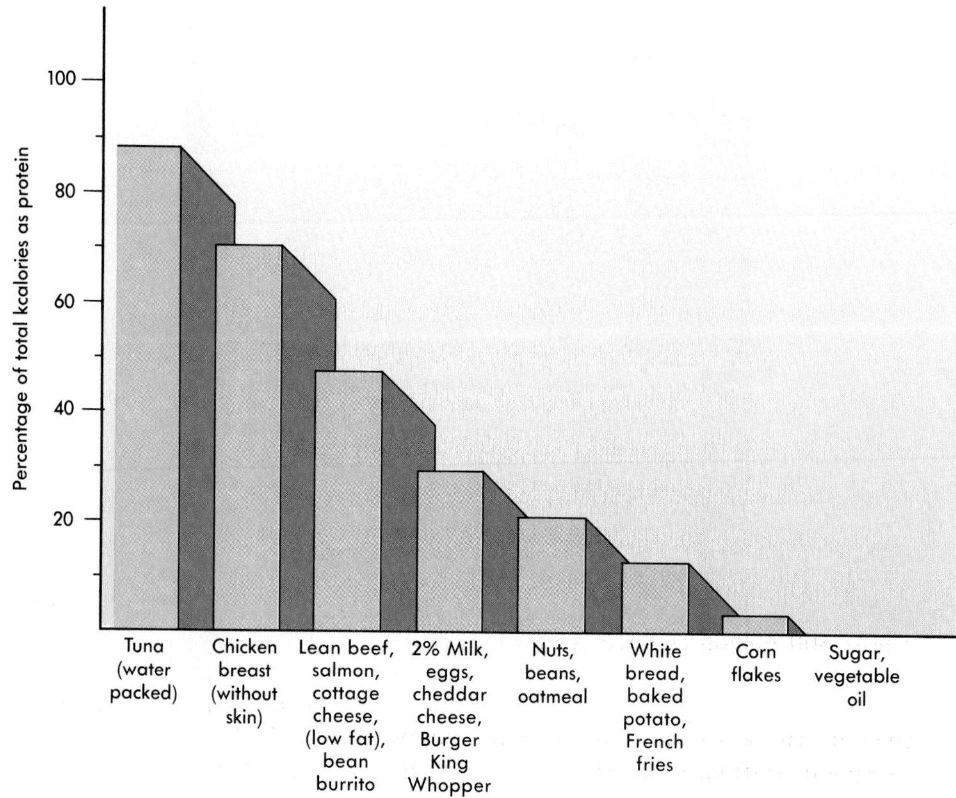

Figure 5-9 Percent of kcalories as proteins in foods. Water-packed tuna provides almost all kcalories as proteins.

It is always wise to consider the documented benefits against the risks when self-prescribing supplements.

The amino acids most likely to be low in a diet are lysine, methionine, threonine, and tryptophan. Table 5-2 lists plant foods that are characteristically low in these amino acids, although new strains of high-lysine and high-tryptophan corn are now available, as well as other improved grains. These strains yield better protein quality. The amino acids most likely to be toxic when consumed in large amounts are methionine and tyrosine. The potential for amino acid imbalances and toxicities are too great to recommend that any be taken individually as supplements. As a case in point, recently an unexpected increase in the number of cases of eosinophilia-myalgia syndrome have been reported.[2] Through careful detective work, many of these cases were associated with the consumption of the amino acid, tryptophan. Eventually, it was discovered that this may be the result of a contaminant introduced into the tryptophan supplement preparation. The supplement was recommended primarily to women as a tranquilizer and sleeping preparation; note that no actual benefit was ever demonstrated. If a diet is low in an amino acid, nutrition experts recommend finding a good food source to supply it.[9]

Protein Deficiency Conditions

protein-energy malnutrition (PEM) A condition resulting from regularly consuming insufficient amounts of kcalories and protein. The deficiency eventually results in body wasting and an increased susceptibility to infections.

In nonindustrialized areas of the world, people often eat diets low in kcalories and protein. Such diets stunt growth and increase susceptibility to disease. A person who eats too little protein and energy food can develop symptoms of undernutrition, usually called **protein-energy malnutrition (PEM)** but also referred to as protein-calorie malnutrition (PCM). Although the number of people who show PEM is

Table 5-7 Factors contributing to protein-energy malnutrition in young children

1. Younger children's relative needs for protein and kcalories (per kilogram of body weight) are greater than those of older family members.
2. Diets that are of low-energy density (often high in fiber and unappealing), low in protein, and not fed frequently enough.
3. Not enough food for the family as a result of poverty, inequity, insufficient land to farm, and food distribution within the family.
4. Infections (viral, bacterial, and parasitic) may cause lack of appetite, reduced food intake, poor nutrient absorption and utilization, or result in nutrient losses.
5. Famine due to droughts, natural disasters, wars, and civil disturbances.
6. Inappropriate formula preparation and weaning practices; inappropriate use of infant formula in place of breastfeeding in poor families or areas with unsanitary water supply.

difficult to determine because of inability to reach areas of occurrence and variation in interpretation of definitions, the World Health Organization (WHO) estimates at least 500 million children worldwide suffer from PEM. Common factors that contribute to PEM, especially in the young child, are listed in Table 5-7. In the United States and other industrialized countries, cases of PEM exist in hospitals where it may be secondary to other conditions, such as AIDS, tuberculosis, malabsorption syndromes, kidney and liver ailments, cancer, and anorexia nervosa.

marasmus A disease that results from consuming a grossly insufficient amount of protein and kcalories; one of the diseases classed as protein-energy malnutrition. The infant or adult will have little or no fat stores, little muscle mass, and poor strength. Death from infections is common.

In its milder form it is difficult to tell if a person with PEM is suffering primarily from a poor intake of kcalories, protein, or both. As the disease progresses and depending in part on the age of onset, the symptoms are primarily those of general starvation (**marasmus**) or those of not meeting protein needs in the face of high requirements (**kwashiorkor**). Still, similarities can be seen in both disorders (Figure 5-10).[12]

KWASHIORKOR

Kwashiorkor is a word from Ghana that means "the disease that the first child gets when the new child comes." From birth the infant is usually breastfed. By the time the child reaches 1 to 1.5 years, the mother is probably pregnant or has already given birth again, and breastfeeding is no longer possible for the first child. This child abruptly switches from nutritious breast milk to native starchy roots and gruels. These foods have low protein densities compared with total kcalories. The foods are also often so bulky and full of plant fibers that it is difficult for the child to eat enough of them to meet energy needs. At the same time infections and parasites are most likely present, which in turn raise energy and protein needs.[12] So these children have their energy needs at best met only marginally, while at the same time their protein needs are unmet, especially when needs are increased by the infections and marginal energy intakes. Probably many vitamin and mineral needs as well, are far from being met. Feeding famine victims starchy roots, such as cassava (tapioca), creates the same problem.

kwashiorkor A disease occurring primarily in young children who have an existing disease and consume generally a marginal amount of kcalories and considerably insufficient protein in the face of high needs. The child generally suffers from infections and exhibits edema, poor growth, weakness, and an increased susceptibility to further illness.

The major symptoms of kwashiorkor are apathy, listlessness, failure to grow and gain weight, and withdrawal from the environment. These symptoms are often added on top of the results of other diseases present, including the infections and parasites that typically precipitate the disease. This can make conditions such as measles, a disease that normally makes a healthy child ill for only a week or so, a severely debilitating and even fatal disease. Further symptoms of the disease are changes in hair color, flaky skin, fat infiltration in the liver, and massive edema in the abdomen and legs. The presence of edema with some subcutaneous fat still present is the

Figure 5-10 A schema for classifying undernutrition. The presence of subcutaneous fat (directly underneath the skin) is a diagnostic key.

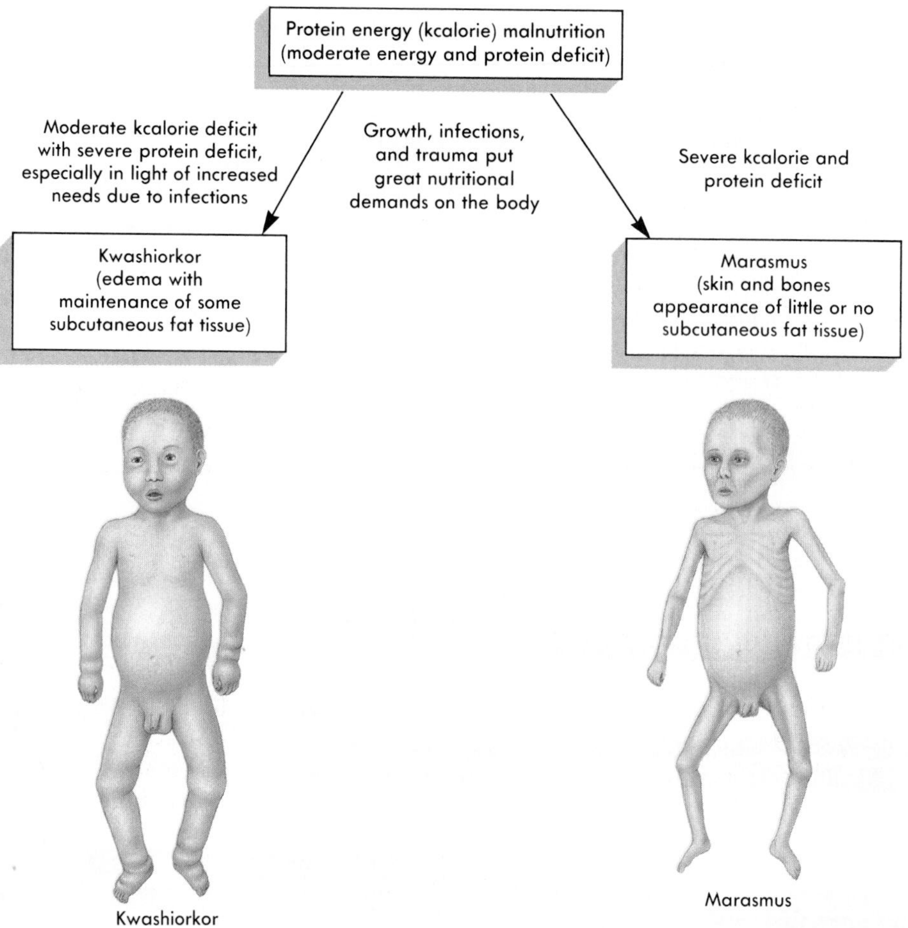

hallmark of kwashiorkor (Figure 5-10). In addition these children hardly move. If you pick them up, they don't cry. When you hold them, you feel the plumpness of edema, not muscle and fat tissue.

We can explain many of these signs of kwashiorkor based on what we know about proteins. Proteins play important roles in fluid balance, immune function, and production of tissues such as skin and hair. We should not expect a child with an insufficient protein intake to grow and mature normally. And they don't!

If a child with kwashiorkor is helped in time—if infections are treated and if the child is fed a diet ample in protein, kcalories, and other essential nutrients—the disease symptoms reverse. The child begins to grow again and may even show no signs of the previous condition, aside perhaps from shortness of stature. However, by the time many of these children reach a hospital or care center, they already have severe infections. In spite of the best care, they still die. Or, if they survive, they return home and repeat the cycle.

MARASMUS

Marasmus typically occurs as an infant starves to death. Greatly insufficient amounts of protein, kcalories, and other nutrients are consumed.[12] The condition is also generally referred to as protein-energy malnutrition, especially when experienced by older children and adults. The word marasmus means "to waste away." Infants (and adults) do just that. They have the "skin and bones" appearance that appears on posters from relief agencies (Figure 5-10). Little or no subcutaneous fat is present. Infants with this condition generally were either not breastfed or stopped breastfeeding in the early months. The weaning formula was then probably improperly

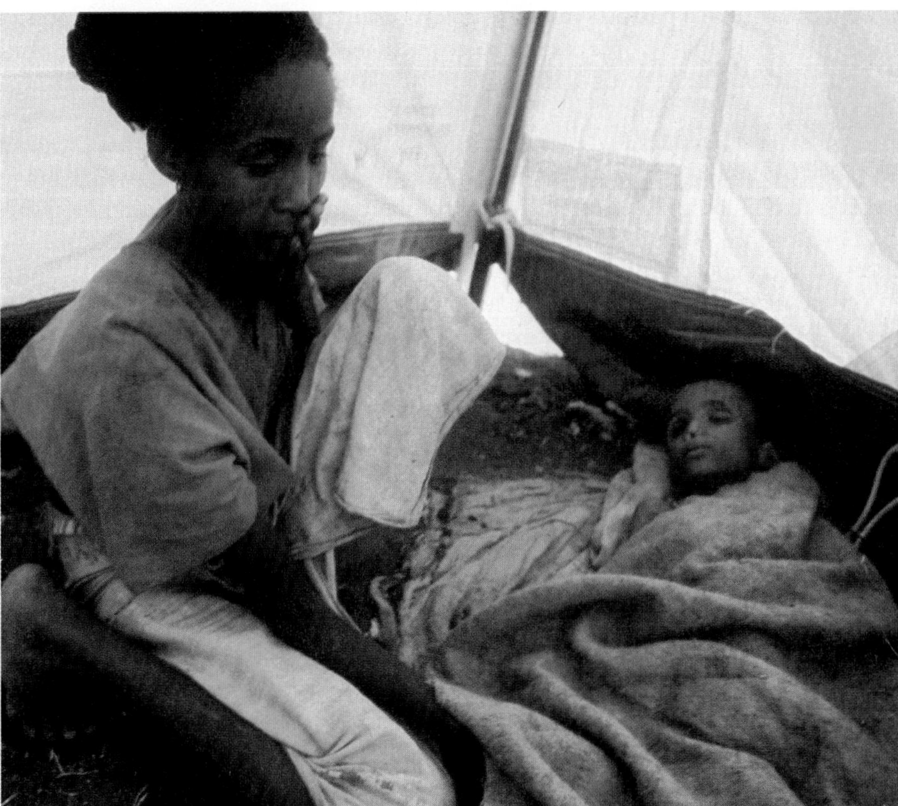

Figure 5-11 The tragedy of poverty and illness.

prepared, partly because of poor water supplied and partly because the parents lacked money to afford sufficient formula for the child's needs. The latter problem most likely led the parents to dilute the formula to provide more feedings. All this does is provide more water for the infant, but the parents do not realize that.

Marasmus in infants commonly occurs in the large cities of poverty-striken countries. In the cities it is often necessary to bottle-feed because the infant must be cared for by others when the mother is working or away from home. When people are poor and sanitation is lacking, bottle-feeding often leads to marasmus. An infant with marasmus requires large amounts of kcalories and protein—like a premature infant—and unless the child receives them, full recovery from the disease may never occur. Most brain growth takes place between conception and the child's first birthday. In fact, the brain is growing at its most rapid rate at birth. If the diet does not support brain growth during the first months of life, the brain may not grow to its full adult size. This reduced or retarded brain growth may lead to some diminished ability to function.

Both kwashiorkor and marasmus wreak havoc on infants and children; mortality rates in poorer countries are often 10 to 20 times higher than in the United States.[16] Over 40,000 infants worldwide die of starvation each year. This high mortality rate in part encourages the high birthrate in poorer countries: If a mother wants four children, she had better have ten to make sure four survive. The overload makes infant mortality much more likely. The problem is further fueled by politics and war. In all, the circumstances often create an intolerable environment for raising children (Figure 5-11). Better food availability and improved sanitation would greatly improve the health of many children worldwide. Chapter 20 looks at the issue of undernutrition worldwide in more detail.

KWASHIORKOR AND MARASMUS MALNUTRITION IN THE HOSPITAL

Kwashiorkor can result in the hospital when a patient is fed primarily glucose intravenously for many days. This may happen when a slow recovery from surgery prevents the use of a person's intestinal tract. In addition, a person may feel too sick to eat much, in spite of the increased nutrient needs caused by the disease state present. Intravenous feeding meets kcalorie needs to some extent but provides little or no protein. The person develops edema, and often the immune function is diminished, leaving the patient at great risk for infections. One of the best markers for kwashiorkor is a person's serum albumin level. When it falls below 3.5 grams per 100 milliliters, the person is at risk. By the time the serum albumin level falls to 2.2 grams per 100 milliliters, the person is at a very high risk for infections and disease associated with this state.

Studies have demonstrated that a hospital patient with a low body weight, a low serum albumin level, and a low white blood cell (especially lymphocyte) count is at a four to six times greater risk for complications and death than is a patient with normal levels for those three factors. The lymphocyte count is a good monitor for immune function. In the last 15 years nutrition support teams have been formed in hospitals. One of their missions is to ensure that patients receive enough oral or intravenous nutrition support to enable them to meet their needs for proteins, carbohydrates, and other nutrients.

Marasmus occurs in a hospitalized patient when a person simply does not receive enough kcalories and other nutrients. This can be the cause in anorexia nervosa, cancer, and some intestinal disorders. The person either does not eat enough food or does not absorb enough nutrients from the intestinal tract to meet nutritional needs. Muscle, vital organ tissue, and fat stores waste away, and the person eventually looks like "skin and bones." Death from starvation or heart failure can then result. A hospitalized person may also have mixed kwashiorkor-marasmus. This is characterized by edema in a person with greatly diminished fat stores.

CONCEPT CHECK

If a person regularly consumes insufficient energy and a marginal amount of protein, protein-energy malnutrition (PEM) develops. The person with kwashiorkor, a severe form of this disease, suffers decreased immune function, edema, weakness, and increased susceptibility to infections. Young children after weaning are especially susceptible to kwashiorkor, especially if they are exposed to infections. This increases their nutritional needs. Marasmus is another severe form of PEM. This condition results when people—especially infants—continually receive too little food, notably not enough protein or kcalories. Symptoms that develop include muscle wasting, absence of fat stores, and weakness. Both an adequate diet and treatment of infections or other diseases must be offered if health is to be restored in both cases. This is true whether one is an adult suffering from cancer or an infant suffering from famine; the symptoms of both kwashiorkor and marasmus are seen in these situations.

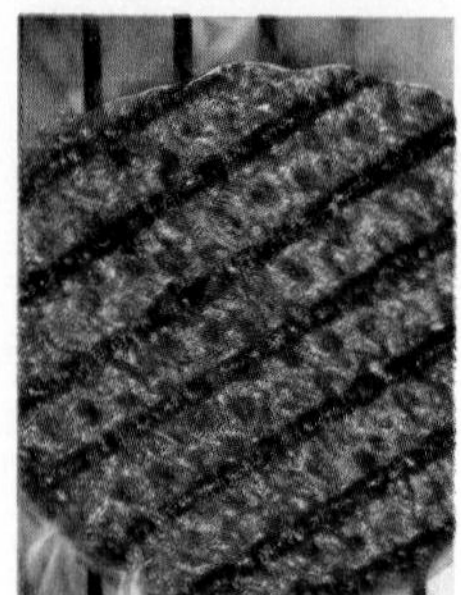

Summary

1. Amino acids are the building blocks of protein. They contain nitrogen in the form of an amine group. Of the 20 types of amino acids found in food, nine are essential in the diet and 11 can be synthesized by the body if amine groups from extra amino acids are available.
2. High-quality protein foods contain an ample supply of all nine essential amino acids in sufficient quantity for protein synthesis. This is typical of animal foods. Low-quality protein foods lack good supplies of one or more of the essential amino acids. This is typical of plant foods. Two plant foods can be combined to complement each other's amino acid deficiencies, in turn providing a high-quality protein meal.

3. Individual amino acids bond together to form proteins. The order (sequence) of the amino acids is important. This order determines the ultimate form and thus the function of the protein. The three-dimensional shape that the protein eventually forms is dictated by the sequence. This structure can be unfolded—denatured—by treatment with heat, acid or alkaline solutions, and other processes. Then the protein can no longer function as intended.
4. Proteins form essential body constituents, such as muscle contractile tissue, connective tissue, transport proteins, visual pigments, enzymes, hormones, and immune bodies. Proteins also provide a source of carbons that can be synthesized into glucose.
5. Protein quality can be measured by determining the extent to which the body can retain the nitrogen contained in the protein absorbed. This ratio of nitrogen retention to nitrogen absorption is called biological value. The ability of a food to support the growth of rats is also a measure of protein quality and is known as the protein efficiency ratio. In addition, the balance of essential amino acids in a food can be compared to an ideal pattern. The ability to match the ideal pattern is referred to as a chemical store. It predicts the ability of the body to retain in tissues the food protein eaten.
6. The RDA for protein for adults is 0.8 grams per kilogram of desirable body weight. For a 70-kilogram (156-pound) person this corresponds to 56 grams of protein per day. The average American man consumes about 90 grams of protein per day; women consume closer to 70 grams of protein per day. Thus our diets generally supply ample protein.
7. Animal proteins are the most nutrient-dense sources of protein. Plant foods generally contain less than 20% of their kcalories as protein. Contrast that to water-packed tuna, which contains over 80% of its kcalories as protein. Still, plant proteins can provide ample protein to a diet as these are consumed as part of a varied diet.
8. Protein- and energy-deficiency conditions include kwashiorkor and marasmus. These two diseases are difficult to separate and either results from insufficient energy intake and a marginal protein intake (kwashiorkor) or from a poor intake of both protein and kcalories (marasmus). Infections, which increase nutritional needs, can tip the balance between health and illness, especially when the diet is limited to a few high-carbohydrate, low-protein foods. Variations of these diseases appear in hospitalized people in America.

Study Questions

1. Discuss the relative importance of essential and nonessential amino acids in the diet. Why is it important to replace essential amino acids lost from the body in the diet?
2. What are four of the functions of proteins? How does the structure of a protein relate to its functions?
3. Why is the quality of a protein important? What foods provide high-quality protein?
4. What is the significance of preventing protein-energy malnutrition in children worldwide?
5. What characteristics of a vegetarian diet could contribute to the improvement of the American diet?

REFERENCES

1. ADA Reports: Position of The American Dietetic Association: vegetarian diets, *Journal of The American Dietetic Association* 88:351-355, 1988.
2. Belongia EA and others: An investigation of the cause of the eosinophilia-myalgia syndrome associated with tryptophan use, *New England Journal of Medicine* 323:357, 1990.
3. Blum M and others: Protein intake and kidney function in humans: its effect on normal aging, *Archives of Internal Medicine* 149:211, 1989.
4. Clark N: How to pack a meatless diet full of nutrients, *The Physician and Sportsmedicine* 19:31, 1991.
5. Dwyer JT: Nutritional consequences of vegetarianism, *Annual Review of Nutrition* 11:61, 1991.
6. Eaton SB, Shostak M, Konner M: *The paleolithic prescription*, New York, 1988, Harper and Row.
7. Farley D: Vegetarian diets, *FDA Consumer*, May 1992, p 21.
8. Fukagawa NK, Young VR: Protein and amino acid metabolism and requirements in older persons, *Clinics in Geriatric Medicine* 3:329, 1987.
9. Herbert V: L-tryptophan, *Nutrition Today*, March/April 1992, P 27.
10. Herbert V: Vitamin B-12: plant sources, requirements, and assay, *American Journal of Clinical Nutrition* 46:852, 1988.
11. Lappe FM: *Diet for a small planet*, New York, 1987, Ballantine Books.
12. Latham MC: Protein-energy malnutrition. In Brown ML, editor: *Present knowledge in nutrition*, Washington, D.C., 1990, International Life Sciences Institute-Nutrition Foundation, pp 39-46.
13. Miller DR and others: Vitamin B-12 status in a macrobiotic community, *American Journal of Clinical Nutrition* 53:524, 1991.
14. National Institute of Nutrition (Canada): Risks and benefits of vegetarian diets, *Nutrition Today* March/April 1990, p 27.
15. Nieman DC and others: Dietary status of Seventh-Day Adventist vegetarian and non-vegetarian elderly women, *Journal of The American Dietetic Association* 89:1763, 1989.
16. Olson RE: World food production and problems in human nutrition, *Nutrition Today* Jan/Feb 1989, p 15.
17. Resnicow K and others: Diet and serum lipids in vegan vegetarians: a model for risk reduction, *Journal of The American Dietetic Association* 91:447, 1991.
18. Robertson L and others: *The new laurel's kitchen*, Berkeley, Calif, 1986, Ten Speed Press.
19. Rudman D: Kidney senescence: a model for aging, *Nutrition Reviews* 46:209, 1988.
20. Spencer H and others: Do protein and phosphorus cause calcium loss?, *Journal of Nutrition* 118:657, 1988.
21. Young VR: Kinetics of amino acid metabolism: nutritional implications and some lessons, 1987 McCollum Award Lecture, *American Journal of Clinical Nutrition* 46:709, 1987.

SUGGESTED READINGS

For more details on amino acid metabolism and protein needs see the review by Young. His research on protein needs spans many years and has led to much of our understanding of this topic. To learn more about the possible health benefits of vegetarianism see the review by Dwyer and the article by Farley. These articles cover essentially every possible effect of a vegetarian versus an omnivorous diet. See also the article by Nieman and others. Finally, an excellent vegetarian cookbook is that by Robertson and others. In addition, this book contains an easy to understand discussion of nutrition as it applies to vegetarianism.

TAKE ACTION

How much protein do you eat?

How much protein do you eat in a typical day? Look at the nutrition assessment you completed at the end of Chapter 2. Review it closely. Find the figure indicating the amount of protein you consumed during your 1-day record. Write it in the space below:

Total Protein ____________________

Let's compare this to your RDA for protein. Find your desirable weight in pounds from the height-weight table on the inside cover of this book. Choose a mid-range value. Divide it by 2.2. This will give you your desirable weight in kilograms. Next multiply that by 0.8 grams per kilogram of body weight. This will indicate your RDA for protein. Write it in the space below:

RDA for Protein ____________________

How does your consumption compare to your RDA?

____

____

____

If you consumed either more or less than the RDA, what foods could you add, subtract, or eat more or less of? (Look at the foods you ate.)

____

____

____

____

Was most of your protein from animal or plant sources?

____

____

NUTRITION PERSPECTIVE

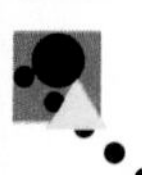

Vegetarianism

The practice of vegetarianism goes back to the time of the Greek philosophers, yet today it is new to many people. Vegetarianism has sparked the interest of men and women for centuries. Throughout human history vegetarianism has changed from being a necessity for some people to being a personal option. Historically, vegetarians have been people particularly interested in philosophy, religion, or science. Today vegetarianism in this country usually appeals to a younger segment of people.[5]

As nutrition science has grown, our ability to plan adequate vegetarian diets has improved. If you choose to be a vegetarian, you can be confident you can meet your nutritional needs by following a few basic rules. Recent studies of all causes of death show that mortality rates are lower for vegetarians than for nonvegetarians.[15] Diet, healthy lifestyles (leanness, not smoking, abstinence from alcohol and drugs, and increased physical activity), and social class selection bias probably all account for these findings.

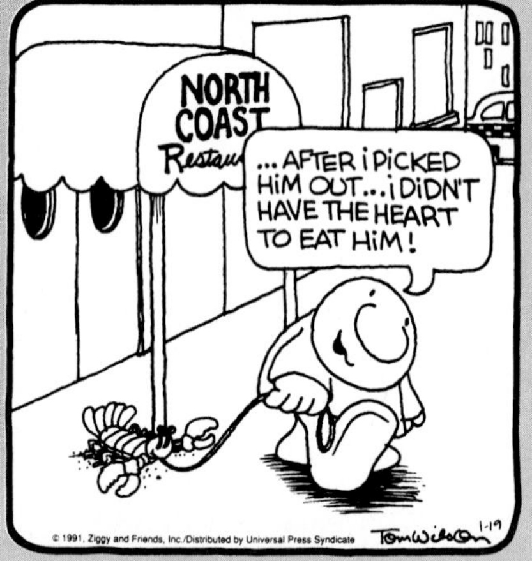
ZIGGY®
NORTH COAST Restau
...AFTER I PICKED HIM OUT...I DIDN'T HAVE THE HEART TO EAT HIM!
© 1991, Ziggy and Friends, Inc./Distributed by Universal Press Syndicate
TomWilson 1-19

Figure 5-12 Ziggy.

WHY DO PEOPLE PRACTICE VEGETARIANISM?

People choose vegetarianism for a variety of reasons. Some think it is more ethical not to kill animals for food (Figure 5-12). Religious orders, such as Hindus and Trappist monks, eat vegetarian meals as a practice of their religion. In the United States many Seventh Day Adventists base their practice of vegetarianism on Biblical texts and believe it is a healthier way to eat.

People might choose vegetarianism because they want to eat fewer pesticides. By eating plants, animals concentrate the pesticides that plants take up. The greater variety of plants a person eats, the less chance that person has of eating a food highly concentrated in pesticides. A person might also become a vegetarian after realizing that animals are not efficient protein factories. It turns out that animals use much of the protein they eat for maintenance rather than for synthesizing new muscle tissue. A cow eats 21 pounds of plant protein for every pound of meat protein it produces. The ratio for pigs is 8 to 1, and 5 to 1 for chickens.[11] Food animals do sometimes eat grasses that humans cannot eat. However, they also eat grains fit for human consumption.

People might eat vegetarian diets because these encourage a high intake of carbohydrates, vitamin A, vitamin E, beta-carotene, vitamin C, magnesium, and fiber, while limiting cholesterol and saturated fat intake.[17] If this rationale sounds similar to the Dietary Guidelines covered in Chapter 2, it is. And some people might pursue vegetarianism because meat is expensive.

Food Planning

There are a variety of vegetarian styles. **Vegans** eat only plant foods. **Fruitarians** eat primarily fruits, nuts, honey, and vegetable oils. **Lacto-vegetarians** eat dairy products and plant foods. **Lacto-ovo-vegetarians** eat dairy products, eggs, and plant foods. **Lacto-ovo-peso-vegetarians** eat dairy products, eggs, and fish, as well as plant foods. The wider the variety of foods eaten, the easier it is to meet nutritional needs.

vegan A person who eats only plant foods.

fruitarian A person who primarily eats fruits, nuts, honey, and vegetable oils.

lacto-vegetarian A person who consumes plant products and dairy products.

lacto-ovo vegetarian A person who consumes plant products, dairy products, and eggs.

lacto-ovo-peso vegetarian A person who consumes plant products, dairy produces, eggs, and fish.

The practice of eating no animal protein separates the vegans and fruitarians from all other vegetarian styles. Including some animal protein in a diet makes diet planning much easier. Most vegetarians consume at least dairy products, if not dairy products and eggs. A four-food-group plan has been developed for both lacto-vegetarians[18] and vegans (Table 5-8). The plans have a protein group that includes nuts, grains, legumes, and seeds. There is also a vegetable group and a fruit group. Lacto-vegetarians then add a milk and/or eggs group.

NUTRITION PERSPECTIVE

You will recognize some similarities as well as some differences between these plans and the typical Guide to Daily Food Choices pattern for **omnivores**. The key to this plan is seeking protein sources in foods other than meats. It's not enough to just cut out meat and to eat everything else. One really needs to search for good quality plant proteins to replace the meat in the diet. That is where the nuts, grain, legumes, and seed group comes in; they become the new "meat" group. For example, instead of having just a muffin for breakfast, have a muffin with peanut butter. Rather than having just greens in a salad for lunch, include some chick-peas or three-bean salad.[4] Overall, by following the food plan in Table 5-8, it should be no problem for vegetarians to obtain an adequate diet.

omnivore A person who consumes both plant and animal food sources.

The Vegan

The vegan has to do some special diet planning.[7] We just outlined a basic approach to the diet, but more consideration is needed. First, it is a good idea to purchase some vegetarian cookbooks. These provide numerous ideas for nutritious ways to creatively use plant foods. A real effort must be made to eat grains and legumes to obtain good quality protein. Then if kcalorie needs are met, protein needs should also be met. A wide variety of protein sources, including the excellent ones just mentioned, should provide **complementarity** of individual amino acids to yield a complete protein diet. In other words, the deficiences in essential amino acid content

complementarity of proteins A situation in which two food protein sources make up for each other's lack in specific essential amino acids, such that together they yield complete protein.

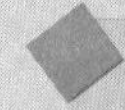

Table 5-8 A four-food-group plan for lacto-vegetarians and vegans. This yields about 1600 to 1800 kcalories. Increase number of servings or add other foods to meet higher energy needs

	Servings		
Group*	Lacto-vegetarian	Vegan‡	Key nutrients supplied
Grains†, legumes, nuts and seeds	6 or more	10 or more, including 2-3 servings of legumes and 1 serving of nuts/seeds	Protein, thiamin, niacin, vitamin B-6, folate, vitamin E, zinc, magnesium, and fiber
Vegetables	3 or more (include one dark green or leafy)	4 or more (include one dark green or leafy)	Vitamin A, vitamin C, folate
Fruits	2 or more	2 or more	Vitamin A, vitamin C, folate
Milk	2 or more	—	Protein, riboflavin, vitamin D, vitamin B-12, and calcium

*Base serving size on those listed in the Guide to Daily Food Choices (see Chapter 2).
†One serving of vitamin and mineral enriched breakfast cereal (≥25% U.S. RDA) is recommended.
‡A calcium-fortified food, such as orange juice or soy milk, is needed unless a calcium supplement is used.

NUTRITION PERSPECTIVE

Vegetarianism—cont'd

in one food protein are made up by the essential amino acid content of another food protein in the meal. Furthermore, the vegan needs to make sure some good sources for riboflavin, vitamin D, vitamin B-12, calcium, iron, and zinc are consumed (Table 5-9).

Riboflavin can be obtained by eating green leafy vegetables, whole grains, yeast, and legumes. Most vegans do eat these foods. Note that the major source of riboflavin in the American diet is milk, which has been omitted from the vegan diet. Vitamin D can be obtained by regular sun exposure. Otherwise, a supplement containing vitamin D should be considered. Vitamin B-12 only naturally occurs in animal foods, but plants may contain soil or microbial contamination that provide some vitamin B-12. However, the vegan should find a more reliable source of vitamin B-12.[10] Examples are fortified soybean milk and soy proteins or special yeast grown on media rich in vitamin B-12 (check the label). Note that by the time a vitamin B-12 deficiency is diagnosed, much nerve damage due to the deficiency can take place[13] (see Chapter 13 for details).

To obtain calcium, the vegan could consume fortified soy milk or fortified orange juice. Tofu, green leafy vegetables, and nuts also contain calcium, but it is either not well absorbed or not very plentiful. Calcium supplements are another possibility.

For iron the vegan can consume whole grains, dried fruits, and legumes. The iron in these foods is not as well absorbed as that found in animal foods, but a good source of vitamin C consumed with these foods can greatly enhance the iron absorption. Thus an excellent recommendation is to include a source of vitamin C in every meal that contains an adequate source of iron from plant foods (see Chapters 13 and 15).

The vegan can find zinc in whole grains and legumes. The phytic acid present in whole grains limits absorption; it is best if the grains are leavened, as in bread, to reduce the influence of phytic acid (see Chapter 15). Of all these nutrients, sufficient calcium is the most difficult to consume (Table 5-9).

Veganism in childhood deserves special attention.[7,14] The sheer bulk of a plant-based diet may make it difficult for a child to consume sufficient kcalories to meet energy needs. This is needed to allow dietary protein to be used for synthetic, rather

Table 5-9 Nutrients likely to be low in the diet of a total vegetarian (vegan)

Nutrient	Plant sources
Vitamin D	Fortified margarines, fortified breakfast cereals
Riboflavin	Whole and enriched grains, leafy vegetables, mushrooms, beans, nuts, seeds
Vitamin B-12	Fortified breakfast cereals, fortified yeast, fortified soy milk
Iron	Whole grains, prune juice, dried fruits, beans, nuts, seeds, leafy vegetables
Calcium	Fortified soy milk*, tofu, almonds, dry beans, leafy vegetables, some fortified breakfast cereals, flours, and certain brands of orange juice*
Zinc	Whole grains, wheat germ, beans nuts, seeds

*Fortified soy milk and fortified orange juice are the best sources.

NUTRITION PERSPECTIVE

than energy, needs. Concentrated sources of kcalories should be included in the diet of a child vegan to avoid this problem. This should be the key concern as a varied diet is followed. Most vegan meals mix complementary foods like beans and rice or bread and peanut butter, so protein is rarely a problem, as long as the child is getting enough kcalories. Examples of energy-rich foods include fortified soy milk, nuts, dried fruits, cookies with vegetable oils, and fruit juices.

Anyone trying vegetarianism should realize that a healthful diet does not happen automatically. It takes some planning and common sense. We keep stressing the importance of eating a wide variety of foods. This is especially important for the vegetarian.

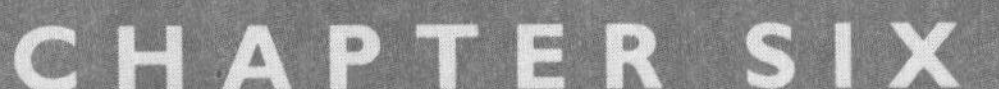

CHAPTER SIX

Digestion and Absorption

***M**erely ingesting foods doesn't nourish you. In many cases you must first break down the nutrients contained in the foods, and in all cases you must absorb them. Only then can nutrients be taken up by the bloodstream and distributed to all of your body's cells.[3] The major parts of the body involved in this process are the gastrointestinal tract, pancreas, liver, and gallbladder.*

We can take our digestion and absorption system for granted because most of the processes involved are autonomic; that is, they control themselves. We don't decide when the pancreas will secrete digestive enzymes into the small intestine, what the liver will do with absorbed glucose, or how quickly foodstuffs will be propelled down the intestinal tract. Hormones, hormone-like compounds, and nerves control these functions. We have two choices: How well to chew food and when to eliminate the stool. Those are voluntary responses. Thus while you go about your daily routine—playing tennis, working in a laboratory session, walking from class to class, and eating lunch—many digestive reactions and functions automatically occur in your digestive tract. Let's examine these processes.

NUTRITION AWARENESS INVENTORY

Here are 15 statements about digestion and absorption. Answer them to test your current knowledge. If you think the answer is true or mostly true, circle T. If you think the answer is false or mostly false, circle F. Use the scoring key at the end of this book to compute your total score. Take the test again after you have read this chapter. Compare the results.

1. T F The process of digestion always begins in the mouth.
2. T F Nutrients that are absorbed directly into the bloodstream from the digestive tract go to the liver first.
3. T F The small intestine is longer than 8 feet (2.5 meters).
4. T F Mucus kills most bacteria that enter the stomach.
5. T F The colon is another name for the large intestine.
6. T F Fruit and meat should not be eaten together if both are to be digested fully.
7. T F Many stomach enzymes work less efficiently in the small intestine.
8. T F The inside of the small intestine has a thick layer of mucus to protect it from ulcer development.
9. T F The presence of bile is required if all of the foods within the digestive tract are to be fully digested.
10. T F The liver, gallbladder, and pancreas are all organs through which food passes during digestion.
11. T F The large intestine is responsible for a great portion of the absorption of nutrients we eat.
12. T F Glucose requires energy to be absorbed, whereas fat does not.
13. T F Peristalsis utilizes a coordinated muscle action.
14. T F Malabsorption of some foods results in bacterial gas production in the colon.
15. T F The entire gastrointestinal tract normally contains a large and thriving population of bacteria.

The Physiology of Digestion

The **gastrointestinal (GI) tract** is a long tube stretching from the mouth to the anus. This tube, also known as the alimentary canal, is in one sense "outside" the body. It is partitioned from the body in such a way that nutrients must pass through the walls of the tube for absorption into the bloodstream. Just eating a food is not enough—the nutrients must also be absorbed.[3] As we will describe, certain diseases may hamper absorption, in turn denying the body of some of the ingested nutrients.

The GI tract is a very complex system that performs a variety of physiological functions: movement (motility), secretion, digestion, absorption, elimination, and nutrient production.[12] (Nutrient production refers to the synthesis of vitamins by bacteria that live in the intestine.) In this chapter we discuss the most important aspects of GI physiology from a nutritional viewpoint. You can find a more detailed discussion of all the organs and processes involved in a physiology textbook.

gastrointestinal (GI) tract The main sites in the body used in digestion and absorption of nutrients. It consists of the mouth, esophagus, stomach, small intestine, large intestine, rectum, and anus.

THE FLOW OF DIGESTION

Let's begin by reviewing the major parts of the body used in digestion. In the mouth, glands produce **saliva**. Saliva contains enzymes that break down carbohydrates, as well as **mucus** that lubricates the foods. Chewing also breaks up solid food into smaller, more manageable pieces. This increases the surface area of the food, thus allowing more efficient and greater digestive action by enzymes. In addition, saliva contains **lysozyme**, which kills bacteria by rupturing "foreign" cellular membranes.

The tongue contains taste receptors for sweet, salty, sour, and bitter tastes.[11] The sweet and salt receptors are near the tip of the tongue, and the sour and bitter receptors are near the base. A variety of diseases and drugs can alter the sense of taste[10]; adding more spices and flavorings to foods can help in these cases.

The mouth and stomach are connected by a "food tube," the esophagus. At its top is a valvelike flap of tissue, the epiglottis, that prevents food from being swallowed into the trachea (wind pipe). During swallowing, food eventually lands on the

saliva A watery fluid produced by the salivary glands in the mouth; it contains lubricants, enzymes, and other substances.

mucus A thick fluid secreted by glands throughout the body. It contains a compound that has both a carbohydrate and protein nature. This acts as both a lubricant and a means of protection for cells.

lysozyme A substance produced by a variety of cells in the body that can destroy bacteria by rupturing its cellular membrane.

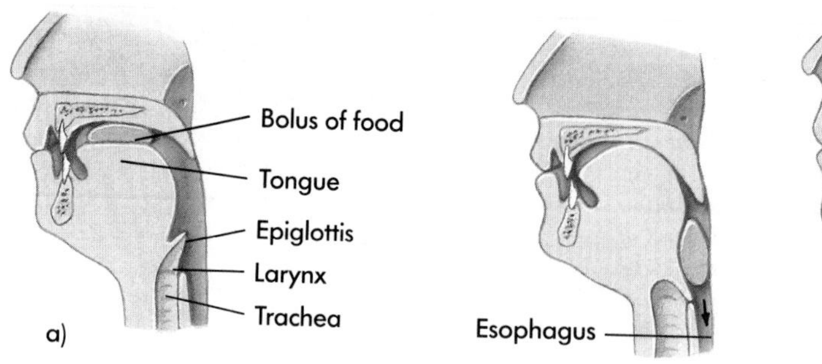

Figure 6-1 The process of swallowing. **A,** During swallowing, food cannot normally enter the trachea because the epiglottis closes over the larynx. **B,** The arrow shows that this allows food to head down the esophagus. **C,** When a person chokes, food becomes lodged in the trachea, in turn blocking air flow to the lungs. The food should have gone down the esophagus, thus preventing choking.

At autopsy, the small intestine muscles relax, allowing the jejunum and the ileum to lengthen to about 11 feet (3.4 meters) each. The small intestine then is about 23 feet (7.1 meters) long, a figure often cited in textbooks.

GI tract flow
Mouth
↓
Esophagus
↓
Stomach—4-cup capacity (1 liter). Food stays 2 to 3 hours.
↓
Small intestine—duodenum, jejunum, ileum—10 feet (3.1 meters) long; food stays 3 to 10 hours.
↓
Large Intestine (colon)—cecum, ascending colon, transverse colon, descending colon, sigmoid colon—3½ feet (1.1 meters) long; food can remain up to 72 hours.

epiglottis. When that happens, the epiglottis covers the larynx (the opening of the trachea) and breathing automatically stops. These involuntary responses ensure that swallowed food will travel only down the esophagus, helped along by its muscular contractions and gravity (Figure 6-1).

As the food exits the esophagus, it passes through the diaphragm that separates the abdominal and cardiac cavities of the body to enter the stomach. This is essentially a holding tank with about a 4 cup (1 liter) capacity. The stomach continues the body's digestive processes by secreting acid and enzymes and then slowly churning them into the food. A meal usually leaves the stomach within 2 to 3 hours of eating. Solids take longer than liquids to leave the stomach, and a fatty meal generally leaves later than a meal containing mostly protein or carbohydrate.[16]

The stomach empties into the small intestine, which is coiled below it in the abdomen (Figure 6-2). The small intestine is divided into three sections: The duodenum is the first foot (1/3 meters); the jejunum is the next 4 feet (1.3 meters); and the ileum is the last 5 feet (1.6 meters). Due to this total length, the small intestine can only be considered small because of its narrow diameter. Most digestion is completed in the jejunum with the help of enzymes made by intestinal cells and the pancreas.

Muscular contractions in the small intestine constantly mix the food, enhancing digestive action. A meal remains in the small intestine about 3 to 10 hours.

The small intestine empties its contents into the large intestine, or colon. This organ measures about 3 1/2 feet (1.1 meters) and is separated into five sections: the cecum, ascending colon, transverse colon, descending colon, and sigmoid colon. Bacteria in the colon digest some leftover plant fibers; otherwise little digestion occurs.[4] However, there is no need for it—about 95% of total digestion occurs in the small intestine. The remaining food that reaches the colon is mostly indigestible. This resides in the colon for about 24 to 72 hours before elimination from the body.

The end of the colon is attached to the rectum, which itself is connected to the anus. These final sections work with the colon to prepare the stool for elimination.

The liver, which provides **bile** to aid fat digestion and absorption, is connected to the gallbladder; the gallbladder stores this bile until it is needed for digestion.[12] A duct leading from the gallbladder connects with a duct from the pancreas. This organ provides critical enzymes as well as other products for use in digestion. The output from the pancreas merges with that of the gallbladder before all of it enters the duodenum for digestive purposes. Thus the liver, pancreas, and gallbladder work with the GI tract but are not part of it.

GASTROINTESTINAL CONTROL VALVES: SPHINCTERS

hormone A compound with a specific synthesis site that, when secreted into the bloodstream, will act to control the function of cells in its target organ or organs. Hormones can be either proteinlike (such as insulin) or fatlike (such as estrogen).

A **sphincter** is a circular muscle arrangement (as seen in the mouth) that acts as a valve to regulate passage or flow of materials.[3] A variety of these valves, sphincters, are located throughout the intestinal tract. Sphincters respond to stimuli from nerves, **hormones**, hormonelike compounds, and the amount of pressure that builds up around them. The flow of food through the esophagus is controlled by the upper and lower esophageal sphincters. The lower esophageal sphincter (also known as

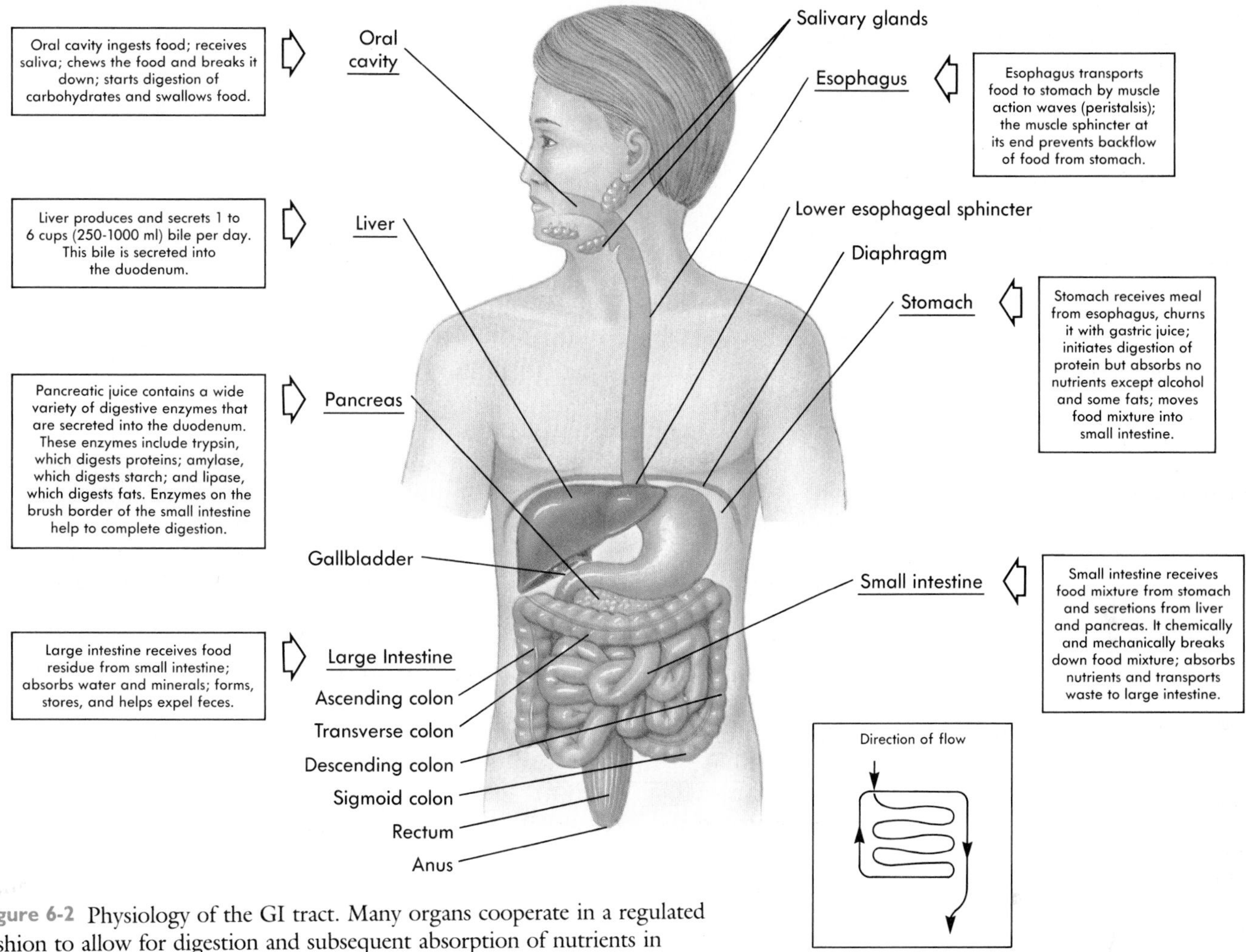

Figure 6-2 Physiology of the GI tract. Many organs cooperate in a regulated fashion to allow for digestion and subsequent absorption of nutrients in foods.

the cardiac sphincter due to its proximity to the heart) is important for preventing backflow (reflux) of stomach contents up into the esophagus. The stomach contents are highly acidic, and if these come in contact with the esophagus, they can cause a pain known as **heartburn**. Coffee, alcohol, and nicotine can weaken the hormonally induced tension of the lower esophageal sphincter and thus are likely to cause heartburn in some people (see the Nutrition Perspective).

The pyloric sphincter, which is located at the base of the stomach, controls the movement of acidic stomach contents into the small intestine. The pyloric sphincter allows the stomach contents to squirt only a few milliliters (about a teaspoon) at a time into the small intestine. This slow rate allows bicarbonate ions (HCO_3^-) from the pancreas to efficiently neutralize the hydrogen ions (H^+) coming from the stomach contents.[5] This neutralization is critical in order to reduce the risk of acid erosion of the small intestine, and in turn a possible **ulcer** (again, see the Nutrition Perspective).[1]

At the end of the gallbladder duct is the sphincter of Oddi. When the hormone cholecystokinin (CCK) stimulates the gallbladder to contract during digestion, the sphincter of Oddi relaxes and allows the contents of the gallbladder to enter the duodenum.[13]

The ileocecal valve forms the end of the small intestine.[21] This sphincter prevents the contents of the large intestine from backing up into the small intestine. Thus

heartburn A pain emanating from the esophagus due to stomach acid backing up into the esophagus and irritating the tissue in that organ.

ulcer Erosion of the tissue lining in either the stomach (gastric ulcer) or upper small intestine (duodenal ulcer). The general condition in either area is often termed a "peptic" ulcer.

Figure 6-3 Levels of human biological organization. We are as simple as a collection of atoms and as complex as a single organism.

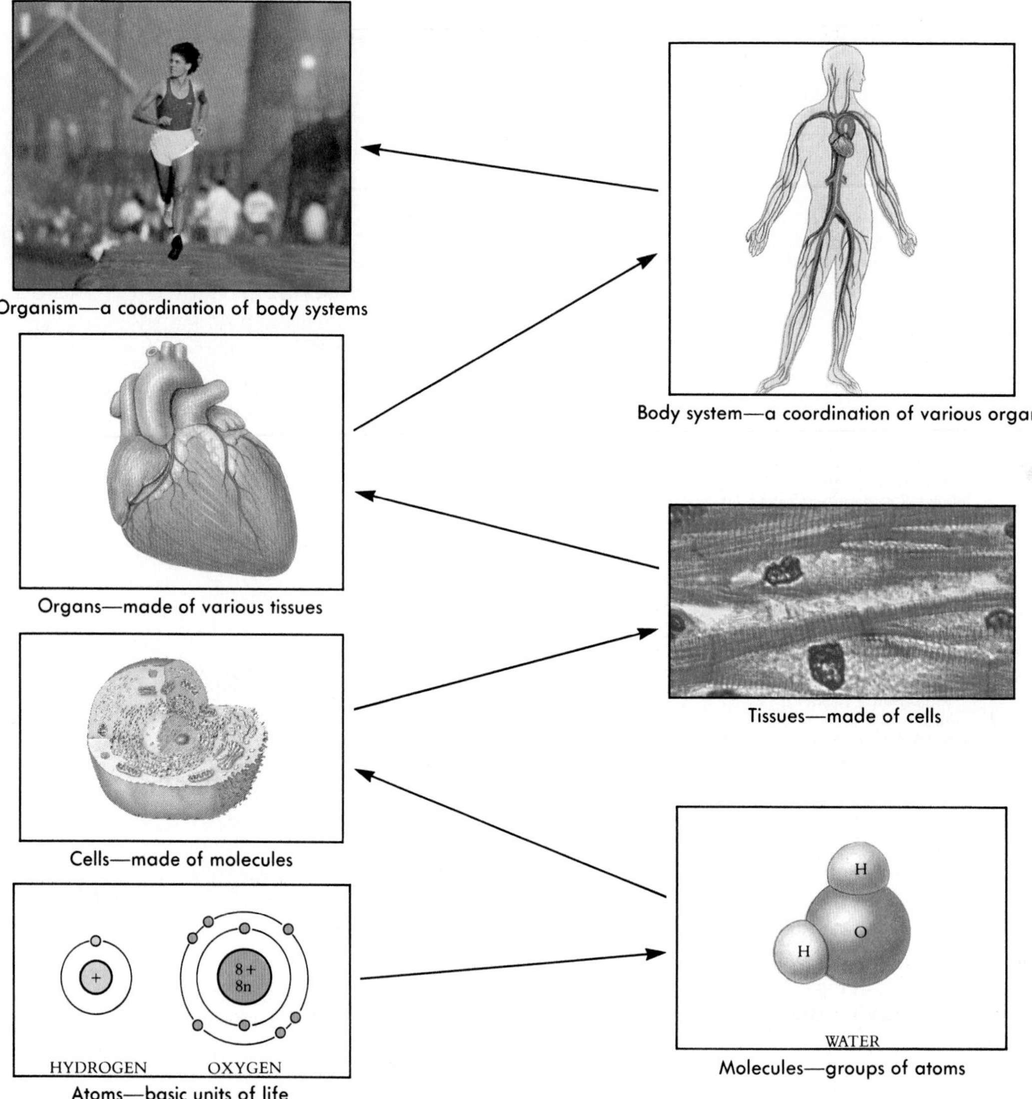

bacteria from the large intestine are prevented from invading and colonizing the small intestine. It is important for the small intestine to have a relatively low concentration of bacteria because these can compete for nutrients, in turn absorbing nutrients before the body can. These bacteria also tend to break down the bile supplied by the gallbladder; in this case the bile can then neither help in the digestion of dietary fat nor be reabsorbed and used again. In turn, poor digestion and absorption of fat can then result. In addition, unresorbed bile entering the colon acts as a powerful **laxative,** often producing diarrhea. The bacteria present in the large intestine do contribute to intestinal function and even nutrient digestion—like soluble fibers—but these large amounts of bacteria need to be kept out of the small intestine.

At the end of the colon are two anal sphincters, one under voluntary control. Once a child is toilet-trained, he or she can fairly well determine when to relax the sphincter, and when it should remain constricted.

Thus sphincters along the intestinal tract perform important functions. Without them we would suffer more heartburn, ulcers, and diarrhea.

GASTROINTESTINAL MUSCULARITY: MIXING AND PROPULSION

Food is propelled down the GI tract partly by a process called **peristalsis**. After swallowing, this coordinated squeezing and shortening occurs in the esophagus in the form of two waves of muscle action closely following each other. In the stomach,

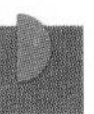

Body Systems Used in Digestion and Absorption

The body is composed of millions of **cells.** Each is a self-contained, living entity (see Chapter 7 for a drawing of a typical cell). When cells of the same type work together for a common purpose, bound together by intercellular substances, they form **tissues** such as bone, cartilage, muscle, and nerve. Often two or more tissues combine in a particular way to form more complex **organs,** such as skin, kidneys, and the liver. At still higher levels of coordination, several organs can cooperate for a common purpose to form an **organ system,** such as the respiratory system or the digestive system. The human body is a coordinated unit of many such organ systems (Figure 6-3).

Every cell in the human body performs a specialized job. A cell's master plan for work and for the necessary machinery to do that work is all encoded into the cell's genetic material, the **DNA** (deoxyribonucleic acid). The DNA acts as a blueprint for synthesizing specific proteins—often enzymes—required to perform specific tasks. Even though most cells in the same organism contain the same DNA information, cells throughout the body are programmed differently. As the embryo forms, different parts of the DNA become active in different cell types. For example, the intestinal cells make digestive enzymes, while in the bone marrow, cells that make the oxygen-carrying protein hemoglobin are active.

Chemical reactions occur all the time in every living cell: The synthesis of new substances is balanced by the breaking down of older ones. For this turnover to occur, a cell requires a continuous supply of energy. Most cells also need oxygen to extract this energy from nutrients for cell use. Cells also need water, the medium in which they live. They further need building blocks, especially the materials they can't make themselves—the essential nutrients supplied from food. These substances enable the tissues—composed of individual cells—to function properly.

An adequate supply of all nutrients to all body cells results from a healthful diet. But to ensure optimal use of these nutrients by cells, the following systems, in addition to the digestive system, also must work efficiently.

Circulatory system

The blood travels two basic routes. It circulates between the right side of the heart and the lungs (the pulmonary circuit) and between the left side of the heart and all other body parts (the systemic circuit) (Figure 6-4). The heart is a muscular pump that normally contracts and relaxes 50 to 90 times per minute while the body is at rest. This continuous pumping action keeps blood moving through the body.

The circulatory system distributes nutrients from digestion and oxygen from the air we breathe to all body cells. All blood goes to the lungs to pick up oxygen and release carbon dioxide. The oxygenated blood then returns to the heart to be pumped to all other body tissues. In the capillaries, cells exchange nutrients and wastes with the blood—cells empty their waste products into the blood and take nutrients from it. Capillaries—networks of tiny blood vessels—serve every region of the body via individual capillary beds, which are only one cell layer thick. Nutrients, gases, and other substances can pass through capillary cells both into and out of other body cells.

The lymphatic system is a second system of circulatory vessels that serves the body; it carries lymph, the clear fluid formed between cells. This fluid filters into tiny lymphatic vessels, which compose a one-way network that funnels lymph from all over the body into two large lymphatic vessels that empty into major veins returning to the heart. As you will see, lymphatic vessels that serve the small intestine have an important role in nutrition.[12]

Excretory system

The kidneys, digestive tract (we cover this later in this chapter), skin, and lungs all remove wastes from the body. For example, as blood passes through the kidneys, body wastes like urea are removed for excretion and put into the urine. Excess intakes of water-soluble nutrients and other substances are also filtered and excreted in that manner. So, if the body already has enough vitamin C, for example, the kidneys screen the extra amount out of the blood and redirect it into the urine. The skin excretes body wastes through the pores along with perspiration. The lungs remove the carbon dioxide produced during metabolism of carbohydrates, fats, and proteins, and exhale it into the air.

Storage systems

The human body must maintain reserves of nutrients. Otherwise, we would need to eat continuously. Storage capacity varies for each different nutrient. Most fat is stored at sites designed specifically for this—adipose (fat) tissue. Short-term storage of glucose occurs in muscles, liver, and blood. The many vitamins and minerals stored in the liver make animal liver a concentrated food source of nutrients. Other nutrient stores are found in individual cells themselves.

During a period of dietary deficiency some nutrients are obtained by breaking down tissues that contain high concentrations of needed nutrients. Calcium is taken from bone and protein is taken from muscle. Neither bones nor muscles are meant to act as nutrient reserves. Rather, nutrient losses in cases of dietary deficiency harm these tissues.

Control systems

The endocrine (hormone) and nervous systems form two control mechanisms that greatly influence nutrient use in the body.[7,13] The hormone insulin helps regulate blood glucose levels, and thyroid hormones help regulate the body's metabolic rate. Nerves influence acid secretion in the stomach and regulate GI tract muscle action. The senses of sight, hearing, touch, smell, and taste all use nerve pathways to communicate such information—the availability of food or the need for it, for example—to the brain. Some nutrients are important in nerve functioning, especially the vitamins thiamin and niacin.

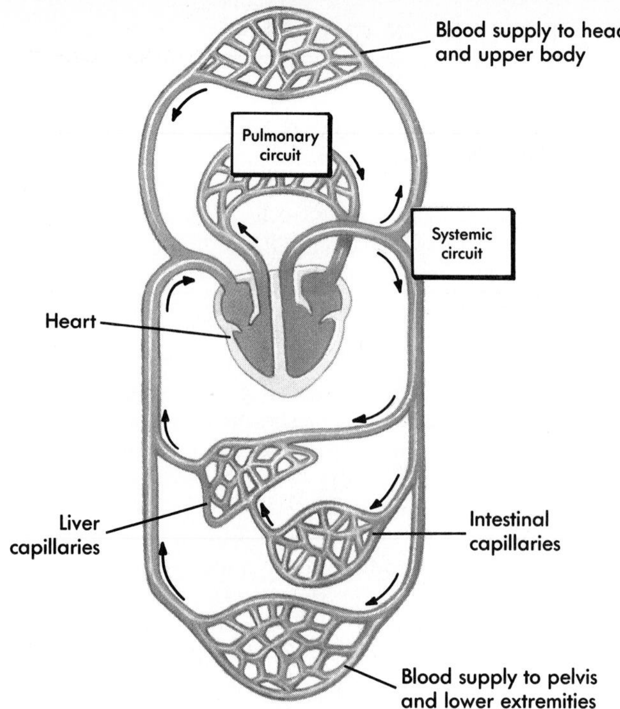

Figure 6-4 Blood circulation throughout the body. This drawing represents the route blood takes through the two circuits that begin and end at the heart. The red color indicates blood that is richer in oxygen; the blue color is for blood carrying more carbon dioxide.

peristaltic waves create a mixing and grinding action as often as three times per minute during digestion. The stomach wall is composed of three opposing muscle layers (circular, diagonal, and longitudinal), which in combination enable the stomach to contract in enough directions to fully churn and mix the meal with the gastric juices.

By far, the most prominent peristalsis occurs in the small intestine, where contractions occur about every 4 to 5 seconds.[12] One group of muscles forms a circular pattern around the GI tract (Figure 6-5). They constrict behind and relax in front of the ingested food. This moves the food down the intestinal tract. At the same time, muscles lying lengthwise down the tract contract to make it shorter. Just image a large snake after it has consumed its prey to visualize the process. The colon has very sluggish peristalsis, employing occasional **mass movements** to help eliminate the stool.

ENZYMES IN DIGESTION

Enzymes speed up digestion by facilitating chemical reactions (making the reactions more likely to happen). Recall from earlier chapters that most enzymes are proteins and work by bringing certain molecules in close proximity and then creating an environment favorable for the intended chemical reaction. This environment primarily consists of lowering the amount of energy needed to allow the reaction to proceed (Figure 6-6). Almost every reaction in the body requires an enzyme to hasten its occurrence. This is especially true for digestion. Furthermore, individual enzymes usually act only on a specific substance (like a lock and key mechanism); enzymes that recognize table sugar (sucrose) will ignore milk sugar (lactose).

It is critical that the activities of the enzymes used in digestion are controllable. Not only must they be readily activated when needed, they must be inactivated when not needed. Enzymes are not always able to distinguish between the proteins, carbohydrates, and fats coming from food, and these same materials that exist as components of bodily tissues. In essence, it is possible to digest your own digestive tract.[1] Within the digestive tract the mechanisms of activation are varied. Enzyme activation is usually very dependent on pH, as well as the presence of key vitamins and minerals. Digestive enzymes that work in the acid environment of the stomach will not work well in the alkaline environment of the small intestine. The body also stores enzymes as zymogens, an inactivated form usually requiring the removal of some minor part for activation.

Enzyme nomenclature is actually simple. The prefix of the enzyme name indicates the target; the suffix is "ase." For example, lipase is the enzyme that digests certain lipids.

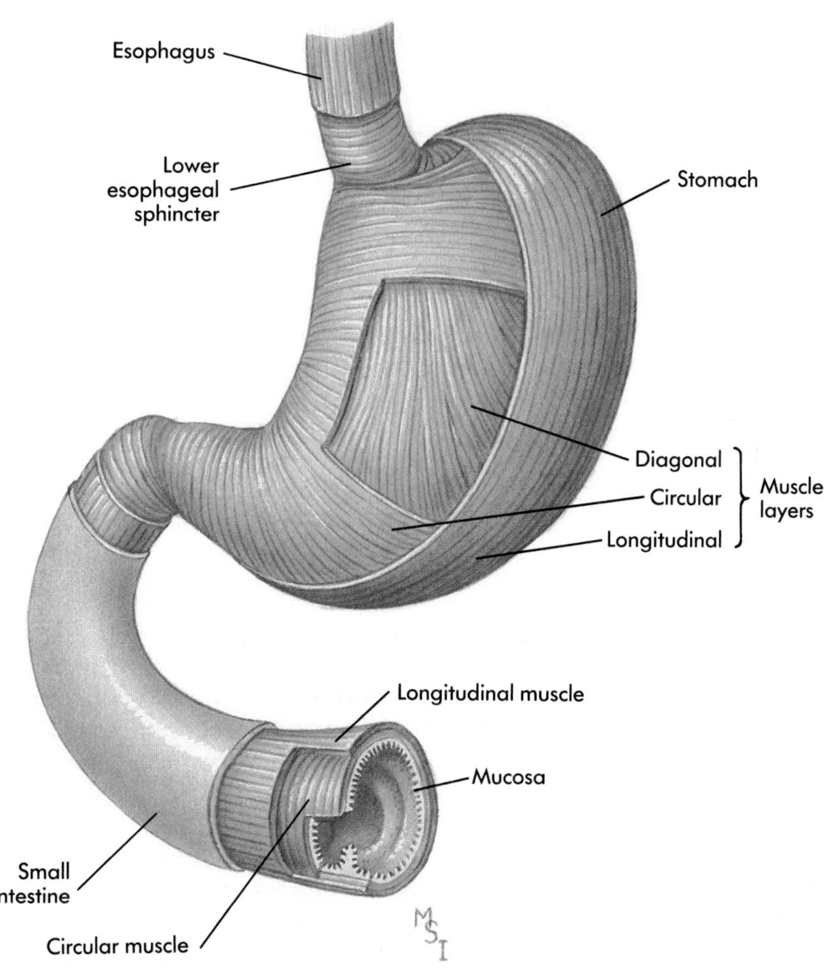

Figure 6-5 Muscularity of the GI tract. Having muscles arranged in different directions is a key to the function of both the stomach and intestinal tract.

Most digestive enzymes are made by the pancreas and small intestine. A few are made by the mouth and stomach.[3]

When either the small intestine or the pancreas is diseased, important enzymes may not be produced in adequate quantities. This scarcity can result in poor digestion and, consequently, very poor absorption. In such cases, the foodstuffs travel into the large intestine instead of being absorbed into the bloodstream. They are metabolized in the large intestine into acids and gas by bacteria present there. The person's stool will look foamy and greasy due to the gases trapped in the stool and the undigested fat present. A person with intestinal malabsorption also will often have a distended abdomen due to intestinal gas present.[9] Whenever digestion and absorption are hampered, the body pays a price. Insufficient enzyme production or insufficient time for complete enzyme action is often at the root of these problems.

People who have pancreatic disease, which is often found in those with cystic fibrosis, may not produce sufficient enzymes for digestion. In cystic fibrosis, excess production of mucus may block the release of the enzymes from the pancreas. This results in malabsorption of nutrients and associated discomfort. Such a person can consume replacement enzymes with meals. Some forms are coated to protect against destruction by stomach acid.

CONCEPT CHECK

The gastrointestinal (GI) tract includes the mouth, esophagus, stomach, small intestine, large intestine (colon), rectum, and anus. Associated with the GI tract are the liver, gallbladder, and pancreas. Together these organs perform the digestion and absorption needed to both extract nutrients from food and funnel them into the bloodstream. In the GI tract, a coordinated muscular activity called peristalsis propels food from the esophagus to the anus. During this journey, enzymes produced by the mouth, stomach, pancreas, and small intestinal cells digest the food so that the nutrients present can be absorbed. The lag time from ingesting food to the eventual elimination of the remains from the body is usually about 1 to 3 days.

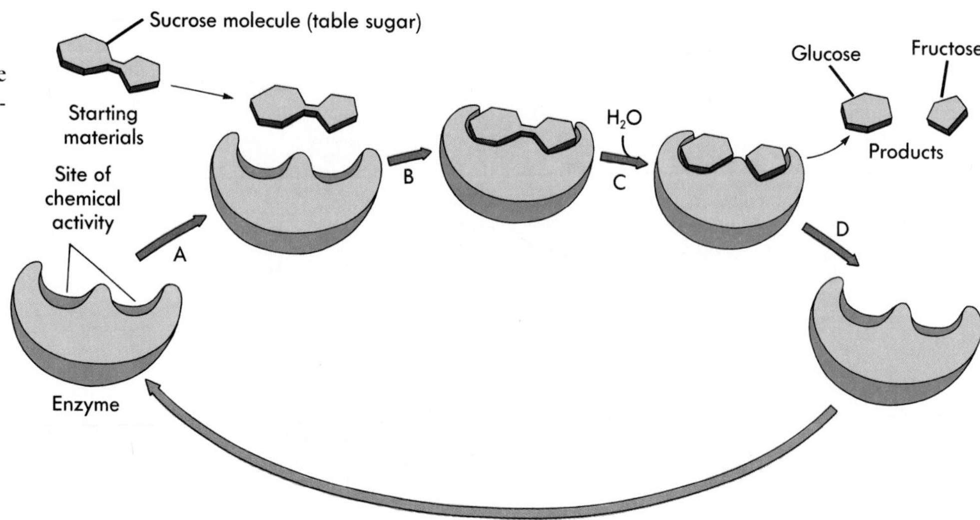

Figure 6-6 A model of enzyme action. With some enzymes, the reaction can go both ways. Sometimes energy in the form of ATP is needed to allow the enzyme to push the reaction in the forward direction.

Digestion—Nutrient By Nutrient

A good way to study digestion of food is to track a single food from the time it enters the mouth until it is either absorbed into the bloodstream or eliminated in the stool. We will use banana bread as an example and start with proteins present since these are the main energy-yielding nutrients digested by the stomach. As you will see, nutrients such as proteins, fats, and carbohydrates in the banana bread are digested at different sites along the GI tract and by different means. Specific enzymes do the work, while nerves, hormones and hormonelike substances control the process.

Digestion actually begins before we start eating. Cooking food can be viewed as a first step in digestion. Cooking unfolds (denatures) proteins and softens tough connective tissues in meats as well as in the fibrous tissue of plants, such as broccoli stalks. When starches are heated, the starch granules present swell as they soak up water, making them much more easy to digest and absorb. All of these effects of cooking make the food easier to chew, swallow, and break down during later digestion and absorption. As you will see in Chapter 19, cooking also makes many foods, such as meats, fish, and poultry, much safer to eat.

PROTEIN DIGESTION

We noted the digestion of the protein in the banana bread—coming mostly from the eggs and milk ingredients—begins in the stomach. The chief cells of the stomach secrete **pepsin**, a major enzyme used for this process. Pepsin attacks all proteins and breaks them down into shorter units, called **peptones**. Pepsin does not completely separate the protein into amino acids because it can break only a few of the many types of bonds found in protein molecules. Thus it has limited activity.

Pepsin is stored in the chief cells of the stomach as pepsinogen, its inactive zymogen form. These cells, along with parietal (acid-forming) cells and mucus-forming cells, lie in gastric pits in the stomach. If pepsin were not stored as an inactive enzyme, it would digest the stomach glands while waiting to be secreted from the pits. Once pepsinogen enters the stomach's acidic environment (pH between 1 and 2), part of the enzyme is broken off, in turn forming the active enzyme pepsin. This storage of the inactive form of pepsin is just one way the stomach prevents **autodigestion** (digesting itself).

The release of pepsin is controlled by the hormone **gastrin**. Just thinking about food or chewing food stimulates the vagus nerve. The vagus nerve, in turn, will

pepsin A protein-digesting enzyme produced by the stomach.

peptones A partial breakdown product of proteins.

autodigestion Literally, "self-digestion." The stomach limits autodigestion by covering itself with a thick layer of mucus and producing enzymes and acid only when needed for digestion of foodstuffs.

gastrin A hormone that stimulates enzyme and acid secretion by the stomach.

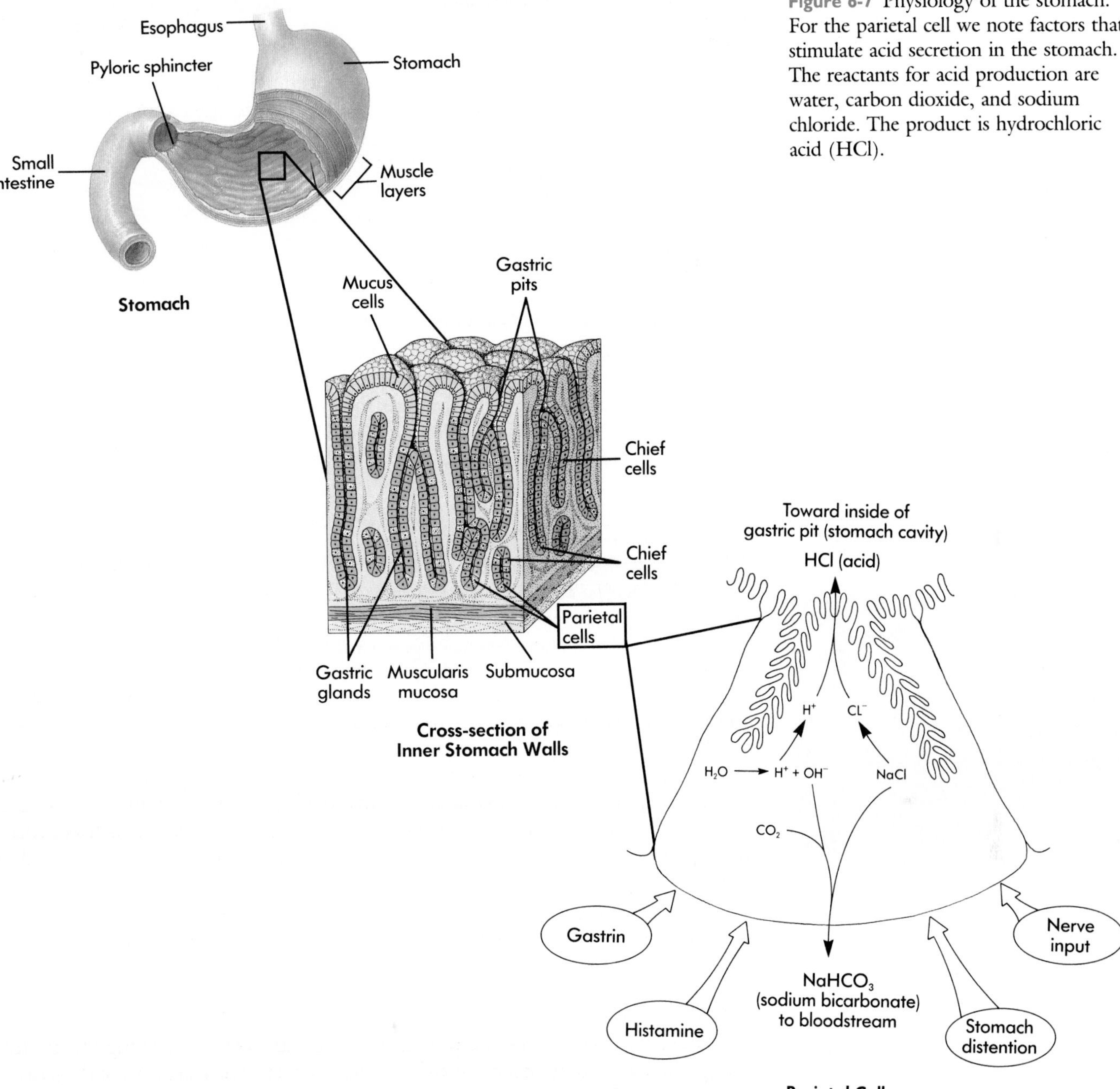

Figure 6-7 Physiology of the stomach. For the parietal cell we note factors that stimulate acid secretion in the stomach. The reactants for acid production are water, carbon dioxide, and sodium chloride. The product is hydrochloric acid (HCl).

"prime" the stomach for the forthcoming meal by stimulating special gastrin-producing cells in the base of the stomach.[7] Gastrin then signals the chief cells in the stomach to begin producing pepsinogen.[13] Now enzymes will be ready when the meal arrives. This is another means by which the stomach prevents autodigestion. Pepsin is present in the stomach only when food enters or is about to reach the stomach because gastrin is released only at those times.

Gastrin also strongly stimulates the stomach's parietal cells to produce acid. In addition, stomach distention or stretching due to the presence of food and a breakdown product of proteins called **histamine** stimulate the parietal cells. When stimulated, the parietal cells produce hydrochloric acid (HCL) from water, carbon dioxide, and chloride ions (Figure 6-7).[20] This hydrochloric acid, in turn, activates pepsin, improves the absorption of iron and calcium, keeps the stomach essentially bacteria

histamine A breakdown product of the amino acid histidine that stimulates acid secretion by the stomach.

free, and inactivates plant and animal hormones that might otherwise act in the body. The parietal cells also produce intrinsic factor, a compound needed for vitamin B-12 absorption.

Since gastrin is released only when we eat or think about eating, acid production follows this same pattern. Furthermore, as the stomach's pH approaches 2, gastrin release stops. Note that we just described several other ways the stomach is protected from autodigestion. The first involves acid production: Acid is produced only when food is present; and secondly only enough is made to aid in digestion of the food that is present. The final barrier against autodigestion is the thick layer of mucus the stomach secretes.[12] The mucus lines the inside of the stomach, insulating it from the acid and pepsin produced for digestion.

PROTEIN DIGESTION CONTINUES IN THE SMALL INTESTINE

The partially digested proteins now move with the rest of the nutrients and other substances in the banana bread from the stomach into the small intestine. The acidic mixture squirts at a slow rate through the pyloric sphincter, which separates the stomach from the upper small intestine (duodenum). All the liquids consumed have combined with the acid produced by the stomach to create a very watery food mixture, called **chyme**. As soon as the chyme squirts into the duodenum, bicarbonate ions (HCO_3^-) made in the pancreas neutralize the acid. This process is coordinated by the hormone **secretin**, which is made in the walls of the upper portion of the small intestine.[13] Acid entering the duodenum causes secretin release. Secretin then stimulates the pancreas to release bicarbonate ions[5] as well as causes a reduction in stomach peristalsis (motility).

chyme A mixture of stomach secretions and partially digested food.

secretin A hormone that causes bicarbonate ion release from the pancreas.

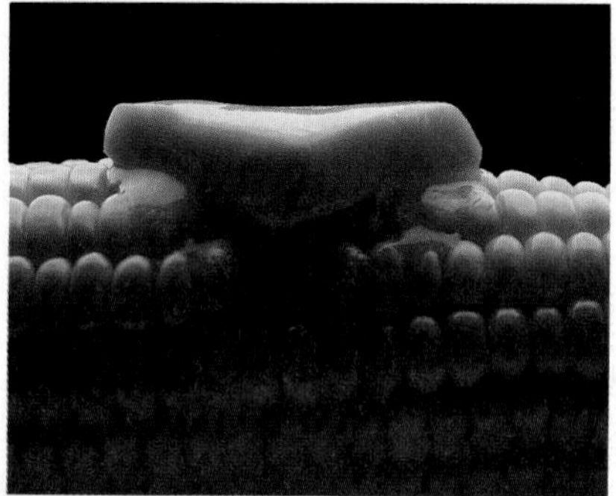

Fat digestion relies on input from many organs—notably the pancreas, gallbladder, and small intestine.

The neutralized chyme is now approximately pH 5 to 7, rather than pH 2 to 3. If the acid chyme is not neutralized, it will eat into the wall of the duodenum. This could eventually lead to an ulcer.[18] Note that unlike the stomach, the small intestine is not protected from acid by a thick layer of mucus. This is because the small intestine must absorb most of the products of digestion, and absorption cannot occur through a thick layer of mucus. Therefore that mode of protection would be impractical. The stomach absorbs only small amounts of alcohol and certain fats; thus a thick layer of mucus poses no problem. The duodenum is protected instead by quick neutralization of the acidic chyme and the constant shedding of its cell lining.

Once in the small intestine, the peptones (and any fats accompanying the incoming peptones produced from a meal) will trigger the release of the hormone cholecystokinin (CCK) from the walls of the small intestine. CCK, in turn, travels through the bloodstream to its target organs, the pancreas and the gallbladder.

The pancreas is responsible for the production and storage of a multitude of digestive enzymes. Among those enzymes are the protein-breaking enzymes: **trypsin**, chymotrypsin, and carboxypeptidase.[12] They are released into the small intestine in their inactive zymogen forms. On arrival, the intestinal enzyme, enterokinase, cleaves the tail portion off of trypsinogen to form trypsin. The now activated trypsin in turn cleaves the tail portions off of both chymotrypsin and carboxypeptidase. In addition, trypsin actually goes back and cleaves the tail portion off of other trypsinogens, creating more of itself. Together these digestive enzymes divide the peptones into short **peptides** and amino acids. As we will cover in a later section, eventual digestion of all the peptides into amino acids then occurs inside the absorptive cells of the small intestine.[3]

trypsin A protein-digesting enzyme secreted by the pancreas to act in the small intestine.

peptides A few amino acids bonded together (often two to four).

FAT DIGESTION

The tongue produces lingual **lipase**, an enzyme that digests fat (lingual refers to the tongue).[8] This enzyme acts primarily on short- and medium-chain fats, such as those found in butter fat. The actual digestion occurs while the fats are in the stomach because lingual lipase requires an acid environment to function. The stomach pro-

lipase Fat-digesting enzymes; lingual lipase is produced by the tongue, gastric lipase by the stomach, and pancreatic lipase by the pancreas.

duces a similar gastric lipase (gastric refers to the stomach). The action of both of these enzymes, however, is usually dwarfed by pancreatic lipase action in the small intestine. Long-chain fats, such as those found in common vegetable oils, must generally wait for intestinal digestion.

Thus the digestion of fat from the vegetable oil, milk, and other ingredients in the banana bread mostly takes place in the small intestine.[19] The hormone **cholecystokinin (CCK)**, that acts to release enzymes for protein digestion, also simultaneously acts to release lipase from the pancreas for fat digestion. In the small intestine, this pancreatic lipase digests the fats into smaller breakdown products, namely monoglycerides and fatty acids. Pancreatic lipase enters the small intestine in a concentration 1000 times greater than needed. This "overkill" makes fat digestion very rapid and thorough given the right circumstances. The "right" circumstances include the presence of bile from the gallbladder. Also released in response to CCK, bile helps to **emulsify** the digestive products of lipase action by forming water-soluble micelles (like a dishwashing detergent breaks up oil spots in dishwater). This improves digestion and absorption because large fat globules break down into smaller ones. This increases the total surface area for lipase action.[3]

Fats and proteins in the chyme also stimulate the release of the hormone **gastric inhibitory peptide (GIP)** from the walls of the upper small intestine.[12] Release of stomach contents into the small intestine is slowed by GIP (Table 6-1). Both the hormones secretin and GIP then help keep the stomach from overwhelming the upper small intestine with chyme. This helps explain why fats in a meal cause a feeling of fullness: the chyme remains in the stomach longer, and so we feel full longer. On the other hand, hunger returns quickly after a low-fat meal.

cholecystokinin (CCK) A hormone that stimulates enzyme release from the pancreas and bile release from the gallbladder.

emulsify To suspend fat in water by isolating individual fat drops using sheets of water molecules to prevent the fat from coalescing.

gastric inhibitory peptide (GIP) A hormone that slows gastric motility and stimulates insulin release from the pancreas.

Table 6-1 Hormones that regulate the digestive tract[17]

Hormone	Origin	Stimulus to secretion	Action
Gastrin	Pyloric region of the stomach	Food and other substances in the stomach, especially proteins, caffeine, spices, alcohol; nerve input	Stimulates flow of stomach enzymes and acid Stimulates contraction of lower esophageal sphincter
Gastric inhibitory peptide	Duodenum, jejunum	Fats, protein	Inhibits secretion of stomach acid and enzymes; reduces stomach motility
Cholecystokinin (CCK)	Duodenum, jejunum	Food, especially fat and protein in duodenum	Causes contraction of gallbladder and flow of bile to duodenum; causes secretion of enzyme-rich pancreatic juice and bicarbonate-rich pancreatic fluid
Secretin	Duodenum, jejunum	Acid chyme; peptones	Causes secretion of bicarbonate-rich pancreatic fluid and reduces stomach motility

Table 6-2 Summary of digestive enzymes

Secretion origin	Enzyme	Substrate	Major end products
Salivary glands	Salivary amylase	Starch, glycogen	Maltose and dextrins
Lingual glands	Lingual lipase	Short-chain triglycerides, medium-chain triglycerides	Fatty acids, monoglycerides
Stomach glands	Pepsin	Protein	Peptides, peptones
	Gastric lipase	Short-chain triglycerides, medium-chain triglycerides	Fatty acids, monoglycerides
Pancreas	Trypsin	Protein, peptides	Polypeptides, smaller peptides
	Chymotrypsin	Protein, peptides	Same as trypsin, more coagulating power for milk
	Carboxypeptidase	Polypeptides	Smaller peptides, free amino acids
	Pancreatic amylase	Starch, glycogen, dextrins	Maltose
	Lipase	Triglycerides	Monoglycerides, free fatty acids
Intestinal wall	Aminopeptidase	Peptides	Amino acids, smaller peptides
	Maltase	Maltose	Glucose
	Sucrase	Sucrose	Glucose, fructose
	Lactase	Lactose	Glucose, galactose
	Enterokinase	Trypsinogen	Trypsin

CARBOHYDRATE DIGESTION

amylase Starch-digesting enzymes from the salivary glands or pancreas.

dextrin Partial breakdown products of starch that contain few to many glucose molecules. These appear as starch is digested into many units of maltose.

Digestion of the large carbohydrates—starches—coming mostly from the flour in the banana bread begins as these mix with saliva during the chewing of food. Saliva contains an enzyme called salivary **amylase**. This enzyme breaks down starch (a chain of thousands of glucose units) into many small sugar units called maltose (merely two glucose units bonded together). You can observe this conversion while chewing a saltine cracker. Prolonged chewing of the cracker causes the taste to become more sweet as some starch is broken into the sweeter sugars.

Salivary amylase does not work in an acidic environment. Once food moves down the esophagus into the stomach, the stomach's acidity halts further salivary amylase action, and consequently starch digestion. However, salivary amylase is not that important because pancreatic amylase in the small intestine will finish what salivary amylase does not finish in the mouth (Table 6-2).

When the carbohydrates are in the intestine, the pancreas releases its amylase to continue the digestion of the starches from the **dextrin** phase into maltose. The original carbohydrates from the banana bread are now present as monosaccharides (glucose and fructose) as well as disaccharides (maltose, lactose, and sucrose). Eventually all the disaccharide (double sugar) forms will be digested to their monosaccharide (single sugar) forms by specialized enzymes called disaccharidases. These enzymes are synthesized by and attached to the cells of the small intestine. Maltose is acted on by maltase to produce two glucose molecules. Sucrose (table sugar) is acted on by sucrase to produce glucose and fructose. Lactose (milk sugar) is acted on by lactase to produce glucose and galactose. The single sugars are then absorbed (Figure 6-8).[12]

When considering carbohydrate digestion, it is important to remember that the needed digestive enzymes come from both the pancreas and cells of the intestinal wall. Intestinal diseases can interfere with the production of the intestinal wall enzymes. Such conditions may interfere with the efficient digestion of the sugars maltose, lactose, and sucrose. If these carbohydrates are not fully digested, they will

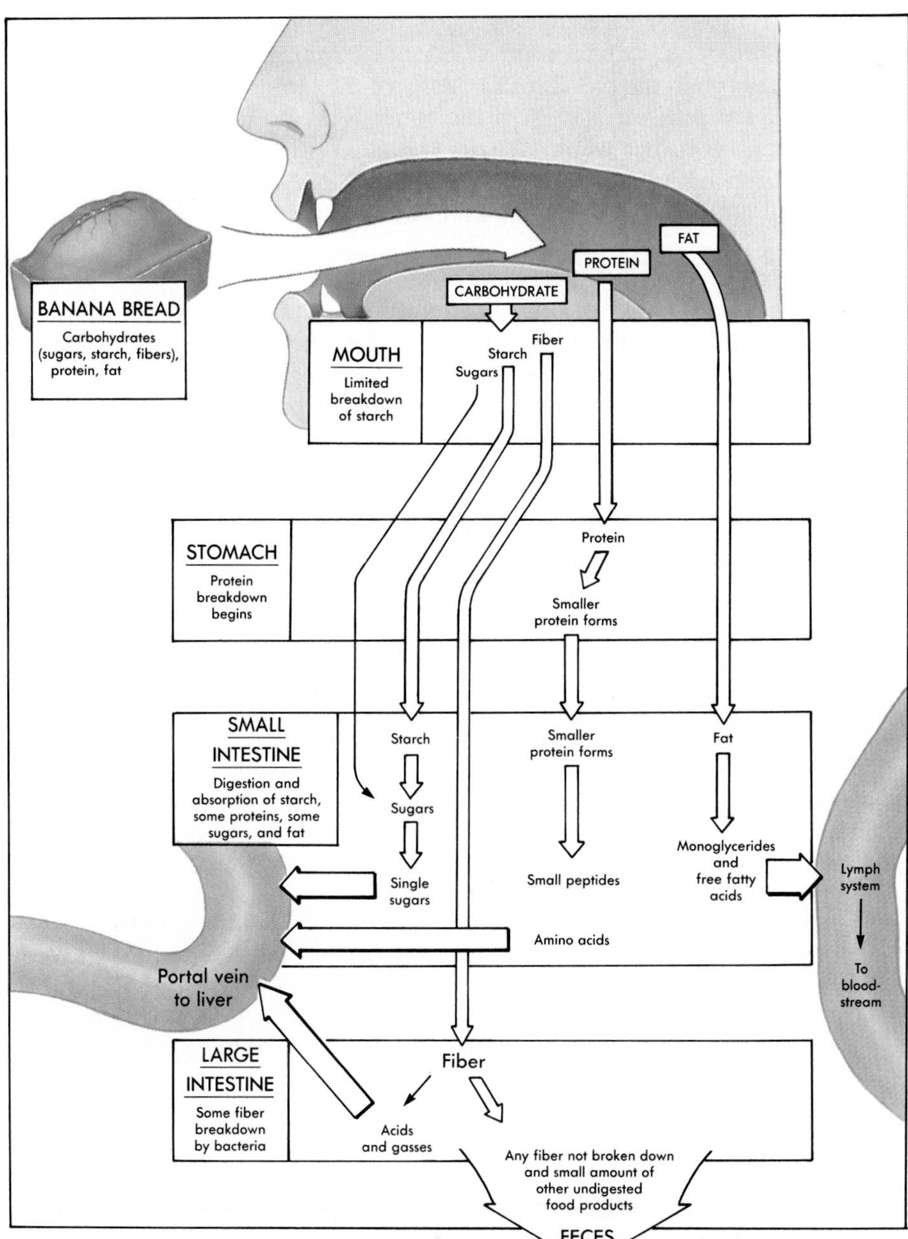

Figure 6-8 Digestion in practical terms. Many enzymes contribute to the digestion of foods, such as seen in this example of banana bread. Absorption is via the bloodstream and the lymphatic system.

not be absorbed. When they end up in the colon, the bacteria present will use the sugars to produce acid and gas, causing abdominal discomfort. People recovering from intestinal disorders, such as diarrhea or bacterial infections, may need to especially avoid lactose for a few weeks because of possible temporary lactose intolerance. Two weeks will give time for the small intestine to again begin producing enough lactase enzyme to allow for lactose digestion.[9]

HORMONES—A KEY TO ORCHESTRATING THIS DIGESTIVE PROCESS

We have now seen the four true hormones that regulate the GI tract: gastrin, secretin, cholecystokinin, and gastric inhibitory peptide (Table 6-1).[13] In order to be a true hormone, a compound must have a specific synthesis site from which it must enter the bloodstream to reach its target organ or organs. Of the four true digestive tract hormones, gastrin may seem confusing. Its site of synthesis as well as its target organ are both the stomach, but it does first enter the bloodstream before acting.

Many other hormonelike compounds also control important aspects of GI function. These compounds diffuse from cells or nerve endings to nearby cells, rather than traveling through the bloodstream. Many of the hormonelike compounds are found in both the intestine and the brain. When a person thinks about eating or prepares to eat, his or her whole GI tract begins to prime itself for action. Hormonelike substances participate in this "priming." The cells that make all these hormones and hormonelike compounds are scattered throughout the GI tract.[3]

DIGESTION—A FURTHER RECAP

After reading this section on the interrelationships of the digestive process and its regulatory mechanisms, it should be clear to you that the digestive tract can readily meet the demands placed on it. The response to any ingested foodstuff is directly related to the nutritional makeup and amount of that particular foodstuff. Foods generally contain a mixture of macronutrients as well as vitamins and minerals; therefore it makes sense that multiple enzymatic responses to the small intestine are the rule, not the exception. The popular contention of fad dieters that ingestion of certain combinations of foods, such as meats and fruits together, hinders the absorptive process does not make sense in light of what we know about physiology and with respect to our collective experiences of eating this type of meal.

CONCEPT CHECK

Digestion is the process by which foodstuffs are broken down into smaller and more simple forms. Therefore, it begins with cooking; heat and moisture unfold proteins, swell starch granules, and soften tough fibrous tissues in plants. Enzymes produced in the mouth begin to digest starch. The stomach primarily digests protein, producing breakdown products called peptones. The small intestine is the major site of all digestion. There, peptones separate into small peptides and amino acids, carbohydrates yield single sugars, and fats form monoglycerides and free fatty acids. Peristaltic muscle contractions in the stomach and small intestine constantly mix the food, enhancing the digestive process. Enzymes used for digestion in the small intestine come from the pancreas and the cells lining the intestinal wall. Fat digestion is aided by bile, which is produced by the liver and later released by the gallbladder.

The Physiology of Absorption

Most nutrient absorption occurs in the small intestine and colon. The small intestine can absorb about 95% of the kcalories it receives in the form of protein, carbohydrate, fat, and alcohol. Only water, small amounts of alcohol, certain types of fats, and glucose are absorbed by the mouth and/or stomach. Some minerals, water, and short-chain fatty acids (produced by bacterial action) are absorbed in the colon.

THE SMALL INTESTINE: SITE FOR MOST NUTRIENT ABSORPTION

absorptive cells A class of cells that cover the surface of the villi (fingerlike projections in the small intestine) and participate in nutrient absorption.

The incredible surface area of the small intestine greatly contributes to efficient absorption. The wall of the small intestine is folded, and within the folds are fingerlike villi projections (Figure 6-9). The "fingers" trap foodstuffs between each other to enhance absorption. Each villi "finger" is made up of numerous **absorptive cells**, and each of these cells has a brush border, or microvilli, cap.[3] The intestinal enzymes are then often found on the glycocalyx, hairlike projections that cover the surface of the microvilli. All these folds, fingers, and indentations in the small intestine increase surface area 600 times beyond that of a simple tube.

ABSORPTIVE CELLS

The absorptive cells are produced in open ended pits (called crypts) buried deep into the wall of the small intestine. The cells migrate up from the crypts to the tip

EXPERT OPINION

Gastroquackery

STEPHEN BARRETT, M.D.

The importance of "regularity" to overall health has been greatly overestimated for thousands of years. Ancient Egyptians associated feces with decay and used enemas and laxatives liberally. In more recent times, this concern has been embodied in the concept of "autointoxication" and has been promoted by warnings against "irregularity."

The theory of "autointoxication" states that stagnation of the colon (large intestine) causes toxins to form that are absorbed and poison the body. Some proponents depict the colon as a "sewage system" that becomes a "cesspool" if neglected. Other proponents state that constipation causes hardened feces to accumulate for months (or even years) on the walls of the colon and block the colon from absorbing or eliminating properly. This, they say, causes food to remain undigested and wastes from the blood to be reabsorbed by the body.

Around the turn of the twentieth century many physicians accepted the concept of autointoxication, but it was abandoned during the 1930s after scientific observations proved it wrong. Among other things, direct observation of the colon during surgical procedures found no evidence that hardened feces accumulate on the intestinal walls.

Today we know that most of the digestive process takes place in the small intestine, from which nutrients are absorbed into the body. The remaining mixture of food and undigested particles then enters the large intestine, which can be compared to a 60-inch-long hollow tube. Its principal functions are to transport food wastes from the small intestine to the rectum for elimination and to absorb minerals and water. Careful observations have shown that the bowel habits of healthy individuals can vary greatly. Although most people have a movement daily, some have several movements each day while others can go several days or even longer with no adverse effects.

Despite these facts, some chiropractors, naturopaths, and assorted food faddists claim that "death begins in the colon" and that "90% of all diseases are caused by improperly working bowels." The practices they recommend include fasting, periodic "cleansing" of the intestines, and colonic irrigation. Fasting is said to "purify" the body. "Cleansing" can be accomplished with a variety of "natural" laxative products. Colonic irrigation is performed by passing a rubber tube through the rectum for a distance of up to 20 or even 30 inches. Warm water—often 20 gallons or more—is pumped in and out through the tube, a few pints at a time, to wash out the contents of the colon. (An ordinary enema uses about a quart of fluid.) Some practitioners add herbs, coffee, enzymes, wheat or grass extract, or other substances to the enema solution.

The danger of these practices depends on how much they are used and whether they are substituted for necessary medical care. Whereas a 1-day fast is likely to be harmless (though useless), prolonged fasting can be fatal. "Cleansing" is unlikely to be physically harmful, but the products involved can be expensive.

Colonic irrigation—which also can be expensive—has considerable potential for harm. The process can be very uncomfortable, since the presence of the tube can induce severe cramps and pain. If the equipment is not adequately sterilized between treatments, disease germs from one person's large intestine can be transmitted to others. Several outbreaks of serious infections have been reported, including one in which contaminated equipment caused amebiasis in 13 people, six of whom died following bowel perforation. Cases of heart failure (from excessive fluid absorption into the bloodstream) and electrolyte imbalance have also been reported.

The popular diet book *Fit for Life* (1986) is based on the notion that when certain foods are eaten together, they "rot," poisoning the system and making the person fat. To avoid this, the authors recommend that fats, carbohydrates, and protein foods be eaten at separate meals, emphasizing fruits and vegetables because foods high in water content can "wash the toxic waste from the inside of the body" instead of "clogging" the body. These ideas are utter nonsense.

Although laxative advertisements warn against "irregularity," constipation should be defined not by the frequency of movements but by the hardness of the stool. Ordinary constipation usually can be remedied by increasing the fiber content of the diet, drinking adequate amounts of water, and engaging in regular exercise. If the bowel is basically normal, dietary fiber increases the bulk of the stool, softens it, and speeds transit time. Defecating soon after the urge is felt also can be helpful because if urges are ignored, the rectum may eventually stop signalling when defecation is needed. Stimulant laxatives (such as cascara or castor oil) can damage the nerve cells in the colon wall, decreasing the force of contractions and increasing the tendency toward constipation. Thus people who take strong laxatives whenever they "miss a movement" may wind up unable to move their bowels without them. A medical doctor should be consulted if constipation persists or represents a significant change in bowel pattern.

Dr. Barrett, who practices psychiatry in Allentown, Pennsylvania, edits Nutrition Forum Newsletter and is a board member of the national Council Against Health Fraud. In 1984 he received the FDA Commissioner's Special Citation Award for Public Service in fighting nutrition quackery. His 27 books include Health Schemes, Scams, and Frauds [Consumer Reports Books 1990] and the college textbook Consumer Health—A Guide to Intelligent Decisions, edition 4 (Mosby-Year Book, 1989.)

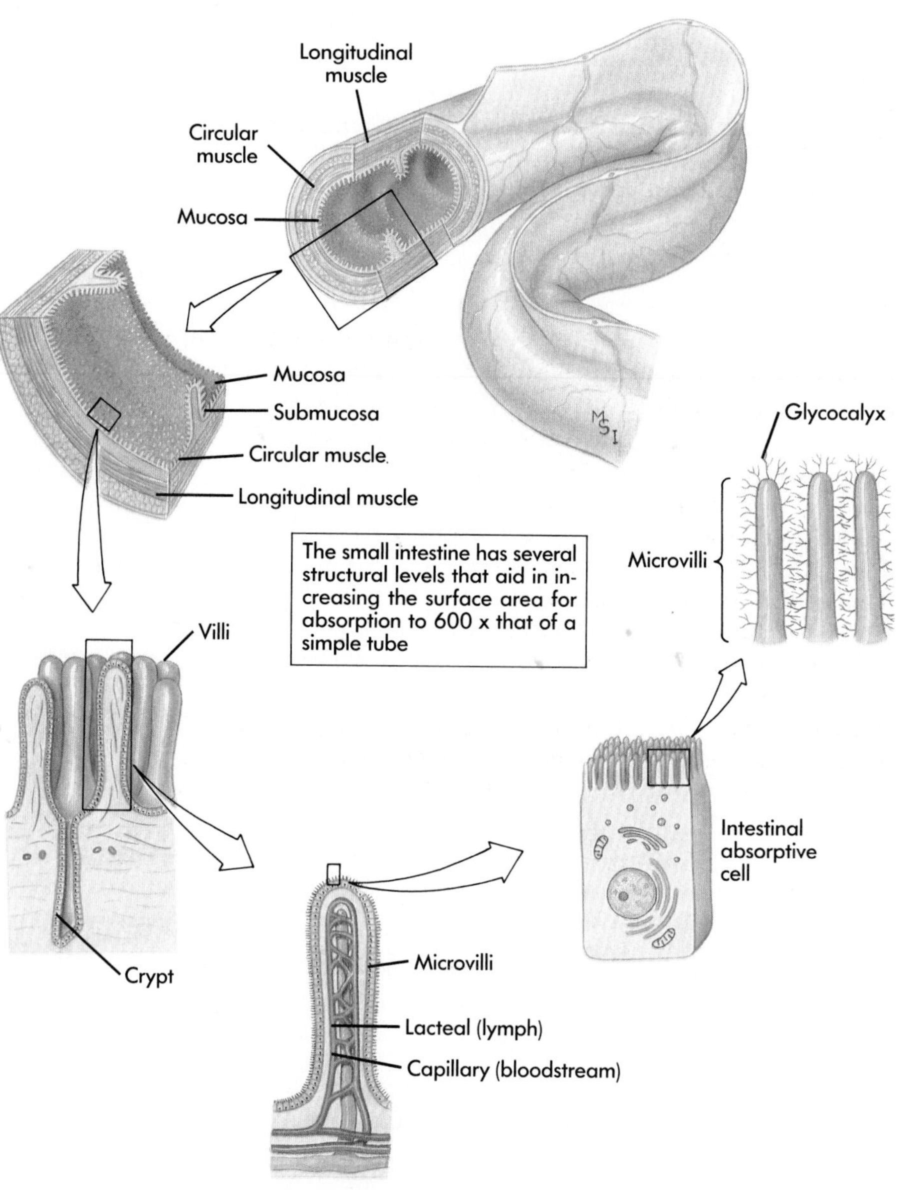

Figure 6-9 Organization of the small intestine. The small intestine has several structural levels that aid in increasing the surface area for absorption to 600 times that of a simple tube.

One cancer treatment uses medications (chemotherapy) to prevent rapid cell growth. This can stop tumor cells from growing. However, chemotherapy also affects body cells that normally have a rapid turnover, such as the absorptive cells of the intestinal villi. Because the cells of the villi are affected, people on these medications usually develop diarrhea as a side effect.

of the villi. As the cells migrate, they mature, and their absorption efficiency increases. By the time they reach the top of the villi, however, they have been partially degraded by digestive enzymes that have been acting on them. They are then ready to be sloughed off. Newly formed absorptive cells are constantly produced, and these march up from the crypts to replace the dying ones.

The journey from the crypt to the top of the villi takes 2 to 5 days for each absorptive cell. Thus these cells have a very short life span. This short life span probably serves as an important adaptive mechanism. Absorptive cells face a harsh environment due to contact with the enzymes, bacteria, and various toxins found in the small intestine. Contact with alcohol also reduces the integrity of the intestinal lining. Therefore constant formation of a new intestinal lining essentially becomes a biological necessity.

Since cell production requires many nutrients, groups of cells with a great need for constant reproduction will have a correspondingly great need for nutrients. With the same logic, one can predict that the small intestine will rapidly deteriorate during a nutrient deficiency or in semistarvation.[9] In addition, researchers have shown that the products of digestion and the hormones associated with the digestive process have a direct growth-promoting action on the cells of the small intestine. The absorptive cells in the small intestine are healthier when GI tract hormones and digestive products are present.

If a disease causes the villi to lie down, the surface area in the small intestine decreases and so malabsorption often results. This is what happens in celiac disease (also called gluten-induced enteropathy). A person having this disease shows an allergic response to a protein, called gluten, found in wheat, rye, oats, and barley. To prevent attacks the person must avoid eating those grains.

TYPES OF ABSORPTION

The small intestine uses four basic types of absorption processes: **passive, facilitative, active,** and **phagocytosis/pinocytosis.**[12] Passive absorption occurs when nutrients enter the absorptive cells without any need for a carrier or energy expenditure. To allow for this, the wall of the intestine must be permeable to the nutrient, and the nutrient must be present in a higher concentration in the intestinal contents than in the absorptive cells. The difference in concentration drives passive absorption. Water and some minerals are passively absorbed.

Facilitative absorption involves a carrier molecule to shuttle the nutrients from the **lumen** of the small intestine into the absorptive cells, but no energy is expended. Again, a concentration difference drives the reaction. Facilitative absorption takes place for the simple sugar fructose, which mostly arises from the digestion of table sugar (sucrose).

Active absorption uses a carrier and expends energy in the process. The single sugars glucose and galactose, amino acids, and other nutrients are actively absorbed (Figure 6-10). Adenosine triphosphate (ATP) is the energy source (see Chapter 7

passive absorption Absorption that requires permeability of the substance through the wall of the small intestine, as well as a favorable concentration gradient higher in the intestinal contents than in the absorptive cell.

facilitated absorption Absorption where a carrier shuttles substances into the absorptive cell but no energy is expended. A concentration gradient higher in the intestinal contents than in the absorptive cell drives the absorption.

active absorption Absorption using a carrier and expending ATP energy. In this way the absorptive cell can absorb nutrients, such as glucose, against a concentration gradient.

phagocytosis/pinocytosis Forms of active absorption in which the absorptive cell forms an indentation in its membrane and particles or fluids entering the indentation are then engulfed by the cell.

lumen The inside cavity of the GI tract.

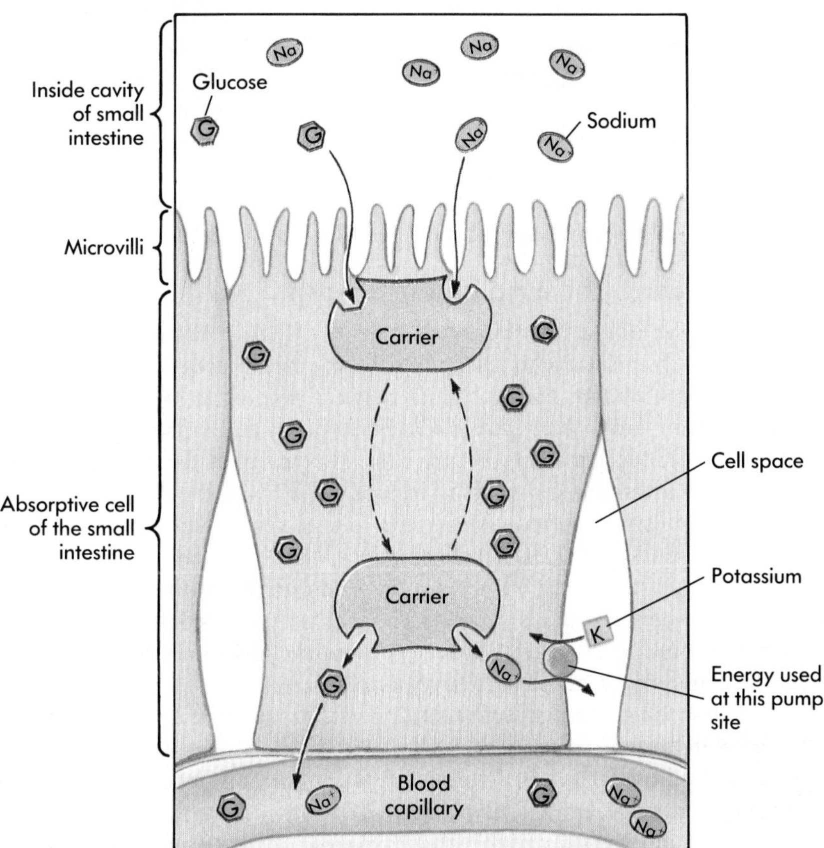

Figure 6-10 Active absorption of glucose. Glucose and sodium pass across the cell membrane of the intestinal absorptive cell in a carrier-dependent, energy-requiring process. The energy is used for maintaining a low concentration of sodium in the cell. Once inside the absorptive cell, glucose can exit by facilitated diffusion down its concentration gradient and enter the bloodstream.

A

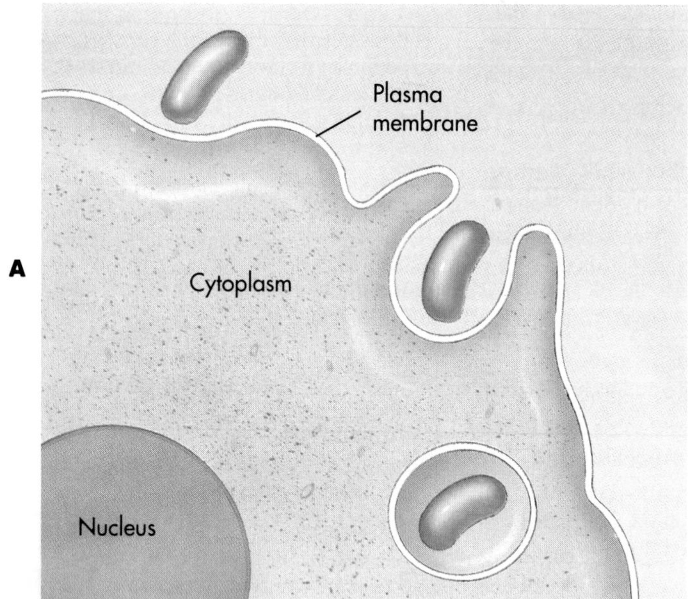

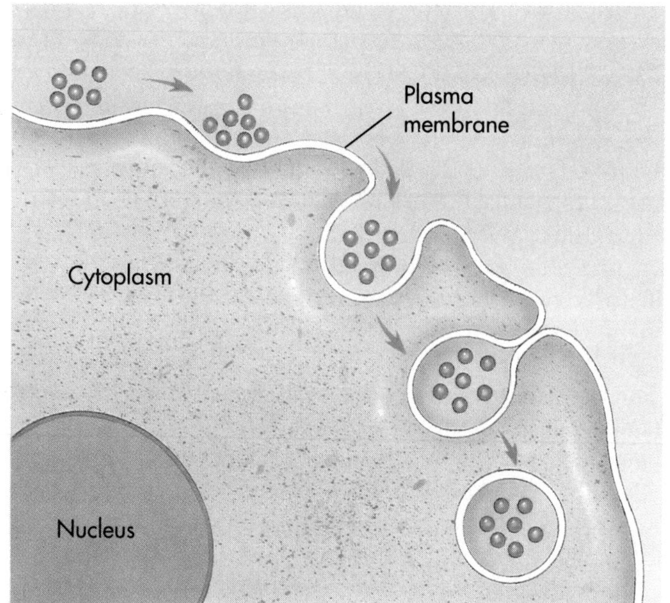

B

Figure 6-11 Phagocytosis—"cell eating"—and pinocytosis—"cell driving." Cells take in substances using a variety of methods, including uptake of whole particles via phagocytosis and liquids via pinocytosis.

If the pump for glucose absorption does not work, much of the glucose in the intestine will not be absorbed. The unabsorbed glucose will draw water into the small intestine, causing diarrhea. This is essentially what happens in cholera. The cholera bacterium poisons the glucose pump, resulting in massive diarrhea. If a person with cholera is not given adequate fluid support while infected, he or she will quickly become dehydrated and die.

for a discussion of ATP).[12] Using this energy, absorptive cells on the villi can even take up a substance in low concentration, such as glucose, from the intestinal contents. Since the bloodstream constantly bathes the absorptive cells, their relative concentration of glucose is high. The absorptive cells will then always have a greater internal concentration of glucose than the intestinal contents. Therefore the ability to absorb glucose against a concentration gradient is critical.

A second type of active absorption by absorptive cells involves the processes of phagocytosis (literally cell eating) and pinocytosis (literally cell drinking). These involve the absorptive cells literally engulfing compounds or liquids. A cell can indent its cellular membrane. When particles or fluids move into the indentation, the cell surrounds and engulfs them (Figure 6-11). This occurs when an infant absorbs antibodies from its mother's milk.

PORTAL AND LYMPHATIC CIRCULATION

The villi in the intestine are drained by two different circulation systems—portal and lymphatic. The nutrients select one of these two systems based on their solubility in either water or fat. The nutrients that are soluble in water (such as proteins, carbohydrates, short-chain fatty acids, B vitamins, and vitamin C) but insoluble in fat will use the bloodstream (Figure 6-8). Blood leaves the heart through arteries, travels to the intestine, and ends up in capillary beds inside the villi. The blood then leaves the capillary beds and collects into a large vein called the **portal vein** (Figure 6-4). This vein leads directly to the liver. Most veins in the body return blood directly back to the heart. However, by going directly to the liver the portal vein enables the liver to process absorbed nutrients in the blood it carries before they enter the general circulation of the bloodstream.[12] Blood flow used for absorption accounts for 30% of the heart's total output.

portal vein Capillaries from the intestine and stomach drain into a large portal vein that leads to the liver.

lymphatic system System of vessels that can accept large or fat-soluble particles, such as chylomicrons, and eventually pass them into the bloodstream.

The other circulatory system that drains the villi is the **lymphatic system.**[21] The lymphatic vessels carry particles that are either very fat soluble (such as long-chain fatty acids and the fat soluble vitamins A, D, E, and K) or too large to pass through the capillaries into the bloodstream (such as large proteins that escape from the bloodstream and chylomicrons formed after the absorption of fat). After substances enter the lymphatic system, they are squeezed through its spongelike vessels by muscular activity. The lymphatic vessels from the intestine drain into the thoracic duct, which stretches from the abdomen to the neck. This duct is connected to the bloodstream via a large vein near the neck.

enterohepatic circulation A continual recycling of compounds between the small intestine and the liver; bile acids are one example of a recycled compound.

ENTEROHEPATIC CIRCULATION

During meals bile circulates about twice through the liver, moves to the gallbladder, travels through the small intestine into the portal vein, and then returns to the liver. This cycling is called **enterohepatic circulation**. Approximately 98% of the bile is recycled. Only 1% to 2% of the bile ends up in the colon and is eliminated in the stool.[12]

As discussed in Chapter 4, a common way to control very high blood cholesterol levels is to consume resins that bind bile and draw its constituents into the feces. This treatment reduces bile's enterohepatic circulation. The liver is then forced to make new bile rather than use recycled bile. The building block for bile synthesis is cholesterol. The liver must take this cholesterol out of the bloodstream to make new bile, thus lowering the blood cholesterol level.

Some cancer cells also travel through the lymph. When cancer is found in the body during surgery, the surgeon will examine the lymph nodes closest to the site of the cancer to see if it has traveled from the original site to other sites in the body. If cancer cells are found in the lymph nodes, they have probably already spread to other organs in the body.

CONCEPT CHECK

The small intestine is the major site for nutrient absorption. Numerous folds and fingerlike projections increase the surface area 600 times that of a simple tube. This provides a large area for nutrient absorption. Absorptive cells have a life span of 2 to 5 days, and so the lining of the small intestine is constantly being renewed. These cells can perform passive absorption, promoted by a concentration gradient; facilitative absorption, promoted by a concentration gradient plus a carrier; and active absorption, which uses energy in addition to a carrier to work against a concentration gradient. Absorptive cells can also engulf compounds and liquids (phagocytosis/pinocytosis). The products of absorption, if water soluble, pass into the portal vein and enter the liver. The products of fat digestion mostly enter the lymphatic system. Some participants in digestion, such as bile, are reabsorbed after use in the small intestine and returned to the liver, only to be sent back again to the small intestine during another bout of digestion. This circulation is called enterohepatic circulation.

Absorption: Step By Step

Absorption of all the energy-yielding nutrients occurs simultaneously. We separate the absorption of each here for simplicity.

PROTEIN ABSORPTION

Small peptides and amino acids—breakdown products of the egg and milk protein in the banana bread—are actively absorbed into the absorptive cells of the small intestine (Figure 6-12). Few whole proteins are absorbed.[6] The small peptides are then broken down into individual amino acids inside the cells, as we mentioned earlier. The amino acids travel to the liver via the portal vein. There they are either combined into protein, converted into glucose or fat, used for energy needs, or released into the bloodstream.

FAT ABSORPTION

Most of the products of fat digestion—in our case primarily from the vegetable oil and milk in the banana bread—have by now been reduced to mere fatty acids and monoglycerides (glycerol backbones with single fatty acids attached). These are passively absorbed as such into the absorptive cells.[19] One key characteristic of fatty acids and monoglycerides affects the manner of their absorption. If the chain length of a fatty acid is less than 12 carbon atoms (a short- or medium-chain variety), it

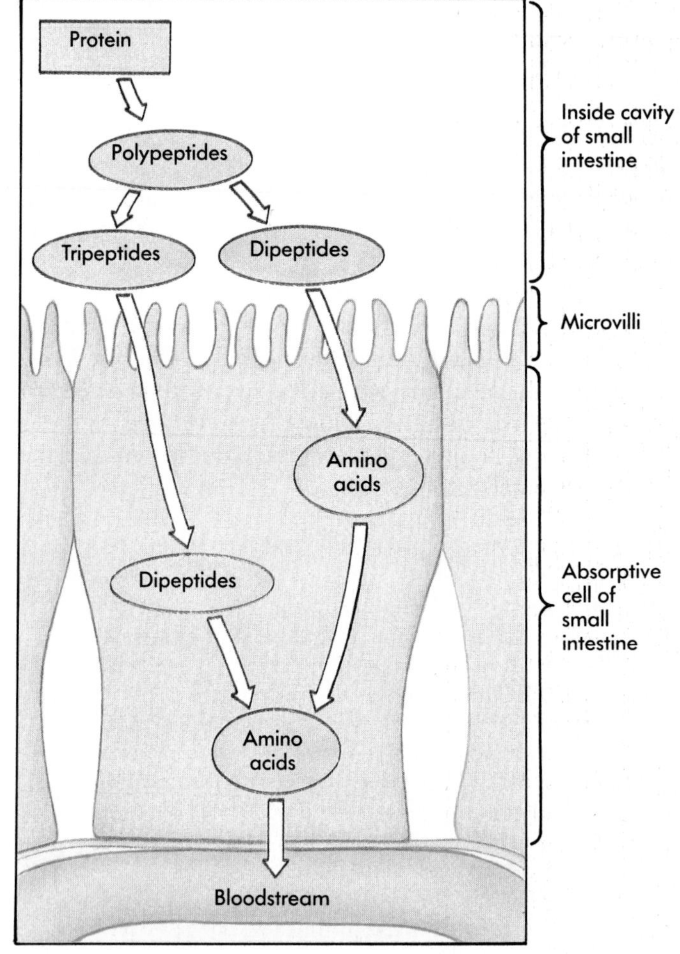

Figure 6-12 Final protein digestion. This takes place in the absorptive cells of the small intestine. In a sodium-dependent, energy-requiring process much like that for glucose absorption, all of the end-products of protein digestion are broken down on the microvilli and within the absorptive cell to amino acids. These are sent to the bloodstream.

is water soluble and so will probably travel as such through the portal vein to the liver. If the fatty acid is a long-chain variety (16 or more carbon atoms), then it must eventually be reformed into a triglyceride molecule and be absorbed via the lymphatic system (Figure 6-13).

The stomach is capable of limited absorption of short-chain fatty acids.[3] These will be present mainly as a result of the action of lingual lipase on foods that contain high amounts of short-chain fats (like butter or milk fat).

The major by-products of lipid digestion are long-chain free fatty acids and monoglycerides. As noted above, these are resynthesized into triglycerides in the villi. The triglycerides are then combined with cholesterol and other substances and covered with a protein coat. This collective structure of fat and protein is termed a lipoprotein, or as in this specific case, a chylomicron. This chylomicron is what actually enters the lymphatic system and eventually the bloodstream to carry most of the absorbed fat from the banana bread.

Note that cholesterol in foods often comes attached with a fatty acid. Enzymes from the pancreas break off this fatty acid, yielding the cholesterol itself. About 60% of this is then absorbed.

CARBOHYDRATE ABSORPTION

Finally, we come to the sugars. In the banana bread, sugars occur naturally in the fruit, are added as table sugar, and are formed as by-products of earlier starch digestion in the mouth and small intestine. As we mentioned, fructose follows facilitative absorption as it is taken up by the absorptive cells. Glucose and galactose (its close relative) are actively pumped into the absorptive cells of the villi. These are transported along with sodium during active absorption (Figure 6-10).[12] The energy used in the process is actually needed to pump the sodium ion back out of

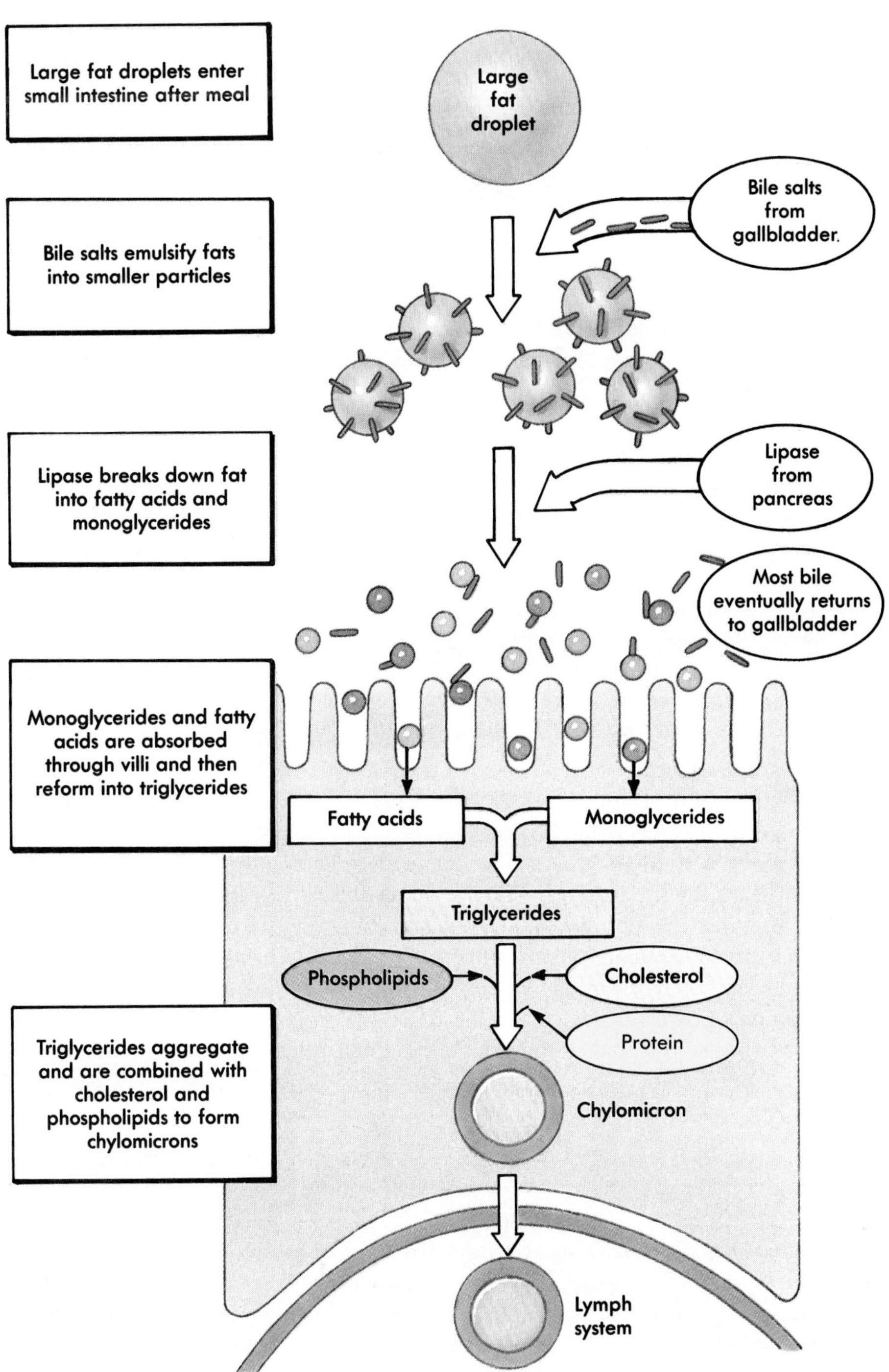

Figure 6-13 A simplified look at fat absorption. Triglycerides made up of long-chain fatty acids primarily form monoglycerides. These are absorbed using bile and then reformed into triglycerides in the absorptive cells. The triglycerides are then formed into chylomicrons and enter the lymphatic system. Note that short-chain fatty acids pass directly into portal circulation. These do not lead to chylomicron formation (see Figure 6-8).

Figure 6-14 Frank and Ernest.
Reprinted by permission of NEA, Inc.

FRANK & ERNEST® by Bob Thaves

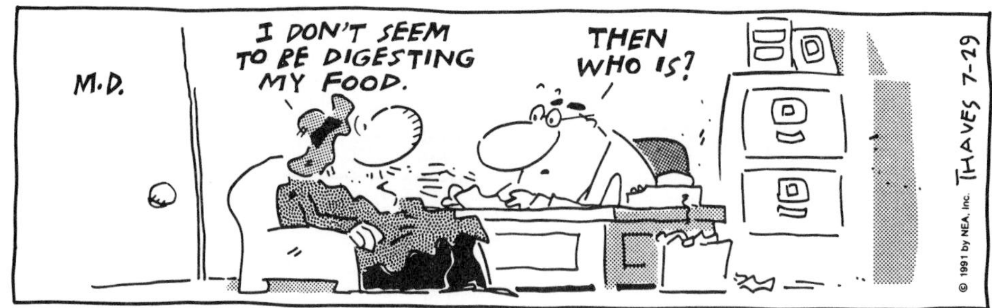
M.D.
I DON'T SEEM TO BE DIGESTING MY FOOD.
THEN WHO IS?
THAVES 7-29
© 1991 by NEA, Inc.

the absorptive cell. Once glucose, galactose, and fructose enter the villi, they are transported via the portal vein to the liver. The liver then exercises its metabolic options—glycogen production, fat production, energy use, or direct release into the bloodstream.

THE LARGE INTESTINE COMPLETES ABSORPTION

The small intestine is responsible for 85% to 90% of the water absorbed from the GI tract. This absorption can reduce the 9 liters the GI tract receives (2 liters of dietary fluid plus 7 liters of GI tract secretions) to about 1.5 liters. Nevertheless, as the intestinal contents leave the small intestine, some water remains. The remnants of digestion entering the colon consist mostly of water, along with some minerals and undigested food fibers. This is often referred to as feces. Again, only a minor amount (5%) of carbohydrate, protein, and fat have escaped absorption (Figure 6-14).

The colon absorbs primarily the minerals sodium and potassium, along with some water. This occurs mostly in the first half of the colon. The unabsorbed water now amounts to only about 200 milliliters. Short-chain fatty acids made from both the metabolism of some plant fibers and undigested starches are also absorbed in the colon, along with some vitamins synthesized by bacteria, such as vitamin K and biotin.[17] By the time the feces in the colon have passed through the first two thirds of its length, they are semisolid. The feces remains in the colon until peristaltic waves and mass movements push it into the rectum for elimination.

The presence of feces in the rectum powerfully stimulates defecation.[12] This process involves powerful muscular reflexes in the sigmoid colon and rectum, as well as relaxation of the anal sphincters. What remains in the stool are undigestible plant fibers, tough connective tissues from animal foods, and bacteria from the colon (Figure 6-15).

The colon has a large diameter and no villi.

CONCEPT CHECK

In protein absorption peptides and amino acids are actively absorbed into the absorptive cells and broken down into amino acid forms. These enter the portal vein en route to the liver. During fat absorption, the breakdown products are passively absorbed into the absorptive cells. These products are mostly resynthesized into triglycerides and combined with cholesterol, protein, and other substances to yield a chylomicron. Chylomicrons enter the lymphatic system and eventually the bloodstream. In carbohydrate absorption the single sugars glucose and galactose are actively absorbed into the absorptive cells; however, fructose follows facilitated absorption, a process in which a carrier is used but no energy is expended. These single sugars then travel via the portal vein to the liver. In the colon, further water and mineral absorption occurs. The remaining contents form the stool and consist primarily of undigestible plant fibers and bacteria.

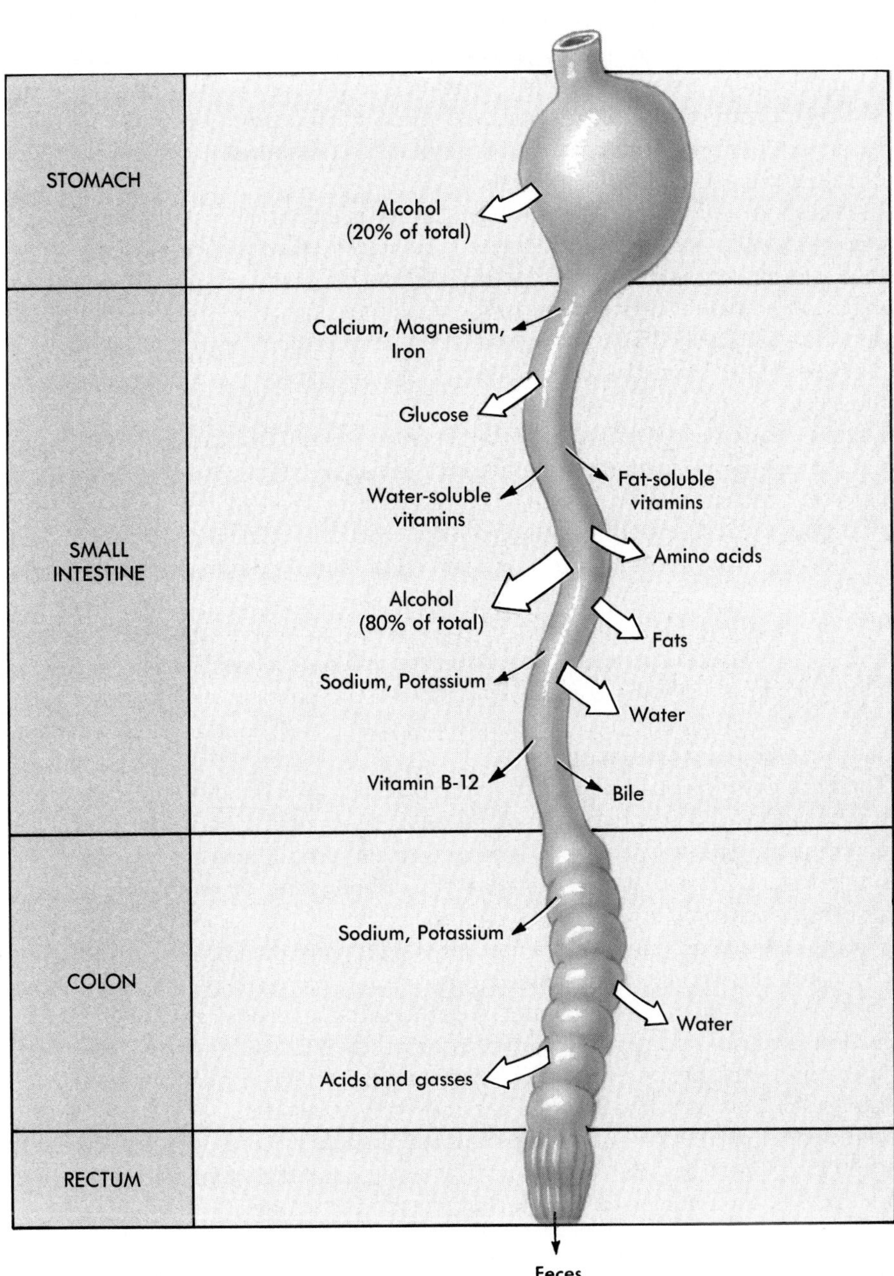

Figure 6-15 Major sites of absorption along the GI tract. The size of the arrow indicates the relative amount of absorption at that site.

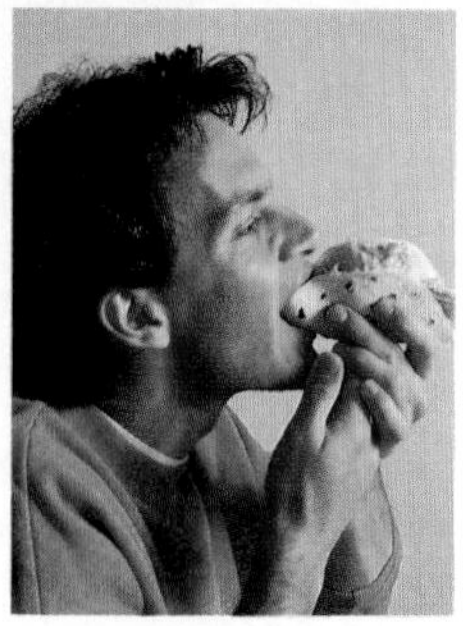

Summary

1. The gastrointestinal (GI) tract consists of the mouth, esophagus, stomach, small intestine, large intestine (colon), rectum, and anus. Most absorption of nutrients occurs in the small intestine.
2. The liver, gallbladder, and pancreas participate in digestion and absorption. Products from these organs enter the small intestine. The enzymes and bile that are supplied play important roles in digesting protein, fat, and carbohydrates.
3. Along the GI tract are valves (sphincters) that control the flow of foodstuffs. Muscular contractions, called peristalsis, propel the foodstuffs down the GI tract. A variety of nerves, hormones, and hormonelike compounds control the activity of sphincters and peristaltic motions.
4. In digestion, the mouth chews food to break it into smaller parts, thereby increasing surface area. Enzyme activity is enhanced when the surface area of the food is increased. Some starch digestion also occurs in the mouth. Much protein digestion occurs in the stomach. In the small intestine carbohydrate and protein digestion are finished and fat digestion begins in earnest. Some plant fibers are digested by the bacteria present in the colon; undigested plant fibers end up in the feces.
5. Digestive enzymes are secreted by the pancreas, mouth, stomach, and cells forming the wall of the small intestine. Pancreatic enzyme release is controlled by the hormone cholecytokinin (CCK). The presence of food in the small intestine stimulates the release of this hormone. Bile needed for fat digestion is synthesized by the liver, stored in the gallbladder, and released in digestion due to the action of CCK.
6. The major absorptive sites consist of fingerlike projections in the small intestine called villi. The absorptive cells that cover the villi have a life span of 2 to 5 days. Thus the intestinal lining continually renews itself. Absorptive cells can perform passive, facilitated, and active absorption, as well as phagocytosis/pinocytosis, another type of active absorption.
7. The products of protein digestion—amino acids and peptides—are actively absorbed into the absorptive cells of the villi. Most of the end products of fat digestion are passively absorbed here as well and rebuilt into triglycerides. The single sugars glucose and galactose, from carbohydrate digestion, are actively absorbed; facilitated absorption is used for fructose.
8. Water-soluble compounds in the absorptive cells enter the portal vein and travel to the liver. Fat-soluble compounds are incorporated into chylomicrons and enter the lymphatic system, which eventually connects to the bloodstream. Some factors used in digestion, such as bile, are reabsorbed by the small intestine, sent back to the liver, and again sent to the small intestine to act in further digestion of foodstuffs. This recycling is called enterohepatic circulation.
9. In the colon, final water and mineral absorption takes place, as well as absorption of products from bacterial breakdown of some plant fibers. Once the feces enter the rectum, the impetus for eventual elimination is strong.

Study Questions

1. Describe the nervous and hormonal interactions involved in the "priming" of the digestive tract.
2. Depict the hormonal and physiological mechanisms by which the health and absorptive abilities of the cells of the small intestine are protected.
3. Outline the possible results that could occur throughout the digestive tract if a person has a completely diseased pancreas.
4. Describe why the small intestine is better suited to carry out the bulk of the absorptive process compared to the other organs of the digestive tract.
5. Explain how each of the following nutritive elements—the three main monosaccharides, long- and short-chain fatty acids, amino acids and water—are absorbed by each of their own particular physiological mechanisms.

REFERENCES

1. Anonymous: Ulcers—screaming or silent, watch with care, *FDA Consumer*, June 1990.
2. Bienenstock J: Mucosal barrier functions, *Nutrition Reviews* 42:105, 1984.
3. Caspray WF: Physiology and pathophysiology of intestinal absorption, *American Journal of Clinical Nutrition* 55:299S, 1992.
4. Cramer T: When do you need an antacid, *FDA Consumer*, Jan/Feb 1992, p 19.
5. Feldman M: Bicarbonate, acid, and duodenal ulcer, *New England Journal of Medicine* 316:408, 1987.
6. Gardner MLG: Gastrointestinal absorption of intact proteins, *Annual Review of Nutrition* 8:329, 1988.
7. Giduck SA and others: Cephalic reflexes: their role in digestion and possible roles in absorption and metabolism, *Journal of Nutrition* 117:1191, 1987.
8. Hamosh M: Lingual and gastric lipases, *Nutrition* 6:421, 1990.
9. Hermann-Zaidins MG: Malabsorption in adults: etiology, evaluation, and management, *Journal of The American Dietetic Association* 86:1711, 1986.
10. Lewis R: When smell and taste go awry, *FDA Consumer*, Nov 1991, p 29.
11. Mattes RD, Mela DJ: The chemical senses and nutrition, *Nutrition Today*, May/June 1988.
12. Mayes PA: Digestion and absorption. In Murray RK and others, editors: *Harper's biochemistry*, East Norwalk, Conn, 1990, Appleton and Lange.
13. Nicholl CG and others: The hormonal regulation of food intake, digestion, and absorption, *Annual Review of Nutrition* 5:213, 1985.
14. Ohning G, Soll AH: Medical treatment of peptic ulcer disease, *American Family Physician* 39:257, 1989.
15. Peterson W: Helicobacter Pylori and peptic ulcer disease, *New England Journal of Medicine* 324:1043, 1990.
16. Quimby GF and others: Active smoking depresses prostaglandin synthesis in human gastric mucosa, *Annals of Internal Medicine* 104:616, 1986.
17. Sandine WE: Roles of bifidobacteria and lactobacilli in human health, *Contemporary Nutrition* 15(1), 1990.
18. Soll AH: Pathogenesis of peptic ulcer and implications for therapy, *New England Journal of Medicine* 322:909, 1990.
19. Thomson ABR: Intestinal aspects of lipid absorption, *Nutrition Today*, July/Aug 1989, p 16.
20. Wolf MM, Soll AH: The physiology of gastric acid secretion, *New England Journal of Medicine* 319:1707, 1988.
21. Wilson JD and others: *Harrison's principles of internal medicine*, ed 12, New York, 1991, McGraw-Hill.

SUGGESTED READINGS

The article by Caspray is a clearly represented description of digestion and absorption. The chapter by Mayes in *Harper's biochemistry* is a step-by-step review of digestion and absorption that includes many tables, figures, and chemical structures of the most important participants. This is one of many excellent books by Appleton and Lange. Finally, the article by Hermann-Zaidins provides a comprehensive look at malabsorption (which is the result when this fine system we have discussed goes awry).

TAKE ACTION

Are you taking care of your digestive tract?

Humans rarely think about the health of their digestive tracts. There are symptoms we need to notice as well as habits we need to practice in order to protect its appropriate function. The following assessment is designed to get you to examine your habits and symptoms associated with the health of your digestive tract. The Nutrition Perspective will help you see why these habits are important to examine. Put a "Y" in the blank to the left of the question to indicate yes and an "N" to indicate no.

1. Are you currently experiencing greater than normal stress and tension? ______
2. Do you have a family history of digestive tract problems (like ulcers, hemorrhoids, diverticulosis, constipation, lactose intolerance)? ______
3. Do you experience pain in your stomach region about 2 hours after you eat? ______
4. Do you smoke cigarettes? ______
5. Do you take aspirin frequently? ______
6. Do you experience the gnawing pain of heartburn in your upper chest at least once per week? ______
7. Do you frequently lie down after eating a large meal? ______
8. Do you drink alcoholic beverages with your meals more than two or three times per week? ______
9. Do you experience abdominal pain, bloating, and gas about 30 minutes to 2 hours after consuming milk products? ______
10. Do you often have to strain while having a bowel movement? ______
11. Do you drink less than 6 to 8 cups of water or fluid per day? ______
12. Do you exercise aerobically (jog, swim, briskly walk, row, stair climb) less than 20 to 30 minutes, three times per week? ______
13. Do you eat a diet relatively low in dietary fiber (recall dietary fiber is found in liberal quantities in whole fruits, vegetables, legumes, nuts and seeds, whole grain breads, and cereals)? ______
14. Do you frequently experience diarrhea? ______
15. Do you frequently use laxatives or antacids? ______

Interpretation

Add up the number of yes answers you gave and record the total in the blank to the right. ______

If your score is from 8 to 15, your habits and symptoms put you at risk of experiencing digestive tract problems in the future. Take particular note of the habits to which you answered "yes." In the future, consider trying to cooperate more with your digestive tract. ▲

NUTRITION PERSPECTIVE

When the Digestive Processes Go Awry

The fine-tuned organ system we call the GI tract can develop problems. Knowing about these likely problems can help you avoid them.

Ulcers

An unfortunate sign of success can be an ulcer. About 1 in 50 adults develop ulcers each year.[1] For some people, stress and tension greatly excite the nerves that control the stomach. This in turn increases acid secretion by the stomach's parietal cells. More tension means more acid, and eventually the acid erodes through the mucous layer in the stomach and into the stomach tissue. This specific case will result in a gastric ulcer. Acid can also erode the tissue lining the duodenum. This specific case will result in a duodenal ulcer. A peptic ulcer is the general term to refer to either of these two cases.

Some people are more susceptible to ulcers than others because of a decreased ability of their stomach and intestinal cells to protect themselves from acid. In addition, recent research suggests that an infection by bacteria (specifically *Helicobacter pylori*) is likely an important provoker of ulcers.[15]

Most ulcers in young people occur in the duodenum; in older people they occur mostly in the stomach. The typical symptom of an ulcer is pain about 2 hours after eating. Digestive acids that work on a meal irritate the ulcer after most of the meal has moved to the jejunum area of the small intestine.

The primary risk in having an ulcer is the possibility of it eating entirely through the stomach or intestinal wall. The GI contents could then spill into the body cavities, causing a massive infection, called peritonitis. In addition, an ulcer may erode a blood vessel, leading to massive blood loss (hemorrhage). For these reasons we should not ignore early warning signs of ulcer development.[1]

In the past, milk and cream therapy—the Sippy diet—was used to help cure ulcers. Today we know that milk and cream are two of the worst foods for an ulcer. The calcium in these foods stimulates gastrin, the hormone that increases stomach acid secretion. Thus this therapy actually inhibits ulcer healing.[14]

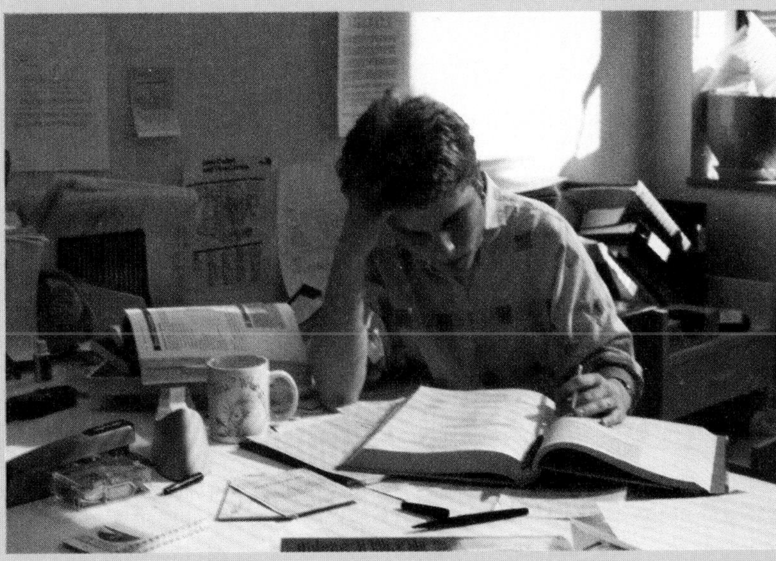

Stress can bring on an ulcer in some of us.

NUTRITION PERSPECTIVE

When the Digestive Processes Go Awry—cont'd

Today, antacid medications are a first line of medical treatment for ulcers. Added to these is a class of medicines called **H_2 blockers**. These include, but are not limited to, cimetidine (Tagamet), ranitidine (Zantac), and famotidine (Pepcid). They prevent histamine-related acid secretion in the stomach and gastrin release (Figure 6-7).[14] The stomach cells produce histamine, and the diet supplies histamine from the breakdown of the amino acid histidine. By preventing histamine from increasing acid secretion, the H_2 blockers greatly speed up ulcer healing and so have greatly reduced the need for surgical treatment. Agents that coat the ulcer, such as sucralfate (Carafate), are also commonly used today.

The person with an ulcer should also stop smoking, if practiced, and minimize the use of aspirin and other aspirin-like compounds.[14,16] These practices reduce the mucus secreted by the stomach. This combination of therapies, along with the use of antacids as needed, has so revolutionized ulcer therapy that changing one's diet is of minor importance today (Table 6-3). Current diet-therapy approaches recommend simply avoiding foods that increase ulcer symptoms.

Is stomach acid also an enemy for those not prone to ulcers? The answer is no. The acid in the stomach enhances our ability to absorb iron, calcium, and vitamin B-12. Acid also minimizes bacterial growth in the stomach; the stomach is essentially bacteria free because of its high acid content. Bacteria in food are quickly destroyed by the acid. This reduces the risk of these bacteria either forming cancer-causing agents or leading to food poisoning (see Chapter 19). Thus acid production by the stomach is an important part of the physiology of digestion and absorption. Ideally one should not take a medication that hampers it.[4] This means that despite their usual presence alongside the breath mints in a convenience store, antacids should not be used excessively.

Heartburn

Some people are very susceptible to heartburn. This gnawing pain in the upper chest is caused by the (reflux) of acid from the stomach into the esophagus. Unlike the stomach, the esophagus has no mucous lining to protect it. The acid quickly erodes the lining of the esophagus, causing pain. An important dietary measure for avoiding heartburn is to eat smaller meals, and especially meals that are low in fat.[4] Fatty

Table 6-3 Recommendations to prevent ulcers and heartburn from recurring

Ulcers

1. *Stop smoking, if you are now a smoker.*
2. Avoid aspirin, ibuprofen, and other aspirin-like compounds.
3. Avoid coffee, tea, and alcohol (especially wine).
4. Limit pepper, chili powder, and other strong spices, if this helps.
5. Eat nutritious meals on a regular schedule.
6. Chew foods well.
7. Lose weight if you are now overweight.

Heartburn

1. Wait about 3 hours after a meal before lying down.
2. Don't overeat at mealtime.
3. Observe the recommendations for ulcer prevention.

NUTRITION PERSPECTIVE

meals remain in the stomach longer than low-fat meals. The large volume of food and secretions that remain in the stomach create pressure in the stomach that can force the stomach contents up into the esophagus.

There are several other measures one may take to prevent heartburn. If one smokes cigarettes, the person is advised to stop.[14] In addition, it is best not to lie down after eating and to avoid foods and other substances that can specifically contribute to heartburn, such as chili powder, onions, garlic, peppermint, caffeine, alcohol, and chocolate. Each person must discover what bothers him or her and tailor the diet accordingly.

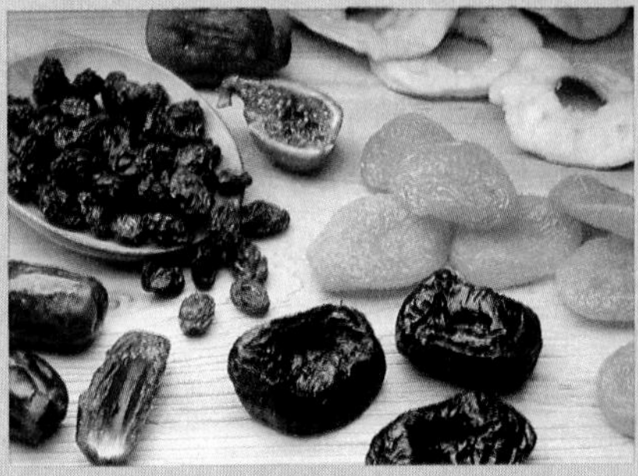

Eating dried fruit is an excellent way to increase your dietary fiber intake.

Certain physical conditions can lead to heartburn. For example, both pregnancy and obesity result in increased production of estrogen and progesterone. These hormones relax the lower esophageal (cardiac) sphincter, making heartburn more likely. A pregnant women may find it helpful to eat more frequent but smaller meals until she delivers her child. The obese person should slim down to a more healthy weight so that blood levels of these hormones decrease. Adipose (fat) tissue turns circulating hormones into estrogen. Thus the more adipose tissue one has, the more estrogen is produced.

Heartburn that recurs several times a week for a month should be investigated by a physician. Long-standing heartburn may require aggressive medical therapy because it can lead to alteration in the cells of the esophagus, which in turn increases the risk of a rare form of cancer.[21]

Constipation and Laxatives

Difficult or infrequent evacuation of the bowels is known as constipation. It is caused by a slow movement of fecal material through the large intestine. As fluids are increasingly absorbed during their extended time in the large intestine, the stool becomes dry and hard. Constipation can result when people regularly inhibit their normal bowel reflexes for long periods of time. People tend to ignore normal urges when it is inconvenient to interrupt occupational or social activities. Muscle spasms of an irritated large intestine can also slow the movement of feces and contribute to constipation. Even medications, such as antacids, can cause constipation.

Constipation is difficult to diagnose. Normal stool frequency ranges from 3 to 12 times per week. However, definitions of "normal" vary from person to person. The best guide for recognizing constipation is the presence of unusually hard, dry stools at infrequent intervals—not a general prescription of "once a day." Any sudden, prolonged changes in stool frequency should be evaluated by a physician. This may be a warning that a more serious intestinal disorder is developing.[21]

Eating dietery fiber, such as those found in whole grain breads and cereals, is the best alternative for treating typical cases of constipation. Dietary fibers stimulate peristalsis by drawing water into the colon and helping form a bulky, softer stool. A person with constipation should also drink more fluids along with the dietary fiber. Eating dried fruits can also help stimulate the bowel. In addition, the person may need to develop more regular bowel habits; allowing the same time each day for a bowel movement can help train the large intestine to respond routinely. Finally, relaxation facilitates regular bowel movements, as does regular exercise.

Laxatives also can lessen constipation. They work either by irritating the intestinal nerve junctions in order to stimulate the peristaltic muscles, or by drawing water into the intestine to enlarge the stool. A larger stool stretches the peristaltic muscles, making them rebound and then constrict. Regular laxative use, especially of the irritating varieties, can decrease muscle action in the large intestine, causing more

NUTRITION PERSPECTIVE

When the Digestive Processes Go Awry—cont'd

future constipation. The GI tract in time can actually become dependent on laxatives for its function. Thus it is unwise to use laxatives routinely, although people in certain circumstances—those who are bedridden or quite elderly—may need periodic help from laxatives to relieve constipation.

Perhaps you have heard that taking laxatives after overeating prevents fat gain from the excess kcalories. It is true that you may temporarily feel lighter after using a laxative because laxatives hasten emptying of the large intestine and increase fluid loss. Note, however, that most laxatives do not actually hurry the passage of food through the small intestine, where digestion and most nutrient absorption take place. As a result, laxatives do not prevent one from getting the kcalories normally obtained without using the laxative.

Hemorrhoids

Hemorrhoids, also called piles, are swollen veins of the rectum and anus. The blood vessels in this area are subject to intense pressure, especially during bowel movements. Added stress to the vessels from pregnancy, obesity, prolonged sitting, violent coughing or sneezing, or straining during bowel movements can lead to a hemorrhoid. Hemorrhoids can develop unnoticed until a strained bowel movement precipitates symptoms. These may include pain, itching, and bleeding. Itching, caused by moisture in the anal canal, swelling, or other irritation is perhaps the most common symptom. Pain, if present, is usually aching and steady. Bleeding may result from a hemorrhoid and may appear in the toilet as a streak in the feces. The blood is bright red. The sensation of a mass in the anal canal after a bowel movement is symptomatic of an internal hemorrhoid that protrudes through the anus.

Anyone can develop a hemorrhoid. Pressure from prolonged sitting or exertion is often enough to bring on symptoms, although diet, lifestyle, and possibly heredity play a role. If you think you have a hemorrhoid, you should consult your physician. Rectal bleeding, although usually caused by hemorrhoids, may also indicate other problems, such as cancer.[21] Your physician may also suggest a variety of self-care measures. Pain can be lessed by warm, soft compresses or sitting in a tub of warm water for 15 to 20 minutes. Dietary recommendations are the same as those for treating constipation. Over-the-counter remedies also can offer relief of symptoms. Americans spend an estimated $200 million annually on these products to treat hemorrhoids. Ask your physician for advice.

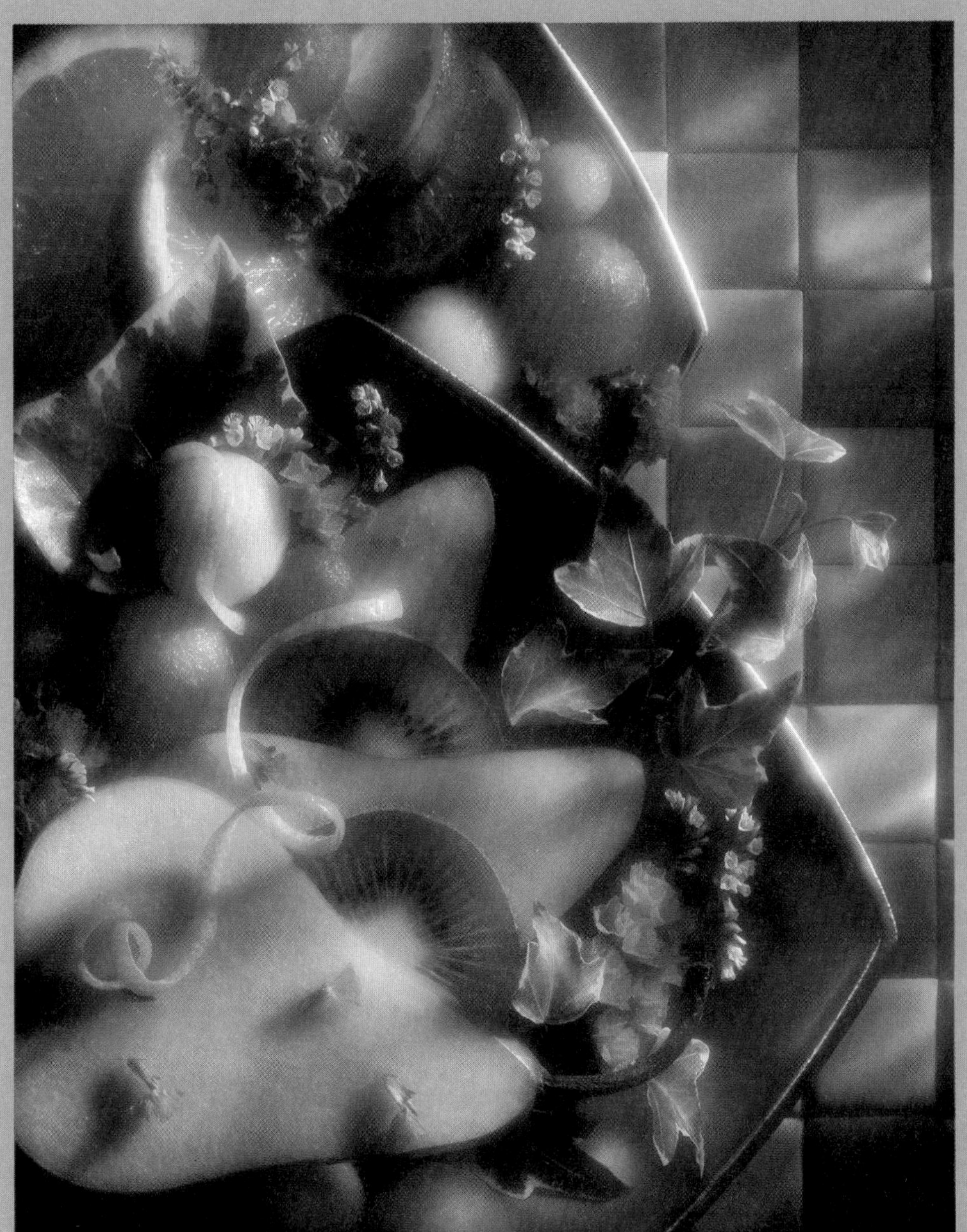

PART THREE

Energy Production and Energy Balance

CHAPTER SEVEN

Metabolism

Metabolism refers to the entire network of physical and chemical processes involved in maintaining life. It encompasses all of the sequences of chemical reactions that occur in the body. These reactions enable us to release and use energy from foods, convert one substance into another, and prepare the products for excretion. More than 1000 different kinds of chemical reactions take place in a simple single-cell bacterium.[7]

Studying metabolism can help us understand other nutrition concepts. Understanding metabolism clarifies how proteins, carbohydrates, fats, and alcohol interrelate. It shows how the carbons in protein molecules become the carbons of glucose, and why carbons of most fatty acids cannot become the carbons of glucose. Second, studying metabolic pathways in the cell sets the stage for examining the roles of vitamins and minerals. Most vitamins function as coenzymes. Most minerals function as cofactors. By their natures, these compounds—coenzymes and cofactors—promote enzyme function and so contribute to important metabolic reactions in the cell. The functions of vitamins and minerals are easier to understand when you are familiar with the basic metabolic processes in the cell.

NUTRITION AWARENESS INVENTORY

Here are 15 statements about metabolism. Read them to test your current knowledge. If you think the statement is true or mostly true, circle T. If you think the statement is false or mostly false, circle F. Use the scoring key at the end of the book to compute your total score. Take this test again after you have read the chapter. Compare the results.

1. T F Carbohydrates can be used for energy needs and fat storage.
2. T F Fats can be used for energy needs and fat storage.
3. T F Eating protein doesn't lead to fat formation.
4. T F The brain gets the energy it needs mostly in the form of glucose.
5. T F Fasting increases blood ketone levels.
6. T F Drink all the alcohol you want, it will never turn to fat.
7. T F The B vitamins thiamin, niacin, and riboflavin participate in energy metabolism.
8. T F Protein metabolism requires vitamin B-6.
9. T F Iron and copper play key roles in energy production in the body.
10. T F Carnitine is used for carbohydrate metabolism.
11. T F Ketones are formed primarily from glycerol.
12. T F Mitochondria supply most of the energy within the cell.
13. T F Acetyl-CoA plays a central role in energy metabolism.
14. T F Plants obtain energy from photosynthesis.
15. T F When fasting, we use proteins to synthesize glucose via a process called gluconeogenesis.

Metabolism

anabolic Describes the building of compounds.

catabolic Describes the breaking down of compounds.

A metabolic progression of chemical reactions from the starting to ending point is called a pathway. **Anabolic** pathways result in the building of compounds. The chemical elements and compounds used to form the new compounds are called building blocks. Conversely, **catabolic** pathways result in the breakdown of compounds into small units. For example, catabolism of glucose results when it is broken down via metabolic pathways into carbon dioxide (CO_2) and water (H_2O). Almost every step in any pathway depends on an enzyme for the necessary chemical reaction to occur.

adenosine triphosphate (ATP) The main energy currency for cells; ATP energy is used to promote ion pumping, enzyme activity, and muscular contraction.

Overall, energy metabolism occurs in three stages.[7] In the first stage large molecules in food, such as proteins, starches, and triglycerides, are broken down during digestion and absorption into smaller units, such as amino acids, monosaccharides, and free fatty acids. In the second stage of metabolism these smaller compounds are further degraded to units of a central two-carbon compound, called acetic acid. In the third stage this two-carbon compound is degraded into carbon dioxide and water molecules. The electrons released during this process are donated to oxygen atoms, with the energy released driving the synthesis of **adenosine triphosphate (ATP)**. ATP is a storage form of energy that cells use. Chapter 6 focused on the first stage of metabolism; let's now examine the last two stages.

THE CELL—PRIMARY SITE FOR METABOLISM

The cell is the basic unit of body structure, and it is where most metabolic reactions occur (Figure 7-1). A quick review of cell structure will aid in the understanding of metabolism.

The cell is surrounded by a membrane that controls the passage of nutrients and other substances in and out of it. Within the cell is fluid called the cytosol. Within the cytosol are organelles, which are small bodies that perform specific metabolic functions. The names and activities of the various cell parts follow below:[4]

Cell membrane: This double-layered structure is composed of lipids and protein and contains channels to admit specific molecules into the cell; receptors that bind hormones and other compounds that send signals into the cell; and protein markers on the outside of the cell membrane that allow the immune system to recognize it as a human cell, as opposed to an invading bacterium.

Nucleus: This spherical structure is bound by its own double membrane. Within the nucleus are chromosomes, which are long threads of DNA that contain hereditary

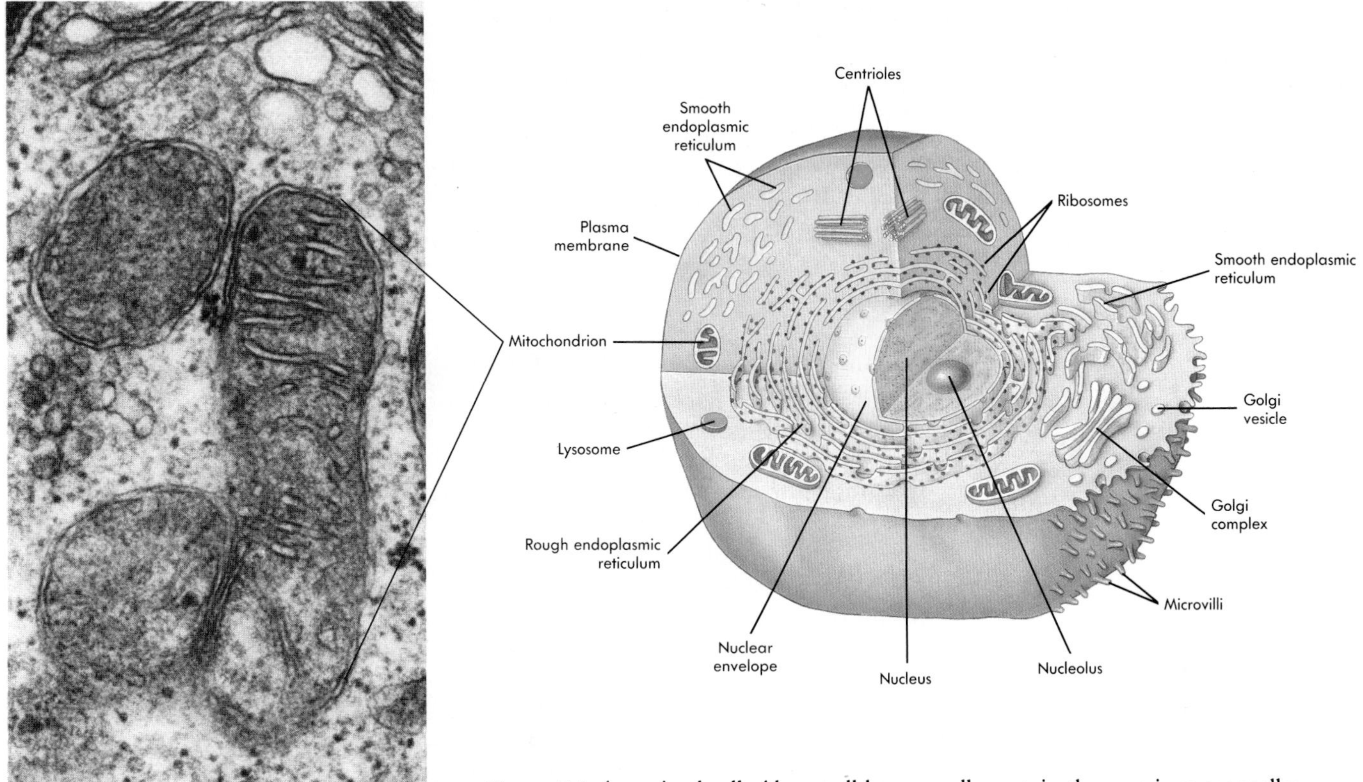

Figure 7-1 An animal cell. Almost all human cells contain these various organelles.

information for directing cell protein synthesis and cell reproduction. Inside the nucleus is a nucleolus. Here a type of RNA (ribosomal RNA) is synthesized that eventually helps assemble ribosomes (see below).

Mitochondria: These have their own outer membrane and an inner membrane that is highly folded. The mitochondria are the major sites of energy production in the cell. Mitochondria also synthesize important cell components, such as carbon skeletons for nonessential (dispensable) amino acids.

Endoplasmic reticulum: This network of internal membranes serves as a communication network within the cell. Small granules called ribosomes cover parts of the outside of the endoplasmic reticulum, known as the rough endoplasmic reticulum; protein is synthesized at these granules. Fat is synthesized in other areas of the endoplasmic reticulum, namely, the smooth endoplasmic reticulum.

Golgi complex: This consists of stacks of flattened structures that both package proteins for export from the cell and help form other cell organelles. Budding off the golgi complex are golgi vesicles, which are fluid-filled sacs destined either for other parts of the cell or for excretion from the cell.

Lysosomes: These small bodies contain digestive enzymes that break down worn out cell parts and other cell debris. A lysosome is prevented from digesting the entire cell because each maintains a very high acidity, which inhibits the digestive enzyme action. When a lysosome fuses with a particle that is to be digested, the acidity in the lysosome then falls, promoting digestive enzyme activity.

Cytosol: This is essentially the fluid inside the cell in which the various organelles are suspended. That fluid plus all organelles (minus the nucleus) is called the cytoplasm.

Storage forms of energy: These occur as glycogen granules and lipid droplets.

Peroxisomes: These carry enzymes, such as catalase, that can break down peroxides and alcohol.

Let's now review energy metabolism in general. Later we will identify the types of metabolic pathways and where they occur in the cell.

To be accurate we must say that energy is released or transferred; energy cannot be produced via metabolism. Energy can be neither created nor destroyed; it is simply transferred around the planet.

ENERGY FOR THE CELL

The energy that runs your body is captured in the chemical bonds of carbohydrate, protein, and fat molecules, as well as in alcohol. Originally this energy is a product of photosynthesis. Plants use energy from the sun to produce glucose and other organic (carbon-containing) compounds. In doing so they trap solar energy in the form of energy that is generated from the sharing of electrons in chemical bonds. Thus a result of the reactions in photosynthesis yields compounds with more energy contained in the chemical bonds of the product than the building blocks, carbon dioxide and water, provided. And the energy for this uphill process comes from the sun.

The body then transforms this electron energy trapped in the carbohydrates, fats, and proteins into other forms: chemical energy to transform carbohydrates to fats; mechanical energy to propel muscular movements; electrical energy to drive nerve transmissions; and osmotic energy to maintain ion balance between cells.[7] The by-products are carbon dioxide and water. The flow of chemical energy from ingested foodstuffs throughout the body, in the first analysis, is then eventually and irretrievably dissipated to the environment as heat. Thus in human respiration we start with glucose and through an elaborate process convert it to carbon dioxide and water. This process results in the release of energy, which in turn allows energy-requiring pathways to function. We rely on plants to convert solar energy into a form we can use, and then eventually lose this energy to the environment (Figure 7-2).

Each covalent bond between the atoms of molecules in foods (carbons, hydrogens, oxygens, and so on) represents potential energy through the sharing of electrons. In every amino acid, glucose, and fatty acid molecule are many sites where solar energy is stored as chemical energy. One function of metabolism is to convert this chemical energy into a form that human cells can use.

Note that many chemical reactions in the body could not occur without the addition of outside energy that food supplies. The outside energy permits compounds, such as glucose, to be transformed into end products, such as glycogen, the storage form of glucose. And while glucose molecules themselves contain the energy needed, this form of food energy neither provides us with the right amount of energy for a chemical reaction nor with a form that our cells can use directly. Human cells must always convert the chemical energy stored in the bonds of foodstuffs into a more appropriate form. A glucose molecule contains over 100 times more energy than required to drive an individual chemical reaction in a cell. A triglyceride molecule contains about 500 times more energy than is needed.[7] So a cell must have a means of breaking down the glucose and fatty acid molecules to both release and then convert the chemical energy trapped in them into usable and smaller energy packets.

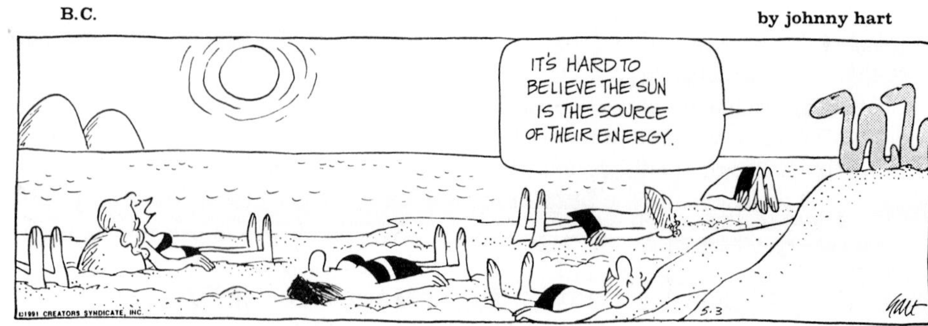
B.C.
by johnny hart
IT'S HARD TO BELIEVE THE SUN IS THE SOURCE OF THEIR ENERGY.
©1991 CREATORS SYNDICATE, INC.

Figure 7-2 B.C.

Reprinted by permission of Creators Syndicate, Inc.

ADENOSINE TRIPHOSPHATE (ATP)

The form of energy that cells generally use is ATP. Every body cell makes ATP to help meet energy needs. To release the energy in ATP, cells split it into adenosine diphosphate (ADP) plus Pi (Figure 7-3). The Pi stands for the inorganic phosphate group that can be added to or split from the larger molecule. In other words, adenosine triphosphate is split into adenosine diphosphate plus a free phosphate group. Splitting ADP into adenosine monophosphate (AMP) plus Pi also yields energy. Muscles do that during intense exercise when ATP is in short supply.

Breaking the bond between either the first and second phosphate group or between the second and third phosphate group on ATP releases energy. This form of energy resembles the energy released when a bond is broken between a carbon and a hydrogen in a glucose molecule. But unlike the energy released from breaking the bonds between a carbon and hydrogen, ATP energy can be used by cells. Energy released when breaking typical chemical bonds releases heat, but unless it also forms ATP, the energy cannot be used directly to promote cellular activity. Enzyme action, ion pumping, or muscle contractions are the three processes human cells need this energy for.[7] Only ATP energy or its derivatives can be used directly for energy by the cell. Thus the energy released from breaking carbon-hydrogen bonds in a glucose molecule is one of the actual "foods" used to make ATP.

Pathways in every cell combine ADP and Pi to form ATP. This process captures chemical energy from food between the phosphate groups of ATP (Figure 7-3). An enzyme can then break that bond to release the energy for driving metabolic reactions. ATP itself is very stable. It takes an enzyme to unlock the energy that ATP stores.

A resting cell has a high ATP concentration. An active cell has some ATP in it, as well as much ADP plus Pi. When a cell is active, it is constantly breaking down ATP in one part of the cell while rebuilding it in another part. An exhausted cell—a muscle cell, for example—will have a very high concentration of ADP and a very low concentration of ATP. When that happens, cell activity grinds to a halt. This state in turn stimulates metabolic processes that produce ATP. Only by resynthesizing needed ATP can the cell ready itself to go again. At rest a person's cells recycle ADP plus Pi to ATP and then reverse the cycle, reusing small amounts over and

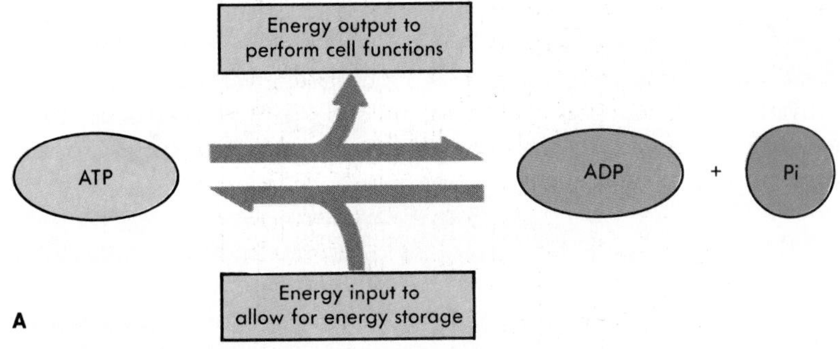

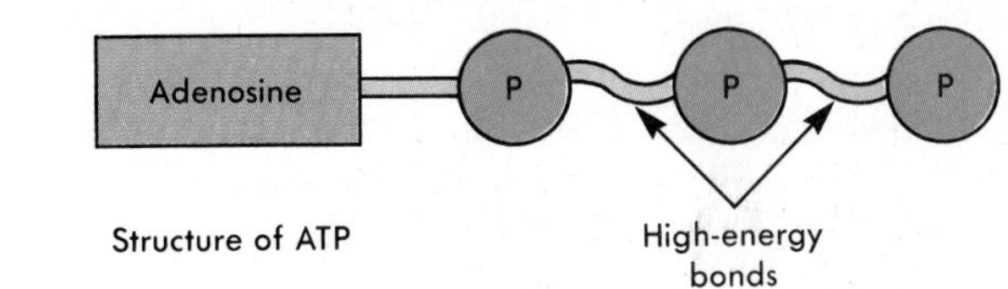

Figure 7-3 ATP stores and yields energy. ATP is the high-energy state, while ADP is the lower-energy state—some energy has been released to form the molecule. When ATP is broken down to ADP + Pi, energy is released for cell use. When energy is trapped by ADP + Pi, an ATP molecule can be formed. Thus ATP represents a storage form of energy for cell use.

Throughout this chapter we simplify many metabolic pathways by including only the most important steps. We mainly want you to understand the overall picture of metabolism. Future courses will cover the pathways step-by-step, enzyme-by-enzyme.

over. The amount of ATP used would be the equivalent of about 40 kilograms (88 pounds) per 24 hours if reuse was impossible. During physical activity, ATP use can reach the equivalent of 0.5 kilograms (1.1 pounds) per minute.[7]

Think about that the next time you race after a bus. When you finally sit down, you are exhausted. You breathe hard, and your heart races. Your muscle cells have used up most of their ATP and other high-energy compounds. While you rest, muscle cells begin to use the energy released from metabolism of foodstuffs to resynthesize ATP. Of course, this is done by fusing together the ADP and Pi created during the breakdown of ATP. If you sit long enough, you can then race to your class using the newly formed ATP.

Carbohydrate Metabolism

Let's now look at how ATP is generated in a human cell. All life forms have only two means for synthesizing ATP—using fuel molecules to supply the energy or trapping light energy by means of photosynthesis. You can do only the former. The easiest place to begin studying ATP generation in human cells is with carbohydrate metabolism. Next we'll look at fat metabolism and protein metabolism, and along the way we'll take a brief look at alcohol metabolism. Again, all of these compounds can be used to synthesize ATP.

GLYCOLYSIS

glycolysis The breakdown of glucose into pyruvate (lactate) molecules.

Glycolysis literally means "breaking down glucose." The glycolysis pathway, found in the cytosol of the cell, has a dual role: it degrades monosaccharides to generate energy, and it provides building blocks for synthesizing needed cell compounds, such as glycerol for triglyceride synthesis. Before glycolysis can begin, a cell must obtain glucose molecules. Only liver and muscle cells store glucose to any extent. Recall that glucose is stored as glycogen. The liver and muscle cells break down the glycogen into a form of glucose; other body cells take glucose from the bloodstream. To allow for this the body maintains a fairly constant level of glucose in the bloodstream. A few types of cells, such as liver cells, can even produce their own glucose from amino acids (see a later section in this chapter on gluconeogenesis). In these ways every body cell has glucose available to it.

Acids commonly lose a hydrogen ion at the pH level found in human cells (pH 7.4). When that ion is lost, the name of the acid is changed by dropping the reference to acid and adding an "ate" ending. Thus lactic acid becomes lactate and pyruvic acid becomes pyruvate.

The net result of glycolysis is the splitting of the six-carbon compound glucose into two units of a three-carbon compound called pyruvic acid (pyruvate) (Figure 7-4).[6] Some cells then convert pyruvate into lactic acid (lactate). But, for the most part, pyruvate is the end point of glycolysis. To begin glycolysis, glucose has a phosphate group added to it, which makes glucose more reactive. Glucose is now ready to participate in subsequent reactions.

The newly formed glucose-phosphate compound eventually has another phosphate group added to it, and then it splits into two three-carbon compounds. These are then converted through a variety of steps into two molecules of the three-carbon compound pyruvate. Thus in glycolysis a cell starts with a six-carbon glucose molecule and ends up with two molecules of the three-carbon compound pyruvate.

SO WHERE IS THE ATP?

In glycolysis, one ATP molecule is used to add the first phosphate group to glucose; another ATP molecule is used to add the second. So to begin glycolysis, a cell uses two molecules of ATP energy. As the two three-carbon molecules are converted into pyruvate, each one generates two ATP molecules, for a total of four. The net energy produced thus far from glycolysis renders four ATP molecules minus two ATP molecules used, or two net ATP molecules. There are more to come; this represents only about 6% of the ATP possible from one glucose molecule.

NAD is actually NAD^+, indicating it has one unpaired electron. By picking up two electrons and one hydrogen ion, NADH ends up with no charge. The extra electron provides electron balance in the molecule. We will ignore the charge on NAD to simplify the discussion.

As glucose breaks into two pyruvate molecules, four hydrogen atoms (containing a total of four electrons) are released. The hydrogen atoms are picked up by a carrier

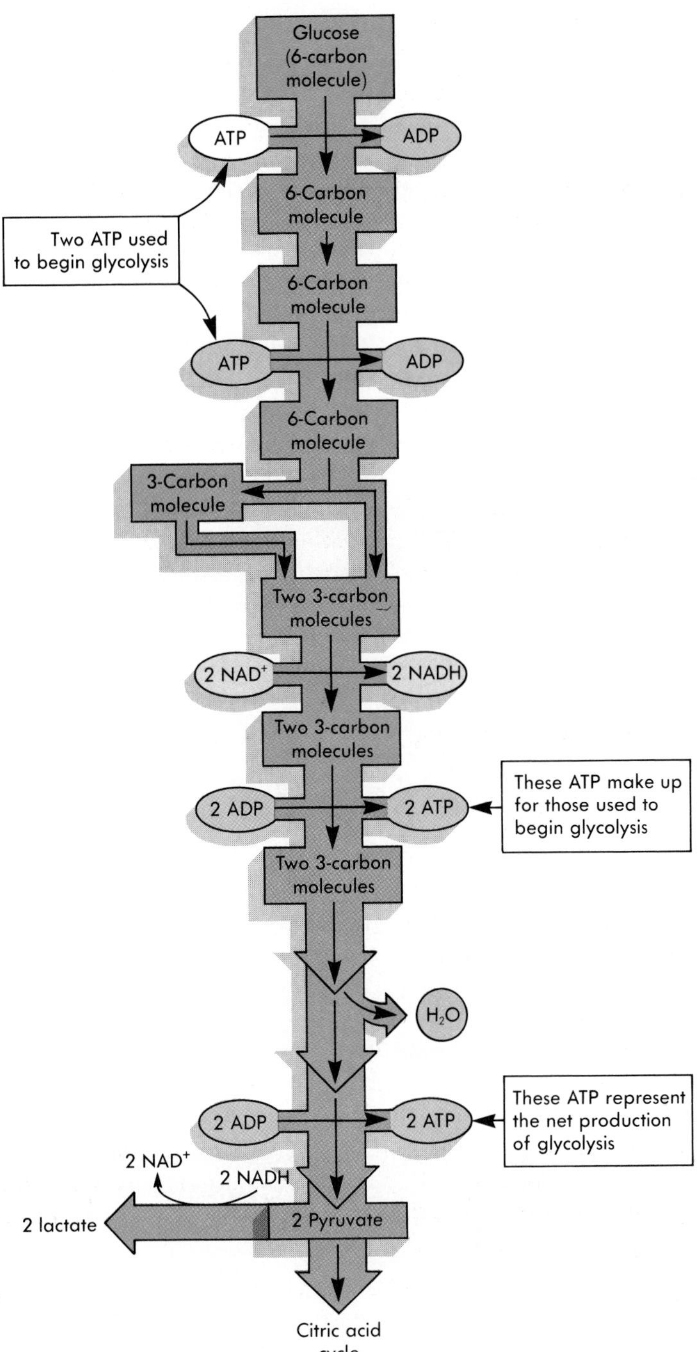

Figure 7-4 Glycolysis simplified. The process begins with one glucose and ends with two pyruvate ($C_3H_4O_3$). Some ATP is produced by the process and the four hydrogens released are captured by NAD. Note that any NADH is paired with a hydrogen ion (but not depicted).

called nictotinamide adenine dinucleotide (NAD). The vitamin niacin forms part of the NAD molecule. Each NAD accepts two electrons but only one hydrogen ion. Thus an end result of glycolysis is also the synthesis of two NADH molecules.

Chemical energy stored in the electrons of NADH can eventually be turned into ATP energy. So NADH is a form of potential energy for the cell; as chemical energy is released from the carbon-hydrogen bonds originally present in glucose, NADH traps some of it. A cell must then convert the energy in NADH into ATP energy. Later we will show how that happens.

Concerning other monosaccharides, much of the fructose from food is metabolized by the liver into successively different compounds that eventually yield a three-carbon compound in the glycolysis pathway. Pyruvate is then eventually formed.[6] Any galactose from foods is converted into a glucose-phosphate compound. Glycolysis can then proceed.

LACTATE PRODUCTION

Some body cells lack the oxygen-requiring (aerobic) pathway for converting NADH energy into ATP energy. The red blood cell is an example. As a red blood cell converts glucose into pyruvate, NADH molecules build up in the cell. Eventually the NAD concentration falls too low for glycolysis to continue because most of the NAD molecules present are in the form of NADH.

To compensate, a red blood cell reacts pyruvate with an NADH molecule and a free hydrogen ion to form lactate (Figure 7-4). In the process, NADH turns into NAD. This process allows the red blood cell to resupply itself with NAD.[6] Exercising muscles produce lactate for the same reason (see Chapter 10). The production of lactate allows the glycolytic pathway to have a supply of NAD readily available.

Regenerating NAD by using lactate represents a fermentation reaction. Some yeasts produce alcohol (ethanol) instead of lactate to regenerate NAD in anaerobic conditions. This is likewise a fermentation reaction.

ATP is needed to begin glycolysis, but future ATP synthesis replaces that used in the beginning reactions and supplies extra for cell use. Since the entire pathway does not use oxygen, it is referred to as an anaerobic process. Again, this pathway yields only about 6% of the potential ATP molecules per glucose molecule. But for some cells—red blood cells, for example—it is the only method for making ATP. The lactate is released into the bloodstream and picked up primarily by the liver.

CONCEPT CHECK

Carbohydrate metabolism begins when a cell either forms glucose from glycogen or takes glucose from the bloodstream. Glucose is then degraded through a sequence of steps into two pyruvate molecules. The pathway, called glycolysis, yields NADH, a potential form of energy, and ATP, an actual energy source for a cell. Both fructose and galactose can also be metabolized via glycolysis to pyruvate molecules. Pyruvate then is either broken down further or converted into lactate. Red blood cells perform the later reaction. The conversion of pyruvate to lactate allows the cell to reform NADH back into NAD. This supports the needs for NAD by glycolysis. NADH can also be turned into NAD via oxygen-requiring pathways found in most cells.

THE CITRIC ACID CYCLE

The two pyruvate (or lactate) molecules formed at the end of glycolysis still contain a lot of stored energy. Pyruvates pass from the cell cytosol into the mitochondria. A cell then uses a pathway found there to extract the remaining energy from those pyruvates to form more ATP; it uses the citric acid cycle.[6] Before the citric acid cycle can begin, however, pyruvate must lose a carbon dioxide group to form acetyl-CoA. This reaction is irreversible, which has important metabolic consequences that we will soon explore. As pyruvate is converted into acetyl-CoA, another NADH molecule is produced, and in turn more potential ATP molecules are produced. The conversion of pyruvate requires the vitamin thiamin. Carbohydrates in the diet increase thiamin needs. Now you know why.

Acetyl-CoA is basically the two-carbon compound acetic acid, which gives the bite to vinegar. Attached to it is a large coenzyme A (CoA) molecule. CoA contains the vitamin pantothenic acid. The CoA molecule activates acetic acid like the way a phosphate group activates glucose. Without a CoA molecule attached, acetic acid will not participate in the first reaction of the citric acid cycle.

Other names of the citric acid cycle are the tricarboxylic acid cycle (TCA cycle) and the Krebs cycle, named after Hans Krebs, the scientist who described it.

The citric acid cycle is an elegant sequence of chemical reactions that cells use to convert carbons into carbon dioxide. Acetyl-CoA adds two carbons to the cycle, and then two carbons are lost as carbon dioxide. In the process, the cell makes more NADH and other related molecules, which can eventually yield many ATP molecules.

The Crossroads of Metabolism

MURRAY L. KAPLAN, PH.D.

In the ancient world, people said that all roads lead to Rome. In the present era of world events, it may appear that all roads lead to Washington, D.C. and the New York City corridor. But in the flow of cellular metabolic activity that is central to all living forms—from bacteria to man—the central hub is not Times Square, but pyruvate and acetyl-CoA. Glycolysis, gluconeogenesis, the citric acid cycle, fatty acid oxidation, fatty acid synthesis, ketogenesis, and transamination and deamination of some amino acids all meet at or near the pyruvate acetyl-CoA hub. These pathways are nearly universal in all cellular life forms, from the simplest to the most complex. The universality of these biochemical pathways is a marvel of animal metabolism.

Cell metabolism appears as a puzzle to those first exposed to the myriad of pathways. To put this mirage into perspective, one approach is to examine the historical development of metabolism and metabolic pathways.

The scientific study of animal energy metabolism starts with Antoine Lavoiser, a French chemist of the late eighteenth century who studied chemical combustion. He noted that animal combustion was identical in principle to burning carbon-containing substances in that consumption of oxygen was required. He was among the first to note that the level of animal oxygen consumption changed with physical activity and the ingestion of food. This observation preceded the understanding of animal bioenergetics or thermodynamics, the elucidation of the pathways of metabolism, or the role of yeast in the fermentation of sugar in grape juice to either alcohol or to acetic acid. Essentially no one understood what happened between the starting material of food or a particular ingredient—grape juice—and the end products of carbon dioxide, alcohol, or acetic acid.

Nearly 100 years later, Louis Pasteur discovered that microbes were responsible for the fermentation of grape juice to either wine or wine vinegar. This provided an opportunity to study chemical reactions in living systems. It was also known by then that the amount of energy required to completely combust glucose to carbon dioxide in one step would be incompatible with life. The concept arose that smaller intermediate steps must be present. Within a few years, biologists, such as Embden and Meyerhof, elucidated the intermediate step beteen glucose and the products, pyruvate, lactate, and ethanol.

During this era of the late nineteenth and early twentieth centuries, others determined the caloric value of different foodstuffs. They found that the physiological energy values were not identical to the total chemical energy available. This also indicated the possible existence of steps in animal energetics that differed significantly from the chemical combustion of carbon-containing material.

In the late nineteenth century, Claude Bernard, a French physiologist, challenged the then prevalent belief that the only source of blood glucose was dietary carbohydrate. He found that glucose was fairly constant in the blood of dogs fed either starch or meat meals, or fasted. He also discovered that the stored form of animal starch, which he named glycogen, was found in the liver. Today we know the glycogen he discovered serves as a source of blood glucose in those metabolic conditions when dietary carbohydrate is unavailable. He also concluded that protein could be a source of the stored glycogen and blood glucose when dietary carbohydrate is absent, a process he termed gluconeogenesis.

An immediate result of Bernard's work was the concept of a fixed "milieu interieur" (internal environment). This was later expanded in the 1920s by Walter B. Cannon as he developed the concept of a self-regulating internal environment or homeostasis.

Another, more long-reaching, consequence of Bernard's work was the search by subsequent researchers to elucidate the steps between glycogen and the release of blood glucose, and the regulation of this process by diet, hormones, and physiological state. Consequently, the metabolic flow from glycogen to glucose-1-phosphate to glucose-6-phosphate to glucose was elucidated. The subsequent activation of glycogen phosphorylase from inactive to active form by hormonal control was also discovered as part of this quest by several research groups. This helped us to understand the processes by which we maintain a fairly constant blood glucose level.

The elucidation of the citric acid cycle in the 1930s by Hans Krebs and the subsequent discovery of its role in gluconeogenesis can be viewed as part of this process to understand the steps and their regulation between starting mateials and final products. Likewise, the pathways of fatty acid oxidation and entry of the acetyl-CoA generated by this process into the citric acid cycle is important to understand the oxygen-dependent oxidation of fatty acids as alternative sources of fuel for metabolic energy. We now know that high rates of fatty aicd oxidation usually inhibit the glycolysis pathway. We also know that fatty acids can serve as a source of fuel when glucose is limiting and can promote gluconeogenesis or ketogenesis. This illustrates the beauty in the coordination of these pathways, like the different parts in a muscial score. Many of the specific steps in this coordination were discovered as recently as the 1960s.

If we can understand the larger picture of basic interconversions of the simple foodstuffs—carbohydrate, fat, and protein—then the specifics of the myriad of metabolic pathways can be viewed as a "road map." The historical perspective merely shows that we are trying to understand how we get from point A to point M. If we first understand the "road map," then we can perhaps understand how to direct the "traffic patterns," or to regulate metabolic flow through a specific pathway. Metabolic disease, such as diabetes, involves abnormal "traffic patterns." Future work by many investigators will continue to unravel the regulation of the "traffic patterns" through the pathways or "road maps."

Dr. Kaplan is a professor in the department of Food Science and Human Nutrition, Iowa State University, Ames, Iowa, 50011. He has spent much of his career studying cellular metabolism in a number of obese animal models.

To begin the citric acid cycle, acetyl-CoA combines with a four-carbon compound (oxaloacetic acid, or oxaloacetate) to form a six-carbon compound (citric acid, or citrate) (Figure 7-5).[6] The CoA molecule is released. Recall that the portion of acetyl-CoA that interests us, the acetic acid, had two carbons. The basic function now of the citric acid cycle is to take this six-carbon citrate molecule and turn it back into a four-carbon oxaloacetate molecule. In the process, two carbon dioxide molecules are lost. More important, however, the process also produces potential ATP in the form of NADH and other compounds.

Overall, the citric acid cycle begins and ends with the same compound, oxaloacetate. The pathway adds two carbons as acetic acid to oxaloacetate. As the citric acid cycle reactions occur, two carbons from carbon dioxide are lost, and the process ends where it started. As citrate is turned back into oxaloacetate, three more NADH molecules are formed. Another hydrogen carrier, flavin adenine dinucleotide (FAD), forms $FADH_2$. FAD contains the vitamin riboflavin. Finally, guanosine triphosphate (GTP, which is analogous to ATP) is made from GDP and Pi.

GTP can be used to synthesize ATP.

Converting citrate back into oxaloacetate requires a variety of reactions in this citric acid cycle. However, the important thing to remember is that two carbons enter the citric acid cycle as acetyl-CoA, and two carbons are then lost as carbon dioxide. These steps help ensure that the beginning and ending compounds are the same: oxaloacetate.

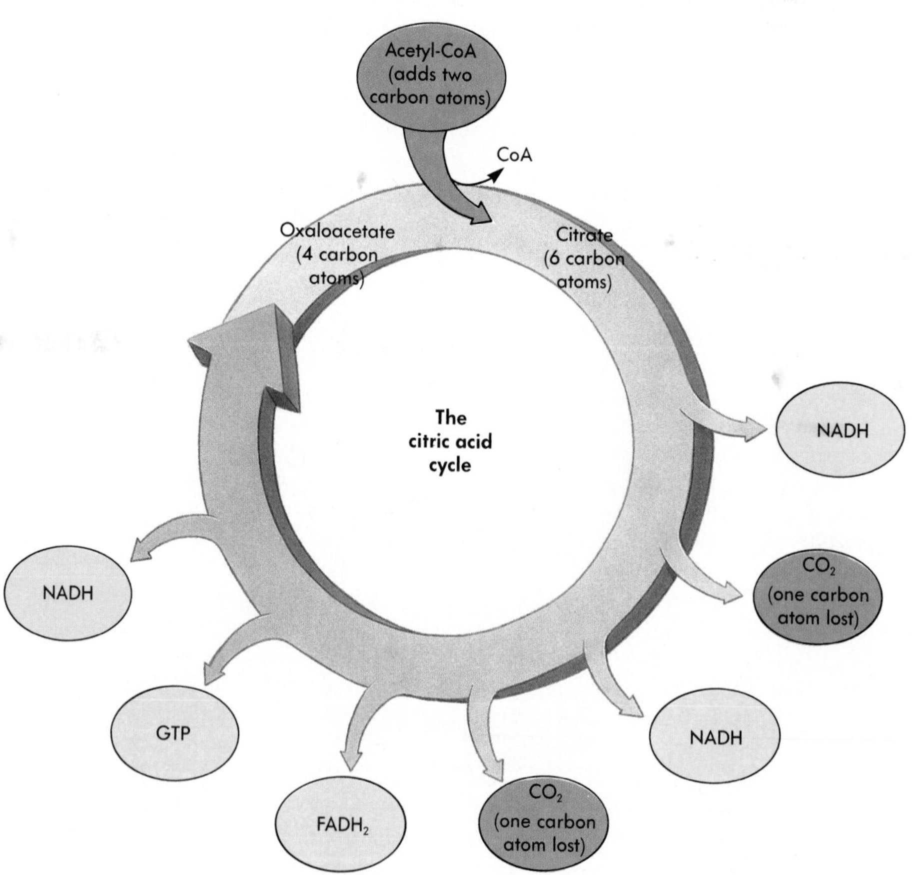

Figure 7-5 The citric acid cycle simplified. Four carbons as oxaloacetate combine with two carbons from acetyl-CoA to form a six-carbon compound called citrate. The six-carbon compound then is reformed into the original four-carbon compound, oxaloacetate, with a net loss of two carbons as carbon dioxide. The pathway thus begins and ends with the same compound—oxaloacetate. This makes it a cycle.

To review we started with the six-carbon glucose, passed through the three-carbon pyruvate to the two-carbon acetyl-CoA, and ended up with carbon dioxide. We have taken all the carbons in glucose and turned them into carbon dioxide. The carbon dioxide eventually leaves through the lungs. In the process, we have made ATP molecules directly using both glycolysis and the citric acid cycle, as well as NADH molecules and $FADH_2$ molecules. These latter molecules can be "cashed in" for ATP in the electron transport chain.

We have accomplished what we set out to do; we took some of the energy in the chemical bonds of glucose and turned it into ATP. In doing that, we converted the energy in foodstuffs into a form that cells can use rather than just converting the energy into heat, as would have happened if we had burned the food with a match. In engineering terms, we captured about 40% of the chemical energy in glucose and eventually stored it in a useful form for later use, namely ATP.[7] The rest escaped as heat via all the reactions where ATP, GTP, NADH, or $FADH_2$ were not made. This same 40:60 ratio applies for energy metabolism of fatty acids and amino acids. That's fairly efficient when you consider that an automobile engine captures only about 10% of the chemical energy in gasoline.

ELECTRON TRANSPORT CHAIN

During the metabolism of protein, carbohydrate, fat, and alcohol, cells generate NADH and $FADH_2$. Most cells can "cash in" these compounds for ATP. The pathway that performs this exchange is called the **electron transport chain.** The process, located in the mitochondria, is called oxidative phosphorylation (Figure 7-6). Both iron and copper are needed for this process.

electron transport chain A series of reactions using oxygen that converts NADH and $FADH_2$ molecules into free NAD and FAD molecules, yielding water and ATP.

Basically, in the electron transport chain NADH donates its chemical energy to an FAD derivative, called flavin mononucleotide (FMN). As the high-energy NADH becomes the low-energy NAD form, the reaction liberates some energy to form one ATP molecule and to yield $FMNH_2$ as well. The $FMNH_2$, through a series of steps that uses other electron carriers called **cytochromes**, donates its electrons to oxygen.[7] Water, two more ATP molecules, and a free FMN molecule are formed. Thus the net result of the electron transport chain is the production of ATP and water. Although we can describe this process, there are still questions about how it actually works.

cytochromes Electron-transfer compounds that participate in the electron transport chain.

The electron transport chain represents the **aerobic** side of metabolism, since it uses oxygen. Although oxygen does not participate directly in the citric acid cycle,

aerobic Requiring oxygen.

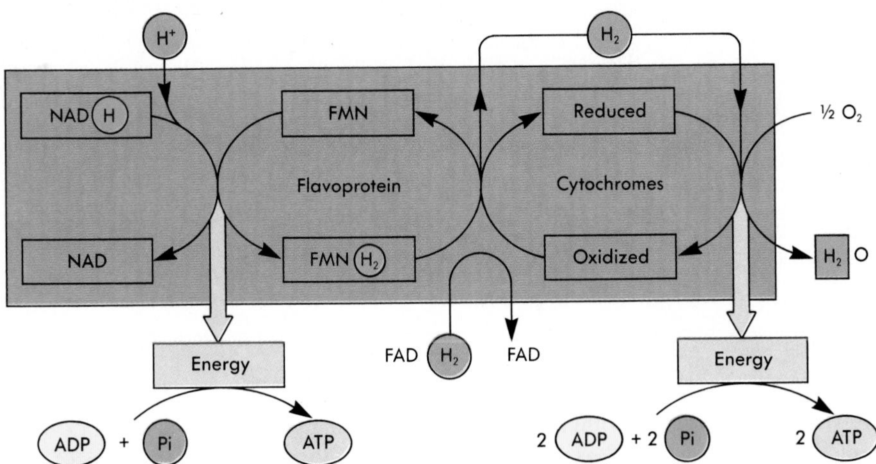

Figure 7-6 Electron-transport chain. NADH and $FADH_2$ transfer their electrons to electron carriers located on a mitochondrial membrane. The energy yielded by the entire process is used to generate ATPs. The electrons and hydrogen ions combine with oxygen to form water (H_2O).

the cycle operates only under aerobic conditions because the NADH and $FADH_2$ produced can be regenerated into NAD and FAD only by the eventual transfer of their stored electrons to oxygen. The citric acid cycle has no way to recycle NADH and $FADH_2$ analogously to the way that anaerobic glycolysis uses lactate; oxygen is a necessity. This is ultimately why oxygen is essential to life: We must have a final acceptor of the electrons and hydrogen ions generated from the breakdown of energy-yielding nutrients. Without oxygen, most of our cells are unable to extract enough energy from energy-yielding fuels to sustain life.

You already know that two by-products of cell metabolism are carbon dioxide and water. You now know where the carbon dioxide and water come from. The carbon dioxide comes from the citric acid cycle and most of the water comes from the electron transport chain (Figure 7-7). In this metabolism, energy is produced in the forms of heat and ATP. That is the essence of metabolism. Cells need to release and then trap as much energy bound in foods as possible, and in a useful form. The body cannot afford to lose all energy as heat. Some heat is necessary for warming the body, but the body also needs mobilizing energy. Glycolysis, the citric

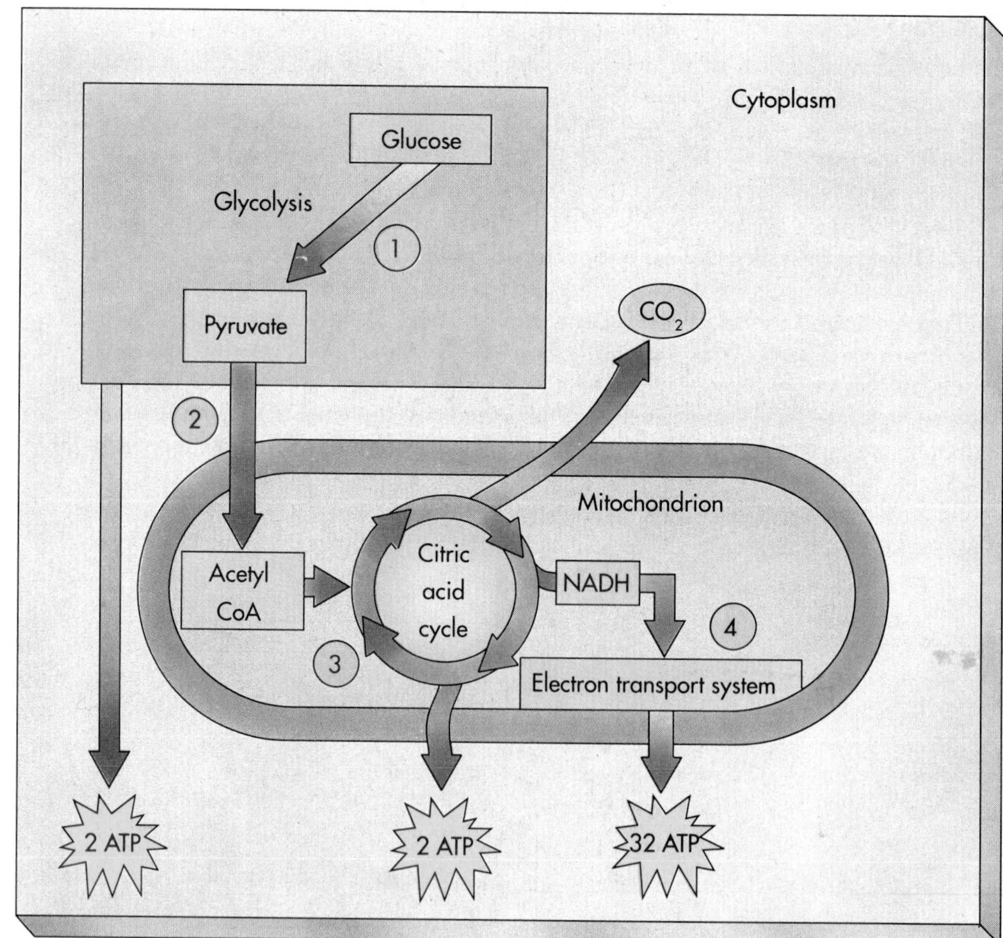

Figure 7-7 An overview of glucose metabolism. The citric acid cycle and the electron transport chain are located within the mitochondria, and glycolysis occurs in the cytoplasm. *1,* In glycolysis, each glucose molecule is broken down into two molecules of pyruvate. *2,* These enter a mitochondrion and, in turn, *3,* the citric acid cycle. All three carbons of pyruvate eventually yield three carbon dioxide molecules. *4,* Chemical energy produced by the citric acid cycle is then transferred to the electron transport chain, which is located in the membranes of the mitochondria. Most of the ATP that results from glucose metabolism is formed at this stage. Water is also a by-product. About 60% of the energy in glucose is lost as heat; 40% of the energy is captured as ATP energy.

acid cycle, and the electron transport chain accomplish many things. The greatest feat of these processes, however, is that they enable cells to capture the chemical energy in food as ATP energy. ATP energy then acts as the cellular energy currency. In effect, it allows cells to get up and do what needs to be done.

GLYCOGEN METABOLISM

Glycogen synthesis uses a form of glucose to eventually add more glucose molecules to an existing glycogen molecule.[6] This provides liver and muscle cells with a short-term storage form of glucose in the cytosol for future needs. Later, when glucose is needed, glycogen breakdown yields glucose as a glucose-phosphate compound. This then eventually begins glycolysis. An enzyme in glycogen breakdown uses a form of vitamin B-6.

CONCEPT CHECK

In the citric acid cycle the two-carbon acetate molecule (in the form of acetyl-CoA) reacts with a four-carbon compound (oxaloacetate) to form a six-carbon compound (citrate). The cycle then, through numerous reactions, causes citrate to lose two carbon dioxide molecules, eventually yielding oxaloacetate, the starting material. This oxaloacetate molecule can then combine with another acetyl-CoA molecule to begin the process again. The NADH and $FADH_2$ molecules produced in the citric acid cycle donate their electrons and hydrogen ions to the electron transport chain, yielding free NAD and FAD molecules, water, and numerous ATP molecules.

Fat Metabolism

LIPOLYSIS: FAT BREAKDOWN

Lipolysis is part of the process of splitting—breaking down—fat (lipid). It represents the breakdown of triglycerides into free fatty acids and glycerol. The further breakdown of the fatty acids for energy production is called fatty acid oxidation, since the donation of electrons to oxygen is the ultimate reaction in the process. This latter pathway takes place in cell mitochondria and peroxisomes, but only mitochondria can use the energy released to form ATP.

lipolysis The breakdown of triglycerides to glycerol and fatty acids.

Almost all fatty acids in nature are composed of an even number of carbons, usually 16 or 18 carbons. The first step in converting the energy in a fatty acid into ATP energy (fatty acid oxidation) is to clip off all carbons, two at a time, from the fatty acid. These two-carbon clips form acetyl-CoA. The process of converting a free fatty acid into many acetyl-CoA molecules is called **beta-oxidation**. During beta-oxidation, NADH and $FADH_2$ are produced. So, as with glucose, a fatty acid is eventually degraded into the two-carbon compound acetyl-CoA. Some of the chemical energy is also trapped, in this case as NADH and $FADH_2$.

beta-oxidation The breakdown of a fatty acid into numerous acetyl-CoA molecules.

The acetyl-CoA then enters the citric acid cycle and is broken down into carbon dioxide molecules, just as with glucose. Thus a breakdown product of glucose and fatty acids use a common pathway—the citric acid cycle—as both compounds yield acetyl-CoA.[7]

No matter how many carbons a fatty acid contains, it will usually be broken down into acetyl-CoA molecules. Occasionally a fatty acid has an odd number of carbons. Then the cell forms many acetyl-CoA molecules, plus one three-carbon compound, propionyl-CoA. The propionyl-CoA enters the citric acid cycle directly, bypassing acetyl-CoA. It can then go on to form carbon dioxide and other products.

CARBOHYDRATE AIDS FAT METABOLISM

In addition to its role in energy production, the citric acid cycle provides compounds that leave the pathway and enter biosynthetic pathways, such as those used to make the red blood cell protein hemoglobin. This means that even though oxaloacetate is reused in the cycle, a minimum level of it must be constantly replaced because the compounds removed from the citric acid cycle for biosynthetic reactions prevent the complete cycle back to oxaloacetate.[7] One source of this additional oxaloacetate is pyruvate, a carbohydrate. Glucose is an original source. So as fatty acids create acetyl-CoA, carbohydrates like glucose can keep the concentration of pyruvate high to help allow the concentration of oxaloacetate to stay high in the citric acid cycle. This then allows acetyl-CoA to yield carbon dioxide. We could say fats tend to burn in a "fire of carbohydrate." Overall the whole pathway for fatty acid oxidation just works better when carbohydrate is available.

ketone bodies Products of acetyl-CoA metabolism containing three to four carbons: they are acetoacetic acid, beta-hydroxybutyric acid, and acetone.

KETOGENESIS: PRODUCING KETONES

Ketone bodies—also called ketones—are products of incomplete fatty acid oxidation. Hormonal imbalances, chiefly inadequate insulin production to balance the amount of glucagon produced by the body, allows some key metabolic conditions to develop that lead to ketosis:[6]

1. Fatty acids from storage of fat cells flood into the bloodstream. The bulk of these fatty acids are taken up by the liver.
2. Fatty acid oxidation to acetyl-CoA is encouraged rather than fatty acid synthesis and ultimate release of triglyceride into the bloodstream.

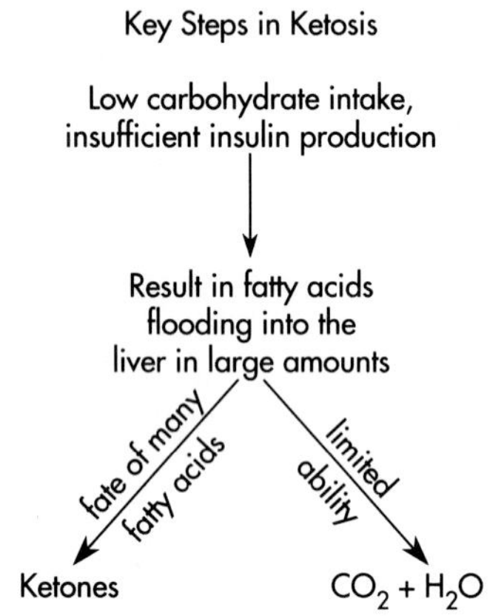

Key Steps in Ketosis

Low carbohydrate intake, insufficient insulin production

↓

Result in fatty acids flooding into the liver in large amounts

fate of many fatty acids → Ketones

limited ability → $CO_2 + H_2O$

In addition, as the liver takes up the fatty acids and degrades them into acetyl-CoA, a limited ability to push these through the citric acid cycle also exists. This is partly because metabolism of fatty acids to acetyl-CoA yields much ATP, and high ATP levels slow citric acid activity in liver cells. Essentially there is no need to use the citric acid cycle—the main role of which is to extract energy from compounds for ATP synthesis—when the cells have plenty of ATP already.

Overall, then, these changes encourage the liver cells to join two acetyl-CoA molecules together to form a four-carbon compound. This compound is further metabolized and eventually secreted into the bloodstream as the ketone acetoacetic acid and related compounds.

Cells pick ketones like acetoacetic acid and turn them back into acetyl-CoA. These molecules are then pushed through the citric acid cycle to form ATP. One of the ketones formed leaves the body via the lungs, giving the person in ketosis a characteristic "fruity" breath.

KETOSIS IN FASTING

When a person fasts, insulin production falls. Again, this causes fatty acids to flood into the bloodstream and eventually to form ketones, as we just discussed. Further encouraging ketone production is the fact that liver cells must use much oxaloacetate to produce a glucose supply for the brain, red blood cells, and part of the kidney.[6] These cells need glucose to function. But now ample amounts of oxaloacetate will be generally unavailable in the liver cells for reacting with acetyl-CoA in the citric acid cycle. This relative scarcity of oxaloacetate—found in people in states of semi-starvation and on low-carbohydrate diets—encourages diversion of acetyl-CoA from the citric acid cycle to form ketone bodies. In essence, ketone production will take place whenever lots of fat oxidation must take place at the same time that glucose availability is limited. Heart muscle and some parts of the kidney then turn to ketone bodies for fuel. Given a few days, the brain also begins to metabolize ketones for energy.

KETOSIS IN DIABETES CAN BE HARMFUL

The main problem in insulin-dependent forms of diabetes is that not enough insulin is produced to allow for normal carbohydrate and fat metabolism. We just discussed that without sufficient insulin, much ketone production occurs. If the level of ketone bodies rises too high in the bloodstream, the excess pours into the urine, pulling sodium and potassium ions with it. Eventually it causes ion imbalances to mount in the body. The problem usually occurs only in ketosis caused by diabetes; in fasting, blood ketone levels usually do not rise high enough.

LIPOGENESIS: BUILDING FATTY ACIDS

Lipogenesis is the formation of fat (lipid). The pathway is found in the cytoplasm of liver cells. Ingested glucose or protein that the body does not use immediately can be stored as triglyceride. Most carbohydrate is stored as glycogen, but the total amount can be only about 350 grams in the body. Some protein resides in amino acid pools in the body, but that also does not amount to much (Figure 5-3). Thus a lot of glucose and amino acid molecules are left over from a large meal, some of their carbons are used to synthesize fatty acids. This process requires ATP and the vitamins biotin, niacin, and pantothenic acid.[7]

lipogenesis The building of fatty acids using derivatives of acetyl-CoA molecules.

Since net ATP is used, lipogenesis is an energy-losing proposition for a liver cell. Note that kcalories of fat consumed in excess of needs will result in almost the same kcalories stored as fat. However, a kcalorie excess of carbohydrate will result in less than the same amount of kcalories stored as fat. The energy cost of lipogenesis is the difference. This has implications for weight regulation (see Chapter 8).

In lipogenesis, the liver begins with carbons from glucose and the carbon skeletons of amino acids that are metabolized into acetyl-CoA. Cells in the liver in effect then bond the acetate parts of acetyl-CoA molecules together in a series of steps to eventually form a 16-carbon saturated fatty acid, palmitic acid. This 16-carbon fatty acid can later be lengthened to an 18- or 20-carbon chain. The fatty acids are then joined (esterified) to a form of glycerol (produced during glycolysis) to yield a triglyceride. The triglyceride is later released as a very low density lipoprotein, or VLDL (see Chapter 4 for a review if needed). Cells then use the synthesized fat for energy production, or it is stored in fat cells along with excess dietary fat intake.

CONCEPT CHECK

Fatty acids are degraded into numerous acetyl-CoA molecules. These molecules participate in the citric acid cycle and electron transport chain to eventually yield carbon dioxide, water, and much ATP. To synthesize fat, a cell binds numerous acetate molecules (donated by a derivative of acetyl-CoA) together to form a fatty acid. Three fatty acids can then react with a form of glycerol to yield a triglyceride. If liver cells are limited in the ability to perform lipogenesis, such as in cases of uncontrolled diabetes, the large amounts of acetyl-CoA resulting from rapid fatty acid oxidation tends to form into ketone bodies. These ketone bodies enter the bloodstream and are eventually metabolized to carbon dioxide and water (after being converted back into acetyl-CoA) by various body cells.

Protein Metabolism

Protein metabolism begins after proteins are degraded into amino acids. Then, to burn an amino acid for fuel, cells first split off the amino group ($-NH_2$) in the processes called deamination and transamination that we covered in Chapter 5. These pathways often require a form of vitamin B-6 to function. Deamination and transamination leave a carbon skeleton, which can usually directly enter the citric acid cycle in the mitochondria. However, some carbon skeletons must enter the pathway at acetyl-CoA (Figure 7-5).[6] In addition, often a cell must first metabolize the carbon skeleton into another compound or compounds before the parts can enter the citric acid cycle. So different parts of an amino acid carbon skeleton may enter at various points in the pathway. Any part of the skeleton that can bypass acetyl-CoA and enter the citric acid cycle directly can eventually become part of glucose. You'll see how shortly.

GLUCONEOGENESIS: PRODUCING NEW GLUCOSE MOLECULES

The starting material for gluconeogenesis is oxaloacetate, which is derived primarily from the carbon skeletons of some amino acids. Alanine is the major amino acid that is used for this purpose. Remember, oxaloacetate is the primary compound needed to keep the citric acid cycle running. The entire gluconeogenesis pathway is present only in liver cells and some kidney cells. The four-carbon oxaloacetate loses a carbon dioxide molecule and converts to the three-carbon compound. This then basically reverses the path back through glycolysis to form glucose (Figure 7-8). Some steps in gluconeogenesis are simply a reversal of glycolysis reactions, but others are variations of glycolysis. This entire process requires ATP as well as forms of the vitamins biotin, riboflavin, niacin, and B-6.

Carbon skeletons of amino acids that enter directly into the citric acid cycle or become pyruvate are called glycogenic amino acids. This indicates that these carbons can become the carbons of glucose. Any parts of carbon skeletons that become acetyl-CoA are called ketogenic because these atoms cannot become parts of glucose molecules.

Let's trace the path of gluconeogenesis by converting glutamic acid, an amino acid, into glucose. Glutamic acid is first deaminated to form its carbon skeleton. This enters the citric acid cycle directly and is converted by stages into oxaloacetate. Oxaloacetate loses a carbon dioxide molecule and then reverses through glycolysis to form glucose. Since a three-carbon compound is used, a cell actually needs two of them to form a six-carbon glucose molecule. So a cell needs two glutamic acid molecules to eventually form one glucose molecule.

Recall from Chapter 3 that if there is an insufficient amount of carbohydrate in your body, the liver and kidneys are forced to make it from body protein to support the energy needs of your brain and red blood cells.[6] We have just described one way that can happen. Liver and kidney cells start with carbon skeletons of some

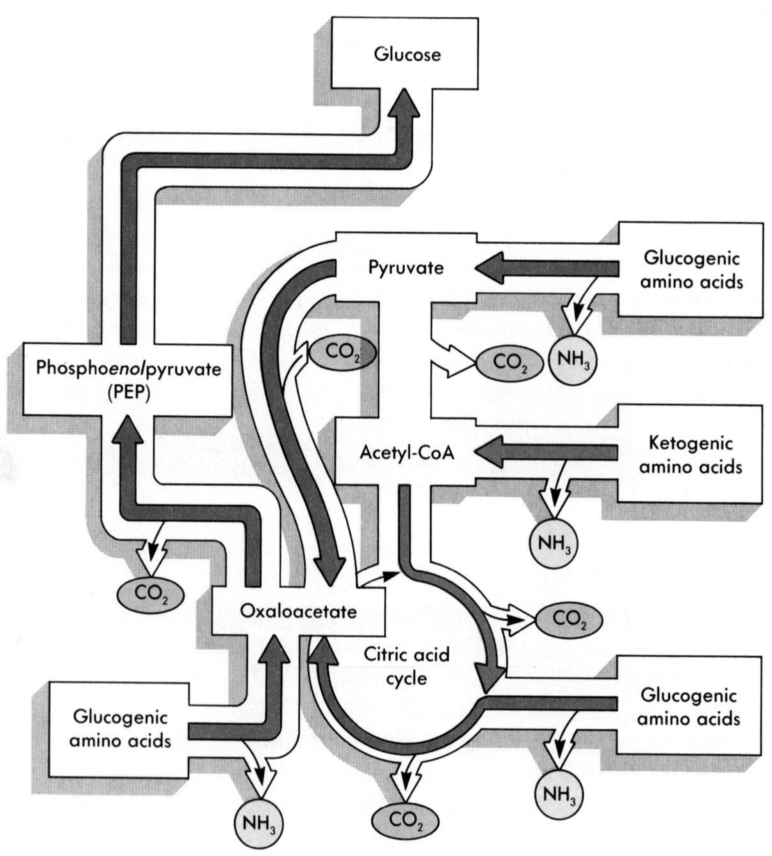

Figure 7-8 Gluconeogenesis. Glycogenic amino acids can yield net glucose while ketogenic amino acids cannot. The deciding factor is whether the amino acid yields a "new" oxaloacetate molecule during metabolism.

amino acids that can directly enter the citric acid cycle. These are converted to oxaloacetate, then to a three-carbon compound, and finally to glucose. Over many weeks, the need for constant gluconeogenesis brought on by semistarvation with respect to carbohydrate and protein leads to a wasting away of body protein. This in turn severely compromises health and eventually contributes to death if carried on long enough, usually about 50 to 70 days of total fasting.

Also, it is worth noting that as fasting is prolonged (beyond a few days), the body's total metabolic rate decreases to limit the drain on energy stores. And as we mentioned, eventually the central nervous system no longer depends entirely on glucose as an energy source. It converts to the use of ketones. In long-term fasting, gluconeogenesis then diminishes; fatty acids in turn provide about 90% of the total energy expenditure of the body.

CAN WE HAVE GLUCONEOGENESIS FROM FATTY ACIDS?

Let's try to turn a typical fatty acid into glucose. A fatty acid with an even number of carbons—again, the typical form in the body—breaks down into many acetyl-CoA molecules. The step between pyruvate and acetyl-CoA is irreversible. Acetyl-CoA can never reform into pyruvate once the carbon dioxide molecule is lost. The only option for acetyl-CoA, besides forming fatty acids or ketones, is to combine with oxaloacetate in the citric acid cycle. However, two carbons of acetyl-CoA are added at the beginning of the citric acid cycle, and two carbons are subsequently lost when citrate converts back to the starting material, oxaloacetate. So when we arrive at oxaloacetate, no carbons are left to turn into glucose. Trying to convert typical fatty acids into glucose is then impossible: it cannot be done.

The only part of a triglyceride that can become glucose is the glycerol portion and any propionyl-CoA that is formed from odd-chain fatty acids. Glycerol enters into the glycolysis pathway, and propionyl-CoA directly enters the citric acid cycle. Both then can flow backward through the citric acid cycle and through the process of gluconeogenesis to convert to glucose. Neither of these compounds yields much glucose, since we form little propionyl-CoA and only about 10% of a triglyceride is glycerol.

Some plants have a metabolic pathway that allows them to convert fatty acids into glucose, known as the glyoxalate pathway.

DISPOSING OF EXCESS AMINO GROUPS

The breakdown of amino acids yields amino groups ($-NH_2$) that then form ammonia (NH_3). The ammonia must be excreted because its buildup is toxic for cells. The liver prepares the amino groups for excretion in the urea cycle. During the urea cycle, two ammonia groups react through a series of steps with carbon dioxide molecules to form urea ($H_2N\overset{\displaystyle O}{\overset{\|}{C}}NH_2$) and water (Figure 7-9).[6] Urea is then excreted in the urine.

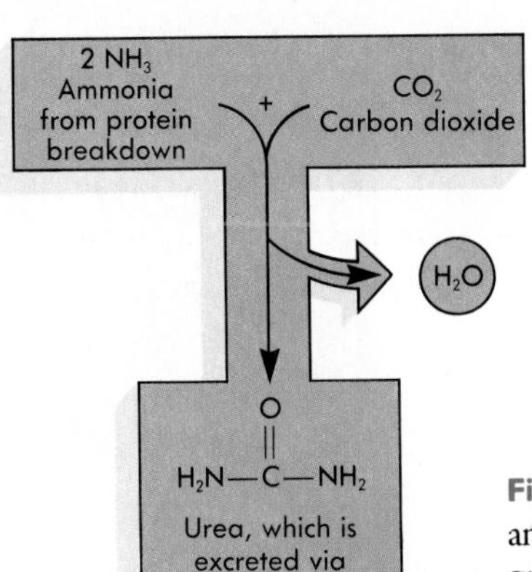

Figure 7-9 Disposal of excess amino groups. The amino groups, as ammonia, form part of urea. This is excreted via the urine. The amino groups originally came from amino acids that went through transamination with ultimate deamination to yield the free amino group.

CONCEPT CHECK

In the process of losing an amino group, individual amino acids form carbon skeletons. Many carbon skeletons can be further metabolized so that they enter either the citric acid cycle or glycolysis pathway. If so, the carbons can be pushed through gluconeogenesis to ultimately form new glucose molecules. If the carbon skeleton enters metabolism as acetyl-CoA, glucose production is not possible. The amino groups go on to form part of urea. This is excreted from the body via urine.

NUTRITION FOCUS

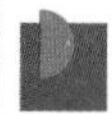

Alcohol Metabolism

Alcohol is still another substance that can supply energy for the body: 7 kcalories per gram. The liver metabolizes most of the alcohol consumed. A social drinker who weighs 150 pounds and has normal liver function metabolizes about 7 to 14 grams of alcohol per hour (100 to 200 milligrams per kilogram of body weight per hour).[6] This is about 8 to 12 ounces of beer or half an ordinary-sized drink. When the rate of alcohol consumption exceeds the liver's metabolic capacity, the blood alcohol content rises and symptoms of intoxication appear.

Pathways for alcohol metabolism

Alcohol at low doses first reacts with NAD to form the compound acetaldehyde. The enzyme used is alcohol dehydrogenase (Figure 7-10).[2] This enzyme requires the mineral zinc for activity. Acetaldehyde is then converted into acetyl-CoA. Both reactions yield an NADH molecule. The acetyl-CoA enters the citric acid cycle, and the NADH, $FADH_2$, and GTP molecules produced in the citric acid cycle can then be used to generate ATP.

In structure, the end of ethanol with the hydroxyl group (−OH) resembles a carbohydrate. But since it breaks down directly into acetyl-CoA, alcohol carbons cannot support glucose production. So alcohol is metabolized more like a fat than like a carbohydrate, and thus is considered a fat in metabolic terms.

When a person drinks a lot of alcohol, the enzyme alcohol dehydrogenase cannot keep up with the demand to metabolize all of it into acetaldehyde. For this and other reasons, another enzyme system in the liver begins metabolizing alcohol. This system is called the microsomal ethanol oxidizing system (MEOS).[2] The MEOS is usually used by the liver to metabolize drugs and other "foreign" compounds. The liver registers excessive molecules of alcohol as foreign compounds, and thus the MEOS kicks in. Once the MEOS is active, alcohol tolerance increases because the rate of alcohol metabolism increases.

There are two interesting aspects about this use of the MEOS. First, instead of forming NADH as does alcohol dehydrogenase, the MEOS uses NADPH, a compound analogous to NADH. Now, instead of yielding "potential" ATP molecules from the first step in alcohol metabolism, the MEOS uses "potential" ATP molecules. This helps explain why people with alcoholism do not gain as much weight as expected from the amount of kcalories they consume via alcohol. High doses of alcohol are inefficiently used by the liver because they require energy for the first metabolic step. The person with alcoholism basically wastes some alcohol kcalories by inducing this alternate metabolic pathway.[2] Liver damage from alcohol, such that other metabolic pathways are hampered, also is implicated in the loss of kcalories associated with high alcohol use.[1,2]

The use of the MEOS also increases the potential for an overdose of alcohol. While the MEOS system is metabolizing alcohol, it has a reduced capacity to metabolize drugs, such as many sedatives. If high amounts of alcohol and these sedatives are mixed, the user may lapse into coma and die. The liver is not able to break down the sedatives in the body fast enough. Alcohol itself is toxic in high quantities. Mix it with sedatives and an extremely toxic combination results. Nutrient deficiencies associated with excess alcohol intake also are likely. We discuss these possible negative health implications in detail in Chapter 18.

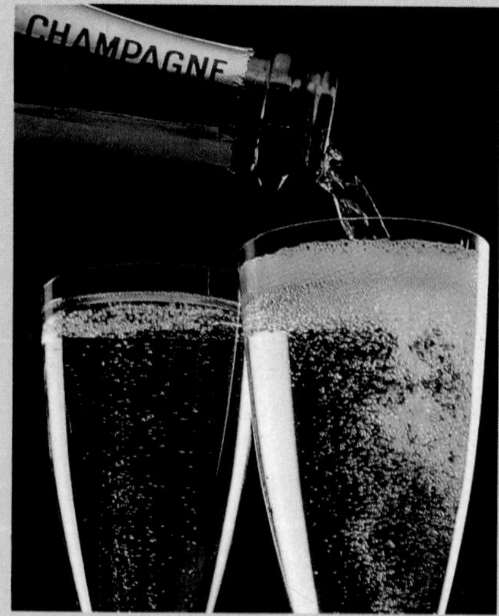

Alcohol is metabolized most like a fat as compared to carbohydrate or protein.

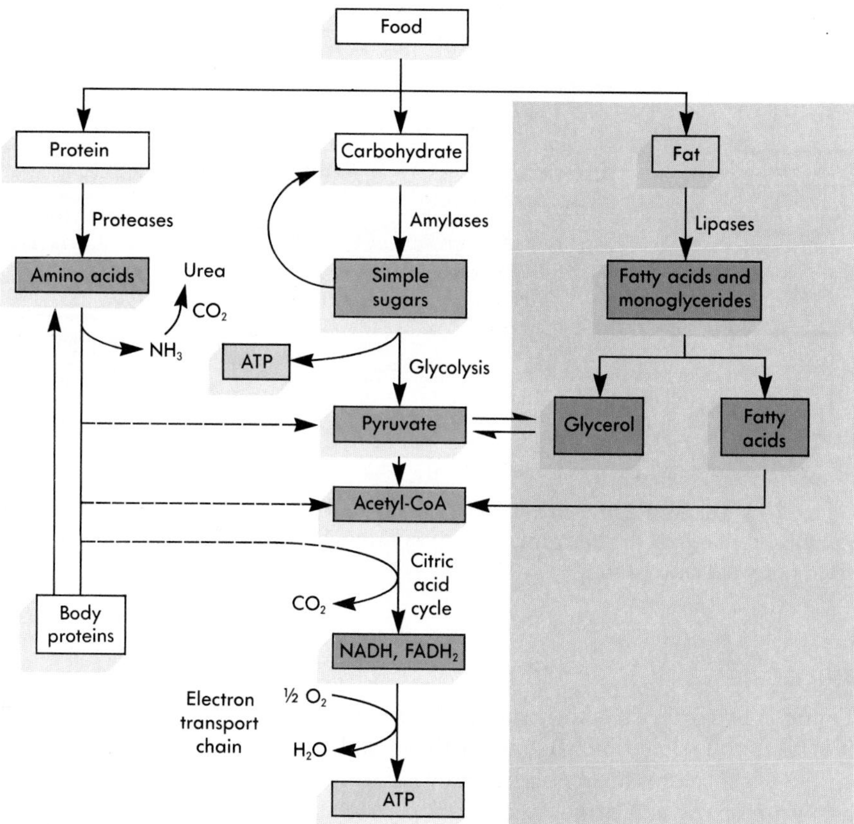

Figure 7-12 The fate of food. In terms of sources for energy production, most food consists of carbohydrate, protein, and fat. During digestion, protein is broken down into amino acids, carbohydrate is broken down into single sugars, and fats are primarily broken down to fatty acids and monoglycerides. Various forms of these compounds then eventually enter a common metabolic pathway—the citric acid cycle.

In all, acetyl-CoA plays a central role in energy metabolism. No matter what type of diet you eat—high carbohydrate, high protein, or high fat—all energy metabolism passes through the acetyl-CoA stage. It is the common denominator that links all human diets (Figure 7-12).[7]

REGULATING METABOLISM

Metabolism is regulated by various means. Enzymes are the key stimuli for metabolic pathways; both their presence and rate of activity are critical to reactions and processes along the pathways. Synthesis of enzymes themselves and their activity levels are somewhat controlled by cells and by the products of the reactions in which the enzymes participate. Hormones also serve as regulators of metabolic processes, as we have shown for insulin throughout this chapter. The ATP concentration in the cell likewise serves to regulate metabolism. Generally, high ATP concentrations decrease energy-yielding reactions and promote synthetic reactions, which then use ATP. High ADP concentrations, on the other hand, stimulate activity of energy-yielding pathways.[6] A still further factor in regulating metabolism is the liver itself, both because it contains such a variety of enzymes and most nutrients pass through it, providing an opportunity for metabolism there (Figure 7-13).

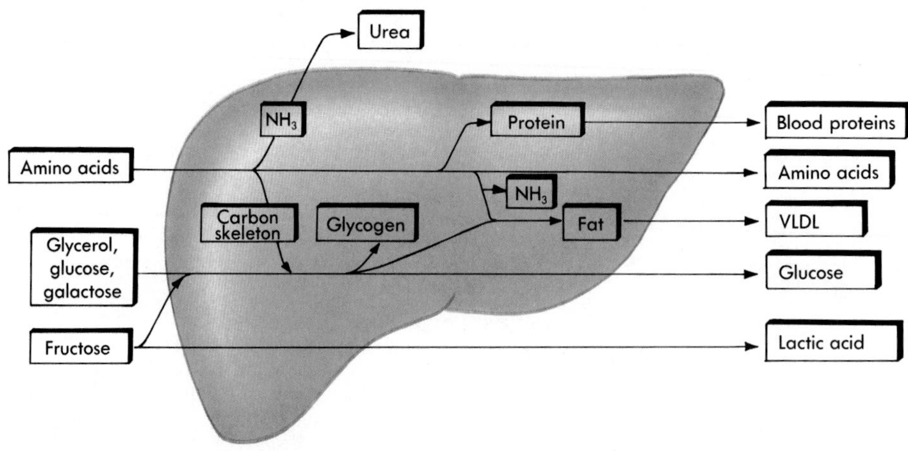

Figure 7-13 The liver is the crossroads for many nutrient interconversions. Most nutrients after absorption into the body must first pass through the liver. What leaves the liver is often not what entered it.

EPILOGUE

Figure 7-11 summarizes the major pathways we have considered. Don't be surprised if it takes you some time to grasp it thoroughly. It illustrates a complicated system within which a lot is taking place. Study it part by part. Consider reading this chapter again tomorrow and maybe again in 2 or 3 days until it begins to fit together.

You now know more about what happens in a cell than most people ever know. Knowledge is power. You can use this power right away to understand how vitamins and minerals function. You can better see how thiamin, niacin, riboflavin, biotin, pantothenic acid, and vitamin B-6, as well as the minerals magnesium, iron, and copper, play important roles in the metabolic cycles (Figure 7-14). This introduction sets the stage for Chapters 12 through 15. You can also use this knowledge to debunk fad diet claims, such as the touted long-term safety of low-carbohydrate diets. Future classes in nutrition, nursing, biology, physiology, biochemistry, pharmacy, and medicine should also be a little easier, because all of them build on this subject of metabolic pathways.

CONCEPT CHECK

Glycolysis takes place in the cytosol of the cell; the citric acid cycle and electron transport chain occur in the mitochondria. Fatty acids break down in the mitochondria, and they are synthesized in the cytosol. The urea cycle and gluconeogenesis take place in both parts of the cell. Hormonal balance, enzyme activity, and need for ATP energy all influence the rate at which these metabolic pathways operate. Since many metabolic pathways converge at acetyl-CoA, it represents a central compound in energy metabolism. Regardless of the diet, whether high protein, high fat, or high carbohydrate, the processes used to release the energy from those diets usually include acetyl-CoA.

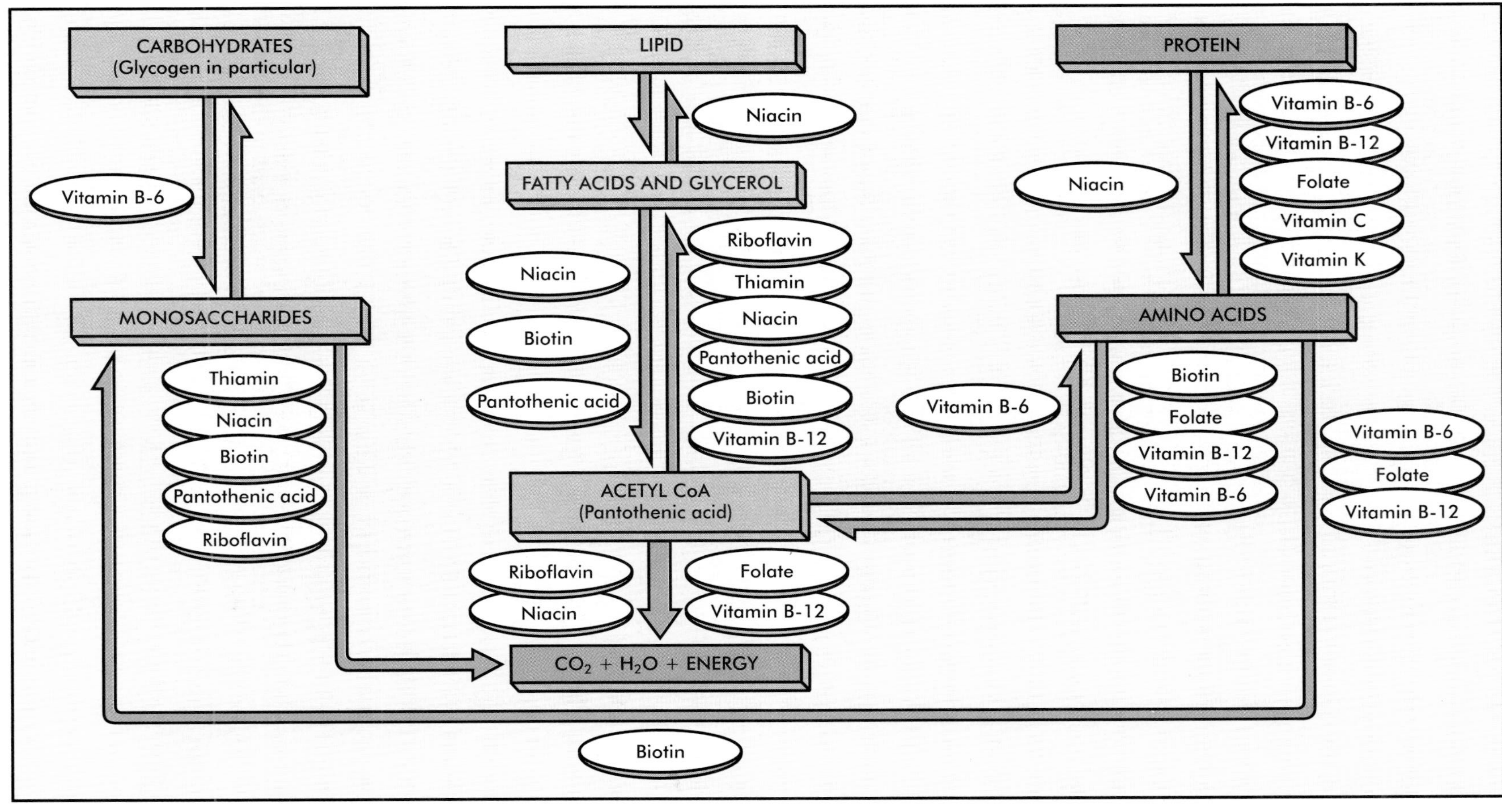

Figure 7-14 Many vitamins and minerals participate in the metabolic pathways. As you can predict, many widespread health problems can develop from nutrient deficiencies since so many key pathways depend on nutrient input.

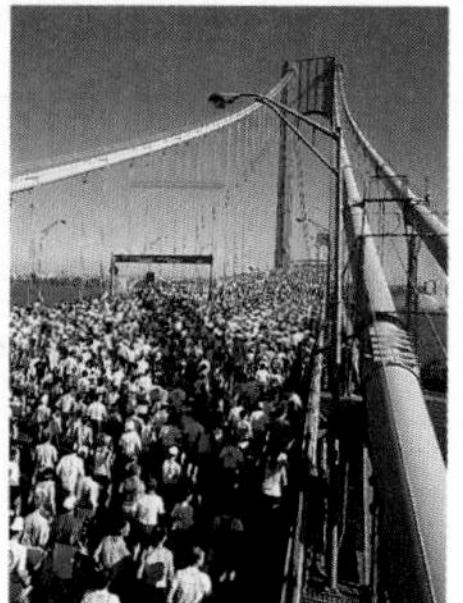

Summary

1. A cell is the basic unit of structure in the body. Within the cell membrane is a nucleus to direct protein synthesis and cell division, mitochondria to produce usable forms of energy, golgi bodies to package cell products, an endoplasmic reticulum whose various areas are involved in protein and fat synthesis, and storage granules of glycogen and droplets of fat.
2. ATP is the major form of energy for cellular metabolism. As ATP is breaking down into ADP plus Pi, energy is released from the Pi bond. This energy is used to pump ions, promote enzyme activity, and contract muscles. All energy available to humans ultimately comes from solar energy. Plants capture solar energy using photosynthesis. Human metabolic pathways are able to extract that energy from foodstuffs and convert it into ATP energy.
3. In glycolysis, glucose is degraded into two pyruvate molecules, yielding NADH (a storage form of energy) and ATP. Pyruvate can then proceed to other metabolic pathways to form carbon dioxide and water or to react with NADH to form lactate. In both pathways, NADH is eventually reformed into NAD, which is needed to continue glycolysis.
4. In the citric acid cycle, the acetyl-CoA is formed when a carbon dioxide molecule is lost from pyruvate. Acetyl-CoA is then pushed away through many metabolic steps, eventually yielding two more carbon dioxide molecules. In this way the citric acid cycle accepts two carbons from acetyl-CoA and yields two carbons as carbon dioxide. In the process, NADH, $FADH_2$, and a form of energy that can yield ATP directly (GTP) are formed. The NADH and $FADH_2$ then enter the electron transport chain to yield numerous ATP molecules and water molecules by combining oxygen with the electrons and hydrogen ions released.
5. In fatty acid breakdown, two-carbon fragments are clipped off of a fatty acid, yielding multiple acetyl-CoA molecules. These then use the citric acid cycle and electron transport chain to yield ATP energy, carbon dioxide, and water. In fat synthesis, acetate molecules (in the form of a acetyl-CoA derivative) are combined to yield a fatty acid, primarily the 16-carbon palmitic acid. These fatty acids can then react with a form of glycerol to yield a triglyceride.
6. During starvation and uncontrolled diabetes, more acetyl-CoA molecules tend to be produced in the liver than can be metabolized to CO_2 plus H_2O. These acetyl-CoA molecules are turned into ketone bodies. Ketone bodies flood into the bloodstream and are metabolized by other tissues after being turned back into acetyl-CoA.
7. Amino acids can lose their amino group to form a carbon skeleton. These skeletons then can be metabolized into compounds that enter the citric acid cycle, eventually yielding energy. Some carbon skeletons can also be formed into oxaloacetate, a compound found in the citric acid cycle, which in turn can be converted to glucose. The process of converting carbon skeletons of amino acids into glucose is part of gluconeogenesis. Acetyl-CoA molecules, and thus fatty acids, cannot participate in gluconeogenesis.
8. Glycolysis occurs in the cytosol of a cell, and the citric acid cycle and electron transport chain occur in the mitochondria. Fatty acid breakdown occurs in the mitochondria, and fatty acids are synthesized in the cytosol. The synthesis of urea and the pathway for gluconeogenesis both take place partly in the cytosol and partly in the mitochondria.
9. Acetyl-CoA is a pivotal player in cell metabolism because carbohydrates, proteins, amino acids, and fatty acids all can yield acetyl-CoA during their metabolism. The coordination of various metabolic pathways allows the carbons of glucose to become the carbons of fatty acids and the carbons of amino acids to become the carbons of glucose.
10. The vitamins thiamin, niacin, riboflavin, biotin, pantothenic acid, and B-6 and the minerals magnesium, iron, and copper play important roles in the metabolic cycles.

Study Questions

1. Many vitamins and minerals are used in the process of energy metabolism. List three instances in which this is the case by naming the vitamin or mineral and its role.

2. Why do cells specifically need ATP energy?

3. Explain how an ample ATP concentration is maintained in a cell. What is the key stimulus to ATP production?

4. If a person misses a meal, will ingesting a large amount of alcohol "make up" for all the kcalories lost? Why or why not?

5. What is the common denominator compound of the many pathways of energy metabolism (citric acid cycle, glycolysis, beta-oxidation, etc.)? Why is this considered a key metabolic player in the body's chemical processes?

REFERENCES

1. Lands WEM, Zakhari S: The case of the missing calories, *American Journal of Clinical Nutrition* 54:47, 1991.
2. Lieber CS: Perspectives: do alcohol calories count? *American Journal of Clinical Nutrition* 54:976, 1991.
3. Lieber CS: Alcohol, liver, and nutrition, *Journal of the American College of Nutrition* 10:602, 1991.
4. Linder MC: *Nutritional biochemistry and metabolism,* New York, 1991, Elsevier Science Publishing.
5. Montgomery R and others: *Biochemistry: a case oriented approach,* ed 5, St. Louis, 1990, Mosby–Year Book.
6. Murray RK and others: *Harper's biochemistry,* Norwalk, Conn, 1990, Appleton & Lange.
7. Stryer L: *Biochemistry,* ed 3, New York, 1988, WH Freeman.

SUGGESTED READINGS

Two excellent biochemistry references that are particularly useful for more detailed discussions of metabolism are those by Murray and others and by Stryer.

TAKE ACTION

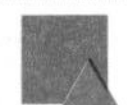

A friend is very overweight and describes to you his method of weight loss. He fasted completely for 1 week and then initiated a strict kcalorie-restricted diet of 400 to 600 kcalories daily under a physician's supervision. He receives these kcalories by drinking a liquid formula product for breakfast, skipping lunch, and eating a small dinner consisting of 3 ounces of protein, ½ cup of vegetables, 1 cup of fruit, and two starch items (a small potato, a piece of bread, etc.). He has also been taking carnitine supplements because he believes they help him burn fat more quickly. He has lost approximately 50 pounds in 6 months.

Based on your knowledge of energy metabolism, answer the following questions he poses:

1. During the fasting stage, what were most likely my sources of energy for my body's cells? What processes happened to provide glucose for my red blood cells? brain? kidneys?
2. Once I began the low-kcalorie phase, how did the metabolic processes in my body most likely change from the fasting state? Do I need to take the carnitine supplements?

Possible answers

1. While fasting, gluconeogenesis supplied the glucose needed for brain, red blood cell, and kidney use. The carbons used came mostly from body protein, leading to a decrease in lean body mass. Ketone production from fatty acid breakdown increased, leading to higher ketone levels in the blood and greater ketone use by many types of body cells. Insulin levels fell, leading to glycogen depletion in the liver and flooding of fatty acids from fat storage into the bloodstream. This later became the major energy-yielding fuel for the body.
2. During the low-kcalorie phase insulin levels in the body rose and carbohydrate intake increased. This would lead to a reduction in ketone production and a sparing of some body protein for use in gluconeogenesis. The body would switch from using primarily fat for energy to more of a mixture of carbohydrate and fat. However, although this use of fat requires carnitine, the body can make what it needs. A carnitine supplement is not needed. ▲

NUTRITION PERSPECTIVE

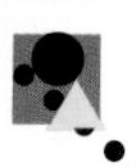

Homeostasis is the Overriding Theme of Body Metabolism

homeostasis A series of adjustments that act to prevent change in the internal environment of the body.

All living things maintain a fairly constant internal environment that is quite different from their surroundings, with more of certain chemical compounds and less of others. **Homeostasis** is the result of the dynamic processes by which an organism maintains this constant internal environment despite changes in the external environment.[4] "Homeo" is Greek for "same" and "stasis" is Greek for "staying." This is a major function of most organs in the human body. Examples of homeostatic effects include regulation of blood pressure, blood glucose levels, and body temperature. In terms of the whole body, the liver is an especially important organ for providing nutritional homeostasis.

Homeostasis plays a vital role in the body because tissues and organs can function efficiently only within a narrow range of conditions. Note that the range of temperatures in which life is possible is a tiny fraction of those found in nature. Cooler temperatures favor preservation of cellular structure, but slow the rates of the chemical reactions carried out by cells. Higher temperatures accelerate chemical reactions, but also may disrupt the structures of the proteins and other large molecules within cells in the human body. Furthermore, each cell of the body is surrounded by a small amount of fluid, and the normal function of that cell depends on the maintenance of its fluid environment within a narrow range of conditions, including volume, temperature, and chemical content. If the fluid surrounding cells deviates from homeostatic ranges, the cells, and possibly the individual, may die.

Methods for Maintaining Homeostasis

Intake and Output. One key aspect of the maintenance of homeostasis requires that the intake of substances, such as water and various ions, must equal their elimination. Ingestion of water and various ions adds them to the body; whereas excretion by organs, such as the kidneys and liver, or to a lesser degree, by the skin, removes them from the body. The regulation of water and ion balance involves the coordinated participation of several organ systems.[6] The kidneys, along with the respiratory, integumentary (skin), and gastrointestinal systems, regulate these parameters. The nervous and endocrine systems coordinate the activities of these systems.

Negative Feedback. An important homeostatic mechanism used for regulation of most conditions is negative feedback. "Negative" means that any deviation from a normal value is resisted or negated.[6] Negative feedback does not prevent variation, but intead maintains that variation within a normal range (Figure 7-15). When a certain factor varies from its optimum set point, automatic regulatory mechanisms act to counterbalance the disturbance and reestablish the internal equilibrium. For example, when the body overheats, sweating is stimulated until the temperature returns to normal. Similarly, when the level of oxygen in the blood is low, breathing is stimulated; when blood pressure falls, heart rate increases.[6]

Passive and Active Transport. Much exchange between cells and their immediate surroundings occurs by diffusion (see Chapter 6), a process in which individual molecules move if there is a concentration gradient—a difference in the concentration of the substance over a distance. However, some substances are actively transported across the cell membrane. The concentration of other substances (e.g., various ions) in the numerous fluid compartments in the body are determined by these transport processes. Virtually all cells contain a high concentration of potassium and low concentrations of sodium, chloride, magnesium, and calcium.[6] Most large molecules (e.g., proteins) that are synthesized within the cell remain within the cell.

Some substances must be exchanged with the environment. In particular, the production of chemical energy in most cell types requires that oxygen and nutrients

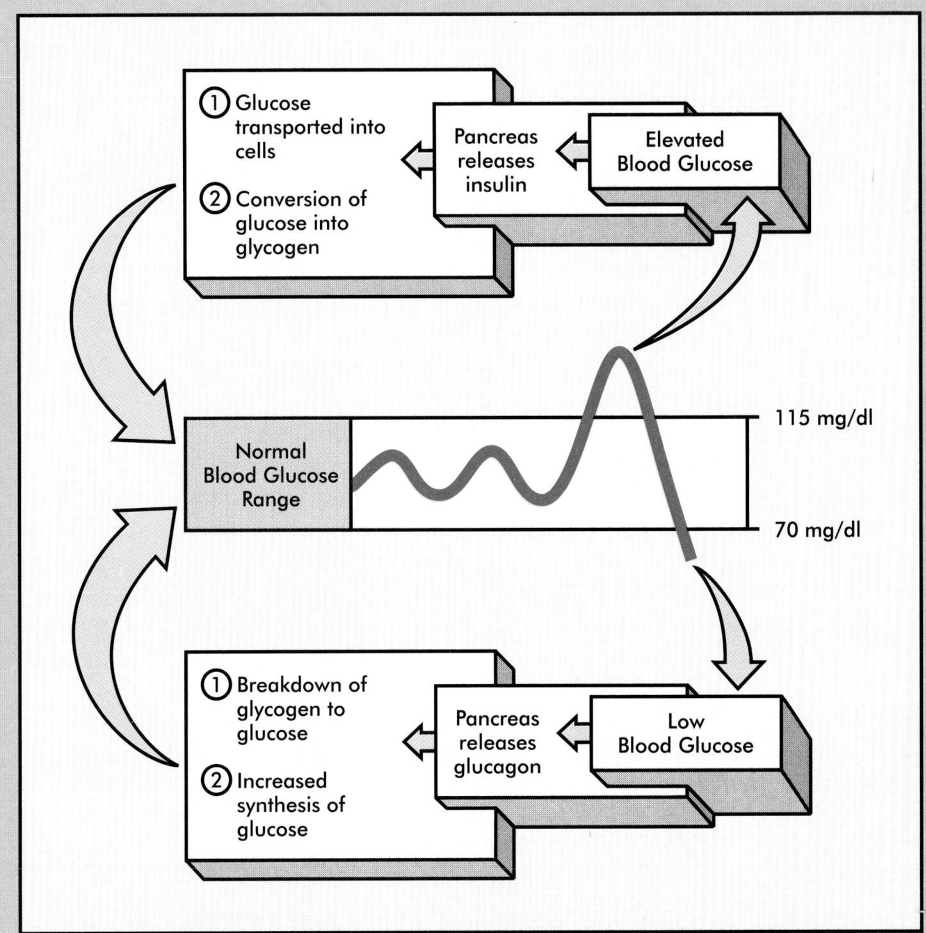

Figure 7-15 Negative feedback. Values for the condition, in this case blood glucose, fluctuate above and below a normal value within a normal range. As long as the values remain within the normal range, homeostasis is maintained. Negative feedback using the various factors involved in the maintenance of one's blood glucose level can correct abnormal levels—those outside the homeostatic range.

reach the interior of cells and that carbon dioxide and other chemical end products be transferred to the environment. In the circulatory system, blood is rapidly moved between the respiratory system, where gases are exchanged; the kidney, where nongaseous wastes and excess fluid and solutes are removed; and the digestive system, where nutrients are absorbed.

Rapid transport of the substances within the internal environment by blood flow overcomes the diffusional limit on large body size of humans. The volume of fluid outside cells in the human body is about one third the volume of that inside cells. The possession of a circulatory system makes it possible for this relatively small fluid volume outside cells to serve a much larger fluid pool that forms part of every cell.[3]

Hormone and Nerve Input. The endocrine system is a key component in the adaptation of the human organism to changes in the internal and external environment. Specific endocrine cells usually grouped in glands sense a "disturbance" and respond by secreting hormones into the bloodstream. These special molecules are

NUTRITION PERSPECTIVE

Homeostasis is the Overriding Theme of Body Metabolism—cont'd

carried via the circulation to various tissues, where they act on their target cells. As a result, the target cells respond in a manner that usually opposes the direction of change that evoked the secretion of the hormone. This helps restore the organism to its original stable state. For example, when blood glucose levels increase, insulin is released by the pancreas. This hormone promotes changes that cause the blood glucose level to fall, such as glucose uptake by fat cells and glycogen synthesis by the liver (Figure 7-15).[7] In addition to having a fundamental role in maintaining homeostasis, the endocrine system also helps to initiate, mediate, and regulate the processes of growth, development, maturation, reproduction, and aging.

The endocrine system may act independently of or may be integrated with the nervous system, which is another major component in the organism's adaptability to internal or external change. The principle of chemical homeostasis and the fundamental relationship of the endocrine system to the nervous system are well illustrated by the response of the organism to an abrupt lowering of the plasma concentration of glucose (hypoglycemia) (Figure 7-15). Because a supply of glucose helps sustain brain function, hypoglycemia cannot be tolerated for long. Endocrine cells in the pancreas respond to hypoglycemia by secreting a hormone called glucagon that stimulates the release of stored glucose from the liver. Nerve endings and adrenal glands release the hormone epinephrine, which also acts on the liver to release stored glucose and directs other tissues to reduce glucose utilization. Finally, other neurons in the hypothalamus also sense hypoglycemia and, via combined neurocrine and endocrine pathways, stimulate the adrenal cortex to secrete the hormone cortisol.[6] This hormone augments synthesis of glucose in the liver to help maintain a supply in case initial stores become depleted. Together these endocrine and neural responses to hypoglycemia raise plasma glucose levels back to normal.

Homeostatic Versus Chemical Individually

Overall, there is a great deal of individual variability in the whole body and tissue content of individual chemical compounds, from proteins to sugars to trace minerals. But the variability in biochemical and chemical constitution of individuals is largely confined to substances inside cells. In contrast, there is a great deal of effort on the part of the body to maintain a constancy in the fluid environment outside cells. It is here that the term "homeostasis" most aptly applies. This fluid composes nearly 20% of the total body weight and includes blood. Accordingly, most compounds in the blood are maintained within a fairly narrow range. Sodium and potassium concentrations typically stay within a very narrow range; the range for glucose and protein is a bit wider, but still shows considerable regulation.

How Constant is Constant?

Although homeostatic parameters, such as blood pressure, are maintained within a set range, the range also can change in a beneficial manner. For example, during exercise the normal ranges for blood pressure and heart rate are increased significantly, resulting in increased delivery of blood to muscle cells. This increases oxygen and nutrient delivery to the muscle cells, which is required to maintain their increased rate of activity. Overall then, homeostasis is an overriding characteristic of the human body, with fine-tuning available to respond to various body stresses.

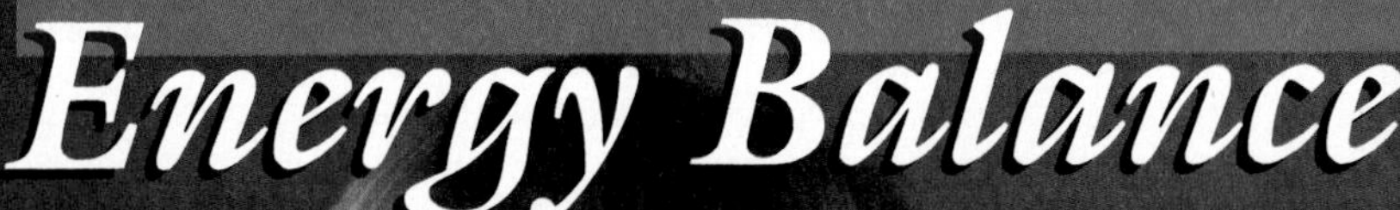

CHAPTER EIGHT

Energy Balance

Maintaining energy balance—regulating kcalorie intake so that it matches output—contributes to our health and well-being. Many adults in America maintain a healthy body weight by balancing their energy intake and output. Achieving that balance and then maintaining it is an important goal for everyone who is interested in good health. Adulthood can be a time of creeping weight gain that eventually turns into obesity. Currently about 29% of adult Americans aged 25 through 74 are overweight (27% of men and 30% of women).[3] The highest proportion of overweight people is found in men ages 45 to 54 years (31%) and in women ages 65 to 74 years (39%). This disorder then increases the likelihood of many health problems.

In this chapter we will discuss health problems related to obesity, review the major concepts underlying the theories of energy balance, and define the various types of obesity and outline how to assess these. Since obesity is a major health problem in America, it is important for us all to understand more about the forces that lead to it. Prevention of this problem is the most important goal.[1] High-fat diets and inactivity are two key causes, but still others need to be considered.[8,11]

NUTRITION AWARENESS INVENTORY

Here are 15 statements about energy balance. Answer them to test your current knowledge. If you think the answer is true or mostly true, circle T. If you think the answer is false or mostly false, circle F. Use the scoring key at the end of the book to compute your total score. Take this test again after you have read this chapter. Compare the results.

1. T F Hunger sensations are partially regulated by the liver.
2. T F Adipose cell size regulates eating on an hour-to-hour and day-to-day basis.
3. T F Total energy needs can be accurately estimated using the RDA.
4. T F The energy required to keep the resting body alive represents basal metabolism.
5. T F Brown adipose tissue is more active in adults than in infants.
6. T F That some obese people live past 80 years of age suggests that obesity probably doesn't affect longevity.
7. T F Excess body fat is a more important measure of risk for poor health than is excess body weight.
8. T F Men and women tend to add most fat to their bodies in the abdomen.
9. T F Health problems related to obesity begin when a person weighs about 20% over desirable weight.
10. T F The more muscle tissue one has, the higher the resting metabolism.
11. T F During physical activity, obese people burn more kcalories than lean people.
12. T F Adult obesity in men is usually tied to childhood obesity.
13. T F The major cause of obesity in America is low thyroid hormone levels.
14. T F Most obesity is due to constant overeating.
15. T F Hunger sensations often change during a meal.

Energy Intake: The First Half of Energy Balance

Energy balance depends on kcalorie input and kcalorie output. This balance then influences energy stores, primarily in adipose tissue (Figure 8-1). Let's look at the factors affecting these relationships.

Many forces influence when and what we eat.[6] Organs—like the liver and brain—interact with hormones, hormonelike factors, the nervous system, and other aspects of body physiology to influence eating behavior. Social forces—culture, work schedule, and income to name a few—act in both separate and interrelated fashions with the more physiological influences to also affect eating behavior. A good example of this potential interrelationship is mood. When depressed, some people eat, while other people do not feel like eating. This tendency, given either choice, influences hormonal balance in the body. This in turn can go on to affect when and what we eat. On the other hand, eating dessert after a more-than-filling dinner because it comes with the restaurant meal is more a social response with respect to eating. It is hard to pass up a free dessert.

Our intent here is not to confuse the issue of what influences when and what we eat. We just want to make it clear at the outset that a variety of forces—many of which are intertwined and work in concert—influence this (Figure 8-2). From a survival point of view, this redundancy of forces is an important attribute of feeding behavior. Because nutrients are so vital to the body, it is critical that many factors are able to encourage us to eat. However, the system is not perfect. Body weight can fluctuate. But as you will see in this chapter, both some powerful "built-in" and more "social" stimuli are at work directing your food intake[7] (Figure 8-3).

WHAT ACTUALLY IS HUNGER?

The when and what questions surrounding feeding behavior can be used to categorize the major influences as primarily internal or external with respect to the body. The physiological influences supplied by the liver and subconscious brain would be

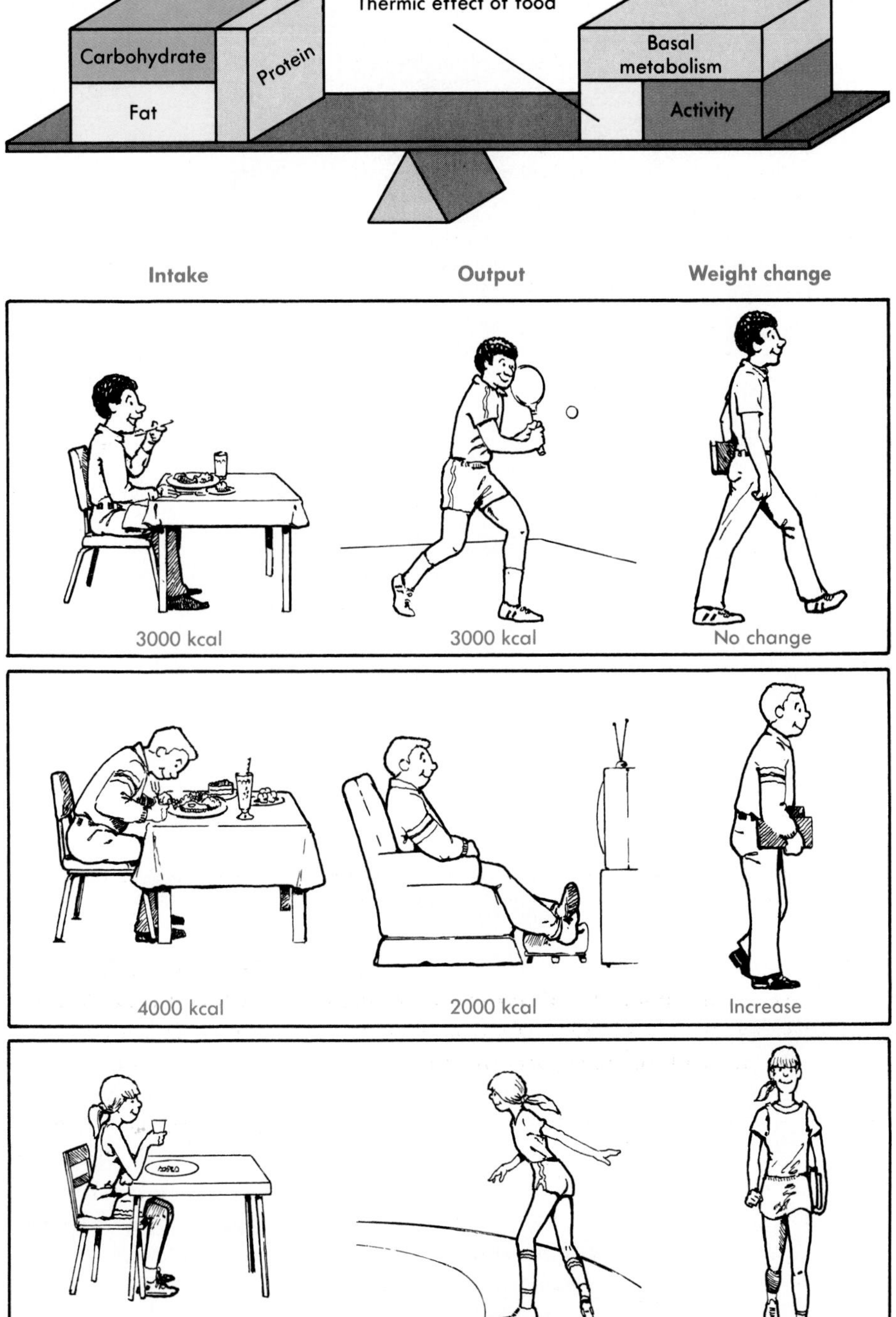

Figure 8-1 A model for energy balance. This model incorporates the major variables that influence energy balance. Alcohol is an additional source of energy for some of us. A fourth form of energy use, adaptive thermogenesis, also contributes to energy balance.

part of the internal network, while eating a piece of cake because it is someone's birthday would be due to external forces—the social setting rather than a physiological response was the key reason the cake was eaten.

hunger The primarily physiological drive to find and eat food. This is mostly driven by internal cues to eating.

Internal forces are linked to what is called **hunger.** For our purposes then, let's define hunger as the primarily physiological forces that encourage us to find and eat food. It stirs the question "When can I eat?"[7] This state is mostly produced by "negative" internal factors, like low blood levels of needed nutrients.[26] External

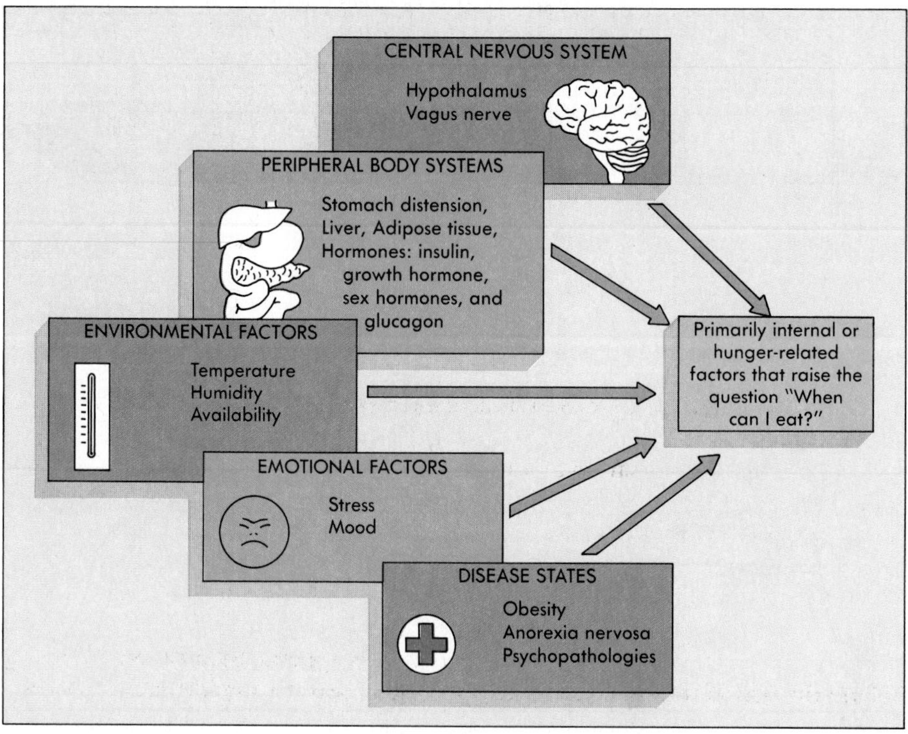

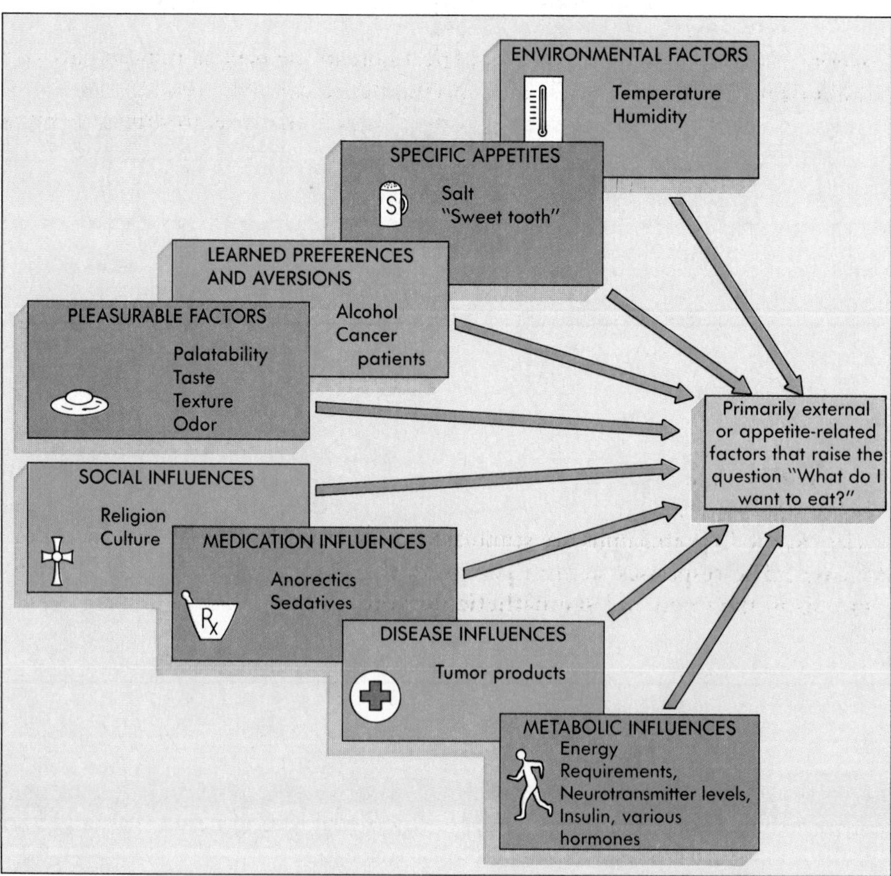

Figure 8-2 A model incorporating many factors that influence satiety. Note that there is some overlap between influences on hunger and appetite. Feeding is regulated by a group of complex and interrelated processes.

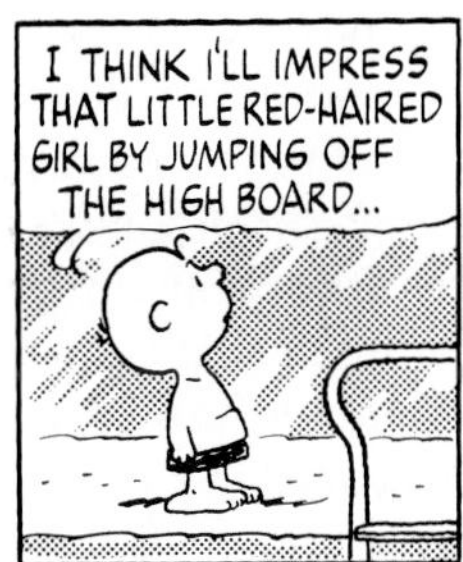
I THINK I'LL IMPRESS THAT LITTLE RED-HAIRED GIRL BY JUMPING OFF THE HIGH BOARD...
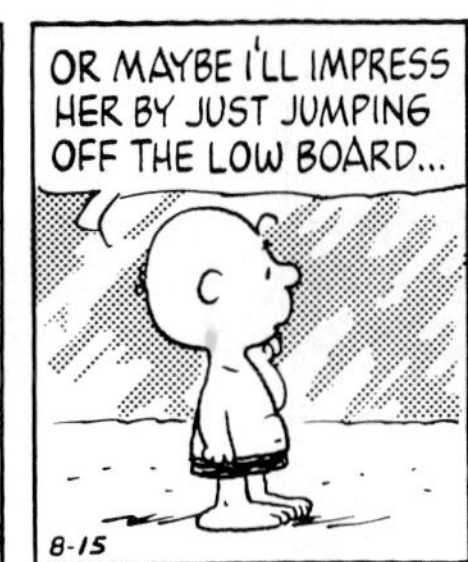
OR MAYBE I'LL IMPRESS HER BY JUST JUMPING OFF THE LOW BOARD...
8-15
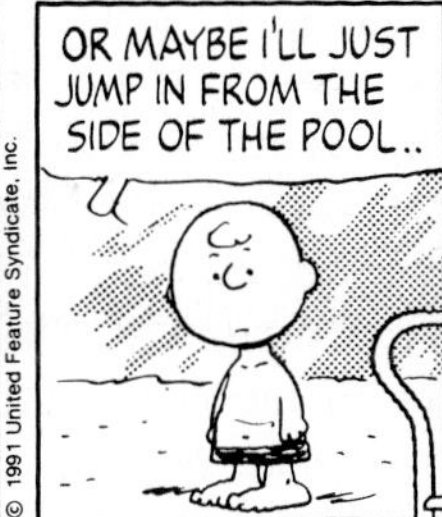
OR MAYBE I'LL JUST JUMP IN FROM THE SIDE OF THE POOL..
© 1991 United Feature Syndicate, Inc.
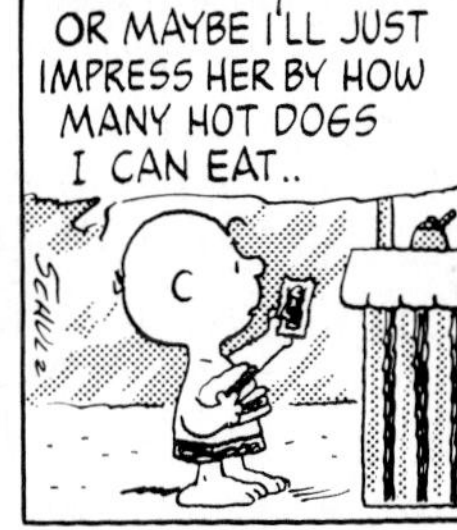
OR MAYBE I'LL JUST IMPRESS HER BY HOW MANY HOT DOGS I CAN EAT..

Figure 8-3 Peanuts.

Reprinted by permission of UFS, Inc.

factors like stress and current environmental temperature also have a role in hunger. Fulfilling this stimulation to eat, and thereby extinguishing the negative stimuli, should lead to a state of **satiety,** meaning the desire to eat ceases, at least for a short time. As you might imagine, together these states—hunger and satiety—and the forces that regulate them greatly influence body weight.

satiety A state in which there is no longer a desire to eat.

At times when internal forces are not driving us to eat, as in the case of just having eaten a large meal, a variety of external forces may influence us to eat, such as consuming another serving of a luscious piece of pie. The question now is more "What do I want to eat?"[7] We will use the term appetite to describe the motive behind this action. In essence, appetite refers to signals that guide dietary selection. You want a piece of pie, you don't want an onion. That process is very different from the rumblings of stomachs that haven't had anything in them for hours, or the feelings of faintness or light-headedness from not eating (i.e., hunger signals). Appetite is mostly based in the psychological state of the person, but can have some physiological dimensions, such as a specific desire for salty foods (Figure 8-2). Furthermore, these forces mostly are "positive" signals that arise to stimulate eating, such as the memory of how good mocha cheesecake tasted the last time you had it.

A CLOSER LOOK AT INTERNAL FORCES INVOLVED IN SATIETY REGULATION

Internal (e.g., physiological) forces, like the levels of nutrients in the blood, neurotransmitter production, levels of circulating hormones and medications, gastrointestinal distention, adipose cell size, and level of physical activity, can affect hunger and satiety (Figure 8-2). Let's look at these forces.

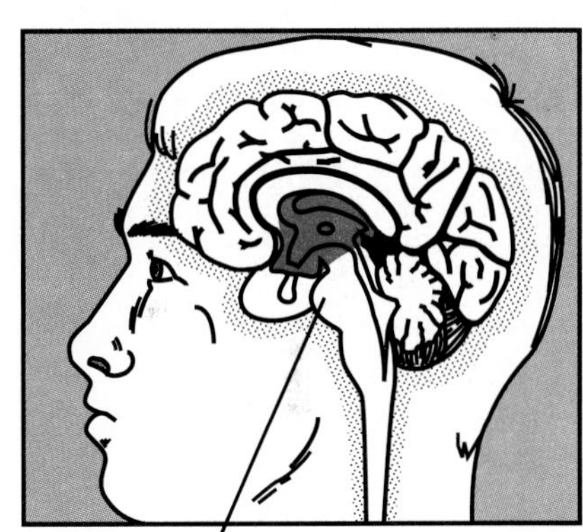

THE HYPOTHALAMUS CONTRIBUTES TO A SATIETY REGULATION

The hypothalamus, a part of the brain, plays a key role in feeding behavior because it helps regulate satiety. Research has shown that when specific groups of cells (called nuclei) in the hypothalamus are stimulated or destroyed, satiety either increases or decreases. The responses stem in part from the changes in both neurotransmitter synthesis in the brain and **sympathetic nervous system** activity.[6] Overall, as sympathetic nervous system activity declines, food intake increases. The opposite is also true.

sympathetic nervous system Part of the nervous system that regulates involuntary vital functions, including the activity of the heart muscle, smooth muscle, and glands. The sympathetic nervous system specifically accelerates heart rate, constricts blood vessels, and raises blood pressure. The parasympathetic nervous system slows heart rate, increases intestinal peristalsis and gland activity, and relaxes sphincters.

Various brain nuclei can be destroyed by specific chemicals, surgery, and certain forms of cancer. When certain cells are destroyed, laboratory animals (and humans) continue to eat until they become quite obese. When other cells are destroyed, animals lose the desire to eat and eventually lose weight. Note that either response is actually quite complex because many nuclei in the vicinity of the destroyed region influence these hypothalamic responses.[26]

THE PRESENCE OF NUTRIENTS IN THE BLOOD

Accumulating evidence from studies on the regulation of hunger—especially from those using laboratory animals—suggests that an underlying hunger for food is never totally absent. After a meal, glucose, fatty acids, amino acids, and other energy-yielding compounds increase in the bloodstream. At this point, and especially as monosaccharides and amino acids are metabolized by the liver, hunger is temporarily shut off.[26] The brain registers satiety. Several hours after eating, when the concentrations of these compounds in the bloodstream begin to fall and the body must begin to pull fuel from body stores, hunger returns. This is because satiety is no longer registered by the metabolism of the energy-yielding compounds just eaten. In other words, feeding signals begin to dominate again. The liver plays a key role in this latter process.

Hunger signals change even while we eat. At the beginning of a meal, we typically consume a variety of foods. By the end of a meal, food choices usually narrow. Consider the last time you went to a buffet. The first trip to the food table you may have chosen some meat, pasta, salad, and something to drink. When you went back, you probably steered toward the cake, pie, and ice cream. Although this may be partly influenced by social custom, and so by mostly appetite cues, research with laboratory animals suggests that this action is also partly physiological. As nutrients are absorbed, the liver and surrounding organs communicate with the brain and change subsequent food choices.[6]

NEUROTRANSMITTER PRODUCTION

histamine A neurotransmitter synthesized from the amino acid histidine that appears to decrease hunger and food intake.

serotonin A neurotransmitter synthesized from the amino acid tryptophan that appears to both decrease the desire to eat carbohydrates and induce sleep.

Studies with rats have shown that deprivation of kcalories and protein may affect neurotransmitter production. Rats placed in a condition of protein-energy malnutrition have a significant decrease in hunger and food intake. It is thought that this is caused by an increase in the production of the neurotransmitter **histamine** in the brain. This is supported by the fact that when rats are given the drug metoprine, which raises brain histamine levels, there is a significant reduction in food intake.[15] Changes in **serotonin** production—another brain neurotransmitter—has also been linked to intake of various nutrients, especially carbohydrate. High levels can calm one's mood and induce sleepiness.

Therefore the presence or lack of certain dietary factors can affect hunger and satiety partly through their effect on neurotransmitter function. It appears then that nutrients or their lack in the blood, as well as variation in neurotransmitter production, are involved in short-term satiety regulation—hour-to-hour and day-to-day. It is an interesting thought that what a person eats can affect mood, behavior, and future food intake.

HORMONAL REGULATION OF FEEDING

endorphins Natural body tranquilizers that may be involved in the feeding response, as well as functioning in pain reduction.

Many hormones, drugs, and hormonelike compounds affect feeding behavior and satiety[3] (Table 8-1). After a meal, blood concentrations of cholecystokinin (CCK), secretin, gastrin, and other hormones increase. These and various other hormone-related compounds increase satiety.[5]

On the other hand, **endorphins,** the body's natural pain killers, and the hormones cortisol and insulin all lead to increased feeding. The presence of cortisol is especially significant if animals are genetically prone to developing obesity. Insulin probably affects both hunger and satiety.[26] As insulin increases liver metabolism of energy-yielding compounds, it promotes satiety. However, after insulin has done its job throughout the body, concentrations of energy-yielding compounds in the bloodstream are low, which causes hunger to return. In general, then, the body's hormonal balance influences the tendency to feel hungry or satiated.

We also see from Table 8-1 that medications like tranquilizers, antidepressants, and cortisone can increase hunger. Others, like antihistamines, often taken to quell pesky allergy symptoms, can increase satiety.

See Chapter 6 to review the role of CCK in digestion, especially in the release of enzymes, bile, and other substances from the pancreas and gallbladder.

GASTROINTESTINAL DISTENTION

As you could logically guess, increased pressure in the stomach and intestines, caused almost notably by food and drink, can increase satiety, especially large meals. In

Table 8-1 Hormones, hormone-like compounds, and medications that affect feeding behavior[8]

Increase food intake	Decrease food intake
Insulin*	Insulin*
Endorphins	Cholecystokinin (CCK)
Norepinephrine	Bombesin
Cortisol	Serotonin
Neuropeptide Y	Calcitonin
Galadin	Glucagon
Tranquilizers	Somatostatin
Antidepressants	Vasoactive inhibitory peptide (VIP)
Growth hormone-releasing hormone	Cortiocotropin-releasing factor
	Thyrotropin-releasing factor
	Neurotensin
	Amphetamines
	Antihistamines
	Fenfluramine
	Tumor necrosis factor (cachectin; a factor produced by immune cells)
	Nicotine
	Histamine
	Dehydroepiandrosterone
	Enterostatin

*Insulin leads to satiety as energy-yielding compounds are being put into use and storage. Once the energy-yielding nutrients fall in concentration in the bloodstream and their rate of liver metabolism slows, hunger returns. Since insulin action leads to both energy nutrient use and eventual depletion from the bloodstream, it needs to appear in both columns.

experiments with animals the hormone CCK and **gastrointestinal distention** appear to work together to quell hunger.

gastrointestinal distention Expansion of the walls of the stomach or intestines due to pressure caused by the presence of gases, food, drink, or other factors.

ADIPOSE CELL SIZE

Let's say your adipose cells have a size considered normal for the general population. One line of research suggests that adipose cells make a protein called adipsin, which reduces sensations of hunger. As your cells get larger, a lot of **adipsin** would be produced, shutting off hunger and decreasing the likelihood that the cells will continue to grow larger. In contrast, if fat is lost from those normal-sized cells the production of adipsin would be reduced, increasing sensations of hunger. This would promote increased food intake and the filling of these cells.

adipsin A protein that appears to be made by adipose cells and acts as a communication link between adipose cells and the brain.

In addition, as adipose cells get larger, they tend to become resistant to insulin.[9] Insulin stimulates fat uptake and storage in adipose cells. As these cells get larger they become less responsive to insulin, leading to less fat storage. In these ways adipose cells can to some degree limit their size. Current research suggests that the size of adipose cells is involved in the long-term regulation of satiety, over months and years. For more information on adipose cells and their link to obesity see the Expert Opinion by Dr. Jules Hirsch and the Nutrition Perspective at the end of this chapter on the set-point theory.

LEVEL OF PHYSICAL ACTIVITY

Does physical activity increase or decrease hunger in humans, and in turn food intake? Studies show varying results, and there is much controversy surrounding this issue. It appears that lean individuals do compensate for increased energy ex-

EXPERT OPINION

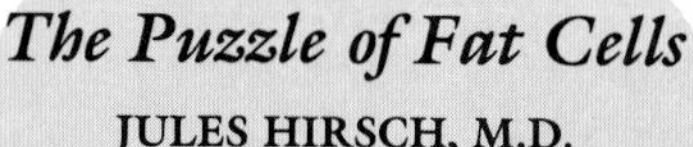

The Puzzle of Fat Cells

JULES HIRSCH, M.D.

All the fat (triglyceride) that causes either overweight or obesity is stored in a special tissue called adipose tissue. There is a large amount of adipose tissue even in people of normal weight. For example, a healthy, nonobese 68-kilogram (150-pound) man might carry as much as 9 kilograms (20 pounds) of fat. If he were to enter the ranks of the obese by gaining 13 kilograms (30 pounds), most of the weight gain would be an increase in the amount of stored fat, to roughly 18 kilograms (40 pounds). Some of the weight gain would be in nonfatty tissue, but the majority would be fat.

Adipose tissue and its cells

Like all tissues, adipose tissue is composed of many cells. Some are capillaries or fibroblasts that nourish and hold the characteristic cells (adipocytes) in place. About half the adipose tissue in an average person lies in subcutaneous depots just beneath the skin; the remainder mostly is in deeper depots found in the abdomen.

Small samples of fat can be safely and easily obtained for scientific study by slipping a small needle just beneath the skin, much as one might do to obtain a blood sample. When the fat is examined under the microscope, it's clear that there are numerous round fat cells. These small cells are practically invisible to the naked eye; it would take several hundred lined up in a row to make 1 inch.

By volume, roughly 90% of the cell is a single droplet of fat. The central oil droplet in each adipocyte is surrounded by a thin rim of cytoplasm (the protoplasm of a cell outside the nucleus) with the usual active cellular machinery. Although a nucleus is present in each cell, it is rare to find adipocytes dividing. So this tissue "turns over" very slowly, if at all, in adults—in sharp contrast to the rapidly dividing cells found in the liver, bone marrow, and the gastrointestinal tract.

The triglyceride in the oil droplet is released under the action of a particular enzyme known as hormone-sensitive lipase. The enzyme reacts to norepinephrine, epinephrine, and other hormones found in the bloodstream. When activated, this enzyme leads to the release of the fatty acids and glycerol. The tissue can also take up fatty acids, relink them with glycerol, and deposit this fat within the cell. The hormone insulin and the level of blood glucose help control the rate of fatty acid uptake and release from adipose tissue. This cycle of fat breakdown and reconstruction happens quite rapidly, thereby assuring that fatty acids and glycerol are always present in the bloodstream, even during fasts.

Larger cells—and more of them

An average fat cell contains about a half microgram (half a millionth of a gram) of triglyceride. To store the many pounds of fat present, it takes roughly 30 billion adipocytes in a normal, nonobese person. In all persons who become obese, these billions of cells tend to get larger. And the grossly obese are apt to have an even greater number of them; that is, morbidly obese people, who are more than double their desirable weight, are likely to have more and larger fat cells.

It is notable that with weight reduction the main change in adipocytes is a decrease in size. Fat cells, once filled with fat, do not disappear easily or at all in the adult state. Thus the formerly obese person persists in having a higher than normal cell number. Whether or not this increased number would ever disappear if the weight were kept down for many years remains arguable. Most evidence indicates that it wouldn't.

There is debate as to whether the increased number of small fat cells found in formerly obese individuals is implicated in the frequent weight regain. Is there such a thing as a starved fat cell? If so, how does this starved cell inform headquarters—the central nervous system with its feeding centers—that more food should be consumed and this obesity restored? These matters are under study, but there is as yet no proof that such signals from fat cells can influence food intake and the presence of absence of obesity.

Many studies have shown that neither animals nor humans are born with their full complement of fat cells. During various stages of growth and development, fat cells increase in number, and to some degree in size. In general, fat cells tend to be made early in life, and the change in number dwindles over time. Yet, it has been shown that fat cells in experimentally overfed animals not only enlarge but also can increase in number. These cells, once formed, do not readily disappear.

Frontiers in obesity research

An exciting chapter from obesity research has been the demonstration that the thin rim of cytoplasm in the adipocyte does more than release and take up fatty acids. It also is responsible for the synthesis of proteins. One of these, known as lipoprotein lipase, is an enzyme that leaves the fat cells and is transported to a nearby capillary, where it functions to break down triglycerides and make them available for deposit in adipose tissue. The amount of this special enzyme increases during abundant feeding and obesity and tends to decrease during starvation. What role this seesawing plays in shuttling fat in and out of adipocytes and in the control of fat cell size is yet to be delineated. Another enzyme, adipsin, has recently been found to be made in fat cells and secreted into the bloodstream. Adipsin amounts are unusually low in certain obesities that occur genetically in rodents. What role this enzyme has, if any, in the production and perpetuation of obesity is yet to be defined.

Fat cells remain somewhat of a puzzle. We know that they are the cells for fat storage in the body and that in the obese they are always enlarged and sometimes more numerous than in leaner persons. But their metabolic activity, influence on body weight regulation, and the steps in their development still remain central questions for the study of human nutrition.

Dr. Hirsch is professor of medicine and senior physician at Rockefeller University.

penditure and adjust food intake upward to maintain their body composition. However, in many obese individuals energy expenditure, hunger, and food intake appear to be independent. Obese people at least don't seem to have increased hunger and food intake after exercise than would normally be expected.

EXTERNAL FORCES THAT AFFECT SATIETY

We have examined primarily physiological forces that influence hunger and satiety. These have been termed internal forces, raising the question "When can I eat?" Let's now look at psychological and environmental forces that influence eating behavior in more appetite-related ways (Figure 8-2). Again, these raise the question "What do I want to eat?"[7]

Psychological factors, like emotional states and personal beliefs, can affect our desire to eat. As we mentioned before, depressed individuals may have decreased or increased hunger. This could be the result of past experiences, when eating made them feel better or worse during a crisis. Eating or not eating may have become conditioned to experiences of stress in life. Personal beliefs, such as "eating chocolate makes me feel better" or "food will make me fat and I must avoid it at all costs," can steer us toward or away from eating.

Environmental factors, such as availability of food, time of day, social obligations, characteristics of a specific food, and temperature and humidity can influence hunger. Have you ever wondered why supermarkets are so cold? This may increase hunger and the likelihood of you buying more food. In addition, those environmental factors that get paired time-wise with eating can later, by themselves, elicit us to eat. If you have always eaten lunch at noon, you are likely to desire food at that time each day, even if no physiological forces are driving you to eat.

Social customs, peers, and authority figures can influence the desire to eat. Concern about appearance when on a date can influence the food choices one might make. A woman concerned about looking "petite" may choose a smaller portion of food than when alone. We also are likely to eat more at a meal when with a large group of people than when with a few people.

Taste, texture, temperature, color of the food, previous experiences with food, as well as the variety provided, can influence food intake. Sour and bitter flavors may decrease a person's willingness to eat. Many people would be "turned off" by coffee that has become cold even if the caffeine is desired. Providing a greater variety of foods at a meal can stimulate greater food intake than a monotonous presentation. Visual and taste stimulation also can cause something called cephalic phase responses by the body. Saliva will flow and digestive hormones and insulin are released in response to seeing and initially tasting that favorite hamburger. These responses are likely to play a role in promoting food intake.

In the United States food intake is stimulated to a greater extent by appetite-related forces rather than hunger-related forces. Instead of attending to internal signals, like a full stomach, we are more likely to eat primarily because food intake has been associated with social acts, such as dinnertime, watching television, or mere availability.

PUTTING HUNGER AND SATIETY INTO PERSPECTIVE

Next time you wonder why you are eating, you will know numerous physiological and more social forces are involved. Cells in the brain, oral cavity, stomach, intestine, liver, and other organs; hormones (insulin and cortisol) and neurotransmitters (serotonin and histamine); and family customs, habits, and religion all influence food intake. Though appetite-related forces probably predominate in humans who have foods available, hunger-related forces predominate in laboratory animals. Keep track of what drives you to eat during the next few days—whether appetite related or hunger related.

CONCEPT CHECK

Hunger is the primarily physiological or internal desire to find and eat food. Appeasing it should leave you in a satiated state—you have no further desire to eat. Satiety is influenced by hunger-related (internal) factors like the brain, adipose tissue, livers, other organs, various hormones, and hormonelike compounds. Food intake is also affected by appetite-related (external) forces like social custom, time of day, palatability, and others. Americans probably respond more to external appetite-related forces rather than hunger-related ones in choosing when and what to eat.

Energy Use: The Other Side of Energy Balance

We have examined some stimuli for consuming energy. Now let's look at the other side of the relationship—energy output.

ENERGY USE BY THE BODY

The body uses energy for four general purposes; **basal metabolism, thermic effect of food,** and physical activity are the most important (Figure 8-1). A fourth use—adaptive thermogenesis—is heat production during long-term caloric excess or exposure to cold temperatures.

Basal Metabolism

Basal metabolism represents the minimum energy it takes to keep the resting, awake body alive. This includes maintaining a heart beat, respiration, temperature, and other functions.[20] It does not include energy needs for activity or digesting foods. Basal metabolism amounts to about 1 kcalorie per kilogram of body weight per hour in men and 0.9 kcalorie per kilogram of body weight per hour in women (or roughly 1 kcalorie per minute).

To determine a person's basal metabolic rate (BMR), he or she must just have woken up, be in a warm room, stay as relaxed as possible, and must not have eaten for at least 12 hours. Oxygen consumption (and usually carbon dioxide output) is measured for approximately 20 to 30 minutes. This then would be used to calculate kcalorie use (see the section on indirect calorimetry). A less accurate value, the **resting metabolic rate** (RMR), is derived when measuring energy use under less stringent conditions. The person has not eaten for at least a few hours and is at rest. RMR is often slightly higher than BMR; however, these often differ by less than 3%. The terms BMR and RMR often are used interchangeably.

About 75% to 80% of basal metabolism depends on the amount of **lean body mass.**[20] The tissues involved—especially heart, liver, brain, and kidney—show high metabolic activity at rest, and so greatly influence kcalorie needs in that state. Other influences on basal metabolism are gender (males have higher rates because of a higher lean body mass), temperature (fever increases metabolic rate), thyroid hormone levels, age, starvation, surface area (tall people have more surface area than short, stubby people and so have a higher metabolic rate due to corresponding heat loss), and pregnancy (Table 8-2).

A low-kcalorie intake decreases BMR about 10% to 20% (about 150 to 300 kcalories per day). This reduction makes continued dieting success even harder (see Chapter 9). In addition, it is hard to maintain a desirable body weight as we age because BMR declines approximately 2% every 10 years after age 30. This is mostly caused by a slow and steady decrease in actively metabolizing cells, which is due to aging (see Chapter 18). However, people who remain active into their elderly years do not show such a great decline in basal metabolism because lean body mass is better maintained.

basal metabolism The minimum energy the body requires to support itself when resting and just awakened. To have basal metabolic rate (BMR) measured, a person must fast for the previous 12 hours and must be maintained in a warm, quiet environment during the measurement. It amounts to roughly 1 kcalorie per minute, or about 1400 kcalories per day.

thermic effect of food The increase in metabolism occurring during the digestion, absorption, and metabolism of energy-yielding nutrients. This represents 5% to 10% of kcalories consumed.

resting metabolic rate The number of kcalories used during rest, without stringently controlling recent physical activity.

lean body mass Body weight minus fat storage weight equals lean body mass. This includes organs like the brain, muscles, and liver, as well as blood and other body fluids.

Table 8-2 Factors that increase and decrease basal metabolism

Increase	Decrease
Muscle mass (fat-free mass)	Age (primarily if lean body mass decreases)
Fever	Reduction in energy intake
Recent food intake	Genetics
Ovulation	
Surface area	
Recent exercise	
Thyroid hormone level	
Trauma	
Epinephrine	
Male gender (greater lean body mass)	
Pregnancy	
Genetics	

Within the general population there is a variation in BMR of about 25% to 30%.[21] In addition, BMR usually accounts for about 70% of daily energy expenditure in sedentary people.

Thermic Effect of Food

Thermic effect of food (TEF) represents the amount of extra energy used by the body during digestion, absorption, metabolism, and storage of energy-yielding nutrients.[20] It is equivalent to 5% to 10% of total kcalories consumed. To supply the body with 100 kcalories, a person must eat between 105 and 110 kcalories. The process of digestion, absorption, and metabolism uses the extra 5 to 10 kcalories to modify the nutrients so that they are more available for use. Given a daily kcalorie intake of 3000, the thermic effect of food would use 180 to 300 kcalories. The value for the thermic effect of food for either a pure-carbohydrate or pure-protein diet is higher than that for a pure-fat diet. This is true because it takes less energy to turn absorbed fat into fat stores than glucose into glycogen or amino acids into protein. Large meals have shown higher values for TEF compared to the same amount of food eaten over many hours.

Other names for the thermic effect of food include specific dynamic action and diet-induced thermogenesis.

Physical Activity

Body energy also fuels physical activity. Physical activity is the aspect of energy expenditure over which we have the most control. The biggest difference in energy use among people is due to different activity levels. Some people are very active physically and others are very sedentary. Together, basal metabolism and the thermic effect of food represent about 80% of total energy use. This means that physical activity accounts for roughly 20% of energy expenditure in sedentary people.

Energy used for physical activity includes expenditures for sports, such as handball and bicycling, and for everyday activities. Using stairs rather than the elevator, parking your car in the most distant lot, and standing in a bus rather than sitting all increase physical activity and hence energy use. Studies show that people who fidget and can't sit still use more energy (an extra 100 to 800 kcalories per day in one study) than those who are generally quite relaxed.[21] As we will discuss in Chapter 9, the rates of obesity in America are alarming. We do not eat so many more kcalories than people did at the turn of this century, but as a group we are considerably less active. This inactivity contributes to our increased rates of obesity.

Because most of the energy for physical activity is converted to heat, this contributor to energy expenditure is often called the thermic effect of exercise.

adaptive thermogenesis Adaptive energy expended, resulting in the heat thermogenesis production, due to exposure to cold environmental conditions or overfeeding.

brown adipose tissue A specialized form of adipose tissue that produces large amounts of heat by metabolizing energy-yielding nutrients without synthesizing much ATP. The energy released simply forms heat.

Adaptive Thermogenesis

Adaptive thermogenesis is energy expended that is expressed as heat production due to exposure to stimuli, such as cold environmental conditions and overfeeding. Heat is produced without work being done. This subject has produced much controversy and interest. Much of the work on this topic deals with the fact that when people were overfed in some studies, they did not gain the amount of weight that might be expected.

In many animals—including humans to an undetermined extent—adaptive thermogenesis is linked to the presence of **brown adipose tissue.** Most fat is stored in white adipose tissue. Brown adipose tissue is less than 1% of body weight in humans. This tissue represents a specialized form of fat storage found primarily in the shoulder area. For hibernating animals it is a main source of heat during their long winter sleep. The brown tint derives from (1) the ample content of arteries and veins that supply the tissue with blood, (2) the numerous mitochondria that are present to allow for enhanced energy metabolism, and (3) myoglobin that is part of the structural material and present for oxygen transport.

Brown adipose tissue yields heat by failing to form much ATP during the metabolism of energy-yielding nutrients. Most energy is simply lost as heat. Thus these cells have the ability to make a lot of heat and, in turn, "waste" a lot of potentially useful energy.

Decreased activity of brown adipose tissue during overfeeding and cold adaptation is associated with obesity in rats. Researchers are not in agreement, but there is some evidence that impaired adaptive thermogenesis due to abnormalities in the functioning of brown adipose tissue may be a factor in human obesity. Activation of some arms of the nervous system (sympathetic nervous system) in response to overfeeding and cold may be the link between these stimuli and activity of brown adipose tissue. Drugs like ephedrine, caffeine, and nicotine increase energy expenditure partially through their ability to increase the activity of the sympathetic nervous system.[6] They appear to increase adaptive thermogenesis and reduce hunger.

Currently the extent to which brown adipose tissue is both present and operative in humans has not been clearly determined. If you touch an infant's back, you can feel the heat produced by the brown adipose tissue. Sensitive instruments can demonstrate hotter spots around the shoulder area of adults, as well. However, it is difficult to determine how much heat production this represents in adults. Although it is unlikely that brown adipose tissue serves a pivotal role in weight regulation in adults, information is too sketchy to permit any definite conclusions. It is estimated that overall, adaptive thermogenesis represents about 10% of energy use.

CONCEPT CHECK

There are four factors that contribute to energy expenditure. Basal metabolism represents the minimum amount of energy needed to maintain a body in a resting state. The amount of a person's basal metabolism depends greatly on the amount of lean body mass, amount of surface area, and thyroid hormone levels. The thermic effect of food represents the additional energy needed to digest, absorb, and process absorbed nutrients. This corresponds to about 5% to 10% of total kcalorie use. Physical activity represents energy use above what is needed for basal metabolism and the thermic effect of food. Adaptive thermogenesis is heat production in response to cold or overfeeding. This phenomenon may be linked to the presence of brown adipose tissue. In a sedentary person, 80% of energy is used for basal metabolism and the thermic effect of food; the remainder is used for physical activity and adaptive thermogenesis.

Determining Energy Use by the Body

DIRECT AND INDIRECT CALORIMETRY

There are two primary ways to measure the amount of energy the body uses: **direct calorimetry** and **indirect calorimetry.** When using direct calorimetry, a person is put into an insulated chamber and the heat released is calculated by measuring the increase in the temperature of a layer of water surrounding the chamber. Recall that a kcalorie is defined as the amount of heat it takes to raise the temperature of 1 liter of water 1° Celsius. By measuring temperature of the water surrounding the direct calorimeter before and after the study, the number of kcalories used can be determined. This method resembles that of using the bomb calorimeter to measure the kcalorie content of a food (see Chapter 1). Direct calorimetry works because all the energy used by the body eventually leaves as heat.

direct calorimetry A method to determine energy use by the body by measuring heat that emanates from the body, usually using an insulated chamber.

indirect calorimetry A method to measure the energy output by the body by measuring oxygen uptake (and often carbon dioxide output as well) by the body, and then using formulas to convert that gas exchange into kcalorie use.

Older direct calorimeters were quite large, about the size of a small room. Newer calorimeters are the size of a phone booth or even smaller, about the size of a space suit. Nevertheless, few studies use direct calorimetry, mostly because of its expense and complexity.

In using indirect calorimetry, instead of measuring heat, a technician measures either a person's oxygen uptake or oxygen uptake plus the carbon dioxide produced (Figure 8-4). There is a predictable relationship between the body's use of energy and its use of oxygen or carbon dioxide output. For example, when burning a mixed diet of carbohydrate, fat, and protein, the body uses 1 liter of oxygen to burn about 4.85 kcalories. Generally, this mixture of nutrients is just the fuel the body uses.

Instruments used to measure oxygen consumption (and often carbon dioxide output too) for indirect calorimetry are widely available. They can be mounted on carts and rolled up to a hospital bed or carried in backpacks while a person plays tennis or jogs. Tables showing the amount of energy used to perform various exercises rely on indirect calorimetry to calculate their figures (see Appendix L).

The newest approach to indirect calorimetry has a person consume isotopically labeled water ($^2H_2{}^{18}O$).[23] A technician measures the ^2H_2O and the $H_2{}^{18}O$ later found in body fluids, such as urine. Using these values and some formulas, total carbon dioxide (CO_2) output per day can then be estimated. This CO_2 value then can be converted into energy use, just as is done with oxygen use in indirect calorimetry. Both ^2H and ^{18}O represent stable isotopes of hydrogen and oxygen; special equipment can measure them.

This isotope method is quite accurate but also very expensive. With wider use, we expect it to soon extend our knowledge of variation in energy use by people over entire day-long periods. This information may further reveal why some people can more easily regulate their body weight than others.

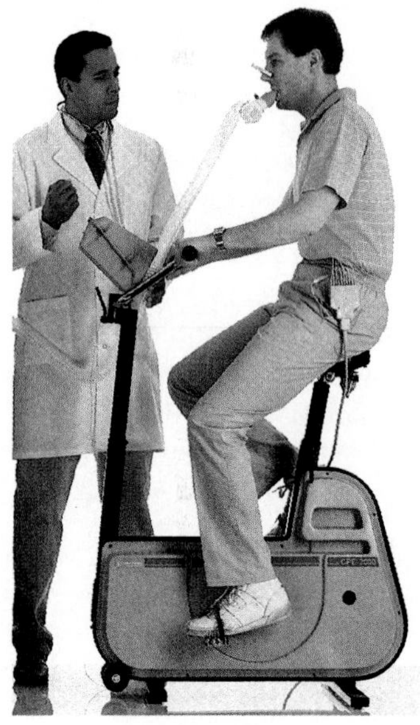

Figure 8-4 Indirect calorimetry. This method can be used to measure energy output during daily activities.

ESTIMATING ENERGY NEEDS

A variety of formulas can estimate the body's resting energy needs (see Appendix J). The **Harris-Benedict equation,** widely used by registered dietitians for hospitalized patients, considers weight, height, and age. The Nutrition Focus on page 246 illustrates how to use the Harris-Benedict equation. The value for resting energy needs is then increased by predetermined factors to reflect a patient's degree of illness. That value then gives total energy needs. Owen and others have published standards for resting energy needs based on weight alone.[18] Still other formulas are based on a person's lean body mass. The equations apply to both normal-weight and overweight people. All of these formulas yield reasonable estimates.

Total energy needs can be roughly estimated using the RDA. This provides average values for people who perform light activity (see inside cover). Another rough estimate uses a person's weight and activity level. Sedentary energy needs are set at 9 to 10 kcalories per pound. The value is then decreased by 100 kcalories for every 10 years of age over age 30. Light activity starts with 12 to 13 kcalories per

Harris-Benedict Equations An equation that predicts resting metabolic rate based on a person's weight, height, and age.

NUTRITION FOCUS

Calculating Energy Use

The following illustrates how to estimate energy expenditure using the previous information given. You will notice that adaptive thermogenesis is not included because of limited knowledge regarding its contribution.

Bill weighs 154 pounds (70 kilograms), is 5′9″ tall (175 centimeters), 35 years of age, and is involved in moderate muscular activity each day.

Basal metabolism

Use the value: 1.0 kcal/kg body weight/hour for **MEN.**
0.9 kcal/kg body weight/hour for **WOMEN.**

For Bill:

1. multiply his weight in kilograms by the appropriate value for men.
   70 kg × 1 kcal/kg/hour = 70 kcal/hr.
2. multiply kcalories used in an hour by hours in a day.
   70 kcal/hr × 24 hr/day = 1680 kcal/day.
   Basal Metabolism = 1680 kcal/day.

Physical activity

Select one of the following categories based on the amount of muscular activity performed in a day.

sedentary activity (mostly sitting): add 20% to 40% of BMR.

light activity (a clerk involved in a daily walking program): add 55% to 65% of BMR.

moderate activity (a teacher involved in daily vigorous exercise): add 70% to 75% of BMR.

heavy activity (a mail carrier who walks the route or an adult involved in a daily exercise program): add 80% to 100% of BMR.

For Bill doing moderate activity:

1. take 70% of his basal metabolism.
   1680 kcal/day × .70 = 1176 kcal/day.
   Physical activity = 1176 kcal/day.

Thermic effect of food

A quick way to approximate this is to take 10% of the sum of the BMR and physical activity kcalories.

For Bill:

1. 1680 kcal/day + 1176 kcal/day = 2856 kcal/day.
2. 2856 kcal/day × .10 = 286 kcal/day.
   Thermic effect of food = 286 kcal/day.

Total energy use

Sum the kcalorie contributions from each factor.

For Bill:

1680 kcal/day + 1176 kcal/day + 286 kcal/day = 3142 kcal/day.

Total energy use = 3142 kcal/day.

Calculating Resting Energy Use Using Harris-Benedict Equations

Remember that previously we estimated Bill's total energy use. Let's calculate Bill's resting energy expediture using the appropriate Harris-Benedict Equation that can be found in Appendix N and compare it to the amount of basal metabolism we determined for him.

Harris-Benedict equation:

66.5 + 13.8 (weight in kilograms) + 5 (height in centimeters) − 6.76 (age in years)

Bill weighs 70 kilograms, is 175 centimeters tall, and is 35 years of age. Therefore Bill's resting energy expenditure is as follows:

66.5 + 13.8 (70 kg) + 5 (175 cm) − 6.76 (35) = 1671 kcal/day.

Resting Energy Use = 1671 kcal/day

Now compare this to the estimate of basal metabolism of 1680 kcal/day we determined previously. You can see that the values are not very different.

pound; heavy activity starts at 20 kcalories per pound; values are then adjusted for age.

A simple method for tracking your energy expenditure, and so energy needs, is to use the forms in Appendix E and the table that lists the energy costs of a variety of activities in Appendix L. The values account for energy use due to basal metabolism, the thermic effect of food, as well as physical activity. Begin by taking an entire 24-hour period and list all activities done, including sleep. Record the number of minutes you spent doing each activity. The total minutes should equal 1440 minutes (24 hours). Next record the energy cost for each activity in kcals per minute, based on your weight in kilograms (pounds ÷ 2.2). Multiply the energy cost by the minutes. This gives the kcalories expended for each activity. Total the activity kcalories. This will give your estimated energy expenditure for the day.

CONCEPT CHECK

Energy use by the body can be measured by direct calorimetry as heat given off, and by indirect calorimetry as oxygen uptake (with or without carbon dioxide output). Energy needs, both resting and total, can be estimated using formulas based on factors such as a person's weight, height, and age, or simply on a person's weight.

Energy Imbalance

If energy intake exceeds expenditure over a period of time **obesity** is likely to result. In this content, medical experts believe that a healthy weight for a person should not be based primarily on body weight, but rather on the total amount of fat in the body, the location of body fat, and the presence or absence of weight-related medical problems.[4]

obesity A condition characterized by excess body fat. In clinical settings it is usually defined as a body mass index above 30 or weighing 20% above desirable weight.

DEFINING OBESITY—OVERWEIGHT VERSUS OVERFAT

Obesity can be defined using several different approaches. Here we will consider definitions based on body fat, body weight for height, fat distribution, and age of onset. Again, the focus on the amount and location of fat is the key consideration.

Using Body Fat

References to the risks of being overweight actually refer only to people who are overfat. Body fat can range from 2% to upwards of 70% of body weight. In this regard, men having over 25% body fat and women having over 30% body fat are considered obese. More desirable figures are 15% to 18% body fat for men and 20% to 25% fat for women. Women need more body fat because some "sex-specific" fat is associated with their reproductive functions. This extra fat is normal and therefore is factored into calculations of body composition (Figure 8-5).

A variety of methods can be used to determine how much fat a person contains.[12] The most widely used method measures skinfold thicknesses. Over half of body fat lies directly under the skin. Clinicians use a special caliper to measure this fat layer. The amount of fat under the skin (subcutaneous) in turn reflects the fat composition

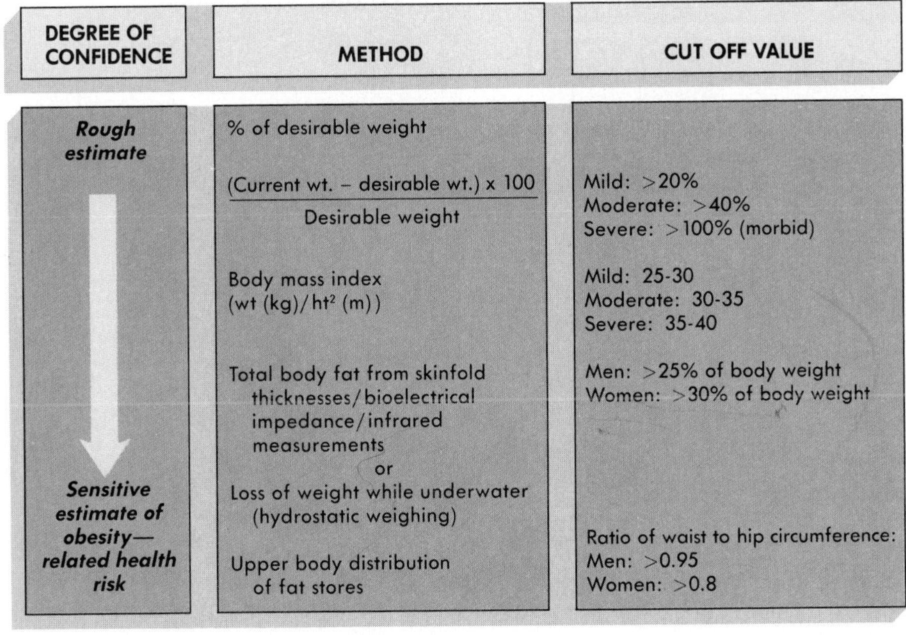

DEGREE OF CONFIDENCE	METHOD	CUT OFF VALUE
Rough estimate	% of desirable weight (Current wt. – desirable wt.) x 100 / Desirable weight	Mild: >20% Moderate: >40% Severe: >100% (morbid)
↓	Body mass index (wt (kg)/ht² (m))	Mild: 25-30 Moderate: 30-35 Severe: 35-40
	Total body fat from skinfold thicknesses/bioelectrical impedance/infrared measurements or Loss of weight while underwater (hydrostatic weighing)	Men: >25% of body weight Women: >30% of body weight
Sensitive estimate of obesity—related health risk	Upper body distribution of fat stores	Ratio of waist to hip circumference: Men: >0.95 Women: >0.8

Figure 8-5 Diagnosing the extent of obesity to predict health risk. If one is obese by any of these measures and has an android distribution of fat stores, the risk of complications is more likely than if the fat distribution is gynecoid. Convert height and weight values to metric units before performing the BMI calculation.

bioelectrical impedance A method to estimate total body fat that measures the impedance (resistance) of a low-energy electrical current by the body; the more fat storage a person has, the more impedance to electrical flow will be exhibited.

underwater weighing A method to estimate total body fat by weighing individuals under water; the more fat a person has the less he or she will weigh under water.

of the body. Better methods use three or four skinfold measurements taken throughout the body to estimate total body fat (Figure 8-6). With practice, these measurements take less than 10 minutes, and the body fat values that are calculated end up quite accurate. Very obese people are hard to measure, however, due to the size of the skinfolds.

Clinicians have recently begun to measure body fat storage using **bioelectrical impedance** (Figure 8-7). This technique uses a low-energy electrical current. Fat resists the flow of electricity. Thus the more fat storage a person has per inch of height, the more resistance. Bioelectrical impedance analyzers convert body electrical resistance into an estimate of the percentage of body fat. The test takes only about 5 minutes.

Another new method for estimating body fat uses infrared light interactions with the fat and protein in arm muscle. A device the size of a flashlight is held on the biceps muscle. Total body fat is then estimated after 2 seconds of infrared exposure.

Skinfold thicknesses and bioelectrical impedance methods were developed using body fat values determined by **underwater weighing** for comparison. Comparing a person's weight on land to that person's weight underwater can yield a very accurate estimate of body fat. This works because adipose tissue is less dense than lean tissue,

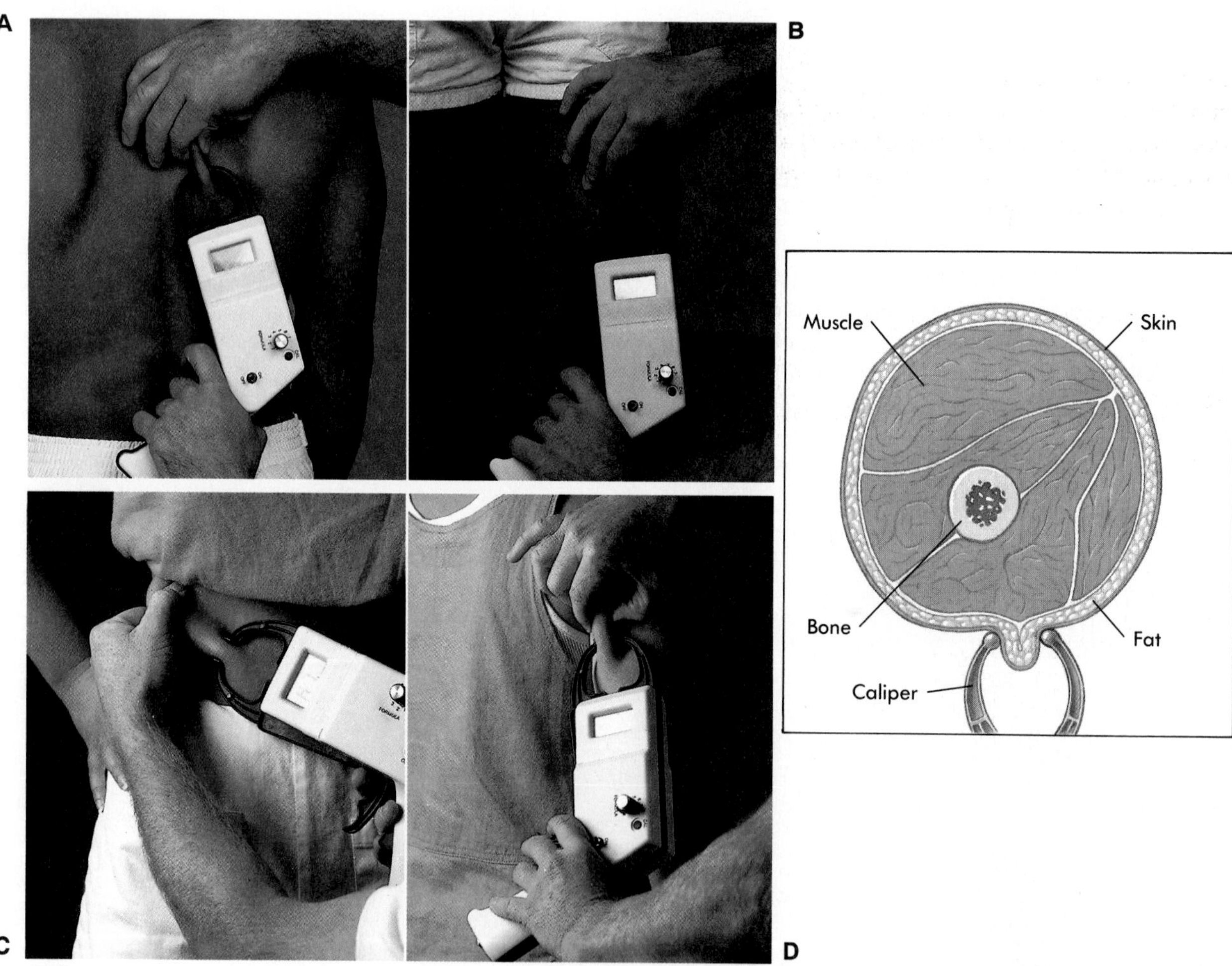

Figure 8-6 Skinfold measurements. Using a proper technique, calibrated equipment, and standards, skinfold measurements can be used to accurately predict body fat content in about 20 minutes. Commonly measured skinfolds are **A,** subscapular, **B,** thigh, **C,** suprailiac, and **D,** triceps.

and so the more adipose tissue in a body, the less a person weighs when submerged (the more he or she tends to float). This is one of the most accurate ways to measure body fat, but it requires expensive equipment that is not widely available.

Using Body Fat Distribution

Calculating distribution of fat stores, in addition to the amount of fat, is also instrumental in assessing obesity—especially for predicting health risks[4] (Figure 8-5). Obese people can be categorized as **android** or **gynecoid** (sometimes called gynoid) (Figure 8-8). Android obesity is the characteristic male obesity with a large abdomen (pot belly) and small buttocks and thighs (apple appearance). High blood testosterone and cortisol levels, as well as increased sympathetic nervous system activity levels, are thought to encourage upper body fat deposition.[3] Fat storage in this area appears to be easier to lose than in the thigh area.

android obesity The type of obesity in which fat is stored primarily in the abdominal area; defined as a waist-to-hip circumference ratio greater than 0.95 in men and 0.8 in women; closely associated with a high risk of heart disease, hypertension, and diabetes.

gynecoid obesity Obesity in which fat storage is primarily located in the buttocks and thigh area.

Gynecoid obesity is the typical female obesity pattern showing a moderate abdomen and much larger buttocks and thigh area (pear appearance). Women tend to have this type of obesity. A low blood-cortisol level and high estrogen level relative to the testosterone level encourage this type of development. The cells in this area contain more lipoprotein lipase, the enzyme that pushes fat from the bloodstream into fat cells. Furthermore, progesterone, a female hormone, increases the action of lipoprotein lipase in the lower torso region.[3] Thus there are biological reasons why men tend to primarily have android fat distribution and women tend to primarily have gynecoid fat distribution.

A ratio of waist circumference (at the level of the umbilicus with stomach relaxed) to maximum hip circumference greater than 0.95 in men and 0.8 in women indicates android obesity. The android form of obesity is associated with more heart disease, hypertension, and diabetes than is gynecoid obesity.[4] This may be because adipose tissue in the abdominal area more greatly resists the action of insulin, in turn increasing the risk of developing diabetes. In addition, fats released from this site appear rapidly in the liver. This in turn interferes with the liver's ability to clear fat from the bloodstream. This can lead to further insulin resistance. The development of diabetes then leads to an increased risk for heart disease and hypertension. Data from the Honolulu Heart Study show that an android shape can increase health risks in men even if they are not obese. Overall, studies suggest women with gynecoid

35 : 38

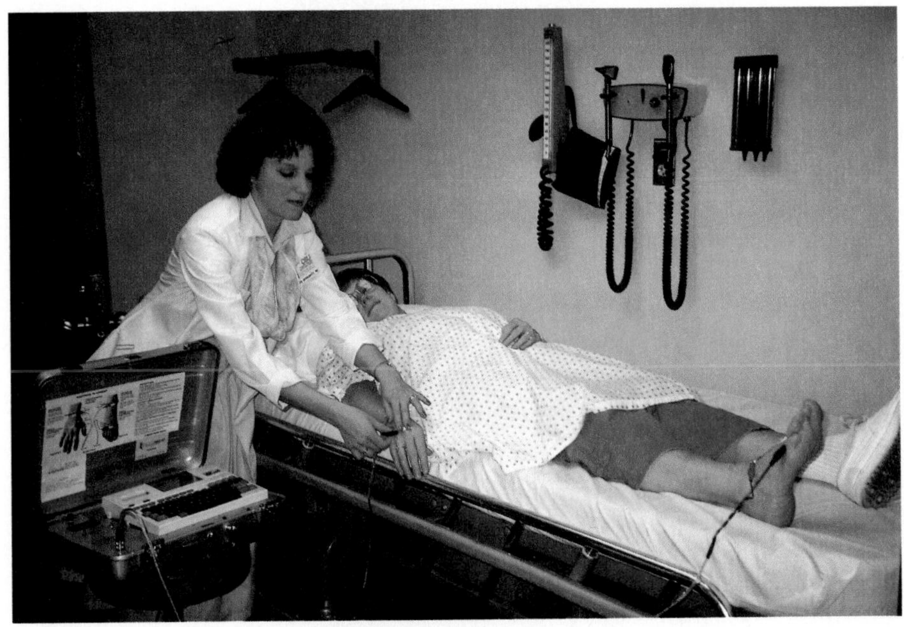

Figure 8-7 Bioelectrical impedance. This method can accurately be used to estimate total body fat in less than 5 minutes.

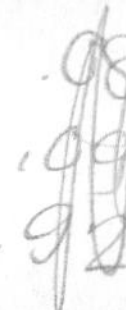

fat distribution must be 20 pounds more obese than men with an android shape to show the same health risks.[4] Note that only a small percentage of women have android obesity.

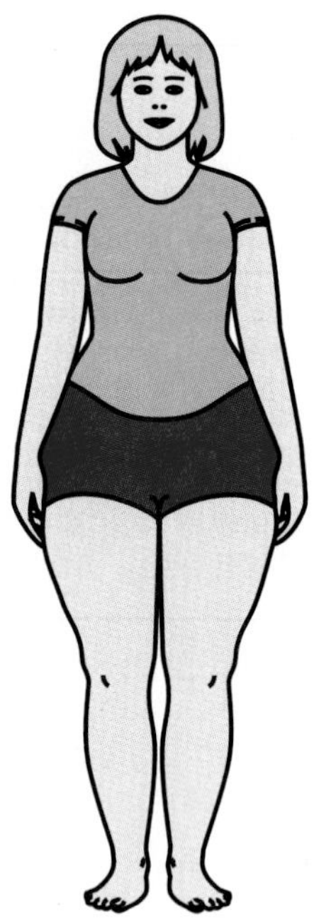

Lower body obesity (gynecoid obesity)

Using Weight for Height

Another way to define obesity is to calculate the **body mass index.** This is a person's weight in kilograms divided by height in meters squared. It represents the best way to assess health risk from obesity using height-weight values.[4] Figure 8-9 presents a graph for determining body mass index (BMI) if a person knows his or her weight and height. Just draw a straight line between your height and weight. What is your body mass index? For instance, a 70-kilogram man who is 1.78 meters tall has a body mass index of: $70/(1.782)^2 = 22$. This particular value represents a low risk for mortality.

Figure 8-10 shows that health risks from obesity for men and women begin when the body mass index exceeds about 25. At a value of about 27, the risk for diabetes or hypertension begins to rise. A body mass index above 30 poses an even greater risk for health problems and is often used as the cutoff for obesity. About 10% to 14% of Americans exceed this value. A body mass index above 40 represents quite a high risk for health problems.

Notice that the graph in Figure 8-10 is curvilinear rather than linear. As one reaches a higher body mass index, health risk increases even more. Thus health risk increases at an even greater rate than does body mass index.

The concept of body mass index is convenient to use because the cutoff values apply to both men and women, and no complicated table is needed. A practical approach is to consider a BMI between 25 and 30 of little concern if health problems

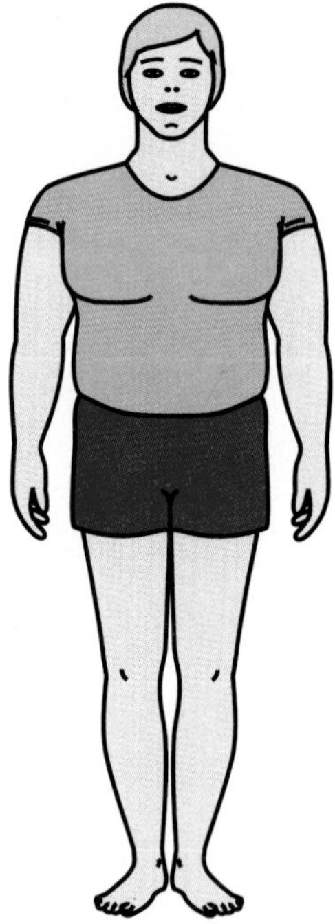

Upper body obesity (android obesity)

Figure 8-8 Body fat distribution. Gynecoid and android obesity. The android form brings higher risks for ill health associated with obesity.

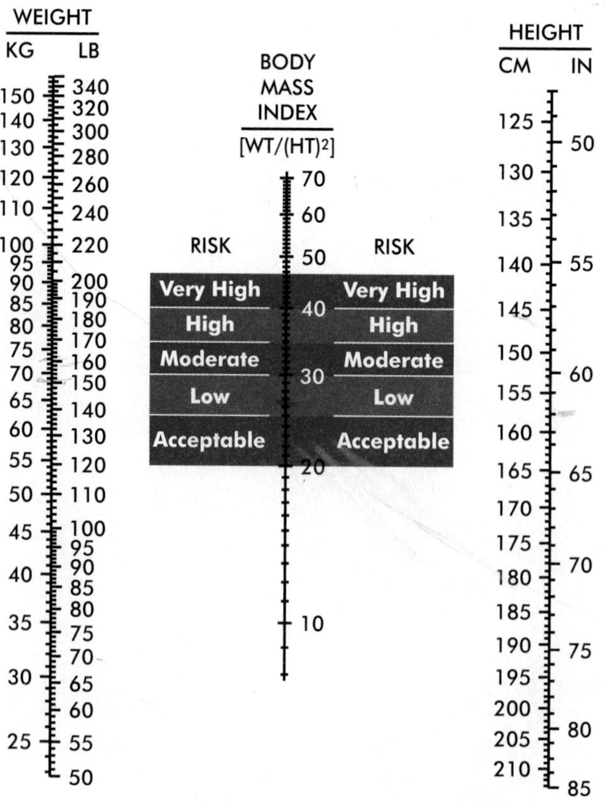

Figure 8-9 A quick way for determining BMI. Lay a straightedge across the figure, connecting your weight and height values. The point where the straightedge crosses the BMI line is the BMI in metric units (kg/m²).

are not present and one does not have an android appearance.[4] A value greater than 30 should be cause for concern. Note also that any body weight for height is actually a crude measure because we are concerned about overfat, not simply overweight (obese) individuals. However, overfat and overweight (obese) conditions almost always appear together; the husky athlete is the exception. We focus in clinical settings on body weight for height mainly because these are easier to measure than total body fat.

Overweight also can be defined as weighing 10% more than desirable body weight, the latter being based on height-weight tables.[16] Obesity is then defined as weighing 20% more than desirable body weight.

To further define obesity, weighing 20% to 40% more than desirable body weight represents mild obesity, weighing 41% to 99% more than desirable body weight represents moderate obesity, weighing more than twice desirable body weight represents severe obesity (morbid) obesity. In the United States and Canada about 90% of cases of obesity are of the mild form. This condition carries little health risk. About 0.2% of cases are severe: this condition carries a twelvefold increase in health risk.

Desirable body weight in a clinical setting is usually based on the current Metropolitan Life Insurance Table (see inside cover). This table lists for any height the weight that is associated with a maximum life span. The table does not tell what weight will make one the healthiest while alive. It simply lists the weight most associated with longevity.

As a clinical tool, the Metropolitan Life Insurance Table is valuable. In 1985 a conference of physicians and research scientists supported its use.[16] However, nagging problems remain. The table's data are derived only from purchasers of life insurance. This results in underrepresentation for poor people and many minorities. People who smoke are included in the Table, and they often have both lower body weights and earlier ages of death because of their increased risk for lung cancer and heart disease. This distorted representation may mean that the table overesti-

When looking at Figure 8-10 you will see an increased risk of disease at very low values of body mass index. This is often termed a "J" shape phenomenon. This increased risk of disease at a low body mass index mostly reflects the poor health of lean people who smoke, but significant underweight does carry some health risks of its own. We discuss these in Chapter 9.

What is a BMI of 30?

Height (feet)	Body weight (pounds)
5′	152
5′1″	165
5′2″	175
5′6″	186
5′8″	198
5′10″	201
6′	221
6′2″	233

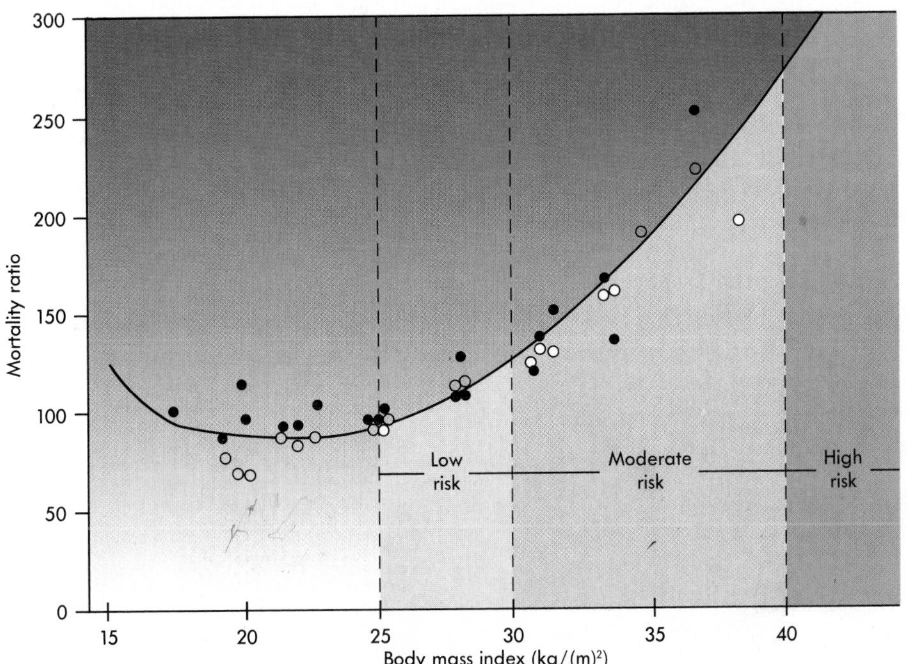

Figure 8-10 The relationship between body mass index and death rates (1.0 equals normal death rate). Solid circles show men and open circles show women. A healthy body weight is a BMI of 19 to 25 under age 35 and 21 to 27 after age 35.

The term desirable body weight was first used in 1959 by the Metropolitan Life Insurance Company. At that time it replaced the term ideal body weight. The 1983 tables used neither the terms desirable nor ideal. Both are commonly seen in medical literature. The tendency today is to use the term desirable or healthy rather than ideal.

mates the best weight for maximum longevity. In addition, body weight was only determined at the time the insurance policy was purchased. No follow-up weights were recorded. A positive point is that the table does not include insured persons with significant diseases, such as heart disease, cancer, and diabetes.

We mention this controversy because it helps put the desirable weight figure listed by the Metropolitan Life Insurance Table into perspective. If you weigh slightly more—or less—than the range listed but show no ill health, it is not necessarily cause for alarm. In addition, the weight ranges listed in the table do not guarantee health when alive. They simply attempt to maximize the chances of living as long as possible.

The weight and height values in the Metropolitan Life Insurance Table assume one is wearing clothes and shoes. Note also that the table refers only to people under 60 years of age. It is not clear if overweight or obesity in elderly people follows the same pattern of association with disease as it does in younger people. Some fat gain is to be expected as we age—about 2 pounds per decade after age 30 is reasonable, but the person should not exceed a BMI of 27 (see Chapter 18). An overweight elderly person may have already avoided the typical causes of death, such as stroke, heart disease, and cancer, to which obesity contributes. The fact that they have survived into their 70s and 80s could suggest that they are more resistant to the effects of obesity than people who have already succumbed.[4]

The height-weight table published with the *Dietary Guidelines For Americans* also allows for some weight gain in the adult years and is included in Chapter 18.

The Metropolitan Life Insurance Table adjusts for small-, medium-, and large-frame sizes. Methods for estimating frame size use measurements of wrist width or elbow breadth (see Appendix K). Either method yields similar estimates.[17] However, although these methods exist, frame size was never measured in the men and women used to develop the Metropolitan Life Insurance Table. Researchers at the Metropolitan Life Insurance Company simply estimated that 25% of people are small framed, 50% of people are medium framed, and 25% of people are large framed based on other studies. They then arbitrarily put the weight data into small-, medium-, and large-frame categories based on those percentages.

Therefore frame size may not be that important to these estimates. You can consider obviously small and thin people as having a small frame, and obviously big and bulky people who have large bones as having a large frame. Consider everyone else as having a medium frame.

One method for estimating desirable body weight is often called the Rule-of-Thumb (ROT) Method. To use it, allow 100 pounds for the first 5 feet for women and then add 5 pounds for every inch thereafter. A desirable body weight in men starts with 106 pounds for the first 5 feet and then adds 6 pounds for every inch thereafter. Other similar formulas exist.

Using Age of Onset

Obesity can be classified as juvenile-onset, adult-onset, or endocrine-onset (Table 8-3). The latter includes obesity caused by relatively rare hormonal abnormalities and rare genetic disorders.

Table 8-3 Types of obesity

Juvenile-Onset:	Hyperplastic—increased fat cell number Hypertrophic—larger fat cells
Adult-Onset:	Mainly hypertrophic About 80% to 90% of obesity is adult-onset
Endocrine:	Hypothyroidism, hypercorticoidism, brain tumors, Prader-Willi syndrome, Turner's syndrome, and others.

When obesity develops in infancy or childhood (especially during puberty), the person develops more adipose cells, and each adipose cell grows greatly. When obesity develops in adulthood, the person usually ends up with a normal number of adipose cells, but each cell contains a large amount of fat. Adipose tissue consisting of a large number of cells shows **hyperplasia,** and adipose tissue consisting of large cells shows **hypertrophy.** Juvenile-onset obesity tends to be both hyperplastic and hypertrophic. Adult-onset obesity tends to be mainly hypertrophic, but in cases of extreme obesity can be both hyperplastic and hypertrophic.[4]

hyperplasia An increase in cell number.

hypertrophy An increase in cell size.

There has been concern for the last 20 years that in cases of juvenile-onset obesity it is more difficult for a person to lose weight and keep it off than with the adult-onset type of obesity. This is because the increased number of fat cells accompanying juvenile-onset obesity may increase the body's resistance to greatly reducing fat stores. The Expert Opinion discusses this idea. It is clear that the longer one is obese, the more difficult it is to correct the problem.

The Individual Path to Obesity

Many paths lead to obesity, and each person with obesity has unique characteristics and problems. The clinician must tailor treatment to deal with these different problems. Some possible characteristics of obese people that clinicians can use to begin to understand more about their clients, besides using body fat content, body weight for height measures, body fat distribution, and age of onset, include family history of obesity, current energy expenditure, fasting blood glucose levels, and the extent of erroneous nutrition beliefs. The variety of this list illustrates the many possible complications of an individual case of obesity.

From our previous discussion, you also can imagine that dysfunctions associated with the hunger-related (internal) or appetite-related (external) forces that affect satiety may promote overeating. Lower than normal energy expenditure could result from impairment of one or a combination of the four contributors to energy use. Therefore you can see that the reasons for an individual being obese can be complex. Its multiple causes often make obesity a very heterogeneous disorder. As we discuss in Chapter 9, it requires consideration for individual treatment plans.

HEALTH RISKS ASSOCIATED WITH OBESITY

Many health problems are associated with obesity. These include an increased risk in surgery, noninsulin-dependent (adult-onset) diabetes, hypertension, heart disease, arthritis, gallstones, pregnancy risks, early death, and various forms of cancer—such as colon, rectal, and prostate cancer in men and breast, uterine, and ovarian cancer in women.[4] Possible explanations of why obesity causes these disorders are listed in Table 8-4. Again, an android pattern of fat distribution raises the risk even more for these disorders.

Before we go on, let's step back and look at an important concept. Most Americans with obesity show relatively low health risks because these people have mild forms of obesity. On a population-wide basis, the cutoff for obesity of a body mass index of 30 or greater than 20% of desirable weight is important with respect to disease prevention in our society. On an individual basis, however, some nutritionists argue that this amount or somewhat more may not necessarily show negative health effects. The extra body fat can set the stage for future disease, but even that is not guaranteed for a specific person.

This suggests that the individual, in conjunction with his or her physician, is best equipped to establish whether a need for weight reduction exists, based on fat distribution patterns, family history for obesity-related disease, and current health status.[4] Still, health planners would like us all to avoid even mild obesity since this could help reduce the extent of chronic disease in our population as a whole, and in turn the associated expense to our nation.

Table 8-4 Health problems associated with excess body fat

Health problem	Partially attributed to:
Surgical risk	Increased anesthesia needs and greater risk of wound infections
Pulmonary disease	Excess weight over lungs
Adult-onset diabetes	Enlarged fat cells, which then poorly bind insulin and also poorly respond to the message insulin sends to the cell
Hypertension	Increase miles of blood vessels found in the fat tissue; however, no validated cause is yet known
Coronary heart disease	Increases in serum cholesterol and triglyceride levels, as well as a decrease in physical activity
Bone and joint disorders	Excess pressure put on knee, ankle, and hip joints
Gallbladder stones	An increase in cholesterol content of bile
Skin disorders	The trapping of moisture and microbes in fat folds
Various cancers	Estrogen production by fat cells; animal studies suggest excess energy intake encourages tumor development
Shorter stature (in some forms of obesity)	An earlier onset of puberty
Pregnancy risk	More difficult delivery and increased anesthesia needs (if the latter is used)
Early death	A variety of risk factors for disease listed above

The greater the degree of obesity, the more likely and the more serious these health problems generally become. They are much more likely to appear in people who show an android fat distribution pattern and/or are greater than twice desirable body weight.

CONCEPT CHECK

Obesity refers to a state of excessive body fat storage. In a clinical setting this usually corresponds to 20% over desirable body weight as predicted by the 1983 Metropolitan Life Insurance Table or a body mass index over 30 (calculated as weight in kilograms divided by height in meters squared). Ideally, obesity is defined as a body fat percentage greater than 25% in men and 30% in women. The actual amount of a person's body fat storage can be estimated using skinfold thicknesses or bioelectric impedance. Fat storage distribution further defines an obese state as android or gynecoid. Obesity in general leads to an increased risk for heart disease, some types of cancer, hypertension, adult-onset diabetes, bone and joint disorders, and some digestive disorders. The risks for some of these diseases are especially high if the fat storage is in an android distribution.

Energy Use in Obesity

Do obese and normal-weight people differ in terms of energy use? Is there something inherent in an obese person that causes more or less efficient energy use than in a lean person? For some obese people that is probably the case. It is clear that some laboratory and farm animals more efficiently turn food energy into fat storage[13] (Figure 8-11). Farmers once selected cows and hogs based on their ability to acquire

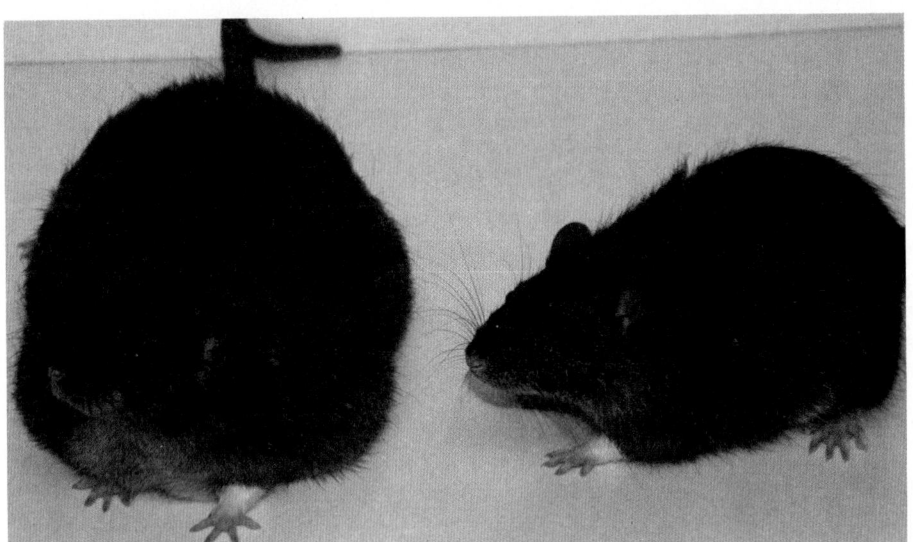

Figure 8-11 A rat with genetic obesity. No matter what type of diet the animal on the left eats, it will make more fat than the normal rat on the right. Genetics can have a powerful effect on the body composition of animals.

fat. Today we know that eating too much animal fat can increase the risk for heart disease, so farmers now select animals that acquire more lean and less fat tissue.

We humans are not so fortunate. Our parents did not choose each other based on genetic counseling. Some of us likely inherited a tendency for leanness and others a tendency for obesity. There is no way to determine which kind of person you are without extensive testing of your resting and total energy needs. However, a person who is constantly struggling to maintain body weight probably has some genetic component to the weight problem.[21] Unfortunately, nothing can be done to change genetic background. Nevertheless, we should all keep in mind that genetic differences do exist, and these can create a greater body weight struggle for some people than for others.

DIFFERENCES IN BASAL METABOLISM

Basal metabolism tends to be higher in obese people because their extra fat stores require the addition of extra lean tissue, such as connective tissue, for support. The more lean tissue one has, the higher one's total basal metabolism is.[20] Basal metabolism of an obese person would appear to be less if expressed as kcalories per pound, because adipose tissue has a low metabolic rate. However, when comparing two people, the obese person will have a higher total basal metabolism. Still, it doesn't take many more kcalories to maintain an obese state, just as it doesn't take many extra kcalories per day to become obese (as we discuss in Chapter 9).

THERMIC EFFECT OF FOOD IN OBESITY

Thermic effect of food is lower in some obese people than in those at desirable weights.[3] This could be partially caused by insulin resistance of adipose cells, a characteristic often present with obesity. Thus the thermic effect of eating carbohydrate will be decreased in the obese person because not enough insulin action is available to promote normal carbohydrate metabolism. It is not known, however, if this is a cause or merely a consequence of obesity.

ENERGY USED IN PHYSICAL ACTIVITY

Obese people burn more kcalories in activity than do lean people because their extra body weight requires more energy to perform muscular activity. Nevertheless, many obese people use fewer total kcalories in an activity because they are less active. Studies of obese teenagers showed that when they played tennis they avoided rigorous activity. Studies using obese adults show that they also perform weight-bearing exercises, such as walking, less vigorously.[2] Recent studies have shown an association between hours of television watching and obesity in children, adolescents, and adults. Long hours of watching television can mean a very sedentary lifestyle.[11] A key component to either treating or preventing obesity often is increasing the person's physical activity level.[25]

DEFICITS IN ADAPTIVE THERMOGENESIS

It has previously been stated that some obese adults may have deficits in heat production in response to stimuli like overfeeding. This could be caused by less sympathetic nervous system activity or deficiencies in brown adipose tissue. Several drugs are being examined with the intent of trying to increase adaptive thermogenesis in obese people.[4]

Why Obesity Develops—Nature Versus Nurture

Both genetic traits and psychological influences can increase the risk for obesity. These two very different types of influences give rise to a "nature versus nurture" question concerning causes of obesity.

HOW INFLUENTIAL IS NATURE IN CONTRIBUTING TO OBESITY?

Identical twins raised apart tend to have similar weight gain patterns. Having been raised apart reduces the effect of nurture—what a person learns about eating habits and nutrition. If one twin is obese, the other is usually obese.

As stated before, we think it is reasonable to assume that some people inherit a **thrifty metabolism**. Genetically obese mice and rats are good examples of animal species destined to become obese (Figure 8-11). Both species are much more efficient than the normal animal at turning energy intake into fat storage.[13] Genetically obese rats and mice even make fat at the expense of synthesizing muscle tissue, which indicates how genetically prone they are to fat deposition and eventual obesity. Certain tribes of Native Americans also have a great tendency to develop obesity.[20]

"thrifty" metabolism A metabolism that characteristically conserves more kcalories than normal, such that the risk of weight gain and obesity is enhanced.

A very thrifty metabolism in a person would require less energy for body maintenance and activity. In earlier times, when food supplies were scarce, a thrifty metabolism would be a great advantage. Today, with food so readily available, a thrifty metabolism requires high physical activity and wise food choices to balance energy intake with output.

One important variable in this efficiency equation could be the degree to which food energy can be turned into ATP energy. We cannot measure small differences in energy efficiency between people. In the long run, however, even a 1% or 2% difference in ability to turn food energy into ATP energy could mean massive weight gain or relative weight maintenance. People with thriftier metabolic systems may more readily convert food energy into ATP energy, leaving extra kcalories to contribute more fat stores each day throughout their lives.

Current research suggests that some families tend more toward low resting metabolic rates than do others.[21] The families with lower resting metabolic rates also show higher rates for obesity. Even after adjusting for the amount of fat a person has, research shows that resting metabolic rate can vary as much as 30% between leaner and more obese families.

So if you feel you have a thrifty metabolism, chances are that you inherited aspects of that characteristic. A child with no obese parent has only a 10% chance of becoming obese. With one obese parent, the child has about a 40% chance of becoming obese. A child who has two obese parents has about an 80% chance of becoming obese.

It can be argued that these probabilities are due to the way a child is raised. Fraternal twins show less variation in weight than two unrelated people. This supports the theory promoting the effects of environment, while the close association of body weights between identical twins supports the theory promoting a genetic explanation. This just shows how complicated it is to separate nature influences from nurture influences when searching for the causes of obesity.

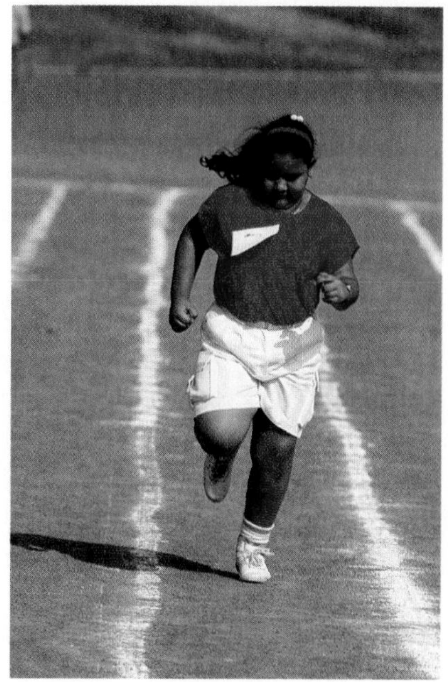

A child who is still obese after 5 years of age often faces a battle against obesity for the rest of his or her life.

DOES NURTURE HAVE A ROLE?

As we just discussed, nurture—how a person is raised—can also strongly influence obesity. Family members often have similar eating habits, make similar food choices, and have similar degrees of fatness. They may find solace in being part of a "clan." This is true even for husbands and wives, two people who have no genetic commonality. So the environment in which a person is raised or now lives can influence food habits and ultimately fatness.

Obesity is related to socioeconomic status in America. Men and women in lower socioeconomic groups are more likely to be obese than people in upper socioeconomic groups. This is especially true for women.[14]

Gender also influences obesity risk. Adult obesity in women can often be tied to childhood obesity, but the same does not hold true for men. Men tend to become obese after age 30, probably as they become more financially successful and therefore more sedentary. This is probably the best evidence for a critical role of nurture in obesity. If nature is an important reason for obesity in men, obesity should be present much earlier in life.

Early research suggested that infant feeding practices may influence a child's chance to become obese in later life. Specifically, it was thought that both bottle feeding, as well as an early introduction of solid foods (before the age of 6 months), encouraged the infant to gain too much weight. This then increased the chance of becoming obese. However, many recent studies reexamining this issue show that very little relationship exists between feeding practices, or even obesity in infancy, and obesity in childhood. The exception could be the infant who gains weight very rapidly in the first 6 weeks of life. Most overweight or obese infants become normal weight schoolchildren.

If a child remains obese at 5 years of age or has become obese by 5 years of age, immediate attention is necessary. Obesity in childhood is highly related to obesity in adulthood, especially in females. We discuss this further in Chapter 17.

NATURE AND NURTURE TOGETHER

In summary, both nature and nurture influence the tendency for obesity (Table 8-5). We can view the development of obesity as nurture allowing nature to be expressed. Some people may begin with a lower rate for energy metabolism. When these people are put into an inactive environment that is full of both high-kcalorie foods and social reinforcement, they are nurtured into expressing their natural tendency for obesity[10] (Figure 8-12). This can be seen as speculation on our part, but it is a reasonable assertion.

We feel it is important for everyone to try to determine his or her own risk for obesity and to discover what specific factors in their lifestyle contribute to this risk. Only then can a person make an individual plan to reduce the risk for obesity. We will talk more about that plan in Chapter 9.

Keep in mind also that although one may be fatter than he or she would like to be, a small amount of extra fat may pose no significant health risk, especially if in a gynecoid distribution.[4] We discussed this idea earlier. That information may help a person put weight loss into perspective. Knowing that weight loss is difficult and that current body weight poses no serious health threat, some people may decide to just stay at their current weight and simply work to not gain any more. That alone would be a positive step for some people, as the odds of a young adult (i.e., college student) gaining about 10 to 15 pounds of body fat by ages 35 to 40 is high.

Table 8-5 What encourages some of us to develop excess body fat stores?

Factor	Reason for increase
Age	Excess body fat is more common in adults and middle-aged individuals.
Gender	Females have more fat.
Positive energy balance	Especially important if over a relatively long period.
Composition of intake	High-fat intake and preference for sugary, fat-rich foods may be contributing factors.
Physical activity level	Low or decreasing level of activity affects body fat stores.
Resting metabolic rate	A low value with respect to lean body mass is linked to weight gain.
Thermic effect of food	Low for some obesity cases.
Use of fat for energy	Poor fat utilization is linked with body fat gain.
Ratio of fat to lean tissue	A high fat-mass–to–lean body-mass ratio is correlated with weight gain.
Adipose-tissue lipoprotein lipase activity	High in obese individuals and remains high (perhaps even increases) with weight loss.
Variety of social and behavioral factors	Obesity is associated with socioeconomic status, familial conditions, network of friends, pattern of leisure activities, television time, smoking habits, alcohol intake, etc.
Undetermined genetic characteristics	These affect energy balance particularly via the energy expenditure components, the deposition of the energy surplus as fat or as lean tissue, and the relative proportion of fat and carbohydrate use by the body.

Modified from Bouchard C: Current understanding of the etiology of obesity: genetic and nongenetic factors, *American Journal of Clinical Nutrition* 53:1561S, 1991.

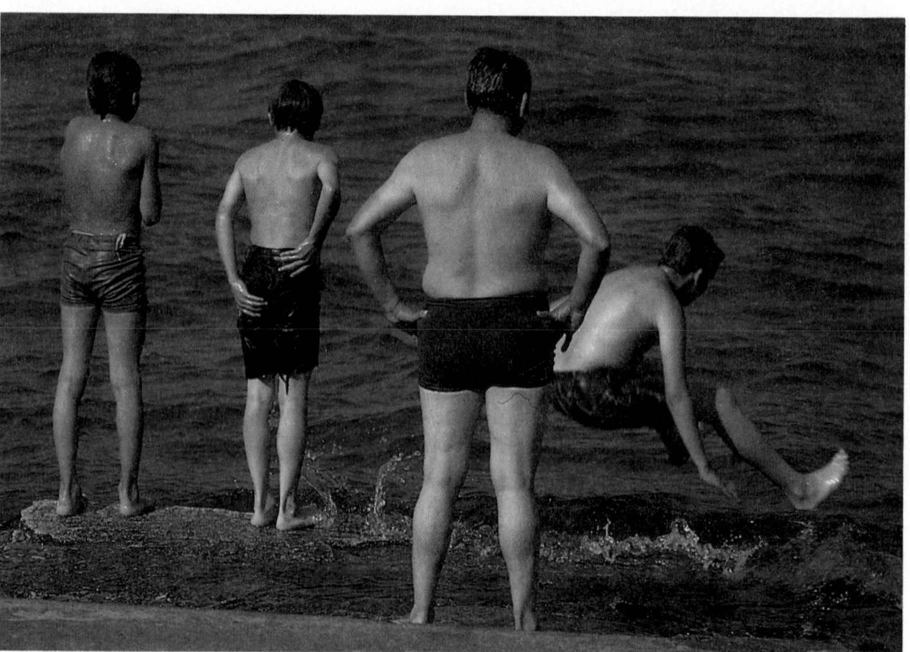

Figure 8-12 Nature versus nurture. Is the difference in body fat due to nature or nurture, or both?

CONCEPT CHECK

Genetic background plays a role in the cause of obesity. Body fat distribution and degree of basal metabolism is partially genetically determined. Nurture is also important. Family members often have similar eating habits, similar activity levels, and similar degrees of fatness. In addition, men tend to develop obesity after age 30 and women tend to develop it throughout their childhood and adult years. Putting both factors together we can speculate that a proper nurturing state may allow a genetic tendency for obesity to either be expressed or overcome.

Summary

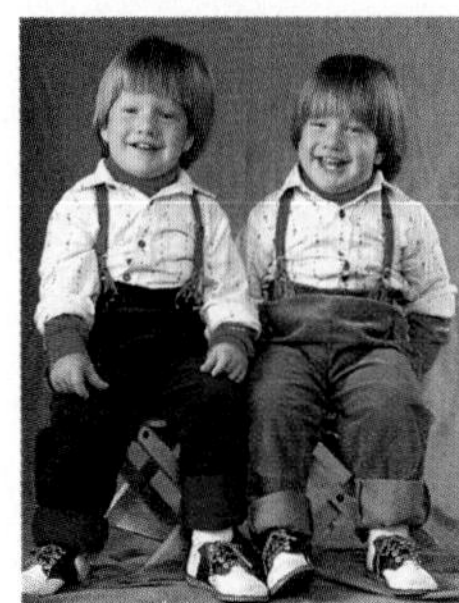

1. Groups of cells in the hypothalamus affect hunger, the primarily physiological desire to find and eat food. These cells may monitor blood glucose and other nutrients and read low levels as a signal to promote feeding.
2. A variety of internal (hunger-related) and external (appetite-related) forces affect satiety. Hunger forces like low levels of certain nutrients in the blood combine with appetite forces like easy availability of food to promote feeding.
3. The major determinants of food intake in America are probably appetite-related forces because food is so readily available to most of us that the more physiological influences that affect eating often are suppressed or ignored.
4. Energy use by the body can be accounted for by basal metabolism, the thermic effect of food, physical activity, and adaptive thermogenesis. Basal metabolism represents the minimum energy needed to keep the resting body alive. It is primarily affected by lean body mass, surface area, and thyroid hormone levels. The thermic effect of food represents the increase in metabolism to facilitate the digesting, absorbing, and processing of nutrients recently consumed. Physical activity represents energy use that is not related to the other two categories. Adaptive thermogenesis is heat production caused by exposure to overfeeding or a cold environment. It is possible that brown adipose tissue is the active heat-producing tissue that is the basis for this. About 80% of energy use goes for basal metabolism and the thermic effect of food.
5. Energy use by the body can be measured directly from heat output or indirectly by measuring oxygen uptake and/or carbon dioxide output. Energy use by the body can be estimated using formulas based on various combinations of body weight, height, lean body mass, and age.
6. Obesity is usually defined as total body fat percentage over 25% in men and 30% in women. A body mass index (weight ÷ height^2 in metric units) over about 30 also represents obesity. Being 20% over desirable body weight as based on the 1983 Metropolitan Life Insurance Table is a further measure of obesity.
7. Fat distribution partially determines the prediction of health risks due to obesity. An android fat storage distribution, in which the waist-to-hip circumference ratio is greater than 0.95 in men or greater than 0.8 in women, suggests higher risks of hypertension, heart disease, and diabetes associated with obesity.
8. Genetic factors influence the tendency to obesity. Basal metabolism and body fat distribution both have genetic links. How one is raised (or nurtured) also influences the tendency for obesity, since family members often develop similar eating habits and activity patterns. Essentially, obesity can be viewed as nurture allowing nature to be expressed.

Study Questions

1. After reexamining the internal and external forces associated with hunger, satiety, and food intake, propose five hypotheses for the development of obesity.

2. Knowing the four contributors to human energy expenditure, propose four hypotheses for the development of obesity solely based on the classes of energy expenditure.

3. John walks into his physician's office and his body status is assessed using the 1983 Metropolitan Life Insurance Table. Provide one advantage and one problem associated with using this table.

4. Describe the best method of defining obesity in a clinical setting. Why is this the best?

5. What are the two most convincing pieces of evidence that both genetic and environmental factors play significant roles in the development of obesity?

REFERENCES

1. Berdanier CD, McIntosh MK: Weight loss—weight regain: a vicious cycle, *Nutrition Today,* Sept/Oct 1991, p 6.
2. Blair D, Buskirk ER: Habitual daily energy expenditure and activity levels of lean and adult-onset and child-onset obese women, *American Journal of Clinical Nutrition* 45:540, 1987.
3. Bouchard C: Current understanding of the etiology of obesity: genetic and nongenetic factors, *American Journal of Clinical Nutrition* 53:1561S, 1991.
4. Bray GA: Pathophysiology of obesity, *American Journal of Clinical Nutrition* 55:488S, 1992.
5. Bray GA: Peptides affect the intake of specific nutrients and the sympathetic nervous system, *American Journal of Clinical Nutrition* 55:265S, 1992.
6. Bray GA: Treatment for obesity: a nutrient balance/nutrient partition approach, *Nutrition Reviews* 49:33, 1991.
7. Castonguay TW, Stern JS: Hunger and appetite. In Brown ML, editor: *Present knowledge in nutrition,* Washington, DC, 1990, International Life Sciences Institute.
8. Dattilo AM: Dietary fat and its relationship to body weight, *Nutrition Today,* Jan/Feb 1992, p 13.
9. DiGirolami M: Cellular, metabolic, and clinical consequences of adipose mass enlargement in obesity, *Nutrition* 7:287, 1991.
10. Drewnowski A and others: Taste preferences in human obesity: environmental and familial factors, *American Journal of Clinical Nutrition* 54:635, 1991.
11. Gortmaker SL and others: Inactivity, diet and the fattening of America, *Journal of The American Dietetic Association* 90:1247, 1990.
12. Jensen MD: Research techniques for body composition assessment, *Journal of The American Dietetic Association* 92:454, 1992.
13. Johnson PR and others: Animal models of obesity: genetic aspects, *Annual Review of Nutrition* 11:325, 1991.
14. Kahn HS, Williamson DF: Is race associated with weight change in U.S. adults after adjustment for income, education, and marital factors? *American Journal of Clinical Nutrition* 53:1566S, 1991.
15. Mercer LP and others: Histidine, histamine and the neuroregulation of food intake, *Nutrition* 6:273, 1990.
16. National Institutes of Health Consensus Development Conference Statement: Health implications of obesity, *Annals of Internal Medicine* 103:1073, 1985.
17. Nowak RK, Schulz LO: A comparison of two methods for the determination of body frame size, *Journal of The American Dietetic Association* 87:339, 1987.
18. Owen OE: Regulation of energy and metabolism. In Kinney JM and others, editors: Nutrition and metabolism in patient care, Philadelphia, 1988, WB Saunders.
19. Owen OE and others: Oxidative and nonoxidative macronutrient disposal in lean and obese men after mixed meals, *American Journal of Clinical Nutrition* 55:630, 1992.
20. Ravussin E, Bogardus C: A brief overview of human energy metabolism and its relationship to essential obesity, *American Journal of Clinical Nutrition* 55:242S, 1992.
21. Ravussin E and others: Reduced rate of energy expenditure as a risk factor for body-weight gain, *The New England Journal of Medicine* 318:467, 1988.
22. Rumpler WV and others: Energy-intake restriction and diet-composition effects on energy expenditure in men, *American Journal of Clinical Nutrition* 53:430, 1991.
23. Schoeller DA, Fjeld CR: Human energy metabolism: What have we learned from the doubly labeled water method? *Annual Review of Nutrition* 11:355, 1991.
24. Schutz Y and others: Role of fat oxidation in the long-term stabilization of body weight in obese women, *American Journal of Clinical Nutrition* 55:670, 1992.
25. Simms EAH: Storage and expenditure of energy in obesity and their implications for management, *Medical Clinics of North America* 73:97, 1989.
26. Stricker EM, Verbalis JG: Control of appetite and satiety: insights from biologic and behavioral studies, *Nutrition Reviews* 48:49, 1990.

SUGGESTED READINGS

The articles by Bray represent a good overview of energy balance issues, from feeding to health risks from obesity. Stricker and Verbalis provide a clear account of the primarily internal factors that influence food intake. Ravussin and Bogardus provide a fascinating account of energy use, drawing on the work with Pima Indians in Arizona.

TAKE ACTION

Am I a candidate for weight loss?

Determine the following two indicators of your body status: body mass index and waist-to-hip ratio

Body Mass Index

Record your weight in pounds: ______________ lbs.
Divide your weight in pounds by 2.2 lbs. to determine your weight in kilograms: ______________ kg.
Record your height in inches: ______________ in.
Divide your height in inches by 39.3 to determine your height in meters: ______________ m.
Calculate your Body Mass Index using the following formula:
BMI = weight (kg) ÷ [height $(m)^2$] BMI = ______________ kg ÷ ______________ $[m^2]$ = ______________.
Take a tape measure and measure the circumferences of your waist (at the belly button with stomach relaxed) and hips (widest point).
Circumference of waist = ______________ in.
Circumference of hips = ______________ in.
Calculate your waist-to-hip ratio using the following formula:
Circumference of waist ÷ circumference of hips.
Waist-to-hip ratio = ______________ in. ÷ ______________ in. = ______________.

Interpretation

1. When BMI is greater than 25, health risks from obesity begin, especially if one has an android appearance. It would be especially advisable to attempt weight loss under your physicians guidance if your BMI exceeds 30. Does yours exceed 30? Yes ______________ No ______________
2. If greater than 20% above desirable weight, a waist-to-hip ratio greater than 0.95 in men and 0.8 in women indicates android (upper body) obesity. This is associated with an increased risk of heart disease, hypertension, and diabetes. If appropriate, does your ratio exceed the standard appropriate for your gender? Yes ______________ No ______________

Application

From what you've learned in this chapter, what changes in eating and exercise habits could you make to lose weight, if needed?

____

____

____

____

____

NUTRITION PERSPECTIVE

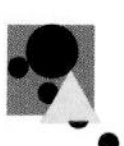

Do You Have a Set Point for Body Weight?

William Bennett and Joel Gurin popularized the "set point theory of weight maintenance" in 1982 by publishing their book, *The Dieter's Dilemma*. This theory espouses the notion that body weight is closely regulated. It is proposed that humans have a genetically predetermined body weight or body fat level that the body attempts to defend at all costs. Some scientists suggest that the hypothalamus monitors the amount of body fat in humans and tries to keep that level constant over time. This level is referred to as a "set point." We have already seen in this chapter that the protein produced by adipose cells, adipsin, may form the communication link between adipose cells and the brain that allows for this regulation.

Analogies to the tight regulation of blood pressure and body temperature are used to support this concept. One researcher has described the set point as a coiled spring; the further you stray from your usual weight, the harder the force acts to pull you back to that weight.

The major studies in humans cited to support the set point theory demonstrate that volunteers who lost weight through starvation later ate in a way to regain weight back to their original level or a little higher. In addition, prisoners with no history for obesity found it hard to gain weight, and after being asked to gain weight, quickly returned to their previous weight when they returned to their previous habits.[25] Note also that after an illness, a person regains lost weight.

There also is sound physiological evidence that body weight tends to be regulated. If one reduces energy intake, the blood level of a thyroid hormone (T_3) falls, causing the metabolic rate to fall.[3] Due to these changes, the body resists further weight loss. In addition, the lower body weight decreases the energy cost of each future weight-bearing activity, and the total energy used by lean tissues falls because some of these tissues are also lost. Furthermore, the enzyme used by adipose cells and muscle cells to pull in fat from the bloodstream (lipoprotein lipase) often increases its activity.

A pound of fat storage gained or lost represents about 2700 kcalories either gained or lost.[18] The fat itself represents 3500 kcalories per pound, but as fat *storage* is lost or gained, so is lean support tissue. This has a much lower energy value, and so the net kcalorie transfer is closer to 2700, accounting for both changes in the fat itself and lean support tissue. Using this 2700 figure you can calculate the various numbers listed in this section.

If a person overeats, in the short run the metabolic rate tends to increase. This causes some resistance to further weight gain. People often recognize the body's resistance to weight loss when dieting but do not think much about the resistance to weight gain after eating a big holiday meal. However, in the long run our resistance to weight gain is much less than our resistance to weight loss. When a person gains weight and stays at that weight for a while, the body will tend to defend that weight.[3]

Let's explore set point regulation of weight in concrete terms. The amount we eat varies from day to day. Daily energy intake varies from about 20% below to 20% above a person's 28-day average energy intake (about 400 kcalories). In comparison, even as little as a 2% (40 kcalorie) over-consumption of energy per day, if continued for 20 years, could result in an 108-pound gain in fat stores. This significant effect from such a small error points out how easy it is to follow the road to obesity. But, the average weight gain between the ages of 18 and 54 years is only 15 to 20 pounds. It appears that some powerful forces encourage a balance of overeating with undereating. Thus, in the long run, daily energy imbalances cancel each other, with high-kcalorie intake days balancing the low-kcalorie intake days. When also considering that over a 35-year period an adult eats about 35 tons of food (yielding 30 million kcalories), the ability to regulate weight, though imperfect, is again still quite impressive.

Arguments against the set point theory cite the fact that during pregnancy women slowly increase body weight and fat with little fight to maintain this trend. Also, an average person's weight does not remain constant throughout adulthood; it usually increases slowly, at least until old age. This means that one must be able to shift their set point. They also argue that if an individual is placed in a different social, emotional, or physical environment weight can become markedly higher or lower and will be maintained. These arguments would say that humans, rather than having a set point determined by genetics or number of adipose cells, actually settle into a particular stable weight based on an interaction between nature and nurture influences.

Other researchers argue that the concept of a set point can actually undermine the therapy for those who are obese. The idea that one's body will strongly resist the maintenance of weight loss can be discouraging and depressing. Obese individuals may fall victim to a self-fulfilling prophecy. A person may believe that maintenance will be so hard or impossible that he or she may give up at the slightest lapse or weight gain. Many experts who specialize in obesity treatment would rather not accept the set point theory until it has been clearly validated.

In the final analysis, we must bear most of the responsibility for weight maintenance ourselves.[3] The odds are against the likelihood that—even with a set point helping us—we can avoid creeping weight gain in adulthood without great attention being given to this tendency. Ideally this includes following a diet moderate in fat content and a lifestyle rich in opportunities for physical activity.

CHAPTER NINE

Weight Control

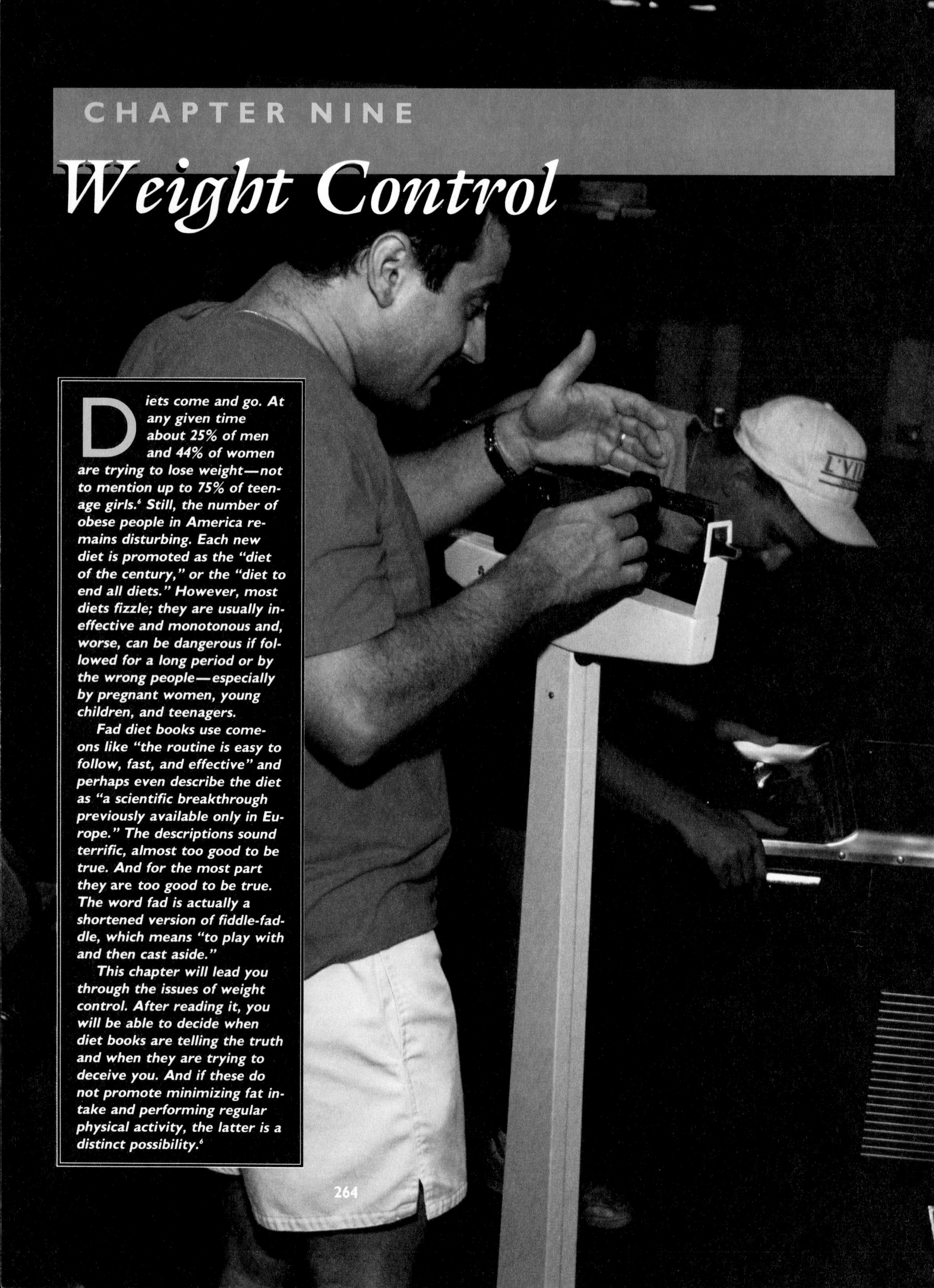

Diets come and go. At any given time about 25% of men and 44% of women are trying to lose weight—not to mention up to 75% of teenage girls.[6] Still, the number of obese people in America remains disturbing. Each new diet is promoted as the "diet of the century," or the "diet to end all diets." However, most diets fizzle; they are usually ineffective and monotonous and, worse, can be dangerous if followed for a long period or by the wrong people—especially by pregnant women, young children, and teenagers.

Fad diet books use come-ons like "the routine is easy to follow, fast, and effective" and perhaps even describe the diet as "a scientific breakthrough previously available only in Europe." The descriptions sound terrific, almost too good to be true. And for the most part they are too good to be true. The word fad is actually a shortened version of fiddle-faddle, which means "to play with and then cast aside."

This chapter will lead you through the issues of weight control. After reading it, you will be able to decide when diet books are telling the truth and when they are trying to deceive you. And if these do not promote minimizing fat intake and performing regular physical activity, the latter is a distinct possibility.[6]

NUTRITION AWARENESS INVENTORY

Here are 15 statements about weight control. Answer them to test your current knowledge. If you think the answer is true or mostly true, circle T. If you think the answer is false or mostly false, circle F. Use the scoring key at the end of this book to compute your total score. Take this test again after you have read this chapter. Compare the results.

1. T F Physical activity is more important than diet in losing weight.
2. T F Scientists understand little about the psychology of weight regain after weight loss.
3. T F Weight-loss diets should contain at least 1000 kcalories per day.
4. T F Success rates of weight-loss programs are reasonably good.
5. T F Rapid weight loss is likely to mean the loss of muscle tissue.
6. T F A weight-loss program should include changes in behavior.
7. T F A weight-loss program should encourage one to not eat meat right after consuming milk products.
8. T F The best foods to emphasize for weight loss are high-carbohydrate foods.
9. T F Eating a low-fat diet for weight control is impractical.
10. T F Changing habits is the single most important factor in keeping weight off.
11. T F Stimulus control refers to controlling factors that encourage eating.
12. T F You can lose 1 pound of fat storage each week by burning 200 extra kcalories per day beyond your normal activity.
13. T F Most obese children become obese adults.
14. T F A 20-minute brisk walk burns up about 100 kcalories.
15. T F Morbid obesity is defined as 100 pounds over desirable weight.

Treatment of Obesity

The year 2000 Health Objectives for the United States include some directed at the reduction in the number of obese individuals, currently estimated at about 34 million.[15] To do that, the National Institutes of Health (NIH) has suggested three specific actions:

1. Teach 90% of all adults that increasing physical activity while decreasing energy intake is the best way to lose weight.
2. Get 90% of the adults already at acceptable or desirable body weights to remain that way.
3. Motivate 90% of overweight Americans to adopt a plan to reduce energy intake and increase physical activity, ultimately attaining and then maintaining a desirable weight.

Improving the health of people in America—and of others in most of the Western World—hinges on the possibility of reducing obesity rates. Reducing present rates of obesity would be one powerful tool to provide a more healthful and fuller life for many people.

SOME BASIC PREMISES

Let's focus on three important principles concerning weight loss for adults (see Chapter 17 for weight-loss suggestions for children).

First, the body resists weight loss. We discussed this in Chapter 8. Thyroid hormone levels, and consequently basal metabolism, drop during weight loss.[4] This drop makes it difficult to lose weight. Recent studies also show that activity of the enzyme lipoprotein lipase increases in adipose cells after weight loss.[8] This enzyme is responsible for removing fat from lipoproteins and absorbing it into adipose cells (see Chapter 5). So after dieting, the body can more efficiently perform the uptake of fat from the bloodstream for storage.

When you read brochures or research reports about specific diet plans, ask not only whether the people lost weight but also whether they maintained that weight loss for a period of a year or more. If the weight loss was not maintained, then the entire dieting program was in vain.

Second, preventing obesity should be emphasized, since curing the disorder is very difficult. Nutrition experts strongly endorse this point.[5] Only about 5% of those who diet actually lose weight and remain at that weight. A weight-loss program should be considered successful only when its subjects remain at their lower weight for 3 to 5 years. Some programs have slightly higher success rates than 5%, as do people who simply lose weight on their own without enrolling in any supervised plan. But overall the statistics are grim and we should pay attention to this fact. Dieting today often results in weight gain next month, creating yo-yo weight swings. And there are negative health consequences associated with this form of weight cycling, such as an increased risk for body fat deposition and heart disease.[16]

Third, the weight should be lost from fat storage, not from muscle and other lean tissues. Rapid weight loss at the start of a diet program often represents fluid lost due to a decreased salt intake, and loss of glycogen from the liver and muscles. Much muscle tissue may be lost as well. People are fooled when they weigh themselves after starting a fad diet. They have lost weight, but very little of it represents fat loss. Any loss of lean tissue will mean a decrease in basal metabolism, and so a decrease in overall kcalorie expenditure.

Note that some books use 3500 kcalories per pound of fat gained or lost, but 2700 kcalories per pound of fat storage is a closer estimate. As mentioned in Chapter 8, this is because when fat tissue is gained or lost, the lean support tissue also lost—muscle, connective tissue, blood supply, and other body components—is mostly water and therefore contains few kcalories. When a lot of fat tissue and some lean tissue is lost, the net result is approximately 2700 kcalories exchanged per pound of fat storage.

WISHFUL SHRINKING—WHY IT CAN'T BE MOSTLY FAT

We know that rapid weight loss cannot be mostly fat loss because of the high-kcalorie deficit needed to lose fat tissue. Body fat itself contains about 3500 kcalories per pound. Fat storage—body fat tissue plus support tissues—represents approximately 2700 kcalories per pound.[17] To lose 1 pound of fat storage per week, energy intake must then be cut by approximately 400 kcalories a day (2700/7 = 386). Diets that promise 10 to 15 pounds weight loss per week cannot ensure that the weight loss will be from fat storage alone. Producing a kcalorie deficit sufficient to lose that amount of fat storage is simply not practical. So what is lost rapidly is not only fat, but lean tissue and water.

A SOUND WEIGHT-LOSS DIET—WHAT TO LOOK FOR?

A sound behavioral weight-loss program should include three components: control of kcalorie intake, especially fat intake; changing problem food habits; and increased physical activity.[10] Focusing on just eating fewer kcalories represents a difficult path to success, as we will show. Specifically, look for the following characteristics:[6,25]

1. The eating plan should meet nutritional needs, except for kcalories. To do that, it should follow the Guide to Daily Food Choices, emphasizing low-fat choices.
2. Slow and steady weight loss, as opposed to rapid weight loss, should be stressed. A loss of 1 to 2 pounds per week of fat storage is desirable.
3. The eating plan should allow adaptations to individual habits and tastes. No rigid rituals—such as only eating fruits in the morning or not eating meat after milk products—should be required.
4. The eating plan should minimize hunger and fatigue. To do this, it should contain at least 1000 kcalories per day. Even so, when kcalories are kept between 1200 to 1500 per day, consuming sufficient vitamins and minerals is difficult, especially for young women. If the eating plan calls for fewer kcalories than this per day, it should recommend either fortified foods (breakfast cereals, for example) or a balanced vitamin and mineral supplement (see Chapter 12 for advice on using supplements).
5. The eating plan should contain readily obtainable foods. There is no magical food that can speed weight loss. If a diet suggests that there is—whether ginseng, tofu, or garlic—look elsewhere for advice.
6. The eating should be socially acceptable. It should allow the person dieting to attend parties, eat at restaurants, and participate in normal daily activities.
7. The program should help change problem eating habits. It should promote reshaping food habits and lifestyle to make weight loss, and then weight maintenance, possible and so thwart further weight gain. Maintenance should be a key concern of any plan—it must be essentially a lifetime focus.[24] A 150-pound person should reduce kcalories, exercise, and start eating like a 130-pound person to become a 130-pound person. But once the weight is lost, he or she can't go

back to what was eaten as a 160-pound person. The program should also focus on changing obesity-promoting beliefs and rallying healthy social support.

8. The program should inprove overall health. It should emphasize regular physical activity, proper rest, stress reduction, and other healthy changes in lifestyle.
9. The program should insist that the person see a physician before starting if the person has existing health problems, plans to lose weight as quickly as possible, or is over 35 years of age and plans to perform substantially greater than usual physical activity.

Controlling Energy Intake

A goal of losing 1 to 2 pounds of fat storage per week usually requires an energy intake of 1000 to 1600 kcalories per day for women and 1600 to 2000 kcalories

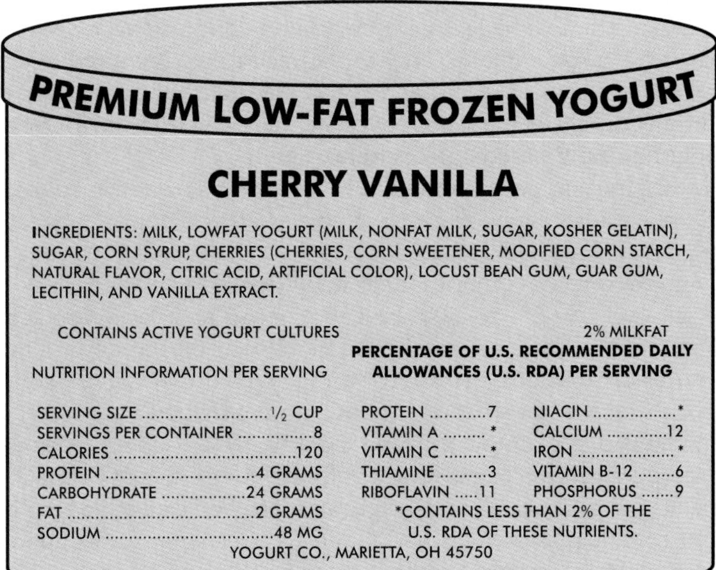

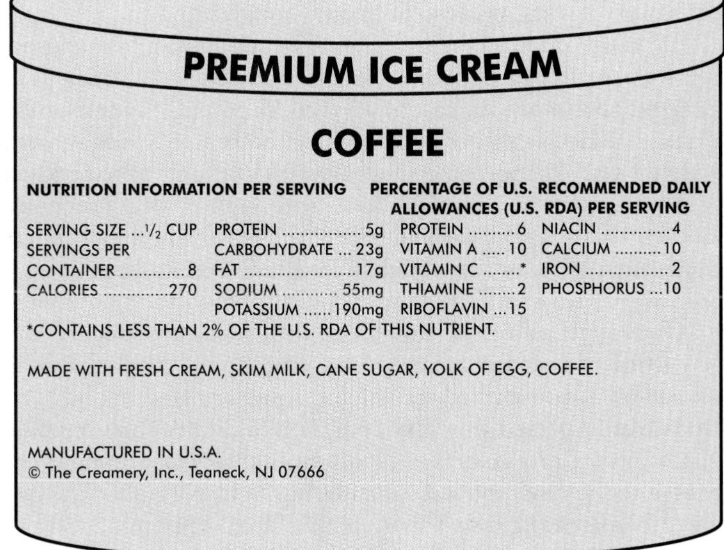

Figure 9-1 Reading labels helps guide one to low-fat food choices. Which frozen dessert represents the best choice for a person on a weight-loss diet?

for men. The range for each gender arises because of the range in physical activity that may be performed. Traditionally dieters have counted kcalories. There is a growing call to count fat mostly, assuming kcalorie control will follow. For kcalorie counters, active people should use the higher energy allowances listed.

Another approach to setting energy needs is to allow 10 kcalories per pound of desirable weight for sedentary people and 13 kcalories per pound for active people. Then subtract 400 kcalories for each pound per week of fat tissue loss desired. For example, an active 160-pound woman who should weigh 140 pounds and wants to lose 1 pound per week could start with 1820 kcalories (13 × 140) and then subtract 400 kcalories. This yields about 1400 kcalories for her diet. Both methods are useful.

In any case, a dieter should not try to eat fewer than 1000 kcalories daily: that causes so much hunger that the person will probably not be able to stick to the plan. A better idea would be to first increase activity level, which could then allow at least 1000 kcalories to be eaten.

Using the exchange system and label reading are two ways for a dieter to monitor energy intake (Figure 9-1). See the menu patterns listed in Table 2-7 for some possible exchange system approaches. Another method is to write down food intake throughout the day and then calculate energy intake from food tables in the evening, adjusting future food choices as needed.

Minimizing fat intake is a very important goal when trying to lose body fat.[18] Recent studies show that diets as low as 20% of kcalories as fat are well tolerated, especially when high in complex carbohydrates and fiber. Adequate satiety is achieved with less total fat kcalories. One study showed that when diets were lowered from a fat level of 40% to 30% and then to 20% of kcalories, subjects compensated slightly. This means that they ate more food on the lower-fat diet. However, the end result was that the lower-fat diet provided far fewer kcalories, allowing the people on the lower-fat diet to lose more weight.

An eating plan that contains 20% to 30% kcalories as fat permits a person to incorporate most commonly eaten foods into the diet.[13] Even subtle changes in food habits can promote desired weight loss. The best eating plan is always one the person can continue practicing throughout life. Changing habits appropriately is the key to both losing weight and maintaining a desirable weight.

Thus the best foods to eat when trying to lose weight are those high in complex carbohydrates and low in fat.[14] Recall carbohydrates provide less than half as many kcalories as fat. A weight-loss diet should include at least 150 grams of carbohydrate daily to prevent ketosis and reduce the risk of bingeing on large amounts of food, particularly sweets, because of intense hunger.

Table 9-1 addressed the question of what foods are appropriate for a weight control plan. Table 9-2 shows how to start saving kcalories.

Most people need to lose fewer than 50 pounds. By consuming a low-fat, lower-kcalorie eating plan these people should be able to achieve a desirable body weight within 1 year. It took time to gain weight. It takes time to lose it.

Starting out on the wrong foot, with limited food selections and rapid weight loss, can sabotage a person's effort to lose weight by encouraging the bingeing and feelings of failure that often accompany those types of dieting approaches (Figure 9-2).

restraint A feeling that occurs as a result of restricted food intake, often associated with the belief that there are good and bad foods.

One suggested reason for failure with restrictive diets is the sense of **restraint** people feel.[22] They feel limited in the amount and types of food they can eat. Often a trade-off is constructed, classifying some foods as "good" and others as "bad." One violation of the diet will be considered a failure. This exerts considerable pressure on the dieter. All it takes is one small emotionally disturbing event or environmental change to "release" the individual trying to lose weight. The person eats a little of the forbidden food, feels a sense of relief from restraint, and has a binge. This leads them to classify themselves as failures and the weight loss attempt is abandoned. Later we address how to avoid this trap.

Table 9-1 What can I eat?

Minimum servings*	Food group	Some suggestions
6	Breads, cereals, rice and pasta	Emphasize whole grains. Breads, yes; avoid those high in fat and sugar. Cereals with little or no sugar. Rice and pasta—but watch out for the sauces and second helpings.
2	Fruits	All except avocados and olives; don't add sugar or whipped cream.
3	Vegetables	All kinds, but go easy on butter, margarine, and other sauces or toppings high in fat. Avoid fried vegetables.
2	Meat, poultry, fish, eggs, dry beans, and nuts	Lean parts of meat; poultry without skin; fish. Broil, roast, simmer. Avoid items that are breaded and fried. Eggs, dry beans, nuts, peas, and tofu are good alternates.
2	Milk, yogurt, and cheese	Skim or low-fat milk and low-fat cheeses. Low-fat and nonfat plain yogurt.
Limit, but include at least one teaspoon of vegetable oil incorporated into foods per day.	Fats, oils, and sweets	Watch out for these. They provide kcalories and little else—not what dieters want. Use spices and herbs instead of sauces, butter, and other fats. For dessert, try fresh fruit or choose baked products made with less fat and sugar—angel food cake, for example. Drink coffee or tea without cream or sugar; use lowfat milk.

*Based on the Guide to Daily Food Choices. This is an excellent plan if the dieter can still lose weight with the kcalories alloted. Otherwise, servings from breads, cereals, rice, and pasta can decrease to four. Adapted from: USDA Home and Garden Bulletin No. 232-2, 1986.

Table 9-2 Saving kcalories: ideas to help get started

Check out the following kcalorie-saving ideas. Then think of other changes to help cut kcalories.

Instead of:	Try:	Kcalories saved:
3 ounces well-marbled meat (prime rib)	3 ounces lean meat (eye of round)	140
½ chicken breast, batter-fried	½ chicken breast broiled with lemon	175
½ cup beef stroganoff	3 ounces lean roast beef	210
½ cup home-fried potatoes	1 medium baked potato	65
½ cup green bean–mushroom casserole	½ cup cooked green beans	50
½ cup potato salad	1 cup raw vegetable salad	140
½ cup pineapple chunks in heavy syrup	½ cup pineapple chunks canned in juice	25
2 tablespoons bottled French dressing	2 tablespoons low-calorie French dressing	150
1/7 9-inch apple pie	1 baked apple	185
3 oatmeal-raisin cookies	1 oatmeal-raisin cookie	125
½ cup ice cream	½ cup ice milk	45
A Danish pastry	Half an English muffin	150
1 cup sugar-coated corn flakes	1 cup plain corn flakes	60
1 cup whole milk	1 cup 1% low-fat milk	45
7-fluid-ounce gin and tonic	6-fluid-ounce wine cooler made with sparkling water	150
1-ounce bag potato chips	1 cup plain popcorn	120
1/12 8-inch white layer cake with chocolate frosting	1/12 angel food cake, 10-inch tube	185
Regular beer	Light beer	40

Adapted from: USDA Home and Garden Bulletin No. 232-2, 1986.

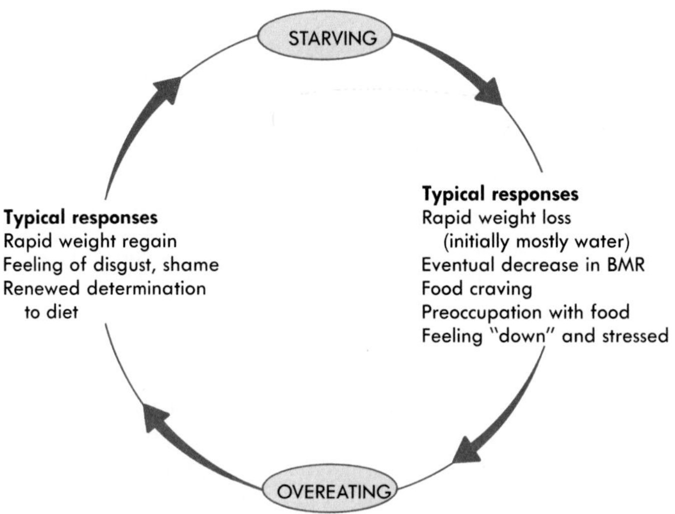

Figure 9-2 A poor start often leads to a poor finish. When considering dieting to lose weight, changing habits is often the key.

CONCEPT CHECK

Key points to consider when attempting to lose weight include: (1) The body resists weight loss; (2) emphasis should be placed on preventing obesity, since curing this disorder is very difficult; (3) weight should be lost from fat stores, not mostly from lean tissues. Appropriate weight loss programs have the following characteristics in common: (1) They meet nutritional needs—this can be evaluated by checking for mostly low-fat and nonfat choices from the Guide to Daily Food Choices; (2) they can adjust to accommodate the person's habits and tastes; (3) they emphasize readily obtainable foods; (4) they promote changing habits that lead to overeating; (5) they encourage an increase in physical activity; (6) they help people change obesity-promoting beliefs and rally healthy social support.

Behavior Modification—Changing Problem Habits

Controlling energy intake and dietary fat are important steps in a weight-loss program. A key for allowing this to happen is behavior modification. Table 9-3 lists behavior modification principles for weight loss. Basically, each person must decide which behaviors contribute to obesity and then find ways to modify those behaviors.[9] In essence, a person's lifestyle and environment should be reshaped so that weight maintenance—rather than weight gain—is the overwhelming thrust, and self-control is not constantly being tested.

To do this, a person should consider the events that cause him or her to start eating, factors that influence food choices, and factors associated with stopping eating. Psychologists often use terms like **chain-breaking, stimulus control, contingency management,** and **self-monitoring** when discussing behavior modification.[9] This terminology helps place the problem in perspective and organize the entire intervention strategy into manageable steps.

Chain-breaking deals with separating behaviors that tend to occur together; for example, snacking on chips and peanuts while watching television. While these activities do not have to occur together, they often do and need to be clearly separated.

Stimulus control involves controlling factors that encourage eating. That may mean hiding irresistible food in the back of the refrigerator, taking the light bulb out of the refrigerator, moving foods from the counter into cabinets, or avoiding the path by a certain vending machine on the way to class.

Contingency management focuses on planning ahead for responses to possible pitfalls and high-risk situations. One strategy, for example, is to rehearse what to say when people press food on you and what to do when irresistible foods are within arm's reach at a party.

Self-monitoring, a key practice in behavior modification, usually begins with keeping a diary of foods eaten and the circumstances that lead to eating. The record can reveal general patterns that provide a better understanding of eating habits (see Take Action in Chapter 1). Self-monitoring is an efficient way to spot problems in eating habits, especially times of unconscious overeating. Self-monitoring can be a persuasive means of encouraging people to adopt new habits to counteract unwanted behaviors. These new habits might include limiting eating to only one place in the house. That could reduce snacking in front of the television and in the kitchen while preparing meals. People who eat very rapidly should put down their utensils while chewing. This practice slows the rate of eating and helps the hormone cholecystokinin (CCK) to signal a natural satiety response. It also gives the stretch receptors in the stomach time to signal fullness. Both of these actions naturally encourage us to stop eating. People who tend to eat anything available can stop purchasing foods they cannot resist.

chain-breaking Breaking the link between two or more behaviors that encourage overeating, such as snacking while watching television.

stimulus control Altering the environment to minimize the stimuli for eating, for example, removing foods from sight and storing them in kitchen cabinets.

contingency management Forming a plan of action to respond to an environment where overeating is likely, such as when snacks are within arm's reach at a party.

self-monitoring A process of tracking foods eaten and conditions affecting eating; actions are usually recorded in a diary, along with location, time, and state of mind. This is a tool to help a person understand more about his or her eating habits.

cognitive restructuring Changing negative, self-defeating, or pessimistic thoughts that undermine weight-control efforts to those that are positive, optimistic, and supportive of weight control.

Current discussions of behavior modification for obesity also include **cognitive restructuring,** social support, providing rewards, and relapse prevention as other helpful strategies. Cognitive restructuring is a strategy for helping individuals change negative, self-defeating, or pessimistic thoughts. Individuals are trained to change thoughts that promote being obese. Thoughts like, "I hate exercise and can never enjoy it," or "I can't have any fun if I don't eat a luscious dessert when I go out with my friends" can undermine a weight control program. By challenging and stopping these thoughts, as well as substituting more appropriate thoughts, adhering to a weight-control program will be easier. Self-talk that reminds us of our achievements, both with weight loss and with other activities in life, helps increase our self-esteem and likelihood of success.

Healthy social support is helpful in weight control.[3] Helping others understand how they could be supportive can make weight control easier. Family and friends can provide praise and encouragement. A weight-control professional can keep the person accountable and help him or her learn from difficult situations. Long-term contact with a professional can be quite helpful for weight-loss maintenance. Groups of individuals attempting to lose weight or maintain losses can provide empathetic support.

Table 9-3 Behavioral principles of weight loss

Stimulus control

Shopping

1. Shop for food after eating—buy nutritious foods
2. Shop from a list; do not buy irresistable "problem" foods
3. Avoid ready-to-eat foods; let others who want them buy them and store them

Plans

1. Plan to limit food intake
2. Substitute exercise for snacking
3. Eat meals and snacks at scheduled times; don't skip meals
4. Don't accept inappropriate foods offered by others

Activities

1. Store food out of sight, preferably in the freezer so that compulsive eating is discouraged
2. Eat all food in the same place
3. Remove food from inappropriate storage areas in the house
4. Keep serving dishes off the table, especially sauces and gravies
5. Use smaller dishes and utensils
6. Avoid being the food server
7. Leave the table immediately after eating

Holidays and parties

1. Drink fewer alcoholic beverages
2. Plan eating habits before parties
3. Eat a low-calorie snack before parties
4. Practice polite ways to decline food
5. Don't get discouraged by an occasional setback

Eating behavior

1. Put fork down between mouthfuls
2. Chew thoroughly before swallowing
3. Leave some food on the plate
4. Pause in the middle of the meal
5. Do nothing else while eating (read, watch television)

Some obese individuals reward or comfort themselves with food. It is important that food not be used for these purposes. Instead one needs to learn to cope adequately in other ways with the normal daily hassles and the stresses and strains of life. Too often we use eating like some people use alcohol or other drugs—to deal with such difficulties. Eating becomes a way of self-medicating or avoiding having to face stressful circumstances. Finding alternative methods to cope with stress is important for keeping the weight off.[9]

The main criteria for effective rewards or outlets for stress are that they be of value and can be frequently given. Music tapes or compact discs, clothing, and tickets to sporting events or concerts can serve as effective rewards, based on the preferences of the individual. A system of rewards can increase the likelihood that a person will exhibit appropriate weight-control behaviors in the future.

relapse prevention A set of strategies used by people to help prevent and cope with weight control lapses.

Relapse prevention is a series of strategies for helping people on diets and on weight maintenance programs to anticipate and cope with problems.[24] A person attempts, with advanced planning, to prevent slips, called lapses, and deal with them when they do occur. A lapse is one mistake, but a relapse is total abandonment of the weight-control program. An individual who is unprepared for a lapse may interpret it as failure and abandon weight-control efforts.

Table 9-3 Behavioral principles of weight loss—cont'd

Reward

1. Solicit help from family and friends. Help family and friends provide this help in the form of praise and material rewards
2. Utilize self-monitoring records as basis for rewards
3. Plan specific rewards for specific behaviors (behavioral contracts)

Self-monitoring

Diet diary

1. Note time and place of eating
2. List type and amount of food eaten
3. Record who is present and how you feel

Nutrition education

1. Use diet diary to identify problem areas
2. Make small changes that you can continue
3. Learn nutritional values of foods
4. Decrease fat intake; increase complex-carbohydrate intake

Physical activity

Routine activity

1. Increase routine activity
2. Increase use of stairs
3. Keep a record of distance walked each day

Exercise

1. Begin a mild exercise program; increase the exercise very gradually
2. Keep a record of daily exercise

Cognitive restructuring

1. Avoid setting unreasonable goals
2. Think about progress, not shortcomings
3. Avoid imperatives like "always" and "never"
4. Counter negative thoughts with rational restatements

Table 9-4 Tactics for managing eating behavior

Many things can trigger inappropriate eating behavior. But effective tactics can be used to gain control of eating. Here is a list of tactics, organized by problem area, that have proved effective for many people. These add to the suggestions in Table 9-3. Decide which tactics might be most effective in helping you gain control of your eating behavior. Then, make them part of a behavior change strategy. While it would be desirable to have the will-power to not eat high-fat foods, most people find that the best alternative is to avoid the temptations.

Buying and storing food

Avoid aisles of problem food in the grocery store
Don't pretend it's for the children or company
Inventory the kitchen and pantry, then give away or discard problem foods

Cooking, preparing, and serving food

Broil, bake, or poach—don't fry
Substitute low-fat and low-kcalorie ingredients
Don't sample while cooking
Plan menus
Measure portions
Let others get their own snacks, desserts, and second helpings

Eating food

Drink plenty of water
Drink little or no alcohol
Eat more complex carbohydrates (vegetables, grains, legumes)
Avoid high-fat foods
Eat three meals a day
Replace impulse snacking with planned, healthy snacks. Keep low-fat snack foods close at hand, especially during peak snacking periods.

Coping with problem food

Make problem food temporarily off-limits, but not permanently forbidden
Plan to eat a little of a problem food under "safe" conditions (where you can't binge)

Eating out in restaurants

Choose a restaurant that allows healthy food choices
Ask the waitress not to put bread and butter on the table before the meal
Request no butter and no sauce on vegetables or entree
Choose a broiled entree
Request water with a meal
Request salad dressing on the side or bring your own
Don't look at the dessert list or dessert tray

Coping with others

Ask co-workers not to offer food
Instead of eating to be polite, thank the person offering food and decline firmly
Just say "No, thank you, I've had enough. It was declicious, and I'm full."

Coping with emotions

Avoid people and situations that upset you
Go for a walk or use other exercises to unwind
Lighten up, don't take it all so seriously
Join a support group or seek counseling

Managing your body

Exercise regularly
Get adequate rest

Adapted from Nash JD: Maximize your body potential, Palo Alto, Calif., 1986, Bull Publishing Co.

Relapse often starts with a high-risk situation, like going on vacation. Most people don't recognize when they are at high risk for relapse, and just "one slip" becomes a series of lapses that lead to complete relapse into "old behaviors." The first "lapse" should be a signal to the person that he or she is stressed, having interpersonal conflicts, and is not coping adequately with everyday events. This is a high-risk situation. One or two slips is not fatal. Healthful behavior can be recovered if the potential for relapse is planned in advance and even expected. The following are some helpful strategies for relapse prevention:

Identify high-risk situations—If and when you backslide, ask yourself if you are in a high-risk situation. This should help you to focus on the event rather than feel guilty about backsliding.

Mentally rehearse a response to a backsliding behavior—Imagine yourself backsliding and see yourself taking positive action to recover. Rehearse a response to as many potential lapses as you can think of.

Remember your goals—Remind yourself of the reasons for making the commitment to change your behavior and of the hard work that has gone into achieving progress.

Stay calm when errors are made—Take charge immediately. Ask for help if you need it.

In conclusion, dieters must analyze their own particular behavior shortcomings, and then should sensitize themselves to facets of their lifestyle that make dieting difficult.[9] Is snacking, compulsive eating, or overeating at each meal a constant problem? Then specific problems must be addressed. There are many options for changing shopping and eating behaviors (Tables 9-3 and 9-4). It is best to integrate many strategies and tactics in a behavior plan. In a later section on the behavior change process we will specifically discuss how to do this.

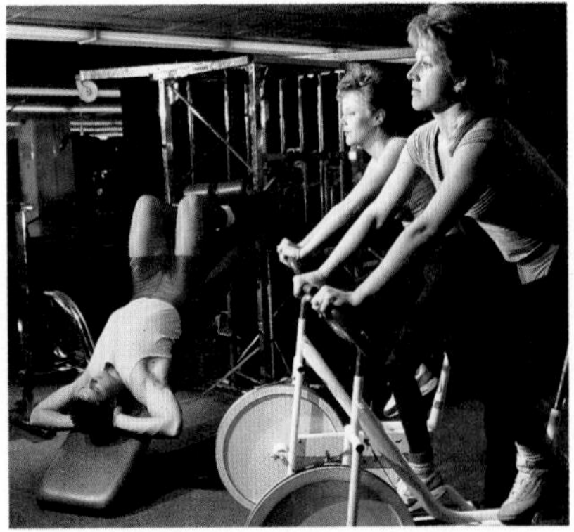

Regular physical activity is one component of a healthy weight-loss plan.

CONCEPT CHECK

Several facets of behavior can be modified to improve conditions for losing weight. One behavior area that requires change involves breaking habit chains that encourage overeating, such as snacking while watching television. Another tactic is to modify the environment to reduce temptations; for example, put foods into cupboards to keep them out of sight. Planning how to handle and refuse food temptations is another strategy. In addition, rethinking attitudes about eating—for example, substituting pleasures other than food as a reward for coping with a stressful day—can be important for altering undesirable eating behavior. Advanced planning to prevent and deal with lapses is vital, as well as rallying healthy social support. Finally, careful observation and recording of eating habits in a diary can reveal subtle behaviors that lead to overeating.

Physical Activity—Another Key to Weight Loss

Engaging in regular physical activity is very important for all people, and especially those who are trying to lose weight. We use many more kcalories in activity than at rest. Burning only 200 to 300 extra kcalories per day—above and beyond the normal activity level—can eliminate about a half pound of fat storage per week: that's about 25 pounds of fat loss in a year. Adding any of the activities given in Figure 9-3 to your lifestyle will allow you to burn an extra 200 kcalories; note that sitting is not a recommended "activity." Duration and regular performance—not necessarily intensity—are the keys to success with this approach to weight loss.

The easiest way to increase physical activity is to make it part of a daily routine. Experts recommend an hour of brisk walking every day. One can try to incorporate

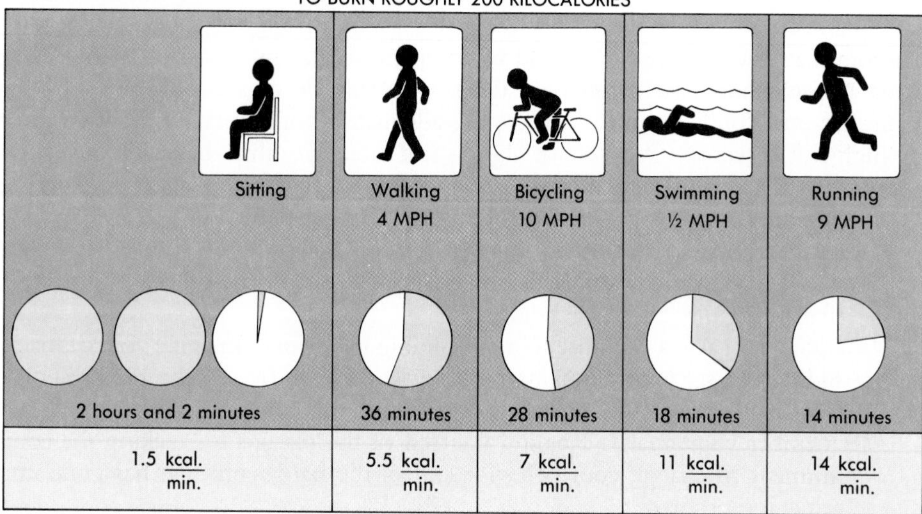

Figure 9-3 Exercise improves any diet. Weight loss will occur because we burn so many more kcalories than at rest. Each of these activities will burn approximately 200 kcalories.

Before embarking on a program of regular physical activity, it might be useful to have your body fat percentage measured by bioelectrical impedance or by a skinfold thickness test. These measurements would enable you to track not only weight changes in dieting but also fat mass versus lean mass changes. Many people find their weight does not change as rapidly as their fat mass changes because some fat mass is replaced by lean tissue due to the exercise.

this, along with stair climbing, in the daily routine. A simple trick is to park your car farther from school or the shopping mall so you can walk farther.

Besides using energy, increased physical activity has the added advantage of reducing the stress and boredom of a diet. It takes the dieter out of the house and away from snacks. Eventually, increased physical activity can lead to modest increases in muscle mass as well. Having more lean tissue raises basal metabolism so that, even while sitting quietly, one burns a few more kcalories than when the same body contained a higher proportion of fat tissue.

Recent studies suggest that activity does not cause the body to raise kcalorie use for hours after an activity, as was earlier thought. Nevertheless, the extra energy used in physical activity, coupled with any increase in muscle mass, can pay dividends. Exercise can also help blunt the loss of muscle mass when on a weight-loss diet. Whatever means of increasing physical activity is chosen, the activities should be ones the dieter enjoys so that the person will practice them regularly. They should also be convenient, within the dieter's budget, and should provide options for bad weather. Note that people who participate in a program of behavior modification plus aerobic exercise lose significantly more weight than those involved in behavior modification alone.

Once a regular program of physical activity is established, the rate of weight loss often begins to diminish. One cause of this slower weight loss is the lowered body weight, which reduces the energy cost of activity. At this point one's activity level should be increased. The dieter could consider walking 15 minutes more or doing more stair climbing each day to receive the same exercise benefit.

EXERCISE—AN ADDED BENEFIT IS HEART HEALTH

cardiovascular Referring to the heart and blood vessels.

One goal in exercising might be to increase **cardiovascular** fitness. To achieve that it is best to increase the heart rate to 70% of the maximum rate for about 30 minutes per day at least 3 days per week. This maximum heart rate is generally estimated as 220 − current age. For lower intensity activities, like brisk walking, 40 to 60 minutes duration might be warranted. When following this exercise prescription, it is important to use at least 5 minutes to both warm up and cool down.

While heart health is a laudable goal, obese people may find it easier to concentrate on losing weight first. When the goal is weight loss, again the key word is duration—not intensity. A day's total physical activity should last long enough to burn 200 to 300 extra kcalories (compared to just staying at rest). To get an idea of how long that takes for different exercises, see Figure 9-3 and Appendix L.

The Behavior Change Process

We have seen the components of an effective weight-control program. Now let's look at the process an obese person can go through to integrate these components into life and in turn make behavior changes that will lead to weight loss.[3,9]

When a person recognizes that his or her obesity is a problem, the next step is to develop a **receptive framework** for learning more about the problem. This might involve evaluating the costs and benefits of changing behavior—perhaps balancing the time and effort exercising requires plus sacrificing some favorite foods against the benefits of lowering weight, decreasing health risks, and feeling and looking better. The person must accept personal responsibility for correcting the problem.

receptive framework The process by which a person opens for learning and responds to learning more about a problem—it usually involves seeking more information about the issue from books and people.

Considering earlier experiences, the would-be changer must decide whether the change is feasible. Can his or her lifestyle accommodate the new goal? Can the person continue the new behaviors for the rest of his or her life? By reading about and speaking with others who have worked on similar health projects, a person might find the changes less threatening. Here the credibility of a health professional can be critical. Where the change may at first appear to demand too much sacrifice or seem impossible, a health professional can possibly provide the information and encouragement necessary to start the change process.

CHARTING A PLAN FOR CHANGE

The next step is the development of a behavioral weight-control plan. A good plan evolves. It is based on rational, deliberate decisions and trial and error methods. It is built after considering and evaluating many options. While a person can't know all possible strategies and tactics before beginning, a good plan incorporates the information at hand. Revisions will be necessary and are expected.

In planning to control weight a person needs to know that the typical restrictive diet not only fails to produce the desired results for most people, but also can produce undesired results, such as fatigue and depression. More effective weight control programs lead people away from severe dieting and toward raising their activity levels. So it's best to know (1) what programs are available, (2) how up-to-date is their information, and (3) how effective are their methods before choosing a program. Useful information about programs can be found by visiting clinic programs; reading health and nutrition books on weight control; and speaking with registered dietitians, physicians, and other health professionals.

GATHERING BASELINE DATA

A next step in creating a personal plan for weight control is to observe present eating behavior and activity patterns, noting strengths and weaknesses. Monitoring eating behaviors is a good beginning exercise—as we mentioned recording meals and snacks in a diary may reveal eating patterns previously unnoticed. Let's assume that you want to adjust habits to control weight and are working to lower your fat intake as one means of doing that. In a diary, you might want to list some—or all—of the following: foods eaten and portion sizes, percentage of fat in the foods eaten, intensity of hunger, time, location, and activity performed at the same time as eating (such as watching television), whether you were influenced by the social aspects of eating with others, and your feelings at the time (we have included a blank facsimile for your use in Appendix E).[9]

A review of the diary, like the one from Chapter 1, might reveal how the external environment and internal cues work together to affect nutrition and health habits. This is the time to look for patterns, identifying positive decisions and needed changes. You might classify food choices as "can't give up," "desirable," and "neutral." Patterns might suggest which food habits should be easy to change and which may be difficult to change. Eating habits may be paired with another activity; you may find that you eat mostly while visiting with friends, while in an angry mood, or perhaps after 6 P.M. Subtle associations can influence eating habits and be the starting point for behavior changes.

Sensory appeal—flavor, appearance, and odor—and habit usually drive both our intended and actual food choices. Of secondary significance in choosing foods to eat are health value, expediency, social influence, kcalorie value, and cost.

SETTING ATTAINABLE GOALS

Once behaviors that need changing have been identified, goals can be developed. As a result of the baseline assessment maybe the person discovers that he or she needs to eat more low-fat foods, remove tempting foods from the house, and institute a regular exercise program. These will serve as the basis for establishing goals.

Good weight-control goals should be measurable, short-term, specific, and based on observable behaviors. A goal like, "I will walk briskly for 30 minutes, four times this week," fulfills these criteria. Two to three goals should be pursued at a time. Pursue each one for at least 3 weeks to give each a chance at becoming a habit. New goals then can be set as possible. It is vital that goals not be vague and solely linked to the bathroom scale; for example, "I will lose 30 pounds in 12 weeks" is not a valuable behavioral goal. Behavioral goals are particularly helpful when they emphasize concrete changes in lifestyle. As these goals are achieved, your lifestyle will be changed as well. At the end of a week a person can evaluate to what degree the goals were achieved and gain reinforcement from something that has been done.

Those trying to lose weight should not try to pursue too many goals in a short period of time or they might be overwhelmed. Pursuing a limited number of goals each week will lead to greater progress in behavior change over the long term, as long as the goals are modified as the person makes progress.

It can help to attach rewards to achievement of current goals. These rewards can reinforce the behaviors that have been practiced. If a person achieves his or her exercise goals maybe he or she would buy a new novel, go to the movies, or allow time for a bubble bath.

Success at changing behavior is strongly tied to a person's commitment; the greater the personal dedication, the greater the chances of success.[3] Examine the goals you have set. Are they worth pursuing? Are health benefits greater than the sacrifices to be made? Some people can ignore persistent arthritis in the knees—which is magnified through the condition of overweight—because they derive great pleasure from eating. Others may love eating ice cream and chips and dips but finally realize that the price is too high; they realize the benefits of losing the weight added from immoderate snacking would eventually be greater than the momentary pleasure of continuing their present behavioral patterns. They understand that in changing their eating habits, they would feel better about themselves, could move around more easily, would feel less anxious in public, and would limit some future health problems.

WORKING OUT THE DETAILS

Once goals are established and the changer discovers personal strengths and weaknesses in pursuing them, it is time to set details of the plan. Some nutrition knowledge is necessary, and the information contained in this book is a good place to start. If you feel unable to work out a plan, professional help is also available.

So let's say you want to eat low-fat dinners 5 nights during the week. You must do the research to find recipes for low-fat dinners, get the ingredients, and allow time to prepare them. If you want to exercise 4 days per week during the winter, you may have to research area fitness centers to see when they are open, if the hours are convenient to you, if they have the kind of equipment that you need, and how much it will cost. These are the kinds of details that must be worked out to achieve the goals that have been set.

MEASURING PROGRESS

There are a few good ways to measure progress while participating in a weight-control program. The first is to track on a weekly basis whether the two to three

NUTRITION FOCUS

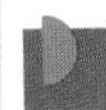

Breaking Behavior Chains

by James Ferguson M.D.

We are creatures of habit. All of our behaviors are linked, one to the next. Much like the chain that holds a boat to its anchor, our behavior chains can anchor us to relatively fixed conditions, like obesity. The behavior chain is a series of interconnected habitual behaviors.

The following is a good example of a behavior chain: Consider the businesswoman who comes home after a hard day at work. She puts down her briefcase, picks up the paper, turns on the television, sits down, gets up and looks in the refrigerator, grabs a snack, again sits in front of the television, and, afterward, eats a meal. After dinner, she sits down to watch television, gets bored, walks into the kitchen, browses through the refrigerator, eats a piece of cheesecake, wanders back to the television, feels guilty about the snack, and assuages her guilt with another piece of cheesecake. The initial event, such as stress or boredom, can seem innocuous, but the ending is always the same—extra kcalories.

How many eating situations in your life can you describe in terms of behavior chains? A study of the series of linked events suggests a strategy for eliminating extra habitual eating or snacking. Break the chain! It's hard to just say no. The easy way to break the chain is to substitute an alternate activity. The earlier the chain is broken, the better and the easier it is to cut kcalories. Once the snack touches your taste buds, it's too late. When that cheesecake is only a gleam in your eye or, even better, a "pregleam" the awareness that you are headed for something to eat makes it easier to break the chain.

The way to cast off your chains is to identify them, pinpoint the weak links, break them, and substitute another behavior. Using alternate activities sounds easy, but it's hard to do on the spur of the moment. Figure 9-4 shows you how to use a diagram to identify the links in your behavior chains. It also gives you the opportunity to list substitute activities that can be used to break the links in the chain.

If your behavior chain is broken at any point, it will probably not continue. (The businesswoman's final behaviors—eating, feeling guilty, eating—probably won't occur.) The earlier in the chain you substitute a nonfood link, the easier it is to intervene.

Four types of behaviors can be substituted in an ongoing behavior chain:

1. Fun activities (grabbing your mate, taking a walk, reading a book)
2. Necessary activities (cleaning a room, balancing your checkbook)
3. Incompatible activities (taking a shower)
4. Urge-delaying activities (setting a kitchen timer for 20 minutes before allowing yourself to eat)

Using activities to interrupt behavior patterns that lead to inappropriate eating can be a powerful means of changing eating habits. This technique can also be useful when you are eating in response to environmental as well as to internal cues for eating, such as television advertisement for food or a hunger pang that you feel at an odd time after a meal or before going to bed. If it's pushing you to eat, substitute!

Dr Ferguson is a nationally prominent psychiatrist who specializes in weight control. He is the author of many books, including Habits, Not Diets.

behavioral goals were accomplished and to what degree. This should help the person modify goals and update goals.

When people are attempting to lose weight they would like to see changes in their body composition. Just weighing oneself daily or weekly would not be recommended because weight can vary based on a number of factors besides fat gained or lost. A better way to track progress is to also use tape measurements of areas of the body like the neck, waist, upper thigh, and upper arm. These measurements are closely related to body fat changes. Monitoring changes in waist or clothing size is an additional way to track long-term progress. Finally, changes in fitness level and health are good indicators of progress. Percentage of body fat, determined by measuring skinfolds, can even be another way to monitor changes. Rather than just setting a goal weight, it would be better for an individual to change his or her lifestyle and see ultimately where weight settles.

Keeping records of diet, activity, changes in body fat or weight, blood pressure, serum cholesterol levels, and clothing size over time can help a person track weight-loss progress. Seeing progress over time will be reinforcing by itself to someone trying to lose weight.

ALTERNATE ACTIVITY SHEET:

SUBSTITUTE ACTIVITIES

Pleasant activities
1. Singing/washing hair
2. Reading comics/biking
3. Sewing/calling a girlfriend

Necessary activities
1. Ironing
2. Vacuuming
3. Straightening apartment

Situations when used
1. Wanted ice cream—delayed with bath
2. Wanted wheat thins—cleaned up apt.
3. Wanted snack—went for walk
4. Wanted cookies—did dishes first
5. Saw leftovers—went for bike ride
6. Tempted by cookies—set timer
7. Wanted snack—read comics

BEHAVIOR CHAIN

Identify the links in your eating response chain on the following diagram. Draw a line through the chain where it was interrupted. Add the link you substituted and the new chain of behaviors this substitution started.

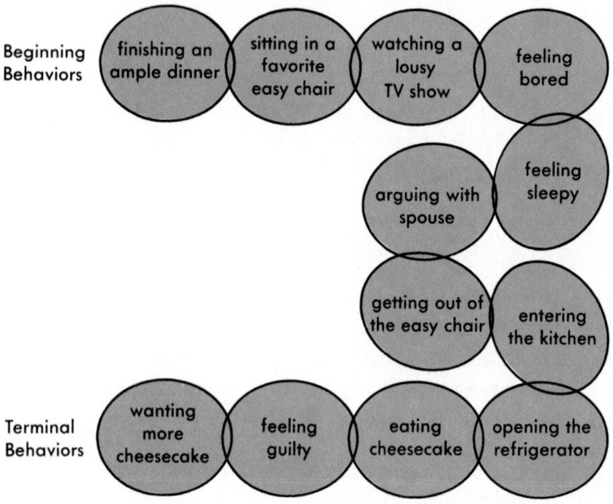

Beginning Behaviors: finishing an ample dinner — sitting in a favorite easy chair — watching a lousy TV show — feeling bored — feeling sleepy — arguing with spouse — getting out of the easy chair — entering the kitchen — opening the refrigerator — eating cheesecake — feeling guilty — wanting more cheesecake :Terminal Behaviors

ALTERNATE ACTIVITY SHEET:

SUBSTITUTE ACTIVITIES

Pleasant activities
1. ______
2. ______
3. ______

Necessary activities
1. ______
2. ______
3. ______

Situations when used
1. ______
2. ______
3. ______
4. ______
5. ______
6. ______
7. ______

BEHAVIOR CHAIN

Identify the links in your eating response chain on the following diagram. Draw a line through the chain where it was interrupted. Add the link you substituted and the new chain of behaviors this substitution started.

Beginning Behaviors

Terminal Behaviors: Guilt — Eating

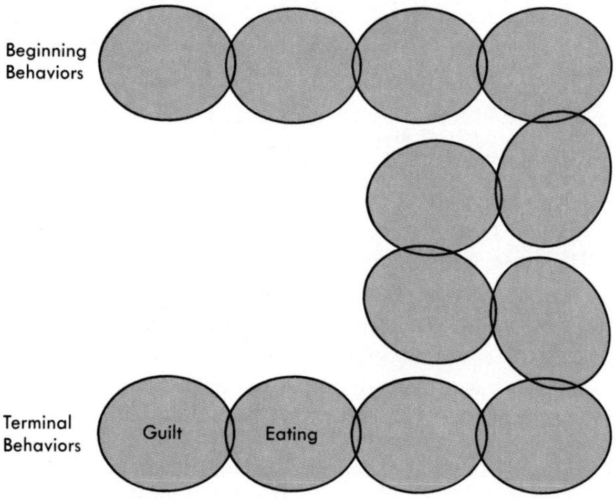

Figure 9-4 Identifying behavior chains is a good tool for understanding more about your habits and pinpointing ways to change unwanted habits.

MAKING IT OFFICIAL

People often find it helpful to develop a behavioral contract to encourage follow-through.[9] The contract could list goal behaviors and objectives, mileposts for measuring progress, and regular rewards for meeting the terms of the contract. Positive reinforcement contributes more to successful behavior change than negative reinforcement. Initially, the focus should be on positive behaviors, then on positive results. Positive behaviors, such as regular exercise, eventually lead to positive outcomes. It may take months to see the effects. Look at the example of a behavior contract for weight loss in Table 9-5. When you have finished your contract, sign it in the presence of some friends to publicly affirm it. Contracts can help promote adherence to the program.

BEING ASSERTIVE WITH OTHERS

When you wish to change yourself, you are likely to get feedback from people who may support the planned changes, but some may prefer to keep things the way they are. They may try to dissuade you from your plan. Even you may have days or moments when you try to talk yourself out of your plan. We all respond to others'

Table 9-5 Behavioral contract

Name Chris Willer

Goal
I agree to spend at least 20 minutes eating.
(specify behavior)

under the following circumstances: in my home, during dinner
(specify where, when, how much, etc.)
5 times per week

Substitute behavior and/or reinforcement schedule I will reward myself at the end of week if I fulfill my goal.

Environmental planning
In order to help me do this, I am going to (1) arrange my physical and social environment by eat more dinners at home, place a timer set for 20 minutes on the dinner table.

and (2) control my internal environment (thoughts, images) by put a note on the refrigerator reminding me.

Reinforcements
Reinforcements provided by me daily or weekly (if contract is kept):
rent one of my favorite VCR movies at the end of the week.
Reinforcements provided by others daily or weekly (if contract is kept):
will ask me at the end of the week if I achieved my goal and if so will complement me.

Social support
Behavior change is more likely to take place when other people support you. During the quarter/semester please meet with the other person at least three times to discuss your progress.
The name of my "significant helper" is: Shawn Jones

This contract should include:
1. Baseline data (one week)
2. Well-defined goal
3. Simple method for charting progress (diary, counters, charts, etc.)
4. Reinforcements (immediate and long-term)
5. Evaluation method (summary of experiences, success, and/or new learnings about self).

From Davis TM: Instructor's Resource Guide to accompany *Core concepts in health* by PM Insel and WT Roth. Mountain View, Calif., 1988, Mayfield Publishing Co.

opinions, especially about ourselves. We like approval, generally, and are influenced by others to behave in certain ways. One problem in undertaking behavior change is to be strong enough to behave in a chosen manner when others encourage—unconsciously or not—behavior inappropriate to the desired goal.

A certain amount of "psyching yourself up" is sometimes necessary to enable you to pursue your goals—in spite of others' expectations. Almost everyone benefits from some assertiveness training when it comes to changing behaviors. Here are a few things you might consider:

- No one's feelings should be hurt if you say, "No, thank you," firmly and repeatedly, when others try to dissuade you from a plan. Rather, ask them—and yourself—why they want you to eat their way. Your needs are as important as someone's else's.

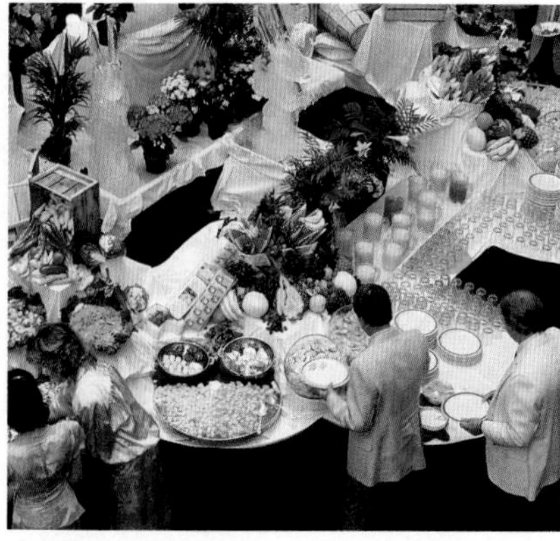

A contingency management plan might consist of learning to eat only healthful foods at a party, or eating a small snack beforehand.

- You don't have to order "big" to accommodate anyone—your mother, business clients, or the chef. Ordering "big" just because someone else is paying for the meal is a trap.
- When entertaining, you can serve lighter, more healthful low-fat meals. You might have to try some new recipes, but that will be a useful step en route to changing your overall approach to cooking.
- Dealing with parties and social occasions built around food is possible but difficult. You can plan celebrations around a hike or a tennis court, rather than around cake and ice cream. When you must attend parties where food is everywhere, you can eat before you go, take low-kcalorie foods with you, and converse far from the food table.
- Learn ways to handle "put-downs"—inadvertent or conscious. The most effective response may be to communicate feelings honestly, without hostility. Tell criticizers that they have hurt your feelings, that you are working to change your habits, and that you would really like their understanding and support.
- Fostering feelings of self-worth will facilitate the ability to change behavior. Getting rid of the habit of self-criticism requires strong self-retraining. Create and memorize lists of strengths, giving credit where deserved. Practice forgiving yourself. Lower unrealistic expectations. Practice stopping negative thoughts about yourself. Purposely switch to positive thoughts.
- Help change the family diet. The best situation is when the whole family wants to eat healthfully. The cook can influence that a great deal. There is extra effort involved in finding and developing new recipes and learning substitutions and shortcuts to cutting fat or kcalories. But the information exists in good cookbooks and recipes and is becoming more widespread as people get more excited about health and good nutrition. If you are not the cook and are living at home with parents, perhaps you could make arrangements to do your own cooking. If you live in a residence hall, you can make careful choices in dining.

FOLLOWING THE PLAN

Once you determine your weight-control plan and, perhaps, write a contract, it is time to implement the plan. To begin, plan a trial of at least 6 to 8 weeks. Thinking of a lifetime commitment can be overwhelming. Remember that you win the game one point at a time. Aim for a total duration of 6 months of new activities before giving up. It is difficult to overcome the inertia of 20, 30, 40 or more years. More than once you may have to persuade yourself of the value of continuing the behavior-change program. You may even backslide. That is not totally disastrous, if you can learn to manage your thinking. Focus on reducing, but not necessarily extinguishing, undesirable behaviors; it is usually unrealistic to say you will never eat chocolate ice cream again. Better to say you will not eat chocolate ice cream as regularly as before.

In all, cultivate a long-term vision for a nutrition and health plan. Forgive occasional indiscretions. Focus on behaviors that have been established and performed day after day. An occasional lapse does not justify a relapse, and certainly not a collapse. Especially watch for rationalization, the attempt to fool oneself—distorting information and denying facts to support wishful thinking are ways to rationalize. Trying to justify backsliding by saying "I can't do it" when you have done it for 4 months already is rationalizing. You don't fool even yourself.

REEVALUATING THE PLAN

After you have practiced a program for several months, reevaluating it may clarify some issues. Are you accomplishing your goals and making progress? If you aren't accomplishing your goals, how must you change your plan? Are there other behaviors that need to be changed that haven't been addressed? These are all pertinent questions. The plan should be modified as needed.

A RECAP

When experts on weight loss pool their collective experience, they identify certain factors that characterize success and failure in weight loss:[3,9,11]

Success is encouraged by:

1. Increased physical activity and moderation in fat/kcalorie intake.
2. Feeling a sense that he or she is in control of personal destiny.
3. Motivation to succeed.
4. Focusing on improved health status to spur short-term success.
5. Social support via family/friends.
6. Sustained vigilance in pursuit of one's goals—this is a lifetime pursuit.
7. Reasonable goals that promote gradual change to improve one's odds of success.
8. Keeping track of one's weight.

Failure is encouraged by:

1. Negative feelings.
2. Out-of-control social situations, such as a family life or lifestyle that constantly challenges the person's will to succeed.
3. Reverting to old habits.

CONCEPT CHECK

Once a person decides to lose weight a series of steps are warranted for effective behavior change. The behavior change process involves: (1) charting a plan; (2) collecting baseline data; (3) setting attainable goals; (4) working out the details of the plan; (5) measuring progress; (6) making it official by drawing up a contract; (7) being assertive with others; (8) following the plan; and (9) reevaluating the plan. This process will increase the chances of losing weight and keeping it off in the future.

Professional Help for Weight Loss

The first professional to see for advice about a weight-loss program is the family physician. Doctors are best equipped to assess overall health and the appropriateness of a weight-loss plan.[6] The physician will probably refer the person to a registered dietitian for a specific plan and for answers to diet-related questions. Registered dietitians are uniquely qualified to help design a weight-loss plan because they understand both food composition and what food means to people. Exercise physiologists can provide advice on an exercise program.

Many communities have a variety of weight-loss organizations. These may include self-help groups, such as Take Off Pounds Sensibly and Weight Watchers. Other programs, such as NutriSystem, Diet Center, and Physicians Weight Loss Center among others, are often less desirable for the average dieter. These programs are generally expensive, mainly because of their requirements for intense counseling and/or mandatory diet foods and supplements.

Spot-reducing using diet and exercise is not possible. Exercise may firm the tissue by tightening the muscles present, but the fat will decrease only as other fat stores in the body generally decrease. "Problem" local fat deposits can be reduced in size, however, using suction lipectomy. Lipectomy simply means surgical removal of fat. A pencil-thin tube is inserted into an incision in the skin and the fat tissue, such as that in the buttocks and thigh area, is suctioned off. This procedure, developed in the early 1980s, carries risks such as infection, large depressions in the skin, and blood clots that can lead to kidney failure. Also, it is often quite painful. It is not designed to help a person lose 30 to 40 pounds, but rather about 4 pounds per treatment. It can be used as part of cosmetic surgery by an experienced physician to help a person reduce localized fat deposits that are very diet-resistant. Costs range from $300 to $6000 per body site.

TREATING MORBID OBESITY

Morbid obesity refers to the status of a body at least 100 pounds over desirable body weight, body mass index greater than 39, or twice one's desirable body weight.[2] Few obese people have morbid obesity, currently about 1.5 million in the United States. But those who do suffer the most severe obesity-related health problems. More drastic treatment measures may be used in these cases if the more conservative plan—reducing kcalorie and especially fat intake, increasing physical activity, and modifying behavior—has failed.

EXPERT OPINION

Very Low Calorie Diets in the Treatment of Obesity

BY JUDY LOPER, PH.D., R.D., L.D.

Both the public and professionals have been searching for an effective treatment for obesity. In the early 1970s research in Boston and Cleveland examined the use of supplemental fasting for the treatment of morbid obesity. Since that time the popularity, composition of the regimens, and the public's perception of this method of weight control has varied. Many diet plans have evolved.

In the late 1970s, there were 58 deaths reported among obese adults using "liquid protein" diets. These diets provided 300 to 500 kcalories per day and contained protein of low biological value (collagen or gelatin). No medical supervision accompanied these very low calorie diets, as they were self-prescribed. These deaths were thought to be linked to the inadequate amino acid composition and low amounts of potassium and other minerals. Overall, this contributed to considerable loss of muscle mass, including heart muscle.

Today's medically supervised very low calorie diets

Very low calorie diets (VLCDs) today supply 400 to 800 kcalories per day. They are designed to promote considerable weight loss while preserving lean body mass. To do this, these diets provide 70 to 100 grams per day of high-quality protein (egg or milk) either (1) in a powdered formulation that must be mixed with water or a low kcalorie fluid or (2) in the form of lean meat, fish, or fowl. The liquid forms of the diet often contain 30 to 120 grams of carbohydrate and supplemental vitamins and minerals, including potassium. These are added to promote retention of lean body mass and minimize some medical complications. The VLCD of lean meat generally contains 1.2 grams of protein per kilogram of desirable body weight and very little carbohydrate. Extra vitamins and minerals are given along with this diet as well. These VLCDs promote weekly weight losses of about 3 pounds in women and 4 pounds in men.

Indications for the VLCD

There are a limited number of therapeutic alternatives in the treatment of the excessively obese patient. Most programs that use the VLCD limit the use of it to persons who are 30% or greater above desirable body weight. Many of these patients have concurrent health problems (i.e., hypertension, diabetes, hyperlipidemia, arthritis, sleep apnea, and coronary heart disease). Even with a modest weight loss on a VLCD, many of these medical problems can be minimized or reduced.

Contraindications

Contraindications for the VLCD are pregnancy or lactation, acute substance abuse, recent myocardial infarction (within 3 months), renal or hepatic failure, cerebrovascular disease (stroke), and transient ischemic disease. Other medical conditions might warrant extra screening or monitoring. The presence of risk factors (i.e., coronary heart disease, diabetes, hypertension, etc.) should not necessarily be contraindicated for starting patients on the VLCD. These are the patients who will most likely benefit.

Medical monitoring

Medical monitoring by experienced physicians includes initial screening, laboratory work, an electrocardiogram, physical examination, and body composition analysis. Safe use of these diets includes medical monitoring through refeeding and weight maintenance. Lab work and serum electrolytes are checked every other week during the period of rapid weight loss. Electrocardiograms may be done periodically.

The length of time a patient should diet is dependent on the patient's initial weight, medical history, and the rate of weight loss. Twelve to 16 weeks of a VLCD has been shown to be safe; some studies have reported safe use for longer than that.

The program

A comprehensive VLCD program includes behavior modification, nutrition education, plus some cognitive therapy (see Chapter 11 for examples) and exercise instruction. Reports of the effectiveness of the VLCD without behavior modification and nutrition education are dismal. Preparation for refeeding and maintenance needs to be made early. Some programs use the "open-group" approach in which a patient stays on the VLCD until he or she reaches goal weight. Then the patient refeeds gradually back to a regular food diet. Other programs use the "closed-group" approach in which a group of patients start the program together, and they stay on the same time sequence for weight loss, refeeding, and maintenance. In this program the fast may be limited to 12 weeks. Some physicians may provide the medical monitoring out of their offices without the help of ancillary personnel, such as the registered dietitian, exercise physiologist, and psychologist. This is not thought to be as effective as multidisciplinary care.

Medical benefits

Use of VLCDs leads to favorable changes in serum LDL cholesterol, glucose tolerance, and blood pressure, just like other weight-loss approaches. Many people after losing even a modest amount of weight can reduce or even discontinue use of medications for managing high blood pressure, diabetes, and heart disease. With the VLCD, patients can see these changes rather quickly. Other patients have noted improvement in symptoms of arthritis and in sleep apnea.

EXPERT OPINION

Very Low Calorie Diets in the Treatment of Obesity—cont'd

Irresponsible use of VLCDs

Unsupervised use of VLCDs is dangerous. This includes the use of powdered diets that can be purchased at health food stores and in the supermarket, and are self-administered. Careful physician scrutiny must be part of the process.

VLCDs can have some temporary side effects like dizziness, muscle cramping, headaches, cold intolerance, and constipation or diarrhea. When quickly identified and medically managed, these problems can be easily corrected or minimized.

Studies are now underway exploring the risk of gallstones and VLCD-linked weight loss. Note that people are at risk for gallstones just by being obese (1% risk). Results of some of the studies show up to a 4% risk of developing symptomatic gallstones from various VLCDs. One mechanism that has been hypothesized for gallstone formation when dieting is incomplete contraction of the gallbladder during meals due to a low dietary fat content. Other factors that correlate with increased risk of gallstone formation include the female gender, estrogen use, cigarette smoking, age, elevated serum triglycerides, low HDL cholesterol level, and recent abdominal surgery. This again points to the necessity of medical monitoring when on the VLCD.

Those people who diet without medical monitoring risk having short-term complications turn into ones that are more serious, like cardiac dysfunction and potassium depletion. Another problem when one buys these diets in stores is the uncertainty of the adequacy of their composition. Currently there are formulas being promoted by the media that are to be used as replacements for not more than two meals per day. Misuse of these can have dangerous consequences. Their unsupervised nature opens the door to abuse, such as skipping the balanced meals that are supposed to accompany the diet plan.

Individuals also need to be wary of physicians prescribing very low calorie diets who are untrained in their proper use. Some physicians prescribe and supervise these diets to make extra money, but have minimal training in clinical nutrition or the medical aspects of weight control.

A final inappropriate use of VLCDs is by people who are mildly overweight. Mildly overweight individuals have less fat stores and may tend to lose more lean body mass than the more obese person who follows a VLCD. Less drastic weight loss methods are generally more appropriate for this population group.

Overall weight loss

Overall weight loss with very low calorie diets has been substantial. In one study with a period of 13 to 14 weeks, 66% of males and 49% of females lost 40 pounds (18 kilograms) or more. In comparison to behavior therapy alone, the weight loss on a very low calorie diet was nearly double. There is no question that adherence to a very low calorie diet produces dramatic weight-loss results.

Maintenance of weight loss

The biggest criticism of weight-loss programs in general is the dismal experience of patients being unable to maintain their weight loss. There are very little data in the literature for these weight-loss programs, whether they be commercial programs or programs administered by health professionals.

Some large clinical trials have elucidated some results of the very low calorie diets. In one study, of the patients who completed treatment, successful weight maintenance (defined as maintaining 60% or more of the lost excess weight at 18 months) was achieved in 46% of the patients at the 18 month follow-up. In another study patients had kept off, on average, two thirds of the weight that was lost during treatment on follow-up after 85 weeks.

These results of the VLCD should be compared to other various weight-loss programs, especially commercial programs. There needs to be some standards on what defines success and what criteria is best to measure this success. One thing is clear from these studies; multidisciplinary care appears to improve long-term results. In addition, those patients who complete treatment have a better chance of maintaining the weight that they have lost.

Some, but not all programs, offer a maintenance phase and an ongoing maintenance program. Ideally, follow-up should be long-term and should include further reinforcement of eating, exercise, and lifestyle habits conducive to weight maintenance.

In recent years the American Medical Association and the American Dietetic Association have approved the responsible use of the very low calorie diets. The benefits of the very low calorie diet, if monitored properly and if part of a comprehensive program, include substantial weight loss, coupled with the associated improvements in some medical and psychosocial problems. However, weight reduction is only the first goal of any program; the second goal is long-term maintenance of the reduced weight. More techniques and research need to be forthcoming in this area.

Dr. Loper practices dietetics in Columbus, Ohio and has many years of experience working with people following VLCD therapy.

Table 9-6 Summary of popular dietary approaches to weight control

Approach and examples	Characteristics and possible negative health consequences
Moderate caloric restriction	
The Setpoint Diet Slim Chance in a Fat World Weight Watcher's Diet The American Heart Assoc. Diet Mary Ellen's Help Yourself Diet Plan The Beyond Diet Nutripoints	Usually 1000-1800 kcal per day Reasonable balance of macronutrients Encourage exercise May employ behavioral approach None Weaknesses: if vitamin and mineral supplement used and permission of family physician is granted
Macronutrient restriction	
Low carbohydrate:	
Atkin's Diet Revolution Calories Don't Count Wild Weekend Diet Miracle Diet for Fast Weight Loss Drinking Man's Diet Woman Doctor's Diet for Women The Doctor's Quick Weight Loss Diet (Stillman's) The Complete Scarsdale Medical Diet Four Day Wonder Diet	Less than 100 grams carbohydrate per day Weakness: ketosis; poor exercise capacity due to poor glycogen stores in the muscles; excessive animal fat intake
Lowfat:	
The Rice Diet Report The Macrobiotic Diet (some versions) The Pritikin Diet The Tokyo Diet The Palm Beach Lifelong Diet The James Coco Diet The 35+ Diet 7-Week Victory Diet Fat to Muscle Diet T-Factor Diet Fit or Fat Two Day Diet Complete Hip and Thigh Diet The Maximum Metabolism Diet The Pasta Diet The McDougall Plan	Less than 20% of calories from fat Limited (or elimination of) animal protein sources, all fats, nuts, seeds Weakness: little satiety; flatulence, possibly poor mineral absorption from excess fiber; limited food choices → deprivation
Novelty diets	
Dr. Abravanel's Body Type and Lifetime Nutrition Plan (or his other books) Dr. Berger's Immune Power Diet	Promote certain nutrients, foods, or combination of foods as having unique, magical, or previously undiscovered qualities

Diets may be listed in more than one category if multiple characteristics apply.

Table 9-6 Summary of popular dietary approaches to weight control—cont'd

Approach and examples	Characteristics and possible negative health consequences
Novelty diets—cont'd	
Fit for Life The Rotation Diet The Hilton Head Metabolism Diet The Junk Food Diet The Beverly Hills Diet Dr. Debetz Champaign Diet Sun Sign Diet F-Plan Diet Fat Attack Plan The Ultrafit Diet The Princeton Plan The Diet Bible Bloomingdale's Diet The Love Diet Eat to Succeed The Underburner's Diet Eat to Win	Weaknesses: malnutrition; no change in habits → relapse; unrealistic food choices → leading to possible bingeing
Very low calorie diets	
Optifast Cambridge Diet The Last Chance Diet Genesis Medifast New Direction HMR Ultrafast	Less than 800 kcalories per day Also known as protein-sparing modified fasts Weakness; organ tissue loss—especially from the heart; low serum potassium level → heart failure; expense → must be under close physician scrutiny; kidney stones; gout
Formula diets	
U.S.A. (United Sciences of America), Inc. Optifast Genesis Cambridge Diet Herbalife The Last Chance Diet Slimfast	Can help people who find it easier not to eat whole foods while dieting to lose weight Based on formulated or packaged products Weaknesses; many are very low kcalorie diet regimens (see above) No change in habits → increased chance of relapse; expensive; constipation
Premeasured diets	
Nutrisystem Jenny Craig	Most food supplied in premeasured servings to take much of the decision-making out of the process of eating Weaknesses: expensive; may not allow for easy sound eating later

Stomach Surgery

gastroplasty Surgery on the stomach to limit its volume to approximately 50 milliliters, which is the size of a shot glass.

The most common surgical procedure for treating morbid obesity today involves modifying the stomach by **gastroplasty,** also known as stomach stapling. The goal is to reduce the size of the stomach to approximately 50 milliliters, the size of a shot glass. That prevents overeating, except with liquids. Overeating solid foods would result in rapid vomiting. One of two specific surgical procedures is commonly used, either a vertical-banded gastroplasty or a Roux-en-Y gastric bypass.[12] The latter surgical procedure is more effective, but is more technically difficult as well. The smaller stomach slows the rate of eating while promoting more rapid satiety. About 75% of patients with morbid obesity eventually loses 50% of body weight after this surgery, and they can maintain much of that weight loss over time. This dramatic loss occurs because they can eat only small amounts of food throughout the day. So they are forced to do what was difficult to do before—eat less.

Stomach surgery for weight loss is costly and often not covered by medical insurance. There is also nothing magical about the surgery. The person does not awaken from anesthesia thin. Instead, torturous months must be endured while weight loss occurs. Thus the surgery should not be seen as an easy answer to obesity. The procedure is analogous to jaw-wiring to prevent overeating, but is more effective.

Very Low Calorie Diets

very low calorie diet (VLCD) Also known as a protein-sparing modified fast (PSMF), this diet allows the consumption of 400 to 800 kcalories per day, generally in a liquid form. Of this, about 30 to 120 grams are made up of carbohydrate; the rest is mostly high-biological value protein.

If more traditional diet changes have failed, treating morbid obesity with **a very low calorie diet (VLCD)** is possible. Commercial programs include Optifast and Medifast. Some researchers believe people with body weights greater than 30% above desirable weight are also appropriate candidates.[23] The diet allows a person to eat 400 to 800 kcalories per day, often in liquid form.[21] (These diets were known earlier as protein-sparing modified fasts.) Of this amount, about 30 to 120 grams are carbohydrates. The rest is high biological value protein, supplying about 70 to 100 grams per day. This low-carbohydrate intake often causes ketosis, which may decrease appetite. However, the main reasons for weight loss are the few kcalories allowed and the absence of food choice. About 3 to 5 pounds can be lost per week: men tend to lose at a higher rate than do women. Weight regain has been a nagging problem with this type of therapy to date.

Very low calorie diets should not be used with infants, children, teenagers, pregnant women, or elderly people. In addition, people with diseases such as gout, active heart disease, hypertension, and diabetes are advised to be cautious with this approach.

CONCEPT CHECK

When a person is faced with morbid obesity and previous failures with conservative weight loss strategies, other options can be considered. Either surgery to reduce the volume of the stomach to approximately 50 milliliters, or a very low calorie diet consisting of 400 to 800 kcalories per day may be used.

Fad Diets—Why All the Commotion?

Many overweight people try to treat themselves using the latest fad diet book. But, as you will see, most of these diets do not help, and some can actually harm those who follow them (Table 9-6).

You may wonder why fad diet books exist at all. Why doesn't the government put a stop to them? Many contain blatant misinformation. However, the FDA concerns itself only when products are suspected of doing serious harm, as in the case of earlier forms of liquid protein diets. The FDA is too busy to pursue every new fad diet plan. So, concerning fad diet books, ancient advice is still valid: "Let the buyer beware." Responsibility rests with the authors and publishers, who want to sell a lot of books, earn a lot of money, and know there is little risk involved. Making outrageous claims sells more books than writing "eat less fat and exercise

35 Pounds of Fat.

DR. EDISON'S OBESITY PILLS AND REDUCING TABLETS CURED MRS. MANNING.

No Other Remedies But Dr. Edison's Reduce Obesity—Take No Others.

SAMPLES FREE—USE COUPON.

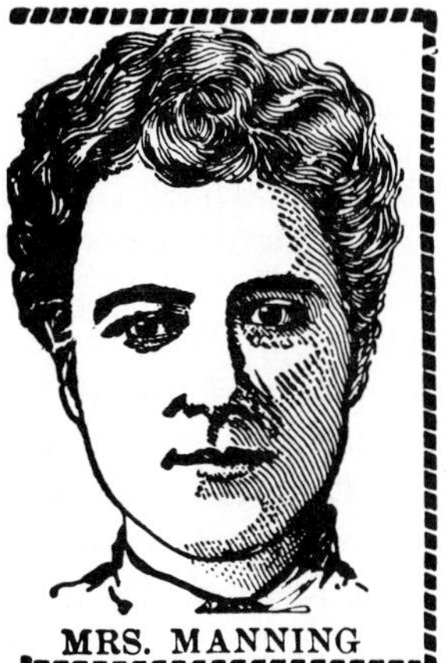

Mary Hyde Manning, one of the best known of Troy's, New York, society women, grew too fleshy, and used Dr. Edison's Obesity Remedies. Read the letter telling of her reduction and restoration to health:—"In six weeks I was reduced 35 pounds, from 171 to 136, by Dr. Edison's Obesity Pills and Reducing Tablets. I recommend these remedies to all fat and sick men and women."

The following well-known men and women have been reduced by DR. EDISON'S OBESITY REMEDIES:

Mrs. H. Mershon, 156 South Jackson St., Lima, O., 148 lbs.
Mrs. Josephine McPherson, 7916 Wright St., Chicago, 42 lbs.
Rev. Edward R. Pierce, 410 Alma St., Chicago, 42 lbs.
C. C. Nichols, 145 Clark St., Aurora, Ill., 36 lbs.
Mrs. W. Davlin, Whitemore, O., 149 lbs.
W. H. Webster, 618 2d Ave., Troy, N. Y., 26 lbs.
J. M. McKinney, 4504 State St., Chicago, 30 lbs.
Mrs. J. M. McKinney, 4504 State St., Chicago, 33 lbs.
Mrs. A. Walker, 1104 Milton Place, Chicago, 20 lbs.

Figure 9-5 Quackery has been with us for ages. Even at the turn of this century, people wanted to believe that fat could be lost without changing habits.

more." Diet quackery has existed for many years (Figure 9-5). Dr. Stephen Barrett discusses the psychology behind diet quackery in the Nutrition Perspective for this chapter.

HOW TO RECOGNIZE A FAD DIET

On pages 266 and 267 in this chapter we listed criteria for evaluating weight-loss programs in regards to their safety and effectiveness. In contrast, fad diets typically share some different common characteristics.[20] We list a few here:

1. They promote quick weight loss. As mentioned before, this loss is primarily due to glycogen, sodium, and lean muscle mass depletion. All lead to a loss of body water.
2. They limit food selections and dictate specific rituals, such as only eating fruit for breakfast.
3. They use testimonials from famous people and tie the diet to well-known cities, such as Beverly Hills and New York.
4. They bill themselves as "cure-alls." Whatever the type of obesity or whatever a reader's specific strengths and weaknesses, these diets claim to work for everyone.
5. They often recommend expensive supplements. Some of these supplements can be harmful because of high doses of vitamin A, vitamin D, vitamin C, or vitamin B-6 (pyridoxine).
6. No attempts are made to permanently change eating habits. The dieter follows the diet until the desired weight is reached and then reverts to old eating habits. Eat rice for a month, lose weight, and then return to old habits.

It is illegal in the United States to falsely represent worthless or dangerous cures and medical devices. Thus U.S. citizens can use their rights under federal law to have the FDA pursue a seller of a dangerous fad diet in an attempt to have it removed from the bookshelves.

7. They are generally critical of and skeptical about the scientific community. They suggest that physicians and registered dietitians do not really want people to lose weight. They encourage people to look outside the medical establishment for correct advice.

Probably the cruelest characteristic of fad diets is that they essentially guarantee failure for the dieter. These diets are not designed for permanent weight loss. Habits are not changed, and the food selection is so limited that the person cannot follow the diet for more than 1 or 2 weeks. Although dieters assume they have lost fat, they have actually lost mostly muscle and other lean tissue mass. As soon as they begin eating normally again, the lost tissue is replaced. In a matter of weeks, most of the lost weight is back. The dieter appears to have failed, when actually the diet has failed. This whole scenario can add more blame and guilt to the psyche of the dieter—and that is very unfortunate. If someone needs help losing weight, professional help is the answer. That is something fad diets rarely offer.

TYPES OF FAD DIETS

Low-Carbohydrate Approaches

This is the most common form of fad diet. The low-carbohydrate intake forces the liver to perform gluconeogenesis (see Chapters 3 and 7). The source of carbons for gluconeogenesis is protein tissue. Thus a low-carbohydrate diet results in protein tissue loss, as well as urinary loss of essential ions, such as potassium. Since protein tissue is mostly water, the person loses weight very rapidly. When a normal diet is resumed, the protein tissue is rebuilt and the weight is regained.

There is nothing special about a low-carbohydrate diet in terms of weight loss. If the diet is also low in kcalories, then it is likely to result in weight loss. But a low-carbohydrate diet by itself does not result in more weight loss than any other type of diet.

Diet plans that use a low-carbohydrate approach are the Dr. Atkinson Diet Revolution, Dr. Stillman's Calories Don't Count Diet, the Scarsdale Diet, the Drinking Man's Diet, Four Day Wonder diet, and the Air Force Diet. When you see a new fad diet advertisement, look first to see how much carbohydrate it contains. If breads, cereals, fruits, and vegetables are extremely limited, you are probably looking at a **ketogenic** diet.

ketogenic A name often given to diets that lead to the production of ketones by the liver due to a low carbohydrate intake.

Low-Fat Approaches

The very low-fat diet turns out to be a very high-carbohydrate diet. These diets contain approximately 5% to 10% of kcalories as fat. The most notable is the Pritikin Diet. This approach is not harmful, but it is extremely difficult to follow. People get bored with this type of diet very quickly because many of their favorite foods cannot be eaten. The dieter primarily eats grains, fruits, and vegetables, and most people cannot do this for very long. Eventually, the person will want some foods higher in fat or protein. Thus the person is bound to suffer a lapse, then a relapse, and probably a collapse. These diets are just too atypical of our usual diet to follow consistently. A popular diet marketed recently, the T-Factor Diet, focuses on restricting fat but is a more moderate approach than the Pritikin diet.

Novelty Diets

A whole variety of diets are built on gimmicks. The Rotation Diet, for example, rotates the amount of kcalories ingested in an attempt to prevent the usual drop in basal metabolism associated with dieting. A woman is supposed to eat 600 kcalories per day for 3 days, then 900 kcalories per day for 4 days, and then 1200 kcalories per day for 7 days, repeating this cycle over and over again. For men, the levels are 1200, 1500, and 1800 kcalories. No scientific data show that this diet works or even how it could work. Diets calling for fewer than 1000 kcalories are suspect because of their low-nutrient content. Thus it must be considered a fad diet.

Other novelty diets emphasize one food or food group and exclude almost all others. A rice diet was designed in the 1940s to lower blood pressure; now it has resurfaced as a weight-loss diet. The first phase consists of eating only rice and fruit until you cannot stand them any longer. Another novelty diet is the egg diet. You eat all the eggs you want. On the Beverly Hills Diet you eat mostly fruit.

The rationale behind these diets is that you can eat only eggs, or fruits, or rice for so long. You will soon become bored and, in theory, will reduce your energy intake. However, chances are that you will abandon the diet entirely before you lose much weight.

Since the 1960s grapefruits have been touted for their supposed unique ability to cause weight loss (Figure 9-6). As far as we know this is bunk. To add appeal to a grapefruit diet, proponents even suggest adding several "diet aids": lecithin to help release fat from the tissues, vitamin B-6 to act as a diuretic, vinegar to provide potassium, and kelp to stimulate the thyroid glands. In the 1980s we had an entirely new product, Herbalife. This contains herbs high in caffeine; caffeine stimulates the metabolic rate. None of these aids is very effective. None of them are substitutes for moderating food intake, modifying behavior, and increasing activity.

The most bizarre of the novelty diets propose that "food gets stuck in your body." Fit for Life and the Beverly Hills Diet are examples. The supposition is that food gets stuck in the intestine, putrefies, and creates toxins that invade the bloodstream and cause disease. This is utter nonsense (see Chapter 6). Nevertheless, the same idea has been promoted in health food books since the 1800s. Today, Fit for Life suggests meat eaten with potatoes will not be digested, and to only consume fresh fruit before noon. These recommendations are absurd. They are gimmicks that appear controversial but are really designed to sell books. If weight loss does occur, it is because the books use such complicated rules and rituals that, by the time you have figured out what you can eat, it is the wrong time to eat it!

Finally, we should mention some commercial schemes used to sell diet books. Books describing the allergy approach to dieting, for instance, suggest that current diseases, including obesity, are due to food allergies. Supposedly, once your food allergies are found and treated, you will no longer have the disease. However, we know of no research that supports the claim that 30% of people have food allergies, as suggested in Dr. Berger's Immune Power Diet Book. In addition, see the Sun Sign Diet if you believe in astrology, the Champagne Diet if you need a drink, or the Body Type and Lifetime Nutrition Diet if you have a "dominant" gland.

Numerous other gimmicks for weight loss have come and gone and are likely to resurface. If in the future an important aid for weight loss is discovered, you can feel confident that major journals will report the finding, such as the Journal of The American Dietetic Association, the Journal of the American Medical Association, or the New England Journal of Medicine. You don't need to rely on paperback books or newspaper advertisements.

CONCEPT CHECK

Fad diets characteristically promote quick weight loss and limited food selections, use testimonials from famous people, bill the plan as a cure-all, include expensive supplements, and show little concern for permanently changing food habits. Typical approaches include low-carbohydrate regimens, low-fat regimens, and novel approaches, which often consist of complex food-combining rules or a focus on one type of food, such as rice or fruit.

Medications to Aid Weight Loss

Over-the-counter medications that claim to facilitate weight loss sell briskly. Some can be effective, but so far none can substitute for the basic approach we have outlined in this chapter to promote weight loss. Diet aids include fiber pills, **phenylpropanolamine,** and benzocaine. Phenylpropanolamine is an epinephrine-like drug that can cause a slight decrease in food intake. Benzocaine numbs the tongue, so a person tends to eat less.

phenylpropanolamine An over-the-counter stimulant that has a mild appetite-reducing effect.

Fiber pills can increase bulk in the stomach and ideally lead to satiety. A recent study showed that only soluble-type fiber, the type found in beans and oats, was

Figure 9-6 Garfield.
Reprinted by permission of UFS, Inc.

GARFIELD

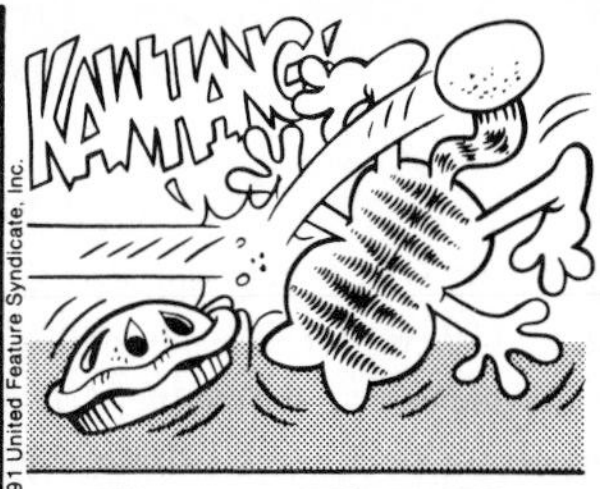

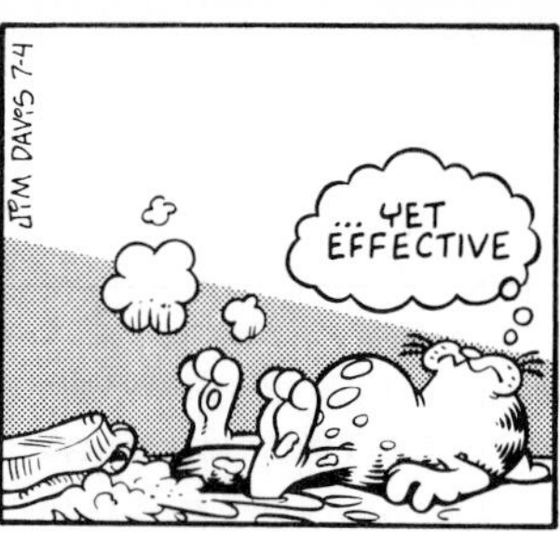

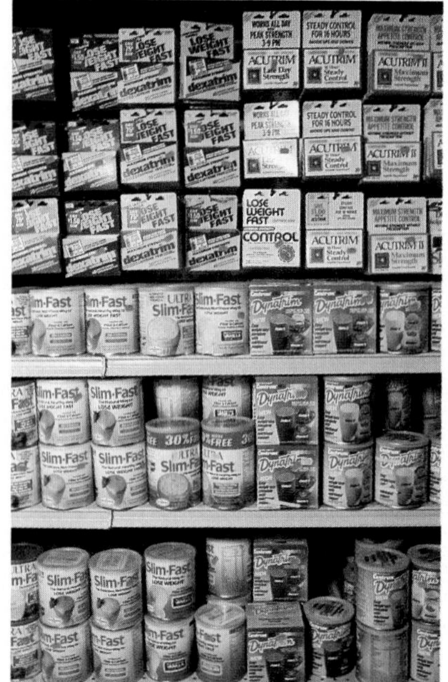

Money spent on over-the-counter diet pills would be better spent on exercise clothes.

effective in decreasing food intake. Bran fiber, such as that found in fiber pills, was not effective. However, when the people in the study took enough soluble fiber (23 grams) incorporated into crackers to decrease food intake, they also experienced significant intestinal gas.

Regarding prescription medications, physicians sometimes prescribe amphetamines for weight loss.[1] Amphetamines cause a person to eat less, but they are also possibly addictive. In addition, amphetamines can increase heart rate and nervousness and lead to insomnia. Thyroid hormone preparations were once popular, but these caused significant loss of lean tissue.

Fenfluramine, fluoxetine, and related medications have been prescribed by physicians to promote weight loss. These drugs increase the action of serotonin in the brain, which may lead to less food craving, especially for high-carbohydrate foods (see Chapter 8). Rapid weight gain after discontinuing the drug is a problem. Addition of behavior therapy to this approach may improve weight maintenance.[7]

Another class of experimental medications that reduce food intake are the opiate-antagonists, such as naloxone and naltrexone. These drugs cause a significant decrease in food intake in animals, but the results from human studies are very discouraging. Development of related drugs is continuing.

Overall, in skilled hands, prescription medications can aid weight loss.[1] However, they do not supplant the need for more conservative approaches of reducing kcalorie and fat intake, modifying problem behaviors, and increasing activity.

Putting Weight Loss into Perspective

A disturbing fact about dieting for weight loss is that often the weight is regained.[27] People may end up heavier after their diet-and-regain cycle than when they began. Based on this information, it appears that dieting itself can promote obesity. Thus dieting should not be undertaken lightly. As we noted earlier, if a person is not highly motivated and does not have the needed social support, dieting for weight loss should be delayed until a more appropriate time.

Would-be dieters should choose and follow diet plans that are appropriate for them. There is a smorgasbord of options: lowered kcalorie and fat intakes, behavior modification, increased physical activity, and group and/or individual counseling. Many tools are effective, but some will be more useful than others, depending on the dieter's lifestyle, personality, and motivation. To discover which techniques promote the best chance of losing weight and maintaining the loss, the person must explore his or her own strengths and weaknesses. Overall, in terms of both health and self-esteem, the life of the dieter should improve as weight is lost.[27]

CONCEPT CHECK

Over-the-counter drugs do not dramatically improve the prospects for weight loss. The focus still remains a reduction in kcalorie intake, modification of problem eating behaviors, and increased physical activity. A dieter should realize that weight loss is difficult and thus should only be attempted when there is a strong commitment to weight loss. A physician must guide any use of prescription diet medications.

Treating Underweight

Underweight can be caused by a variety of factors like anorexia nervosa, cancer, infectious diseases, digestive tract disorders, and excessive physical activity. Genetic background may have also lead to a higher resting metabolic rate and/or a slight body frame.[19] As you can see in Figure 8-10, underweight is also associated with increased death rates, especially when associated with smoking cigarettes. This is surprising to some people because most of the time we hear about the risks of obesity, but not underweight. In our society being underweight is much more socially acceptable than being obese.

underweight Body weight for height about 15% to 20% of desirable weight, or a body mass index below about 19. These cutoffs are less precise than for obesity since less of this condition has been undertaken.

Underweight is sometimes a problem that requires medical intervention. Underweight can increase the risk of a woman delivering a low birth weight baby (see Chapter 16), lead to complications in surgery, and slow recovery after illness. A physician should be consulted to rule out hormonal imbalances, depression, or other hidden disease in underweight people. Treatments for underweight adults use several different approaches:

1. Gradually increase consumption of kcalorie-dense foods, especially those higher in fat, with particular emphasis on vegetable fats. These are best eaten at the end of a meal so that they don't cause early satiety. Low-fat cheeses, dried fruit, bananas, nuts, and granola are good kcalorie sources, as these have a potential for a low content of saturated fat (read the label).
2. Avoid diet soft drinks and other substitutes for good energy sources.
3. Keep a daily food record and review it weekly to see whether higher kcalorie food choices could be made (see the left side of Table 9-2 for some possible choices).
4. Set a goal of eating high-kcalorie snack foods each day, such as sweetened yogurt, nuts, bananas, avocados, granola, raisins, and fruit juices.
5. Consider reducing physical activity. If the person remains very lean, a body-building program might be considered, incorporating weight lifting to increase muscle development.
6. Avoid fluids with meals to prevent premature satiety.
7. Don't overdo fiber consumption, which can lead to premature satiety.
8. To some degree, accept a genetic tendency for underweight.

If these efforts fail to achieve the desired weight, they at least should prevent health problems associated with being underweight. Because of our cultural and societal emphasis on thinness, we are likely to see more problems with underweight in the future.

Summary

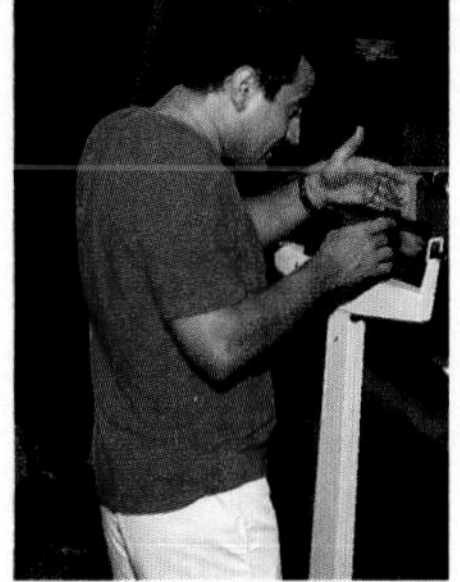

1. When considering a treatment for obesity, three points should be remembered: (1) The body resists weight loss; (2) the emphasis should be on preventing obesity, since curing the disorder is very difficult; (3) weight loss on a diet should represent a loss of fat storage and not the loss of muscle and other lean tissues.

2. A sound weight-loss diet should meet the dieter's nutritional needs by emphasizing low-fat food choices from the Guide to Daily Food Choices; it should adapt to the person's habits, consist of readily obtainable foods, strive to change poor eating habits, recommend regular physical activity, and insist the person see a physician if weight is to be lost rapidly or if the person is over 35 years of age and plans to perform substantially greater physical activity than usual.

3. A pound of adipose tissue lost or gained represents approximately 2700 kcalories. Thus if energy output exceeds energy intake by about 400 kcalories per day, a pound of fat storage can be lost per week. Decreasing the intake of high-fat foods is probably the best way to obtain this kcalorie deficit, along with increasing physical activity.
4. Behavior modification is a vital part of a weight-loss program because the dieter may have many habits that encourage overeating, and so discourage weight maintenance. Specific behavior modification techniques, such as stimulus control and self-monitoring, can be used to help change those problem behaviors.
5. Increasing physical activity is a vital part of a weight-loss program; the focus should be on duration rather than intensity. Ideally, approximately 200 to 300 kcalories should be expended in vigorous activity each day.
6. It is important to have a personal behavior-change plan to lose weight and keep it off. Assessing commitment and behaviors is an important first step. After that, goals should be established with appropriate rewards. These goals should be written in a contract and witnessed by significant others.
7. Treatment of morbid obesity includes stomach surgery to reduce stomach volume to approximately 50 milliliters, or very low calorie diets, containing 400 to 800 kcalories per day. Both these procedures should be reserved for people who have failed at more conservative approaches to weight loss. They require medical supervision.
8. Fad diets are easy to recognize. They often promote rapid weight loss, have limited food selections, offer testimonials from famous people, are billed as "cure-alls," include expensive supplements, and make little or no attempt to permanently alter food habits. General criticism of and skepticism about the scientific community is also common.
9. Fad diets can be classed as low-carbohydrate approaches, low-fat approaches, and novel approaches. The latter category includes diets with complex food-combining rituals and those that focus on one type of food to the exclusion of most others, such as rice or fruit.
10. Medications to aid weight loss that are available over-the-counter in drug stores include phenylpropanolamine, benzocaine, and fiber pills. None of these, however, can substitute entirely for a good diet, behavior, and physical activity plan.

Study Questions

1. What are the major psychological and physiological problems associated with rapid weight loss?
2. When searching for a sound weight-loss program, what six characteristics would you look for?
3. You are following a nutritional plan for weight loss. What are five specific ways you could save kcalories?
4. Describe the term behavior modification. Relate it to the terms stimulus control, self-monitoring, chain breaking, relapse prevention, and cognitive restructuring. Give examples of each of the latter.
5. Describe the type of physical-activity plan you would suggest for someone who is obese.
6. Give four characteristics of fad diets.

REFERENCES

1. Bray GA: Drug treatment for obesity, *American Journal of Clinical Nutrition* 55:538S, 1992.
2. Bray GA: Pathophysiology of obesity, *American Journal of Clinical Nutrition* 55:488S, 1992.
3. Brownell KD: *The LEARN program for weight control,* Philadelphia, 1989, KD Brownell.
4. Burgess NS: Effect of a very-low-calorie diet on body composition and resting metabolic rate in obese men and women, *Journal of The American Dietetic Association* 91:430, 1991.
5. Canadian Dietetic Association: Obesity: a case for prevention, *Journal of the Canadian Dietetic Association* 49:11, 1988.
6. Council on Scientific Affairs, American Medical Association: Treatment of obesity, *Journal of the American Medical Association* 257:1323, 1988.
7. Darga LL and others: Fluoxetine's effect on weight loss in obese subjects, *American Journal of Clinical Nutrition* 54:321, 1991.
8. Eckel RH, Yost TJ: Weight reduction increases adipose tissue lipoprotein lipase responsiveness in obese women, *Journal of Clinical Investigation* 80:992, 1987.
9. Ferguson J: *Habits, not diets: the secret to lifetime weight control,* Palo Alto, Calif, 1988, Bull Publishing Co.
10. Fitzwater SL and others: Evaluation of longterm weight changes after a multidisciplinary weight control program, *Journal of The American Dietetic Association* 91:421, 1991.
11. Frankel RT, Yang M: *Obesity and weight Control,* Rockville, Md, 1988, Aspen Publishers.
12. Gastrointestinal surgery for severe obesity: National Institutes of Health Consensus Development Conference Statement, *American Journal of Clinical Nutrition* 55:615S, 1992.
13. Gorbach SL and others: Changes in food pattern during a low-fat dietary intervention in women, *Journal of The American Dietetic Association* 90:802, 1990.
14. Kendall A and others: Weight loss on a lowfat diet: consequence of the imprecision of the control of food intake in humans. *American Journal of Clinical Nutrition* 53:1124, 1990.
15. Kuczmarski RJ: Prevalence of overweight and weight gain in the United States, *American Journal of Clinical Nutrition* 55:495S, 1992.
16. Lissner L and others: Variability of body weight and health outcomes in the Framingham study, *New England Journal of Medicine* 324:1839, 1991.
17. Owen OE: Regulation of energy metabolism. In Kinney JM and others, editors: *Obesity in nutrition and metabolism in patient care,* Philadelphia, 1988, WB Saunders.
18. Pi-Sunyer FX: Effect of the composition of the diet on energy intake, *Nutrition Reviews* 48:94, 1990.
19. Ravussin E, Bogardus C: A brief overview of human energy metabolism and its relationship to essential obesity, *American Journal of Clinical Nutrition* 55:242S, 1992.
20. Rock CL, Coluston AM: Weight-control approaches: a review by the California Dietetic Association, *Journal of The American Dietetic Association* 88:44, 1988.
21. Seim HC, Rigden SR: Approaching the protein sparing modified fast, *American Family Physician* 42(5):51S, 1990.
22. Stunkard AJ, Wadden TA: Restrained eating and human obesity, *Nutrition Reviews* 48:78, 1990.
23. Wadden TA and others: Responsible and irresponsible use of very-low-calorie diets in the treatment of obesity, *Journal of The American Dietetic Association* 263:83, 1990.
24. Westover SA, Lanyon RI: The maintenance of weight loss after behavioral treatment, *Behavior Modification* 14:123, 1990.
25. Willard MD: Obesity: types and treatments, *American Family Physician* 43(6):2009, 1991.
26. Wing R: Behavioral treatment of severe obesity, *American Journal of Clinical Nutrition* 55:545S, 1992.
27. Wooley SC, Garner DM: Obesity treatment: the high cost of false hope, *Journal of The American Dietetic Association* 91:1248, 1991.

SUGGESTED READINGS

Excellent reviews on treating obesity by reducing kcalorie intake and modifying behavior can be found in the article by the Council on Scientific Affairs of the American Medical Association and the article by Rock and Coulston. The book by Brownell is also an excellent reference for behavior modification. Together these articles provide a detailed account of all conservative options available for losing weight. The article by Wing contains numerous suggestions for behavior modification practices. The article by Seim and Rigden is an excellent review on the use of very low calorie diets. In addition, see the article written by Wadden and others on this subject.

TAKE ACTION

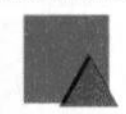

Is the TTFV Lipoloss Weight-Loss Plan for You?

Read the following discussion of the TTFV Lipoloss Weight-Loss Plan. See if it is one you would want to follow.

I. Do you want to turn your body into a high-powered fat burner? Try the TTFV Lipoloss Weight Loss Plan, scientifically proven to be the quickest and most permanent fat loss miracle in America. The nutritional part of the TTFV Plan consists of eating 800 kcalories of delicious tuna, turkey, fruits, and vegetables. Combine the fruits with the turkey and the vegetables with the tuna to achieve the greatest lipoloss effect (remember, lipo means fat).

We encourage at least 30 minutes of aerobic exercise—brisk walking, jogging, swimming, or biking—three to five times per week. And we haven't forgotten those diet-wrecking urges and cravings. Fight them with our high-fiber Urgesmasher Wafers. These wafers fill you up, fighting the gnaw of hunger.

If you have any health problems, see your physician for approval and clearance for regular exercise. Overall, with the TTFV LipoLoss Plan you can lose 3 to 5 pounds each week and enjoy a variety of tasty food.

Now rate this diet based on the following questions: a perfect score of 100 points indicates a good weight-loss plan. For every "no" answer to the questions below subtract the appropriate points.

1. Will the diet meet all nutritional needs with a wide variety of foods? IF NOT, SUBTRACT 10 POINTS.
2. Does the program stress slow and steady weight loss of about 1 to 2 pounds per week rather than rapid loss? IF NOT, SUBTRACT 10 POINTS.
3. Is the diet tailored to individual habits and tastes, diminishing feelings of deprivation? IF NOT, SUBTRACT 10 POINTS.
4. Does the plan avoid rigid rituals such as eating fruits only in the morning or not eating meat after milk products? IF NOT, SUBTRACT 10 POINTS.
5. Does the diet minimize hunger and fatigue by containing at least 1000 kcalories per day? IF NOT, SUBTRACT 10 POINTS.
6. Does the diet include readily obtainable foods, with no special products to buy to speed weight loss? IF NOT, SUBTRACT 10 POINTS.
7. Is the diet socially acceptable, allowing the dieter to attend parties, eat at restaurants, and participate in normal daily acitivity. IF NOT, SUBTRACT 10 POINTS
8. Does the plan promote changes in eating habits and lifestyle so that weight maintenance will be possible? IF NOT, SUBTRACT 10 POINTS.
9. Does the plan emphasize regular physical activity? IF NOT, SUBTRACT 10 POINTS.
10. Does the plan encourage the dieter to see a physician before starting if the person has existing health problems, wants quick weight loss, is over 35 years of age, or plans to perform vigorous physical activity? IF NOT, SUBTRACT 10 POINTS.

Now, having assessed the TTFV Lipoloss Weight Loss Plan, how many points would you give it? SCORE________

Would you choose this weight loss plan if you were attempting to lose fat and keep it off? Yes________ NO________

Ask yourself the following questions based on the food record you kept in Chapter 1:

II. WHAT ARE SOME SIGNIFICANT THINGS YOU NOTICED ABOUT YOUR EATING HABITS?

Do you spend at least 20 minutes eating?

Do you eat your food mostly as meals or snacks?

Do you eat most of your meals standing up, watching television, or sitting down?

Do you eat most of your food out, in the cafeteria, in your room, or at your house?

How do the people you spend time with affect your eating habits?

How do your eating habits vary with your feelings?

Now that you've closely examined your eating habits, consider drafting a plan to change one of them:

1. Choose one habit you would be willing to change. Example: To spend at least 20 minutes eating your meals.
2. Use a behavioral contract as in Table 9-6 to outline your behavior-change plan. Remember to make your goal specific and measurable. Have a significant other sign and witness it.
3. Start by trying to fulfill your contract for a week. Then reevaluate its appropriateness. Make sure to reward yourself for completing it. ▲

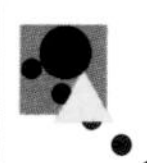

Ten Common Misconceptions About Quackery By Stephen Barrett, M.D.

Misconception 1: Quackery is Easy to Spot

Quackery is far more difficult to spot than most people realize. Modern promoters use scientific jargon, which can fool people unfamiliar with the concepts being discussed. Even health professionals can have difficulty in separating fact from fiction in fields unrelated to their expertise.

Misconception 2: Personal Experience Is the Best Way to Tell Whether Something Works

When you feel better after having used a product or procedure, it is natural to give credit to whatever you have done. This effect can be misleading, however, because most ailments resolve by themselves, and those that don't can have variable symptoms. Even serious conditions can have sufficient day-to-day variation to enable quack methods to gain large followings. In addition, taking action often produces temporary relief of symptoms (a placebo effect). For these reasons, scientific experimentation is usually necessary to establish whether health methods actually work.

Misconception 3: Most Victims of Quackery Are Gullible

Individuals who buy one diet book or "magic" diet pill after another are indeed gullible. And so are many people who follow whatever health fads are in vogue. But the majority of quackery's victims are merely unsuspecting. People tend to believe what they hear the most. And quack ideas—particularly those regarding nutrition—are everywhere. Another large group of quackery's victims is composed of individuals who have serious or chronic diseases that make them feel desperate enough to try anything that offers hope.

Alienated people—many of whom are paranoid—form another victim group. These people tend to believe that our food supply is unsafe, that drugs do more harm than good, and that doctors, drug companies, large food companies, and government agencies are not interested in protecting the public. Such beliefs make them vulnerable to those who offer foods and healing approaches alleged to be "natural."

Misconception 4: Quackery's Victims Deserve What They Get

This misconception is based on the feeling that people who are gullible should "know better" and therefore deserve whatever they get. This feeling is a major reason why journalists, enforcement officials, judges, and legislators seldom give priority to combat quackery. As noted earlier, however, most victims are not gullible. Nor do people deserve to suffer or die because of ignorance or desperation.

Misconception 5: Quacks Are Frauds and Crooks

Quackery is often discussed as though all its promoters were engaged in deliberate deception. This is untrue. Promoters of mail-order quackery are almost always hit-and-run artists who know their products are fakes but hope to profit before the Postal Service shuts them down. But most promoters of quackery sincerely believe in what they do.

Most people think of quackery as being promoted by quacks, charlatans, or others who are deliberately taking advantage of others. Actually, most of it is promoted by victims of quackery who share their misinformation and personal experiences with others. Quackery is also involved in misleading advertising of nonprescription drugs. Again, no "quack" is involved—just hype from an advertising agency.

NUTRITION PERSPECTIVE

Ten Common Misconceptions About Quackery—cont'd

Misconception 6: Most Quackery Isn't Dangerous

Quackery can seriously harm or kill people by inducing them to abandon or delay effective treatment for serious conditions. Although the number of people harmed in this manner cannot be determined, it is not large enough or obvious enough to arouse a general public outcry. Most victims of quackery are harmed economically rather than physically. Moreover, many people believe that an unscientific method has helped them. In most cases, they have confused cause-and-effect and coincidence. But sometimes an unproven approach actually relieves symptoms by lowering the person's tension level.

Misconception 7: "Minor" Forms of Quackery Are Harmless

Quackery involving small sums of money and no physical harm is often viewed as harmless. Examples are "nutrition insurance" with vitamin pills and wearing a copper bracelet for arthritis. But their use indicates confusion of the part of the user and vulnerability to more serious forms of quackery. There is also harm to society. Money wasted on quackery would be better spent for research, but much of it goes into the pockets of people who are spreading misinformation and trying to weaken consumer protection laws.

The Feingold diet—based on the notion that food additives cause children to be hyperactive—is an example of quackery whose potential harm is underestimated. Although the diet itself is harmless, it is probably harmful to teach children that the way they behave depends on what they eat rather than on what they feel. Also, social development can be jeopardized if eating habits subject children to ridicule or lead them to avoid group activities where forbidden foods are served.

Misconception 8: The Media Are Reliable

Most people believe that statements about health issues "wouldn't be allowed" if they weren't true. Some media outlets do achieve great accuracy. But most are willing to publish sensational viewpoints that they believe are newsworthy and will increase their audience. Radio and television talk shows abound with promoters of quackery. Even exposés on questionable methods are often "balanced" by including testimonials from satisfied customers.

There is a widespread public belief that if something isn't legitimate, publications and broadcast outlets would not allow it to be advertised. Although most outlets have some limitations, few screen out misleading advertisements for health products.

Misconception 9: Government Protects Us

Although various government agencies are involved in fighting quackery, most don't give it sufficient priority to be effective. Moreover, the agencies involved do not have a coordinated plan to maximize their effectiveness.

Misconception 10: Quackery's Success Represents Medicine's Failure

It is often suggested that people turn to quacks when doctors are brusque with them, and that if doctors were more attentive, their patients would not turn to quacks. It is true that this sometimes happens, but most quackery does not involve medical care. Blaming medicine for quackery is like considering the success of astrology the fault of astronomy. Some people's desires exceed what scientific health care can provide.

Dr. Barrett, a practicing psychiatrist and consumer advocate, is coauthor/editor of 22 books including *Vitamins and "Health" Foods: The Great American Hustle* and *Consumer Health*. In 1984 he received the FDA Commissioner's Special Citation Award for Public Service in fighting nutrition quackery.

CHAPTER TEN

Nutrition for Fitness

***A**thletes invest a lot of time and effort in training. Because they are often seeking ways to modify their diets to improve their performances, athletes make easy targets for purveyors of nutrition misinformation. Still most athletes don't want to miss out on any advantages, whether real or perceived, that might give them the winning edge. Proper diet choices are a key ingredient to top-notch performance.[6] Nutrition knowledge helps open the door to victory.*

Once muscles have nutrients available to them, what determines the type of fuel muscles will use? The athlete does, to an extent, depending on how physically fit he or she is and how hard one performs. Physical fitness—defined as the ability to do moderate to vigorous activity without undue fatigue—affects fuel use. A proper diet that supplies the fuel muscles need also has an effect. We will discuss this in detail later in the chapter.

In this chapter you will discover how physical fitness benefits the entire body: It is an essential ingredient in achieving maximum health.[16] Benefits include improvement in several aspects of heart function, less injury, better sleep habits, and improvement in body composition (less body fat, more muscle mass).[21] Exercise also can reduce stress and positively affect blood pressure and blood sugar regulation, as well as aid in weight control.[10] And there is another basic reason to be physically fit, of course: It's fun, it feels good, and it even lessens the strain of such daily activities as housework and yardwork. Let's now look at these concepts further.

NUTRITION AWARENESS INVENTORY

Here are 15 statements about nutrition and fitness. Read them to test your current knowledge. If you think the statement is true or mostly true, circle T. If you think the statement is false or mostly false, circle F. Use the scoring key at the end of the book to compute your total score. To review, take this test again later, and especially before tests.

1. T F A cell can use the energy stored in carbohydrate to fuel a muscle's energy demands without further modification.
2. T F Carbohydrates can be used for energy needs, but fat cannot.
3. T F Complete metabolism of carbohydrate does not require oxygen.
4. T F Carbon dioxide is a by-product of energy metabolism.
5. T F Even when athletes are getting RDA quantities of vitamins and minerals in the diet, it has been shown that supplements of vitamins and minerals will increase athletic performance.
6. T F There are really no disadvantages for an athlete who attempts to lose weight durning the competitive season.
7. T F It is particularly important for athletes to consume protein and amino acid supplements because it is hard for them to get enough through their diets.
8. T F A large portion of carbohydrate food like starches or fuits should be consumed within 2 hours after an exercise bout to maximize glycogen synthesis because this is when glycogen synthesis is the greatest.
9. T F Sportstype drinks like Gatorade are not significantly better beverages for fluid replacement than water for the everyday athlete. However, for endurance athletes they may be advantageous.
10. T F Caffeine use has improved athletic performance in some cases.
11. T F A target heart rate for general, routine exercise is 80% to 95% of maximum heart rate.
12. T F Cool-down exercises are not as important as a good warm-up.
13. T F Thirst is a good guide for fluid replacement after hard exercise.
14. T F It is a good idea to eat lots of carbohydrate before a 100-meter dash.
15. T F Anabolic steroids are illegal ergogenic aids for athletes.

Fueling Muscles

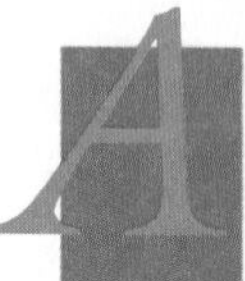

As you found out in Chapter 7, cells can't directly use the energy released from breaking down glucose or fat. Rather, the energy must first be stored in a special form, called **adenosine triphosphate (ATP).**

adenosine triphosphate (ATP) The main energy currency for cells. ATP energy is used to promote ion pumping, enzyme activity, and muscular contraction.

ADENOSINE TRIPHOSPHATE (ATP)

To store chemical energy, our cells make ATP. Conversely, to release energy from ATP for cell use, cells partially break down ATP to ADP and Pi. This then releases usable energy for cell functions. Essentially, ATP is the immediate source of energy for body functions—this includes locomotion.[27] The overall goal of any fuel use then—carbohydrate, fat, or protein—is to make ATP.

A resting muscle cell only has a small amount of ATP that can be used. If no resupply of ATP were possible, this stored ATP could keep the muscle working maximally for only about 2 to 4 seconds. Fortunately, there are several types of chemical compounds—phosphocreatine (PCr), carbohydrates, fats, and proteins—that can be broken down to release enough energy to make more ATP.[17] Cells actually must constantly use and then reform ATP, over and over again.

PHOSPHOCREATINE IS THE FIRST LINE OF DEFENSE FOR RESUPPLYING ATP IN MUSCLES

phosphocreatine (PCr) A high-energy compound that can be used to reform ATP from ADP.

The instant that breakdown products of ATP begin to accumulate in the contracting muscle, an enzyme is activated to split **phosphocreatine (PCr).** This is another high-energy compound stored in a muscle cell, in addition to ATP. Muscles use

ATP and various amino acids to make PCr. The P released from PCr immediately combines with ADP to resupply ATP; thus, PCr + ADP → Cr + ATP (Figure 10-1). This releases the energy needed to reform ATP.[27] If no other source of ATP resupply were available, PCr could probably maintain maximal muscle contractions for about 10 seconds. But since other ATP sources kick in, PCr ends up the major source of energy for all events lasting up to about 1 minute (Table 10-1).

The main advantages of PCr is that it can be activated instantly and can replenish ATP at rates fast enough to meet the energy demands of the fastest and most powerful sports events, including jumping, lifting, throwing, and sprinting actions. The disadvantage of PCr is that there is not enough of it made and stored in the muscles to sustain a high rate of ATP resupply for more than a few minutes. Many attempts have been made over the years to improve the muscle ATP and PCr stores by dietary means, but none have worked.[17]

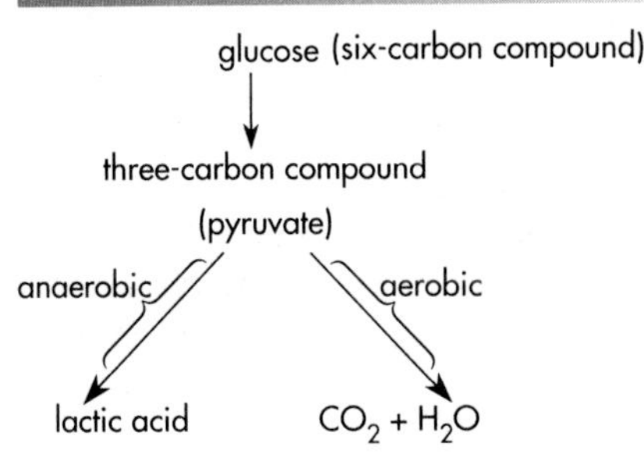

USING GLUCOSE AS A MUSCLE FUEL—GLYCOLYSIS

Anaerobic Glycolysis

Recall from Chapter 7 that when glucose breaks down, the resulting three-carbon compound, called pyruvate, follows either of two main routes. When oxygen supply is limited (**"anaerobic"**) or when the exercise is intense (e.g., running 400 meters or swimming 100 meters), the three-carbon compound pyruvate accumulates in the muscle and is converted to **lactic acid.** This conversion of glucose to lactic acid is called anaerobic **glycolysis** ("glyco" means sugar and "lysis" means breakdown). A few ATP are directly formed in the pathway. Carbohydrate is the only fuel that can be used for this process.[27]

The advantage of anaerobic glycolysis for the muscle is that, other than PCr breakdown, it is the fastest way to resupply ATP. Anaerobic glycolysis provides most of the energy for events ranging from about 30 seconds to 2 minutes. The reason for this is that some of the steps in fat utilization simply cannot occur fast enough to meet the ATP demands of short-duration, high-intensity exercise. If fat

anaerobic Not using oxygen. Anaerobic activities use muscle groups at high intensities that exceed the body's capacity to supply energy using only oxygen-requiring pathways.

lactic acid A three-carbon acid formed during anaerobic cell metabolism; a partial breakdown of glucose; also called lactate (see Chapter 7).

glycolysis The pathway that results in the breakdown of glucose into two three-carbon molecules.

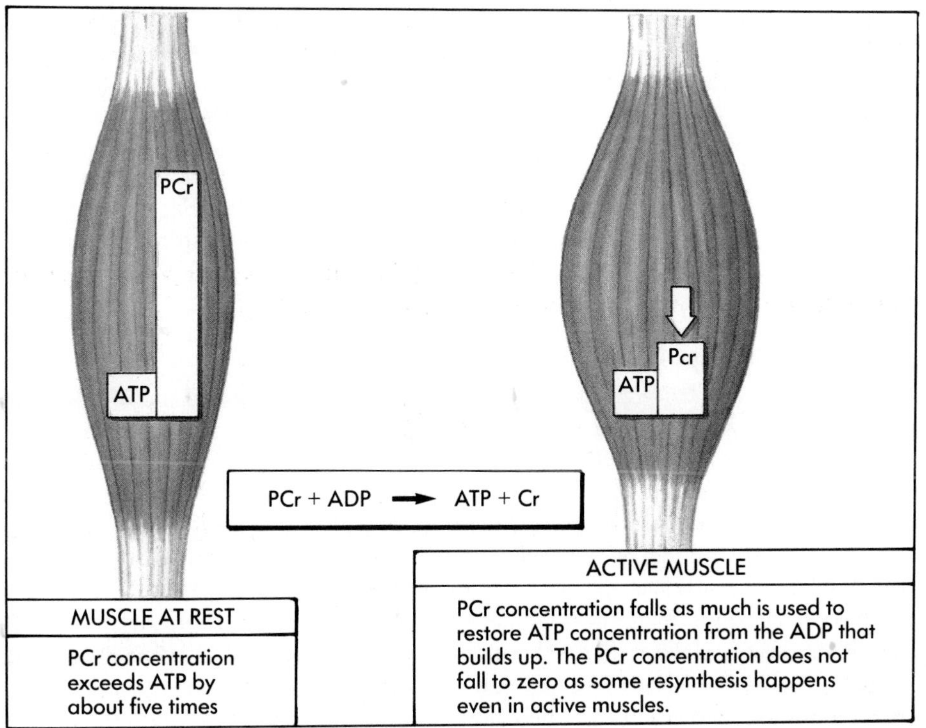

Figure 10-1 Quick energy for muscle use includes a supply of creatine-phosphate (PCr). This can rapidly replenish ATP stores as activity begins. Phosphocreatine can be nearly totally depleted in maximally contracting human forearm mucles in less than 60 seconds. It takes 4 minutes of rest to replenish half the PCr and 7 minutes to replenish 95% of the PCr. Similarly, it takes about 7 minutes of rest to replenish 95% of the PCr depleted with repeated knee extensions against resistance.

Table 10-1 Energy systems for muscle cell use

System	When in use	Example of an exercise
ATP	At all times	All types
Phosphocreatine (PCr)	All exercise initially; extreme exercise thereafter	Shotput, jumping
Anaerobic glycolysis (carbohydrate)	High intensity exercise, especially lasting 30 seconds to 2 minutes	200-yard (200-meter) run for time
Aerobic glycolysis (carbohydrate)	Exercise lasting 2 minutes to 4 to 5 hours; the higher the intensity (such as running a 6-minute mile), the greater the use	Basketball, swimming, jogging
Aerobic fat use	Exercise lasting more than a few minutes; greater amounts are used at lower levels of exercise intensity	Long-distance running, long distance cycling; 70%-90% of fuel use in a brisk walk is fat
Aerobic protein use	Low levels during all exercise; moderate levels in endurance exercise, especially when carbohydrate fuel is lacking	Long-distance running

The fuel mix in exercise sustained over 1 hour or more is 60%-80% fat, 15%-30% carbohydrate, and up to 10% protein. As intensity increases, carbohydrate use climbs to about 40% and protein use to about 15%. Fat use falls accordingly.

were the only available fuel, we would be unable to carry out exercise more intense than a fast walk or jog. High-caliber sports events would be out of the question.[17]

The two major disadvantages of anaerobic glycolysis are (1) this high rate of ATP production cannot be sustained for long events, and (2) the rapid accumulation of lactic acid greatly increases the acidity of the muscle. This acid inhibits the activities of key enzymes in the glycolysis **pathway;** this then slows anaerobic ATP production, and in turn causes fatigue.

pathway A metabolic progression of individual steps from starting materials to ending products, like $C_6H_{12}O_6$ (glucose) + O_2 →→→ CO_2 + H_2O.

For the most part, the lactic acid accumulates in active muscle cells until it is released into the bloodstream. From there the liver picks the lactic acid up and resynthesizes it into glucose. Glucose then can reenter the bloodstream where it is available for cell uptake and breakdown. The heart also can use the lactic acid directly for its energy needs, as can less active muscle cells situated near active ones.[8]

aerobic Using oxygen. Aerobic activities use large muscle groups at moderate intensities. This permits the body to use oxygen to supply energy and to maintain a steady rate for more than a few minutes.

Aerobic Glycolysis

If there is plenty of oxygen available in the muscle (**aerobic** state) and the exercise activity is of moderate to low intensity (e.g., jogging or distance swimming), the bulk of the pyruvate produced from the breakdown of glucose can be shuttled to the **mitochondria** of the cell. There it is further **metabolized** into carbon dioxide and water. This is known as aerobic glycolysis because the breakdown of glucose takes place with the aid of oxygen. About 95% of the ATP made from glucose metabolism is formed "aerobically" in mitochondria (Figure 10-2).

mitochondria Structure inside most cells, including muscle cells. These are the main sites of energy production in a cell. Mitochondria also contain the pathway for burning fat for fuel, among other metabolic pathways.

metabolism Chemical reactions that occur in the body, enabling cells to release energy from foods, convert one substance into another, and prepare end products for excretion.

Aerobic glycolysis supplies ATP more slowly than does anaerobic glycolysis, but again more energy is released. Furthermore, this slower rate of aerobic energy supply can be sustained for hours. Accordingly, aerobic glycolysis makes a major energy contribution to sports events lasting anywhere from about 2 minutes to 4 or 5 hours (Table 10-1).

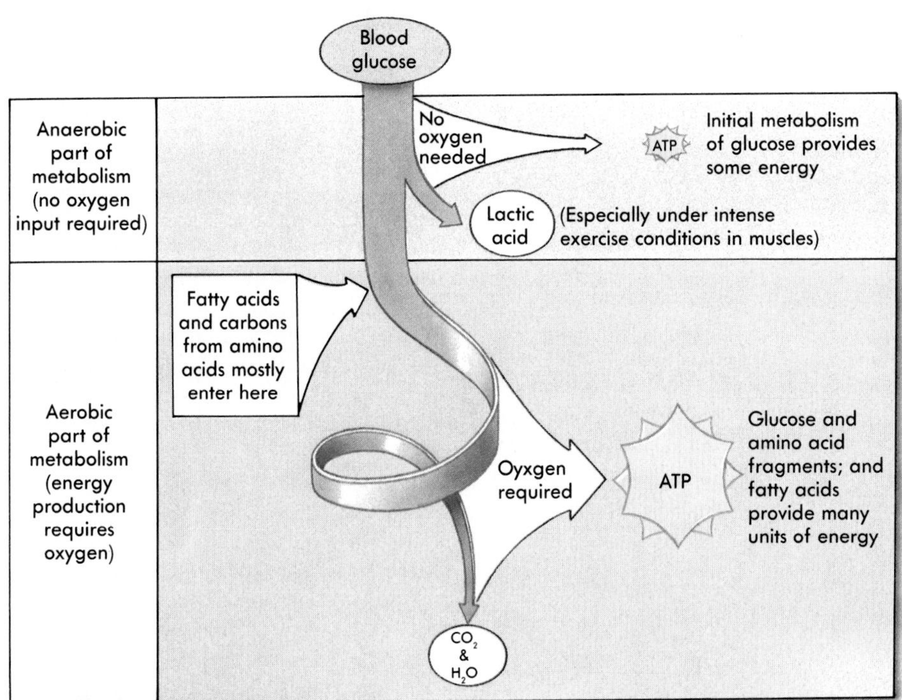

Figure 10-2 Carbohydrate, fat, and protein fuel can all supply ATP energy for the muscle cell.

IMPORTANCE OF GLYCOGEN VERSUS BLOOD GLUCOSE FOR CARBOHYDRATE FUEL

It is important to note that muscle glycogen, the temporary storage form of glucose in the muscles, is the preferred fuel for both anaerobic glycolysis and for aerobic glycolysis in fairly intense muscular activities that last for less than about 2 hours. For these activities, the depletion of this glycogen fuel in the muscle can cause fatigue. Diets high in carbohydrate can be used to build up muscle glycogen stores in advance of competition, thereby forestalling fatigue and improving endurance.[8] Dr. David Lamb discusses how to do this in his Expert Opinion.

As exercise duration increases beyond about 20 to 30 minutes, blood glucose becomes increasingly important as a fuel for glycolysis. This use of glucose from the bloodstream can spare the glycogen, saving it in the muscle for sudden bursts of effort that may be required, such as a sprint to the finish in a marathon race. Because it is important to maintain high concentrations of glucose in the bloodstream for prolonged exercise, many investigations have studied various types of carbohydrate feedings immediately before and during exercise in hopes of maximizing glucose supply.[25] We will also look at this issue in a later section.

CONCEPT CHECK

ATP is the main form of energy that cells use. Metabolic pathways use food energy to form ATP. Carbohydrate metabolism to form ATP begins as glucose becomes available from the bloodstream or from glycogen breakdown. In a muscle cell, each glucose is broken down through a series of steps to yield either lactic acid or carbon dioxide (CO_2) plus water (H_2O). When glucose is broken down into carbon dioxide and water, this is called aerobic glycolysis since oxygen is used. The conversion of glucose to lactic acid is called anaerobic glycolysis as no oxygen is used. This latter process allows the cell to quickly reform ATP and supports the demand for energy during intense exercise, as does phosphocreatine (PCr).

Ergogenic Aids: Some Substances can Enhance Athletic Performance

DR. DAVID LAMB

Manipulating one's diet for better performance has a long history. As long as 30 years ago, American football players were encouraged on hot practice days to "toughen up" for competition by liberally consuming salt tablets before and during practice and by not drinking water. Now it is widely recognized that this practice can be fatal. Today's athletes are as likely as their predecessors to experiment—artichoke hearts, bee pollen, dried adrenal glands from cattle, seaweed, freeze-dried liver-flakes, gelatin, and ginseng are just some of the worthless substances now used by athletes in hopes of gaining an "ergogenic" (work-producing) edge.

Still, modern-day athletes can benefit from recently-documented scientific evidence that a few dietary substances do have ergogenic properties. These ergogenic aids include sufficient water, lots of carbohydrate, and a balanced and varied diet that follows suggestions in the Guide to Daily Food Choices. Protein and amino acid supplements are presently not on the list. The average American apparently eats plenty of protein, athletes included.

Clearly, it is not possible to change average athletes into champions simply by altering diets. This means nutrient supplements require careful evaluation. Use should be designed to meet a specific dietary weakness, such as a poor iron intake. These and other aids whose benefit is often dubious and which nonetheless can pose health risks must be given close scrutiny before use. The risk-benefit ratio of these ergogenic aids especially needs to be examined. Athletes must stay on guard against false promises.

Carbohydrate loading

For athletes who compete in events lasting 90 to 120 minutes or longer or in shorter events repeated in a 24-hour period, it is often advantageous to undertake a **"carbohydrate-loading"** regimen to maximize muscle glycogen stores. One possible regimen includes a gradual reduction or "tapering" of exercise intensity and duration, coupled with a gradual increase in dietary carbohydrate as a percentage of energy intake. The procedure can begin 6 days before competition, with the athlete completing a hard workout lasting about 60 minutes. Workouts for the next 4 days then last about 40, 40, 20, and 20 minutes, respectively, with exercise intensities being progressively reduced each day. On the final day before competition, the athlete rests.

The dietary carbohydrate on the first 3 days of this regimen (about 450 grams) contributes 45% to 50% of energy intake. This rises to 65% to 75% carbohydrate (about 600 grams per day) for the last 3 days leading up to competition. This carbohydrate-loading technique usually increases muscle glycogen storage by 50% to 85% over usual conditions (i.e., when a typical amount of carbohydrate is consumed [46% of kcalories]). The greater carbohydrate stores then often result in improved athletic endurance.

A potential disadvantage to carbohydrate loading is that along with the glycogen, some water is also stored in the muscles. The water adds body weight and may cause muscle stiffness. For some people, this makes carbohydrate loading an unfeasible practice. Athletes considering carbohydrate loading should try it during training (and well before an important event) to experience its effects on performance. They can then determine if it is worth the effort.

Carnitine supplementation

The majority of the energy stored in the body for muscle use is found in fat. During physical activity, fatty acids are released from the fat depots into the bloodstream and travel to the muscles, where they are taken into each cell and "aerobically" broken down to carbon dioxide and water. These fatty acids must enter the cell's mitochondria before they can be broken down. The fatty acids are mostly transported from the fluid portion of the cell into the mitochondria using a transport system that contains a compound called carnitine. Athletes sometimes take carnitine supplements hoping carnitine will help them burn fat faster in exercise. But since our cells can make carnitine quite easily, carnitine supplements provide no reliable benefit.

Bicarbonate loading

We have noted that muscles that contract vigorously during athletic performance produce lactic acid. Lactic acid buildup inhibits the activity of enzymes involved in energy metabolism, and may lead to early fatigue. In the 1930s, athletes' attempts to counter this lactic acid accumulation by ingesting small doses of **sodium bicarbonate** (a base) failed to improve their athletic performances. On the other hand, more recent experiments using large doses of bicarbonate (300 milligrams per kilogram body weight) that were consumed 1 or 2 hours before exercise generally showed improved strenuous performance lasting 2 to 10 minutes. About 20 minutes of warm-up has typically preceded the exercise performance in these experiments. The bicarbonate loading apparently speeds the removal of lactic acid from contracting muscle cells and increases sodium levels in body fluids to help reduce acidity. Unfortunate side effects of large doses of sodium bicarbonate are nausea and diarrhea, often at unpredictable times. For this reason, bicarbonate loading has so far not become popular with athletes.

Caffeine supplementation

Drinking 2 to 4 cups of coffee (4 to 9 milligrams of caffeine per kilogram body weight) or using caffeine suppositories about 1 hour before an endurance competition (lasting more than 2 hours) enhances performance in some, but not all, athletes. The effect is less apparent in athletes who have ample stores of glycogen or are highly trained. The reason for the overall effect is not well established; sparing of muscle glycogen by increasing the use of fatty acids for muscle fuel, psychological effects, or enhancement of glycolysis in muscle all deserve consideration. However, some athletes experience changes in heart rhythm, nausea, or lightheadedness that can actually impair performance. Olympic officials view caffeine as a drug and do not condone its use. They consider a body level of caffeine exceeding the equivalent of 5 to 6 cups of coffee illegal.

Ergogenic Aids: Some Substances can Enhance Athletic Performance—cont'd

Use of anabolic steroids

Public attention focused on the use of anabolic **steroids** when Ben Johnson, winner of the gold medal for the 100-meter dash in the 1988 Olympic Games, was disqualified. Johnson took anabolic steroids regularly as part of his training regimen. These steroids are used by athletes to enhance performance in a variety of sports, most commonly "strength sports," such as football, wrestling, weight lifting, and certain track-and-field events. Steroids have also been used by swimmers and cyclists and are often used by male and female body builders and even nonathletic high school students in an attempt to "get big."

Steroids are synthetic versions of male sex hormones that promote two types of effects: masculinization (**androgenic** effect) and growth promotion (anabolic effect).[11] Athletes have taken these drugs, often in doses 10 to 30 times normal androgen output, to increase muscle size, strength, and performance; note that no reliable cardiovascular benefit has been found.

Although they often can increase muscle mass and strength, steroid use is unsafe and, in athletics, illegal. In the United States their possession without a prescription is a federal crime. The consequences of steroid use also can occasionally be devastating depending on the dose. The practice can cause growth plates in bones to close prematurely (thus possibly limiting the adult height of a teenage athlete); produce bloody cysts in the liver; accelerate the development of heart disease; and lead to high blood pressure, sterility, and many other detrimental physical effects.[26] Psychological consequences vary from increasing aggressiveness, drug dependence (addiction), withdrawal symptoms such as depression and sleep disturbances, and mood swings to decreased sex drive, depression, and even "roid-rage" (violence attributed to steroid use).[9] Some football players consider the increased aggressiveness an additional benefit.

Athletes often begin to use steroids during high school, and occasionally as early as junior high school. Many serious athletes must make a hard choice—to not use steroids and face a large field of artificially endowed opponents or to use the drugs and risk side effects and legal sanctions.

Growth hormone injections

There is too little scientific information available on the effects of **growth hormone** on muscle mass and strength in athletes to allow firm conclusions to be made about this drug. However, it is known that the skin, tongue, and bones of the jaw, fingers, and toes may grow abnormally under growth-hormone stimulation. Abusing growth hormone may increase height if consumed at critical ages, but uncontrolled growth of the heart and other internal organs and even death are also potential consequences. All in all, use of growth hormone is dangerous—it requires careful monitoring by a physician. Arginine and ornithine supplements, basically amino acids, a new rage among body builders, are promoted as growth-hormone boosters.[15] Current evidence suggests that any increase in growth hormone after consuming amino acids is rather modest and probably of little physiological consequence.

Blood doping

Injecting red blood cells into the bloodstream—known as **blood doping**—is used to try to enhance aerobic capacity. In this procedure, an athlete donates at least 2 pints of blood at least 6 weeks before the event and freezes the cells while the body makes more blood to replace it. Then, a day or two before competition, the frozen red cells are thawed and reinfused into the veins; the added cells elevate the total red blood cell count and hemoglobin concentration above normal.

A simpler, faster, but more dangerous way to "blood dope" is to inject a synthetic form of the hormone called erythropoietin. Erythropoietin is secreted by the kidney to stimulate red blood cell production by the bone marrow. Erythropoietin can increase the concentration of red cells so greatly that blood clots develop in the lungs or brain, leading to strokes that can paralyze or kill. It is widely speculated in the medical community that erythropoietin abuse is responsible for a sudden dramatic increase in deaths of young competitive cyclists in Europe over the last few years.[1]

Admissions by world-class athletes—including members of the victorious U.S. cycling team in the 1984 Olympics—that they used blood doping to reduce race times continue to stimulate questions about both sports ethics and how well the procedure actually works. Several studies confirm an aerobic benefit to the athlete as a result of blood doping, but the potential negative health consequences, especially with erythropoietin abuse, are very serious. It is also an illegal practice under Olympic guidelines.

Phosphate loading

Contrary to beliefs of many athletes and coaches, phosphate pills do not always improve performance or efficiency of heart function during endurance events. Some studies have suggested that loading phosphate for 4 days increased the levels of a metabolically important phosphate compound, **diphosphoglycerate (DPG),** in red blood cells. These studies also showed that increased levels of DPG potentially improved the delivery of oxygen to muscles and reduced work by the heart during vigorous exercise. We now know that rigorously trained athletes already have high levels of DPG in their red blood cells. Thus, although a single dose of phosphate can induce blood chemistry changes, it does not reliably improve the ability to perform endurance exercise, nor does it necessarily increase the efficiency of aerobic metabolism.

Summing up

Although many claims of ergogenic effects in athletes are unfounded, the exceptions we've described are based on systematic scientific investigations. This is not to say that there are no other potentially ergogenic substances but such aids are not scientifically verified.

Dr. Lamb is Professor and Director of the Exercise Physiology Laboratory, School of Health, Physical Education, and Recreation, at Ohio State University.

FUELING MUSCLES USING FAT

The majority of the stored energy is found in the fatty acids of stored triglycerides. When fat stores in various fat deposits in the tissues are broken down for energy, one triglyceride molecule first yields three fatty acids and a glycerol. The fatty acids are released from the fat depots into the bloodstream and travel to the muscles, where they are taken into each cell's cytosol. These fatty acids must enter the cell's mitochondria before they can be "aerobically" broken down into carbon dioxide and water. Recall from Chapter 7 that the mitochondria produce most of the ATP supply for a cell. The fatty acids are mostly transported from the cytosol into the mitochondria using a transport system that contains a compound called **carnitine.**[27] Athletes sometimes take carnitine pills hoping it will help them burn fat faster in exercise. But since our cells can make carnitine quite easily, carnitine supplements provide no reliable benefit.[17]

carnitine A compound used to shuttle fatty acids into the mitochondria of a cell. This allows for the fatty acids to be burned for energy.

The rate at which muscles use fatty acids is partly dependent on the concentration of fatty acids in the bloodstream. In other words, the more fatty acids that are released from fat stores into the bloodstream, the more fat will be used by the muscles. Recently, athletes have attempted to raise their blood concentrations of fatty acids by consuming caffeinated beverages.[28] This practice actually can increase fatty acid release from the fat depots, and so can be helpful to some athletes (see the Expert Opinion).

As we just mentioned, fat is ultimately not a very useful fuel for intense, brief exercise, but it becomes progressively more important as an energy source as exercise becomes increasingly prolonged, especially when exercise remains at a low or moderate (aerobic) rate (Table 10-1).

The advantage of fat as a fuel source over other sources of energy is that it provides tremendous stores of energy in a relatively lightweight form. For a given weight of fuel, fat supplies more than twice as much energy as carbohydrate. On the basis of ATP produced per carbon atom, fat also comes out ahead of carbohydrate. The aerobic breakdown of a six-carbon glucose molecule yields 36 to 38 ATP (ratio of about 6 ATP to 1 carbon atom), whereas an 18-carbon fatty acid molecule produces 147 ATP (ratio of about 8.2 ATP to 1 carbon atom).[27] In addition, when energy is needed for a long duration of exercise or physical labor, a body's reserves of carbohydrate are too small to sustain work, but there is almost always an overabundance of fat that can be called on.

However, carbohydrate is more efficient than fat in a very important comparison: the amount of ATP produced per unit of oxygen consumed. It takes six O_2 molecules to produce 38 ATP molecules during the aerobic breakdown of a molecule of glucose (ratio of about 6 ATP to 1 O_2 molecule), whereas 26 O_2 molecules are needed to produce 147 ATP molecules from an 18-carbon fatty acid (ratio of about 5.7 ATP to 1 O_2 molecule). In this comparison, carbohydrate is more efficient in terms of oxygen consumed per ATP molecule produced. Thus in situations when an athlete's maximal performance would be limited by the activity of oxygen-requiring pathways (as in competitive endurance exercise), it is important that muscle cells also are able to use carbohydrate as long as the carbohydrate supply, especially muscle glycogen, lasts.

During very lengthy activities, such as a triathalon, ultramarathon, manual labor in a foundry, or even sitting at a desk for 8 hours a day, fat supplies about 70% to 90% of the energy required. Overall, keep in mind that the only fuel we eat that can support "fast-paced" (anaerobic) activity is carbohydrate; slow and steady (aerobic) activity uses all three energy sources, i.e., carbohydrate, fat, and protein.[6]

DOES THIS MEAN WE USE PROTEIN TO FUEL PHYSICAL ACTIVITY?

Protein—actually amino acids—are used for fueling muscles, but this contributes only about 6% to both the body's general energy needs, and also for the typical energy needs of exercising muscles. However, proteins can contribute significantly to energy needs in endurance exercise, perhaps as much as 10% to 15%, especially as carbohydrate stores in the muscle are exhausted. We easily eat enough to supply this amount of fuel. Protein or amino acid supplements are not needed.[23] Contrary to what many athletes believe, protein is used less for fuel in resistance types of exercise (i.e., weight lifting) than for endurance exercise (i.e., running). The primary fuels for weight lifting are phosphocreatine (PCr) and carbohydrate.

CONCEPT CHECK

Fat is a key aerobic fuel for muscle cells, especially at low exercise intensities. At rest muscles burn primarily fat for energy needs. On the other hand, little protein is used to fuel muscles. It supplies about 6% of energy needs, and at perhaps 10% to 15% of energy needs during endurance events.

The Body's Response to Exercise

We have discussed how muscle cells obtain the ATP energy needed to do work. Let's now focus on how muscles and related organs adapt to an increased workload.

TRAINING—THE BODY ADAPTS TO THE DEMAND

Repeated aerobic exercise produces beneficial changes in the heart and blood vessels that are responsible for delivering oxygen to the mitochondria of the muscles. Because it uses more oxygen, the body responds to training by producing more red blood cells and total blood volume. The heart, a muscle itself, enlarges and strengthens. Each contraction empties the heart's chambers more efficiently.[18] Now more blood is pumped with each beat. As exercise increases the heart's efficiency, its rate of beating at rest and during submaximal exercise is lower. This is an index of fitness—a lower heart rate is seen as fitness increases. In addition, oxygen can be delivered more easily through the blood vessels of the muscles to the mitochondria because the number of capillaries in the muscles increases after exercise training.

After a period of aerobic training, muscle cells contain more and larger mitochondria. The muscles can then more efficiently fuel themselves from fatty acid stores as these changes enable muscle cells to produce more ATP using oxygen-requiring pathways. This includes the pathway used to burn fat for fuel. These changes in mitochondrial function allow for greater intensity during aerobic exercise. The athlete can now train harder and longer at an "aerobic" pace. Furthermore, a 20% to 50% improvement in muscle glycogen stores seen with training allows for larger carbohydrate sources to be available for muscular work.

MEASURING EXERCISE CAPACITY

There is more oxygen in the air we inhale than in the air we breathe out. Oxygen taken up by the mitochondria to help produce ATP energy accounts for this difference. The amount of oxygen consumed by the mitochondria of the body tissues is directly related to the ATP requirement during exercise. Every atom of oxygen consumed results in the production of two to three ATP molecules in the electron transport system of the mitochondria. Thus oxygen consumption indicates how hard a person is exercising. The harder the muscles work, the more oxygen they demand.

The more physically fit a person is, the more work the muscles and body can do, and the more oxygen the person can consume. The maximum volume of oxygen one can consume (**VO_2 max**) is calculated by measuring oxygen consumption while exercising, say running on a treadmill. The treadmill speed and/or grade is gradually increased until the subject becomes fatigued. The point right before total exhaustion

VO_2 max Maximum volume of oxygen consumed per unit of time during exercise.

NUTRITION FOCUS

Designing a Training Program

Getting started

A gradual increase to regular physical activity is recommended for all healthy persons. But if one is 35 or older, has been inactive for many years, or has an existing health problem, the American College of Sports Medicine recommends talking to a physician first. Health problems that require medical evaluation before beginning an exercise program are obesity, heart disease (or family history of it), high blood pressure, diabetes (or family history), shortness of breath after mild exertion, and arthritis. Although vigorous exercise involves minimal health risks for those in good health, far greater risks exist for those who are inactive.[4]

A basic exercise program should begin with warm-up exercises, primarily to increase blood flow and warm the muscles. This reduces risk of injuries. Then activities to increase muscular strength, endurance, and flexibility are done. Cool-down exercises finish the program. Table 10-2 shows how to design a cardiovascular workout program. Fitness target heart rates for adults are about 60% to 90% of one's predicted maximum heart rate (220 − current age) (Figure 10-3).[22]

To determine whether you are in the target exercise zone, learn to count your pulse. Placing your hand over the heart is a simple method. However, since clothing may obscure the beat, it is best to lightly put pressure on either large artery at the side of your neck. A full pulse can also be felt at the wrist or inside the bend of the elbow. Count the pulse immediately on stopping exercise because the rate changes very quickly once exercise is slowed or stopped. Find the beat within a second and count for 10 seconds. Multiply this number by six to obtain the count for a minute. Do not count for the whole minute, or even for 15 seconds, because the fall-off after exercise is too fast.

When to exercise and how much is enough?

The easiest way to increase physical activity is to make it part of a daily routine, just as we make time for other regular activities, such as studying. The best time to exercise might be when you need an energy pick-me-up or when you need a break from work. Rather than giving up the whole idea when obstacles impede an exercise program, strive to use small spaces of time. As you have fun and reap the benefits of exercise, the time devoted to exercise tends to grow. Aim for 30 minutes of exercise at 60% to 70% of your maximum heart rate three to four times a week to start.[22] As you progress, increase heart rate to 70% to 90% of maximum heart rate. It's fine to try pushing past a little fatigue, but when arms or legs start shaking uncontrollably, it's time to ease up. Note that ignoring pain can almost guarantee an injury.

Find several pleasurable ways to exercise. Start off gradually and work up to longer times. Doing too much too fast is a quick way to extinguish your enthusiasm and determination. Combine walking and swimming, tennis and jogging, or attend an aerobics class. A new trend in exercising is cross-training, in which a variety of exercises are incorporated into a fitness program. For example, instead of jogging for 30 minutes, a person may swim for 15 minutes and then jog for 15 minutes. By adding variety to your program, it not only keeps you mentally fresh, but it also strengthens different muscle groups and reduces risk of injury. Variety also keeps it interesting. An exercise partner may offer additional motivation.

Search for an exercise that suits you: heel-to-toe brisk walking is recommended for just about everyone. To ease into a regular aerobic exercise routine, start by walking. Begin with 30 to 45 minutes of brisk walking 5 days a week. After a few weeks, if you find yourself feeling more energetic, speed up to a jog or start an aerobic dance program. More than most other forms of exercise, walking lends itself to sharing, socializing, and enjoying nature. And because it's so easy and pleasurable, you're likely to continue including it in your routine long after you've dropped more exotic or strenuous sports.

More vigorous exercise for overweight persons should be non–weight-bearing activities such as swimming and bicycling. If you do jog or run, or do aerobic dance, pace yourself so that you are able to talk comfortably without becoming short of breath. At this point lactic acid production remains low, so muscle fatigue from that will be minimized. It is best for a beginner to switch from brisk walking to jogging and back again every couple of minutes. Gradually, the amount of walking time can be decreased while jogging time is extended. Jogging or running may be stressful on knees; it is very important to select proper shoes and to use an appropriate running surface, such as a track.

Whatever the means chosen for increasing physical activity, the activities should be enjoyable. This way they can become routine. Keep in mind convenience, cost, and options for bad weather so that when motivation wanes, you are not adding any further obstacles.

Setting an exercise prescription

Exercise output can be quantified in terms of METs and is often done so in the cardiovascular rehabilitation setting.[22] METs represent essentially a ratio of energy use in exercise to energy use at rest. A person at rest burns about 1 kcalorie per kilogram body weight per hour. This by definition is one MET. A 70-kilogram man then would be expending 10 METs if he was cycling at a rate of 700 kcalories per hour.

$$\frac{700 \text{ kcalories per hour}}{(1 \text{ kcalorie per kilogram} \times 70 \text{ kilograms}} = 10 \text{ METs}$$

As we mentioned, MET units are often used to set exercise prescriptions for rehabilitation programs, such as for people recovering from a heart attack. Table 10-3 on page 312 lists MET units for various physical activities.

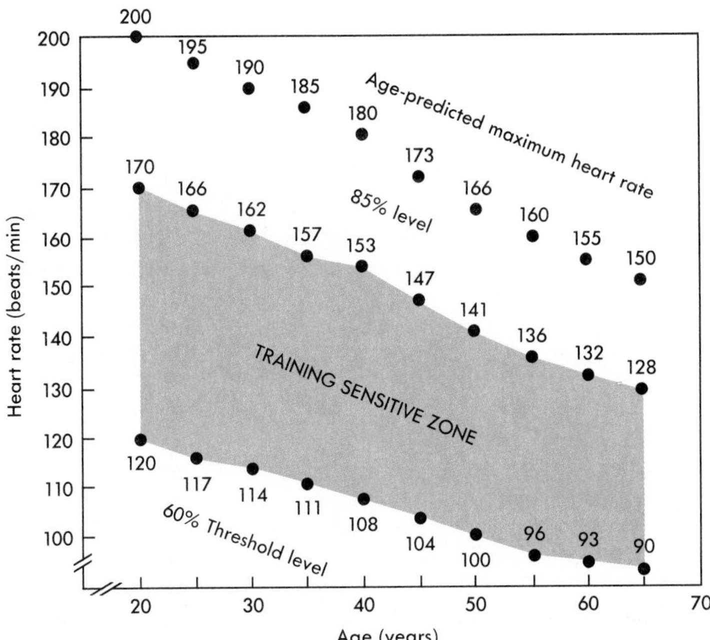

Figure 10-3 Target heart rate for cardiovascular fitness. These rates balance the need for cardiovascular stimulation with those of safety.

is VO_2 max. This is the most oxygen that one can use.[17] While each person's VO_2 max is unique, it can usually improve 15% to 20% or even more with exercise training.

When discussing an exercise intensity, it is usually best to express that intensity as a percentage of VO_2 max. Low intensities (fast walk) require approximately 30% to 50% of VO_2 max; moderate intensities (fast jog) require 50% to 65% VO_2 max; high intensities (3-hour marathon pace) use 70% to 80% VO_2 max; and very high intensities (sprints) use 85% to 150% of VO_2 max. (The extra 50% is accounted for by the anaerobic production of ATP in both PCr breakdown and anaerobic glycolysis.)

FUEL USE IN EXERCISE—A CLOSER LOOK

The fuel used for a specific workload is determined by the intensity (portion of VO_2 max used) and duration of exercise. The availability of certain energy-yielding pathways in a cell—notably the citric acid cycle and electron transport system—depends on the workload and how much work has been done already (Table 10-1). Because these concepts are highly complex, we will only summarize them briefly.

Rest and Low Level Workloads

Muscle cells—either resting or during low workloads such as a brisk walk—primarily burn fat for fuel because the supply of ATP generated from fat metabolism easily can sustain that workload. Fuel use is about 70% to 90% fat; the rest comes mostly from carbohydrate metabolized in the mitochondria using the citric acid cycle and electron transport system. (Chapter 7 reviews these metabolic systems.) Also, while a muscle cell is busy making ATP using fat energy, it cannot easily make ATP using glucose energy; high concentrations of ATP and other substances produced during fat metabolism in the cell inhibit important enzymes used in glycolysis.[27] On the other hand, there is no such inhibition for use of the citric acid cycle and electron transport system. This tips the balance toward using fat to form ATP energy.

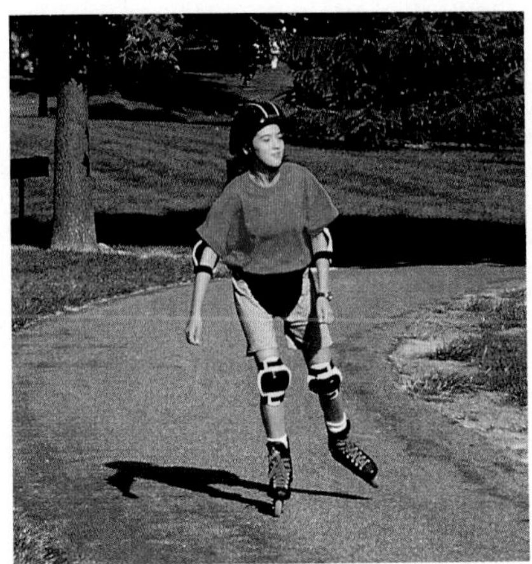

The idea is to stay physically active throughout one's life.

Brief and Maximally Intense Exercise

Intense exercise, such as running 200-meter sprints, requires maximum effort and cannot be sustained. In fact, this exercise is so intense that it may last for no more than 30 seconds. For such workloads muscles use PCr and some anaerobic glycolysis. During short bursts of maximally intense work (up to about 10 seconds), the supply

Table 10-2 Your exercise prescription

Fitness component	Definitions	Activity
Flexibility	The ability to bend without injury; it is dependent on elasticity of muscles, tendons, ligaments, and conditions of joints.	Stretches will enhance flexibility. They should be held for at least 10 seconds. Never use bouncy, choppy, or painful stretches that twist or put pressure on joints.
Strength	The ability to work against resistance.	Using few repetitions (8-12 per set), with weights as heavy as is safely possible, will increase strength.
Muscle Endurance	The ability of a muscle to sustain effort over a period of time.	Repetitive exercises, such as push-ups, pull-ups, sit-ups.
Cardiovascular Endurance	The ability of the cardiovascular system to sustain effort over a period of time; it should involve larger muscle groups and be performed at 65%-80% of maximum effort.	Activities include fast walking, jogging, swimming, bicycling, and stair climbing. These can provide the needed sustained, submaximal work if the exercise is performed at appropriate pace.

The plan

WARM-UP: 5-10 minutes of stretching the whole torso. Start with smaller muscle groups (arms) and work towards larger muscle groups (legs and abdomen).

5-10 minutes more of exercises, such as walking, slow jogging or any slow version of anticipated activity. Low-level movement literally warms up muscles so that muscle filaments slide more easily over one another and will gradually bring heart rate up to target level.

WORKOUT: 20 or more minutes of rhythmic continuous activity 3-4 times a week. Pace should be set so that exercise raises heart rate to within target range. Modify pace or workload as necessary so that the heart rate reaches and does not exceed target range. A good rule of thumb is that you should be able to still converse. "Huff-puff" indicates increased lactate production. Popular aerobic conditioning activities include brisk walking, jogging, swimming, cycling, cross-country skiing, and aerobic dance. Activities such as basketball and racquetball provide a good workout, but because the heart rate jumps up high and then drops and then goes up again, it does not condition the heart as rhythmic continuous activities do. Exercises that develop muscular strength and endurance can follow the aerobic session or alternate with them on different days. Resistance exercises, such as weight training or calisthenics, encourage muscle maintenance and are particularly important in weight-reducing diets in order to maintain muscle mass.

COOL-DOWN: Follow a reverse pattern of warm-up: 5-10 minutes of low-level activity and 5-10 minutes of stretching. The same exercises performed during warm-up are appropriate. The cool-down is essential to the prevention of injury, soreness, and unnecessary drop in blood pressure.

of PCr is depleted rapidly from muscle tissue as it reforms ATP. The PCr system is also used as muscle contractions begin after a rest to reinitiate activity. However, in prolonged exercise at moderate intensity, PCr is not as critical because other cell pathways are available for ATP replenishment.[22]

Moderately Intense Exercise

When someone exercises hard and sustains it for more than a few minutes—for example, running a 6-minute mile—fat metabolism via the citric acid cycle and electron transport system cannot keep pace with the cell's ATP demands. Both anaerobic and aerobic glycolysis must kick in to help. This is partly because the electron transport system in each mitochondrion takes a few minutes to shift into high gear. That being the case, the ATP concentration at the start of exercise in muscle cells drops, and ADP concentration in muscle cells increases. The PCr system kicks in, but fades fast. Now the low ATP concentration in the muscle cells allows important enzymes in the glycolytic process to speed up. Glycogen in the muscle then breaks down into glucose, which undergoes glycolysis to form pyruvate. Carbohydrate ends up supplying 80% to 90% of the fuel used. Much of this pyruvate forms lactate. Because so little ATP energy is produced for each glucose molecule in anaerobic glycolysis, this type of glycolysis must proceed very rapidly in muscle cells to be of much value. This results in the production of many lactate molecules.

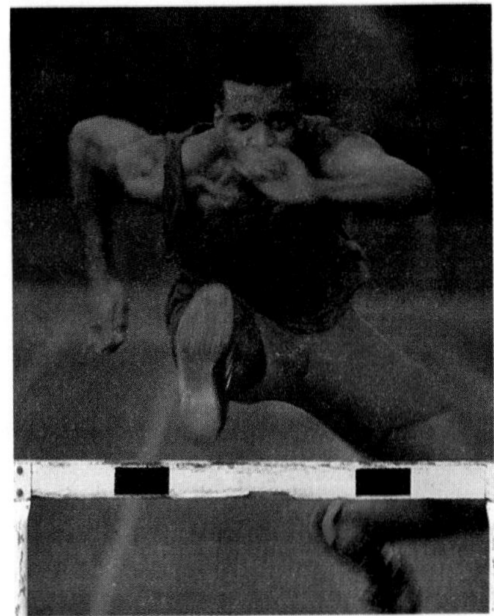

Short athletic events are fueled by creatine phosphate and carbohydrate.

The lactate option is most active for the first minute of exercise. After that, aerobic pathways kick in as well to keep up with ATP demands.

It has long been assumed—incorrectly—that lactate accumulation in muscle and blood always meant that muscle was anaerobic (deprived of oxygen) during exercise. We now know that lactic acid is formed and removed continuously and frequently at all times, even when muscles are at rest; only the amount of total production varies.[8]

If a person starts exercising regularly four or five times a week, he or she will experience a "training effect." At the start the person might be able to exercise for 20 minutes before tiring. Months later exercise can be extended to an hour before the person feels tired. During the months of training, muscle cells have produced more mitochondria and so can burn more fat. That means the person will produce less lactate during exercise. Since lactate contributes to muscle fatigue, the less lactate produced, the longer the person will be able to exercise. Part of the training effect derives also from the increased aerobic efficiency of heart and muscles that we described earlier.[7] However, when you consider only metabolism, a very important result of training is the increased number of mitochondria in the muscle cells, resulting in less dependence on the lactate system for energy production.

Endurance Exercise

Endurance exercise, such as walking or cycling, often involves moderate effort sustained over 1 or more hours. Muscles can continue to metabolize fat via the citric acid cycle and electron transport system for about 60% to 80% of energy needs at these moderate workloads, but aerobic glycolysis using carbohydrate also plays a role (about 15% to 30%), along with protein fuel (up to 10%). However, less lactate builds up in endurance exercise than during high-intensity activities because the slower rate of glucose metabolism can be handled by the oxygen-requiring processes in the mitochondria.

As intensity increases, such as in a 3-hour marathon run at 70% VO_2 max, muscles use about a 60:40 ratio of fat to carbohydrate.[17] When carbohydrate fuel (glycogen) in muscles is eventually used up, it is difficult to maintain the high initial workload unless blood glucose concentrations are elevated by carbohydrate feedings. Athletes call this condition "hitting the wall." So, when levels of exertion meet or exceed 70% of VO_2 max for more than an hour, an athlete (like a long distance runner or cyclist) should consider increasing the amount of carbohydrate stored in muscles and blood.[24] The Expert Opinion discussed how to do this.

Power Food: What Should an Athlete Eat?

Athletic training and genetic makeup are two very important determinants of athletic performance. A good diet won't substitute for either factor, but as we have hinted, diet can further enhance and maximize an athlete's potential. More importantly, a poor diet can certainly harm performance.[14]

HOW MUCH FOOD ENERGY DOES AN ATHLETE NEED?

Athletes need varying amounts of food energy, depending on his or her body size, current body composition, and the type of training or competition being considered. A small person may need only 1700 kcalories daily to sustain normal daily activities without losing body weight. A large muscular man may need 4000 kcalories. These are only estimates. Consider these starting points that need to be individualized by trial and error for each athlete. Kcalories required for sports training or competition have to be added to this energy needed just to carry on normal activities (see Table 10-3). An hour of bowling, for example, requires few kcalories in addition to those required to sustain normal daily living. On the other extreme, 12-hour endurance bicycle races over mountains can require an additional 4000 kcalories per day. Therefore, some athletes may need as much as 7000 kcalories daily just to maintain body weight while training, whereas others may need 1700 kcalories or less.

How can we know if an athlete is getting enough energy from food? The first step is to estimate the athlete's body fat percentage by measuring skinfold thicknesses,

Table 10-3 Approximate energy costs of various activities in MET units and Kcalories per hour for a 150-pound (68-kilogram) person

Activity	MET units*	Kcal/hour
Aerobics—heavy	8.0	544
Aerobics—medium	5.0	340
Backpacking	9.0	612
Basketball—vigorous	10.0	680
Bicycling (5.5 MPH)	3.0	204
Calisthenics—heavy	8.0	544
Canoeing (2.5 MPH)	3.3	224
Cleaning	3.5	236
Cycling (13 MPH)	9.7	659
Dressing/showering	1.6	106
Eating (sitting)	1.36	93
Football—touch	7.0	476
Horseback trotting	5.1	346
Ice skating (10 MPH)	5.8	394
Jogging—medium	9.0	612
Jogging—slow	7.0	476
Racquetball—social	8.0	544
Roller skating	5.1	346
Running or jogging (10 MPH)	13.2	897
Skiing (10 MPH)	8.8	598
Swimming (.25 MPH)	4.4	299
Tennis	6.1	414
Volleyball	5.1	346
Walking (3.75 MPH)	4.4	299
Water skiing	7.0	476
Weight lifting—heavy	9.0	612
Writing (sitting)	1.7	118

*By definition, lying at rest is 1 MET. These are approximate values.
Modified from Mosby Diet Simple, N-Squared Computing, Salem, Oregon, 97302

bioelectrical impedance, or using the underwater weighing technique (see Chapter 8). Body fat should be in the desirable range, i.e., about 4% to 12% for most male athletes and 10% to 20% for most female athletes.[13] The next step is simply to monitor body weight changes on a daily or weekly basis. If body weight starts to fall, food energy should be increased; if weight rises, and it is due to increases in body fat, the athlete should be encouraged to eat less.

If the body composition test shows that the athlete has too much body fat, the athlete should eat about 200 to 500 fewer kcalories per day until the desirable fat percentage is achieved while maintaining a regular exercise program. Reducing fat intake is the best nutrient-related approach. On the other hand, if the athlete needs to gain weight, an additional 200 to 500 kcalories per day will eventually lead to the needed weight gain. A mix of carbohydrate and fat is advised, coupled again with exercise to make sure this gain is mostly from lean tissue, and not mostly added fat stores.

Rapid Weight Loss by Dehydration

Wrestlers, boxers, judo players, and oarsmen often try to lose weight so that they can be certified to compete in a lower weight class. This helps them gain a mechanical advantage over an opponent of smaller stature. Most of the time, this weight is lost a few hours before stepping on the scale for weight certification. Athletes can lose up to 22 pounds (10 kilograms) of body water in 1 day by sitting in a sauna, exercising in a plastic sweat suit, and/or taking diuretic drugs that speed water loss from the kidneys. Losing as little as 3% of body weight by dehydration can sometimes adversely affect endurance performance.[17] A pattern of repeated weight loss or gain of more than 5% of body weight by dehydration carries some risk of kidney malfunction and heat illness. Dehydration also causes a reduction in blood volume, increases body temperature, and may cause heat cramps or heat exhaustion.

This habit of losing weight by dehydration is common in sports such as interscholastic and intercollegiate wrestling. This means most competitors probably face an opponent who has gone through the same misery to gain an "advantage." If an athlete wishes to compete in a lower body weight class and has enough extra fat stores, that athlete should begin a gradual, sustained reduction in food energy intake long before the competitive season starts. In so doing, the athlete will have a presumably healthier body composition (less fat) and can avoid the potentially harmful and certainly misery-creating effects of severe dehydration. If an athlete has no extra body fat he should be discouraged from attempting to compete at a lower body weight class. It is important for coaches and trainers to be aware of the decreased performance and serious side effects of severe dehydration.

GENERAL PRINCIPLES FOR MEETING OVERALL NUTRIENT NEEDS IN THE TRAINING DIET

Anyone who exercises regularly, including the dieter, needs to consume a diet that includes moderate to high amounts of carbohydrates.[5] This should be about 55% to 70% of total kcalories, rather than our typical 46%. Endurance athletes should meet the higher value. Fat intake should then fall from our typical 38% of total kcalories to 15% to 30%. Protein should make up the rest of the energy—about 10% to 15% of total intake. This yields a training table plate of about two thirds carbohydrate-rich foods and one third protein-rich foods.

All athletes should consume a variety of foods, adhering to the Guide to Daily Food Choices (see Chapter 2). Numerous selections of starches and fruits will help maintain adequate muscle glycogen stores and especially replace glycogen losses from the previous day. Triathletes and marathoners should consider eating close to 600 grams of carbohydrates a day and even more if necessary to (1) prevent chronic fatigue and (2) load the muscles and liver with glycogen.[19] This is especially important when performing multiple training bouts in a day, such as swim practices, or heavy training on successive days, as in cross-country running.[6] Table 10-4 can

It cannot be emphasized enough that any nutrition strategies should be tested out during practice and trial runs before being used in a meet or key event. An athlete should never try a new food or beverage on the day of competition. Some food items or beverages may not be tolerated well, and the day of competition is not the time to find that out.

help plan a 600-gram carbohydrate intake. This is based on the exchange system, which we covered in Chapter 2. As mentioned there, this is a very useful tool for planning all types of diets. Reference no. 20 provides still another tool to aid in the planning of a high carbohydrate diet.

Table 10-5 provides an example of a high-carbohydrate diet. Note that one does not have to give up any specific food. The diet focus just must turn to more of the best—high-carbohydrate foods—and away from the rest—concentrated fat sources.[6]

Sports nutritionists emphasize the difference between a high-carbohydrate meal and a high-carbohydrate/high-fat meal. Before endurance events, such as marathons or triathalons, some athletes attempt carbohydrate loading by eating potato chips, French fries, banana cream pie, and pastries, assuming these foods contain carbo-

Table 10-4 Grams of carbohydrate in typical foods

Starchy vegetables, breads, and cereals—15 grams carbohydrate per serving
One serving:

½ cup dry breakfast cereals*	1 small baked potato
½ cup cooked breakfast cereals	½ bagel
½ cup cooked grits	½ English muffin
⅓ cup cooked rice	1 slice bread
½ cup cooked pasta	¾ ounce pretzels
¼ cup baked beans	6 saltine crackers
½ cup corn	2 four-inch-diameter pancakes
½ cup beans	2 taco shells

Vegetables—5 grams carbohydrate per serving
One serving:

½ cup cooked vegetables
1 cup raw vegetables
½ cup vegetable juice
Examples: carrots, green beans, broccoli, cauliflower, onions, spinach, tomatoes, vegetable juice

Fruits—15 grams carbohydrate per serving
One serving:

½ cup fresh fruit	12 cherries or grapes
½ cup fruit juice	½ grapefruit
¼ cup dried fruit	1 nectarine
1 small apple	1 orange
4 apricots	1 peach
½ banana	1-¼ cup watermelon

Milk—12 grams carbohydrate per serving
One serving:

1 cup milk
8 ounces plain low-fat yogurt

Sweets—15 grams carbohydrate per serving
One serving:

½ slice cake	½ cup ice cream
2 small cookies	¼ cup sherbet
3 ginger snaps	

*Note the carbohydrate contents of dry cereals vary widely. Check the label of the ones you choose and adjust serving size accordingly.
Modified from *Exchange Lists for Meal Planning* by the American Diabetes Association and American Dietetic Association, 1986, Chicago, American Dietetic Association.

hydrate.[6] They do contain carbohydrate, but they also contain a lot of fat. Reading nutrition labels can more reliably guide high-carbohydrate food choices. Better food choices are pasta, rice, potatoes, bread, and many breakfast cereals. Sports drinks appropriate for carbohydrate loading, such as GatorLode or Exceed High Carbohydrate Source, can also help. Following a moderate dietary fiber intake during the final day is a good precaution to reduce the chances of bloating and intestinal gas during the next day's event.

Table 10-5 A 600-gram carbohydrate diet

4000 kcalories:

623 grams of carbohydrates	(61% of kcalories)
139 grams of protein	(14% of kcalories)
118 grams of fat	(26% of kcalories)

Menu	Carbohydrate (grams)
Breakfast	
1 orange	14
2 cups oatmeal	50
1 cup skim milk	12
2 bran muffins	48
Snack	
¾ cup chopped dates	98
Lunch	
Lettuce salad:	
1 cup romaine lettuce	2
1 cup garbanzo beans	45
½ cup alfalfa sprouts	5.5
2 Tablespoon French dressing	2
3 cups macaroni and cheese	80
1 cup apple juice	28
Snack	
2 slices whole-wheat toast	26
1 teaspoon margarine	—
2 Tablespoon jam	14
Dinner	
2 ounce turkey breast (no skin)	—
2 cups mashed potatoes	74
1 cup peas and onions	23
1 banana	27
1 cup skim milk	12
Snack	
1 cup pasta with	33
2 teaspoon margarine and	—
2 Tablespoon parmesan cheese	—
1 cup cranberry juice	36
TOTAL	628 grams

A carbohydrate: protein: fat ratio of 60:15:25 is a good goal when planning a diet to aid athletic performance.

MUSCLE-BULKING DIETS

During muscle-building regimens, athletes should consume 1 to 1.5 grams of protein per kilogram (0.5 to 0.7 grams per pound) of body weight every day. This range goes from slightly above to about double the protein RDA (0.8 grams per kilogram of desirable body weight).[23] Anyone eating a variety of foods can easily meet the higher amounts. Thus these athletes can follow the diet plan we have outlined for athletes in general. For example, a 123-pound (53-kilogram) woman can consume close to her upper range of 80 grams of protein by eating 4 ounces of chicken (one chicken breast) and 3 ounces of beef (a small lean hamburger), and drinking 3 glasses of milk during a single day. And this does not even include the protein in the grains or vegetables she will also eat. A 180-pound (77-kilogram) man needs only to consume 6 ounces of chicken (a large chicken breast), and a 6-ounce can of tuna, and drink 3 glasses of milk during a day to obtain close to his upper range of 115 grams of protein.

Many athletes eat many more protein-rich foods as they meet their energy needs (Table 10-5). Again, we see that protein supplements are not needed for athletes because their diets typically exceed even the most generous protein recommendation.

Athletes who either feel they must significantly limit their energy intake or are vegetarians should determine how much protein they eat; they should make sure it equals at least 1 gram per kilogram of desirable body weight. Skimping on protein is not any better than is the use of protein supplements.

VITAMINS AND MINERALS

Athletes usually consume many kcalories, and so they tend to consume plenty of vitamins and minerals. The B-vitamins and minerals, such as iron and copper, are especially needed to support energy metabolism (Table 10-6). If a low-energy intake—less than 1200 kcalories—is needed, athletes should pay very close attention to their vitamin and mineral intake. A focus on nutrient-dense foods, such as low-fat and nonfat milk, broccoli, tomatoes, oranges, strawberries, whole grains, lean beef, kidney beans, turkey, fish, and chicken, is a good idea. Vitamin and mineral fortified foods (e.g., many breakfast cereals) also can be used. Vitamin and mineral intakes greatly exceeding the RDA are not needed. Note that vitamin and mineral supplements supply no known **ergogenic** (work-producing) benefit. They only benefit the body when a medically diagnosed deficiency exists![28]

ergogenic Work-producing. An ergogenic aid is a physical, mechanical, nutritional, psychological or pharmacological substance or treatment that is intended to directly improve exercise performance.

Iron

Athletes, especially female and adolescent athletes, should focus special attention on iron intake. Iron losses in sweat, increased iron requirements for the enhanced red blood cell production associated with athletic fitness, foot-strike destruction of red blood cells (red cells are broken by trauma created as these pass through the foot as it strikes the ground during exercise), and iron loss during menstruation in women's iron stores. When this iron is not replenished, it can eventually lead to iron-deficiency anemia and markedly impaired endurance performance. Although true anemia (noted as a depressed blood hemoglobin concentration) is quite rare among athletes, it is a good idea, especially for adult women athletes, to have the blood hemoglobin levels checked regularly and to monitor dietary iron intake. Vegetarian female athletes should be especially careful to watch iron status. If blood iron levels are consistently low, the use of iron supplements by an athlete may be advisable. Iron supplements can improve athletic performance if the athlete is truly anemic, but they have no effect when the athlete simply has low blood levels of iron that have not resulted in anemia.

Long distance runner, Alberto Salazar, was experiencing problems sleeping and performance impairment until it was found to be due to his low iron intake and related iron-deficiency anemia. Thus men and women are at risk, and both should regularly monitor iron status.

Calcium

Athletes, especially women who are attempting to lose weight by restricting their intake of dairy products, can have marginal or low dietary intakes of calcium. This

Table 10-6 Vitamins and minerals: Function and usage with regard to exercise

Vitamins and minerals	Exercise-related function	Proposed benefit to performance	Effects of supplementation in excess of RDA/ESADDI
Thiamin	Carbohydrate metabolism	Enhances endurance performance	Does not enhance performance
Riboflavin	Energy metabolism	Enhances aerobic performance	Does not enhance performance
Niacin	Energy metabolism	Enhances energy metabolism	May impair performance by reducing fatty acid release
Vitamin B-6	Formation of hemoglobin	Enhances exercise performance	Does not enhance performance
Pantothenic acid	Energy metabolism	Enhances aerobic performance	Unclear research results to date
Vitamin B-12	Red blood cell development	Enhances endurance performance	Does not enhance performance
Folate	Cell synthesis; red blood cell formation		No studies available
Biotin	Fat and glycogen synthesis		No studies available
Vitamin C	Antioxidant	Prevents tissue damage; speeds repair	Well-controlled studies show no effect
Vitamin A	Antioxidant	Prevents tissue damage; speeds repair	Enhanced performance unlikely
Vitamin D	Bone mineral metabolism	Bone formation during muscle building	Does not affect work performance; may affect muscle building (one study), but needs likely do not exceed the RDA. Note excess intakes can be toxic
Vitamin E	Antioxidant	Prevents tissue damage; speeds repair	Does not enhance performance; may reduce exercise damage caused by breakdown in fat structure in cell membranes
Zinc	Carbohydrate, fat, and protein metabolism; tissue repair	Repair of exercise damage	Enhances some measures of muscle performance after 2 weeks (one study), but the dose was too high to be safely consumed on a regular basis (nine times the male RDA)
Copper	Red blood cell synthesis; energy metabolism	Enhances aerobic performance	Studies not available
Chromium	Carbohydrate metabolism; increases effects of insulin	Delays fatigue	Studies not available
Selenium	Antioxidant	Protects against exercise damage; delays fatigue	Studies not available
Iron	Oxygen transport and delivery	Reduces fatigue; enhances endurance	No effect on performance in nonanemic or non-iron-deficient subjects

From Clarkson PM: Vitamins and trace minerals. In Lamb DR and Williams M, editors: *Perspectives in exercise science and sports medicine*, vol 4, Ergogenics: Enhancement of exercise and sport performance, Indianapolis, 1991, Benchmark Press.

practice does not contribute to optimum bone health. Of still greater concern are women athletes who have stopped menstruating as a result of arduous exercise training that has interfered with the normal secretion of the reproductive hormones. Disturbing reports show that female athletes who do not menstruate regularly have far less dense spinal bones—in other words, less calcium present—than both non-athletes and female athletes who menstruate regularly.[12]

Researchers have clearly documented the importance of regular menstruation for the promotion of bone maintenance. Current studies imply that a woman runner who does not menstruate regularly may also have a higher risk for the development of a **stress fracture.** Female athletes whose menstrual cycles become irregular should consult a physician to ascertain the cause. Decreasing the level of training and/or increasing energy intake and body weight often restores regular menstrual cycles. If irregular menstrual cycles persist, severe bone loss and osteoporosis may result. Extra calcium in the diet does not necessarily compensate for this loss of menstruation, but inadequate dietary calcium can make matters worse.

stress fracture A fracture that occurs from repeated jarring of a bone. Common sites include bones of the foot.

PRE-EVENT MEAL

A light meal (300 kcalories) should be eaten 2 to 4 hours before an endurance event to top off muscle and liver glycogen stores and prevent hunger during the event. Added to this is extra fluid, as described in the next section. The foods in the overall meal then should consist primarily of carbohydrate, contain little fat or dietary fiber, and include a moderate amount of protein. Good choices are spaghetti, bagels, muffins, bread, and breakfast cereals with low-fat or nonfat milk. Liquid meal replacement formulas, like Carnation Instant Breakfast, also can be used. Foods rich in dietary fiber should be eaten the previous day to help clear the bowels before the event, but they should not be eaten the night before. Foods to avoid are those that are fatty or fried, such as sausage, bacon, sauces, and gravies. A meal high in carbohydrate is quickly digested, promotes normal blood glucose levels, and avoids the need to dip right away into glycogen stores. If an athlete feels a pre-event meal harms performance, eating a high-carbohydrate diet the day and night before can help meet the same goal.[6]

Consuming carbohydrate an hour or so before competition was previously thought to adversely affect performance because it increases insulin release, and insulin causes blood glucose to fall. However, we know now that such feedings do not cause premature fatigue nor decrease endurance for most people. In fact, recent studies show positive benefits of this type of pre-event feeding.[25] However, there are some athletes who are extremely sensitive to an insulin surge. Thus athletes should experiment with pre-event carbohydrate feedings to see if their performance is adversely or positively affected.

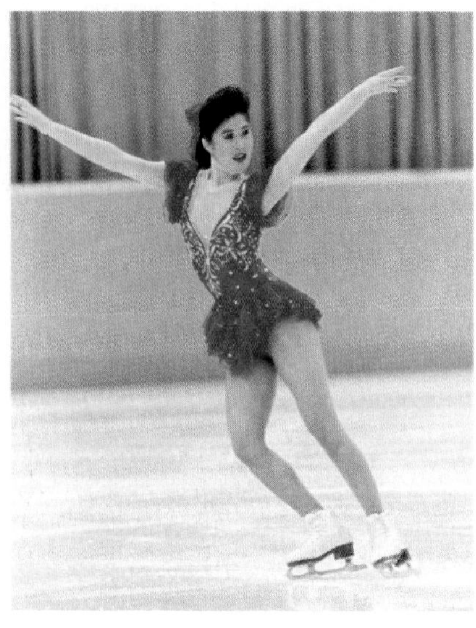

Hard training requires a hard look at one's diet—can it make the grade?

MAXIMIZING BODY FLUIDS AND ENERGY STORES DURING EXERCISE

Athletes need enough water to maintain the body's ability to regulate its internal temperature and so keep itself cool.[3] Most energy released during metabolism appears immediately as heat. Unless this heat is quickly dissipated, heat cramps, heat exhaustion, or deadly heat stroke may ensue. Sweat evaporating from the skin helps remove this heat from the body. Sweat rates during prolonged exercise range from 3 to 8 cups (750 to 2000 milliliters) per hour. To keep the body from becoming dehydrated, fluid intake during exercise, when possible, should be adequate to minimize body weight loss, and even be practiced in the wintertime when sweating can go unnoticed. However, most athletes find it very uncomfortable to replace more than about 75% to 80% of this sweat loss during exercise.

By experimenting, athletes can determine how much fluid they require to maintain weight and how much fluid intake they can tolerate without experiencing stomach cramps. This determination will be most accurate if the athlete is weighed before and after a typical workout. For every 1 pound (½ kilogram) lost, 2 cups (0.5 liter) of water should be consumed during exercise or immediately afterward.

Thirst is not a reliable indicator of fluid need, especially in winter. By relying on thirst alone, an athlete might take 48 hours to replenish fluid loss. After several days of practice, the increasing fluid debt can begin to impair performance. By the time one feels thirsty, the person may have lost 3% of body weight through sweat.

A good rule of thumb is to drink beverages freely up to 2 hours before an event. Don't worry about thirst. Then consume 1 to 2 cups (0.25 to 0.5 liters) of these fluids (like water, diluted fruit juice, or sports drinks) about 15 minutes before a sports event. This is called hyperhydration. The extra fluid in the body will be ready to replace sweat losses as needed. Next, consume approximately 1 to 1.5 cups of fluid (preferably at refrigeration temperature on hot days to also help cool the body) each 15 minutes for events that last longer than 30 minutes. If the weather is hot and/or humid, even more fluids may be required. The athlete need not worry that gradual consumption of fluids will cause bloating or impair performance. But skipping fluids will almost certainly cause problems! The Nutrition Perspective discusses whether this fluid should be a sports-type drink.

Alcohol and caffeine both have a dehydrating effect on the body, so fluids containing them should not be part of any hydration plan for exercise.

CARBOHYDRATE INTAKE DURING RECOVERY FROM EXERCISE

A large portion of the day's carbohydrate-rich foods should be consumed within 2 hours after a training exercise bout, and the sooner the better. This period of time is when glycogen synthesis is the greatest.[24] Athletes who are training hard can consume a simple sugar candy, sugared soft drink, fruit juice, or a sports-type carbohydrate supplement right after training as they attempt to reload their muscles with glycogen.

Fluid and **electrolyte** (i.e., sodium and potassium) intake is also an essential component of the athlete's recovery diet. This helps reestablish normal levels of body fluids as quickly as possible. This is especially true if two workouts a day are followed and if the environment is hot and humid.

electrolytes Compounds that break down into ions in water and, in turn, are able to conduct an electrical current. These include sodium, chloride, and potassium.

CONCEPT CHECK

All athletes would do well to plan a diet following the Guide to Daily Food Choices. High-carbohydrate foods should be emphasized, and these should dominate the pre-event meal. Additional protein intake above a usual American intake is not necessary. Nutrient supplements should be taken only to correct actual nutrient deficiencies. Fluid should be consumed as liberally as possible before, during, and after an event.

Summary

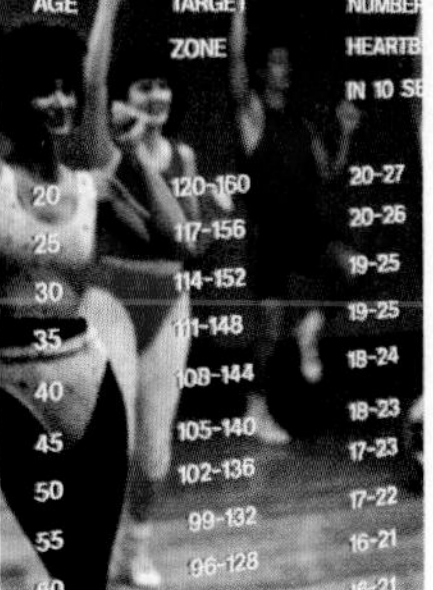

1. ATP is the major form of energy used for cellular metabolism. Human metabolic pathways extract that energy from foodstuffs and convert it into ATP.
2. In glycolysis, glucose is broken down into a three-carbon compound (pyruvate), yielding in addition some ATP. The three-carbon compounds can then proceed to other aerobic pathways to form carbon dioxide (CO_2) and water (H_2O), or anaerobic pathways to form lactic acid.
3. A gradual increase to regular physical activity is recommended for all healthy persons. If one is over age 35, it is recommended that he or she consult a physician first. A basic exercise program should begin with warm-up exercises to increase blood flow and warm the muscles and end with cool-down exercises. A good exercise program includes 30 minutes of activity at 60% to 70% of your maximum heart rate three to five times a week.

4. VO_2 max is a measure of the maximum volume of oxygen one can consume per unit of time. Oxygen consumption is measured by exercising the subject at an increasing pace and workload until fatigue occurs. The oxygen consumed right before total exhaustion is VO_2 max. Each person's VO_2 max is unique and usually improves with exercise training.
5. At low workloads, muscle cells mainly use fat for fuel. For intense exercise of short duration, muscles use phosphocreatine (PCr) for energy. For more sustained intense activity, muscle glycogen breaks down into lactic acid. For endurance exercise, fat and carbohydrate are used as fuels; carbohydrate is used increasingly as activity intensifies. Little protein is used to fuel muscles.
6. Anyone who exercises regularly needs to consume a diet that is moderate to high in carbohydrates and that follows the suggestions of the Guide to Daily Food Choices. Weekend athletes would be well advised to do the same, as the many health benefits experienced add to those from the exercise.
7. Athletes should consume enough fluid to both minimize loss of body weight and ultimately restore pre-exercise weight.

Study Questions

1. How does greater physical fitness contribute to more efficient usage of oxygen? Explain the process.
2. ATP is a continuously supplied fuel source. Describe how ATP is maintained in the muscle, from immediately after initiation of exercise to long distance endurance exercise. Incorporate VO_2 max into your answer.
3. What is the difference between anaerobic versus aerobic exercise? At what point is the switch made from mostly anaerobic to mostly aerobic fuel metabolism? Explain why aerobic metabolism is increased by a regular exercise routine.
4. Based on your knowledge of protein, why is it unnecessary to supplement the diet of an athlete with specific amino acids, often touted as beneficial to exercise? Explain the best way for a 90-kilogram male to receive the recommended amount of protein for muscle building.
5. You are a sports nutrition expert; answer the following questions:
   a. Mr. K is running a 20-kilometer race tomorrow and asks your advice on fluid recommendations for before and during the event. What will you tell him?
   b. An athlete comes to you and asks your advice on a supplement sold in the local sporting goods store that contains specific vitamins, minerals, and amino acids. Will this really help peak his or her performance? What are your recommendations?

REFERENCES

1. Adamson JW, Vaprek DV: Recombination erythropoietin to improve athletic performance, *The New England Journal of Medicine* 324:698, 1991.
2. Astrand P: Physical activity and fitness, *American Journal of Clinical Nutrition* 55:1231S, 1992.
3. Barr S, Costill D: Water: Can the endurance athlete get too much of a good thing? *Journal of The American Dietetics Association* 89:1629, 1989.
4. Blair SW and others: Physical fitness and all-cause mortality, *Journal of the American Medical Association* 262:2395, 1989.
5. Burke L, Read R: Sports Nutrition: approaching the nineties, *Sports Medicine* 8:80, 1989.
6. Clark N: *Nancy Clark's sports nutrition guidebook: eating to fuel your active lifestyle,* Champaign, Ill, 1990, Leisure Press.
7. Costill D: *Inside running: basics of sports physiology,* Indianapolis, 1985, Benchmark Press.
8. Costill D: Carbohydrates for exercise: Dietary demands for optimal performance, *International Journal of Sports Medicine* 9:1, 1988.
9. Council on Scientific Affairs: Medical and nonmedical uses of anabolic-androgenic steroids, *Journal of the American Medical Association* 264:2923, 1990.
10. Hagen RD: Benefits of aerobic conditioning and diet for overweight adults, *Sports Medicine* 5:144, 1988.
11. Hallagan JB and others: Anabolic-androgenic steroid use by athletes, *The New England Journal of Medicine* 321:1042, 1989.
12. Highet R: Athletic amenorrhea: An update on etiology, complications and management, *Sports Medicine* 7:82, 1989.
13. Hoffman CJ, Coleman E: An eating plan and update on recommended dietary practices for the endurance athlete, *Journal of The American Dietetic Association* 91:325, 1991.
14. Hultman E: Nutritional effects on work performance, *American Journal of Clinical Nutrition* 49:949, 1989.
15. Jacobson BH: Effect of amino acids on growth hormone release, *The Physician and Sportsmedicine* 18(1):63, 1990.
16. Kavanagh T, Shephard RJ: Can regular sports participation slow the aging process? Data on Masters athletes, *The Physician and Sportsmedicine* 18(6):94, 1990.

17. Lamb D: *Physiology of exercise: responses and adaptatations,* New York, 1984, MacMillan Press.
18. Lavie CJ and others: Exercise and the heart, *Postgraduate Medicine,* 91:130, 1992.
19. Lindeman AK: Eating and training habits of triathletes: a balancing act, *Journal of The American Dietetic Association* 90:993, 1990.
20. Moses K, Manore NM: Development and testing of a carbohydrate monitoring tool for athletes, *Journal of The American Dietetic Association* 91:962, 1991.
21. National Research Council, Committee on Diet and Health: *Diet and Health,* Washington, D.C., 1989, National Academy Press.
22. Nieman David C: *Fitness and sports medicine: an introduction,* Palo Alto, Calif, 1990, Bull Publishing Company.
23. Paul G: Dietary protein requirements of physically active individuals, *Sports Medicine* 8:154, 1989.
24. Sherman M, Lamb D: Nutrition and prolonged exercise. In Lamb D, Murray R, editors: *Perspectives in exercise science and sports medicine: prolonged exercise,* Indianapolis, 1988, Benchmark Press.
25. Sherman WM and others: Carbohydrate feedings 1 h before exercise improves exercise performance, *American Journal of Clinical Nutrition* 54:866, 1991.
26. Shroyer JA: Getting tough on anabolic steroids: can we win the battle, *The Physician and Sportsmedicine* 18(2):106, 1990.
27. Stryer L: *Biochemistry,* ed 3, New York, 1988, WH Freeman.
28. Williams MH: Nutritional ergogenic aids and athletic performance, *Nutrition Today,* Jan/Feb 1989, p 7.

SUGGESTED READINGS

Paul reviews the question of protein needs for athletes. The article contains ample support for the recommendation that athletes should spend more time worrying about carbohydrate intake than protein intake. Williams reviews the use of ergogenic substances to enhance performance. Together with the Expert Opinion by Lamb, this article provides a detailed examination of this topic. The article by Hallagan and others reviews anabolic steroid use from a physician's standpoint. The information should cause an athlete to step back and carefully weigh the consequences of steroid use. Finally, Clark provides a practical approach to planning diets for athletes in her book. She is an experienced nutrition counselor, and the many helpful hints she gives reflects her varied experiences.

TAKE ACTION

Are you measuring up to the numbers?

In this chapter several key nutrients were highlighted in our discussion of exercise performance. Some of the guidelines mentioned (which aren't only guidelines for athletes, but those for maintaining general good fitness) were as follows:

- *eat a moderate to high amount of carbohydrates (55% of total kcalories)*
- *athletes should eat a minimum of 1 gram of protein per kilogram body weight*
- *consume the RDA for vitamins and minerals*
- *make sure iron and calcium intake is at RDA levels, especially in women*

Review the results of the dietary assessment you completed in Chapter 2. Remember that you assessed 1 day's food intake. Now answer the following questions (even if you are not an athlete):

1. What percentage of your kcalories were from carbohydrate? Was your intake 55% of your total kcalories or greater?

____

2. Were you eating at least 0.8 grams of protein per kilogram body weight? If you are an athlete are you getting about 1 gram per kilogram body weight?

____

3. Did you consume at least the RDA for all vitamins and minerals assessed? For which ones were you below the RDA?

____

____

4. Were you consuming the RDA for iron and calcium?

____

5. What can you do to improve your dietary intake to promote general fitness, and if you are an athlete, to promote maximum performance in your chosen event(s)?

____

____

NUTRITION PERSPECTIVE

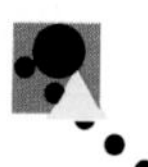

Sports Drinks: Are They Necessary?

A question that often arises is whether to drink water or a sports-type carbohydrate-electrolyte drink, like Bodyfuel, Exceed, Gatorade, or 10-K, during competition. For sports that require less than 30 minutes of exertion, replacing the water lost in sweat is the primary concern because losses of body carbohydrate stores and electrolytes (sodium, chloride, potassium, and other minerals) are not usually too great in such activities. Electrolytes are lost in sweat, but the quantities lost in exercise of brief to moderate duration can be easily replaced later by consuming normal foods, such as orange juice, potatoes, or tomato juice.

Water is certainly cheaper than a sports drink. But sports-type drinks can taste better than water, which may make one drink more often—a clear benefit for fluid replenishment. In addition, the carbohydrate in these drinks quickly replace carbohydrate used up during practice or competition. The sodium present also aids glucose absorption.

For endurance athletes (i.e., those whose sports demand exertion for longer than 30 minutes) the discussion of sports drinks becomes more critical. Beverages for the endurance athlete must provide water for hydration, electrolytes to both enhance water and glucose absorption from the intestine and to help retain blood volume, and carbohydrate to provide energy.[25] Beyond 60 to 90 minutes of exercise, electrolyte replacement becomes increasingly important.

Prolonged exercise results in large sweat losses, and some of the fluid for sweating comes from the bloodstream. If plain water is used to replace the fluid losses in the blood, the concentration of essential electrolytes in the bloodstream may become too diluted. This makes it important to include small amounts of sodium and potassium in a sports drink to help maintain blood volume.

Including carbohydrates in sports drinks also has been found to delay fatigue in endurance exercise.[25] In exercise at intensities of a 3-hour marathon pace, ingesting carbohydrate improves endurance, presumably by either preventing great drops in blood glucose levels or by providing an outside source of glucose for muscle use.

The amount of carbohydrate recommended for consumption about 15 minutes before endurance exercise is 1 to 2 cups of a 10% to 20% solution of carbohydrate (10 to 20 grams of carbohydrate per 100 milliliters of water), such as GatorLode or Exceed High Carbohydrate Source. Once exercise begins, ½ to 1 cup of a 5% to 8% carbohydrate solution (5 to 8 grams per 100 milliliters of fluid) should be consumed every 15 to 20 minutes. This is the carbohydrate concentration of typical sports drinks (check the label to be sure).

glucose polymers Carbohydrate sources used in some sports drinks that consist of grouping of a few glucose molecules together.

Some beverage labels mention **glucose polymers** (glucoses linked together in short chains). Solutions containing glucose polymers were initially thought to empty from the stomach faster than solutions containing glucose. We now know that there's little difference in stomach emptying times between sports drinks containing glucose polymers and those containing simple sugars such as glucose or sucrose. Furthermore, comparisons of drinks containing glucose polymers (more properly known as maltodextrins), glucose, or sucrose show that all of these carbohydrates have similar positive effects on exercise performance and physiological function as long as the concentrations of carbohydrate are in the 5% to 8% range. The exception to this rule is drinks whose only carbohydrate source is fructose. Fructose is absorbed from the intestine more slowly than glucose and often causes bloating or diarrhea.

Overall then the decision to use a sports drink hinges primarily on the duration of the activity. As the duration of continuous activity begins to total 30 minutes or longer, the advantages from use of a sports drink over plain water begin to emerge.

CHAPTER ELEVEN

Anorexia Nervosa and Bulimia

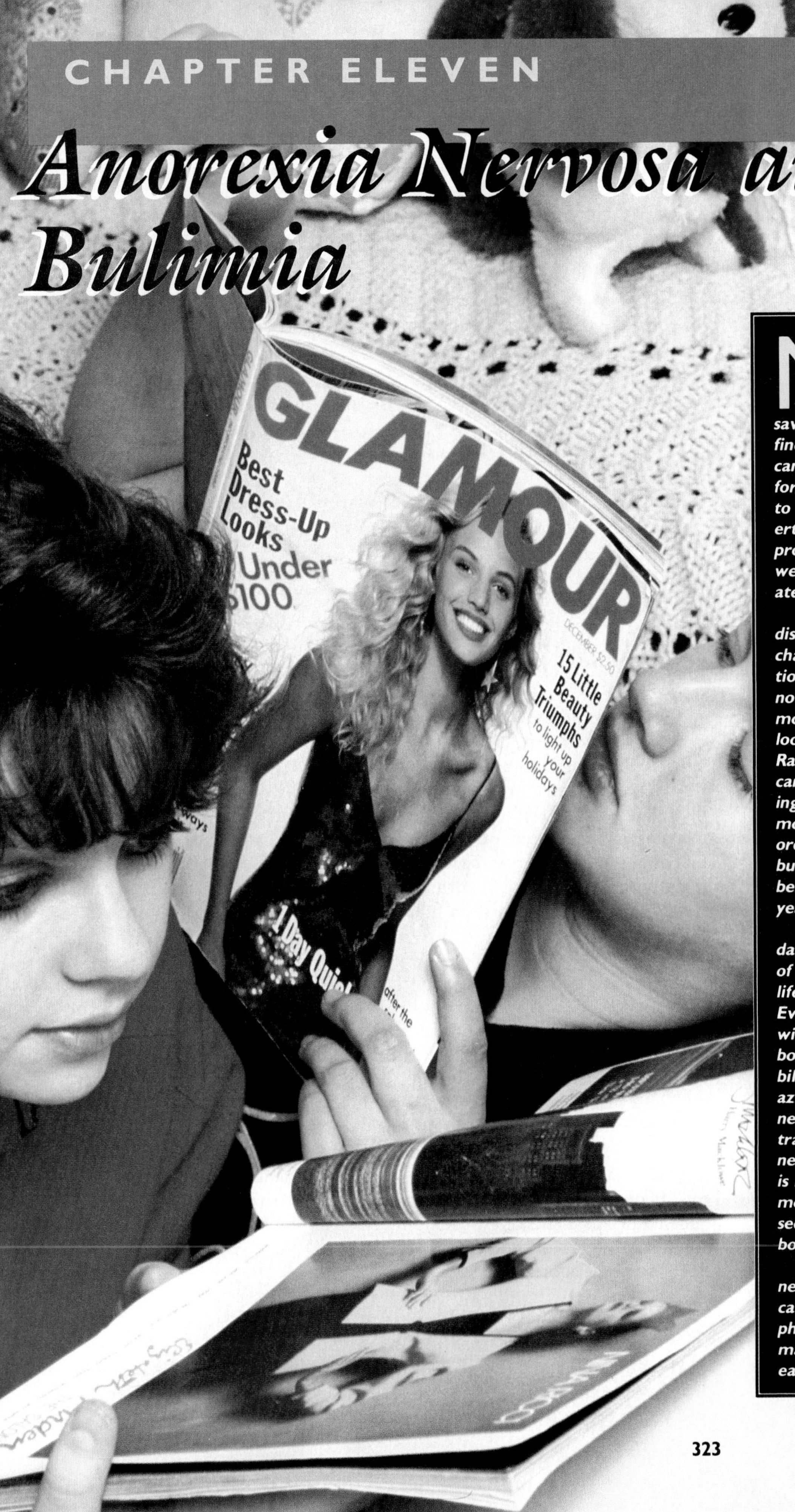

Most of us occasionally eat until we're stuffed and uncomfortable. Faced with savory and tempting foods, we find that they taste so good we can't stop eating. Usually we forgive ourselves, vowing not to overeat the next time. Nevertheless, many of us have problems controlling our weight, and it is usually associated with overeating.

In stark contrast, the eating disorders we explore in this chapter involve severe distortions of the eating process. It is not dieting for a week on mostly grapefruits in order to look good in a bathing suit. Rather, these eating disorders can develop into life-threatening conditions.[9] And what's most alarming about these disorders, anorexia nervosa and bulimia, is the increasing number of cases reported each year.

We live in a society of abundant food, and although some of us regularly exercise, our lifestyles are fairly sedentary. Everyday we are bombarded with images of the "ideal" body. Television programs, billboard advertisements, magazine pictures, movies, and newspapers tell us that an ultra-slim body will bring happiness, love, and even success. It is hard not to compare the media images with our own, seemingly less than perfect, bodies.

Some people are quite vulnerable to these messages, because of both psychological and physical reasons. These people may be more likely to develop eating disorders.[17]

NUTRITION AWARENESS INVENTORY

Here are 15 statements about eating disorders. Read them to test your current knowledge. If you think the statement is true or mostly true, circle T. If you think the statement is false or mostly false, circle F. Use the scoring key at the end of the book to compute your total score. Take this test again after you have read the chapter. Compare the results.

1. T F Human societies deal irrationally with food.
2. T F Eating disorders are widespread in Western society.
3. T F People with anorexia nervosa have an intense fear of losing weight.
4. T F Bulimic people often induce vomiting to control their weight.
5. T F People with anorexia nervosa are often overachievers.
6. T F People with anorexia nervosa have a distorted view of their own bodies.
7. T F People with bulimia are aware that their eating patterns are abnormal.
8. T F People with bulimia are easy to identify because of their openness about their problem.
9. T F American society favors the lean and angular look.
10. T F The real problem underlying eating disorders is how people feel about themselves.
11. T F People with eating disorders are often perfectionists.
12. T F Eating disorders are easier to treat at early stages.
13. T F Bingeing is characteristic of bulimia.
14. T F Treatment of bulimia emphasizes the immediate return to a strict diet.
15. T F Baryopobia is a new eating disorder found in children.

We All Need to Eat

Eating—a completely instinctive behavior for animals—serves an extraordinary number of psychological, social, and cultural purposes for humans. We already mentioned in Chapter 1 that eating practices may take on religious meanings; identify bonds among cultural, ethnic, and family groups; and be a means of expressing hostility, affection, prestige, and class values. Similarly, providing, preparing, and distributing food may be a means of expressing love or hatred, or even power in family relationships. Given these possibilities, it is not surprising that some eating behaviors take on unusual and strange rituals, progressing from (1) normal responses to hunger and satiety cues through (2) obsessive weight loss to (3) a full-blown eating disorder.

Progression for eating habits—from ordered to disordered

Attention to hunger and satiety signals
Limitation of energy intake to restore weight to a healthful level
↓
Some "disordered" eating habits begin as weight loss is attempted
↓
Clinically evident eating disorder can be recognized

FOOD CAN REPRESENT MUCH MORE THAN NUTRIENTS

From birth we link food with personal emotional experiences. An infant associates milk with security and warmth, and so the bottle or breast becomes a source of comfort as well as food. We are further exposed to the use of foods as rewards. Here are some typical statements heard at the dinner table:

"You can't play until you clean up your plate."
"I'll eat the broccoli if you let me watch TV."
"If you love me, you'll eat what I fixed for dinner."

On the surface, this practice appears harmless enough, but, eventually, both caregivers and children can build behavior patterns that use foods to achieve unstated goals. Food, then, can take on a much larger role. At the extreme—when food is regularly used as a tool of expression rather than simply as a source of nutrients—it can contribute to disordered eating patterns. At their worst, these patterns form the links to later anorexia nervosa.

anorexia nervosa An eating disorder involving a psychological loss of appetite and self-starvation, resulting in part from a distorted body image and various social pressures associated with puberty.

bulimia An eating disorder in which large quantities of food are eaten at one time (bingeing) and then purged from the body by vomiting, use of laxatives, or other means.

Two Common Types of Eating Disorders

Anorexia nervosa and **bulimia** (sometimes called bulimia nervosa) have been written about for centuries, at least as far back as the Middle Ages. Anorexia nervosa is characterized by extreme weight loss, poor and distorted body image, and an irrational, almost morbid, fear of obesity and weight gain. The term anorexia alone implies a loss of appetitie, which may be a side affect of certain diseases or varied medical treatments. Denying one's appetite more accurately describes anorexia nervosa. By rough estimate, approximately 1 of every 100 (1%) girls between the ages of 12 and 18 years suffers from anorexia nervosa.[10] It occurs less commonly among adults. And fewer men are affected, partly because the ideal image for men is big and bulky. Men in weight-control sports, such as wrestling or judo may practice bulimia,[28] but poor self-esteem and other psychological problems don't seem to be the cause of this behavior. Most of these athletes dehydrate themselves and vomit so that they can compete in lower weight classes. On the other hand, people with anorexia nervosa typically see themselves as fat even though they are extremely thin.

Models, ballet dancers, and gymnasts are groups of people with long-standing histories of disordered eating patterns and anorexia nervosa. Earning their living often depends on maintaining ultra-slim bodies.

Bulimia means "ox hunger," or being as hungry as an ox.[12] It is characterized by episodes of bingeing followed by attempts to purge the food from the body, usually by vomiting, fasting, taking diuretics, or using laxatives. People with this disorder may be difficult to identify because they keep their binge-purge behaviors secret and their symptoms are not obvious. Researchers think that approximately 2% to 8% of adolescent and college-age women suffer from this disorder. A growing number of male athletes also report these practices,[7] especially swimmers, wrestlers, and track participants. "Get thin and win" is a slogan heard around gyms.[28]

The Diagnostic and Statistical Manual of Mental Disorders (DSM III-R) of the American Psychiatric Assocaition lists specific criteria for diagnosing these disorders (Table 11-1).[21] Anorexia nervosa and bulimia overlap considerably, such that a

Table 11-1 Diagnostic criteria for anorexia nervosa and bulimia nervosa

Anorexia nervosa	Bulimia nervosa
A) Refusal to maintain body weight over a minimal normal weight for age and height, for example, weight loss leading to maintenance of body weight 15% below that expected; or failure to make expected weight gain during period of growth, leading to body weight 15% below that expected.	A) Recurrent episodes of binge eating (rapid consumption of a large amount of food in a discrete period of time).
B) Intense fear of gaining weight or becoming fat, even though underweight.	B) A feeling of lack of control over eating behavior during the eating binges.
C) Disturbance in the way in which one's body weight, size or shape is experienced. The person claims to "feel fat" even when emaciated, believes that one area of the body is "too fat" even when obviously underweight.	C) The person regularly engages in either self-induced vomiting, use of laxatives or diuretics, strict dieting or fasting, or vigorous exercise to prevent weight gain.
D) In females, absence of at least three consecutive menstrual cycles when otherwise expected to occur (primary or secondary amenorrhea). (A woman is considered to have amenorrhea if her periods occur only following hormone administration, such as estrogen.)	D) A minimum average of two binge eating episodes a week for at least 3 months.
	E) Persistent overconcern with body shape and weight.

From Diagnostic and Statistical Manual for Mental Disorders, DSM III-R.

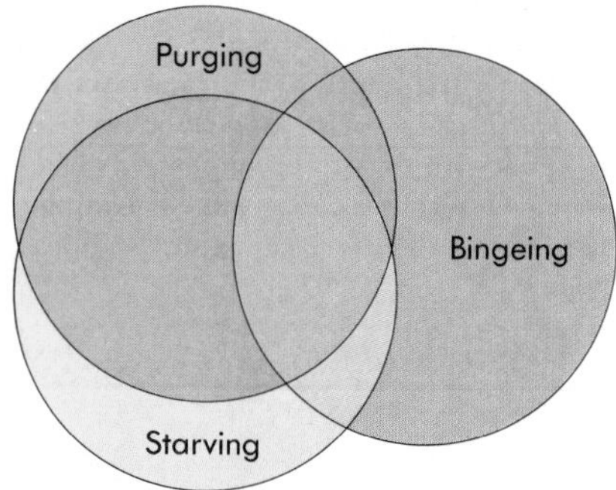

Figure 11-1 The overlap of eating disorders. A combination of binge eating, purging, and/or starving can be found in both anorexia nervosa and bulimia.

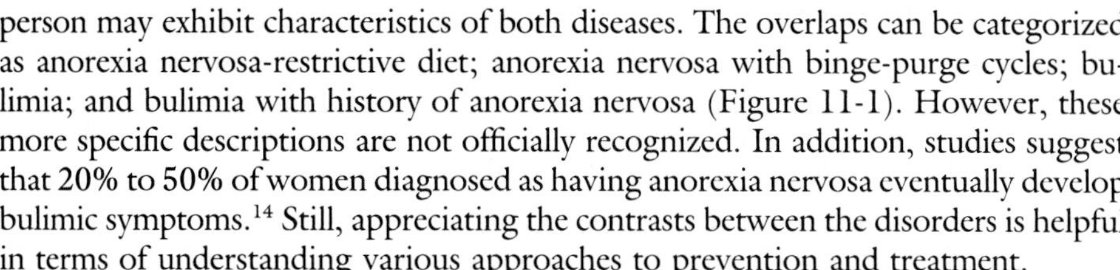

person may exhibit characteristics of both diseases. The overlaps can be categorized as anorexia nervosa-restrictive diet; anorexia nervosa with binge-purge cycles; bulimia; and bulimia with history of anorexia nervosa (Figure 11-1). However, these more specific descriptions are not officially recognized. In addition, studies suggest that 20% to 50% of women diagnosed as having anorexia nervosa eventually develop bulimic symptoms.[14] Still, appreciating the contrasts between the disorders is helpful in terms of understanding various approaches to prevention and treatment.

Table 11-2 lists some characteristics of people with anorexia nervosa and bulimia. Do you know someone who is at risk? If so, a professional diagnosis, coupled with professional help, is needed. The sooner help begins the better.[20] The first step is to rule out other diseases, such as cancer, gastrointestinal disease, schizophrenia, and depression. If an eating disorder is diagnosed, the person should consider immediate treatment. The best a friend can do is to lead the person to treatment. Professional help is often available at student health centers and student guidance/counseling facilities on college campuses. We need to be cautious of "diagnosing" eating disorders in friends and family members. A number of diagnostic criteria must be met before this is possible, and only a professional is equipped to do so.

There are no simple causes or solutions to eating disorders. They are rooted in multiple causes—biological,[30] psychological, and social—that are eventually manifested partly through disordered eating.[17] Stress especially may have a strong role in the development of eating disorders. An underlying commonality seems to be the lack of appropriate coping mechanisms as individuals begin to reach adolescence and young adulthood (Figure 11-2).

In the Nutrition Perspective we review some sociological aspects of eating disorders. From that perspective you might develop further insights on why the disorders develop and how some people are more susceptible than others.

Table 11-2 Some characteristics of eating disorders. These can be used as a tool for group discussion to help people discover their risks. Having some of these characteristics does not diagnose the disease but should cause a person to reflect on their eating habits and related concerns.

Characteristics of anorexia nervosa	Characteristics of bulimia
• Rigid dieting causing dramatic weight loss	• Secretive binge eating; never overeating in front of others
• False body perception—thinking "I'm too fat," even when emaciated; relentless pursuit of thinness	• Eating when depressed or under stress
• Rituals involving food, excessive exercise, and other aspects of life	• Bingeing followed by fasting, laxative abuse, self-induced vomiting, or excessive exercise
• Maintenance of rigid control in lifestyle; security found in control and order	• Shame, embarrassment, deceit, and depression; low self-esteem and guilt (especially after a binge)
• Feeling of panic after a small weight gain; intense fear of gaining weight	• Fluctuating weight resulting from alternate bingeing and fasting (± 10 lbs or 5 kg)
• Feelings of purity, power, and superiority through maintenance of strict discipline and self-denial	• Loss of control; fear of not being able to stop eating
• Preoccupation with food, its preparation, and observing another person eat	• Perfectionism, "people pleaser"; food is the only comfort/escape in an otherwise carefully controlled and regulated life
• Helplessness in the presence of food	• Erosion of teeth, swollen glands
• Lack of menses after what should be the age of puberty	• Purchase of syrup of ipecac

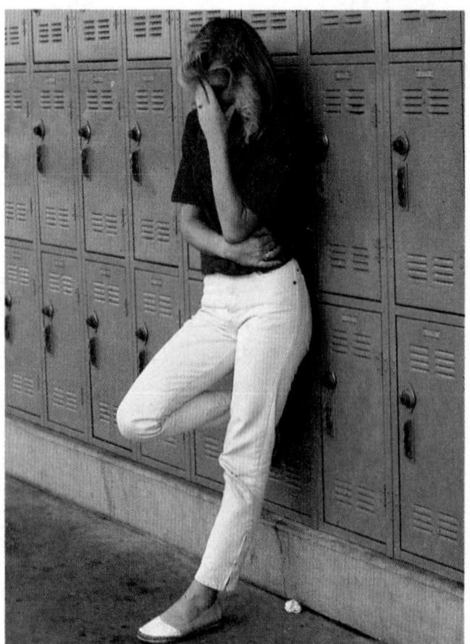

Figure 11-2 The stress of crossing from childhood into adulthood may trigger anorexia nervosa.

Anorexia Nervosa

Anorexia nervosa evolves from a dangerous mental state to an extremely dangerous physical condition. People suffering from this disorder think they are fat and intensely fear obesity and weight gain. They lose much more weight than is healthy. Recent studies indicate that 3% to 8% of people with anorexia die prematurely—from suicide, heart ailments, and infections.[23] About half of those who survive it recover within 6 years; the rest simply exist with the disease. The longer one suffers from anorexia nervosa, the poorer the chances for complete recovery. A young patient with a short episode and a cooperative family has a better outlook. Prompt and vigorous treatment with close follow-up improves the chances.[9]

Anorexia may begin as a simple attempt to lose weight. A comment from a well-meaning friend or relative suggesting that the person seems to be gaining weight or is too fat may be all that is needed. The stress of having to maintain a certain weight to look attractive or competent on a job can set off a problem. Physical changes associated with puberty, the stress of leaving childhood, or losing a friend may also trigger extreme dieting (Figure 11-3). Leaving home for boarding school or college or starting a job can reinforce the desire to make oneself more "socially acceptable." Still, looking "good" does not necessarily help a person deal with anger, depression, low self-esteem, or past experiences with sexual abuse. If these issues are pushing the disorder and are not resolved as weight is lost, the individual may intensify efforts to lose weight "to look even better" rather than working through unresolved psychological concerns.

A person with anorexia nervosa may use the disorder to gain attention from the family, sometimes in hopes of holding the family together.

All in all, adolescence is a period of turbulent sexual and social tensions. Teenagers seek—and are often expected—to establish separate and independent lives. While declaring independence they seek acceptance and support from peers and parents, and react intensely to how they think others perceive them.[9] At the same time, their bodies are changing, much of it beyond their control. Adolescents often lack appropriate coping mechanisms for the stress of teen years. The attempt to take charge of their lives sometimes results in exercising extreme control over the body. Genetic factors also appear to play a role in anorexia nervosa; usually both identical twins—rather than only one—develop the disorder.[10]

Once dieting begins, a person developing anorexia nervosa does not stop. The results are long periods of semistarvation practiced rigidly, almost with a vengeance, in a relentless pursuit of thinness.[23] Anorexia may eventually lead to bingeing on large amounts of food in a short time, then purging. Purging occurs primarily through vomiting, but laxatives, diuretics, fasting, and exercise are also used. Thus a person with anorexia nervosa may exist in a state of semistarvation, or may alternate periods of starvation with periods of bingeing and purging.[4]

PROFILE OF A PERSON WITH ANOREXIA NERVOSA

A person with anorexia nervosa refuses to eat. That behavior is the hallmark of the disease, whether or not other practices such as binge-purge cycles, appear. The person is usually a girl from the middle or upper socioeconomic class. Perhaps her mother also has distorted views of a desirable body shape and acceptable food habits. The girl is often described by parents and teachers as "the best little girl in the world." She is competitive and often obsessive.[4] Her parents set high standards for her. At home, she may not allow clutter in her bedroom. Physicians note that after a physical examination, she may fold her examination gown very carefully and clean up the examination room before leaving. Even though such behaviors may be apparent, it takes a skilled professional to tell the difference between anorexia nervosa and other common adolescent complaints, such as delayed puberty, fatigue, and depression.[9]

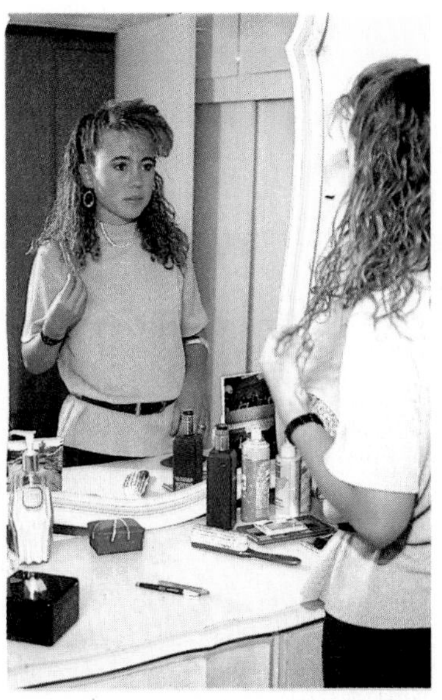

Figure 11-3 Self-image can be ever-changing. For those with eating disorders, the difference between the real and desired body image may be too difficult to accept.

A common thread underlying many, but not all, cases of anorexia nervosa is conflict within the family structure, especially rooted in an overbearing mother.[16,22] When family expectations are always too high, resulting frustration leads to fighting. Overinvolvement, rigidity, overprotection, and denial also typically appear in the daily transactions of such families.[9] Often the eating disorder allows the person to exercise control over an otherwise powerless existence. Consider the parents who do not believe their teenager mature enough to make decisions. She disagrees, and if the situation is very tense, may turn to purging or starving as a way to show her power. "You may try to control my life, but I can do anything I want with my body."

In the words of one young woman: "I couldn't get angry, because it would be like destroying someone else, like Mother. It felt like she would hate me forever. I got angry through anorexia nervosa. It was my last hope. It's my own body and this was my last ditch effort."

EARLY WARNING SIGNS

A person developing anorexia nervosa will exhibit important warning signs. At first, dieting becomes the life focus.[20] The person may feel, "The only thing I am good at is dieting. I can't do anything else." This innocent beginning often leads to very abnormal eating habits, such as cutting a pea in half before eating it. An anorectic woman may cook a large meal and watch others eat it but refuse to eat any herself. As the disease progresses, she narrows her own food choices considerably. For someone developing anorexia nervosa these practices say "I am in control." The anorectic person may be hungry but denies it. She is driven by the belief that good things will happen for her if she just becomes thin enough. It becomes a question of willpower.

Soon the anorectic person becomes irritable and hostile and begins to withdraw from family and friends. School performance generally crumbles. The person refuses to eat out with family and friends, thinking, "I won't be able to have the foods I want to eat," or "I won't be able to throw up afterward." The person also tends to be excessively critical of herself and others. Nothing is good enough. Because it cannot be perfect, life appears meaningless and hopeless. A sense of joylessness colors everything.

As stress increases in an anorectic person's life, sleep disturbances and depression are common. For a female these problems, coupled with low body weight and diminished fat stores, can cause menstrual periods to stop.[7] This may be the first sign of the disease a mother notices. Parents, teachers, friends, and coaches need to be aware of the early warning signs of anorexia nervosa. As we stated earlier, this disease is much easier to treat when caught at an early stage. If not treated right away, it quickly leads to self-destruction.

NUTRITION FOCUS

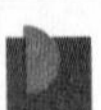

Anorexia Nervosa: A Case Study

At fifteen Alma had been healthy and well-developed, had menstruated at age 12, was 5 feet 6 inches tall, and weighed 120 pounds. At that time her mother urged her to change to a school with higher academic standing, a change she resisted. Her father suggested that she should watch her weight, an idea that she took up with great eagerness, and she began a rigid diet. She lost rapidly and her menses ceased. That she could be thin gave her a sense of pride, power, and accomplishment. She also began a frantic exercise program, would swim by the mile, play tennis for hours, or do calisthenics to the point of exhaustion. Whatever low point her weight reached, Alma feared that she might become too fat if she regained as little as an ounce.

At age 20 when she came for consultation, she looked like a walking skeleton, scantily dressed in shorts and a halter top, with her legs sticking out like broomsticks, every rib showing, and her shoulder blades standing up like little wings. Alma insisted that she looked fine and that there was nothing wrong with being so skinny.

From Brunch H: *The golden cage: the enigma of anorexia nervosa,* Cambridge, Mass, 1978, Harvard Univ Press.

Ultimately, an anorectic person eats very little food; 300 to 600 kcalories daily is not unusual. In place of food the person may consume up to 20 cans of diet soft drinks each day. Once a person loses more than 15% of normal body weight, there is a great risk for life-time suffering of anorexia nervosa. After losing more than 25% of body weight, a cure becomes very difficult, hospitalization is almost always necessary, and premature death is more likely.[6]

PHYSICAL SIGNS AND SYMPTOMS

Rooted in the emotional state of the victim, anorexia nervosa produces profound physical effects. A typical medical description reveals a reluctant young woman and a frantic family.[9] The anorectic person is often 20% to 40% below desirable body weight and appears to be skin and bones. This state of semistarvation disturbs many body systems as it forces the body to conserve as much energy as possible. Hormonal responses to semistarvation then can cause an array of predictable effects:[6]

- Lowered body temperature due to a loss of fat insulation and slower basal metabolism, the latter caused by decreased synthesis of active thyroid hormone and loss of lean body mass.[5]
- Decreased heart rate as metabolism slows, leading to easy fatigue, easy fainting, and an overwhelming need for sleep.
- Iron-deficiency anemia from poor nutrient intake, which leads to further weakness.
- Rough, dry, scaly, and cold skin from a poor nutrient intake and anemia.
- Low white blood cell count due to a poor nutrient intake, especially protein and zinc. This condition increases the risk of infection, a cause of death in some anorectic people.
- Loss of hair caused by a poor nutrient intake.
- Appearance of **lanugo,** downy (fine) hairs on the body that trap air, insulating against heat loss and replacing some insulation lost with the fat layer.
- Constipation from semistarvation and laxative abuse.
- Low blood potassium (hypokalemia) because of a poor nutrient intake, possibly vomiting, and the use of some types of diuretics. This increases the risk of heart rhythm disturbances, another leading cause of death in anorectic people.
- Loss of menstrual periods because of low body weight, low fat content, and the stress of the disease. Periods cease when body weight drops to around 100 pounds or less. Accompanying hormonal changes cause a loss of bone mass and increase the risk of osteoporosis (see Chapter 14).
- Eventual deterioration of teeth due to frequent vomiting. Poor dental health and loss of bone mass can be lasting signs of the disease, even if the other physical and mental problems are resolved.
- Poor outcome of pregnancy, such as poor fetal growth and development, especially if a woman begins pregnancy in an anorectic state.

A person with anorexia nervosa is psychologically and physically ill and needs help.

lanugo Fine, textured, soft hair that appears after a person has lost much body fat due to semistarvation. The hair stands erect and traps air, acting as insulation to the body to replace the insulation usually supplied by body fat.

CONCEPT CHECK

Anorexia nervosa is an eating disorder characterized by semistarvation. It is found primarily, but not exclusively, in adolescent girls, starting at or around puberty. An anorectic person dwindles essentially to "skin and bones," but often thinks he or she is fat. Semistarvation produces hormonal and other changes that can lower body temperature, slow the heart rate, decrease immune response, stop menstrual periods, and contribute to hair loss. It is a very serious disease that often produces lifelong consequences. It can end with premature death.

TREATMENT OF ANOREXIA NERVOSA

Anorectic persons often sink into shells of isolation and fear. They deny that a problem exists. Frequently, friends and family members meet in a group with the person to confront the problem in a loving way. They present evidence of the problem and encourage entrance into treatment immediately. Treatment then should include a team of physicians, registered dietitians, psychologists, and other health professionals working together. Often the ideal setting is an inpatient eating disorders clinic in a medical center,[20] as this location can take the person away from many environment influences that encourage the disorder.

Once the medical team has gained the cooperation of the anorectic person, they work together to restore a sense of balance, purpose, and future. As we said, anorexia nervosa usually is rooted in psychological conflict. However, a person who has been barely existing in a state of semistarvation can not focus on much besides food. A psychiatrist can not counsel a starving person. Dreams and even morbid thoughts about food will interfere with therapy until sufficient weight is regained.

Nutrition Therapy

The first goal of therapy then must be increasing the person's food intake. Enough weight must be gained to raise the basal metabolism to normal and to reverse as many physical signs of the disease as possible. Food intake is designed to first minimize or stop any further weight loss. Then the focus shifts to restoring regular food habits. After this is accomplished, the expectation can be switched to slow weight gain, from 1 to 4 pounds (0.5 to 2 kilograms) each week until weight exceeds 90% of preillness weight. A starting point for energy intake can be set by the Harris-Benedict equation or the Boothby and Berkson Food Nomogram (see Appendix J). Once weight maintenance is established, a reasonable goal would be a weekly increase of 200 kcalories as treatment progresses. Weight gain is not the sole goal of treatment but rather a prelude to fuller engagement in psychological issues.[22] The medical team should stress that patients will not be abandoned after they gain weight.

One critical goal at early stages of treatment is to allow the person a feeling of control over his or her life.[4] Only when the patient knows exactly what to expect can this be achieved. Unanticipated weight gain at this stage of treatment—even when caused by fluctuating menstrual fluids after periods resume—can easily set up a feeling of being completely out of control.

Experienced professional help is the key. An anorectic person may be on the verge of suicide and near starvation. Today suicide is the most common cause of death in these people.[23] In addition, anorectic people are often very clever and resistant. They may try to hide weight loss by wearing many layers of clothes, putting coins in their pockets, and drinking numerous glasses of water. Also, health professionals should measure and compare weight for height to standards—not merely rely on sight—because our assessments of "thin" are distorted by the very thin models in advertisements.

Psychological Therapy

Once the physical problems are addressed, the therapist should try to determine how dieting became such a dominant force, knowing that it usually signals a deeper emotional illness.[20] To heal, the anorectic person must reject the sense of accomplishment associated with an emaciated body. If therapists can discover reasons for the disorder, they can develop strategies to restore normal weight and eating habits by resolving psychological conflicts.

A key aspect of psychological treatment is showing the person how to regain control of some facets of his or her life and how to cope with tough situations. Therapists work to help people accept setbacks, and to regard these setbacks as opportunities to learn more about themselves rather than as sources of depression and frustration. Counselors can also provide background literature to clarify the issues of the disease and to encourage greater participation in the treatment. Furthermore, the counselor can lead the individual to focus on positive health goals, such as consuming more potassium, dietary fiber, and calcium. As eating evolves into a normal routine, the person can turn to previously neglected activities.

Family therapy is important in treating anorexia nervosa.[4] It focuses on the role of the illness among family members, how individual family members react, and how their behavior might unknowingly contribute to the abnormal eating patterns. Therapy involves all family members relevant to the behavior problem. Frequently, a therapist finds family struggles at the heart of the problem. As the disorder resolves, the person has to relate to family members in new ways in order to gain the attention previously tied to the disease.[20] The family needs to help the young person ease into adulthood and to accept its responsibilities as well as its advantages.

Self-help groups for anorectic and bulimic people, as well as their families and friends, represent nonthreatening first steps into treatment. Individuals also can attend meetings to get a sense of whether they really do have an eating disorder problem.

With professional help, many people with anorexia nervosa can again lead normal lives. They then do not have to depend on unusual eating habits to cope with daily problems. As a young woman recovering from anorexia nervosa said, "I have lost a specialness that I thought it gave me. I was different from everyone else. Now I know that I'm somebody who's overcome it, which not everybody does." Although they are not totally cured, they do recover a sense of normalcy in their lives. There are no set answers or approaches; each case is different.[9] There is also no specific pharmacological agent used to treat anorexia nervosa. Increasing intake of food is considered the drug of choice. Medications used typically depend on the physician's preference and the patient. Tranylcypromine sulfate (Parnate), imipramine (Tofranil), amitriptyline (Elavil), desipramine (Norpramin), and lithium carbonate (Lithane) are useful mainly when depression accompanies the disorder. Chlorpromazine (Thorazine) has been shown to decrease anxiety about eating.[29]

Still, establishing a strong relationship with either a therapist or another supportive person is a key to recovery.[20] The anorectic person needs to feel understood and accepted by another person, then he or she can begin to build a sense of self and exercise some autonomy.

CONCEPT CHECK

Treatment of anorexia nervosa first requires a person to be brought back from a semistarvation state. Once weight gain allows normal basal metabolism to be maintained, psychotherapy can begin to uncover the causes of the disease and to help the person develop skills needed to return to a healthy life. Family therapy is an important component in the many stages of treatment for the person recovering from anorexia nervosa.

Bulimia

One of your best friends may practice bulimia without your knowledge. The person may feel desperate, yet will go to great lengths to keep it secret. This eating disorder involves episodes of bingeing followed by attempts to purge the food. College-age students practice it most commonly.[27] Susceptible people may have both biological factors and lifestyle patterns that predispose them to becoming overweight. As teenagers, these people probably tried many weight-reduction diets. Now as young adults their fear of gaining weight is overwhelmed by periods of real hunger.

Like people with anorexia nervosa, those with bulimia are usually female and successful. They are usually at or slightly above a normal weight. Females with bulimia are more likely to be sexually active than those with anorexia nervosa, and are usually somewhat older. The person with bulimia may think of food constantly.

Men, especially athletes, are increasingly likely targets of bulimia as they attempt to maintain a certain weight.

The major difference from anorectics is that the bulimic person turns to food during a crisis or problem, not away from it. Also, unlike those with anorexia nervosa, people practicing bulimia know their behavior is abnormal.[20] These people often have very low self-esteem and are depressed. The world sees their competence, while inside they feel out of control, ashamed, and frustrated.

Bulimic people tend to be impulsive. It has been suggested that part of the problem may actually arise from an inability to control responses to impulse and desire.[13] Some studies have demonstrated that bulimic people tend to come from "disengaged" families, ones that are loosely organized. Roles for family members are not clearly defined. Too little protection is given for family members and rules are very loose. This is in contrast to anorectic people who come from "engaged" families where roles are too well defined.

Pinpointing the number of people who practice bulimia is difficult if the strictest medical guidelines are followed. These guidelines specify that to be diagnosed as bulimic a person must vomit at least twice a week for 3 months. Approximately 2% to 8% of college-age women fit this description.[7] However, many people with bulimia lead secret lives. There is often really no way to tell just by looking that someone has this disorder. Usually it is practiced in isolation. Estimates of cases come largely from self-report and may therefore be unreliable. The problem, especially of milder cases, may be much more widespread than we think.

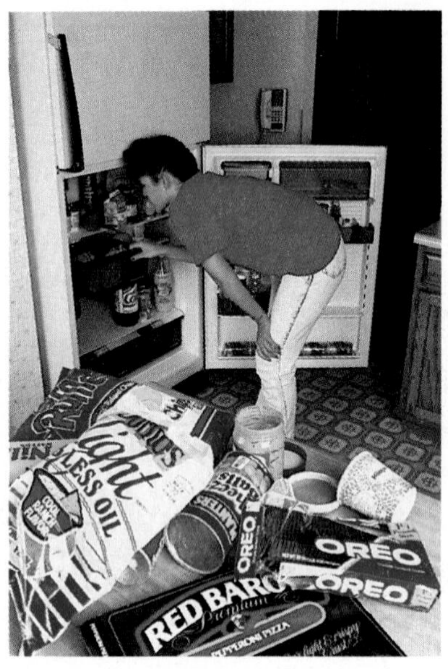

Figure 11-4 The binge-purge cycle. It can lead to a sense of helplessness.

Among sufferers of bulimia, binges often alternate with attempts to rigidly restrict food intake. Elaborate "food rules" are common. One frequently encountered rule is to avoid eating sweets. Thus, if even one cookie or donut is consumed, the person may feel that he or she has broken a "rule" and must "get rid of" the objectionable food. Usually this leads to further overeating, both because it is easier to regurgitate a large amount of food than a small amount, and because "having blown it," a decision is made to "go all the way" and start over tomorrow.

Binge-purge cycles may be practiced daily, weekly, or at other intervals.[11] A special time is often set aside. Most bingeing occurs at night when other people are less likely to interrupt, and usually lasts from 30 minutes to 2 hours. A binge can be triggered by a combination of stress, boredom, loneliness, and depression. It often follows a period of strict dieting, and so can be linked to intense hunger. The binge is not at all like normal eating and, once begun, seems to propel itself. The person loses control. Bulimic people often report that they do not taste or enjoy the food once the binge has started (Figure 11-4).

Foods chosen for a binge are usually convenience foods—cakes, cookies, pies, ice cream, donuts, and pastries. As much as 20,000 or more kcalories might be eaten in a binge.[7] Purging follows in hopes that weight gain will be blunted. Vomiting, laxatives, fasting, and exercise are possible approaches. But even when vomiting follows the binge very quickly, 20% to 33% of the kcalories taken in are still absorbed. Even more kcalories are absorbed when laxatives are used for purging. And essentially all the kcalories are absorbed when the other purging methods are used. People are mistaken in thinking that there will be no caloric cost as long as they vomit or use laxatives soon after a binge.

Since people starting bulimia may use their fingers to induce vomiting, bite marks around the knuckles are a characteristic sign of this disorder. Therefore, it is important for physicians to routinely examine the hands of young people. Once the disease is established, however, a person often can vomit simply by contracting the abdominal muscles. Vomiting may also occur spontaneously.

People practicing bulimia are not proud of these behaviors. After a binge, they usually feel guilty and depressed. Over time they feel hopeless about their situations. Compulsive lying and drug abuse can further intensify these feelings. All this just makes things worse (Figure 11-5). If a person has just started a binge when somebody comes to visit, the response may be, "Get out of my house." The person distances herself from friends and family, becoming more preoccupied with bingeing and purging, an activity that takes up a lot of time.

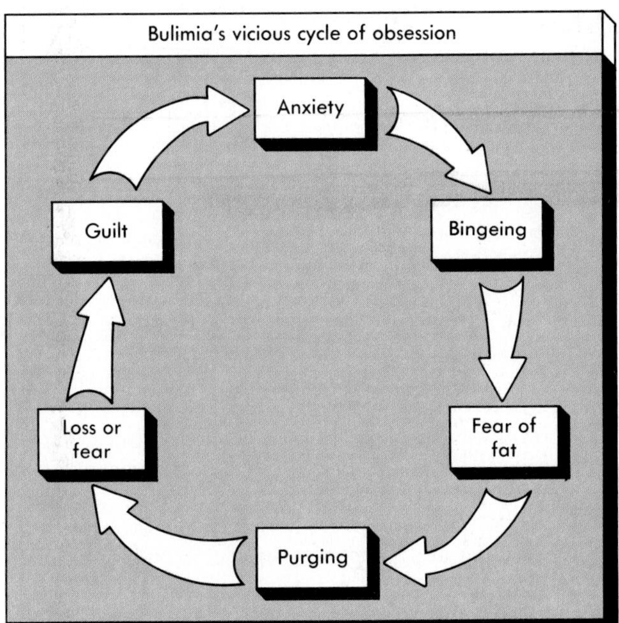

Figure 11-5 Bulimia's vicious cycle of obsession.

HEALTH PROBLEMS STEMMING FROM BULIMIA

Most health problems in bulimia arise from vomiting, if practiced. While vomiting is the most effective way of purging, it is also the most physically destructive method.

- Repeated exposure to the acid in vomit demineralizes teeth. The person complains of painful teeth that are sensitive to heat, cold, and acids. Eventually, the teeth may severely decay, erode away from fillings, and finally fall out. Dental professionals are sometimes the first health professionals to notice signs of bulimia.[18]
- Blood potassium levels can drop significantly with regular vomiting or use of certain diuretics. This can disturb the heart's rhythm and even produce sudden death.
- Salivary glands may swell due to infection and irritation from the vomit. A link between the swelling and hormonal changes is also suspected.
- The person may even suffer from stomach ulcers and bleeding and tears in the esophagus.
- Constipation may result from frequent laxative use.
- Ipecac syrup, also used to induce vomiting, is poisonous to the heart, liver, and kidneys. It has caused accidental poisoning when taken repeatedly.
- Cuts on the fingers from their use to induce vomiting. This poses little health risk, but again can be used by clinicians in accessing whether bulimic habits are present in a suspected case.

In all, bulimia represents a potentially debilitating health risk.

Tooth decay seen in a bulimic patient.

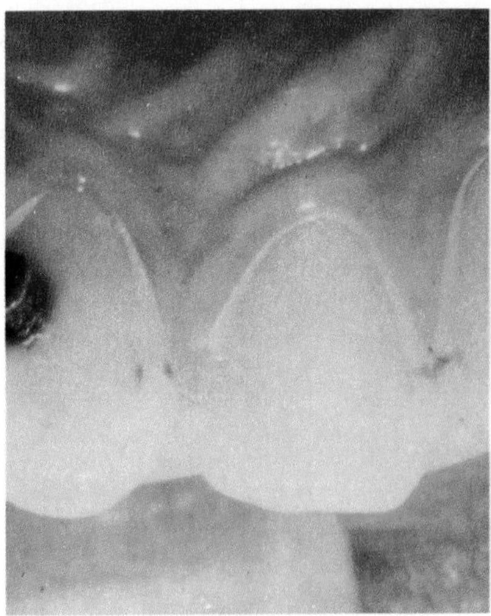

TREATMENT OF BULIMIA

Therapy for bulimia, as for anorexia nervosa, requires a team approach. Treatment should last at least 15 to 20 weeks. Clinicians have yet to agree on the best method. Generally, psychotherapy aims primarily to help a person with self-acceptance and to be less concerned with body weight.[20] Therapy focuses on correcting typical bulimic behaviors, such as the "all or none" thinking: If I'm not perfect, I'm a failure, so one slip-up—one cookie—justifies a binge. The person might be asked to role play a scientist testing assumptions and beliefs about food and weight. Patient and therapist together examine the validity of such beliefs. The premise for this therapy is that if abnormal attitudes and beliefs can be altered, normal eating will follow.[20] In addition, the therapist guides the person to establish behaviors that will minimize

NUTRITION FOCUS

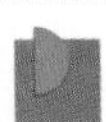

Thoughts of a Person With Bulimia

I am wide awake and immediately out of bed. I think back to the night before when I made a new list of what I wanted to get done and how I wanted to be. My husband is not far behind me on his way into the bathroom to get ready for work. Maybe I can sneak onto the scale to see what I weigh this morning before he notices me. I am already in my private world. I feel overjoyed when the scale says that I stayed the same weight as I was the night before, and I can feel that slightly hungry feeling. Maybe **IT** will stop today; maybe today everything will change. What were the projects I was going to get done?

We eat the same breakfast, except that I take no butter on my toast, no cream in my coffee, and never take seconds (until Doug gets out the door). Today I am going to be really good, and that means eating certain predetermined portions of food and not taking one more bite than I think I am allowed. I am very careful to see that I don't take more than Doug. I judge by his body. I can feel the tension building. I wish Doug would hurry up and leave so I can get going!

As soon as he shuts the door, I try to get involved with one of the myriad of responsibilities on my list. I hate them all! I just want to crawl into a hole. I don't want to do anything. I'd rather eat. I am alone; I am nervous; I am no good; I always do everything wrong anyway; I am not in control; I can't make it through the day, I know it. It has been the same for so long.

I remember the starchy cereal I ate for breakfast. I am into the bathroom and onto the scale. It measures the same, BUT I DON'T WANT TO STAY THE SAME! I want to be thinner! I look in the mirror, I think my thighs are ugly and deformed looking. I see a lumpy, clumsy, pear-shaped wimp. There is always something wrong with what I see. I feel frustrated, trapped in this body, and I don't know what to do about it.

I float to the refrigerator, knowing exactly what is there. I begin with last night's brownies. I always begin with the sweets. At first I try to make it look like nothing is missing, but my appetite is huge and I resolve to make another batch of brownies. I know there is half of a bag of cookies in the bathroom, thrown out the night before, and I polish them off immediately. I take some milk so my vomiting will be smoother. I like the full feeling I get after downing a big glass. I get out six pieces of bread, toast one side in the broiler, turn them over, load them with pats of butter, and put them under the broiler again until they are bubbling. I take all six pieces on a plate to the television and go back for a bowl of cereal and a banana to have along with them. Before the last toast is finished, I am already preparing the next batch of six more pieces. Maybe another brownie or five, and a couple of large bowls full of ice cream, yogurt, or cottage cheese.

My stomach is stretched into a huge ball below my rib cage. I know I'll have to go into the bathroom soon, but I want to postpone it. I am in never-never land. I am waiting, feeling the pressure, pacing the floor in and out of the rooms. Time is passing. Time is passing. It is getting to be the time.

I wander aimlessly through each of the rooms again, tidying, making the whole house neat and put back together. I finally make the turn into the bathroom. I brace my feet, pull my hair back, stick my finger down my throat, stroke twice, and get up a huge pile of food. Three times, four, and another pile of food. I can see everything come back. I am glad to see those brownies because they are SO fattening. The rhythm of the emptying is broken, and my head is beginning to hurt. I stand up feeling dizzy, empty, and weak. The whole episode has taken about an hour.

bingeing. Examples of these behaviors are eating regular meals and using alternate methods—rather than food—to cope with stressful situations.[2] Group therapy is often useful. As in cases of anorexia nervosa, if a person enters treatment in a state of starvation, psychotherapy will be delayed.

One goal of therapy is to help a bulimic person accept as normal some depression and self-doubt. As with anorexia nervosa there is no specific medication used to treat bulimia.[1] Therapists may prescribe antidepressant medications, such as amitriptyline (Elavil) and tranylcypromine (Parnate), to combat some depression associated with bulimia. That often also works to reduce bingeing in early phases of treatment.[29] The medication fenfluramine (Pondimin) may also be used in an attempt to curb appetite.

Nutritional counseling can help correct misconceptions about food.[3] This entails teaching the person about bulimia and its consequences, focusing on its extreme means of weight control. In early stages it may be best for the person with bulimia to avoid eating binge foods or weighing him- or herself. The primary goal is to develop a normal eating pattern so that food choices become more mechanical. Some nutrition specialists achieve this goal by encouraging daily meal planning. Using the exchange system is helpful as it enables a person with bulimia to more accurately assess the energy content of different foods. The person needs to understand that no food, when eaten in moderation, is necessarily fattening; the exchange system convincingly demonstrates that by listing kcalorie contents.

Nutritional counseling emphasizes setting up regular eating habits rather than stopping the bingeing and purging.[3] Usually a food diary is kept throughout treatment. This helps the person monitor food intake as well as feelings that accompany binge-purge cycles. Alternate coping strategies can then be tried. A therapist might use such information to identify events that seem to trigger binge episodes.

Regular eating habits should help the binge-purge cycle stop by itself. The person should be discouraged from following strict food rules. Stressing the maintenance of healthful eating habits is a key to helping a person regain nutritional perspective.

Bulimia is a serious health problem. If not treated, grave medical complications can result. Since relapse is likely, therapy should be long term.[20] People with bulimia can be very depressed and are at a high risk for suicide. That is why they need professional help.

Preventing Eating Disorders

Parents, friends, and professionals working with young adults should consider the following advice for preventing eating disorders:

1. Discourage restrictive dieting, meal skipping, and fasting.
2. Provide information about normal changes that occur during puberty.
3. Correct misconceptions about nutrition, normal body weight, and approaches to weight loss.
4. Carefully phrase weight-related recommendations and comments (Figure 11-6).

Our society as a whole can benefit from a fresh focus on healthful food practices and a healthful outlook toward foods.

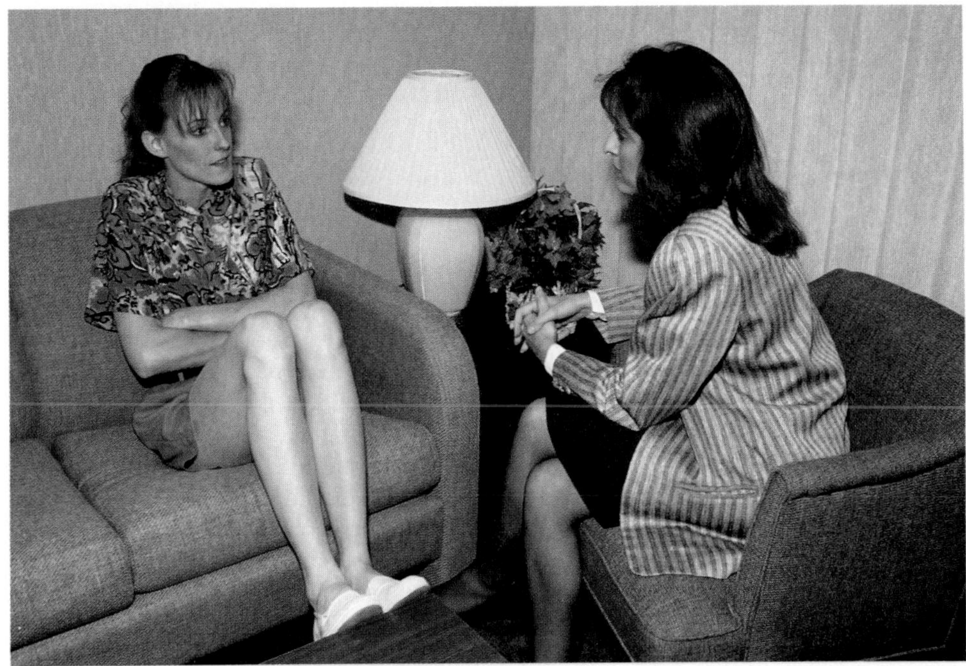

Figure 11-6 A psychologist cannot council a starving person—issues surrounding food intake must be addressed early in therapy.

EXPERT OPINION

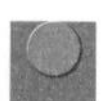

Compulsive Overeating

BY JEFF HARRIS, DHSC, RD

It is 11:00 P.M., and Marge is sitting alone in the kitchen before a half gallon of gourmet chocolate-chocolate chip ice cream as she frequently does when individuals in her family take advantage of her. As she eats large spoonfuls of the cold, flavorful food she becomes emotionally numb and in a sense feels she has removed herself from her frustrating, anger-provoking situation. Yes, she will awaken and feel the guilt of having finished the whole half gallon, but for the moment it feels good to get away from those uncomfortable and painful feelings. This is an example of compulsive overeating.

The term, compulsive overeating, has been a confusing one. It has been used in many ways, of which some make it synonymous with bulimia nervosa, while other uses suggest simply regularly eating large portions of food. In fact the term is not defined in the *Diagnostic and Statistical Manual of Mental Disorders* (DSM III-R), the major guide for making psychological diagnoses. However, many professionals that deal with eating disorders see it as a distinct eating problem. It is expected that the next edition of the DSM, due for release in early 1993, will contain a diagnosis recognizing frequent binge eating behavior not accompanied by purging.

Compulsive overeating can be viewed as eating to avoid feeling and dealing with emotional pain.[26] It is performed without regard to biological need for nutrients and done in a repeated, ritualized fashion to induce a sense of well-being, numbness, or freedom from anxiety. When defined in this way it does generally meet the DSM III-R criteria for obsessive compulsive disorder. For some people the behavior pattern is expressed as continually eating food throughout a defined period of time (grazing), and for others, cycles of bingeing interspersed with normal eating. For example, one person who has a stressful or frustrating job comes home from work every night and eats continually (grazes) until bedtime. Another person might be eating normally most of the time, but when an emotional setback occurs he or she eats large quantities of food.

Compulsive overeating is different from anorexia nervosa, and particularly bulimia nervosa, because it doesn't necessarily involve a persistent concern with body shape, weight, and thinness. Bulimic people may compulsively overeat to alleviate emotional pain, but the disorders are not synonymous. Compulsive overeating doesn't necessarily involve eating the large quantities of food that bulimic people eat, nor the purging and periods of starvation.[24] In addition, not all obese people compulsively overeat, so obesity and this disorder aren't necessarily associated. Obesity can be a result of trying to numb emotional pain with food but is not necessarily an outcome. Some studies have confirmed that some obese individuals do not necessarily overeat.

Compulsive overeating has been classified by many as an addiction to food because a psychological dependence is involved.[26] There is an attachment to the behavior, a drive to continue it, a sense of limited control over it, and a need to continue it despite negative consequences. Food is used to reduce stress, produce feelings of power and well-being, avoid feelings of intimacy with others, and avoid life problems.

Why is compulsive overeating a problem? This behavior results in people who never learn to appropriately express and deal with their feelings. In addition, rather than face their problems, they choose to eat instead. They continue to do the things that perpetuate the experience of frustration, anger, and pain. Walt may be frustrated regularly because of his lack of assertiveness, but he eats to deal with his frustration rather than learning to share it with someone and practice assertiveness training. His frustration will continue because he will not change his behavior and become more assertive. Another reason the compulsive behavior is a problem is that the person feels that he or she cannot control the behavior pattern and there is a sense of life being out of control. In addition, the result of compulsive overeating

Baryophobia

baryophobia A disorder associated with a poor growth rate in a child because parents underfeed the child in an attempt to prevent development of obesity and heart disease.

Baryophobia, literally "the fear of becoming heavy," is a relatively new disorder.[25] The term applies to children or young adults who grow slower and less than the norm. Decreased growth in a child usually reflects disease. If no hormonal or other abnormality can be found, the possibility of baryophobia should be investigated.

This disorder occurs when parents put their children on the same low-fat, high-carbohydrate diet that adults follow. Adults do this in an attempt to prevent their children from developing obesity or heart disease later in life. Today's parents, themselves frequently harassed by weight problems, are determined to free their children from that ordeal. Well-intended efforts to prevent obesity can lead them to severely restrict food intake of their children. The child doesn't get enough

EXPERT OPINION

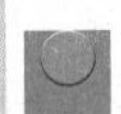

Compulsive Overeating—cont'd

is often an increase in negative feelings. Eating two large pizzas and half a cake would result in many people feeling guilty, embarrassed, and ashamed. So it is definitely a pattern that needs to be changed.

How do people develop this dysfunctional eating behavior? At least in the United States, during childhood we are often comforted with food. Jane is given crackers or candy to soothe her grumpiness. Bobby, when he is crying, is promised a treat. Jill is frustrated over her inability to be assertive at school and is comforted with milk and cookies. Individuals who compulsively overeat often grow up in families that do not address feelings in healthy ways. The parents nurture and comfort their children with food rather than engage in a healthy exchange of self-disclosure of feelings and potential solutions. After awhile people do not eat because they are hungry and to satiate physical needs, but in response to emotional needs and pain. Those that become compulsive overeaters grow up nurturing others (instead of themselves), avoiding their feelings, and take little time for themselves. They do not know how to satisfy their personal and emotional needs in healthy ways. They turn to food for their needs to be met.

Studies show that compulsive overeaters often come from alcoholic families and were objects of sexual abuse. In these dysfunctional families emotions aren't dealt with effectively; substances are used to cope. Individuals in the family have learned to live in a pattern of covering for the alcoholic person and nurturing him or her at the expense of his or her personal needs.

How can compulsive overeaters overcome their disorder? The individual must learn to eat in response to biological signals (hunger) rather than emotions and external factors like time of day or the presence of food. Experts often have compulsive overeaters keep a record of their level of physical hunger throughout the day and at the beginning and end of every meal. These individuals learn to eat just until a prescribed level of fullness is reached at each meal. Diets must be avoided, in that food deprivation can promote an experience of more disruptive emotions and a greater sense of unmet needs. Diets will encourage more intense problems with compulsive overeating.

Compulsive overeaters must learn to identify their personal needs that are unmet. They must find healthy ways to satisfy these needs. As these people experience more psychological, emotional, and spiritual fulfillment, food decreases in importance. The tendency to nurture others at the expense of their own needs must be identified and faced. New patterns of behavior will need to be developed to let others take responsibility for their own needs, while the compulsive overeater addresses his or her own.

Healthy ways to express emotion must be explored. Often these individuals will need to be shown how to identify their emotions in given situations and appropriately share them. Learning simple phrases to say to oneself can help individuals stop themselves from overeating when the desire is strong.

Lastly, Overeaters Anonymous is a self-help group that has been devoted to help overeaters achieve recovery. Participation in this program has been helpful for many. Each chapter attempts to supply an environment of encouragement and accountability to overcome this eating disorder. Their philosophy is similar to Alcoholics Anonymous.

It is estimated that compulsive overeating is much more prevalent than anorexia nervosa or bulimia nervosa. Next time you find yourself running to some candy bars when times are stressful, consider asking yourself how you could better address the emotions you are feeling.

Dr. Harris is an Associate Professor of Health at West Chester University in West Chester, PA. His research interests include various aspects of obesity and eating disorders and their treatment.

kcalories to maintain an adequate growth rate. In young adults, the low-kcalorie diet may be self-imposed to avoid a perceived risk of obesity.

In these cases, counseling is needed. The parents or the young adult need to be informed of the nutrient requirements and weight-gain patterns for the age group involved. The parents will learn that including some sweets and higher-fat foods in a young person's diet is appropriate. The diet can still minimize saturated fat, a more important focus in a diet designed to reduce the risk of heart disease. Supplying adequate kcalories, protein, and other nutrients is the key to promoting growth—height and weight—in child and young adult years, and it can be done in a healthful manner.

CONCEPT CHECK

Bulimia is characterized by episodes of bingeing followed by purging, usually by vomiting. Vomiting is very destructive to the body, often causing severe dental decay, stomach ulcers, irritation of the esophagus, and blood potassium imbalances. Treatment using nutrition counseling and psychotherapy attempts to restore normal eating habits, help the person correct distorted beliefs about diet and lifestyle, and find tools to cope with the stresses of life. Although not recognized as an eating disorder, compulsive overeating is characterized by frequent binge eating (without purging) to avoid feeling and coping with emotional pain. Baryophobia describes a situation where a young child fails to grow properly because he or she is underfed by the parents, often with intention of reducing the risk for obesity or heart disease.

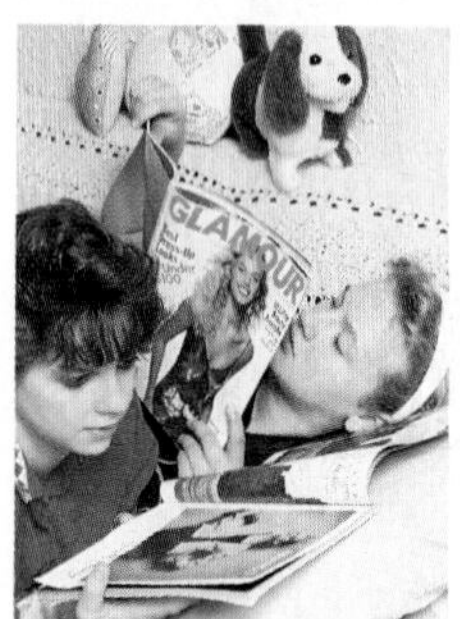

Summary

1. The person with anorexia nervosa is usually a girl around the age of puberty who begins to diet but then finds it difficult to stop. She is generally a perfectionist and a high achiever, often described as the "best little girl in the world." Some cases are seen in men.
2. Warning signs for anorexia nervosa include abnormal food habits, such as cutting a pea in half before eating it or cooking a large meal and watching others eat. Later, school performance crumbles, the person often refuses to eat out with family and friends and develops a very critical and joyless nature.
3. Physical effects of anorexia nervosa include decreases in body temperature and heart rate, iron-deficiency anemia, a low white blood cell count, hair loss, constipation, low blood potassium level, and the loss of menstrual periods. A person with anorexia nervosa is physically very ill.
4. Treatment of anorexia nervosa includes increasing food intake to at least support basal metabolism and then to allow for gradual weight gain. Psychological counseling attempts to help the person establish regular food habits and to find means of coping with the life stresses that led to the disorder. Hospitalization may be necessary.
5. Bulimia is characterized by bingeing on up to 20,000 or more kcalories at one sitting, and then purging by vomiting, laxative use, exercise, or other means. Both men and women are at risk. Vomiting as a means of purging is especially destructive to the body; it can cause severe tooth decay, stomach ulcers, irritation of the esophagus, low blood potassium levels, and other problems. Bulimia poses a serious health problem and is associated with significant risk of suicide.
6. Treatment of bulimia includes psychological as well as nutritional counseling. During treatment, the person learns to accept him/herself and to cope with problems in ways that do not involve food. Regular eating patterns are developed as the bulimic person begins to plan meals in an informed, healthy manner.
7. Compulsive eating represents bingeing behavior that is not linked to purging. Emotional problems are often at the root of this disordered form of eating. Treatment should address deeper emotional issues in addition to restoration of regular eating habits.
8. Baryophobia describes a condition where children are underfed by parents in an attempt to limit risk of future disease, such as obesity or heart disease. Growth failure—weight and height gains—can result if nutrient intake is not increased to appropriate levels.

Study Questions

1. What, in your opinion, is a healthful attitude toward food and eating?

2. What are the key differences between anorexia and anorexia nervosa. What are common manifestations of anorexia nervosa? If you knew someone who you thought had this psychological eating disorder, what would you do?

3. List the detrimental physical and psychological side effects of bulimia. Describe important goals of psychological and nutrition therapy in treatment of bulimia.

4. How might parents significantly contribute to the development of an eating disorder? Share an attitude that perhaps a parent of yours displayed that may not have been conducive to developing a normal relationship to food.

5. Based on your knowledge of good nutrition and sound dietary habits, answer the following questions:

   a. How could poor eating habits, such as those exhibited in a binge/purge cycle, cause significant nutrient deficiencies? Describe the major nutrient deficits associated with bulimic behavior.

   b. How can significant nutrient deficits contribute to major health problems in later life? Elaborate on the nutrient deficiencies that you listed in part **a** and their long-term effects.

REFERENCES

1. Alger and others: Effect of a tricyclic antidepressant and opiate antagonist on binge-eating behavior in normal weight bulimic and obese, binge-eating subjects, *American Journal of Clinical Nutrition* 53:865, 1991.
2. Anonymous: Orderly dieting and disordered eating: a case report, *Nutrition Reviews* 49:16, 1991.
3. ADA Reports. Position of the American Dietetic Association: Nutrition intervention in the treatment of anorexia nervosa and bulimia nervosa, *Journal of The American Dietetic Association* 88:68, 1988.
4. Beresin EV and others: The process of recovering from anorexia nervosa, *Journal of The American Academy of Psychoanalysis* 17:103, 1989.
5. Casper RC and others: Total daily energy expenditure and activity level in anorexia nervosa, *American Journal of Clinical Nutrition* 53:1143, 1991.
6. Comerci GD: Medical complications of anorexia nervosa and bulimia nervosa, *Medical Clinics of North America* 74:1293, 1990.
7. Farley: Eating disorders require medical attention, *FDA Consumer,* March 1992, p 27.
8. Feldman W and others: Culture versus biology: children's attitudes toward thinness and fatness, *Pediatrics* 81:190, 1988.
9. Field HL: Eating disorders, *Comprehensive Therapy* 15:3, 1989.
10. Goldbloom DS and others: Anorexia nervosa and bulimia nervosa, *Canadian Medical Association Journal* 140:1149, 1989.
11. Greene GW and others: Dietary intake and dieting practices of bulimic and non-bulimic female college students, *Journal of the American Medical Association* 90:576, 1990.
12. Health and Public Policy Committee, American College of Physicians: Eating disorder: anorexia nervosa and bulimia, *Nutrition Today,* March/April 1987, p 29.
13. Kirkley BG, Burge JC: Dietary restriction in young women: issues and concerns, *Annals of Behavioral Medicine* 11:66, 1989.
14. Kreipe RE and others: Long-term outcome of adolescents with anorexia nervosa, *American Journal of Diseases of Children* 143:1322, 1989.
15. Miller KD: Compulsive overeating, *Nursing Clinics of North America* 26:699, 1991.
16. Larson BJ: Relationship of family communication patterns to eating disorder inventory scores in adolescent girls, *Journal of The American Dietetic Association* 91:1065, 1991.
17. Mackenzie M: The pursuit of slenderness and addition to self-control: an anthropological interpretation of eating disorders. In Briggs GM, editor: *Nutrition update,* vol 2, New York, 1985, John Wyley & Sons, p 173.
18. Monehen R: Anorexia nervosa, bulimia, and the dental assistant, *Dental Assistant,* July/Aug 1989, p 19.
19. Morris A and Others: The changing shape of female fashion models, *International Journal of Eating Disorders* 8:593, 1989.
20. Mynors-Wallis LM: The psychological treatment of eating disorders, *British Journal of Hospital Medicine* 41:470, 1989.
21. Nicholi AM, editor: *The new Harvard guide to psychiatry,* Cambridge, Mass, 1988, Harvard University Press.
22. Omizo SA: Anorexia nervosa: psychological considerations for nutritional counseling, *Journal of The American Dietetic Association* 88:49, 1988.

23. Patton G: The course of anorexia nervosa, *British Medical Journal* 299:139, 1989.
24. Mount R and others: An obsessive-compulsive view of obesity and its treatment, *Journal of Clinical Psychology* 46:68, 1990.
25. Pugliese MT and others: Fear of obesity: a cause of short stature and delayed puberty, *The New England Journal of Medicine* 309:513, 1983.
26. Riley EA: Eating disorders as an addictive behavior, *Nursing Clinics of North America* 26:715, 1991.
27. Stensland SH, Sobal J: Dietary practices of ballet, jazz, and modern dancers, *Journal of The American Dietetic Association* 92:319, 1992.
28. Thornton JS: Feast or famine: eating disorders in athletes, *Physician and Sportsmedicine* 18:116, 1990.
29. Tolstoi LC: The role of pharmacotherapy in anorexia nervosa and bulimia, *Journal of The American Dietetic Association* 89:1640, 1989.
30. Uhe AM and others: Potential regulators of feeding behavior in anorexia nervosa, *American Journal of Clinical Nutrition* 55:28, 1992.

SUGGESTED READINGS

The articles by Comerci and Field provide a detailed medical perspective of eating disorders. These articles contain numerous references for further reading. The article by Thornton provides an interesting account of eating disorders in athletes. The article by Omizo demonstrates a registered dietitian's perspective on the treatment of eating disorders. This topic is further developed in the position paper by The American Dietetic Association. In total, all these references supply a detailed account of the causes, development, and treatment for these disorders.

Aside from our formal reference list, in this chapter we also want to provide you with less technical sources to give you more insight into eating disorders. These include:

HOT LINES

Bulimia Anorexia Self Help/Behavior Adaptation Support and Healing (BASH), PO Box 39903, St. Louis, MO 63139, 1-800-762-3334 or 314-567-4080

Available 24 hours, this is a treatment and research center for eating (anorexia, bulimia, overweight) and mood (depression, anxiety, phobias, panic attacks) disorders. It will provide assistance and information.

American Anorexia/Bulimia Association, Inc. 133 Cedar Lane, Teaneck, New Jersey 07666, 201-836-1800

This group can refer a person to a treatment center near the person's home.

BOOKS

Kano S: *Making peace with food,* New York, 1989, Harper and Row.

Vredevelt P, Whitman J: *Walking a thin line,* Portland, Ore, 1985, Multnomah Press.

Levenkron S: *Treating and overcoming anorexia nervosa,* New York, 1982, Charles Scribner's & Son.

NEWSLETTER

NAAS Quarterly Newsletter, 1925 East Dublin Granville Rd., Columbus, Ohio 43229, 614-436-1112.

Material is appropriate for professional and personal use. Ten back issues and "Overview of Eating Disorders" can be ordered for $10.00. A current subscription also is available through NAAS membership.

TAKE ACTION

A self-evaluation on the risk of developing an eating disorder

Table 11-1 of this chapter lists the criteria for the eating disorders anorexia nervosa and bulimia. These criteria are repeated below. Put an "X" in the space before statements that describe your characteristics and lifestyle. Respond as honestly as possible.

_______ 1. You refuse to keep your body weight over a minimal normal weight for age and height.
_______ 2. You intensely fear gaining weight or becoming fat, even though you are underweight.
_______ 3. You feel fat even though you are quite thin.
_______ 4. If you are female, you have missed at least three consecutive menstrual cycles.
_______ 5. You have recurrent episodes of binge eating.
_______ 6. You feel out of control over eating behavior during the eating binges.
_______ 7. You regularly either self-induce vomiting, use laxatives or diuretics, diet strictly or fast, or vigorously exercise to prevent weight gain.
_______ 8. You engage in a minimum average of two binge eating episodes a week.
_______ 9. You have a persistent overconcern with body shape and weight.

Questions 1 through 4 pertain to anorexia nervosa and 5 through 9 to bulimia.

COMPLETE THIS ACTIVITY BY ANSWERING THE FOLLOWING QUESTIONS:

1. After having completed this checklist, do you feel that you might have an eating disorder or the potential to develop one?

____

____

2. Do you think some of your friends might have an eating disorder?

____

____

3. What counseling and education resources exist in your area or on your campus to help with a potential eating disorder?

____

____

4. If a friend had an eating disorder, what do you think would be the best way to assist him or her in getting help?

____

____

If you would like more information you can contact the following national self-help groups:

American Anorexia/Bulimia Association, Inc.
418 East 76th Street
New York, New York 10021
212/734-1114

Anorexia Nervosa and Associated Disorders, Inc.
P.O. Box 7
Highland Park, IL 60035
708/831-3438

Anorexia Nervosa and Related Eating Disorders, Inc.
P.O. Box 5102
Eugene, OR 97405
503/344-1144 ▲

NUTRITION PERSPECTIVE

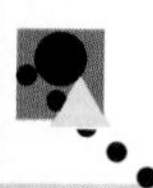

Eating Disorders: A Sociological Perspective

We evaluate ourselves in many ways. One way is based on body image. We identify our bodies with ourselves and judge our bodies as we think others see us, knowing that our appearance affects their opinions of us.

Early in life, we learn to recognize what "acceptable" and "unacceptable" body types look like. Of all attributes that constitute attractiveness, body weight is probably perceived as the most important, partly because it is an aspect we feel we can control somewhat.

Yet body weight is probably the aspect of image that dissatisfies us most. Fatness has been ranked as the most dreaded deviation from our cultural ideals of body image, the one most derided and shunned, even among schoolchildren.[8]

Women, in particular, are likely to diet because they have very strong feelings about what is an acceptable size and weight. In general, though, these women aren't technically obese. Rather, they diet to correct some perceived flaw or because they simply feel they should weigh less than they do now.

A Glamour magazine survey with 30,000 respondents indicated that 80% of the survey participants were ashamed of their bodies. This dissatisfaction focuses primarily on the desire for lower weight and smaller thighs, hips, buttocks, and waists (typical sites of greatest fat deposition in sexually mature women).[13]

Changing times

The "full-bodied" woman as a cultural ideal did not survive into the twentieth century. Over the course of this century, a woman's "ideal" body form has become thinner and thinner, despite the natural physical maturation of a woman's body to soft, rounded shapes. Our passion for thinness may have its roots in the Victorian era, which specialized in denying "unpleasant" physical realities, such as appetite and sexual desire.[17] Flappers of the 1920s cemented a trend for thinness (Figure 11-7). Over the past 20 years, the ideal has gradually moved toward a thinner, more angular and muscular body shape. Female models for women's magazines have become taller, thinner, and more "tubular" in that bust and body circumferences have decreased compared to waist size.[19] At the same time, the population as a whole has gained weight. The same holds true for men in general; a lean, slightly muscular physique characterizes men in advertisements and movies.

In the past women also used undergarments to mold their bodies into the latest acceptable body shape. By the 1960s, the trend was to diet to reshape the body through weight loss.

Researchers have linked this preference for a lean, muscular body type to the recent surge in eating disorders. As the more full-figured woman (earth mother) is being replaced by the ultra-thin malelike woman, our preoccupation with obesity and the number of people with eating disorders have increased. It appears that the cultural pressures toward thinness are stretching the physiological capabilities of many women and men. Given the natural variability in rates for resting metabolism, our easy access to food, and increasingly sedentary lifestyles, it is no surprise that some of us gain weight. People predisposed to eating disorders for either biological or emotional reasons may be nudged "over the edge" by this change in social values.

The pursuit of power

Today, society views obesity as a failure of control, willpower, competence, and productivity, all social ideals of the 1980s and 1990s. At stake is social acceptance and even access to scarce resources, such as good jobs or an attractive spouse. Whether we like it or not, our appearance says a lot about us. The question implicit in our society's values is this: If a person cannot control him- or herself enough to stay slim, can that person supervise employees, organize the work day, and reliably bear heavy responsibilities?

NUTRITION PERSPECTIVE

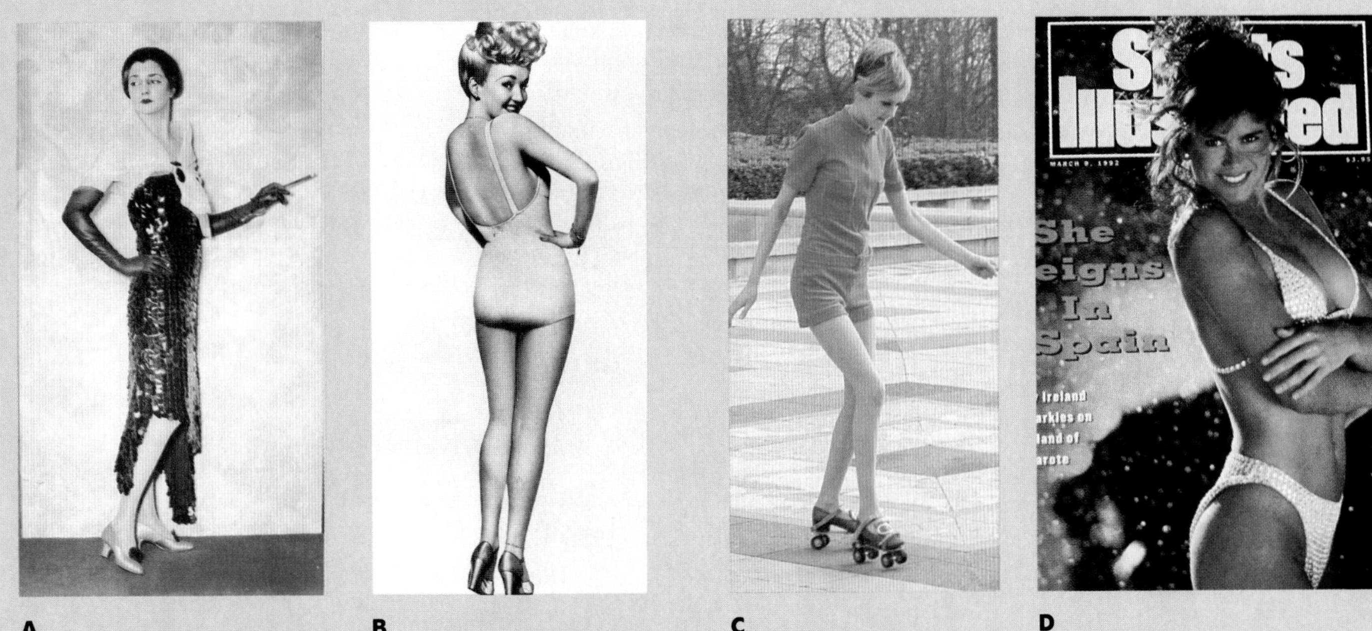

Figure 11-7 The changing views of desirable body weight. American society has imposed varying stereotypes for desirable body weight, especially for women. **A,** The svelte flapper of the 1920s. **B,** The "thin but curvaceous" look of the 1940s. **C,** Ultra-thin was in during the 1960s. **D,** Lean and well-toned physiques grace magazine covers of the 1980s and 1990s.

Mixed messages

On top of the pressure for thinness, we receive mixed messages. Half the advertisements in women's magazines may be for diets, and the other half for tasty foods. Movie and television stars are almost always perfect physical specimens. Yet television advertisements encourage us to visit our local fast-food restaurant. There you can buy a hamburger, French fries, and a milk shake, totaling about 1200 kcalories—about the amount of energy our daily resting metabolism uses—without even leaving the car.

New pressures

Divorce now ends about one half of all marriages. This increases the stress on children and adolescents, who, like adults, may turn to food. Considering other prevalent stresses—alcoholism in the family, school and work pressures, and crowded urban conditions—many of us face family and social environments that encourage us to find a pressure release valve. That valve may be food.

Thin is in!

All in all, fat has lost favor in our society. Today's myth is that thin people are better than obese people—more competent, healthier, and more strong willed.

Eating disorders are usually only a symptom of greater emotional trauma in a person's life. When psychiatrists are able to dig deeper, they find that eating disorders mask serious questions of self-worth, family struggles, and sometimes fears of puberty and the future.[12] The real illnesses are not the eating disorders—though they eventually contribute to poor health—but rather, the way people feel about themselves. And negative self-images are reinforced by current social values.

NUTRITION PERSPECTIVE

Eating Disorders: A Sociological Perspective—cont'd

Eventually, by severely restricting kcalories for long periods of time, people with anorexia nervosa greatly compromise their nutritional status, impair their reproductive systems, retard growth, and put themselves at risk for osteoporosis and even death. The harm produced by milder, shorter periods of diet restriction is not clear. Evidence, however, suggests that even moderate diet restriction, if continued, contributes to the risks for various anemias, pregnancy complications, low birth weight infants, and may reduce bone density and metabolic rate. It may also impair growth in children and young adolescents. The percentage of adolescents and young adults who significantly restrict kcalories is not known. But at least two problems, iron-deficiency anemia and pregnancy complications, are significant problems in this age group.

Glimmers of Hope

For women there are some glimmers of hope. Feminists are beginning to point out that true liberation means being free to find your natural weight. Women who combine careers and motherhood are saying that they have more important things to worry about; fashion leaders are tolerating more curves; exercise programs are encouraging walking rather than jogging. Working out to feel good, rather than just touting the glory of burning kcalories, is now emphasized. Writers, therapists, and some registered dietitians are working to help women accept and love their bodies.

What is the difference between people who can accept themselves—even with a few more pounds than the glamorous people weigh—and those who chronically diet and feel dissatisfied? Perhaps it is the willingness to recognize that satisfaction with appearance comes from within, not from what they see in the mirror or what someone else tells them (Figure 11-8). The challenge facing Americans today is achieving a healthy body weight without excessive dieting. This means adopting and maintaining sensible eating habits, a physically active lifestyle, and realistic and positive attitudes and emotions, while practicing creative ways to handle stress.

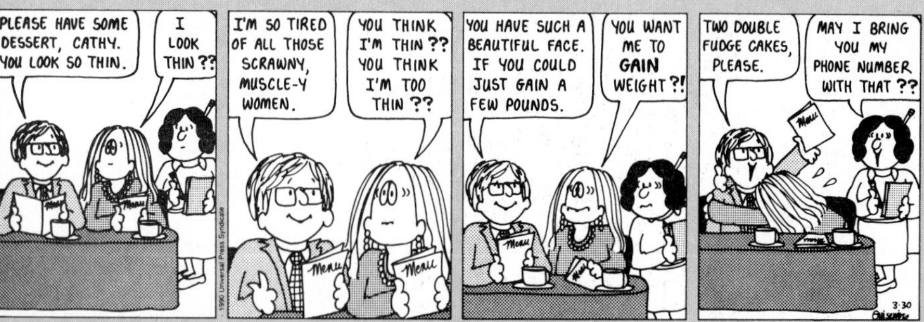
cathy®
by Cathy Guisewite
PLEASE HAVE SOME DESSERT, CATHY. YOU LOOK SO THIN.
I LOOK THIN??
I'M SO TIRED OF ALL THOSE SCRAWNY, MUSCLE-Y WOMEN.
YOU THINK I'M THIN?? YOU THINK I'M TOO THIN??
YOU HAVE SUCH A BEAUTIFUL FACE. IF YOU COULD JUST GAIN A FEW POUNDS.
YOU WANT ME TO GAIN WEIGHT?!
TWO DOUBLE FUDGE CAKES, PLEASE.
MAY I BRING YOU MY PHONE NUMBER WITH THAT??

Figure 11-8 Cathy.

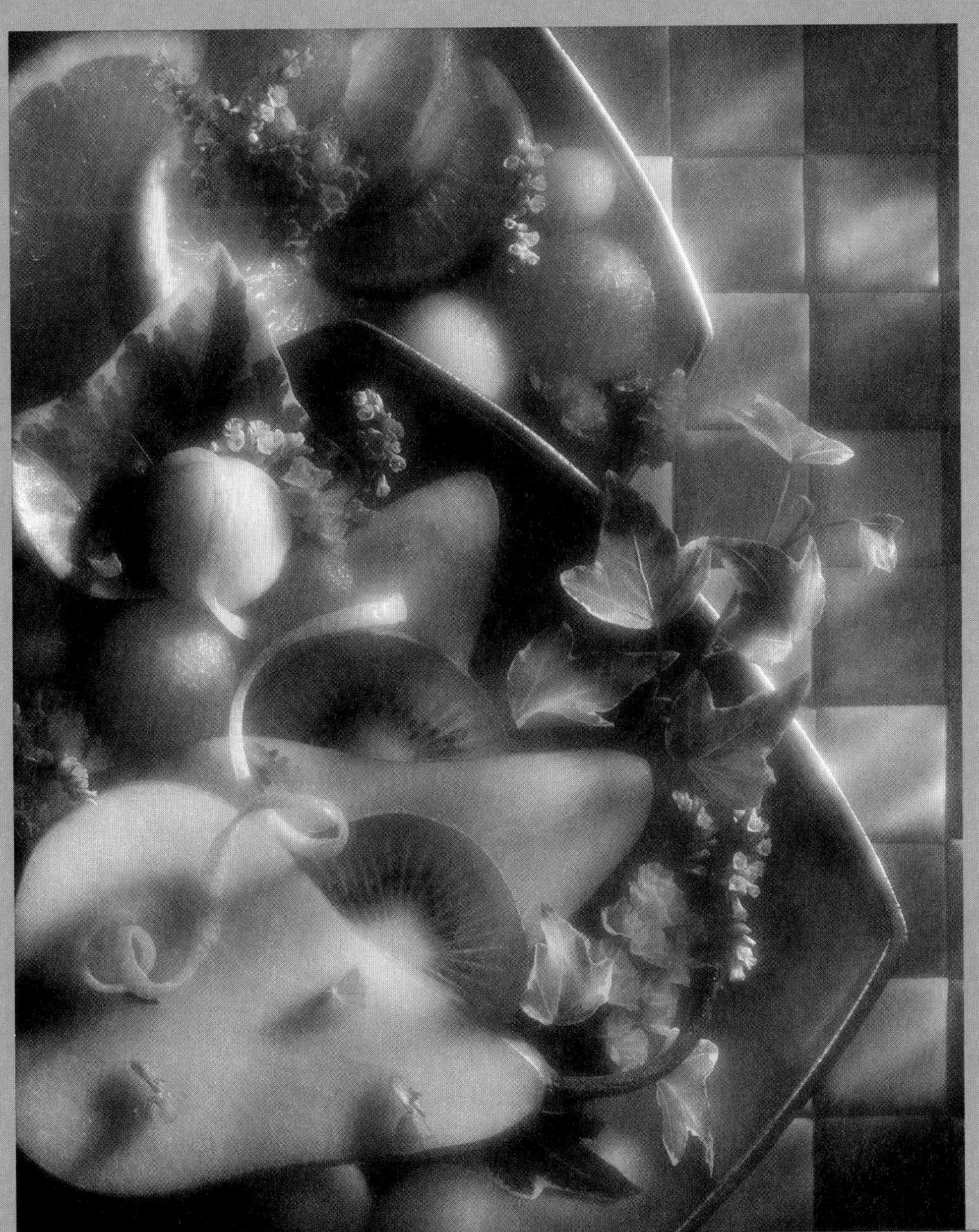

PART FOUR

The Vitamins and Minerals

CHAPTER TWELVE

Vitamins in General and the Fat-Soluble Vitamins A, D, E, and K

When it comes to vitamins, we often hear "If a little is good, then more must be better." Many people believe that consuming vitamins far in excess of their needs provides them with extra energy, protection from disease, and prolonged youth. Up to about 40% of adults in certain areas of the United States take vitamin supplements.[19] This helps fuel the fire in what has become a multibillion dollar industry.

In stark contrast, our total vitamin needs to prevent deficiency symptoms are really quite small. In general, we require about a total of 1 ounce (28 grams) of vitamins for every 150 pounds (70 kilograms) of food we consume. Most plants can synthesize all of the vitamins they need. Abilities of animals to make vitamins varies. For example, the guinea pig, like the human, is one of the very few species of animals that is unable to synthesize its own supply of vitamin C.

As we noted in Chapter 1, vitamins themselves yield no energy for the body. Instead, they facilitate energy-yielding chemical reactions and promote body growth and development. Vitamins A, D, E, and K dissolve in fat, while the B vitamins and vitamin C dissolve in water. In addition, the B vitamins and vitamin K function as parts of coenzymes (i.e., molecules that help enzymes function). Let's now look more closely at the vitamins—important contributors to health, and so to life.

NUTRITION AWARENESS INVENTORY

Here are 15 statements about vitamins in general and fat-soluble vitamins in particular. Answer them to test your current knowledge. If you think the answer is true or mostly true, circle T. If you think the answer is false or mostly false, circle F. Use the scoring key at the end of the book to compute your total score. Take this test again after you have read the chapter. Compare the results.

1. T F There is a danger of deficiency if a vitamin is missing in your diet for 3 days.
2. T F Vitamin K is the least efficiently excreted of all the fat-soluble vitamins.
3. T F People who use mineral oil as a laxative at mealtimes are susceptible to fat-soluble vitamin deficiencies.
4. T F Fat-soluble vitamins are generally more easily lost in cooking than are the water-soluble vitamins.
5. T F It is extremely unlikely that all vitamins have been discovered.
6. T F Vitamin D improves calcium absorption.
7. T F Vitamin A is important for night vision.
8. T F Toxic levels of vitamin A may appear at five times RDA amounts.
9. T F Vitamin D can be considered a hormone.
10. T F Foods in general can be fortified with Vitamin D by exposure with ultraviolet light.
11. T F Vitamin E is an enzyme required by several energy-producing reactions.
12. T F Vitamin K is important for blood clotting.
13. T F Antibiotic use can provoke a vitamin K deficiency.
14. T F Vegetables are good sources of vitamin K.
15. T F A safe dosage for a vitamin supplement is generally 50% to 150% of the U.S. RDA.

Vitamins—A Vital Part of a Diet

By definition, vitamins are organic (carbon-containing) substances that are needed in small amounts in the diet (organic micronutrients) for use in important metabolic reactions in the body. Humans either can not make the vitamin at all or can not make it rapidly enough to always meet their needs. For this reason we must rely on our diets to supply vitamins. Notable exceptions are the conditional status of vitamin D (which may be synthesized by the skin in the presence of sunlight), niacin (which may be synthesized from the amino acid tryptophan) and vitamin K and biotin (which may be synthesized by the bacteria in the colon). For the definition to truly fit, lack of a specific vitamin for a prolonged period of time must cause a deficiency disease that—if caught in time—is quickly cured when the vitamin is resupplied.

Doses of vitamins well above the RDA also have been proven useful as medicinal agents in a small number of diseases. For example, high doses of niacin are an accepted part of blood cholesterol-lowering treatment for appropriately selected individuals. Other various medical applications of vitamins for the prevention or treatment of nondeficiency diseases await further studies.[25] At this time any claims concerning vitamin supplement use, especially if in excess of U.S. RDA values, should be looked at cautiously because many unproven claims have been, and are continually, made.

Vitamins for the human diet come from both plant and animal foods. Whether isolated from foods or synthesized in the laboratory, vitamins are the same chemical compounds and work equally well in the body. Claims in health-food literature that "natural" vitamins isolated from foods are more healthful than those synthesized in a laboratory are unfounded. Some vitamins exist in several related forms that differ in chemical or physical properties. Vitamin E, for example, has alpha and gamma forms. These forms exist both in nature and in synthesized vitamin supplements. It is important to consume the specific vitamin forms that the body can use; we will point out those forms throughout the next two chapters.

Vitamins—A Historical Perspective

The structure and chemical formula of the first known vitamin (thiamin) was determined in 1937. The last known vitamin (vitamin B-12) was characterized in 1948. Before this, knowledge that certain foods, or more appropriately, that components within certain foods were capable of curing ills (brought on by what we now know were vitamin deficiencies) were part of written history. The link between foods containing vitamin A and vision had been known since ancient Egyptian times, when topical application of juice extracted from liver was used as a cure for night blindness. Native Americans in the United States used pine needle extracts to cure scurvy, the vitamin C deficiency disease. During the fifteenth and sixteenth centuries, it was observed that the disease scurvy developed during long sea voyages when few fruits and vegetables were eaten. British scientists later discovered that lime juice cured the scurvy. Using this knowledge, the British navy used the lime to develop a healthier work force and in turn went on to dominate seas worldwide.

As we just noted, the twentieth century brought key breakthroughs in the field of vitamins. These actually began in the early 1900s when Casimir Funk isolated a chemical substance he called "vitamine." This term came from the root phrase "vital amine" (an amine is a compound with a carbon bonded to a nitrogen). This later became the term vitamin that we use today. In the 1920s, scientists fed a variety of foods to mental patients suffering from the disease pellagra and found that the disease was curable by foods high in protein and yeast. By the 1930s, scientists had both isolated vitamin C by extracting it from lemon juice and had cured a pellagra-like disease seen in dogs, called blacktongue, using nicotinic acid. Today we call that substance niacin. In addition, the chemical structure of the many vitamins were deduced.

Knowledge in this area of vitamins is by no means complete—research marches ahead, as we will point out. You may wonder if there are still more vitamins lurking in foods, waiting to be discovered. After all, knowledge of their structures and formulas is only about 6 decades old. Though some optimistic researchers hope to discover one more vitamin,[3] most scientists are confident that all vitamins needed by humans have been discovered; we can already maintain human life for years on total parenteral nutrition if it is properly designed and the person is closely monitored. In this case a person receives all nutrients by vein. No food needs to be eaten. By receiving close medical monitoring in conjunction with protein, carbohydrate, fat, all the known vitamins, and the essential minerals in this manner, a person can continue not only to live but to build new body tissue, have a baby, heal wounds, and fight existing diseases. Experiences with total parenteral nutrition also have reinforced scientific evidence concerning the importance of all known vitamins for human health.

Fat-Soluble Versus Water-Soluble Vitamins

Overall, fat-soluble vitamins are not readily excreted from the body, while water-soluble vitamins are. This occurs partly because the water in cells dissolves water-soluble vitamins and flushes them out of the body via the kidneys. Notable exceptions are the fat-soluble vitamin K and the water-soluble vitamin B-12; vitamin B-12 is stored much more readily than vitamin K. Vitamins in foods should be consumed daily, but an occasional lapse in the intake of water-soluble vitamins should cause no harm. It takes an average person 10 days to develop the first symptoms of a thiamin deficiency and 20 to 40 days for a vitamin C deficiency to develop when these vitamins are completely lacking in the diet.

Because fat-soluble vitamins are not readily excreted, some can build up in the body and cause toxic reactions. And while toxic reaction from an excessive intake of any vitamin is theoretically possible, toxicities of fat-soluble vitamins A and D are observed most frequently.[1] Isolated reports in the scientific literature show that vitamin E and the water-soluble vitamins B-6 and niacin also can be toxic, but only when consumed in very high amounts (50 to 100 times the RDA). So except for vitamin pill use, these three vitamins are unlikely to cause toxic symptoms. In comparison, vitamins A and D can cause toxicity with long-term use at just five to ten times typical RDA values.

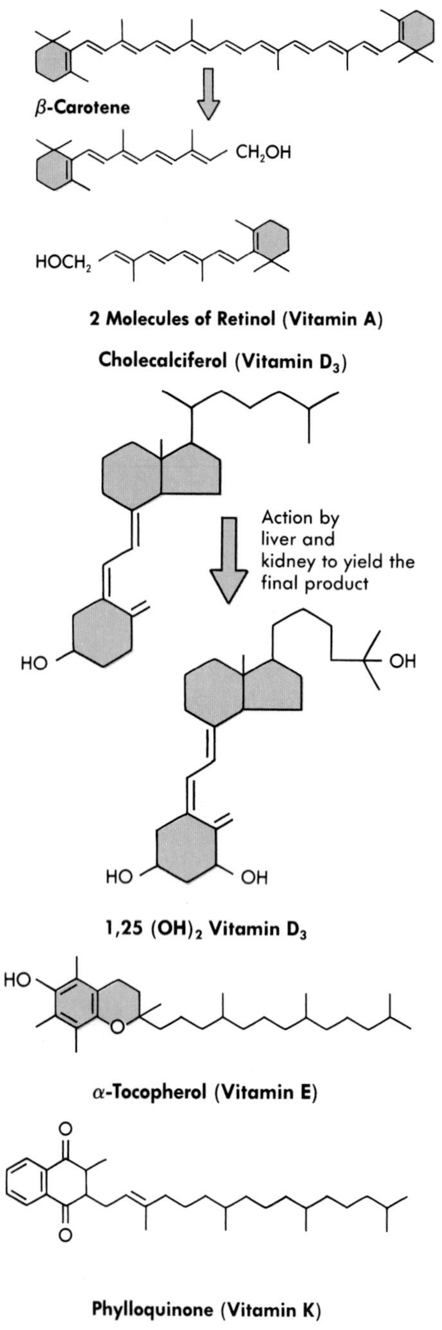

Regular use of a "one-a-day" type of multivitamin and mineral supplement usually yields less than two times the RDA and is therefore unlikely to cause toxicity problems. A noted exception to this results during pregnancy when vitamin A toxicity is possible (see p. 356 for a discussion). But consuming many vitamins, especially highly potent sources of vitamins A and D, can cause problems. In the 1930s fish oils, such as cod liver oil, became sources of vitamin toxicity because of their very high concentrations of vitamins A and D. Today major sources of vitamin toxicity are found in grocery, drug, and health-food stores,[20] where very concentrated forms of vitamin A and vitamin D are sold. See the Nutrition Perspective to find out whether you should take a vitamin supplement, and if so, how to do so safely.

FAT MALABSORPTION AND ITS EFFECTS ON VITAMIN NEEDS

People who experience fat malabsorption—for example, those with cystic fibrosis, celiac disease, or Crohn's disease—also can experience fat-soluble vitamin malabsorption.[30] Unabsorbed fat carries fat-soluble vitamins to the colon and into the feces. Such a person is especially susceptible to a vitamin K deficiency because it is more readily excreted than other fat-soluble vitamins. People who use mineral oil as a laxative at mealtime are also susceptible to fat-soluble vitamin deficiencies. The mineral oil collects fat-soluble vitamins and pulls them into the colon and on into the feces. Some B vitamins (such as folate) and minerals (such as calcium and magnesium) are also susceptible to malabsorption during intestinal disease.

VITAMIN LOSSES IN COOKING

Water-soluble vitamins can be lost in cooking due to heat, alkalinity, and leaching into the cooking water. Steaming, stir-frying, microwaving, or simmering vegetables in minimal moisture allows them to retain most of the B vitamins and vitamin C (see Chapter 13). Although baking soda is sometimes added to vegetables during cooking to make them greener, or to beans to make them softer, it is not a good nutritional practice: the alkalinity destroys much of the thiamin and vitamin C found in the vegetables. Cooking losses for most other vitamins are generally less likely. Important examples will be discussed as we review specific vitamins, and in the Nutrition Focus in Chapter 13.

The Fat-Soluble Vitamins—A, D, E, and K

Let's turn to the fat-soluble vitamins—A, D, E, and K. Figure 12-1 shows their chemical structures.

β-Carotene

CH_2OH

$HOCH_2$

2 Molecules of Retinol (Vitamin A)

Cholecalciferol (Vitamin D_3)

Action by liver and kidney to yield the final product

HO

OH

HO OH

1,25 $(OH)_2$ Vitamin D_3

HO

α-Tocopherol (Vitamin E)

O

O

Phylloquinone (Vitamin K)

Figure 12-1 The fat-soluble vitamins.

ABSORPTION OF FAT-SOLUBLE VITAMINS

The vitamins A, D, E, and K in the diet are absorbed along with dietary fat. When fat absorption is efficient—that is, the actions of bile salts and the enzyme lipase in the small intestine promote adequate digestion and there is adequate absorptive capacity from a healthy intestinal wall—about 40% to 90% of the fat-soluble vitamins are absorbed. As we just mentioned, diseases or medications that hamper fat absorption decrease absorption of fat-soluble vitamins as well, especially vitamins E and K. Supplements, taken under a physician's guidance, may then be appropriate (see the Nutrition Perspective).

The fat-soluble vitamins, once absorbed, are then packaged in the chylomicrons with other dietary fats and travel through the lymphatic system, eventually reaching the bloodstream. They are then carried by the chylomicrons and other lipoproteins

(VLDLs and LDLs) to target cells.[5] As the blood lipoproteins are metabolized by cells lining the bloodstream, the lipoprotein remnants (remains) are picked up by the liver. In this way the fat-soluble vitamins contained in the remnants also enter the liver, which is a major storage site, especially for vitamin A. Other carriers in the bloodstream also help distribute vitamins A and K.

CONCEPT CHECK

Fat-soluble vitamins—A, D, E, and K—are generally less readily excreted and less likely to be lost in cooking than are the water-soluble vitamins—B vitamins and vitamin C. When a person ingests a vitamin-free diet, the first deficiency signs will be due to lack of thiamin and appear after about 10 days. This shows that even water-soluble vitamins persist to some extent in the body, and so an occasional inadequate daily consumption should be of no health concern. It is prudent, however, to regularly consume foods rich in both water-soluble and fat-soluble vitamins. Fat malabsorption decreases fat-soluble vitamin absorption; this has the greatest effect on the status of vitamin E and K in the body. Fat-soluble vitamins pose the greatest risk of toxicity, especially vitamins A and D. Water-soluble vitamins known to show toxic effects are vitamin B-6 and niacin, but only at very high doses.

Vitamin A

Vitamin A deficiency is the leading cause of nonaccidental blindness in the world.[4] The good diets readily available to most American children place them at little risk for developing this deficiency. However, children in less-developed nations are especially susceptible to vitamin A deficiency because their poor intakes and stores of the vitamin fail to meet the high needs of rapid childhood growth. Over 500,000 children in poorer nations of the world become blind each year because of vitamin A deficiency, and many die shortly thereafter because of infections. Today, widespread deficiencies of vitamin A constitute one of the most important public health problems in developing countries.

In the United States, the leading cause of blindness in adults is diabetes; in children it is accidents.

Vitamin A comes in a variety of forms: retinal (aldehyde form), retinol (alcohol form), retinoic acid (acid form), and others ready for our use (preformed). These are found in the diet in animal products; the various forms can be converted into each other to some extent.[28] As a family, these compounds are called **retinoids.**

retinoids Chemical category for preformed vitamin A; one source is animal foods.

Vitamin A activity in the diet is also present in the form of the common carotenoid plant pigments, such as beta-carotene. These are also called provitamin A (Figure 12-1). Carotenoids, actually the original source of all vitamin A, must first be converted to the retinoid form if we are to use them for vitamin A functions. Over 600 carotenoids are found in nature; 50 of them have potential vitamin A activity, and so serve as provitamin A. The most potent form is beta-carotene.

Carotenoids are only absorbed with 40% efficiency, about half of that seen for preformed vitamin A. In the intestinal cells, most carotenes are split in two, potentially yielding two molecules of vitamin A. About 30% of carotenoids are absorbed intact and deposited as such into adipose cells. This gives the characteristic yellow-orange tone to the skin of people who are especially fond of carrot juice.

The retinoids and the provitamin A carotenoids as a group yield what is generically referred to as vitamin A. Almost all vitamin A (greater than 90%) is stored in the liver.

Functions of Vitamin A

Vitamin A performs many important functions in the body. Its importance to night and color vision is perhaps its best-known role.

THE VISUAL CYCLE

The sensory elements of the retina consist of the cones and the rods. The cones are responsible for the visual processes occurring under well-lit circumstances and translate objects into a color image. The rods are responsible for the visual processes that occur in the absence of light and translate objects into black and white images.

To participate in vision, one form of vitamin A—retinal—combines with a protein in the eye, called opsin, forming rhodopsin[28] (Figure 12-2). This rhodopsin is critical to the night vision capabilities of the rods. When light strikes rhodopsin, retinal undergoes a structural change (11-cis retinal is converted into all-trans retinal) and is lost from the protein portion of the rhodopsin molecule (called opsin). This then alters the structure of rhodopsin, which in turn allows ions to enter cells in the eye. The change in ion balance in the cell membranes of the eye stimulates nerve fibers. This signals the brain that light is striking the eye.

Thus when light strikes the eye, rhodopsin is altered, in turn signaling a message to the brain. The bulk of the visual processes also then switch from the rods to the cones. Note that in bright light so much rhodopsin is broken down that not much is available to initiate signals to the brain. This allows the eyes to become "adapted" to bright light. Conversely, in a dark room more rhodopsin is produced, making the retina more light sensitive.

See Appendix B for a description of cis and trans isomer forms.

The cells in the eye recover from a flash of light by first turning the all-trans retinal back into the 11-cis form, and then by resynthesizing rhodopsin. This series of actions constitutes the visual cycle. Not all retinal can be recycled: a certain amount is lost and must be replaced by retinol from the bloodstream. When reaching the eye, retinol is converted to retinal (the form required for forming rhodopsin), allowing the rods to continue to provide night vision.[28]

If an adult's diet is deficient in vitamin A for many years, the retinol level in the bloodstream decreases. In children, body stores are naturally lower, and so low retinol levels in the bloodstream will appear sooner. When retinol in the bloodstream is insufficient to replace that lost from the visual cycle, the cells in the eye recover from flashes of light more slowly. Night blindness increases, and the ability to adapt

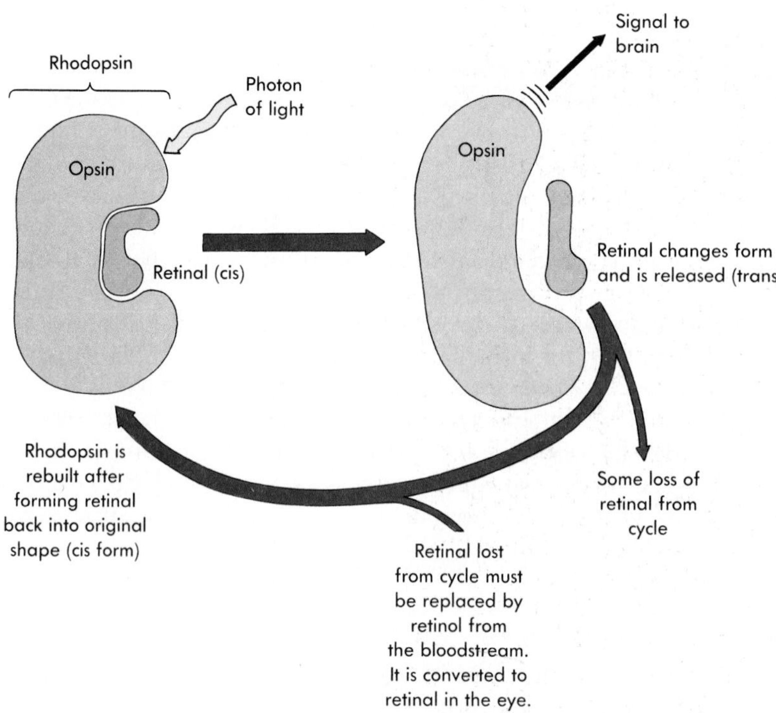

Figure 12-2 Vitamin A participates in the visual cycle. Light (photons) hits rhodopsin. This causes retinal to change form, and so it is released from opsin. Opsin then changes shape and allows the ion balance in the retina membrane to change. This ion change signals "light" to the brain.

to darkness decreases. It now takes longer to see light again once it has already struck the eye, such as after seeing headlights of an oncoming car. An injection of vitamin A into the bloodstream can cure night blindness in a matter of minutes!

HEALTH AND MAINTENANCE OF CELLS

Vitamin A is very important for the maintenance of mucus-forming cells and the synthesis of various **mucopolysaccharide** substances. Without vitamin A, mucus-forming cells deteriorate and no longer synthesize mucus, a much-needed lubricant used throughout the body. In addition, the cells then make a hard protein, called keratin, which is typically found in hair and nails. The organ first affected by this loss of mucus-synthesizing capacity are the eyes, especially the cornea. Mucus in the eye serves several critical functions. It is required for the lubrication of the eye surface and the washing away of dirt and other particles that land on the eye.[4] In addition, mucus also contains an enzyme—lysozyme—that will degrade many foreign substances, most notably bacteria.

mucopolysaccharides Substances containing protein and carbohydrate parts, as found in bone and other organs.

In a vitamin A deficiency, the surface of the eye dries out, partly because of a lack of mucus production. This drying out develops in conjunction with the night blindness. The compromised protection of the eye will eventually allow dirt particles to scratch the dry surface of the eye. Bacteria then invade the scratch and cause an infection. White blood cells arrive at the infection site and make matters worse by synthesizing digestive enzymes that attack the eye itself. The lesions that develop on the eye as a result of this attack are first referred to as Bitot spots. Soon enough the infection spreads from one Bitot spot to the entire surface of the eye, eventually leading to blindness (Figure 12-3). This disease process is called **xerophthalmia,** which means "dry eye."[4] As stated earlier, this leads to blindness in millions of people throughout the world each year. Worldwide attempts to reduce this problem have included distribution of large doses of vitamin A twice yearly, as well as supplementing sugar and monosodium glutamate with vitamin A. These food vehicles are used because they are commonly consumed by the populations of less-developed nations.

xerophthalmia Literally "dry eye." A cause of blindness that results from a vitamin A deficiency. The specific cause is a lack of mucus production by the eye, which then leaves it more vulnerable to surface dirt and bacterial infections.

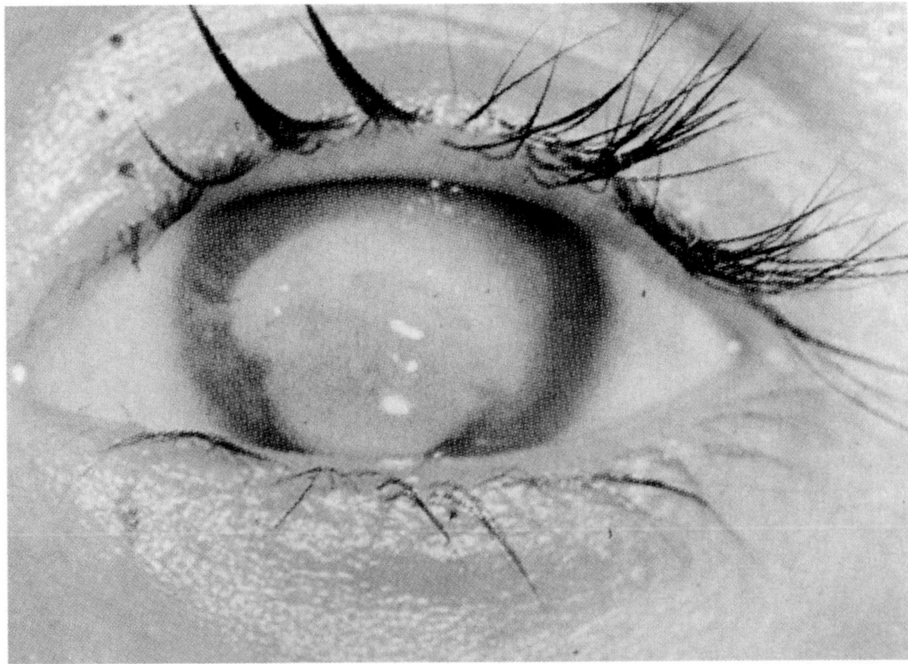

Figure 12-3 A vitamin A deficiency can eventually lead to blindness. Note the severe scar on this eye.

IMMUNE FUNCTION

The many results of vitamin A deficiency—insufficient mucus production in the intestines and lung cells, poor general health of many types of cells, and reduced activity of some immune cells, such as T-lymphocytes—leave a person very vulnerable to infections. That is why night blindness in children is accompanied by two to three times the normal risk for respiratory tract infections and corresponding mortality, and heightens the risk of dying from measles.[9]

GROWTH AND DEVELOPMENT

Vitamin A, specifically retinoic acid, is necessary for the growth.[33] The development of cells, specifically in the area of cellular differentiation, also relies on vitamin A nutriture. Cellular differentiation is the process by which specific regions of a cell's genetic material are expressed. The cell then produces specific proteins needed for that cell type. Now the cell can assume its specific role within a tissue, and in turn the body. Vitamin A travels into a cell and interacts with the DNA by attaching to special binding proteins in the cell nucleus to make this differentiation happen.[36] This effect of vitamin A is most easily demonstrated with laboratory animals; for example, vitamin A deficient animals cannot reproduce. Vitamin A can also help synthesize mucopolysaccharides that also influence cell metabolism.

Other types of growth are also enhanced by vitamin A. The resorption of old bone, which precedes deposition of new bone, requires bone cells that may be stimulated by vitamin A. The synthesis of some components of bone requires vitamin A (the later section on vitamin D and Chapter 14 contain more information about bone metabolism).

epithelial cells The surface cells that line the outside of the body and all external passages within it.

oxidizing agent In one sense, a substance capable of capturing an electron from another compound (see Appendix B).

CANCER PREVENTION

The ability of retinoids to influence cell development, coupled with their ability to increase immune system activity, could make these a valuable tool in the flight against cancer, especially skin, lung, bladder, and breast cancer. Researchers have been encouraged by animal studies, and also by the fact that most forms of cancer arise from cells that are influenced by vitamin A, known as **epithelial cells.** Active research with humans using forms of vitamin A is now under way in many centers in America. However, wait for those findings before embarking on personal experimentation with vitamin A as toxicity is a possible result. The Guide to Daily Food Choices is still the best nutrition tool for reducing cancer risk (see Chapter 13).

Carotenoid precursors of vitamin A, especially beta-carotene (in green and yellow vegetables) and lycopene (in tomatoes), may also help prevent cancer because they are excellent antioxidants.[6] The many double bonds present in some carotenoid molecules make them effective traps for free oxygen atoms and peroxides. These are two of many **oxidizing agents** that can probably initiate the cancer process.[18] (The section on vitamin E reviews the roles of antioxidants in greater detail.) Some evidence shows that regular consumption of vegetables high in carotenes decreases risk of lung cancer in smokers.[27] However, much more investigation is needed in this area before specific recommendations regarding carotenes and cancer prevention—other than eating fruits and vegetables regularly—can be made.

BETA-CAROTENE SOURCES FOR YOUR DIET

VEGETABLES:	FRUITS:
Spinach	Cantaloupe
Sweet potatoes	Mango
Carrots	Papaya
Butternut and Hubbard squash	Apricots
Collard greens	Nectarines
Dandelion greens	Peaches
Kale	
Turnip greens	
Beet greens	
Red peppers	
Swiss chard	
Bok choy	
Mustard greens	
Tomatoes	
Broccoli	

NOTE: Foods are ranked according to beta-carotene content from highest to lowest

VITAMIN A IN FOODS

Vitamin A in foods exists in the two forms already discussed: animal (preformed vitamin A) and plant (provitamin A). Preformed vitamin A is found in liver, fish oils, fortified milk, and eggs. Margarine is also fortified with vitamin A, but we don't eat enough to make it a significant source. Provitamin A carotenoids are mainly found in dark green and orange vegetables and some fruits. Carrots, spinach, squash, broccoli, papayas, and apricots are examples of such sources. About 50% of the vitamin A in our diets comes from animal (preformed vitamin A) sources; the rest comes as provitamin A.

Table 12-1 Good food sources of vitamin A activity, ranked by nutrient density

Food	Serving size to yield 333 RE*	Kcalories needed to yield 333 RE
Fried beef liver	1/9 ounce	4
Whole carrot	1/6 each	10
Baked sweet potato	1/6 each	16
Baked butternut squash	1/6 each	17
Cooked spinach	1/4 cup	20
Romaine lettuce	2.5 cups	23
Chopped green onions	1/3 cup	33
Cooked tomatoes	1 cup	40
Cantaloupe	1/4 each	43
Cooked turnip greens	1/2 cup	50
Mango	1/2 each	58
Papaya	2/3 each	64
Apricots	3 2/3 each	67
Cooked broccoli	1 1/3 cups	70
Cooked mustard greens	1/2 cup	83
Cooked asparagus	2 1/3 cups	98
Skim milk	2 1/3 cups	207
2% milk	2 1/3 cups	273

*1/3 of Adult male RDA

Note how few kcalories you need to consume to obtain the RDA if you choose the right vegetables and fruits. Other good but higher kcalorie vitamin A sources include liverwurst, nectarines, swordfish, pumpkin, and watermelon.

The major contributors of vitamin A—either preformed or provitamin A—to our diets are liver, carrots, eggs, tomatoes, vegetable soups, whole milk, and greens. Foods providing the highest nutrient density (per kcalorie) for vitamin A are carrots, liver, spinach and other greens, sweet potatoes, yellow squash, and romaine lettuce (Table 12-1). Several extremely rich sources of vitamin A, which are rarely consumed in the United States, are the oils from the livers of shark, marine fish, and mammals, such as polar bears. Note the concentrations of vitamin A in polar bear liver are often so great that its consumption can prove dangerously toxic and possibly deadly, as was seen in the nineteenth century by early explorers of the North Pole.

Not all the carotenoids in fruits and vegetables yield vitamin A; an example is lycopene in tomatoes.

Beta-carotene accounts for some of the yellow-orange color of carrots. Such a yellow-orange color is often masked, however, by dark-green chlorophyll pigments in vegetables such as broccoli. These foods then also have provitamin A. Consuming a varied diet rich in green vegetables and carrots ensures sufficient sources for meeting vitamin A needs.

RETINOL EQUIVALENTS (RE)

Most nutrient levels in foods were formerly expressed in crude **international units (IU).** These were usually based on the different growth rates animals showed when fed different amounts of a specific nutrient or food. Today we can precisely measure nutrient quantities, and so milligrams (1/1000 of a gram) and micrograms (1/1,000,000 of a gram) have replaced international units. Some food labels still show the older IU values for nutrients because the U.S. RDA is based on the RDAs from 1968, which used the IU system. The current RDAs do not.

international unit (IU) A crude measure of vitamin activity often based on the growth rate of animals. Today these units have been replaced by more precise microgram quantities.

For vitamin A, the new unit of measurement is the retinol equivalent (RE), which is basically 1 microgram of retinol. In this system, 6 micrograms of beta-carotene equals 1 microgram of vitamin A activity. In addition, 12 micrograms of

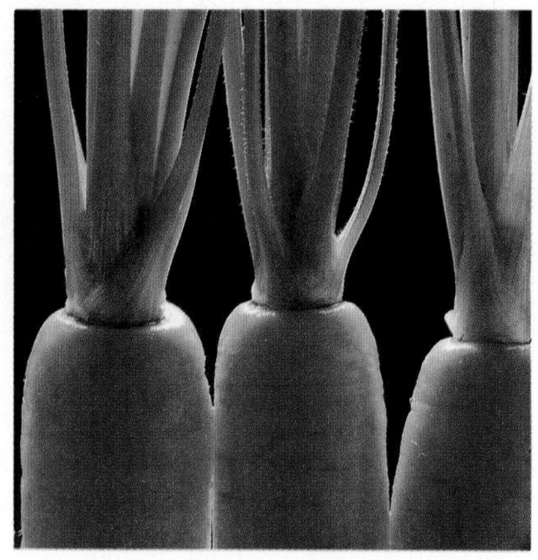

Carrots are a rich source of beta-carotene. Make them a regular part of your diet.

Conversion Values for Vitamin A

Compound with vitamin A activity	Micrograms	=	RE	=	IU
Retinol	1.0		1.0		3.3
Beta-Carotene	6.0		1.0		10.0
other carotenoids (alpha-, delta-, etc)	12.0		1.0		10.0
Mixture of both preformed and provitamin	—		1.0		5.0

any other provitamin A carotenes (alpha, delta, or others) are needed to yield 1 microgram of vitamin A activity. Total retinol equivalents (RE) in a food are then calculated by adding the actual weight of retinol (preformed vitamin A) within a food to the adjusted weight values for the provitamin A carotenoids also found within that same food (see above).

Relative to preformed vitamin A, the beta-carotene measurement is divided by 6 to compensate for both its poorer absorption and its incomplete conversion into vitamin A. The other carotene measurements are divided by 12 because these forms are not so active as the beta form. Actually, these values—6 and 12—are our best educated guesses, based on incomplete knowledge.

A good translation formula for older IUs to newer REs equates 1 RE of vitamin A to 5 IU of vitamin A if based on a mixture of preformed and provitamin A. Otherwise, 3.3 IU of preformed vitamin A alone equals 1 RE.

RDA FOR VITAMIN A

The current RDA for vitamin A for adults is 1000 RE for men and 800 RE for women. (Throughout the next four chapters, refer to the inside cover for vitamin recommendations for other ages and to Appendix D for Canadian recommendations.) The recommendation approximates the average intake for adult men and women in the United States. In the older system, the RDA value is 5000 IU for men and 4000 IU for women.

Most adults in the United States have liver reserves that are three to five times greater than they need to provide for good health. The use of supplements of vitamin A by most people is then completely unnecessary.[8]

AMERICANS AT RISK FOR A VITAMIN A DEFICIENCY

Measuring serum vitamin A levels is one way to assess a person's status. However, this is an insensitive measure since serum levels do not fall until vitamin A stores in the liver are very low.

Poor vitamin A status may be seen in preschool children who do not eat enough vegetables. The urban poor, the elderly, and adults who have alcoholism or who have liver disease (which limits vitamin A storage) can also show poor vitamin A status, especially with respect to stores. Finally, children with severe fat malabsorption, as in cases of celiac disease and cystic fibrosis, may also show a vitamin A deficiency.

Parents and other caregivers often encourage their children to eat vegetables. Besides contributing to good food habits, this practice helps them take in enough vitamin A. Adults provide important role models for children, and adults can positively influence children's eating habits by eating as they want the children to eat.

TOXICITY FROM EXCESSIVE VITAMIN A

teratogen An agent that causes physical defects in a developing fetus.

As we mentioned, toxicity symptoms from excessive vitamin A can appear with long-term supplement use at just ten times the RDA (Figure 12-4). Three kinds of vitamin A toxicity exist: acute, chronic, and **teratogenic** (causing fetal deformities). Acute toxicity is caused by the ingestion of one very large dose of vitamin A or of several large doses taken over several days. The signs of acute toxicity are largely manifestations of central nervous system abnormalities. Once the dosing is stopped, these signs disappear. Extraordinarily large doses, however, can cause death.

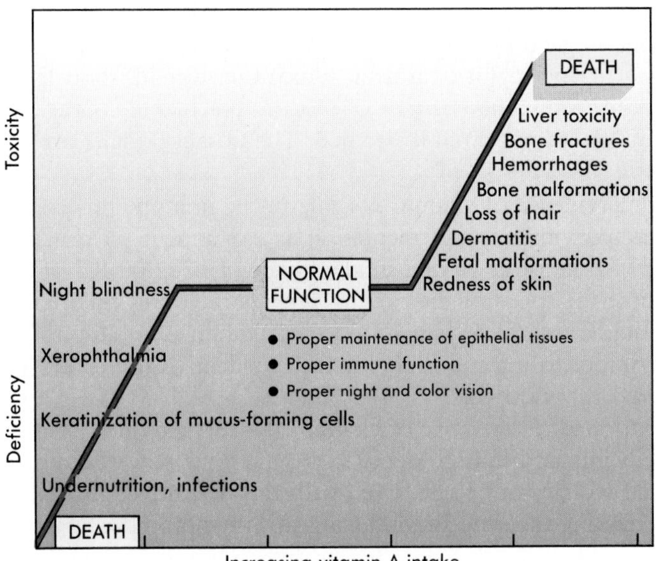

Figure 12-4 Consuming the right amount of vitamin A is critical to overall health. A very low (deficient) and a very high (toxic) vitamin A intake can produce damaging symptoms and even lead to death. The severity of effects and the intake range vary for individuals.

Chronic toxicity, which is much more common than acute toxicity, results from ingesting excessive doses of vitamin A on a regular basis during a period of weeks to years.[1] The symptoms range in infants and adults from bone pain, loss of appetite, headache, dry skin, and hair loss to increased liver size and vomiting. Treatment is simply to withdraw the supplement. Symptoms then decrease over the next few weeks to a month as blood levels fall to normal range. However, permanent damage to the liver, bones, and eyes, as well as recurrent joint and muscle pain, can occur.

A few individuals suffer signs of chronic vitamin A toxicity on relatively low daily intakes of vitamin A; for example, less than six times the adult male RDA. Such persons probably suffer from vitamin A intolerance, which seems to have a genetic basis and often is exacerbated by other clinical problems. These cases, although rare, are nonetheless worthy of note. In addition, the elderly as a group are more susceptible to toxic reactions than younger people.

The most serious and tragic effects of hypervitaminosis A are teratogenic, most notably birth defects. Vitamin A and its related medicinal forms, all-trans retinoic acid (tretinoin) and 13-cis retinoic acid (isotretinoin), have long been known to cause abortion and birth defects in experimental animals. The risk was recently highlighted in a study of a group of pregnant women taking large doses of isotretinoin for acne. Their offspring showed birth defects in the head, probably because neural crest cells, which are important in the development of the head and brain, are known to be very sensitive to excess amounts of vitamin A. Only a few cases of a clear relationship between birth defects and excessive intakes of vitamin A, as distinguished from medicinal forms, such as isotretinoin, have been reported.

Carotenoids in great amounts from foods will not readily result in toxicity. Their rate of conversion into vitamin A (retinol) is relatively slow. In addition, the efficiency of carotene absorption from the small intestine decreases markedly as the oral intake increases. Thus nature protects us from any serious toxic effects from dietary carotenes.

If someone consumes large amounts of carrots (in the form of carrot juice, for example) or if infants eat a great deal of squash, the high carotene levels in the bloodstream that result can turn skin a yellow-orange color. The result is termed **hypercarotenemia** (or just carotenemia). Recall "hyper" means high and "emia" means in the bloodstream. The person appears to have jaundice, but unlike a case of jaundice, the sclerae (whites of the eyes) are white (instead of yellow) and the liver does not enlarge. Again, this is thought to cause no harm.

hypercarotenemia High level of carotene in the bloodstream, usually caused by a diet high in carrots or squash, or by taking beta-carotene supplements.

MEDICINAL USAGE OF LARGE VITAMIN A DOSES

In children, one single dose of 60,000 RE has been used for the possible prevention of vitamin A deficiency. This treatment, which causes mild, short-lived side effects in some children, is common as part of medical practice in countries where foods high in vitamin A are not often consumed. The dosage should last the child for 3 to 6 months.

In addition, evidence of vitamin A's role in the immune processes has recently led researchers to examine supplementation as a treatment for childhood infection and disease.[9,33] Administration of a single dosage of 120,000 RE of vitamin A was found to double the speed of the healing process in young children with measles. More interestingly, the researchers found that vitamin A's ability to greatly reduce infant susceptibility to infection may be independent of the child's present status with respect to other nutrients.

Recently, derivatives of vitamin A have been put into creams (Retin-A) that manufacturers claim will reduce some effects of aging on the skin. Note that if one is already deeply wrinkled, these creams won't be the answer. In addition, limiting sun exposure and using sun blocks are much better preventive measures.

As we mentioned, a derivative of vitamin A—13-cis retinoic acid (Accutane)—is an oral medicine used in high doses to treat serious acne. Taking high doses of vitamin A itself would not be safe. Even with this derivative, physicians walk a fine line between treating the acne and inducing toxic symptoms. The person must also limit sun exposure because skin is quite sensitive to sunburn when this drug is used. Furthermore, as noted, women must not be pregnant or become pregnant while using this medication because it carries a very high risk for causing fetal malformations.

CONCEPT CHECK

Vitamin A in the diet comes in two forms: retinoids (preformed vitamin A) and carotenoids (provitamin A). Vitamin A is important for maintaining vision and mucus-forming cell activity in the body, ensuring the health of the immune system, and directing aspects of growth and development. Carotenoid intake is associated with a reduced risk of developing some forms of cancer. Major food sources of vitamin A include liver, carrots, eggs, tomatoes, milk, and many vegetables. Americans most at risk for poor vitamin A status are preschool children, because of insufficient intakes or fat malabsorption, and adults with alcoholism. Vitamin A can be quite toxic, even at dosages only about ten times the RDA, especially during pregnancy.

Vitamin D

Vitamin D has a somewhat questionable status as a vitamin. Unlike the other vitamins, vitamin D is also a hormone. It is considered a hormone because, in the presence of sunlight, skin cells are capable of synthesizing a sufficient supply of vitamin D for the body (Figure 12-5). This vitamin D is then metabolically activated to its final hormone form by other tissues and then ultimately delivered to its target organs, primarily the bones, kidneys, and intestine. The amount of sun exposure needed to produce vitamin D depends on the darkness of the skin: young light-skinned people need approximately 15 minutes a day in the sun, while dark-skinned people need more sun exposure. The process is also more efficient in younger people than in the elderly.[35]

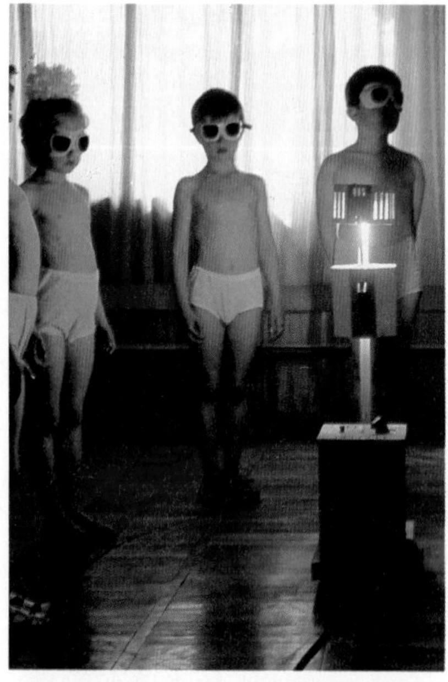

Figure 12-5 Who's got the tanning oil? Russia endures a long winter. These kids are exposed to a quartz lamp to provide the vitamin D synthesis they would normally experience from playing outdoors.

Anyone who does not receive enough sunshine to make vitamin D must have a dietary source of vitamin D. For these people, vitamin D is actually a vitamin. To discover why the vitamin nature of vitamin D is emphasized more than its hormonal nature see the Nutrition Focus on the history of vitamin D.

SYNTHESIS OF VITAMIN D

The starting product for vitamin D synthesis in the body is 7-dehydrocholesterol, a derivative of cholesterol (Figure 12-6). In a two-step process, sunshine (specifically, ultraviolet light with a wavelength of 282 nanometers) first strikes the skin and opens up a ring on the 7-dehydrocholesterol molecule. The compound produced will then slowly convert itself in the second step into vitamin D (cholecalciferol) over a span of 36 hours.[35]

Staying too long in the sun causes the skin to make, in addition to vitamin D, other related compounds, such as lumisterol. These other products probably protect us from making too much vitamin D, which otherwise could then result in

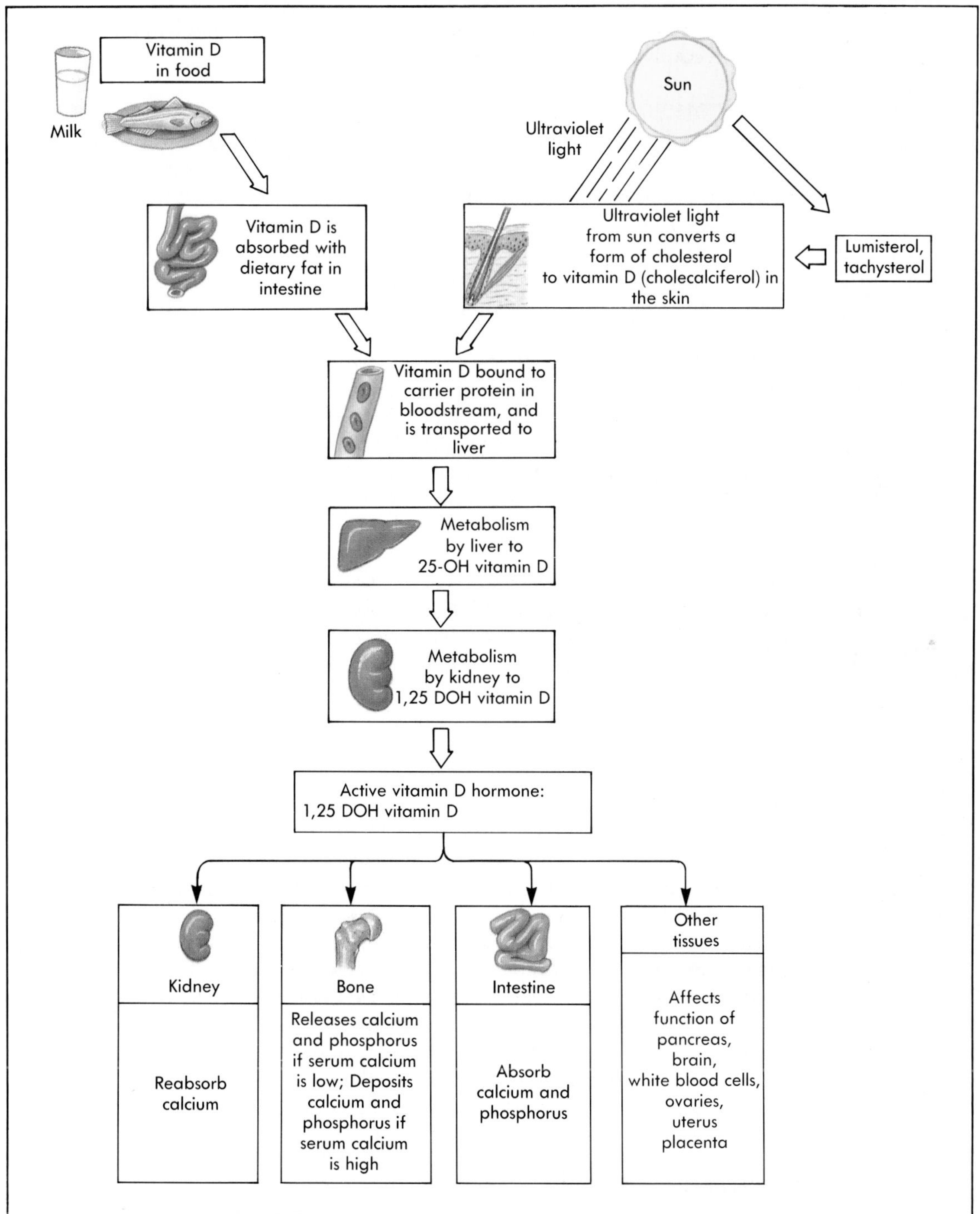

Figure 12-6 The many facets of vitamin D metabolism. Note that when made by the body using sunshine, vitamin D is actually a hormone.

vitamin D toxicity, Over time, these other compounds can be converted back into vitamin D.

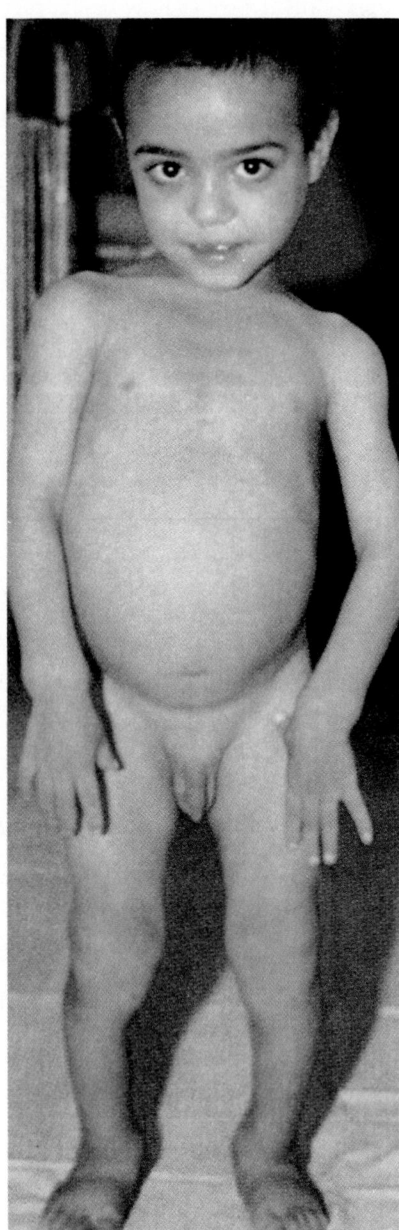

Figure 12-7 The bowed legs of rickets—the vitamin D deficiency disease.

FORMING THE ACTIVE VITAMIN D HORMONE

To form the active hormone, vitamin D has to have two hydroxyl groups (-OH) added to it. The liver adds the first hydroxyl group to form 25-hydroxy vitamin D. The second hydroxyl group is then added primarily by the kidney to form 1,25-dihydroxy vitamin D. The final compound formed depends on which type of vitamin D begins the process. The animal form (the one humans make), cholecalciferol (or D_3), makes 1,25-dihydroxy cholecalciferol, known as **calcitriol.** The plant form of vitamin D, ergosterol (or D_2), yields 1,25-dihydroxy ergocalciferol. Both compounds work effectively in humans.

FUNCTIONS OF VITAMIN D

The classical function of the vitamin D hormone calcitriol is to help regulate calcium and bone metabolism. To do this, it performs a variety of functions: Vitamin D helps regulate absorption of calcium and phosphorus from the intestine, it reduces kidney excretion of calcium, and it helps regulate the amount of calcium in the bones.

The vitamin D hormone calcitriol probably increases calcium and phosphorus absorption in the small intestine by means of two separate mechanisms. In one process, calcitriol travels into the nucleus of the intestinal cell to direct the DNA to synthesize a variety of calcium-transport proteins, including one that binds calcium.[23] These proteins then increase calcium and phosphorus absorption from the intestine. In the other process, calcitriol alters the characteristics of intestinal cell membranes, allowing more passive calcium absorption into the intestinal cells. Researchers think this second mechanism must be at least partially responsible for enhanced calcium absorption. This is because after calcitriol treatment, calcium absorption increases even before the calcium-binding proteins appear in the cell.[2]

RICKETS AND OSTEOMALACIA

The net result of calcitriol action is to increase calcium and phosphorus deposition in bones. Without adequate calcium and phosphorus deposition, bones weaken and bow under pressure. When these symptoms occur in a child, the disease is called **rickets** (Figure 12-7). Symptoms of rickets include enlarged head, joints, and rib cage, a deformed pelvis, and bowed legs.

The diets of infants, particularly, and of others as well, should contain a food or supplement source of vitamin D if sufficient exposure to sunlight is not possible. This is especially important for breast-fed infants in their first 6 months of life and for elderly people. Note that both human milk and cow's milk are not naturally good sources of vitamin D. Store-purchased milk is fortified—the vitamin D is added. Today, rickets is most commonly associated with fat malabsorption, as is seen in children with cystic fibrosis.

Rickets in adults is called **osteomalacia,** which means "soft bones." It can cause fractures in the hip, spine, and other bones. (Do not confuse this with the disease osteoporosis, which we discuss in Chapter 14). Osteomalacia in adults most likely occurs in people with kidney, stomach, gallbladder, or intestinal disease (especially when most of the intestine has been removed), and with cirrhosis of the liver. These diseases affect both vitamin D metabolism and calcium absorption. Combinations of sun exposure and/or treatment with calcitriol can be used in these cases.

calcitriol The active hormone form of vitamin D (1,25-dihydroxy vitamin D)—not to be confused with calcitonin, the hormone that also affects calcium utilization.

rickets A disease characterized by softening of the bones due to poor calcium deposition. This deficiency disease arises from lack of vitamin D activity in the body.

CALCITRIOL, PARATHYROID HORMONE, AND CALCITONIN: A BALANCE

The vitamin D hormone calcitriol works in conjunction with parathyroid hormone and the hormone calcitonin to maintain the critical homeostasis with respect to

NUTRITION FOCUS

Solving the Rickets Mystery

Rickets was first described in England about 1650. The "English disease" spread throughout Europe in the years following, mostly due to the pall of coal smoke that flooded Europe during the Industrial Revolution. In the early 1800s a German town called Wezlar was described as follows: "The children must sit indoors, which ends in death, or if they continue to live, they develop thick joints, cease to be able to walk, and have deformed legs. The head becomes large and even the vertebral column bends. It comes to pass that such children sit often for many years without being able to move; at times they cease to grow and are merely a burden to those about them."

As early as 1888, researchers noted that animals in the London Zoo contracted rickets, while those in the wild never did. This gave rise to the hypothesis that rickets was due to confinement. The long, cold winter months in Europe kept people indoors, and this was thought to bring on rickets. Physicians in Germany noted that children that were born in the fall and then died in the spring had rickets, while those who were born in the spring and then died in the fall were free of the disease.

When the English missionary Theobald Palm traveled to Japan in 1890, he was struck by the absence of rickets among the Japanese compared with the children of England and Scotland. He, too, deduced that rickets was caused by confinement, especially by isolating the children from the benefits of sunlight.

By early 1900s, it became increasingly clear to many physicians that sunlight had the power to prevent and cure rickets. However, there was no way to provide this sunlight during the long European winters. Then in 1919, a Berlin physician tried the light from a mercury-vapor quartz lamp—which includes the ultraviolet wavelengths—on four cases of advanced rickets in children. He found that this exposure completely cured rickets within 2 months.

In 1924, other researchers found that ingesting linseed, cottonseed, or yeast radiated with ultraviolet wave lengths cured rickets. It became increasingly clear that there was a relationship between sunlight and rickets. To further make that point, scientists showed that the incidence of rickets was closely tied to residing in the major smoke-filled industrial areas of England, and was not found as frequently in rural areas.

Vitamin D becomes a vitamin

In 1919, Sir Edward Mellanby showed that a particular diet could cause rickets in dogs. He then found that cod liver oil could cure the rickets. He hypothesized that a substance or "vitamine" in cod liver oil cured rickets.

The idea that rickets was due to a vitamin deficiency reflected the tenor of the times. Casimir Funk and others had recently established the "vitamine" theory—that substances vital to health were contained in foods. The British Medical Research Committee was excited about this work on rickets and in turn endorsed the notion that rickets was a nutritional deficiency disease.

Is vitamin D a vitamin?

It is clear that sunlight alone, irrespective of diet, can cure rickets. But because of the early influence of important researchers, such as Mellanby, and powerful organizations, such as the British Medical Research Committee, people now think of vitamin D as primarily a vitamin. As mentioned at the outset of this chapter, vitamin D is not a vitamin for many people. It is a vitamin for the homebound and shut-in, and maybe for people who live in very northern climates (especially the elderly) and who receive little sunlight in the wintertime. But many of us in the temperate world can make enough vitamin D every sunny day that we step outside.

serum calcium levels and bone mineralization (see Chapter 14 for a detailed description of bone mineralization).[14]

When serum calcium levels are low, the parathyroid gland releases parathyroid hormone to increase the synthesis of the active vitamin D hormone (calcitriol) via the two step process involving both the liver and kidneys. The calcitriol will, in turn, bind to DNA in bone-resorbing cells to activate them, in addition to reducing calcium loss in the kidneys. The net effect of both of these actions is to increase serum calcium. When these hormonal actions eventually raise serum calcium, further production of parathyroid hormone decreases, and this in turn reduces further calcitriol synthesis[26] (Figure 12-6).

On the other hand, if serum calcium levels are high, the thyroid gland releases the hormone calcitonin. Calcitonin signals the kidneys to add a hydroxyl group to vitamin D at a position that will inactivate it. The kidneys hydroxylate the 25-hydroxy cholecalciferol that was produced in the liver at the "24" position instead

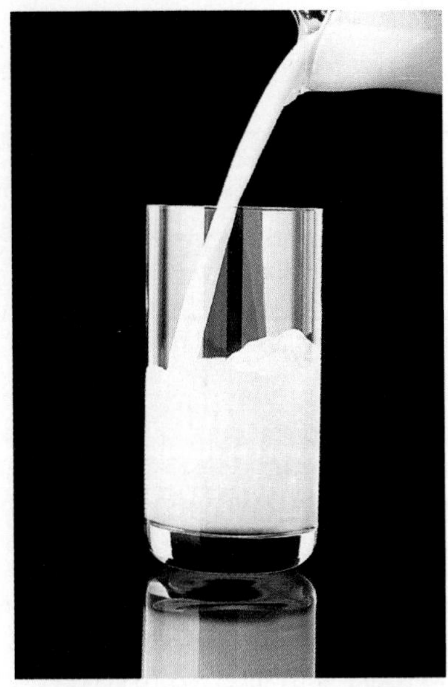

Milk is often fortified with vitamin D, which is important especially for people who receive little sun exposure.

of the more active "1" position, forming 24,25-dihydroxy D_3. In addition, calcitonin inhibits bone demineralization by halting the action of the bone-resorbing cells. Together, these actions lower serum calcium levels.

AN EVEN LARGER ROLE FOR VITAMIN D?

It was once thought that vitamin D's only significant role was in regulating calcium metabolism. However, recent research is on the brink of ushering in a new era concerning vitamin D's known functions. The vitamin D hormone calcitriol may ultimately control part of the differentiation of all the cells within its range of target tissues. Again, differentiation is a maturation process by which a cell produces specific proteins in effort to assume a final and specific function within a tissue. Calcitriol is capable of influencing differentiation and function in cells of the intestine, skin, immune system, and bones.[26] More interestingly, vitamin D is capable of influencing differentiation in some cancer cells, such as skin cancer cells, bone cancer cells, and breast cancer cells. However, it is not yet entirely clear how vitamin D regulates this differentiation or how significant its action may be on tissues, other than those actions associated with its classical roles. In any event, these findings certainly have awakened interest in a vitamin about which we used to think we knew almost everything.

VITAMIN D IN FOODS

When exposure to sunshine does not create vitamin D sufficient to meet a person's needs, fatty fish (fish oils) and fortified milk serve as the most nutrient-dense sources (Table 12-2). In the United States, milk is fortified with 10 micrograms (400 IU) per quart, and in Canada the amount is 9 micrograms (360 IU) per quart. Eggs, butter, liver, and many fortified breakfast cereals contain vitamin D, but require too great a serving size to be considered significant sources. There are so few foods containing vitamin D that food tables rarely list sources.

RDA FOR VITAMIN D

The RDA for adults for vitamin D varies from 5 to 10 micrograms per day (200 to 400 IU per day). Recall that young light-skinned people can make this amount of vitamin D in about 15 minutes of sun exposure on just the face and hands.[35]

AMERICANS AT RISK OF VITAMIN D DEFICIENCY

Studies suggest that particular groups—elderly people, infants that are only breast fed, or anyone else who both stays inside most of the day and ingests little or no

Table 12-2 Food sources of vitamin D, ranked by nutrient density

Food	Serving size to yield* 3.33 micrograms	Kcalories needed to yield 3.33 micrograms
Eel, smoked	1/12 ounce	5
Cod liver oil	1/3 teaspoon	15
Herring	1/2 ounce	30
Baked salmon	1 ounce	63
Tuna fish	1 1/2 ounce	90
Sardines	1 2/3 ounces	100
Milk (fortified, skim)	1 1/3 cups	120
Margarine	2 tablespoons	203
Wheaties cereal	3 ounces	330

*1/3 of Adult RDA (higher limit)

Aside from fish and fortified milk, no other foods are good kcalorie bargains for vitamin D.

vitamin D—are at risk for developing a vitamin D deficiency.[14] These people need either a predictable amount of sun exposure or a regular food (or supplemental) source of vitamin D.[10,31] People who suffer from severe fat malabsorption, such as children with cystic fibrosis, should concentrate on getting their vitamin D from the sun.

Measuring the serum 25-hydroxy cholecalciferol is the best way to assess vitamin D status in the body.

VITAMIN D RESISTANCE

Some human bodies resist the action of vitamins, including vitamin D. Resistance to vitamin D can be caused either by a lack of calcitriol synthesis in the kidney or by an inability of calcitriol to bind to **receptors** throughout the body. In both cases, the treatment is a large daily dose of calcitriol. This treatment works fine in the first case, but is not so successful in the other.

receptor A site on or in a cell where compounds (such as hormones) bind. Cells that contain receptors for a specific compound are affected by that compound.

TOXICITY OF VITAMIN D

Vitamin D is a very toxic substance. An intake of just five times the RDA can be toxic in children if consumed regularly. Anyone who needs to supplement the diet should consider a dosage not higher than the RDA, 5 to 10 micrograms per day. Consuming more than 25 micrograms (1000 IU) of vitamin D per day requires close scrutiny by a physician. The main symptom of toxicity is overabsorption of calcium, and eventual calcium deposits in the kidneys and other organs. The person will also suffer the typical symptoms of **hypercalcemia**—weakness, loss of appetite, diarrhea, vomiting, mental confusion, and increased urine output. Calcium deposits in organs cause local cell death. Additional symptoms will then result from this cell death.

hypercalcemia A high level of calcium in the bloodstream that can lead to loss of appetite, calcium deposits in organs, and other health problems.

CONCEPT CHECK

Vitamin D is a vitamin only for people who fail to produce enough from sunlight. Using a form of cholesterol, most people can synthesize adequate vitamin D by the interaction of sunlight on their skin. The vitamin D is later activated by the liver and kidneys to form the active hormone, calcitriol. This compound increases calcium absorption in the intestine and works with other hormones to maintain proper calcium metabolism in bones and other organs in the body. Calcitriol also appears to be an important regulator of cell differentiation in many areas of the body. Significant food sources of vitamin D are fish oils and fortified milk. Vitamin D is quite toxic; intakes greater than five times the RDA should be consumed only with a physician's guidance. Sun exposure likely poses no risk of vitamin D toxicity.

Vitamin E

Popular health food literature attests to many benefits of vitamin E, only some of which have been shown to be true for humans. A vitamin E deficiency in laboratory animals can result in muscular dystrophy, fetal resorption, and impotence. The link between vitamin E deficiency and fetal resorption in rats, noted in 1922, gave vitamin E its chemical name tocopherol, which means "to bring forth birth." However, although vitamin E is able to cure some human medical problems, that does not include any of these conditions.

What we call vitamin E is actually a family of compounds—the **tocopherol** series and the tocotrienol series. Various forms exist for both these major types of vitamin E. Some forms are more active than others, as you will soon see.

tocopherols The chemical name for some forms of vitamin E.

FUNCTIONS OF VITAMIN E

Vitamin E is one of the body's fat-soluble antioxidants; vitamin C is one water-soluble counterpart.[11] As noted earlier, an antioxidant has the ability to step between

Antioxidants: They Just Don't Get Any Respect!

PAUL B. ADDIS, PH.D.

One of the most exciting areas of research nowadays is that of antioxidants, including vitamin E and the provitamin A compound called beta-carotene. Other antioxidants include the water-soluble vitamin C and the synthetic antioxidants, such as BHA and BHT. Evidence strongly suggests that antioxidants, known to protect foods from development of rancidity, may also protect the body from harmful chemical reactions and possibly improve your long-term health.

At the outset I must clarify an important point. The RDAs for vitamins, including the antioxidants, are set to prevent nutritional-deficiency diseases, maintain some stores, but nothing more. In this discussion, we are considering the use of antioxidants to prevent cancer, coronary heart disease (CHD), and other diseases, usually of the chronic variety. Dietary supplementation with beta-carotene will not make you see better but may help you resist the development of CHD. Some would describe this as the use of nutrients as drugs (nutriceuticals). Keep in mind the objectives of the RDA and suggested levels of supplement intake discussed later are clearly different.

Antioxidants function chiefly to protect us and our food supply from the ravages of oxygen. How can this be? Oxygen is the most vital element in our environment; we can live for a year without vitamin A in our diet but only about 4 to 5 minutes without oxygen. How can something so vital be so toxic? The answer in part lies in the fact that under the right conditions oxygen becomes much more reactive, forming active oxygen species. These include singlet oxygen, hydrogen peroxide, superoxide anion radical, and hydroxyl radical. Other major compounds include ozone (O_3) and nitrogen-oxygen combinations that are important components of air pollutants. These compounds, sometimes working together with some common metals like copper, iron, and cobalt, attack an important group of tissue constituents—notably lipids—creating a number of deleterious effects. Stress, anesthesia, anticancer drugs, pain killers, and even normal energy metabolism also will release free radicals in varying amounts. Evidence of free-radical damage to DNA is seen commonly in urine as excretion of altered genetic material occurs simultaneously with DNA repair.

Active oxygens attack firstly the polyunsaturated fatty acids, important components of phospholipid-rich cell membranes. Secondly, cholesterol, vitamins, and even nonlipids like proteins can be destroyed. The end products of these complex reactions are usually toxic to cells (cytotoxic). Some of these reaction products can react with DNA and therefore are considered carcinogenic.

Fortunately, a considerable amount of protection exists in the body in the form of antioxidants and certain enzymes, like glutathione peroxidase, catalase, and superoxide dismutase. These react directly with active oxygens or peroxides to reduce their reactivity and thereby help protect cells. Antioxidants like BHA, BHT, and vitamin E supply an electron (actually a hydrogen radical, $H^{\bullet}$) to stabilize free radicals. Vitamin C helps to regenerate vitamin E. Still other antioxidants, "chelators," tie up certain metals so that they cannot catalyze oxidation. With all of the foregoing protecting mechanisms available, do already healthy people need further protection in the form of supplementation?

First consider that CHD and cancer are the two biggest causes of death in the United States. Some types of cancer are related to free-radical production and most antioxidants are anticarcinogenic compounds for some types of cancer. A practical fact is that eating foods rich in vitamin C does appear to reduce the risk of cancer and that the vitamin C itself is the most likely component to explain this observation.

Antioxidants and CHD is an exciting new area of research that shows much promise. A great deal of evidence exists that supports the idea that lipid oxidation products are damaging to coronary arteries and that antioxidants help prevent such damage. Such arterial damage is the forerunner to atherosclerosis and CHD. It now appears that LDL must first undergo oxidation before plaque accumulations can occur. Because LDL is the primary carrier of fat-soluble vitamins it seems logical that antioxidant vitamin supplementation can fortify LDL with antioxidant power and increase resistance of LDL to oxidation. Epidemiological evidence has supported the concept that elevated dietary and serum levels of antioxidants are associated with reduced risk of CHD.

One key aspect of CHD virtually ignored by the media is the function of platelets. These blood clotting agents create blood clots that trigger the heart attack by lodging in arteries partially blocked by plaque. Again, antioxidants to the rescue! Vitamin E reduces the tendency of platelets for form clots.

Overall, the risks of antioxidant supplementation are virtually nonexistent if some knowledge and common sense are applied. Vitamin E toxicity has been noted in rats but at a level equivalent to a 100-kg (220-pound) man taking 13 pounds of pure vitamin E in a month! Likewise, people taking extremely high levels of vitamin C and beta-carotene are at risk for various disagreeable effects.

Conditions that might suggest the use of supplemental antioxidants include smoking, living in a smoggy environment and a familial risk for CHD and/or cancer. Since life itself is associated with free-radical production, everyone could benefit.

How much to take? First, I should state that I do not recommend general supplementation of vitamins and minerals. Given that, and after much study on my part and consultation with learned colleagues, I have come to a recommendation that is simple, inexpensive, and reasonable. First, be sure to eat a lot of fruits, vegetables, and whole-grain foods. Second, 1 to 2 grams of vitamin C, 50 to 100 milligrams of vitamin E, and 20 milligrams of beta-carotene per day may offer some additional protection. Smokers may need more.

Dr. Addis is a Professor of Food Science and Technology and a Professor of Nutrition and Dietetics at the University of Minnesota. His research involves antioxidants and oxidation of food constituents.

Supplemental Antioxidants: No proven panacea

DONALD B. McCORMICK, PH.D.

It is clear that many natural compounds have different actions when consumed in amounts significantly above those levels associated with basic physiologic needs in healthy individuals. However, this pharmacologic loading often proves harmful, even for compounds that are essential nutrients when provided at lower levels. Classic examples include vitamins A, D, and B-6; most of the minerals; and even macronutrients, especially fats. Such findings should lead us to exercise some caution with nutrient supplementation. In spite of this, there are those who would push for ingestion of levels of nutrients well above that found in typical well-balanced diets.

By far the majority of us seem able to live healthy lives by eating a variety of foods that provide more than ample quantities of nutrients. There is, however, a fraction of our population who for medical reasons, namely those with impaired absorption or problems of utilization, do require higher than normal dietary levels—supplements—of certain nutrients. Because of the examples of such uncommon but justified needs for supplement use, the lack of detailed knowledge that any given individual has for his or her specific nutrient needs, and the misunderstandings about RDAs and similar population-based recommendations, there is impetus for those with an insecurity borne of uncertainty to take supplements. Probably at least half of American adults have taken some nutrient supplements, often a multivitamin or vitamin-trace element mix, to be "on the safe side" in regards to their perception of what is needed for best health. Some commercial interests have indeed capitalized on this public concern for health, and the supplement business now runs into billions of dollars.

As stated by the *Surgeon General's Report on Nutrition and Health* (1988), nutrient supplements are usually safe in amounts corresponding to the RDAs, but such values are already set "to provide maximum benefit consistent with safety." It follows that there is no reason to believe larger doses will improve health in already healthy people, and excess is known to be harmful in some. This is reiterated by the *Diet and Health Report* (1989) from the Food and Nutrition Board, which again suggests that for the normal person "there are no demonstrated benefits of self supplementation beyond these (RDA) allowances." Nonetheless, vitamin supplements have been perceived by some in the public (and obviously the vitamin industry) as an ideal form of dietary self-therapy, and supplements continue to be so regarded (however correctly or incorrectly) in the prevention and even cure of certain chronic and age-related diseases.

The general antioxidant behavior of the fat-soluble vitamin E group, carotenoids including beta-carotene (a provitamin A form), and water-soluble vitamin C (L-ascorbic acid) is drawing renewed attention. This is because some of the process of aging and perhaps some age-related diseases, such as cancer and coronary heart disease may, in part, reflect oxidative damage to body constituents. The extrapolation of these possibilities has even led to fraudulent products sold for health promotion. These latter include superoxide dismutase (to enhance our ability to destroy harmful superoxide anion) and nucleic acids (to replace the damaged gene material). The fact that such ingested materials are broken down during digestion and cannot reach the intended area within cells to achieve what is claimed does not bother hucksters interested in sales.

In fairness, however, there is some mounting evidence that antioxidant vitamins and precursors may be able to provide some protection against oxidative stress, which in turn may be causally related to some disease processes. It may be instructive to consider a few such studies that point the way to encouraging possibilities, while at the same time emphasizing the incomplete stage of our knowledge in this area.

An eight-year study of over 87,000 women in the United States suggested a modest reduction in risk of heart attack by those taking more than 100 mg of vitamin E compared to those with intakes of 30 milligrams or less (RDA for adults is 8 to 10 milligrams). There was also a decrease in risk of stroke and heart attack from those on daily beta-carotene intakes of more than 15 to 20 milligrams compared to those with less than 6 milligrams per day. The investigators noted, however, that a randomized trial of such antioxidants will be needed to obtain conclusive evidence of a role in prevention of cardiovascular disease. As for the effect of the natural dietary antioxidants on cancer, data regarding vitamin E and beta-carotene as single agents in cancer care are too preliminary for conclusive evaluation. Even with vitamin C, where consumption of adequate amounts may be useful in prevention of certain tumors, such as gastric cancer that can be caused by nitrosamines, optimal dosage has not yet been proven to be higher than that achievable by consumption of a well-balanced diet containing foods rich in vitamin C, such as vegetables and fruits. Again, more studies are needed before overly zealous consumption of supplements is warranted.

Several unfortunate cases of self-prescribed "diet therapy" should serve to warn us of possible dangers. For example, administration of high levels of vitamin E can exacerbate blood coagulation defects in vitamin K-deficient individuals, including those who are given a vitamin K antagonist as medication to decrease chances for clots and ongoing risk of cardiovascular events. High amounts of vitamin C pose a risk for those who tend to overstore iron (hemochromatosis). Vitamin C can enhance the absorption of iron, as well as inhibit copper absorption.

From all of the above, it would seem more prudent to recognize we must learn more before any scientifically secure recommendation can be made about what, if any, supplementation is useful. Until then, most of us would be better served to abide by the proven recommendation of obtaining our nutrients by eating in moderation a variety of healthy foods.

Dr. McCormick is Fuller E. Callaway Professor and Chairman, Department of Biochemistry, Emory University School of Medicine, Atlanta, GA.

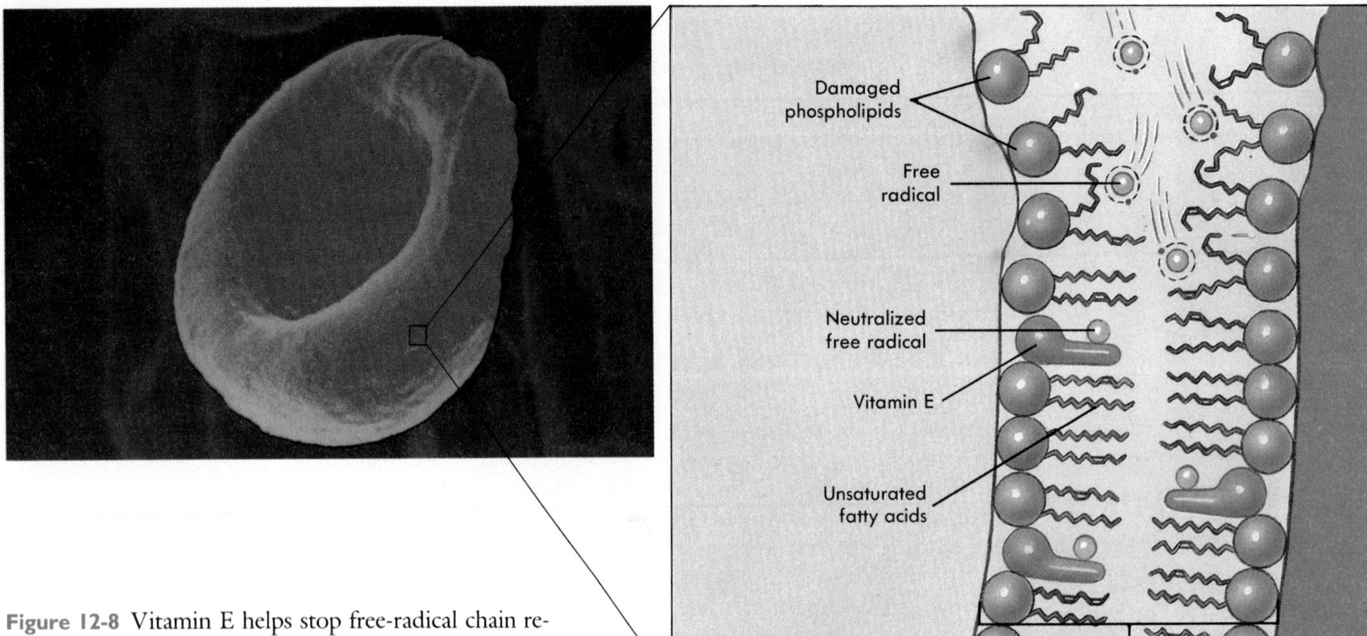

Figure 12-8 Vitamin E helps stop free-radical chain reactions. This should happen before much cell damage takes place, such as in a red blood cell membrane.

a compound seeking electrons and the compound's target molecule, such as a fatty acid in a cell membrane (Figure 12-8). Acting as an antioxidant, vitamin E resides in cell membranes and donates electrons (actually derivatives of hydrogen) to an electron-seeking compound, thus neutralizing it.[21] This then protects other molecules or parts of the cell from an attack by the electron-seeking compound.

free radical Short-lived form of compounds that exists with unpaired electrons. This imbalance causes it to have an electron-seeking nature, which can be very destructive to electron-dense areas of a cell, such as the DNA and cell membranes.

If vitamin E does not step in, the electron-seeking compound can pull electrons from cell membranes, DNA, and other electron-dense cell parts.[11] That either alters the cell DNA, which may increase the risk for cancer, or injures the cell membrane, possibly causing cell death and acceleration of the aging process.

One group of electron-seeking compounds likely to be found in cells are **free radicals.** These short-lived forms of compounds exist in a state in which an oxygen or carbon atom in the molecule contains an unpaired electron in its outer shell. Consequently, it seeks an electron to fill the missing space.[21] The special chemical natures of oxygen and carbon atoms allow them to readily form a free-radical structure. Often a free radical is generated by breaking a chemical bond in which each breakdown product takes an electron. That yields two compounds, each having one unpaired electron in an end atom of the molecule.

Free radicals are a necessary result of cell metabolism. But because free radicals cause chain reactions, it is very important for vitamin E to buffer their assault on cell membranes to prevent significant cell destruction. Within minutes, one free radical can generate thousands of others; a small amount of cell destruction can lead to great destruction.[21] Enzyme systems in the cell, such as superoxide dismutase, aid vitamin E in neutralizing free radicals. Vitamin E, when in action, is broken down itself and typically a derivative form is excreted. Some vitamin E can be recycled by the action of other antioxidants, such as vitamin C.

High levels of vitamin E are found in the lungs, which is good because oxygen is concentrated there. The lung needs protection from the oxygen. People who smoke need even more vitamin E because of the oxidant stress that smoking puts on the lung. A recent study, however, showed that even when consuming 240 times the adult RDA, smokers still had lower vitamin E concentrations in their lung fluids. Thus the safest way to protect the lungs is to not smoke.

PROTECTING RED BLOOD CELL MEMBRANES

A deficiency of vitamin E causes breakdown (hemolysis) of red blood cells, especially in infancy. The polyunsaturated fatty acids in the red blood cell membrane are very sensitive to attack by free radicals. Since vitamin E can neutralize these agents, it can protect the red blood cell membrane from damage.

Red blood cell hemolysis is common in premature infants for two reasons. First, they did not receive sufficient vitamin E from their mothers. Second, the rapid growth of the premature infant, coupled with the high oxygen concentration found in infant incubators, greatly increases the stress on red blood cells, raising the risk of free-radical damage. Special formulas and supplements for premature infants compensate for their lack of vitamin E. These products can reduce hemolysis of red blood cells and other deficiency symptoms, such as some eye disorders. But vitamin E treatment does not totally prevent the vitamin E-related disorders of prematurity. Hemolysis of red blood cells also occurs in adults who are deficient in vitamin E.

One way to assess the vitamin E status of a person is to incubate a sample of red blood cells with peroxide. After 3 hours the extent of red blood cell destruction is measured. A newer method uses the same procedure but instead measures the amount of a breakdown product of polyunsaturated fatty acids. These tests can be used in addition to measuring the serum vitamin E level.

OTHER ROLES FOR VITAMIN E

Vitamin E can help improve vitamin A absorption if the dietary intake of vitamin A is low. Vitamin E may also reduce platelet aggregation[29] and oxidation of the blood lipoprotein LDL, thereby lowering risk of heart disease.[13] Current studies are evaluating this possibility. In these cases vitamin E acts to protect carbon-carbon double bonds in the lipoprotein from damage. Vitamin E can also help protect the carbon-carbon double bonds in dietary unsaturated fatty acids. In addition, vitamin E is needed for iron metabolism in the cell and the maintenance of nervous tissues and immune function, again functioning in an antioxidant capacity.[15] In this role it may also reduce the risk of developing cataracts in the eye. [29,34]

Related to vitamin E's abilities as an antioxidant are its abilities to detoxify compounds, specifically substances that initiate the formation of free radicals. These include, but are not limited to ozone, lead and mercury, and compounds particularly toxic to the liver, such as benzene and carbon tetrachloride.[24]

Vitamin E has been promoted as an antiaging vitamin. This is because as cells age, they accumulate lipid breakdown products called lipofuscin (ceroid pigments). These appear as the brown spots on the skin, often called "liver spots." The ceroid pigments may then eventually reduce cell metabolism and lead to cell death. Unquestionably, consuming the RDA for vitamin E is important for minimizing lipid destruction by free radicals and, in turn, maintaining cell health. However, there is no clear evidence that supplementation beyond this amount reduces aging.

We suggest that if you really want to prevent the effects of aging, you begin by following the Guide to Daily Food Choices, see your physician regularly (for early diagnosis of health problems), don't smoke, limit your alcohol intake, maintain a desirable body weight, and stay physically active. These factors have a much greater influence on the rate of aging of Americans than does vitamin E.

Some of the mystery surrounding vitamin E stems from our incomplete understanding of this family of compounds. Many functions of vitamin E depend on its antioxidant ability. But others, such as the maintenance of male sexual function in rats, are unrelated to its antioxidant system. When questions persist concerning a vitamin's function, promoters of fad diets and health-food zealots are quick to suggest that the mystery powers of such vitamins can cure a myriad of diseases or provide other physical benefits. Such is the case with vitamin E.

THE MINERAL SELENIUM CAN SPARE SOME OF THE NEED FOR VITAMIN E

An enzyme in cells—**glutathione peroxidase**—converts peroxides into harmless forms of alcohols and water, in turn reducing the peroxide load in a cell. Peroxides tend to form free radicals. So with a decreased peroxide load, the tendency to form free radicals likewise decreases. Consequently the need for vitamin E decreases because fewer free radicals will be made.[11] Glutathione peroxidase may also regenerate vitamin E by donating electrons to it. The cellular enzyme catalase also helps destroy peroxides, specifically hydrogen peroxide.

glutathione peroxidase A selenium-containing enzyme that can destroy peroxides. It acts in conjunction with vitamin E to stabilize free radicals. Its activity may mask a vitamin E deficiency somewhat.

The enzyme glutathione peroxidase contains the mineral selenium. Adequate levels of selenium in the diet allow this enzyme to function at full speed, destroying

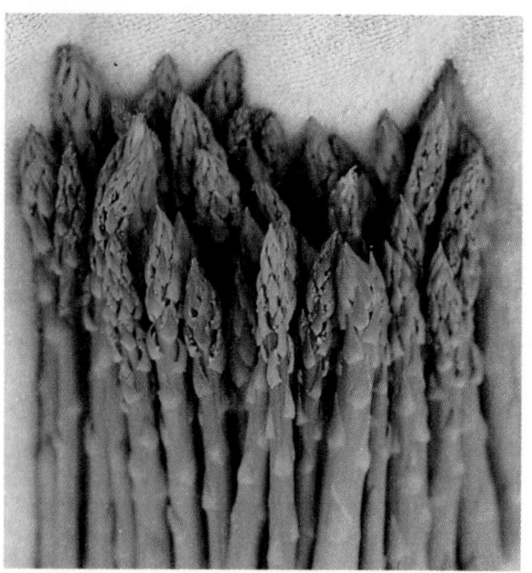

Asparagus is a nutrient-dense source of vitamin E.

peroxides, thereby sparing some of the need for vitamin E. Thus an adequate dietary intake of selenium reduces the need for vitamin E, whereas low selenium intake in the diet increases it.

VITAMIN E IN FOODS

The most nutrient-dense food sources of vitamin E are plant oils, some fruits and vegetables, such as peaches and asparagus, and margarine[20] (Table 12-3). In addition, grain meals, such as oatmeal and wheat germ, are good sources. However, in other grains the vitamin E is often lost in the milling process, and is not returned, such as in white flour. Animal fats have practically no vitamin E.

One reason to eat a variety of foods is to obtain the vitamin E spread throughout selections from the Guide to Daily Food Choices. A diet rich in fruits and vegetables, along with a tablespoon of plant oil in foods eaten each day, is especially effective in supplying an ample amount of vitamin E.

The actual vitamin E content of a food depends on how it was harvested, processed, stored, and cooked because vitamin E is very susceptible to destruction by oxygen, metals, light, and especially repeated use of oils in deep-fat frying. For healthy people, a varied diet supplies the vitamin E they need. Selenium, which spares the need for vitamin E, is found in cereals, meats, and seafoods.

Overall, the likelihood of finding signs of a vitamin E deficiency in the United States among healthy nonsmokers is very low. The Expert Opinions in this chapter discuss whether just trying to prevent deficiency symptoms is a sufficient course to take with this vitamin. It is important to note that beneficial effects of vitamin E and other antioxidants in counteracting free radical damage in biological systems will be most apparent only when viewed on a long-term basis, since free radical-related damage to cells needs to occur over time to be evident.

RDA FOR VITAMIN E

The RDA for adults for vitamin E is 10 milligrams per day for men and 8 milligrams per day for women. This is about how much we usually eat each day, but some adults show lower intakes. Eating more fruits and vegetables would be a good low-calorie way for these people to obtain vitamin E. To convert from the older IU

Table 12-3 Good food sources of vitamine E, ranked by nutrient density

Food	Serving size to yield 3.33 milligrams*	Kcalories needed to yield 3.33 milligrams
Wheat germ oil	⅓ teaspoon	14
Corn oil†	1 teaspoon	40
Wheat germ	1½ tablespoons	45
Sunflower oil	½ tablespoons	50
Soybean oil	½ tablespoons	50
Safflower oil	1½ teaspoons	60
Cooked asparagus	1⅙ cups	60
Cottonseed oil	2 teaspoons	80
Canned peaches	1 cup	118
Peanut oil	1 tablespoon	120
Margarine	1⅓ tablespoons	233
Peanuts, roasted	1½ ounces	240
Oatmeal (cooked)	3 cups	550

*⅓ of Adult male RDA.
†Vitamin E is in other plant oils as well; these are just some examples.
This shows how important a tablespoon of oil a day is to our diets. For other sources of vitamine E, either the serving size and/or the kcalorie cost is too great.

system, 10 milligrams equals about 15 IU. A variety of forms of vitamin E exist. The RDA is based on alpha-tocopherol equivalents. Beta-tocopherol, delta-tocopherol, and gamma-tocopherol are not as active. Once a food's content is calculated in alpha-tocopherol equivalents, this amount can be called vitamin E.

In 1980, the RDA for vitamin E was decreased from previous recommendations. However, the U.S. RDA still uses the older 1968 value (20 milligrams). So current food labels, because they are based on a percentage of the older, larger value, understate the vitamin E contribution of foods. New labeling guidelines will soon correct this as RDI replace U.S. RDA (see Chapter 2).

Diets high in polyunsaturated fatty acids need to contain more vitamin E to protect all the double bonds present. So when consuming more vegetable oils, a person needs to also consume more vitamin E. Luckily, plant oils high in polyunsaturated fatty acids are also often high in vitamin E; thus things usually balance out. One exception is highly unsaturated fish oils. Used in greater amounts lately by some people in supplement form, these often contain very little vitamin E.

AMERICANS AT RISK FOR A VITAMIN E DEFICIENCY

Vitamin E deficiency is most likely to be found in people with a fat malabsorption syndrome, especially when accompanied by low serum selenium levels. Still, the effects or symptoms of a vitamin E deficiency may remain hidden for years. When the symptoms do appear they are likely to take the form of increased red blood cell fragility and subtle neurological disorders affecting the spinal cord and the retina.[15] In addition, recent studies indicate a link between low vitamin E levels and an increased risk for gastrointestinal and other cancers. This was found to be especially true for men and women with low serum selenium levels.[17]

By far those running the greatest risk for a vitamin E deficiency are premature infants or infants born with a fat-malabsorption condition—like cystic fibrosis. The neurological symptoms will appear rapidly and will only be partially reversible if not treated quickly. And as previously mentioned, these infants may also become anemic due to the increased fragility of their red blood cell membranes.

TOXICITY OF VITAMIN E

Vitamin E is relatively nontoxic. Some studies show that amounts in excess of approximately 500 milligrams per day of vitamin E can cause nausea, weakness, headache, diarrhea, and fatigue. In addition, excessive amounts of vitamin E can antagonize vitamin K's role in the clotting mechanism, especially if taken in conjunction with anticoagulant medications (see the following section on vitamin K). However, other studies show that intakes up to 800 milligrams may be safe for months in people who are not taking anticoagulant medicines. People with diseases such as phlebitis, in which blood clots form easily, may sometimes benefit from large supplements of vitamin E, but should follow such a regimen under the careful eye of a physician. Otherwise, hemorrhages may result.

CONCEPT CHECK

Vitamin E functions primarily as an antioxidant. It can donate electrons to electron-seeking compounds, such as free radicals. By neutralizing free radicals, vitamin E helps prevent cell destruction, especially the destruction of red blood cell membranes. The breakdown of red blood cell membranes occurs with a vitamin E deficiency. The best sources of vitamin E are plant oils. The more plant oils consumed, the more vitamin E needed to protect the double bonds found in plant oils. However, the vitamin E content in plant oils is usually high. One reason to eat a variety of foods is to obtain the vitamin E spread throughout selections from typical foods, especially fruits and vegetables. For adults, people who smoke or show long-term fat malabsorption run the biggest risk of a vitamin E deficiency. In the former case, the best therapy is to stop smoking. Supplements are not that helpful.

Vitamin K

Vitamin K is vital for blood clotting. The K stands for koagulation, as it is spelled in Denmark. This is because a Danish researcher, Dam, first noted the relationship between vitamin K and blood clotting.

phylloquinone A form of vitamin K that comes from plants.

The family of compounds known as vitamin K include **phylloquinone** from plants and the menaquinones found in fish oils and meats. The menaquinones are also synthesized by bacteria in the human small intestine (Figure 12-1).

prothrombin A blood protein needed for blood clotting that requires vitamin K for its synthesis.

FUNCTIONS OF VITAMIN K

Vitamin K contributes specifically to the synthesis of several blood-clotting factors, including **prothrombin**(Figure 12-9). Vitamin K is needed for adding carbon dioxide molecules to these compounds, specifically on the amino acid glutamic acid (glutamate). This forms gamma-carboxyglutamate. In turn, these gamma-carboxyglutamate molecules give the protein its calcium-binding potential. This is an important ability if prothrombin is to participate in the blood-clotting cascade.[32] Vitamin K also adds carbon dioxide molecules to glutamate residues on proteins found in the bones, muscles, and kidneys, in turn imparting calcium-binding potential to those organs.

A deficiency of vitamin K most likely occurs when a person takes antibiotics or has severe fat malabsorption.[7,32] Antibiotic use destroys many bacteria in the intestines that normally account for half the vitamin K absorbed. It is critical to establish a vitamin K deficiency does not exist before a person undergoes surgery, otherwise excess bleeding is likely.

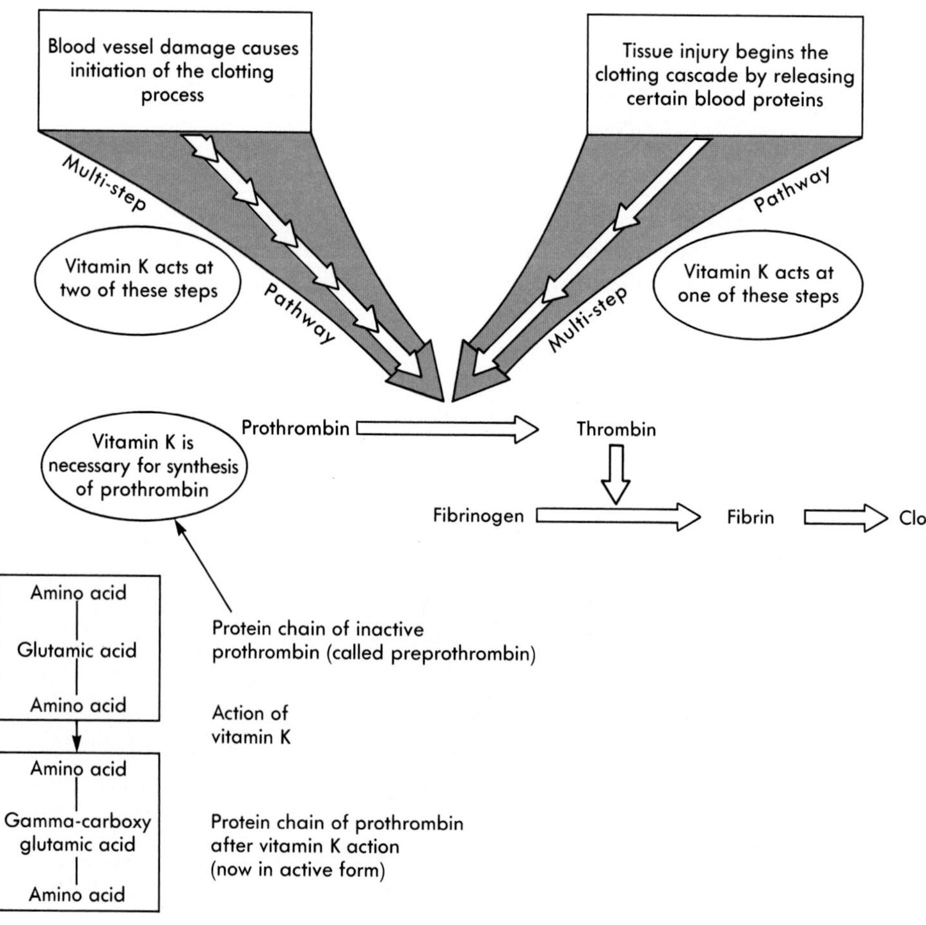

Figure 12-9 Forming a blood clot. This requires the participation of vitamin K in both the intrinsic and extrinsic blood clotting pathways.

Physicians use vitamin K's link to blood clotting to a practical advantage. Because the structure of vitamin K resembles those of the drugs dicumarol and warfarin, the drugs can antagonize the action of vitamin K and so act as potent anticoagulants. People who tend toward increased blood clotting greatly benefit from these drugs. However, people taking these medications must be warned against consuming supplements of vitamin K and foods especially rich in vitamin K, since that would reduce their action.

The most reliable clinical sign of a vitamin K deficiency is an increase in blood clotting or prothrombin formation time. The latter is a measure of how quickly prothrombin in the blood can form a clot. In addition, today the actual vitamin K and prothrombin levels in the bloodstream can be measured.

FOOD SOURCES OF VITAMIN K

The most nutrient-dense food sources of vitamin K are green, leafy vegetables, other vegetables such as peas, broccoli, and green beans, and liver (Table 12-4). Vitamin K is yet another reason to consume a diet rich in vegetables. Most vitamin K consumed in a day is gone by the next. However, vitamin K is so abundant in the diet that there is low risk of suffering a deficiency. Vitamin K is quite resistant to cooking losses.

Not much vitamin K is found in human milk. In addition, an unborn child is not well adapted to store vitamin K, nor has the gastrointestinal bacteria that adults can rely on to synthesize vitamin K. So at birth, infants run the risk of poor blood clotting and eventual hemorrhage due to a lack of vitamin K. To prevent this possible vitamin K deficiency condition, physicians routinely treat infants at birth with a form of vitamin K. This protection is intended to last until the infant's intestinal bacteria begin to synthesize vitamin K.

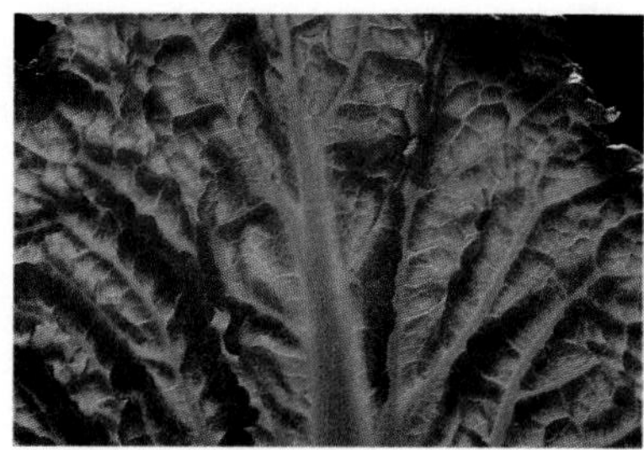

Green leafy vegetables supply much vitamin K.

RDA FOR VITAMIN K

The RDA vitamin K for adults is 60 to 80 micrograms per day. Our diets contain 300 to 500 micrograms per adult per day of vitamin K, so again a deficiency is very unlikely. However, excessive amounts of the fat-soluble vitamins A and E are known to antagonize the actions of vitamin K. Vitamin A is thought to interfere with the absorptive processes concerning vitamin K. Vitamin E's mechanism of antagonism, on the other hand, is not yet well understood. In either case, supplements of these vitamins poses a risk to vitamin K status.

Toxicity from vitamin K is highly unlikely because, although it is fat soluble, as noted before, it is readily excreted by the body. One medicinal form of vitamin K, menadione, can lead to toxicity. Symptoms include jaundice and a type of anemia.

Table 12-4 Good food sources of vitamin K, ranked by nutrient density

Food	Serving size to yield 27 micrograms*	Kcalories needed to yield 27 micrograms
Cooked turnip greens	2 teaspoons	3.3
Cooked kale	2 teaspoons	3.3
Cooked spinach	2 teaspoons	3.3
Cooked green peas	2 teaspoons	3.3
Raw cabbage	⅓ cup	5
Cooked green beans	1 tablespoon	5
Cooked broccoli	2 tablespoons	8.3
Fried beef liver	1 ounces	66.7

*⅓ of Adult male RDA

Make a serving of green vegetables a regular part of your diet to get a concentrated and low kcalorie source of vitamin K. Other sources include brussels sprouts, asparagus, lettuce, cauliflower, tomatoes, and eggs.

CONCEPT CHECK

Vitamin K is important for blood clotting because it imparts a calcium-binding ability to certain blood proteins, such as prothrombin. To do this, vitamin K helps add a carbon dioxide molecule to the amino acid glutamate in a protein molecule. About half the vitamin K we absorb every day comes from bacterial synthesis in the intestines and about half from the diet. The amount in the diet alone is generally about five times higher than our needs. Thus, except for newborns, a deficiency of vitamin K is unlikely, even though it is readily excreted from the body. Table 12-5 reviews fat-soluble vitamins.

Table 12-5 Summary of the fat-soluble vitamins, their functions, deficiency conditions, and food sources

Vitamin	Major Functions	Deficiency Symptoms	People Most at Risk	Dietary Sources	RDA	Toxicity Symptoms
Vitamin A (retinoids) and provitamin A (carotenoids)	1. Vision, light and color 2. Promote growth 3. Prevent drying of skin and eyes 4. Promote resistance to bacterial infection	1. Night blindness 2. Xerophthalmia 3. Poor growth 4. Dry skin (keratinization)	People in poverty, especially preschool children (still very rare) in the United States	Vitamin A Liver Fortified milk Provitamin A Sweet potatoes Spinach Greens Carrots Cantaloupe Apricots Broccoli	Females: 800 RE* (4000 IU†) Males: 1000 RE* (5000 IU†)	Fetal malformaltions, hair loss, skin changes, pain in bones
D (chole- and ergo-calciferol)	1. Facilitate absorption of calcium and phosphorus 2. Maintain optimum calcification of bone	1. Rickets 2. Osteomalacia	Breastfed infants, elderly shut-ins	Vitamin D–fortified milk Fish oils Tuna fish Salmon	5-10 micrograms (200-400 IU)	Growth retardation, kidney damage, calcium deposits in soft tissue
E (tocopherols, tocotrienols)	1. Antioxidant: prevent breakdown of vitamin A and unsaturated fatty acids	1. Hemolysis of red blood cells 2. Nerve destruction	People with poor fat absorption (still very rare)	Vegetable oils Some greens Some fruits	Females: 8 Alpha-tocopherol equivalents Males: 10 Alpha-tocopherol equivalents	Muscle weakness, headaches, fatigue, nausea, inhibition of vitamin K metabolism
K (phyllo- and menaquinone)	1. Helps form prothrombin and other factors for blood clotting	1. Hemorrhage	People taking antibiotics for months at a time (still quite rare)	Green vegetables Liver	60-80 micrograms	Anemia and jaundice

*Retinol equivalents.
†International units.

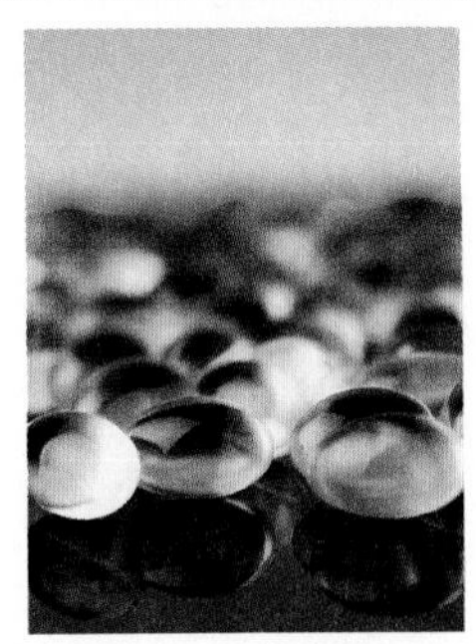

Summary

1. Vitamins are organic (carbon-containing) compounds needed for important metabolic reactions in the body. They yield no energy themselves to the body. Instead they contribute to many energy-yielding chemical reactions in the body, thereby promoting growth, development, and maintenance. Vitamins A, D, E, and K are fat soluble, while the B vitamins and vitamin C are water soluble. Fat-soluble vitamins are excreted less readily from the body and are less susceptible to cooking loss than are water-soluble vitamins.
2. Some fat-soluble vitamins pose a potential for toxicity. Vitamins A and D are especially likely to build up to toxic levels. The water-soluble vitamins B-6 and niacin can also induce toxic symptoms, but only at very high doses in comparison to their RDA.
3. Fat-soluble vitamins are absorbed along with dietary fat. They travel through the lymphatic system into the bloodstream and interact with certain lipoproteins. In disease states in which fat digestion is poor or when lipoprotein synthesis is hampered, fat-soluble vitamin status may be compromised, especially with vitamins E and K.
4. Vitamin A consists of a family of compounds: retinal, retinol, and retinoic acid. A plant derivative known as beta-carotene, along with other carotenoids, yields vitamin A after metabolism by the intestine or liver. Vitamin A contributes to the maintenance of vision, the proper development of cells (especially mucus-forming cells), and proper immune function. Vitamin A is found in liver, fish oils, and fortified milk; carotenoids are especially plentiful in dark green and orange vegetables and in some fruits.
5. Americans at risk for poor vitamin A status are children with poor fat absorption and adults with alcoholism. Vitamin A can be quite toxic when taken at just five to ten times the RDA. High vitamin A intakes are especially dangerous during pregnancy because they can lead to fetal malformations.
6. Vitamin D is usually a hormone rather than a vitamin. It can be synthesized by the skin using sunshine and a form of cholesterol. This vitamin D is then metabolized by the liver and kidney to yield the active hormone, calcitriol. Calcitriol is important for calcium absorption from the intestine, and with other hormones it helps regulate bone metabolism. Vitamin D in foods is found in fish oils and fortified milk. Vitamin D can be a very toxic substance. An intake just two and a half to five times the RDA, if taken regularly, can be toxic in children. Anyone who feels a need to use a supplement should consult a physician first.
7. Vitamin E primarily functions as an antioxidant. By donating electrons to electron-seeking compounds, it neutralizes them. One group of electron-seeking compounds, known as free radicals, can cause widespread cell destruction, both to cell membranes and to DNA, if not stabilized. Vitamin E is plentiful in plant oils. Fruits and vegetables are another good source. The more plant oils one consumes, the more vitamin E one needs, but this need is usually met by those same plant oils. Fish oils, in contrast, often contain little vitamin E.
8. Vitamin K contributes to blood clotting; it imparts calcium-binding capability to certain blood proteins by adding carbon dioxide molecules to the amino acid glutamate in proteins. About half the vitamin K absorbed each day comes from bacterial synthesis in the intestine; the other half comes from foods, primarily green leafy vegetables. Vitamin K is readily excreted from the body, but our daily intake from diet alone is about five times our need.

Study Questions

1. Why do fat-soluble vitamins tend to be much more toxic to the body than the water-soluble vitamins?
2. Why do the carotenoids pose much less of a threat for vitamin A toxicity than preformed vitamin A?
3. What signs of a particular vitamin deficiency might one expect an elderly person confined to a nursing home to display. Why?
4. Why is it critical for a surgeon to know the vitamin K status of a patient before operating?
5. In a child with either unattended or undetected cystic fibrosis, what fat-soluble vitamin deficiencies will be highly likely. Why?

REFERENCES

1. Anonymous: Iatrogenic liver disease from vitamin A, *Nutrition Reviews* 49:309, 1991.
2. Anonymous: Nongenomic effects of vitamin D, *Nutrition Reviews* 49:306, 1991.
3. Anonymous: Is pyrroloquinoline quinone a cofactor derived from an undiscovered vitamin? *Nutrition Reviews* 46:139, 1988.
4. Bauernfeind JC: Vitamin A deficiency: a staggering problem of health and sight, *Nutrition Today,* March/April 1988, p 34.
5. Bjorneboe A and others: Absorption, transport and distribution of vitamin E, *Journal of Nutrition* 120:233, 1990.
6. Burton GW: Antioxidant action of carotenoids, *Journal of Nutrition* 119:109, 1989.
7. Carlin A, Walker WA: Rapid development of vitamin K deficiency of an adolescent boy receiving total parenteral nutrition following bone marrow transplantation, *Nutrition Reviews* 49:181, 1991.
8. Council on Scientific Affairs: Vitamin preparations as dietary supplements and as therapeutic agents, *Journal of the American Medical Association* 257:1929, 1987.
9. Coutsoudis A and others: Vitamin A supplementation reduces measles morbidity in young African children: a randomized, placebo-controlled, double-blind trial, *American Journal of Clinical Nutrition* 54:890, 1991.
10. Dawson-Hughes B and others: Effect of vitamin D supplementation on wintertime and overall bone loss in healthy postmenopausal women, *Annals of Internal Medicine* 115:505, 1991.
11. Di Mascio PD and others: Antioxidant defense systems: the role of carotenoids, tocopherols, and thiols, *American Journal of Clinical Nutrition* 53:194S, 1991.
12. Diplock AT: Antioxidant nutrients and disease prevention: an overview, *American Journal of Clinical Nutrition* 53:189S, 1991.
13. Gey KF and others: Inverse correlation between plasma vitamin E and mortality from ischemic heart disease in cross-cultural epidemiology, *American Journal of Clinical Nutrition* 53:326S, 1991.
14. Haddad JG: Vitamin D—solar rays, the milky way, or both? *The New England Journal of Medicine* 326:1213, 1992.
15. Howard LJ: The neurologic syndrome of vitamin E deficiency: laboratory and electrophysiologic assessment, *Nutrition Reviews* 4:169, 1990.
16. Hussey GD, Klein M: A randomized, controlled trial of vitamin A in children with severe measles, *The New England Journal of Medicine* 323:160, 1990.
17. Knekt P and others: Vitamin E and cancer prevention, *American Journal of Clinical Nutrition* 53:283S, 1991.
18. Krinsky NI: Effects of carotenoids in cellular and animal systems, *American Journal of Clinical Nutrition* 53:238S, 1991.
19. Medeiros DM and others: Long-term supplement users and dosages among adult westerners, *Journal of The American Dietetic Association* 91:980, 1991.
20. Murphy SP and others: Vitamin E intakes and sources in the United States, *American Journal of Clinical Nutrition* 52:361, 1990.
21. Packer L: Protective role of vitamin E in biological systems, *American Journal of Clinical Nutrition* 53:1050S, 1991.
22. Park YK and others: Characteristics of vitamin and mineral supplement products in the United States, *American Journal of Clinical Nutrition* 54:750, 1991.
23. Pike JW: Vitamin D_3 receptors: structure and function in transcription, *Annual Reviews of Nutrition* 11:189, 1991.
24. Pryor WA: Can vitamin E protect humans against the pathological effects of ozone in smog? *American Journal of Clinical Nutrition* 53:702, 1991.
25. Pryor WA: The antioxidant nutrients and disease prevention—what do we know and what do we need to find out? *American Journal of Clinical Nutrition* 53:391S, 1991.
26. Reichel H and others: The role of the vitamin D endocrine system in health and disease, *The New England Journal of Medicine* 320:980, 1989.

27. Robertson JM and others: A possible role for vitamins C and E in cataract prevention, *American Journal of Clinical Nutrition* 53:346S, 1991.
28. Ross CA: Vitamin A: current understanding of the mechanisms of action, *Nutrition Today,* Jan/Feb 1991.
29. Salonen JT and others: Effects of antioxidant supplementation on platelet function: a randomized pair-matched, placebo-controlled, double-blind trial in men with low antioxidant status, *American Journal of Clinical Nutrition* 53:1222, 1991.
30. Sauberlich HE: Vitamins—how much is for keeps? *Nutrition Today,* Jan/Feb 1987, p 20.
31. Sherman SS and others: Vitamin D status and related parameters in a healthy population: the effects of age, sex and season, *Journal of Clinical Endocrinology and Metabolism* 71:405, 1990.
32. Sutie JW: Vitamin K and human nutrition, *Journal of The American Dietetic Association* 92:585, 1992.
33. Tarwotjo I and others: Xerophthalmia and growth in preschool Indonesian children, *American Journal of Clinical Nutrition* 55:1142, 1992.
34. Varma SD: Scientific basis for medical therapy of cataracts by antioxidants, *American Journal of Clinical Nutrition* 53:335S, 1991.
35. Webb AR, Holick MF: The role of sunlight in the cutaneous production of vitamin D3, *Annual Reviews of Nutrition* 8:375, 1988.
36. Wolf G, Phil D: The intracellular vitamin A-binding proteins: an overview of their functions, *Nutrition Reviews* 49:1, 1991.

SUGGESTED READINGS

The article by the Council on Scientific Affairs of the American Medical Association reviews current recommendations for vitamin and mineral supplement use and is particularly detailed. The article by Bauernfeind outlines the result of vitamin A deficiency, which worldwide is a much more serious problem. The articles by Packer and Pryor together give a good account of our current knowledge concerning antioxidants—nutrients under great scrutiny at this time. Finally, Sutie reviews vitamin K nutrition. This article contains numerous references for further research.

TAKE ACTION

Measuring your vitamin intake against the RDAs

This activity requires you to reexamine the nutritional assessment you did for Chapters 1 and 2. You recorded all the foods and drinks you consumed for 1 day and their quantities. Then you assessed your intake by recording the total amounts of nutrients you consumed. You were then asked to compare your nutrient intake to certain standards. Many of the standards you used were the 1989 RDAs found on the inside front cover of this book. Take your completed assessment and look at your intakes of vitamins A, E, C, B-6, B-12, and thiamin, riboflavin, niacin, and folate. Record these numbers in the table below. Next, record the RDAs for each of these nutrients off your assessment. Then, record the percentage of the RDA you consumed for each vitamin. Lastly, place a +, −, or = in the space provided reflecting an intake higher than, lower than, or equal to the RDA.

VITAMIN	INTAKE	RDA	% OF RDA	+, −, =
A				
E				
C				
THIAMIN				
RIBOFLAVIN				
NIACIN				
B-6				
FOLATE				
B-12				

ANALYSIS

1. Which of your vitamin intakes equaled or exceeded the RDA?

___

2. Which if your vitamin intakes were below the RDA?

___

3. What foods could you eat to improve your dietary intake of vitamins in low amounts in your diet? (Review sources of certain vitamins in this chapter and the next.)

___

___

NUTRITION PERSPECTIVE

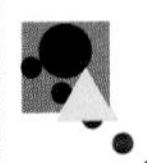

Vitamin Supplements—Who Needs Them?

Our opinions about vitamins have changed since the turn of the century when Casimir Funk first coined the term from the words "vital amine" (an amine has a carbon atom bonded to a nitrogen atom). As you might have already noticed from some of the vitamin structures shown in this chapter, not all vitamins are actually amines. Thus Funk was somewhat incorrect in his terminology. In these early years, vitamins were first a curiosity. They then became the subject of intense scientific scrutiny and research.

Today, vitamins are promoted as cure-alls by many health food enthusiasts and consumed as supplements by as many as 40% of adults in certain areas of the United States. Supplements are such big business, in fact, their sales more than doubled between 1976 and 1986 from $1.2 billion to almost $3 billion.

Should you take a vitamin and mineral supplement? To answer that question, you first need to look closely at your diet. Does it follow the Guide to Daily Food Choices outlined in Chapter 2, especially emphasizing low-fat dairy products, lean meats, whole grains, leafy and dark green vegetables, fruits containing vitamin C, and some vegetable oil? If so, men are probably meeting their needs; some women (those with heavy menstrual flows) may still need more iron. Secondly, do you regularly consume a fortified breakfast cereal? Most breakfast cereals have extra vitamins and minerals added (Figure 12-10).

Nutrition scientists generally agree that most people can obtain the vitamins and minerals they need if they eat a healthy diet.[8] We think you should start there first. Improve your diet where needed, using Chapter 2 for guidance. After that, consider whether you need a supplement. We advise talking to your doctor as well, who may refer you to a registered dietitian.

Recently a panel of scientists from the American Institute of Nutrition and the American Society for Clinical Nutrition suggested a few cases in which vitamin and mineral supplementation should be considered:

- Women with excessive bleeding during menses may need extra iron.
- Women who are pregnant or breast-feeding may need extra iron, folate, and calcium.
- People with very low kcalorie intakes need the range of vitamins and minerals.
- Some vegetarians may need extra calcium, iron, zinc, and vitamin B-12.
- Newborns, under the direction of a physician, need a single dose of vitamin K.

People with specific other illnesses or diseases, such as vitamin-resistance diseases, and those who use certain medications may require supplementation with specific vitamins and minerals under the direction of a physician. Examples of medications requiring supplemental vitamins or minerals would be thiazide diuretics, which often require extra potassium, and the treatment of osteoporosis, which may require extra vitamin D.

Supplementation during illness and drug therapy needs to be directed by a physician because the use of some vitamin and mineral supplements can cause harm by themselves and may counteract the actions of certain medications. Vitamin B-6 can counteract the action of L-dopa (used in treating Parkinson's disease) and isoniazid (used in treating tuberculosis). High intakes of vitamin E can inhibit vitamin K metabolism, and therefore increase the action of anticoagulants, such as warfarin.

Which supplement should you choose?

If you decide to take a vitamin and mineral supplement, which one should you choose? We suggest following the guidelines set forth by the Council on Scientific

GOLDEN CRUNCH CEREAL

NUTRITION INFORMATION

SERVING SIZE: 1.2 OZ. (1 OZ. CEREAL WITH 0.2 OZ. NUTS AND FRUIT; 33.1 g, ABOUT 1/2 CUP)

SERVINGS PER PACKAGE: 13

	CEREAL, NUTS & FRUIT	WITH 1/2 CUP VITAMINS A & D SKIM MILK
CALORIES	120	160*
PROTEIN, g	3	7
CARBOHYDRATE, g	25	31
FAT, TOTAL, g	2	2*
UNSATURATED, g	2	
SATURATED, g	0	
CHOLESTEROL, mg	0	0*
SODIUM, mg	170	230
POTASSIUM, mg	115	320

PERCENTAGE OF U.S. RECOMMENDED DAILY ALLOWANCES (U.S. RDA)

PROTEIN	6	15
VITAMIN A	15	20
VITAMIN C	**	2
THIAMIN	25	30
RIBOFLAVIN	25	35
NIACIN	25	25
CALCIUM	2	15
IRON	25	25
VITAMIN D	10	25
VITAMIN E	20	20
VITAMIN B_6	25	25
FOLIC ACID	25	25
VITAMIN B_{12}	20	30
PHOSPHORUS	8	20
MAGNESIUM	8	10
ZINC	20	25
COPPER	4	6
PANTOTHENATE	20	25

*2% MILK SUPPLIES AN ADDITIONAL 20 CALORIES, 2 g FAT, AND 10 mg CHOLESTEROL.
**CONTAINS LESS THAN 2% OF THE U.S. RDA OF THIS NUTRIENT.

INGREDIENTS: WHOLEWHEAT, BROWN SUGAR, WHOLE OATS, ALMONDS, WHOLE BARLEY, DRIED APPLES, CORN, RICE, WHEAT BRAN, PARTIALLY HYDROGENATED SOYBEAN AND/OR COTTONSEED OIL, SALT, CORN SYRUP, WHEY, MALT FLAVORING, CINNAMON. **VITAMINS AND MINERALS:** IRON (FERRIC PHOSPHATE), VITAMIN E (ALPHA TOCOPHEROL ACETATE), NIACINAMIDE, ZINC (OXIDE), CALCIUM PANTOTHENATE, VITAMIN B_6 (PYRIDOXINE HYDROCHLORIDE), VITAMIN B_2 (RIBOFLAVIN), VITAMIN A (PALMITATE; PROTECTED WITH BHT), VITAMIN B_1 (THIAMIN HYDROCHLORIDE), FOLIC ACID, VITAMIN D, AND VITAMIN B_{12}.

Figure 12-10 The fortification levels for various vitamins and minerals in a typical breakfast cereal. Note three fat-soluble vitamins are included.

NUTRITION PERSPECTIVE

Vitamin Supplements—Who Needs Them?—cont'd

Definitions for supplements

supplement—to enhance nutrient intake (50% to 150% of the RDA).

therapeutic agent—used under medical supervision to correct a nutrient deficiency (two to ten times the RDA).

pharmacological dose—megadose (usually greater than ten times the RDA).

Affairs of the American Medical Association.[8] They recommend that a supplement contain no more than 50% to 150% of the adult U.S. RDA (or RDI) for vitamins A, D, E, and C, folate, thiamin, riboflavin, niacin, vitamin B-6, and vitamin B-12. They do not recommend that this supplement contain biotin or pantothenic acid (because a deficiency is so unlikely) and vitamin K (because it can disturb anticoagulant therapy). For minerals, we suggest using the same guideline, 50% to 150% of the U.S. RDA (or RDI) as an upper limit, or up to 100% of the estimated safe and adequate daily dietary intake (see the inside cover). All of these guidelines are usually observed in your basic one-a-day type vitamin, but read the label to be sure. For example, the amount of nutrient in one tablet of a typical B-complex product can range from 33% of the U.S. RDA for biotin to 6670% or more for thiamin—not what we consider a balanced formulation.

A balanced formulation in a multivitamin and mineral supplement is important. Balance will minimize the chance of vitamin and mineral competition as well as possible accompanying toxicity problems. For example:

- High amounts of vitamin C can cause overabsorption of iron and lead to iron toxicity in susceptible people. Consuming high amounts of vitamin C may also inhibit copper absorption, in addition to decreasing the ability of certain diagnostic tests to assess the development of diabetes or colon cancer.
- Large amounts of vitamin E inhibit vitamin K metabolism.
- Large amounts of fish oil can lead to a decrease in blood clotting.
- Excessive zinc intake can inhibit copper absorption.
- Excessive fluoride exposure in childhood may stain and even weaken the teeth (see Chapter 15).
- Large amounts of folate can mask symptoms of a vitamin B-12 deficiency, therefore preventing the early diagnosis of a potentially life-threatening condition. Large doses of folate, approximately 100 times the RDA, can also inhibit the action of anticonvulsants. Patients with epilepsy who require anticonvulsant therapy jeopardize their health if they also consume many folate supplements.

These are more reasons to discuss vitamin and mineral supplementation beyond the RDA or ESADDI with a physician and registered dietitian. Only then can you appropriately evaluate whether supplementation is in your best interest. We will discuss these and other potentially toxic effects of vitamin and mineral overuse further in Chapters 13 to 15. For now, keep in mind that the intake level set by the Food and Nutrition Board for vitamins or minerals, as outlined in RDA and ESADDI values, is important for good health. But that does not suggest that taking higher doses (greater than 1.5 times the U.S. RDA) will be safe, nor necessarily more beneficial. In fact, the chances are great that as doses increase, toxic symptoms will eventually result.

Surveys of people who use vitamin and mineral supplements find that they generally consume multivitamin and mineral preparations. About 60% of the supplement market consists of these.[22] For single supplemental doses, iron, vitamins E and C, and calcium are the most common. Some supplementation may be appropriate if it is designed to counteract a limited food intake when dieting (below about 1200 to 1400 kcalories/day) or possibly to retard some bone loss with calcium supplements (see Chapter 14). But most supplementation practices, such as using vitamin E to treat arthritis, are inappropriate.

Note that unless the Food and Drug Administration (FDA) has evidence that a supplement is inherently dangerous or marketed with illegal claims, it will not regulate it closely (see the section in Chapter 13 on folate for a major exception).

NUTRITION PERSPECTIVE

FDA is in fact prevented from doing so by the Proxmire Amendment to the 1938 Food, Drug, and Cosmetic Act. In addition, FDA has limited resources and has to act on one supplement at a time. Injuries can likely occur before FDA can do anything about a reformulation of a supplement. So Americans cannot rely on the federal government to protect them from vitamin and mineral supplement overuse. People have to know what they are doing and preferably rely on the advice of physicians and registered dietitians for guidance.

Today a popular practice in Japan is to consume tonics that are promoted as producing high energy and greater health. These tonics are often laced with ethanol, caffeine, nicotine-derivatives, and vitamins, along with bizarre substances, such as extract of cobra and essence of seal. This practice has not invaded America, but keep an eye out for it. Remember that Americans can not blindly trust any supplement, since FDA has limited jurisdiction over them. Nor do most people even need supplements. This situation is a prime example of "let the buyer beware."

It may not be many years before the concept of the RDA is broadened, with one daily recommendation for a nutrient designed to prevent known vitamin deficiency diseases and a higher value recommended to optimize the disease-preventing properties of these nutrients, as is the case with antioxidant nutrients.[27] Currently, it remains very controversial among knowledgeable scientists to suggest that taking vitamin pills in addition to eating a healthy diet might be beneficial to already healthy people.

CHAPTER THIRTEEN

The Water-Soluble Vitamins: B Vitamins and Vitamin C

As defined in the last chapter, vitamins are essentially carbon-containing compounds that the body must obtain, although in only small amounts, to maintain health. In this case obtain means either ingested or produced by bacteria in the intestine. The latter is true, however, in only a few cases.

The B vitamins and vitamin C play critical roles in cell metabolism. The B vitamins form coenzymes, which are compounds that enable specific enzymes to function. Many metabolic pathways in a cell could not function without those coenzymes. Vitamin C acts directly to promote its functions. Every student of nutrition should understand how the body uses these vitamins to function, what foods supply them, and how either a deficiency or toxicity affects the body.

At the end of this chapter we discuss vitamin-like compounds. People may need these substances under certain unusual circumstances, and for this reason they have generated quite a bit of interest. However, they cannot be called vitamins because the average healthy person does not need to consume them. The term vitamin is reserved for a compound that is truly an essential part of the diet, one that is able to cure a disease caused by its lack if supplied in time. This fact is often given little attention by health-food enthusiasts, who often misuse the term vitamin to promote an unproven nutrition claim.

NUTRITION AWARENESS INVENTORY

Here are 15 statements about water-soluble vitamins. Answer them to test your current knowledge. If you think the answer is true or mostly true, circle T. If you think the answer is false or mostly false, circle F. Use the scoring key at the end of the book to compute your total score. Take the test again after you have read the chapter. Compare the results.

1. T F Thiamin needs are related to the amount of fat intake.
2. T F Thiamin is found in high quantities in pork.
3. T F White rice itself is a good source of niacin.
4. T F Milk is a good source of riboflavin.
5. T F A deficiency in riboflavin suggests a concurrent deficiency in thiamin, niacin, and vitamin B-6.
6. T F Physicians should investigate the possibility of poor absorption of vitamin B-12 in their elderly patients.
7. T F Using an amino acid, the body can make the vitamin niacin.
8. T F A niacin deficiency causes severe skin inflammation.
9. T F High doses of nicotinic acid can lower serum cholesterol levels.
10. T F Alcohol decreases the absorption of vitamin B-6.
11. T F Excessive supplementation of vitamin B-12 may mask a folate deficiency.
12. T F Vitamin B-12 is present only in animal foods.
13. T F A deficiency in vitamin C causes pinpoint hemorrhages in the skin.
14. T F Vitamin C enhances iron absorption.
15. T F Vitamin C can prevent the common cold.

The B Vitamins

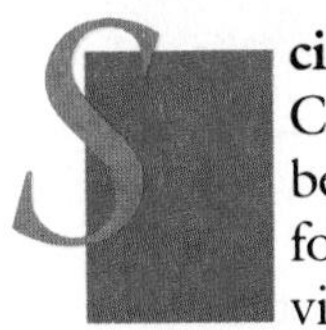

Scientists began to identify the substances we call the B vitamins and vitamin C around the turn of this century. Deficiency diseases, such as scurvy, beriberi, pellagra, and pernicious anemia, had caused enormous suffering for centuries. Once scientists discovered that the problems arose because vital substances—vitamins—are missing from the diet, the diseases were dramatically cured.

For the most part, as the vitamins were discovered they were named alphabetically, A, B, C, D, E, and so on. Later many substances originally classified as vitamins were found not to be essential for humans and were dropped from the list. This explains the many gaps in the alphabetical listing. Other vitamins, thought at first to be only one chemical form, turned out to be many forms, so the alphabetical name had to be broken down by numbers (e.g., B-6, B-12). The only numbers we still use for the B vitamins are B-6 and B-12. Nutritionists no longer refer to thiamin as vitamin B-1, riboflavin as vitamin B-2, or niacin as vitamin B-3 (Figure 13-1).

After ingestion, the B vitamins are first broken down from their coenzyme forms into free vitamins in the stomach and small intestine. The vitamins are then absorbed, primarily in the small intestine. About 50% to 90% of B vitamins in the diet are typically absorbed. About 80% to 90% of vitamin C is absorbed when consumed at RDA levels. Once inside cells, needed coenzyme forms are resynthesized. Because we make them when needed, we don't need to consume the coenzyme forms.

The B-Vitamin and Vitamin C Status of Americans

The focus of this chapter is generally on the water-soluble vitamin status as found among Americans. (For a more detailed discussion of worldwide nutritional deficiencies, refer to Chapter 20). Status of the B vitamins and vitamin C in the United States is generally good. Our diets allow us a plentiful and varied supply of many natural as well as enriched sources of the water-soluble vitamins. At worst, some Americans are on the verge of marginal vitamin status. The long-term effects of existing in that state are as of yet unknown. It is likely the such a state merely leads to fatigue or other bothersome and unspecific symptoms.

It is the rare exception that we develop any of the more serious deficiency diseases

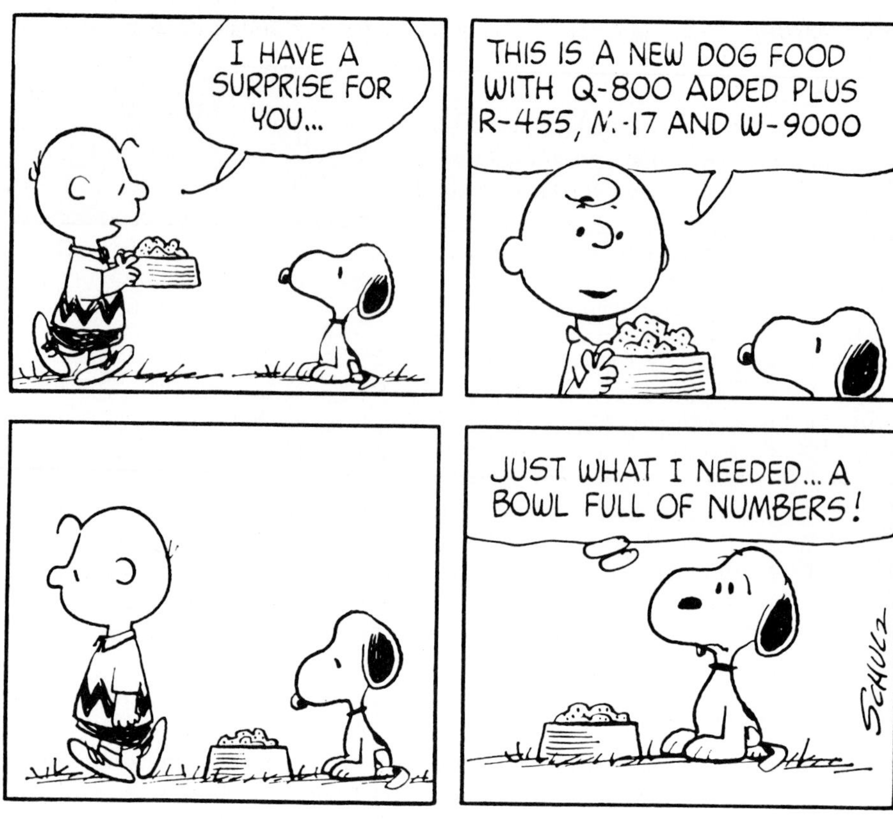
I HAVE A SURPRISE FOR YOU...
THIS IS A NEW DOG FOOD WITH Q-800 ADDED PLUS R-455, M.-17 AND W-9000
JUST WHAT I NEEDED... A BOWL FULL OF NUMBERS!
SCHULZ

Figure 13-1 Peanuts.
Reprinted by permission of UFS, Inc.

due to a poor diet alone. People with alcoholism, however, are an exception. The extremely poor diets of some Americans associated with prolonged alcoholism in combination with an alcohol-induced alteration of vitamin absorption and metabolism make these people very susceptible to some serious nutrient deficiencies.[5] We cover this in detail in the Nutrition Perspective in Chapter 18.

Thiamin

beriberi The thiamin deficiency disorder characterized by muscle weakness, loss of appetite, nerve degeneration, and sometimes edema.

Beriberi—the thiamin deficiency disease—is traditionally found among those populations for whom polished (white) rice is a dietary staple. Brown rice, which has its bran and germ layer intact, is a good source of thiamin. White rice has had its bran and germ layer removed, thus rendering it a poor source of thiamin. However, thiamin is often replaced during the enrichment process for rice and other grains available in the United States, so beriberi is rarely found here.

Thiamin is a compound made up of two rings connected by a mutual attachment to a carbon group. The bonds to this mutual carbon between the two rings are easily broken by prolonged cooking of food, in turn destroying function of the vitamin. This is also true if food is cooked in alkaline solutions, such as cooking green beans in baking soda and water to maintain the fresh green color. The name thiamin comes from the sulfur (thio-) and nitrogen (amine) groups in the molecule. Note that in modern spelling the "e" has been dropped from thiamin, although FDA retains it in food labeling.

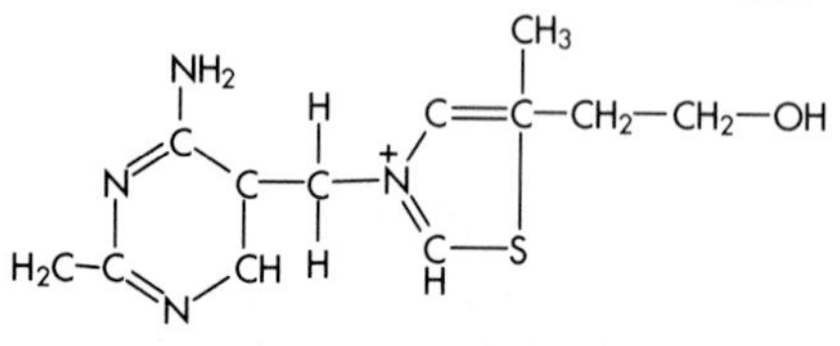

Thiamin

Thiamin has two phosphate molecules added to form the coenzyme (thiamin pyrophosphate).

FUNCTIONS OF THIAMIN

Thiamin, like other B vitamins, must form into a coenzyme to function in aiding enzyme reactions in the body (Figure 13-2). The thiamin coenzyme is called thiamine pyrophosphate (TPP). A key thiamin-related reaction is one in which TPP plus an enzyme form a complex to allow for the loss of a carbon dioxide molecule from a larger molecule. An example of this reaction is the conversion of pyruvate to acetyl-CoA during carbohydrate metabolism to prepare pyruvate to enter the citric acid cycle. This conversion is critical if aerobic metabolism of glucose is to be sustained.[29] The body can bypass much of the need for this mechanism for a while by using mostly fat for fuel. But eventually the body will pay a price in terms of health. TPP also plays an active yet poorly understood role in nerve function. It is thought that TPP may aid in the synthesis of neurotransmitters (such as acetylcholine), aid in the energy production needed by the highly active nerve tissue, and regulate nerve-impulse transmission.

An alternate metabolic pathway for carbohydrate found in some cells, the hexose monophosphate shunt, also uses TPP.[26] This pathway allows cells to make the monosaccharide ribose for RNA. In addition, TPP participates in reactions in which carbon dioxide molecules are removed from some amino acids. Although thiamin is used by a variety of cellular metabolic pathways, the most important pathway is its link with carbohydrate metabolism.

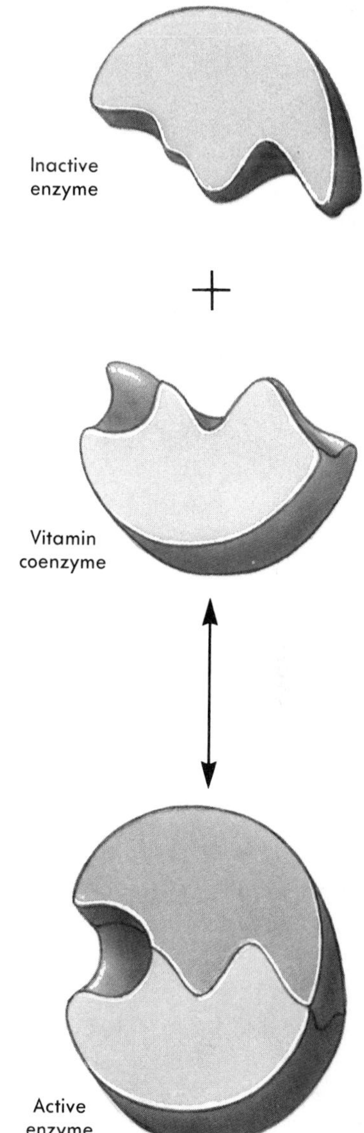

Figure 13-2 The enzyme-coenzyme interaction. The B vitamins form coenzymes—these are compounds that enable specific enzymes to function.

BERIBERI

As we noted earlier, the thiamin deficiency disease is called beriberi. This means "I can't, I can't" in Sinhalese. The signs and symptoms include weakness, loss of appetite, irritability, nervous tingling throughout the body, poor arm and leg coordination, and deep muscle pain in the calves. A person with beriberi often develops an enlarged heart and sometimes severe edema (a variant known as "wet" beriberi).

Bodily functions associated with brain and nervous action are often quick to show signs of a thiamin deficiency. This is because brain and nerve cells convert pyruvate into acetyl-CoA and then push the acetyl-CoA through the citric acid cycle to obtain ATP energy. The thiamin coenzyme TPP participates in these metabolic pathways. Nerve tissues are highly active and place great demands on the citric acid cycle to provide the energy it requires.

Symptoms of depression and weakness can be seen after only 10 days on a thiamin-free diet. This shows how poorly our bodies store thiamin. Thus it is best to consume ample thiamin from foods daily. Also, note that although the symptoms of beriberi are due to a thiamin deficiency, they can also be partly due to concurrent B-vitamin deficiencies. This is possible because the B-vitamins are often found in the same foods, so a poor amount of one B vitamin in a diet may mean other B-vitamins are deficient as well.

THIAMIN IN FOODS

Foods containing a very high nutrient density of thiamin are pork products and sunflower seeds. Whole grains (wheat germ), enriched grains, green beans, organ meats, peanuts, dried beans, and other seeds are also good sources. However, aside from pork products, there is really no one excellent source to provide thiamin in our diets. The foods we eat—especially meat, milk products, and grains—tend to contribute small amounts of thiamin (Table 13-1). Following the Guide to Daily Food Choices is a reliable way to obtain enough thiamin.

Major individual contributors of thiamin to our diets are white bread and rolls, crackers, pork, hot dogs, luncheon meat, cold cereals, orange juice, and dairy products. White bread, bakery products, and cereals are usually enriched with thiamin. They serve as important sources because people eat them so often. Laboratory-animal studies show that the thiamin in these products is as available as that found in whole grains. Some fish and shellfish contain an enzyme called thiaminase, which destroys thiamin. Fortunately, cooking inactivates thiaminase.

Enzyme activities in red blood cells that require vitamins to function can be used to test vitamin status. The tests are categorized as functional biochemical tests. Enzyme tests are available for thiamin (transketolase), riboflavin (glutathione reductase) and vitamin B-6 (aminotransferase) status.

RDA FOR THIAMIN

The RDA for thiamin for adults is approximately 1.5 milligrams per day for men and 1.1 milligrams per day for women. (Throughout the rest of this chapter refer

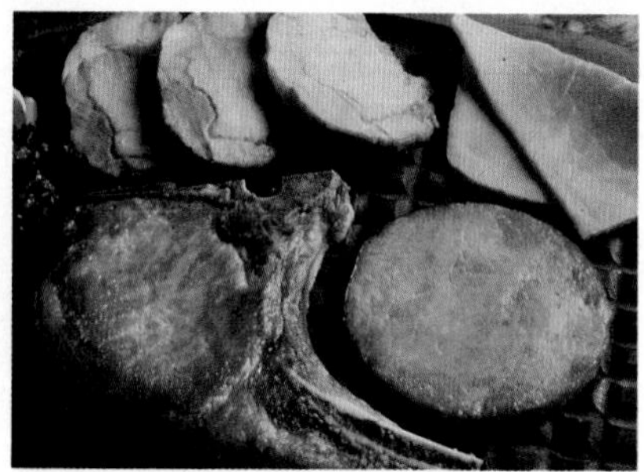

Pork is a good source of thiamin.

Table 13-1 Good food sources of thiamin, ranked by nutrient density

Food	Serving size to yield .5 milligrams*	kcalories needed to yield .5 milligrams
Brewers yeast	½ tablespoon	10
Ham, canned roasted	2 ounces	84
Wheat germ, raw	⅓ cup	90
Cooked Canadian bacon	3 pieces	113
Sunflower seeds, dry	⅙ cup	123
Pork chop, broiled	2 ounces	156
Watermelon	1⅓ slices	195
Oatmeal, cooked	1⅔ cups	248

* ⅓ RDA for adult male, ages 19 to 24 years.
Sunflower seeds, pork, and ham yield much thiamin for both a limited serving size and kcalorie cost. Other foods contain small amounts, but they add up as servings from the Guide to Daily Food Choices are consumed.

to the inside cover for vitamin recommendations for other age groups and to Appendix D for Canadian recommendations.) The U.S. food supply yields approximately one-and-a-half times the RDA for thiamin per person per day, but that does not consider the thiamin lost in food preparation and in cooking.

The more carbohydrate consumed and the greater one's energy output, the more thiamin one needs for metabolic needs. The RDA can even be expressed in terms of energy intake: 0.5 milligrams of thiamin per 1000 kcalories but no less than 1 milligram per day if a person is on a low-kcalorie diet. No cases of toxicity have been associated with consumption of vitamin supplements of thiamin.

AMERICANS AT RISK FOR A THIAMIN DEFICIENCY

Some groups of people, such as the poor and the elderly, may barely meet their needs for thiamin. A diet dominated by highly processed and unenriched foods, sugar, fat, and alcohol also creates a potential for a thiamin deficiency. Women should be especially careful to consume good sources of thiamin. Their average intakes barely meet the RDA.

When physicians see a person suffering from unexplained delirium in the emergency room, they must consider whether it may be caused by a thiamin deficiency due to alcoholism. The treatment is an injection of thiamin. Dietary supplementation will not suffice because thiamin is only slowly absorbed, especially in a person with alcoholism.

People with alcoholism are at great risk for thiamin deficiency because absorption and use of thiamin is profoundly diminished by alcohol consumption. Furthermore, the poor diet that often accompanies severe alcoholism makes matters worse. Recall that thiamin is very poorly stored in the body. If an alcohol binge lasts 1 to 2 weeks, the person may quickly deplete already poor stores of thiamin. Thiamin deficiency in alcoholism can lead to a combination of symptoms, including mental confusion, memory loss, and poor nervous system control of arms and legs.

Riboflavin

Clinicians have great difficulty identifying true riboflavin deficiencies because clinical signs and symptoms are not specific for riboflavin. Other B vitamin deficiencies, such as thiamin, vitamin B-6, and folate, also cause similar effects. In addition, an isolated riboflavin deficiency probably does not exist. A riboflabin deficiency would likely occur with deficiencies of niacin, thiamin, and vitamin B-6, as these nutrients are often found in the same foods.

Riboflavin is a three-ringed structure with a monosaccharide-like compound (ribitol) attached. The name riboflavin comes from its yellow color—flavus means "yellow" in Latin. Riboflavin forms the coenzymes flavin mononucleotide (FMN) and flavin adenine dinucleotide (FAD). Riboflavin is present as FMN and FAD in food, except in enriched grain products, where riboflavin is present as the vitamin itself. All these forms are well used by the body.

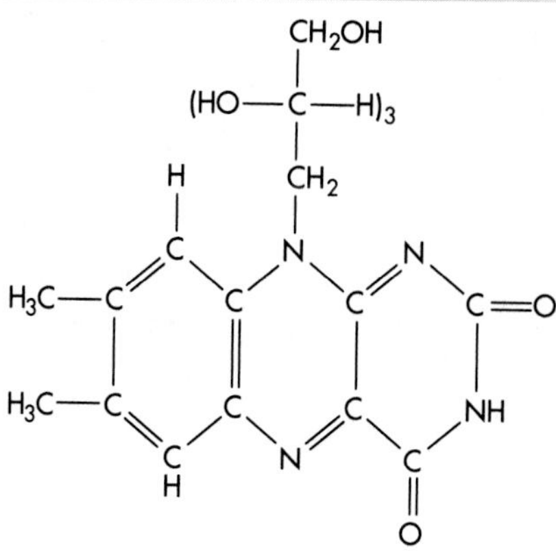

Riboflavin

FUNCTIONS OF RIBOFLAVIN

The coenzymes of riboflavin participate in many cellular metabolic pathways. Both the citric acid cycle and the pathway for breaking down fatty acids (beta-oxidation) use FAD to form $FADH_2$. The electron transport chain in the mitochondria uses these coenzymes and FMN and $FMNH_2$, as well.[26] In all these examples, the coenzymes act first as electron and hydrogen ion acceptors and then as electron and hydrogen ion donors. When cells form ATP using aerobic pathways, or fatty acids are broken down and burned for energy, the coenzymes of riboflavin are used. Some vitamin metabolism also requires riboflavin.

RIBOFLAVIN DEFICIENCY

Early symptoms associated with a riboflavin deficiency (technically called **ariboflavinosis**) include inflammation of the mouth and tongue. This is later followed by dermatitis, cracking of tissue around the corners of the mouth (cheilosis), various eye and nervous system disorders, and confusion (Figure 13-3). The first symptoms of a deficiency are inflammation of the mouth and tongue. The complete picture of deficiency symptoms develops after approximately 2 months of consuming a riboflavin-poor diet (consuming one fourth of the RDA).

ariboflavinosis A condition resulting from a lack of riboflavin. The "a" stands for "without," and "osis" stands for "a condition of."

RIBOFLAVIN IN FOODS

The most nutrient-dense sources of riboflavin are liver, mushrooms, spinach and other green leafy vegetables, and low-fat and nonfat milks (Table 13-2). Lean meats, poultry, and eggs are also good sources.

One quarter of the riboflavin in our diets comes from milk and milk products. Riboflavin is a major contribution of the milk, yogurt, and cheese group of the Guide to Daily Food Choices. Including dairy products in your diet is the best guarantee for a good riboflavin intake. The rest of our riboflavin intake typically comes mostly from enriched white bread, rolls, and crackers, as well as meats. For

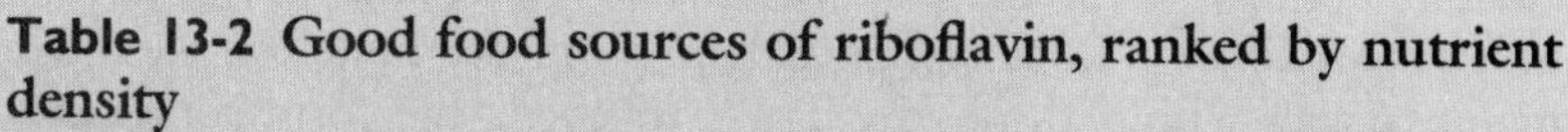

Table 13-2 Good food sources of riboflavin, ranked by nutrient density

Food	Serving size to yield .57 milligrams*	kcalories needed to yield .57 milligrams
Beef liver, fried	½ ounce	31
Brewers yeast	2 tablespoons	46
Mushroom pieces, cooked	1¼ cups	53
Spinach, cooked	1⅓ cups	55
Broccoli, cooked	1⅔ cups	81
Nonfat milk + solids	1⅓ cups	120
Braunschweiger sausage	1⅓ pieces	120
1% low-fat milk	1⅓ cups	137
Buttermilk	1½ cups	147
Oysters, Eastern	1⅓ cups	213
Whole milk	1½ cups	216
Cottage cheese, low-fat	1⅓ cups	273
Steak, beef	5⅓ ounces	315
Pork, roasted	5⅓ ounces	373

* ⅓ RDA for adult male, ages 19 to 24 years.
By eating vegetables and drinking milk, the riboflavin needs are easily met using very few kcalories.

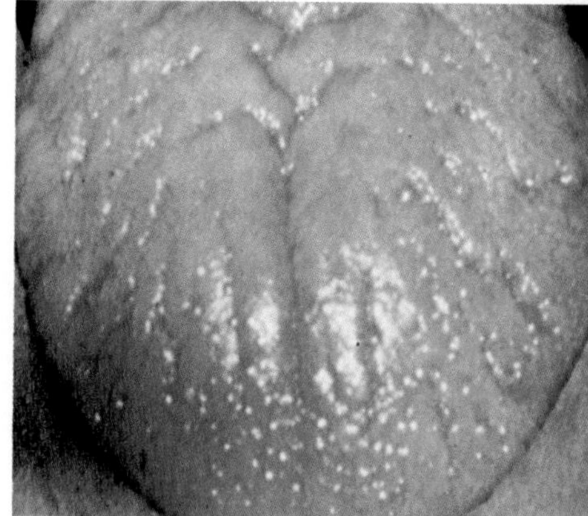

Figure 13-3 An inflamed tongue (glossitis) can signal a vitamin deficiency. A painful and inflamed tongue can be seen in a niacin, vitamin B-6, riboflavin, folate, or vitamin B-12 deficiency. Often more than one deficiency may be the cause. Since other medical conditions can also cause glossitis, the person needs a further evaluation before a nutrient deficiency can be established.

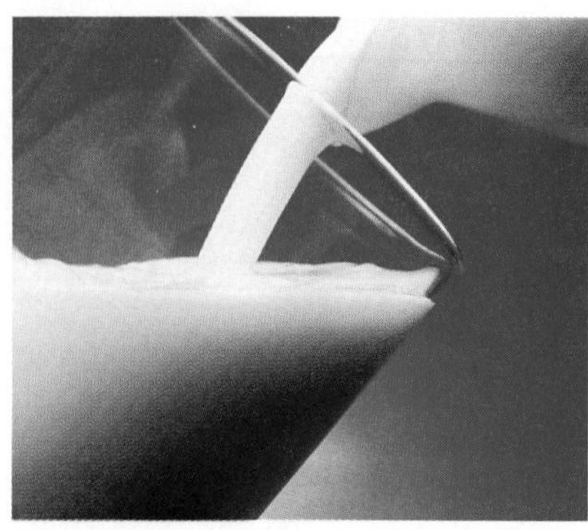

Milk products are our major sources of riboflavin.

some people, high meat consumption partially offsets a low intake of dairy products in terms of meeting riboflavin needs.

Riboflavin is very stable at room temperatures used to both pasteurize milk or reheat foods in a microwave. However, its sensitivity to light causes riboflavin to break down rapidly when exposed to ultraviolet radiation. To protect milk products from light, paper and plastic cartons—not glass—work well.

RDA FOR RIBOFLAVIN

The RDA for riboflavin for adults is 1.4 to 1.7 milligrams per day for men and 1.2 to 1.3 milligrams per day for women. Another way of expressing the RDA is 0.6 milligrams per 1000 kcalories but no less than 1.2 milligrams per day. On average, we consume the RDA for riboflavin. Athletes may need extra riboflavin because of their increased use of fat for fuel (the metabolic pathways use FAD), and their greater use of all the energy-yielding pathways in the cell. However, the RDA will still suffice according to the Food and Nutrition Board. There are no specific signs or symptoms that indicate riboflavin toxicity is a concern.

AMERICANS AT RISK FOR A DEFICIENCY OF RIBOFLAVIN

Riboflavin deficiencies are rare; however, some people barely consume an adequate amount. This is especially true for those who do not regularly consume milk and milk products. People with alcoholism also risk riboflavin deficiency because they often eat very nutrient-poor diets. We suggest that if you do not regularly use milk and milk products, you should search for another adequate dietary source of riboflavin. Enriched breakfast cereals are a good choice.

Niacin

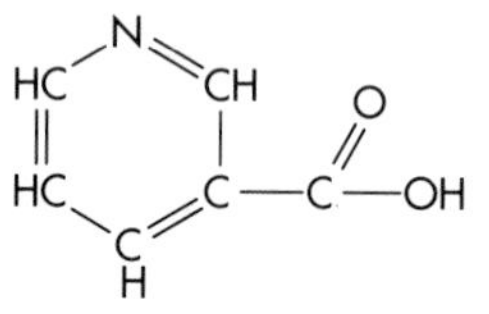

Nicotinic acid

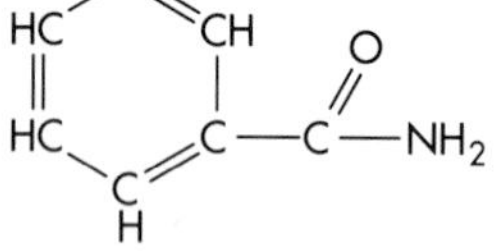

Nicotinamide

The symptoms associated with pellagra—the niacin deficiency disease—include a reddened inflammation of the skin where the sun strikes, diarrhea, dementia, and hallucinations. These have been described in humans since the fourteenth century. The first official record of pellagra was made by the Spanish physician Casal in 1735. It was named mal de la rosa or "red sickness." The typical redness appearing around the neck was called "Casal's necklace."

The vitamin niacin actually exists in two forms—nicotinic acid (niacin) and nicotinamide (niacinamide). Both compounds perform the functions we attribute to the vitamin niacin within the body. The two coenzyme forms of niacin are nicotinamide adenine dinucleotide (NAD) and nicotinamide adenine dinucleotide phosphate (NADP).

FUNCTIONS OF NIACIN

The coenzyme forms of niacin, NAD and NADP, function in many cellular metabolic pathways, especially those used when ATP is being formed. NAD is used first in glycolysis and the citric acid cycle as an electron and hydrogen ion acceptor and then in the electron transport chain as an electron and hydrogen ion donor.[26]

Synthetic pathways in the cell—those that make new compounds—often use NADPH, a reduced form of NADP (see Appendix B for a review of oxidation and reduction.) This is especially true for the pathway for fatty acid synthesis. Cells that synthesize a lot of fatty acids, such as those in the liver and female mammary glands, have higher concentrations of enzyme systems needed to synthesize NADPH than do cells that do not synthesize fat, such as muscle cells.

PELLAGRA

Since almost every cellular metabolic pathway uses either NAD or NADP, a niacin deficiency causes widespread damage in the body. The entire collection of symptoms is known as pellagra, which means "rough" or "painful skin." The effects of the disease are known as the three "D's"—dementia, diarrhea, and dermatitis (Figure

13-4). Death is then likely to follow. Early symptoms include poor appetite, weight loss, and weakness.

Pellagra decimated corn-eating populations of southern Europe beginning in the 1700s, partly because corn is low in available niacin (see page 388). Pellagra then spread to the southeastern United States. The first cases of pellagra in the United States may have been described as early as 1864, but certainly by 1902 to 1906 the outbreak of pellagra in the southeastern United States had begun.[7] Note that this has been the only widespread vitamin deficiency disease to reach epidemic proportions in the United States. By 1918 over 200,000 people in the United States had pellagra, and many of these people ended up with such severe dementia that they were relegated to spend the rest of their lives in mental institutions. Over 10,000 Americans died of pellagra in 1915.

Even as late as 1930, there were still 200,000 cases of pellagra in the United States. And discovering the cure for pellagra—niacin—in the late 1930s still did not lead to its eradication. Poverty and poor diets were still at the root of the problem. It took the prosperity of milltowns and farmers in the southeastern United States following World War II, along with the enrichment of refined grains in 1941, to deal the final blow to the epidemic.

An important link in the pellagra story was supplied in 1948 when researchers showed that the amino acid tryptophan was converted into niacin in the body. This helped explain the earlier finding by researchers that diets high in protein, but not high in niacin, also cured pellagra. Pellagra is still found today throughout Southeast Asia and Africa, associated with those diets very low in protein and niacin.

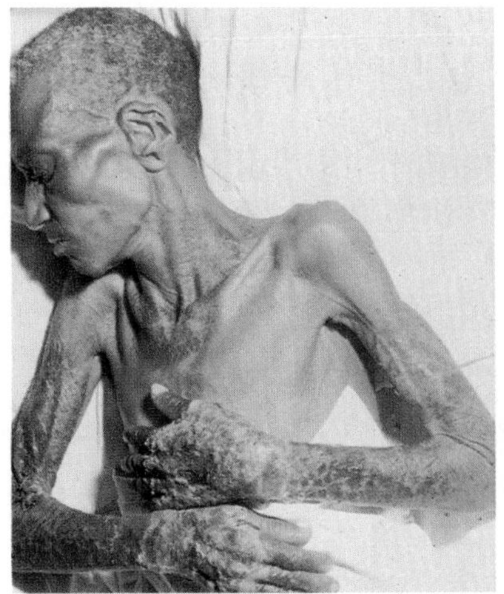

Figure 13-4 The dermatitis of pellagra. Dermatitis on both sides of the body (bilateral) is a typical result of pellagra. Sun exposure worsens the condition.

NIACIN IN FOODS

The most nutrient-dense sources of niacin are mushrooms, wheat brain, tuna (as well as some other fish), chicken, asparagus, and peanuts (Table 13-3). Most niacin in our diets comes from enriched white bread, rolls, crackers, and breakfast cereals (niacin is added as part of the enrichment process); beef, chicken, and turkey. Niacin is very heat stable; little is lost in cooking.

Niacin status can be determined by measuring the amount of its breakdown product, N-methyl nicotinamide, in the urine. Low amounts suggest poor status.

Table 13-3 Good food sources of niacin, ranked by nutrient density

Food	Serving size to yield 6.3 milligrams*	kcalories needed to yield 6.3 milligrams
Mushroom pieces, cooked	1 cup	36
Wheat bran	½ cup	47
Brewers yeast	2 tablespoons	47
Tuna, canned	1⅓ ounces	61
Chicken breast, roasted	¼ each	71
Beef liver, fried	1½ ounces	90
Pink salmon, canned, raw	2⅔ ounces	106
Halibut, broiled w/butter and lemon juice	2⅓ ounces	109
Salmon, broiled/baked	3⅓ ounces	154
Sardines, canned	4 ounces	161
Turkey, roasted	4 ounces	187
Peanuts, dried unsalted	1⅓ ounces	240
Lamb chops	3⅓ ounces	267
Peanut butter	3⅓ ounces	280
Steak, beef	5⅓ ounces	317
Hamburger, lean	4 ounces	317

* ⅓ RDA for adult male, ages 19 to 24 years.

Mushrooms, chicken, beef, pork, and salmon supply ample niacin within both a reasonable serving size and kcalorie cost.

Besides the preformed niacin found in protein foods, each 60 milligrams of extra dietary tryptophan (leftover after protein synthesis) may be converted within the body to yield approximately 1 milligram of niacin.[26] This conversion requires participation from riboflavin and vitamin B-6 coenzymes. We can assume that 1% of dietary protein is tryptophan. Therefore to estimate the number of milligrams of niacin supplied by dietary protein, just divide extra grams of dietary protein intake by six; based on the equation below:

$$1 \text{ gram protein} \times \frac{1 \text{ mg tryptophan}}{100 \text{ mg protein}} \times \frac{1 \text{ mg niacin}}{60 \text{ mg tryptophan}} = \frac{\text{grams}}{6}$$

About half the niacin we use is produced by this process. Animal proteins (except gelatin) are especially rich in tryptophan. Food tables list only preformed niacin content. Therefore they often underestimate the total niacin contribution in protein foods since protein in foods contributes niacin from the conversion of tryptophan.

Niacin in corn is bound by a protein, so it is poorly absorbed. Soaking corn in an alkaline solution such as lime water (water and calcium hydroxide) releases bound niacin and renders it more usable. Hispanic populations soak corn in lime water before making tortillas. The soaking treatment is one reason that Hispanic populations rarely suffer from pellagra, unlike Europeans and Caucasian and African Americans. Unaware of the importance of soaking the corn in lime water, Spanish explorers failed to inform the Europeans how to prepare corn properly when they brought it back from the New World.

RDA FOR NIACIN

The RDA for niacin for adults is 15 to 19 milligrams per day for men and 13 to 15 milligrams per day for women. The difference in muscle mass between the genders accounts for the difference in recommendations. The RDA is expressed as niacin equivalents to account for niacin received intact from the diet, as well as that synthesized from tryptophan.

Our food supply contains approximately 1.4 times the RDA (26.8 milligrams of niacin) per person per day, without considering the contribution from tryptophan. As long as you follow the Guide to the Daily Food Choices, developing a niacin deficiency is highly unlikely. People with alcoholism are generally the only population group to show niacin deficiency, primarily because of a poor intake of food sources rich in niacin.

TOXICITY OF NIACIN

Intakes of 100 milligrams or more of nicotinic acid can lead to an increase in blood flow to the skin, causing a general blood vessel dilation or "flushing" of the body. Headache and itching also may result. Such an excessive intake is sometimes used, under a physician's guidance, as a relatively safe and inexpensive means to lower elevated blood cholesterol levels.

CONCEPT CHECK

The B vitamins thiamin, niacin, and riboflavin are all important in the diet to derive energy in the metabolism of carbohydrates, proteins, and fats. Enriched grains are adequate sources of all three vitamins. Otherwise, pork is an excellent source of thiamin; milk is an excellent source of riboflavin; and protein foods in general, such as chicken, are excellent sources of niacin. Deficiencies of all three vitamins can occur with alcoholism, and of the three, a thiamin deficiency is the most likely. Only niacin shows toxicity symptoms when consumed in high doses.

Pantothenic Acid

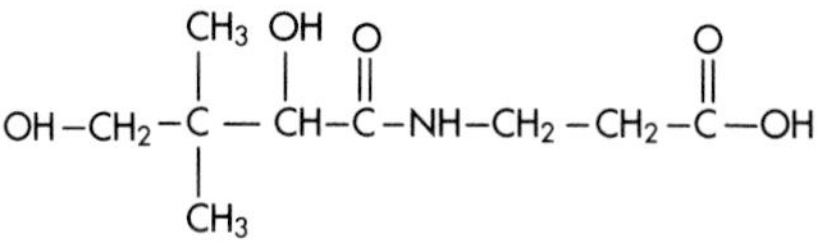

Pantothenic Acid

Pantothenic acid is far too widespread in foods to ever allow for a nutritional deficiency. In addition, humans are somewhat resistant to deficiency due solely to dietary origin, requiring periods of greater than 12 weeks to display any symptoms. A full-blown deficiency is so rare that it has possibly only been observed during World War II. Prisoners in the Philippines and Japan displayed a "burning foot" syndrome described by numbness and tingling in the toes and burning and shooting pains in the feet, in addition to other mental and neurological symptoms.

FUNCTIONS OF PANTOTHENIC ACID

Pantothenic acid forms part of coenzyme A. To do so the vitamin must combine both with a part of ATP and with the amino acid cysteine. This last addition provides the sulfur atom, which is the "business end" of the coenzyme.

By forming coenzyme A (CoA), pantothenic acid allows many important metabolic actions of the citric acid cycle to take place.[34] In fact, CoA must be added to the pathways of carbohydrate and fat metabolism for the eventual products to enter the citric acid cycle. This is because the CoA molecule is needed to make these molecules much more reactive. Coenzyme A is also used in the beginning steps of fatty acid synthesis.

Pantothenic acid also forms a part of a compound called the acyl carrier protein. This attaches to fatty acids and shuttles them through the pathway designed to increase their chain length.[34]

Based on its widespread availability in the food supply, research in the area of pantothenic acid deficiency has had to require subjects to consume an antagonist capable of artificially inducing a deficiency state. When the antagonists are given, people suffer from tingling hands, fatigue, headache, sleep disturbances, nausea, and abdominal distress.

PANTOTHENIC ACID IN FOODS

"Pantothen" actually means "from every side" in Greek, reflecting its ample supply in foods. Nutrient-dense sources of pantothenic acid are mushrooms, yeast, liver,

Table 13-4 Good food sources of pantothenic acid, ranked by nutrient density

Food	Serving size to yield 2.3 milligrams*	kcalories needed to yield 2.3 milligrams
Raw mushrooms	1½ cups	27
Brewers yeast	3⅓ tablespoons	76
Fried beef liver	1½ ounces	91
Broccoli, cooked	2⅓ cups	114
Cooked lobster	4⅔ ounces	211
Cooked eggs	3⅔ each	213
1% milk	3 cups	270
Cooked chicken, roasted	1½ cups	331
Wheat bran	3⅔ cups	335
Blue cheese	4⅔ ounces	476
Baked salmon	7⅓ ounces	420
Peanuts, oil-roasted	⅔ cup	626
Dates	1⅔ cups	815
Pecans	1 cup	1010

* ⅓ of top range of ESADDI.
Some vegetables supply the greatest nutrient density, but nuts and meats offer the most reasonable serving size relative to their nutrient density.

peanuts, and eggs (Table 13-4). Other good sources are meat, milk, and many vegetables. Because pantothenic acid is not added to enriched grains, these are not especially good sources of the vitamin.

ESADDI FOR PANTOTHENIC ACID

The estimated safe and adequate daily dietary intake (ESADDI) for pantothenic acid is 4 to 7 milligrams per day for adults. Recall this is not a true RDA, but a range of acceptable intakes included in the RDA publication (see Chapter 2). Current adult intakes are about 6 milligrams of pantothenic acid per person per day.

A deficiency of pantothenic acid might occur in cases of alcoholism in which a very nutrient-deficient diet is consumed. However, the symptoms would probably be hidden among deficiencies of thiamin, riboflavin, vitamin B-6, and folate, so the pantothenic acid deficiency might be unrecognizable. There is no known toxicity level for pantothenic acid.

Biotin

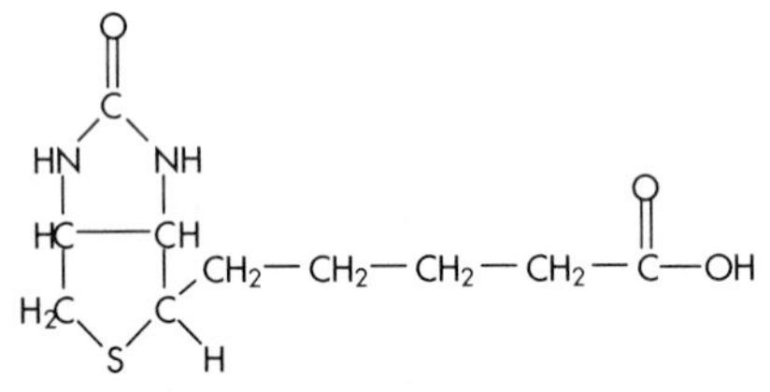

Biotin

Biotin is commonly found in two forms—the free vitamin itself and biocytin, an inactive form that is simply biotin with the amino acid lysine attached.[23] Occasionally, infants are born with a genetic defect that leaves them very low levels of the enzyme biotinidase (about 1 in 8000 to 12,000 births). This is needed to turn biocytin into biotin. These infants develop biotin deficiency symptoms. Clinicians debate whether infants should be screened at birth for a biotinidase deficiency, as they are for phenylketonuria (see Chapter 5). If a deficiency is found, the infant is treated with 50 to 200 times the ESADDI for biotin.

Both forms of biotin are absorbed. Cleavage of the lysine group is essential for active function but not for biotin absorption. It even appears that the form best absorbed is the biocytin form, not free biotin. Cleavage of the lysine group from biocytin via biotinidase can occur in several places, such as in the lumen of the small intestine. The enzyme needed is found in the pancreatic juices released for protein digestion. Biotinidase activity is also evident in the blood, and as such, is capable of cleaving absorbed biocytin to biotin where and when needed.

FUNCTIONS OF BIOTIN

Biotin acts as a coenzyme in fat and carbohydrate metabolism. Specifically, it is an integral part of certain enzymes used for adding carbon dioxide molecules to other compounds.[23] Two biotin-dependent enzymes are critical in preventing the depletion of key compounds of the citric acid cycle. Without biotin, these compounds may not be sufficiently replenished, so the citric acid cycle could not run effectively. As a result, lactic acid (an anaerobic byproduct of glycolysis) levels within the blood would rise as aerobic glucose metabolism is slowed. It is postulated that increased lactic acid levels within the central nervous system are the basis for the neurological disorders—depression, lethargy, hallucinations, and numbness of the extremities—that accompany a severe biotin deficiency.

In addition, another biotin-dependent enzyme contributes the carbon dioxide groups needed to synthesize fatty acids. In a biotin deficiency a person will also show signs similar to an essential fatty acid deficiency—scaly inflammation of the skin, hair loss, and even loss of eyelashes and eyebrows if it occurs in infancy. Biotin also aids in the breakdown of some amino acids, participates in the synthesis of one of the two types of bases (purines) used in constructing DNA and RNA, and aids in the metabolism of the three-carbon fatty acids so that they can enter the citric acid cycle.

BIOTIN IN FOODS

Cauliflower, egg yolks, yeast, liver, peanuts, and cheese are the most nutrient-dense sources of biotin (Table 13-5). Fruits are generally poorer sources. It is likely that

Table 13-5 Good food sources of biotin, ranked by nutrient density

Food	Serving size to yield 33.3 micrograms*	kcalories needed to yield 33.3 micrograms
Brewers yeast	2 tablespoons	47
Cooked cauliflower	1 cup	53
Egg yolk	1⅓ each	84
Cooked beef liver	1½ ounces	93
Cheese, American	1⅔ ounces	157
Wheat bran	1⅓ cups	206
Canned sardines	5⅓ ounces	257
Broiled chicken, roasted	7⅓ ounces	412
Peanut butter	⅓ cup	500
Baking chocolate	3⅔ ounces	518
Peanuts	3⅓ ounces	575

* ⅓ of top range of ESADDI; bacterial synthesis in the intestinal tract probably also yields some biotin. Egg yolks, liver, and cheese provide the most reasonable balance of kcalorie cost and serving size. Cauliflower, peanut butter, and chicken are probably the best choices if a low cholesterol, low saturated fat intake is followed.

intestinal synthesis of biotin by bacteria supplies at least part of our needs, as evidenced by the rather rare incidence of biotin deficiency. In fact, we excrete more biotin than we consume. However, questions remain about the actual bioavailability of that biotin synthesized by the intestinal flora. Some researchers think it might be bound inside the bacteria and therefore unavailable.[23] In any event, if a person lacks a large part of the small intestine or needs to take antibiotics for many months, special attention should be paid to eating good food sources of biotin.

A protein called **avidin** in raw egg whites can bind biotin and inhibit its absorption. Feeding many raw egg whites to animals leads to the classic "egg white injury" deficiency symptoms as described previously. An occasional raw egg in eggnog is of no concern because it would take a regularly daily consumption of 12 to 24 raw eggs to produce a biotin deficiency. In cases of alcoholism, however, biotin deficiency symptoms resulting from raw eggs have been reported in people with a regular consumption of just three raw eggs a day. These people probably had very poor diets. In any event, one must still exercise caution when consuming raw eggs due to the danger of food-borne illness from *Salmonella* bacteria (see Chapter 19).

avidin A protein found in raw egg whites that can bind biotin and inhibit absorption; cooking destroys avidin.

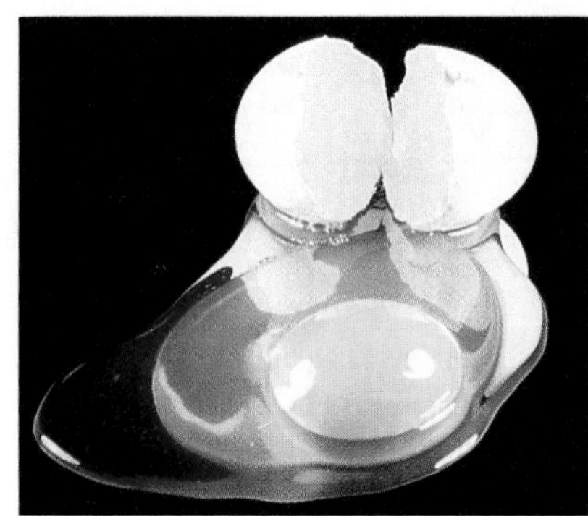

Egg yolks are a nutrient-dense source of biotin.

ESADDI FOR BIOTIN

The ESADDI for biotin is 30 to 100 micrograms per day for adults. Our food supply is thought to contain 100 to 300 micrograms per person per day. It is important to avoid a biotin supplement that exceeds the ESADDI, unless a physician recommends it. We know very little about this vitamin, especially its potential for toxicity.

AMERICANS AT RISK FOR A BIOTIN DEFICIENCY

As previously mentioned, a biotinidase deficiency may lead to a severe deficiency if undetected in an infant. Signs and symptoms may appear within a few months of life and begin with a skin rash and hair loss. The person will eventually develop neurological disorders, and infants and children will show impaired growth.

People on long-term anticonvulsant drugs may run the risk of a biotin deficiency. Several of these drugs may directly inhibit intestinal uptake of biotin or block the biotinidase enzyme action.

A diet designed to decrease the risk of heart disease, calling for less egg and organ meat consumption, may end up to be low in biotin. Again, current thinking is that bacterial synthesis of biotin in the intestine probably compensates for the difference between our biotin needs and what our diets supply, but we can't be absolutely sure. Seeking alternate food sources is a wise measure.

One problem in assessing biotin status is that there is no accurate measure for it.[23] To complicate matters, the symptoms of an overt biotin deficiency are rather general and (like the other B vitamin deficiencies) are difficult to pin to the lack of any one specific vitamin.

Vitamin B-6

Vitamin B-6 (represented by pyridoxol)

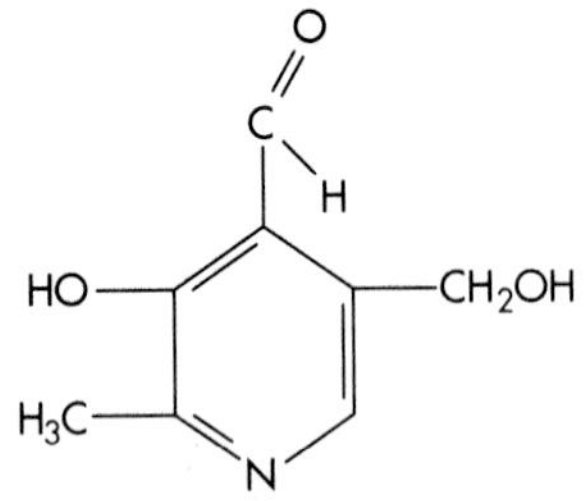

Pyridoxal

In the 1950s, infants fed oversterilized commercial formulas developed Vitamin B-6 deficiency symptoms, most notably, convulsions. Heat had destroyed vitamin B-6 in the formulas, possibly contributing to the infants' decreased ability to synthesize neurotransmitters—a key function of vitamin B-6. Today, manufacturers are more careful to maintain adequate vitamin B-6 levels in formulas.

Vitamin B-6 is actually a family of compounds: pyridoxal, pyridoxine, and pyridoxamine. All three forms can be changed to the active vitamin B-6 coenzyme, pyridoxal phosphate (PLP). The general vitamin name is pyridoxine.

FUNCTIONS OF VITAMIN B-6

Vitamin B-6 is needed for the activity of more than 50 enzymes involved in carbohydrate, protein, and fat metabolism.

Protein Metabolism

The most important function of vitamin B-6 concerns protein because the metabolism of every amino acid requires the active coenzyme PLP.[26] This includes transamination reactions (see Chapter 5). Essentially, the PLP coenzyme combines with an enzyme requiring its assistance to ease the splitting of the amine group from an amino acid.

If vitamin B-6 were missing from the body, every amino acid would become an "essential" (indispensable) amino acid—that is, every amino acid would have to be supplied by the diet. Under normal circumstances, we can make 11 of the 20 types of amino acids our bodies need. None of that synthesis would be possible without the vitamin B-6 coenzyme. Thus poor protein and overall cell synthesis, as evidenced by skin changes (dermatitis) and a sore tongue, occurs with vitamin B-6 deficiency.

Vitamin B-6 status can be assessed by measuring the amount of coenzyme PLP in the bloodstream.

Blood Cell Synthesis

The vitamin B-6 coenzyme is important for the synthesis of the hemoglobin ring structure, the oxygen-carrying part of the red blood cell. As expected, an anemia condition, resembling iron-deficiency anemia, occurs in a vitamin B-6 deficiency (see Chapter 15). Vitamin B-6 is also necessary for the synthesis of white blood cells, major players in the immune system.

Neurotransmitter Metabolism

As we just mentioned, the syntheses of many key neurotransmitters—serotonin, gamma amino butyric acid (GABA), and norepinephrine—requires the active vitamin B-6 coenzyme. These compounds allow nerve cells to communicate with each other. As one might expect, a deficiency of vitamin B-6 will result in neurological disorders, such as depression, headaches, confusion, and even convulsions.[20]

The link between vitamin B-6 and neurotransmitters suggested to some researchers that vitamin B-6 might be helpful in the treatment of **premenstrual syndrome.** This disorder appears in some women a few days before a menstrual period begins and is characterized by depression, irritability, anxiety, headache, bloating, and mood swings. Researchers thought that increasing vitamin B-6 intake might increase the synthesis of serotonin, and in turn decrease the depression and confusion associated with premenstrual syndrome.

premenstrual syndrome A disorder found in some women a few days before a menstrual period begins. It is characterized by depression, anxiety, headache, bloating, and mood swings.

Table 13-6 Good food sources of vitamin B-6, ranked by nutrient density

Food	Serving size to yield .67 milligrams*	kcalories needed to yield .67 milligrams
Brewers yeast	1⅔ tablespoons	42
Spinach, cooked	1½ cups	62
Broccoli, cooked	2 cups	97
Banana, peeled, slices	⅔ cup	106
Salmon, broiled/baked	3 ounces	147
Watermelon	1 slice	147
Chicken breast, roasted	⅔ whole	200
Cantaloupe	1 each	202
Tuna, water packed	9 ounces	205
Turkey	4⅔ ounces	233
Sunflower seeds, oil-roasted	⅓ cup	315
Beef liver, cooked	6 ounces	392

* ⅓ RDA for adult male, ages 19 to 24.

Some vegetables provide more vitamin B-6 per kcalorie than meat and fish, but the serving size for many vegetables presents quite a challenge, and the vitamin B-6 present is often less absorbable. Thus meats, fish, and poultry are ultimately our best sources of vitamin B-6.

However, researchers now know that vitamin B-6 is not only a questionable treatment for PMS,[10] it also has a great potential for toxicity.[1] Some women have suffered toxic side effects of vitamin B-6 (see the section on B-6 toxicity) in attempting to treat themselves for premenstrual syndrome. The cause of PMS is not well-understood, but a better nutrition-related approach to treatment is to eat a nutrient-rich diet; decrease alcohol, caffeine, nicotine, and salt use to decrease nervousness, depression, and bloating; and increase exercise to stimulate relaxation. If that therapy is not helpful, women with premenstrual syndrome should seek a physician's advice, in which antidepressant or hormonal therapy may be tried.[30] They should definitely avoid the widely available PMS "cures" that are sold primarily in drug stores and by mail-order.

VITAMIN B-6 IN FOODS

The most nutrient-dense sources of vitamin B-6 are some fruits and vegetables, such as bananas, cantaloupe, broccoli, and spinach (Table 13-6). Protein foods, especially meat, fish, and poultry (vitamin B-6 is stored in muscles) are also good sources. In addition, the vitamin B-6 present in animal foods is often more readily absorbable than that in plant foods.[21] This makes meats, fish, and poultry our best sources of vitamin B-6. Note that vitamin B-6 is not part of the enrichment process. If it were, we would probably see breads, cakes, and cookies listed as major sources, although these do provide some vitamin B-6 to our diets. Food tables listing vitamin B-6 sources often do not provide a complete picture of its availability for many foods because measuring this vitamin in foods is difficult.[31]

RDA FOR VITAMIN B-6

The RDA for vitamin B-6 for adults is 2 milligrams per day for men and 1.6 milligrams per day for women. The RDA is set high in response to high protein intakes found in the United States. The more protein eaten, the more vitamin B-6 needed. The recommendations can also be expressed as 0.016 milligrams of vitamin B-6 per gram of protein. This corresponds to 2 milligrams per 126 grams of protein—approximately twice the RDA for protein for adult men. Our consumption of vitamin B-6 is 2.06 milligrams per person per day, or about the RDA.

Athletes may need more vitamin B-6 because of their increased use of glycogen for fuel (glycogen metabolism requires vitamin B-6), their increased use of amino

Some Mysteries Surrounding Vitamin B-6

JIM LEKLEM, PH.D.

Vitamin B-6 is considered to be one of the water-soluble micronutrients our body needs. While it is a "micro" nutrient, this unique vitamin can be viewed as a "sleeping giant" in nutrition. There are several new and some rediscovered areas of research that are awakening a new view of vitamin B-6.

The perspective of this nutrient as being water-soluble suggests it is not retained or stored. In fact, recent studies have shown that we store this vitamin in muscle tissue. About 170 milligrams of vitamin B-6 is found in the human body, with a majority in muscle bound to glycogen phosphorylase enzyme in the active coenzyme form, pyridoxal phosphate (PLP). Because vitamin B-6 is stored, we would assume that in times of a dietary deficiency of vitamin B-6 these muscle stores are used. Research has shown that this is not the case in rats or humans. Rather, the stores appear to be used in times of energy deficit. This is consistent with the role PLP plays in a process called gluconeogenesis. In this process, PLP aids in the breakdown of certain amino acids such that their carbon skeletons are ultimately converted to glucose.

One of the areas where the interplay between kcalorie need and storage of vitamin B-6 may play a role is exercise. We have observed that vitamin B-6 metabolism is altered during exercise. Blood levels of PLP increase during exercise and then decrease significantly after exercise. We have also observed under conditions of strictly controlled intakes of vitamin B-6 that there is an increased excretion of the major metabolite of vitamin B-6 in trained as compared to untrained women. Increased urine levels of this metabolite also occur with exercise as compared to no exercise in trained men. These observations indicate that there is a 5% to 7% increased loss of vitamin B-6 with strenuous exercise, such as cycling or running. Based on these limited number of studies, athletes may need slightly more vitamin B-6 than persons who are sedentary.

Recent research has revealed a new and exciting role for vitamin B-6 as a possible modulation of steroid hormone action. Vitamin B-6, as PLP, interacts with steroid hormone receptor proteins in the body. As a result of this reaction of PLP with the receptors, hormone action is reduced. In studies in rats, when there is a deficiency of vitamin B-6, the effects of glucocorticoid hormones are enhanced. We must await further research to reveal to what extent the action of these types of hormones is influenced by nutritional status of vitamin B-6, or by an excess intake of vitamin B-6, which could occur with use of vitamin B-6 supplements.

In some cases vitamin B-6 supplements are consumed by people in an attempt to prevent certain disorders or to treat a given clinical condition. Premenstrual syndrome (PMS) and **carpal tunnel syndrome,** respectively, are two examples. Is vitamin B-6 effective for either of these syndromes?

Of the 12 studies in which vitamin B-6 supplements have been used to treat PMS, only three had some beneficial effect. The remaining nine studies found ambiguous or no positive effect of vitamin B-6. In all these studies, the amount of vitamin B-6 the women took ranged from 50 to 500 milligrams per day. In addition, the length of time the women took the supplement varied, as did the number of subjects. A more important consideration is that many of the studies were not designed as double-blind placebo controlled trials. This complicates the interpretation of the results because there may have been a placebo effect. Until more well-controlled studies are conducted, it is not possible to conclude that vitamin B-6 supplements alleviate the symptoms of PMS. If vitamin B-6 is effective in treating PMS, it may do so via a modulation of hormone action.

Similarly, the benefits of using vitamin B-6 to treat carpal tunnel syndrome is open to question. The same problems present in the studies of treating PMS with vitamin B-6 are seen for the few studies in which vitamin B-6 supplements have been used to treat carpal tunnel syndrome. This syndrome is thought to affect people whose jobs involve repetitive motion that adversely impacts the carpal tunnel, an opening in the wrist through which tendons, nerves, and blood vessels pass. Of seven studies in which vitamin B-6 was used to treat this syndrome, five showed some modest improvement in certain symptoms. The one controlled study showed variable effect. Several of these studies were not double-blind, placebo-controlled trials and criteria for improvement of symptoms varied between studies. Thus there is no strong evidence for a benefit of vitamin B-6.

While supplemental doses of vitamin B-6 may prove to be of benefit in some clinical conditions, maintenance of optimal vitamin B-6 status is a key to health and well-being. To obtain optimal amounts of vitamin B-6 from foods, one should choose foods containing adequate amounts that are in a form which is highly available. A form of vitamin B-6 that is present in plant foods is linked with glucose. This form is called pyridoxine glucoside. In both animals and humans, there is incomplete absorption of this form, and that which is absorbed in this form is not readily used by cells. Animal foods do not contain glucose-linked vitamin B-6. Plant foods such as soybeans, peanuts, carrots, potatoes, wheat bran, and raisins contain 25% or more of the total vitamin B-6 in the food in that form. These foods are still good sources of vitamin B-6, but in individuals who have a low intake of vitamin B-6, such as women and elderly, consumption of these foods at the expense of animal sources may adversely affect their vitamin B-6 nutrition. At the risk of being redundant, or of using a phrase which may anger the sleeping giant, meeting RDA levels for vitamin B-6 from a variety of foods—both animal and plant sources—would be prudent.

Dr. Leklem, a Professor in the Department of Nutrition and Food Management at Oregon State University, focuses his research efforts on vitamin B-6.

acids for fuel, and their high protein intakes. Still the protein foods in their diets should supply any extra vitamin B-6 needed.

Before deciding to take a supplement of vitamin B-6, or any supplement to treat a disorder, make sure that double-blind studies published in medical journals, such as the ones we cite in the references, support your decision. Then discuss your plans with your physician. To review the characteristics of a double-blind study, see Chapter 1.

AMERICANS AT RISK FOR VITAMIN B-6 DEFICIENCY

Numerous studies show that about 35% to 40% of adolescent, adult, and elderly women have poor vitamin B-6 intakes below RDA levels.[28] However, since the vitamin B-6 values of many foods are not known, intake is likely greater. Therefore it is possible that true intakes are better than we think. Routine multivitamin supplement use, which women commonly follow, helps out as well. Moreover, the basis for the vitamin B-6 RDA assumes a daily intake of over 100 grams of protein. Women, on average, consume only 70 grams of protein daily and thus will often have lower needs for B-6 than the RDA suggests. Still, there is concern that the vitamin B-6 status for some women is poor. The Expert Opinion discusses controversies surrounding vitamin B-6 status.

People with alcoholism are susceptible to a vitamin B-6 deficiency because acetaldehyde, a metabolite formed in ethanol metabolism, can displace the active coenzyme form of vitamin B-6 from its enzyme, in turn increasing its tendency to be broken down. In addition, alcoholism decreases the absorption of vitamin B-6 and decreases the synthesis into its active form. Cirrhosis and hepatitis (both of which may accompany alcoholism) also disable liver tissue from actively metabolizing vitamin B-6, which decreases synthesis of its active form.

TOXICITY OF VITAMIN B-6

Intakes of 2 to 6 grams of vitamin B-6 per day for 2 to 40 months can lead to irreversible nerve damage.[1] Use, or more appropriately stated, misuse of these high doses of vitamin B-6 have occurred in women attempting to treat themselves for PMS and in body builders. Symptoms include walking difficulties and hand and foot numbness. Some nerve damage in individual sensory neurons is probably reversible, but damage to the ganglions (where many nerve fibers converge) is probably permanent.

CONCEPT CHECK

Pantothenic acid and biotin both participate in metabolism of carbohydrate and fat. A deficiency of either vitamin is unlikely; pantothenic acid is found widely in foods, and our need for biotin is probably partially met by synthesis from intestinal bacteria. Vitamin B-6 is important for protein metabolism, neurotransmitter synthesis, and other key metabolic functions. Headache, anemia, nausea, and vomiting can result from a vitamin B-6 deficiency. Women, in general, should evaluate vitamin B-6 intake and consume a diet rich in vitamin B-6, using animal protein sources and plant foods, such as broccoli, spinach, and bananas. Doses of vitamin B-6 in excess of about 100 times the RDA can cause nerve destruction.

Folate

A common form of cancer therapy provides a vivid example of the effects of a folate deficiency. This vitamin is needed for DNA metabolism. A cancer drug, methotrexate, closely resembles folate. Because of this resemblance, when methotrexate is taken in high doses, it substitutes for and so hampers folate metabolism. DNA synthesis then decreases throughout the body as the body acts as if it is deficient in folate. Since cancer cells are among the most rapidly dividing cells in the body, their growth is affected first by the decrease in DNA synthesis. However, other rapidly dividing cells, such as intestinal cells and skin cells, are also affected by poor DNA synthesis. As one might expect, typical side effects of methotrexate therapy then mirror those of a folate deficiency (e.g., hair loss).

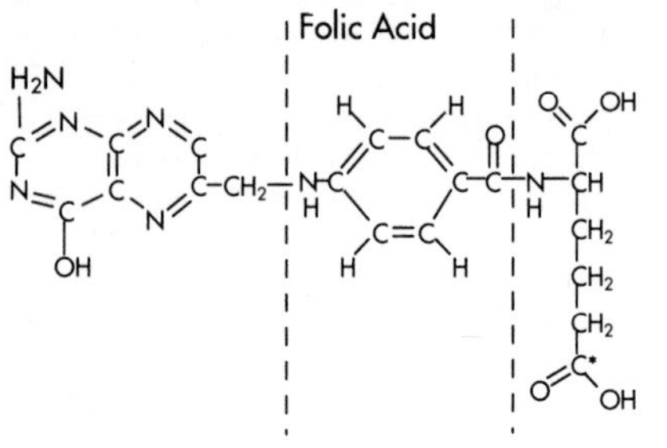

Folic Acid

H_2N ... CH_2 ... N ... C ... OH

Pteridine **Para-aminobenzoic acid** **Glutamate**

***Polyglutamate bonds form at this carbon**

What we call folate today was known earlier as either folic acid or folacin. Today, the term folate is preferred because it encompasses the variety of food forms of the vitamin. Only a few food forms are in the true folic acid configuration, but vitamin supplements often contain this form.

Folate is built of three parts—a pteridine group, para-aminobenzoic acid (PABA), and glutamic acid (an amino acid). If one glutamate molecule is present, it is in the folic acid form. However, in foods, over three quarters of the folate molecules have more than one glutamate added. These are known as the **polyglutamate** forms.[2]

ABSORPTION OF FOLATE

Absorption of folate occurs with both the monoglutamate (folic acid) and the polyglutamate forms. Approximately 85% of true folic acid (the monoglutamate form) is absorbed, and 20% to 70% of the polyglutamate forms are absorbed. All but the last glutamate molecule must eventually be released during absorption. The cells that line the small intestine accomplish that using the **conjugase** enzyme system present.[2] After absorption, most folate is stored in the liver. Thus liver is quite a good dietary source of folate. Once inside the body's cells, all folate forms are quickly converted to the active coenzyme tetrahydrofolic acid (THFA).

FUNCTIONS OF FOLATE

When it participates in metabolic reactions, the acitve coenzyme forms of THFA are always accepting or donating single-carbon molecules. Transfers of single-carbon molecules are needed for the synthesis of DNA and RNA, as well as for the metabolism of various amino acids and their derivatives.

Single carbon molecules include methyl groups ($-CH_3$), formyl groups ($-CH=O$), methylene groups ($-CH_2-$), and methynyl groups ($-CH=$).

Probably the most important role of folate is to contribute to the formation of the purine and pyrimidine bases used in RNA and DNA. As we just mentioned, a deficiency of folate will first affect those cell types with actively reproducing DNA—those cells with a short life span and rapid turnover rate. Thus one of the first major deficiency signs to appear are changes in the early phases of red blood cell synthesis. The precursor cells cannot divide to become mature red blood cells because they cannot form new DNA. The cells grow larger and larger because they can still synthesize enough protein and other cell parts to make new cells. But when it is time for the cells to divide, there is insufficient DNA to form two nuclei. The cells then remain in a large immature form, known as a **megaloblast.** Megaloblasts may mature to abnormally large and fragile red blood cells, called **macrocytes.**

Since the bone marrow of a folate-deficient person produces mostly immature megaloblast cells, few mature red blood cells (erythrocytes) arrive in the bloodstream. Since fewer mature red blood cells are present, oxygen-carrying capacity decreases, causing anemia.[12] In short, a folate deficiency causes megaloblastic anemia.

The changes in red blood cell formation occur after 7 to 16 weeks on a folate-free diet, depending on the folate stores of the person. Serum levels of folate fall even before that. White blood cell formation is also affected, but not as much as red blood cell formation. In addition, cell division throughout the entire body is disrupted. We focus primarily on red blood cells because they are easy to examine. Clinical signs and symptoms of folate deficiency also include inflammation of the tongue, diarrhea, poor growth, mental confusion, and problems in nerve function.[16]

conjugase An intestinal enzyme system that enhances folate absorption by removing glutamate molecules from polyglutamate forms.

megaloblast A large, immature red blood cell that results from a cell's inability to divide when it normally should.

macrocyte A greatly enlarged mature red blood cell; they have short life spans.

FOLATE IN FOODS

Green leafy vegetables (the term folate is derived from the Latin word folium, which means foliage), organ meats, sprouts, other vegetables, and orange juice are the most nutrient-dense sources of folate (Table 13-7). In fact, 1 cup of orange juice contains about 100 micrograms of folate, which is approximately one half of the RDA. While orange juice is promoted for its vitamin C content, an added benefit of orange juice is its substantial folate contribution. The vitamin C in the juice also reduces folate destruction. Grain products also supply some folate to our diets.

Table 13-7 Good food sources of folate, ranked by nutrient density

Food	Serving size to yield 66.7 micrograms*	kcalories needed to yield 66.7 micrograms
Brewers yeast	½ teaspoon	5
Spinach, fresh chopped	½ cup	7
Romaine lettuce, chopped	1 cup	8
Spinach, cooked	¼ cup	10
Turnip greens, cooked	⅓ cup	11
Asparagus, cooked	⅓ cup	16
Broccoli, cooked	½ cup	29
Beets, cooked	⅔ cup	31
Orange juice	½ cup	68
Wheat germ, raw	¼ cup	73
Cantaloupe melon	½ each	78
Beef liver, fried	1⅓ ounces	82
Liver, beef	1½ ounces	126
Beans, pinto	½ cup	133
Sunflower seeds, oil-roasted	½ cup	175

* ⅓ RDA for male adults.

Spinach, asparagus, broccoli, and orange juice are some good nutrient-dense folate sources. Other fruits and vegetables also contribute to total dietary folate.

Food processing and preparation destroy 50% to 90% of the folate in food. Folate is very susceptible to destruction by heat. This underscores the importance of regularly eating fresh fruits and lightly cooked vegetables—or raw when appropriate—as part of the Guide to Daily Food Choices regimen.[2] Vegetables are best cooked quickly in minimal water—steaming, stir-frying, or microwaving.

RDA FOR FOLATE

The RDA for folate for adults is 180 to 200 micrograms per day. These figures approximate the current folate content of the food supply in the United States, which is approximately 225 micrograms per day per person (not accounting for losses in preparation and cooking).[28]

AMERICANS AT RISK FOR FOLATE DEFICIENCY

Folate deficiencies sometimes appear in pregnancy. Pregnant women need extra folate to meet the greater cell division rate, and therefore greater DNA synthesis, for themselves and the fetus. Today prenatal care often includes vitamin and mineral supplements enriched with folate to compensate for extra pregnancy needs. This is one important reason why women need to see their physicians early in pregnancy. They need to increase the folate sources in their diet and/or start their folate supplements as soon as possible if these are deemed necessary (see Chapter 16).

Young women in general often register low serum folate values. It is important for women to seek good sources of folate that they enjoy eating, and then eat those foods regularly. Folate deficiencies also often occur in alcoholism. In fact, signs of a folate-related anemia often tip off a physician to the possibility of alcoholism. Alcohol disrupts folate absorption, probably by inhibiting the conjugase enzyme system in the small intestine that is needed for efficient absorption.

TOXICITY OF FOLATE

There are no documented symptoms of folate toxicity, probably because it is difficult to consume large doses of folate. This is because in the United States FDA limits the amount of folate in nonprescription vitamin supplements to 400 micrograms when no statement of age is listed on the label. When age-related doses are listed, there can be no more than 100 micrograms for infants, 300 micrograms for children, or 400 micrograms for adults. Therefore consuming a large amount of folate would require eating many, many vitamin pills.

FDA regulates potency of folate supplements because consuming excessive amounts of folate can mask a vitamin B-12 deficiency. The metabolism of folate and B-12 are linked, as we will soon discuss. Regularly consuming excessive amounts of folate could prevent the appearance of an early warning sign of vitamin B-12 deficiency—the alteration in blood cell formation, resulting mainly in macrocytic anemia.[16] For unrelated reasons, a B-12 deficiency may ultimately lead to paralysis and death. Thus early detection and treatment of a folate deficiency is critical. Considering the danger associated with overzealous supplementation and that only about 100 micrograms of folate are even required to treat a deficiency, FDA's strict limits on folate content of supplements seems very appropriate.

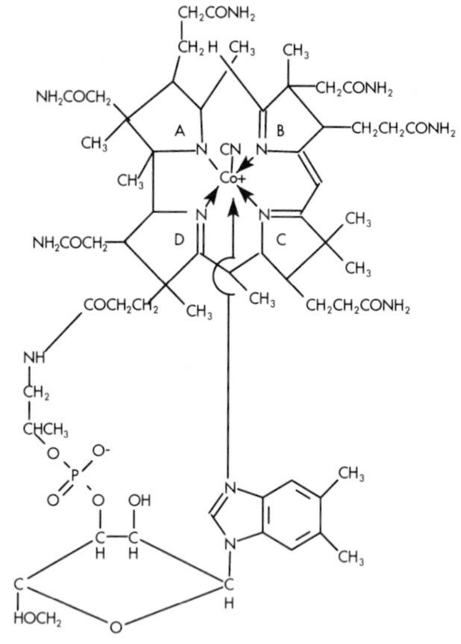

Vitamin B-12
(represented by cyanocobalamin)

Vitamin B-12

Vitamin B-12 is present only in animal foods. While plants do not contain vitamin B-12, bacteria and soil contamination of vegetables and the process of fermentation contribute very little to a diet. This is an important consideration for the vegan's diet. Supplement sources, as we covered in Chapter 5, must be consumed to maintain long-term health. Animals, such as cows and sheep, obtain vitamin B-12 from either bacterial synthesis in their multiple stomachs (rumen) or from soil they ingest while eating and grazing. All vitamin B-12 compounds are synthesized exclusively by bacteria, fungi, and other lower organisms. This makes soil a rich source of vitamin B-12.

What we call vitamin B-12 is actually a family of compounds all containing a cobalt center. They form the active coenzymes, such as methylcobalamin and 5-deoxyadenoxylcobalamin.

ABSORPTION OF VITAMIN B-12

R-protein A protein produced by the salivary glands that enhances vitamin B-12 absorption possibly by protecting it during its passage through the stomach.

intrinsic factor A proteinlike compound produced by the stomach that enhances vitamin B-12 absorption.

Vitamin B-12 in food enters the stomach and is liberated from other materials by digestion, especially by the digestive action of stomach acid. Within the stomach, the free vitamin B-12 then binds with a substance called **R-protein.** Produced by salivary glands in the mouth, researchers think binding with R-protein functions to prevent bacteria in the small intestine from absorbing and using the vitamin B-12. The R-protein/vitamin B-12 complex travels to the small intestine, where the pancreatic enzyme trypsin removes the R-protein (Figure 13-5).[16]

Once vitamin B-12 is free again, it binds to **intrinsic factor,** a type of protein made by the stomach's acid-producing parietal cells. The resulting intrinsic factor/vitamin B-12 complex travels to the last portion of the small intestine, the ileum. Ileum cells absorb vitamin B-12 and transfer it to a special blood transport protein, transcobalamin II. This vitamin-protein complex enters the circulation and is taken up by the liver, bone marrow, and other tissues. Note that while the microbial populations within our own intestines are capable of producing vitamin B-12, they are located beyond the point of vitamin B-12 absorption. Otherwise we would be able to use the vitamin B-12 produced by the bacteria in the colon, and would not necessarily require food sources of the vitamin.

Using this complex system, approximately 30% to 70% of dietary vitamin B-12 is absorbed, depending on the body's need for it. Failure in any of the links found in the absorptive chain of events will result in an ability to only absorb 1% to 2% of dietary vitamin B-12.

Vitamin B-12 absorption can be disrupted by inefficient synthesis of intrinsic factor, a genetic deficiency in R-protein synthesis, a lack of trypsin synthesis by the pancreas, poor binding of the intrinsic factor/vitamin B-12 complex in the ileum, or the absence of an ileum or stomach. In addition, a host of other variants prevents vitamin B-12 absorption, including surgical removal of key parts of the stomach, bacterial overgrowth of the small intestine, and tapeworm infestations.

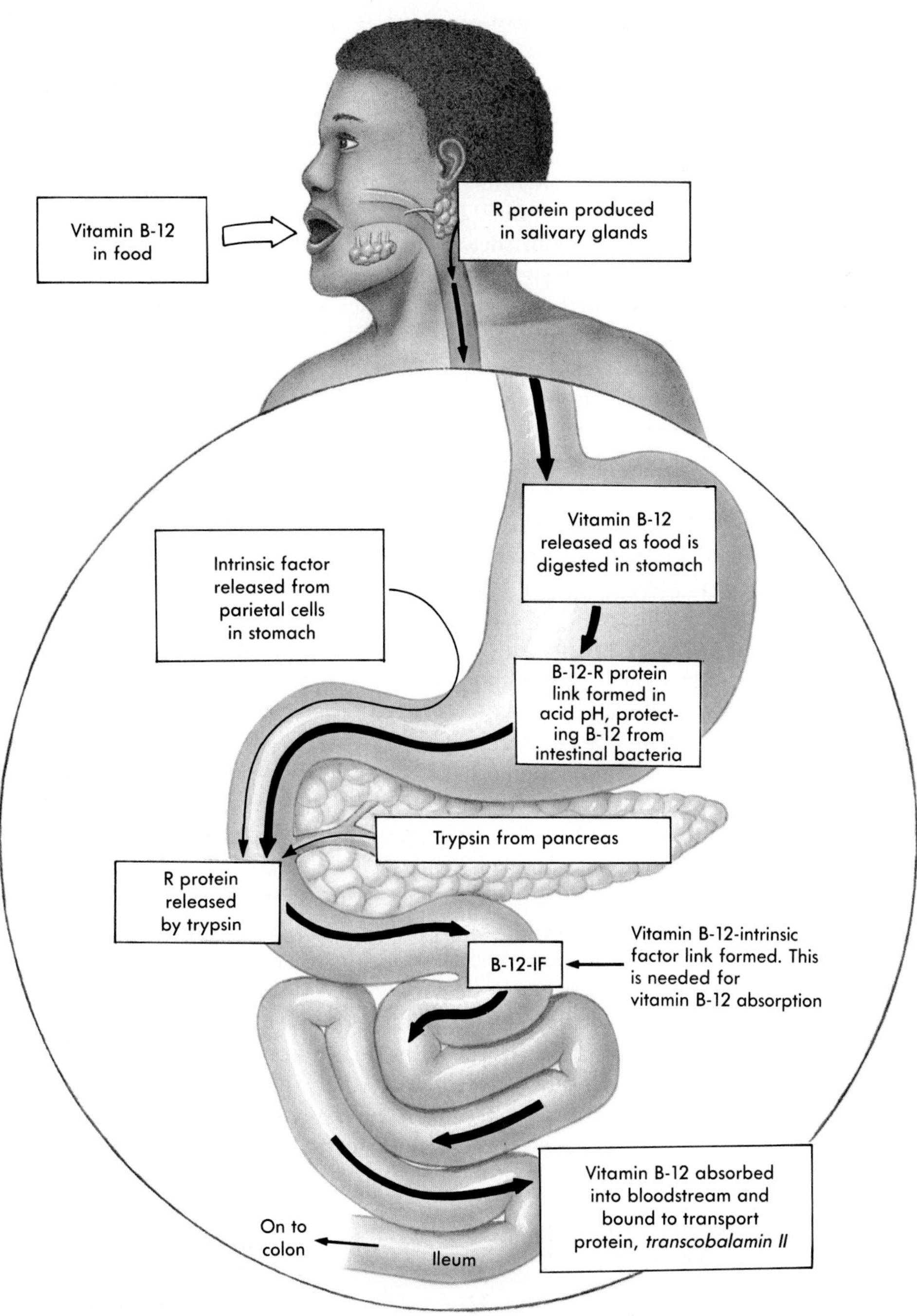

Figure 13-5 Absorption of vitamin B-12. Many factors and sites in the GI tract participate.

Once a defect in absorption is established, the person must then take monthly injections of vitamin B-12 to bypass the need for absorption, use a vitamin B-12 nasal gel (nasal absorption does not require the intrinsic factor), or take very potent vitamin B-12 supplements weekly (300 times the RDA). Ninety-five percent of all cases of vitamin B-12 deficiencies in healthy people in the United States result from a defect in vitamin B-12 absorption, rather than from inadequate intakes.

In the 1920s, researchers noted that they could cure a vitamin B-12 deficiency with massive amounts of liver or with concentrated water extracts of liver. In this case, the researchers cured a vitamin B-12 absorption defect by providing enough vitamin to allow simple diffusion to suffice. No R-protein/intrinsic factor system was needed.

FUNCTIONS OF VITAMIN B-12

Vitamin B-12 participates in a variety of reactions. Probably its most important function is in folate metabolism. Once the folate coenzyme is bonded to a methyl group ($-CH_3$), a form of vitamin B-12 is needed to remove the methyl group. Without vitamin B-12, the folate coenzymes are quickly bound by methyl groups.

The cell then has insufficient free folate coenzymes for metabolic needs. This shortage inhibits other important metabolic reactions, such as DNA synthesis, from taking place in the cell. Thus a vitamin B-12 deficiency contributes to a secondary folate deficiency. In this way the metabolism of vitamin B-12 and of folate are closely intertwined.[16]

Another vital function of vitamin B-12 is maintaining the myelin sheaths that insulate nerve fibers from each other. People with vitamin B-12 deficiencies show patchy destruction of the myelin sheaths, especially those surrounding the spinal cord. While the actual cause is unknown, alterations in the ability of vitamin B-12 to aid in the addition of a methyl group to homocysteine (to convert it to the amino acid methionine) may be a contributing factor. Whatever the cause, this destruction eventually causes paralysis, and even death.

Another important function of vitamin B-12 is its ability to aid in the rearrangement of carbon atoms in derivatives of three-carbon chain fatty acids so that they can eventually enter the citric acid cycle.[16]

pernicious anemia The anemia that results from a lack of vitamin B-12 absorption; it is pernicious because of associated nerve degeneration that can result in eventual paralysis.

PERNICIOUS ANEMIA

In the past, the inability to absorb vitamin B-12 eventually led to death. Researchers in midnineteenth century England noted a form of anemia that caused death within 2 to 5 years of initial illness. They called this **pernicious anemia** (pernicious literally means "leading to death"). Clinically, the anemia looks much like a folate-deficiency anemia. You can probably guess why—the folate/vitamin B-12 connections. Many macrocytes (abnormally large and immature red blood cells) are seen in the bloodstream. Thus the vitamin B-12 anemia is called a macrocytic anemia.

Strictly speaking, a lack of vitamin B-12 in the diet alone cannot cause pernicious anemia. It can only result from a decreased ability to absorb vitamin B-12.[18] Otherwise, it would take too long to develop significant nerve destruction from a strict dietary lack. Once pernicious anemia is noted, an injection of vitamin B-12 reverses changes in red blood cell synthesis and other clinical signs in 1 to 2 days.

Pernicious anemia and its accompanying nerve destruction often occurs in elderly people. The average age of occurrence in whites is 68 years. In African-Americans and Hispanics it appears about a decade sooner. As stomach parietal cells age, they lose their ability to synthesize the intrinsic factor needed for vitamin B-12 absorption. Current research suggests that this failure is due to an autoimmune reaction—people make white blood cells and other factors that attack their own parietal cells. Because parietal cells make acid, pernicious anemia is often accompanied by a decrease in stomach acid production, a condition called **achlorhydria.**

achlorhydria Decrease in stomach acid primarily due to age-associated loss of acid-producing stomach cells.

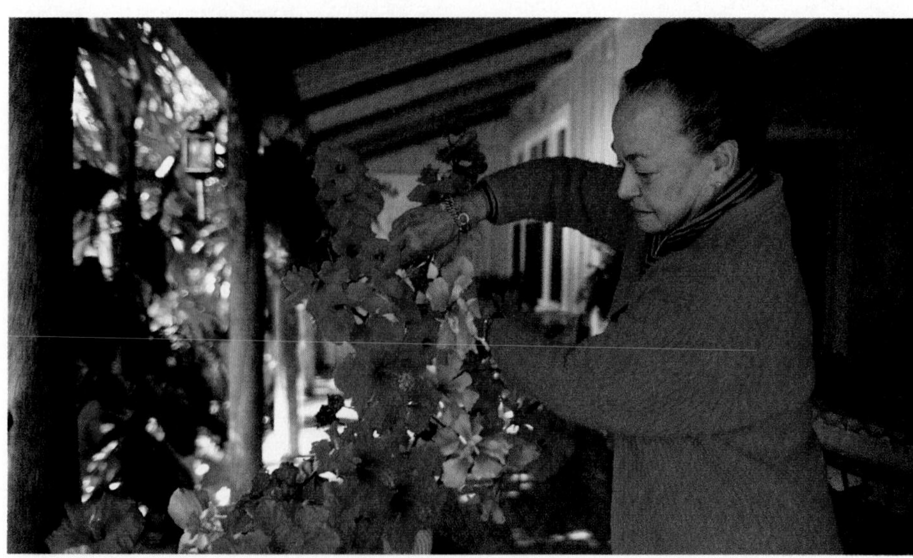

Due to poor vitamin B-12 absorption, older adults face a greater risk for pernicious anemia than those that are younger.

Table 13-8 Good food sources of vitamin B-12, ranked by nutrient density

Food	Serving size to yield 0.67 micrograms*	kcalories needed to yield 0.67 micrograms
Beef liver, fried	1/50 ounce	1
Oysters	½ each	3
Clams, canned	2 teaspoons	50
Roast beef	½ ounce	22
Egg	½ each	47
1% milk, low-fat	½ cup	60
Frankfurter, beef	1 each	80
Ham, baked	2½ ounces	117

* ⅓ RDA for adults.
Many types of animal protein provide ample vitamin B-12 within a reasonable energy intake.

Besides anemia, clinical signs and symptoms of pernicious anemia include weakness, sore tongue, back pain, apathy, and tingling in the extremities.[16] It takes about 3 years for symptoms of nerve destruction to develop.

VITAMIN B-12 IN FOODS

The most nutrient-dense sources of vitamin B-12 are the organ meats, especially the liver, kidneys, and heart. Into the above grouping, one may also include hot dogs because they contain many organ meat scraps. Additional sources are clams, oysters, beef, pork, eggs, and milk (if not over-processed; for example, sterilizing a bottle of infant formula or milk for over 10 minutes). Again, plant foods naturally contain no vitamin B-12.

RDA FOR VITAMIN B-12

The RDA for vitamin B-12 for adults is 2 micrograms per day. Our food supply yields approximately 8 micrograms of vitamin B-12 per person per day. This high intake provides the average meat-eating person with 2 to 3 years' storage of vitamin B-12 in the liver. Thus if you eat animal foods regularly and can absorb vitamin B-12, a vitamin B-12 deficiency is highly unlikely.

It takes approximately 20 years of consuming a diet essentially free of vitamin B-12 for a person to exhibit nerve destruction caused by a deficiency. However, as mentioned before, it takes only approximately 2 to 3 years to see the same nerve destruction if a person develops an inability to resorb vitamin B-12. That difference is mostly due to the ability of the body to reclaim vitamin B-12 it secretes into the small intestine if absorption is possible. Supplements of vitamin B-12 are virtually nontoxic.

AMERICANS AT RISK OF A VITAMIN B-12 DEFICIENCY

As we mentioned, vegans who eat no animal products should find a source of vitamin B-12. Options include a vitamin supplement, fortified soy milk, and special yeast grown in media rich in vitamin B-12. Otherwise, a vitamin B-12 deficiency is possible. The elderly are at risk for developing pernicious anemia. Regular physical examinations should especially look for enlarged red blood cells, low blood levels of vitamin B-12, and nervous tingling in the extremities.[18]

People who regularly consume excessive amounts of vitamin C supplements (just ten times the RDA) need to beware of its effect on vitamin B-12. Although the exact mechanism has yet to be determined, the antioxidant action of vitamin C may be capable of reducing the food availability of vitamin B-12 by converting it to a biologically inactive form.

CONCEPT CHECK

Folate is needed for cell division because it is tied to RNA and DNA synthesis. A folate deficiency results in anemia, as well as diarrhea, inflammation of the tongue, and poor growth—all signs of poor cell division. Folate is found in fresh vegetables and organ meats. It is important to emphasize "fresh" and "lightly cooked" with vegetables, because much folate is lost during cooking. Folate needs during pregnancy are especially high. Otherwise, a deficiency appears most often in alcoholism. Vitamin B-12 is necessary for folate metabolism. Without dietary vitamin B-12, folate deficiency symptoms, such as anemia, develop. In addition, vitamin B-12 is necessary for maintaining the nervous system; paralysis can develop from a vitamin B-12 deficiency. Vitamin B-12 is found only in animal foods; meat eaters generally have a 3- to 5-year supply stored in the liver. However, vitamin B-12 absorption may decline in the elderly years, requiring monthly injections.

Vitamin C

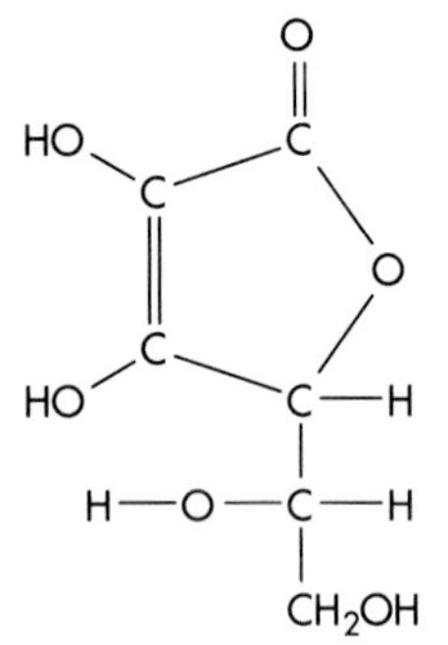

Vitamin C (ascorbic acid) is a puzzling vitamin. It is found in all living tissues, and most animals are capable of synthesizing their own supply from glucose. Only humans (as well as other primates), guinea pigs, birds, and few fish cannot make their own vitamin C and must obtain it from dietary sources. What is strange is that animals that synthesize vitamin C often make quite a lot of it. For instance, a pig produces 8 grams per day (though we do not benefit from it when we eat pork, since it is lost in processing). This amount is over 130 times our human RDA of 60 milligrams, and even 60 milligrams appears to be quite a generous intake for humans. As little as 10 milligrams daily can prevent scurvy, the vitamin C deficiency disease. Why some animals make so much vitamin C, while a few other animals, including humans, appear to need so little, has fueled much controversy surrounding this vitamin.

Ascorbic acid

ABSORPTION AND METABOLISM OF VITAMIN C

Absorption of vitamin C occurs in the small intestine by means of a specific transport system. The efficiency of the absorptive mechanism is related specifically to the amount of vitamin C available in a given load. About 80% to 90% of vitamin C is absorbed when a person consumes between 30 and 120 milligrams of it per day. If someone ingests 6 grams per day, absorption efficiency drops to about 20%. A common side effect of high vitamin C intake is diarrhea. The unabsorbed vitamin C stays in the small intestine and attracts water until it finally causes diarrhea.

Vitamin C can be reversibly altered (oxidized) to form dehydroascorbic acid. When vitamin C is broken down in the body, dehydroascorbic acid is irreversibly converted into diketogulonic acid. This acid may then be broken down into oxalic acid and other products. When high levels of vitamin C are consumed, most of it is excreted in the urine as vitamin C itself or a slight derivative. Oxalic acid is a major breakdown product or metabolite at low doses (about 100 milligrams).

FUNCTIONS OF VITAMIN C

reducing agent In one sense, a compound capable of donating electrons (also hydrogen ions) to another compound (see Appendix B).

Vitamin C performs a variety of very important cell functions. It does this primarily by being a nonspecific **reducing agent.** In one sense, a reducing agent is a substance capable of donating electrons (or hydrogen ions) (see Appendix B for a review of oxidation and reduction). By primarily acting on metal ions, especially iron in the Fe^{+2} state, vitamin C uses its abilities as a reducing agent to maintain metal ions in their active form.

Collagen Synthesis

Probably the most notable role of vitamin C is in developing the structural integrity of the three protein chains that are eventually woven together like a rope to form the fibrous protein called collagen. Collagen is present wherever tissues require strengthening, especially in those tissues with a protective, connective or structural function. Collagen fibers are critical to the maintenance of bone and blood vessels, and to heal wounds.

To be more specific, vitamin C is responsible for maintaining the active form of an iron atom that is critical to function of the enzymes involved in collagen synthesis. These enzymes in turn add a hydroxyl group (−OH) to the amino acid proline within the three protein chains discussed previously. In addition, these enzymes add a hydroxyl group to the lysine amino acids (also found on the protein chains), enabling them to cross-link the three chains of collagen together. The hydroxyl additions to these two types of amino acids are found all along these three chains of collagen, and are critical for providing collagen with its characteristic strength.

As expected, a deficiency in vitamin C results in widespread and disastrous changes in tissue metabolism and structure throughout the body. The deficiency disease is known as scurvy. The first symptoms of scurvy appear after about 20 to 40 days of no vitamin C intake and include weakness and pinpoint hemorrhages (petechiae) around hair follicles on the back of the arms and legs (Figure 13-6). In addition, gums bleed and joints become painful. Other symptoms of scurvy include opening of previously healed wounds, bone pain, fractures, and diarrhea. Most of these symptoms are linked to poor collagen structure.

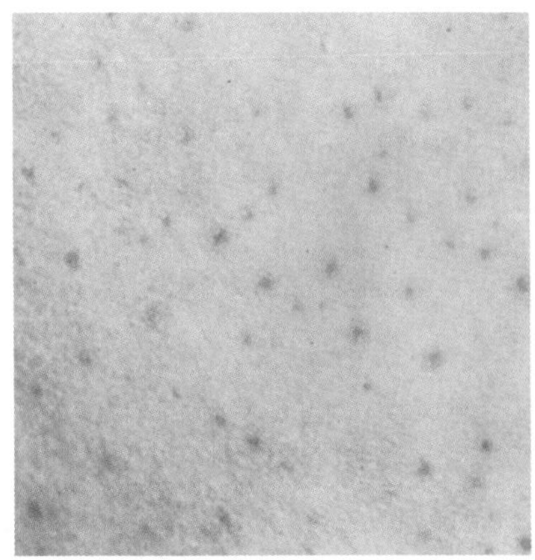

Figure 13-6 Pinpoint hemorrhages of the skin—an early stage of scurvy. The spots are caused by slight bleeding into hair follicles. The person will also often show poor wound healing—all signs of poor collagen synthesis.

Antioxidant

Because of its ability to act as a reducing agent, vitamin C is one of the cell's water-soluble antioxidants. Recall that vitamin E is a fat-soluble antioxidant in the cell membrane. Using its antioxidant capabilities, vitamin C can reduce the formation of carcinogenic nitrosamines in the stomach, minimize destruction of vitamin A, and also keep the folate coenzymes intact to prevent their destruction. Vitamin C is thought to be effective in helping prevent certain cancers,[4] as well as cataracts in the eye, probably because of its antioxidant capabilities.

Scurvy was the bane of sailors throughout the nineteenth century. On long sea voyages a captain often lost half or more of his crew to scurvy. From 1556 to 1857, more than 114 scurvy epidemics were reported in Europe. Soldiers in the U.S. Civil War died of scurvy. In 1740, Dr. James Lind, working aboard the HMS Salisbury, showed that citrus fruits—two oranges and one lemon a day—could cure scurvy. Fifty years after Lind's discovery, rations for British sailors included limes to prevent scurvy. That is why the British today are often called "limeys."

Enhancing Iron Absorption

Vitamin C is important for iron absorption. Among its roles in this process, vitamin C keeps iron in the Fe^{+2} form. This conversion renders the iron much more soluble in the small intestine's alkaline environment, and thus increases iron absorption. To produce this effect, about 50 milligrams of vitamin C (about 4 ounces of orange juice) must be consumed at the same meal with the iron.

Increasing vitamin C intake is very beneficial if one has poor iron stores. However, some people suffer from a disease characterized by an over-storage of iron (hemochromatosis; see Chapter 15). These people are actually harmed if, by increasing their vitamin C intake, they likewise increase their iron absorption. This is just one of many examples in which recommending a vitamin intake above the RDA may have conflicting results. Some people may benefit, whereas others may be injured.

Synthesis of Vital Cell Compounds

Vitamin C is necessary for the synthesis of thyroxine—the thyroid hormone—as well as epinephrine, carnitine, norepinephrine, serotonin, bile acids, steroid hormones, and the purine bases used for DNA synthesis. The synthesis of these compounds requires the addition of hydroxyl groups.

Vitamin C is vital for the function of the immune system, especially for the activity of certain cells (lymphocytes) in the immune system.[17] In addition, vitamin C is used by chemical-detoxifying mechanisms in cells. Thus both disease states and drug use can increase the need for vitamin C, but we don't know how much vitamin C intake above the RDA to prescribe.

Vitamin C status is assessed by its concentration in white blood cells. A diet history of limited fruit and vegetable consumption also suggests a deficiency.

Table 13-9 Good food sources of vitamin C, ranked by nutrient density

Food	Serving size to yield 20 milligrams*	kcalories needed to yield 20 milligrams
Green peppers, whole, raw	⅓ each	4
Cauliflower, cooked	⅓ cup	9
Bok choy cabbage, cooked	½ cup	9
Broccoli, cooked	⅓ cup	9
Strawberries, fresh	¼ cup	11
Mustard greens, cooked	⅔ cup	12
Brussel sprouts, cooked	⅓ cup	12
Papaya, whole fresh	1/9 each	13
Romaine lettuce, chopped	1½ cups	14
Grapefruit pink/red	½ each	16
Cantaloupe	1/12 each	17
Orange, fresh, medium	⅓ each	17
Asparagus, cooked	½ cup	18
Orange juice, fresh	⅙ cup	18
Tomato juice, canned	½ cup	19
Grapefruit white	½ each	20
Grapefruit juice, fresh	⅓ cup	20
Spinach, cooked	½ cup	21
Tomato, whole raw	1 each	22
Sauerkraut canned	⅔ cup	25
Cooked peas	⅔ cup	71
Baked potato	1 medium	95
Sweet potato	1 medium	100

* ⅓ RDA for adults.
All these foods provide ample vitamin C within both a limited serving size and kcalorie cost. Emphasize these fruits and vegetables for a nutritious diet.

VITAMIN C IN FOODS

The most nutrient-dense sources of vitamin C are green peppers, cauliflower, broccoli, cabbage, strawberries, papayas, and romaine lettuce (Table 13-9). Citrus fruits, potatoes, and other green vegetables are also good sources of vitamin C. The five to nine servings of combined fruits and vegetables from the Guide to Daily Food Choices should easily provide enough vitamin C. The major contributors of vitamin C to our diets are oranges and orange juice, grapefruit and grapefruit juice, tomatoes and tomato juice, fortified fruit drinks, tangerines, and potatoes. Note that the isoascorbate (erythorbate) that is used as a food preservative in fruits and vegetables has no vitamin C value.

Vitamin C is easily lost in processing and cooking. Juices are good foods to fortify with vitamin C because their acidity reduces vitamin C destruction. Vitamin C is very unstable when in contact with heat, iron, copper, or oxygen.

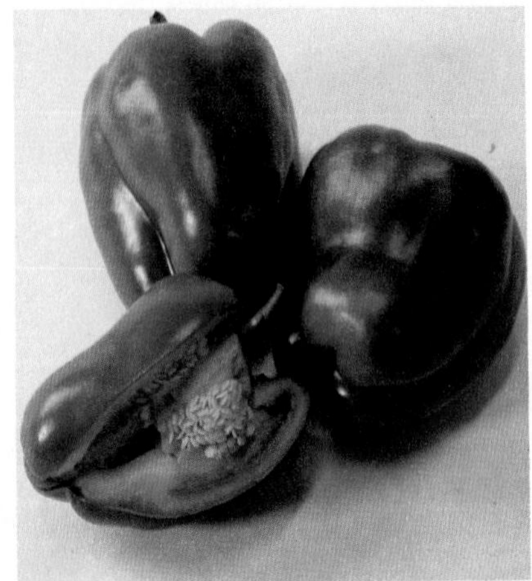

Many people may be surprised to learn that green peppers are a good source of vitamin C.

RDA FOR VITAMIN C

The RDA for vitamin C for adults is 60 milligrams per day. The current RDA publication suggests cigarette smokers consume 100 milligrams per day because they greatly stress their lungs. Our food supply yields about twice the adult RDA (120 milligrams) of vitamin C per day, of which approximately 82 milligrams is derived naturally from foods. The rest comes from food supplements. So it is likely that nearly all of us are meeting our daily need for vitamin C.

AMERICANS AT RISK FOR VITAMIN C DEFICIENCY

Today vitamin C deficiency appears mostly in people with alcoholism who eat nutrient-poor diets and in elderly men who eat poorly. Studies show that 14% to 20% of adult and elderly men have low serum vitamin C levels. Men are more susceptible than women because they are less apt to consume vitamin supplements.

Smokers generally have lower vitamin C stores.[32] Recent findings show that smokers may need as much as 200 milligrams of vitamin C daily in order to meet their needs and to maintain a serum level of vitamin C equal to that of nonsmokers consuming the 60 milligram RDA. This is a troubling finding since only 27% of smokers even consume as much as 100 milligrams daily of vitamin C.

Worldwide, scurvy is associated with poverty. It is especially common in infants who are fed boiled milk (all forms of milk are poor sources of vitamin C) and not provided with a good food source of vitamin C or a supplement.

TOXICITY OF VITAMIN C

Vitamin C is probably not toxic when consumed in amounts less than 1 to 2 grams, aside from the concern that some vitamin B-12 destruction can take place. Regularly consuming more than that can cause stomach inflammation, diarrhea, overabsorption of iron, oxalate kidney stones, and possibly "rebound" or "withdrawal" scurvy. What may happen in "rebound" scurvy is that the body, when receiving a high vitamin C intake, develops enzyme systems to rapidly metabolize it. If one abruptly reduces the intake to normal, the enzyme systems take a while to readjust. Thus if a person has a history of a high vitamin C intake, slowly tapering the intake is recommended.[25]

Keep in mind that most vitamin C consumed in large doses just ends up in the stool or the urine. The body is totally saturated at intakes of 150 milligrams per day. In any event, maladies such as common colds are rarely severe enough, nor last long enough, to merit megadose vitamin C therapy. Consuming vitamin C may decrease a cold's severity somewhat, so we see no reason to discourage people from drinking a few glasses of orange juice when they have a cold. If it doesn't help them physically, it may help them psychologically. Psychological effects can often work wonders. However, there is no striking evidence from double-blind studies that large amounts of vitamin C greatly decrease the severity or duration of a cold.[37]

In addition, no credible evidence suggests that a dose even as high as 10 grams a day will cure colon cancer. Early studies suggesting this role for vitamin C megadoses were too poorly controlled to be credible.[27] If people with cancer want to dabble with large doses of vitamin C, they should alert their physician, primarily because high doses of vitamin C can change reactions to medical tests for diabetes or blood in the stool. Physicians may misdiagnose conditions when large doses of vitamin C are consumed without their knowledge.

Now that we have discussed the vitamins, see Table 13-10 for a review.

CONCEPT CHECK

Only guinea pigs, monkeys, some birds and fish, and humans need dietary vitamin C. It is used mainly to help synthesize collagen, a major connective tissue protein. A vitamin C deficiency, known as scurvy, causes many changes in the skin and gums, such as small hemorrhages. This is due to poor collagen synthesis. Vitamin C also improves iron absorption and is involved in synthesizing certain hormones and neurotransmitters. Citrus fruits, green peppers, cauliflower, broccoli, and strawberries are good sources of vitamin C. As with folate, fresh or lightly cooked foods are important to emphasize, since loss of vitamin C in cooking can be high. At doses greater than about 33 times the RDA (2 grams), vitamin C can lead to diarrhea. These high doses do not prevent the common cold or cure cancer; however, consuming the RDA of vitamin C is part of the overall approach to good health.

Table 13-10 A summary of the water-soluble vitamins

Name and coenzyme	Major functions	Deficiency symptoms	Deficiency risk conditions
Thiamin; TPP	Glycolysis, citric acid cycle, and hexosemonophosphate shunt activity; nerve function	Beriberi; nervous tingling, poor coordination, edema, heart changes, weakness	Alcoholism, poverty
Riboflavin; FAD and FMN	Citric acid cycle and electron transport chain activity; fat breakdown; drug-detoxifying pathways	Ariboflavinosis; inflammation of mouth and tongue, cracks at corners of the mouth, eye disorders	Possibly people on certain medications if no dairy products consumed
Niacin; NAD and NADP	Glycolysis, citric acid cycle, and electron transport chain activity; fat synthesis, fat breakdown	Pellagra; diarrhea, bilateral dermatitis dementia	Severe poverty where corn is the dominant food; alcoholism
Pantothenic acid; Coenzyme A, acylcarrier protein	Citric acid cycle; fat synthesis, fat breakdown	Tingling in hands, fatigue, headache, nausea	Alcoholism
Biotin, biocytin	Glucose production; fat synthesis; purine (part of DNA, RNA) synthesis	Dermatitis, tongue soreness, anemia, depression	Alcoholism
Vitamin B-6, pyridoxine and other forms; PLP	Protein metabolism; neurotransmitter synthesis; hemoglobin synthesis; many other functions	Headache, anemia, convulsions, nausea, vomiting, flaky skin, sore tongue	Adolescent and adult women; people on certain medications; alcoholism
Folate (folic acid); THFA	DNA and RNA synthesis; amino acid synthesis; choline synthesis	Anemia, inflammation of tongue, diarrhea, poor growth, mental disorders	Alcoholism, pregnancy, use of certain medications
Vitamin B-12 (cobalamins)	Folate metabolism; nerve function	Macrocytic anemia, poor nerve function	Elderly due to poor absorption; vegans
Vitamin C (ascorbic acid)	Collagen synthesis; hormone and neurotransmitter synthesis	Scurvy; poor wound healing, pinpoint hemorrhages, bleeding gums, edema	Alcoholism, elderly men living alone

Vitamin-Like Compounds

The various vitamin-like compounds—choline, carnitine, inositol, taurine, and lipoic acid—are necessary to maintain proper metabolism in the body. They can be synthesized by the body, but that often occurs at the expense of important nutrients, such as essential amino acids. The needs for these compounds also can increase in times of rapid tissue growth, as is the case with the premature infant.

There is no concern that these vitamin-like compounds are needed by the average healthy adult. But more research is needed for certain disease states, specifically concerning their addition to infant formulas and total parenteral nutrition solutions. Presently, manufacturers often add these vitamin-like compounds to infant formulas.

CHOLINE

$$HO-CH_2-CH_2-\overset{\oplus}{N}(CH_3)_3$$

Choline

Choline is widely distributed within the plant and animal kingdoms. So much choline naturally occurs in the diet that a deficiency is hardly possible. Choline has a very simple structure. It can be built in the liver using carbon atoms from the amino acids methionine and serine, along with the help of folate and vitamin B-12. If enough choline is not in the diet, the body can normally make the rest if enough methionine-containing protein is eaten.[33]

Table 13-10 A summary of the water-soluble vitamins—cont'd

Adult RDA or ESADDI	Dietary sources	Toxicity
1.1-1.5 milligrams	Sunflower seeds, pork, whole and enriched grains, dried beans, peas, brewers yeast	None possible from food
1.2-1.7 milligrams	Milk, mushrooms, spinach, liver, enriched grains	None reported
15-19 milligrams	Mushrooms, bran, tuna, salmon, chicken, beef, liver, peanuts, enriched grains	Flushing of skin at intakes > 100 milligrams
4-7 milligrams	Mushrooms, liver, broccoli, eggs; most foods have some	None
30-100 micrograms	Cheese, egg yolks, cauliflower, peanut butter, liver	Unknown
1.8-2 milligrams	Animal protein foods, spinach, broccoli, bananas, salmon, sunflower seeds	Nerve destruction at doses > 100 milligrams
180-200 micrograms	Green leafy vegetables, orange juice, organ meats, sprouts, sunflower seeds	None, nonprescription vitamin dosage is controlled by FDA
2 micrograms	Animal foods, especially organ meats, oysters, clams (not natural in plants)	None
60 milligrams	Citrus fruits, strawberries, broccoli, greens	Doses > 2 grams causes diarrhea and can alter some diagnostic tests

Choline forms part of the emulsifier lecithin (actually called phosphatidylcholine) and the neurotransmitter acetylcholine, as well as other compounds. Lecithins are widely distributed in blood lipoproteins, cell membranes, and bile. The name choline actually comes from "chole," which means bile.

A choline-free diet in animals can cause a choline deficiency, of which a major symptom is a fatty liver. Animals evidently cannot make enough to supply all their needs. However, this type of fatty liver is not the same type as that seen in human alcoholism. Attempts to treat alcoholic fatty liver in humans with high doses of choline or lecithin have failed. Scientists have attempted to treat some neurological disorders, such as Alzheimer's disease and other forms of senile memory loss, with lecithin. Despite the highly active research in this area, it is still too early to say if persons with these problems can benefit from that treatment.

We consume probably 400 to 900 milligrams of choline per day. Doses as high as 20 to 30 grams per day have been administered. The side-effects include a "fishy" body odor, especially when choline itself, rather than lecithin, is used. Gastric distress, vomiting, and diarrhea may also result. There is some concern that these high doses of choline may also increase the risk of developing stomach cancer, since choline can be metabolized to compounds that then form the powerful carcinogens known as nitrosamines.

NUTRITION FOCUS

Preserving Vitamins in Food

Substantial amounts of vitamins in foods can be lost from the time a fruit or vegetable is picked until it is eaten. The water-soluble vitamins, particularly thiamin, vitamin C, and folate, can be destroyed with improper storage and excessive cooking. Heat, light, exposure to the air, cooking in large amounts of water, and alkalinity are all factors that can destroy vitamins. The sooner the food is eaten, the less chance of nutrient loss.

In general, if the food is not to be eaten within a few days, freezing is the best method to retain nutrients. In fact, frozen vegetables and fruits are often better than supermarket "fresh." This is because such foods are often frozen immediately after harvesting. As part of the freezing process, vegetables are quickly blanched in boiling water. This destroys the enzymes that would otherwise degrade the vitamins. "Fresh" food often lingers in the grocery store or at home for a while before being eaten.

Below are some tips to aid in preserving the vitamins in food:

- Keep fruits and vegetables cool. Enzymes in foods begin to degrade vitamins once the fruit or vegetable is picked. Chilling reduces this process, so refrigerating these foods until they are consumed is important.
- Refrigerate foods in moisture-proof containers. Nutrients keep best at temperatures near freezing, at high humidity, and away from exposure to air.
- Avoid trimming and cutting fruits and vegetables into small pieces when possible. The greater surface exposed speeds vitamin breakdown by oxygen. Keep in mind that the outer leaves of lettuce and other greens have higher values of vitamins and minerals than the inner, tender leaves or stems. The skins of potatoes, apples, and carrots for example, are higher in vitamins and minerals than the center part.
- To retain the high levels of nutrients in vegetables, microwave cooking, steaming, or using a pan or wok with very small amounts of water and a tight-fitting lid are best. The less contact with water, and the shorter the cooking time, the more nutrients retained. Whenever possible, cook fruits or vegetables in their skins.
- Minimize reheating food. This reduces the vitamin content.
- Don't add baking soda to the water when cooking vegetables to enhance the green color. The alkalinity destroys much vitamin C, thiamin, and other vitamins.
- Store canned goods in a cool place. To get maximum nutritive value from the canned goods, whenever possible, serve any liquid packed with the food. Canned foods vary in the amount of nutrients lost, largely due to differences in storage time and canning processes.
- Keep milk cold, covered and away from strong light. Riboflavin is lost in direct light. Note, however, that pasteurizing raw milk does not destroy the main nutrients we look to milk products to provide—protein, riboflavin, and calcium, among others.

$$CH_3-\overset{\oplus}{N}(CH_3)_2-CH_2-CH(OH)-CH_2-C(=O)-OH$$

Carnitine

CARNITINE

With the help of vitamin B-6, liver cells make carnitine using the amino acids lysine and methionine. People with very low protein intakes, such as people with kwashiorkor (see Chapter 5), appear to have lower levels of carnitine in the bloodstream. Thus it is important to eat an adequate amount of protein to supply the building blocks needed for making this compound. There is concern that people with cirrhosis of the liver may need carnitine supplements because carnitine is made in the liver. (See the Expert Opinion in Chapter 10 to see if this is also true for athletes.)

Carnitine in the cell primarily shuttles long-chain fatty acids from the cytosol into the mitochondria so that fatty acids can be burned to provide energy. Carnitine also shuttles the breakdown products of some amino acids into the mitochondria.[8]

In addition, carnitine has displayed pharmaceutical usefulness in the removal of compounds that can build to toxic levels in people with inborn errors of metabolism. Dosages at approximately 10 times those of dietary intake have been shown to improve the condition of persons with progressive muscle disease and cardiomyopathy.

Meat and dairy products are the main sources of carnitine. We consume about 100 to 300 milligrams per day. Vegetarian diets are very low in carnitine because it is not found in plant foods. However, vegetarians show normal blood levels of carnitine. Consequently, it is doubtful that carnitine is necessary in the diet of healthy people.[15] In times of recovery from disease or serious trauma, carnitine supplements may be important.

INOSITOL

The roles of inositol within the cell membrane appear to be involved with the recognition and transfer of stimuli. This transfer of information may be important to the function of neurotransmitters and hormones. Such a role might explain why such high phosphatidylinositol concentrations are found within the brain and its structures.

There are nine forms of inositol. The one used by humans is called myo-inositol. Inositol has a structure similar to that of glucose. In fact, we make inositol from glucose. As part of phosphatidylinositol, it also is found in high concentrations in cell membranes.

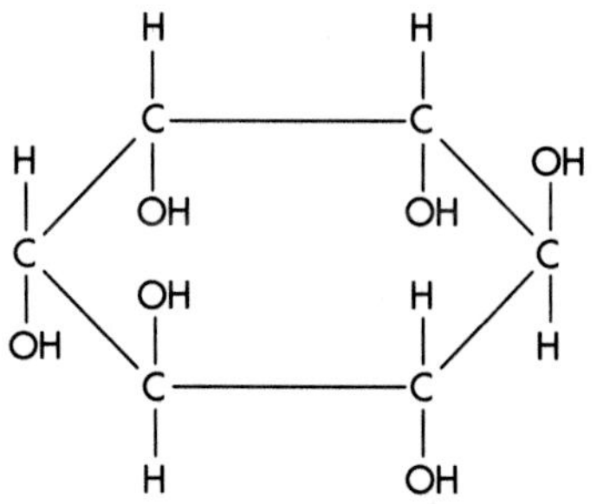

Inositol also forms a basic part of phytic acid, a compound that binds minerals in plant foods, such as wheat bran. In animal foods it may be found as the inositol or phosphatidylinositol forms. In either form, it is widely found in both plant and animal products. The average American diet provides about 1 gram of inositol per day, and our kidneys are capable of synthesizing 4 grams of inositol a day.

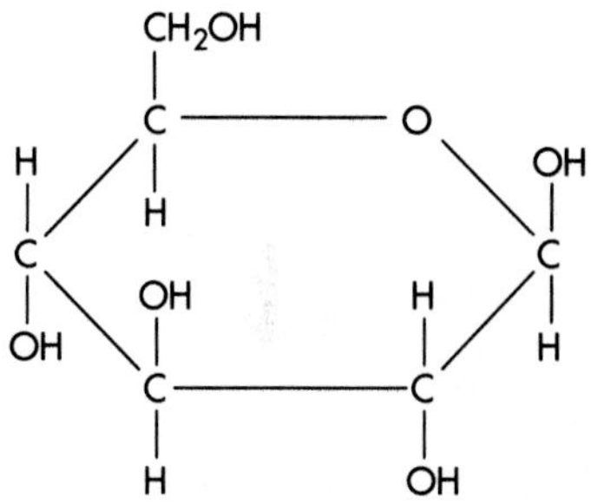

Myo-Inositol

Glucose

TAURINE

Taurine performs many vital functions. It forms part of some bile acids, is necessary for nerve function, and is important for vision. It is synthesized from the amino acids methionine and cysteine and is found only in animal foods. Taurine looks like the amino acid glycine except for the substitution of a sulfur-containing group. It is the only free amino acid readily found in nature (others are combined into proteins).

No clear cases of taurine deficiencies have been diagnosed in vegans, and again it is not found in plants. Thus it appears that healthy people need not worry about consuming taurine. Synthesis by the body apparently meets our needs.

During rapid growth we seem to need more taurine. Once growth rates level off in adulthood, the need for taurine decreases.[11] Premature infants now have taurine added to their formulas, primarily because the taurine concentration in human milk is very high.

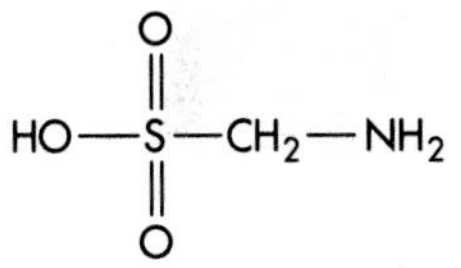

Taurine

LIPOIC ACID

Lipoic acid is used in reactions in which a carbon dioxide molecule is lost, as when pyruvate is converted into acetyl-CoA. Health-food stores sell this compound, but our bodies readily make lipoic acid.

BOGUS VITAMINS

A variety of bogus vitamins is promoted by health-food enthusiasts. None of these compounds is important in human nutrition. Some may increase growth in less complex forms of life, so vitamin hucksters try to pass them off as necessary for humans.

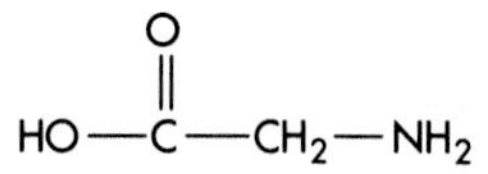

The list of these pseudo-vitamins changes frequently. The following list shows some of the more persistent pseudos:[16]

Paraaminobenzoic acid—Recall that this compound is part of folic acid. If people consume this drug in conjunction with sulfa antibiotics, they can defeat the effect of the antibiotic.

Laetrile—This cyanide-containing compound, wrongly labeled "vitamin B-17," is promoted as a cure for cancer, but FDA does not recognize it as a legitimate therapy.

Bioflavonoids—These compounds, wrongly labeled "vitamin P," include rutin and hesperidin. They were originally thought to be more effective than vitamin C

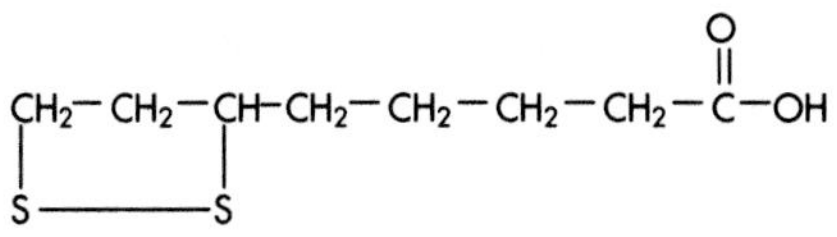

Glycine

Lipoic acid

alone for treating fragile blood vessels in scurvy. Today, there is no recognized nutritional or medical need for bioflavonoids, although they may enhance vitamin C absorption.

Pangamic acid—This bogus compound, wrongly labeled "vitamin B-15," has no link to nutrition and deserves no attention.

Other compounds will come and go in the next few years. Again, since people have been maintained for years on parenteral feedings containing all the known essential nutrients without developing deficiency symptoms, it is unlikely that any vitamin remains to be discovered. You can be sure that if a "new" compound has the potential to be a vitamin, the Food and Nutrition Board of the National Academy of Sciences will closely examine it. If it then appears with the rest of the nutrients that have an RDA or ESADDI, you can be confident the compound can be called a vitamin and is worth your attention.

CONCEPT CHECK

A variety of vitamin-like compounds are found in the body. They can be synthesized by cells using common building blocks, such as amino acids and glucose. In disease states, synthesis may not meet bodily needs, and therefore dietary intake can be crucial. The need for choline, carnitine, and taurine in certain conditions, such as for premature infants or in total parenteral nutrition, are current areas of research.

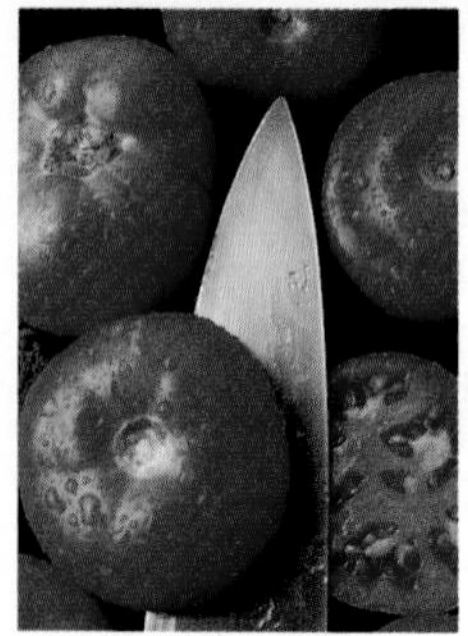

Summary

1. Thiamin has a key role in carbohydrate metabolism. A deficiency will impair nervous system functions, primarily because nervous tissues use mostly carbohydrate for energy. Deficiencies are most likely in alcoholism. Pork, dried beans, and enriched grains are excellent sources of thiamin.
2. Riboflavin participates in the metabolism of all energy-yielding nutrients because it plays key roles in the citric acid cycle, electron transport chain, and fat breakdown. An isolated deficiency will result in mouth and tongue inflammation, but is quite unlikely. Dairy products and enriched grains are good sources of riboflavin.
3. Niacin is a key nutrient used in many pathways for metabolism of energy-yielding nutrients. A deficiency results in severe skin lesions, dementia, diarrhea, and eventually, death. Alcoholism and the poor diets consumed by the impoverished can lead to a deficiency. High niacin concentrations are found in protein foods we commonly consume.
4. Pantothenic acid participates in many aspects of cell metabolism, including fat metabolism and the citric acid cycle. A deficiency is unlikely since (as its name implies) it is widely found in foods.
5. Biotin participates in glucose production and fat synthesis and contributes to DNA synthesis as well. A deficiency results in anemia and inflammation of the skin and tongue. It may appear with alcoholism. Synthesis by intestinal bacteria probably suffices for some of our needs and adds to the biotin found in eggs, cheese, and peanuts.
6. Vitamin B-6 forms a vital role in protein metabolism, especially in the synthesis of nonessential (dispensable) amino acids. It also participates in the synthesis of neurotransmitters and performs other metabolic roles. Headaches, anemia, nausea, and vomiting result from a deficiency. Some women are likely to have poor vitamin B-6 stores. Regular consumption of animal protein foods, cauliflower, and broccoli provides needed vitamin B-6. Destruction of nervous system tissues appears from high doses, specifically starting at 100 times the RDA.

7. Folate plays an important role in RNA and DNA synthesis. Signs of poor cell division, such as anemia, tongue inflammation, diarrhea, and poor growth, appear in a deficiency. Pregnancy puts high demands for folate on the body. Otherwise, a deficiency occurs most likely in alcoholism. Excellent food sources are leafy vegetables, organ meats, and orange juice. Since the amount of folate lost in cooking can be great, dietary emphasis should be on lightly cooked vegetables.
8. Vitamin B-12 is needed for metabolizing folate and maintaining the insulation surrounding nerves. A deficiency results in anemia (because of its relationship to folate) and nerve degeneration. Poor absorption of vitamin B-12 often occurs in the elderly. In these cases, monthly injections of the vitamin can be used. For others, a deficiency is unlikely because it is present in high concentrations in animal foods, which constitute a major part of our diets. Vitamin B-12 does not occur in plant foods, except through minor soil contamination. Vegans need to find a supplemental source.
9. Vitamin C is needed mainly to synthesize collagen, a major protein used in building connective tissue. A vitamin C deficiency results in scurvy, which is evidenced by poor wound healing, pinpoint hemorrhages in the skin, and bleeding gums. Vitamin C also enhances iron absorption and is needed for the synthesis of some hormones and neurotransmitters. Fresh fruits and vegetables, especially citrus fruits, are generally good sources. Since the amount of vitamin C lost in cooking is high, the dietary emphasis—as with folate—should be on fresh or lightly cooked vegetables. Deficiencies often occur in people with alcoholism and in elderly men whose diets lack enough fruits and vegetables. High doses of vitamin C often cause diarrhea.
10. A variety of vitamin-like compounds are found in the body. Cells synthesize them using common building blocks, such as amino acids and glucose. In disease states, synthesis may not meet needs, and therefore dietary intake becomes more critical. The need for choline, carnitine, and taurine in some conditions, such as for premature infants or for total parenteral nutrition, are current areas of research.

Study Questions

1. Name the vitamins for which needs will increase during increased energy expenditure and explain why.
2. For what vitamins does the body have an endogenous source (originating within the body). Describe those sources.
3. Explain why individual B vitamin deficiencies generally are so rare in the United States. Describe an incidence where one might occur.
4. Although folate is not known to have any toxic effects, the FDA limits the amount that may be found in supplementary forms. Why?
5. Since the deficiency disease of vitamin C is so severe, is it a good idea for Americans to take excess supplementation in efforts to avoid such a deficiency? Do the benefits of vitamin C supplementation above and beyond the RDA outweigh any negative consequences? Discuss these two questions, especially in light of what was covered in Chapter 12.
6. What distinguishes the vitamin-like compounds from the actual vitamins? Does their role within the body warrant any special attention at all?

REFERENCES

1. Albin RL and others: Acute sensory neuropathy-neuronopathy from pyridoxine overdose, *Neurology* 37:17, 29, 1987.
2. Bailey LB: Evaluation of a new Recommended Dietary Allowance for folate, Journal of the American Dietetic Association 92:463, 1992.
3. Birt DF: The influence of dietary fat on carcinogenesis: lessons from experimental models, *Nutrition Reviews* 48:1, 1990.
4. Block G: Vitamin C and cancer prevention: the epidemiologic evidence, *American Journal of Clinical Nutrition* 53:270S, 1991.
5. Blocker DE, Thenen SW: Intestinal absorption, liver uptake, and excretion of 3 H-folic acid-deficient, alcohol-consuming nonhuman primates, *American Journal of Clinical Nutrition* 46:503, 1987.
6. Burton GW: Antioxidant action of carotenoids, *Journal of Nutrition* 119:109, 1989.
7. Carpenter K: Comment on Goldberger J, Wheeler GA: Experimental pellagra in the human subject brought about by a restricted diet, *Nutrition* 6:357, 1990.
8. Carroll JE: Carnitine deficiency revisited, *Journal of Nutrition* 117:1501, 1987.
9. Carroll KK: Dietary fats and cancer, *American Journal of Clinical Nutrition* 53:1064S, 1991.
10. Casey V, Dwyer JT: Premenstrual syndrome: theories and evidence, *Nutrition Today,* Nov/Dec 1987, p 4.
11. Chesney RW: Taurine: is it required for infant nutrition? *Journal of Nutrition* 118:6, 1988.
12. Clark NG and others: Treatment of iron-deficiency anemia complicated by scurvy and folic acid deficiency, *Nutrition Reviews* 50:134, 1992.
13. Comstock GW and others: Prediagnostic serum levels of carotenoids and vitamin E as related to subsequent cancer in Washington County, Maryland, *American Journal of Clinical Nutrition* 53:260S, 1991.
14. Dwyer JT: Unproven nutritional remedies and cancer, *Nutrition Reviews* 50:106, 1992.
15. Feller AJ, Redman D: Role of carnitine in human nutrition, *Journal of Nutrition* 118:541, 1988.
16. Herbert VD: "Folic acid" and "vitamin B-12" and "Pseudovitamins." In Shils ME, Young VR, editors: *Modern Nutrition in health and disease,* ed 7, Philadelphia, 1988, Lea & Febiger.
17. Jacob RA and others: Immunocompetence and oxidant defense during ascorbate depletion of healthy men, *American Journal of Clinical Nutrition* 54:1302S, 1991.
18. Karnad AB, Krozser-Hamati A: Pernicious anemia: early identification to prevent permanent sequelae, *Postgraduate Medicine* 91:231, 1992.
19. Knekt P and others: Vitamin E and cancer prevention, *American Journal of Clinical Nutrition* 53:283S, 1991.
20. Kretsch MJ and others: Electroencephalographic changes and periodontal status during short-term vitamin B-6 depletion of young, nonpregnant women, *American Journal of Clinical Nutrition* 53:1266, 1991.
21. Leklem JE: Vitamin B-6: of reservoirs, receptors and requirements, *Nutrition Today,* Sept/Oct 1988, p 4.
22. Malone WF: Studies evaluating antioxidants and B-carotene as chemopreventives, *American Journal of Clinical Nutrition* 53:305S, 1991.
23. Marshall MW: The nutritional importance of biotin—an update, *Nutrition Today,* Nov/Dec 1987, p 26.
24. Masse PG: Nutrient intakes of women who use oral contraceptives, *Journal of The American Dietetic Association* 91:1118, 1991.
25. Maye ST and others: Rebound effect with ascorbic and in adult males, *American Journal of Clinical Nutrition* 48:379, 1988.
26. McCormick DB: "Thiamin," "riboflavin," "niacin," "vitamin B-6," "pantothenic acid," and "biotin." In Shils ME, Young VR, editors: *Modern nutrition in health and disease,* ed 7, Philadelphia, 1988, Lea & Febiger.
27. Moertel CG and others: High-dose of vitamin C versus placebo in a treatment of patients with advanced cancer who have had no prior chemotherapy, *The New England Journal of Medicine* 312:137, 1985.
28. Nutrition Monitoring Division, Human Nutrition Information Service: Nationwide Food Consumption Survey: *Nutrition Today,* May/June 1986, pp 18, 23; Nov/Dec 1986, p 31; Sept/Oct 1987, p 36.
29. Oriot D and others: Severe lactic acidosis related to acute thiamine deficiency, *Journal of Parenteral and Enteral Nutrition* 15:105, 1991.
30. Reid RL: Premenstrual syndrome, *The New England Journal of Medicine* 324:1208, 1991.
31. Reynolds RD: Determination of dietary vitamin B-6 intake: is it accurate? *Journal of The American Dietetic Association* 90:799, 1990.
32. Schectman G and others: Ascorbic acid requirements for smokers: analysis of a population survey, *American Journal of Clinical Nutrition* 53:1466, 1991.
33. Sheard NF, Zeisel SH: Choline: an essential dietary nutrient? *Nutrition* 5:1, 1989.
34. Song Wo: Pantothenic acid: how much do we know about this B-complex vitamin?, *Nutrition Today,* March/April 1990, p 19.
35. Stahelin HB and others: B-carotene and cancer prevention: the Basel Study, *American Journal of Clinical Nutrition* 53:265S, 1991.
36. Tubiana M: Human carcinogenesis—introductory remarks, *American Journal of Clinical Nutrition* 53:223S, 1991.
37. Truswell AS: Ascorbic acid, *The New England Journal of Medicine* 315:709, 1986.
38. Weisburger JH: Nutritional approach to cancer prevention and emphasis on vitamins, antioxidants, and carotenoids, *American Journal of Clinical Nutrition* 53:226S, 1991.
39. Zeigler RG: Vegetables, fruits, and carotenoids and the risk of cancer, *American Journal of Clinical Nutrition* 53:251S, 1991.

SUGGESTED READINGS

McCormick reviews our current understanding of many water-soluble vitamins in the textbook by Shils and Young. Casey and Dwyer discuss premenstrual syndrome and the possible role of nutrition—including vitamin B-6—in its treatment. Truswell provides an updated look at vitamin C therapy for the common cold. Carpenter comments on the search for the cause of pellagra. Reading the reprint of the original 1915 report that accompanies the article is a must if you want a glimpse into early vitamin research. Weisburger reviews in detail how certain vitamins in the diet might be linked to lower cancer risk.

TAKE ACTION

Spotting fraudulent vitamin claims

Visit a health-food store and browse through their magazines. How many statements about vitamins can you find that you consider fraudulent? Record at least four below. Discuss these statements with your friends and explore their point of view.

1. ______________________________

2. ______________________________

3. ______________________________

4. ______________________________

NUTRITION PERSPECTIVE

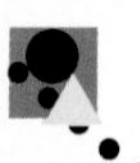

Nutrition and Cancer

Cancer is the second leading cause of death for adults in America. Cancer is actually many diseases; different types of cells are affected, and many different causes contribute to cancer (Figure 13-7). The factors leading to skin cancer are different from those leading to breast cancer, and their treatments also differ. Each of us needs to look seriously at cancer in general and at the risk we have of getting it.

Cancer is essentially an abnormal and uncontrollable growth of cells or tissues.[36] This typically leads to death if untreated. Most cancers take the form of tumors, although not all tumors are cancers. A tumor is simply a mass of new tissue that serves no physiological purpose. It can be benign, like a wart, or malignant, like most lung cancers; the terms malignant tumor and malignant neoplasm are synonymous with cancer.

Benign tumors are made up of cells similar to the surrounding normal cells and are enclosed in a membrane that prevents them from penetrating other tissues. They are dangerous only if their physical presence interferes with bodily functions. A benign brain tumor, for example, can cause death if it blocks the blood supply to the brain. In contrast, a malignant tumor, or cancer, is capable of invading surrounding structures, including blood vessels, the lymph system, and nerves. It can also spread, or metastasize, to distant sites via the blood and lymphatic circulation, and so produce invasive tumors in almost any part of the body. A few cancers like leukemia, or cancer of the blood, don't produce a mass and so aren't properly called tumors. But since the leukemic cells do have the fundamental property of rapid and inappropriate growth, they are still malignant and therefore represent cancer.

Both genetics and life-style play a strong role in the risk for developing cancer. Cancer tends to occur in some families more than in others. Thus persons within certain families are said to be genetically predisposed or at risk for developing certain types of cancer. This is especially the case with colon cancer. However, lifestyle (environment) is also a critical factor. We know this because rates of cancer differ around the world. The Japanese, for example, have higher rates of stomach cancer

Figure 13-7 Cancer is actually many diseases. Numerous types of cells and organs are its target.

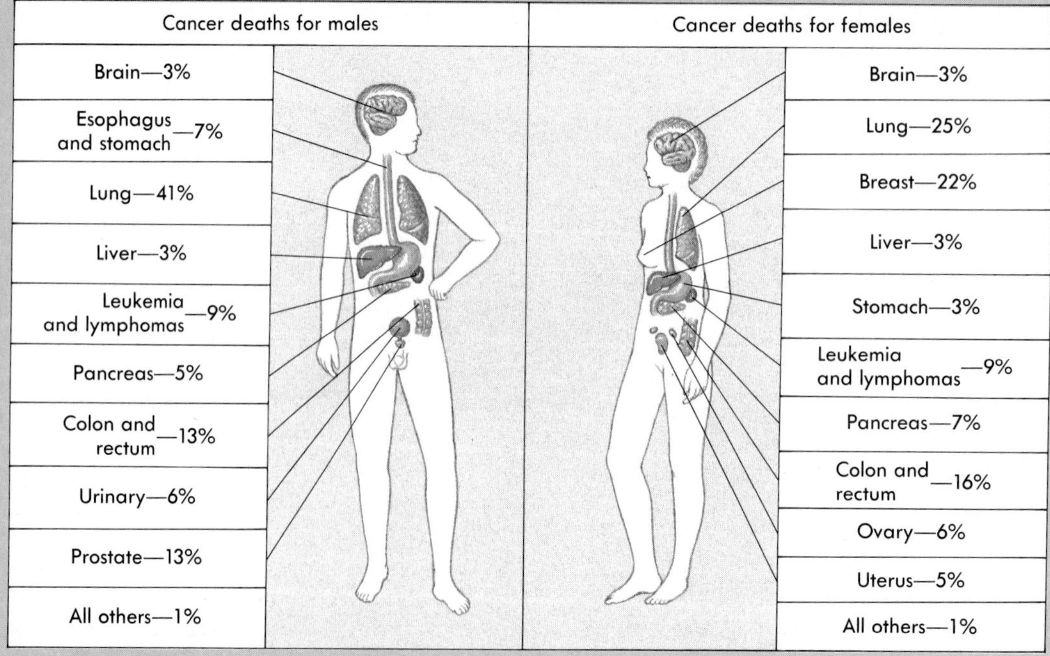

NUTRITION PERSPECTIVE

and Americans tend to have a higher rate of colon cancer. When Japanese people immigrate to the United States, their rates for stomach cancer decrease but their rates for colon cancer increase.[9] Women who have more children show a reduced risk for endometrial cancer. Poor people show high cancer risks, possibly due to generally inadequate health care.

Although we have little control over our genetic risks for cancer, we have a great deal of choice in deciding the risks determined by our lifestyles, especially with regard to smoking and alcohol intake. It is well established that one third of all cancer cases in the United States are due to smoking tobacco. In addition, it has become increasingly apparent (as we shall soon discuss) that dietary factors constitute many pieces in the cancer puzzle.[38] Once again, it seems that poor diet choices we make today cause us to pay tomorrow.

Mechanisms

To understand how to prevent cancer we first need to examine how cancer develops in the body. The process begins with an alteration in DNA, the genetic material in the cells. The DNA is altered so that the cell no longer responds to normal physiological controls. The cell can now dictate its own rate of growth and is not inhibited from growing at the expense of the cells around it. There are many ways to alter DNA. A substance or phenomenon capable of altering DNA and in turn causing cancer is known as **genotoxic carcinogen** or **initiator** (Figure 13-8). The alteration requires from only minutes to days to occur.

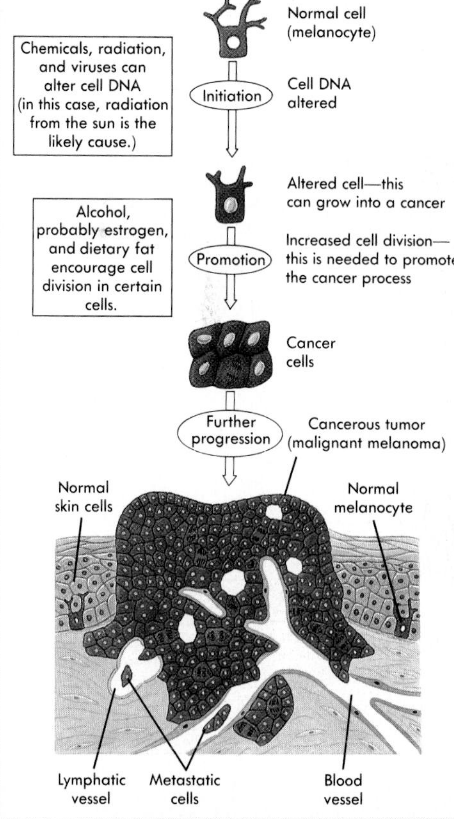

Figure 13-8 Progression from a normal cell to a tumor. The ball of cells is a developing tumor. As the mass of cells grows, it can invade surrounding tissues and eventually penetrate into lymphatic vessels and blood vessels. These vessels carry metastatic cancer cells throughout the body, where they can form new tumors.

Radiation from the sun can cause DNA to bind to itself or break into pieces. This is often how skin cancer begins. The altered skin cells may then begin to grow out of control and result in cancer.

DNA can be altered by chemicals, especially multiringed chemicals, such as aflatoxin and benzo(a)pyrene (see the structure of cholesterol on page 103 for an example of a multiringed structure). Aflatoxin is formed when mold is present in peanuts and peanut butter. FDA regulates how much aflatoxin can be present in peanut butter (see Chapter 19). Rejecting moldy foods is one way you can avoid possible carcinogens. Benzo(a)pyrene is found in charcoal-broiled foods. These multiringed compounds can insert themselves into DNA and cause breaks and other changes.

A third agent that can alter DNA is viruses. Viruses can insert their **genes** into human cells and eventually into the human genetic material. If the genes promote growth (so-called **oncogenes**), then the cell may begin to grow out of control.

Human cells contain their own growth-promoting oncogenes. Scientists think that viruses capable of inducing oncogenic activity in us have previously infected humans and taken oncogenes from the human cells. The viruses then can multiply and reinfect other humans. When a growth-promoting gene from one human is placed in another human by a virus and later turned on, the newly infected cell may be able to grow autonomously. Other genes, called tumor suppressors, prevent the abnormal growth. When mutation causes the tumor suppressors to not work normally, then a natural control on cell growth is removed. Evidence suggests that it may take one or more oncogenes plus the mutation of one or more suppressor genes for a tumor to develop.

Thus the three basic means of altering DNA are through radiation, chemicals, and viruses. However, having a cell with altered DNA does not guarantee cancer. Special enzymes travel up and down the DNA to repair breaks and changes in it. The repair enzymes may find alterations caused by chemicals or radiation and fix them before the altered cell divides to begin its growth.

NUTRITION PERSPECTIVE

Nutrition and Cancer—cont'd

Epigenetic carcinogens

Anything that increases the rate of cell division decreases the chance that the repair enzymes will find the altered part of the DNA. Once a cell multiplies and incorporates its newly altered DNA into its genetic instructions, the cell no longer realizes that the DNA is altered.

Compounds that increase cell division are called **promoters**, or **epigenetic carcinogens**. They are thought to promote cancer by either decreasing the time available for repair enzymes to act or by encouraging cells with altered DNA to develop and grow. Development and growth of these altered cells may take up to 10 to 30 years. We know this because increased lung cancer rates lagged about 30 years behind the increase in cigarette smoking and asbestos exposure that began during World War II. Common promoters are estrogen, alcohol, and probably high levels of dietary fat. Bacterial infections in the stomach are also suspected agents.

Once a cell with altered DNA has multiplied, there is still no guarantee that cancer will result. First, a stage of progression must occur where the cell mass increases to an extent that it can significantly affect body metabolism. During this initial stage of growth, the immune system may find the altered cells and destroy them. In addition, the cancer cells also may be so defective that their own DNA limits their ability to grow, and they die anyway.

Diet and cancer

Cancer quackery aside, a generally nutritious diet, as well as other factors related to diet and life-style, can reduce your risk of cancer initiation and promotion (Table 13-11).[14] For example, maintain a desirable body weight and practice regular physical activity. Both obesity and physical inactivity are linked to an increased risk for many types of cancer.

Obesity in fact is related to all major forms of cancer except lung cancer. Obesity-related forms include breast cancer, colon cancer, **endometrial** cancer, and **prostate** cancer.[9] The link probably occurs because adipose tissue can synthesize estrogen from other hormones in the bloodstream, and high levels of estrogen in the bloodstream promote cancer. A long-standing excess energy intake may also promote cancer. When animals are fed diets high in fat or total kcalories, they tend to experience more cancer, especially in the colon and breast.[3] The effect is most apparent when a carcinogen is used to initiate the cancer process, and then a high-fat or high-kcalorie diet is used to promote cancer development. Thus fat and kcalories usually are not considered initiators of cancer, but promoters.

The National Cancer Institute believes there is a sufficient link between dietary fat and cancer, especially breast cancer, to warrant encouraging Americans to eat less fat. It recommends decreasing dietary fat consumption to about 20% to 30% of total kcalories. Some nutritionists, however, believe that this agency has over-reacted to the fat and cancer issue. Epidemiological evidence relates fat to cancer, but the evidence is not strong. The question of how much fat can be eaten while minimizing the risk of cancer is not settled. To be on the safe side, moderating fat intake is a reasonable goal to help reduce cancer risk.

A stronger link between diet and cancer concerns total kcalories in the diet. If a rat or mouse is treated with a carcinogen for either breast cancer or colon cancer and then is allowed a typical kcalorie intake versus a reduced kcalorie intake, the animals with a low kcalorie intake will have about a 40% reduction in tumor yield compared with the animals consuming a typical intake.[3] The amount of fat in the

NUTRITION PERSPECTIVE

Table 13-11 Food constituents having a suspected role in cancer

Nutrient	Dietary sources	Action*
Possibly protective agents in foods		
Vitamin A	Liver, fortified milk, fruits, vegetables	Encourages normal cell development
Vitamin E	Whole grains, vegetable oil, green leafy vegetables	Antioxidant
Vitamin C	Fruits, vegetables	Antioxidant; can block conversion of nitrites and nitrates to potent carcinogens
Folate	Fruits, vegetables, whole grains	Encourages normal cell development
Selenium	Meats, whole grains	Part of the glutathione peroxidase antioxidant system
Carotenes	Fruits, vegetables	Many are antioxidants
Indoles, Phenols	Vegetables, especially cabbage, cauliflower, and brussels sprouts	May reduce carcinogen activation
Dietary fibers	Whole grains, fruits, vegetables, beans	May bind carcinogens in the stool, decrease stool transit time, thus lowering risk of colon and rectal cancer
Calcium	Diary products, green vegetables	Slows cell division in the colon, binds bile acids and free fatty acids
Omega-3 fatty acids	Cold-water fish	May inhibit tumor growth
Soy products		Phytic acid present may bind carcinogens in the intestinal tract

Food agent	Sources	Actions*
Possibly carcinogenic agents in foods		
Fats	Meats, milk and milk products, vegetable oils	Excessive body fat is linked to increased synthesis of estrogen and other sex hormones, which in excess themselves may increase the risk for cancer
Alcohol	Beer, wine, liquor	Contribute to cancers of the throat, liver, and bladder and possibly the breast. Increased cell turnover is the main mechanism
Nitrites, nitrates	Cured meats especially ham, bacon, and sausages	Under very high temperatures will bind to amino acid derivatives to form nitrosamines, potent carcinogens
Multi-ringed compounds:		
Aflatoxin	Formed when mold is present on peanuts and other grains	Multiringed compounds may alter DNA structure and inhibit its ability to properly respond to physiologic controls
Benzo-a-pyrene	Charcoal-broiled foods, especially meats	Aflatoxin is linked to liver cancer; benzo-a-pyrene is linked to stomach and other intestinal cancers

*Many of the actions listed for these possibly protective agents are speculative and have only been verified by animal studies.

NUTRITION PERSPECTIVE

Nutrition and Cancer—cont'd

diet is not important, as long as the low kcalorie diet is about 70% of the usual kcalorie intake of the animals.

The mechanism behind this effect of total kcalorie intake is probably hormonal. The kcalorie-restricted animals have higher levels of the hormone cortisol and lower levels of the hormone prolactin than the animals allowed to feed at will. This hormonal state inhibits tumor growth, while higher prolactin levels and lower cortisol levels increase tumor growth. The restricted diet may also lower serum estrogen levels. As noted, this hormone can promote cancer.

Can we use this evidence from animals? We don't want to suffer from cancer, but very few of us want to eat only 70% of our usual kcalorie intake. While there is a strong link between some types of cancer and obesity, this evidence has been insufficient to convince many of us to slim down to more desirable body weights. It is a much bigger task to reduce kcalories to 70% of usual intake. So while the data obtained from animal studies are interesting, nutritionists do not know how to derive any practical use from their meaning. In addition, once cancer is present, kcalorie restriction is no longer helpful.

Antioxidants may be anticarcinogens

Many single nutrients are promoted as keys to preventing cancer. They are called anticarcinogens (Table 13-11). The most important ones are beta-carotene (a plant form of vitamin A), vitamin E, vitamin C, and selenium.[13,19,22,35] All four of these nutrients function as or contribute to antioxidant systems in the body. These antioxidant systems help prevent the alteration of DNA by electron-seeking substances. Beta-carotene is strongly linked to a decrease in lung cancer risk in smokers.[6] In addition, both prospective and retrospective studies suggest that vegetable and fruit intake may reduce the risk of cancers of the mouth, pharynx, larynx, esophagus, stomach, colon, rectum, bladder, and cervix. These foods are normally rich in beta-carotene and vitamin C, plus supply dietary fiber and vitamin E. Note that the antioxidant vitamin E also helps protect unsaturated fatty acids from damage by electron-seeking compounds.[19] A diet that follows the Guide to Daily Food Choices, so that fruits, vegetables, and plant oils are eaten daily, is rich in these nutrients.[39]

Is dietary fiber an anticancer agent?

In Chapters 4 and 6 we mentioned the possible role of fiber in preventing colon cancer. Fiber (specifically insoluble fiber) may do this by decreasing transit time so that the stool is in contact with the colon for a shorter period of time. This would reduce the contact of carcinogens with the colon wall. Soluble fibers may bind bile acids and so block some recycling of these by the body. Bile acids are thought to contribute to cancer risk by irritating the colon cells, and in turn increasing cell division. In addition, dietary fiber (specifically the insoluble fiber lignin) may be able to increase the binding and excretion of the sex-linked hormones testosterone and estrogen from within the intestines. This is of importance because of the links between excessive amounts of sex hormones and certain types of cancers, specifically prostate and colon cancer. However, the evidence regarding the importance of fiber in preventing colon cancer is still inconclusive. For now the recommendation to eat 20 to 35 grams a day is probably best. Liberal use of whole grains, fruits, and vegetables should suffice to yield this amount.

Calcium is also linked to a decreased risk for developing colon cancer. As with fiber, the evidence is inconclusive. Some studies show that calcium decreases the growth of cells in the colon; therefore it probably decreases the risk of a genetically

NUTRITION PERSPECTIVE

Table 13-12 General dietary recommendations to reduce the risk of cancer*

1. Avoid obesity.
2. Reduce fat intake to 30% of total kcalories.
3. Eat more higher-fiber foods, such as fruits, vegetables, and whole-grain cereals.
4. Include foods rich in vitamins A, E, and C, as well as carotenes in the daily diet.
5. If alcohol is consumed, do not drink excessively.
6. Use moderation when consuming salt-cured, smoked, and nitrite-cured foods.

*The National Cancer Institute (U.S.) endorses all the above but warns not to exceed 35 grams of dietary fiber intake.
The American Cancer Society endorses all the above, but sets no percentage for fat intake, and adds a recommendation to include cruciferous vegetables in the diet (cabbage, broccoli, and brussels sprouts). These may decrease carcinogen activation.
The Canadian Dietetic Association generally endorses all of the above, but the specific language differs.

altered cell developing into a cancer. Calcium may also bind free fatty acids and bile acids in the colon so they are less apt to interact with cells there and cause cancer. We need more research before calcium can be promoted as a cancer-preventing agent. Nevertheless, there are many important reasons for consuming the RDA for calcium. We will discuss those in Chapter 14.

A bottom line?

Table 13-12 lists a variety of changes you can make in your diet to possibly reduce your risk for cancer. Start by making sure your diet is not excessive in energy or total fat and is rich in fruits, vegetables, whole grains, beans, and low-fat dairy products. In other words, follow the Guide to Daily Food Choices. In your effort to eat more fruits and vegetables, consider the following suggestions:

- Use fresh or canned fruit as a topping for puddings, yogurt, hot or cold cereal, and frozen deserts.
- Put raisins, grapes, apple chunks, pineapple, grated carrots, zucchini, or cucumber into coleslaw, chicken, or tuna salad.
- Toss raw or steamed vegetables into potato salad, pasta, or rice. Try broccoli or cauliflower florets, mushrooms, peas, carrots, corn, or peppers.
- Be creative at the salad bar; try fresh spinach, leaf lettuce, red cabbage, sprouts, zucchini, yellow squash, cauliflower, peas, mushrooms, or red or yellow peppers.
- Pack fresh or dried fruit for snacks away from home instead of grabbing a candy bar or going hungry.
- On sandwiches, lettuce and tomato are just the beginning. Add slices of cucumber or zucchini, bean sprouts, spinach, carrot slivers, or snow peas.
- Try one or two vegetarian meals per week, such as beans and rice or pasta, or spaghetti squash and tomato sauce.
- When daily protein intake is more than required, reduce the meat, fish, or poultry in casseroles, stews, and soups by one third to one half and add more vegetables.
- In the refrigerator, keep a bowl of fresh vegetables handy for snacks.
- Choose 100% fruit or vegetable juices instead of sodas.
- Have a bowl of fruit on hand.

NUTRITION PERSPECTIVE

Nutrition and Cancer—cont'd

A current nationwide study under way in the United States to reduce colon cancer risk employs a diet with fat at 20% of kcalories and five to eight servings of fruits/vegetables per day. This diet also aims for about 30 grams of dietary fiber in the diet. In addition, if you are going to drink alcohol or consume pickled, smoked, and charcoal-broiled foods, do so in moderation. And finally, we remind you again that one third of all cancer cases are due to cigarette smoking. Therefore a priority in avoiding cancer is avoiding cigarette usage—and even avoiding usage of smokeless tobacco varieties (chewing tobacco).

Note also that if a cancer is left untreated, it can spread quickly throughout the body. This makes the eventual result of death much more likely. Thus early detection is critical. Aids to early detection include the seven warning signs of cancer:

1. a change in bowel or bladder habits
2. a sore that does not heal
3. unusual bleeding or discharge
4. a thickening or lump in the breast or elsewhere
5. indigestion or difficulty in swallowing
6. an obvious change in a wart or mole
7. a nagging cough or hoarseness

There are still other ways to detect cancer early. Colo-rectal examinations for adults of both genders and Papanicolaou tests and regular breast examinations for women are recommended by the American Cancer Society.

CHAPTER FOURTEEN

Water and the Major Minerals

Water—the most versatile medium for all kinds of chemical magic—constitutes the major portion of our bodies. Without water, our life processes would cease in a matter of days. We operate on about 2 quarts (2 liters) of water daily, and it should be replenished daily because the body does not store water well. We experience this constant demand for water as thirst.

Because water dissolves many nutrients, it enables minerals and other chemicals to react in the body. Among other uses, it lubricates joints and serves as a vehicle to transport minerals and other substances throughout the body. In addition, water is a key means of controlling body temperature and removing waste products.

Minerals, like water, are vital to health. As free atoms, they are considered inorganic because they are not bonded to carbon atoms. Minerals are key players in body metabolism, muscle movement, body growth, and water balance, among other wide-ranging processes. We are not sure that all the minerals found in our bodies—for example, vanadium and tin—are necessary to sustain human life. Some minerals, such as lead and cadmium, may be found in humans only as a contaminant. The mere presence of a mineral in our bodies is not proof that we need it. Nevertheless, we know that some mineral deficiencies can cause severe health problems. For this reason the study of minerals is critical to understanding human nutrition.

NUTRITION AWARENESS INVENTORY

Here are 15 statements about water and the major minerals. Answer them to test your current knowledge. If you think the answer is true or mostly true, circle T. If you think the answer is false or mostly false, circle F. Use the scoring key at the end of the book to compute your total score. Take the test again after you have read this chapter. Compare the results.

1. T F Water is an electrolyte.
2. T F "Major" minerals are more important to health than "trace" minerals.
3. T F Vitamins often need minerals to help perform metabolic reactions.
4. T F Plant foods are usually the best sources of minerals.
5. T F You can survive longer without food than without water.
6. T F When water evaporates from your skin, you feel cooler, because evaporating water takes heat with it.
7. T F The estimation of dietary water needs is 1 milliliter per kcalorie burned by the body.
8. T F You can never drink too much water.
9. T F Sodium is often added to processed foods.
10. T F Mineral absorption is greatest when consumed in conjunction with a high-fiber diet.
11. T F A preference for salty foods is partially learned.
12. T F Most foods in the same food group, such as milk and cheese, contain similar amounts of sodium.
13. T F Perspiration has a lower sodium concentration than blood.
14. T F Calcium supplements can prevent osteoporosis.
15. T F Salt is "bad" for most people.

Water

To appreciate how minerals operate, the nature of water and its characteristics must be understood. Water is the base of operations for minerals, and it is the chief constituent of the human body composition. An adult can probably survive about 8 weeks without eating food (depending on fat stores), but only a few days without drinking water. This is not because water is more important than energy, protein, vitamins, or minerals, but rather because we can neither store nor conserve water as well as we can store the other components of our diet.

Water has some fascinating properties. Its molecular structure is highly polar (meaning the positive charges tend to align themselves to one end and the negative charges to the other end). Because of this, it can dissolve most substances. It expands as it freezes so that a jar full of water cracks when in the freezer. Water has a high heat capacity; it takes much more energy to heat water than it does to heat fat. Therefore, foods with high water content heat up and cool down slowly. Compare the time it takes to heat water with the time it takes to heat butter in a microwave oven. Because water requires so much energy to change from a liquid to a gas, it forms an ideal medium for removing heat from the body. We will discuss that shortly.

OSMOSIS—A KEY INTERACTION OF MINERALS AND WATER

Osmosis occurs where a semipermeable membrane separates two bodies of fluid. In this case, semipermeable means water can pass through the membrane but particles cannot. In the body, these particles are usually ions, and the membranes are cell membranes. If the number of particles in both compartments is the same, then osmosis works to equalize the amounts of water in each compartment.

osmotic pressure The exerted pressure needed to keep particles in a solution from drawing liquid across a semipermeable membrane.

Figure 14-1 illustrates osmosis. Adding particles to a compartment increases its particle concentration. Since particles cannot easily pass through the membrane, water shifts from the diluted compartment to that with a high ion concentration. The term **osmotic pressure** refers to the amount of force needed to prevent dilution of the compartment with a higher ion concentration. Examples of osmosis are sugar pulling fluid from strawberries, a salty salad dressing wilting lettuce, and red blood cells swelling or shrinking when put into different solutions with various salt concentrations.

THE FLUID OF LIFE

Since all life comes from water, it is not so surprising that we carry so much of it around with us. Looking at our constituents alone, humans are not much more than an organized bag of seawater—between 50% and 70% of our body weight is made up of water. Lean muscle tissue is made up of about 73% water. The more body fat, the less body water a person has. As fat content increases, the percentage of lean tissue decreases in the body and total body water then drifts down toward 50%.

All this water is strictly compartmentalized to add greater order and control to its presence within the body. Controlling water movement throughout the body allows specific variations of ion concentrations and conditions to exist within a tiny space.

Intracellular and Extracellular Fluid

Water migrates in and out of body cells. When functioning inside cells, water is known as the **intracellular fluid.** When outside the cells, water is known as the **extracellular fluid.** Extracellular fluid is further divided into **interstitial fluid**—water between cells—and **intravascular fluid**—water in the bloodstream (Figure 14-2). Interstitial fluid forms an important transport link between tissue cells and the bloodstream.

The ratio of intracellular to interstitial to intravascular water is about 25 : 14 : 3.[20] Water shifts freely from one compartment to another. For example, if blood volume falls, water can shift from the areas both inside and around cells to the bloodstream to increase blood volume. On the other hand, if blood volume increases, water can shift out of the bloodstream into cells and the areas between them.

The body controls the amount of water in each compartment mainly by controlling the ion concentrations in each compartment. Ions are charged particles. Because of its polar nature, water follows sodium, potassium, chloride, phosphate, magnesium, calcium, and other ions. In a water molecule, the oxygen atom tends to be more negative and the hydrogen atoms tend to be more positive. The slightly negative oxygen atom is attracted to positive sodium and potassium ions, and the slightly positive hydrogen atoms are attracted to negative chloride and phosphate ions. By shifting ions in and out of the cellular compartments, the body can maintain a desirable amount of water in each compartment. Where ions go, so goes water.

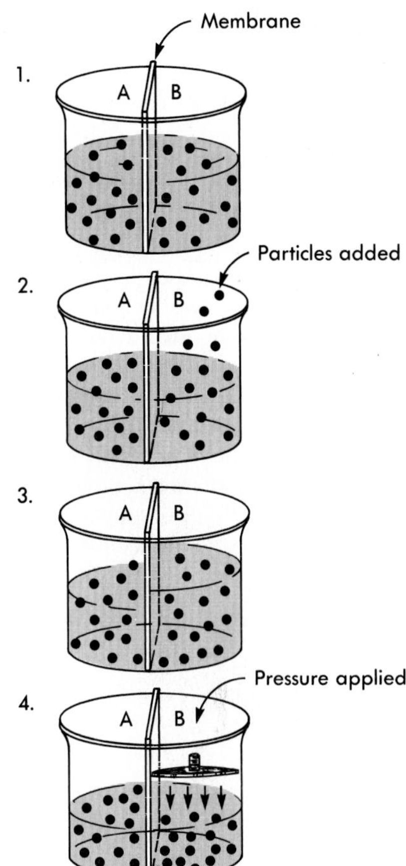

Figure 14-1 A graphic representation of osmosis and osmotic pressure. *1.* Equal number of particles on both sides allows equal amounts of water. *2.* Now additional particles are added to *side B,* but the particles cannot flow across the membrane. *3.* Water can flow across the membrane, and so it flows to *side B* where there are more particles. The volume of water becomes greater on *side B,* causing the concentrations on *sides A* and *B* to again become equal. *4.* If physical pressure (such as a pump) compressed the fluid on *side B* to restore the original volume, that pressure would equal the osmotic pressure exerted by the added particles.

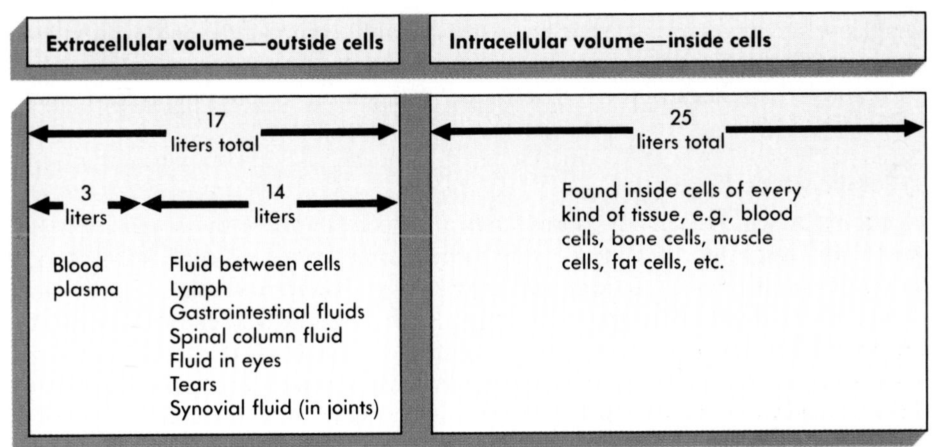

Figure 14-2 The fluid compartments in the body.

intracellular fluid Fluid contained within a cell.

extracellular fluid Fluid present outside the cells; it includes intravascular and interstitial fluids.

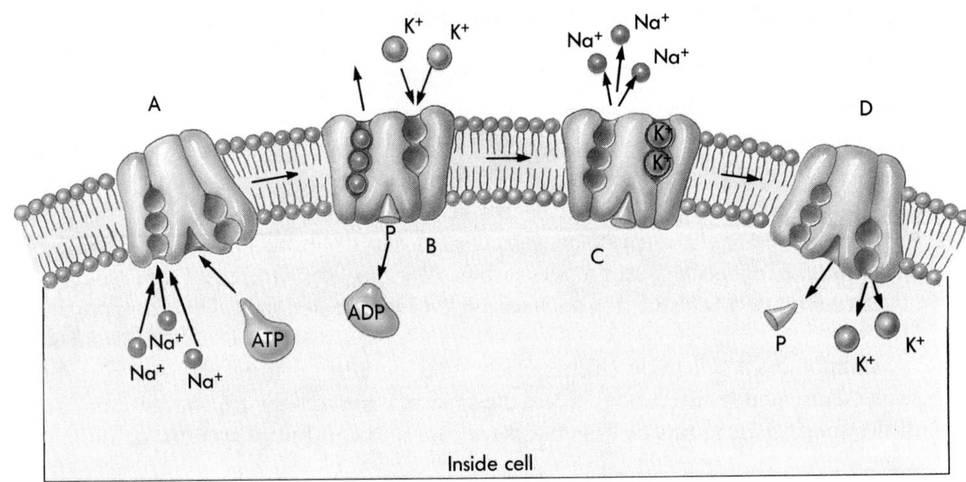

Figure 14-3 Schematic diagram of the sodium (Na^+) and potassium (K^+) pump cycle. **A,** Three Na^+ ions bind from inside the cell. **B,** The pump protein is activated by ATP. **C,** Activation causes a change of the protein form. This results in a decrease in the affinity of Na^+ binding sites and an increase in affinity of K^+ binding sites. The three Na^+ ions are then released to the outside of the cell. **D,** Two K^+ ions occupy the K^+ binding sites, and the pump protein releases the phosphate donated from ATP and returns to its original conformation. The affinity of the K^+ binding sites decreases, and that of the Na^+ increases. The K^+ ions are released to the cell. The pump is now ready to bind three Na^+, and the cycle starts again.

Water and Ions in the Body—a Balancing Act

Adding water—instead of particles—to a compartment dilutes its ion concentration, and so the compartment will in turn tend to donate water to more concentrated compartments nearby. All of this is caused by the osmotic tendency to equalize the ion concentrations across membranes.

Cell membranes differ slightly from this model. Cell membranes contain an extremely sophisticated system for gatekeeping. Selectively permeable to many ions, they have pumping mechanisms that constantly draw potassium ions into the cell and pump sodium ions out (Figure 14-3). Energy is used by this sodium-potassium pump to drive each of these two electrolytes against their concentration gradient. This pumping action, in effect, leaves cell membranes permeable to water, but not to many ions.[20] Ions, such as sodium, may cross into the cell, but the cell quickly pumps them back out.

Positive ions, such as sodium and potassium, pair with negative ions, such as phosphate and chloride. Intracellular water volume depends primarily on intracellular potassium and phosphate concentration. Extracellular water volume depends primarily on the extracellular sodium and chloride concentration.

Besides balancing the ion concentrations between the inside and outside of cells, the body must also balance ion charges. If a negative ion enters a cell, a positive ion also must enter the cell or another negative ion must leave it.

FUNCTIONS OF WATER

Because of its unique chemical and physical characteristics, water plays several key roles in our life processes. Two major roles of water involve chemical reactions. For example, water serves as a solvent for many chemical compounds, and it provides a medium in which many chemical reactions occur. It also actively participates in chemical reactions, such as the reaction used in digestion to split one maltose into two glucoses.

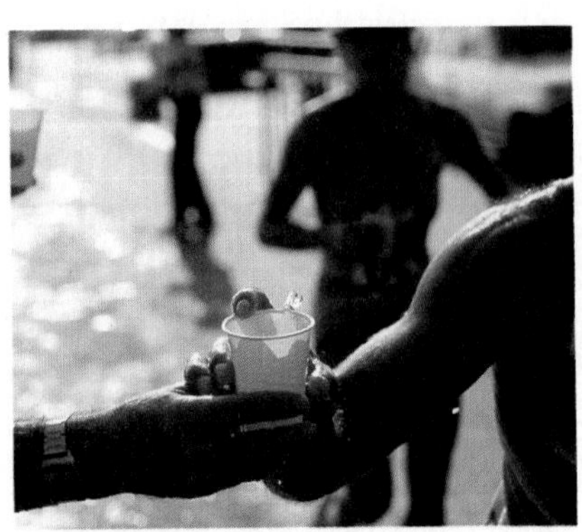

It is important to drink plenty of water, especially when you exercise vigorously.

Temperature Regulation

One means by which the body looses fluids is via perspiration—the evaporation of water through skin pores. Whether due to hard work, fever, exposure to heat, or merely normal metabolic reactions, an elevation of temperature within the body can only be tolerated within a very small range. As the level of heat energy contained within the body goes up, water (due to its high specific heat) in the surrounding tissues will absorb any excess heat energy. When the water absorbs enough heat energy, it will evaporate through the pores in the skin, in turn cooling the environment it leaves behind. Each liter of perspiration lost represents approximately 600 kcalories of energy lost from the skin and surrounding tissues.[20]

Recall from Chapter 7 that 60% of the chemical energy in food is turned directly into body heat. Only 40% becomes ATP energy, and even that energy eventually leaves the body in the form of heat. The otherwise resultant rise in body temperature if this heat could not be dissipated would prevent enzyme systems from functioning efficiently. Perspiration is the primary way to prevent a rise in body temperature.

Humans tolerate hot, dry climates far better than they do hot, humid climates, because dry climates allow perspiration to work as it should. In hot, humid climates, not all perspiration can evaporate: some of it simply rolls off the skin or soaks into clothing. This perspiration does little to cool the body because water must evaporate to do its job. And so people just feel hot and sticky.

Removal of Waste Products

Water is an important vehicle for ridding the body of waste products. Most unwanted substances in the body are water soluble, and can leave the body via the urine. In addition, liver metabolism may sometimes convert fat-soluble compounds into water-soluble compounds so that they too can be excreted in the urine.

A major body waste product is urea, made from the amine groups (-NH_2) of amino acids. The more protein eaten, the greater the necessity for excreting nitrogen (in the form of urea) in the urine. Likewise, the more sodium consumed, the more sodium excreted in the urine. Total urine production is primarily determined by protein and sodium chloride (salt) intake. More fluid output is needed as we need to excrete more of these compounds.[20] By limiting excess protein and sodium intakes it is possible to limit urine output—a useful practice, for example, in space flights.

A healthy urine volume totals at least 1 to 2 liters (1 to 2 quarts) per day. More than that is healthy, but less—especially less than 600 milliliters (2½ cups)—forces the kidneys to form a very concentrated urine. The heavy level of ion concentration also increases the risk of kidney stone formation in susceptible people. Kidney stones are simply minerals and other substances that have precipitated out of the urine and eventually lodge in kidney tissues.

Lubrication and Miscellaneous Functions

Water helps form the lubricants found in knees and other joints of the body. It is the basis for saliva, bile, and **amniotic fluid**. Amniotic fluid acts as an important shock absorber surrounding the growing fetus before birth. Ion concentrations vary in each fluid compartment to accommodate specific needs.

amniotic fluid Fluid contained in a sac within the uterus. This surrounds and protects the fetus during its development.

insensible losses Fluid losses that are not perceptible to the senses, such as losses through lungs, feces, and skin (an exception is heavy perspiration).

WATER NEEDS

Water needs for adults are roughly estimated as 1 milliliter per kcalorie burned. This works out to 2.4 liters (10 cups) for a 2400-kcalorie energy output. Of this, about 1 liter is due to typical water losses from a total of the lungs (400 milliliters or 1⅔ cups), feces (150 milliliters or ⅔ cup), and skin (500 milliliters or 2 cups) (Figure 14-5). Since people are not normally aware of these water losses, they are called **"insensible"** water **losses.**

The loss of only 150 milliliters of water from feces per day is an incredible feat, considering that in addition to the 2000 milliliters of water (8 cups) added through the diet, about 8000 milliliters (33 cups) enter the gastrointestinal (GI) tract daily via secretions from the stomach, intestine, pancreas, and other organs.[20] Not too surprisingly, severe diarrhea (such as may be the case with viral or bacterial infections) can result in water losses as high as 1 liter per hour.

We consume about 1 liter (4 cups) of water per day in various liquids (Figure 14-4). Foods supply another liter of fluid, and water as a by-product of metabolism provides approximately 350 milliliters (1½ cups). This yields a total of about 2.4 liters (10 cups). Note that this is very similar to estimates of water needs based on 1 milliliter per kcalorie burned, based on a typical energy output.

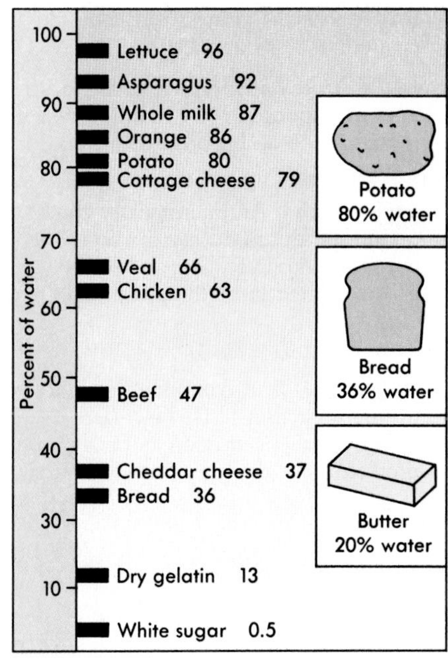

Water content of various foods (percent of total weight).

Thirst

If a person doesn't consume enough water, the body first signals so by registering thirst. Still, this is not a sensitive signal of fluid depletion. It kicks in somewhat after you should have begun replenishing your losses. The hypothalamus in the unconscious brain communicates to higher brain centers that the person needs to drink.[20] However, the thirst mechanism is not always reliable, especially during illness, in elderly years, and when participating in vigorous athletic events. We have already

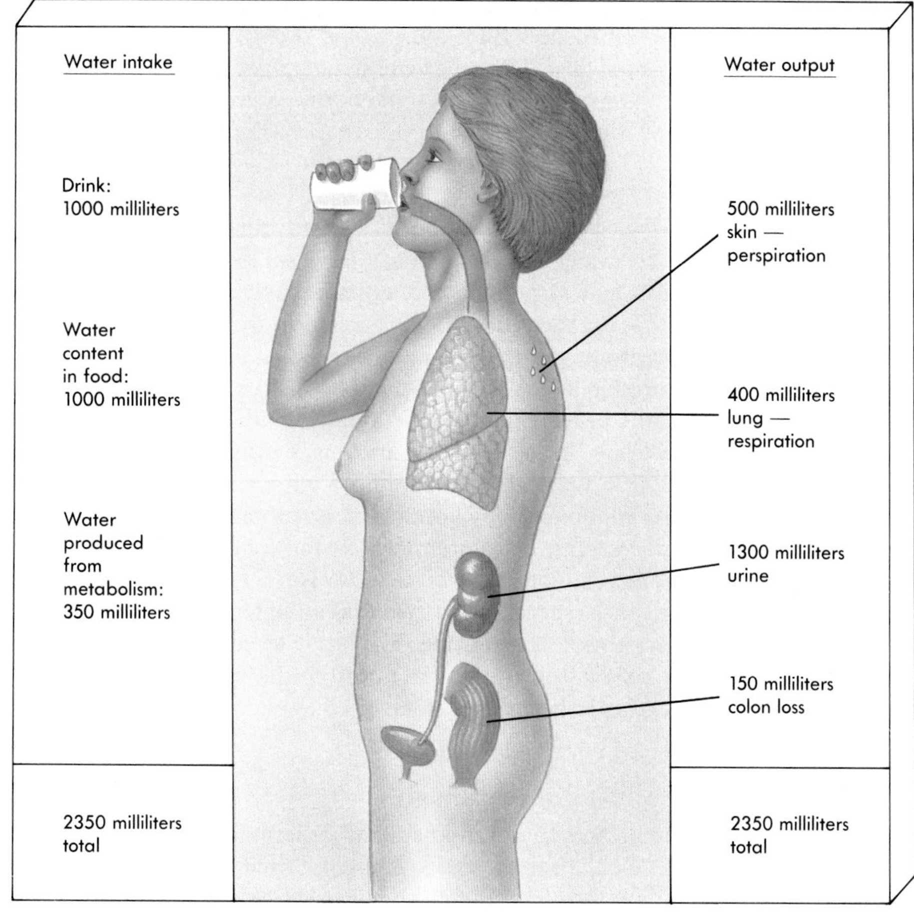

Figure 14-4 Water balance—intake versus output. We maintain body fluids at an optimum level by adjusting water intake and output. Most water comes from the liquids. Some comes from the moisture in more solid foods, and the remainder is manufactured in metabolism. Water output includes that via lungs, kidneys, skin, and bowels.

mentioned in Chapter 10 that athletes should weigh themselves before and after training sessions to determine their rate of water loss and thus their water needs. Children who are ill, especially those with fever, diarrhea, and increased perspiration, need to be reminded to drink plenty of fluid. Elderly people in general, and especially those in hospitals and nursing homes, also should have fluid intake and output monitored. One other situation that demands extra fluid for the body is a long airplane flight: a traveler can lose approximately 1.5 liters (6 cups) of water during a 3-hour flight. The dehumidified air in the airplane is so dry that excessive "insensible" perspiration and evaporation occur.

antidiuretic hormone (ADH) A hormone secreted by the pituitary gland that acts on the kidneys to cause a decrease in water excretion.

renin An enzyme formed in the kidneys in response to low blood pressure; it acts on a blood protein to produce angiotensin I.

angiotensin I An intermediary compound, produced during the body's attempt to conserve water and sodium; it is converted in the lungs to angiotensin II.

angiotensin II A compound produced from angiotensin I. This increases blood vessel constriction and triggers production of the hormone aldosterone.

What if the Thirst Message is Ignored?

When the body registers a shortage of available water, fluid conservation increases. The pituitary gland releases **antidiuretic hormone (ADH)** to force the kidneys to conserve water.[20] As its name implies, ADH slows diuresis (urine flow).

In addition, as fluid volume drops in the bloodstream, blood pressure falls. This fall initiates a sequence of reactions beginning in the kidneys. Signaled by highly sensitive pressure receptors, the kidneys release an enzyme called **renin.** Renin, in turn, activates a circulating blood protein called angiotensinogen to form the compound **angiotensin I.** Angiotensin I is converted in the lungs to **angiotensin II.** That triggers the adrenal gland to release more of the hormone aldosterone, in turn signaling the kidneys to retain more sodium and therefore more water[20] (Figure 14-5). Remember that water always follows ions. Thus low blood pressure, through this roundabout measure using the kidneys, causes increased water conservation in the body.

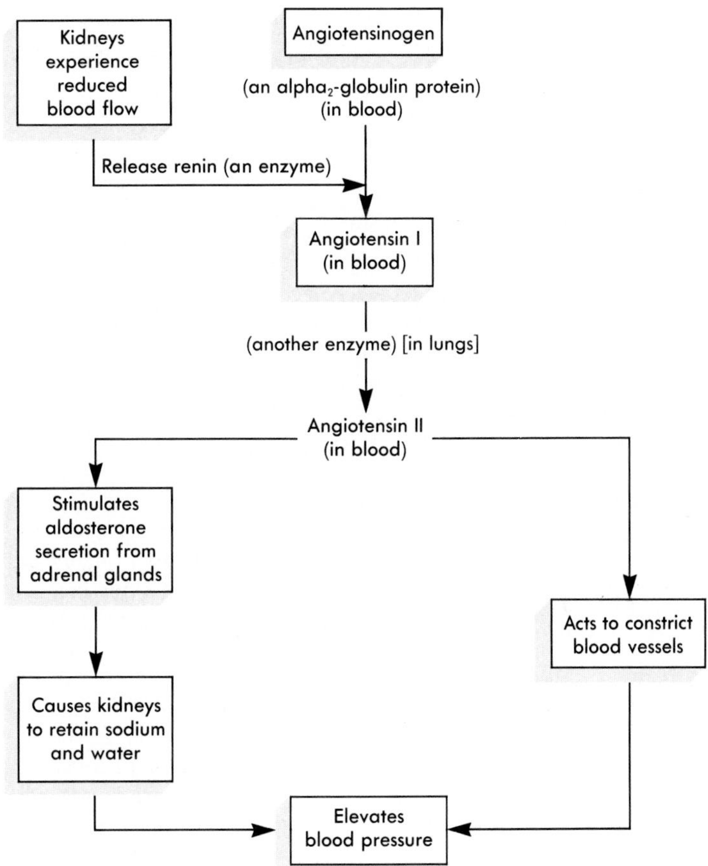

Figure 14-5 The renin-angiotensin system. This is one regulator of blood pressure.

The effectiveness of ADH and aldosterone is limited. Fluid is constantly lost via the insensible routes—feces, skin, and lungs. Those losses, too, must be replaced. In addition, urine can become only so concentrated. Eventually, if fluid is not consumed, the body becomes dehydrated and suffers ill effects, possibly constipation and kidney stones.

Alcohol inhibits the action of ADH. One reason people feel so bad the day after heavy drinking is that they are very dehydrated. Even though they may have consumed a lot of liquid in their drinks, they have lost even more liquid because alcohol has inhibited ADH.

The Effects of Dehydration

By the time a person loses 2% of body weight in fluids, he or she will be thirsty. At a 4% loss of body weight, muscles undergo a significant drop in strength and endurance. By the time body weight is reduced by 10% to 12%, heat tolerance is decreased and the person feels very weak. At a 20% reduction, the person may lapse into a coma and soon die (Figure 14-6).

CONCEPT CHECK

Since the body can neither readily store nor entirely conserve water, we can survive only a few days without it. Water functions as a solvent, a medium for chemical reactions, a thermoregulator, and a lubricant. Water constitutes 50% to 70% of body weight and is prevalent in lean tissue, intracellular and extracellular fluid, urine, and all other body fluids. For adults, water needs can be estimated as 1 milliliter per kcalorie burned. Thirst is the body's first sign of dehydration. If a thirst mechanism is faulty, as it may be with illness or vigorous exercise, hormonal mechanisms also help conserve water. Too much water in a diet can be toxic.

NUTRITION FOCUS

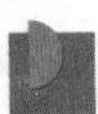

Bottled Water—Is It Worth the Cost?

These days it is common to see 5-gallon bottles of water being delivered to homes. Grocery store shelves are now stocked with all kinds of bottled waters—over 600 brands are available in the United States alone. As people become increasingly more concerned with their health, they gravitate towards purchases they perceive as being healthy ones. Enterprising individuals in the bottled water industry have managed to turn this behavior into a $2 billion a year business. It is an institution in Europe, as popular as soft drinks are in the United States.

Varieties of bottled water vary depending on their source, mineral content, and carbonation. All bottled waters must list the source of water on the label. This can include wells, spas, springs, geysers, and quite often the public water supply.

Many people choose bottled water over tap water because they doubt the safety of public drinking water. The Environmental Protection Agency (EPA) is responsible for tap water quality. Under the Safe Water Drinking Act, all public drinking water supplies are monitored for contaminants such as bacteria, various chemicals, and some toxic metals (such as lead and mercury). Some bottled water meets these same standards, but not all. FDA and private inspections of these products are less frequent than tests done on municipal utilities.

A recent EPA poll also showed that 21 out of 50 bottlers surveyed revealed their source as the public supply—essentially a filtered version of the same source of tap water found in many homes. On the other hand, bottled waters derived from springs and wells may lack potentially helpful minerals (like fluoride, calcium, and magnesium) and may be vulnerable to the same groundwater contamination as the public supply.

By most standards, bottled water ranges from moderately expensive to expensive. In many cases you are paying for water that is not much different from tap water. Some consumers may not care about the extra cost because they prefer the taste of bottled water. But they should not think that just because they buy their water off the shelf rather than drink what comes out of the faucet that they are necessarily taking an extra step to safeguard their health. If your use of bottled water stems from concern about the safety of your tap water, have it tested by your local health department. The laboratory fee will be comparatively insignificant to an otherwise expensive alternative.

WATER—IS IT POSSIBLE TO GET TOO MUCH OF A GOOD THING?

Too much water—whatever greatly exceeds the kidney's ability to excrete it—can be toxic, but an excessive amount would have to normally approach many liters (quarts) each day. Most people have little risk of drinking too much water. Problems do accompany some disease states and mental disorders, such as schizophrenia. Excessive drinking of water then can quickly overwhelm the kidneys' capacity to excrete it. Water then accumulates in the body, causing headache, blurred vision, cramps, and eventually convulsions.

Minerals—A Preliminary Look

major mineral A mineral vital to health that is required in the diet in amounts greater than 100 mg per day.

trace mineral A mineral vital to health that is required in the diet in amounts less than 100 mg per day.

Minerals are categorized as major and trace minerals based on the amount humans need per day. Generally speaking, if we require 100 milligrams (1/50 of a teaspoon) or more per day of a mineral, it is considered a **major mineral**; otherwise, it is considered a **trace mineral.** Using this basis, calcium and phosphorus are major minerals and iron and zinc are trace minerals. The total of all trace minerals in the body is less than 15 grams (1/2 ounce). Nevertheless, trace minerals, such as iron and zinc, are very important. The small amount needed does not necessarily reflect a mineral's nutritional importance.

The metabolic roles of minerals vary considerably. Some, such as magnesium and manganese, enable enzymes to function. Minerals also act as key parts to important body compounds. For example, iodine is a component of the hormone thyroxine, and iron is a component of hemoglobin in the red blood cell.

Some minerals, such as sodium, potassium, calcium, and chloride, are electrolytes. These are positive or negatively charged ions that, by maintaining electrical balance throughout the body, aid in water balance, the transmission of nerve impulses and muscle contraction, as well as perform a multitude of other important roles. Finally,

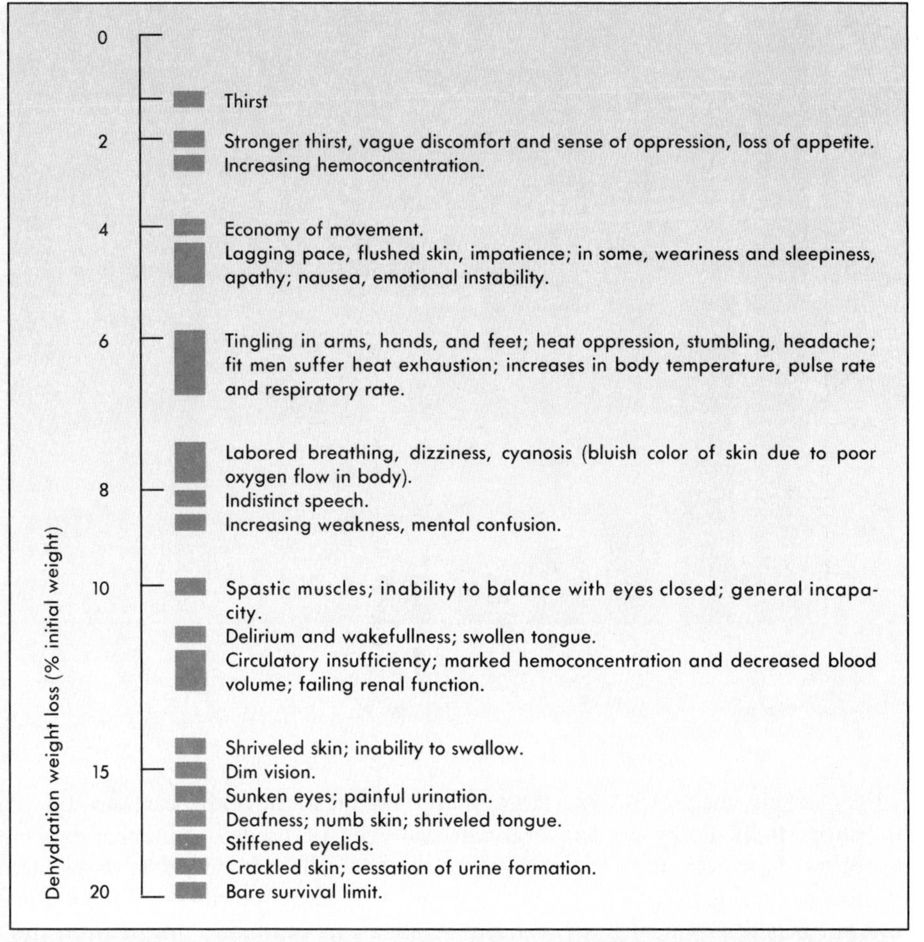

Figure 14-6 The effects of dehydration. These range from thirst to death.

some minerals, such as calcium and phosphorous, have critical roles in the growth, development, and structural integrity of bones (Figure 14-7). At all levels—cellular, tissue, organ, and whole body—minerals clearly play important roles in maintaining body functions.

MINERAL BIOAVAILABILITY

Although one may obtain the entire gamut of minerals from dietary sources, individual variation makes it difficult to determine exact amounts that are available for absorption from a specific food. While minerals may be present in a food, they are not **bioavailable** unless the body can absorb them. The ability to absorb minerals from a diet depends on many factors. A value listed in a food composition table is just a starting point for estimating the true contribution a food makes to our mineral needs. A significant factor determining the degree to which a mineral may be absorbed is the physiological need for that mineral at the time of consumption. Other factors are discussed below.

bioavailability The degree to which the amount of an ingested nutrient is absorbed and so is available to the body.

Mineral-Mineral Interactions

Many minerals have similar molecular weights and charges (valences). Magnesium, calcium, iron, and copper can exist in the +2 valance state. Having similar size and the same charge causes these minerals to compete with each other for absorption, and so they affect each other's bioavailability. Nutritionists caution people against taking individual mineral supplements, unless a medical condition specifically warrants it, because an excess of one mineral can hamper the absorption and metabolism of other minerals.

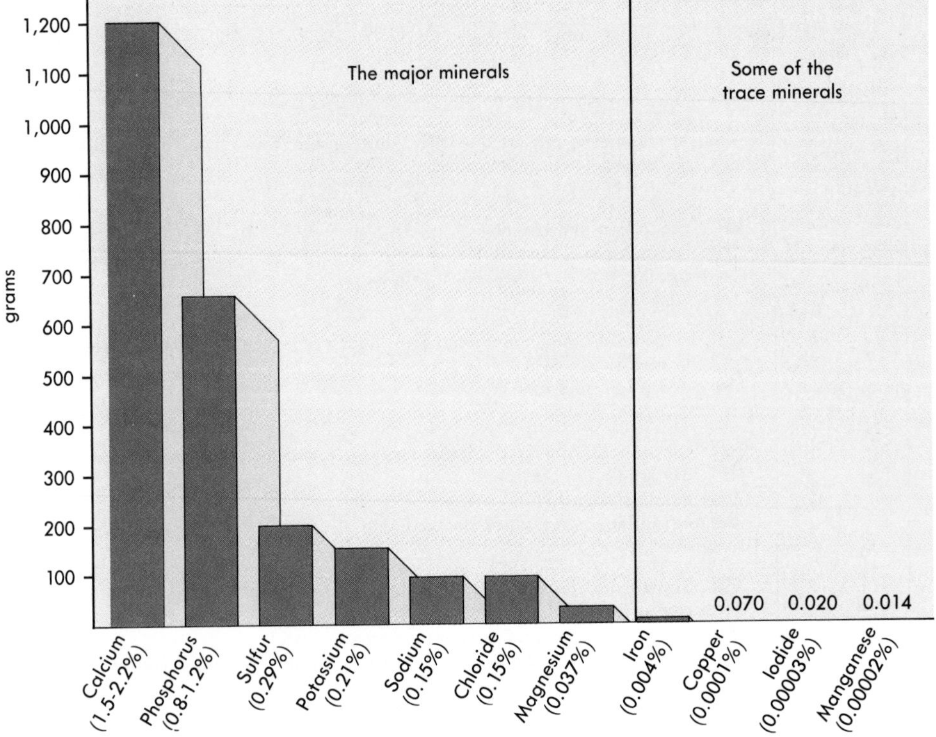

Figure 14-7 A list of minerals found in a 130-pound (60-kilogram) person. The percent figures represent percentage of body weight. Other trace minerals of nutritional importance include chromium, fluoride, molybdenum, selenium, and zinc.

For example, the presence of a large amount of zinc in the body decreases copper absorption. If medically needed, oral zinc can even be used to minimize copper absorption. However, mineral interactions are generally not desirable, as we are only now beginning to see with the recent surge in calcium supplementation. Despite hopes for benefits from such use, calcium supplements can reduce magnesium and iron absorption.

Vitamin-Mineral Interactions

When consumed in conjunction with vitamin C, iron absorption improves greatly. The vitamin D hormone calcitriol improves calcium absorption. Many vitamins require specific minerals to act as key components in their structure and function. For example, the thiamin coenzyme requires magnesium or manganese to function efficiently.

Fiber-Mineral Interactions

Mineral bioavailability can be affected by nonmineral dietary substances as well. Phytic acid (phytate) in grain fibers binds minerals, limiting their absorption, as does the oxalic acid in spinach and other vegetables. High-fiber diets are known to decrease the absorption of iron, calcium, zinc, magnesium, and probably other minerals. In diets that contain more than 35 grams of dietary fiber, decreased mineral absorption may occur to a problematic extent. We know very little about the long-term effects of very high-fiber diets on mineral status in the body. Recognizing this, scientists are actively researching the area. We advise you not to overconsume dietary fiber—stick to the recommendation of up to 35 grams per day unless under a physician's close scrutiny.

Spinach contains plenty of calcium, but only about 5% of it can be absorbed because of the vegetable's high concentration of oxalic acid. Usually, about 30% of calcium is absorbed from foods.

If grains are leavened with yeast, as they are in bread, enzymes produced by the yeast can break some of the bonds between phytic acid and minerals. This increases mineral absorption. The zinc deficiencies found among some Middle Eastern populations can be attributed partly to low dietary zinc and partly to their use of unleavened breads. Phytic acid binds so much of the zinc from unleavened breads that little is absorbed (see Chapter 15).

FOOD SOURCES OF MINERALS

Although plant foods are among the best sources of trace minerals such as copper, molybdenum, selenium, and chromium; in general, the best dietary mineral sources are animal products, especially seafoods. This is mainly because minerals in animal tissues are more concentrated than in plant tissues. As an animal eats plants year after year, minerals from the plants concentrate in the animal's body tissues. Likewise, sea animals, such as clams, oysters, and shrimp, concentrate the minerals found in seawater as they drink copious amounts of water throughout their lives. Minerals in animal foods are also more bioavailable than in plant foods because there are less mineral-binding substances in animal foods than in plant foods.

A diet devoid of animal products is very likely to be marginal in minerals, such as iron, zinc, and calcium. A key exception is magnesium, which is far more plentiful in plant than in animal sources. Otherwise, some plants are good, but not excellent, sources of many minerals. Vegans need to be aware of this and regularly choose good plant sources of minerals (see Chapter 5).

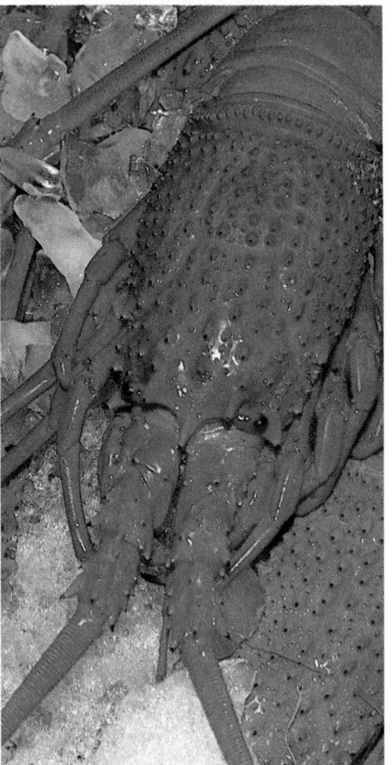

The mineral content of a food reflects the environment the food source was raised in. The mineral content of seafood reflects the mineral content of seawater.

MINERAL TOXICITY

Minerals can be quite toxic. As we cover each of the minerals in detail, it will become clear that toxicity is yet another reason to carefully consider the use of mineral supplements. Miners have suffered the ill-effects of minerals, especially from manganese. Selenium also can cause many toxic side effects (see Chapter 15).

CONCEPT CHECK

Many minerals are vital to health, though our needs for some remain uncertain. The bioavailability of minerals depends on many factors, including a body's need for the mineral and the mineral's interaction with fiber as well as other minerals. Taking an individual mineral supplement can greatly affect the absorption and metabolism of others. Animal products are generally rich sources of minerals because animals concentrate the minerals they consume from plants. Some minerals are potentially toxic. This is another reason to carefully consider any dietary mineral supplementation.

Major Minerals

We have discussed some general characteristics of water and briefly how it interacts with minerals in the body. Now let's review the individual properties of the major minerals.

Sodium

We both crave and fear sodium (Na) and its primary dietary source, table salt. Some of this fear is warranted, and some is not.

FUNCTIONS OF SODIUM

Almost all dietary sodium is absorbed. Its role within the body is primarily as the major positive ion in extracellular fluid. As such, it is a key electrolyte for retaining water in that compartment. Fluid balance throughout the body depends partly on the various sodium concentrations found in body water compartments.

Nerve Conduction

Sodium ions are important for nerve conduction. Impulses are transmitted down the nerve by sodium ions rushing into nerve cells. This reverses the charge of the cell membrane—**depolarizes** it—as the positive sodium ions rush in. The resulting electrical current produced travels from nerve cell to nerve cell. After the electrical wave passes through a nerve cell, sodium ions are pumped back out of the cell and

depolarize To create a neutral or uncharged condition.

potassium ions are pumped back in.[20] This process requires ATP energy—one molecule of ATP for each combination of three sodium ions pumped out and two potassium ions pumped in. When the ions regain their usual concentrations, the net charge along the membranes returns to its resting electrical value and the nerve cell is ready to "fire" again.

To assess sodium, potassium, chloride, calcium, magnesium, or phosphorus status in a person, serum levels can be measured. We will point out other methods, often more sensitive, when appropriate.

SODIUM BALANCE IN THE BODY

A low-sodium diet, coupled with high perspiration losses or diarrhea, can deplete the body of sodium. This state can lead to muscle cramps, nausea, vomiting, and dizziness and eventually to shock and coma. The kidneys are the major organs to respond to this depletion. They begin a variety of reactions that eventually triggers the release of the hormone aldosterone, as previously mentioned (Figure 14-5). Aldosterone then increases sodium retention by the kidneys.

Even in cases of high rates of perspiration, sodium depletion in the body is very unlikely because our diets contain ample sodium. Only when weight loss from perspiration exceeds 6 pounds (2.7 kilograms) should sodium losses raise concern. Even then, merely salting foods—not a salt tablet—is needed. Perspiration has only two thirds the sodium concentration of blood (about 2 grams of sodium per liter of perspiration versus 3 grams per liter for blood). And although perspiration tastes salty on the skin, it is not because perspiration is highly concentrated in sodium: rather, in evaporating from the skin, water leaves concentrated sodium behind.

When evaluating condiments, sauces, and seasonings, look first for the word sodium. The following are high in sodium: onion salt, celery salt, garlic salt, seasoned salt, baking powder, sea salt, salad dressings, pickles, soy sauce, steak sauce, barbecue sauce, meat tenderizer, baking soda, salt pork, brine, chili sauce, catsup, mustard, worcestershire sauce, bouillon, monosodium glutamate (MSG), and relish.

SODIUM IN FOODS

About one third to one half the sodium we consume is added during cooking or at the table (Table 14-1). Most of the rest is added during food manufacturing. Most foods naturally contain little sodium; milk is one exception. The more made-from-scratch cooking one has in his or her diet, the more sodium control one has. Major contributors of sodium to our diets (partly due to the frequency of consumption) are white bread, rolls, hot dogs, lunch meats, cheese, soups, and spaghetti with tomato sauce. Other foods especially high in sodium are tomato-based products in general, salted snack foods, French fries, potato chips, sauces, and gravies. Remember, you can not always rely on the salty taste of a food as a measurement for actual sodium content—tomato-based products are a prime example. Not too surprisingly, many condiments also contain large amounts of sodium—salt makes many foods taste better.

If we ate only unprocessed foods and added no salt, sodium intake would be about 500 to 1000 milligrams per day. By comparing that range with our typical intakes—3000 to 7000 milligrams—it is clear that food processing and cooking contributes a considerable amount to our dietary sodium.

A nutrition label lists a food's sodium content. In addition, a number of descriptive terms are used on labels, such as "sodium free" (less than 5 milligrams

Table 14-1 Sodium content of food varies with method of preparation

½ Cup of cooked peas	Sodium content of ½ cup of peas (milligrams)
Fresh	2
Frozen	70
Canned	185
Frozen with 2 tablespoons of cheese sauce	205
Frozen with 2 tablespoons of hollandaise sauce	310

sodium), "very low sodium" (35 milligrams or less per serving), "low sodium" (145 milligrams or less per serving), and "reduced sodium" (a 75% reduction in sodium content). The terms "unsalted," "no salt added," or "without added salt" on labels describe food products processed without salt when it normally would be used. Many medicines contain sodium, and they must be limited if dietary sodium is restricted. Similarly, when sodium is severely restricted, contributions from tap water (especially softened water) must be considered.

MINIMUM SODIUM REQUIREMENTS

The minimum sodium requirement for health as set by the 1989 RDA committee is 500 milligrams per day for adults. (Throughout this chapter, see the inside cover for other age groups and Appendix D for Canadian recommendations. Chapter 2 reviews the concept of minimum requirements for health.) This is a generous amount considering that we really need only about 100 milligrams per day.

Table salt is 40% sodium and 60% chloride. So our range of intake of 3 to 7 grams of sodium per day translates to 7.5 to 18 grams of salt (1½ to 3½ teaspoons).[19] Note a teaspoon of salt contains about 2 grams of sodium (a teaspoon of most dry substance equals approximately 5 grams).

Most humans can adapt to various dietary salt levels. For most of us, today's sodium intake is simply tomorrow's urine output. However, approximately 10% to 15% of American adults are sodium sensitive. For these people, high-sodium intakes contribute to hypertension (high blood pressure), and lower sodium diets (about 2 grams or ½ teaspoon daily) often help in correcting the hypertension[13] (see the Nutrition Perspective on Minerals and Hypertension). Scientific groups generally suggest that all adults limit daily sodium intake to 2.4 to 3 grams, mostly to limit the risk of developing hypertension.

If you have hypertension, you should try to reduce your sodium intake. If you don't have hypertension, you might still consider slowly reducing your intake to build good habits for the future, but no study confirms that this will prevent hypertension. If your daily sodium intake range is already within 2 to 3 grams, you are doing enough. See Table 14-2 to estimate your sodium intake.

LOWERING YOUR SODIUM INTAKE

If you choose to lower your sodium intake, you can eventually adapt to a low-sodium diet. At first foods will taste quite bland, but eventually you will perceive more flavor and your tongue will have a lower salt threshold. (The tongue's salt receptors will be triggered by less salt.)

By slowly reducing dietary sodium and substituting garlic, oregano, lemon juice, and other herbs and spices, you can eventually consume a flavorful diet that has only 2 to 3 grams of sodium daily. Many newer cookbooks can guide you to excellent recipes for flavorful low-salt foods. Except for yeast breads, omitting salt from food preparation can still yield an excellent product. For some people, this low-sodium approach to eating makes the difference between normal and high blood pressures.

CONCEPT CHECK

Sodium is the major positive ion of the extracellular fluid. It is important for maintaining fluid balance and conducting nerve impulses. Sodium depletion is unlikely since our diets have abundant sources and most sodium consumed is absorbed. The more foods we prepare at home, the more control we have over our sodium intakes. The minimum sodium requirement for health per day for adults is 500 milligrams. The average American consumes 3 to 7 grams daily. About 10% to 15% of the population is sensitive to sodium in the diet. In these people, hypertension can develop as a result of high intakes. To reduce the effects of hypertension, they can limit sodium intake to 2 to 3 grams per day, as suggested by scientific groups. This practice may also reduce the risk for future hypertension to those who are currently normotensive, but we don't have the scientific evidence to support this claim.

Table 14-2 A guide to sodium content of foods

Foods	Approximate sodium content (in milligrams)
Breads, cereals, and grain products:	
Cooked cereal, pasta, rice, unsalted	Less than 5 per ½ cup
Ready-to-eat cereal	100-360 per ounce
Bread, whole-grain or enriched	110-175 per slice
Biscuits and muffins	170-390 each
Vegetables:	
Fresh or frozen vegetables, cooked without added salt	Less than 70 per ½ cup
Vegetables, canned or frozen with sauce	140-460 per ½ cup
Fruit:	
Fruits (fresh, frozen, or canned)	Less than 10 per ½ cup
Milk, cheese, and yogurt:	
Milk and yogurt	120-160 per cup
Buttermilk, salt added	260 per cup
Natural cheeses	110-450 per 1-½ ounces
Cottage cheese, regular and low-fat	450 per ½ cup
Process cheese and cheese spreads	700-900 per 2 ounces
Meat, poultry, and fish:	
Fresh meat, poultry, fish with fins	Less than 90 per 3 ounces
Cured ham, sausages, luncheon meat, frankfurters, canned meats	750-1,350 per 3 ounces
Fats and dressings:	
Oil	None
Vinegar	Less than 6 per tablespoon
Prepared salad dressings	80-250 per tablespoon
Unsalted butter or margarine	1 per teaspoon
Salted butter or margarine	45 per teaspoon
Salt pork, cooked	360 per ounce
Condiments:	
Catsup, mustard, chili sauce, tartar sauce, steak sauce	125-275 per tablespoon
Soy sauce	1,000 per tablespoon
Salt	2,000 per teaspoon
Snack and convenience foods:	
Canned and dehydrated soups	630-1300 per cup
Canned and frozen main dishes	800-1400 per 8 ounces
Nuts and popcorn, unsalted	Less than 5 per ounce
Salted nuts, potato chips, corn chips	150-300 per ounce
Deep-fried pork rind	750 per ounce
Hamburger with bun	450-750 each
French fries, salted	200 per 20
Fried chicken	50 per drumstick
Hot dog with bun	750 each

From USDA Home and Garden Bulletin No. 232-6, April 1986.

Potassium

Potassium (K) performs many of the same functions as sodium, but it operates inside rather than outside cells. It is also associated more with lowering—rather than raising—blood pressure.[28] We absorb about 90% of the potassium we eat. Once inside the cell, much of the potassium is bound by phosphate ions and proteins. Some of these proteins are enzymes that function more efficiently when potassium ions are present. The intracellular fluid contains 95% of the potassium in the body. Potassium participates in fluid balance and nerve transmission. After the transmission of a nerve impulse, when sodium ions are pumped back out of the nerve cell, potassium ions are pumped back into the nerve cell.

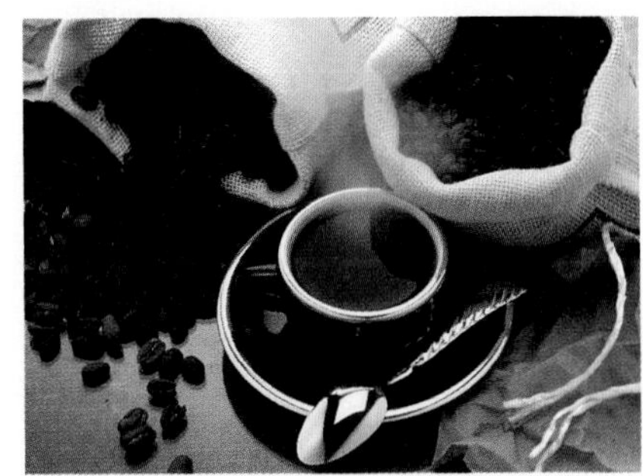

Coffee is a major contributor of potassium to our diets, primarily because so much coffee is consumed.

RESULTS OF A POTASSIUM DEFICIENCY

A potassium deficiency is more likely than a sodium deficiency because we generally do not add potassium to foods. Such deficiencies occur in some disease states, such as when long bouts of vomiting and diarrhea deplete potassium stores. A continually poor food intake, as may be the case in alcoholism, can also result in a potassium deficiency.

A low blood potassium level (hypokalemia) is a life-threatening problem. Results often include a loss of appetite, muscle cramps, confusion and apathy, and constipation. Eventually, the heart will beat irregularly, decreasing its capacity to pump blood.[20]

POTASSIUM IN FOODS

Leafy and other vegetables are all nutrient-dense sources of potassium (Table 14-3). Milk, whole grains, dried beans, and meats are also good sources of potassium. Major contributors of potassium to the U.S. diet include coffee, tea, milk, potatoes (French fries and other potato products), and orange juice. Bananas also are an excellent source.

MINIMUM POTASSIUM REQUIREMENTS

The minimum potassium requirement for health for adults is 2000 milligrams (2 grams) per day. Our diets supply enough potassium if a variety of foods is eaten. Intakes in the United States average 2 to 4 grams per day; women consume amounts near the lower intake level.

AMERICANS AT RISK FOR A POTASSIUM DEFICIENCY

People who take potassium-wasting diuretics, such as thiazides and furosemide, need to monitor their potassium intakes carefully. These medicines are used chiefly to control hypertension (see the Nutrition Perspective), but in the process deplete body potassium, along with other ions. Water follows the excreted ions, eventually reducing blood volume and blood pressure. In such cases, high-potassium foods, such as fruits, fruit juices, and vegetables, are good additions to a diet. In more serious deficiencies, potassium chloride supplements may even be recommended by a physician.

Several other groups are at risk for potassium deficiency and need blood potassium levels monitored. These groups include persons with anorexia nervosa or bulimia. Poor diets and losses from vomiting cause the problem. People on very low calorie diets (protein-sparing modified fasts) or who just eat very little food (as we mentioned for people with alcoholism) are also at risk, as well as heavily exercising athletes. These people can avoid the detrimental side effects of low potassium levels by consuming potassium-rich food sources.

TOXICITY OF POTASSIUM

If kidneys function normally, typical intakes of dietary potassium are not toxic. When kidneys function poorly, potassium levels build up in the bloodstream

Table 14-3 Good sources of potassium, ranked by nutrient density

Food	Serving size to yield 667 milligrams*	kcalories needed to yield 667 milligrams
Spinach, cooked	1 cup	40
Lima beans	½ cup	40
Zucchini squash, cooked	1⅓ cups	42
Asparagus, cooked	1 cup	45
Winter squash, baked	⅔ cup	62
Cantaloupe	⅓ each	75
Orange juice	1 cup	117
Potato, baked	⅔ each	160
Pinto beans	⅔ cup	177
Bananas	1 each	212
Kidney beans	1½ cups	220

* ⅓ Minimum adult requirement.
A diet rich in vegetables and fruits provides ample potassium.

(creating a condition called hyperkalemia) and inhibit heart function by causing slowed heartbeats. This eventually can cause the heart to stop beating. Consequently, in cases of reduced kidney function, close monitoring of potassium intake is critical.

Chloride

Chlorine (Cl) is a very poisonous gas. Public water utilities often rely on this gas to kill bacteria in water supplies. Consequently many water-borne diseases are rare in America.

Chloride, an ionic form of chlorine, forms an important negative ion for the extracellular fluid. These ions are a component of the hydrochloric acid produced by the parietal cells in the stomach and are also used during immune responses as white blood cells attack foreign cells. Nerve impulse conduction also employs chloride ions.[20] Most of the body's chloride is excreted by the kidneys; some is lost in perspiration.

A chloride deficiency is unlikely because our dietary sodium chloride intake is so high. Frequent and lengthy bouts of vomiting, if coupled with a nutrient-poor diet, can contribute to a deficiency because stomach secretions contain chloride. In 1978 to 1979, not enough chloride was added to a brand of infant formula. Infants who consumed it suffered severe convulsions and other health problems, clearly showing what can happen when the need for a nutrient normally abundant in our diets is not given adequate attention.

CHLORIDE IN FOODS

A few fruits and some vegetables are naturally good sources of chloride. However, most chloride comes from the addition of salt to food. If we know a food's salt content, we can predict closely its chloride content (sodium content x 1.5). Naturally occurring sodium or chloride doesn't significantly affect this calculation.

MINIMUM CHLORIDE REQUIREMENT

The minimum requirement for health for adults for chloride is 700 milligrams per day. Assuming that the average American consumes at least 7.5 grams of salt daily, that yields 4.5 grams (4500 milligrams) of chloride, a more than abundant intake of this ion.

TOXICITY OF CHLORIDE

The chloride ion itself may be an important part of the blood pressure–raising action of sodium. Together, then, the sodium and chloride components of salt are implicated in the high rates of hypertension in the United States. One researcher has suggested that chloride supplies a negative ion that allows the body to retain the positive sodium ion. Since chloride ions tend to remain in the body, they trap the positive sodium ions to balance the equation. The result is the same either way: For hypertension, control salt intake.

CONCEPT CHECK

Potassium has functions similar to those of sodium, except it is the main positive ion of intracellular, not extracellular, fluid. Potassium is vital to fluid balance and nerve transmission. A potassium deficiency caused by poor intake, persistent vomiting, or use of certain diuretics can lead to loss of appetitie, muscle cramps, confusion, and heart arrhythmias. Leafy vegetables, melons, tomatoes, and potatoes are rich sources of potassium. A risk of toxicity accompanies impaired kidney function. Chloride is the major negative ion of extracellular fluid. It functions in digestion as part of hydrochloric acid, in nerve impulse transmission, and in immune system responses. Deficiencies are unlikely because dietary sodium chloride intake is so high.

Calcium

Calcium (Ca) is clearly the most abundant mineral found within the body (Figure 14-7). It amounts to nearly 1200 grams, or about 40% of the total mass of all the minerals combined. Nearly 99% of the calcium found within the body acts to strengthen the teeth and bones. However, the remaining 1% circulating within the bloodstream is not to be discounted for it does play important roles in the function of each cell. Growth and bone development in laboratory animals is closely tied to calcium intake. This link is seen in humans,[15] too, but we can probably better adapt to a low calcium intake.

ABSORPTION OF CALCIUM

Calcium is absorbed primarily in the upper part of the small intestine (duodenum), because calcium requires a pH below six to stay in solution. The duodenum tends to be a favorable environment for absorption because it takes time for the acidic stomach contents to be fully neutralized by bicarbonate released from the pancreas (see Chapter 6). In addition, calcium absorption within the upper small intestine depends on the active vitamin D hormone calcitriol. Some additional calcium absorption occurs throughout the lower small intestine.

In normal adults consuming 400 to 1000 milligrams of calcium, absorption varies from about 25% to 40%. An average value is 30%. The upper limit of absorption is seen in children during active periods of skeletal growth—absorption may be as great as 75% of dietary calcium intake. During pregnancy, absorption may be as high as 60% of intake. Young people in general tend to absorb calcium better than older people.[30] This is especially true when one considers postmenopausal women—calcium absorption in this case is very poor. Exhibiting the lower limit of calcium absorption, these women may absorb as little as 20% of dietary calcium.

The female sex hormone estrogen plays a key role in the absorption of calcium, and after menopause the levels of this crucial hormone plummet. Fortunately, estrogen therapy (in a supplementary form of the hormone itself) has shown to increase the synthesis of calcitriol, which in turn, increases calcium absorption.

Many cumulative factors enhance calcium absorption, such as the acidic environment of the upper small intestine; the presence of the vitamin D hormone (calcitriol), parathyroid hormone, dietary glucose, and lactose; and normal intestinal

Table 14-4 Absorption of calcium from the intestinal tract

Factors favoring absorption	Factors hindering absorption
Acid nature of upper intestinal tract	Alkaline reaction in lower intestinal tract
Normal digestive activity and motility of intestinal tract	Large amounts of dietary fiber
Dietary calcium and phosphorus in about equal amounts	Laxatives or any circumstances that induce diarrhea or hypermotility of the intestine
Vitamin D	*Great* excess of phosphorus or magnesium in proportion to calcium
Need for higher amounts by the body, as during pregnancy	Phytate, oxalic acid, and unabsorbed fatty acids: they all bind calcium in the intestine
Low calcium intake	Vitamin D deficiency
Parathyroid hormone	Menopause
Lactose	Old age
Glucose	Tannins in tea

motility (flow) (Table 14-4). Factors limiting calcium absorption include large amounts of phytate, fiber, magnesium, or phosphorus in the diet, and tannins in tea; a vitamin D deficiency; menopause; diarrhea; and old age.

One problem in setting the RDA for calcium is predicting the extent to which calcium will be absorbed. The RDA is based on an estimated 30% to 40% absorption. Some people absorb calcium more efficiently than that, and others less efficiently. Less efficient absorption raises needs. However, deciding who is consuming sufficient calcium to accommodate body needs—such as when they are not consuming the RDA—is not practical. That requires measuring calcium absorption, a complex task.

Bone loss caused by insufficient calcium in the diet proceeds slowly.[23] Only after many years are clinical signs apparent. By not meeting the RDA for calcium, some people, especially women, may be setting the stage for future bone fractures. But, because we don't know how efficiently individuals absorb calcium, we often cannot predict those at high risk for bone loss, and so for whom this poses a problem.

REGULATING SERUM CALCIUM

Each cell has a critical need for calcium, as we will discuss. This is probably the reason humans have such excellent hormonal systems to control blood calcium levels. A normal blood calcium level can be maintained despite a poor calcium intake. The bones, however, pay the price. This makes serum calcium levels generally a poor measure of calcium status. In addition, measuring bone density over short periods isn't much more useful, because changes in bone density develop very slowly (see the Nutrition Focus on Calcium and Osteoporosis).

As discussed in Chapter 12, when the serum calcium level falls, the parathyroid gland releases parathyroid hormone. This hormone increases calcium absorption by increasing synthesis of calcitriol. It also increases the kidney's retrieval of calcium before possible urine excretion. In addition, parathyroid hormone causes increased calcium release from bones via increased osteoclast (bone-breakdown cells) activity. In all, then, parathyroid hormone action increases the serum calcium level.

When serum calcium levels are too high, the thyroid gland secretes the hormone calcitonin. Calcitonin decreases calcium loss from bones via decreased osteoclast activity and decreased synthesis of the calcitriol. This causes the calcium level in the blood stream to fall into the normal range.

Bone Structure—How Calcium Fits Into The Picture

The role of calcium as it pertains to bone is easily the most recognizable function of the mineral. To better understand the role calcium plays within bone structure, it is important to understand the varying levels of structural sophistication found within the bone and how those levels are maintained.

MICROSTRUCTURE OF BONE

Within a bone itself are found two vital cell types, each integral to maintaining bones. Despite its "dead" appearance, bone is very metabolically active.

Osteoclast Cells

These bone cells are continually breaking down the bone network. In essence, osteoclasts break down bone in areas where it is not needed. These osteoclasts are very active when a diet is deficient in calcium because their action (triggered by parathyroid hormone) releases calcium from the bone so it can enter the bloodstream. Remember, a supply of calcium is vital to all cells, not just to bone cells.

Osteoblast Cells

Bone also contains osteoblast cells. These cells secrete a collagen protein matrix that forms the support structure of bone. They then secrete bone mineral, which strengthens the bone. This mineral matures and eventually approaches the composition of $Ca_{10}(PO_4)_6OH_2$, called **hydroxyapatite.**

BONE CELL INTERPLAY DURING STRUCTURAL MODIFICATION

Bone turnover refers to a cycle of bone breakdown by the osteoclasts and then bone rebuilding by the osteoblasts. In this way, bone is remodeled when necessary.[23] Before new bone can be built, the old bone in that area must be partially broken down.

During human growth, total osteoblast activity exceeds osteoclast activity, so we make more bone than we break down. In the first year of life, all bones in the body are rebuilt. In the young adult, 15% to 30% of the skeleton is rebuilt each year, with more bone being built in areas put under high stress. A right-handed tennis player, for example, will build more bone in that arm in comparison with the left arm.

BONE MACROSTRUCTURE

Bone macrostructure consists of two primary levels that interact to form quite an engineering marvel of strength.

Cortical bone. The outer surface of an entire bone is composed of a very dense type of bone, called cortical (compact) bone. The shafts of bones, such as those of the arm, are almost entirely cortical bone.

Trabecular bone. Trabecular (spongy) bone is found in the ends of the bones, inside the spinal vertebrae, and inside the flat bones of the pelvis. Trabecular bone forms an internal scaffolding network for a bone (Figure 14-8). It supports the outer cortical shell of the bone, especially in heavily stressed areas, such as joints.

DETERMINANTS OF BONE STRENGTH

Density

Bone strength is determined primarily by its density. The more densely packed the bone crystals are, the stronger the bone structure. Total bone mass refers to the weight of bone in the body, while bone density reflects how densely packed the crystals are in a particular bone. The denser the bone the stronger it is.

Bone Repair Rate

The next important determinant of bone strength is the rate at which the bone can heal itself. **Microfractures,** so small they cannot be seen on an x-ray or any type of

hydroxyapatite A compound composed of calcium and phosphate that is deposited into the bone protein matrix to give it strength and rigidity.

cortical bone Dense, compact bone that composes the outer surface and shafts of bones.

trabecular bone The spongy, inner matrix of bone found primarily in the spine, pelvis, and ends of bones.

microfractures Small fractures, undetectable by x-rays or other bone scans, that may occur constantly in bones.

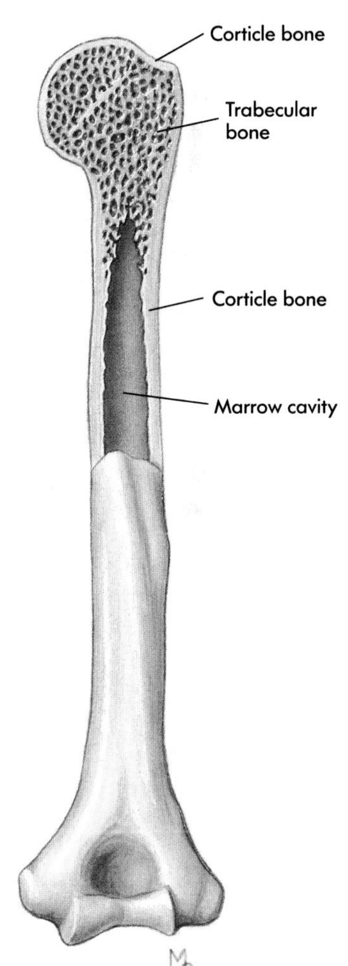

Figure 14-8 Cortical and trabecular bone. Cortical bone forms the shafts of bones and outer mineral covering. Trabecular bone supports the cortical bone in various bones of the body, as in the bone pictured.

EXPERT OPINION

Nutrition and Peak Bone Mass

VELIMIR MATKOVIC, M.D., PH.D.

The human skeleton develops through infancy and childhood to a peak bone mass during late adolescence or the early twenties. Thereafter, bone loss gradually occurs, resulting eventually in a bone mass value that increases fracture risk after minimal or moderate trauma. Research suggests that the main determinants of osteoporotic-related fractures are the peak bone-mass level reached at skeletal maturity and the subsequent rate of bone loss.

Peak bone mass

Since bone mass is a principal determinant of fracture risk, a high bone mass at skeletal maturity is considered important protection against age-related bone loss. Besides well-known factors influencing body stature, such as protein and zinc intake, very little is known about the mechanisms for increasing peak bone mass. Peak bone mass is clearly the result of age, gender, and probably other genetically determined factors. We do know that men have higher bone mass values than women, and that blacks have heavier skeletons than whites. As a direct consequence, men and blacks have a lower incidence of fractures than other populations. Peak bone mass could also be related to calcium nutrition.

The ages between 9 and 20 years are critical for achievement of peak bone mass. From birth until about age 20 years, bones grow rapidly. After this period, the skeleton constantly remodels itself throughout life. The adolescent growth spurt is probably the most important period for bone growth. That is when bone mineral content is increasing at the rate of about 8.5% per year.

The average male begins his growth spurt at around 12 years of age, reaching his maximum velocity in height growth at about 14 years of age. At this time, he will be growing at nearly twice his childhood or preadolescent rate. His growth will be almost completed by age 18. Females begin puberty approximately 2 years earlier (at 8 to 10 years of age) and reach maximum velocity in height growth around 12 years of age. Cessation of linear growth in girls will be around age 16 years. There is about a 2% increase in body length thereafter in both boys and girls, extending to the early twenties of the young adult period. This increase is accounted for primarily by continued vertebral growth. Peak skeletal bone mass, based on skeletal weight measurements, is then achieved by the beginning of the third decade.

Total body calcium is also greatest at about age 20 years. The external diameter of tubular (cortical) bones peaks by the age of 20 years in males, and a few years earlier in females. Bone mineral content of the forearm also approaches its highest level by the beginning of young adulthood, indicating once again that adolescence can be a critical period for cortical peak bone mass formation. There are few data regarding changes in trabecular bone mass in the adolescent period, but present literature suggests that peak bone mass for the vertebral column has been achieved by the age of 20 years. Postmortem data, using bone ash measurements and compressive strength measurements, indicate an increase in the vertebrae values after the beginning of

bone scan, are constantly developing in bone.[9] These microfractures must be knitted back together with collagen protein and bone crystal. Otherwise, they can accumulate and eventually allow for a major fracture.

Integrity of the Trabecular Bone Network

The third important element of bone strength is the trabecular bone network inside the bone. It is especially critical for the trabeculae to extend continuously—without breaks—throughout its sites in the bone. Any break weakens the support of the outer edge of the bone and increases the risk for bone fracture.

Of those three factors—bone density, rate of self-healing, and integrity of the trabecular support—the only one that can be measured when the bone is inside a person is bone density. The bone density value can predict fracture risk, but it cannot account for other factors that also determine bone strength. Not all people with low bone density suffer fractures, and some people with high bone densities do suffer fractures, probably because these other factors come into play, as well.

EXPERT OPINION

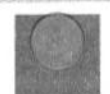

Nutrition and Peak Bone Mass—cont'd

the third decade and a decline thereafter. Bone mineral density in the lower spine and pelvic area also declines after its maximum at about the age of 20 years in both males and females.

Calcium and bone density

Experiments with laboratory animals show that a calcium deficiency can influence either peak bone mass formation and/or the subsequent rate of bone loss and eventually lead to osteoporosis. In the majority of the experiments, animals were fed a low-calcium diet during the growing period and skeletons were examined when the animals reached adulthood. The results indicated that calcium deficiency can cause osteoporosis by decreasing peak bone mass formation, rather than affecting later adult bone mass. Experimental calcium deficiency can cause growth retardation in animals, affecting bone volume and decreasing bone density (bone mass per bone volume). Despite a large body of information obtained from additional animal studies, we have no clear-cut evidence that skeletons of growing humans will react to inadequate calcium intake in the same way.

It is clear from human studies that malnutrition certainly can lead to growth retardation, and conversely, correction of the nutritional deficit may in some instances return growth to normal. At present, we don't know if there is adequate "catch-up mineralization" of the skeleton, particularly after the growth spurt period.

A study I performed of the calcium intake, bone mass, and fracture rates in two populations in Croatia, revealed that people who consume higher amounts of calcium throughout their lifetimes (1000 to 1200 milligrams/day) had denser skeletons and lower hip fracture rates than people with lower calcium intakes (400 to 500 milligrams/day). Since differences were present at the age of 30 years, this study suggests calcium is probably more important to peak bone mass formation, rather than to protect people from bone loss.

Adolescent females in the United States often have poor calcium intake compared with their calcium needs for skeletal growth. To satisfy their need for a high skeletal retention (up to 400 milligrams per day), supply enough to replace unavoidable calcium excretion into the urine, and account for variable absorption efficiency, calcium intake during adolescence should exceed 1200 milligrams per day. The current RDA is 1200 milligrams per day and probably is not enough for all adolescents. Support for this recommendation is added by the recent report that postmenopausal women who had decreased dairy product consumption during adolescence had decreased bone mass in the postmenopausal period. Also some recent clinical trials showed positive effects of calcium supplementation on bone mass during growth and skeletal consolidation.

Conclusion

Late childhood and adolescence represents the ideal time to build a dense skeleton, and both laboratory animal and human research points to an adequate calcium intake as an inportant goal. A calcium intake of about 1500 milligrams per day in adolescence should represent a critical objective in diet planning.

Dr. Matkovic is Associate Professor of Physical and Internal Medicine at The Ohio State University. His main research interest is in osteoporosis and calcium nutrition.

OSTEOPOROSIS

Failure to maintain enough bone mass in the body eventually results in **osteopenia,** which means "little bone." When a person has osteopenia, and no cause can be found—such as osteomalacia, the use of certain medications, or cancer tumors—the diagnosis is osteoporosis.[23] Osteoporosis can be further classified as Type I (postmenopausal), which appears in the years right after menopause, and Type II (senile), which is found in people of advanced ages.

Bone composition in osteoporosis is essentially normal. The bone may contain some extra sodium, but basically there is just less bone throughout the body. Because these bones have lesser substance, osteoporosis can lead to fractures in old age, as well as to loss of teeth. Recall from Chapter 12 that in osteomalacia the bone is abnormal because it is poorly calcified.

ADDITIONAL FUNCTIONS OF CALCIUM

Bone formation and maintenance are major roles for calcium in the body. However, the importance of calcium in the body does not stop there.

NUTRITION FOCUS

Calcium and Osteoporosis

Widespread advertising has made it almost impossible for women to ignore osteoporosis. Its crippling effect on elderly women is now recognized as a medical emergency. The disease affects 25 million people in the United States, mostly older women, and is taxing our health-care system. This results primarily from the costs related to the 1.5 million associated bone fractures (approximately about $10 billion a year). When scientists estimate the exercise and dietary patterns of humans living at the end of the Stone Age, they find calcium intake was twice that of contemporary humans and needs for physical exertion were also greater than at present. Bony remains from that period suggest that Stone Age humans developed a greater peak bone mass in young adulthood and experienced less age-related bone loss than do humans in the twentieth century.[6] Does this tell us something?

How bone density, age, and gender fit into the picture

The question of how and why osteoporosis takes place is largely a matter of one's bone density. The reason this is primarily a concern of women is that for the most part, they make less bone than men, lose it at a faster rate, and live longer. Thus women start their adult years with less bone and have a longer time to lose it. And possibly for that very reason, about one third of women will eventually experience osteoporosis-related fractures.

Although adult stature is reached and most bone mass is developed in the teen years,[15,24] the skeleton continues to accumulate mass until age 30 years to 35 years, at least so long as the diet supplies sufficient calcium. The actual amount built is quite variable among women. Bone loss, especially in trabecular areas (the inner parts of flat bones, vertebrae, and bone ends), begins around age 30 years in women. The rate of bone loss between age 30 years and menopause (approximately age 50 years) is typically slow and continuous. It often speeds up at menopause and continues at a high rate for the next 5 to 10 years. By age 65 years, bone-loss rate has fallen to about the same rate as before menopause.[14]

Osteoporosis leads usually to fractures in the hip, spine, and wrist. The slender, inactive woman who smokes is more susceptible to osteoporosis, but any woman who lives long enough can suffer from the disease. As women age into their 80s and 90s, osteoporosis becomes the rule—not the exception. The spine fractures commonly found in cases of women with osteoporosis cause considerable pain and deformity and decrease physical ability (Figure 14-9). Furthermore, osteoporosis is not only debilitating, it can be fatal. Between 12% and 20% of all elderly persons who suffer hip fractures eventually die from fracture-related complications.[17]

Can osteoporosis be prevented?

As no cure currently exists for osteoporosis-related fractures, preventing this disease is very important. Since 1985, estrogen replacement therapy has been recommended at menopause to prevent osteoporosis.[29] It is also used to reduce symptoms of menopause. Studies to date show that estrogen replacement at menopause virtually stops further bone loss in women. Thus it is reasonable to assume that estrogen replacement therapy will eliminate risk for significant osteoporosis in women who begin it right after menopause and take it for the rest of their lives. However, we really need long-term studies to be sure. This therapy, given the low levels of hormone administered, is relatively safe, but does require the watchful eye of a physician. Estrogen replacement therapy also reduces the risk of heart disease in women, probably by raising blood HDL cholesterol levels.

Is estrogen therapy the only answer?

Some women cannot take estrogen because they have estrogen-sensitive breast and uterine tumors. Other therapies, such as taking the active vitamin D hormone calcitriol or the hormone calcitonin, are available and quite effective. But for these women—and other women—will increasing calcium intake substitute for taking either estrogen or other medications?

Studies from the United States and Denmark have found that taking even 2000 milligrams of extra calcium (equal to 7.5 glasses of milk) does not prevent bone loss seen in the 10 or so years after menopause in the spine, hip, or wrist as successfully as estrogen replacement therapy does. Extra dietary calcium more effectively reduces bone loss in the total skeleton than doing nothing at all.[3] But a high calcium intake may be no better for reducing bone loss in the spine than just meeting the RDA. However, increasing calcium intake to 1500 milligrams per day can reduce the dose of estrogen needed to prevent bone loss. Overall, for most women it is not estrogen versus calcium but probably estrogen plus calcium that constitutes the most effective treatment.

Are all women at risk?

About one third of all women experience osteoporosis-related fractures in their lifetimes. Some women just do not live long enough to suffer from osteoporosis. They may experience bone loss, but their bones still remain strong enough throughout their lives. This is especially true of women who die before the age of 75 years.

In addition, some women have much denser bone than others. They probably built more bone when they were young, and so they can endure greater bone loss without experiencing more fractures. Also, some women may more easily adapt to lower-calcium diets.

Actually, the reason for such variation in bone density and fracture risk in women at any age still needs more research. However, numerous factors, such as physical activity,

NUTRITION FOCUS

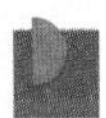

Calcium and Osteoporosis—cont'd

calcium intake throughout life, ability to adapt to low-calcium diets, and fluoride intake, are associated with higher bone density values in some studies (Table 14-5).[29] On the other hand, a lack of regular menstruation, premature menopause, use of certain medications, excess sodium in the diet (because it pulls calcium into the urine with it), and prolonged bed rest are all associated with low bone density values in women. We can't focus only on calcium when discussing this disease—many factors are involved.

Am I at risk?

Medical and nutritional recommendations concerning osteoporosis are best made when the individual status of a person is known. The bone density of a person's spine, hip, and wrist can aid decisions. Special bone densitometers are available in medical centers for these measurements. Unfortunately, these density measurements don't reveal anything about bone architecture. Recall that bone relies on its mineral density, trabeculae crossbracing, and its ability to heal microfractures for its strength.[9] So a bone-density measurement tells part of the story, not the whole story.

A plan for fracture prevention

Prevention of osteoporosis focuses on two main strategies: increasing bone mass by the time full skeletal maturity is reached (again about 30 to 35 years of age) and reducing age-related bone loss.

As women mature from young children to their elder years, different strategies for preventing osteoporosis are needed. Young women should see a physician at any sign of irregular menstruation and pursue an active lifestyle that includes sun exposure and weight-bearing exercise. Greater muscle mass is linked to greater bone density, as this keeps tension on bone.[11] Note that exercise does not prevent the bone loss associated with irregular menstruation. Regular menstruation is the overwhelming key to bone maintenance in young women, as evidenced by poor bone density in nonmenstruating female athletes.

Meeting the RDA for calcium is also important.[18] Recall early humans both ate lots of calcium and performed much physical activity.[6] If foods from the milk and cheese group are not usually consumed, it is wise to find another calcium source. Note that the average calcium intake of American women today is less than 700 mg/day from age 20 years to 50 years and less than 500 mg/day from age 50 years on. On any given day, one woman in four gets less than 300 mg of calcium. And most teenage girls and young women currently consume less than two thirds the RDA.[2]

Avoidance of smoking and alcoholism are also important.[16] Alcohol is toxic to bone cells. Smoking and alcoholism are probably two major undiagnosed and unrecognized causes of osteoporosis today. Moderation in caffeine intake is also advised.[12]

At menopause, women need to discuss estrogen replacement therapy with a physician. They also need to accurately track their height. A decrease of more than 1 inch from premenopausal values is a sign that significant bone loss is taking place. If a plan to prevent osteoporosis is not in effect, a loss in height is the signal to see a physician and establish a plan.

Elderly women need to stay as physically active as possible and meet the RDA for calcium. These two goals alone can slow bone loss in one's advanced years. They also need to minimize the risk for falls, especially by limiting their use of alcohol and medications, both of which might disturb coordination. Regular sun exposure and consuming food sources of vitamin D are also good ideas.[29]

Table 14-5 Factors associated with bone maintenance versus bone loss

Maintenance	Loss	
Normal menses	Lack of menses	Alcoholism
Estrogen replacement	Amenorrhea	Cigarette smoking
African descent	Early menopause	Slender figure
Thiazide diuretics	Glucocorticoid use	Bed rest (months)
Physical activity*	Hyperparathyroidism	Dietary fiber
Dietary Calcium	Hyperthyroidism	High sodium intake
	Thyroid hormone replacement	Anorexia nervosa

*The degree of effect remains to be established.

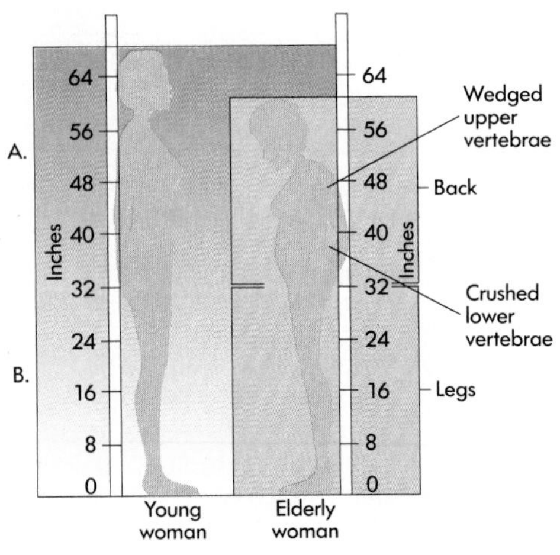

Figure 14-9 A loss of height and distorted body shape are common signs of osteoporosis. Monitor your adult height changes to detect early osteoporosis.

tetany A state marked by sharp contraction of muscles and failure to relax afterward; usually caused by abnormal calcium metabolism.

calmodulin A cell protein that, once bound to calcium, can influence the activity of some enzymes in the cell.

Blood Clotting

Calcium is essential for blood clotting. It participates in a reaction whereby prothrombin contributes to the synthesis of fibrin so that a blood clot can form. Without sufficient calcium in the bloodstream, blood will not clot.

Muscle Contraction

Calcium is critical for muscle contraction. It allows the proteins in muscles, actin and myosin, to interact properly during muscle contraction. If the blood calcium level falls below a certain level, muscles cannot relax after contraction. The body then stiffens and shows signs of **tetany.**

Nerve Transmission

Normal nerve transmission requires calcium. It permits the release of neurotransmitters, as well as the flow of ions in and out of nerve cells. Tetany can also occur when nerve transmission fails because insufficient calcium is available.

Cell Metabolism

Finally, calcium helps regulate metabolism in the cell by participating in the **calmodulin** system. When calcium enters a cell (often because of hormone action) and binds to the protein calmodulin, the protein/calcium complex formed then goes on to regulate the levels of activity for various enzymes, including those that synthesize glycogen.

OTHER POSSIBLE BENEFITS OF CALCIUM IN THE DIET

Besides contributing to bone strength, dietary calcium may reduce the risk of colon cancer.[10] It appears that a high calcium content in the stool can bind free fatty acids and bile acids found there. These compounds, when unbound, tend to irritate the colon. The irritation may increase cell turnover and in turn increase the risk of cancer (see Chapter 13). A daily dietary calcium supplement of 1250 milligrams reduces cell turnover in the colon. High calcium levels in the colon may also increase the tendency of cancer cells in the colon to clump together, and so decrease their tendency to metastasize to other areas. Calcium intakes of 1 gram or more per day may also slightly decrease blood pressure, compared to intakes of 400 milligrams or less per day (see the Nutrition Perspective).

Both these areas of calcium research—colon cancer and high blood pressure—are new areas of research. Thus practical dietary recommendations stemming from this research—other than meeting the RDA—are not yet established.

CALCIUM IN FOODS

Dairy products, such as milk and cheese, provide most of the calcium in our diets. The exception is cottage cheese because most calcium is lost during production. White bread, rolls, crackers, and other foods made with milk products are secondary contributors. The most nutrient-dense calcium sources are green leafy vegetables (Table 14-6). However, much calcium in these vegetables is not absorbed because of the presence of oxalic acid. That makes nonfat milk the best nutrient-dense source of calcium because of its high bioavailability and low kcalorie value. The new calcium-fortified versions of orange juice are close competitors. Soybean curd (tofu) is also a good source of calcium if it is made with calcium carbonate (check the label).

One reason the Guide to Daily Food Choices contains a milk, yogurt, and cheese group is to supply calcium to the diet. In addition, the group provides protein, vitamin A, vitamin D, riboflavin, potassium, and magnesium. People who do not like milk can use products made with milk, such as chocolate milk, yogurt, cheese, and ice cream. All forms of milk, yogurt, and cheese allow about the same degree of calcium absorption.[22] We hesitate to recommend either cheese or ice cream because they are usually high in saturated fat. However, some low-fat cheeses and ice milks

Table 14-6 Good sources of calcium ranked by nutrient density

Food	Serving size to yield 267 milligrams*	kcalories needed to yield 267 milligrams
Turnip greens, cooked	1⅓ cups	40
Spinach, cooked	1 cup	40
Beet greens, cooked	1⅔ cups	67
Broccoli, cooked	1½ cups	69
1% low-fat milk	¾ cup	83
Romano cheese	¾ ounce	83
Parmesan cheese	¼ cup	89
Shrimp, boiled	3 ounces	91
Buttermilk	1 cup	100
Swiss cheese	1 ounce	107
Muenster cheese	1⅓ ounce	139
Sardines, canned w/ bones	2⅔ ounce	167

* ⅓ RDA for adults 25 years of age.
Green leafy vegetables supply the fewest kcalories, but the calcium in nonfat milk is more bioavailable. So nonfat milk is actually the best nonfortified food source.

are good calcium sources and have a low saturated-fat content. Bones in canned fish, such as salmon and sardines, also supply calcium.

To review options for dairy product use in lactose intolerance, see Chapter 6.

CALCIUM SUPPLEMENTS

Calcium supplements can be used by people who don't like milk or cannot incorporate either enough milk products or foods made with milk into their diets. Calcium carbonate, the form commonly found in antacid tablets, is the type of supplement usually recommended. It contains 40% calcium. For elderly people who have lost much of their stomach acidity, calcium citrate—which is acidic itself—is a better choice for use between meals.[30] If a calcium supplement is taken with meals this is not an issue since meals induce acid secretion in the stomach. The lower percentage of calcium in calcium citrate, however, requires a greater number or size of pills. These supplements should be taken in divided doses with meals so that the acid produced by the stomach can aid digestion and absorption.

We hesitate to encourage calcium supplement use before one tries to improve his or her diet, even though supplements are as well absorbed as milk calcium. We know that many people have difficulty adhering to a supplement regimen, and calcium supplements themselves can reduce the absorption of other minerals, such as iron. Regular food habits can likely be integrated more easily into a routine than can remembering to take several pills a day.

Some calcium supplements are poorly digested because they do not readily dissolve. To test a supplement for this, put one in 6 ounces of cider vinegar. Stir every 5 minutes. It should dissolve within 30 minutes.

Taking 1000 milligrams of calcium in the form of calcium carbonate or calcium citrate is most likely safe. There appears to be no risk from a high dietary calcium intake. Foods supply a natural balance of other minerals, in addition to calcium, in turn decreasing the likelihood of mineral imbalance.

RDA FOR CALCIUM

The RDA for calcium for adults is 800 milligrams per day. The current RDA extends the 1200 milligram level used in teenage years to age 25, in hopes that these higher calcium intakes will help women build and maintain a higher bone mass. There is reason to believe that this may be a good idea. At 800 milligrams a day, young adult women have enough calcium to maintain bone, but some may not have enough to keep building more bone.[15,18]

A recent National Institutes of Health (NIH) committee also recommended that postmenopausal women who do not take estrogen replacements consume 1500

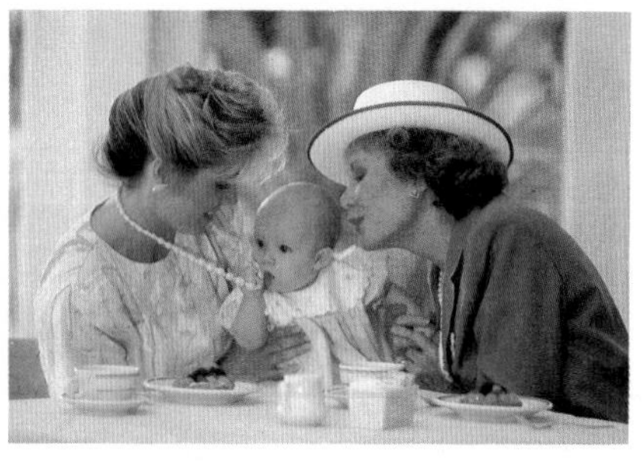

As a woman enters different stages of life, her calcium needs change.

milligrams of calcium daily (equivalent to 5 cups of milk). However, some research shows that even this amount will not be enough for these elderly women. The second Nutrition Focus provided some help in sorting out this controversy.

AMERICANS AT RISK OF A CALCIUM DEFICIENCY

We noted earlier the average calcium intake of women ranges from approximately 500 to 700 milligrams per day.[19] Intakes average 800 to 900 milligrams per day for men. About 25% of women consume less than 300 milligrams per day. So women's diets tend to be deficient in calcium, while men's do not. Men eat more food in general to support their higher kcalorie outputs, and that accounts for part of the difference. An easy way for women to increase calcium intake is to increase activity level and in turn their food consumption.

To estimate your calcium intake, use the rule of 300s. Give yourself 300 milligrams to start with. This accounts for small amounts of calcium provided by a moderate kcalorie intake from foods scattered throughout the diet. Add to that another 300 milligrams for every cup of milk or yogurt or 1.5 ounces (45 grams) of cheese.

If you eat a lot of tofu, almonds, or sardines, food composition tables will give you a more accurate account of your calcium intake. Our shortcut method underestimates calcium intake, especially in the case of vegans. It is important for vege-

Table 14-7 Meeting calcium needs of an adult (> age 24 years) following a vegan diet

Food choice	kcalories	Calcium
Breakfast		
1 cup orange juice (calcium-fortified)	110	240
1 bran muffin	125	60
herbal tea	—	—
Lunch		
sandwich:		
2 T. peanut butter	190	10
2 T. jam	110	10
2 sl. whole-wheat bread	140	40
2 oatmeal raisin cookies	120	10
1 fresh peach	40	5
1 cup apple juice	120	15
Dinner		
2 bean burritos (no cheese)	500	135
2 cups romaine lettuce	20	40
½ tomato	10	5
2 T. oil and vinegar dressing	140	5
1 cup sliced raw carrots	30	20
½ cup orange juice (calcium-fortified)	55	120
Snack		
trail mix:		
¼ cup almonds	202	100
¼ cup raisins	123	20
¼ cup chocolate peanuts	220	50
Totals	2250	885

For adolescents and young adults, the goal of 1200 milligrams of calcium could be met with inclusion of snacks of calcium-fortified foods, such as some brands of ready-to-eat breakfast cereals, or using other types of calcium-fortified beverages—certain brands of apple juice and soy milk are two possibilities.

tarians to focus on eating good plant sources of calcium as well as on the total amount of calcium ingested (Table 14-7).

TOXICITY OF CALCIUM

The major risk from taking excess calcium supplements is development of one form of kidney stones. A good rule of thumb is that calcium intake should not exceed 2500 milligrams per day.[5] Any more leads to much calcium in the urine. This can increase kidney stone risk, especially in people who tend to form them. The body absorbs calcium less efficiently as calcium intake increases, but overzealous use of calcium supplements can overwhelm the control of absorption.

If calcium/antacid supplements and milk intake together become exceedingly high, a milk-alkali syndrome can result. With this condition, serum calcium climbs so high that calcium precipitates into tissues all over the body, causing local tissue death. Sticking to an intake of 1500 to 2500 milligrams, however, poses essentially no risk for developing this problem.

CONCEPT CHECK

About 99% of calcium in the body is found in the bones. Aside from its critical role in bone, calcium also functions in blood clotting, muscle contraction, nerve transmission, and cell metabolism. Calcium requires a slightly acid pH and the vitamin D hormone calcitriol for efficient absorption. Factors that reduce calcium absorption include large amounts of dietary fiber, decreased estrogen levels, and excess magnesium or phosphorus. Serum calcium level is regulated by parathyroid hormone and calcitonin and does not closely reflect daily intake or bone stores. Osteoporosis is bone loss with no outward cause. Women are particularly at risk for osteoporosis because they make less bone than men, lose it faster, and live longer. Dairy products are the best food sources of calcium. Supplemental forms, such as calcium carbonate, are well-absorbed. However, supplements may interfere with the absorption of other minerals. Overzealous supplementation can also result in the development of one form of kidney stones.

Phosphorous

The body absorbs phosphorus (P) quite efficiently and can increase absorption from 60% to 90% as body needs vary. This high absorption rate plus its wide availability in foods makes phosphorus a lesser concern in diet planning than calcium. The active vitamin D hormone calcitriol enhances phosphorus absorption, as it does for calcium. Excretion by the kidneys is primarily responsible for maintaining body levels. This is unlike calcium, where in addition to regulation by excretion, changes in the rates of absorption are also very important.

FUNCTIONS OF PHOSPHORUS

Phosphorus plays many important roles in the body. It is a component of enzymes, adenosine triphosphate (ATP), cell membranes, and the bone mineral hydroxyapatite. About 85% of phosphorus in the body is found in bone. The rest circulates freely in the bloodstream and operates inside cells. No deficiency disease is currently associated with a poor phosphorus intake, but a poor intake may contribute to bone loss in elderly women.

PHOSPHORUS IN FOODS

Milk, cheese, bakery products, and meat provide most of the phosphorus in our diets. Cereals, bran, eggs, nuts, and fish are also good sources (Table 14-8). About 20% to 30% of dietary phosphorus comes from food additives, especially those found in baked goods, cheeses, and processed meats, as well as in soft drinks (about 75 milligrams per 12-ounce serving). Phosphorus is one of the most difficult nutrients to limit in the diet because it is found in so many foods.

Table 14-8 Good sources of phosphorus, ranked by nutrient density

Food	Serving size to yield 267 milligrams*	kcalories need to yield 267 milligrams
Cereal, bran	⅓ cup	54
Skim milk	1 cup	74
Milk, 2%	1 cup	120
Cheese, American	1⅓ ounces	134
Salmon, broiled	3 ounces	150
Sardines, canned in oil w/bones	2 ounces	176
Trout, cooked	3⅓ ounces	192
Eggs, yolks	3 each	194
Cheese, Swiss	1⅔ ounces	207
Liver, calf, fried	2⅔ ounces	217
Wheat flour, whole	⅔ cup	217
Herring, smoked, kippered	3⅔ ounces	223
Chicken, light meat	4 ounces	227
Cheese, Colby	2 ounces	230
Enriched wheat flour	⅔ cups	260
Turkey, roasted	4⅔ ounces	270
Almonds, dried	⅓ cup	283
Pork loin	4 ounces	283
Beef	4 ounces	316
Nuts, mixed, shelled	½ cup	374

* ⅓ RDA for adults 25 years of age.
Phosphorus is more widely distributed than calcium in the Guide to Daily Food Choices. Diet soft drinks are another nutrient-dense choice.

RDA FOR PHOSPHORUS

The adult RDA for phosphorus is the same as that for calcium—800 milligrams per day. Our diets provides 1000 to 1500 milligrams of phosphorus per day.[19] Thus deficiencies of phosphorus are unlikely in adults, especially when considering its highly efficient absorption.

AMERICANS AT RISK FOR A PHOSPHORUS DEFICIENCY

Marginal phosphorus status can be found in premature infants, vegans, people with alcoholism, elderly people on nutrient-poor diets, cases of long-standing diarrhea, and people who use aluminum-containing antacids daily (usually as part of the treatment for peptic ulcers, kidney failure, or kidney dialysis therapy). These types of antacids bind phosphorus in the small intestine. If a low dietary phosphorus intake is suspected, the diet's phosphorus content should be calculated.

TOXICITY OF PHOSPHORUS

If serum phosphorus levels are too high, the phosphate ions bind calcium, which leads to tetany and convulsions. Inefficient kidney function can cause such detrimentally high levels. However, there is no known toxicity in healthy adults associated with phosphorus consumption. Formerly, scientists believed that a high phosphorus intake coupled with a low calcium intake led to bone loss. Recent research casts doubt on the importance of the calcium to phosphorus ratio in a diet, as long as the RDA for calcium is met.[27] If not met, then a high phosphorus intake may compound the bone loss from a poor calcium intake.

Table 14-9 Good sources of magnesium, ranked by nutrient density

Food	Serving size to yield 117 milligrams*	kcalories needed to yield 117 milligrams
Spinach, cooked	⅔ cup	27
Beet greens, cooked	1 cup	40
Wheat bran	⅔ cup	50
Broccoli, cooked	1 cup	50
Tofu (soybean curd)	3⅓ ounces	75
Shrimp, boiled	3⅔ ounces	125
Wheat germ, raw	½ cup	150
Popcorn, air popped	5 cups	150
Sunflower seeds, dry	¼ cup	192
Blackeyed peas, cooked	1 cup	223
Cashews	1⅔ ounces	267
Kidney beans	1⅓ cups	307

* ⅓ RDA for adult male.
Plant foods provide the most nutrient-dense sources of magnesium.

Magnesium

Magnesium (Mg) is best found in plant, rather than animal, products. Magnesium in the plant pigment chlorophyll and iron in hemoglobin in the red blood cell both serve similar roles in respiration. We absorb about 30% to 40% of the magnesium in our diets, but absorption efficiency can increase to 75% if our intakes of magnesium are low. The active vitamin D hormone calcitriol may enhance magnesium absorption.

FUNCTIONS OF MAGNESIUM

Bone contains 60% of the body's magnesium. We do not know if this magnesium is of functional significance or if it is just stored there. The rest circulates in the blood and operates inside cells. Over 300 enzymes use magnesium as an activator. Without magnesium, many enzymes would function less efficiently. In addition, magnesium binds to ATP to form "active ATP." A magnesium ion bridges between the second and the last phosphate groups on an ATP molecule.

Proper nerve function and cardiac function require magnesium.[25] Animals deficient in magnesium become very irritable. Eventually, if the deficiency becomes severe, the animals suffer convulsions and often die. In humans, a magnesium deficiency causes an irregular heartbeat, which is sometimes accompanied by weakness, muscle pain, disorientation, and seizures. However, a magnesium deficiency develops very slowly because we have large stores. A link between magnesium deficiency and sudden heart attacks has been observed,[21] and its use in therapy for acute myocardial infarction is advocated by leading cardiologists. There is no test for magnesium deficiency both sufficiently accurate and available for use in routine clinical practice.[25]

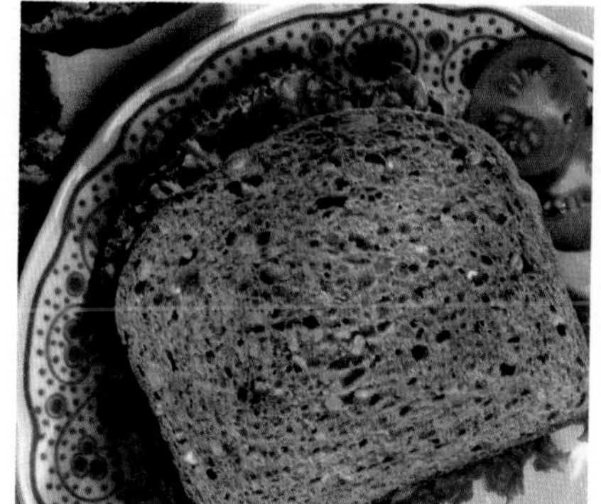

Not only are whole grain breads high in dietary fiber, they are excellent sources of magnesium.

MAGNESIUM IN FOOD

Good food sources for magnesium are whole grains (wheat bran), broccoli, squash, beans, nuts, and seeds (Table 14-9). Magnesium is one reason why registered dietitians emphasize the importance of whole grains and vegetables in a diet; these are excellent magnesium sources. Dairy products, chocolate, and meats also contribute magnesium to the diet. "Hard" tap water often contains a high concentration of magnesium and so can be considered a source.

RDA FOR MAGNESIUM

The adult RDA for magnesium is 350 milligrams per day for men and 280 milligrams per day for women. Our diets supply about 350 milligrams of magnesium per persom per day (about 120 milligrams per 1000 kcalories). Adult men consume an average of 330 milligrams daily, while women consume an average of 200 milligrams daily.[19] The low intake for women causes concern, especially because many women have increased calcium consumption in response to fear of osteoporosis. We have mentioned that as calcium in the diet increases, magnesium absorption decreases. We suggest women find some good sources of magensium that they like, and eat them regularly.

AMERICANS AT RISK FOR A MAGNESIUM DEFICIENCY

A magnesium deficiency is possible if one uses thiazide diuretics because they increase magnesium loss in the urine. In addition, heavy perspiration for weeks in hot climates and long-standing diarrhea or vomiting cause significant magnesium loss. Alcoholism also increases the risk of a deficiency because dietary intake may be poor, and alcohol increases magnesium excretion in the urine. The disorientation and weakness from alcoholism is similar to that seen when magnesium is low in the blood. Presently, we have more questions than answers about the role of magnesium in human diseases. Again, assessing magnesium status is tedious, and even then, difficult to determine.

To perform a sensitive measure of magnesium status in the body, first, a large dose is given. Then, total magnesium excretion in the urine must be measured over 24 hours. This is not a practical test, and so is not often performed.

TOXICITY OF MAGNESIUM

Magnesium toxicity does not occur in healthy people who eat typical foods. Toxicity is associated with kidney failure because the kidneys primarily regulate serum magnesium levels. A high serum magnesium level leads to weakness, nausea, and eventual malaise.

Sulfur

Sulfur (S) is a component of many important compounds in the body, such as the amino acids methionine and cysteine and the vitamins biotin and thiamin. Sulfur participates in acid-base balance in the body and is an important part of the drug-detoxifying pathways found in the liver. Finally, disulfide bridges, which occur when two sulfur atoms bind to each other, give important stability to many protein molecules (see Chapter 5).

We actually do not need to consume sulfur directly in our diets. Proteins supply the sulfur we need, so sulfur is naturally a part of a healthful diet. Sulfur compounds are also used to preserve foods (see Chapter 19).

CONCEPT CHECK

Phosphorus absorption is quite efficient and is enhanced by the active vitamin D hormone calcitriol. Urinary excretion maintains body levels. Phosphorus aids enzyme function and is part of ATP molecules and cell membranes. No deficiency symptoms caused by poor intake have been reported. Good food sources include dairy products, baked goods, and meat. The RDA is met by most of us. Magnesium is found mostly in plant sources where it functions in chlorophyll. Magnesium is important to humans for nerve and cardiac function and is a cofactor for many enzymes. People on thiazide diuretics and people with alcoholism are at risk of developing a deficiency. Toxicity is mainly found in people with kidney failure. Sulfur is a component of certain vitamins and amino acids. It plays an important role in drug-detoxification and protein structure. Our diets naturally supply sulfur via the protein and vitamins normally consumed.

Oxygen

Oxygen (O) is in a class by itself; it is not a nutrient in a dietary sense but is still vital for sustaining life. We use oxygen for aerobic respiration in the electron transport chain. In addition, some cellular metabolic reactions incorporate oxygen directly into compounds. About 21% of air is oxygen, a vital resource on which we all depend. All oxygen in the atmosphere either is produced by plants and microbes that perform photosynthesis or is released by chemical breakdown in rocks. Nutritionists are sometimes accused of forgetting that the lungs are a part of our physiological machinery. Breathing is so much more automatic than eating, that it is easy to forget just how essential oxygen is to our overall well-being.

• • •

See Table 14-10 for a review of the major characteristics of water and the minerals we have covered so far.

Table 14-10 A summary of water and the major minerals

Name	Major functions	Deficiency symptoms	People most at risk	RDA or minimum requirement	Dietary sources	Results of toxicity
Water	Medium for chemical reactions, removal of waste products, perspiration to cool the body	Thirst, muscle weakness, poor endurance	Infants with a fever, elderly in nursing homes	1 milliliter per kcalorie burned*	As such and in foods	Probably only in mental disorders, headache, blurred vision, convulsions
Sodium	A major ion of the extracellular fluid, nerve transmission	Muscle cramps	People severely restricting sodium to lower blood pressure (250-500 milligrams/day)	500 milligrams	Table salt, processed foods	High blood pressure in susceptible individuals
Potassium	A major ion of intracellular fluid, nerve transmission	Irregular heart beat, loss of appetite, muscle cramps	Use of potassium-wasting diuretics, poor diets seen in poverty and alcoholism	2000 milligrams	Vegetables, fruits, milk	Slowing of the heart beat, seen in kidney failure
Chloride	A major ion of the extracellular fluid, acid production in stomach	Convulsions in infants	No one, probably, if infant formula manufacturers control product quality adequately	700 milligrams	Table salt, some vegetables	High blood pressure in susceptible people when combined with sodium
Calcium	Bones, teeth, blood clotting, nerve transmission, muscle contractions, cell regulation	Poor intake probably increases the risk for osteoporosis	Women in general, especially those who consume few dairy products	800 milligrams (1200 milligrams ages 11-24)	Dairy products, canned fish, leafy vegetables, tofu, fortified orange juice	Very high intakes may cause a form of kidney stones in susceptible people

Continued.

Table 14-10 A summary of water and the major minerals—cont'd

Name	Major functions	Deficiency symptoms	People most at risk	RDA or minimum requirement	Dietary sources	Results of toxicity
Phosphorus	Bones, teeth, metabolic compounds such as ATP, ion of intracellular fluid	Probably none; poor bone maintenance possible	Elderly consuming very nutrient-poor diets, total vegetarians? alcoholism?	800 milligrams (1200 milligrams ages 11-24)	Dairy products, processed foods, soft drinks	Induces high levels of parathyroid hormone in kidney failure; poor bone mineralization if calcium intakes are low
Magnesium	Bones, enzyme function, nerve and heart function	Weakness, muscle pain, poor heart function	People on thiazide diuretics	Men: 350 milligrams Women: 280 milligrams	Wheat bran, green vegetables, nuts, chocolate	Causes weakness in kidney failure
Sulfur	Part of vitamins and amino acids, drug detoxification, acid-base balance	None	No one who meets their protein needs	None	Protein foods	None likely

*Just an approximation; best to keep urine volume greater than 1 liter (4 cups).

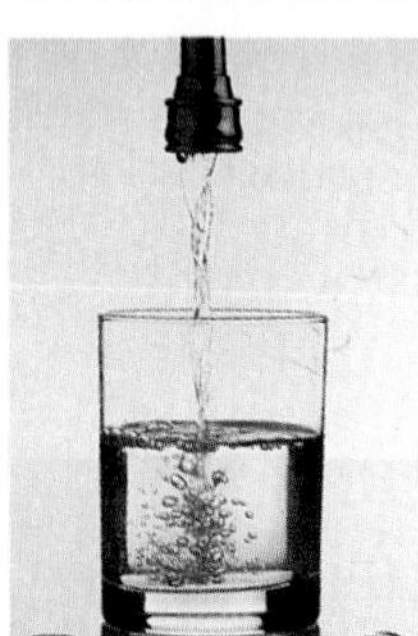

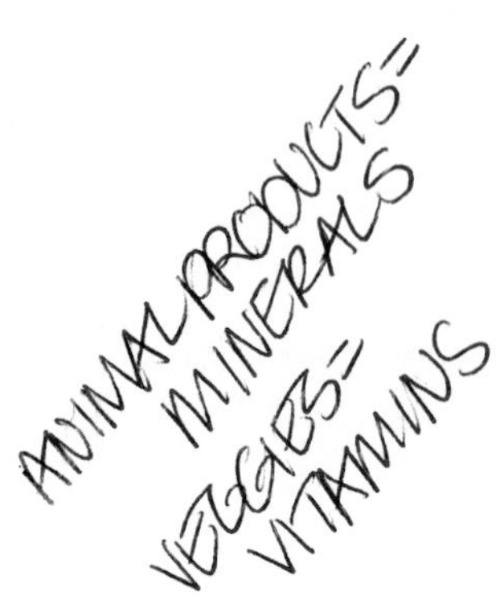

Summary

1. Many minerals are vital for sustaining life. For humans, animal products typically are the best sources of most minerals. Supplements exceeding 150% of the U.S. RDA should be taken only under a physician's supervision, since toxicity and deleterious nutrient interactions are a real possibility.
2. Water constitutes 50% to 70% of the human body. Its unique chemical properties enable it to function as a solvent, a medium for chemical reactions, a thermoregulator, and a lubricant. It also helps regulate the acid-base balance in the body. For adults, daily water needs are estimated at 1 milliliter per kcalorie burned.
3. Sodium, the major positive ion of the extracellular fluid, is vital in fluid balance and nerve impulse transmission. Our diets provide abundant sodium through processed foods and table salt. About 10% to 15% of the population is sodium sensitive and is at risk for hypertension from consuming excessive sodium.
4. Potassium, the major positive ion of the intracellular fluid, functions similarly to sodium. Milk, fruits, and vegetables are good sources.
5. Chloride is the major negative ion in extracellular fluid. It functions in digestion as part of gastric hydrochloric acid and in nerve and immune function. Table salt supplies most of the chloride in our diets.
6. Calcium forms a vital part of bone structure and is also very important in blood clotting, muscle contraction, and nerve transmission. Calcium absorption is enhanced by stomach acid and calcitriol. Dairy products are important calcium sources.
7. Osteoporosis is defined as bone loss with no apparent cause. Women are particularly at risk and should maintain adequate calcium intake and regular exercise. Estrogen replacement at menopause is currently the most accepted way to stop significant adult bone loss in women.

8. Phosphorus aids enzyme function and forms part of ATP molecules, numerous metabolites, and cell membranes. It is efficiently absorbed, and deficiencies are rare, although there is concern about the intake of elderly women. Good food sources are dairy products, bakery products, and meats.
9. Magensium is the only mineral found mostly in plants, where it functions in chlorophyll. For humans, magnesium is important for nerve and heart function and as a cofactor to many coenzymes. Good food sources are whole grains (bran), vegetables, nuts, and seeds.
10. Sulfur is incorporated into certain vitamins and amino acids. Its ability to bond with other sulfur atoms enables it to stabilize protein structure.

Study Questions

1. Within what physiological system do sodium, potassium, chloride, and calcium interact. What are the individual roles of those minerals within that system?
2. What is the relationship between sodium and water and how is that relationship monitored as well as maintained in the body?
3. Why, specifically, is there relatively little concern for chloride deficiency in the United States?
4. What might you need to tell to a 12-year-old child about the importance of consuming enough calcium?
5. Phosphorous is second only to calcium in terms of mineral content within the body. Name two ways in which phosphorous and calcium are alike, and then name two ways in which they differ.

REFERENCES

1. Aloia JF and others: Relationship of menopause to skeletal and muscle mass, *American Journal of Clinical Nutrition* 53:1378, 1991.
2. Anderson JB: Dietary calcium and bone mass throughout the life cycle, *Nutrition Today,* March/April 1990, p 9.
3. Andon MB and others: Spinal bone density and calcium intake in healthy postmenopausal women, *American Journal of Clinical Nutrition* 54:927, 1991.
4. Australian National Health and Medical Research Council: Fall in blood pressure with modest reduction in dietary salt intake in mild hypertension, *Lancet* 1:399, February 25, 1989.
5. Chesnut CH: Osteoporosis and its treatment, *The New England Journal of Medicine* 326:406, 1992.
6. Eaton SB, Nelson DA: Calcium in evolutionary perspective, *American Journal of Clinical Nutrition* 54:281S, 1991.
7. Fackelmann KA: The African gene? *Science News* 140:254, 1991.
8. Fishman JA: Control of hypertension through lifestyle and nutrition, *Topics in Clinical Nutrition* 3:47, 1988.
9. Frost HM: The pathomechanics of osteoporosis, *Clinical Orthopedics and Related Research* 200:198, 1985.
10. Garland CF and others: Can colon cancer incidences and death rates be reduced with calcium and vitamin D? *American Journal of Clinical Nutrition* 54:193S, 1991.
11. Garraway WM, Whisnant JP: The changing pattern of hypertension and the declining incidents of stroke, *Journal of the American Medical Association* 258:214, 1987.
12. Hernandez-Avila M and others: Caffeine, moderate alcohol intake, and risk of fractures of the hip and forearm in middle-aged women, *American Journal of Clinical Nutrition* 54:157, 1991.
13. Houston MC: Sodium and hypertension, *Archives of Internal Medicine* 146:139, 1986.
14. Lindsay R and others: Bone mass and body composition in normal women, *Journal of Bone and Mineral Research* 7:55, 1992.
15. Matkovic V, Heaney: Calcium balance during human growth: evidence for threshold behavior, *American Journal of Clinical Nutrition* 55:992, 1992.
16. Mazess RB, Barden HS: Bone Density in premenopausal women: effects of age, dietary intake, physical activity, smoking, and birth-control pills, *American Journal of Clinical Nutrition* 53:132, 1991.
17. Papazian R: Osteoporosis treatment advances, *FDA Consumer,* April 1991.
18. Peacock M: Calcium absorption efficiency and calcium requirements in children and adolescents, *American Journal of Clinical Nutrition* 54:261S, 1991.
19. Pennington JAT and others: Nutritional elements in U.S. diets: results from the total diet study, 1982-1986, *Journal of The American Dietetic Association* 89:659, 1989.

20. Randal HT: Water, electrolytes, and acid-base balance. In Shils ME, Young VR, editors: *Modern nutrition in health and disease,* ed 7, Philadelphia, 1988, Lea & Febiger.
21. Rasmussen HS and others: Influence of magnesium substitution therapy on blood lipid composition in patients with ischemic heart disease, *Archives of Internal Medicine* 149: 1050, 1989.
22. Recker RR and others: Calcium absorbability from milk products and imitation milk and calcium carbonate, *American Journal of Clinical Nutrition* 47:93, 1988.
23. Riggs BL: Overview of osteoporosis, *The Western Journal of Medicine,* Jan 154:63-77, 1991.
24. Sentipal JM and others: Influence of calcium intake and growth indexes on vertebral bone mineral density in young females, *American Journal of Clinical Nutrition* 54:425, 1991.
25. Shils ME: Magnesium in health and disease, *Annual Reviews of Nutrition* 8:429, 1988.
26. Singh RB and others: Effect of diet and weight reduction in hypertension, *Nutrition* 6:297, 1990.
27. Spencer H and others: Do protein and phosphorus cause calcium loss? *Journal of Nutrition* 118:657, 1988.
28. Tobian L: Potassium and hypertension, *Nutrition Reviews* 46:273, 1988.
29. Wadlaw GM, Barden HS: Osteoporosis—summary of the 19th Steenbock Symposium, *Nutrition Today,* Sept/Oct 1989, p 30.
30. Wood RJ, Serfaty-Lacrosniere C: Gastric acidity, atrophic gastritis, and calcium absorption, *Nutrition Reviews* 50:33, 1992.

SUGGESTED READINGS

For an excellent review of osteoporosis, see the review article by Riggs. Wardlaw and Barden's article looks at the latest research in the area of osteoporosis. Houston's article covers various issues surrounding sodium and hypertension. The article by Fishman shows how lifestyle changes can help control hypertension. Finally, Shils' article is a good look at magnesium, a mineral whose role in overall health nutritionists continue to question.

TAKE ACTION

Working for denser bones

In the second Nutrition Focus, you learned some significant information about the disease OSTEOPOROSIS.

The disease affects 25 million people in the United States. One third of all women experience fractures due to it. It leads to 1.5 million bone fractures per year. In addition, 12% to 20% of all elderly persons who suffer hip fractures die from complications.

This is a disease you can do something about. Some risk factors cannot be changed, but others can. Let us see to what degree you are doing the things that can help prevent this debilitating disease. Answer "yes" or "no" to the following by placing an "x" in the appropriate box.

	YES	NO
1. Do you drink fortified milk regularly or average at least 30 minutes of sun exposure per day on at least your face and hands to get enough vitamin D?	______	______
2. Do you regularly engage in weight-bearing exercise (e.g., jogging, walking, etc.)?	______	______
3. If you are a woman, do you experience regular menstruation?	______	______
4. Do you avoid smoking cigarettes?	______	______
5. Do you avoid regular consumption of large amounts of alcohol?	______	______
6. Do you consume milk and cheese regularly, or substitute other sources to meet your RDA for calcium and phosphorous?	______	______

Use your diet analysis from Chapter 2 to see how you should have answered the last question on that particular day. The more "yes" answers you have, the more you are actively doing to preserve your bone density for the future. Also remember that this is not just a valuable consideration for women. If men plan to live well into their 80s and 90s, they too can be at risk for osteoporosis. ▲

NUTRITION PERSPECTIVE

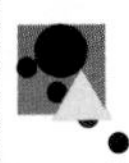

Minerals and Hypertension

More than 35 million Americans suffer from hypertension. American Heart Association statistics show it kills about 31,000 people each year.

Blood pressure is expressed by two different numbers. The higher number represents systolic blood pressure, which is the pressure in the arteries when the heart actively pumps blood. The second value is for diastolic pressure, which is the artery pressure when the heart is relaxed. Normal systolic blood pressure values vary from 100 to 140 millimeters of mercury (mm Hg). Normal diastolic blood pressure values varies from 60 to 90 mm Hg. A high diastolic pressure shows a strong relationship to various diseases, as does a high systolic pressure.

Hypertension is defined as sustained high blood pressure, usually with systolic pressure exceeding 140 mm Hg or diastolic blood pressure exceeding 90 mm Hg. Most hypertension (90% to 95%) has no apparent cause. It is called primary or essential hypertension. Kidney disease often causes the other 5% to 10% of cases and is known as secondary hypertension.

About 30% of adults have primary hypertension. This is called a "silent" disease because, unless blood pressure is measured periodically, no one knows it is developing.

A physician usually does not treat hypertension with medication until the diastolic blood pressure measures at least 95 mm Hg (or the systolic blood pressure reaches 160) on three or more occasions. The health risks of drug intervention in cases of only mild hypertension may outweigh any possible benefits gained from the drugs. But any value over 90 mm Hg is actually too high and deserves dietary and lifestyle interventions.

Hypertension	
Mild	Diastolic 90 to 140 mm Hg Systolic 140 to 159 mm Hg
Moderate	Diastolic 105 to 114 mm Hg Systolic ≥160 mm Hg
Severe	Diastolic ≥115 mm Hg

Why control hypertension?

Hypertension needs to be controlled mainly to prevent heart disease, kidney disease, and strokes. All three diseases are much more likely to be found in people with hypertension than in people with normal blood pressure.[11]

People with hypertension need to be diagnosed and treated as soon as possible. We now know the value of aggressively treating hypertension. In the last 20 years, blood pressure values have fallen, as have the number of strokes.

Causes of high blood pressure

A variety of factors affect blood pressure. Blood pressure usually increases as a person ages. Some increase is due to atherosclerosis (see Chapter 4). As plaque builds up in the arteries, the arteries become less flexible and cannot expand. When vessels remain rigid, blood pressure remains high. Eventually the plaque begins to choke off blood supply to the kidneys, decreasing their ability to control blood volume, and in turn, blood pressure.

Obesity often is associated with high blood pressure, especially in women. High insulin levels associated with insulin-resistant fat cells are one reason for this. Insulin increases sodium retention in the body and speeds atherosclerosis. Inactivity also is associated with hypertension. If an obese person can lose weight and become more physically active, exercising three to four times a week, blood pressure often returns to normal. A weight loss of as little as 10 pounds can help.[26] Often a minor change in lifestyle such as this can greatly reduce, or even eliminate, the need for medications.[8]

High blood pressure is more likely to be seen in African-Americans than in whites, and African-Americans are more likely to suffer from the ill effects than whites. These also appear earlier in life in African-Americans.[7] In addition, alcohol

NUTRITION PERSPECTIVE

Minerals and Hypertension—cont'd

has a greater tendency to raise blood pressure in African-Americans than it does in whites.

Finally the enzyme renin, and some hormonelike compounds, affect blood pressure (Figure 14-5). Medications are available to reduce the effect of the renin-angiotensin system.

Sodium and blood pressure

Sodium intake tends to increase blood pressure. The average American intake of 3 to 7 grams can elevate blood pressure, particularly in those who are susceptible to the effect. However, nutritionists believe that only some of the 30% of Americans with hypertension are very susceptible to sodium-linked hypertension. So sodium in the diet is not a problem for everyone, even among people with hypertension. Nevertheless, in populations that eat 1500 milligrams or less of sodium daily, hypertension is rare.

Groups of people who migrate from a developing to an industrialized nation and adopt a Western diet and lifestyle gradually do develop a level of hypertension characteristic of the new country. However, dietary changes would likely affect not only sodium intake, but also intakes of potassium, calcium, protein, fat, dietary fiber, alcohol, and probably almost all other nutrients as well. Furthermore, changes in physical activity, obesity, psychosocial stresses, and numerous other environmental factors make it impossible to single out any one factor as being causative. Although some researchers recommend that all people with hypertension reduce sodium intake, ideally dietary advice should be decided on an individual basis, once the response to treatment is verified (Figure 14-10).

If a person has hypertension, it is a good idea to reduce sodium.[4] Approximately 2 grams of sodium daily is the point at which sodium restriction usually improves hypertension, but this is a hard diet to follow. While an intake less than that may lower blood pressure even more, people find it very difficult to retrict sodium intake so severely for any length of time. Physicians usually resort to a combination of medication and a moderate sodium restriction (4 grams) to help in patient compliance.

Calcium and blood pressure

Since 1983 there has been debate concerning whether calcium intake can affect blood pressure. Careful studies show that about 50% of people register slightly lower blood pressures when they consume at least the RDA for calcium per day, as compared to one third to half that amount. Systolic blood pressure is affected more than diastolic blood pressure. It is reasonable for a person with hypertension to

Figure 14-10 Beetle Bailey

BEETLE BAILEY

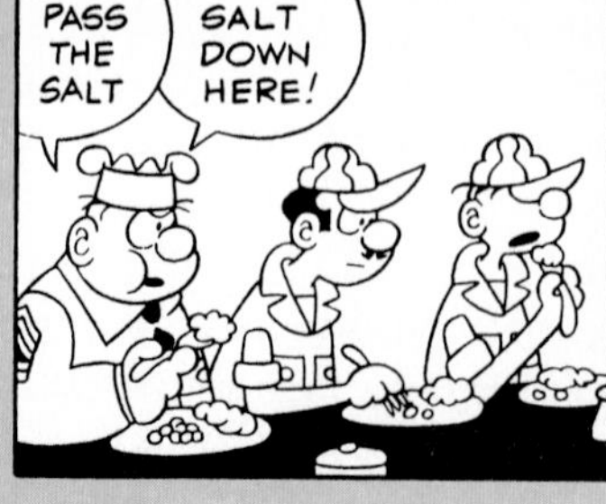
PASS THE SALT
SALT DOWN HERE!

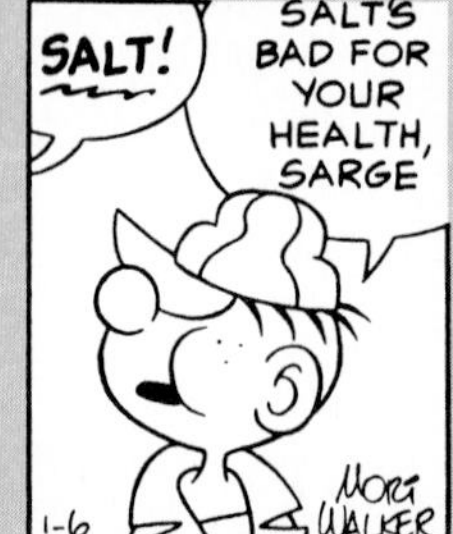
SALT!
SALT'S BAD FOR YOUR HEALTH, SARGE
1-6
MORT WALKER
© 1989 King Features Syndicate, Inc. World rights reserved

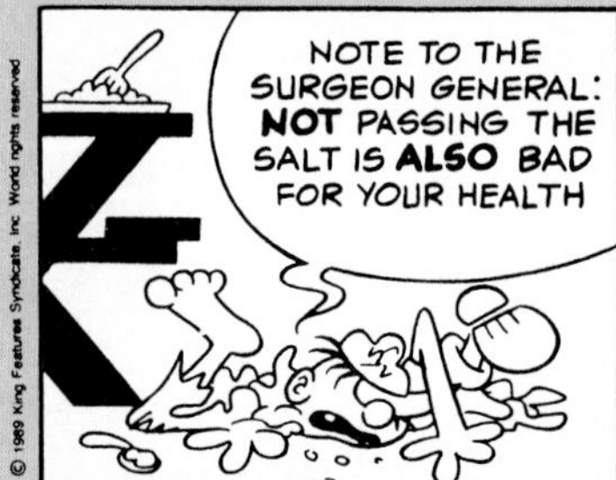
NOTE TO THE SURGEON GENERAL: NOT PASSING THE SALT IS ALSO BAD FOR YOUR HEALTH

experiment, in consultation with a physician, by increasing calcium intake to see if that produces a benefit worth the trouble and expense.

Potassium, magnesium and hypertension

Similarly to calcium, potassium supplementation has been shown to moderately decrease blood pressure in those currently consuming far below the recommended levels.[28] In addition, this effect of potassium supplementation is only seen in those patients not on a sodium-restricted diet. Magnesium is capable of lowering blood pressure if rapidly infused, but as a means of sustained hypertension therapy it is ineffective.

Preventing hypertension

To prevent hypertension we recommend maintaining an active lifestyle and a healthy body weight. Regular exercise is a key component. Epidemiological evidence suggests that a low-sodium diet may lead to less hypertension in later life.[13] You can decide if you want to restrict sodium in your diet now, or simply wait until hypertension develops. Hypertension does develop in many adults, especially in those with family histories of hypertension, but there are no studies to clearly guide the decision of when to restrict sodium in the diet. For many people, it probably takes decades of high sodium intake to result in sodium-induced hypertension. Without a readily available test for sodium sensitivity, some scientists feel it is prudent for all adults to keep sodium intake to about 2 to 3 grams/day. Limiting alcohol use is also very important. A reduction in stress adds to the list of preventive measures.

In addition, we suggest consuming a diet outlined by the Guide to Daily Food Choices, especially one rich in fruits and vegetables. This provides ample potassium, calcium, and magnesium—all of which help contribute to normal blood pressure values (Table 14-11). Even if drugs are still needed, a proper diet and life-style approach can often reduce the dosage, and in turn the expense and side effects of medications. Nutritional therapy is a key to treating hypertension.

Table 14-11 A nutritional plan to minimize hypertension risk

1. Attain and maintain a healthy body weight.
2. Incorporate regular physical activity into one's lifestyle.
3. Meet the RDA for calcium, phosphorus, and magnesium.
4. Consume alcoholic beverages in moderation, if at all.
5. Consume moderate to scant amounts of sodium.

CHAPTER FIFTEEN

The Trace Minerals

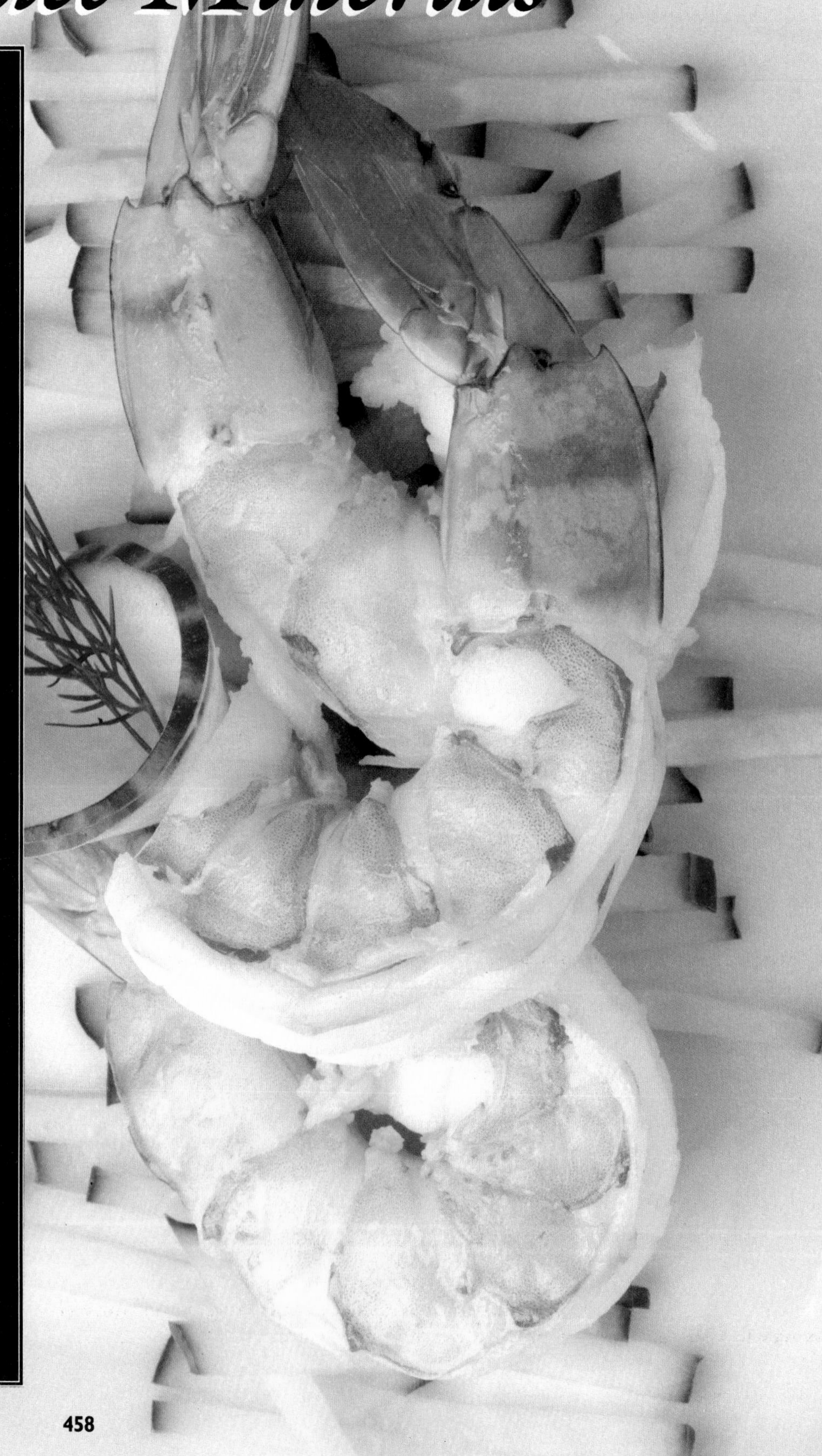

Trace minerals constitute less than 1% of all minerals in your body. As noted in Chapter 14, a trace mineral is defined as one for which our daily nutritional need is less than 100 milligrams. Grouping them together this way, however, is too simplistic because trace mineral functions and their means of absorption and metabolism all vary. For example, the body carefully regulates absorption of iron, copper, and zinc, but not selenium and iodide. So selenium and iodide levels in the body depend more on the mineral content of a food eaten. The trace minerals are also very interactive; the abundance of one mineral in the diet and body can affect the absorption and metabolism of several others.

Of all trace minerals, iron raises the most concern in menu planning, and so is a major focus of this chapter. Iron deficiency anemia is the most prevalent nutritional problem in the world today.[29] In the United States about 10% of all infants—and 20% of poor infants—are estimated to be deficient in iron at some point in their first two years of life. This can cause later learning difficulties.[19] Diminished levels of iron in adults can affect work capacity and increase the chances of acquiring and dying from infection.

Information about trace minerals is perhaps the most rapidly expanding area of knowledge in nutrition. With the exception of iron and iodide, the importance of trace minerals to humans has been recognized only within the last 30 years, since most of your parents were in school. Let's examine some of these new findings.

NUTRITION AWARENESS INVENTORY

1. T F Trace mineral deficiencies often are difficult to detect.
2. T F Some trace minerals can interfere with the absorption of other minerals.
3. T F Trace mineral concentrations in plants usually depend on the trace mineral concentrations in the soil in which the plants are grown.
4. T F Enriched grains contain less of many trace minerals than whole grains.
5. T F Iron is the only nutrient with a higher RDA for adult women than for adult men.
6. T F Iron is easily excreted from the body when consumed in excess.
7. T F Zinc is important to the growth of children.
8. T F Zinc can be assessed using hair analysis.
9. T F High doses of zinc supplements can reduce immune function.
10. T F Copper plays an important role in iron metabolism.
11. T F A copper deficiency could result from consuming too much zinc.
12. T F The ultimate sources of most of our iodide intake are unprocessed foods.
13. T F Fluoride inhibits the growth of the bacterium that causes dental caries.
14. T F Consuming excess chromium supplements is not dangerous since there is little chance of chromium toxicity.
15. T F The terms iron deficiency and anemia are synonymous, and so interchangeable.

Here are 15 statements about trace minerals. Answer them to test your current knowledge. If you think the answer is true or mostly true, circle T. If you think the answer is false or mostly false, circle F. Use the scoring key at the end of the book to compute your total score. Take this test again after you have read this chapter. Compare the results.

Trace Minerals

Discovering the importance of each trace mineral to humans is a fairly recent and still unfolding drama that, in some cases, reads like a detective story. As recently as 1961, scientists linked dwarfism in villagers in the Middle East to a zinc deficiency.[25] Other researchers recognized that an obscure form of heart disease in an isolated area of China was linked to a selenium deficiency. In the United States some trace mineral deficiencies were first observed in the late 1960s to early 1970s when they were not added to synthetic formulas used in total parenteral nutrition.[28] The lack of early human research means our understanding of trace mineral metabolism still relies mostly on knowledge of farm and laboratory animal nutrition.

Researching our **trace mineral** needs is difficult because we need only minute amounts. Highly sophisticated technology is required to measure such small amounts in both food and body tissues. Rigorous protocols are required to produce a deficiency in animals. (All animal research referred to in this text was conducted with farm and/or laboratory animals.) They must be raised in ultraclean environments. Their diets must be carefully produced from individual essential nutrients to ensure that no mineral contamination occurs. Stainless steel and plastic cages must be used so that the animals do not obtain any trace minerals, such as zinc, from chewing on the cages. Minerals must sometimes even be filtered from the air, and the water must be as free of minerals as possible. In addition, glassware used for chemical analysis may need to be rinsed repeatedly in acid to eliminate trace mineral contamination; sometimes only plastic bottles are appropriate.

trace mineral A mineral vital to health that is required in a diet in amounts less than 100 milligrams per day.

Because producing most trace mineral deficiencies in laboratory animals requires so much effort, overt human deficiencies are unlikely, considering all our mineral sources in food, air, and water. However, for some trace minerals, such as iron, zinc, copper, and chromium, there is considerable concern that marginal dietary intakes do occur and mild deficiencies go undetected.

NUTRITION FOCUS

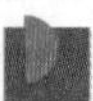

Hair Analysis for Trace Mineral Assessment?

For the last 20 years researchers have been experimenting with hair analysis as a way of assessing trace mineral status in the body. After a clump of hair is clipped close to the scalp, the first 2 inches are digested in acid and trace mineral content is measured.

Hair analysis immediately encounters some problems. Hair is contaminated by air pollution and by the shampoos, conditioners, dyes, and bleaches that people use on their hair. Hair treatments can substantially change the trace mineral content of hair. In the laboratory, slight changes in the method of washing and heating the hair before analysis can even make results from different laboratories difficult to compare. Only trained scientists with experience can produce reliable results.

The next problem is that there are insufficient standards with which to compare the results. So, once the results of the analyses are obtained, we often don't know what they mean. There is insufficient research to show that subtle changes in trace mineral content of hair actually reflect subtle changes in trace mineral content in the body.

There are, however, some possibilities for hair analysis. It can be used to establish an environmental toxicity from arsenic and, under controlled research conditions, it may also be a good method for measuring zinc status. However, at this time, there are many questions about hair analysis, and so its place should be only in the research laboratory.[16] There is no evidence that hair analysis is useful for routine human nutrition assessment at this time.

Commercial laboratories throughout America perform hair analysis. For about $25 to $50 they will analyze a hair sample, and some even send an impressive computer printout listing the mineral content of the hair. Some even list your vitamin status based on the hair analysis. There is no evidence that hair can predict vitamin status. The report may also predict the mineral status of the body and perhaps even include a few pages of health recommendations, including a catalog of supplements that will "restore" health.

A noted scientist sent samples of hair from two women to 13 commercial laboratories around the country. Reported results varied significantly from laboratory to laboratory for the same sample. Considering that scientists are having a difficult time determining the role of hair analysis, it is improper for laboratories to use this as a nutrition assessment tool for the average person. Reputable scientists suggest hair analysis is still in the experimental phase and not ready for clinical applications.

SETTING NUTRIENT NEEDS FOR TRACE MINERALS

The difficulty in measuring trace mineral nutrition in humans makes setting RDAs for them problematic. Most trace minerals have only an estimated safe and adequate daily dietary intake (ESADDI); only a few trace minerals have an RDA.

The major method used to set trace mineral nutrient needs is the balance study. The same basic technique used for nitrogen balance studies works for minerals. (See Chapters 2 and 5.) Researchers try to determine the lowest mineral intake that meets all mineral losses from urine, feces, hair, skin, perspiration, menses, and so on. These studies are very expensive to perform and often inconclusive because laboratory results frequently contradict each other. In addition, a balance study tells only the level of dietary intake needed to maintain a specific **pool** of the mineral in the body, but this pool does not necessarily represent the amount needed to maintain the best health.

pool The amount of a mineral stored within the body that can be easily mobilized when needed.

There are further problems in setting nutrient needs for trace minerals. Symptoms often appear only with severe deficiencies. We lack knowledge of subtle signs of most trace mineral deficiencies, so we cannot always detect when people are compromising their health. They may consume just enough of a mineral to prevent obvious symptoms from being expressed. Besides lacking sensitive clinical signs, we also often lack sensitive laboratory assays to measure trace minerals. The main factor limiting chromium research today is the lack of a sensitive measure of it in body tissue and fluids.

A final complication is that trace minerals interact with each other.[6] An overabundance of zinc or iron in the body can interfere with absorption of the other minerals. Thus, to set the RDA for zinc, nutrition scientists must estimate the amounts of iron and other minerals that will be consumed to predict how much zinc the body will actually absorb. Overall then, quite a lot of scientific judgement must go into setting desired intakes for trace minerals.

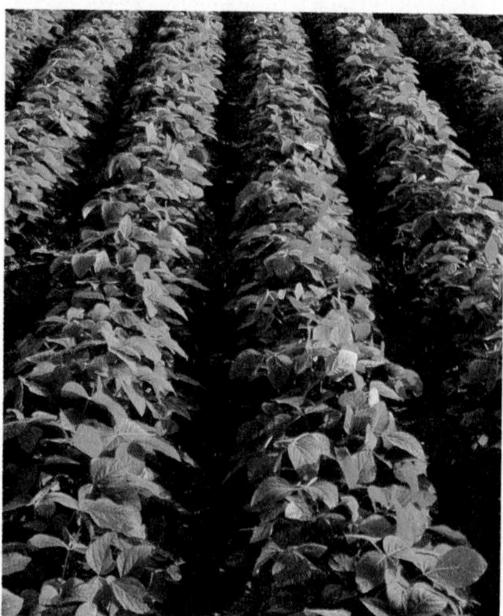

The trace mineral content of plant foods reflects the trace mineral content of the soil in which they are grown.

Trace Minerals in Foods

The trace mineral content of plants depends primarily on trace mineral concentration in the soil. Because soil concentrations of trace minerals vary greatly, food composition tables can give misleading values for trace mineral contents of plant foods. This is not as true for foods from animals because animals often eat a variety of plant products and are often shipped from one area to another during their growth, processing, and finishing in a feed lot. They then can consume foods from multiple soil conditions.

The bioavailability of trace minerals is another issue in planning diets. Finding a mineral-rich food does not ensure that you can absorb a particular mineral from it. Many factors in food inhibit mineral absorption. Mineral absorption from some plant foods often amounts to only 3% to 6% of the total present.[8] In general, animal sources of minerals are superior because they show more efficient absorption. Animal sources also often contain factors that enhance mineral absorption, even for those trace minerals supplied by plant foods in a meal.[29]

Throughout this book we repeatedly recommend eating a variety of foods. By doing that you eat plants and animals that have derived nutrients from a variety of soils, and you thus maximize your chances of consuming an adequate amount of trace minerals. In addition, it is best to consume as many minimally processed foods as possible. Generally, the more refined a food—consider white flour—the lower its content of trace minerals. As far as minerals are concerned, the enrichment process adds only the trace mineral iron. The selenium, zinc, and copper lost when grains are refined are not replaced.

We need far more research on trace minerals. Much has been and is being done. But because many questions remain, we caution you to be very careful when considering using trace mineral supplements. You can easily harm your body by using these types of supplements.

Iron

The importance of dietary iron (Fe) has been recognized for centuries. The Persian physician Melampus in 4000 B.C. gave iron supplements to sailors to compensate for the iron lost from bleeding during battles. As we noted earlier, today iron deficiency anemia is the most common nutrient deficiency worldwide. Twenty-five percent of all infants and two thirds of children and women of childbearing age in most developing nations are estimated to suffer from iron deficiency;[29] one third of them have the more severe form of the disorder, anemia.[29]

Iron is the only nutrient for which adult women have a greater RDA than adult men. It is found in every living cell; total body content is about 5 grams (1 teaspoon).

ABSORPTION AND DISTRIBUTION OF IRON

The body uses several mechanisms to regulate iron absorption. Controlling absorption is important because the body cannot easily eliminate excess iron once it is absorbed. Iron absorption from foods varies from about 3% to 40%, depending on a variety of factors (Table 15-1).

The form of iron in foods greatly influences its absorption. Iron that is still part of the **hemoglobin** and **myoglobin** molecules in animal flesh (40% of total iron present), called **heme iron**, is absorbed over twice as efficiently as the simple elemental iron, known as **nonheme iron**. Nonheme iron is also present in animal flesh, eggs, milk, vegetables, grains, and other plant foods.

About 10% to 15% of iron in the American diet is heme iron, and usually 25% to 35% is absorbed. Nonheme iron makes up the rest, and usually 2% to 20% is absorbed. That makes animal flesh, especially red meat and pork, the best source of

hemoglobin The iron-containing part of the red blood cell that carries oxygen to the cells and carbon dioxide away from the cells. It is also responsible for the red color of blood.

heme iron Iron provided from animal tissues as hemoglobin and myoglobin. Approximately 40% of the iron in meat is heme iron; it is readily absorbed.

nonheme iron Iron provided from plant sources and animal tissues other than hemoglobin and myoglobin. Nonheme iron needs to be ionized before absorption and is less efficiently absorbed than heme iron.

Table 15-1 Dietary factors that affect iron absorption

Increase	Decrease
Vitamin C	Phytate (in dietary fiber)
Acid in the stomach	Oxalates
Heme iron	Tannins (in tea)
High body demand for red blood cells (blood loss, high altitude, physical training, pregnancy)	Full body stores
Low body stores	Excess of other minerals* (Zn, Mn, Ca)
Meat protein factor (MPF)	Lack of stomach acid
	Some antacids

*Especially when taken as supplements.

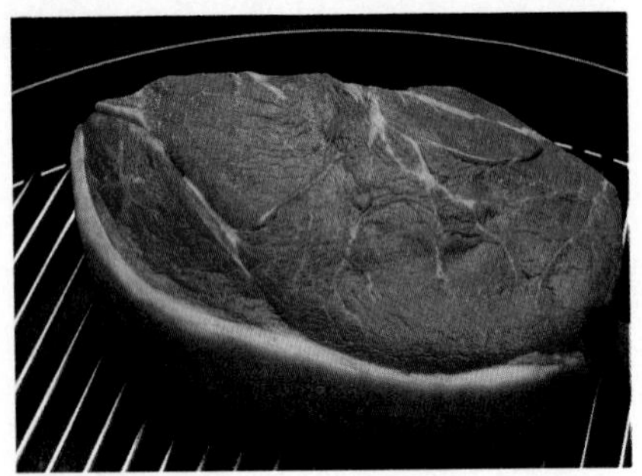

Red meat is a major source of iron in the American diet.

iron in our diets, considering both iron content and the increased efficiency of absorption for the iron present in the heme form.

Consuming heme iron and nonheme iron together increases nonheme iron absorption. One of several possible nonheme absorption facilitators may be a protein factor in meat. This factor appears to consist of amino acids that bind iron and enhance its absorption.[20] Overall, eating meat with vegetables and grain products enhances the absorption of the nonheme iron present.

Organic acids, such as vitamin C, can increase nonheme iron absorption by changing Fe^{+3} (ferric form) to Fe^{+2} (ferrous form).[30] The ferrous form of iron is better absorbed, as this is the only form of iron that can bind tightly to transport proteins. Consuming more foods rich in vitamin C is particularly desirable if dietary iron is inadequate or serum iron levels are low. When using an iron supplement, it's a good idea to take it with a glass of orange juice.

Several dietary factors interfere with our ability to absorb iron. Phytic acid (phytate) and other factors in grain fibers and oxalic acid (oxalate) in vegetables can all bind iron, reducing its absorption.[26] A long-term consideration if you increase dietary fiber intake above 35 grams per day is the tendency for fiber components to bind iron (and other trace minerals), in turn decreasing absorption. Tannins found in tea also reduce iron absorption. When trying to rebuild iron stores it is a good idea to reduce tea consumption, particularly at mealtimes. Finally, high doses of calcium supplements also bind much iron—an important disadvantage to weigh when choosing calcium supplements instead of regularly consuming dairy products.[7] On a total diet basis, a meal plan designed to enhance iron absorption can do so about 2.5 times better than one that contains many inhibitors of iron absorption.

The most important factor influencing iron absorption is the body's need for it.[9] In a deficiency state, nonheme iron absorption can increase about tenfold, and heme iron absorption can increase twofold. When iron stores are adequate, the main blood protein that carries iron, called transferrin, is full (saturated). This condition reduces iron transfer from the intestinal cells to the bloodstream. The iron remains in the intestinal cells in the protein-bound form called **ferritin**. When intestinal cells are sloughed at the end of their 2 to 5 day life cycle, the iron returns to the intestinal tract for excretion.

ferritin A protein compound that serves as the storage form of iron in the blood and tissues.

When iron stores are low, transferrin in the bloodstream readily binds more iron, shifting it from ferritin stores in intestinal cells into the bloodstream. The iron itself is then deposited mostly in the liver, reforming ferritin. By this means—under normal circumstances—iron is absorbed only if needed. This block against excess iron absorption is termed a "mucosal block" (Figure 15-1).

Heme iron is absorbed intact into the intestinal cell. The iron released then combines with the nonheme sources of iron. Some of this iron pool will be bound by transferrin and ushered directly into the bloodstream, depending on body needs.

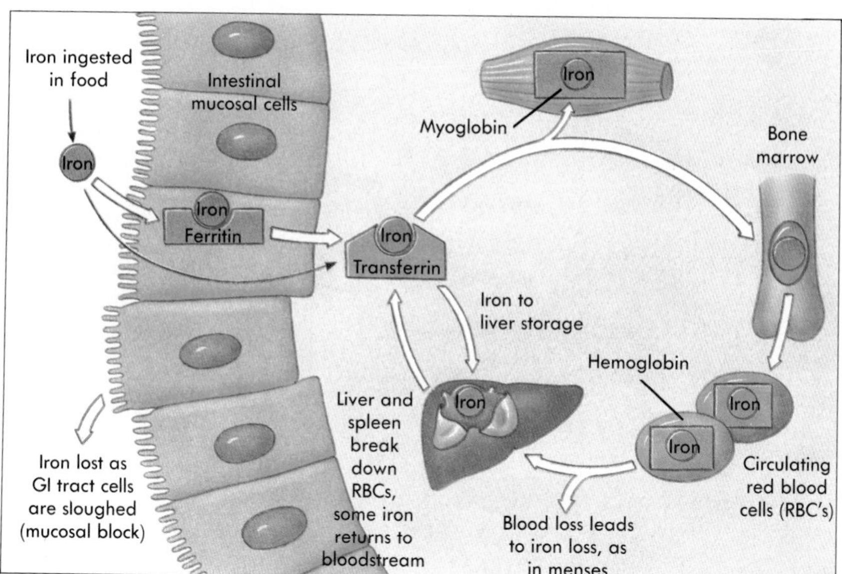

Figure 15-1 Iron absorption and distribution. Iron binds with a protein to form ferritin when stored in cells. If the intestinal absorption cells are shed before iron is absorbed from them, the iron is not absorbed into the bloodstream. This is one way the body can limit overabsorption of iron.

The rest forms ferritin in the intestinal cells. This gives us a short-term form of iron storage for intestinal cells. First, however, the copper-containing protein called **ceruloplasmin** first converts Fe^{+2} to Fe^{+3} so that it can bind to apoferritin. Thus copper metabolism and iron metabolism are closely linked.[14] Eventually, the iron is either absorbed or sloughed off with the intestinal cell.

ceruloplasmin A blue, copper-containing protein component of plasma that converts Fe^{+2} (ferrous form) to Fe^{+3} (ferric form) so that it can bind with apoferritin.

Most iron in the body is present in the hemoglobin molecules in the red blood cells (Figure 15-2). Some iron is stored in the bone marrow, and a small portion goes to other body cells or to the liver for storage in the form of ferritin. As liver concentration of ferritin increases, it is partly digested by the liver cells, and the iron forms a more insoluble product called **hemosiderin.**[15] As iron is needed, it can be mobilized and enter the bloodstream from body stores (with the help of ceruloplasmin). If dietery intake is inadequate, these iron stores become depleted. Only then do signs of an iron deficiency appear.

hemosiderin An insoluble iron-protein compound in the liver. Hemosiderin stores iron when the amount in the blood exceeds the storage capacity of ferritin.

FUNCTIONS OF IRON

Iron forms part of hemoglobin in red blood cells and myoglobin in muscle cells. Iron is also necessary for the synthesis in the mitochondria of cytochromes used for the electron transport chain and for other metabolic systems found elsewhere. Iron is used to synthesize some enzymes and is needed for immune function (see the Nutrition Perspective entitled "Nutrients and Immunity"). Iron is involved in the synthesis of the protein collagen and contributes to drug detoxification pathways in the liver. In addition, iron is found in an enzyme vital to the production of a host of neurotransmitters, including serotonin, norepinephrine, and epinephrine, as well as dopamine.

A key attribute of iron is its ability to both take up and release oxygen atoms and electrons. This allows it to participate in carrying oxygen in the bloodstream and in transferring electrons in the electron transport chain of the cell mitochondria.

Hemoglobin molecules in red blood cells carry oxygen from the lungs to cells, and carry back some carbon dioxide (CO_2) from cells to the lungs for excretion (Figure 15-2). Bone marrow cells in adults synthesize red blood cells when stimulated by the hormone **erythropoietin**, which comes from the kidneys. Erythropoietin is released in response to a decrease in oxygen concentration in the bloodstream, blood loss, or carbon monoxide binding to red blood cells.

erythropoietin A hormone secreted by the kidneys that enhances red blood cell synthesis and stimulates red blood cell release from bone marrow.

As a red blood cell matures in the bone marrow, it expels its nucleus, which contains DNA. That limits its life span to approximately 120 days because without DNA the red blood cell can't direct new protein synthesis to replace worn out cell parts, such as enzymes. A rapid cell turnover such as this puts great nutrient demands on the body, and iron is one of those greatly demanded nutrients.

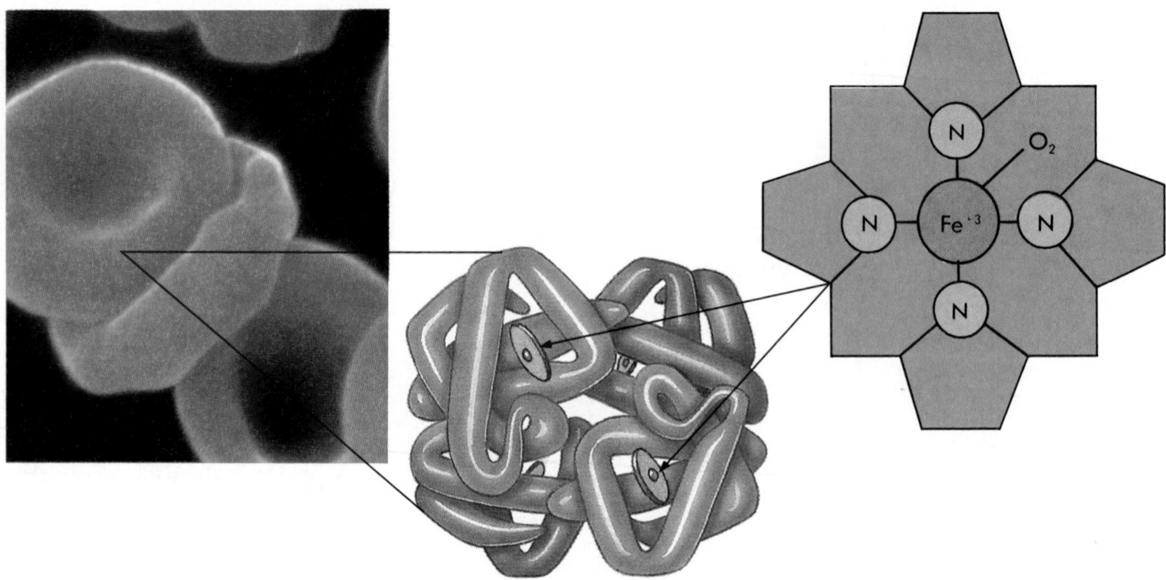

Figure 15-2 Most iron in the body is present in the hemoglobin molecules in the red blood cells. Iron gives hemoglobin the ability to carry oxygen.

IRON-DEFICIENCY ANEMIA

If neither the diet nor body stores can supply the iron needed for hemoglobin synthesis, red blood cell synthesis is reduced. Eventually, the red blood cell number falls so low that the amount of oxygen carried in the bloodstream is decreased. Such a person has anemia, which is essentially a decreased oxygen-carrying capacity of the blood.[29] While there are many types of anemia, the major type found worldwide is iron-deficiency anemia. About 30% of the world's population is anemic, and about half of those cases are due to an iron deficiency.

hematocrit The percentage of total blood volume occupied by red blood cells.

In iron-deficiency anemia, the percentage of red blood cells in the blood (**hematrocrit**) falls below 34% to 37%. In addition, the hemoglobin concentration in the bloodstream falls below 10 to 11 grams per 100 milliliters of blood. A variety of diseases can reduce hemoglobin and hematocrit values, but usually, if both are reduced, the person has iron-deficiency anemia. If the volume of each red blood cell is also reduced, this is further evidence of anemia. Probably about 8% of Americans have iron-deficiency anemia.

More of us are iron deficient—as evidenced by poor iron stores—than have iron-deficiency anemia. Probably about 30% of women in the United States have scant or no iron stores. Their blood hemoglobin values are still normal, but they have no stores to draw from in times of pregnancy or illness.

Life stages during which iron-deficiency anemia often appears are infancy, preschool years, and puberty for both males and females. Women are also more vulnerable during childbearing years when menses occurs. In addition, anemia is also often found in pregnant women, as we will discuss in Chapter 16. These life stages are singled out because either growth, with the resulting expansion of blood volume and muscle mass, increases iron needs, or total kcalorie intakes make it difficult to consume enough iron. Note that iron deficiency during pregnancy can prove dangerous. The risk of maternal and infant death, and premature birth are significantly increased.

Much anemia in the Mediterranean area, Southeast Asia, and other parts of the world is due to a group of diseases called thalassemia. This genetic disease causes a person to synthesize incorrect forms of hemoglobin. The red blood cell then lacks the usual ability to carry oxygen.

Clinical symptoms of iron-deficiency anemia include pale skin and brittle finger nails, which can eventually turn up into a spoon shape. The person suffers fatigue, poor temperature regulation, loss of appetite, and apathy. Insufficient iron for the synthesis of red blood cells and cytochromes may cause the fatigue.

EXPERT OPINION

Do Marginal Mineral Intakes Pose Health Threats?

DR. ROBERT DiSILVESTRO

Nutrition textbooks usually discuss mineral insufficiencies primarily in terms of overt deficiency symptoms. In other words, poor iron intake is said to cause anemia; magnesium deficiency is said to produce tetany, and so on. This approach emphasizes the best understood information. On the other hand, you should be aware that researchers are examining the nutritional state occurring when enough mineral is consumed to prevent deficiency, but not enough to reach recommended levels. This is referred to as marginal intake.

Exact definitions for marginal and deficient intakes do not exist. There is no specific percentage of an RDA, or of an estimated safe and adequate daily dietary intake (ESADDI), that is labelled marginal or deficient. Generally, intakes are called deficient when they produce symptoms traditionally associated with a given mineral deficiency. Intakes are called marginal when they do not produce these symptoms, but are still somewhat lower than recommended intakes. To some nutritionists, the latter might be 50% of the RDA, but to others it might be another percentage. Ideally, nutritionists would like to say that marginal intake is that which poses health risks. However, we do not yet fully know what those risks are, or how much mineral consumption is needed to prevent them.

Addressing this issue is not as easy as it may seem. For one thing, mineral needs will vary between individuals and can even vary for one individual under different circumstances. Another problem is that many of the sympoms that might be associated with marginal mineral intake are influenced by a variety of factors. Possible symptoms include poor growth; suboptimal immune function; fatigue and increased risk of degenerative diseases, such as cancer, cardiovascular disease; and osteoporosis. It can be difficult to determine how much, if any, marginal mineral intakes contribute to these conditions.

One approach is to assess the mineral status of groups of people, and then compare their status with the incidence of a given health problem. For instance, copper status could be compared to serum cholesterol as one test of whether marginal copper status can contribute to risk of cardiovascular disease. Researchers generally like to use blood tests to assess mineral status. Unfortunately, the blood tests currently used are not reliable for every mineral under every circumstance. For instance, serum concentrations of the copper protein ceruloplasmin are sometimes used to assess copper status, but these values can also be influenced by other factors. Thus the researcher can't always tell what the true mineral status of a person really is.

Some progress has been made in relating marginal mineral intakes to health problems. For example, moderately low zinc intake by children has been found to limit growth. Also, moderately low iron consumption, though not producing anemia, has been shown to cause fatigue and reduce work capacity. We can safely say that these two consequences of marginal mineral intake do exist, but we cannot yet say how widespread either of these problems are. Evidence has accumulated concerning other possible effects of marginal mineral consumption, but the evidence is not yet considered conclusive. Examples include calcium with osteoporosis, magnesium with high blood pressure, and copper with cardiovascular disease.

Some insight into possible consequences of marginal mineral consumption is coming from studies in experimental animals. For instance, work in rats suggests that immune function may be among the most susceptible of body systems. Another emerging concept is that marginal mineral intake poses its worst threat when combined with physiological stress, such as infection, inflammation, toxin exposure, drug therapies, and certain genetic makeups. This speculation seems reasonable, but actual research is just beginning.

Most studies to date concerning marginal mineral intake by humans or experimental animals have focused on single minerals. This represents the simplest approach to such research. Eventually, researchers must also examine marginal intake of one mineral in combination with marginal intake of another mineral, or of some vitamin. If a person's diet is marginal in one nutrient, then it could also be marginal in another nutrient.

In summary, marginal mineral consumption occurs in humans and negative effects have been found. However, the full range of health threats and the extent to which they actually occur are not yet understood. Further research should help answer many of the questions we currently have on this topic. ●

Dr. DiSilvestro is an associate professor in the Department of Human Nutrition and Food Management at The Ohio State University. His research focuses primarily on copper metabolism.

Researchers have shown that poor iron stores can also decrease learning ability, work performance, and immune status even before a person is actually anemic.[19] This may be due to poor function of the electron transport system—the cytochromes in this system contain iron. Thus it makes sense to maintain good iron stores so that the body is able to respond to critical times for iron needs, such as during blood loss from disease, an increased need for blood synthesis when moving to a higher altitude, or the demands of pregnancy. Overall, iron deficiency remains one of our most common and easily preventable deficiencies.[29] Efforts must continue to efficiently identify the individuals still suffering the effects and treat them.

CAUSES OF IRON-DEFICIENCY ANEMIA

Blood loss due to intestinal and blood-borne parasite infections is a common additional cause of anemia in poverty, especially when people do not wear shoes. Parasites, such as hookworms, can easily penetrate the soles of the feet and enter the bloodstream. Although hookworm disease has been largely eradicated in the United States and other industrialized nations, it continues to plague more than one fifth of the world's population.

A poor dietery intake of iron can lead to iron-deficiency anemia. Other causes include chronic blood loss from heavy menses, ulcers, hemorrhoids, and colon cancer, among others. Iron-deficiency anemia in men is usually due to ulcers, colon cancer, or hemorrhoids. The donation of 1 pint (0.5 liter) of blood represents a loss of 250 milligrams of iron. It generally takes several months to replace that iron. So it is wise, especially for women, to limit blood donations to two or three times a year. Remember that many people are iron deficient without showing symptoms of anemia. It takes a long time for iron-deficiency anemia to develop. Inefficient absorption from the predominantly vegetarian diets of most people in poor countries worldwide is a primary cause of iron deficiency.[29] For these people meat is expensive and consumed in small quantities or not at all. Iron deficiency and anemia eventually affect the majority of individuals in such populations.

MEASURING IRON STATUS

free erythrocyte protoporphyrins (FEP) Immature red blood cells released from the bone marrow. An increased serum level of FEP reflects a decreased ability to make red blood cells and suggests iron-deficiency anemia. Lead poisoning also raises blood FEP levels.

microcytic Literally means "small cell." Red blood cells that are smaller than normal.

hypochromic Pale red blood cells lacking sufficient hemoglobin due to an iron-deficiency. Hypochromic cells have a reduced oxygen-carrying ability.

The most sensitive measure of iron storage in the body is the serum ferritin level. If the serum ferritin level is low, iron stores in the liver are low.[33] Because most extra iron is stored in the liver, low liver stores indicate that total body storage is also low.

As iron deficiency proceeds, total iron-binding capacity of the blood increases. Many iron-binding sites on the blood proteins become free, leaving more room than usual for extra iron to bind. At the same time, the bone marrow, which synthesizes red blood cells, begins releasing immature red blood cell products called **free erythrocyte protoporphyrins (FEP)**. Finally, as the iron deficiency worsens, hemoglobin and hematocrit values fall (Figure 15-3). The red blood cells will now be very small and pale. We refer to this as a **microcytic** (small cell) **hypochromic** (pale) anemia. Only very severe cases of iron deficiency reach this point.

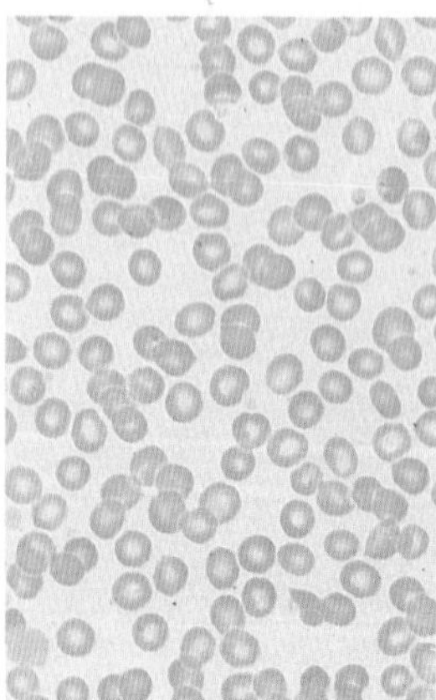

A

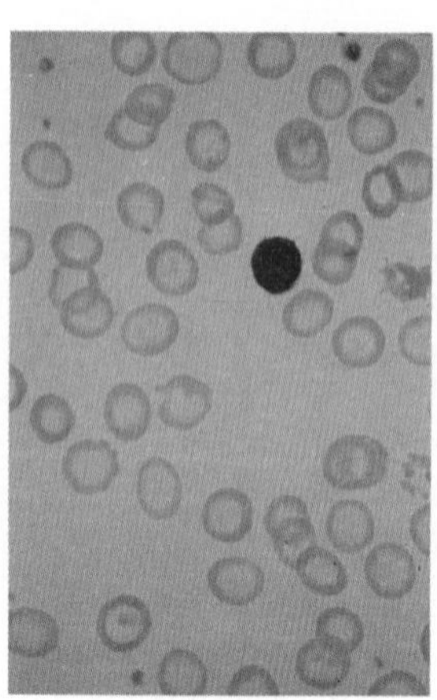

B

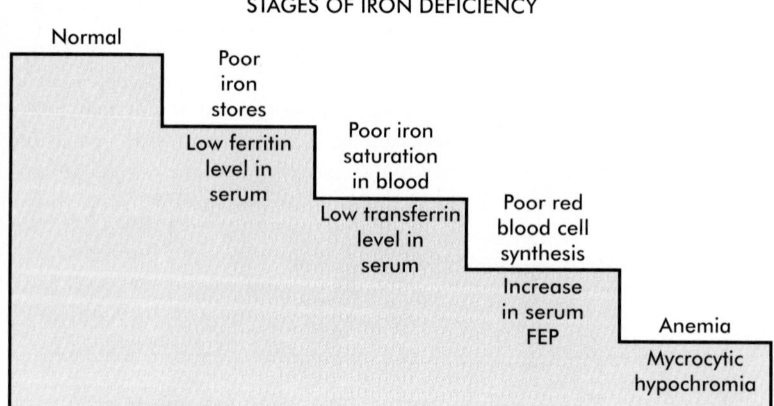

Figure 15-3 Iron-deficiency anemia. **A,** Normal cells; both cell size and color are normal. **B,** Iron-deficient cells; both cell size and color are decreased. The loss of color stems from the lower amount of the pigment hemoglobin.

TREATING IRON-DEFICIENCY ANEMIA

To speed the cure of iron-deficiency anemia, medicinal forms of iron, such as ferrous sulfate, need to be ingested. A physician should also find the cause so that the anemia does not recur. A good diet may prevent iron-deficiency anemia, but medicinal iron is a better cure (Figure 15-4). This iron should be given to increase the hemoglobin and hematocrit values and to replace depleted iron stores. This treatment usually involves 200 milligrams of iron as ferrous sulfate per day for 6 to 12 months. If this dose upsets the stomach, it can be reduced and the time of treatment extended. A vitamin C source consumed with the supplement is advised to enhance absorption.

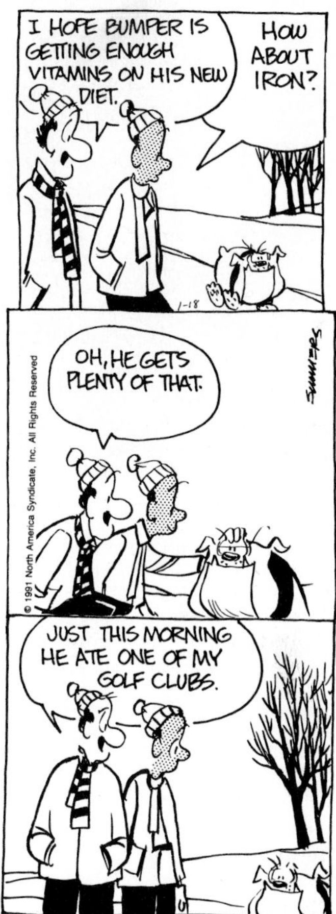
I HOPE BUMPER IS GETTING ENOUGH VITAMINS ON HIS NEW DIET.
HOW ABOUT IRON?
OH, HE GETS PLENTY OF THAT.
JUST THIS MORNING HE ATE ONE OF MY GOLF CLUBS.
© 1991 North America Syndicate, Inc. All Rights Reserved

Figure 15-4 The Middletons.

IRON IN FOODS

The most nutrient-dense iron sources are spinach, oysters, liver, peas, and legumes (Table 15-2). However, total iron content of foods and nutrient density are not the only considerations when choosing dietary iron sources. Serving size and bioavailability are probably more important. For example, although spinach is iron rich, the body can absorb only very little of it. Animal sources contain some heme iron, the most bioavailable form. These are our best iron sources. The major iron sources in our diets are animal sources—beef steak, roasts, and hamburger. The next greatest sources are bakery products—white breads, rolls, and crackers. Most of this iron is added to refined flour to enrich it. Today, about 25% of the iron in the U.S. food supply comes from enriched bakery products. But there is debate about the value of iron enrichment; only about 3% of this iron is absorbed, both because of the form used and because other substances in flour bind iron.

The use of iron-fortified formulas and cereals in the Special Supplemental Food Program for Women, Infants, and Children (WIC) in the United States is probably a major contributor to decreasing rates of iron-deficiency anemia in preschool children (see Chapters 16 and 17). Milk is a very poor source of iron. A common cause of iron-deficiency anemia in children is an over-reliance on milk, coupled with an insufficient meat intake. An additional possible iron source is cooking utensils. When acidic foods, such as tomato sauce, are cooked in iron pots and frying pans, some iron from the cookware is taken up by the food.

RDA FOR IRON

The body needs to absorb about 0.9 milligrams daily for men and 1.4 milligrams daily for women. The adult RDA for iron is 10 milligrams daily for men and 15

Table 15-2 Good sources of iron, ranked by nutrient density

Food	Serving size to yield 5 milligrams*	kcalories needed to yield 5 milligrams
Spinach, cooked	1 cup	30
Oysters, raw	¼ cup	40
Sauerkraut, canned	1⅓ cups	65
Green peas, cooked	2 cups	105
Beef liver, fried	3 ounces	175
Braunschweiger sausage	2 slices	190
Kidney beans, cooked	1 cup	190
Lima beans, cooked	1 cup	220
Navy beans, cooked	1 cup	220
Steak, beef	5 ounces	280
Prune juice	2 cups	310
Pot roast	4⅓ ounces	350

* ⅓ of the RDA for adult females, ages 11-50 years.
Bioavailability must be considered, as well as nutrient density. Due to the presence of heme iron and the meat protein factor, liver and meat are superior sources of iron compared with plants.

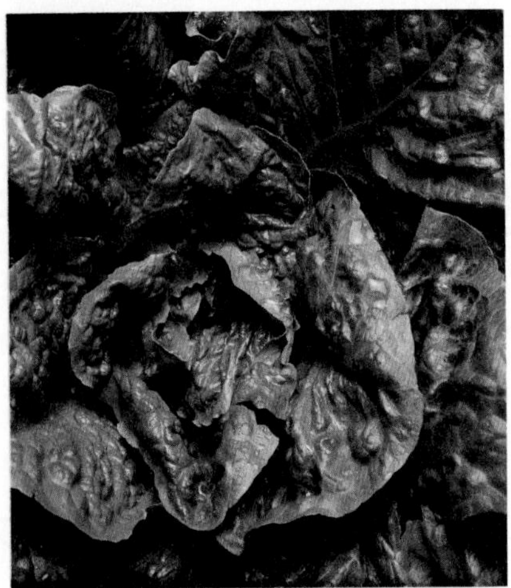

Spinach is rich in iron but the bioavailability of iron from spinach is low.

milligrams daily for women (throughout the rest of this chapter see the inside cover for other age groups and Appendix D for Canadian recommendations). The RDA value assumes that about 10% of dietary iron is absorbed. If iron absorption exceeds that, less dietary iron is needed.

The higher RDA for women is primarily due to menstrual blood loss. This leads to about 15 milligrams of iron lost per month. Women who menstruate more heavily and longer than the "average" menstruation need even more dietary iron, and those who have lighter and shorter flows may need less iron. The variation in menstrual blood loss makes it difficult to set an RDA for iron for women.

By recording dietary intakes from a variety of women, we find that most women do not consume 15 milligrams of iron daily. The average value is closer to 11 milligrams per day.[24] Of course, not all women need 15 milligrams of iron daily because the RDA is set high enough to meet the needs of most women. In addition, varied amounts of menstruation plus wide differences in iron absorption (recall it varies with need) further complicates evaluating a dietary intake. The RDA for a person absorbing 20% of dietary iron could be half that of the person absorbing 10% of it.

Thus a registered dietitian who finds that a person is not consuming the RDA for iron should be concerned, but not alarmed. This person should try to consume a diet that meets the RDA for iron. But whether a lower intake is actually harming this person's health is difficult to determine. Although we have very sensitive measures of iron stores in the body, we lack the knowledge to translate this information into predictors of health status.

AMERICANS AT RISK FOR AN IRON DEFICIENCY

As stated earlier, an iron deficiency is most common when iron needs greatly exceed normal intake—during infancy, preschool years, and puberty and during the child-bearing years for women. Pregnancy and disease also increase iron needs and therefore the risk for deficiency. Repeated pregnancies pose a special challenge to women to maintain adequate iron stores.

Our diet contains about 5 to 7 milligrams of iron per 1000 kcalories. Thus men generally achieve a good iron status because a daily energy intake of 2000 to 3000 kcalories meets their RDA for iron. Most women, on the other hand, have difficulty eating 3000 kcalories daily while maintaining desirable weight. They then have difficulty consuming 15 milligrams of iron daily unless they seek out nutrient-dense forms of iron for their diets, such as is found in fortified breakfast cereals. If that does not suffice, a supplement should be used. Iron-deficiency anemia, and especially poor iron stores, is not just a disease of the poor; it cuts across all social strata. Vegans should pay special attention to their intakes.

"RUNNER'S ANEMIA"

runner's anemia A decrease in the blood's ability to carry oxygen found in athletes that may be caused by iron loss in perspiration, red blood cell destruction due to the impact of exercise, or increased blood volume and iron needs.

Athletes incur a special type of anemia called **runner's anemia** as we discussed in Chapter 10. Three possible factors contribute to it: additional iron losses via increased perspiration, red blood cell destruction (hemolysis) from trauma of the red blood cells being flattened as they pass through the foot when it strikes the ground during exercise, and the increase in blood volume associated with athletic fitness. Runner's anemia can decrease sports performance and so should be avoided. Athletes should have their hemoglobin levels and other iron status indicators monitored, and they should attempt to meet their iron needs by either dietary means or iron supplementation.

TOXICITY OF IRON

Although iron deficiency is a common problem, an overabundance of iron can also be a serious problem because it is toxic. Even a large single dose of iron can be life-threatening. Iron pills and vitamin supplements containing iron commonly poison children. Smaller doses (but still greater than what is needed) over a long period can also cause problems. A form of iron toxicity has been observed in an African tribe that brews beer in iron pots. Repeated blood transfusions also can lead to iron toxicity.

Iron toxicity also accompanies the genetic disease called **hemochromatosis**. This result is also called hemosiderosis if it develops without a genetic link, such as from repeated blood transfusions. People with hemochromatosis overabsorb iron, and throughout time the amount of iron in their bodies builds up to high levels, especially in the bloodstream and liver.[13] Some iron also deposits in the muscles, pancreas, and heart. If not treated, the excess iron deposited contributes to severe organ damage, especially in the liver and heart. Diabetes and a bronze skin pigmentation also are possible outcomes. Researchers think that about one of ten Americans has one of the two genes needed to cause hemochromatosis. About 1 in 2000 of us may have both hemochromatosis genes and therefore the disease, although more cases may be present but just missed because of failure to diagnose it.[15]

hemochromatosis A disorder of iron metabolism characterized by increased absorption, saturation of iron-binding proteins, and deposition of hemosiderin in the liver tissue.

Probably the only factor keeping many people with hemochromatosis from experiencing serious effects of the disease is that they consume such a low amount of iron. For many years some nutrition interest groups have recommended increasing iron enrichment in grains to decrease the incidence of iron-deficiency anemia. However, for people with hemochromatosis, that could increase the numbers who actually develop disease symptoms.

Elevated serum iron levels or transferrin saturation levels suggest the presence of hemochromatosis. In the future, you will probably notice a more aggressive approach in screening for hemochromatosis. This is because with appropriate treatment, such as frequent bleeding and the use of medications to bind iron in the bloodstream to increase urinary excretion, the disease process can be stopped, and the person can live a healthy and normal life.[15] A first sign of hemochromatosis is arthritis-like symptoms, such as painful joints.

Excess iron in the blood may lead to enhanced oxidation of LDL cholesterol and so speed development of atherosclerosis. This is a new area of research but nevertheless suggests cautious use of iron supplements unless a need is documented.

CONCEPT CHECK

Iron absorption depends on its form and the body's need for it. Absorption is controlled by a "mucosal block," but excess iron intake can override the control, leading to toxicity. Iron absorption increases in the presence of vitamin C and decreases in the presence of large amounts of calcium and some components of grain fiber, such as phytate. Iron is most important in synthesizing hemoglobin and myoglobin and supporting immune function. An iron deficiency can cause decreased red blood cell synthesis, which can lead to anemia. It is particularly important for women of childbearing age to consume adequate iron, primarily to replace that lost in menstrual blood. Good sources include red meat, pork, enriched grains and cereals, and oysters.

Zinc

Although zinc (Zn) has been recognized as an essential nutrient in animals since the early 1900s, zinc deficiency was first recognized in humans in the early 1960s in Egypt and Iran. The deficiency was determined to be the cause of growth retardation and poor sexual development in many people. Curiously, the zinc content was fairly high in their diets. However, the customary diet contained almost exclusively unleavened bread and little animal protein. Unleavened bread is very high in phytates and other factors that decrease zinc bioavailability. Yeast fermentation of bread, as is done in a typical loaf of bread, reduces the effect of phytate by tenfold. In addition, parasite infestation and the practice of eating clay also contributed to severe zinc deficiency.[25]

In the United States, zinc deficiencies were first observed in the early 1970s in hospitalized patients on total parenteral nutrition. Zinc was not added to the intravenous solutions, but the protein source in the solutions was based on milk protein or blood fibrin, which are naturally rich in zinc. When the solutions were changed

Figure 15-5 Zinc and copper absorption. Both influence the absorption of the other. The short life span of the intestinal absorptive cells also influences absorption.

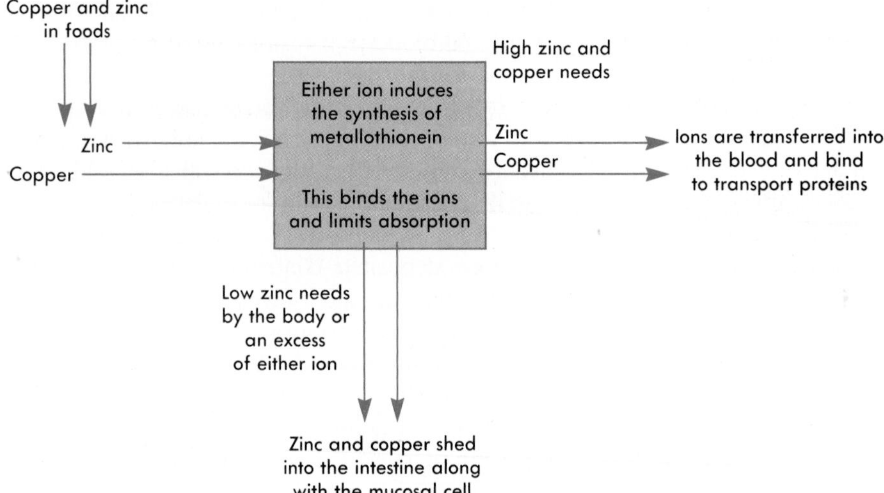

to include mostly synthetic amino acids as the protein source in the 1970s, deficiency symptoms quickly developed. This source of protein is very low in zinc content.

ABSORPTION OF ZINC

Like iron, zinc absorption is influenced by foods ingested. About 25% to 40% of dietary zinc is absorbed; the higher figure is more likely when animal protein sources are used and the body's zinc needs are elevated. Zinc absorption, despite extensive study, is not clearly understood, but probably involves a compound that works in the intestine to help transport zinc into the intestinal cells.

metallothionein A protein that binds and regulates the release of zinc and copper (and other positive ions) in intestinal and liver cells.

When zinc is absorbed into intestinal cells, it induces the synthesis of the protein **metallothionein**. This binds zinc in much the same way that ferritin binds iron. If zinc is not transferred to the bloodstream from the intestinal cells within 2 to 5 days, it is sloughed off along with the cell and excreted.[32] Thus a "mucosal block" works against overabsorption of zinc and iron (Figure 15-5). However, if large doses of zinc are taken, it overrides the mucosal block. Luckily for overconsumers, zinc is also excreted via the pancreas to the intestinal tract, unlike iron.

Zinc intakes worldwide are generally poor. Supplementary iron competes with zinc for absorption, and toasting cereals also reduces zinc absorption as it binds with flour constituents. Because most people worldwide rely on cereal grains for their source of protein, kcalories, and zinc, finding adequate zinc sources and maintaining adequate zinc intakes are a problem. And since zinc and iron are most available from the same foods, zinc and iron deficiencies occur together in populations of the less-developed countries. Therefore, it would seem prudent to consider individuals with iron deficiency at very high risk of zinc deficiency. Overall, more research on zinc status is needed worldwide.

FUNCTIONS OF ZINC

Over 200 enzymes require zinc as a cofactor for optimum activity. Adequate zinc intake is necessary to support many bodily functions, such as:

- nucleic acid and protein metabolism, wound healing, and growth
- proper immune function (intakes in excess of the RDA do not provide any extra benefit to immune function)
- proper development of sexual organs and bone
- storage and release of insulin
- prostaglandin synthesis

A recent study emphasizes the importance of zinc for growth. Children recovering from malnutrition gained weight much faster when they consumed zinc supplements containing approximately three times the RDA, under a physician's guidance.[31]

Table 15-3 Good sources of zinc, ranked by nutrient density

Food	Serving size to yield 5 milligrams*	kcalories needed to yield 5 milligrams
Oysters, raw	2 tablespoons	10
Wheat germ, raw	½ cup	125
Crab meat, canned	1 cup	125
Shrimp, boiled	5 ounces	150
Sirloin steak, lean	3 ounces	175
Beef liver, fried	3½ ounces	213
Beef pot roast, lean	3 ounces	225
Lamb chop	4 ounces	250
Corned beef, canned	4 ounces	253
Turkey, all meat roasted	5½ ounces	275
Blackeyed peas, cooked	1½ cups	316

* ⅓ Adult male RDA.
Seafoods are good, readily bioavailable sources of zinc.

Two important enzymes that require zinc are carbonic anhydrase and alcohol dehydrogenase. Carbonic anhydrase helps balance acids with bases in the blood and aids stomach acid production. Alcohol dehydrogenase breaks down alcohol.

Aside from poor growth, symptoms of zinc deficiency include an acnelike rash, diarrhea, lack of appetite, reduced sense of taste and smell, hair loss, mental confusion, delivery of a low birth weight baby in pregnant women, and poor sexual development in children and adolescents (Figure 15-6).[25] Poor learning ability may result, as zinc deficiency can be a cause of impaired neuropsychological function among children, as is seen in iron deficiency. A persistent rash, especially in the presence of a poor diet, should prompt a clinician to evaluate zinc status in a person.

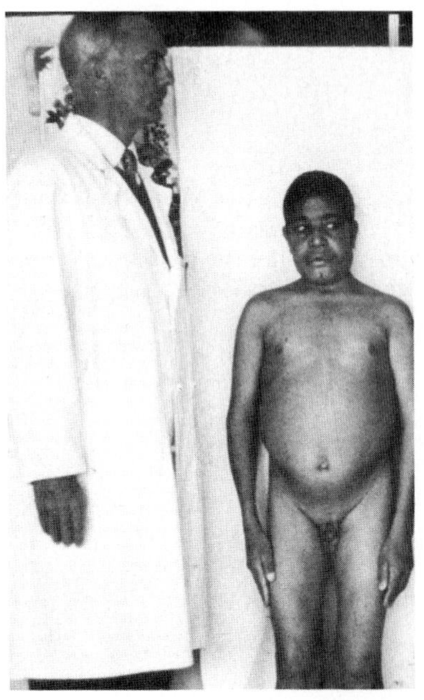

Figure 15-6 An example of zinc deficiency. An Egyptian farm boy, age 16 years and 49 inches tall, with dwarfism and poor sexual development associated with a zinc deficiency.

ZINC IN FOODS

In general, protein-rich diets are also rich in zinc. The most nutrient-dense sources of zinc are oysters, shrimp, crab, beef, turkey, greens, and mushrooms (Table 15-3). As with iron, nutrient density is not the only issue; bioavailability is probably more important. Animal foods, such as lean meats, poultry, and dairy products, are our best zinc sources because zinc from animal sources is neither bound by phytates, nor so affected by local soil conditions. Animal foods supply almost half our zinc intake, but their cost makes zinc a very expensive nutrient. Still, we shouldn't discount good plant sources of zinc, such as whole grains, peanuts, and beans, however, because studies show that they can deliver substantial amounts of zinc to body cells. Zinc is not part of the enrichment process, so refined flours are not a good source.

RDA FOR ZINC

The adult RDA for zinc is 15 milligrams daily for men and 12 milligrams daily for women. The average adult American intake of zinc is 8 to 12 milligrams daily.[24] This raises concern that some people have marginal intakes. Still, there are no indications of moderate or severe zinc deficiencies in an otherwise healthy adult population. Strong homeostatic control of absorption and excretion can maintain persons in zinc balance with intakes lower than those furnished by typical diets of Americans. However, the long-term effects of such intakes are not known.

AMERICANS AT RISK FOR A ZINC DEFICIENCY

Zinc deficiencies are most commonly found in hospital patients with severe malabsorption. Sickle-cell disease increases zinc needs by destroying massive amounts of red blood cells, which contain a great deal of zinc. In addition, people with alcoholism, elderly people, and vegans can be deficient in zinc because of either a

A rare disease, acrodermatitis enteropathica, results from an inherited inability to absorb zinc. Symptoms in infants include rash, hair loss, depressed immune response, poor sense of taste, lack of appetite, and poor growth. This disease can be treated with supplements of zinc in amounts of about twice the RDA.

poor overall nutrient intake or a diet low or absent in animal foods.[25] Greater zinc intake in these people can sometimes increase their appetite and sense of taste. In the United States, symptoms of zinc deficiency have been observed in groups of middle-income and low-income children with poor growth. As we mentioned, supplementation with zinc then improved growth and appetite.

The link between zinc and appetite, taste acuity, wound healing, and immune response underscores zinc's importance in the diets of elderly people. Immune status is often depressed in elderly people. Because of poorly fitting dentures or low-income status, elderly people may not eat enough animal products. This reduces zinc intake.

Although there are probably many cases of marginal zinc status in America, we lack a sensitive marker for zinc status. The body must be very zinc depleted for clinical tests to register a deficiency. Assessment of zinc status is difficult because serum zinc levels do not reflect body stores, and no test using a zinc-containing enzyme is accepted.

TOXICITY OF ZINC

A high consumption of zinc works against iron and copper absorption. Recall that iron, copper, and zinc can all exist with a +2 valance. Oversupplementation with zinc can cause a copper deficiency.[12] One study has shown that zinc supplements at approximately three to five times the RDA can reduce HDL cholesterol levels by about 15%.[3] In that case, excess zinc may interfere with copper metabolism. That is disturbing for two reasons. First, low HDL cholesterol levels are associated with an increased risk of developing heart disease (see Chapter 4). Second, it is common for people who take zinc supplements to consume this amount. So some Americans, by unwittingly lowering their HDL cholesterol levels, may be increasing their risk for developing heart disease—even though they think that supplementing zinc in the diet contributes to overall health. Again, this shows why mineral supplements should not be consumed except under close scrutiny of a physician. Zinc intakes over 2 grams daily also result in diarrhea, cramps, nausea, vomiting, and sometimes depresses immune system function.

Copper

Copper (Cu) is a part of certain enzymes, contributes to the activity of other enzymes, and aids in iron metabolism.

FUNCTIONS OF COPPER

Copper increases iron absorption by helping form a protein called ceruloplasmin (also known as ferroxidase).[14] As we said earlier, this compound helps mobilize iron by converting Fe^{+2} into Fe^{+3}. To cross cell membranes (intestinal and other body cells) any FE^{+2} must be converted to Fe^{+3}. Thus ceruloplasmin can enable iron to leave the intestinal cells and sites of iron storage in the liver and bind to the protein transferrin in the bloodstream. The iron is then transported to bone marrow and other cells, aiding needed hemoglobin synthesis.

Copper is part of an enzyme that cross-bonds collagen—a connective tissue protein—and elastin. In a copper deficiency, blood vessels in laboratory animals rupture because collagen is not available to form the important connective tissue network needed to strengthen blood vessels.

Copper also is part of enzymes that synthesize norepinephrine and dopamine, two neurotransmitters. In addition, copper-containing enzymes help in myelination (insulation) of the nervous system, cholesterol metabolism, and the scavenging of electron-seeking (free radical) compounds. One of the body's major free radical scavengers, the enzyme superoxide dismutase, can contain copper and zinc. Finally, copper is important for proper immune system function and blood clotting.[14]

Symptoms of copper deficiency include anemia, low white blood cell count (specifically, the neutrophils), bone loss, increased serum cholesterol levels, poor

Table 15-4 Good sources of copper, ranked by nutrient density

Food	Serving size to yield 1 milligram	kcalories needed to yield 1 milligram
Oysters, raw meat	½ ounce	7
Lobster	2½ ounces	75
Brewer's yeast	3½ tablespoons	90
Liver, beef or calf, fried	1½ ounces	90
Cocoa powder, low-fat	1¼ ounces	90
Molasses, blackstrap	3½ tablespoons	150
Wheat germ, toasted	¾ cup	270
Sunflower kernels, dry hulled	2 ounces	290
Brazil nuts, shelled	½ cup	345
Beans, red kidney, dry, cooked	2 cups	450
Walnuts, English	¾ cup	480
Pecans	¾ cups	550

For comparison, the adult ESADDI is 1.5 to 3 milligrams.
Oysters, lobster, nuts, seeds, and beans are good sources of copper.

growth, and heart disease.[4,10] Frank copper deficiency has been linked to heart disease in laboratory animals. Note, however, experts in the heart disease field do not list copper deficiencies as even a minor cause of heart disease in Western society.

COPPER IN FOODS

Copper is primarily found in liver, cocoa, legumes, nuts, and whole-grain breads and cereals (Table 15-4). It is not added to breakfast cereals since it speeds fat breakdown in the product (Figure 15-7). Milk is also a very poor source of copper. About 25% to 40% of dietary copper is absorbed. Food tables often list few values for copper, and even those values may not be reliable because soil conditions greatly affect the copper content of plant foods.

ESADDI FOR COPPER

Copper has an estimated safe and adequate daily dietary intake of 1.5 to 3 milligrams daily for adults. Studies of young men show a minimum intake should be 1.3 milligrams daily. Our average intake is about 1 milligram daily.[24] Women generally have marginal intakes. Even so, the copper status of adults in America appears to be fine, though this may be because we lack sensitive measures for copper status, causing some cases of marginal deficiencies to be missed.

Several groups of people at the greatest risk for a copper deficiency include premature infants, infants recovering from malnutrition on a diet dominated by milk (which is a poor source of copper), people recovering from intestinal surgery (during which time copper absorption decreases), and people on long-term total parenteral nutrition when insufficient copper is added. Use of large doses of antacids may also bind enough copper in the intestine to cause a deficiency.

A copper deficiency can result from overzealous supplementation of zinc, since zinc can hamper copper absorption (Figure 15-5).[12] Zinc increases the synthesis of the protein metallothionein, which binds them both—but particularly copper—in the intestinal cells, reducing future transfer into the bloodstream.

TOXICITY OF COPPER

Copper tends to cause vomiting at single doses greater than 10 to 15 milligrams. When copper is used to treat a deficiency, it must be given in divided doses to limit

RAISIN SQUARES

NUTRITION INFORMATION
SERVING SIZE: 1 OZ. (28.4 g, ABOUT 1/2 CUP)

SERVINGS PER PACKAGE: 16

	CEREAL	WITH 1/2 CUP VITAMINS A & D SKIM MILK
CALORIES	90	130*
PROTEIN, g	2	6
CARBOHYDRATE, g	23	29
FAT, TOTAL, g	0	0*
UNSATURATED, g	0	
SATURATED, g	0	
CHOLESTEROL, mg	0	0*
SODIUM, mg	0	65
POTASSIUM, mg	110	310

PERCENTAGE OF U.S. RECOMMENDED DAILY ALLOWANCES (U.S. RDA)

PROTEIN	4	15
VITAMIN A	**	4
VITAMIN C	**	2
THIAMIN	25	30
RIBOFLAVIN	25	35
NIACIN	25	25
CALCIUM	**	15
IRON	45	45
VITAMIN B_6	25	25
FOLIC ACID	25	25
VITAMIN B_{12}	25	35
PHOSPHORUS	8	20
MAGNESIUM	6	10
ZINC	10	15
COPPER	2	4

*2% MILK SUPPLIES AN ADDITIONAL 20 CALORIES, 2 g FAT, AND 10 mg CHOLESTEROL.
**CONTAINS LESS THAN 2% OF THE U.S. RDA OF THIS NUTRIENT.

INGREDIENTS: WHOLE WHEAT, RAISINS, BROWN SUGAR, GLYCERIN.

VITAMINS AND MINERALS: IRON, NIACINAMIDE, ZINC (OXIDE), VITAMIN B_6 (PYRIDOXINE HYDROCHLORIDE), VITAMIN B_2 (RIBOFLAVIN), VITAMIN B_1 (THIAMIN HYDROCHLORIDE), FOLIC ACID, AND VITAMIN B_{12}.

TO KEEP THIS CEREAL FRESH, BHT HAS BEEN ADDED TO THE PACKAGING.

MADE BY XXY COMPANY
BATTLE CREEK, MI 49016, U.S.A.
© 1984 BY XXY COMPANY
® XXY COMPANY

Figure 15-7 Breakfast cereals are better sources of iron and zinc than copper. This is because adding copper would speed fat breakdown in the product.

An inherited condition known as Menkes' kinky hair syndrome is characterized by slow growth, brain degeneration, kinky white hair, and low serum copper levels. This condition results from a defect of copper absorption and incorporation into proteins, such as ceruloplasmin. Supplemental copper is given in an attempt to partially reverse this condition.

this effect. An inherited condition called Wilson's disease results in accumulation of copper in the liver, brain, kidneys, and cornea of the eye. If recognized early, treatment that binds copper in the bloodstream and increases its excretion in the urine can prevent damage to these tissues and reduce the mental degeneration commonly seen in active cases.

CONCEPT CHECK

Similar to iron absorption, zinc absorption is regulated by a mucosal block. Both animal protein sources and increased body needs lead to increased zinc absorption. Iron competes with zinc for absorption. Zinc functions as a cofactor for many enzymes and is important for growth, immune function, and sense of taste. Beef, seafood, and whole grains are good food sources. Copper functions mainly as part of enzymes and other compounds involved in iron metabolism, cross-bonding of collagen, myelination of nerve cells, and neurotransmitter synthesis. A deficiency can result in a form of anemia. Good food sources of copper are liver, legumes, and whole grains.

Selenium

Selenium (Se) exists in many ionic forms. Most selenium in foods is bound to the amino acid derivatives of methionine and cysteine. These forms are readily absorbed from the diet. There appears to be no physiological control of how much we absorb, so selenium has a high toxic potential.

We have now seen that the absence of many nutrients from the diet can lead to anemia:

- **Vitamin E deficiency can lead to hemolytic anemia (see Chapter 12).**
- **Vitamin K deficiency, especially coupled with use of antibiotics, can lead to blood loss and so to hemorrhagic anemia (see Chapter 12).**
- **Vitamin B-6 deficiency can lead to microcytic anemia (see Chapter 13).**
- **Folate deficiency can lead to a megaloblastic anemia (see Chapter 13).**
- **Vitamin B-12 malabsorption can lead to macrocytic anemia (see Chapter 13).**
- **An iron deficiency can lead to microcytic hypochromic anemia.**
- **A copper deficiency can lead, although rarely, to a secondary iron-deficiency anemia, as copper aids in iron metabolism.**

FUNCTION OF SELENIUM

Currently the only clearly understood role for selenium is as cofactor for the activity of a major form of the enzyme glutathione peroxidase.[18] Each enzyme molecule can have four seleniums attached to it. This enzyme participates in a system that metabolizes peroxides into less toxic alcohols and water. In Chapter 12 we discussed how important this action of glutathione peroxidase is; peroxides tend to become free radicals that can then attack and break down cell membranes, causing cell death. In this regard selenium is important for protecting heart cells against oxidative damage. Selenium might also aid immune function via activity of glutathione peroxidase.

Recall that vitamin E also functions to prevent attacks on cell membranes by free radicals. Thus vitamin E and selenium work together. Selenium participates in an enzyme system that prevents free radical production by reducing peroxide concentration in the cell; and vitamin E stops the action of free radicals once they are produced. So an adequate selenium intake spares some of the body's need for vitamin E.

At one time, high dietary levels of selenium were considered carcinogenic, but after further studies, this is in doubt. Today's understanding is in fact that selenium's role in reducing free radical production gives it a potential for reducing cancer. In Chapter 13 we discussed how electron-seeking compounds can alter DNA. Alterations in DNA are known to cause cancer. By reducing the concentration of free radicals, it appears that an adequate selenium intake could be an important cancer prevention measure. Animal studies in this area are encouraging, and scientists hope results of human studies currently under way will clarify selenium's role in cancer prevention. Until then, recommending selenium supplementation to possibly prevent cancer in humans is premature. Selenium may have yet other metabolic functions, but none have been firmly established.

Selenium deficiency symptoms in animals and humans include muscle pain, muscle wasting, and heart disease. Farm animals in areas with low selenium soil concentrations, such as New Zealand and Finland, and humans in some areas of China develop characteristic muscle and heart disorders associated with poor selenium

Table 15-5 Good sources of selenium, ranked by nutrient density

Food	Serving size to yield 23 micrograms*	kcalories needed to yield 23 micrograms
Tuna, canned in water	1 ounce	42
Whole-wheat bread	1 slice	80
Ham, roasted, cooked	3 ounces	130
Egg noodles	⅔ cup	140
Eggs, poached	2 each	145
Oatmeal, cooked	1 cup	170
White bread	2 slices	210
Hamburger with bun	3½ ounces	230
Beef, sirloin steak, cooked	4 ounces	320
Chicken, meat, cooked	6½ ounces	350
Meat loaf, beef and pork	5 ounces	350

* ⅓ Adult male RDA.
Meats, bread and grain products, and eggs are good sources of selenium.

intake.[23,27] Other factors may also contribute. These same symptoms are noted when insufficient selenium is added to total parenteral nutrition solutions.

Selenium is now the focus of much research. The FDA has limited supplemental doses in studies to 200 micrograms per day, based on our lack of knowledge of this mineral.

SELENIUM IN FOODS

Fish, meats—especially organ meats—eggs, and shellfish are good animal sources of selenium. Grains and seeds grown in soils containing selenium are good plant sources. Major selenium contributors to our diet are tuna, beef, white bread, chicken, eggs, noodles, and milk (Table 15-5). Since we eat a varied diet supplied from many geographic areas, it is unlikely that selenium deficiency in the soil in a few areas will cause a selenium deficiency in our diets. But the difference in selenium content of foods grown throughout the United States makes it difficult to get a true selenium value for any food, such as whole-wheat bread.

RDA FOR SELENIUM

The RDA for selenium is 55 to 70 micrograms daily for adults. About 40 micrograms daily probably represents our minimum needs. Our diets likely include enough selenium, since the average intake is 80 to 130 micrograms daily. However, we do not have sensitive measures of selenium status, and cannot accurately distinguish between a good and a marginal status.

TOXICITY OF SELENIUM

Excess selenium can be toxic. Daily intakes as low as 2 to 3 milligrams (just 35 times the RDA) can cause toxicity symptoms if taken for many months. These symptoms include a garlicky odor of the breath, hair loss, nausea and vomiting, and a general weakness. Rashes and cirrhosis of the liver may also develop. Selenium illustrates the saying: "It's the dose that makes the poison."

Animals show selenium toxicity symptoms if they eat plants containing high selenium levels. Some plants naturally concentrate selenium from the soil. Birds who live in water polluted with selenium leached from nearby fields also have exhibited toxicity symptoms.

Iodide

Iodine (I), present in food as iodide and other nonelemental forms, was linked to the presence of an enlarged thyroid gland (goiter) during World War I. Men drafted from the Pacific Northwest and the Great Lakes region of the United States had a much higher rate of goiter than men from other areas of the country. The soils in these areas are very low in iodide content. Researchers in Ohio then fed a large group of children low doses of iodide in the 1920s for 4 years. They found iodide could prevent goiter in children. That finding led to the addition of iodide to salt beginning in the 1920s.

Many times the term Iodine (I_2) is used instead of iodide (I). The ion iodide is what is essential in the diet. The element iodine itself is quite poisonous. To emphasize this point, we will use the term iodide exclusively.

Today, many nations, such as Canada, require iodide-fortification of salt. In the United States, salt can be purchased either fortified or plain. By law, the label on a salt container sold in the United States must clearly state if iodide is present or not. Some areas of Europe, like northern Italy, have very low iodide levels in the soil but have yet to adopt the practice of fortifying salt with iodide. People in these areas, especially women, still suffer from goiter, as do people in areas of Central America, South America, and Africa. About one billion people worldwide are at risk of iodide deficiency.[11]

FUNCTION OF IODIDE

The thyroid gland actively accumulates and traps iodide from the bloodstream to support its hormone synthesis. Thyroid hormones, such as thyroxine, are synthesized from the amino acid tyrosine and iodide and help regulate metabolic rate, growth, and development, in addition to promoting bone and protein synthesis.

Structure of thyroxine.

If a person's iodide intake is insufficient, the thyroid gland enlarges as it attempts to take up more iodide from the bloodstream. The hormone that stimulates thyroid hormone production, **thyroid-stimulating hormone**, also stimulates the growth of the thyroid gland. Usually, enough thyroid hormone is made to limit production of thyroid-stimulating hormone. However, in an iodide deficiency, insufficient thyroid hormone is produced to shut off the synthesis of this hormone. The constant release of thyroid-stimulating hormone by the pituitary gland causes continual growth of the thyroid gland, eventually producing a greatly enlarged thyroid gland, or **goiter**[11] (Figure 15-8). Goiters have been described in people as far back as 3000 B.C., usually in women.

goiter An enlargement of the thyroid gland; this can be caused by a lack of iodide in the diet

Goiters are also associated with the consumption of large amounts of raw turnips and rutabagas. These vegetables contain compounds called **goitrogens**, which inhibit the function of the thyroid gland, and in turn, thyroid hormone synthesis. However, goitrogens are not an important cause of goiter since they are destroyed by cooking and the foods they are found in do not often play an important role in human diets.

If a woman consumes an iodide-deficient diet during the early months of her pregnancy, her infant may be born with short stature and develop mental retardation. Maternal iodide needs take precedence over fetal needs. This stunted growth is referred to as **cretinism**. Cretinism appeared in the United States before the program for iodide fortification of table salt began. Today, cretinism still appears in Europe, Africa, Latin America, and Asia. In these areas iodinated vegetable oil is being used in an attempt to decrease iodide deficiency.[11]

cretinism Stunting of body growth and mental development that results from inadequate maternal intake of iodide during pregnancy.

FOOD SOURCES OF IODIDE

Saltwater fish, seafood, iodized salt, molasses, and some plants contain various forms of iodide, especially plants grown near the sea. Sea salt found in health food stores, however, is not a good source, since the iodide is lost during processing. A half teaspoon of iodide-fortified salt (about 2 grams) supplies the adult RDA for iodide (the actual fortification level in the United States is 76 micrograms of iodide per gram of salt).

The ocean is the source of most iodide naturally present in our diets. As ocean mist blows onto nearby land, iodide becomes part of the soil. Plants that grow in that soil accumulate the iodide.

RDA FOR IODIDE

The RDA for iodide for adults is 150 micrograms daily. Probably the minimum intake to prevent goiter is 50 micrograms per day. Most of us consume much more

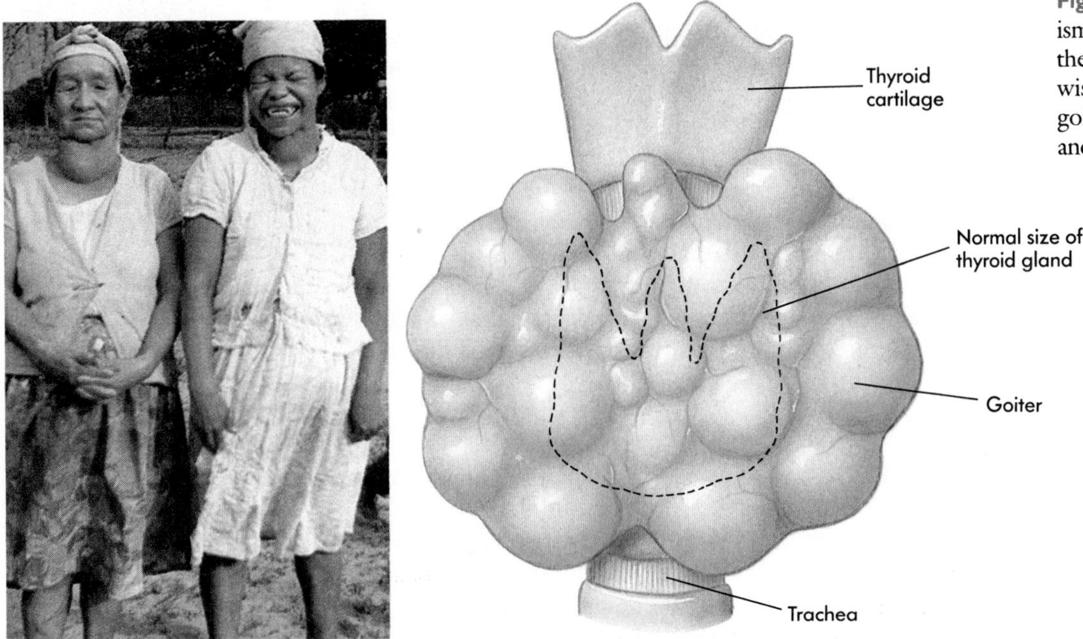

Figure 15-8 Goiter and cretinism in Bolivia. The mother on the left is goitrous, but otherwise normal. The daughter is goitrous, mentally retarded, and a deaf mute.

iodide (consumption is estimated to be at least 300 micrograms per day) than the RDA. This is because of its use: (1) as a sterilizing agent in dairies and restaurants, (2) as a dough conditioner in bakeries, (3) in food colorants, and (4) in iodized salt. So there is no need for concern about insufficient iodide intake here unless dietary sodium intake must be kept below 500 milligrams per day. However, these types of low-sodium diets are rarely used today.

TOXICITY OF IODIDE

Reports in scientific literature raise concern about high-iodide intake. Levels up to 1 milligram (6.6 times the RDA) per day appear to be safe. However, when very high amounts of iodide are consumed, thyroid hormone synthesis is inhibited, as in a deficiency. A "toxic goiter" results. "Toxic goiter" can appear in people who eat a lot of seaweed, since some seaweeds contain as much as 1% iodide by weight. Total iodide intake then can add up to 60 to 130 times the RDA. Manufacturers are working to reduce unnecessary iodide use in dairies, restaurants, and bakeries.

Fluoride

Dentists in the early 1900s noticed a lower rate of dental caries in the southwestern United States. These areas naturally contained high amounts of fluoride (F) in the water. The levels were sometimes so high that small spots on the teeth, called **mottling**, appeared. Even though these mottled teeth were quite discolored, they contained very few dental caries. After experiments showed that fluoride in the water did indeed decrease the rate of dental caries, controlled fluoridation of water in parts of the United States began in 1945.

mottling Discoloration or marking of the surface of teeth due to fluorosis.

Those people who grew up drinking fluoridated water generally have 50% to 70% fewer dental caries than people who did not drink fluoridated water as children. Dentists can provide fluoride treatments, and schools can provide fluoride tablets, but it is much less expensive and more reliable to simply put fluoride in a community's drinking water. Neither all state nor all private water sources contain enough fluoride. When in doubt, contact your local water plant, or have the water in your home analyzed for fluoride content. If it doesn't supply the recommended amount—1 part per million parts of water (1 ppm)—talk to your dentist about the best means for children to obtain the needed fluoride.

fluorapatite A tooth crystal containing fluoride ions that make the tooth relatively acid resistant.

FUNCTIONS OF FLUORIDE

Dietary fluoride during bone and teeth development aids the synthesis of **fluorapatite** crystals, rather than hydroxyapatite crystals (see Chapter 14). Only fluoride taken internally, whether in drinking water or dietary supplements, can strengthen developing teeth to resist decay. Once the teeth have erupted, they're beyond help from ingested fluoride. Fluorapatite crystals strongly resist acid, so teeth containing fluorapatite crystals are very resistant to dental caries. Fluoride also inhibits the growth of bacteria that cause dental caries (see Chapter 3 for a review of the development of dental caries).

For both children and adults, fluoride applied to the surface of the teeth can add some protection against dental caries. Dietary fluoride also improves growth rate in mice, but scientists are not sure if fluoride is actually necessary for growth in humans.

FLUORIDE IN FOODS

Tea, seafoods, seaweed, and some natural water sources are the only good food sources of fluoride. Most of our fluoride intake comes from water-fortification, toothpaste, and fluoride treatments performed by dentists. No evidence shows that water fluoridation in the United States at present levels is harmful.

ESADDI FOR FLUORIDE

The estimated safe and adequate daily dietary intake of fluoride for adults is 1.5 to 4 milligrams daily. The American Dental Association and the American Academy of Pediatrics recommend 0.25 milligrams per day up to age 1 year, 0.5 milligrams for ages 2 and 3 years, and 1 milligram after age 3 years and until the teen years. This range of intake provides the benefits of resistance to dental caries without causing mottling of the teeth.

TOXICITY OF FLUORIDE

A fluoride intake greater than 6 milligrams daily can mottle teeth during a developmental stage. High fluoride intake in adults does not cause mottling. In addition, when fluoride intakes reach 20 milligrams daily during tooth development, the tooth structure is weakened and can crumble. This is called fluorosis and appears in humans and other animals.

High doses of fluoride (20 or more milligrams per day) were used experimentally in adults to treat severe osteoporosis. This practice has recently been questioned for any real benefit because the bone formed has poor structural strength.[17] These dosages also can cause significant side effects, such as stomach upset and bone pain.

CONCEPT CHECK

Selenium is important for the activity of glutathione peroxidase, an enzyme that reduces the concentration of peroxides, lessening the free radical load in the body. In this way, selenium spares some of the need for vitamin E. A deficiency results in muscle and heart disorders. Organ meats, eggs, fish, and grains are good selenium sources; however, the selenium content in plants depends on the selenium concentration in the soil. A high selenium intake is potentially toxic. Iodide is vital in the synthesis of thyroid hormones. A prolonged insufficient intake will cause the thyroid gland to enlarge, resulting in a goiter. The use of iodized salt has virtually eliminated this condition in the United States. Fluoride incorporated into teeth during development makes them resistant to acid and bacterial growth, in turn reducing the chance of developing dental caries. Most of us get adequate amounts via water fortification and toothpaste. A high fluoride intake during tooth development can lead to spotted, or mottled, teeth.

Chromium

The importance of chromium (Cr) in human diets had been recognized only in the past 20 years. There is much we do not understand about this mineral, but chromium deficiency may be related to both diabetes and coronary heart disease.

FUNCTIONS OF CHROMIUM

The most studied function of chromium is the maintenance of normal glucose uptake into cells.[1,21] Researchers are not sure how chromium does this. Early work suggested that it formed a glucose tolerance factor with the vitamin niacin, but that is no longer accepted. Our current understanding is that chromium forms a type of complex that appears to help insulin bind to cells.

In both animals and man, a chromium deficiency is characterized by impaired glucose tolerance and elevated serum cholesterol and triglyceride levels. The mechanism by which chromium influences cholesterol metabolism is not known, but may involve enzymes that control cholesterol synthesis. Chromium deficiency appears in people maintained on total parenteral nutrition not supplemented with chromium and in children with malnutrition. Since sensitive measures of chromium status are not available, marginal chromium deficiencies may go undetected.

FOOD SOURCES OF CHROMIUM

Overall, there is little data regarding chromium values of foods. Egg yolks, whole grains (bran), and meats are good sources. Yeast is also a source. Fruits, vegetables, many seafoods, highly processed foods, and drinking water are generally poor sources. The ultimate chromium level in foods is closely tied to local soil content of chromium. To provide yourself with a good chromium intake, choose whole grains, as opposed to refined grains, when possible.

ESADDI FOR CHROMIUM

The estimated safe and adequate daily dietary intake of chromium is 50 to 200 micrograms daily. Average adult intakes are closer to 30 micrograms a day.[1] This is currently a concern of researchers in the area of study. Marginal to low chromium intakes in the elderly may contribute to their increased risk for developing diabetes. Studies show that chromium intakes of less than 20 micrograms per day may be detrimental to a significant portion of the population that has marginally elevated blood glucose. Some research also shows that an intake at the high end of the ESADDI, or slightly above, may raise HDL cholesterol levels. More studies are needed on this effect. Chromium toxicity has been reported in people exposed to industrial waste and in painters using art supplies with a very high chromium content. Liver damage and lung cancer can be the result.

Manganese

It is easy to confuse the mineral manganese (Mn) with magnesium (Mg). Their names are similar, and in a few metabolic pathways they often substitute for each other.

FUNCTIONS OF MANGANESE

Manganese is a cofactor for certain enzymes, such as pyruvate carboxylase, an important enzyme in carbohydrate metabolism.[2] Manganese is also important in bone formation. No human deficiency symptom is associated with a low manganese intake. Animals on manganese-deficient diets show changes in physiological functions, such as alterations in brain function, bone formation, and reproduction. If human diets were low in manganese, these problems would probably appear as well. As it happens, our need for manganese is very low, and our diets tend to be quite high in manganese.

Table 15-6 A summary of the major trace minerals

Mineral	Major functions	Deficiency symptoms	People most at risk	RDA or ESADDI	Dietary sources	Results of toxicity
Iron	Part of hemoglobin, myoglobin and cytochromes; used for immune function.	Low serum ferritin levels; small, pale red blood cells; low blood hemoglobin and hematocrit values.	Infants, preschool children, adolescents, women in child-bearing years, some endurance athletes.	Men: 10 milligrams. Women: 15 milligrams.	Meats, spinach, seafood, broccoli, peas, bran, enriched breads	Toxicity is seen when children consume 200-400 milligrams in iron pills, and in people with hemochromatosis. In this case people overabsorb iron.
Zinc	Part of over 200 enzymes. These include enzymes involved in growth, immunity, alcohol metabolism, sexual development, and reproduction.	Skin rash, diarrhea, decreased appetite and sense of taste, hair loss, poor growth and development, poor wound healing.	Vegetarians, the elderly.	Men: 15 milligrams. Women: 12 milligrams.	Seafoods, meats, greens, whole grains	Reduces iron and copper absorption; causes diarrhea, cramps, and depressed immune function.
Copper	Aids in iron metabolism; part of many enzymes, such as those involved in protein metabolism and hormone synthesis.	Anemia, low white blood cell (neutrophil) count, poor growth.	Infants recovering from malnutrition, intestinal surgery patients, and overzealous supplementation of zinc.	1.5-3 milligrams	Liver, cocoa, beans, nuts, whole grains, dried fruits	Vomiting; nervous system disorders.
Selenium	Aids in peroxide metabolism, as is part of gluthathione peroxidase.	Muscle pain, muscle weakness, heart disease.	Unknown.	55-70 micrograms.	Meats, eggs, fish, milk, seafoods; whole grains	Nausea, vomiting, hair loss, weakness, liver disease.

Table 15-6 A summary of the major trace minerals—cont'd

Mineral	Major functions	Deficiency symptoms	People most at risk	RDA or ESADDI	Dietary sources	Results of toxicity
Iodide	Part of thyroid hormone.	Goiter; poor growth in infancy when mother is deficient in pregnancy.	No one in the United States, as salt is usually fortified.	150 micrograms.	Iodized salt, white bread, saltwater fish, dairy products.	Inhibition of function of the thyroid gland.
Fluoride	Increases resistance of tooth crystal to acidic erosion.	Increased risk of dental caries.	People in areas where water is not fluoridated and dental treatments do not make up for this lack of fluoride.	1.5-4 milligrams.	Fluoridated water, toothpaste, dental treatments, tea, seaweed.	Stomach upset, mottling (staining) of teeth during development.
Chromium	May increase action of the hormone insulin.	High blood glucose levels after eating.	People on total parenteral nutrition, and perhaps elderly people with adult-onset diabetes mellitus.	50-200 micrograms.	Egg yolks, whole grains, pork	Due to industrial contamination, not dietary excess.
Manganese	Part of some enzymes, such as those involved in carbohydrate metabolism.	None in humans.	Unknown.	2-5 milligrams.	Nuts, rice, oats, beans.	Unknown in humans.
Molybdenum	Part of enzymes, such as xanthine dehydrogenase.	None in humans.	Unknown	75-250 micrograms.	Beans, grains, and nuts.	Unknown in humans.

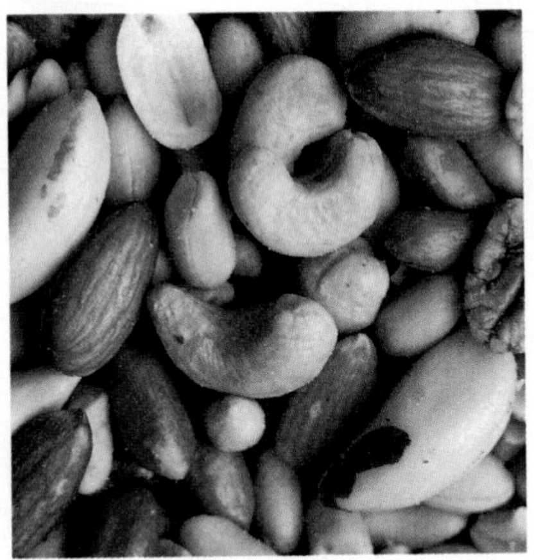
Nuts are a good source of manganese.

MANGANESE IN FOODS

Good food sources of manganese are nuts, rice, oats and other whole grains, beans, and leafy vegetables. The estimated safe and adequate daily dietary intake of manganese is 2 to 5 milligrams daily. Studies of young men show that an intake of 3.5 milligrams per day meets their manganese needs. Manganese is toxic at high doses, as evidenced by toxicity that appears in miners of manganese.

Molybdenum

Molybdenum (Mo) is notable for its interactions with iron and copper, especially inhibition of copper absorption.

FUNCTIONS OF MOLYBDENUM

Several enzymes, including **xanthine dehydrogenase** and a related form, xanthine oxidase, require molybdenum. The oxidase form of the enzyme is produced from the dehydrogenase form during tissue injury. No molybdenum deficiency has been noted in a person consuming a normal diet, though deficiency symptoms have appeared in people on total parenteral nutrition. These symptoms include increased heart and respiration rates, night blindness, mental confusion, edema, and weakness.

xanthine dehydrogenase An enzyme containing molybdenum and iron that functions in the formation of uric acid and the mobilization of iron from liver ferritin stores.

MOLYBDENUM IN FOODS

Good food sources of molybdenum include beans, whole grains, and nuts. The estimated safe and adequate daily dietary intake for molybdenum is 75 to 250 micrograms per day. A minimum intake for good health is probably about 80 to 115 micrograms per day. When consumed in high doses, symptoms of molybdenum toxicity in animals include weight loss and decreased growth.

Other Trace Minerals

A variety of minerals are found in the body for which researchers are still trying to justify a human need. We probably consume too much of these minerals to suffer a deficiency, and if truly needed they are required by few enzymes or metabolic systems. We briefly note them here because as more research is reported, these may achieve more importance. If you have a concept of their roles in the body, you can put new research into perspective. And you can refute the need for widespread use of supplements based on what we know now.

BORON

Boron (B) is an important growth factor for plants. Research in the early 1980s suggested that boron in humans is involved in the metabolism of steroid (cholesterol-containing) hormones, such as the vitamin D hormone calcitriol and the estrogens.[22] Good sources of boron include noncitrus fruits, leafy vegetables, nuts, and beans. Meats and fish are poor sources. Adults need about 0.5 to 1 milligram daily. Human intakes vary widely.

NICKEL

Plants and animals need nickel (Ni) for the activity of certain enzymes, and perhaps for iron metabolism.[22] Humans have never shown a deficiency of nickel when consuming a normal diet. Good food sources of nickel include nuts, beans, grains, and chocolate. Researchers estimate adults need less than 100 micrograms of nickel per day. Our diets supply much more than this.

VANADIUM

Vanadium (V) aids in the activity of some enzymes, such as those involved in sodium and potassium transport in the red blood cell.[22] To produce a vanadium deficiency in animals, researchers need to use an ultra-clean environment. Even the air must be filtered. Good food sources of vanadium include shellfish, mushrooms, and grain products. Researchers estimate adult vanadium needs are less than 10 micrograms per day. Our dietary intakes exceed this amount, so humans do not run a risk for a vanadium deficiency.

ARSENIC

While arsenic (As) is a very poisonous compound, animals need it in small amounts to metabolize protein and amino acids, especially methionine and taurine.[22] Researchers estimate adults need about 12 micrograms per day. There is no known human deficiency of arsenic. Food sources include fish, grains, and cereal products.

POSSIBLE ESSENTIAL MINERALS

We can add lithium, silicone, tin, cadmium, and cobalt (Li, Si, Sn, Cd, and Co, respectively) to the list of minerals that humans possibly need. Animal data suggest that human needs are possible, but this is unconfirmed. Of course, we need cobalt in the form of vitamin B-12, and there is some speculation that dietary cobalt may be synthesized into vitamin B-12 in the human intestines by bacteria. However, this is not known. For cobalt needs, food sources of vitamin B-12 should be the focus.

CONCEPT CHECK

Chromium may act to increase the action of the hormone insulin. The amount of chromium found in food depends on soil content. Vegetable oils, whole grains, and egg yolks are some of the better sources. Manganese is a component of bone and many enzymes, including those involved in glucose production. Since our need for it is low, deficiencies are rare. Good food sources are nuts, rice, oats, and beans. Molybdenum is a component of enzymes. Deficiencies appear only with total parenteral nutrition. Beans, grains, and nuts are good sources. The needs for some other trace minerals, such as boron, nickel, arsenic, and vanadium, have not been fully established in humans. They are required in such small amounts that our current diets are probably adequate.

See Table 15-6 to review what we have covered on trace minerals.

Summary

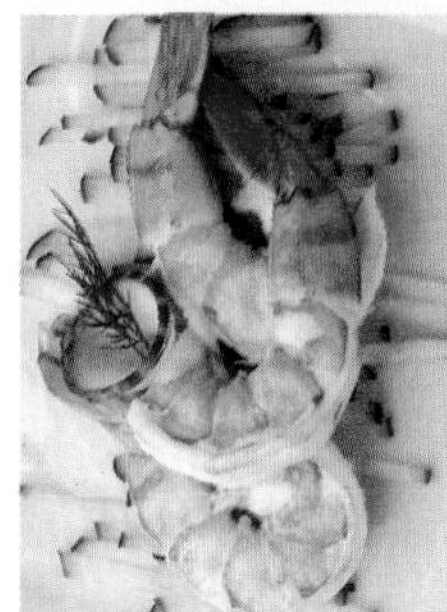

1. Some trace mineral deficiencies are difficult to detect in humans and were first observed in small geographically isolated groups or in patients on total parenteral nutrition. Eating a variety of foods maximizes your chances of consuming adequate amounts of trace minerals. Supplementing with trace minerals is potentially harmful, since so many questions remain regarding daily needs and interactions.
2. Iron is the only nutrient for which the RDA is greater in adult women than men because of women's iron losses that occur during menstruation. Iron absorption depends mainly on the form of iron present and the body's need for it. Heme iron from animal sources is better absorbed that the nonheme iron obtained primarily from plant sources. Consuming vitamin C simultaneously with iron will increase nonheme absorption.
3. The main function of iron is for synthesizing hemoglobin and myoglobin. It is also important in the synthesis of some enzymes, cytochromes, and in the action of the immune system. A prolonged low iron intake can lead to decreased production of red blood cells, and in turn reduced ability of the blood to carry sufficient oxygen. Such a condition is called iron-deficiency anemia and may result in fatigue, apathy, and decreased learning ability.

4. Foods rich in iron include beef, oysters, broccoli, and liver. Other sources are spinach and enriched breads and cereals. However, iron from plant sources is not well absorbed. Iron toxicity usually results from a genetic disorder called hemochromatosis. This disease causes overabsorption and accumulation of iron, which can result in severe liver and heart damage.
5. Zinc functions as a cofactor for over 200 enzymes that are important for growth, development, immune function, wound healing, and taste sensation. A zinc deficiency results in poor growth, loss of appetite, poor mental function, reduced sense of taste and smell, hair loss, and a persistent rash.
6. Zinc is best absorbed from animal sources, especially when body needs are high. A mucosal block in the intestinal cells regulates zinc absorption in a manner similar to that of iron. Both iron and copper compete with zinc for absorption, especially when all are consumed as supplements. The most nutrient-dense sources of zinc are oysters, shrimp, crab, and beef. Good plant sources are whole grains, peanuts, and beans.
7. Copper is important for iron metabolism, collagen cross-bonding, nerve cell myelination, and scavenging of free-radicals. A copper deficiency can result in microcytic, hypochromic anemia and rupture of blood vessels. Copper is found mainly in liver, cocoa, legumes, and whole grains. Milk is a poor source. Soil content greatly affects the copper content in plants.
8. The most important role of selenium is as a cofactor in the glutathione peroxidase system, which reduces the production of free radicals. In this way, selenium reduces the need for vitamin E, whose role is to neutralize free radicals once they are produced. Muscle pain, muscle wasting, and heart disease may result from a selenium deficiency. Meats, especially organ meats, eggs, fish, and shellfish, are good animal sources of selenium. Good plant sources include grains and seeds. Selenium is potentially toxic because there is no physiological control on the amount absorbed. Symptoms of toxicity are a garlicky breath odor, hair loss, weakness, nausea, and vomiting.
9. Iodide forms part of the thyroid hormones. A lack of dietary iodide results in the development of a goiter. Iodized salt is a good food source. Fluoride incorporated into teeth during development makes them resistant to dental caries. Most Americans receive the bulk of their fluoride from fluoridated water and toothpaste.
10. Chromium may help increase the action of insulin. Meats and whole grains are good sources of chromium. Manganese and molybdenum contribute to the activity of various enzymes. Deficiencies are rarely seen for all three of these nutrients. The body's need for other trace minerals is so low that deficiencies are uncommon.

Study Questions

1. Minerals in the diet are likely to interact with each other. Provide two examples of this for trace minerals.
2. Describe how a "mucosal block" lessens the risk of developing an iron or zinc toxicity state.
3. Outline the histories of iodide and fluoride in human nutrition—from epidemiological observations to dietary intervention.
4. Relate the role of two nutrients to immune function, including at least one trace mineral.
5. Describe what is meant by a marginal deficiency state with respect to trace minerals. What two factors make studying this state of health difficult?

REFERENCES

1. Anderson RA and others: Supplemental-chromium effects on glucose, insulin, glucagon, and urinary chromium losses in subjects consuming controlled low-chromium diets, *American Journal of Clinical Nutrition* 54:909, 1991.
2. Anonymous: Manganese deficiency in humans: fact or fiction? *Nutrition Reviews* 46:348, 1988.
3. Black MR and others: Zinc supplements and serum lipids in young adult white males, *American Journal of Clinical Nutrition* 47:970, 1988.
4. Castillo-Duran C, Uauy R: Copper deficiency impairs growth in infants recovering from malnutrition, *American Journal of Clinical Nutrition* 47:710, 1988.
5. Chandra RK: 1990 McCollum Award Lecture. Nutrition and immunity: lessons from the past and new insights into the future, *American Journal of Clinical Nutrition* 53:1087, 1991.
6. Clydesdale FM: The relevance of mineral chemistry to bioavailability, *Nutrition Today,* March/April 1989, p 23.
7. Cook JD and others: Calcium supplementation: effect on iron absorption, *American Journal of Clinical Nutrition* 53:106, 1991.
8. Cook JD and others: Assessment of the role of nonheme-iron availability in iron balance, *American Journal of Clinical Nutrition* 54:717, 1991.
9. Cook JD: Adaptation in iron metabolism, *American Journal of Clinical Nutrition* 51:301, 1990.
10. Danks DM: Copper deficiency in humans, *Annual Reviews of Nutrition* 8:235, 1988.
11. Dunn JT: Iodine deficiency—the next target for elimination? *The New England Journal of Medicine* 326:267, 1992.
12. Fosmire GJ: Zinc toxicity, *American Journal of Clinical Nutrition* 51:225, 1990.
13. Gable CB: Hemochromatosis and dietary iron supplementation: implications from U.S. mortality, morbidity, and health survey data, *Journal of The American Dietetic Association* 92:208, 1992.
14. Johnson MA, Kays SE: Copper: its role in human nutrition, *Nutrition Today,* Jan/Feb 1990, p 6.
15. Kinney TB, DeLuca SA: Idiopathic hemochromatosis, *American Family Physician* 44:873, 1991.
16. Klevay LM and others: Hair analysis in clinical and experimental medicine, *American Journal of Clinical Nutrition* 46:233, 1987.
17. Kleerekoper M, Balena R: Fluorides and osteoporosis, *Annual Reviews of Nutrition* 11:309, 1991.
18. Levander OA: Scientific rationale for the 1989 Recommended Dietary Allowance for selenium, *Journal of The American Dietetic Association* 91:1572, 1991.
19. Lozoff B and others: Long-term developmental outcome of infants with iron deficiency, *The New England Journal of Medicine* 325:687, 1991.
20. Monsen ER: Iron nutrition and absorption: dietary factors which impact iron bioavailability, *Journal of The American Dietetic Association* 88:786, 1988.
21. Morris BW and others: The trace element chromium—a role in glucose homeostasis, *American Journal of Clinical Nutrition* 55:989, 1992.
22. Nielsen FH: Nutritional requirements for boron, silicon, vanadium, nickel, and arsenic: current knowledge and speculation, *FASEB Journal* 5:2661, 1991.
23. Oldfield JE: Some implications of selenium for human health, *Nutrition Today,* July/Aug 1991, p 6.
24. Pennington JAT and others: Nutritional elements in U.S. Diets, *Journal of The American Dietetic Association* 89:859, 1989.
25. Prasad AS: Discovery of human zinc deficiency and studies in an experimental human model, *American Journal of Clinical Nutrition* 53:403, 1991.
26. Reddy MB, Cook JD: Assessment of dietary determinants of nonheme-iron absorption in humans and rats, *American Journal of Clinical Nutrition* 54:723, 1991.
27. Robinson MF: Selenium in human nutrition in New Zealand, *Nutrition Reviews* 47:99, 1989.
28. Sanstead HH: Discovery of zinc deficiency in patients receiving total parenteral alimentation, clinical correlations, *Nutrition* 5:21, 1989.
29. Scrimshaw NS: Iron deficiency, *Scientific American,* Oct 1991, p 46.
30. Siegenberg D and others: Ascorbic acid prevents the dose-dependent inhibitory effects of polyphenols and phytates on nonheme-iron absorption, *American Journal of Clinical Nutrition* 53:537, 1991.
31. Simmer K and others: Nutritional rehabilitation in Bangladesh—the importance of zinc, *American Journal of Clinical Nutrition* 47:1036, 1988.
32. Taylor CM and others: Homeostatic regulation of zinc absorption and endogenous losses in zinc-deprived men, *American Journal of Clinical Nutrition* 53:755, 1991.
33. Tershakovec AM, Weller SC: Iron status of inner-city elementary school children: lack of correlation between anemia and iron deficiency, *American Journal of Clinical Nutrition* 54:1071, 1991.

SUGGESTED READINGS

To learn more about iron metabolism and iron deficiency see the articles by Cook and others, as well as the one by Scrimshaw. Then, look at the article by Kinney and DeLuca to learn more about hemochromatosis. This will allow you to see both sides of iron—its essential and toxic natures. To learn more about copper, see the article by Johnson and Kays. Then review the article by Levander on selenium. These articles provide an excellent background on these two exciting trace minerals. Finally, Nielsen discusses our current knowledge for some of the more misunderstood trace elements, providing a window into our needs for future nutrition research.

TAKE ACTION

How does your trace mineral intake measure up?

To complete this activity you must reexamine the nutritional assessment you did for Chapter 2. Compare your intake of selective minerals to their RDA or ESADDI, using the completed assessment you did when you analyzed your nutritional intake for 1 day. In the table below, for each mineral, record your intake, the RDA or ESADDI, the percentage of the RDA or ESADDI you consumed, and a +, −, or =, indicating an intake higher, lower, or equal to the RDA or ESADDI.

MINERAL	INTAKE	RDA or ESADDI	% of RDA or ESADDI	+, −, =
Iron				
Zinc				
Selenium				
Copper				

Analysis

1. Which of your mineral intakes equaled or exceeded the RDA or ESADDI?

____

2. Which of your intakes were below the standard for your age and gender?

____

3. What foods or cooking practices could be emphasized or deemphasized to modify your weaknesses?

____

____

____

____

____

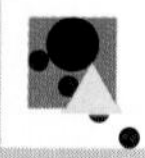

Nutrients and Immunity

We have frequently mentioned the importance of good nutrition for proper immune function in this book. Early humans were plagued by famine, infections, and death. Many of us now, due to better nutrition, can avoid that cycle. Some of us, striving for optimum nutrition, even go too far; excess quantities do not further boost immunity and can in fact decrease it. Let's review some major components of the immune system—the skin, intestinal cells, and white blood cells—and consider how nutrient intake affects each component (Figure 15-9).

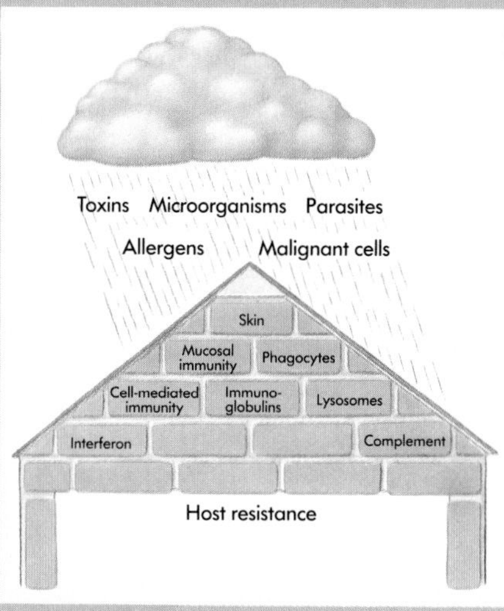

Figure 15-9 Host protective factors. The immune system has many "arms"—all are influenced by nutrient intake.

Skin

The skin forms an almost continuous barrier surrounding the body. Invading microorganisms have difficulty penetrating the skin. However, if the skin is split by lesions, bacteria can easily penetrate this barrier.[5] Nutrient deficiencies that reduce the health of the skin include those of essential fatty acids, vitamin A, niacin, and zinc. Vitamin A deficiency also decreases gland secretions in the skin, which contain enzymes that kill bacteria. Recall that in a vitamin A deficiency, a bacterial infection of the eye is often seen (see Chapter 12).

Intestinal Cells

The cells of the intestines form an important barrier to invading microorganisms. Not only are the cells closely packed together, but also antibody-producing cells are scattered throughout the intestinal tract. These antibodies bind invading microorganisms, preventing them from entering the bloodstream. The production of these antibodies is low during protein and vitamin A undernutrition.

In undernutrition, the intestinal cells break down so that microorganisms more easily enter the body and cause infections. Two common results are diarrhea and bacterial infections of the bloodstream.[5] To protect the health of the intestinal tract, an adequate nutrient intake is necessary, especially of protein, vitamin A, vitamin B-6, folate, vitamin B-12, vitamin C, zinc, and other nutrients needed for intestinal cell synthesis and maintenance.

White Blood Cells

Once a microorganism enters the bloodstream, white blood cells attack it. A variety of white blood cells participate in this response, including **neutrophils, B-lymphocytes, T-lymphocytes,** and macrophages. As a group, together with specialized proteins called **complements,** these cells make antibodies to bind to microorganisms, engulf and digest them, and then create a template (memory) that allows future recognition of the organism. Recognition allows more rapid attacks in the future (see Figure 15-10).

neutrophil The major form for white blood cells, comprising 55% to 65% of their total number.

β-lymphocyte White blood cells processed by liver and spleen tissues that are responsible for antibody production.

T-lymphocyte White blood cells processed by the thymus gland and responsible for recognition of foreign substances (such as bacteria) in the body.

complement A group of serum proteins involved in immune responses, such as phagocytosis and destruction of bacteria.

Your nutrient intake affects these white blood cells and protein factors. Some white blood cells live only a few days. Their constant resynthesis requires a steady nutrient input. The immune system needs iron to produce an important killing factor that is used; it needs copper for the synthesis of neutrophils; and it needs adequate amounts of vitamin C, protein, vitamin B-6, folate, and vitamin B-12 for general cell synthesis and, later, cell activity. Zinc and vitamin A are also needed for the overall growth and development of the immune cells.[5]

A deficiency of any of these nutrients compromises the ability of the white blood cells and the complement protein system to seek and destroy invading microorganisms. In addition, during undernutrition, the thymus gland shrinks. This is the place where T-lymphocytes mature before they enter the bloodstream.

One proof that nutrition is important to immune status is the body's response to microorganisms; microorganisms normally present in the body usually cause disease only in severely undernourished people.[5] A good example is measles. Your parents probably have had this viral infection and survived. (You were probably vaccinated against measles.) However, many undernourished children who contract it die. Thus

Nutrients and Immunity—cont'd

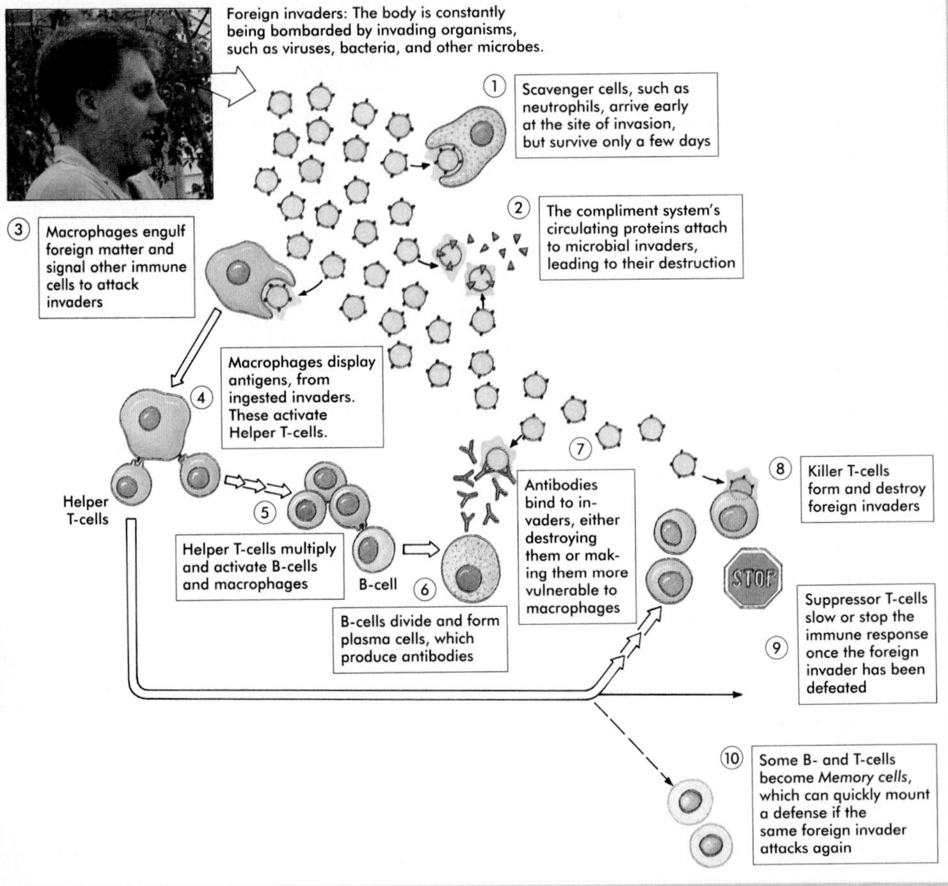

Figure 15-10 Biological warfare. The body commands a wide assortment of defenders to reduce the danger of infection and help guard against repeat microbial infections.

In the early 1970s, physicians began feeding patients with major body burns much sooner then they had in the past. This earlier feeding dramatically reduced the number of infections (by 80%) that burn patients suffered and thus greatly improved their chances of surviving. A major reason for this improved survival is the earlier supply of nutrients to support immune function.

the presence of microorganism in the body does not guarantee its triumph over the immune system, but if a person's health is already compromised through undernutrition, the chances of a destructive microorganism winning are greater.

The white blood cell count, especially the number of T-lymphocytes and β-lymphocytes in the blood, can predict the chances of either complications or death in hospitalized patients. When the lymphocyte count is low, disease and death are much more likely. In the future, when you see poorly nourished people in hospitals, at a senior citizen center, or your neighborhood, remember that their poor nutrient intake is compromising not only the function of their liver, kidneys, and other organs, but also their immune systems.

A Note of Caution

Many studies show that a good nutritional status is associated with good immune status. However, other studies also show that an overabundance of certain nutrients can actually harm the immune system. High intakes of polyunsaturated fatty acids and vitamin E have been implicated in a decreased immune response in mice. Excess intakes of zinc (300 milligrams per day for 6 weeks) also appear to decrease immune function.[12] This decrease may be partially due to zinc's interference with copper absorption. The copper deficiency contributes to decreased synthesis of neutrophils, a class of white blood cells.

The message here is that eating a balanced diet will help you maintain the health of all components of the immune system. Your body needs this defense to continuously protect you from environmental pathogens. However, consuming nutrients in excess of needs is not going to boost the immune system to even higher abilities. In fact, this may harm certain aspects of immune function.

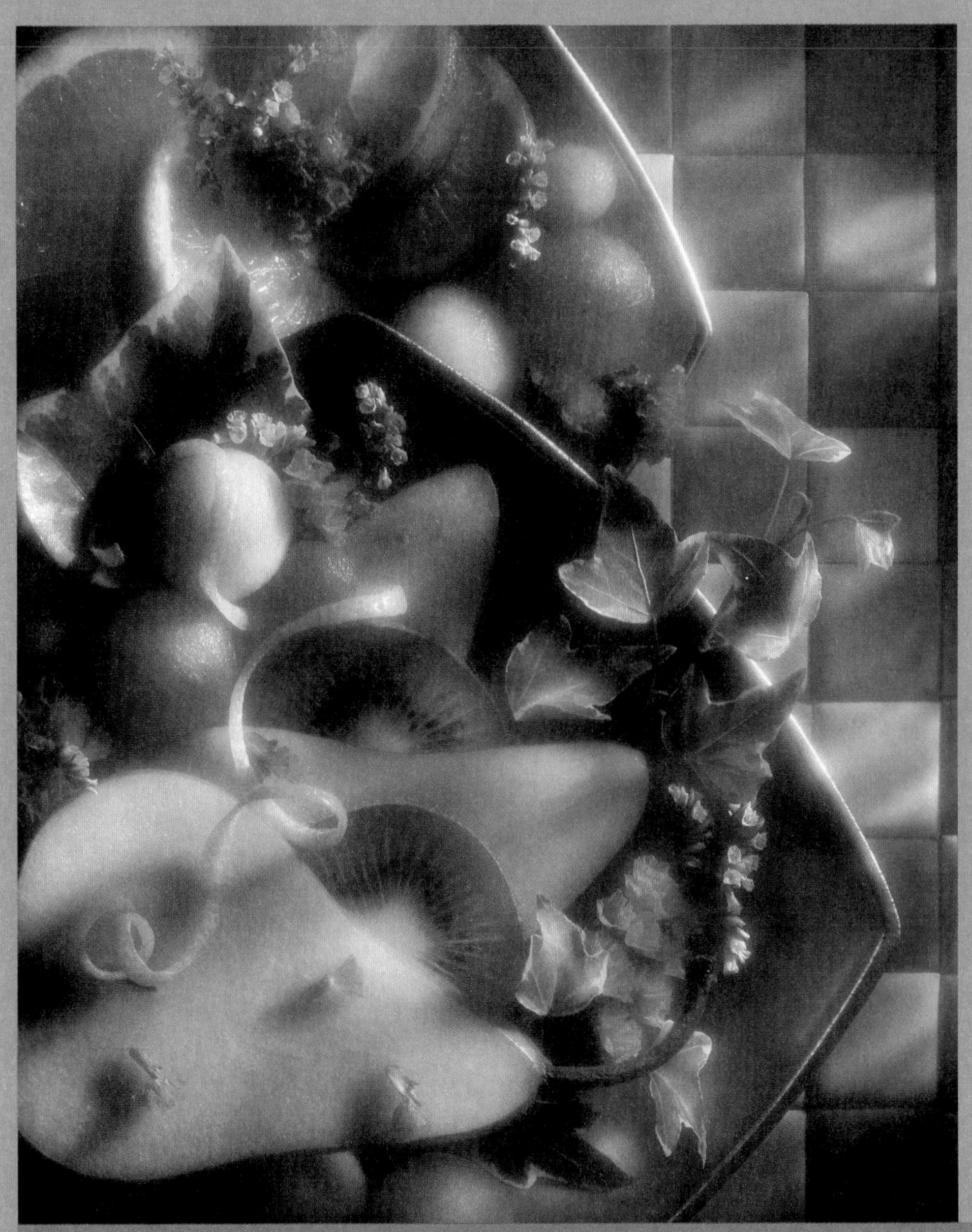

PART FIVE

Nutrition Applications in the Life Cycle

CHAPTER SIXTEEN

Pregnancy and Lactation

Pregnancy can be one of the most special times in a parent's life. Along with the responsibility of shaping a child's health and personality comes the exhilaration of contributing to a new life. This is an especially important time for nutrition to come into focus. We should be very receptive to nutrition information, striving to do everything possible to maximize the chances of turning the dream of a healthy baby into reality.

The reality, however, is that the infant mortality rate in the United States is higher than that of 21 other industrialized nations. In the United States 40,000 infants per year die before their first birthday. One of three pregnant women receives inadequate prenatal care, and in recent years 73,000 women annually received no prenatal care. These are alarming statistics for our country with its high per capita expenditure for health care.[5]

Producing a healthy baby is not just a matter of luck. While some aspects of fetal and newborn health are beyond our control, conscious decisions about social, health, and nutritional factors affect the baby's health and future. What we do can directly relate to the likelihood of having a healthy newborn, while at the same time not tearing away at the mother's health.[22] *Let's examine what contributes to making a healthy pregnancy for both mother and baby more than just a dream.*

NUTRITION AWARENESS INVENTORY

Here are 15 statements about pregnancy and lactation. Answer them to test your current knowledge. If you think the answer is true or mostly true, circle T. If you think the answer is false or mostly false, circle F. Use the scoring key at the end of the book to compute your total score. Take this test again after you have read the chapter. Compare the results.

1. T F Infants weighing less than 5.5 pounds (2500 grams) at birth are more likely to have medical problems than those weighing more than 2500 grams.
2. T F The most crucial time for fetal development is during the last 13 weeks of pregnancy.
3. T F Nutritional factors are more important than genetic factors in determining birth weight.
4. T F Pregnant women have increased energy needs.
5. T F Most women should gain about 25 to 35 pounds during pregnancy.
6. T F Poor food choices during pregnancy are more common than low-kcalorie intakes in developed countries.
7. T F Pregnant women know instinctively what to eat.
8. T F Mineral needs increase during pregnancy.
9. T F Pregnancy can precipitate a form of diabetes.
10. T F Breast-fed infants suffer fewer respiratory infections than formula-fed infants.
11. T F A major barrier to breast-feeding is often a lack of information.
12. T F Mothers who must take medications that pass into the milk should check with their doctor before continuing to breast-feed.
13. T F The placenta is the site of oxygen and nutrient transfer from the mother to the fetus.
14. T F Most miscarriages occur during the first trimester.
15. T F Cow's milk can be substituted for human milk when an infant is 2 to 3 months old.

Prenatal Growth and Development

The life of an embryo begins when an egg and sperm unite. A baby is born about 40 weeks later. This first form of life grows through the **embryo** stage and is known as a fetus after 8 weeks of development. The mother nourishes this offspring via a **placenta** that forms in her uterus. The placenta serves to accommodate growth and development of the offspring throughout gestation (Figure 16-1). Many times a woman does not suspect she is pregnant during these first few weeks, and often does not seek medical attention until after the first 3 months (first **trimester**).

embryo The developing human life form during the second to eighth week after conception.

placenta An organ formed in a women only during pregnancy that secretes hormones and makes possible the transfer of oxygen and nutrients from the mother's blood to the fetus, as well as removal of fetal wastes.

trimester The normal pregnancy of 38 to 42 weeks is divided into three, 13- to 14-week periods, called trimesters.

Even without fanfare, the embryo grows and develops daily. For that reason, the health and nutritional habits of a woman several years before pregnancy and while she is trying to become pregnant—or has the potential of becoming pregnant—are particularly important. For example, a history of anorexia nervosa or bulimia does not set the stage for a healthy pregnancy. Since prepregnancy dietary habits can affect the health of a newborn, good nutrition is especially critical during a woman's childbearing years.[6] We know that certain nutritional deficiencies, use of certain medications (even aspirin), other drugs, and alcohol can all cause detrimental effects in the growing embryo, and later in the fetus. This is true for the weeks before the woman realizes she is pregnant. Much research suggests that an adequate vitamin and mineral intake in the months before conception and during pregnancy may help prevent birth defects, such as neural tube defects.[9] For these reasons, it is important for parents to be aware of the role nutrition plays in the development of a healthy baby.

The view that life begins at conception currently is a topic of much controversy and debate.

The time to focus on good nutritional and other health habits, then, is before a woman becomes pregnant. Maternal nutrition should be a focus during all phases of reproductive life—from childhood to menopause—to ensure that all women are in good health (including good nutritional status) at the time of conception. Good habits can then be carried into pregnancy, thereby providing optimum health and nutrition from before conception until birth.

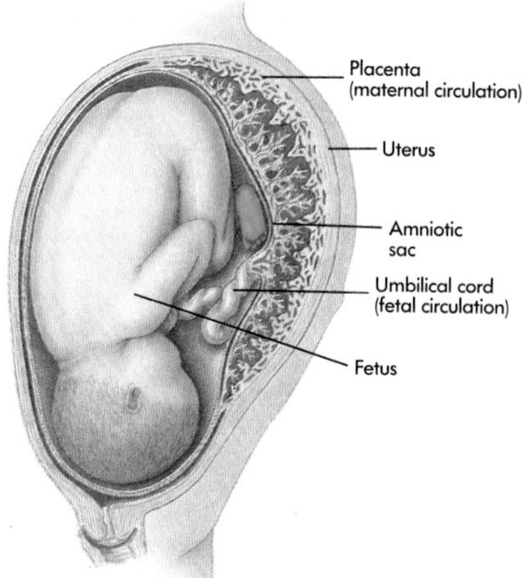

Figure 16-1 The fetus in relation to the placenta. This is the organ through which nourishment flows to the fetus.

FETAL GROWTH

Fetal growth begins with a rapid increase in cell number (hyperplasia). This type of growth dominates fetal development. The newly formed cells then begin to grow larger (hypertrophy; see Chapter 8 to review these terms). Further growth and development of the fetus is then a combination of hyperplasia and hypertrophy. At about 3 weeks, cells begin to form specialized organs and body parts. By the end of 13 weeks, the heart is complete and beating, most organs are formed, and the fetus can move (Figure 16-2).

At any stage of development an insult (injury) to the fetus caused by nutritional deficiencies, medications and other drugs, radiation, trauma, or other factors can alter or arrest the specific phase of growth and development in progress. Some effects—like cleft palate and missing limbs—can last a lifetime. The most critical time for fetal development is the first trimester, especially weeks two through eight. During this period most premature terminations of pregnancy occur. Currently, about one third of all pregnancies result in spontaneous abortion, often so early that the woman does not realize she was pregnant. These usually result from a genetic defect or fatal error in fetal development.

During this first trimester, then, a woman must be especially careful to avoid substances that may harm the developing fetus. Vitamin A, for example, when taken in large doses by the mother can result in serious fetal malformations. In addition, development is so rapid during the first trimester that if a nutrient essential to development is not sufficiently supplied, the growing fetus may be affected even before the mother shows deficiency signs. Even though many women experience loss of appetite and nausea during the first trimester, adequate nutrition is still extremely important.

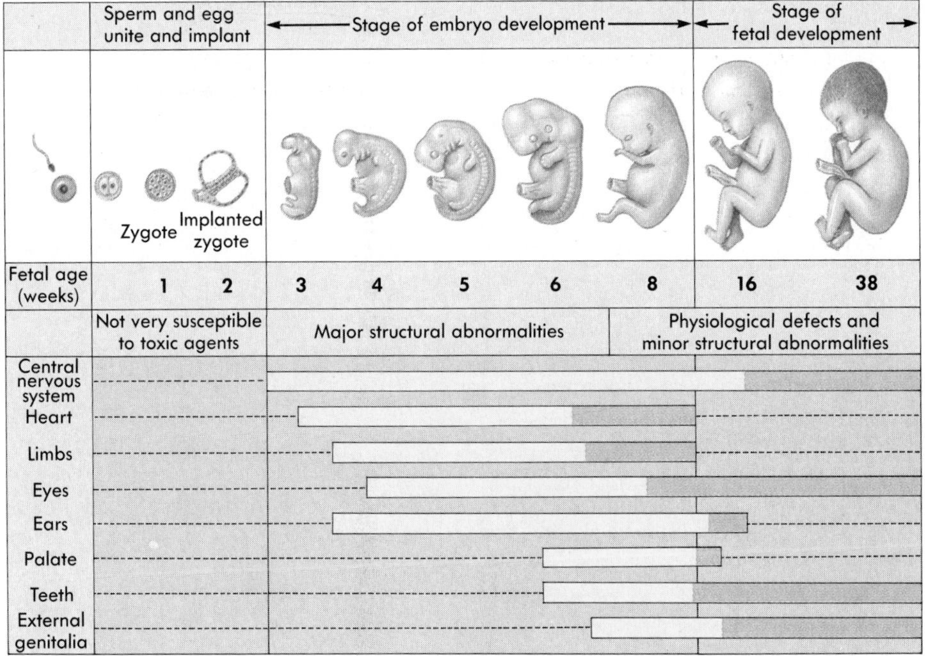

Figure 16-2 Vulnerable periods of development. The most serious damage from exposure to toxins is likely to occur during the first 8 weeks after conception. The lighter bars indicate the time of greatest risk to the organ. As the chart shows, however, damage to vital parts of the body—including the eyes, brain, and genitals—also can occur during the last months of pregnancy.

THE SECOND TRIMESTER

By the beginning of the second trimester, a fetus weighs about 1 ounce. Arms, hands, fingers, legs, feet, and toes are fully formed. The fetus has ears and is beginning to form tooth sockets in its jawbone. During this phase of development organs continue to grow and mature, and a physician can detect a heart beat. Most bones will be distinctly evident throughout the body. Eventually the fetus begins to look more like a baby. It might suck its thumb and it may kick strongly enough to be felt by the mother.

THE THIRD TRIMESTER

gestation The time of fetal growth from conception to birth; a period of about 40 weeks.

premature An infant born before 38 weeks of gestation.

By the beginning of the third trimester, a fetus weighs approximately 2 to 3 pounds. After about 28 to 30 weeks of **gestation**, there is a good chance of survival for a **premature** infant if cared for in a nursery for high-risk newborns.[31] However, the infant will be deficient in mineral and fat stores normally accumulated in the last month of gestation. This and other medical problems complicate nutritional care. At 9 months, the fetus weighs about 7 to 8 pounds (about 3.5 kilograms) and is about 20 inches long (about 50 centimeters). There is an especially large soft spot

EXPERT OPINION

What Do I Really Have to Give up When I'm Pregnant?

BONNIE WORTHINGTON-ROBERTS, Ph.D., R.D.

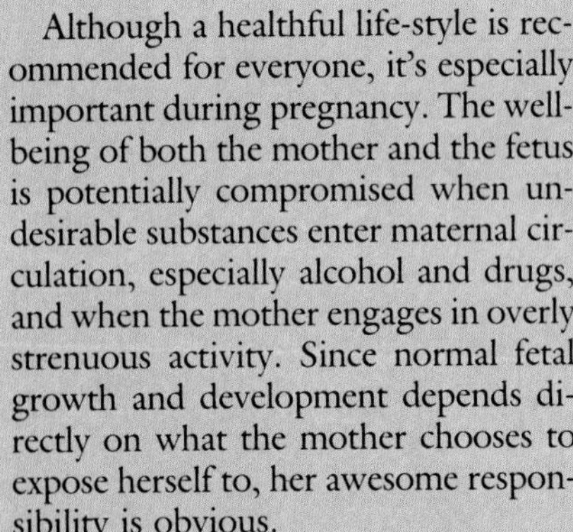

Although a healthful life-style is recommended for everyone, it's especially important during pregnancy. The well-being of both the mother and the fetus is potentially compromised when undesirable substances enter maternal circulation, especially alcohol and drugs, and when the mother engages in overly strenuous activity. Since normal fetal growth and development depends directly on what the mother chooses to expose herself to, her awesome responsibility is obvious.

Smoking

It's widely known that smoking during pregnancy increases the risk of both premature delivery and low birth weight. (It is also suspected of increasing the risk of congenital malformations, sudden infant death, and childhood cancer.) These serious problems are believed to be related to the physiological, biochemical, and/or hormonal effects of nicotine, carbon monoxide, and possibly other compounds present in cigarette smoke. Significant dietary deficits have not been identified in pregnant women who smoke.

Exercise

Physical activity during pregnancy is generally advocated, especially for women who have been quite active before pregnancy. Not surprisingly, pregnant women who are involved in regular exercise programs have shown an improved self-image during pregnancy and higher fitness scores by their delivery date. But as was covered in the chapter, common sense is in order. Clearly, what needs to be exercised is basically moderation, especially during the last trimester.

Diet

Caffeine

There are very few dietary restrictions for pregnant women. Alcohol is a well-known exception, as is discussed in the Nutrition Perspective. The potential danger of caffeine use during pregnancy also deserves consideration. This has been debated for quite some time. Although evidence so far doesn't justify recommending abstinence during pregnancy, several recent epidemiological studies have come up with some provocative findings. In one case, moderate-to-heavy caffeine users were found to have a significantly greater risk of spontaneous abortion during the late first and second trimesters than women who used less caffeine. Moderate caffeine use was defined as consumption of at least 150 milligrams of caffeine per day, which is equivalent to no more than about 1.5 cups of coffee daily. A second study concluded that the risk of low birth weight rose as the level of daily caffeine use increased. The risk was more than 4.5 times greater for women who consumed more than 300 milligrams of caffeine daily than for women who used no caffeine at all. Even though additional research is needed to confirm these observations, it seems justifiable at this point to advocate moderation in caffeine consumption during pregnancy.

Food additives

Unfortunately, some pregnant women are frightened by rumors that various food additives cause abnormal fetal development. This fear is largely unjustified. True, we don't know the cause of most birth defects and, theoretically, some substances in the food supply may be problematic, but there's no proof of such relationships. Regulations currently enforced by the FDA mandate in the upper head (fontanel) where the bones of the skull are growing together. It takes about 12 to 18 months for that soft spot to close.

Although a mother's decisions, practices, and precautions during pregnancy contribute to the health of the fetus, she cannot guarantee the fetus good health. Some genetic and environmental factors are beyond her control. Professionals should not foster an unrealistic illusion of control.

What is a Successful Pregnancy?

Defining a successful pregnancy is difficult, and no specific standards have been spelled out. As we noted at the outset, protection of the mother's physical and emotional health must be a goal. As for the infant, two commonly stated goals are: (1) a gestation period longer than 37 weeks and (2) a birth weight greater than 5.5 pounds (2500 grams).[15] The longer the gestational age, the more time is provided for fetal lungs to develop. Sufficient lung development is critical for survival. By 37 weeks, fetal lungs are well developed, and other medical problems occur less often.

Infants born before 37 weeks are called premature, or preterm. Infants born after 37 weeks, but who weigh less than 5.5 pounds, are called **small for gestational age (SGA).** This is true for about 1 in 14 infants born in the United States. These infants are more likely than normal-weight infants to have medical complications,

EXPERT OPINION

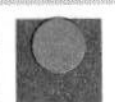

What Do I Really Have to Give up When I'm Pregnant?—cont'd

that any company proposing to introduce a new additive into the U.S. food supply must prove its safety through a series of animal studies. Proof must be provided to the federal government that the proposed new additive causes neither cancer nor birth defects. Many additives that have been used in the American food supply for years are "generally recognized as safe" (see Chapter 19). Ongoing reevaluation of many of these substances has yielded little cause for concern.

Among the additives receiving much attention in the popular press is aspartame (NutraSweet and Equal). This sweetener has now replaced sugar and saccharin in many commercially manufactured products. Many pregnant women have been led to believe that some component of aspartame may adversely affect the fetus. The phenylalanine component has been of special concern as a possible cause of fetal brain damage if maternal exposure is frequent. It is known that high levels of maternal serum phenylalanine (as seen in women with the disease called phenylketonuria) seriously interfere with the normal brain development of the fetus. But it is virtually impossible for a woman without phenylketonuria to maintain high serum levels of phenylalanine. Observations of human subjects have generated no data to support the notion that aspartame use by pregnant women adversely affects the course and outcome of pregnancy. Without such data, it's hardly warranted to recommend that pregnant women abstain from using aspartame-sweetened products.

Nutritional supplements

Nutritional supplements should not be assumed to be benign. Although pregnant women with poor dietary patterns are good candidates for prenatal vitamin/mineral supplements, excessive use of supplements may harm both the mother and the fetus. This is especially true of a high intake of vitamin A by pregnant women, which is associated with producing birth defects. Unfortunately, it is all too easy to consume megadoses of vitamin A; nutritional supplements sold over the counter in grocery and drug stores often contain doses of this vitamin far in excess of the RDA.

If vitamin A in large doses can interfere with normal fetal development, other vitamins may potentially have the same effect. Data supporting this idea, however, are not available. It makes good sense, nevertheless, to be cautious about self-supplementation. The idea that "more of a good thing is better" is foolish. If supplements are used, they should be used under medical guidance.

Unfortunately, there is still much mystery about why some babies develop abnormally or are delivered prematurely. At present, the data suggest that pregnant women should meet their nutritional needs through sensible food choices, avoid alcohol, and use caffeine-containing foods and beverages judiciously. Above all, pregnant women in America should appreciate how lucky they are to have access to a superb food supply. They should delight in knowing that they can provide all the nutrition the fetus needs through wise food choices and, generally, without nutritional supplements.

Dr. Worthington-Roberts is professor of nutritional sciences and chief nutritionist at the Child Development Center at the University of Washington.

such as problems with blood sugar control, temperature regulation, and growth and development in the early weeks after birth.

A definition of a successful pregnancy must also consider the newborn's "quality of life." This consideration includes the newborn's ability to grow, develop, learn, and eventually reproduce. Parents should strive toward producing a baby who is born healthy; on time; and with the mental, physical, and physiological capabilities to take advantage of all that life offers, while also protecting the mother's health.

CONCEPT CHECK

Adequate nutrition is vital both before and during pregnancy to help ensure optimal health of both the fetus and the mother. Fetal organs and body parts begin to develop very soon after conception. The first 13 weeks (first trimester) is a critical period when poor nutrition or drug use can result in birth defects. During the second and third trimesters, organs continue to mature, and very rapid growth occurs. Nutritional insults during the last 7 months of pregnancy can also interfere with fetal growth and affect the newborn's ability to survive. Infants born after 37 weeks of gestation and weighing more than 5.5 pounds (2.5 kilograms) have the fewest medical problems at birth. To reduce the possibility of infant and maternal medical problems or death, those involved must be willing to take all steps necessary to allow the mother to carry her baby in the uterus for the entire 9 months. Good nutrition and health habits aid in this goal.

Meeting Increased Nutrient Needs of a Pregnancy

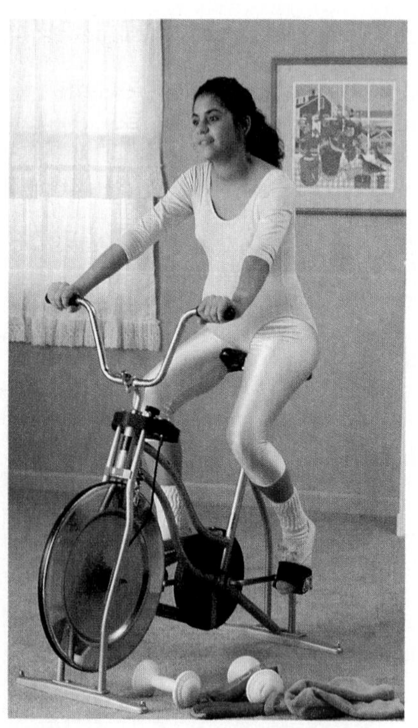

As long as a woman feels comfortable exercising and is under a physician's care, she can continue exercising during her pregnancy.

Dietary advice given to pregnant women by the medical community has varied tremendously over the past century. In the 1950s, a common recommendation was that women restrict weight gain to between 15 and 18 pounds. Severe kcalorie and sodium restrictions were at times also recommended to keep the baby small, in hopes of easing labor and avoiding complications. Few of these practices were based on sound scientific information, and we know now that many of these recommendations are in fact harmful to the mother and fetus.[28]

The first comprehensive scientific report about nutrition and pregnancy, titled *Maternal Nutrition and the Course of Pregnancy,* was issued in 1970 by The National Academy of Sciences. This document remains a landmark source of research information on the role of nutrition in human reproduction. The report was updated in 1990.[22] Both versions emphasize the increased nutritional requirements during pregnancy (not restrictions) and the importance of individual assessment and counseling.

INCREASED ENERGY NEEDS

An average pregnancy requires approximately 300 extra kcalories daily during the second and third trimesters. Kcalories needs during the first trimester are essentially the same as for the nonpregnant woman. This 300 kcalories is equivalent to just 2 cups of low-fat milk and a slice of bread. And so although she may "eat for two," the pregnant woman must not double her normal kcalorie intake. She cannot afford a "Big Mac" for herself and another for the fetus, even during late pregnancy. She will want to seek the highest quality foods to create the best possible health for her child. Many vitamin and mineral needs are increased, but the mother only needs an additional 300 kcalories in the latter two trimesters from which to obtain these nutrients (Figure 16-3).[31]

If a woman is active during pregnancy, the kcalories burned can be added to any extra kcalories needed for pregnancy to balance her energy expenditure. The greater body weight of a pregnant woman requires a higher energy cost for activity. Physicians today recognize the benefits of exercise and encourage women to continue most activities during pregnancy, except scuba diving, downhill skiing, weight lifting, and contact sports, like hockey. Overall, activities that require jumping, jarring

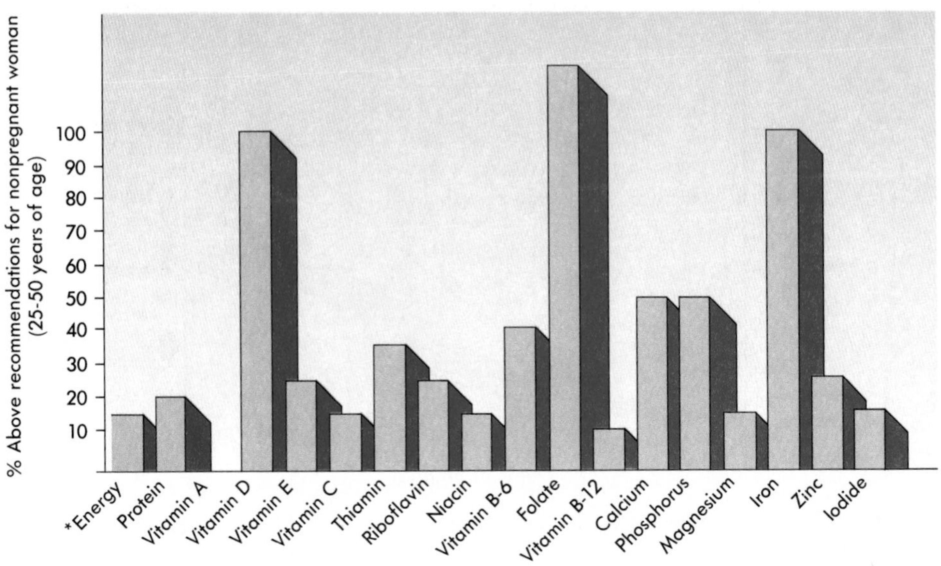

Figure 16-3 Changes in the RDA for pregnancy. During pregnancy, many nutrients are needed in greater amounts than at other times; these include vitamin D, folate, and iron.

motions, or rapid changes in direction should be avoided because of joint instability. In addition, deep flexion or extension of joints—especially deep knee bends—should be avoided because connective tissue is lax during pregnancy. Still, walking, cycling, swimming, and light aerobics are generally appropriate.

Note also that exercise may need to be restricted during high-risk pregnancies. To ensure optimal health for both the mother and baby, pregnant women should first obtain advice regarding exercise limitations from their physicians.

The American College of Obstetrics and Gynecology suggests the following guidelines for exercise during pregnancy:

1. **Do not allow heart rate to exceed 140 beats per minute.**
2. **Avoid exercising in hot, humid weather.**
3. **Discontinue exercise that causes discomfort or overheating.**
4. **Drink plenty of liquids to avoid dehydration and overheating.**
5. **After about the fourth month, don't exercise while lying on one's back.**
6. **Avoid abrupt decrease in exertion (don't just stop and stand around after a hard workout; women should continue exercising, but with less and less vigor, gradually reducing pulse rate).**

RECOMMENDED WEIGHT GAIN

The prenatal diet should allow for approximately 2 to 4 pounds of weight gain during the first trimester, and then a subsequent weight gain of ¾ to 1 pound per week during the second and third trimesters. The total weight gain goal is about 25 to 35 pounds.[27] Adolescents often have smaller babies and are strongly advised to aim for the higher number in this weight range.

For underweight women (body mass index <20) the goal increases to 28 to 40 pounds. And for overweight women (body mass index >26), the goal decreases to 15 to 25 pounds. Obese women (body mass index >29) should strive for the lower value.[22] It may be difficult for someone who has a significant weight problem to understand the need to gain weight during pregnancy, but the goal of this weight gain is to help ensure a healthy baby. Figure 16-4 shows why the weight gain recommendation starts at 25 pounds. It accounts for the total weight of the baby (8 pounds), placenta (1 pound), and amniotic fluid (2 pounds); the mother's increased breast tissue (3 pounds) and increased blood supply (4 pounds); and the increased fat (2 to 8 pounds) and muscle tissue (2 pounds) she needs to support pregnancy and lactation.

A weight gain of about 25 to 35 pounds has repeatedly been shown to yield optimum health for both mother and fetus.[3] This poundage especially reduces the risk for delivering an infant of low birth weight and should yield a birth weight of 7 to 8 pounds. Kcalorie deprivation leading to poor weight gain, such as is seen in famine conditions, is clearly linked to poor outcome of pregnancy.

Weight gain during pregnancy needs regular monitoring, especially in teenage years. Infant birth weights improve if the mother's weight meets the ranges just given. A prenatal weight gain chart can be used to help assess how much the mother's food intake should be adjusted to promote adequate weight gain (Figure 16-5). If a woman deviates from the ideal weight gain pattern, she should be warned of that.

Weight gain pattern in metric units:
first trimester—1 to 2 kilograms
second and third trimesters—350 to 450 grams per week
Total weight gain:
standard—11.5 to 16 kilograms
underweight—12.5 to 18 kilograms
obese—7 to 11.5 kilograms
usual birth weight—3.2 to 3.6 kilograms

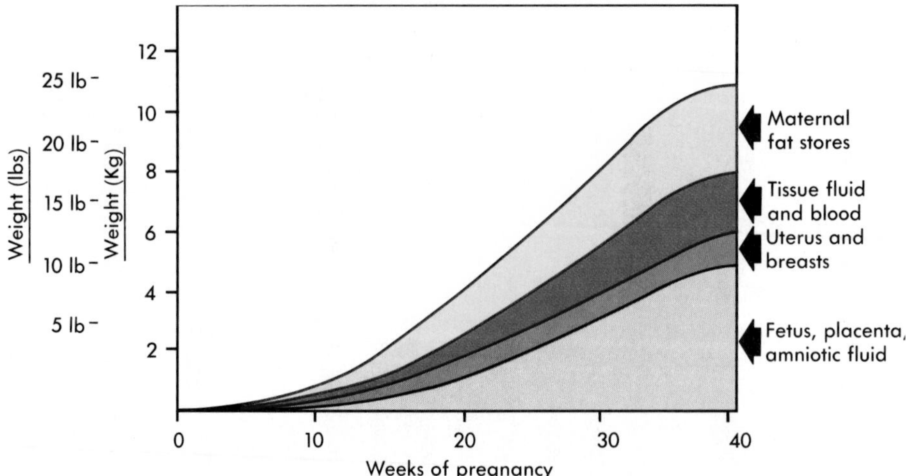

Figure 16-4 The components of weight gain in pregnancy. A weight gain of 25 to 35 pounds is recommended. Note the various components total about 25 pounds.

If she gains too much weight, she should not be encouraged to lose weight in order to get back on the curve. She should simply keep eating her prenatal diet but watch extra kcalories in order to slow the increase in weight and parallel the rise on the prenatal weight gain chart. In other words, the sources of the unneeded kcalories should be found and then minimized. If a woman fails to gain as much weight as she should at a given point in pregnancy, she shouldn't be encouraged to gain the needed weight rapidly. Instead, she should slowly gain slightly more weight than the typical pattern to meet the charted line by the end of pregnancy.

During pregnancy, excess weight gain and poor food choices are more common than an inadequate kcalorie intake. The focus needs to be both on a high-quality diet and reasonable weight gain—neither should be ignored. In the United States, the problem is often how to limit weight gain appropriately—to about 25 to 35 pounds—to prevent the need for significant weight loss after pregnancy. Excessive weight gain increases risk for complications in pregnancy and encourages excess fetal growth, which can increase the risk for birth trauma.[2] Multiple pregnancies with excessive weight gains can contribute to creeping obesity in women. Loose, accommodating maternity clothes designed for comfort do not provide the usual feedback about weight gain, and fluid retention can likewise mask "true" weight gain during pregnancy. Thus careful monitoring by a health professional is desirable.

INCREASED PROTEIN NEEDS

The RDA for protein is increased by 10 grams per day for adults over age 24 and about 15 grams per day under age 24. However, many women already eat the overall recommendation of 60 grams of protein per day. High protein supplements are not recommended because they have been associated with an increased number of premature infants and excessive fetal deaths.

INCREASED CARBOHYDRATE NEEDS

Carbohydrate needs are at least 100 grams per day. This amount prevents ketosis and the interruption of fetal development and brain maturation that may result from ketosis. Most women eat about twice this amount each day.

INCREASED VITAMIN NEEDS

Vitamin needs in general are increased, especially the need for vitamin D and folate (Figure 16-5).

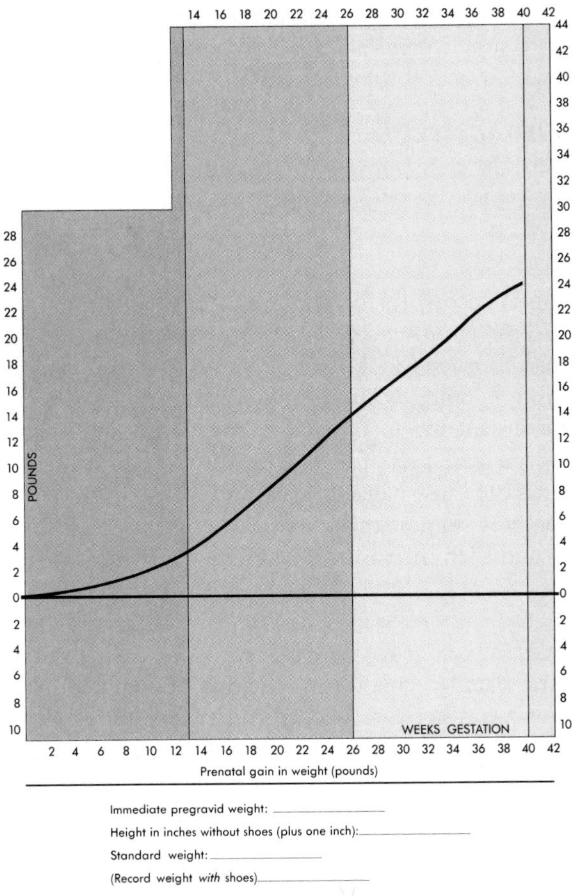

Figure 16-5 A chart for following weight gain in pregnancy. Charting weight gain is a routine, but vital, part of prenatal care.

Vitamin D

Calcium metabolism increases during pregnancy. To facilitate the absorption and distribution of calcium for forming fetal bones, the mother's need for vitamin D doubles to 10 micrograms per day. Pregnant women should get regular sunlight exposure. If that is impossible and insufficient vitamin D–fortified milk is consumed to make up the difference (4 cups or about 1 liter yields 10 micrograms), a pregnant woman should consider a supplement containing 5 to 10 micrograms (200 to 400 IU). The typical prenatal supplement contains this extra amount of vitamin D.

Folate

The synthesis of DNA requires folate. This means the growth of the fetus and mother depends on an ample supply of folate. Red blood cell formation increases in pregnancy, also requiring folate. Serious anemia can result if folate intake is inadequate. The RDA is increased by an additional 220 micrograms of folate, for a recommended total of 400 micrograms per day.

Some women have difficulty consuming sufficient folate to satisfy their pregnancy needs. Recent studies show that some pregnant women consume only about the nonpregnant RDA—250 micrograms per day. However, by choosing foods wisely—for example, folate-rich fruits and vegetables as outlined in the Guide to Daily Food Choices—a woman can meet her needs. This should be a goal for every pregnant woman.

A prenatal vitamin supplement may be used to meet the RDA for folate, especially by women with histories of inadequate folate intake, frequent or multiple births, megaloblastic anemia, or anticonvulsant drug therapy. Today, folate-related anemias do not often occur during pregnancy. Widespread use of prenatal supplements, which supply folate, is probably the major reason. As we noted earlier, if folate intake is deficient during pregnancy, neural tube defects may result. Currently some physicians feel folate supplements should be given before pregnancy to women who have had a child with a neural tube defect.[9]

INCREASED MINERAL NEEDS

Mineral needs generally increase during pregnancy, especially the need for iron, calcium, magnesium, zinc, and fluoride (Figure 16-5).

Iron

So much extra iron is needed for hemoglobin synthesis during pregnancy that the RDA doubles to 30 milligrams a day. A supplement is needed to provide that much iron if sufficient iron-fortified foods, such as breakfast cereals, are not eaten.[22] Eating foods rich in vitamin C along with an iron supplement increases iron absorption. Severe iron-deficiency anemia in pregnancy may lead to premature delivery, low birth weight,[21] and increased risk for fetal death in the first weeks of gestation.

Iron supplements can cause nausea, constipation, and decreased appetite. Because of this some researchers suggest that pregnant women start with 30 milligrams of extra iron per day and then increase their intake only when laboratory tests dictate more is needed.

Today, iron is the only nutrient that the National Academy of Sciences recommends be supplemented during pregnancy.[22] However, physicians routinely prescribe specially formulated prenatal multivitamin and mineral supplements. They may do this because it is easier and quicker to prescribe supplements than to discuss dietary changes. Also, some women are not willing to make changes to improve their diets to meet the increased nutrient needs during pregnancy. The typical prenatal supplement contains many nutrients, including four critical nutrients for pregnancy—iron, folate, vitamin D, and calcium. Under certain conditions, such as poverty, teenage pregnancy, poor maternal diet, and multiple fetuses (twins or more), the use of supplements is prudent.

Pregnancy, in particular, is not a time to self-prescribe vitamin and mineral pills.

Calcium

Calcium is needed during pregnancy to promote adequate mineralization of the fetal skeleton and teeth. Most calcium is required during the third trimester, when skeletal growth is at a maximum and teeth are forming, but extra intake should start immediately. The RDA for calcium in pregnancy increases by 400 milligrams for women over age 24 years. Pregnant teenage women should consume an extra 600 milligrams of calcium per day. The only practical food sources for this calcium belong to the milk, yogurt, cheese group, and calcium-fortified orange juice. Otherwise, calcium supplements are needed. A prenatal supplement generally contains 200 milligrams of calcium.

Zinc

Zinc is an important mineral for supporting growth and development. The RDA for zinc increases from 12 to 15 milligrams per day. The extra protein foods in the diet of a pregnant woman should supply most of this zinc. A poor zinc status in pregnancy increases the risk for having a low-birth-weight infant.

Fluoride

Fluoride in the mothers diet can improve fetal tooth development. Women should ask their dentists if extra fluoride is needed, depending on the local water supply.

IS THERE AN INSTINCTIVE DRIVE IN PREGNANCY TO EAT MORE NUTRIENTS?

Extra needs in pregnancy for folate, iron, calcium, and zinc are the most difficult for women to satisfy. These, then, should be the focus of diet planning for pregnancy.

Before we discuss diet planning, however, one very important misconception about pregnancy needs to be dispelled. Some people believe that mothers instinctively know what to eat and that their drive for pickles or ice cream is dictated by a natural desire to consume needed nutrients. However, no studies support that notion, and if it were true, one would wonder why some women seek out clay, starch, ice, and other nonfood items during pregnancy.[13] There may be a natural instinct to consume the right foods in pregnancy, but we are so far removed from living by instinct that relying on our desires is risky. Good nutritional counseling can focus food choices more reliably.

A Food Plan for Pregnancy

Table 16-1 outlines one approach to a good diet during pregnancy. It includes three or more servings from the milk, yogurt, and cheese group; three servings from the meat, poultry, fish, dry beans, eggs, and nuts group; three servings from the vegetable group; two servings from the fruit group; and six servings from the breads, cereal, rice, and pasta group. Specifically, the servings from the milk, yogurt, and cheese group could include low-fat milk, yogurt, and cheese. These foods supply extra protein, calcium, riboflavin, and magnesium. Servings from the meat, poultry, fish, dry beans, eggs, and nuts group should include both animal and vegetable sources. Besides protein, the animal sources help provide the extra iron and zinc needed, and the vegetable sources help provide much of the extra magnesium needed.

The vegetable and fruit group servings provide vitamins and minerals. One serving from this combination should be a good vitamin C source, and one serving should be a green vegetable or other rich source of folate, such as orange juice. Selections from the breads, cereals, rice, and pasta group should be the whole grains

Table 16-1 A minimum food plan for pregnancy and breast-feeding

Food group	Key nutrients supplied	Number of servings
Milk, yogurt, and cheese: 1 cup; 1½ ounces for cheese	Protein Riboflavin Calcium	3*
Meat, poultry, fish, dry beans, eggs, and nuts: 2-3 ounces meat; 1 cup beans; 2 eggs; ½ cup nuts	Protein Thiamin Vitamin B-6 Iron Zinc	3
Vegetables: ½ cup or ¾ cup raw	Vitamin A Vitamin C Folate Dietary Fiber	3
Fruits: 1 piece generally	Vitamin C Folate Dietary Fiber	2
Breads, cereals, rice, and pasta: 1 slice or ½-¾ cup cooked	B-vitamins Iron Dietary Fiber	6

* Four servings if a teenager.

Table 16-2 A sample diet based on recommendations in Table 16-1

Breakfast

¾ cup raisin bran
4 ounces orange juice
½ cup 1% milk

Snack

2 tablespoons peanut butter
1 slice whole-wheat toast
½ cup plain low-fat yogurt
½ cup strawberries

Lunch

spinach salad with
2 tablespoons oil and vinegar dressing
½ sliced tomato
2 slices whole-wheat toast
1½ ounces of provalone cheese

Snack

4 whole-wheat crackers
1 cup 1% milk

Dinner

3 ounces lean ham
1 cup navy beans
1 cornbread muffin
¾ cup cooked broccoli
1 teaspoon corn oil margarine
iced tea or milk (if teenager)

This diet meets the RDA for pregnancy and lactation for only 1800 kcalories (34 milligrams of iron).

and enriched varieties. Table 16-2 shows this basic diet plan can contain as little as 1800 kcalories and still meet the extra needs of pregnancy, except for iron.

THE PREGNANT VEGETARIAN

The vegetarian woman who becomes pregnant should not necessarily have special nutritional problems if she is a lacto-ovo vegetarian or a lacto vegetarian. A total vegetarian (vegan), on the other hand, must carefully plan a diet that includes sufficient protein, vitamin B-6, iron, calcium, and zinc. A vitamin B-12 supplement is necessary if insufficient vitamin B-12–supplemented foods are eaten. The basic vegan diet listed in Chapter 5 should be supplemented in the grain group, as well as in the beans, nuts, and seeds group to supply more of the necessary nutrients. Since iron and calcium are poorly absorbed from most plant foods, an iron and calcium supplement is probably desirable. The levels provided by a typical prenatal supplement should suffice for iron needs but not for calcium needs; additional calcium supplementation or calcium-fortified orange juice may be necessary.

CONCEPT CHECK

Energy needs increase by an average of 300 kcalories per day during pregnancy during the second and third trimester. Weight gain should be slow and steady up to a total of 25 to 35 pounds for a woman of normal weight. Protein, vitamin, and mineral needs all increase during pregnancy. Vitamin D, folate, iron, calcium, and zinc are nutrients of particular concern. A pregnant woman's diet should be varied and generally include more milk products and more specified fruits and vegetables than a prepregnancy diet. Prenatal supplemental vitamins and minerals are commonly prescribed, but are generally unnecessary, aside from the iron supplied.

The Effect of Nutrition on the Success of Pregnancy

As we have discussed, the growth of the fetus and the changes in the mother's body that occur to accommodate the fetus require extra nutrients and energy. Although pregnancy is a normal process, the sizeable changes in the mother's body pose nutritional stresses for her. Her uterus and breasts grow, the placenta develops, her total blood volume increases, the heart and kidneys work harder, and stores of body fat increase—all in preparation for birth and milk production.[22] The nutrients needed for these "support systems" changes are added to the nutrient needs of both the growing fetus and the mother's own normal physiological functions. For this reason, a growing adolescent faces almost overwhelming nutritional demands during pregnancy.

The specific effects on fetal development of either a marginal intake of nutrients and energy during pregnancy or marginal nutritional stores of the mother at the start of pregnancy are difficult to establish. We noted earlier that a diet containing greatly insufficient kcalories (only 1000 kcalories per day) has been shown to retard fetal growth and development.[29] The mother's body, however, can adapt to the demands of pregnancy in a variety of ways, including increased absorption of nutrients from foods. For some nutrients, such as iron and calcium, the fetus may also use—and deplete—the mother's stores if the diet is not adequate.

Research shows that genetic background can explain very little of the difference in birth weights of infants. Both environmental factors and nutritional factors, such as the mother's weight gain, are much more important.

EARLY RESEARCH SUPPORTS THE IMPORTANCE OF GOOD NUTRITION IN PREGNANCY

During World War II, parts of Russia and much of Holland were blockaded. Food supplies were quickly exhausted. The resulting undernutrition greatly affected infant birth weights of the mothers who were in their second or third trimester at that time. The number of new pregnancies also fell as women's health status weakened. After the blockades were lifted, birth weights and the numbers of new pregnancies quickly rose again to prewar levels.

At the same time, researchers working in Boston noticed that an adequate protein intake was associated with a greater success of pregnancy. It appeared that the mother's diet—not only during pregnancy but also preceding conception—contributed to the health of both mother and infant. Better health care for those who could afford higher protein diets probably also contributed to the well-being of these mothers and infants. Studies in Toronto then showed that dietary supplements and nutritional counseling improved the health of the pregnant mother and yielded a healthier baby. Rates of complications also were reduced.

Researchers in Great Britain then showed that height and social class were more important than dietary intake during pregnancy in predicting the outcome of pregnancy.[6] Supporting this is a recent study of middle class African-American women in Chicago. Their risk of having **low-birth-weight** babies still exceeded that of middle class Caucasians, possibly reflecting the effects of previous generations of poverty.[8] This finding again suggested that long-term nutritional intake is critical to pregnancy outcome.

low birth weight (LBW) Infant weight at birth of less than 5.5 pounds (2.5 kilograms), usually because of premature birth; these infants are at higher risk for health problems.

Later, laboratory animal studies supported the importance of diet during pregnancy. Food deprivation during pregnancy in animals resulted in decreased organ sizes in the pups, even in the brain, which is usually very resistant to nutritional insults. In addition, there was a decrease both in the weight of the placenta and in the number of healthy pups that survived the first weeks of life.

MATERNAL AND INFANT MORTALITY

In the United States, approximately 12 of every 100,000 live births lead to the mother's death (maternal mortality). Nine hundred and seventy infant deaths (age

1 to 365 days) occur for each 100,000 live births (infant mortality). And for African-Americans in the United States the number of infant deaths is double that seen in Caucasians or Hispanics. These statistics are quite saddening. Considerable efforts are being made to reduce both infant and maternal deaths. Good health care and nutritional practices are one key to reducing these deaths. Age over 35 years is not much of a concern if good health care and nutrient intake are assured.[24] Specific nutrition-related factors that affect the health of both the mother and the fetus (infant), aside from a poor diet in general, include:[25]

- **Socioeconomic status**—Poverty, inadequate health care, poor health practices, lack of education, and unmarried status are all related to problems in pregnancy.[20]
- **Obesity**—This leads to an increased rate of high blood pressure and diabetes during pregnancy and to surgical and other complications during delivery. These pregnancies require intense monitoring to reduce the potential risks for both the mother and the infant.
- **Poor, absent, or delayed prenatal care**—This can allow maternal nutritional deficiencies to deprive the fetus of needed nutrients, and/or can increase the risk of fetal damage in the case of chronic diseases, such as hypertension or diabetes. Ideally, prenatal care should start before conception. Still, about 25% of women in the United States receive no prenatal care during the first trimester—a critical time to change habits.
- **Smoking, alcohol consumption, use of some medications, or illegal drug use in pregnancy**—The Nutrition Perspective reviews fetal alcohol syndrome. Smoking is linked to low birth weight in the infant, probably because the fetus is denied needed oxygen when nicotine constricts the arteries, and so the blood supply.[22] There is also a question of an increased risk of birth defects, such as cleft lip and/or palate, as well as increased risk for colds, asthma, and other respiratory problems in the infant.

A recent survey of 36 hospitals throughout the United States found that overall, 11% of women use illicit drugs during pregnancy. The actual range reported from individual hospitals was 0.4% to 27%. In 1989, research at a major hospital in Philadelphia revealed that 15% of 852 women exhibited positive toxicology studies for cocaine or combinations of cocaine, marijuana, and narcotics. This percentage was equally distributed among private and medically assisted patients. Clearly, this is not an issue for poor minorities alone; infants in all socioeconomic and ethnic groups are adversely affected by these agents.

Fetal exposure to cocaine is of special concern. Cocaine abuse has become more widespread in recent years and has been linked to such problems as premature labor, small body and head size, physical malformations, disturbed nervous system development, and poor learning ability in childhood.[18] At birth the infants are quite irritable and may cry incessantly.[7]

- **Pica**—This is the practice of eating nonfood items, such as dirt, starch, ice, or clay, especially while pregnant.[13] Although pica occurs more frequently in populations that have poor iron and zinc status, this practice probably results more from habit, culture, and superstition than from a need for specific nutrients. Eating soil raises the risk of infections from parasites and can cause life-threatening blockages of the intestinal tract. Eating laundry starch should be discouraged because it contains silicon and other toxic compounds. Eating ice may break the teeth.
- **Prenatal ketosis**—There is debate about the extent to which ketosis harms a growing fetus. Ketone bodies are thought to be poorly used by the fetal brain and thus can slow fetal brain development. Researchers stress the need for a pregnant woman not to "crash" diet nor to fast for more than 12 hours. A pregnant woman can develop significant ketosis after only 20 hours of fasting.
- **Inadequate weight gain**—This increases the risk of having a low-birth-weight (LBW) infant.[28]

Women with acquired immune deficiency syndrome (AIDS) should understand that the odds are about one-in-three that the virus will pass to the child and that an infected baby will likely get sick and die within just a few years.

In the United States, 7% to 10% of infants are born with a low birth weight, that is, they weigh less than 5.5 pounds (2.5 kilograms). Low-birth-weight infants

NUTRITION FOCUS

Teenage Pregnancy

Teenage pregnancy is a major cause of infant mortality in the United States. About half a million teenagers give birth to babies in the United States each year. What is sometimes a glorious experience frequently becomes a real problem when adolescents are not ready to be parents—physically, financially, socially, and culturally. Teenage pregnancy poses special health problems for both the mother and child. To accommodate their normal growth even when not pregnant, teenagers need an extraordinary nutrient supply.[1] Women normally continue to grow taller for 2 years after they begin menstruating. Teen pregnancy adds the needs of the growing fetus to those of the growing mother. They both need considerable amounts of nutrients for their growing bodies.

Teen diets—pregnant teens included—vary greatly in nutritional adequacy. Many teens have irregular eating habits, skip meals, snack on low-nutrient foods, and frequently diet. Many of them eat less than two thirds of the RDA for many vitamins and minerals.

Teenagers are more likely than most mothers to be underweight at the beginning of pregnancy and to gain less than 16 pounds during pregnancy. Consequently, teens frequently produce low-birth-weight infants.[20] And these quite vulnerable infants are a major health problem in the United States.

The specific nutrient needs of the pregnant adolescent vary according to their own growth patterns, body build, and exercise habits. That makes it difficult to predict individual needs. But health workers can evaluate the adequacy of a pregnant teenager's diet by checking for appropriate weight gain during pregnancy and appropriate food choices.

To improve pregnancy outcomes and the health of pregnant teenagers, their eating practices should be routinely examined and they should be counseled concerning nutrition during prenatal care.[1] Pregnant teens need information about basic nutrition guidelines: relationship between food and health; issues that affect adequate nutrition and food resources (e.g., participation in the WIC program, which is discussed later in this chapter); kind and amount of food energy needed to support appropriate weight gain; how to select nutrient-rich foods; regular use of prenatal vitamin/mineral supplements; and preparation for breast-feeding or for using infant formulas. They also need to be made aware of the risks involved with smoking, drinking alcohol, or using drugs and medications not approved by their physician.

Complications accompanying teenage pregnancies and the higher rates of low birth weight, illness, and death for their babies were once assumed to result from the mother's biological immaturity. It now appears that the most important factor is the mother's day-to-day health practices (Table 16-3). Regardless of age, teenage mothers with healthy life-styles—those who generally consume balanced diets; gain the recommended amount of weight during pregnancy; and do not smoke, drink alcohol, or use drugs—tend to be healthier and remain healthier than other teen mothers. Their infants also tend to be healthy.

With proper nutrition education and encouragement, teenage mothers might resolve some of the health problems associated with teenage pregnancy.[20] The other major problem related to teenage pregnancy—the impact of pregnancy and parenthood on the mother's education and economic future—remains. Young mothers may be deprived of education that would help them to better jobs and better means of looking after themselves and their children. Few teenagers can successfully care for and support themselves and their children. Thus, ultimately, prevention of teenage pregnancy is generally the best approach.

Table 16-3 Nutrient-related risk factors in teenage pregnancy

- Low pregnancy weight gain
- Low prepregnancy weight for height (or other evidence of poor nutrition)
- Smoking
- Excessive prepregnancy weight for height
- Anemia

Other risk factors suggested by health histories

- Unhealthy life-style (i.e., use of drugs and alcohol)
- Unfavorable reproductive history
- Chronic diseases
- History of an eating disorder

Adapted from the *Journal of The American Dietetic Association* 89:106, 1989.

show a greater risk for infection, illness, disabilities, and death than normal weight infants. Premature birth, poor diet during pregnancy, some medical conditions in the mother, and the abovementioned factors influence an infant's birth weight. Reducing the number of low-birth-weight infants will help reduce the total number of infant deaths.

Education, an adequate diet, and early and consistent prenatal medical care are vital for increasing the chances for producing a healthy baby. Early prenatal care should include a medical examination, dietary advice, laboratory tests, and counseling. The woman should be counseled to avoid x-ray exposure, smoking, vitamin A supplements, certain medications, illegal drugs, and alcohol. If diabetes is present or developing, it must be carefully controlled to minimize complications in the pregnancy.[2] We will address this problem in a later section.

It is best if these examinations and counseling strategies begin before the woman becomes pregnant, but certainly they should begin early in pregnancy. Many problems can develop in pregnancy that a physician can diagnose and quickly treat.

Almost all women need prenatal nutritional counseling, especially those at high risk for nutritional problems (Table 16-4). Food habits cannot be predicted from income, education, or life-style. It is important for all women to review the principles of an adequate diet for pregnancy. While some women already have good nutritional habits, most can still benefit from the prenatal nutrition advice we have provided, including warnings about habits that may harm the growing fetus, such as severe dieting or fasting. Focusing on excellent prenatal care, good nutritional intake, and proper health habits can give the fetus, and later the infant, the best chance of thriving.[22]

U.S. government programs exist to reduce infant mortality by providing high-quality health care and foods designed to alleviate the effects of poverty and poor education. An example of such a program is the Special Supplemental Food Program for Women, Infants, and Children (WIC). This program offers health assessments and foods (or vouchers for foods) that supply high-quality protein, calcium, iron, vitamin A, and vitamin C to pregnant women, infants, and children (to age 5 years) from low-income populations.

Participants' diets have improved markedly on this program, as has the woman's likelihood of having a healthy baby. The WIC program is credited with decreasing the cases of iron-deficiency anemia and low-birth-weight infants within the population it serves. Studies have estimated that every dollar spent on the prenatal component of WIC saves up to four dollars in public health expenditures for the care of low-birth-weight babies.

The WIC program is found throughout the United States and has a trained staff ready to help all who need help in providing a healthful diet in pursuit of a healthy baby. Prenatal women are a priority for this program. Budget constraints force some programs to disenroll children to make space for pregnant women.

Table 16-4 Women generally defined as nutritionally "at risk" during pregnancy

- Women who do not ordinarily consume an adequate diet
- Women carrying more than one fetus
- Women who use cigarettes, alcohol, illegal drugs
- Women with lactose intolerance
- Women who are underweight or overweight at conception or who gain inadequate or excessive weight during pregnancy
- Adolescents
- Women with poor knowledge about nutrition or who have insufficient financial resources to purchase adequate food

CONCEPT CHECK

Infants born after 37 weeks of gestation and weighing more than 5.5 pounds (2.5 kilograms) have the fewest medical problems at birth. Individual mothers and whole societies can attempt to reduce infant and maternal death and medical problems by limiting factors that increase the risk of having a premature or small-for-gestational (SGA) infant. Such contributing factors, besides a poor diet in general, include poor socioeconomic status; obesity; poor, absent or delayed prenatal care; smoking; imprudent medicine use; alcohol consumption; illegal drug use; pica; teenage pregnancy; inadequate prenatal weight gain; and prenatal ketosis. Adequate nutrition can reduce the risk of many medical problems in pregnancy.

Physiological Changes and Resulting Problems in Pregnancy

During pregnancy, the fetus' needs for oxygen, nutrients, and excretion increase the burden on the mother's lungs, heart, and kidneys. Although the mother's digestion and metabolic processes work very efficiently, some discomfort accompanies the changes her body undergoes to accommodate the fetus.

HEARTBURN, CONSTIPATION, AND HEMORRHOIDS

Progestins produced by the placenta relax muscles in both the uterus and the intestinal tract. This often causes heartburn as stomach acid slips up through the lower esophageal sphincter into the esophagus (see Chapter 6). When that happens, the woman should avoid lying down after eating, reduce fat consumption so that foods pass quickly from the stomach into the small intestine, and avoid spicy foods if they are not tolerated. She should also consume liquids between meals to decrease volume and pressure in the stomach.[31] More severe cases may need antacids. This approach has a well-established safety record.

progestins Hormones, including progesterone, that are necessary for maintaining pregnancy and lactation.

Constipation often results from the relaxation of intestinal muscles, especially late in pregnancy as the fetus competes for space with the GI tract. Consuming more water, dietary fiber, and dried fruits and exercising can help a pregnant woman avoid constipation and an often accompanying problem, hemorrhoids.[31] Straining can lead to hemorrhoids, which are more likely to occur during pregnancy anyway because of physiological changes occurring during pregnancy.

EDEMA

Estrogens and progestins combine to cause connective tissue to retain fluid during pregnancy. Blood volume also greatly expands during pregnancy and normally contributes some edema. There is no reason to restrict salt or use diuretics to limit mild edema. Studies have demonstrated that some edema even is linked to a positive pregnancy outcome.[5] However, the edema may limit physical activity late in pregnancy and occasionally require the woman to elevate her feet to control the symptoms. Overall, edema generally spells trouble only if hypertension and the appearance of protein in the urine accompany fluid retention.

MORNING SICKNESS

Nausea is common in the early stages of pregnancy; it is possibly a reaction to pregnancy-related hormones circulating in the bloodstream. Although known as "morning sickness," nausea may occur at any time and persist all day. It is often the first signal to a woman that she is pregnant. Some women partially control mild nausea by eating soda crackers or dry cereal before getting out of bed, avoiding large fluid intakes early in the morning, cooking with open windows to dissipate nauseating smells, eating smaller, more frequent meals, and avoiding foods that increase nausea.[5] Usually, nausea stops after the first trimester, but it can continue throughout the entire pregnancy. In cases of serious nausea, the preceding practices offer little relief. When appetite is severely reduced or vomiting persists, medical therapy is needed.

gestational diabetes A high blood glucose level that develops during pregnancy and returns to normal after birth; one cause is placental production of hormones that antagonize blood glucose regulation.

GESTATIONAL DIABETES

Hormones synthesized by the placenta antagonize the action of the hormone insulin. This antagonism can precipitate **gestational diabetes,** often beginning in weeks 20 to 24, particularly in women with family histories of diabetes.[2] During pregnancy, it is important for women to have regular checks of their urine or blood glucose levels to detect developing diabetes. Once detected, a special diet and sometimes insulin injections are needed. Regular exercise is also helpful. Gestational diabetes often disappears after the infant's birth, but is linked to development of diabetes later in life. Proper control of both gestational diabetes and diabetes present in the mother before pregnancy is extremely important. If not treated, the fetus can grow quite large, often necessitating an early delivery and increasing the risk of birth trauma and malformations, as well as hypoglycemia in the infant at birth.

physiological anemia The normal increase in blood volume in pregnancy that dilutes the concentration of red blood cells, resulting in anemia; also called hemodilution.

ANEMIA

To supply fetal needs, the mother's blood volume expands up to approximately 150% of normal. But the red cell mass expands only 20% to 30% above normal, and this occurs more slowly. This leaves proportionately fewer red cells in a pregnant woman's bloodstream. The lower ration of red blood cells is a condition known as **physiological anemia,** since it is a normal response to pregnancy, rather than the result of poor nutrient intake.[31] If during pregnancy, however, iron stores and/or dietary intake—particularly of iron and folate—is inadequate, resulting anemia may require medical attention. Under the advice of a physician, some women should continue to take iron supplements after birth to rebuild iron stores depleted during pregnancy.

pregnancy-induced hypertension A serious disorder that can include high blood pressure, kidney failure, convulsions, and even death of the mother and fetus. Although exact cause is not known, good nutrition and prenatal care may prevent or limit its severity. Mild cases are known as preeclampsia; more severe cases are called eclampsia. Another term for this disorder is toxemia.

PREGNANCY-INDUCED HYPERTENSION

A high risk to pregnancy results from **pregnancy-induced hypertension.** This disorder, also known in mild forms as preeclampsia and in severe forms as eclampsia, resolves once the pregnancy state ends. Early signs and symptoms include a rise in blood pressure, excess protein in the urine, and fluid retention. More severe results, including convulsions, can occur in the second and third trimesters. Good nutrition such as illustrated in Table 16-1—especially an adequate calcium intake (about 2 grams per day)—may prevent or lessen the disorder.[4] Mild effects can be lessened by bed rest and certain medications. If not controlled, liver and kidney damage, and even death of the mother and fetus, may result. Careful medical attention is needed.

CONCEPT CHECK

Heartburn, constipation, nausea and vomiting, edema, gestational diabetes, and anemia are possible discomforts and complications of pregnancy. Changes in food habits can often ease these problems. Pregnancy-induced hypertension, with high blood pressure and kidney failure, can lead to severe complications, even death to both the mother and fetus, if not treated. A high calcium intake is linked to a reduced risk.

Breast-Feeding

Before the 1900s, if you were not breast-fed by your mother, a "wet nurse" may have breast-fed you. Formula feeding was fraught with complications, primarily because people did not know the importance of sterilizing formulas against bacteria, nor much about the nutritional needs of infants. During the early 1900s, the technology of formula feeding improved. From the 1920s and especially in the 1940s when women worked in armament factories during World War II, more and more babies were fed formulas. Throughout the 1950s and early 1960s, interest in breast-feeding further waned. In the 1970s, breast-feeding enjoyed a resurgence, which has since leveled off.

Recent statistics show that about 52% of middle class women nurse their babies in the hospital; about 29% of poor do so.[16] These figures are well below the recommendations of a U.S. government program, Healthy People 2000, which suggests that 75% of infants be breast-fed at the time of hospital discharge. The same approximate ratio of middle class to poor women remains true after the infant is 4 months old. Those women who choose to breast-feed usually find it an enjoyable and "special" time in their lives and in their relationship with their new baby (Figure 16-6). Bottle feeding using an infant formula is also a nutritious choice, as we will discuss in the next chapter. Note that if a woman decides not to nurse her child, breast weight returns to normal very soon after birth.

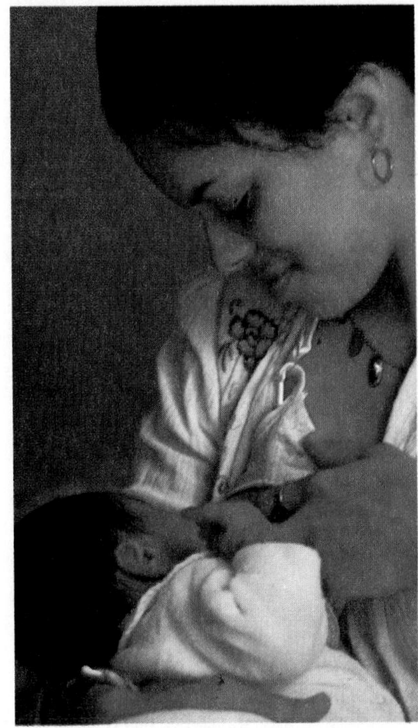

Figure 16-6 Breast-feeding fosters closeness between mother and infant. This is part of the process called bonding, which is part of the normal parent-child nurturing process. Bottle-feeding also allows for this.

PHYSIOLOGY OF LACTATION

Almost all women can breast-feed their children. Major problems are usually due to a lack of information. Anatomic problems in breasts, such as inverted nipples, can be corrected during pregnancy.[17] Breast size is no indication of success in breast-feeding. First-time mothers who plan to breast-feed should learn as much as they can about the process before delivering the baby. Interested women should learn the proper technique, what problems to expect, and how to respond to them. Some physicians recommended that mothers-to-be stimulate their nipples by pulling, twisting, or rolling them between their fingers. This toughens the nipples in preparation for breast-feeding. Familiarity with the overall process of breast-feeding builds the confidence and knowledge necessary for success.

PRODUCING HUMAN MILK

During pregnancy, cells in the breast aggregate to form milk-producing cells called **lobules** (Figure 16-7). Hormones from the placenta stimulate these changes in the breast. After birth, the rise in the maternal production of the hormone prolactin acts to maintain these changes in the breast and in turn enhances the ability to produce milk.[17] During pregnancy, breast weight increases by 1 to 2 pounds.

The hormone **prolactin** also stimulates the synthesis of milk. Suckling stimulates prolactin release. Milk synthesis then occurs as an infant nurses. The more the infant suckles, the more milk is produced. Milk production closely parallels infant demand—in this way even twins can be nursed. Demand is the driving force for milk production.[17]

prolactin A hormone secreted by the mother that stimulates the synthesis of milk.

Most protein found in human milk is synthesized by breast tissue. Some proteins also enter the milk directly from maternal circulation. These proteins include immune factors and enzymes. Long-chain fatty acids, found as triglycerides in human milk, come from the mother's diet. Short-chain fatty acids, also found as triglycerides in breast milk, are synthesized by breast tissue. The monosaccharide galactose is synthesized in the breast, while glucose enters from maternal circulation. Together these monosaccharides form the disaccharide lactose, the main carbohydrate in human milk.

THE LET-DOWN REFLEX

An important brain-breast connection—the **let-down reflex**—is necessary for breast-feeding (Figure 16-8). The brain releases the hormone oxytocin to allow the breast tissues to "let down" or release the milk from storage sites to travel to the nipple area.[31] A tingling sensation signals the let-down reflex shortly before milk flow begins. If the let-down reflex doesn't operate, little milk is available to the infant. The infant gets frustrated, and this can frustrate the mother.

let-down reflex A reflex stimulated by infant suckling that causes the release (ejection) of milk from milk ducts in the mother's breasts.

The let-down reflex is easily inhibited by nervous tension, a lack of confidence, and fatigue. Mothers should be especially aware of the link between tension and a

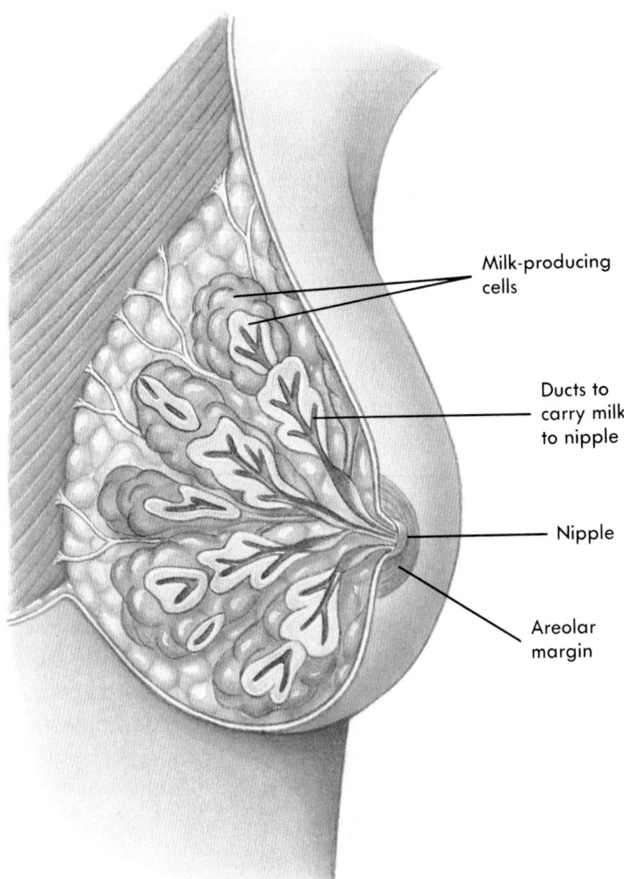

Figure 16-7 The anatomy of the breast. Many types of cells form a coordinated network to produce and secrete human milk.

weak let-down reflex. They need to find a relaxed and supportive environment where they can breast-feed.

After a few weeks, the let-down reflex becomes automatic. The mother's response can be triggered just by thoughts about the baby or by seeing or hearing another baby. But at first, the process can be a bit bewildering. Because she cannot measure the amount of milk the infant takes in, a mother may fear that she is not adequately nourishing the baby. A good standard of comparison for a breast-fed baby is that (1) it should have six or more wet diapers per day and show normal growth; (2) the stool should look like mustard, with one or two stools each day being typical; and (3) the breast should soften during the feeding. If so, enough milk is being consumed.

It generally takes 2 to 3 weeks to fully establish the feeding routine: infant and mother both feel comfortable, the milk supply meets infant demand, and initial nipple soreness disappears. Establishing the routine requires patience, but the rewards are great. The adjustments are easier if supplemental formula feedings are not introduced until breast-feeding is well established, after about at least 3 weeks, but preferably after 2 to 3 months. Then a supplemental bottle or two of infant formula per day is fine. Note that providing water in a bottle during hot weather at earlier ages is fine and often desirable.

The parents need not be concerned that breast-fed infants grow a bit more slowly after about 3 months of age than formula-fed infants.[17] The infant's physician is the best judge of whether the rate of growth of the breast-fed infant is satisfactory. Growth will likely catch up to formula-fed infants by 2 years of age.

COMPOSITION OF HUMAN MILK

Human milk is very different in composition from cow's milk. Unless altered, cow's milk should not be used in infant feeding until the infant is 6 to 12 months old.

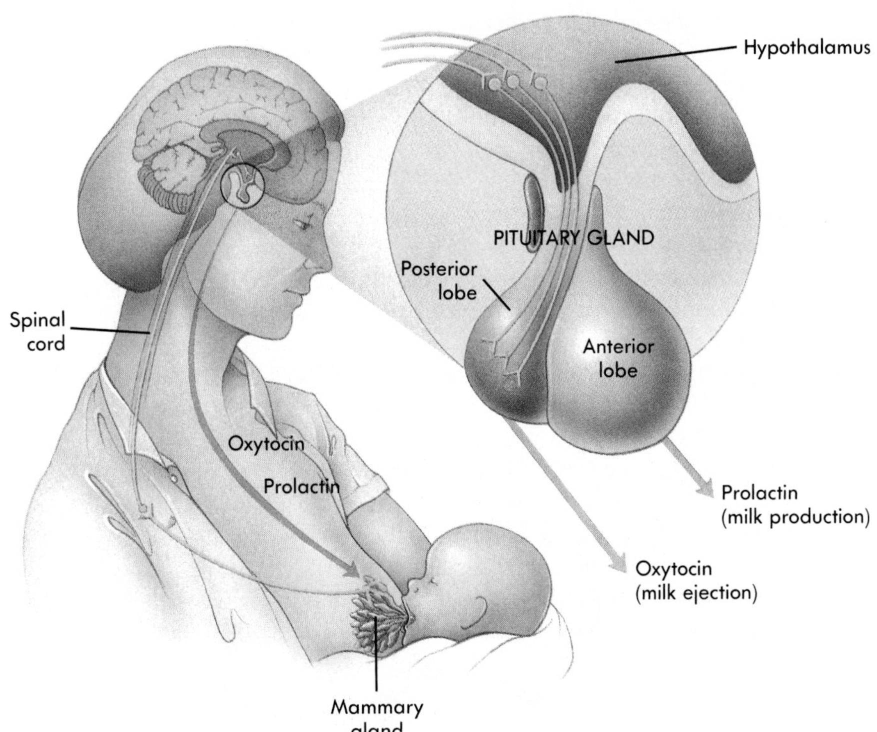

Figure 16-8 The let-down reflex. Stimulation of the nipple by the baby's suckling tires nerves that connect with the hypothalamus. The hypothalamus stimulates the posterior pituitary to release oxytocin, which stimulates milk release from the breast, and the anterior lobe to release prolactin, which stimulates additional milk production.

Many authorities recommend against using cow's milk until the infant is at least 1 year old—it is too high in minerals and protein and does not contain enough carbohydrate to meet infant needs. In addition, the major protein in cow's milk, casein, is harder for an infant to digest than the major protein found in human milk, called lactalbumin.

Colostrum

The first fluid made by the human breast is **colostrum.** This can leak from the breast during pregnancy, and is produced in earnest for a few days to a week after birth. It is yellowish and thick and may appear during late pregnancy. Colostrum contains immune factors (e.g., immunoglobulin A [IgA] and lymphocytes) that supply the infant immunity from some diseases. The immature GI tract of the young infant allows these immune factors to pass unaltered into the bloodstream. These immune factors in turn compensate for the infant's immature immune system in its first few months of life.[19] One reason breast-fed infants have fewer respiratory and intestinal infections than formula-fed infants is the presence of these immune bodies in colostrum and in breast milk.

colostrum The first fluid secreted during late pregnancy and the first few days after birth. This thick fluid is rich in immune factors and protein.

Colostrum has potent laxative properties that help the baby pass **meconium,** a stool produced during fetal life. One compound in colostrum, the ***Lactobacillus bifidus* factor,** encourages the growth of *Lactobacillus bifidus* bacteria. These bacteria limit the growth of potentially toxic bacteria in the intestine, such as *Escherichia coli,* and so promote the intestinal health of the breast-fed infant.

meconium The first thick mucouslike stool passed after birth.

***Lactobacillus bifidus* factor** A protective factor secreted in the colostrum that encourages growth of beneficial bacteria in the newborn's intestines.

Mature Milk

Human milk composition gradually changes until several days after delivery, when it achieves the normal composition of mature milk. Human milk looks very different from cow's milk. Human milk is thin, almost watery, in appearance and often has a slight bluish tinge. It has a number of impressive nutritional qualities:

- **Type of protein**—The lactalbumin proteins present form a soft-light curd in the infant's stomach, easing digestion. The lactoferrin proteins bind iron, reducing the growth of iron-requiring bacteria. Many of these type of bacteria cause diarrhea. The immunoglobulin proteins offer important immune protection. The amino acid composition of the protein is noted for its low concentration of phenylalanine, which the infant has a limited ability to metabolize. Human milk also has a high concentration of the amino acid taurine, which is needed for bile salt synthesis to aid lipid digestion.

- **Lipid**—Lipids in the milk are high in linoleic acid and cholesterol, which are needed for brain growth. Lipase enzymes in the milk improve the intestinal digestion of the lipid.

Human milk changes in fat composition during each feeding. The consistency of milk initially (about 60% of the volume) resembles skim milk. The next amount (about 35% of the total volume) has a greater fat proportion, similar to whole milk. Finally, the remaining milk (about 5% of the total), is essentially like cream, and is usually released 10 to 20 minutes into the feeding.[31] Babies need to nurse long enough (i.e., total of 20 to 40 minutes total) to get the kcalories in this fat-rich milk to be satisfied between feedings and to grow well.

- **Lactose**—The major carbohydrate in breast milk is lactose, which creates an acidic environment in the intestine by stimulating the growth of acid-producing bacteria. It also provides galactose for nerve sheath synthesis.
- **Vitamin D**—Some vitamin D is present in human milk. Nevertheless, it is best to provide a vitamin D supplement for the infant if adequate sunlight exposure cannot be guaranteed (see Chapter 12).
- **Iron**—While human milk is low in iron, about 50% of it is absorbed, compared with 2% to 30% for typical foods. The infant needs another source of iron by the age of 4 to 6 months. By that time, the baby's iron stores, formed in utero, are probably depleted. Some researchers recommend iron supplements by 1 to 2 weeks after birth for breast-fed infants.

A Food Plan for Breast-Feeding Women

Nutrient requirements for a breast-feeding mother change slightly—if at all—from those of the pregnant woman.[23] Overall, the high-quality diet of pregnant women should be continued. Exceptions are decreases in folate and iron needs and increases in vitamin A, vitamin C, niacin, and zinc needs. However, the diet for a breast-feeding woman can be the same as that for a pregnant woman, except that the woman should add an additional serving from the milk, yogurt, and cheese group, especially if she is a teenager (Tables 16-1 and 16-2). The best bet is to eat a balanced diet of at least 1800 kcalories a day that is low in fat but rich in calcium, vitamins, and other minerals from a variety of fruits, grains, and vegetables.

It is important for the woman to drink fluids every time the baby nurses. A high fluid intake encourages ample milk production. If a woman restricts her kcalories too severely, the quantity of milk also decreases. This is not a time to crash diet. Research shows that more than two alcoholic drinks a day also decreases milk output, as does smoking.

Milk production requires approximately 750 kcalories per day.[11] The RDA for energy during lactation is an extra 500 kcalories per day, though this may be too generous when there is a need to lose excess fat acquired during pregnancy. The difference between kcalorie needs and intake (750 versus 500) should allow for slow loss of the 3 to 5 plus pounds of fat accumulated during pregnancy. This shows how practical the link is between pregnancy and breast-feeding. Weight loss of 1 to 2 pounds per month is appropriate. A greater rate of weight loss reduces milk output, as dieting becomes too severe. If the mother continues to breast-feed beyond 4 to 6 months or is physically active, more kcalories will be needed.

Most substances the mother ingests are secreted to some extent into the milk. For this reason, caffeine intake should be limited or avoided and all medications should be checked with a pediatrician. Some mothers believe that some foods, such as garlic and chocolate, flavor the breast milk and upset the infant. If a woman notices a connection between a food she eats and later fussiness in the infant, she could consider avoiding that food. However, she might want to experiment again with it later. Infants become fussy for many reasons, and the suspected ingredient may not be the cause.

CONCEPT CHECK

Recognition of the importance of breast-feeding has contributed to its popularity in the last 20 years. Almost all women have the ability to breast-feed. The hormone prolactin stimulates synthesis of milk by the breast tissue. Some components of human milk come directly from the mother's bloodstream. Infant suckling triggers a let-down reflex that releases the milk. The more an infant nurses, the more milk is synthesized. The nutrient composition of human milk is very different from that of cow's milk and changes as the infant matures. The first fluid, colostrum, is very rich in immune factors. The human milk that appears after 10 to 20 minutes of nursing in each breast resembles cream, being rich in both fat and kcalories. The diet for breast-feeding women is generally similar to that for pregnant women except that additional kcalories and fluids are recommended.

Making the Decision to Breast-Feed

Human milk is tailored to meet infant needs for the first 4 to 6 months of life. The possible exceptions are fluoride, iron, and vitamin D. Although formula-feeding can be satisfying for the infant, mother, and the rest of the family (see Chapter 17), there are many physiological and practical advantages to breast-feeding.

FEWER INFECTIONS

Breast-feeding reduces the general risk of infections to the infant. This partially results from the immune factors in human milk that an infant can use.[12,19] As already mentioned, these reduce the risk of respiratory and intestinal infections. Ear infections are also reduced because infants cannot sleep with a bottle in the mouth, as bottle-fed infants often do. While an infant sleeps with a bottle in its mouth, milk pools in the mouth and backs up through the throat into the **eustachian tubes** and into the ears. This creates a growth media for bacteria. Infant ear infections are a common problem that parents want to avoid to decrease discomfort for the infant and trips to the doctor, as well as to prevent possible hearing loss.

eustachian tubes Thin tubes in the middle ear that open into the throat.

FEWER ALLERGIES AND INTOLERANCES

Breast-feeding reduces the incidence of allergies, especially in allergy-prone infants. Cow's milk contains a number of potentially allergy-causing proteins that are absent from human milk. Breast-feeding also avoids the possibility of infant intolerance of formulas. Formulas sometimes must be switched several times until caregivers find one that the infant thrives on.

CONVENIENCE AND EXPENSE

Breast-feeding frees the mother from time and expense involved in buying and preparing formula and washing bottles. Breast milk is already "prepared" and sterile. There is no measuring or mixing. This allows the mother to spend more time with her baby. Breast-feeding is also less expensive, even when considering the cost of the mother's extra food needs.

On the other hand, if the child is bottle-fed, the mother may be freed to do other things while others feed the baby.

BARRIERS TO BREAST-FEEDING

A lack of role models, widespread misinformation, fear of appearing immodest, and women working away from their children all serve as barriers to breast-feeding.

Misinformation

Probably the major barriers to breast-feeding are misinformation and lack of role models. If a woman is interested in breast-feeding, we suggest that she talk to women who have done it successfully. Experienced mothers can be an enormous help to the first-time mother. She should find a friend she can call on to ask questions. In almost every community, a group called La Leche League offers classes in breast-feeding and advises women who have problems with it, or just have questions. One can check the white pages of the telephone book or ask the local health department for the telephone number.

Returning to an Outside Job

Working outside the home can complicate plans to breast-feed. After 1 or 2 months of breast-feeding, a mother can readily express milk either by breast pump or by hand into a sterile plastic bottle or nursing bag to use in a disposable bottle system. Saving breastmilk requires careful sanitation and rapid chilling. There is a knack to learning how to do this, but the freedom can be worth it. Then others can feed the mother's milk to the infant. If the mother freezes her own milk for later use, she should be cautioned not to thaw the milk in a microwave. The heat can destroy immune factors present and create hot spots that can scald the infant's tongue.

Some women can juggle both a job and breast-feeding, but others find it too cumbersome and decide instead to formula-feed. A compromise—balancing some breast-feedings, say early morning and at night, with formula-feedings during the day—is possible. However, keep in mind that too many supplemental feedings decrease milk production. A schedule of expressing milk and using supplemental formula-feedings is most successful if not initiated until after 1 to 2 months of exclusive breast-feeding. After 2 months, the baby is well adapted to breast-feeding and probably feels enough emotional security and other benefits from nursing that he or she is willing to drink both ways.

The key months for breast-feeding are the first 2 to 3 months of an infant's life. Even a few weeks is of benefit. A longer commitment is better, but the first few months are critically important. During that time human milk provides the antiinfective properties needed until the infant begins to synthesize its own immune factors in high concentrations. Working women can try to find infant day-care centers close to the workplace so that they can visit a few times during the day for feeding. Some businesses have day-care facilities on the premises that enable women to return to work and still breast-feed their children. A combination of breast-feeding and formula-feeding may work. If a woman wants to breast-feed her baby, she has many options.

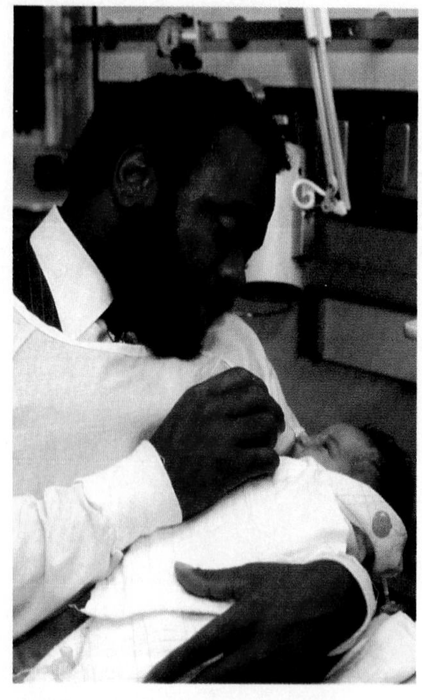

Bottle-feeding is a nutritionally acceptable alternative to breast-feeding when done in a hygienic manner.

Social Reticence

Another barrier for some women is embarrassment when nursing a child in public. Our society historically has stressed modesty and frowned on baring breasts in public—even in so good a cause as nourishing babies. With appropriate clothing, it is possible to nurse quite discreetly.

When is Breast-Feeding not a Good Idea?

Mothers should not breast-feed their infants if they don't want to do so. There are distinct advantages to breast-feeding, but none so great that a woman who decides to bottle-feed should feel she is penalizing her infant.

Infants with the disease phenylketonuria often cannot be breast-fed, and those with galactosemia never can because of the amount of phenylalanine and galactose in human milk (see Chapter 5). Mothers who take medications that pass into the milk and adversely affect the child also should not breast-feed. In addition, a woman who has a serious chronic disease, such as tuberculosis, acquired immune deficiency syndrome (AIDS) or HIV positive, or hepatitis, or who is being treated for cancer, should not breast-feed.

WHAT ABOUT ENVIRONMENTAL CONTAMINANTS?

Some women wonder whether breast-feeding is safe. There is some legitimate concern over the levels of various environmental contaminants in human milk, but the benefits from human milk are very well established, and the risks from environmental contaminants are still largely theoretical. Thus it is probably best to operate with what we know works until sufficiently strong research data dissuades us.

A few measures a woman might take to counteract some known contaminants would be to avoid freshwater fish from polluted waters, carefully wash and peel fruits and vegetables, and remove the fatty edges of meat. In addition, a woman should not try to lose weight rapidly while nursing, because contaminants stored in fat tissue then enter the bloodstream and then the milk. If a woman questions whether her milk is safe, especially if she has lived in an area known to have a high concentration of toxic wastes or environmental pollution, she should ask her local health department for advice.

CAN A PREMATURE INFANT BE BREAST-FED?

There is no clear-cut answer to whether a woman can breast-feed a premature infant. A birth weight about 1500 grams (3½ pounds) is typically one prerequisite. In some cases, human milk is the preferred form of nourishment. It must usually be expressed from the breast and fed through a tube. This type of feeding demands great dedication from the mother. Fortification of the milk with nutrients, such as calcium, phosphorus, sodium, and protein is often needed to match the infant's rapid growth.[17] In other cases, special feeding problems may prevent use of human milk or necessitate some supplementation with formula. Sometimes even total parenteral nutrition is the only option. Working as a team, the pediatrician, neonatal nurse, and registered dietitian guide the parents in this decision.

A NOTE TO FUTURE HEALTH PROFESSIONALS

A precaution for health professionals who counsel mothers who breast-feed infants bears consideration—don't be overly proscriptive.[5] Health-care professionals can scare women away from breast-feeding because the women know they cannot possibly live up to the instructions, so why try? Most women have been so careful during pregnancy that they need to let up a little on dietary advice after the infant is born. Professionals need to stress concern for both continued health and well-being of the mother, as well as for her infant. A compromise is to suggest that mothers follow the recommendations generally, but be more lenient. For example, if she has consumed all the milk and milk products she feels she can tolerate, suggest another source of calcium. If recommendations are too restrictive, health-care professionals will be contributing to the decrease in rate of breast-feeding rather than promoting it.

CONCEPT CHECK

Human milk provides most of an infant's nutritional needs for the first 6 months. Vitamin D, iron, and fluoride may be supplemented. The advantages of breast-feeding over formula-feeding include fewer intestinal, respiratory, and ear infections; fewer allergies and food intolerances; and convenience. Lack of role models, misinformation, and social reticence may dissuade a mother from breast-feeding. A combination of breast-feeding and formula-feeding is possible when a mother is regularly away from the infant. Breast-feeding is not desirable if a mother has certain diseases or must take medication potentially harmful to the infant. The premature infant, depending on its condition, may benefit from consuming human milk.

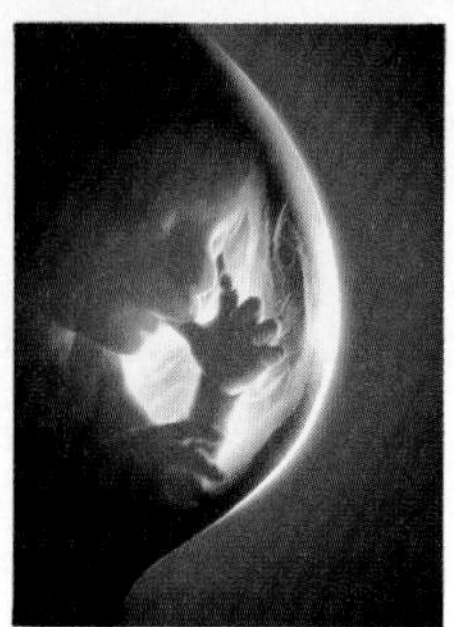

Summary

1. Adequate nutrition is vital during pregnancy to ensure the well-being of both the infant and the mother. Insults due to poor nutrition and some medications can cause birth defects, especially if they occur in the first trimester. Growth retardation and altered development can also occur if these insults happen later in pregnancy.
2. Infants born prematurely (before 37 weeks of gestation) or with low birth weight (less than 5.5 pounds, or 2500 grams) usually have more medical problems at birth than normal infants.
3. Teenage pregnancy requires very careful prenatal and nutritional care. Complications are more common in these pregnancies because of the very high physiological demands and often poor social and economic support.
4. Daily energy needs increase by an average of 300 kcalories during the second and third trimesters of pregnancy. Weight gain should be gradual to a total of 25 to 35 pounds in a normal weight mother.
5. Protein, vitamin, and mineral requirements increase during pregnancy. Extra servings from the milk, yogurt, and cheese group and the meat, poultry, fish, dry beans, eggs, and nuts group of the Guide to Daily Food Choices are recommended. Supplements of iron and folate, in particular, may be needed.
6. Pregnancy-induced hypertension, gestational diabetes, heartburn, constipation, nausea, vomiting, edema, and anemia are all possible discomforts and complications of pregnancy. Nutrition therapy can often help minimize these problems.
7. The popularity of breast-feeding has increased in the past 20 years. Almost all women have the ability to nurse their infants. The nutrient composition of human milk is very different from cow's milk. Colostrum, the first fluid produced by humans, is very rich in immune factors. Mature milk is rich in the protein lactalbumin and in lactose.
8. Advantages of breast-feeding over formula-feeding for the infant include fewer intestinal, respiratory, and ear infections; fewer allergies and food intolerances; and convenience. An infant can be adequately nourished with formula if the mother chooses not to breast-feed. Breast-feeding is not desirable if the mother has certain diseases or must take medication potentially harmful to the infant.

Study Questions

1. What historical evidence establishes the importance of nutrition in pregnancy outcome?
2. Provide three key pieces of advice for a couple who are seeking to maximize their chances of having a healthy baby. Why did you single out those specific factors?
3. What health problems can a woman possibly expect to develop during pregnancy? What nutrition-related advice can you provide to help prevent these problems from developing into serious conditions?
4. Give three reasons why a woman should give serious consideration to breast-feeding her infant.
5. Describe the physiological links that are linked to milk production and release. How does knowing about these help a clinician provide more informed advice to nursing mothers?

REFERENCES

1. ADA reports: Position of the American Dietetic Association: nutritional management of adolescent pregnancy, *Journal of The American Dietetic Association* 89:104, 1989.
2. Abrams RS, Coustan DR: Gestational diabetes uptake, *Clinical Diabetes* 8:19, 1990.
3. Abrams B and others: Maternal weight gain and preterm delivery, *Obstetrics and Gynecology* 74:577, 1989.
4. Belizan JM and others: Calcium supplementation to prevent hypertensive disorders of pregnancy, *The New England Journal of Medicine* 325:1399, 1991.
5. Boyne L: Nutrition in pregnancy, *Nutri-News* 5:10, 1992.
6. Carr-Hill R and others: Is birth weight determined genetically? *British Medical Journal* 295:687, 1987.
7. Chasnoff IJ and others: Cocaine/polydrug use in pregnancy: two year follow-up, *Pediatrics* 89:284, 1992.
8. Collins JW, Jr., Davis RJ: The differential effect of traditional risk factors on infant birthweight among blacks and whites in Chicago, *American Journal of Public Health* 80:679, 1990.
9. Folate supplements prevent recurrence of neural tube defects, *Nutrition Reviews* 50:21, 1992.
10. Gearhart JG and others: Alcoholism in women, *American Family Physician* 44(3):908, 1992.
11. Goldberg GR and others: Longitudinal assessment of the components of energy balance in well-nourished lactating women, *American Journal of Clinical Nutrition* 54:788, 1991.
12. Goldman AS: Immunology of milk and the neonate conference, *Nutrition Today,* Sept/Oct 1991, p 30.
13. Horner RD and others: Pica practices of pregnant women, *Journal of The American Dietetic Association* 91:34, 1991.
14. Iannucci L: The perplexities of pregnancy, *FDA Consumer,* Nov 1990, p 17.
15. Jacobson HN: A healthy pregnancy, the struggle to define it, *Nutrition Today,* Jan/Feb 1988, p 30.
16. Kurinij N and others: Breast-feeding incidents and duration in black and white women, *Pediatrics* 81:365, 1988.
17. Lawrence RA: *Breastfeeding,* ed 3, St Louis, 1989, Mosby–Year Book.
18. Lipschultz SE and others: Cardiovascular abnormalities in infants prematurely exposed to cocaine, *Journal of Pediatrics* 118:44, 1991.
19. Lonnerdal B, Picclano MF: Mechanisms relating lactation and infant nutrient utilization, *Nutrition Today,* May/June 1991, p 32.
20. McGrew MC, Shore WB: The problem of teenage pregnancy, *The Journal of Family Practice* 32:17, 1991.
21. Mitchell MC, Lerner E: Maternal hematologic measures and pregnancy outcome, *Journal of The American Dietetic Association* 92:484, 1992.
22. National Academy of Sciences—Institute of Medicine: *Nutrition during pregnancy,* Washington, D.C., 1990, National Academy of Sciences Press.
23. National Academy of Sciences—Institute of Medicine: *Nutrition during lactation,* Washington, D.C., 1991, National Academy of Sciences Press.
24. Resnik R: The "elderly primigravida" in 1990, *The New England Journal of Medicine* 322:693, 1990.
25. Springer NS and others: Using early weight gain and other nutrition-related risk factors to predict pregnancy outcomes, *Journal of The American Dietetic Association* 92:217, 1992.
26. Streissguth AP and others: Fetal alcohol syndrome in adolescents and adults, *Journal of The American Dietetic Association* 265:1961, 1991.
27. Suitor CW: Perspectives on nutrition during pregnancy, *Journal of The American Dietetic Association* 91:96, 1991.
28. Susser M: Maternal weight gain, infant birth weight and diet: causal sequences, *American Journal of Clinical Nutrition* 53:1384, 1991.
29. Walker ARP and others: Nutrition needs in pregnancy: why is the state of knowledge still speculative? *Nutrition Today,* Nov/Dec 1991, p 18.
30. Waterson EJ, Murray-Lyon IM: Preventing alcohol-related birth damage: review, *Social Science Medicine* 30:349, 1990.
31. Worthington-Roberts B and others: *Nutrition in pregnancy and lactation,* St. Louis, 1989, Mosby–Year Book.

SUGGESTED READINGS

For a more detailed look at nutrition and pregnancy see *Maternal nutrition during pregnancy* by the National Academy of Sciences and the textbook, *Nutrition in Pregnancy and Lactation* by Worthington-Roberts and others. Together these sources contain essentially all the information a health professional needs about nutrition in pregnancy and breast-feeding. The article by Streissguth and others supplies the classic description of the effects of alcohol in pregnancy. Finally, read the position paper by The American Dietetic Association on the nutritional management of adolescent pregnancy. This age group presents a great challenge to health-care professionals because of the simultaneous problems of meeting nutritional needs of growth by the fetus and the teenage mother.

Targeting necessary nutrients for a pregnant woman

In this chapter we mentioned that the nutrient needs hardest to meet during pregnancy are FOLATE, VITAMIN D, IRON, CALCIUM, and ZINC. Refer to Chapters 12 through 15 on vitamins and minerals to find five foods rich in each nutrient. List them next to the appropriate heading below.

NUTRIENT	FOODS	
	1. ______________	4. ______________
Folate	2. ______________	5. ______________
	3. ______________	
	1. ______________	4. ______________
Vitamin D	2. ______________	5. ______________
	3. ______________	
	1. ______________	4. ______________
Iron	2. ______________	5. ______________
	3. ______________	
	1. ______________	4. ______________
Calcium	2. ______________	5. ______________
	3. ______________	
	1. ______________	4. ______________
Zinc	2. ______________	5. ______________
	3. ______________	

Did you list any foods next to more than one nutrient? What are they?

____

Foods rich in more than one of these nutrients would be doubly useful and valuable. Those foods would be ones on which to focus when pregnant.

Are there any reasons why it might be hard for a person to get the needed amount of these nutrients, aside from having generally increased needs during pregnancy?

____

Now, design a diet you would like to follow that meets prenatal nutrient recommendations. Use the foods you selected in the above exercise to plan these meals. Try to show it to a pregnant women. What insights have you gained?

BREAKFAST: ____

LUNCH: ____

SNACK: ____

DINNER: ____

SNACK: ____ ▲

NUTRITION PERSPECTIVE

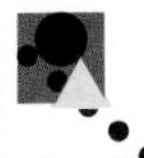

Fetal Alcohol Syndrome

The effect of alcohol use during pregnancy is a very important issue. There is no question that large amounts of alcohol harm the fetus. Over 2000 scientific reports have now appeared that confirm alcohol is a drug capable of producing lifelong disabilities after fetal exposure. Women suffering from chronic alcoholism produce children with a recognizable pattern of malformations called **fetal alcohol syndrome (FAS)** (Figure 16-9). A diagnosis of FAS is based mainly on poor prenatal and infant growth, physical deformities, and mental retardation.[10] Prenatal brain damage may permanently disrupt the ability to concentrate, think abstractly, and function independently, continuing even into adulthood.

fetal alcohol syndrome (FAS) A group of physical and mental abnormalities in the infant that result from the mother consuming alcohol during pregnancy.

The range of abnormalities varies from severe FAS to milder forms showing reduced birth weight, premature birth, behavioral effects, such as poor judgment, distractibility, and difficulty perceiving social cues, as well as poor learning ability in infants of women reporting only social drinking. The latter category is termed fetal alcohol effects.[26] Annually, about 4000 to 7,500 infants are born in the United States with FAS, and about 35,000 are born with fetal alcohol effects. This makes alcohol the leading cause of ***preventable*** birth defects and mental retardation in the United States.[30] Binge drinking is perilous, especially during the first 12 weeks, when signs of pregnancy are few and key aspects of fetal development take place.

Exactly how alcohol causes these defects is not known, but other factors, such as poor nutrition, cigarette smoking (nicotine intake), and other drugs compound the problems. One line of research shows poor cell migration in the brain during early stages of development in the presence of alcohol. In addition, we do not know how much alcohol intake produces these problems. Because of this, many health authorities, including the U.S. surgeon general and the American Medical Association, believe it is best for mothers-to-be to avoid alcohol altogether.

Alcohol reaches the fetal blood at the same concentration as is in the mother's blood within 15 minutes of her drinking. However, the effect on the fetus may be up to 10 times greater. Just one bout of binge drinking can arrest and alter cell division occurring during a critical phase of fetal development. The fetus then may develop with an irreversible defect.

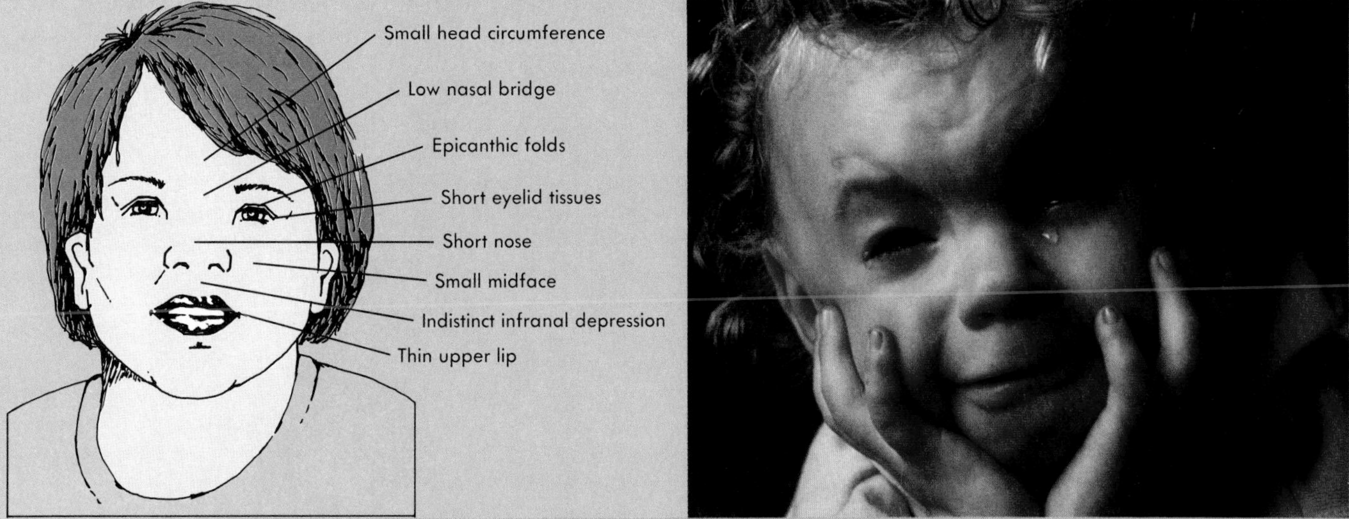

Figure 16-9 Fetal alcohol syndrome. Milder forms of alcohol-induced changes on the fetus and the infant are known as fetal alcohol effects.

NUTRITION PERSPECTIVE

Fetal Alcohol Syndrome—cont'd

Since alcohol has the capacity to adversely affect each stage of fetal development, the earlier in pregnancy that heavy drinking ceases, the greater is the potential for improved outcome. The best course is to consider alcohol an indulgence that can be eliminated until after pregnancy.[14]

Not only is it important for pregnant women to abstain from alcohol during pregnancy, but also when trying to conceive, and anytime the possibility of conception is present. One step in the right direction is the new congressionally mandated warnings about drinking during pregnancy that appear on all alcoholic beverage containers. Recall that many women are not aware they are pregnant until 2 to 3 months after conception, and during that time much fetal growth and development takes place. Considering that pregnancy lasts only 9 months and that parents may spend a lifetime caring for a handicapped child, it is important for parents—especially women—to realize that avoiding alcohol completely during pregnancy is a lesser sacrifice. Although an affected child is still loved, the life that results is needlessly difficult for the child and the family. Since women who drink heavily often respond to supportive therapy focused on abstinence, prenatal care providers have a unique opportunity to intervene and provide benefits for both the mother and her newborn.

CHAPTER SEVENTEEN

Infants, Children, and Teens

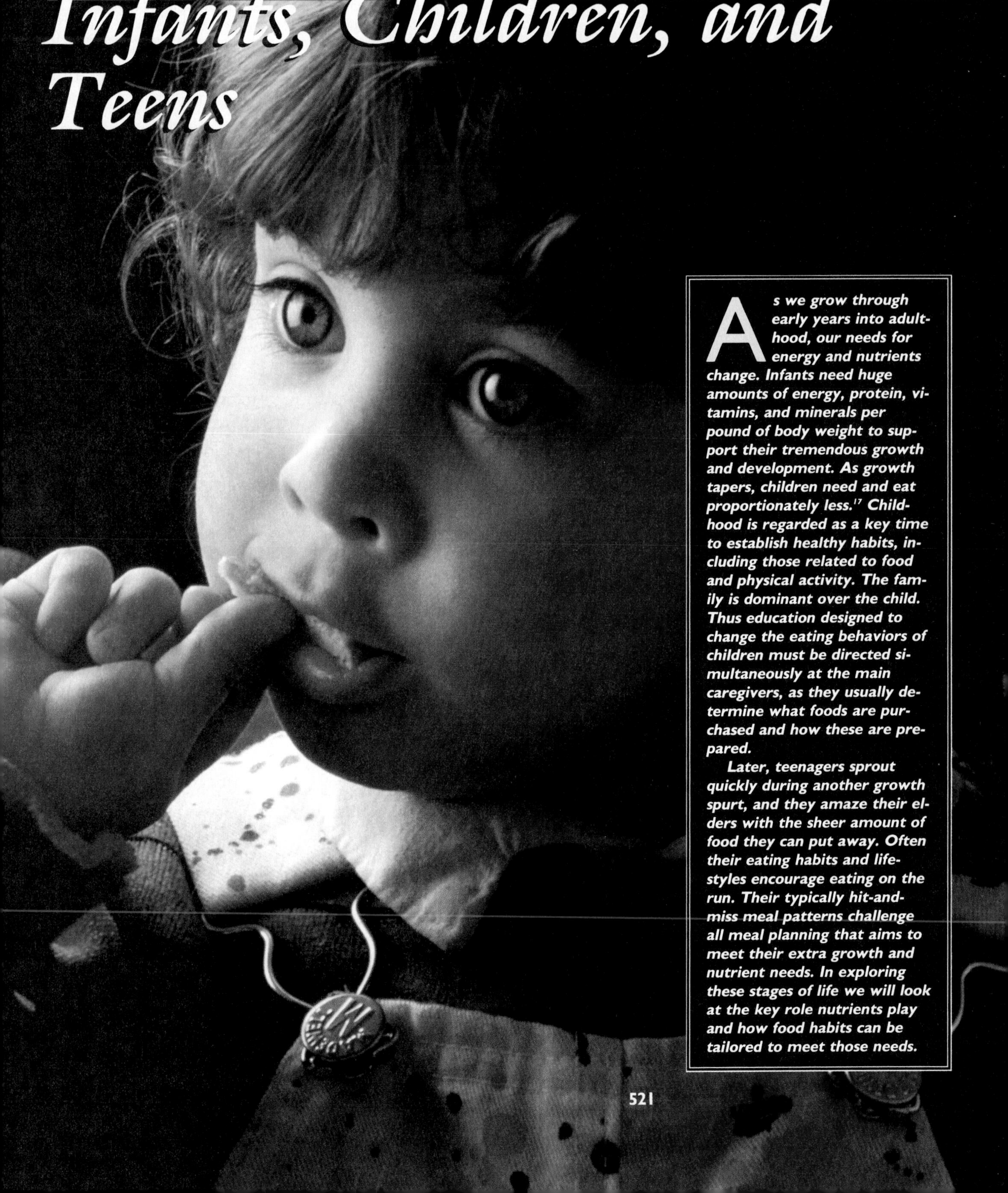

As we grow through early years into adulthood, our needs for energy and nutrients change. Infants need huge amounts of energy, protein, vitamins, and minerals per pound of body weight to support their tremendous growth and development. As growth tapers, children need and eat proportionately less.[17] Childhood is regarded as a key time to establish healthy habits, including those related to food and physical activity. The family is dominant over the child. Thus education designed to change the eating behaviors of children must be directed simultaneously at the main caregivers, as they usually determine what foods are purchased and how these are prepared.

Later, teenagers sprout quickly during another growth spurt, and they amaze their elders with the sheer amount of food they can put away. Often their eating habits and lifestyles encourage eating on the run. Their typically hit-and-miss meal patterns challenge all meal planning that aims to meet their extra growth and nutrient needs. In exploring these stages of life we will look at the key role nutrients play and how food habits can be tailored to meet those needs.

NUTRITION AWARENESS INVENTORY

Here are 15 statements about nutrition for infants, children, and teens. Answer them to test your current knowledge. If you think the answer is true or mostly true, circle T. If you think the answer is false or mostly false, circle F. Use the scoring key at the end of the book to compute your total score. Take this test again after you have read this chapter. Compare the results.

1. T F Consuming low-protein diets in childhood can greatly affect ultimate adult height.
2. T F An infant's length increases by 50% in the first year.
3. T F Brain growth is greatest during the teen years.
4. T F Most obese infants become obese adults.
5. T F Infants have lower energy needs per pound than older children.
6. T F An infant's diet should be very low in fat.
7. T F Infants need solid food by 3 months of age.
8. T F Infants enjoy blander foods than do adults.
9. T F Colic is caused by a gas buildup in the intestinal tract.
10. T F Cow's milk fed during early infancy can cause allergies.
11. T F Iron-deficiency anemia often occurs in infants whose diets are composed mainly of cow's milk.
12. T F It is nutritionally important to put children on a schedule of three meals per day.
13. T F The two most common nutritional problems in childhood are obesity and iron-deficiency anemia.
14. T F Parents should carefully control the amount of food their children eat.
15. T F Acne can be avoided by limiting certain foods in the diet.

Infant Growth and Physiological Development

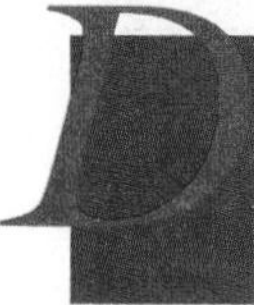

During infancy a child's attitudes toward food and the whole eating process are shaped. Depending on the nutritional knowledge and flexibility of parents and other caregivers, an infant can start life with both an optimum nutritional status that accommodates brain and body growth spurts and a willingness to experiment and try new foods.

THE GROWING INFANT SHOWS GAINS IN WEIGHT AND HEIGHT

Today a variety of different people—parents, grandparents, daycare workers, and others—may have a major role is raising a child. We will tend to use the word parent, but realize many others may be key decision makers.

It seems as though all babies do is eat and sleep during the first few months. There is a good reason for this; rapid growth characterizes infancy. An infant's birth weight is doubled in its first 4 to 6 months and increases three times within the first year. Such growth requires considerable nourishment and sleep. Beyond the first year, growth is slower and more steady; it takes 5 years to double the weight seen at 1 year. An infant's length also increases by 50% in the first year. It then continues to increase throughout preschool and teen years.[17] This growth stops when the bone ends (epiphyses) fuse together, halting further significant linear increases (Figure 17-1).

All this growth requires a generous nutrient intake to support body needs. We know from observing Egyptian mummies that infants were about the same size in 300 B.C. as they are today. However, adult mummies are much smaller than today's adults. Notice from museum collections of the Middle Ages the small sizes of many of the suits of armor. People of the past ate diets that tended to stunt their growth.

In Third World countries today, about half the children are short and underweight for their age. They are simply smaller versions of nutritionally fit children. In these countries, when breast-feeding ceases, children are often left to consume a high-carbohydrate, low-protein diet. This diet supports some growth but does not allow them to achieve their genetic potential. Adequate protein intake is critical for growth. Weight primarily reflects current nutrient intake, while height is a better measure of long-term nutrient intake during childhood.

Infants show a pattern of physiological development in which body water is reduced from about 75% at birth to about 60%, the proportion typical in adults. By 1 year of age an infant's body nitrogen content (and so, protein content) has increased from 2% of body weight at birth to 3%, indicating the infant has synthesized much new lean tissue. A further indication of lean tissue synthesis is an increase in body potassium concentration from infancy to adulthood.[17] Recall from Chapter 14 that potassium is the major positive ion operating inside cells. As children build more cells, they accumulate more potassium.

THE EFFECT OF MALNUTRITION ON GROWTH

In Chapter 16 we described growth as a process of cell division (hyperplasia) and then of cell growth (hypertrophy). The long-term effects of nutritional problems in infancy and childhood depend on the severity, timing, and duration of the nutritional insult to these cell processes, just as they did when the fetus was **in utero.** Poor hypertrophy is reversible. Organs in the process of hypertrophy during a nutritional famine can regain and restore that growth when an adequate diet is resumed.

in utero "In the uterus," or in other words, during pregnancy.

Hyperplasia stopped by a poor diet probably cannot be reversed. If cell division is arrested, an adequate diet later probably will not help much because the appropriate hormonal environment necessary for that cell division will no longer be present. A 15-year-old Central American girl who is 4 feet 8 inches tall cannot attain the adult height of a typical American simply by improving her diet. Once the time for growth ceases (in women this is about 2 years after the onset of menses), a good nutrient intake will help maintain health but will not compensate for lost growth.

ASSESSING INFANT GROWTH AND DEVELOPMENT

Health professionals monitor a child's increases in height, weight, and head circumference, and interpret the records using growth charts. All these parameters are useful indicators of nutritional health. The typical charts contain seven percentile divisions, which represent 90% of children (see Appendix M). A percentile simply represents the rank of the person among 100 age- and gender-matched peers. If Tony, for example, is at the ninetieth percentile height for age, this description means that if you measure 100 representative children of that age, ten children will be taller than Tony, and 89 will be shorter. A child at the fiftieth percentile is considered average. Fifty children will be taller than this child, while 49 will be shorter.

The two growth charts that give the most useful information for children are height-for-age—which assesses linear growth—and weight-for-height—which assesses weight status based on height for prepubertal states. For children under 3 years of age, head circumference-for-age is also a useful measure of growth. Since

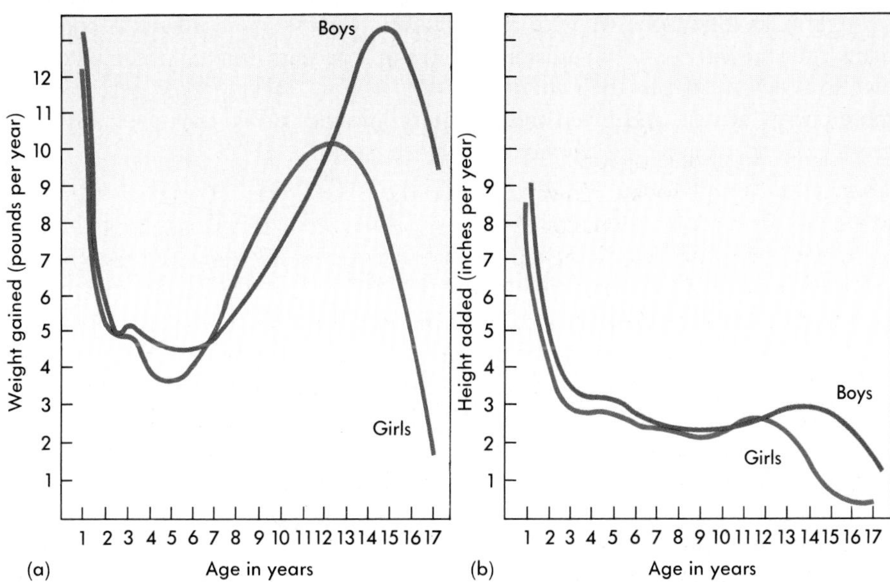

Figure 17-1 Growth rates. **A,** Average gains in weight for girls and boys. **B,** Average additions to height for girls and boys.

children under 2 to 3 years of age are measured with knees unflexed, lying on their backs, the term length is used instead of height.

Individual growth charts are available for both males and females, for ages ranging from 0 to 36 months or 2 to 18 years (see Appendix T). Growth of infants and children should be plotted during their regularly scheduled health checkups. It takes 1 to 3 years for an infant to establish his or her "genetic" percentile. Once this figure is established, such as length-(height-)for-age, the child's measurement should then track along that percentile, but spurts and lulls in growth can also be expected.[23] If the child's growth overall does not keep up with his or her percentile, the physician needs to investigate whether a medical or nutritional problem is impeding the predicted growth.

Infants born prematurely may catch up in growth in 2 to 3 years. This requires that the child jump up in the percentiles. If this occurs—especially in height-for-age—it is usually no cause for alarm. On the other hand, jumping percentiles in weight-for-height can be disturbing if the child approaches the eightieth to ninetieth percentiles. Generally a child at the ninetieth percentile for weight-for-height is considered "overweight." Above the ninety-fifth percentile, the child is considered obese.

BRAIN GROWTH

The rate of brain growth is maximal at birth. Increases in cell number (hyperplasia) cease between 12 and 15 months of age. However, different areas of the brain peak in hyperplasia at different times. When studying the effect of nutritional status on brain development and ultimate intelligence quotient (IQ), it is difficult to separate the effects of nature from nurture. However, studies from Central America suggest that IQ after age 5 years relates more closely with the amount of schooling the child receives than with nutritional intake during childhood.

ADIPOSE TISSUE GROWTH

Since 1970, researchers have speculated that overfeeding during infancy increases adipose tissue cell number (see Chapter 8 for details). This link has been difficult to establish, since researchers can neither see nor count empty adipose cells. Therefore when analyzing an adipose sample from a thin infant, researchers are not sure if they are counting all cells present. It could be that an obese infant has just filled up more cells, while a lean infant has as many cells, but some are hidden (still not filled).

If energy intake is restricted in infancy to decrease adipose tissue hyperplasia, the growth of other organ systems may decrease as well. In addition, no evidence strongly links infant obesity with adult obesity.[17] Most obese infants become normalweight preschoolers. In addition, one thing is certain: Infants need an adequate diet so they can obtain their intended adult height. Taller people necessarily use more energy at rest, and given the sedentary lifestyles of us, they probably have a greater chance of avoiding obesity than shorter people.

CONCEPT CHECK

Growth occurs rapidly during infancy; birth weight doubles in 4 to 6 months and increases by three times within the first year. Other physiological changes during infancy include an increase in lean tissue and a reduction in the percentage of body water. Undernutrition can cause irreversible changes in growth and maturation. Infant and child growth is monitored by tracking body weight, height (or length) and head circumference over time. The most useful growth charts in childhood plot height-for-age and prepubescent weight-for-height. Development of obesity is not desirable in infancy, though there is no strong evidence that an obese infant will become an obese adult.

Infant Nutritional Needs

An infant's nutrient needs differ from adult needs in both amount and proportion, and vary with stages of growth. Fortunately, early needs usually can be met by human milk or formula. Solid foods generally are not needed to supplement these nutrient sources until after 4 to 6 months of age. Even so, the basis of an infant's diet for the first year remains human milk or formula.[17]

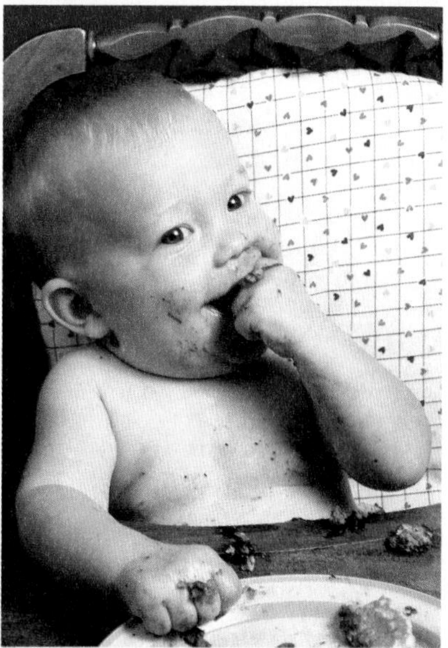

An infant first practices self-feeding at about six to seven months of age.

ENERGY

Daily energy needs in infancy are about 45 to 50 kcalories per pound per day (98 to 108 kcalories per kilogram per day). Based on body weight, this is proportionately two to four times the energy needs of an adult (Figure 17-2). Infants require an easy way to meet their high-energy needs. Either human milk or formula is ideal during the first few months. Both are high in fat and supply about 650 kcalories per 32 ounces of fluid (700 kcalories per liter; Table 17-1). Later, a combination of human milk or formula with solid foods can provide even more energy.

The high energy needs of the infant are primarily driven by rapid growth and a high metabolic rate—the latter in part is because of the ratio of the infant's great surface area to its weight. More surface area allows more heat loss from the skin; energy metabolism is required to replace that heat.

PROTEIN

Daily protein needs vary in infancy from 0.7 to 1 gram per pound of body weight (1.6 to 2.2 grams per kilogram per day). One liter of formula or human milk contains about 13 grams (or 12 grams per quart). About 40% of this protein should be of high quality to contain ample essential amino acids. Total protein intake should not exceed 20% of kcalorie needs. Excess nitrogen and minerals supplied by high-protein diets would overtax the infant's kidney function.

A protein deficiency in infants is unlikely here, except in cases of mistaken feeding practices, such as overdiluting an infant's formula. A protein deficiency may also

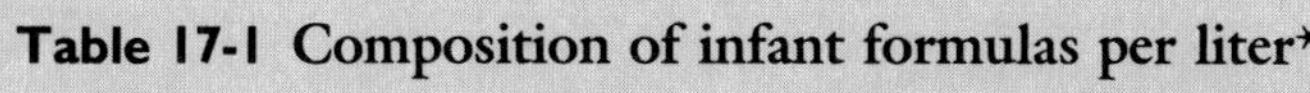

Table 17-1 Composition of infant formulas per liter*

Milk or formula	Kcalories	Protein (grams)	Fat (grams)	Carbohydrate (grams)	Minerals† (grams)
Human milk	750	11	45	70	2
Casein-based formulas					
Similac	680	15.5	36	72	3.3
Enfamil	670	15	38	69	3
SMA	670	15	36	72	2.5
Gerber	670	15	36	72	2.4
Cow's milk					
Whole	670	36	36	49	7
Skim	360	36	1	51	7
Soybean protein-based formulas					
ProSobee	670	20	36	68	4
Isomil	570	20	36	68	4
Nursoy	670	20	36	68	4
Predigested protein					
Nutramigen	670	19	26	90	1.1
Alimentum	670	19	38	70	1.2

* 1 liter equals about 30 fluid ounces.
†Calcium, phosphorus, and other minerals

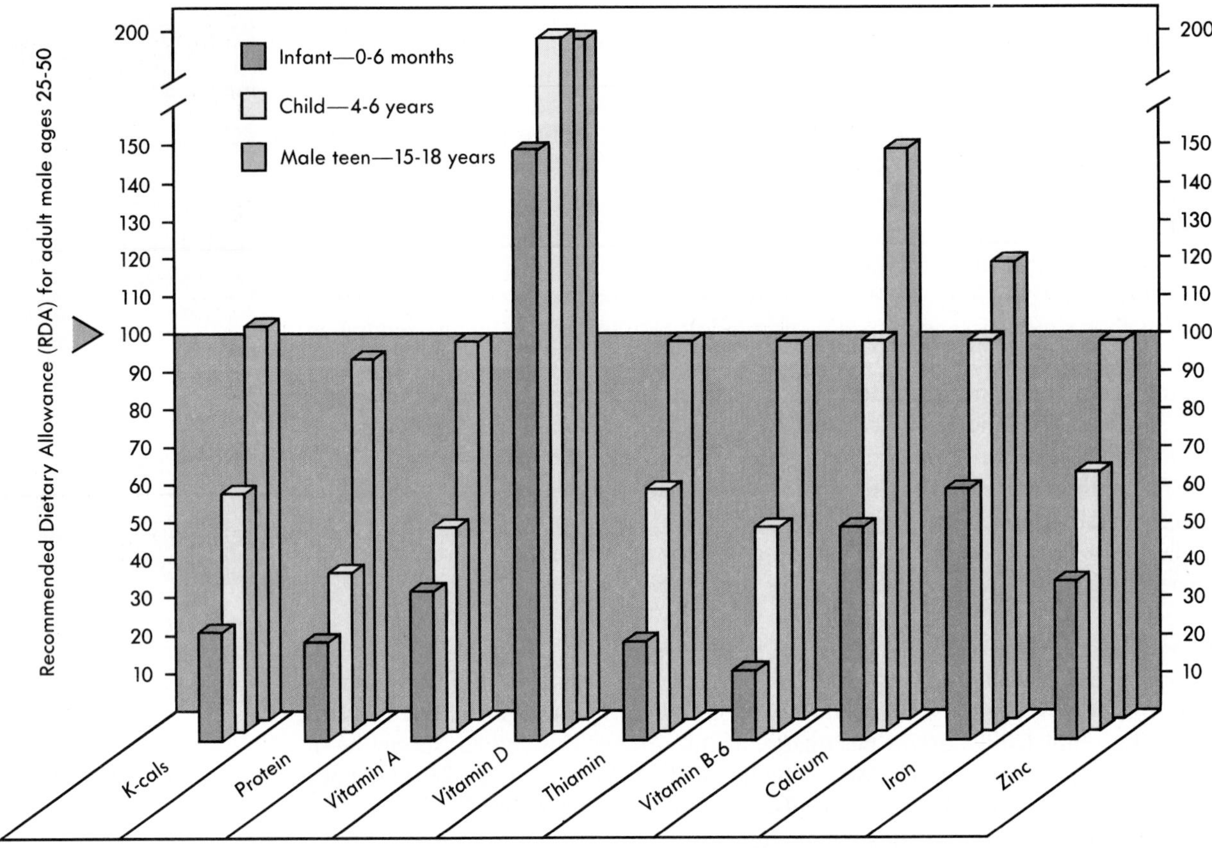

Figure 17-2 RDAs for infants, children, and teens. Compared to energy needs, infants need greater quantities of some nutrients than adults. This is illustrated by comparing the height of the kcalories bar to all other bars for infants. The same comparison can be made for children and teens.

result from allergies. The clinician needs to closely watch infants with allergies because, as foods are eliminated from their diets, they may be offered insufficient protein (see the Nutrition Perspective on Food Allergies and Intolerances).[3]

FAT

Fat should make up about 30% to 50% of an infant's energy intake. More than this amount may lead to poor fat digestion. Both human milk and formula supply about 50% of energy as fat. Essential fatty acids should make up at least 3% of total energy intake. Formulas and human milk do so. Fats are an important part of the infant's diet because they are energy dense. This characteristic helps resolve the dilemma of high energy needs but small stomach capacity.

VITAMINS OF SPECIAL INTEREST

Vitamin K is routinely administered (usually injected) to all infants at birth. This dose lasts until the infant's intestinal bacteria are established and begin to synthesize vitamin K. Formula-fed infants receive the rest of the vitamins they need from the formula. Breast-fed infants, especially dark-skinned ones, should receive a vitamin D supplement if they are not exposed to much sunlight. The time needed in the sun to obtain adequate vitamin D is approximately 15 to 30 minutes per day for white infants and longer for African-Americans. Breast-fed infants whose mothers are total vegetarians (vegans) should receive a vitamin B-12 supplement. Infants who drink goat's milk need supplements of folate and vitamin B-12 since this type of milk is low in bioavailability and/or amounts of these vitamins.

MINERALS OF SPECIAL INTEREST

Iron stores present at birth are generally depleted by the time birth weight doubles, which is around 4 to 6 months of age. For this reason, formula-fed infants should be fed an iron-fortified formula. Breast-fed infants need solid foods to supply extra iron at about 6 months of age. The need for iron is a major consideration in deciding when to introduce solids.[19] Some researchers recommend liquid iron supplements from birth or by 1 month of age for breast-fed infants.

It is important for an infant to receive adequate amounts of iodide and zinc to support growth. Human milk and formula supply these needs if the infant's energy needs are met. In addition, fluoride supplementation may be necessary for breast-fed infants, and for bottle-fed infants where the water supply used in formula preparation does not contain fluoride. Note that formula manufacturers use fluoride-free water in formula preparation. Parents should consult their dentist about the need for extra fluoride.

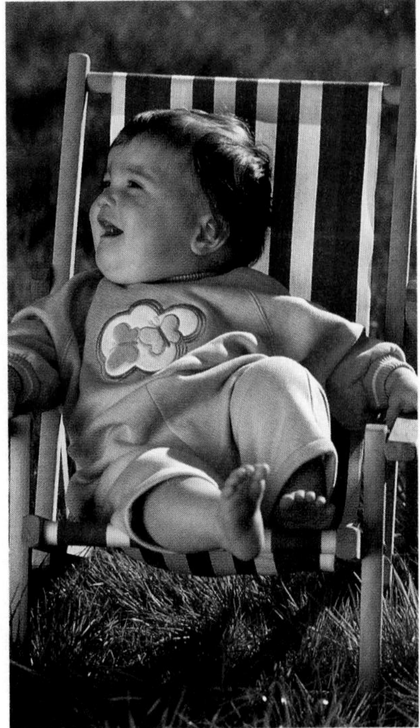

Some sun exposure helps an infant meet vitamin D needs.

WATER

An infant needs approximately 1.5 milliliters of water (fluid) per kcalorie in the diet.[17] The typical consumption of human milk or formula usually meets this need. These yield about 95% of volume as water. However, in hot climates small amounts of supplemental water may be necessary. In addition, diarrhea, vomiting, and fever also often lead to a greater need for supplemental water, under a physicians' guidance. It is important to remember that an infant is easily dehydrated. Dehydration can result in a rapid decrease in kidney function, and the infant may then require hospitalization for rehydration. Keep in mind also that too much supplemental water can be harmful, especially to the brain. It is best to limit supplemental fluids to about 4 ounces per day unless the physician feels a greater need exists because of disease or other conditions. Overall, extreme fluid intakes—either too little or too much—can lead to health problems.

CONCEPT CHECK

Most nutrient needs in the first 6 months are met by human milk or formula. Vitamin D, fluoride, and iron may need to be supplemented for breast-fed infants. Water needs are generally met by the human milk or formula.

FORMULA-FEEDING FOR INFANTS

We discussed breast-feeding in detail in Chapter 16. Let's now focus on formula-feeding. Recall that a major advantage of breast-feeding is providing immune proteins, which impart immune protection to the infant. That advantage is very important, especially in cases of poverty and poor hygiene where safe water supply and proper formula preparation are not likely. However, many parents choose not to breast-feed their infants and opt for formula feeding. Today, formula-feeding is a safe alternative in the United States since high standards for water purity and cleanliness are common.

FORMULA COMPOSITION

Cow's milk, because of its high protein and mineral content, cannot be used in early infancy. It must be altered. Commercially altered forms, known as infant formulas, were first available in 1931. Since 1980 infant formula manufacturers have been required to conform to strict guidelines for nutrient composition and quality set by federal law. Generally, infant formulas contain lactose or sucrose for carbohydrate needs, heat-treated **casein** and **whey** proteins from cow's milk for protein needs, and vegetable oils for fat needs (Table 17-1).[17] Today's formulas are much improved over earlier versions because the new heat-treated casein is easier to digest than the previously used natural forms of casein. Whey proteins are naturally easy to digest,

casein Proteins found in milk that form curds when exposed to acid, and are difficult for infants to digest.

whey Proteins, such as lactalbumin, that are found in great amounts in human milk and are easy to digest.

If an infant does not tolerate a standard formula, the protein source is usually switched to soybean-based protein and the carbohydrate to corn syrup or sucrose. If the soybean-based formula is not tolerated, the next step is to try a predigested (hydrolyzed) protein source, such as found in Nutramigen or Alimentum.

allergy an immune response that occurs when antibodies react with a foreign substance (antigen).

and so many formulas are supplemented with extra whey protein to bring the casein-to-whey ratio closer to that found in human milk.

Formulas contain vitamins and minerals in amounts suggested by the guidelines of the American Academy of Pediatrics. We recommend an iron-fortified formula. Check the container carefully as not all are iron fortified. Research shows that added iron does not lead to intestinal complaints, such as constipation, any more than nonfortified formulas do, though some people believe this misconception.

A variety of specialized formulas exist. These vary in energy content; type of protein, carbohydrate, and fat used; and iron fortification. The variations are responses to the special needs of some normal-term infants, premature infants, infants with **allergies,** infants with higher energy needs, and infants with special metabolic problems, such as those with phenylketonuria (see Chapter 5).

Health food stores often sell formula-type products that can lead unsuspecting parents into thinking they are providing their infants with a complete nutritional formula. Soy Moo, for example, a soy beverage sold in health food stores, should not be confused with soy-based infant formulas. Unlike nutritionally complete infant formulas, this product, and others like it, lack some essential nutrients and can lead to severe nutritional deficiencies in infants. For example, a severely malnourished 5-month-old infant was recently admitted to Arkansas Children's Hospital in Little Rock with symptoms of heart failure, rickets, inflamed blood vessels, and possible nerve damage. According to the hospital, the baby girl had been fed nothing but Soy Moo since she was 3 days old. Because of cases such as this one, parents should consult their physician when choosing an appropriate infant formula.

FORMULA PREPARATION

In the 1950s, it was common to prepare a day's supply of bottles and then sterilize them in boiling water for about 30 minutes. Today, it is often more convenient to prepare bottles one at a time. All utensils should be washed before preparing the formula. Concentrated or powdered formulas are poured into a bottle to which clean, cold water is added (follow label directions). The formula is then warmed, if desired, mixed and fed immediately to the infant. Hot water from the faucet should not be used to make formula since it poses a risk for high lead content (see Chapter 19). Ready-to-feed formula is also available. It is important to note that infant formula should not be heated in a microwave oven. Hot spots can develop that may burn the infant's mouth.

When using a powdered formula it is very convenient to simply have bottles on hand that have the powder added. These then can be quickly diluted with cold water, heated if desired, and fed to the infant. It is safe to refrigerate diluted formula for 1 day. However, formula left over from a feeding should be discarded because it will be contaminated by bacteria and enzymes from the infant's saliva. If well water is used, it should be boiled for a minute or so before making formula, and also should be checked for abnormally high levels of naturally occurring nitrates. These can bind hemoglobin in red blood cells and lead to severe anemia.

Whether bottle-feeding or breast-feeding, it is important to burp a baby after the baby has been given each 1 to 2 ounces (30 to 60 milliliters) and at the end of feeding.[17] Spitting up a bit of milk is normal at this time (be prepared). Once fed, the child should be placed on one side, possibly with a rolled up blanket against its back to support it in this position. If the infant spits up milk, this position will decrease the infant's tendency to inhale the milk and choke.

It is important to stop a feeding when the infant indicates he or she is full. Parents and other caregivers need to pay attention to cues that the infant has had enough. Such cues can include inattention, turning its head away, falling asleep, or becoming playful. Adults should trust the infant's appetite rather than administer a standardized serving size. This includes allowing the infant to refuse some milk in the bottle. Feeding cues are not as much of a concern for breast-fed infants because

Table 17-2 Feeding skills, as with other life skills, take time to develop

Age	Skills to watch for
0-2 months	Can grasp a finger; crying is the only language
2-4 months	Thrashing movements common; these can interfere with feeding
4-5 months	Turns head to voices; begins eye-hand coordination
5-6 months	Sits erect when supported; crawling and finger-feeding begin
6-7 months	Transfers objects from hand to hand; chewing pattern (up and down) begins
7-8 months	Sits erect without support for a minute or so; reaches for, grabs, and closely inspects objects; can hold a bottle and self-feed a cookie
8-10 months	Makes efforts to stand; develops pincer grasp
10-11 months	Takes a few steps with support; mealtimes become more messy as food is something to be explored
11-12 months	Practices self-feeding in earnest; walking becomes more likely; develops likes and dislikes for foods; chewing is better developed; hands bottle to caregiver when finished
12-15 months	Becomes more skilled at walking and self-feeding; inquisitive toddlers explore everything, so household toxins must be safely stored out of reach
21-24 months	Vocabulary builds; food patterns become more individualized

This timeline is just an estimate. Infants vary. A pediatrician should be consulted if caregivers are concerned about an infant's developmental progress.

the mother cannot tell how much milk is left to consume. After about 20 minutes, the baby has probably had enough.

Solid Food Introduction

By 6 to 7 months of age, the infant has learned to grab and transfer objects from one hand to the other (Table 17-2). About this time teeth begin to appear, and the infant begins to handle "finger foods" with some dexterity. Dry toast slices offer hours of enjoyment.

By age 8 to 9 months the infant can push a plate around and play with a drinking cup. He or she can now hold a bottle and self-feed a cracker or piece a toast. This is an important time for the infant to develop self-confidence and self-esteem, so the parents must be patient and supportive with these early feeding attempts.

Around 10 months of age, the infant earnestly practices self-feeding finger foods and drinking from a cup.[17] Feeding time may be very messy. Food is seen as something not only to eat but also to feel, smear, and drop. By the first birthday, an infant's body has developed sufficiently to accommodate crawling, probably walking, and self-feeding. While first attempts at feeding are erratic, the developing child soon takes great pride in doing more things independently. As the child drinks from a cup more frequently, fewer bottle- or breast-feedings are necessary. The mobility of walking should naturally lead to gradual weaning from the bottle or breast. Walking and weaning go together.

INTRODUCING SOLID FOODS

The time to introduce solid foods into an infant's diet hinges on several important factors:[8]

Nutritional need—As noted, iron stores are exhausted by about 6 months of age. Either solid foods or iron supplements are then needed to supply iron if the child is breast-fed or is fed a formula not supplemented with iron. No nutritional needs besides iron make solid foods a necessary dietary component before 6 months of age.

Physiological capabilities—Starch digestion is not very active before 3 months of age. As an infant ages, the ability to digest starch increases. In addition, kidney function is quite limited until about 4 to 6 weeks of age. Until then, waste products from high levels of dietary protein or minerals are difficult to excrete, as we noted earlier.

Physical ability—Before 3 to 4 months of age, the infant practices tongue thrusting. Generally, the child quickly spits out any solid food put on the tongue. It is about 5 or 6 months before an infant can sit up, turn the head away when full, and control tongue thrusting.

Preventing allergies—During the first 3 months of life, absorption of whole proteins is possible—but generally undesirable—through the intestinal tract. Whole protein absorption may set up the child for future allergies, including food allergies.[26] (See the Nutrition Perspective.) Even though most food allergies are to high-carbohydrate foods, like corn and wheat, it is best to minimize the number of all different types of protein sources in a child's diet during these first 3 months to limit chances of developing an allergy.

Keeping these considerations in mind—nutritional need, physiological and physical readiness, and allergy prevention—the American Academy of Pediatrics recommends that solid foods not be introduced until 4 to 6 months of age (Table 17-3). Before that time it is difficult to get the infant to consume much solid food, anyway. This may lead to force-feeding with a feeder (a giant syringe) or to mixing infant cereal with milk and putting that in a bottle. The inconvenience of these practices alone should make one consider whether all the effort is worth it.

Even so, many children are already eating solids by 2 months of age. In a recent study, one half of all African-American infants were consuming solid foods by 2 months of age, mostly infant cereals. Again, this practice is unnecessary nutritionally, tedious for parents, and possibly dangerous for the infant because it increases the risk of allergies and choking. Young infants can easily be frightened when eating with a spoon and may start crying. If feeding proceeds, the crying infant may then take a deep breath during spoon feeding and inhale the food into its lungs.

In general, an infant starting solid foods should weigh at least 13 pounds (6 kilograms) and should be drinking more than 32 ounces (1 liter) of formula daily. Sometimes a rapidly growing infant—one who consumes more than 32 ounces (1 liter) of formula per day—may need solid foods at 4 months of age to meet high energy needs. However, most infants can easily wait until 6 months of age. By this time the infant is ready for solid food and feeding is much easier.

WHY START SOLID FOODS BEFORE 4 TO 6 MONTHS OF AGE?

A common reason offered for introducing solid foods early—before 4 to 6 months of age—is the belief that it helps the infant sleep through the night. However, many studies have shown that sleeping through the night is a developmental milestone for the infant; it has little to do with how much food an infant eats before going to bed. Infants naturally begin sleeping through the night between the ages of 1 to 3 months. Girls generally reach this stage before boys. Filling them with cereal is not going to influence that process in a significant way.

WHICH SOLID FOODS SHOULD BE FED FIRST?

Since the main reason for feeding solids is the need for iron, the first solid foods for infants are usually iron-fortified cereals.[17] Some pediatricians may recommend lean ground (strained) meats for more absorbable forms of iron. If parents wait to 4 to 6 months before introducing solid foods, the type of first food is not an important issue. Before this age, starting with infant cereal is best; rice cereal is the

Table 17-3 One approach for the introduction of semisolid foods and table foods in infancy

Food	Age (Months) 4 to 6	6 to 8	9 to 12
Iron-fortified cereals for infants	Add		
Vegetables		Add strained	Gradually delete strained foods, introduce table foods
Fruits		Add strained	Gradually delete strained foods, introduce chopped, well-cooked, or canned foods
Meats*		Add strained or finely chopped table meats	Decrease the use of strained meats, increase the varieties of table meats
Finger foods such as arrowroot biscuits, oven-dried toast		Add those that can be grasped	Increase the use of small finger foods as the pincer grasp develops
Well-cooked mashed or chopped table foods, prepared without added salt or sugar			Add
Juice by cup			Add

*These can be added first, if the infant begins solid foods at 4 to 6 months of age. At 1 year of age formula or human milk should also be replaced by cow's milk. Modified from Pipes PL: *Nutrition in infancy and childhood*, St. Louis, 1989, Mosby–Year Book.
The shape of the triangle indicates gradual addition or deletion of the food product.

best cereal to begin with because it is least likely to cause allergies. Although yogurt, cottage cheese, strained fruits, and strained vegetables are also well tolerated as early foods because of their consistency, they are not good sources of iron. Once a new food has been fed for 7 days without ill effects, another food can be added to the infant's diet. In the early days, this may be another type of cereal or perhaps a cooked and strained (blended) vegetable, meat, fruit, or egg yolk.

Waiting 7 days between each new food is important because it can take that long for signs of an allergy, such as a rash, asthma, or diarrhea, to develop. It is important not to introduce mixed foods until each component has been introduced separately. Otherwise, if an allergy or intolerance develops, the offending food component will not be easy to identify. Note also that many babies outgrow food sensitivities in childhood. It is probably best not to introduce common allergy-causing foods during infancy. These include egg whites, chocolate, and nuts.

The American Academy of Pediatrics condones, but does not encourage, the use of cow's milk in infancy (up to about 24 ounces or about 0.75 liters daily) if the child is consuming at least one third of total kcalories from solid food. This is usually the case by about 8 to 9 months of age. Overall, however, human milk and/or formula are the best choices, not cow's milk, during the entire first year of life.

A variety of strained foods are available for infant feeding. Parents should read labels on prepared baby foods if they are concerned about sugar or salt in the infant's diet. Single food items are more desirable than mixed dinners and desserts, which are less nutrient dense. Most brands have no added salt, but some fruit desserts have significant amounts of added sugar. Alternately, one can simply grind plain foods from the table—vegetables, fruits, or meats (no seasoning added)—in an inexpensive plastic baby food grinder/mill and feed the food to the infant. Another option is to blenderize large amounts of food, freeze and store it as ice cubes in plastic bags, and then defrost and warm this as needed. Infant foods made at home do not need extra salt or sweeteners. Introduction of a variety of foods should occur throughout this period so that by the end of the first year the infant is consuming a variety of foods listed in the Guide to Daily Food Choices.

Juices and liquids other than water and formula are best given in a cup. Juices fed from a bottle may cause "nursing bottle syndrome." As an infant toys with a bottle, the carbohydrate-rich fluid bathes the teeth, providing an ideal growth media for bacteria. Bacteria on the teeth then makes acids from the carbohydrate, and the acids dissolve tooth structure. In addition, an infant should not be put to bed with a bottle or placed in an infant seat with a bottle propped up for him. As the child lies in bed, fluid (even milk) pools around the teeth, increasing the likelihood of dental caries.

Nursing bottle syndrome—an extreme example of tooth decay. This child was probably often put to bed with a bottle. The upper teeth have decayed almost all the way to the gum line.

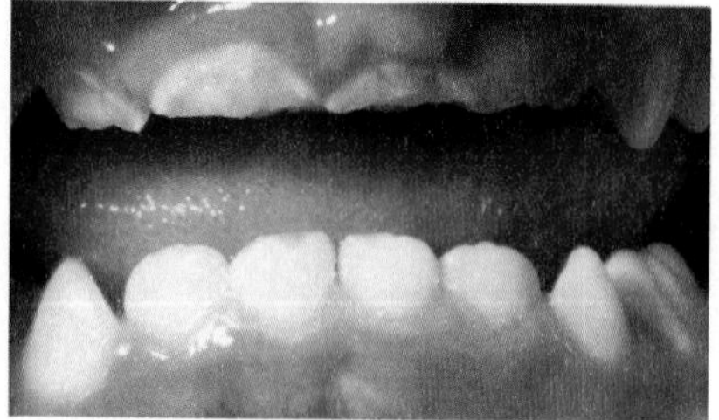

In the early months of solid food introduction, it is quite a challenge just to get the food into the infant, as opposed to on and around the child. Self-feeding skills require coordination and practice and are slow to develop. Also by 9 to 10 months of age, the infant's desire to explore, experience, and play with food further hinders feeding. It is best to relax and take this phase of infant development in stride. Sloppy, friendly mealtimes actually can make good memories about one's infant.

By the end of the first year, finger-feeding becomes more efficient, drinking from a cup improves, and chewing is easier as more teeth erupt.[17] The child's eating becomes neater, but experimentation and a lack of predictability still rule the day.

WHAT NOT TO FEED AN INFANT

Several foods and practices to avoid when feeding an infant are:

Honey and corn syrup—These products may contain spores of *Clostridium botulinum*. The spores can eventually develop into bacteria in the stomach and lead to botulism food-borne illness, which is often fatal in children under 1 year old (see Chapter 19).

Overly salty and overly sweet foods—Infants do not need a lot of sugar or salt added to their foods. They enjoy bland foods, much blander than do adults.

Feeding more than 40 ounces (1.2 liters) of formula or 32 ounces (1 liter) of milk per day—Solid foods should play a greater role in satisfying an infant's increased appetite after 6 to 8 months of age. About 24 to 32 ounces (¾ to 1 liter) of human milk or formula per day is ideal after 6 months of age, with food supplying the rest of energy needs. This is mainly because foods can contain much iron, whereas human milk, cow's milk, and non–iron-fortified formulas do not.

Certain foods that tend to cause choking—These foods include hot dogs, candy, nuts, grapes, coarsely cut meats, raw carrots, apples, and popcorn.

Low-fat or nonfat cow's milk—After 1 year of age, children can drink 2% fat milk since by then they are consuming enough solid foods to meet energy needs. The use of low-fat milk in infancy would provide too many minerals as the infant attempts to meet its energy needs. This would overtax the kidneys. Keep in mind that cow's milk is approximately three times higher in protein and minerals than human milk.

Excessive apple or pear juice—The sorbitol contained in these juices can led to diarrhea because sorbitol is a poorly absorbed sugar.

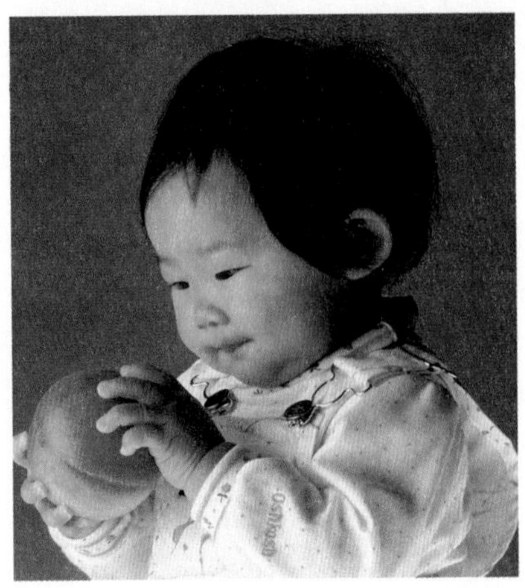

By the end of the first year, self-feeding comes much easier.

WILL INFANTS INSTINCTIVELY EAT A DIET THAT MEETS THEIR NUTRITIONAL NEEDS?

In the 1920s, Dr. Clara Davis investigated this question. She studied a small number of infants and allowed them to choose their own diet from a number of foods, such as milk, eggs, bananas, apples, oranges, and oatmeal. Her work showed that, given a variety of nutritious food choices, infants could choose a healthy diet. She also showed that solid foods were well digested during the ages of 6 months to 1 year. At the turn of the century, it was common to wait at least a full year before feeding solid foods to infants.

Other investigators misinterpreted this original (yet still unreplicated) research, stating that "infants naturally knew what foods to eat." It is probably better stated that given nutritious food choices, infants instinctively chose a balance of foods to meet their needs. We do not know if an infant would act like a mouse or a rat when faced with doughnuts, cookies, cake, and ice cream and gobble them up. Recall from Chapter 8 that when given these food options, rats and mice quickly become obese.

For a recap, here is a summary of infant feeding recommendations:

Breast-fed infants

- Breast-feed for 6 months or more if possible.
- Consider fluoride, iron, and vitamin D supplements.
- Add iron-fortified cereal at about 6 months of age.
- Provide a variety of basic, soft, solid foods after 6 months of age.

Formula-fed infants

- Use infant formula for at least 6 months, preferably an iron-fortified type.
- Give a fluoride supplement if water supply is not fluoridated.
- Add iron-fortified cereal at about 6 months of age.
- Provide a variety of basic, soft, solid foods after 6 months of age.

CONCEPT CHECK

Infant formulas generally contain lactose or sucrose, heat-treated casein and whey proteins from cow's milk, and vegetable oil. Formulas may or may not be fortified with iron. Sanitation is very important in preparing and storing formula. Solid food should not be added to an infant's diet until the child is ready for solid food, which is usually between 4 and 6 months of age. The first solid food given can be iron-fortified infant cereals, with very gradual additions of other foods, one at a time each week. Some foods to avoid giving infants in the first year include honey, low-fat cow's milk, overly salty or sweet foods, and foods that may cause choking.

Nutrition-Related Problems in Infancy

Parents, other caregivers, and clinicians should be aware of a variety of potential feeding problems and certain medical disorders related to infant nutrition.

POTENTIAL FEEDING PROBLEMS

Some potential feeding problems in infancy include:

- Insufficient iron in the diet.
- Avoidance of an entire food group once solid food use is established.
- Use of raw cow's or goat's milk. Raw cow's milk raises the possibility of viral and bacterial contamination (see Chapter 19). Goat's milk is low in folate and vitamin B-12.
- No progression to using a cup by 1 year of age.
- Bottle-feeding past 18 months of age.
- Supplemental vitamin use beyond 150% of an infant's or child's U.S. RDA.

FAILURE TO THRIVE

Occasionally an infant does not grow, in spite of adequate physical health. Physical causes might include poor development of the oral cavity, presence of infections, heart problems, and constant diarrhea associated with intestinal problems. However, about half the infants who show failure to thrive suffer from no apparent disease. About 40% show a combination of medical problems and parental neglect as the cause. In only 6% of the cases is a medical problem the main cause.

Thus the problem of failure to thrive often stems from poor infant-parent interactions. Also, in the majority of these cases, poor child-rearing practices stemming from misinformation, lack of a parent role model, or apathy about the child's welfare form the core of the problem.[17] In essence, the problem arises from the parent's not knowing what to do. Infants need cuddling, and they respond to voices and eye contact, especially at feeding time. Young parents need to be counseled regarding these needs.

Clinicians faced with an infant who is failing to thrive must first determine if the child is consuming enough energy; for infants that is approximately 40 to 50 kcalories per pound of body weight per day. For a breast-fed infant, the clinician needs to make sure that sufficient milk is being consumed. The child should be nursing about six to eight times a day for about 20 minutes a session, have six to eight wet diapers each day, and the mother should have an adequate intake of food and fluid (see Chapter 16). Failure to thrive is not often seen in children older than 2 years of age because they can often get food for themselves. Younger children are limited to what the parents and other caregivers provide.

COLIC

colic Periodic crying in a healthy infant associated with a GI tract gas buildup.

The first time an infant has a lengthy, unexplained crying spell, most parents panic. Crying episodes that do not respond to typical remedies like feeding, holding, and diaper changes, are characteristic of infants who develop **colic.** That includes about 1 in 5 infants, so colic is neither uncommon or abnormal. Late afternoon and early evening can be the most difficult times. The infant may cry continuously. Nighttime sleeping is most always disturbed by crying spells. Again, efforts to soothe a colicky infant—feeding, rocking, and holding—are usually ineffective. The only good news is that colic usually goes away after a few intense months.

We don't know a lot about colic. It appears to be caused by one of two reasons: (1) allergy-causing proteins in formula or human milk, or (2) excess gas buildup in the gastrointestinal (GI) tract due to poor peristalsis.[4] Tucking itself into a ball is a common response to colic by the infant. Painful accumulation of gas in the GI tract may be the reason for this response. The crying is usually not related to feeding, but positioning a colicky baby upright when feeding allows him to more easily expel trapped air by burping. In addition, the infant should be burped regularly during feeding and fed for no longer than 30 minutes. The longer the infant suckles at the bottle or breast, the more air he or she takes in.

Changing the infant's diet from a cow's milk protein-based formula to a predigested protein formula sometimes helps in severe cases of colic. Avoiding dairy products by the breast-feeding mother was found to be helpful in a recent study. In addition, the physician may prescribe medications to calm the child and reduce gas buildup. Overall, the parents need the counsel and support of other adults to ease their distress during this trying period, which often lasts for the first 3 to 4 months. Because a colicky baby is so stressful for parents to handle, hearing from other parents who have experienced similar problems is especially helpful.

DIARRHEA

Diarrhea results from various causes in infancy, including bacterial and viral infections. In the United States, about 500 infants per year die of simple dehydration resulting from diarrhea. To prevent dehydration, infants with diarrhea should be given plenty of fluids. Specialized fluids, such as Pedialyte, are available. This contains glucose, sodium, potassium, chloride, and water. Parents should be cautioned to obtain and follow a pediatrician's recommendations concerning fluid replacement.

Diarrhea is less common with breast-fed infants. The natural immunity provided by human milk reduces the risk of developing diarrheal disease.

Once diarrhea subsides, a bottle-fed infant may be switched to a soy-based, lactose-free formula for 2 weeks. This allows time for the lactase enzyme to again reach a high enough production rate in the intestine to digest the large amount of lactose found in a typical formula.

MILK ALLERGY

Over 25 proteins in milk can lead to allergies. Some of these are inactivated sufficiently by scalding milk. However, some proteins are very heat stable. A "true" milk allergy is actually quite rare and develops in less than 1% of formula-fed infants. However, many infants are switched to soy-based formulas in an attempt to decrease their crying and spitting up. Just because a child thrives better on a soy-based formula does not mean he or she has a true milk allergy.

IRON-DEFICIENCY ANEMIA

Iron-deficiency anemia typically occurs in infants who consume few solid foods and whose diets are dominated by cow's milk, which has little iron.[19] Iron stores are then quickly depleted by the daily demand for new red blood cell synthesis. To prevent iron-deficiency anemia, it is best to start an infant at about 6 months of age on iron-fortified cereals and meats, as well as limit formula or cow's milk to 16 to 25 ounces (500 to 750 milliliters) per day. The infant should also avoid cow's milk for the first year of life because it also tends to cause intestinal bleeding, especially before 3 months of age. If anemia does develop, medicinal iron supplements are advised, under a physician's guidance.

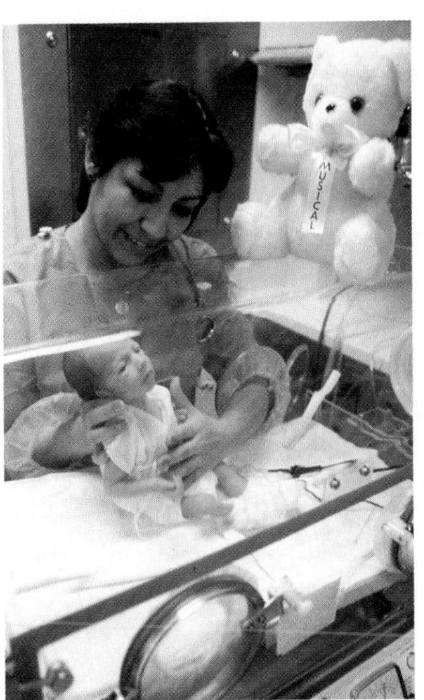

Premature infants have special nutritional needs.

THE PREMATURE INFANT

The premature infant is fed either a specially designed formula or human milk. As noted in Chapter 16, nutrients may be added to human milk to increase its protein, mineral, and energy content. Two amino acids not normally needed in the diet—tyrosine and cysteine—may be essential amino acids for the premature infant. In addition, some vitamins—such as vitamin E—and vitamin-like compounds—such as carnitine—may be helpful additions to this infant's diet.

Because many bacteria require iron to thrive, iron supplementation may be delayed for the premature infant to limit the tendency for bacterial infections. The premature infant must be fed immediately because he or she has little fat or glycogen storage. Body composition of the full-term infant includes about 12% fat, while the composition of the premature infant may include only about 2% fat, depending on gestational age.

DIETARY GUIDELINES FOR INFANT FEEDING

In response to various controversies surrounding infant feeding, experts have written dietary guidelines for infants.[9]

- Build to a variety of foods.
- Listen to your baby's appetite to avoid overfeeding or underfeeding.
- Don't overly restrict fat and cholesterol.
- Don't overdo high-fiber foods.
- Sugar is OK, but in moderation.
- Sodium is OK, but in moderation.
- Babies need more iron, pound for pound, than adults.

These guidelines have been accepted by the American Academy of Pediatrics and The American Dietetic Association. Clinicians may need to provide parents with more specific and practical suggestions to help implement these guidelines. The recommendations in this chapter are also consistent with these guidelines. In essence, the evidence supporting a positive effect of dietary restrictions during infancy to reduce the risk of later obesity or heart disease is equivocal, while the hazards of this approach are well documented.

CONCEPT CHECK

When an infant does not grow properly, this failure to thrive may be due to medical problems, but most likely is due to inappropriate feeding practices. Colic appears to be caused by either allergy-producing proteins in human milk or formula or from gas buildup in the GI tract, and may be reduced by regular burping during feeding. Switching formulas is usually not needed to treat colic. Diarrhea requires additional fluids to prevent dehydration. Allergy to milk proteins is rare, but may require switching to soy-based formula. Introducing iron-containing solid foods at an appropriate time and avoiding cow's milk can generally prevent iron-deficiency anemia in infancy.

Childhood

The rapid growth rate of infancy quickly tapers during the next few years. The average weight gain is only 5 pounds during the second year of life (Figure 17-1). The toddler shows conformational changes, however, as the percentage of body water and fat decreases, while the percentage of lean tissue increases.

As a toddler's growth rate tapers, food habits may change, and feeding problems can appear. One major cause of potential feeding problems stems from the slower growth and accompanying decrease in appetite that characterizes the preschool years. Preschoolers normally have less hunger than they did as infants.

One nutritional challenge at this age is to adapt food choices to the new growth rate. When little food is consumed, the nutrient density of each food choice should be maximized. This usually means watching fat intake while increasing intake of whole grains, fruits, and vegetables. There is no need to decrease fat intake severely, but fatty food choices should not overwhelm more nutritious ones.[12]

Surprisingly, children eat what they are exposed to. At this age, children can eat a well-rounded and healthy diet if one is served to them. Parents provide important role models. If offered whole-grain breakfast cereals, whole-wheat bread, vegetables, salad, and fresh fruits regularly and if they see parents eating these foods, young children accept and eat most of them. A lack of opportunity limits—and possibly deprives—a child's diet.[24]

The preschool years are the best time for a child to start a healthful pattern of living and eating. Self-esteem and successful eating are closely tied. Parents and other caregivers need to be aware of this. A good practice for children is the "one-bite" policy: children should take at least one bite of the foods presented to them. For snacks, parents should decide the options. Children should then be allowed to choose; responsibility for food choice should start early.[5]

HOW TO HELP A CHILD CHOOSE NUTRITIOUS FOODS

Above all, one needs to feed the preschool child affectionately. This is a time for children to experience new foods. It is also a time for them to develop their own likes and dislikes. Preschool children are very unpredictable (Figure 17-3). Be ready for setbacks. If adults can be patient and persevere, children eventually build good food habits.

Research shows that children like certain foods, especially those with crisp textures and mild flavors, and familiar foods. Young children are especially sensitive to and reject hot-temperature foods.

If children see good table manners, they more readily learn good table manners. Using good table manners leads to harmony and a positive environment for learning good nutrition habits. Preschoolers eventually develop skill with spoons and forks and can even use dull knives. But it is also a good idea to allow some finger foods.

CHILDHOOD FEEDING PROBLEMS

Tensions between parents, or between parents and children, often contribute to eating problems. Getting to the root of family problems and creating a more harmonious family atmosphere is an important part of resolving many childhood feeding problems. In addition, parents must often be educated to know what to expect of a preschool child and what goals to set. Following are a few typical problems, their causes, and suggestions for correcting each problem.

"My Child Won't Eat as Much, or as Regularly, as He did as an Infant"

This is to be expected. The growth rate slows from that of infancy, so the child does not need as much food. Parents must often be reminded that they shouldn't expect a 3-year-old child to eat as voraciously as an infant, nor to eat adult-sized portions.[17] Parents should remain calm if the child leaves an entire meal untouched. Overall, for children under age 3 years, 1 tablespoon per year of life of each food is a good guide for serving size. By age 5 years about two thirds of the typical servings in the Guide to Daily Food Choices is a good benchmark. In addition, appetite varies depending on a child's activity level and how the child feels—whether well or sick.

Parents should also be reminded that food likes and dislikes change rapidly in childhood and are influenced by food temperature, appearance, texture, and taste. Again, children usually prefer mild flavors, but there are exceptions to this rule.

"My Child is Always Snacking, Yet She Never Finishes Her Meal"

Children have small stomachs. Offering many small meals is often more successful than limiting children to three meals per day. Actually, three meals per day is just a social custom. There is no nutritional significance to that type of plan. Snacking is fine as long as good dental care, including tooth brushing after snacks, is practiced.

Calvin and Hobbes **by Bill Watterson**

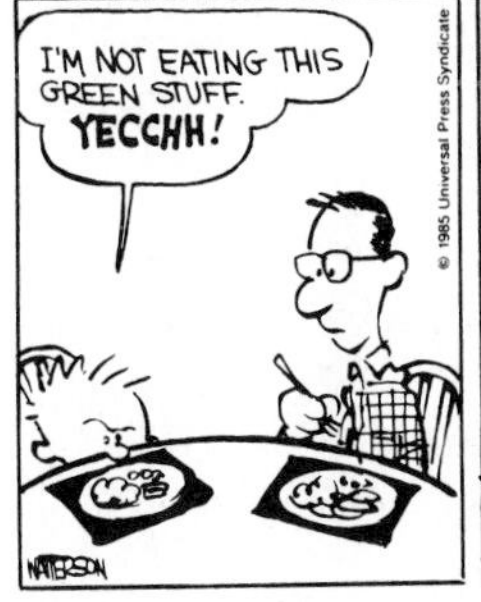
I'M NOT EATING THIS GREEN STUFF. YECCHH!
© 1985 Universal Press Syndicate

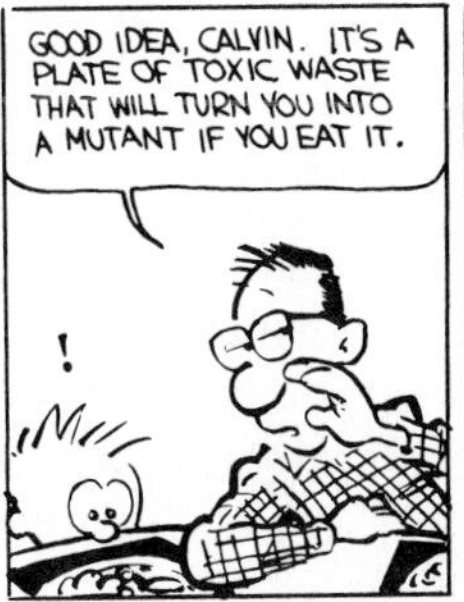
GOOD IDEA, CALVIN. IT'S A PLATE OF TOXIC WASTE THAT WILL TURN YOU INTO A MUTANT IF YOU EAT IT.
!

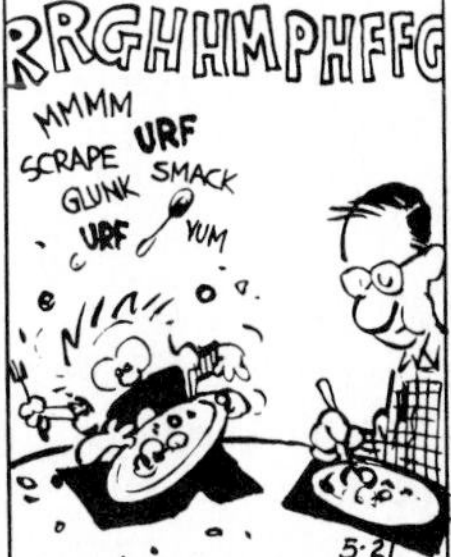
RRGHHMPHFFG
MMMM
URF
SCRAPE
GLUNK
SMACK
URF
YUM

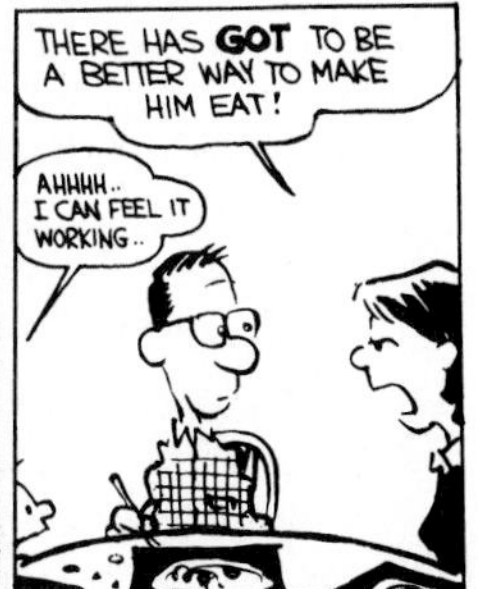
THERE HAS GOT TO BE A BETTER WAY TO MAKE HIM EAT!
AHHHH.. I CAN FEEL IT WORKING..

Figure 17-3 Calvin and Hobbes.

EXPERT OPINION

Helping Children to Eat Well

ELLYN SATTER, M.S., R.D.

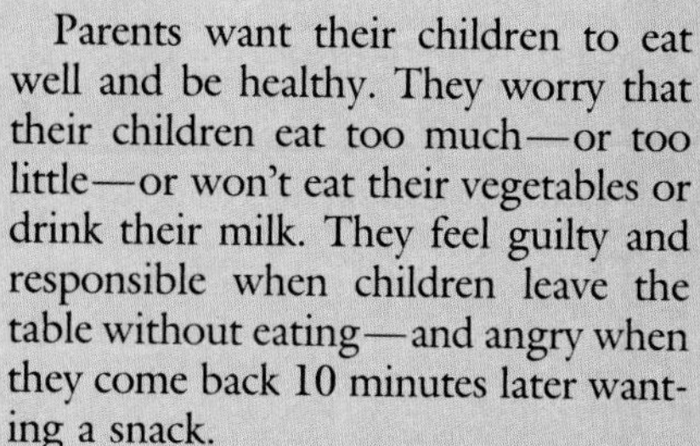

Parents want their children to eat well and be healthy. They worry that their children eat too much—or too little—or won't eat their vegetables or drink their milk. They feel guilty and responsible when children leave the table without eating—and angry when they come back 10 minutes later wanting a snack.

In some families, the dinner table becomes a battleground. Parents turn into reluctant food hustlers, insisting that children eat a regulation "four bites of broccoli before you can have dessert." Children gag. Adults feel pity. They know as one sensitive mother observed, that "when you don't want to eat something, it feels as if it grows in your mouth." Nonetheless, this perceptive mother feels obligated to insist that her son eat his vegetables.

How many bites of broccoli does it take to earn dessert? How do you get yourself out of the position where you have to make such ridiculous rules?

Respect the child's capability

Children have built-in motivators to eat. They get hungry, they are interested in eating, they have hearty appetites for good food, and they are interested in survival. But the way they operate with eating can fool you. Children are wary of new food: if it's new, they often don't like it.

But children do work to master new foods and new eating skills in the same way that they work to master other skills. They see new foods, taste them (needing as many as 15 or 20 attempts), and eventually learn to like them. Keep in mind that a taste is just a taste, and not necessarily a swallow. Toddlers put foods into their mouths, sample them for flavor and texture, and take them out again.

Unfortunately, to adults, these attempts at mastery look very much like rejection. While children are learning to like the new foods, the adults get anxious and try to hurry them along. It doesn't work; bribing backfires. Researchers find that preschoolers who are rewarded for eating a new food are less likely to go back to it later than preschoolers who are allowed to approach the food on their own. In addition, food rewards produce a negative side effect; children who get dessert for eating their vegetables learn to like the dessert more and the vegetables less. Giving a reward for eating a new food is not a good idea. It gives the child the clearest of messages that you don't expect her to learn to like the new food. So she won't.

Children naturally eat a variety of foods. An internal process called sensory specific satiety ensures that they will tire of even favorite foods and eat something different. Adults have the same tendency, but they ignore it. They override their appetites and eat because the food is good for them, or because they paid for it, or to keep them from getting hungry later.

Children know how much they need to eat. They respond to their internal sense of hunger and fullness more strongly than adults do, and they eat the right amount of foods for proper growth. Unlike most adults, they stop when they are full rather than when the food is gone. Their food intake fluctuates considerably from meal to meal and day to day. This is alarming to parents, who often try to train this sensitivity out of their children by encouraging them to eat past satiety or restraining them when they eat heavily.

Whether these tactics succeed depends on the determination of the parent—and the determination of child. Some children submit to parental controls. Others fight back. Children whose parents attempt to overfeed them may be revolted by food and may tend to undereat when they get the chance. Children whose parents attempt to underfeed them may become preoccupied with food and then overeat when they get the chance.

Provide appropriate support

So what are parents to do? They can only provide a variety of attractive, wholesome foods in pleasant surroundings and approach feeding in a positive way. They can't force children to eat.

Maintain structure. Children eat best and are more likely to learn to like a variety of foods if they have regular meals and snacks at predictable times and aren't allowed to panhandle between times. Consistent eating times help children to come to the table hungry and, therefore, more likely to accept the food.

Don't limit the menu to foods the child readily accepts, and don't be a short-order cook. Prepare a variety of foods, then let the child pick and choose from what's available. A meal should include a main dish, a fruit or vegetable, and a starchy food such as potato or rice.

Let the child learn from mistakes. If a toddler gets down from the table having eaten nothing and comes around 5 minutes later begging for a cookie, tell him, "Nothing until snack time." He may feel frustrated, but if you hold firm, the next time he may take his meal more seriously.

Maintain a division of responsibility in feeding

It all boils down to what I call a "division of responsibility in feeding." The parents are responsible for what their child is offered to eat and for setting up a pleasant eating environment. The child is responsible for deciding how much or even whether he or she eats. Children master their eating when adults provide opportunities to learn, give support for exploration, and limit inappropriate behavior.

But kids have their own ways of learning—and eating—so over the short term, it can look as if they are doing poorly. But children will eat, they will learn to like a variety of foods, and they will grow appropriately. Just don't hold your breath.

Ellyn Satter, M.S., R.D., A.C.S.W., a family therapist and specialist in eating disorders is the author of How to Get Your Kid to Eat . . . But Not Too Much, *Palo Alto, Calif 1987, Bull Publishing Co.*

It is really not when one eats, but what one eats, that is important. Nutritious snacks should be readily available (Table 17-4). Then, when the child becomes hungry in midmorning or midafternoon, healthful foods are available. Busy parents should find this idea quite helpful.

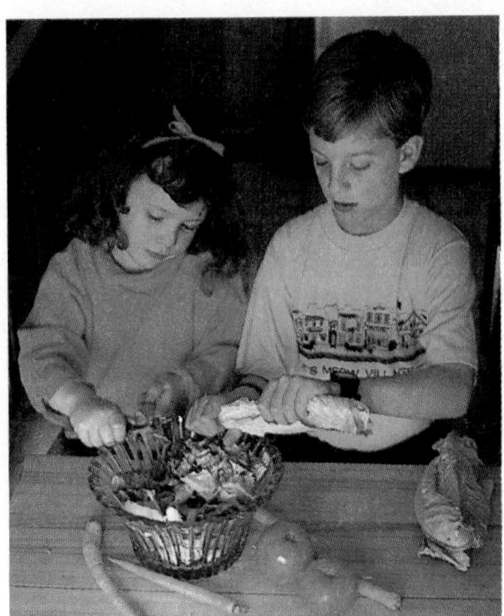

Figure 17-4 Parents can involve children in meal preparation. This helps children to develop an interest in new foods.

"My Child Never Eats His Vegetables"

Everyone dislikes certain foods. Again, the "one-bite" policy can be encouraged and guidelines can be set to discourage fussing over unfamiliar foods. Children eventually learn that they can eat foods they don't particularly like without first gagging, choking, and yelling "Oh gross!" It takes time for a child to become enthusiastic about a new food, but with continual exposure and a positive role model, chances are the child may even grow to like it.

It may work to feed a child vegetables at the start of a meal, when he or she is hungriest. Introduce one new food at a time. Do not make a big deal about serving a new food. Give small portions of unfamiliar foods. Offering new foods with familiar ones is a good idea. A platter of raw or blanched (lightly cooked to soften) carrots, broccoli, green and red peppers, cabbage, and mushrooms eaten as a snack with friends can do a lot to remedy a vegetable problem. Nutritious dips, such as ranch dressing made with mayonnaise, sell vegetables to many children. Finally, letting a child help prepare vegetables may increase their appeal (Figure 17-4). When a child reaches the age at which he or she can safely handle raw vegetables without fear of choking (about 4 or 5 years), offering thin carrot sticks or broccoli flowers can be an option to cooked ones. The child may find the taste and texture more pleasing.

"How Do I Know If My Child is Eating Healthfully?"

The Guide to Daily Food Choices listed in Chapter 2 forms the basis for a healthy diet in childhood. If a child eats the desired servings from those food groups and shows regular increments in height and weight, that is evidence of a good diet. Some nutrients that deserve special attention during childhood are calcium, iron, and vitamins A and C. These nutrients need not be deficient in a child's diet if it includes enough foods from all the food groups—milk, yogurt, and cheese group; meat, poultry, fish, dried beans, eggs, and nuts group; fruit group; vegetable group; and breads, cereals, rice, and pasta group.

Major scientific groups, such as The American Dietetic Association and the American Society for Clinical Nutrition, believe that giving vitamin and mineral supplements is unnecessary for healthy children (see Chapter 12). It is better to focus on good foods, rather than on nutrient supplements. Studies show that many parents offer children conservative amounts of vitamins, so toxicity is unlikely. Still, the practice of giving supplements is unnecessary, especially given today's highly fortified breakfast cereals, which children often eat. However, a nutrient supplement at the RDA level may be needed when a child is ill, especially if the illness is prolonged. In addition, if the child is a total vegetarian (vegan), special consideration should be given to the intake of protein, vitamin B-12, calcium, iron, and zinc.

NUTRITIONAL PROBLEMS IN CHILDHOOD

The two most common nutritional problems in childhood are obesity and iron-deficiency anemia. Childhood obesity is covered in a later Nutrition Focus.

IRON-DEFICIENCY ANEMIA

Childhood iron-deficiency anemia is most likely to occur in children between 6 and 24 months of age.[19] It can lead to poor stamina because the oxygen supply to cells is decreased. Learning ability also may be compromised. However, the incidence of childhood anemia is decreasing. In 1970, about 12% of children ages 18 to 23 months were diagnosed anemic in the United States. By 1984, the figure had dropped to 4%. This decrease is probably due to the increased use of iron-fortified

Table 17-4 Serving nutritious snacks and beverages

Snack suggestions:

Fresh raw vegetables	Serve with a dip of cottage cheese or yogurt blended with dried buttermilk dressing
Celery	Spread with peanut butter and sprinkle on raisins, shredded carrots or nuts finely chopped
Bananas	Dip in sweetened yogurt or spread with peanut butter and roll in coconut, chopped nuts or granola
Crackers or sliced apples	Serve with a dip of peanut butter, honey, nuts, raisins and coconut mixed together
Bagels	Spread with cream cheese or peanut butter and top with chopped bananas, crushed pineapple or shredded carrots
Quick bread or muffins	Make with carrots, zucchini, pumpkin, bananas, nuts, dates, raisins, lemons, squash, and berries
Flour tortillas	Spread with refried beans or canned chili, sprinkle with grated cheese and broil; top with mild salsa
Trail mix	Put together a large batch of cereal, pretzel, and nut mix. Divide into individual plastic bags.
Ready-to-eat cereals	Use brands low in sugar and containing fiber. Serve with raisins.
Pita loaf	Place sliced meat, cheese, lettuce and tomato in open pocket
English muffins or pita bread	Top with spaghetti sauce, grated cheese and meats; broil or bake and cut in fourths
Potato skins	Sprinkle with shredded cheese, broil and top with yogurt and bacon bits
Canned chili	Heat and top with onions, lettuce and tomato; use as dip for Italian or French bread, biscuits or corn bread
Kabobs	Make with any combination of the following: fruit, vegetables and sliced or cubed cooked meat (remove toothpicks before serving)
Popcorn	Serve plain or make three quarts and sprinkle with ¼ c grated cheese and ½ t garlic or onion salt
Parfait	Make with yogurt, fruit and granola
Gelatin	Consider using sugar-free varieties. Add fruit or vegetable juice, vegetables, fruits, or cottage cheese
Frozen fruit cubes	Freeze pureed applesauce or fruit juice into cubes
Fruit fizz	Add club soda to juice instead of serving soft drinks
Fruit shake	Blend milk with fresh fruit (bananas, berries or a peach) and a dash of cinnamon or nutmeg
Yogurt frost	Combine fruit juice and yogurt; add fresh fruit if desired
Hot chocolate	Make hot chocolate or cocoa with milk chocolate and a dash of cinnamon
Seeds	Shelled sunflower seeds
Fish	Tuna fish
Canned soup	Vegetable or minestrone; nice on a cold winter's day.

Adapted from *A food guide for the first five years*, National Meat and Livestock Board, 444 North Michigan Avenue, Chicago. Ill 60611.

formulas and increased iron fortification of breakfast cereals that began in the early 1970s. In addition, the Special Supplemental Food Program for Women, Infants, and Children (WIC) sponsored by the federal government (which also began in the early 1970s) emphasizes the importance of iron-fortified formulas and cereals and distributes these items to infants and preschool children.

Prevention of iron-deficiency anemia in children should center on regular consumption of adequate sources of iron.[19] Iron-fortified breakfast cereals and a few ounces of lean meat are convenient ways to incorporate more iron into a child's diet. The high proportion of heme iron in many animal foods make the iron more readily absorbed than iron from plant foods. In addition, recall that consuming a vitamin C source with any plant or supplemental source of iron aids absorption.

IS CHILDHOOD THE TIME TO START A DIET DESIGNED TO LIMIT THE RISK FOR HEART DISEASE?

Parents may wonder whether it is important to limit children's cholesterol and fat intake to minimize future risk of heart disease. Many health authorities, including the American Academy of Pediatrics, do not recommend low-fat diets for children under 2 years of age. Health authorities, however, do recommend screening children for blood cholesterol levels in families in which early heart disease is common (parents or grandparents diagnosed with heart disease at age 55 or less or found to have high blood cholesterol levels), and then treating children with high blood cholesterol levels using appropriate diet and drug therapy.[11]

Although there may be no reason to put children on low-fat diets at this time, parents can introduce "heart-healthy" habits by limiting a child's exposure to saturated fats. Heart disease often starts in childhood.[20] Fatty streaks in arteries of the heart have been noted in the aortas of some children over 3 years of age in the United States, and these can increase rapidly in extent through adolescence. Fatty streaks are also present in children from many different populations. Autopsies of young military men who died in Korea and Vietnam showed the early signs of plaque buildup in their blood vessels. It is best to encourage foods that have a higher proportion of monounsaturated and polyunsaturated fat. Moderation is the best strategy; overly restrictive diets can be detrimental to overall growth.

The child needs to consume enough energy while also building good health habits that can be carried into the teen years. One strategy is to have them consume milk that is 2% fat after age 1 year and then 1% fat or nonfat after 2 years of age, and to limit the intake of high-fat meats, high-fat cheeses, and butter.[25] Overall, the guidelines do not recommend a decreased consumption of meats or dairy products, specifically milk, but a switch from high-fat meats and whole milk to lean meats and skim or low-fat milk so that adequate kcalories, vitamins, and mineral intakes are maintained.[14]

If current childhood feeding practices aim to follow the most healthful dietary patterns, they should gradually shift away from high-fat diets to those containing ample fruits, vegetables, and grains. If more fruits and vegetables are offered, children's consumption of high-fat foods, such as desserts and many snack foods, will gradually decline. After 2 years of age, many health authorities recommend eating patterns for children that contain no more than 30% of total kcalories as fat and no more than 10% of kcalories as saturated fat. Cholesterol intake should be limited to 300 milligrams per day. Currently children consume a diet in which total fat averages 34% to 36% of total kcalories. Saturated fat averages approximately 14%, with about 200 to 300 milligrams of cholesterol.

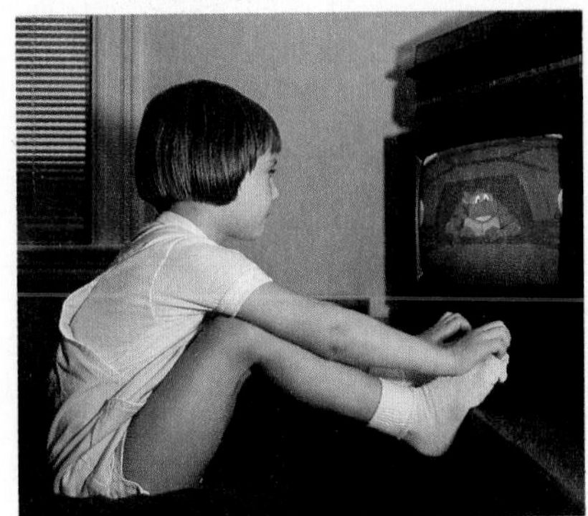

Some children spend too much time in sedentary activities that often include consumption of high-fat snacks.

WHAT ABOUT LOW-SODIUM DIETS FOR CHILDREN?

Scientific data neither confirm nor refute that a reduction in sodium intake reduces the risk of future high blood pressure. Moderation in sodium consumption does help build good health habits for the future—especially if the person later develops hypertension and needs to control sodium intake even more.

NUTRITION FOCUS

Obesity in the Growing Years

There are many potential causes for obesity in the growing years. Recall the nature versus nurture comparison discussed in Chapter 8. Obesity does have a genetic component. Some infants are born with lower metabolic rates; they use energy more efficiently, and in turn have an easier time saving kcalories for fat storage. Some infants are less active than others, and so they use fewer kcalories per day. Research shows a moderate relationship between the amount of hours a child spends watching television and obesity. Today's television generation now glues itself to the tube for an average of 22 hours per week. The average child, then, loses almost an entire day's worth of time that he or she could have been actively playing, and at the same time watches numerous advertisements for poor food choices.[7] Obesity also tends to run in families. We can also expect further environmental influences, such as snacking and high-fat/high-kcalorie food choices, to contribute to childhood obesity.

Obesity in infancy

Infant obesity does not necessarily result in childhood obesity, so parents need not worry excessively. But if an infant is over the ninetieth percentile weight-for-length and is still gaining weight, it may be time to reevaluate the infant's diet and activity patterns. A quick dietary assessment can detect if the infant is consuming about 45 to 50 kcalories per pound of body weight (105 to 115 kcalories per kilogram), the amount recommended for an infant.

The obese infant can be encouraged to crawl and climb more often, and parents can decrease confinement in playpens and walkers. If the infant tends to cry for a bottle, water can be given. It may also be time to switch from a bottle to a cup. Finally, if this infant is still less than 6 months old, decreasing the use of solid foods (if already given) is a good idea. Severe restriction of food or milk is not desirable. Instead, the infant's height should be allowed to catch up to his or her present weight. The overall goal is to moderate weight gain so that the infant is satisfied and yet remains below the ninety-fifth percentile of weight-for-height.

Obesity in childhood

About 40% of obese children become obese adults, and about 70% of obese adolescents become obese adults. Thus the time to strike against obesity is in childhood because there is such a high likelihood that an obese school-age child will become an obese adult (Figure 17-5). In the United States, 15% to 25% of children are overweight and about 15% of adolescents are obese. This incidence of overweight children and adolescents leads not only to an increased chance of later obesity, but also to a decrease in physical fitness and, sooner or later, to other aspects of ill health, as well.

Children over the ninetieth percentile for weight-for-height on growth charts are considered overweight, and those over the ninety-fifth percentile are considered obese. Skinfold thickness can also be measured to assess obesity.

A first approach to treating childhood obesity is assessing the child's activity level. If a child spends much free time in sedentary activities (such as watching television), physical activities should be encouraged. The U.S. government plan Healthy People 2000 endorses this goal for all children.[21] These activities do not necessarily have to be competitive sports. Children should be given opportunities to participate in what they like, such as walking (maybe to and from school), cycling, swimming, and jazz dancing, and then encouraged to do these often.

Moderation in kcalorie intake, especially high-fat/high-kcalorie food choices, is important. Resorting to a weight-loss diet is usually unnecessary. Children have an advantage over adults in losing weight—some stored kcalories can be used by growth. If weight gains can be moderated, height gains may soon catch up. This is one reason why treating obesity in childhood is so desirable. Further growth can contribute to success.[18]

Sometimes weight loss is necessary if a child is still obese after attaining ultimate adult height. Then weight loss should be gradual, perhaps ½ pound per week. The child should be closely monitored to ensure that during this weight loss the rate of growth is normal. It is important that the child's kcalorie intake does not compromise gains in height.

Behavior modification adds a third important component to treating childhood obesity. Children often need to find a new way to relate to foods, especially snack foods. It may be important for children to eat only at the kitchen table. This could stop endless hours of snacking in front of the television.

Parents play a key role in treating childhood obesity.[10] After all, they select and bring the food home. One goal is to keep healthy, nutrient-rich but kcalorie-light snacks on hand. The parents also must help a child turn his or her interest from food consumption toward other interests, such as sports, hobbies, and school. Any management plan for treating childhood obesity must involve the parents. This involvement improves the chances for success.

Parents must remember that the self-esteem of a child is quite fragile. Humiliation does not work; it only makes the child feel worse. Support, admiration, and encouragement are offerings to be emphasized.

Parents also should realize that by denying a child favorite foods, they do not necessarily deny love. The child can have treats, such as candy, in small amounts, not a whole bag. Often parents and children need to develop new ways of relating—those that do not involve food and obesity.

THE IMPORTANCE OF BREAKFAST

In the early school years regular meals, especially breakfast, becomes an important focus. Some research suggests that breakfast helps children learn better in the subsequent hours they spend in school. The energy and nutrients consumed can stimulate attention, energy level, and motivation, yielding better test scores. Athletic performance can be improved as well. This makes sense since depleted carbohydrate stores in the liver can be replenished at breakfast. In spite of this evidence, some researchers dispute the importance of the breakfast meal in learning, saying that it is the more motivated students who eat breakfast rather than eating breakfast that motivates students. In our opinion, it is a good idea to provide breakfast to all students, and especially to otherwise sluggish ones.

To help increase the likelihood of their eating breakfast, children should be encouraged to find breakfast foods they enjoy. These do not have to be traditional foods. Instead, they might be pizza, spaghetti, soups, yogurt with trail mix on top, chili, sandwiches, and shish kebab. Food composition, not social tradition, is the key.

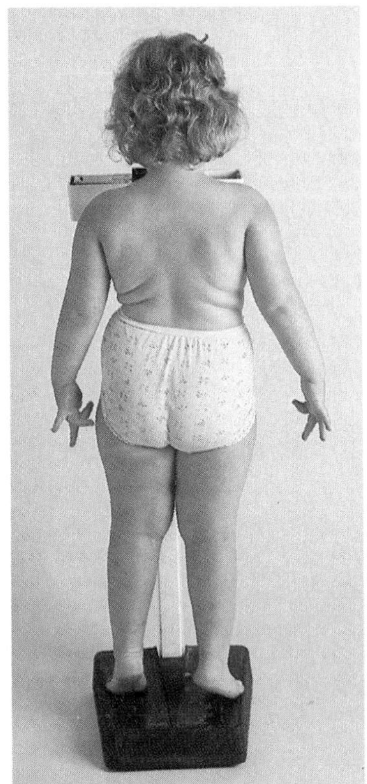

Figure 17-5 Childhood obesity. A female child like this one who is still obese after 5 years of age often faces a battle against obesity for the rest of her life. This age represents an ideal time to intervene with moderation in kcalorie intake and ample opportunities for physical activity.

CONCEPT CHECK

The rapid growth rate of the first year of life slows during the toddler and preschool years. Appetite decreases, necessitating selection of nutrient-dense foods. Adults should select the foods served, but allow the child to decide the amount to eat. Snacking is appropriate if there is careful selection of foods and attention to dental hygiene. Vitamin and mineral supplementation is usually not needed. In childhood, prevention of iron-deficiency anemia should center on regular consumption of good sources of iron. In part, this can be accomplished by providing children with a nutritious, iron-fortified breakfast cereal. Developing "heart-healthy" habits at this age can be seen as good health insurance.

The Teenage Years

A rapid growth spurt begins in most girls between the ages of 10 and 13 years and in most boys between the ages of 12 and 15 years. These growth spurts last about 3 years. Early maturing girls may begin their growth spurt as early as 7 to 8 years of age, while early maturing boys may begin it by 9 to 10 years of age. During this growth spurt, girls gain about 10 inches (25 centimeters) in height and boys gain about 12 inches (30 centimeters). Girls also tend to develop both lean and fat tissue, whereas boys tend to gain mostly lean tissue. This growth spurt provides about 42% to 51% of ultimate adult weight, and 15% to 25% of ultimate adult height (Figure 17-1).

The growth spurt in girls surrounds the onset of menses, called menarche. We have noted before that little further increase in height occurs 2 years after menarche. Because the time for the growth spurt varies during the teen years, it would be ideal to base the RDA at this age on the presence or absence of the growth spurt, rather than on chronological age.

Fortunately, as the growth spurt begins, so does an increase in food intake. Kcalorie needs average approximately 2200 to 2500, based on RDA guidelines. If teens choose nutritious food, they can take advantage of their increased hunger and easily satisfy their nutrient needs.

NUTRITIONAL PROBLEMS OF TEENS

We covered anorexia nervosa and bulimia in Chapter 12. Other nutritional problems are more common during the teen years. A major concern is that many teenage girls stop drinking milk, and therefore may not consume sufficient calcium to allow for

Table 17-5 Guide to daily food choices for adolescents and teens*

	Include at least this many servings daily
Milk, yogurt, and cheese (preferably low-fat or nonfat)	3
Meats, poultry, fish, dry beans, eggs, and nuts	2-3
Vegetables	3-5
Fruits	2-4
Breads, cereals, rice, and pasta (preferably whole grain; otherwise enriched or fortified)	6-11
Fats, oils, and sweets	Use sparingly

*Use serving sizes from Adult Guide to Daily Food Choices.
†Here we define "teen" as a person who has added height in the past year, and is at least 12 years old.
‡This guide should be used through age 24 years.

maximum mineralization of bones through their early twenties. Although this issue is still being researched, many investigators are concerned that young women who do not drink milk are sowing the seeds for future osteoporosis (see Chapter 14).[15] Three servings of the milk, yogurt, and cheese group are recommended per day (Table 17-5). If lactose intolerance is a problem, the two latter choices, along with calcium-fortified fruit juices, are good choices (see Chapter 3). The RDA for calcium increases between ages 11 and 24 years from 800 to 1200 milligrams for males and females. Only about one in six teenage girls consume that amount.

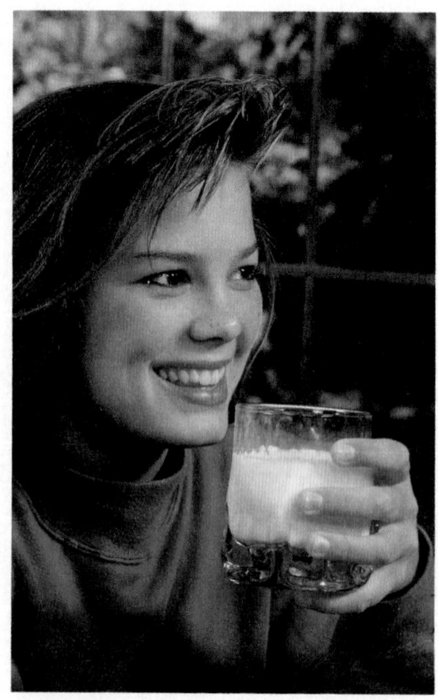

Three to four servings of milk products per day are recommended for teenage girls.

Another concern is iron deficiency. Iron-deficiency anemia appears in girls after the onset of menses and in boys during their growth spurt.[19] About 12% to 14% of teenagers have low iron stores. It is important that teenagers choose good food sources of iron, such as lean meats, whole grains, and fortified cereals. In addition, we have mentioned many times that consuming a vitamin C source with any plant or supplemental source of iron is always a good idea.

Adolescent and teenage girls need to eat good sources of iron (or regularly consume an iron supplement), particularly girls with heavy menstrual flows. Iron-deficiency anemia is not a desirable state for a teen. It can produce an increased tendency for fatigue and decreased ability to concentrate and learn. School performance then may falter.

Another potential problem primarily involves boys during their growth spurt, when food consumption is great. Their great energy needs can accommodate large intakes of saturated fat and cholesterol, especially if they regularly consume hamburgers, French fries, fried chicken, and milk shakes. This high intake of saturated fat and cholesterol can pave the arteries for early coronary heart disease.[20] We believe it is prudent for boys to begin to choose "heart-healthy" foods, using the Dietary Guidelines for Americans for evaluating food choices, especially during the high energy intake years associated with the teen growth spurt.

ACNE AND DIET

Diet appears to have no effect on acne. Though one hears that eating nuts, chocolate, and pizza can make acne worse, scientific studies have been unable to show a strong link between any dietary factor and acne. Teens are simply warned to avoid "trigger foods," assuming that planning a well-balanced diet is still possible.[16] Acne naturally waxes and wanes, and so it falls easy prey to notions about relationships to dietary factors. Acne may be more dormant in summer, since sunlight appears to improve this condition. The effect of artificial ultraviolet light on acne is not so pronounced.

The main culprit of acne is over-activity by the sebaceous glands in the skin.[16] They respond to testosterone, which is mainly a male hormone. This is why men tend to have more serious cases of acne and to a greater extent than do women. Women also secrete testosterone and other **androgen** (testosterone-like) compounds. If produced in large amounts, a woman also may experience serious acne.

One drug dermatologists sometimes prescribe for acne is tretinoin, which is sold under tradenames such as Retin-A. A derivative of vitamin A, tretinoin comes in cream, gel, and liquid forms and is rubbed onto the skin once nightly. It is highly effective for treating blackheads and modestly effective for treating pimples.[16] Tretinoin usually begins to clear up acne in 2 or 3 weeks. Scientists do not know exactly how tretinoin works, but research suggests that it both pushes out the plugs in the ducts beneath the skin and helps prevent their reformation.

The most exciting news for serious acne is probably the introduction of Accutane (13-cis retinoic acid or isotretinoin). This prescription oral medication, another derivative of vitamin A, appears to change the nature of sebaceous gland development. It decreases the production of **sebum** and in turn reduces the number of acne lesions.[16] The medication is especially helpful in treating cases resistant to antibiotic therapy (see Chapter 13 for more information about Accutane). Teens should be cautioned against self-medicating with Vitamin A itself in hopes of curtailing acne. Instead they should rely on advice from their physician. It is the derivatives of vitamin A, not the vitamin itself, that are helpful, and these are only available by prescription. Recall as well that excess dosages of Vitamin A can cause toxicity, so this would also likely be a hazardous choice.

The sebaceous glands surround hair follicles on the face, ears, back, chest, eyelids, and other areas. In these glands are cells that secrete triglycerides, very long-chain fatty acids (waxes), and other lipids. Collectively, these substances are known as sebum. If the sebum blocks a duct in the gland, this can lead to an infection and local pressure, resulting in an acne lesion.

androgen A general term for hormones that stimulate development in male sex organs; testosterone is an example.

sebum Secretion of the sebaceous glands consisting of lipids, waxes, and other triglycerides.

A CLOSER LOOK AT THE DIETS OF TEENAGERS

Teens consume 36% to 37% of kcalories as total fat and 14% as saturated fat. Teenage boys, but not girls, consume more cholesterol than recommended. Teens, especially girls, have been found to consume inadequate amounts of nutrients other than calcium and iron: vitamins A and C, and zinc. Busy schedules, part-time jobs, athletics, and social activities all may interfere with regular mealtimes and adequate nutritional intake. Breakfast is often skipped, which can deprive the teen of sufficient kcalories and nutrients.

The increased responsibility assumed by today's teens for purchasing and preparing food, often without sufficient knowledge to make healthy food choices, is another factor contributing to their susceptibility to nutrition-related problems. In addition, fear of excessive weight gain may cause young girls to limit their energy intake, and this limits their food choices. Overall, if their limited food choices then consist of French fries, soft drinks, and pastries, little room is left for foods that are good nutrient sources. These nutrients are easy to obtain through nutrient-dense food choices based on the Guide to Daily Food Choices.

According to the United States Public Health Service, 7-year-olds to 17-year olds are the heaviest users of diet pills. Moreover, 10-year-olds to 29-year olds suffer the greatest number of serious, sometimes fatal, reactions to an ingredient in several over-the-counter diet pills (phenylpropanolamine). In their effort to succeed, many adolescent athletes are vulnerable to food-related fads and fallacies.

To optimize performance, adolescents in competitive sports also may try to lose body weight by using diuretics, laxatives and diet pills, starvation, and enhanced sweating. These extreme weight loss measures can impair both performance and health. A more realistic approach to diet and exercise is needed (see Chapter 9).

Many teens are also striving to forge an identity by adopting dietary patterns with which their families are unfamiliar—vegetarianism, for instance. The problem is that they may not know enough about a vegetarian diet to keep from developing health problems, such as iron-deficiency anemia.

HELPING TEENS EAT MORE NUTRITIOUS FOODS

Teenagers face a variety of upheavals in their lives. They pursue their independence, experience identity crises, seek peer acceptance, and worry about physical appearance. All these factors affect food choice.

Teens often do not think well in abstractions. They have a hard time relating today's actions to long-term health outcomes. Physicians face this problem in counseling teenagers with diabetes. If diabetes is not controlled in the teenage years, the ultimate life span of a person can be significantly reduced because serious complications tend to happen at a much earlier age. Still, it is hard for clinicians to convince teenagers of this because they often lack a long-term orientation.[22]

OVERCOMING THE TEENAGE "MIND SET"

Clinicians—whether physicians, registered dietitians, or nurses—need to hone their skills when working with teenagers. Topics such as sports nutrition, eating disorders, steroids, and drug and alcohol abuse are typical issues that the clinician may face. These topics, except for drug and alcohol abuse, are usually not the concern of older adult clients.

One strategy for working with teenagers is to stress the importance of nutrition for physical development, fitness, vigor, and health. For boys this can be muscular development. With teenage girls, the focus can be on how to make nutrient-dense food choices that lead to better health while maintaining appropriate weight. It can be explained that beauty is based on the glow of health, and that unhealthy people wither unappealingly, while also sowing the seeds for future medical problems. Good nutrition throughout the growing years builds a healthy foundation. The teen who learns to make food choices consistent with the Dietary Guidelines for Americans gains valuable skills that can last a lifetime.

ARE TEENAGE SNACKING PRACTICES HARMFUL?

As we discussed, the major focus with snacks should be what is eaten. Teens often obtain one fourth to one third of all their energy and major nutrients from snacks. Teenagers can obtain many nutrients from the one to seven or more snacks generally consumed each day. The problem is that many of their food choices are often sweet and high in salt as well. Parents can influence their teens to a considerable degree by modeling nutritious food choices, even in quick-service restaurants. By choosing wisely, like from the salad bar, or grilled plain sandwiches, teens can eat at these restaurants and still consume a very good diet. Other healthful snack choices can include bagels instead of donuts, nonfat frozen yogurt instead of ice cream, low-fat or nonfat milk in place of whole milk, fruit instead of candy, and air-popped popcorn instead of chips. Snacks and quick-service restaurants themselves are not the problem: poor food choices are.[17]

CONCEPT CHECK

Another period of rapid growth occurs during the teen years. Girls generally start this growth earlier than boys. Common nutritional problems in these years arise from poor food choices, and include poor calcium intake in girls, iron-deficiency anemia, and sometimes excessive saturated fat intake. Acne is common among teens but not directly linked to diet. The importance of nutrition may be difficult to impress on this age group. Clinicians must be aware of the implications of the social, psychological, and physical changes that occur during these years.

Summary

1. Growth is very rapid during infancy. Birth weight doubles in 4 to 6 months, and length increases by 50% in that year. An adequate diet, especially protein intake, is very important to support normal growth. Undernutrition can cause irreversible changes in growth and development.

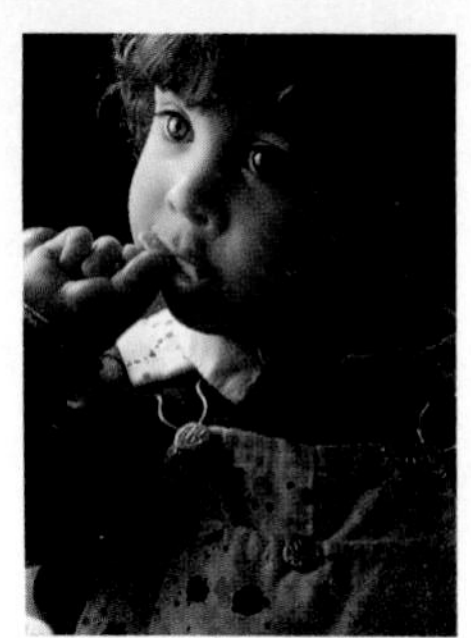

2. Growth in an infant and child is monitored by measuring body weight, height (or length), and head circumference over time. The most useful growth charts measure height-for-age and weight-for-height.
3. Nutrient needs in the first 6 months can be met by human milk or iron-fortified formula. Supplementary vitamin D and iron may be needed in the first 6 months for breast-fed infants, and supplemental fluoride may be needed by all infants.
4. Infant formulas generally contain lactose or sucrose, heat-treated casein and whey proteins from cow's milk, and vegetable oil. Formulas may or may not be fortified with iron. Sanitation is very important when preparing and storing formula.
5. Solid food should not be added to an infant's diet until there is a nutritional need, the GI tract can digest these complex foods, the infant has the physical ability to swallow voluntarily and control tongue thrusting, and the risk of developing food allergies decreases. For most infants, this readiness for solid food occurs between 4 and 6 months of age.
6. The first solid food given should be iron-fortified infant cereals or ground meats, with very gradual addition of other individual foods, perhaps one food per week. Some foods to avoid giving infants in the first year include honey, low-fat cow's milk, overly salty or sweet foods, or foods that may cause choking.
7. Introduction of iron-containing solid food at the appropriate time and avoidance of cow's milk can generally prevent iron-deficiency anemia in later infancy.
8. A slower growth rate in preschool years makes the choice of nutrient-dense foods and a reduction in serving size important. Iron-rich foods, such as lean red meats, are an important part of the Guide to Daily Food Choices at this age. In the teen and young adult years, a focus on adequate iron and calcium in the diet is important, especially for girls.

Study Questions

1. Describe how you would assess whether an 8-month-old infant is consuming a healthy diet.
2. Outline three key factors that should enter in the decision of when to introduce solid foods into an infants diet.
3. Why should obesity in childhood be discouraged? What three factors are likely contributing to this problem in a typical 6-year-old child?
4. Contrast the dietary guidelines issued for infants in this chapter with those for children over 2 and adults listed in Chapter 2. Which guidelines are similar? Do any contradict each other? If so, what would be the reason(s)?
5. Describe three pros and cons for snacking. What is the basic advice for healthy snacking from childhood through teen years?
6. What two nutrients are of particular interest in planning diets for teens? Why does each deserve to be singled out?

REFERENCES

1. Barrett S: Unproven allergies: an epidemic of nonsense, *Nutrition Today,* March/April 1989, p 6.
2. Behrman RE and others: *Nelson textbook of pediatrics,* ed 13, p. 64-67, Philadelphia, 1987, WB Saunders, pp 64-67.
3. Carroll P and others: Guidelines for counselling parents of young children with food sensitivities, *Journal of The American Dietetic Association.* 92:602, 1992.
4. Colon AR and Dipalma JS: Colic, *American Family Physician* 40(6):122, 1989.
5. Forbes GB: Children and food: order amiss chaos, *The New England Journal of Medicine* 324:269, 1991.
6. Gans DA: Sucrose and unusual childhood behavior, *Nutrition Today,* May/June 1991, p 8.
7. Gortmaker SL and others: Inactivity, diet, and the fattening of America, *Journal of The American Dietetic Association* 90:1247, 1990.
8. Hendricks KM, Badruddin SM: Weaning recommendations: the scientific basis, *Nutrition Reviews* 50:125, 1992.
9. Johnson GH: *Dietary guidelines for infants,* Fremont, Mich, 1989, Gerber Products Co.
10. Klesges RC and others: Parental influence on food selection in young children and its relationships to childhood obesity, *American Journal of Clinical Nutrition* 53:859, 1991.
11. Mauer AM: Should there be intervention to alter serum lipids in children? *Annual Review of Nutrition* 11:375, 1991.
12. McNutt K: Are we pickin' on the kids? *Nutrition Today,* May/June 1991, p 42.
13. Metcalfe DD: Diseases of food hypersensitivity, *The New England Journal of Medicine,* 321:255, 1989.
14. Nicklas TA and others: Nutrient adequacy of low fat intakes for children: The Bogalusa Heart Study, *Pediatrics* 89:221, 1992.

15. Peacock M: Calcium absorption efficiency and calcium requirements in children and adolescents, *American Journal of Clinical Nutrition* 54:261S, 1991.
16. Phillips TJ, Dover JS: Recent advances in dermatology, *The New England Journal of Medicine* 326:167, 1992.
17. Pipes PL: *Nutrition in infancy and childhood,* St Louis, 1989, Mosby–Year Book.
18. Rees JM: Management of obesity in adolescence, *Medical Clinics of North America* 74:1275, 1990.
19. Ritchey AK: Iron deficiency in children, *Postgraduate Medicine* 82:59, 1987.
20. Snetselaar L, Lauer RM: Childhood, diet and the atherosclerotic process, *Nutrition Today,* Jan/Feb 1992, p 22.
21. Splett PL, Story M: Child nutrition: Objectives for the decade, *Journal of The American Dietetic Association* 91:665, 1991.
22. Story M and others: Adolescent nutrition: self-perceived deficiencies and needs of practitioners working with youth, *Journal of The American Dietetic Association* 88:591, 1988.
23. Vaughan VC: On the utility of growth curves, *Journal of the American Medical Association* 267:975, 1992.
24. Warwick ZS: Development of taste preferences: implications for nutrition and health, *Nutrition Today,* March/April, 1990, p 15.
25. Wilson DKW, Lewis NM: Weight-for-height measurement and saturated fatty acid intake are predictors of serum cholesterol level in children, *Journal of The American Dietetic Association* 92:192, 1992.
26. Zeiger RS: Prevention of food allergy in infancy, Annals of Allergy 65:430, 1990.

SUGGESTED READINGS

The textbook by Pipes entitled *Nutrition in infancy and childhood* is an excellent source for more details on nutrition issues during the growing years. The booklet produced for health professionals by Gerber Products Company outlines dietary guidelines for infants developed by experts on infant feeding and nutrition. Call the Gerber Products Company in Fremont, Michigan (1-800-4-Gerber). A pamphlet designed by parents is also available. McNutt gives a nice account of controversies in child feeding. Gans specifically covers issues surrounding sugar intake. Finally, Zeiger reviews the steps to take to reduce the risk of food allergy in infancy.

TAKE ACTION

Getting little Billy to eat

Bill is 3 years old, and his mother is worried about his eating habits. He refuses to eat vegetables, meat, and dinner in general. Some days he eats very little food. He wants to eat snacks most of the time. His mother wants him to eat a formal lunch and dinner to make sure he gets all the nutrients he needs. Mealtime is a battle because Billy claims he isn't hungry, but his mother wants him to eat everything served on his plate. He drinks five to six glasses of whole milk per day because that is the one food he adores.

When his mother prepares dinner she makes plenty of vegetables, boiling them until they are soft, hoping this will appeal to Bill. Bill's dad eats his vegetables last, regularly telling the family that he eats them only because he has to. He also regularly complains about how dinner has been prepared. Bill saves his vegetables until last and usually gags when his mother orders him to eat them. Billy has been known to sit at the dinner table for an hour until the war of wills ends. Billy's mother serves casseroles and stews regularly because these are her best dishes. He likes to eat breakfast cereal, fruit, and cheese and will regularly request these foods for snacks. However, his mother tries to deny his requests so he will have an appetite for dinner.

If you were Bill's brother or sister, what would you suggest your mother do to get Bill to eat?

Analysis

1. Give six mistakes Bill's parents are making, contributing to Billy's poor eating habits.

____

____

____

2. Give six strategies they might try to promote good eating habits in Billy.

____

____

____

NUTRITION PERSPECTIVE

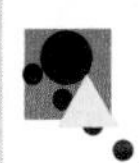

Food Allergies and Intolerances

Adverse reactions to food are commonly reported, in some studies approaching 8% to 33% of people. These occur more frequently in women. The most common ages for adverse food reactions are in infancy and young adulthood. Types of reactions associated with food ingestion are:[13]

- *Classical allergic*—Symptoms include, itching, redness of the skin, asthma, and a runny nose.
- *Gastrointestinal*—Symptoms include nausea, vomiting, diarrhea, intestinal gas, bloating, pain, constipation, and indigestion.
- *General*—Symptoms include headache, skin reactions, tension and fatigue, tremor, and psychological dysfunction.

Foods frequently identified with adverse reactions include milk, alcohol, meat and meat products, vegetables, sugars, cereals, fish and seafood products, fats and oils, eggs, fruits, chocolate, and cheese. About 90% of food allergies are caused by milk, eggs, nuts, and wheat. A family history of allergies greatly increases the risk.

Food Allergies

A food allergy is caused by an immune response to a food substance. **Food sensitivity** is a term often used today to describe reactions milder than distinct allergic ones.[13] The word allergy specifies a disorder of the immune system. Allergens are usually acidlike proteins with a specific configuration. Their typical molecular weight is between 18,000 and 40,000. The actual allergy-producing part of the protein is thought to be present in a series of amino acids that are able to bind to the immunoglobulin IgE.

food sensitivity A mild reaction to a substance in a food that might be expressed as slight itching or redness of the skin.

Normally, proteins foreign to the body—also called antigens—are met by special immune proteins of the immunoglobulin G, A, and M types. These are important factors for immune protection. However, in most people susceptible to allergies, immunoglobulin E also plays a major role. This immunoglobulin is normally found in low concentrations in the body, except when functioning as a natural defense mechanism against parasitic invasions.

When an antigen enters an allergic-prone host for the first time, specific antibodies of the IgE class are formed. These attach to specialized cells, called **mast cells,** which are located primarily in the GI tract. No reaction occurs at the first encounter. However, on subsequent exposures the antigen attaches to the specific IgE proteins on the mast cell. This joining of the mast cell and the antigen leads to a combination of chemical reactions and changes that cause the mast cell to release **histamine,** serotonin, and other chemical factors. These factors then cause the symptoms associated with an allergy.

mast cells Cells that contain histamine and are responsible for some aspects of allergic and inflammatory reactions.

histamine A chemical that causes a variety of effects on the body, such as contraction of smooth muscles, increased nasal secretions, relaxation of blood vessels, and changes in relaxation of airways.

Histamine, in particular, excites various receptors on cells. This causes contraction of smooth muscle, increased permeability and relaxation of blood vessels, nasal secretions, itching, and changes in dilation of the airways.

Why Do Allergies Occur?

A big question concerning food allergies is how intact food proteins (antigens) can cross the natural barriers of the GI tract to interact with the immune system. Considering the thoroughness of the digestive system, it seems that these particles would break down into amino acids that the body could then metabolize with no adverse effects. Evidence now shows that large particles, however, can gain access to the immune system through gaps between intestinal cells. These large particles can enter the lymph system or the capillaries, and eventually be transported via the bloodstream

NUTRITION PERSPECTIVE

Food Allergies and Intolerances—cont'd

to various body sites. Here they can cause a reaction, as is the case when they join specific IgE sites on mast cells.

In a nonallergic person, the immunoglobulin IgA synthesized by intestinal cells acts as a natural barrier against absorption and transportation of large molecules into circulation. This protection doesn't seem to function efficiently for a person with food allergies.

Testing for a Food Allergy

The first step in determining whether a food allergy is present is to record in detail a history of symptoms, time from ingestion to onset of symptoms, most recent reaction, quantity of food needed to produce a reaction, and the food suspected of causing a reaction. A family history of allergic disease can also help. The physician can look for signs of allergy in a physical examination, such as inflammation in the nasal cavity, skin diseases, and asthma (Table 17-6).

Perhaps the best laboratory test for determining what compounds a person is allergic to is the RAST test. This test estimates the amount of IgE present in a person's blood that binds certain food-borne antigens. Skin tests may also be used, where a drop of the antigen is placed on skin that has been scratched or punctured. However, skin tests are often unreliable because they sometimes overdiagnose the presence of a food allergy.

The next step is to eliminate from the diet all tested compounds that appear to cause allergic symptoms, plus all other foods the person's history suggests may cause an allergy. If symptoms are still present, the person can more severely restrict the diet or even use special formula diets that are hypoallergenic.

elimination diet A restrictive diet that systematically tests foods that may cause an allergic response by first eliminating them and then adding them back, one at a time.

anaphylactic shock A severe allergic response that results in lowered blood pressure and respiratory and GI tract distress. This can be fatal.

cytotoxic test An unreliable test to define food allergies that involves mixing whole blood with food proteins.

Once the **elimination diet** yields no symptoms, after about 2 to 4 weeks, then cautious introduction of foods—those which don't cause **anaphylactic shock**—can begin one at a time. Doses of ½ to 1 teaspoon (2.5 to 5 milliliters) are given first. The amount is increased until the dose approximates usual intake. This may be done using a double-blind approach (see Chapter 1), especially when there is a psychological component to the reaction, or when symptoms are vague or ill-defined. Dried foods can be encapsulated and then given to the person.

A bogus method to test for food allergies is the **cytotoxic test.**[1] In this case, food proteins are mixed with whole blood or serum, and then the number of white blood cells broken during the subsequent reaction between the proteins and the blood are counted. This method is quite unreliable in predicting food allergies. We recommend exploring the possibility of food allergies with a physician-allergist instead of relying on a pseudoscientific method such as cytotoxic testing.

Table 17-6 Assessment strategy for food allergies

History to provide detailed description of symptoms, time from ingestion of food to onset of symptoms, most recent reaction, quantity of food necessary to produce a reaction, and suspected foods; includes family history of allergies.
Physical examination for signs of allergy
RAST test to assess immune reactions
Trial elimination diet of suspected foods for 2 to 4 weeks or until symptoms clear
Food Challenge where suspected foods are added to diet, one at a time

Treatment of Food Allergies

Once potential allergens are identified, the best treatment is to avoid them, especially for people with zero tolerance. Cromolyn sodium, a prescription medication given as an inhalant, can limit the extent of the immune reaction in the lungs. This medication limits activity of mast cells.

If a woman is pregnant or breast-feeding, she should avoid any offending foods for her because antigens can cross the placenta, and will be secreted in her milk. Moreover, when food allergies run in the family, women are advised to breast-feed their infants.[26] Formula-fed infants have a greater risk of developing allergies. Breast-feeding should continue for as long as possible, preferably at least 1 year, and early introduction of cow's milk should be avoided. If breast-feeding is not possible, special formulas that contain altered forms of cow's milk proteins are available (such as Nutramigen and Alimentum). These are especially valuable when treating an infant with an allergy to cow's milk.

The American Academy of Allergy and Immunology has a 24-hour, toll-free hot line (1-800-822-ASMA) to answer questions about food allergy and to help direct people to specialists who treat the problem.

A major challenge for the clinician who is treating a person with a food allergy is to make sure that what remains in the diet can still provide the essential nutrients needed.[3] Special care should be taken when removing many potentially offending foods from a child's diet.

Will a Child Always Have the Food Allergy?

The **prognosis** for IgE-related food allergies that occur before 3 years of age is good. About 40% of children outgrow a food allergy. Food allergies diagnosed after age 3 years often are more long lived. Adults have reported reactions that still will appear even after 15 or more years of the first episode.

prognosis A forecast of a disease's problem course.

Except in cases where shock (anaphylaxis) is possible, foods causing allergies may be reintroduced every 6 months or so to see whether the allergy symptoms have decreased, but not before 1 year of age. If so, it indicates that tolerance to a food has developed. People with mild or moderate allergies to several foods may benefit from a diet in which an offending food is eaten every fifth day to encourage a tolerance. If cow's milk sensitivity starts in infancy, the child usually outgrows this sensitivity by 2 to 3 years of age.

Food Intolerances

Besides food allergies, there can be other causes of adverse food reactions known as **food intolerances.** These do not involve the immune system, and so it is important to separate them from typical food allergies. These cases have a higher threshold for the offending food before symptoms occur, and the treatment differs from that for food allergies. Causes of food intolerances can be categorized as:

food intolerance An adverse reaction to food that does not involve an immune response.

- Substances that produce pharmacological (drug) activity, such as tomatoes or pineapples.
- Toxic contaminants, such as bacterial toxins; synthetic compounds, such as tartrazine (F, D, & C yellow no. 5); antibiotics; and insect parts.
- Deficiencies in digestive enzymes, such as lactase.
- Food-borne illness because of improper handling or cooking, as in *Clostridium botulinum* food-borne illness (see Chapter 19).
- Viral and bacterial infections, as in *Salmonella* food-borne illness.

All these conditions can lead to GI symptoms. In addition, anyone can expect to be sensitive to one or more of these causes—not only people with specific changes in their immune system.

Four very common food intolerances are induced by the presence of sulfites in

NUTRITION PERSPECTIVE

Food Allergies and Intolerances—cont'd

wines or heated vegetables, monosodium glutamate in Chinese food, the yellow food dye tartrazine, and tyramine in aged foods, such as cheeses. A sulfite reaction causes flushing, spasms of the airways, and a loss of blood pressure. Evidence of reaction to monosodium glutamate might be an increase in blood pressure, sweating, vomiting, headache, and facial pressure. A reaction to tartrazine includes spasm of the airways, itching, and redness of the skin. About 8% to 15% of people with aspirin intolerance are also intolerant to tartrazine. A final compound, tyramine, can cause high blood pressure in people taking monoamine-oxidase inhibitor medications (for depression).

The basic treatment for food intolerances is to avoid specific offending components. However, this usually does not require total elimination. Again, we need to emphasize that most people are generally less sensitive to factors that cause food intolerances than are allergic people to their offending food components. For instance, a slight amount of sulfites in a glass of wine may be tolerable, whereas a large dose from a chef's salad may cause a reaction. See Chapter 19 on food safety for more details about toxic reactions from foods.

Does Sucrose Have Ill Effects on Children?

Some researchers have suggested that sucrose affects behavior, especially in children. They claim sucrose creates an excited, even antisocial state, which may lead to violence and disruptive behavior. However, almost all researchers and health authorities find that sucrose itself is not the villain.[6] No adequate evidence supports the hypothesis that reactive hypoglycemia caused by sugar consumption commonly causes violent behavior (see Chapter 3). If there is a villain, it is probably the excitement or tension surrounding high-sucrose foods (such as is seen at parties and during Halloween), or the extra attention a child receives when put on a relatively sucrose-free diet. Thus recommendations to lower the amount of sucrose in children's diets in hope of preventing or treating behavioral problems is, at best, premature.

How Many Children Are Sensitive To Food Additives?

In 1973, Dr. R. Benjamin Feingold suggested that food additives caused hyperactivity (now known as a part of the attention deficit disorder) in children. He theorized that because some children are allergic to aspirin-like compounds, and some food additives have aspirin-like structures, such children would also be allergic to certain food additives. Much research followed this proposal. Generally, the research has not supported a strong or predictable association between the consumption of food additives and hyperactivity in children.

The incidence of attention deficit disorder with hyperactivity is approximately 5% to 10% of school-age children; boys are affected four to six times more than girls.[2] Today the leading theory attributes hyperactivity to a chemical imbalance in the part of the brain that controls concentration. The initial identification of hyperactivity in children commonly occurs as they enter nursery or elementary school. Teachers report that these students are uncontrollable, unable to sit still, bother other children, and intrude into other children's activities.

There are many pitfalls in studying this diet-behavior relationship. If parents put a "hyperactive" child on an additive-free diet, it will tend to be a more nutrient-rich diet because it will contain more whole, unadulterated foods. In addition, the child will receive much more attention from the parents, which alone can decrease disruptive behavior.

NUTRITION PERSPECTIVE

The only definitive way to study this relationship is to use a double-blind protocol. A child would be given an additive-free food and then later one full of additives. Both the parents and the child must not know what is in the food. Then researchers would have to score the child's behavior after consuming these foods, again not knowing which foods the child had consumed.

This procedure is much too cumbersome to be used in a school system or by a private pediatrician. Thus many suspected cases of food-linked hyperactivity are not tested in a definitive scientific manner. This is problematic since some diets used for hyperactive children are limited and eliminate more than food additives. Some popular "defined diets" eliminate dietary essentials such as milk, fruit, and some grain products. The more limited the diet, the greater the risk of nutrient deficiency and poor growth.

If an additive-free diet follows the Guide to Daily Food Choices and actually improves a child's attention span and behavior, one may continue with that approach. About 5% to 10% of cases may be helped by this treatment.[2] This does not mean the diet free of additives is the key factor; more attention and other changes could still be the major reason for the behavioral change. Parents must ensure they do not leave the child with a sense of deprivation, nor should they make peer interactions more difficult for their child, without agreement from medical advisors that the special diet and restrictions are worth the effort. In addition, the child should not see behavior as more directed by diet than by how one feels.

Hyperactivity tends to decrease as a child ages. In addition, parents of children whose hyperactivity contributes to an attention deficit disorder syndrome need to be reminded that important behavior therapies can be used to treat this problem. The advice of a pediatrician skilled in this disease should be sought. The general approach to treatment includes behavior management techniques (especially to reinforce structure in one's life), frequent opportunities to dissipate excess energy, education help, and possibly the use of medications.

CHAPTER EIGHTEEN

Nutrition for the Adult and Elderly Years

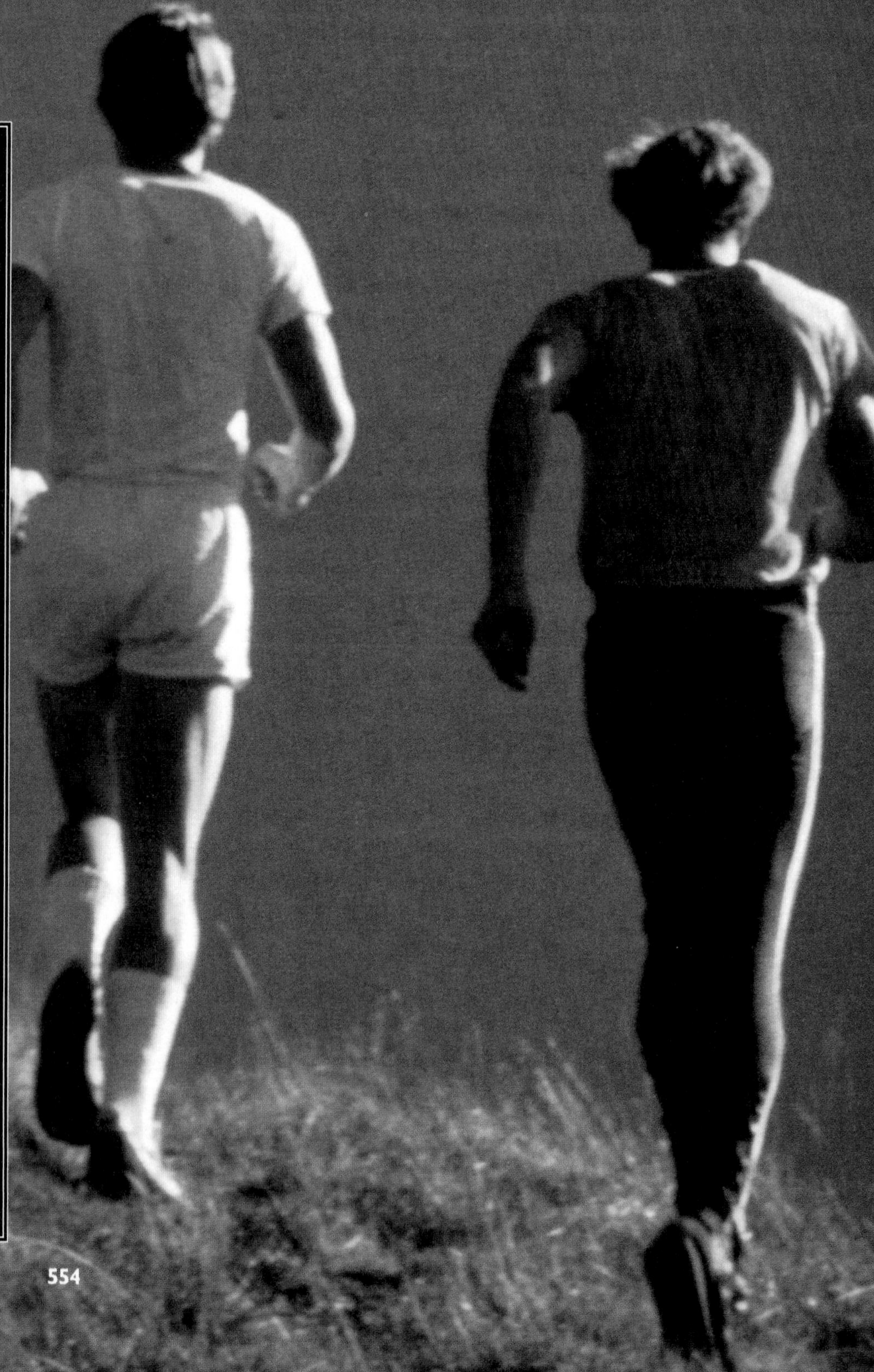

We can now review some major nutrition concepts and put recommended nutrition practices in focus for you. This review can help you tailor information from the previous chapters into a personal nutrition and health plan.

We have noted may times that nutritional recommendations should be individualized because responses to foods are often idiosyncratic. Some of us are very sensitive to the amounts of saturated fat or sodium in our diets; and some have family histories of heart disease, cancer, diabetes, alcoholism, and osteoporosis that may make us more susceptible than others to major chronic diseases. Assuming that you know your serum LDL cholesterol level and total cholesterol to HDL cholesterol ratio, your blood pressure values, your blood glucose level, and your family history for major diseases among Americans, you are now ready to formulate a personal nutrition and health plan.

In this chapter we begin with an overview of nutritional recommendations for adults, and then extend this nutrition knowledge to the special needs of the elderly. Keep in mind that choices made in younger adult years concerning food intake and overall health practices can significantly influence health during your later years.[1]

NUTRITION AWARENESS INVENTORY

Here are 15 statements about nutrition for adults and the elderly. Answer them to test your current knowledge. If you think the answer is true or mostly true, circle T. If you think the answer is false or mostly false, circle F. Use the scoring key at the end of the book to compute your total score. Take this test again after you have read this chapter. Compare the results.

1. T F The maximum age at which people die has increased dramatically.
2. T F Adults should aim to expend about 2000 kcalories per week exercising.
3. T F Medications taken by the elderly can cause nutritional problems.
4. T F The greatest nutritional problem for many Americans is overeating.
5. T F People over age 65 years account for more than half the health-care costs in the United States.
6. T F Optimal diets can stop the aging process.
7. T F The senses of taste and smell usually increase with age.
8. T F Older people often lose their desire for liquids.
9. T F Vitamin B-12 absorption often decreases in elderly people.
10. T F The most frequently occurring intestinal problem in the elderly is constipation.
11. T F An excessive intake of vitamin A supplements in the elderly can cause bone pain and hair loss.
12. T F Poor wound healing should alert a clinician to examine the protein, zinc, and vitamin C intakes of an elderly person.
13. T F An active life-style tends to maintain muscle mass.
14. T F Dietary recommendations made by the American Heart Association could, if followed, substantially reduce blood cholesterol levels in all people.
15. T F People over 65 years of age are quite similar in physical capabilities.

Your Adult Years

While most of us wish for long life, we do not like the thought of poor health in old age. And rightfully so! A long life can be enjoyable if it is productive and relatively free of illness. Rather than suffer the ravages of heart disease, obesity, strokes, diabetes, osteoporosis, and other chronic diseases from age 40 or 60 years until death, we should strive to be as free of disease as possible and to enjoy vitality throughout even our last decade. The focus here is not necessarily on living longer but on living healthier. **Life expectancy** is about at a maximum these days in the United States. Many people spend the majority of these years in a healthy, productive body, while others do not. What better goal to have?

life expectancy The average length of life for a given group of people.

The goal of striving to have the greatest number of healthy years and the fewest years of illness is referred to as **compression of morbidity.**[11] An example of this concept is illustrated in Figure 18-1 for heart disease. Of the three lines shown, the line on the left depicts rapid deterioration in health status, where symptoms of heart disease appear by about age 40 and death occurs at about age 60. In addition, between the ages of 40 and 60 years, symptoms of heart disease—and therefore disability—are present. A healthier life-style follows the middle line pattern. Here, heart disease is postponed so that the first symptoms are not apparent until age 60; severe symptoms occur at age 80, with death following a few years later. The line on the right is the ideal; the disease progresses at such a slow rate that symptoms do not appear throughout a person's lifetime, and therefore the disease process never hampers a person's activities.

compression of morbidity Maintaining good health practices to delay the onset of disabilities due to chronic disease.

Aging is a natural process; body cells age no matter what health practices we follow. But to a considerable extent you can choose how fast you age throughout your adult years. You have some say in the matter (Table 18-1). "Successful" aging is the goal. In light of the many studies showing the ability to even reverse atherosclerosis,[17] we can say age fast or age slow—to some extent the choice is yours.

While there is little doubt as to the benefits of a healthy lifestyle, scientists have also found a strong genetic component to how long we live. When researchers closely examine the genetic and lifestyle backgrounds of long-lived people, they

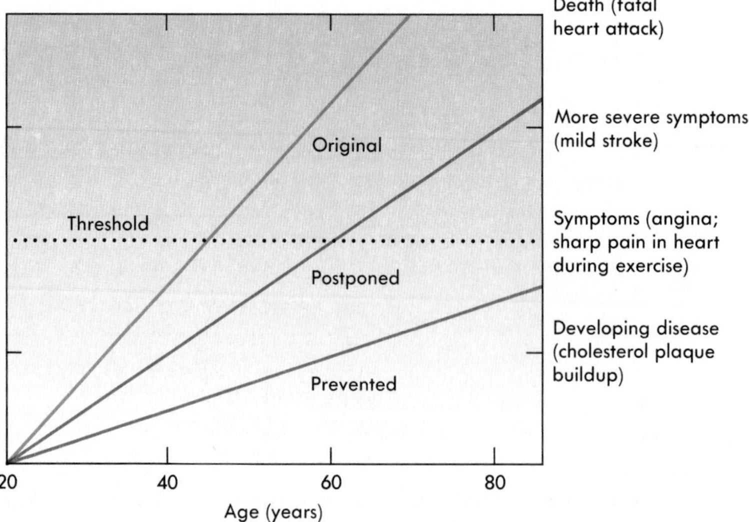

Figure 18-1 "Compression of morbidity." The goal is to postpone sickness in life until one's final days and, in turn, lead as healthy a life as possible. Heart disease is used as an example. Of the three lines shown, the line on the left shows rapid deterioration in health status, where symptoms of heart disease appear by about age 40 and death occurs at about age 60. In addition, between the ages of 40 and 60 years, symptoms of heart disease—and therefore disability—are present. A healthier lifestyle follows the middle line pattern. Here, heart disease is postponed so that the first symptoms are not apparent until age 60; severe symptoms occur at age 80, with death following a few years later. The line on the right is the ideal: the disease progresses at such a slow rate that symptoms do not appear during a person's lifetime, and therefore the disease process never hampers a person's activities.

Table 18-1 What can we expect from good nutrition and health habits?

- Meeting our needs for protein, kcalories, and other essential nutrients by following the Guide to Daily Food Choices helps prevent:
  - Birth defects and low birth weight in pregnancy
  - Poor growth and poor resistance to disease in infancy and childhood
  - Poor resistance to disease in adult years
  - Deficiency diseases, such as cretinism, scurvy, and anemia due to iron or folate deficiency
- Meeting our needs for calcium intake helps prevent:
  - Some adult bone loss, and so lessens the risk for osteoporosis
- Obtaining adequate fluoride and minimizing sugar intake helps prevent:
  - Dental caries
- Eating enough dietary fiber helps prevent:
  - Digestive problems such as constipation and diverticulosis, and possibly colon cancer
- Enough vitamin A and beta-carotene intake in the diet may help reduce:
  - Susceptibility to some cancers, especially in smokers
- An adequate, regular exercise helps prevent:
  - Obesity
  - Noninsulin-dependent (adult-onset) diabetes
  - Heart disease
  - Some adult bone loss
  - Loss of muscle tone
- Moderation in kcalorie intake helps prevent:
  - Obesity and related diseases, such as diabetes, hypertension, cancer, and heart disease
- Limiting sodium intake helps prevent:
  - Hypertension and related disease of the heart and kidney in susceptible people
- Avoiding saturated fat intake helps prevent:
  - Heart disease
- Minimizing alcohol intake helps prevent:
  - Liver disease
  - Fetal alcohol syndrome
  - Accidents
- Moderation in intake of essential nutrients by using supplements wisely, if at all, prevents:
  - Most chances for nutrient toxicities

surmise that genetic background, vigorous physical activity, low-fat diets, and the prevention of overweight may be key factors in longevity. Studies of families, and of twins in particular, provide strong evidence for genetic control of human longevity. Identical twins tend to die at similar ages with similar causes of death. Since identical twins have exactly the same genetic information, this argues that longevity is at least partially hereditary.

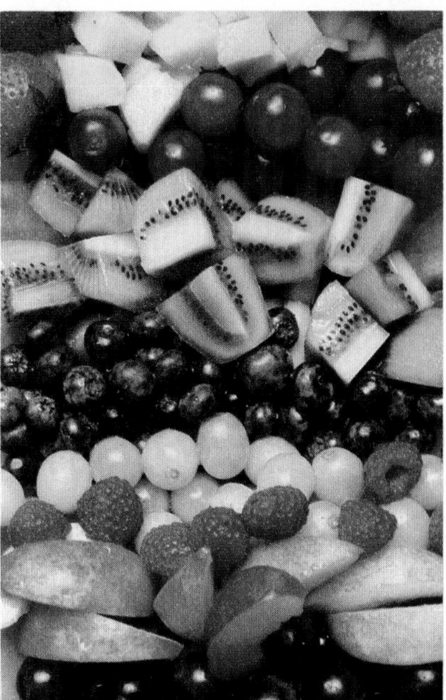

Fresh fruit makes a tasty and healthy dessert.

A BASIC PLAN FOR HEALTH PROMOTION AND DISEASE PREVENTION

Adults can best promote health and prevent chronic disease by practicing the following behaviors:

Consume a proper diet—A varied diet that maintains a desirable weight should be a priority. The Guide to Daily Food Choices in Chapter 2 is a great place to start. Place particular emphasis on consuming whole grains, minimizing fat intake by seeking low-fat and nonfat food choices, and choosing dark green or leafy vegetables regularly[16,23] (Table 18-2).

Exercise—Research suggests that about 2000 kcalories per week should be spent in brisk walking, jogging, swimming, cycling, stair climbing, and other activities that stimulate the cardiovascular system.[18]

Abstain from smoking—Lung cancer, which is primarily due to smoking cigarettes, is the only form of cancer where rates still increase every year.

Limit alcohol intake—Limit alcohol consumption to not more than 1 ounce per day.[16,23] This is approximately equivalent to two 12-ounce beers, two 4-ounce glasses of wine, or one ordinary-sized mixed drink. African-Americans are especially sensitive to the effects of alcohol on blood pressure. Furthermore, women should not consume alcohol during pregnancy.

Limit stress, or learn ways to manage stress more effectively—Practice better time management, relax, listen to music, have a massage, exercise regularly—do your favorite things to reduce stress.

The key to maximizing health is to establish harmony between the physical, mental, psychological, and social states. There is no general formula for achieving this ideal; each of us must juggle and balance personal goals with opportunities and

Table 18-2 Sample diet of nutrient-dense food choices for the elderly that follows the Guide to Daily Food Choices and meets all Recommended Daily Allowances for 1600 kcalories

Breakfast	Lunch
1 cup Crispy Wheat 'n Raisins	Turkey sandwich
1 cup 1% milk	2 slices whole-wheat bread
1 orange	2 ounces roasted turkey breast
tea or coffee, if desired	mustard
	1 banana
Dinner	1 oatmeal raisin cookie
Salad	1 cup 1% milk
1 cup romaine lettuce	
½ cup tomatoes	
2 tablespoons Italian dressing	
¼ cup sunflower seeds	
4 ounces lean roast beef	
½ cup brown rice with au jus	
¾ cup carrot sticks	
1 oatmeal raisin cookie	

NOTE: This diet follows the Guide to Daily Food Choices as it contains at least the following: 2 servings of milk/yogurt/cheese; 2 servings of meat/poultry/fish/dry beans/eggs/nuts; 2 servings of fruits; 3 servings of vegetables; and 6 servings of breads/cereals/rice/pasta.

obstacles encountered. In addition, people who practice health promotion and disease prevention may not necessarily live longer—because of heredity, accidents, or other things outside of their control—but they probably live healthier lives. Thus the quality of their lives is enhanced.[11] It is especially important for health care professionals to develop and follow a plan that emphasizes wellness for themselves. By taking this initiative, they act as positive models for others to follow.

HEALTH OBJECTIVES FOR THE UNITED STATES FOR THE YEAR 2000

Health promotion and disease prevention became a public health strategy in the United States in the late 1970s. In 1979, a variety of health-related areas were highlighted as goals for national efforts in the document *Healthy people: The U.S. Surgeon General's report on health promotion and disease prevention*. Some goals in this document became the 1990 Health Objectives for the nation. Since this time, a new report, *Healthy people 2000,* issued in late 1990 by the U.S. Department of Health and Human Services' Public Health Service, has been released. This report consists of national health promotion and disease prevention objectives for the nation for the year 2000.

The Surgeon General's report states that "for most of us, the more likely problems are overeating—too many calories for our activity levels—and an imbalance in the nutrients consumed."

Healthy people 2000's nutrition-related challenges address the following:

- iron-deficiency anemia
- poor growth in infants and children
- high fat intake
- obesity
- high serum LDL cholesterol levels
- high sodium intakes
- low calcium intakes
- low complex carbohydrate and dietary fiber intakes
- the need for more home-delivered meals for the elderly
- a relative lack of breast-feeding, poor general nutrition knowledge, and the lack of nutrition education
- the need for more food labeling information
- the need for a comprehensive, nationwide, nutritional assessment and monitoring system both in health-care and consumer settings.

DIETARY RECOMMENDATIONS FOR ADULTS

The American Heart Association (AHA) began recommending that adults consume a nutritious diet for maintaining a healthy heart in 1957.[5] Some scientists believe the recommendations should apply to all people over 2 years of age. Table 4-2 listed the latest recommendations by the AHA. Then, in 1977, the Senate Select Committee on Nutrition issued dietary goals for the United States. (We discussed this in Chapter 2.) These goals—actually the revised version published soon after the first edition—are listed in Appendix I. The goals generated controversy in the United States, primarily because they set such specific dietary recommendations for consumption of kcalories, fats, cholesterol, sucrose, sodium, and other dietary factors.

More general dietary guidelines for Americans were published in 1980 (and slightly revised in 1985 and 1990) by a joint commission of the U.S. Department of Agriculture (USDA) and the U.S. Department of Health and Human Services (DHHS). The National Cancer Institute (NCI),[5] the Surgeon General's Office,[23] and most recently, the National Academy of Sciences (NAS)[16] and World Health Organization (WHO)[1] have added to or clarified these dietary guidelines. We reviewed the current dietary guidelines issued by USDA and DHHS in Chapter 2. We list them here with clarifying statements by the other organizations just mentioned:

Chapter 2 also reviews diet planning guidelines issued by the Canadian government for Canadians.

1. **Eat a variety of foods**—Focus on the Guide to Daily Food Choices. The NAS report suggests limiting protein intake to twice the RDA and not taking a nutrient supplement in quantities greater than the RDA in any 1 day. Both the NAS and

What Should I Eat to Live Longer?

DAVID KLURFELD, Ph.D.

The fountain of youth emanates, according to popular culture, from a proper diet. This rosy view stems, in part, from the dietary recommendations made by many scientific groups to reduce the risk of heart disease, cancer, and other chronic illnesses. Implicit in proposed dietary recommendations is the promise of longer life—but how long and for whom?

Cardiovascular disease and cancer account for almost three fourths of all deaths in affluent societies. One reason for this is that many causes of premature death—infections, poor sanitation, and accidents—have been dramatically allayed. This change translates into a life expectancy at birth in the United States of 71 years for men and 78 years for women. In only a few other countries is this life span exceeded—but by no more than a few years—and in most of them the diet is similar to that in the United States. In spite of our highly publicized "killer diet," deaths from heart disease, stroke, and cancer unrelated to tobacco use have all declined significantly over the last 20 years.

We don't know for sure why this drop occurred, but it has been attributed, in part, to less use of tobacco and reductions in hypertension and in serum cholesterol, along with better medical care. These changes in risk factors point to the multifaceted causes of both heart disease and cancer. In addition, since many environmental factors interact with genetic predisposition to a disease, it is incorrect to attribute most of the risk for chronic diseases to diet alone.

Many of the estimates of dietary contribution to the risk of cancer are made by default; that is, cancers that are not traceable to other risk factors are often lumped as being caused by diet. The National Academy of Science's 1989 report on Diet and Health concluded that "the data are not sufficient, however, to quantitate the contribution of the diet to overall cancer risk or to determine the amount of reduction in risk that might be achieved by dietary modification." Nevertheless, this committee and others have proposed a low-fat, high–complex-carbohydrate diet to reduce cancer risk. They point out that in Mediterranean countries the death rates for diet-associated cancers are half those in the United States. But do these people live longer or enjoy better health? There is a conspicuous lack of good data to decide this. Thus to date we cannot reliably estimate the quantitative impact of diet on cancer.

Can we, though, reduce cardiovascular disease by dietary means with some degree of certainty? Probably, according to epidemiologic and animal data. But epidemiology offers only leads—it cannot demonstrate cause and effect. Today, there's little controversy over increased risk of heart disease with elevated levels of serum cholesterol. What is debated is at what point dietary treatment should be supplemented with drugs. And although the consensus recommendation is to reduce cholesterol below 200 milligrams per deciliter (mg/dl), some argue that this is too modest a target, while others contend that it's an unnecessary one. Still, the slope of heart disease versus serum cholesterol is quite steep at the upper levels (over 250 milligrams per deciliter), but very shallow near 220 milligrams per deciliter. So much less benefit, if any, is derived from lowering average cholesterol values.

The Multiple Risk Factor Intervention Trial (MRFIT) data show that at average serum cholesterol levels, there's the least mortality; at higher levels, heart disease increases; and at the lowest levels, there's excess mortality from cancer and other causes. These results (and those from other studies) indicate that a reduction in high serum cholesterol levels is of benefit in preventing heart disease but not in prolonging life.

Both epidemiologic and experimental studies point to specific nutrients that are associated with the incidence of chronic disease. Generally, these nutrients are found in a high-fat, low-fiber diet—a diet that is also an indicator of affluence. There's also a strong statistical correlation between gross national product, telephones, flush toilets, and other signs of wealth and the incidence of cancer and heart disease because life expectancy is longer in more affluent countries. Populations that can afford to eat a lot of fat, sugar, and salt do so because these three dietary components are what make—or what people think make—food taste good. Poor people who eat a lot of starch do so because they cannot afford more nutritious foods. Americans tend to eat far more protein than they need, yet there's little debate over this indulgence as a contributor to essential hypertension—even though it is known that high protein intake increases renal blood flow. Instead, everyone in the country has been told to follow a low-sodium diet when only a minority are hypertensive and some of those are salt sensitive.

A potential explanation for the lack of uniformity in response to dietary factors is that perhaps only some of the population shows elevated serum cholesterol from eating saturated fat, only some people are genetically predisposed to cancer of the colon, while a fortunate few are destined to live long healthy lives no matter what rules they violate. This observation does not necessarily discount the importance of nutrition but suggests that recommendations for dietary modification should not be blanket public health policies, but instead recommendations need to be made on individualized bases—that is, only for those who are at increased risk for killer diseases via family history or the presence of other risk factors.

The explanation that such diets wouldn't hurt may satisfy some, but it's certainly not scientific. The burden of proof should fall on those who suggest major dietary changes rather than on those who question the efficacy of those changes. Although what is written today will surely be outdated in the future, there are two general nutritional rules that will probably make sense over time: (1) eat a variety of foods, and (2) consume all foods in moderation. Boring, perhaps, but advice one can take to heart.

Dr. Klurfeld is associate professor at the University of Pennsylvania School of Medicine and The Wistar Institute.

surgeon general's report encourage everyone to meet their RDA for calcium, especially adolescent girls and women.

2. **Maintain healthy weight**—The midranges of the Metropolitan Life Tables can serve as a standard, or one can use a body mass index range of 19 to 27 (see Chapter 8). Both the NAS and the Surgeon General's report emphasize balancing food intake with regular physical activity.
3. **Choose a diet low in fat, saturated fat, and cholesterol**—The NAS, AHA, WHO, and NCI suggest limiting fat intake to 30% of total kcalories. The NAS report, WHO, and AHA recommend limiting saturated fat to one third of total fat intake (10% of total kcalories) and dietary cholesterol to 300 milligrams per day.
4. **Choose a diet with plenty of vegetables, fruits, and grain products**—Emphasize complex rather than simple carbohydrates. The NAS report suggests five or more servings of vegetables and fruits daily and six or more servings of breads, cereals, and legumes daily. This is consistent with the Guide to Daily Food Choices plan. The WHO intends this to yield the bulk of the 55% of kcalories that they recommend from carbohydrate. The NCI intends this intake to yield 20 to 35 grams of dietary fiber per day.
5. **Use sugars in moderation**—The WHO suggests a limitation of 10% of total kcalories.
6. **Use salt and sodium in moderation**—The WHO and NAS report suggests limiting salt intake to no more than 6 grams per day, which would yield 2.4 grams of sodium. A restriction of this magnitude would require a great change in food habits for many people, such as eliminating processed meats, salted snack foods, most canned and prepared soups, regular cheese, and many tomato-based products.
7. **If you drink alcoholic beverages, do so in moderation**—Both the NAS and Surgeon General's reports recommend not more than two drinks daily, and no alcohol use during pregnancy.

The NCI further recommends moderation in consuming salt-cured, smoked, and nitrate-cured foods. The NAS and Surgeon General's report add a recommendation for obtaining an optimum fluoride intake, particularly during the growing years. Finally, the Surgeon General's report recommends that children, adolescents, and women of child-bearing age consume iron-rich and calcium-rich foods.

These guidelines do not apply equally to everyone. We vary in susceptibility to high serum cholesterol levels, high blood pressure, obesity, and other health problems these guidelines seek to counteract. For instance, in people who have a low energy output, a high sugar intake may be a problem, since they need to consume a nutrient-dense diet. However, for adolescents who have very active lifestyles and practice good dental hygiene, dietary sugar causes no apparent health problems. The same argument applies to sodium; some people are more sensitive to the blood pressure–raising effects of sodium than other people. In addition, no scientific data has shown that typical sodium intakes necessarily produce high blood pressure later in a person who presently has normal blood pressure, although the NAS report cautions this may be true. Overall, you should consider your own health status to apply these guidelines appropriately.

A NOTE OF CAUTION

Based partly on this personal response to diet components, not all nutrition and health researchers agree with the blanket nutrition guidelines set by our major health and science institutions. Most researchers agree on the need for varying food sources in the diet; controlling body weight; reducing dietary total fat and saturated fat for adults; eating more fruits, vegetables, and breads and cereals; and moderating alcohol intake.[5] However, many scientists do not think that general recommendations for the public can be justified for sugar, dietary fiber, salt, and cholesterol. Rather, they believe these recommendations need to be individualized.

It can be argued that while individualized dietary recommendations are best, that approach is too costly for the nation and therefore impractical. If that is indeed the case, general recommendations can be made if these benefit the health of most people while not hampering the health of others. Not all people would benefit equally from following the general recommendations—for example, a reduction in sodium intake—but no one would be harmed. The dietary change could, however, cause some inconvenience, and perhaps for some people require new eating habits.

Nevertheless, we should all consider some of the general dietary recommendations, such as emphasizing low-fat and nonfat dairy products, lean meats and plant proteins, fruits and vegetables, and ample breads and cereals. These recommendations are consistent with the Guide to Daily Food Choices and form the best approach to optimizing nutritional health, based on current scientific knowledge. And overall, a life-style that contains about an hour of physical activity each day combines with a sensible dietary intake to reduce the risk of premature development of almost all the chronic diseases we adults face, including in the elderly.[1]

CONCEPT CHECK

Compression of morbidity is the goal of delaying symptoms and disabilities primarily due to chronic diseases for as many years as possible. A basic plan to promote health and prevent disease includes eating a proper diet, exercising, abstaining from smoking, limiting alcohol intake, and limiting or learning ways to deal with stress more effectively. More specific dietary guidelines direct people to eat a variety of foods; maintain healthy weight; choose a diet low in fat, saturated fat, and cholesterol; choose a diet with plenty of vegetables, fruits, and grain products; use sugars only in moderation; use salt and sodium only in moderation; and, if you drink alcoholic beverages, do so in moderation. Recommendations to pay particular attention to fluoride, iron, and calcium intake during certain life stages are also included. Some scientists believe these guidelines do not necessarily constitute an individual "prescription."

ARE WE FOLLOWING THESE NUTRITION AND HEALTH RECOMMENDATIONS?

Americans generally are trying to follow many recommendations listed above. Saturated fat intake in the form of whole milk and cream has decreased since the mid-1950s. To some extent skim and low-fat milk have replaced them. However, cheese consumption has increased, which is usually a concentrated form of saturated fat. Since 1963, butter, egg, and animal fat consumption have fallen, while use of vegetable fats and oils and fish consumption have increased. All these changes, except the increased cheese consumption, are generally consistent with recommendations to focus on monounsaturated and polyunsaturated fat intake at the expense of saturated fat intake.

Animal breeders are raising much leaner cows and hogs today than in 1950. The demand for chicken has skyrocketed. In fact, a major fast-food chain recently had to delay introducing a new chicken product for several months until enough chickens were available for the day of introduction.

Other aspects of our diet are more mixed. The NHANES II survey in the early 1980s showed that the five major contributors of kcalories to the our diet (in order) are: (1) white bread, rolls, and crackers; (2) doughnuts, cakes, and cookies; (3) alcoholic beverages; (4) whole milk and whole milk beverages; and (5) hamburgers, cheeseburgers, and meatloaf. If the new thrust in diets truly is toward a decrease in alcohol, sugar, and saturated fat intakes, along with increased consumption of fiber, the foods listed above are not the types we would expect to top the list. In terms of sheer frequency, coffee and tea; white bread, rolls and crackers; margarine; whole milk and whole milk beverages; doughnuts, cakes, and cookies; and sugar are still

FRANK & ERNEST® by Bob Thaves

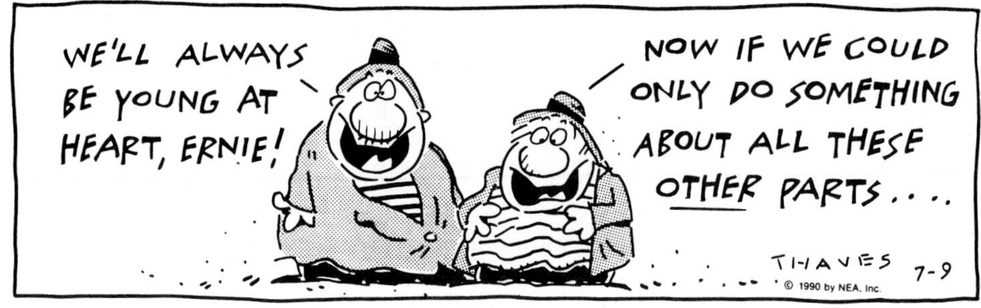
WE'LL ALWAYS BE YOUNG AT HEART, ERNIE!
NOW IF WE COULD ONLY DO SOMETHING ABOUT ALL THESE OTHER PARTS....
THAVES 7-9
© 1990 by NEA, Inc.

Figure 18-2 Frank and Ernest.
Reprinted by permission of NEA, Inc.

the top six food categories most commonly consumed. (Note: the overall diet of Americans may have improved since that study was completed in 1980. NHANES III will soon verify whether that is true.) Our suggestions for improvement would stress low-fat and nonfat milk; whole-wheat bread and whole-grain cereals; lean meat and fish, such as tuna and salmon; and ample selections of fruits and vegetables. What would your list look like?

IS THERE AN IDEAL DIET FOR ADULTS?

There probably is an ideal diet for you, based on your particular nutritional and health status, but there is no single type of diet that provides optimal health for everyone. The Japanese diet is often promoted as a healthful alternative for Americans. At the same time, it has been associated with one of the highest rates of stomach cancer in the world, which offsets its low risk for colon or breast cancer. Death from heart disease is about seven times lower in Japan than in the United States, but life expectancy is only about 3 years longer.

Many cultural dietary patterns encompass the practices recommended by nutrition experts: eating a variety of foods, maintaining a desirable body weight, and maintaining a physically active life-style. For you, the key is to focus on the likely causes of sickness and ultimate death in your life, and to make specific changes to address those causes. Whether these changes include switching to bran cereal, rice, pasta, fish, chicken, broccoli, and bok choy and walking 2 miles five times a week is up to you. These practices all provide a means to further and maintain nutritional and overall health, but are not the only path to this goal. Your overriding consideration should be the overall quality and length of life and how they can be enhanced by dietary and life-style changes[11] (Figure 18-2).

CONCEPT CHECK

Surveys show that Americans are beginning to follow general health recommendations. Some health promotion goals, however, have yet to be met. Scientists do not agree as to the best dietary recommendations for the public. Genetic background, medical conditions, and other life-style practices influence an individual's optimal diet. Many scientists support general dietary recommendations that benefit the health of most people, while not hampering the health of others, but individual plans should be developed when possible.

Nutrition in the Elderly Years

life span The potential oldest age to which a person can survive.

The human **life span** is approximately 120 years. Recently a woman in Florida died at the age of 116. This is about as long as anyone can expect to live. In comparison, the domestic dog has a life span of 20 years, while a rat has a life span of 5 years.

Table 18-3 Changes in the causes of death during this century in the United States. Chronic diseases rather than the infectious diseases, are now the major "killers." AIDS is currently the eleventh leading causes of death.

1900			1989		
Rank	Cause of death	Percent of deaths	Rank	Cause of death	Percent of deaths
1	Pneumonia and influenza	12	1	Heart disease	34
2	Tuberculosis	11	2	Cancer	23
3	Diarrhea and enteritis	8	3	Cerebrovascular disease (strokes)	7
4	Heart disease	8	4	Accidents	4
5	Cerebrovascular disease (strokes)	6	5	Pulmonary (lung) diseases	4
6	Nephritis (kidney disease)	5	6	Pneumonia and influenza	4
7	Accidents	4	7	Diabetes mellitus	2
8	Cancer	4	8	Suicide	1
9	Diphtheria	2	9	Liver disease and cirrhosis	1
10	Meningitis	2	10	Homicide and law enforcement	1

LIFE EXPECTANCY

In 1990 life expectancy in the United States was 73 years for white males and 79 years for white females. For African-Americans the values were 66 years and 74 years, respectively. As we just pointed out, life expectancy hasn't always been this long. For primitive humans it was about 30 to 35 years. It increased to 49 years by medieval times in England, and remained so until the turn of this century in the United States. During the last 80 years, life expectancy for nearly all people has lengthened, mainly because of changes in the principal causes of death.

At the turn of this century, infectious diseases were a common cause of death. Now the number one cause of death in Western societies is heart disease and number two is cancer (Table 18-3). The decline in infant and childhood deaths, coupled with better diets and health care in general have allowed more people to age into their elderly years.[11] Because of all these changes, life expectancy has increased.

Note although life expectancy has increased since 1900, the maximum life span of a human has remained constant.

In 1900, half of all whites died before reaching age 55. In 1940, half were still alive at age 68. Today, 50% are alive at ages exceeding 70 years. About 5% of adults over age 65 are cared for in nursing homes, the rest live independent lives. In the year 2035, about 20% of the population will by 65 years and older, twice as many will reach 65 years as today (Figure 18-3). This age—65 years old—is often listed as the dividing line for when one's elderly years begin, as one can qualify for full social security. Among the older population, the 85+ years group is the fastest growing segment. Between 1986 and 2050, the population aged 85+ years is expected to increase from about 1% to more than 5% of the total U.S. population. This is the first time in history a society will need to deal with such a large elderly population.

THE "GRAYING" OF AMERICA

The aging of our adult population poses some problems. People older than age 65 years account for 11% of the U.S. population, they account for 25% of all pre-

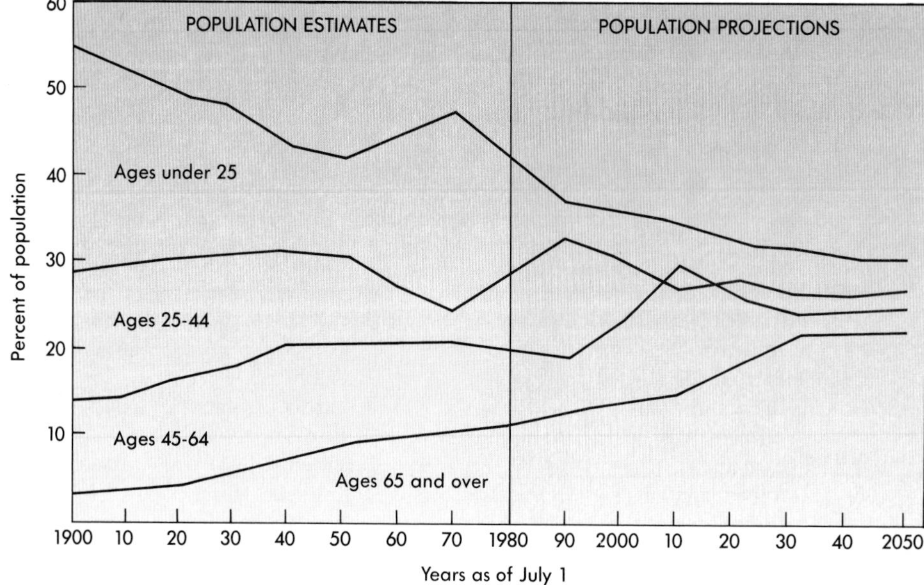

Figure 18-3 Trend in age distribution of U.S. population (including armed forces overseas), 1900-2050. The United States has never had a population with so many elderly people as it now has.

scription drugs used, 40% of acute care hospital stays, and 50% of the federal health budget. Of the elderly, 85% have nutrition-related problems, such as heart disease, diabetes, hypertension, and osteoporosis (Table 18-4).

Compression of morbidity, as suggested at the beginning of this chapter, is an important goal for controlling health care costs in the future, since merely by the increase in our numbers we will require more total health care services as we age. The more independent, healthy years we live, the less we burden our health care system, which will increasingly have to scramble to accommodate a burgeoning elderly population.[3]

WHAT CAUSES AGING?

The process of aging is still a mystery. It is also difficult to design a model for it because so often disease speeds the process. But diseases that commonly accompany old age—osteoporosis and atherosclerosis, for example—are not an inevitable part of aging. Some people do just die of "old age," and not as a direct result of disease. In itself, aging is not a disease.

One view of aging describes it as processes beginning soon after fertilization. When we are young, aging is not apparent because the major metabolic activities are geared toward growth and maturation. We produce plenty of active cells to meet physiological needs. During adolescence and early adulthood, maintenance and homeostasis become the body's major tasks. Eventually, as more cells age and die, homeostatic mechanisms cannot totally adjust to meet physiological demands. Physiological functioning begins to decrease, but organs usually retain enough **reserve capacity** so that for a long time they show no disease. While no symptoms appear, subclinical disease may develop, and if allowed to progress for years, organ function noticeably deteriorates.

reserve capacity The extent to which an organ can preserve essentially normal function, despite decreasing cell number or cell activity.

Cell aging probably results from both automatic cellular changes and environmental influences. Throughout the animal kingdom, aging is predictable. Eventually, cells lose their ability to regenerate needed components, and they die. As more and more cells in an organ system die, organ function decreases. After age 14 months, human brain cells are continually lost, but we have enough reserve capacity to maintain mental function throughout life. There is also a continual loss of **kidney nephrons.** In some people this loss leads to eventual kidney failure, but most of us maintain sufficient kidney function. Thus in aging, there is first a reduction in reserve capacity. Only after that is exhausted does actual organ function decrease.

kidney nephrons Unit of kidney cells that filter wastes from the bloodstream.

Table 18-4 Selected disease conditions associated with aging

Chronic condition	Rate of occurrence per 1000 persons			
	Total	45-64 years	65-74 years	75+ years
Arthritis	131	280	460	508
Hypertension	124	265	408	395
Hearing impairments	91	149	261	381
Heart conditions	83	137	291	339
Visual impairments	35	46	72	136
Deformities or orthopedic impairments	121	175	191	198
Diabetes	26	55	98	92
Diverticula of intestines	8	15	36	45
Asthma	37	32	47	26

Again, why cells age remains a mystery. Whether aging is due mostly to automatic or environmental influences is part of the question. Many theories have been promoted:[13]

Errors in DNA replication—Once enough errors in DNA replication (copying) accumulate, a cell can no longer synthesize the major proteins it needs to function, and therefore it dies.

Aging of the connective tissue—Changes in collagen proteins may decreasae flexibility in key body components and so alter organ function. Wrinkled skin is an apparent result.

Buildup of toxic products—Breakdown products of lipids, such as **lipofuscin,** may hamper normal metabolic processes by clogging cells. You can think of lipofuscin as intracellular "sludge."

Free radical damage—Free radicals attack cells and damage cell membranes and proteins. But a diet rich in antioxidants such as beta-carotene, vitamin C, and vitamin E, can play a role in reducing this type of cell damage (see Chapters 12 and 13).[6] In contrast, consuming cellular enzymes that are designed to break down free radicals and other highly oxidative compounds does not help; ingested enzymes are dismantled during digestion—before they can act in the body. For example, the enzyme **superoxide dismutase,** which is sold by some health-food stores, is made by cells to destroy super oxide negative free radicals (O_2^-). Adding superoxide dismutase to a diet does not help because digestion in the intestine breaks it into amino acids along with other proteins in the diet.

Changes in hormone function—The hormone dehydroepiandrosterone (DHEA), produced by the adrenal glands, is present in extremely high levels in the blood of young adults and falls sharply with age. This has led to speculation that it may play a role in aging. Long-term effects of using products containing this hormone are unknown. FDA has not approved use of DHEA, so any marketing of this drug in the United States is illegal.

Changes in the efficiency of the immune system—The thymus gland, located in the upper chest, is a major component of the immune system. Present at birth, it reaches maximum size during adolescence and is barely visible by age 50. The immune system itself runs along a somewhat parallel track: it is most efficient during childhood and young adulthood. With advancing age it is less able to recognize and counteract foreign substances, such as viruses, that enter

A good example of this aging process is lactase deficiency. For some people, lactase enzyme activity may decline during childhood but, generally, clear symptoms of gas and bloating after milk consumption do not appear until adulthood. Although lactase output decreases in these cases, perhaps from birth, enough enzyme is present to maintain sufficient lactose digestion until adulthood.

lipofuscin (ceroid pigments) Signs of accumulation of lipid breakdown products in cells often seen as brown spots on the skin.

superoxide dismutase An enzyme that can neutralize a superoxide negative free radical.

the body. An adequate diet helps immune function, as we covered in Chapter 15.

autoimmune Immune reactions against normal body cells; self against self.

Autoimmune effects—**Autoimmune** reactions occur when your white blood cells and antibodies fail to distinguish between you and foreign compounds invading your body. White blood cells and antibodies then begin to attack body tissues, as well as foreign compounds. Many diseases, including some forms of diabetes and arthritis, involve an autoimmune response.

Programmed death—In humans, each cell can divide only a limited number of times, about 50. Once this number of divisions occurs, the cell automatically succumbs. As the number of possible cell divisions increases, so does life span. The Galapagos tortoise, whose cells divide about 140 times, has a life span of perhaps 200 years.

Glycosylation of proteins—Blood glucose, especially when chronically elevated as in poorly controlled diabetes, attaches to body proteins. This decreases protein function and can encourage immune system attack on such altered proteins.[15] Eventually, cell health declines.

Most likely, the actual cause of aging is a combination of these events and changes.

CAN DIET STOP THE AGING PROCESS?

No diet can stop aging, but research in this century shows that raising laboratory animals after weaning on low-energy diets—about two thirds the energy they normally consume—greatly slows aging. Animals on these lean rations live about 50% longer than control groups allowed to feed "ad libitum" (at their pleasure) and show much lower rates of cancer.[27]

The key is to restrict only kcalories, not other nutrients. Humans living in semistarvation conditions do not live longer than our typical "Western" life expectancy; their diets are low in kcalories, but also low in proteins, many vitamins, and many minerals.

It is not clear how a low-kcalorie diet increases the life span of animals. Hormonal or immune system changes may be involved, as suggested in Chapter 5. Delaying puberty may also play a key role. Lessening DNA damage in areas that can lead to reducing the activity of cancer-causing genes is also suggested as a mechanism. Researchers doubt that a decreased metabolic rate is the reason.[15] It is clear that the animals grow more slowly, and this may affect their tendency to develop disease. How to apply the findings from these animal studies to humans is unknown. Severe kcalorie restriction, especially for infants, can be dangerous. We must wait for further research before applying this research to the human condition, especially because some processes of aging seen in rats and mice differ from those in humans.

CONCEPT CHECK

While life span has not changed, life expectancy has increased dramatically over the past century. For societies, this means an increasing proportion of the population is, and will be, over 65 years of age. Continually rising health care costs make compression of morbidity very important. Aging may begin before birth and probably results from both automatic cellular changes and environmental influences. Some popular theories about why we age raise these possibilities: errors in DNA replication accumulate and cause cell death; aging of the connective tissue; buildup of lipid by-products, such as lipofuscin; free-radical damage; hormonal and immune system dysfunction; and autoimmune damage. Diet can play a role in slowing some of these processes.

The Effects of Aging on the Nutritional Health of the Elderly

Elderly people vary more in health status among themselves than do any other age group. Physiological age is much more important than chronological age in the elderly years in terms of predicting the nutritional problems of an elderly person. It is necessary to know to what extent a person's physiological capabilities have been affected by aging (Figure 18-4), as well as the extent to which the person shows early warning signs for poor nutritional status (Table 18-5).[7] Let's examine how aging affects some major body systems and how these changes contribute to poor nutritional status. As possible we will note which changes in nutrient intake are needed to counteract problem conditions.

TASTE AND SMELL

Sensitivity to taste and smell usually decreases with aging.[20] About one third to one half of a person's taste buds die by age 70 years. Food companies are carving a niche in the marketplace by capitalizing on this change: by using a variety of flavor enhancers they attempt to make foods tastier for the elderly. But for this group, a poor diet and possibly zinc deficiency can also contribute to a loss of taste. So a poor appetite should never by dismissed as a characteristic of old age. Many causes can be remedied.[9]

DENTITION

About 50% of people over age 50 years have lost all their teeth. Replacement dentures enable some to chew normally, but many elderly people, especially men, have denture problems. A pureed diet is not necessarily the remedy, but the elderly often do require some individual dietary problem-solving to identify which foods need to be modified in consistency, and which can be eaten in a typical state. Surprisingly, many elderly people with no teeth are still able to eat most foods they could before they lost their teeth. For this reason it is important not to assume that a lack of teeth translates into the need for an unappealing pureed or ground diet. When people have problems chewing, nutrient-dense snacks like yogurt, bananas, and peanut butter can help. Sometimes just allowing extra time for feeding and swallowing encourages more eating.

THIRST

Elderly people often partially lose their sense of thirst. They are then more likely to suffer from dehydration, which can lead to confusion. It is important for older adults to consume enough fluids, and if necessary, to be monitored to ensure adequate fluid intake. An approximate fluid recommendation is the same for younger adults, 1 milliliter per kcalorie burned, or about 2 liters per day (8 cups per day). This amount must be adjusted to reflect increased urination due to the use of diuretics,

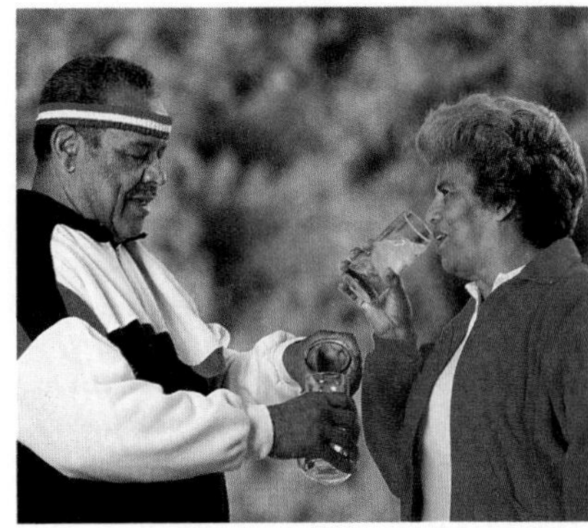

Older people should be careful to maintain an adequate fluid intake.

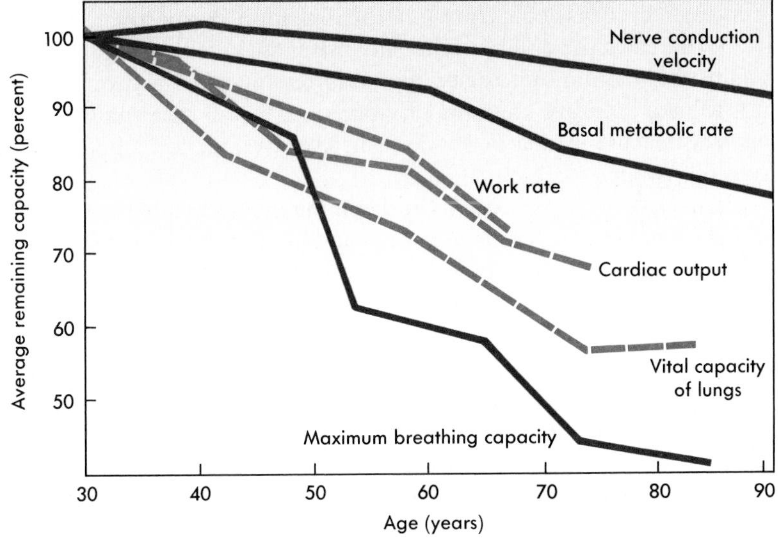

Figure 18-4 The declines in physiological function with aging. Some decline in many body functions are seen in aging, especially in primarily sedentary people.

Table 18-5 Potential easily recognizable warning signals for poor nutritional status

Obesity	Frequent nausea/vomiting
Recent unplanned weight change of ± 3 kg (7 lb)	Diarrhea/constipation
Chewing/swallowing difficulties	High alcohol intake
Poor appetite	Side effects of medication, especially with long-term use
Recent surgery	Skipped meals or drinks
Illness lasting longer than 3 weeks	No food stores
Physical disability, such as those that affect shopping for or eating food	Food wastage/rejection
Lack of sunlight exposure	Lack of fruit, fruit juices, raw or freshly cooked vegetables
Depression/loneliness/social isolation	Low budget for food
Mental confusion	Poor nutritional knowledge
Advanced age (>80 years)	
Dry mouth	

or loss of fluid through other routes, such as from an **ostomy**. Some important signs of dehydration, other than confusion, include dry lips, sunken eyes, increased body temperature, dizziness, decreased blood pressure, constipation, decreased urine output, and nausea.

THE INTESTINAL TRACT

The main intestinal problem for the elderly is constipation.[20] Elderly people generally need to consume more dietary fiber than they did in their youth, approximately 35 grams a day. Fluid intake should also increase to avoid intestinal obstruction resulting from a high fiber intake. However, all age-groups should avoid using mineral oil as a laxative at mealtimes because it binds fat-soluble vitamins.

The reduced synthesis of stomach acid also hampers iron absorption. Factors that further interfere with iron status in the body include: regular use of aspirin, which causes blood loss in the stomach; use of antacids, which may bind iron; and ulcers and hemorrhoids, which also cause blood loss.

Lactase synthesis frequently slows in elderly people. The options for people with lactose intolerance are listed in Chapter 3. A decrease in stomach acid production in the elderly is usually accompanied by decreased intrinsic factor synthesis. These last two changes can lead to poor absorption of vitamin B-12, and in turn, to pernicious anemia. Elderly people should be watched by their physicians for signs of pernicious anemia (see Chapter 13).

LIVER, GALLBLADDER, AND PANCREAS

The liver functions less efficiently in the elderly years. Some decline results from a fat buildup if there is long-standing alcohol consumption. If actual cirrhosis develops, the liver functions even less efficiently (see the Nutrition Perspective). This drop in liver function decreases the ability to detoxify many medications, and also increases the possibility for vitamin A toxicity. For this reason, elderly people should be warned not to take excessive amounts of vitamin A. Recall that vitamin A toxicity causes hair loss, malaise, headache, bone pain, liver dysfunction, and a decrease in white blood cell count.

Gallstones may cause liver problems by damming the fluids intended for secretion through the gallbladder. The fluids then pool and back up into the liver. Gallstones can also hamper fat digestion because less bile is secreted into the small intestine. A low-fat diet may be necessary.

The digestive function of the pancreas may decline in the elderly years, but the pancreas has a large reserve capacity.[20] A sign of a failing pancreas is high blood glucose due to decreased insulin secretion. High blood glucose levels in the elderly can also be caused by insulin resistance, a common result of obesity.[16] Where appropriate, improved nutrient intake, weight loss, and increased physical activity can often improve insulin action.

KIDNEY FUNCTION

Kidneys eventually filter wastes more slowly as they lose nephrons (filters). Kidneys deteriorate in aging partly because of excess dietary protein and, in some cases, excess kcalorie intake. The deterioration significantly decreases their ability to excrete the products of protein breakdown. The ability to convert a derivative of vitamin D into its active hormone state also declines. While an increase in protein intake to 1 gram per kilogram of desirable body weight has been recommended for physically active elderly people, that does not apply to cases where decreased kidney function causes urea, the by-product of protein metabolism, to build up in the bloodstream.

Incontinence—the inability to control the muscle responsible for retaining urine—afflicts up to 20% of the elderly living at home and 75% of those in nursing homes. The embarrassment of having to wear diapers causes many to avoid fluids (resulting in dehydration and constipation), and to become socially isolated.

IMMUNE FUNCTION

With age, the immune system often operates less efficiently, as we mentioned earlier. Adequate protein and zinc intakes are necessary to maximize the health of the immune system. Recurrent sicknesses and poor wound healing are warning signs of deficient protein and zinc intakes. They may be due to insufficient total food or to too few animal proteins in the diet, possibly because meats are difficult to chew. Recall that animal proteins are an excellent source of zinc. On the other hand, overnutrition also appears to be equally harmful to the immune system. For example, obesity and excessive iron and zinc intake can suppress the immune system.

LUNG FUNCTION

Lung efficiency declines somewhat in aging,[3] but especially in elderly people who have smoked tobacco products and continue to smoke. Breathing becomes shallower and faster and more difficult as the number of **alveoli** decreases. Smoking often leads to emphysema and/or lung cancer. The decrease in lung efficiency accompanies a general downward spiral in body function; it leads to decreased physical activity and endurance and frequently to decreased food intake. These eventually hamper the ability to maintain overall health. Besides not smoking, exercise helps prevent lung problems. People need not lose their capacity to breathe deeply as long as sufficient aerobic exercise is a regular practice.[21]

alveoli Small air sacs in the lung.

HEARING AND VISION

Vision and hearing both decline in the elderly years, though hearing impairment occurs mainly in industrial societies with urban traffic, aircraft, loud music, and pile drivers. People differ as to when or if these losses become disabling. Vision and hearing losses can make food shopping difficult. Elderly people may be unable to drive or read food labels. They may also avoid social contacts as much as possible because they can't hear and respond to others. Poor vision may make them afraid to walk for fear of falling. They may need assistance in shopping.[7]

DECREASE IN LEAN TISSUE

Some muscle cells shrink and others are lost as muscles age; some muscles lose their ability to contract as they accumulate fat and collagen. Life-style partially determines the rate of muscle mass deterioration; an active life-style tends to maintain muscle mass, whereas a very inactive one causes a loss of muscle mass.[3]

As lean tissue decreases with age, less energy is used while a person is resting.[26] Accompanying the loss in lean body mass is a continual decline in basal metabolism of about 2% every 10 years from age 30 years. This requires elderly people to choose foods wisely, because while their enegy needs decrease, their needs for most vitamins and minerals do not.

Physical activity is desirable for elderly people because it allows them to eat more food, thereby increasing their chances of consuming an adequate diet. Another advisable practice is to decrease sugar and fat consumption as energy needs fall to increase the diet's nutrient density. An elderly person may need to take a multivitamin and mineral supplement with a physician's guidance if energy intake falls below 1500 kcalories per day (see the Nutrition Perspective in Chapter 12).

NUTRITION FOCUS

Alzheimer's Disease

Alzheimer's Disease has become a dreaded possibility for many people approaching old age. Many of us have had first-hand experience as loved ones have been "lost" to this form of progressive dementia. Although it seems a disease of the times—with more and more people both in nursing homes and in families devoting more time to caring for these people—the disease has been around for quite a while.

In 1907 Dr. Alois Alzheimer documented several cases of what seemed to be early senility. Typical symptoms of the disease included personality changes, unreasonable fears, outbursts, and general forgetfulness. Today, the disease Dr. Alzheimer first described affects about 4 million people over age 65 years in the United States—this includes about 25% of all people over age 85 and 50% of all people in nursing homes.

More reports identifying people with Alzheimer's disease surface every year. Is this a disease of modern society, or has it always been around but we didn't know how to diagnose it? Old age is often accompanied by a general decline in mental function. But what makes Alzheimer's disease different is that it can be diagnosed specifically by the presence of special proteins deposited in tangled masses of nerves in the brain in areas linked to memory and thinking. However, this type of diagnosis can be done only at autopsy, and so it is difficult to know precisely how many cases of dementia in old age are actually the Alzheimer's type. Clinical assessments can be made, based on losses in memory, day-to-day skills, and overall mental health—in the absence of other specific causes of mental disease. As we learn more about the typical course of the disease, these clinical methods of diagnosis have become more reliable.[28]

Causes and physical effects

In general terms, Alzheimer's disease is best described as a progressive brain disorder marked by an inability to remember, reason, or understand what is going on. Age is the primary risk factor. Scientists propose causes including altered cell development, presence of altered brain proteins, and unidentified blood-borne agents. Genetic predisposition is closely linked to a minor form that occurs at about age 40. Aluminum is highly concentrated in abnormal protein accumulations in the brain, but the aluminum is more likely an effect than a cause of the disease. Whether there are other, as yet unknown, causes remains to be seen.

Alzheimer's is a progressive disease. Its course has been divided into three stages, although these can vary in duration and intensity with individuals. Generally, (1) what begins as confusion, depression, anxiety, and short-term memory loss, (2) develops into long-term memory loss, and problems in communication and perception. The individual with Alzheimer's disease may (3) eventually become bedridden and completely dependent. Death is frequently attributable to bacterial infection or pneumonia associated with accidental food inhalation.

Treatment

Today, treatment of Alzheimer's disease is usually limited to the use of antidepressants and other drugs that target related symptoms of the disease. Therapies currently under investigation range from simple aspirin to overlapping doses of potent, synthetically-produced brain chemicals. Attending support groups for the family members is likely helpful. Overall, in order to treat a disease, we generally need to

INCREASES IN FAT STORES

As lean tissue decreases with age, the body often takes on more fat. Some researchers feel that some extra fat stores in the elderly may be fine. Large population studies suggest that in otherwise healthy people, a little fat gain during the adult years does not pose health risks.[10] The booklet accompanying the 1990 Dietary Guidelines allows ranges for healthy body weights at a given height to climb by 11 to 18 pounds once a person is over 35 years of age. The greater amounts are for taller people (Table 18-6). However, obesity is not desirable because it can raise blood pressure and blood glucose levels, as well as make it more difficult to walk and to care for oneself. Staying physically active is one positive step to lessen all these risk factors for chronic disease.[23]

CARDIOVASCULAR HEALTH

cardiac output The amount of blood pumped by the heart.

Cardiac output often drops in elderly people.[21] The decline is usually due to inactivity and resultant poor heart conditioning. This allows fatty and connective tissues to infiltrate the heart's muscular wall. If an elderly person remains physically

NUTRITION FOCUS

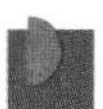

Alzheimer's Disease—cont'd

understand its causes. And unfortunately, we don't yet know as much as we need to about Alzheimer's disease.

Nutrition considerations

The main nutritional goal for people with this disease is a healthy diet that maintains body weight. Forgetfulness may lead to irregular eating habits with associated weight loss. Because one characteristic of Alzheimer's disease is the death of cells that secrete the brain neurotransmitter acetylcholine, scientists once thought that a diet that provided choline and the related compound lecithin might correct this deficit. However, studies have found this to have no effect on Alzheimer's patients. Work proceeds with medications that stimulate production of the neurotransmitter, however.

Abnormal food behaviors, such as gorging, are often seen early in the course of Alzheimer's disease. A craving for sweets may lead to a temporary weight gain that can be managed by offering lower kcalorie snacks and meals.[4] At the other extreme there is often a partial or complete refusal to eat. Frequent, small meals and nutrient-dense snacks using favorite foods when possible may encourage more regular eating. People who are still leading reasonably independent lives may not be able to shop or to remember to eat meals. Congregate feeding programs and home-delivered meals may be helpful during the early stages of disease. Keep in mind that by the time the disease has been diagnosed, some people have already developed nutritional problems.

With the progression of the disease, there is more confusion and distractibility. At this stage, it is wise for others to oversee food planning and mealtimes. Measures should be taken to control distractions, such as television, radio, children, pets, and the telephone, that can disrupt a meal for someone with Alzheimer's disease. Others should monitor food temperatures because victims may ignore discomfort and burn themselves. Tough, crunchy foods that may easily cause choking should be avoided. For those still capable of self-feeding, assistive feeding devices should be used when appropriate: roller-rocker knives, bowls, plate guards, a damp washcloth under the plate to prevent skidding, cups with tops, flexible straws, and large bibs. These are available at medical supply houses. As people with Alzheimer's disease become less able to manage eating by themselves, it becomes more of a challenge for those trying to feed them. They may hold food in the mouth, forget how to eat or to swallow, spit out food, and play with and refuse food.[4]

All of us need to pay attention to dietary recommendations to promote and maintain health. People with Alzheimer's disease may not be able to do this on their own. In later stages of this disease, people may not be tuned into their own needs. The responsibility for providing good nutrition will ultimately fall to family, health-care providers, and nursing home staff. The disease also takes an immense emotional toll on its victims and their family members. However, keep in mind that throughout much of the course of the illness individuals maintain the capacity for giving and receiving love, for sharing warm interpersonal relationships, and for participating in a variety of meaningful activities with family and friends.

The fastest-growing segment of the population is made up of people 85 and older. Thus in the future, Alzheimer's disease could have devastating consequences for our already strained health-care system.

active, cardiac output does not fall, so the decline is not due to an aging process per se.

The dramatic problems of the cardiovascular system associated with aging—heart attack and stroke—are caused primarily by atherosclerosis and high blood pressure. Atherosclerotic plaque accumulates in the arteries, reducing their elasticity and constricting blood flow, which then elevates blood pressure. You already know the main way to limit the build up of atherosclerotic plaque: keep the serum LDL-cholesterol level and total cholesterol/HDL-cholesterol ratio in the desirable range (see Chapter 4).

As for high blood pressure, while a severe sodium restriction works for most people, a mild sodium restriction (4 grams of sodium daily) is not as helpful for people who are not sensitive to salt; it is more effective for "salt sensitive" people. A limit of 2 grams of sodium helps almost all people with hypertension, but that is a difficult diet to plan and follow (see the Nutrition Perspective in Chapter 14).

We can do much to prevent premature heart attack and stroke just be eating nutritiously, walking briskly or exercising regularly, controlling blood pressure, and avoiding smoking.

Table 18-6 Suggested weights for adults

Height*	Weight in Pounds†	
	19 to 34 years	35 years and over
5′0″	97-128‡	108-138
5′1″	101-132	111-143
5′2″	104-137	115-148
5′3″	107-141	119-152
5′4″	111-146	122-157
5′5″	114-150	126-162
5′6″	118-155	130-167
5′7″	121-160	134-172
5′8″	125-164	138-178
5′9″	129-169	142-183
5′10″	132-174	146-188
5′11″	136-179	151-194
6′0″	140-184	155-199
6′1″	144-189	159-205
6′2″	148-195	164-210
6′3″	152-200	168-216
6′4″	156-205	173-222
6′5″	160-211	177-228
6′6″	164-216	182-234

*Without shoes.
†Without clothes.
‡The higher weights in the ranges generally apply to men, who tend to have more muscle and bone; the lower weights more often apply to women, who have less muscle and bone.
From USDA/DHHS: *Dietary Guidelines for Americans,* 1990.

In the early elderly years, excess weight gain is the major problem, while in the later elderly years, weight loss is more of a concern. (It is best to compare an elderly person's weight with his or her previous year's weight.) Weight loss in elderly people often means increased risk of death. It may also indicate increased sickness and poor tolerance of medications.

BONE HEALTH

We discussed the decline in bone density with aging in Chapter 14. Recall that bone loss in women occurs especially in the 10 to 15 years after menopause. Bone loss in men is slow and steady from middle age throughout the elderly years. For women, increasing one's calcium intake to 1500 milligrams per day can help maintain density in the cortical-type bones, but this does not predictably prevent bone loss associated with menopause in the more trabecular bony parts throughout the body. Presently, only estrogen replacement therapy, active vitamin D hormone (calcitriol) therapy, and calcitonin therapy—administered with a physician's guidance—can claim that. From laboratory animal studies we infer that performing weight-bearing exercises also helps sustain bone.[21]

If osteoporosis becomes very severe, the ability of elderly people to exercise, shop, prepare food, and live normally is limited.[22] Thus a further decrease in nutrient intake will likely result. Older adults often eat less and get fewer nutrients than younger adults. There is additional concern that much hidden osteomalacia (vitamin D deficiency) may be present in the elderly population.[8] Osteomalacia occurs primarily from a lack of sun exposure and possibly poor vitamin D synthesis in the skin. If predictable sun exposure is not available, as when the person is homebound, then a source for 10 micrograms of vitamin D (400 IU) per day should be found: fortified milk products or a vitamin supplement.

It is important to encourage elderly women to continue consuming the RDA for calcium and to seriously consider estrogen replacement therapy if they are still within 10 to 15 years of menopause.

Other Factors that Influence Nutrient Needs in the Elderly

Use of certain medications can profoundly affect nutrient needs in the elderly (Table 18-7).[19] Often at this age several medications must be taken for extended time

Table 18-7 Potential drug-nutrient interactions for some commonly used drugs

Drug	Use	Nutrient	Potential side effect
Alcohol	—	Thiamin, vitamin B-6, folate, and zinc	Poor absorption/poor utilization
Antacids (Maalox)	Reduce stomach acidity	Calcium, vitamin B-12 and iron	Decreased absorption due to altered gastrointestinal pH
Anticoagulants (coumadin)	Prevention of blood clots	Vitamin K	Poor utilization
Antihistamines (Benedryl)	Treatment of allergies and nausea; as local anesthetic	—	Weight gain
Beta-blocker (propanolol, Inderal)	Decrease hypertension	(Cholesterol)	Some can increase serum cholesterol levels
Aspirin	Anti-inflammatory, pain reduction	Iron	Anemia from blood loss
Cathartics (laxatives)	To induce bowel movement	Calcium, potassium	Poor absorption
Cholestyramine	Reducing blood cholesterol	Vitamins A, D, E, K	Poor absorption
Cimetidine (Tagamet)	Treatment of ulcers	Vitamin B-12	Poor absorption
Colchicine	Treatment of gout	Vitamin B-12, carotenes, and magnesium	Decreased absorption due to damaged intestinal mucosa
Corticosteroids (prednisone)	Anti-inflammatory	Zinc Calcium	Poor absorption Poor utilization
Furosemide (Lasix)	Potassium-wasting diuretic	Potassium and sodium	Increased loss
Isoniazid (INH)	Tuberculosis	Vitamin B-6	Poor utilization
Neomycin	Antibiotic	Fat, protein, sodium, potassium, calcium, iron, and vitamin B-12	Decreases pancreatic lipase, binds bile salts, and so interferes with absorption
MAO inhibitors (Parnate)	Antidepressant	Tyramine in aged foods	Hypertension caused by poor tyramine metabolism
Phenobarbital	Sedative; treatment of epilepsy	Vitamin D and folate	Reduced metabolism and utilization
Phenytoin (Dilantin)	Treatment of epilepsy	Vitamin D and folate	Reduced metabolism and utilization
Tricyclic antidepressants (Elavil)	Antidepressant	—	Weight gain due to appetite stimulation

Modified from Chernoff R: Aging and nutrition, *Nutrition Today* March/April, 1987, p 4.

periods. Drug-related nutritional problems often can be significant. The most notable ones are an increased need for potassium when consuming some types of diuretics, and increases in food intake when taking some types of antidepressant agents or antibiotics.

About 12% to 14% of elderly people experience significant depression. That, combined with isolation and loneliness as family and friends die, move away, or become less mobile, frequently contributes to disinterest in eating and so to weight loss. Depression can lead to poor appetite, weakness associated with decreased nutrient intake, and then to an even poorer appetite. In the elderly, the resulting poor nutritional state can lead to mental confusion and increased isolation and loneliness. Isolation and loneliness in and of itself is linked to increased death rates in the elderly, especially if the person has no close friends.

The role of nutrition in preserving mental function in the elderly remains unclear. Specific nutritional deficiencies of thiamin, niacin, vitamin B-6, and vitamin B-12,

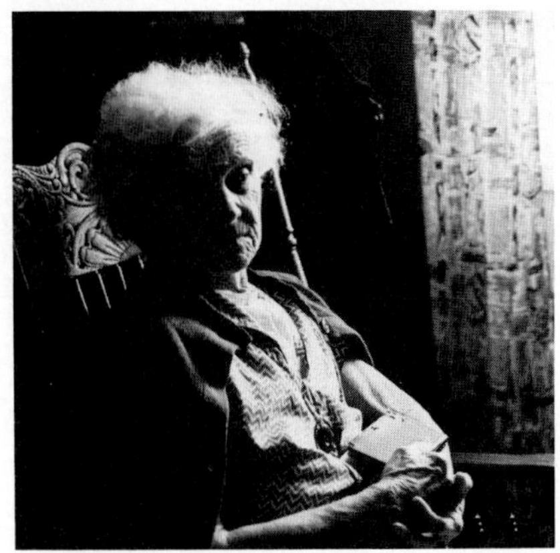

Loneliness and depression can contribute to a lack of appetite.

as well as excessive alcohol use, cause well-recognized central nervous system disorders. However, the subtle effects of a low kcalorie intake that leads to semistarvation are often overlooked.[29] In addition, as mentioned earlier, a poor fluid intake may lead to dehydration and in turn to confusion.

We know mental illness can lead to a poor nutritional state, but the extent to which subtle nutritional deficiences can lead to a poor mental state is not clear. It is important to prevent overt nutrient deficiencies, especially the ones mentioned above. Whether extra intake of specific amino acids, such as tryptophan and tyrosine, or choline can increase brain neurotransmitter synthesis and therefore alter behavior is not established.

Lastly, a variety of other social circumstances can lead to problems: In today's mobile society where the extended family may not be close at hand, there may be no one to assist with the daily needs of the elderly, including shopping for and preparation of meals; transportation may be difficult; Many elderly people are no longer able to drive, do not have ready access to public transportation, may not have the stamina to get to the bus stop, take the bus, get to the final destination and reverse the process. Even if that were physically possible, how many would be strong enough to carry the groceries home?

Some older Americans are too proud to ask for assistance, having been independent all of their lives. Asking for assistance may seem like being on the "public dole." Many are afraid of asking for help in meal preparation for fear of losing their independence or being victimized by those they hire.

CONCEPT CHECK

Nutritional problems of the elderly are related to both the presence of chronic diseases and to the normal decreases in organ function that occur with time. All these organ systems and functions decrease as we age: sense of taste, smell, thirst, hearing, and sight; digestion and absorption; liver, gallbladder, pancreas, kidneys, lungs, heart; and the immune system. In addition, muscle mass (largely due to inactivity) and bone mass often gradually decrease. Diet changes can often help reduce the impact of these results of aging.

Do the RDAs Increase in the Elderly Years?

Currently, the RDAs for nutrients and kcalories includes one category for both men and women who are 51 years of age and older. Scientists know very little about the nutrient needs of the elderly, especially for those over age 75 years. Only during the last few years has much research focussed on this. Our lack of information is reflected in the lack of changes in the RDAs for nutrients for people older than 51 years.

Recently, a noted research team suggested that the current RDA for vitamin A for the elderly is probably too high; the RDAs for protein (for active elderly people), vitamin D, riboflavin, vitamin B-6, and vitamin B-12 are too low; and the RDAs are "about right" for the other nutrients.[24] In this case, the "about right" label may reflect either that studies suggest an RDA is adequate or that we lack sufficient data to make a more definitive statement. Still, a well-planned diet that follows the Guide to Daily Food Choices should meet all nutrient needs of the elderly (Table 18-2). Thus our recommendations for an adult diet also applies in general to the elderly. There is no need to design a unique diet plan.

There is a concern that the RDA for calcium should be increased to help lessen the acceleration of bone loss suffered by elderly women. Iron needs do not increase, since elderly women have no menstrual periods. However, blood loss stemming from ulcers, hemorrhoids, and chronic aspirin use may necessitate an increased iron intake. Recall, though, that the RDAs apply only to healthy people. Elderly people with ulcers and following heavy aspirin use are not covered by the RDA for iron.

Overall then, nutrient needs for the elderly are similar to those for younger adults, but individual modifications are necessary to compensate for specific diseases present.

PLANNING A DIET FOR THE ELDERLY

To supply energy needs for adults 51 years of age or older, the current recommendation is at least 1.5 times daily basal metabolism or about 1950 kcalories per day.[30] The 1989 RDA publication suggests 2300 kcalories for men; for females, the recommendation is 1900 kcalories. Studies show that elderly men eat closer to 1600 to 1900 kcalories, while women eat about 1250 to 1550 kcalories per day. More physical activity could allow for higher energy intakes, and in turn likely improve their diets.[26]

Diet plans for the elderly should focus on vitamin D (and sun exposure), vitamin E, vitamin B-6, vitamin B-12, vitamin C, and thiamin and the minerals iron, calcium, and zinc. It is best if the elderly can increase physical activity level so that they can safely increase food intake. This expands nutrient sources, simplifying the planning of an adequate diet. Also, as mentioned earlier, protein needs are approximately 1 gram per kilogram of desirable body weight (for physically active people), and fluid needs are 1 milliliter per kcalorie burned, or about 2 liters (8 cups) per day. A high-fiber diet can decrease constipation, but fiber intake should be slowly increased to about 35 grams, making sure a glass of water (or other fluid) follows a meal or food high in dietary fiber.

Contrary to what many believe, the majority of elderly people like most foods, including vegetables. There is no need to follow stereotypes suggesting that the group dislikes broccoli because it forms gas or tomatoes because they are too acidic. Eating habits in the later years are individualistic, reflecting region, social class, ethnic group, and life experiences. Individual patterns need to be respected and explored.

Another issue that demands special attention is food preparation for elderly people who live alone. Singles of all ages face problems with food and nutrition;

Table 18-8 Guidelines for promoting healthful eating in later years

- Eat regularly; small frequent meals may be best. Use nutrient-dense foods as a basis for each menu.
- Find out which convenience foods and labor-saving devices can be of help.
- Try new foods, new seasonings, and new ways of preparing foods. Don't just use convenience foods and canned goods.
- Keep some easy-to-prepare foods on hand for times when tired.
- Have a treat occasionally, perhaps an expensive cut of meat or a favorite fresh fruit.
- Eat in a well-lit or sunny area; serve meals attractively; use foods with different flavors, colors, shapes, textures, and smells.
- Arrange things so food preparation and clean-up are easier.
- Eat with friends, relatives, or at a senior center when possible.
- Share cooking responsibilities with a neighbor.
- Use community resources for help in shopping and other daily care needs.
- Stay physically active.
- If possible, take a walk before eating to stimulate appetite.
- When necessary, chop, grind, or blend hard-to-chew foods. Softer, protein-rich foods can be substituted for meat when poor dental function limits normal food intake. Prepare soups, stews, cooked whole-grain cereals, and casseroles.
- If eating movements are limited, cut the food ahead of time, use utensils with deep sides or handles, and obtain more specialized utensils if needed.

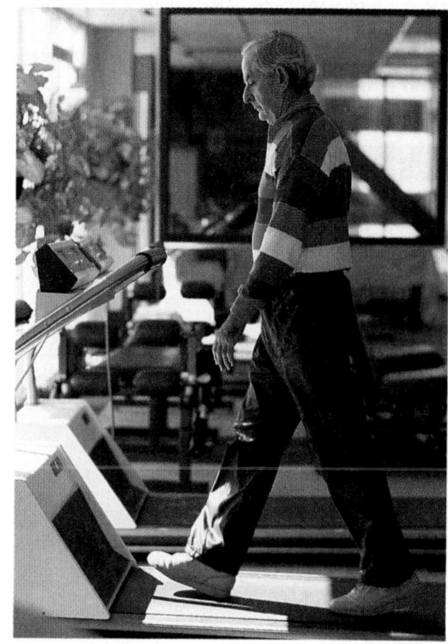

Regular exercise constitutes one step towards preventing premature heart attack and stroke and helps promote healthful eating.

purchasing, preparing, storing, and using foods with minimal waste is challenging. Economy packages of meats and vegetables are normally too large to be useful for a single person. Many singles live in small dwellings, some without kitchens and freezers. Gearing a diet to accommodate a limited budget and facilities requires special considerations. Note that poverty rates are quite high in minority elderly people and widows in general.

Following are some practical suggestions for diet planning for singles.

- If you own a freezer, cook large amounts, divide into individual portions, and freeze. This then allows for quick food production when the desire to cook is low.
- Buy only what you can use: Small containers may be more expensive, but letting food spoil is also costly.
- Ask the grocer to break open a family-sized package of wrapped meat or fresh vegetables.
- Buy only small pieces of fruit—perhaps a ripe one, a medium-ripe one, and a green one—so they will ripen over a period of several days.

The benefits of good nutrition in the elderly are many. It may delay disease progression; improve management of existing diseases; hasten recovery from illnesses; increase mental, physical, and social well-being; and decrease the need for and length of hospitalization.[3] Overall, a good nutritional intake should be a vital part of the health maintenance program for elderly people. Table 18-8 lists a variety of ideas to promote healthful eating in the elderly years. These should focus on presenting nutritious, tasty food in a pleasant, friendly environment.

Community Nutrition Services for the Elderly

Health-care advice and services can come from clinics, private practitioners, hospitals, and health maintenance organizations. Hospice centers, home health care agencies, adult day-care programs, and adult overnight-care programs can supply day-to-day care.

Feeding sick, infirm, and/or mentally confused elderly people is time-consuming and demanding work that requires special training. It is important to look for a poor nutrient intake in these elders, even if they live in nursing home settings.

Nutrition programs for the elderly include congregate meal programs, for which elderly people gather for lunch (age of eligibility is 60 years); home-delivered meals,[2] which deliver meals to homes; food cooperatives; and a variety of clubs and social organizations. The congregate meal and home-delivered meal programs (the latter often called meals-on-wheels) are funded partially by the U.S. government under Title III of the Older Americans Act and through volunteer community efforts. The U.S. government also sets specific standards for home-served meals and for those served in congregate feeding centers. The meals are constructed so they include one third of the RDA. The basic meal pattern is 3 ounces of meat or meat alternative, 1 cup of vegetables (2 or more servings), 1 slice of bread or alternative, 1 teaspoon of butter, 1 cup of milk, and ½ cup of dessert. The social aspect often improves an elderly person's appetite and general outlook.

Studies have found that congregate meal programs can positively influence the nutritional status of otherwise homebound people. Still, both congregate and home-delivered meal programs provide at most one to two meals per day, and usually not every day of the week. So if people come to depend on these meals exclusively, they will be eating too few meals and therefore obtaining inadequate nutrients. One additional problem with home-delivered meals is that they may never be eaten, or if not eaten on delivery but left at room temperature, they may become unsafe to eat later. In spite of the many challenges they face, home delivered and congregate meal programs effectively aid many frail elderly; in many cases waiting lines to gain access to the programs are quite long.

For those elderly who need help shopping for food, special transportation arrangements may be available through a local transit company or taxi service. Elderly people need to be made aware of opportunities available to them in their community.

In this way, they can be assisted in their day-to-day health and nutrition care and, ideally, remain as healthy and free to conduct their own lives independently for as long as possible. Remaining alone and isolated reduces the likelihood that an adequate diet will be eaten. This condition should be avoided.

CONCEPT CHECK

Specific nutrient requirements for the elderly are only now being extensively studied. Diet plans for the elderly should consider decreased physical abilities, presence of drug-nutrient interactions, possible depression, and economic constraints. Particular attention should be paid to sun exposure and intake of vitamin D, vitamin E, thiamin vitamin B-6, vitamin B-12, and vitamin C and the minerals iron, calcium, and zinc. Many services such as congregate meals and home-delivered meal programs are available to assist the elderly population in the United States in obtaining a healthy diet.

Summary

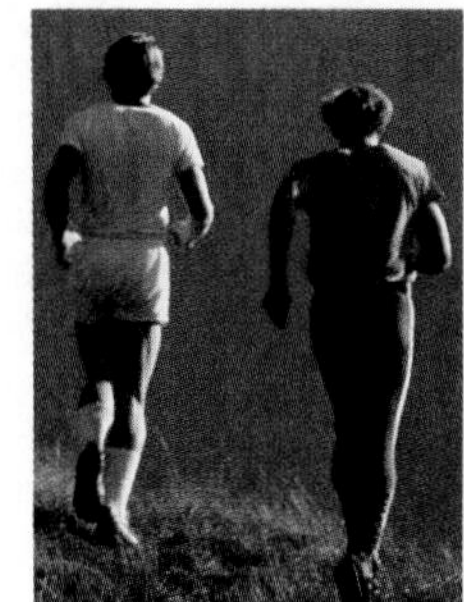

1. "Compression of morbidity" is the goal of delaying symptoms of and disabilities from chronic diseases for as many years of one's life as possible. Good nutritional habits—especially following the Guide to Daily Food Choices and the Dietary Guidelines for Americans—play a role in this process.
2. A basic plan for health promotion and disease prevention includes eating a proper diet that focuses on a variety of foods and moderation in fat intake, exercising regularly, abstaining from smoking, limiting alcohol intake, and limiting stress.
3. The 1990 Dietary Guidelines for Americans recommend that individuals eat a variety of foods; maintain healthy weight; choose a diet low in fat, saturated fat, and cholesterol; choose a diet with plenty of vegetables, fruits, and grain products; use sugars only in moderation; use salt and sodium only in moderation; and, for those who drink alcoholic beverages, do so in moderation. In addition, specific recommendations to reduce cancer risk emphasize moderation in use of cured and smoked meats. Fluoride use can also minimize dental caries.
4. Scientists disagree as to the best diet recommendations for the general public. Genetic background, medical conditions, and other life-style practices influence a person's optimal diet. An overall emphasis on variety in the diet, control of body weight, moderation in total fat and saturated fat intake, eating ample fruits and vegetables, and moderation in alcohol intake has wide support.
5. While life span has not changed, life expectancy has increased dramatically over the past century. For societies this means an increasing proportion of the population is over 65 years of age. Health care costs associated with this trend are increasing, making the goal of compression of morbidity very important.
6. Aging probably begins before birth. This aging likely results from automatic cellular changes and environmental influences, such as DNA damage, free radical reactions, hormonal changes, and alterations in the immune system.
7. Nutritional problems of the elderly are related to the presence of chronic diseases and to the normal decreases in organ function that occur with time. These include loss of teeth, a reduction in senses of taste and smell, changes in gastrointestinal tract function, and deterioration in cardiac and bone health.
8. Specific nutrient requirements for the elderly are only now extensively being studied. Diet plans should be based on the Guide to Daily Food Choices, with consideration for present health problems, decreased physical abilities, presence of drug-nutrient interactions, possible depression, and economic constraints. Specific nutrients, such as vitamin D, vitamin E, thiamin, vitamin B-6, vitamin C, vitamin B-12, iron, zinc and calcium, often deserve special attention in diet planning.

Study Questions

1. Describe the concept of compression of morbidity in terms your parents would understand. Why might it be important that they are aware of this idea?
2. Define the term "reserve capacity" of organs and relate how this tends to hide the early effects of aging.
3. Describe two theories surrounding the causes of aging and note evidence for each in your daily life experiences.
4. List four organ systems that can decline in function in the elderly years, along with a diet/life-style response to each.
5. What three resources in a community are widely available to aid the elderly in maintaining nutritional health?

REFERENCES

1. Anonymous: Diet, nutrition and the prevention of chronic diseases: a report of the WHO study group on diet, nutrition, and the prevention of noncommunicable diseases, *Nutrition Reviews* 49:291, 1991.
2. Asp EH, Darling ME: Home-delivered meal: food quality, nutrient quality, and characteristics of recipients, *Journal of The American Dietetic Association* 88:55, 1988.
3. Carethers M: Health promotion in the elderly, *American Family Physician* 45:2253, 1992.
4. Claggett MS: Nutritional factors relevant to Alzheimer's disease, *Journal of The American Dietetic Association* 89:392, 1989.
5. Cronin FJ, Shaw AE: Summary of dietary recommendations for healthy Americans, *Nutrition Today,* Nov/Dec 1988, p 26.
6. Cutler RG: Antioxidants and aging, *American Journal of Clinical Nutrition* 53:3735, 1991.
7. Davies L, Knutson KC: Warning signs for malnutrition in the elderly, *Journal of The American Dietetic Association* 91:1413, 1991.
8. Delvin EE: Vitamin D nutritional status and related biochemical indices in autonomous elderly population, *American Journal of Clinical Nutrition* 48:373, 1988.
9. Dwyer J: Screening older Americans' nutritional health: future possibilities, *Nutrition Today,* Sept/Oct, 1991, p 21.
10. Fischer J, Johnson MA: Low body weight and weight loss in the aged, *Journal of The American Dietetic Association,* 90:1697, 1990.
11. Fries JF: Strategies for reduction of morbidity, *American Journal of Clinical Nutrition* 55:1257S, 1992.
12. Hegsted DM, Ausman LM: Diet, alcohol, and coronary heart disease in men, *Journal of Nutrition* 118:1184, 1988.
13. Kirkwood TBL: Comparative life spans of species: why do species have the life spans they do? *American Journal of Clinical Nutrition* 55:1191S, 1992.
14. Lieber CS: Alcohol, liver, and nutrition, *Journal of the American College of Nutrition* 10:602, 1991.
15. Masoro EJ: Retardation of aging processes by food restriction: an experimental tool, *American Journal of Clinical Nutrition* 55:1250S, 1992.
16. National Academy of Sciences report on diet and health, *Nutrition Reviews* 47:142, 1989.
17. Ornish D: Can lifestyle changes reverse coronary heart disease? *Lancet* 336:129, 1990.
18. Paffenbarger RS and others: Physical activity, all-cause mortality, and longevity of college alumni, *The New England Journal of Medicine* 314:605, 1986.
19. Roe DA: Therapeutic affects of drug-nutrient interactions in the elderly, *Journal of The American Dietetic Association* 85:174, 1985.
20. Russell RM: Changes in gastrointestinal function attributed to aging, *American Journal of Clinical Nutrition* 55:1203S, 1992.
21. Smith EL and others: Diet, exercise, and chronic disease patterns in older adults, *Nutrition Reviews* 46:52, 1988.
22. Stehlin D: Women and nutrition, *FDA Consumer,* Jan/Feb 1991, p 11.
23. Surgeon general's report on nutrition and health: summary and recommendations, *Nutrition Today,* Sept/Oct 1988, p 22.
24. Suter BM, Russell RM: Vitamin requirements of the elderly, *American Journal of Clinical Nutrition* 45:501, 1987.
25. U.S. Preventive Service Task Force: Screening for alcohol and other drug abuse, *American Family Physician* 40:137, 1989.
26. Vaughan L and others: Aging and energy expenditure, *American Journal of Clinical Nutrition* 53:821, 1991.
27. Walford RL and others: Dietary restriction and aging: historical phases, mechanisms and current directions, *Journal of Nutrition* 117:1650, 1987.
28. Warshaw GA: New perspectives in the management of Alzheimer's disease, *American Family Physician* 42 (Nov):415, 1990.
29. White JV: Risk factors for poor nutritional status in older adults, *American Family Physician* 44(6):2087, 1991.
30. Young VR: Energy requirements in the elderly, *Nutrition Reviews* 50:95, 1992.

SUGGESTED READINGS

The summary of the Surgeon General's report on nutrition and health published in *Nutrition Today* and the summary of the National Academy of Sciences report on diet and health in *Nutrition Reviews* underscore the importance of diet to health maintenance. See Kirkwood's article on the processes of aging to learn more about how body functions decrease over time. The article by Suter and Russell and that by Schneider and others review how nutrient needs change in response to aging. The article by Paffenbarger and others shows the importance of regular physical activity for the maintenance of health. Finally, the article by White and others summarizes the key factors to consider when evaluating the nutritional health of the elderly.

TAKE ACTION

Could you or someone you know have a problem with alcohol?

The Nutrition Perspective discusses ethanol, commonly known as alcohol. This Take Action section sets the stage for that discussion. All adults; including the elderly, should take a careful look at the potential problem excess alcohol use raises. Misuse of alcohol is one of our most preventable health problems. It is a prominent contributor to five of the ten leading causes of death in the United States. The social consequences of alcohol dependency include divorce, unemployment, and poverty. The following questionnaire was adapted from one developed by the National Council on Alcoholism. With this assessment you can examine whether you or someone you know might need help. Answer the following questions by placing an "X" in the appropriate blank.

	YES	NO
1. Do you occasionally drink heavily after disappointment, a quarrel, or under stress?	____	____
2. When you have trouble or feel under pressure, you always drink more heavily than usual?	____	____
3. Have you ever noticed that you're able to handle liquor better than you did when you were first drinking?	____	____
4. Did you ever wake up the "morning after" and discover that you couldn't remember part of the evening before, even though your friends tell you that you didn't pass out?	____	____
5. When drinking with other people, do you try to have a few extra drinks when others won't know it?	____	____
6. Are there certain occasions when you feel uncomfortable if alcohol isn't available?	____	____
7. Have you recently noticed that when you begin drinking, you're in more of a hurry to get the first drink than you used to be?	____	____
8. Do you sometimes feel a little guilty about your drinking?	____	____
9. Are you secretly irritated when your family or friends discuss your drinking?	____	____
10. Have you recently noticed an increase in the frequency of your memory blackouts?	____	____
11. Do you often find that you wish to continue drinking after your friends say they've had enough?	____	____
12. Do you usually have a reason for the occasions when you drink heavily?	____	____
13. When you're sober, do you often regret things you have done or said while drinking?	____	____
14. Have you tried switching brands or following different plans for controlling your drinking?	____	____
15. Have you often failed to keep promises you've made to yourself about controlling or cutting down on your drinking?	____	____
16. Have you ever tried to control your drinking by changing jobs or moving to a new location?	____	____
17. Do you try to avoid family or close friends while you're drinking?	____	____
18. Are you having an increasing number of financial and work problems?	____	____
19. Do more people seem to be treating you unfairly without good reason?	____	____
20. Do you eat very little or irregularly when you're drinking?	____	____
21. Do you sometimes have the "shakes" in the morning and find that it helps to have a little drink?	____	____
22. Have you recently noticed that you can't drink as much as you once did?	____	____
23. Do you sometimes stay drunk for several days at a time?	____	____
24. Do you sometimes feel very depressed and wonder whether life is worth living?	____	____
25. Sometimes after periods of drinking do you see or hear things that aren't there?	____	____
26. Do you get terribly frightened after you have been drinking heavily?	____	____

These are all symptoms that may indicate alcoholism. "Yes" answers to several of the questions indicate the following stages of alcoholism:

Questions 1-8: Early Stage.
Questions 9-21: Middle Stage.
Questions 22-26: Final Stage.

It is vital that people assess themselves honestly. If you or someone you know demonstrates some or a number of these symptoms, it is important that help be pursued. If there is even a question in your mind, go talk to a professional about it. Alcohol abuse is one of the many problems adults face. ▲

NUTRITION PERSPECTIVE

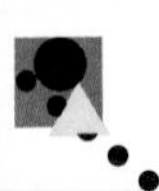

Ethanol—It's Potential to Influence Health

Alcohol is an important issue for all adults to carefully examine. Alcohol, in excess, is by far the most common drug—wrecking families and friendships, and filling jails. In 1990 its use cost American society an estimated 136 billion dollars and more than 65,000 lives, 22,000 of them on highways. From early adulthood through elderly years, the ability of excess alcohol to tear away at nutritional and overall health is enormous (Figure 18-5).

Alcohol Absorption and Action

After someone drinks an alcoholic beverage, their blood level of alcohol rises rapidly. Alcohol, technically known as ethanol, is readily absorbed into the blood from all parts of the gastrointestinal tract. You've probably been warned—with good reason—not to drink on an empty stomach. Alcohol absorption depends partly on the rate of stomach emptying. Food, particularly fat, slows the stomach's emptying rate and stimulates secretions. These dilute the alcohol and slow its absorption into the bloodstream.

Some alcohol is metabolized in the cells lining the stomach. Most of the remaining alcohol is metabolized in the liver. Recall we talked about this process in Chapter 7. About 10% of the ethanol in the body is directly eliminated by diffusion through the kidneys or lungs.[14]

Alcohol affects the brain more than any other organ. Acting as a sedative, alcohol tends to relieve the drinker's anxiety, slur speech and reduce coordination in walking, impair judgment, and encourage uninhibited behavior.[25] Because it lowers inhibitions, alcohol appears to act as a stimulant, but in fact it is a powerful depressant to the body. As William Shakespeare wrote: "It stirs up desire, but takes away the performance." Because it reduces secretion of the body's antidiuretic hormone, alcohol increases urination. It also causes the blood vessels to dilate, releasing body heat.

It is thought that alcohol causes its effects on behavior by acting upon nerve cell membrane activity and the mechanisms that help conduct nerve impulses.

Metabolism

As we noted in Chapter 7, a social drinker who weighs 150 pounds and has normal liver function metabolizes about 7 to 14 grams (the equivalent of ½ to 1 beer, or half an ordinary-sized drink) of alcohol per hour (100 to 200 milligrams of alcohol per kilogram of body weight per hour). When the rate of alcohol consumption exceeds the liver's metabolic capacity, the blood alcohol content rises and symptoms of intoxication appear (Table 18-9).

When a man and woman of similar size drink the same amount of alcohol, the woman retains more alcohol in her bloodstream; women have lower levels of the key alcohol-metabolizing enzyme, alcohol dehydrogenase. Women also cannot metabolize as much alcohol in their stomach cells as men. In addition, women more quickly develop alcohol-related ailments, such as cirrhosis of the liver, than do men with the same drinking history.

As we also covered in Chapter 7, when a person drinks a lot of alcohol, alcohol dehydrogenase in the liver can not break it all down. For this and other reasons, another liver enzyme system begins to metabolize alcohol. The liver usually uses the same system to metabolize medications and other "foreign" compounds. Once the extra system is activated, alcohol tolerance increases since the rate of alcohol metabolism increases.[14]

While the liver is metabolizing alcohol, it cannot as rapidly metabolize medications, such as sedatives. Consequently, high amounts of alcohol mixed with some sedatives may cause a person to lapse into coma and die.

Alcohol and Overall Health

About 32% of all Americans have three drinks or less each week, 22% have two drinks or less a day. Only 11% have more than two drinks a day. Although the

NUTRITION PERSPECTIVE

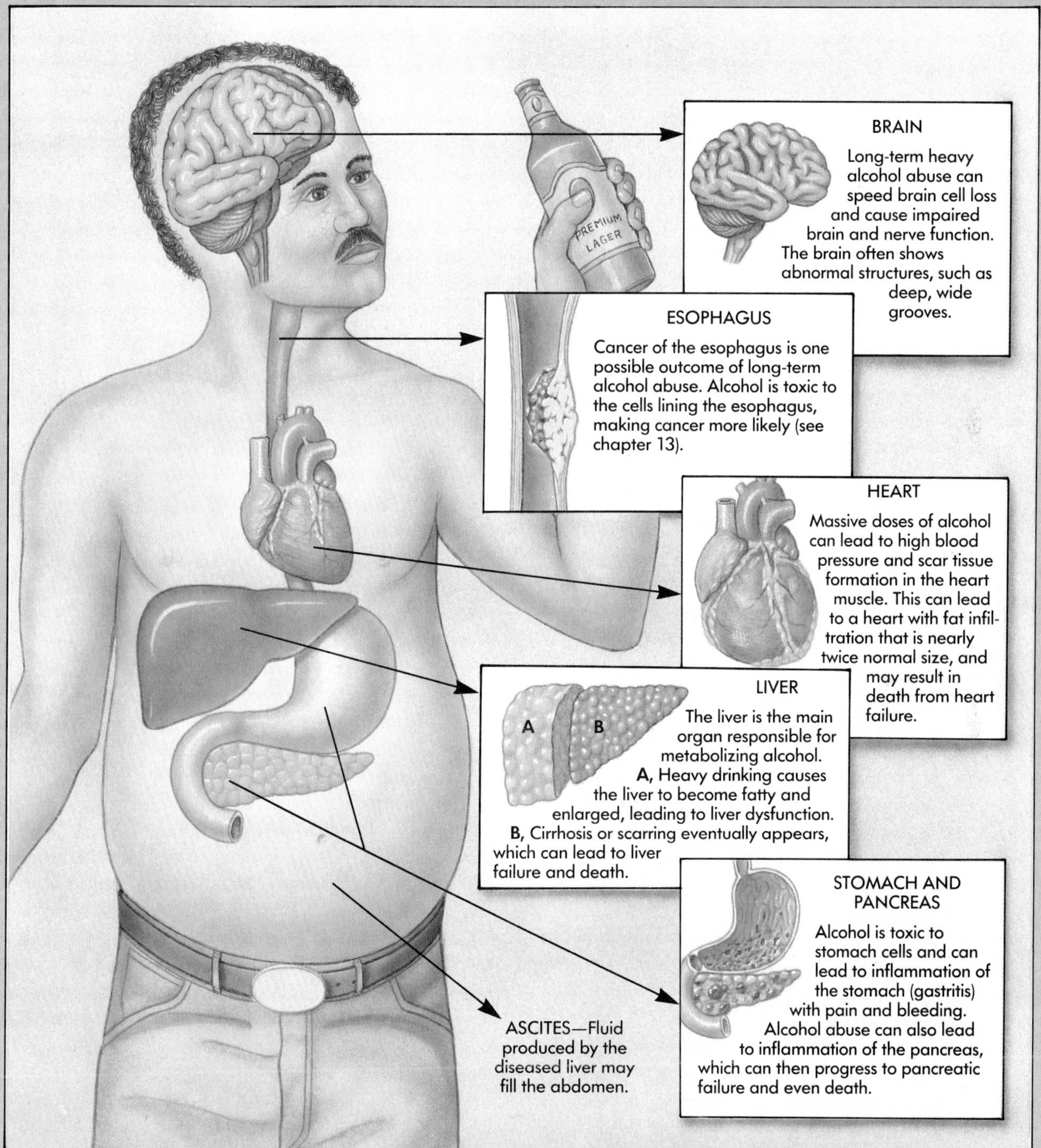

Figure 18-5 What happens to you when you abuse alcohol. The mind-altering effects of alcohol begin soon after it hits the bloodstream. Within minutes alcohol enters the brain, numbing nerve cells. In the heart, cardiac muscles strain to cope with alcohol's depressive action. If drinking continues, alcohol builds in the bloodstream, causing decrements in speech, vision, balance, and judgement. With extremely high levels of alcohol in the blood, respiratory failure becomes a possibility. In the long run, alcohol abuse increases the risk of certain forms of heart disease and cancer—and liver and pancreas failure.

NUTRITION PERSPECTIVE

Ethanol—It's Potential to Influence Health—cont'd

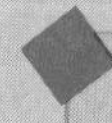

Table 18-9 Blood alcohol levels and symptoms

Level (mg/dl)	Sporadic drinker	Chronic drinker	Hours for alcohol to be metabolized
50 (party level)	Congenial euphoria; decreased tension	No observable effect	2-3
75	Gregarious	Often no effect	
100 (0.1%)	Uncoordinated; legally drunk (as in drunk driving) in most states; a level of 0.08% is legal drunkenness in a growing number of areas in the United States.	Minimal signs	4-6
125-150	Unrestrained behavior; episodic dyscontrol; legally drunk at 0.15% in all states	Pleasurable euphoria or beginning of incoordination	6-10
200-250	Alertness lost; lethargic	Effort required to maintain emotional and motor control	10-24
300-350	Stupor to coma	Drowsy and slow	>24
>500	Some will die	Coma	

Modified from Wyngaarder JB and Smith LH: *Cecil textbook of medicine* Philadelphia 1988, WB Saunders.

public health impact of alcohol abuse is still being calculated, misuse of alcohol is one of the most preventable health problems in the United States. Drinking alcohol excessively contributes significantly to 5 of the 10 leading causes of death in the United States—namely certain forms of cancer, cirrhosis of the liver, motor vehicle and other accidents, suicides, and homicides. Tobacco reacts with alcohol in a way that reinforces its effects in causing esophageal and oral cancer. In addition, excessive alcohol drinking increases the risk of some types of heart disease, high blood pressure (especially in African-Americans), nerve diseases, nutritional deficiencies (discussed later), damage to a pregnant woman's fetus, and many other disorders. A major cause of lasting mental retardation that begins in infancy is fetal exposure to alcohol (see Chapter 16).

Social consequence of dependence on alcohol include divorce, unemployment, and poverty. An estimated 27 million American children are more likely to develop abnormally in psychosocial skills and relationships because their parents abuse alcohol.

All this must tell us—use alcohol cautiously and in moderation, if at all. Drinking even small amounts of alcohol can lead to dependence. Approximately 10% of those who drink alcoholic beverages in the United States suffer from alcoholism. As many as 15 million Americans are estimated to have alcohol problems. Of these, 41% (7.2 million) are alcohol abusers, drinkers who experienced at least one severe or moderately severe consequence of alcohol abuse, such as job loss, arrest, or illness, in a previous year.[25]

The people who drink the most alcohol are those in the 20- to 40-year age group. The practice often begins earlier. In a 1985 survey, 66% of the high school seniors interviewed reported that they had consumed alcohol in the past month and 5% described themselves as daily drinkers.

Table 18-10 Caloric, carbohydrate, and alcohol content of alcoholic beverages

Beverage	Amount (ounce)	Alcohol (grams)	Carbohydrate (grams)	Energy (kcalories)
Beer				
Regular	12	13	14	150
Light	12	10	6	90
Extra light	12	8	3	70
Near	12	2	12	60
Distilled				
Gin, rum, vodka, whiskey	1.5	15	—	105
Brandy, cognac	1.0	11	—	75
Wine				
Red	4	12	1	85
Dry white	4	11	0.5	80
Sweet	4	12	5	103
Sherry	2	9	1.5	75
Port, muscatel	2	7	7	95
Vermouth, sweet	3	12	14	141
Vermouth, dry	3	13	4	105
Manhattan	3	21	2	165
Martini	3	19	1	140
Old-fashioned	3	21	1	180

From Guthrie HA: *Introductory nutrition,* ed 7, St Louis, 1989, Mosby–Year Book.

Studies of adoptees raised by nonalcoholic parents suggest a genetic component in alcoholism. Upon reaching adulthood, the biological children of alcoholic parents have a four-fold greater incidence of alcoholism than biological children of nonalcoholic parents, even where the adopting families had similar patterns of alcohol consumption. Other studies question how strong the genetic component is to this disorder. And children of people with alcoholism account for only a fraction of the alcohol abusers in the United States. Essentially any of us can become addicted if we drink long enough and hard enough.

Cirrhosis. Long-term alcohol use causes fatty liver, alcoholic hepatitis, and cirrhosis. Cirrhosis is a chronic and usually relentlessly progressive disease characterized by fatty infiltration of the liver.[25] Eventually the fat chokes off the blood supply, depriving the liver cells of oxygen and nutrients (Figure 18-6). Liver cells then die and are replaced by connective (scar) tissue. This scarring process is what we call cirrhosis. In the United States, most cases of liver cirrhosis are caused by alcohol consumption. Cirrhosis develops in 12% to 31% of cases of alcoholism. In addition to the amount and duration of alcohol consumption, genetic factors and individual differences determine the body's response to alcohol.

No specific amount of alcohol consumption guarantees cirrhosis of the liver. Rather, some people are very susceptible to its effects, while others are not. One observable pattern is that cirrhosis commonly results from a 15-year consumption of approximately 80 grams of alcohol per day (Table 18-10). This is equivalent to 7 beers per day. Some evidence suggests the dose may be effective when it's as low

NUTRITION PERSPECTIVE

Ethanol—It's Potential to Influence Health—cont'd

as 40 grams a day for men and 20 grams a day for women.[16] Early stages of alcoholic liver injury are reversible, while advanced stages usually are not. The only known prevention for alcoholic cirrhosis is to limit consumption of alcohol.

A nutritious diet can help prevent some complications associated with alcoholism, but usually alcoholism wreaks serious destruction on the body with or without an adequate diet. Lab animal studies show clearly that even when consuming a nutritious diet, alcoholism can lead to cirrhosis of the liver. Still, a poor nutritional status compounds the problem of cirrhosis as it makes the liver more vulnerable to toxic substances by depleting supplies of antioxidants, such as vitamin E and vitamin C.

Alcohol and Nutrition

Nutritional problems in a person with alcoholism result from deficiencies of a variety of nutrients[14]:

Vitamin A deficiency may be caused by a poor diet, or an inability of the liver to produce retinol-binding protein. In addition, the chemical-detoxifying systems in the liver induced by chronic alcohol consumption may hasten the degradation of vitamin A in the liver.

Thiamin deficiency can be caused by decreased thiamin absorption or decreased liver synthesis of the active thiamin coenzyme. People with alcoholism often exhibit nervous system problems similar to those seen in a thiamin deficiency.

Niacin deficiency and resulting pellagra can be caused by a poor diet.

Vitamin B-6 deficiency probably stems from a poor dietary intake of the vitamin and possibly increased break down of the vitamin B-6 coenzyme.

Folate deficiency can be caused by a poor diet and poor nutrient absorption.

Vitamin D deficiency is usually due to the liver's decreased capacity to convert vitamin D into the final useable form. Alcohol also may encourage bone cell dysfunction that diminishes bone formation and reduces bone mineralization. This can lead to osteoporosis.

Vitamin C deficiency may result primarily from a decrease in dietary intake or from altered liver metabolism, or both.

Vitamin K deficiency probably occurs because less of it is synthesized in intestinal bacteria, less is consumed, and less is absorbed.

General Guidelines for Alcohol Use

The Surgeon General's office does not recommend drinking alcohol, and cautions that if adults do they should 1) drink alcohol only in moderation (no more than two drinks a day); 2) avoid drinking any alcohol before or while driving, operating machinery, taking medications, or engaging in any other activity requiring judgment, and 3) avoid drinking alcohol while pregnant.[23] This obviously isn't a plea for teetotalers to start drinking. But we need to point out that people who have a drink or so a day and are not prone to abuse should know that there's nothing wrong with moderate drinking. In fact there are some benefits, such as a reduction in heart disease risk.[12] The reason for this is still unknown. Unfortunately, however, when some of us open the door to alcohol we end up walking into a part of life we wish we never entered.

The National Academy of Science's report on *Diet and Health* also does not recommend alcohol consumption. For those who do drink alcoholic beverages, the committee recommends limiting consumption to the equivalent of less than 1 ounce of pure alcohol in a single day.[16] This is the equivalent of two cans of beer, two small glasses of wine, or one average cocktail. Again, this report suggests pregnant women should avoid alcoholic beverages.

NUTRITION PERSPECTIVE

Do You Have a Problem With Alcohol?

Asking a person about the quantity and frequency of alcohol consumption is an important means of detecting abuse and dependence. The CAGE instrument is popular for use in routine health care.[3]

Another key point to probe is tolerance. Does it take more to make you inebriated than it did in the past? More than one positive response to the CAGE questionnaire is suggestive of an alcohol problem.

Treatment

Once a diagnosis of alcohol abuse or dependence is established, a physician should arrange appropriate treatment and counseling for the patient and family. The drinker must confront the immediate problem of how to stop the drinking. Total abstinence must be the primary goal. For people with alcoholism, there is no such thing as "controlled drinking." A problem drinker cannot return safely to social drinking. The person should enter an Alcoholics Anonymous (AA) program, or one similar, and the spouse into Al-Anon. Success is usually proportionate to participation in AA, other social agencies, religious counseling, and other resources. About 2 years of treatment should be expected.

Current research does not support the generally negative public opinion about the prognosis for alcoholism. In most industrial alcoholism treatment programs, where workers are socially stable and—because of the risk to jobs and pensions—well motivated, recovery rates run at the 70% to 80% level. This remarkably high cure rate is probably accounted for by early detection. Once a person moves from problem drinking to an advanced stage of alcoholism, success rates seldom exceed 40% to 50%. Early identification and intervention remain the most important steps in the treatment of alcoholism.[25]

CAGE Questionnaire to Screen for Alcohol Abuse

C: "Have you ever felt you ought to **Cut** down on drinking?"

A: "Have people **Annoyed** you by criticizing your drinking?"

G. "Have you ever felt bad or **Guilty** about your drinking?"

E: "Have you ever had a drink first thing in the morning to steady your nerves or get rid of a hangover **(Eye-opener)**?"

The medical deterrent drug disulfiram (Antabuse) can be of critical importance in helping the alcoholic to make the essential decision to stop drinking. An early step in alcohol metabolism is blocked by the action of this drug. As a result, a highly toxic alcohol by-product accumulates in the blood, producing prostrating nausea, vomiting, diffuse flushing, and a shocklike reaction.

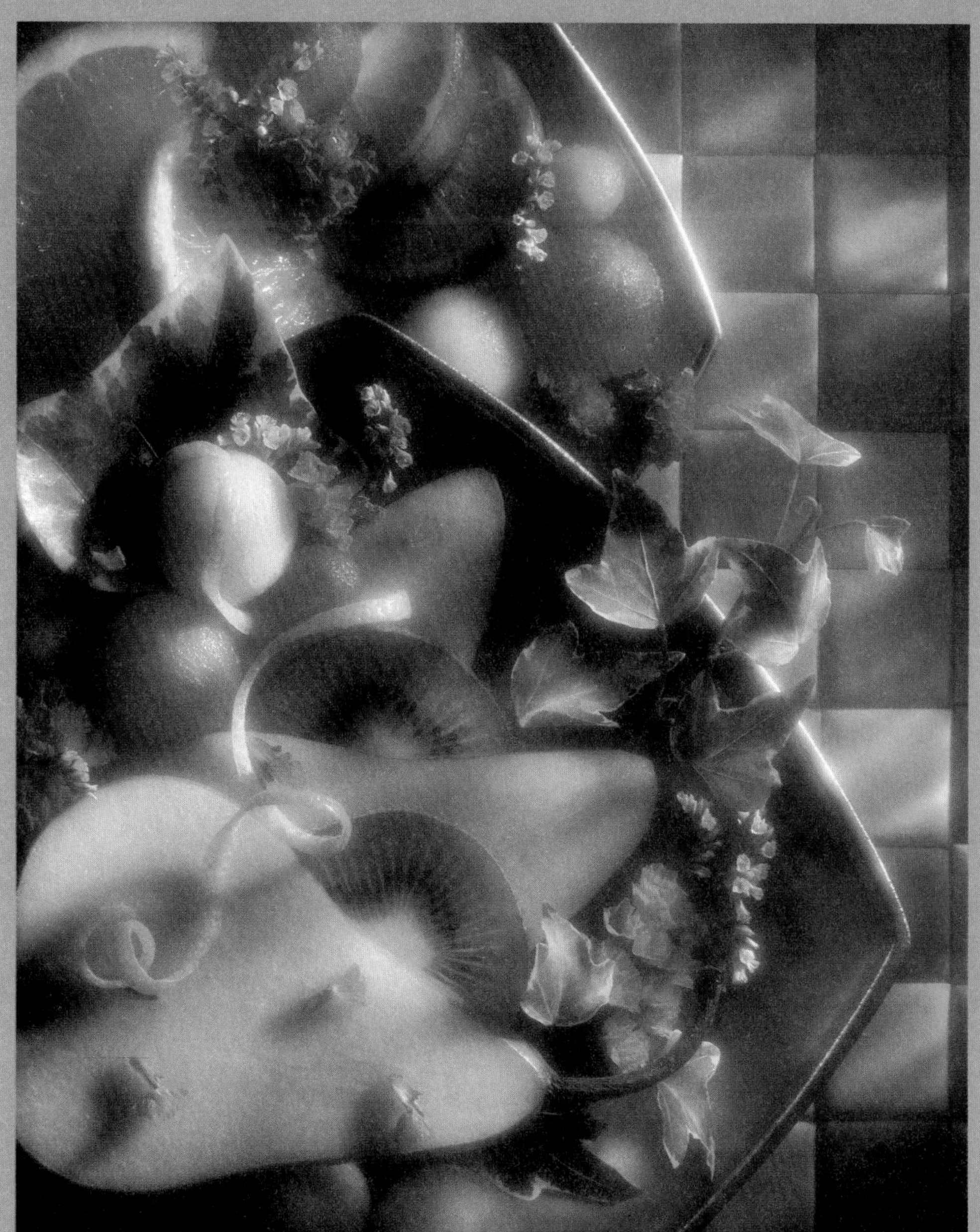

PART SIX

Putting Nutrition Knowledge Into Practice

CHAPTER NINETEEN

Food Safety

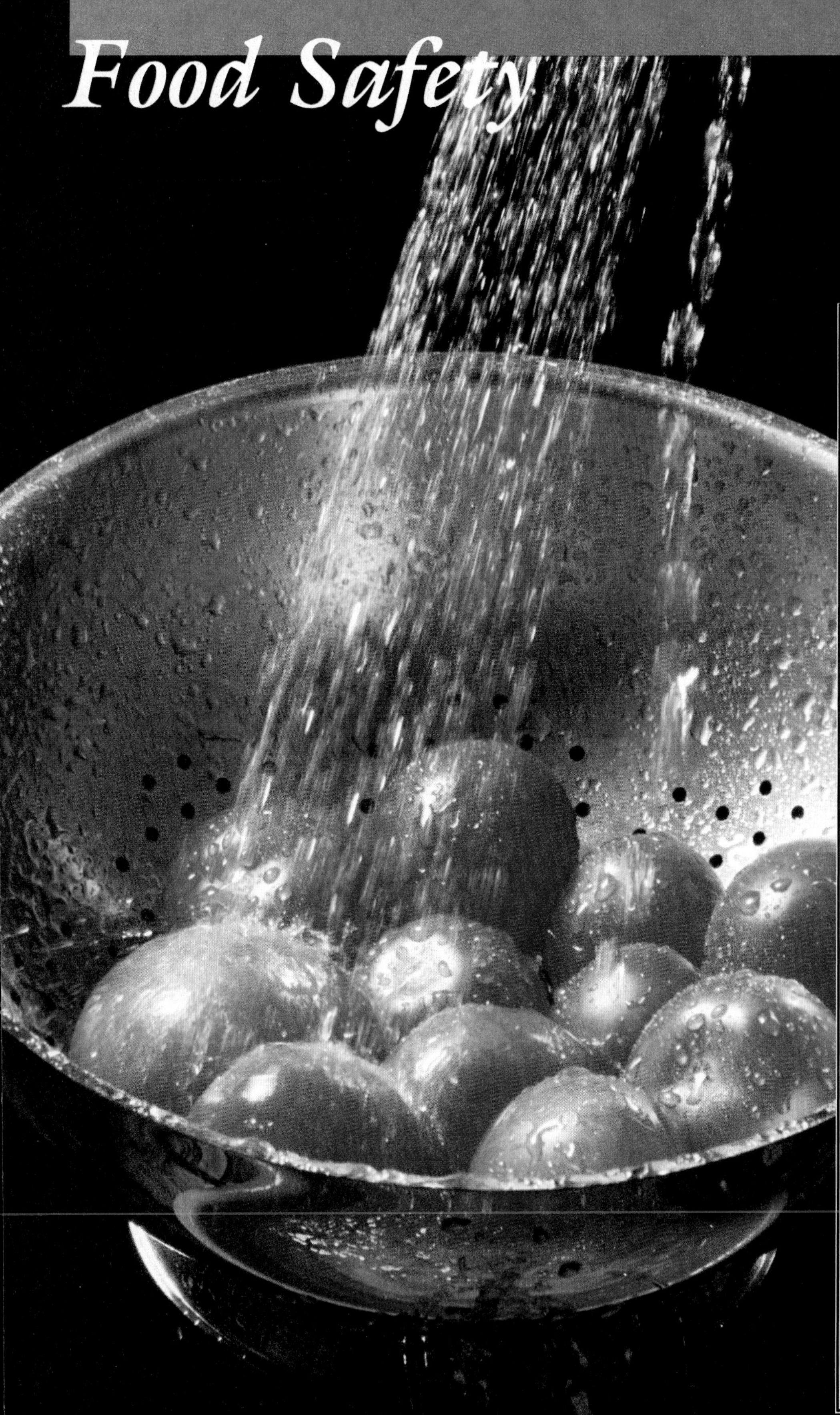

How safe is our food? Scientists and health authorities, whether working independently or for the government, agree that Americans enjoy the safest, most wholesome food supply in the world.[1]

Yet, they also acknowledge that despite the tremendous progress made in food safety throughout the past half century, a health risk from microbes and chemicals is still present in foods.

The greatest short-term health risk from food is microbial contamination from bacteria and, to a lesser extent, from fungi (including molds) and viruses. These microbes in foods can cause food-borne illness. However, regardless of evidence that microbial contamination is by far the major cause of food-related illness in the United States and throughout the world, we seem more concerned about health risks from chemicals in foods. Fully 75% of consumers surveyed in a recent Gallop poll said that pesticide contamination was a major concern to them. In the long run there is some merit to this concern. But on a day-to-day basis, according to the Centers for Disease Control in Atlanta, Georgia, only 2% of all cases of food-related illness in the United States are due to food additives.

We will first discuss food-borne illness, because it is by far the more important issue for our day-to-day health. Then we will cover the use and safety of food additives.

NUTRITION AWARENESS INVENTORY

Here are 15 statements about food safety. Answer them to test your current knowledge. If you think the answer is true or mostly true, circle T. If you think the answer is false or mostly false, circle F. Use the scoring key at the end of the book to compute your total score. Take this test again after you have read this chapter. Compare the results.

1. T F In the United States about one of every ten people suffers a bout of diarrhea from food-borne illness each year.
2. T F You can usually tell from a food's taste, odor, or appearance if that food poses a risk for food-borne illness.
3. T F Imported food does not pose a risk for food-borne illness because of careful inspection on entry into this country.
4. T F Synthetic (man-made) chemicals are more harmful to health than those that occur naturally.
5. T F Exposure to oxygen causes some foods to spoil.
6. T F Food can be preserved by reducing its water content.
7. T F Most kinds of bacteria can cause food-borne illness.
8. T F Most food-borne illness microbes thrive on temperatures between 40° F and 140° F (4° C and 60° C).
9. T F Symptoms of food-borne illness resemble flu symptoms.
10. T F Victims of food-borne illness receive some immunity against future attacks.
11. T F Chickens are a common source for *Salmonella* infections.
12. T F Botulism is the deadliest form of food-borne illness, and the bacteria that cause it are present in soil.
13. T F *Clostridium botulinum,* the bacteria that cause botulism, grows only in the absence of air.
14. T F Eating raw fish can cause serious health problems.
15. T F Alcoholic beverages are free of toxic compounds.

Food-Borne Illness

food-borne illness Sickness caused by ingestion of foods containing toxic substances produced by micrograms.

At the turn of the century, conditions in Chicago's meat-packing industry were sickening. Moldy, spoiled meat was commonly doused with borax to cover up the smell and glycerine was added to make it look fresh. Upton Sinclair outraged the American public with his first-hand account of these deplorable conditions in *The Jungle,* published in 1906. Then, later that year, increasing public pressure forced the passage of the first Food and Drug Act. Federal inspection began to safeguard the public from worm-infested and diseased meat. Food preparation standards also generally improved. Indeed, we have come a long way.

Still, today about one third to one half of all diarrhea cases in the United States—upward of 13 million per year—are due to food-borne microorganisms. Estimates of the yearly number of diarrhea cases caused by food-borne illness vary from about 1 of every 10 persons to 1 of every 35 persons. This costs the U.S. economy from one to ten billion dollars annually. Either way, the presence of microbes in food poses a considerable health risk.

Food contamination presents a unique risk to the elderly, whose poor eyesight and reduced senses of smell and taste make it harder for them to spot spoiled food or dirty utensils. Their reduced appetite can lead in turn to weakened immune system. The elderly face further risks because their stomachs may be low in acid, which destroys harmful bacteria, and because of poor blood circulation, which can prevent antibodies from reaching sites of infection.

Food-borne illness is not always a brief—although distressing—episode of diarrhea. Some individuals, especially children, the elderly, people with alcoholism, and people with underlying health problems, such as cancer and AIDS, can suffer greatly from illnesses caused by certain food-borne microorganisms.[6] Some bouts of food-borne illness are lengthy and lead to rheumatic diseases, food allergies, seizures and other nervous disorders, or other ills.

It is not always possible to tell from taste, smell, or sight that eating a particular food poses a risk for food-borne illness. The main exception to this rule is the uncommon *Bacillus subtilis,* which causes "off flavors" in pastry items. So your last case of the "flu" actually may have been due to a food-borne cause. The symptoms of both flu and food-borne illness are often the same: diarrhea, vomiting, fever, and weakness.

WHY IS FOOD-BORNE ILLNESS SO COMMON?

The risk of having food-borne illness is rising, partly because of efforts by the food industry to increase the shelf life of products. Longer shelf life allows foods to remain at room temperatures long enough for bacteria to multiply sufficiently to cause illness. Some bacteria—for example *Listeria* and *Yersinia*—can grow even at refrigeration temperatures.[23] Partially cooked—and some fully cooked—products pose a special risk because refrigerated storage may only slow, but not prevent, bacterial growth. This is an area of great concern to FDA.

Another factor increasing the risk of food-borne illness arises from changes in the sites of food preparation. During the past decade, the supermarket has become a major food processor offering a variety of prepared foods from the delicatessens, salad bars, fish counters, and bakeries. These foods are usually prepared in central kitchens and shipped to individual stores, often across state lines. Some supermarkets have their own in-store food preparation facilities. Whether the food is prepared in a central location or prepared in-house, if the food handlers have little or no training in safe food preparation, product contamination can occur. Patrons of supermarkets then are subject to food-borne illnesses.

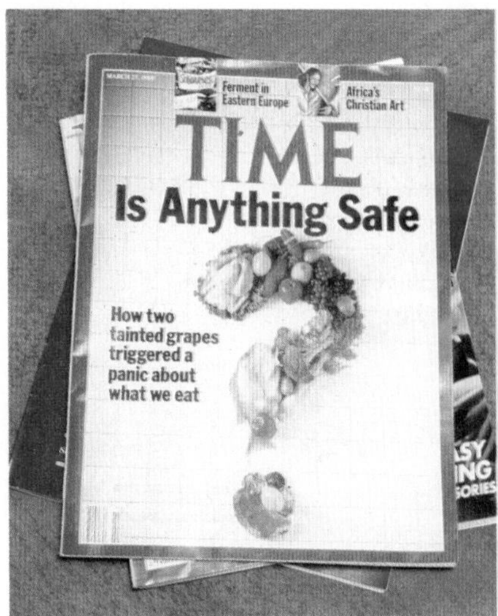

Food safety should be an issue that all of us pay attention to.

In 1985, a malfunction in dairy plant equipment lead to 16,284 confirmed cases of *Salmonella* infections (with at least two deaths) scattered throughout several midwestern states from the consumption of contaminated low-fat milk. In 1987, lettuce shredded in a Texas plant and then placed in large plastic bags was the cause of the largest *Shigella* bacteria outbreak ever reported in the United States. At least 347 people were reported ill. The nutrients released when the lettuce was shredded, coupled with the moist environment provided by the plastic bags, allowed growth and reproduction of the organism. These incidents show in general how one production site can influence the health of a great number of people.

Still another cause of increased food-borne illness in our society is greater consumption of ready-to-eat foods imported from foreign countries. In the past, food imports consisted of mostly raw products processed here under strict sanitation standards. Now, however, imports of processed foods, some of which are contaminated, are on the rise. Two recent examples are cheese from France and seafood from Asia.[15] Note that most imported seafood undergoes no inspection before distribution in the United States.

Finally, reported cases of food-borne disease have increased because of our greater awareness of food as a vehicle for microorganisms, not only those that grow in food but also those merely transmitted by food. Every decade, new diseases are discovered that have their origins in food-borne illness. It was not until 1982 that health officials began to suspect that soft cheeses were the vehicles for the spread of *Listeria monocytogenes*.[23] The list of microorganisms suspected of causing food-borne illness just continues to grow.

FOOD PRESERVATION—PAST, PRESENT, AND FUTURE

For centuries, salt, sugar, smoke, fermentation, and drying have been used to preserve food. Ancient Romans used sulfites to disinfect wine containers and preserve wine. In the age of exploration, European adventurers traveling to the New World preserved their meat by salting it.

Many preservation methods work on the principle of reducing the amount of **free water** in food. Salts and sugar reduce free water by **binding** it, and drying drives off free water. A measure of free water in a food is known as its **water activity.** Most bacteria need a water activity greater than 0.9 to grow. Yeasts can grow at water activity above 0.8, and molds grow at water activity above 0.6. The water activities of typical foods are listed in the margin on p. 592. Using this list, you can now predict why bacteria are a problem in eggs and meat, but not in jam or honey. You can also see that, unless properly treated and stored, dried fruits can still support the growth of molds.

free water The water not bound to the components in the food. This is available for microbial use.

bound water Water that is attached to organic substances. This is not available for microbial use.

water activity A measure of the amount of free water in a food. Most bacteria need a water activity greater than 0.9 to grow, while molds can grow in water activity as low as 0.6.

Foods	Water activity
fruits and vegetables	0.97
eggs	0.96
meats	0.96
cheese, bread	0.96
jam	0.85
honey	0.75
dried fruit	0.70

Some foods with high water activity would be greatly altered by decreasing their free-water content. In these cases, selected bacteria are used to ferment (pickle) or "spoil" the food. Pickles, sauerkraut, yogurt, and wine are all examples of this type of processing. The fermenting bacteria make acids and alcohol, which minimize the growth of other microbes. The acid produced is helpful in preventing the growth of *Clostridium botulinum,* a potential problem in canned foods especially.

Today, we can add **pasteurization,** sterilization, refrigeration, freezing, **irradiation,** canning, and chemical preservatives to the list of food-preservation techniques.[19] Another method for food preservation—**aseptic packaging**—simultaneously sterilizes the product and the package separately, filling the package without recontaminating the product, and sealing so that microorganisms cannot enter. Liquid foods, such as fruit juices, are especially easy to process in this manner. With aseptic packaging, boxes of sterile milk and juices can remain untainted on supermarket shelves, free of microbial growth, for many years. This method of food preservation has the advantage of producing a product at a lower price, with lighter weight and excellent flavor qualities.

pasteurization The process of heating food products to kill pathogenic microorganisms. One method heats milk at 161° F for 20 seconds at least.

irradiation A process whereby radiation energy is applied to foods, creating compounds (free radicals) within the food that destroy cell membranes, break down DNA, link proteins together, limit enzyme activity, and alter a variety of other proteins and cell functions that can lead to food spoilage.

FOOD-BORNE ILLNESS

Current microbiological research has clearly demonstrated that specific toxins produced by bacteria and other microbes cause food-borne illness. These organisms do so in two ways: (1) directly, by invading the intestinal wall and releasing **endotoxin,** as do *Salmonella* organisms or (2) indirectly, by producing an **exotoxin,** as does the *Staphylococcus* bacterium. Many different types of microorganisms cause food-borne illness, especially bacteria such as *Bacillus, Campylobacter, Clostridium, Escherichia, Listeria, Vibrio, Yersinia, Salmonella,* and *Staphylococcus.*[20]

Because each teaspoon of soil contains about two billion bacteria, we are constantly at risk for food-borne illness. Luckily, only a small number of all bacteria actually pose a threat. Determining which microbe has caused food-borne illness depends on identifying the clinical features of the poisoning, the incubation period for the symptoms to appear, and the food source (Table 19-1).

GENERAL RULES FOR PREVENTING FOOD-BORNE ILLNESS

Following a few important rules greatly minimizes the risk for food-borne illness:[11]

- Thoroughly wash hands with hot, soapy water before handling food. It is especially important also to wash hands after handling raw meat, fish, poultry, or eggs.
- When grocery shopping, select frozen foods and perishable foods, such as meat, poultry, or fish, last. Always have these products put in separate plastic bags so that drippings don't contaminate other foods in the shopping cart. Then don't let groceries sit in a warm car; this allows bacteria to grow. Get the perishable foods home and promptly refrigerate or freeze.
- Don't buy or use food from flawed containers that leak, bulge, or are severely dented, nor buy or use food from jars that are cracked or have loose or bulging lids. Do not taste or use food that has a foul odor or any food that spurts liquid when the can is opened. The deadly *Clostridium botulinum* toxin is probably present.
- Make sure counters, cutting boards, dishes, and other equipment are thoroughly cleaned and rinsed before being used. Be especially careful to use hot, soapy water to wash countertops, cutting boards, utensils, and other pieces of equipment that have come in contact with raw meat, fish, poultry, and eggs as soon as possible to rid *Salmonella* bacteria that may be present.
- When thawing foods, do so in the refrigerator for 1 to 3 days, under cold running water or in a microwave oven. Never let frozen foods stay out all day or night, thawing on the counter.
- Carefully wash fresh fruit and vegetables under running water to remove dirt.

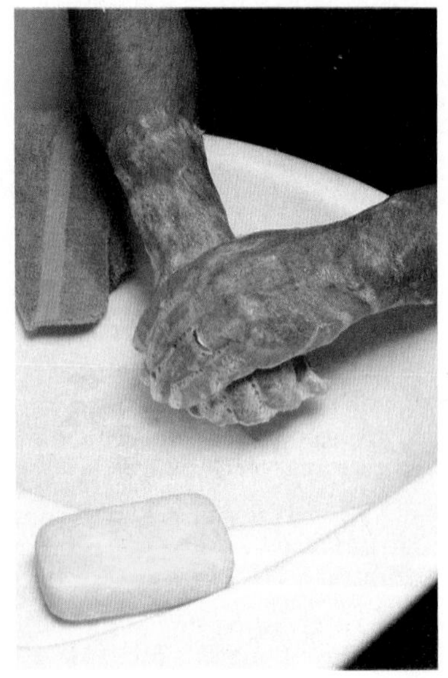

Washing hands should be a first step in preparing food.

- If possible, cut foods to be eaten raw on a clean, plastic cutting board reserved for that purpose. Then clean this cutting board using hot, soapy water. If the same board must be used for both meat and other foods, cut the raw items before cutting any potentially contaminated items, such as meat.
- Cook foods thoroughly, especially beef, fish, and pork (160° F, 71° C), poultry (180° F, 82° C), and eggs (until the yolk and white are hard). A good general precaution is to eat no raw animal products (Figure 19-1).[28] Most chickens are contaminated by *Salmonella;* this is killed by thorough cooking (white flesh, not pink). Many people are poisoned each year by eating raw seafood. It can contain *Vibrio,* which are linked to severe food-borne illness. Undercooked pork can allow infection by the parasite that causes trichinosis. The USDA will answer questions on safe use of animal products (phone: 1-800-535-4555, 10 AM to 4 PM weekdays Eastern time).
- Once a food is cooked, cool it rapidly (to 40° F, 4° C, within 2 hours) if it is not to be eaten immediately. Do this by separating the foods into as many pans as needed to provide a large surface area. Be careful not to recontaminate cooked food by contact with raw meat or juices via hands, cutting boards, dirty utensils, or in other ways.
- Reheat leftovers to 165° F, 74° C; reheat gravy to a rolling boil to kill potential *Clostridium perfringens* bacteria present. Stopping at a good eating temperature is not good enough to kill sufficient bacteria.

Keep hot foods hot and cold foods cold. Avoid time and temperature abuses. Hold food below 40° F (4° C) or above 140° F (60° C) (Figure 19-2). Food-borne illness microbes thrive in more moderate temperatures (60° to 110° F, 16° to 40° C). Some microbes can even grow in the refrigerator, as we pointed out. Do not leave cooked or refrigerated foods, such as meat and salads, at

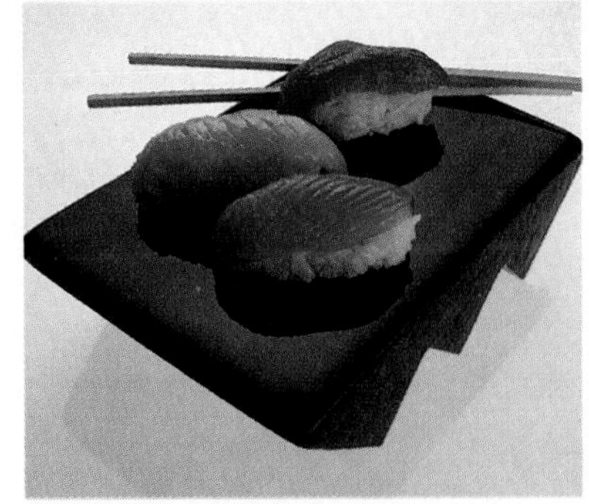

Figure 19-1 Sushi, like all raw fish or meat dishes, is a high-risk food. Animal foods should be cooked thoroughly before eating.

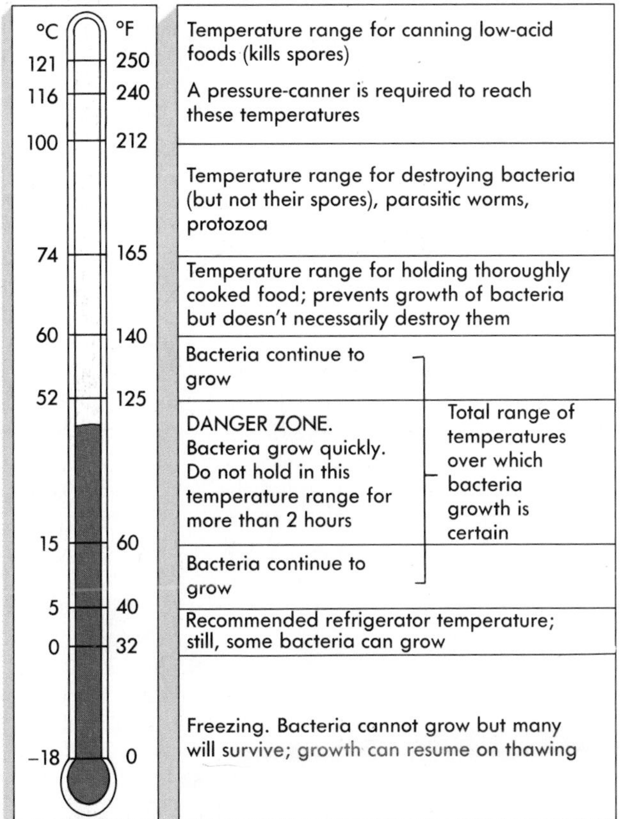

Figure 19-2 Effects of temperature on organisms that cause food-borne illness. (Adapted from *Temperature guide to food safety: food and home notes,* No. 25, Washington, D.C., June 20, 1977, USDA.)

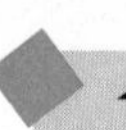

Table 19-1 Organisms that cause food-borne illness: their source, symptoms, and prevention

Organism	Source of illness	Symptoms	Prevention methods
Bacteria			
Staphylococcus aureus	Found in nasal passages and in cuts on skin. Toxin is produced when food contaminated by bacteria is left for extended time at room temperature. Meats, poultry, egg products, tuna, potato, and macaroni salads, and cream-filled pastries are good environments for these bacteria to produce toxin.	Onset: 2-6 hours after eating. Diarrhea, vomiting, nausea, and abdominal cramps. Mimics flu. Lasts 24-48 hours. Rarely fatal.	• Sanitary food-handling practices. • Prompt and proper refrigeration of foods. • Keep cuts on skin covered.
Salmonella	Found in raw meats, poultry, eggs, fish, milk, and products made with these items. Multiplies rapidly at room temperature. The bacteria themselves are toxic.	Onset: 5-72 hours after eating. Nausea, fever, headache, abdominal cramps, diarrhea, and vomiting. Can be fatal in infants, the elderly, and the sick.	• Handling food in a sanitary manner. • Thorough cooking of foods. • Prompt and proper refrigeration of foods. • Watch cross-contamination.
Clostridium perfringens	Found throughout the environment. Generally found in meat and poultry dishes. Multiply rapidly when foods are left for extended time at room temperature. The bacteria themselves are toxic.	Onset: 8-24 hours after eating (usually 12 hours). Abdominal pain and diarrhea. Symptoms last a day or less, usually mild. Can be more serious in older or debilitated people.	• Sanitary handling of foods, especially meat and meat dishes, gravies, and leftovers. • Thorough cooking and reheating of foods. • Prompt and proper refrigeration.
Clostridium botulinum	Found throughout the environment. However, bacteria produce toxin only in low-acid, anaerobic (oxygen-free) environments, such as in canned green beans, mushrooms, spinach, olives, and beef. Honey may carry spores.	Onset: 12-36 hours after eating. Neurotoxic symptoms include double vision, inability to swallow, speech difficulty, and progressive paralysis of the respiratory system. OBTAIN MEDICAL HELP IMMEDIATELY. BOTULISM CAN BE FATAL.	• Using proper methods for canning low-acid foods. • Avoiding commercial cans of low-acid foods that have leaky seals or are bent, bulging, or broken. • Toxin can be destroyed after can or jar is opened by boiling contents hard for 20 minutes, but discard if suspect toxin is present because of off-odors.
Campylobacter jejuni	Found on poultry, cattle, and sheep, and can contaminate their meat and milk. Chief food sources are raw poultry and meat and unpasteurized milk.	Onset: 3-5 days after eating, or longer. Diarrhea, abdominal cramping, fever, and sometimes bloody stools. Lasts 2-7 days.	• Thorough cooking of foods. • Handling food in a sanitary manner. • Avoiding unpasteurized milk.
Listeria monocytogenes	Found in soft cheeses and unpasteurized milk. Resists acid, heat, salt, and nitrate well.	Onset: 4-21 days. Fever, headache, vomiting, and sometimes even more severe symptoms. May be fatal.	• Thorough cooking of foods. • Handling food in a sanitary manner. • Avoiding unpasteurized milk.

Table 19-1 Organisms that cause food-borne illness: their source, symptoms, and prevention—cont'd

Organism	Source of illness	Symptoms	Prevention methods
Bacteria—cont'd			
Yersinia enterocolitica	Found throughout nature; carried in food and water. They multiply rapidly at both room and refrigerator temperatures. Generally found in raw vegetables, meats, water, and unpasteurized milk.	Onset: 2-3 days. Fever, headache, nausea, diarrhea, and general malaise. Mimics flu and appendicitis. May cause gastroenteritis in children.	• Thorough cooking. • Sanitizing cutting instruments and cutting boards before preparing foods that are eaten raw. • Avoidance of unpasteurized milk and unchlorinated water.
Viruses			
Hepatitis A virus	Found in shellfish harvested from contaminated areas and foods that are handled a lot during preparation and then eaten raw.	Onset: 30 days. Jaundice, fatigue. May cause liver damage and death.	• Sanitary handling of foods. • Use of pure drinking water. • Adequate sewage disposal. • Adequate cooking of foods.
Norwalk, Human Rotavirus	Found in the human intestinal tract and expelled in feces. Contamination occurs: 1) when sewage is used to enrich garden/farm soil 2) by direct hand-to-food contact during the preparation of meals, and 3) when shellfish-growing waters are contaminated by sewage.	Onset: 1-3 days. Severe diarrhea, nausea and vomiting. Respiratory symptoms. Usually lasts 4-5 days, but may last for weeks.	• Sanitary handling of foods. • Use of pure drinking water. • Adequate sewage disposal. • Adequate cooking of foods.
Parasites			
Trichinella spiralis	Found in pork and wild game.	Onset: weeks-months. Muscle weakness, fluid retention in face, fever, flulike symptoms.	• Thoroughly cook pork and wild game.
Anisakis	Found in raw fish.	Onset: 12 hours. Stomach infection, severe stomach pain.	• Thoroughly cook fish.
Giardia lamblia	Found most frequently associated with consumption of contaminated water. May be transmitted by uncooked foods that become contaminated while growing or after cooking by infected food handlers. Cool, moist conditions favor organism's survival.	Onset: 1-3 days. Sudden onset of explosive watery stools, abdominal cramps, anorexia, nausea, and vomiting. Lasts usually 1-2 weeks. Especially infects hikers, children, travelers, and institutionalized patients.	• Boil drinking water when camping or water supply is suspected of being contaminated.
Tape worms	Found in raw beef, pork, and fish.	May cause abdominal discomfort, diarrhea.	• Thoroughly cooking of all animal products.
Mycotoxins			
A group of toxic compounds produced by molds, such as aflatoxin B-1 and ergot.	Found in foods that are relatively high in moisture. Chief food sources: beans and grains that have been stored in a moist place.	May cause liver and/or kidney disease.	• Checking foods for visible mold and discarding those that are contaminated. • Proper storage of susceptible foods.

The microwave has one food safety disadvantage. It sometimes leaves cold spots in food. Bacteria can survive in these spots. To avoid risks:
- **Stir and rotate your food for even cooking.**
- **Observe the standing time called for in a recipe or package directions. During the standing time, food finishes cooking.**
- **Use the oven temperature probe or a meat thermometer to check that food is done. Insert it at several spots.**

USDA Food Safety "Musts"
- **Get perishable foods into the refrigerator as quickly as possible after buying them.**
- **Wash raw vegetables thoroughly.**
- **Keep your kitchen or food preparation areas clean.**
- **Wash your hands before preparing food.**
- **Keep hot foods hot and cold foods cold after they are prepared.**

room temperature for more than 2 hours because that provides microbes an opportunity to grow. Store dry food at 60° F to 70° F (16° C to 21° C).
- Avoid coughing or sneezing over foods, even when you are healthy. Cover cuts on hands with a sterile bandage. This helps stop *Staphylococcus aureus* from entering food.
- Make sure the refrigerator stays below 40° F (4° C). Generally keep it as cold as possible without freezing the milk or lettuce.
- Cook stuffing separately from poultry (or wash poultry thoroughly, stuff immediately before cooking, and then transfer the stuffing to a clean bowl immediately after cooking). Make sure the stuffing obtains a temperature of 165° F (74° C). Again, *Salmonella* is the major concern with poultry.
- Consume only pasteurized milk and cheese. This is especially important for pregnant women because very toxic bacteria and viruses that can harm the fetus thrive in unpasteurized milk.[23]
- Completely remove moldy portions of food or don't eat the food. When in doubt, throw the food out. Mold growth is prevented by properly storing foods at cold temperatures and using the foods within a reasonable length of time. When in doubt, throw it out.

Microbes that cause food-borne illness commonly enter food through cross-contamination and grow because they are allowed to thrive in temperatures favorable to them. A recent example was at a large gathering with turkey franks contaminated with *Listeria monocytogenes*. When the franks were later added to the salad, it too became contaminated, causing food-borne illness. Overall, it is important to practice sanitary food-handling procedures when preparing any food.

As one final precaution, watch for safe food-handling techniques when you eat out. Check that foods in a salad bar are iced; custard and pudding pies are chilled; hot foods served on a hot food bar are hot; and vending machines are checked regularly, especially those with sandwiches and milk. Foods stored and served in dormitory cafeterias should be properly handled.

TREATMENT FOR FOOD-BORNE ILLNESS

To offset the effects of diarrhea, drink a lot of fluids.[10] To prevent further contamination, thoroughly wash hands before food handling or eating until the diarrhea disappears. Bedrest speeds recovery. A fever of 102° F (39° C) or greater, blood in the stool, and dehydration from frequent vomiting or diarrhea (a sign of dehydration is dizziness when standing) deserves a physician's evaluation, especially if symptoms persist for more than 2 or 3 days. In cases of suspected botulism poisoning, consult a physician immediately because use of an antitoxin may speed recovery.

USDA specifies three particular situations in which it is vital for consumers to report incidents of food-borne illness to the local health department:
- if the food in question was eaten at a large gathering.
- if the item came from a restaurant, delicatessen, sidewalk vendor, or a kitchen that serves large numbers of people.
- if the suspect food was a commercial product, such as some kind of canned goods or frozen, packaged item.

CONCEPT CHECK

The presence of bacteria and the toxins they produce pose the greatest risk for food-borne illness. In the past, the addition to foods of sugar, salt, and smoke, as well as drying, were used to prevent the growth of microorganisms. Today, we know that cleanliness, keeping hot foods hot and cold foods cold, and cooking foods thoroughly offer additional protection from food-borne illness. Treat all raw animal products, any cooked food, and raw bean sprouts as potential sources of food-borne illness. Symptoms of an attack are similar to those of flu: diarrhea, vomiting, abdominal bloating, and headache. Treatment generally requires only bedrest and extra fluids.

A Closer Look at Microbes That Cause Food-Borne Illness

We noted that finding a food-poisoning agent requires some detective skills. Determining the agent depends on knowing the food source, the incubation time for symptoms, the types of symptoms, and the duration of illness associated with an outbreak. Again, the undesirable results can be either due to a exotoxin produced by the microorganism—called an intoxication—or the presence of the microorganism itself and its endotoxin—called an infection. Let's begin by looking at the characteristics of the major "problem" microbes individually. One general rule: When you exhaust the possibilities, the cause of the illness is probably a virus.

STAPHYLOCOCCUS AUREUS

The organism *S. aureus* causes 20% to 40% of cases of food-borne illness each year. While growing in food, this microbe produces exotoxin that, once ingested, cause nausea, vomiting, diarrhea, headaches, and abdominal cramps. Thus it is classified as bacterial intoxication. Symptoms usually develop within 2 to 6 hours of eating the contaminated food. The person rarely dies, but develops no immunity against future attacks. Bed rest and fluids are generally the only treatment, and recovery takes place usually within 2 to 3 days.[17]

S. aureus bacteria live mainly in the nasal passages and in sores on the skin. These microbes enter food when food handlers sneeze and cough over food or expose food to open skin sores. Once in food it begins to grow. *S. aureus* prefers a warm room temperature near 100° F (38° C). It multiplies rapidly and can release enough exotoxin to cause illness in about 4 hours. This toxin is heat stable, so cooking the food at this point will only kill the bacteria but not inactivate the toxin. The contaminated food will neither appear or taste unusual, nor will any odor be detected.

Common foods associated with intoxications from *S. aureus* are custard, ham, egg salad, cheese, seafood, cream-filled pastries, and milk. Whipped cream standing at room temperature for hours is a typical source. Keeping these and other foods above 140° F (60° C) or below 40° F (4° C) prevents the bacterium's growth, thus preventing production of its toxin. Never leave susceptible foods inside the temperature range of 40° F to 140° F for more than 2 hours. To further prevent this type of food-borne illness, hand cleanliness and sanitation are important, as are directing coughs and sneezes away from food and covering skin cuts with sterile bandages when in contact with food. Note that food-borne infections caused by this microbe are most common during the summer months and at holiday time: November, December, January.

SALMONELLA

There are over 2000 types of *Salmonella* found in the animal kingdom. They have been isolated from poultry, reptiles, livestock, rodents, birds, and humans. Most infections can be traced to contaminated water or food, or the direct fecal-oral route among children. *Salmonella* are found in animal and human feces and enter food via contaminated water, cutting boards, meat products, cracked eggs, and actual bits of feces in food.[17]

Illness in this case is due to the presence of the endotoxin in the bacteria themselves. Symptoms of a *Salmonella* infection are the same as those of *Staphylococcus* intoxications, but they take 6 to 48 hours to develop. Again, bed rest and fluids are the only treatment, and recovery usually occurs within 2 to 3 days. Fatalities are rare. The disease occurs when the microorganism has an opportunity to multiply to a high density in a food, such as eggs, chicken, meat (and meat products), and custard made with contaminated eggs. About 60% of raw chickens are contaminated. Undercooked foods pose a special risk, but thorough cooking kills *Salmonella* bacteria.

To be safe, eggs should be simmered 7 minutes, poached 5 minutes, or fried 3 minutes on each side until the yolk is not runny and the white is firm.[27] No raw eggs should be used in salads or sauces. Hollandaise sauce, often warmed at low

FDA warns us not to consume homemade ice cream, eggnog, and mayonnaise because of the risk of *Salmonella* food poisoning. Commercial forms of these products are safe because they have been pasteurized. This process kills *Salmonella* bacteria. In addition, commercial mayonnaise has enough acid to prevent bacterial growth.

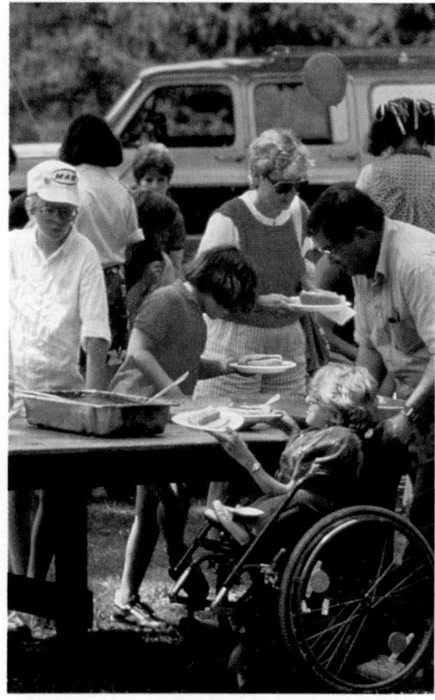

Figure 19-3 A likely target for food-borne illness. Keeping hot foods "hot" and cold foods "cold" is one key to minimize the risk of food-borne illness at picnics. The warm days of summer make this an especially key goal.

heat, is a significant threat. Recent research indicates that not only are cracked eggs at risk for *Salmonella* bacteria infections but also strains of the bacteria may exist inside an intact egg, especially if it has been left at room temperature for a few hours.

Most outbreaks of *Salmonella* infections can be traced to mistakes in food handling in either food establishments, homes, or outdoor gatherings (Figure 19-3). *Salmonella* bacteria need about 8 hours to produce quantities sufficient to cause illness. Observing the temperature precautions for *Staphylococcus* organisms also prevents *Salmonella* bacteria growth.

Salmonella poses a great risk for cross-contamination of foods. In November 1986, five residents of a Windsor, Conn, nursing home died, and 25 others became ill from *Salmonella.* Health officials suspect that a blender used to puree food had previously been used to mix raw eggs and had not been properly cleaned. This reminds us to keep hands and utensils clean when preparing foods; scrub the cutting board with a chlorinated cleanser after contact with raw meat or poultry, and store foods in temperatures either hot or cold enough to prevent bacterial growth. Wooden cutting boards pose a special risk because they are difficult to sanitize. Plastic cutting boards are recommended. Do not allow susceptible foods to stand for more than 2 hours at room temperature and marinate meats in the refrigerator. While acid in a marinade slows bacterial growth, it does not stop it. Finally, thaw foods in the refrigerator, in a microwave oven, or under a stream of cold water—not on the kitchen counter.

CLOSTRIDIUM PERFRINGENS

Clostridia are widely dispersed in soil and water (particularly those contaminated with feces) and in the normal microbial flora in the GI tracts of animals, including humans. They cause a variety of diseases, including food-borne illness. Their ability to survive adverse environmental conditions is due to their ability to form spores.

Clostridium perfringens experiences a rapid rate of growth under favorable conditions. During this time the exotoxin is produced that causes the illness. Clostridium perfringens is called the "cafeteria germ" because most food-borne outbreaks by this organism are associated with the foodservice industry, or with events where large quantities of food are prepared and served. Symptoms of the illness resemble those caused by *Salmonella:* abdominal cramps and watery diarrhea, but without fever or vomiting. Symptoms are seen within 8 to 24 hours after consuming a food product contaminated with large number of the bacteria. Again, bed rest and fluids are the only treatment, and recovery occurs usually within a few days.[17]

C. perfringens is an anaerobic bacterium. The spores it produces are quite resistant to heat. Foods stored in deep serving dishes are especially fertile media for bacterial growth because the centers are isolated from air and stay warm. At temperatures between 70° F and 120° F (21° C to 49° C) spore forms germinate and become bacteria, multiplying quickly to disease-causing levels.

C. perfringens organisms are often found in cooked beef, turkey, gravy, dressing, stews, and casseroles. The best insurance against promoting their growth is to maintain proper holding temperatures and to divide large "leftover" portions into smaller ones. The latter treatment exposes more food to air, reducing the anaerobic conditions. Be especially careful to cook meats completely and cool them rapidly in small containers. Thoroughly reheat leftover meat to 165° F (74° C) before serving. Always bring leftover gravy to a rolling boil. Store cold cuts and sliced meats below 40° F (4° C) and serve them cold.

CLOSTRIDIUM BOTULINUM

Clostridium botulinum bacteria can cause fatal food-borne illness via production of a potent nerve toxin. This anaerobic microbe is present in the soil, and is therefore probably present as a bacterium or spore in all foods. The bacteria release the deadly exotoxin as they grow in food.[17] The toxin binds to nerve endings and prevents release of a neurotransmitter. With transmission of certain nerve impulses blocked, weakness and paralysis result. The death rate, which depends on the amount of toxin consumed, is about 10%, given that modern medical therapies are employed.

Symptoms of botulism appear 1 to 2 days of consuming contaminated foods. These include vomiting, abdominal pain, double vision, and dizziness. Death occurs from respiratory failure as nerve function is profoundly diminished. Diarrhea does not occur. If the person survives, recovery can take months to years. Normally, bed rest and respiratory care are the main therapies. With quick diagnosis, treatment with an antiserum is possible. Although botulism receives much public attention, few cases are reported each year in the United States.

Since *C. botulinum* grows only in the absence of air, it thrives primarily in canned foods, especially improperly home-canned low-acid foods, such as string beans, corn, mushrooms, beets, and asparagus. Recently, other foods with "anaerobic centers," such as potato salad, sauteed onions, stew, and chopped garlic have caused botulism. Cured meats also pose a risk for botulism; however, the nitrates and vitamin C used to preserve the meats are potent inhibitors of its growth. Certain food preservation practices of Alaska natives, especially with dried fish, beaver and whale meat, greatly increase their risk for botulism.

Canned foods pose the main threat for botulism because as the canning process kills all bacteria present and the heat used drives out all oxygen, spores of *C. botulinum* remain intact in the food if insufficient heat is used. When the can or jar cools, the spores germinate into bacteria and the bacteria produce toxin.

Following canning directions explicitly is essential when food is canned at home. Boiling home-canned foods for 10 to 20 minutes before serving is an excellent idea because that destroys any toxin present. In the first few minutes of boiling, smell the food. Heat often brings out the tell-tale sign of botulism odors. If no odor is detected, lower the heat and continue boiling the food for 10 minutes for high-acid foods and 20 minutes for low-acid foods, such as meat and poultry products, peas, beans, and corn.

Commercially canned foods may also harbor botulism. Always check cans carefully. Look for rust on the seams, holes, and swollen sides or tops. Make sure the can sucks in air when opened and the liquid inside is clear, not milky, and does not smell bad. If there are any signs of spoilage, return the can to the store or to the nearest public health department. Whatever you do, DON'T TASTE THE FOOD. ONE STRING BEAN CAN CONTAIN ENOUGH TOXIN TO KILL YOU.

Recently, researchers have noted that botulism poisoning may develop in vivo (inside the living body). Infants between 2 and 9 months of age are at the highest risk, with about 250 cases reported each year. Fortunately, the death rate is low, 1% to 2%. People with poor stomach acid production also are at risk. Bacteria spores germinate in the stomach and produce the exotoxin. For this reason, honey should not be given to young infants because it can contain the spores of this bacteria.

CAMPYLOBACTER JEJUNI

The most common form of bacterial GI tract infections is caused by *Campylobacter jejuni,*[10] leading to about 2 million cases per year in the United States. The disease promotes the destruction of the mucosal surfaces of the jejunum and also the ileum and the colon. *Campylobacter* was established as a human pathogen in 1971. Probably an enormous number of cases of food-borne illness caused by these organisms are unreported because they are difficult to detect in foods. A recent USDA study found that 30% of chickens carried *Campylobacter* organisms.

Nearly all outbreaks of *Campylobacter* illness result in acute intestinal pain with fever, muscle pain, headache, and diarrhea.[20] During the peak of the disease, ten or more bowel movements per day are common, and stools are bloody. Treatment employs antibiotic medications. Cases are associated with raw or inadequately cooked animal foods, including raw milk. Because this organism grows slowly, the onset of symptoms is delayed, occurring 2 to 5 days after intake of contaminated food, although it may take weeks. Most people recover in less than 1 week, and death is

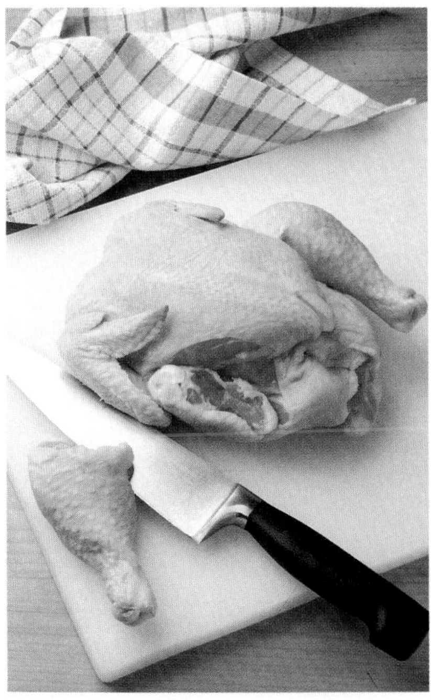

Wooden cutting boards are difficult to sanitize—plastic is preferable.

rare. Recently, the nerve disorder Guillain-Barre syndrome has been linked to infections with *C. jejuni.* In addition, one form of this microbe, *Campylobacter pylori* (also called *Heliobactor pylori*), may be an important cause of stomach ulcers.

Luckily, *Campylobacter* organisms are very sensitive to heat. This trait probably saves us from numerous attacks. Complete cooking of food and careful storage of leftovers at cold temperatures are important ways to prevent its growth.

LISTERIA MONOCYTOGENES

Listeria monocytogenes is a very tough microbe.[23] It resists heat, salt, nitrate, and acidity much better than many other microorganisms. It survives and even grows below refrigeration temperatures of 40° F (4° C). The first documented report of food-borne illness caused by *Listeria* organisms in North America occurred in 1981 in Canada. It was linked to commercially prepared coleslaw. Later, incidents that involved 47 deaths were associated with soft "Mexican style" cheeses. Since pasteurization destroys *Listeria* organisms, reports of milk and cheese products contaminated by these organisms suggest that contamination occurred following pasteurization, probably from addition of raw milk. Although the incidence of listeriosis in the United States is unknown, it appears to be relatively rare, with about 1600 to 1800 cases occurring each year, and about 400 deaths.

Listeria bacteria infections cause mild flulike symptoms, such as fever, headache, and vomiting, about 7 to 30 days after exposure. However, newborn infants, pregnant women, and people with depressed immune function may suffer severe symptoms, including meningitis, spontaneous abortion, and serious blood infections.[17] In high-risk people, 25% of infections may be fatal. Because unpasteurized milk, soft cheeses, and cabbage can be sources of *Listeria,* it is especially important that pregnant women and other people at high risk avoid these products. Recently, raw hot dogs and undercooked chicken have been suspected to be a major source of *Listeria* infections. And as we noted even vegetables like lettuce (and cabbage) can carry these organisms, and once cut, support its growth.

We advise consuming only pasteurized milk products and cooking meat, poultry, and seafood thoroughly to kill this organism. USDA recommends cooking meat to an internal temperature of 160° F (71° C) at the thickest part, and poultry to 180° F (82° C). Avoid eating raw meats; even their juices can contaminate cooked foods. Although *Listeria* organisms can grow at low temperatures, it is still important to keep food refrigerated to slow its growth. Finally, wash fresh produce thoroughly to remove possible contamination.

YERSINIA ENTEROCOLITICA

Yersinia enterocolitica was recognized as a human pathogen in 1939. Food-borne illnesses have been noted since 1976.[20] Foods implicated include water, chocolate milk, reconstituted dry milk, wild and domestic animals, and tofu. Usually the microbe enters the food after pasteurization. Symptoms of an infection occur 24 to 36 hours after eating the contaminated foods and include diarrhea, fever, headache, and severe abdominal pain that mimics appendicitis. (There are cases where unnecessary appendectomies have been performed after *Yersinia* infections.) The disease can last as long as 2 weeks, and even a year or longer in some cases. The disease may also trigger arthritis, inflammation of heart tissue, and blood infections.

Yersinia organisms grow at cold temperatures, so refrigerated storage does not control its growth in food. Therefore sterilization methods, such as sufficient cooking or pasteurization, must occur to destroy this microbe. It is fortunate that the strains of *Yersinia* bacteria primarily associated with human illness do not commonly occur in foods at this time.

OTHER FOOD-BORNE BACTERIA THAT POSE A RISK

Escherichia coli is commonly found in the intestinal tract of humans and other animals. Certain strains are now recognized as food-borne illness microbes.[10] Symptoms include severe abdominal cramps, bloody diarrhea, and kidney failure. Thoroughly cooking meat and avoiding recontamination of meat should protect against illness. Food-borne illness caused by the bacteria *Shigella* is a common childhood disease for those youngsters in day-care centers, nurseries, and custodial institutions. The infection is transmitted by the fecal-oral route, primarily by way of the hands, and to a lesser extent by food and water. Symptoms include abdominal cramps, diarrhea, fever, and bloody stools. There are carriers of *Shigella* who show no effect but represent a potential threat to all who are in their care. Recently, 407 adults who ate at one restaurant were afflicted with Shigella. Handwashing and sanitary food production offer the best protection.

Infections from *Vibrio vulnificus,* a newly identified bacterium, have been linked to eating raw seafood, especially raw oysters.[13] It causes a serious infection that can be fatal in about 50% of cases. Prompt treatment is needed. Eating raw shellfish poses a high risk, as does eating any raw or lightly (partially) cooked seafood. Symptoms include diarrhea, fever, weakness, blood infections, and other serious health problems.

Vibrio cholerae causes a severe form of GI tract infection.[10] Sources of *V. cholerae* are human carriers and infected shellfish. The disease is spread by contaminated water and food. Cholera is usually seen in countries with poor sanitation. Handwashing after defacating is vital to reduce risk. The disease occurs 2 to 3 days after ingesting the contaminated food or water. Symptoms include vomiting and severe watery diarrhea, which can lead to dehydration and cardiovascular collapse. The death rate can be as high as 60%. Treatment consists of replacement of fluids and electrolytes.

VIRUSES

The hepatitis A virus can be transmitted in food, although this route accounts for only a small percentage of the total number of hepatitis A infections. This food-borne agent most often thrives because of unsanitary food handling in restaurants. People have also contracted hepatitis from eating raw or undercooked shellfish—clams, oysters, muscles—harvested from waters contaminated with raw or improperly treated sewage.[17] Symptoms include intestinal problems, weakness, fatigue, jaundice, and sometimes even development of serious liver disease requiring hospitalization. Because symptoms of hepatitis A infection do not usually occur until about 1 to 2 months after eating contaminated food, the source is difficult to identify.

Raw clams and oysters are especially risky to eat because they are filter feeders, a process that concentrates viruses and toxins present in the water as it is filtered for food. It is important to buy oysters and clams only from the most reliable sources. By law, shellfish offered for sale must come from licensed beds, but often they do not. So be careful when you either purchase these foods or harvest them yourself.[16] Check with the local health department if you question the safety of waters in an area. Proper handwashing by foodservice personnel is especially important in restaurants, day-care centers, hospitals, and other institutions to lessen hepatitis outbreaks. Chlorine treatment of drinking water is a reliable means of destroying the virus.

Norwalk viral infections usually cause mild illness with nausea, vomiting, diarrhea, weakness, abdominal pain, loss of appetite, headache, and fever. The virus is found in water and foods, and shellfish and salads are most often implicated. Norwalk viruses are probably responsible for about 30% to 40% of all cases of viral intestinal flu in adults. Recently, an outbreak from contaminated ice occurred in Pennsylvania and Delaware.

Rotaviruses are another important cause of diarrhea; it is a main cause in children.[12] Symptoms appear in 1 to 7 days. Day-care centers are common sites for infections.[10] Thorough, regular handwashing is a necessary and important practice at these sites.

THE FAR SIDE By GARY LARSON

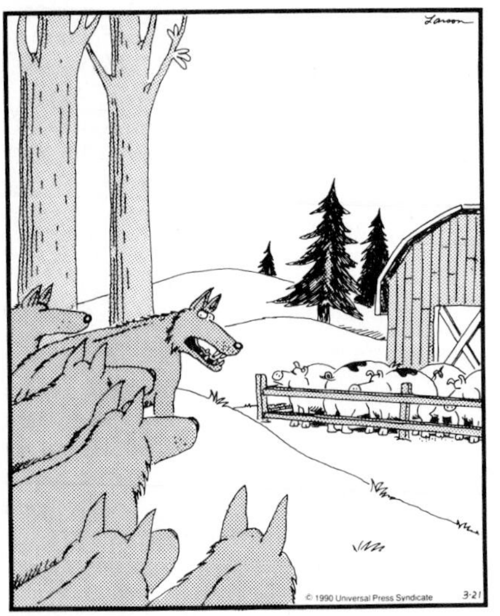

"I say we do it . . . and trichinosis be damned!"

Figure 19-4 The Far Side.

larvae An early developmental stage in the life history of some microorganisms, such as parasites.

PARASITES

Parasites that enter the body through the intestinal tract include some protozoans, flukes, nematodes, roundworms, and tapeworms. In the United States, the parasite most apt to be in the food supply is *Trichinella spiralis*. This tiny organism may be present in raw and undercooked pork and pork products, such as sausage. Trichinosis is rare today, probably because people realize that pork must be cooked thoroughly to kill the nematode worm that causes it and modern sanitary feeding practices have reduced Trichinella in hogs (Figure 19-4). About a hundred cases of trichinosis per year are reported in the United States. However, other cases may be unreported. Besides pork, bear meat and other raw meats are potential sources. The worm is seldom found in commercial meat.

This infection begins with the consumption of meat containing the **larvae.** The larvae are released during digestion in the small intestine. Within 2 days the larvae develop into adult nematodes (worms). New larvae then are produced and move into the blood via the intestinal mucosa. The blood carries the larvae to muscle fibers, where they become resident.[17]

In its early stages, trichinosis is difficult to diagnose. The symptoms in mild cases develop over weeks to months and are usually thought to be flu. If enough larvae are present, muscle weakness, fever, and fluid retention in the face may eventually result. Greater numbers of larvae usually mean more severe symptoms. Thoroughly cooking meat, especially pork, to 170° F (77° C) destroys the larvae.

Anisakis is a roundworm parasite found in larval form in raw fish. They invade the stomach or intestinal tract, causing mild or serious effects.[17] The infection is difficult to diagnose and cannot be treated. A stomach infection is characterized by sudden onset of violent pain within 12 hours of eating raw fish. The larvae may penetrate the stomach lining. Serious stomach pain can continue until the larvae are surgically removed. The fresher the fish, the less likely this disease will occur because larvae move from the fish's stomach to the tissues only after the fish is dead. Thoroughly cooking fish or freezing it for at least 72 hours are reliable methods for eliminating the threat of *Anisakis* disease. Consumption of raw or slightly cooked fish increases the risk for infection, especially from Japanese-style sushi and sashimi.

Other Risks From Fish and Shellfish

Scombroidosis results from an acute allergic reaction to eating spoiled fish. Fish typically implicated are tuna, mackerel, and mahimahi. An affected person develops facial flushing, itching, intestinal upset, and headache within 10 to 60 minutes of consumption. The illness is caused by a toxin found in the muscle of the spoiled fish. Improperly refrigerated fish pose a special problem, and cooking does not destroy the toxin. So it is important to carefully refrigerate and use fresh fish soon after purchasing, especially those mentioned above.

Paralytic shellfish poisoning occurs when toxins produced by microscopic algae, called dinoflagellates, are consumed. These toxins are associated with the phenomenon known as a red tide, which is actually an explosive growth of the dinoflagellates in water. Symptoms, such as respiratory difficulty, appear within 4 hours. It is important that shellfish are harvested in clean waters, uncontaminated by sewage, industrial waste, and high levels of toxic dinoflagellates. An outbreak in Guatemala in 1985 killed 26 people. Because fish and shellfish pose a considerable risk for contamination and so food-borne illness, consider adopting the following practices:

- No consumption of raw fish or shellfish. Sufficient cooking is most important of all when it comes to seafood safety.
- Avoid fish or shellfish with strong odors. This usually indicates spoilage.
- Eat fresh fish or shellfish the day you buy it. If frozen make sure it stays so until eaten.
- When buying a whole fish, make sure it has bright, clear, bulging eyes to ensure freshness.

FUNGI

Mycotoxins are a group of compounds produced by molds growing on food. The best known are the aflatoxins, produced by *Aspergillus flavus*.[17] Aflatoxin B-1 causes cancer in animals and so human exposure is regulated by FDA. The foods most often contaminated with aflatoxins are tree nuts, peanuts, corn, wheat, and oil seeds, such as cottonseed. FDA considers aflatoxins unavoidable contaminants on foods and therefore has set practical limits for aflatoxins in foods and animal feeds.

mycotoxins A group of toxic compounds produced by molds, such as aflatoxin B-1, found on moldy grains.

Cooking and freezing halts fungal growth but does not eliminate mycotoxins already produced. Moldy food should not be eaten, or at least not without discarding the moldy portion and much of the surrounding area. Again, when in doubt, throw the food out. Mold growth is prevented by properly storing foods at cold temperatures and using them within a reasonable length of time.

CONCEPT CHECK

To prevent food-borne intoxications from *Staphylococcus* organisms, cover cuts on hands and avoid sneezing on foods. To avoid *Salmonella* infections, separate raw meats, especially poultry products, from cooked foods. Thoroughly cook meat and poultry products to destroy any *Salmonella* bacteria present. To avoid intoxications from *Clostridium perfringens,* rapidly cool leftover foods and thoroughly reheat them. To avoid intoxications from *Clostridium botulinum,* carefully examine canned foods and don't allow cooked foods to stand for more than 2 hours at room temperature. For other causes of food-borne illness, what we already have mentioned generally applies as well. In addition, carefully handle raw animal products so that their juices do not contaminate other foods; thoroughly cook all foods, especially fish and other seafood; consume only pasteurized dairy products; and thoroughly wash your hands with soap and water after going to the bathroom.

Food Additives

Food additives are used to maintain or increase a food's nutritional value, preserve freshness, enhance flavor or appearance, or aid in processing and/or preparation.

DO WE NEED TO USE FOOD ADDITIVES?

Limiting food spoilage is the major impetus for using additives. Foods spoil in two ways. The first and potentially most serious is the spoilage already discussed, that caused by bacteria, fungi, and other microorganisms. This may lead to food-borne illness and changes in food texture and flavor. Food additives, such as potassium sorbate, are used to maintain the safety and acceptability of foods by retarding microbial growth.

The second and less serious means of food spoilage is through oxygen exposure, which causes undesirable changes in color and flavor. The rust color that appears when apple and peach slices are exposed to air is a good example of this reaction. Antioxidants, which are a group of preservatives, retard the action of oxygen on food surfaces. These preservatives are not necessarily novel chemicals—they include vitamin E, vitamin C, and a variety of sulfites.

Without the use of some food additives, it would be impossible to safely produce massive quantities of foods and distribute them nationwide or worldwide, as is now done. Despite consumer concerns about the safety of food additives, many have been extensively studied and proven safe when FDA guidelines for use are followed.

intentional food additives Additives knowingly (directly) incorporated into food products by manufacturers.

incidental food additives Additives that gain access to food products indirectly from environmental contamination of food ingredients, or during the manufacturing process.

INTENTIONAL VERSUS INCIDENTAL FOOD ADDITIVES

Food additives are classified as those that are either **intentionally** (directly) added to foods or **incidentally** (indirectly) enter foods. Both are regulated by FDA. The latter group includes substances that may be reasonably expected to become components of food through surface contact with equipment or packaging materials. This includes substances that may be formed during processing. Currently over 2800 different substances are intentionally added to our foods. As many as 10,000 other substances incidentally enter our foods.

generally recognized as safe (GRAS) A list of food additives that in 1958 were considered safe for consumption. Manufacturers were allowed to continue to use food additives, without special clearance, when needed in food products. FDA bears responsibility for proving they are not safe, and can remove unsafe products.

THE GRAS LIST

In 1958, all food additives used in the United States and considered safe were put on a **generally recognized as safe (GRAS)** list. Congress reasoned that if knowledgeable scientists regarded a substance as safe, manufacturers did not have to provide additional evidence. As is still the case, FDA was assigned responsibility for providing that a substance did not belong on the GRAS list. Since 1958, some substances on the list have been reviewed. A few, such as cyclamates, failed the review process and were removed from the list. Largely because of expense, many chemicals on the GRAS list have not been rigorously tested. These chemicals have received a low priority for testing mostly because they have long histories of use without evidence of harm and/or because their chemical structures do not suggest they are harmful.

ARE SYNTHETIC CHEMICALS ALWAYS BAD?

Nothing about a natural product makes it inherently safer than a synthetic (man-made) product. Many synthetic products are simply chemicals that also occur in nature. In addition, although humans are responsible for some toxins in foods—synthetic pesticides and industrial chemicals, for example—nature's poisons are often even more potent and prevalent. Dr. Bruce Ames, a noted cancer researcher, suggests that we ingest at least 10,000 times more (by weight) natural toxins produced by plants than we do man-made pesticide residues. This comparison doesn't make man-made chemicals any less harmful, but it does lend perspective.

Consider the familiar food additive baking powder, which is used to make batter rise for cakes, pancakes, and other "quick breads." When manufacturers list potassium acid tartrate, sodium aluminum phosphate, or monocalcium phosphate on the labels

Table 19-2 Key U.S. Food Laws

1906: **Pure Food and Drug Act**—This most importantly defined adulterated foods: those foods containing "any added poisons or other added deleterious ingredient that may render such article injurious to health."

1938: **Federal Food, Drug, and Cosmetic Act**—This provided for exemptions and safe tolerances for substances that, although not desirable in foods, were either necessary in production or unavoidable.

1958: **Food Additives Amendment (and the Color Additives Amendment of 1960)**—These made it necessary for manufacturers to demonstrate the safety of a new food additive before approval by the FDA. The 1958 act also included the Delaney clause: "no additive shall be deemed to be safe if it is found to produce cancer when ingested by man or animals, or if it is found after tests which are appropriate for the evaluation of the safety of the food additives to induce cancer in man or animals."

In contrast to food additives, colors in use before the legislation were allowed continued use only if they underwent further testing to confirm their safety. No GRAS status was given. Of the original 200 provisionally listed color additives, 90 have been listed as safe and the remainder have either been removed from use by FDA or withdrawn by industry.

NUTRITION FOCUS

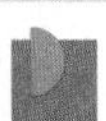

Protecting the U.S. Food Supply

A variety of federal, state, and local agencies in the United States monitors food safety. Table 19-2 lists some key food laws they enforce. Below is a list of some of the agencies involved:

- *The U.S. Department of Agriculture (USDA)*. This agency enforces standards for wholesomeness and quality of meat and poultry through its Food Safety and Inspection Service. USDA also routinely monitors animal foods for antibiotic residues.
- *Bureau of Alcohol, Tobacco, and Firearms*. This agency is responsible for enforcing laws that cover the production, distribution, and labeling of alcoholic beverages—except wine beverages that contain less than 7% alcohol (those are the responsibility of FDA).
- *Environmental Protection Agency (EPA)*. This agency must approve all pesticides before they are sold in the United States. It determines the safety of new pesticide products and sets allowable limits (tolerances) for pesticide residue in foods. For agricultural use, EPA tolerances specify residue limits for about 10,000 pesticide/food combinations involving about 300 active pesticide ingredients. A tolerance is not necessarily the maximum safe level of a pesticide in a food. The EPA sets tolerances no higher than needed for a product's intended use. These limits are then enforced by FDA. EPA also establishes water quality standards, including those for drinking water.
- *Food and Drug Administration (FDA)*. This agency is responsible for ensuring the safety and wholesomeness of most foods sold in interstate commerce (exceptions include meat and poultry products, which are primarily under USDA jurisdiction). FDA also sets standards for specific foods and enforces federal regulations for labeling, food and color additives, food sanitation, and the safety of foods based on laws passed by the U.S. Congress. The agency inspects food plants, imported food products, and mills that make feeds containing medications or nutritional supplements for animals destined for human consumption.

  FDA acts primarily when the public health is endangered or when proper medical care is being discouraged. It regulates products, not people. FDA cannot control what people say, just what is on the label and how a product is promoted. FDA gives low priority to simple economic deception by products.

  To monitor foods for contaminants, FDA routinely samples items that are of dietary importance, such as produce. Foods suspected of illegal residues receive a more intensive evaluation. An important part of FDA's safety sampling is a "market basket" study of foods that typify the American diet. Four times a year, identical purchases of 234 foods, including processed foods, are analyzed for pesticide residues, radioactive elements, toxic metals, and other undesirable substances. Of the few samples found containing illegal pesticide residues, most involve pesticides approved for use on other foods, but not on that particular food. In addition, FDA operates an Adverse Reaction Monitoring System (ARMS) to help serve as an ongoing safety check of all additives. The system monitors and investigates all complaints by individuals or their physicians that are believed to be related to specific foods; food and color additives; or vitamin and mineral supplements.

  Imported foods with illegal residues can be refused entry into the country by FDA. In the case of domestic foods, FDA can impose the sanctions of seizure, injunction, and prosecution.[24]
- *National Marine Fishery Service*. This agency is part of the Department of Commerce. It is responsible for seafood quality and other aspects of fisheries management. It has a voluntary inspection program for fish products, but no mandatory program. This is probably one reason why one fourth of all food-borne illness incidents in the United States involve eating fish and seafood, according to the Centers for Disease Control in Atlanta, Georgia. FDA does inspect seafood processing plants and spotchecks imported fish and seafood. More inspection efforts by government agencies such as these will likely take place in the future, given the significant chance for fish and seafood contamination.[15]
- *State and local government*. States inspect restaurants, retail food establishments, dairies, grain mills, and other food-related establishments within their borders. States have the primary responsibility for milk safety. FDA provides guidelines to state and local governments for regulating dairy products and restaurants.
- *Foreign governments*. Governments of at least 40 nations are now partners with the United States in ensuring food safety through agreements that cover 24 food products, including shellfish. International cooperation is expanding in terms of food inspection and regulatory standards.

The current budgets of government enforcement agencies at all levels limit the number and thoroughness of inspections. So individuals have to assume some responsibility for these protective activities themselves. We must remain alert in cases of apparent abuse, and contact the appropriate government agency to begin correction of the problem.

Today, sugar, salt, corn syrup, and citric acid still constitute 98% of all additives by weight.

of cake mixes, they are referring to baking powder by its chemical names. Baking soda could be listed by its proper name sodium bicarbonate, just as ordinary table salt could be called sodium chloride. The question should not be whether a food additive, such as salt, is a chemical, but rather whether the chemical additive is safe to use.

Vitamin E is often added to food additives to prevent rancidity of fats. This chemical is safe when used within certain limits. However, high doses have been associated with health problems (see Chapter 12). Thus even well-known chemicals we are comfortable using can be toxic in certain circumstances. We see again that an old adage applies: "The dose determines the poison."

TESTING FOOD ADDITIVES FOR SAFETY

no observable effect level (NOEL) This corresponds to the highest dose of an additive that produces no deleterious health effect in animals.

Food additives are tested for safety on at least two animal species, usually rats and mice. Scientists determine the highest dose of the additive that produces no deleterious health effects in the animals. This is called the **no observable effect level (NOEL).** The NOEL is then divided by a number between 100 and 1000 to establish a margin of safety for human use. The 100-fold safety factor is most often used. Thus the highest level of an additive found in a food should be no more than 1/100 of the highest level that produced no apparent deleterious health effects in test animals.[22] Note that the margin of safety for some vitamins and trace minerals is only ⅕ or ⅒. So food additives are subjected to much stricter limits than are essential nutrients, such as selenium and vitamin A.

Delaney clause This clause to the 1958 Food Additives Amendment of the Pure Food and Drug Act in the United States prevents the intentional (direct) addition to foods of a compound that has been also been shown to cause cancer in animals or man.

One important exception appears in this schema for testing food additives. If an additive is shown to cause cancer in test animals or humans, no margin of safety is allowed. The food additive cannot be used because this would violate the **Delaney clause** in the 1958 Food Additive Amendments. This clause prohibits the intentional use of cancer-causing compounds in foods.

In recent years some people have called for "loosening" the Delaney clause to permit use of some weak carcinogens. Advocates of the law point out that in the absence of the Delaney clause, regulators and politicians would be under constant pressure to allow "just a little cancer." Currently, the law stands as originally written.

Recently, the value of animal cancer tests also has been questioned.[21] Research suggests that when rats are fed massive doses of chemicals, as they typically are in the tests, it may be the dose itself, rather than the chemical action, that causes cancer. The scientific community is currently debating which is the best method to test additives to evaluate cancer risk in humans. The question boils down to how to test chemicals efficiently and how to apply data obtained from laboratory animals to humans. Nevertheless, we are struck with our current approach until someone establishes a better method.

Some definitions here might help you:
- **toxicology—The scientific study of harmful substances.**
- **safety—The relative certainty that a substance won't cause injury.**
- **hazard—The chances that injury will result from use of a substance.**
- **toxicity—The capacity of a substance to produce injury at some level of intake.**

Incidental food additives pose a unique problem with respect to cancer. FDA cannot simply ban pesticide residues, various industrial chemicals, and mold toxins from foods, even though they cause cancer. These products are not purposely added to foods—they are present whether we like it or not. FDA sets an acceptable level for these substances in foods. Basically, it establishes a safety margin of one million, which means that during the entire lifetimes of one million people, cancer cases can theoretically increase by no more than one case because of the presence of the agent in food.

OBTAINING APPROVAL FOR A NEW FOOD ADDITIVE

Today, a new substance to be added to foods must undergo strict testing to establish its safety. Manufacturers present information to FDA in the forms of a petition that identifies the new additive, its chemical composition, how it is manufactured, and laboratory methods used to measure its presence in the food supply at levels of intended use. The petition must establish that the proposed laboratory method can actually detect the substance so that FDA can later monitor whether food manufacturers are complying with regulations.

There also must be proof that the additive will accomplish the intended result in a food and that the level sought for use is no higher than is reasonably necessary to do the job intended. Finally, information provided by the petitioner must prove that the additive is safe for its intended use.

Additives cannot be used to hide defective food ingredients, deceive customers, or replace good manufacturing practices. A petitioner must establish that the ingredient is really necessary for producing a specific food product.

COMMON FOOD ADDITIVES

A list of various classes of food additives appears in Table 19-3. Let's look at some of the major examples to understand exactly why food additives are used and to learn more about the specific chemical substances that are used as food additives.

Acidic or Alkaline Agents

Acids, such as calcium lactate, have many uses in foods. They serve as flavor-enhancing agents, preservatives to inhibit microbial growth, antioxidants to prevent discolorization or rancidity, and adjustors of pH. Acids impart a tart taste to soft drinks, sherbets, and cheese spreads. Acids also increase the safety of naturally low-acid vegetables, such as beets.

Alkaline products, such as sodium hydroxide, are used to alter the texture and flavor of foods, like chocolate. In processing, alkaline products are sometimes used to produce a milder flavor by neutralizing the acids produced during fermentation.

Anticaking Agents

By absorbing moisture, compounds such as calcium silicate, ammonium citrate, magnesium stearate, and silicon dioxide keep table salt, baking powder, powdered sugar, and other powdered food products free-flowing. These chemicals prevent the caking, lumping, and clustering that would make powdered or crystalline products inconvenient to use.

Antioxidants

These preservatives help delay discoloration of foods, such as peeled or cut potatoes. They also help keep fats from turning rancid. Two widely used antioxidants are BHA (butylated hydroxyanisole) and BHT (butylated hydroxytoluene). Vitamin E and Vitamin C also are used as antioxidants.

Sulfites have been widely used as antioxidants in foods and drugs for centuries. Sulfites are actually a group of sulfur-based chemicals—sulfur dioxide, sodium sul-

Table 19-3 Food additive categories

Anticaking	Formulation aids: carriers, binders, fillers, plasticizers	Processing aids: clarifying, clouding, catalyst, floculants, filter aids, crystallization inhibitors
Antimicrobial	Fumigants	Propellants
Antioxidants	Humectants	Sequestrants
Color, and adjuncts	Leavening	Solvents and vehicles
Conditioners	Lubricants and release agents	Stabilizers and thickeners
Curing and pickling	Nonnutritive sweeteners	Surface active agents
Dough strengtheners	Nutritive sweeteners	Surface-finishing agents
Drying agents	Oxidizing and reducing agents	Synergists
Emulsifiers	pH control	Texturizers
Enzymes		
Firming agents		
Flavor enhancers		
Flavoring agents		
Flour treating		

From Hegarty V: Decisions in Nutrition, St. Louis, 1988, The CV Mosby Co.

fide, sodium and potassium bisulfite, and sodium and potassium meta bisulfite. Sulfites inhibit the action of the enzyme polyphenyl oxidase, in turn preventing the browning reaction that this enzyme encourages.

Since August 8, 1986, FDA has prohibited use of sulfites on raw fruits and vegetables—an action directed mainly at salad bars. Potatoes were not covered by that regulation. As of January 8, 1987, FDA also requires manufacturers to declare the presence of sulfites on labels of packaged foods containing at least 10 parts per million of sulfites.[14] Labels on wine bottles often list a sulfite warning, and drug companies are required to produce a warning statement on prescription drugs containing sulfites. Some people are very sensitive to sulfites and suffer difficulty in breathing, wheezing, hives, diarrhea, vomiting, abdominal pain, cramps, and dizziness after exposure.

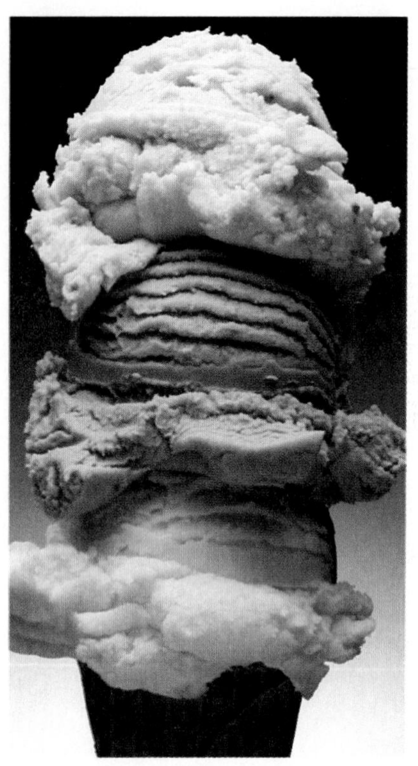

Ice cream often contains added emulsifiers and stabilizers.

Coloring Agents

By law, color additives are tested in a distinct fashion. They are not classified as intentional or unintentional food additives, but are in a class by themselves. Color additives do not improve eating or nutritional qualities, but they do make foods appear more appetizing. No food coloring can be used if it promotes deception of the consumer. They cannot be used to cover a blemish, conceal inferiority, or mislead the consumer in any way.

Controversy has surrounded the use of some of the red food colors, primarily because of their suspected link to cancer.[4] Currently, the safety of using the color additive tartrazine (FD&C yellow No. 5) also is disputed. It is known to cause allergic symptoms, such as hives, itching, and nasal discharge in sensitive individuals. Sensitivity is especially common in people allergic to aspirin. Fortunately, the number of us sensitive to tartrazine is small. Nevertheless, FDA requires manufacturers to list yellow dye No. 5 on labels of any food products containing it.

Emulsifiers

These widely used additives are important in incorporating fat in water-based mediums to improve the uniformity, smoothness, and body of foods such as bakery goods, ice cream, and candies. Emulsifiers also stabilize fat-and-water mixtures so that they do not separate. In mayonnaise, for example, egg yolks act as emulsifiers to prevent the oil from separating from the acids. Lecithin, derived from soybeans, acts as an emulsifier in chocolate and margarine. Monoglycerides and diglycerides, the same by-products found in lipid digestion, are used as emulsifiers in cake mixes.

Extenders

Extenders are used to add texture and bulk to a product. Hydrolyzed protein (HP), hydrolyzed vegetable protein (HVP), hydrolyzed plant protein (HPP), textured protein (TP), texturized vegetable protein (TVP), and texturized plant protein (TPP) are often used in this manner.

Fat Replacements

Fat replacements such as Paselli SA2, Dur-Low, and Sta-Slim 143 are currently in commercial use. These carbohydrate-based products join another major player—Simplesse—covered in Chapter 5. These types of additives provide body to products, like fat-free mayonnaise, primarily by binding water.

Flavors and Flavoring Agents

Naturally occurring and artificial agents can impart more flavor to foods. These agents include extracts from spices and herbs and man-made agents. You are probably familiar with flavors of some spices and of liquid derivatives of onion, garlic, cloves, and peppermint. To meet the demand of industry, manufacturers have developed synthetic flavors that not only accurately resemble natural flavors, but also have the advantage of stability. Often artificial flavors, such as butter or banana flavors, are the components of the natural flavor.

Flavor Enhancers

These substances—monosodium glutamate (MSG), for example—help bring out the natural flavors of foods. Some people are sensitive to MSG and suffer flushing, chest pain, facial pressure, dizziness, sweating, rapid heart rate, nausea, vomiting, and high blood pressure after exposure. Infants are the most sensitive to MSG because they have not yet developed a complete blood-brain "barrier." This means they cannot fully exclude such substances as MSG from the brain. MSG is often used in Chinese food, and thus reactions to it have acquired the name "Chinese restaurant syndrome." The onset of symptoms occurs about 10 to 20 minutes after ingestion and may last from 2 to 3 hours. People who find themselves sensitive to MSG should avoid it.

Humectants

These chemicals, such as glycerol, propylene glycol, and sorbitol, are added to foods to help retain proper moisture, fresh flavor, and texture. They are often used in candies, shredded coconut, and marshmallows.

Leavening Agents

The term leavening means to "make light and porous." The major leavening gases are air, steam, and carbon dioxide. They are used to create light textures in breads, cakes and other baked flour products. Carbon dioxide, the most reliable of the three, is produced by fermentation, a biological process, and chemically by baking powder and baking soda. Baking soda will produce a bitter off-flavored product unless used in the presence of an acid. Baking powders composed of soda plus the acid ingredient.

Maturing and Bleaching Agents

By hastening the aging process of flour, these compounds enable its early use in bread products. Freshly milled flour makes very poor bread because it lacks the qualities necessary to make a stable, elastic dough. When aged for several months, flour gradually whitens and matures to become useful for baking. Chemical changes that take place in the proteins in the flour allow for a better dough structure. Compounds such as bromates, peroxides, and ammonium chloride enhance the natural aging and whitening processes.

Nonnutritive Sweeteners

Currently, saccharin and acesulfame (Sunette) are the only nonnutritive sweeteners used in foods. Recall that aspartame (Nutrasweet) yields energy (see Chapter 3). Saccharin has been found to be a carcinogen only in rats and only if administered over two generations. The cancers are found primarily in the bladder of these animals. Recall that the U.S. Congress has prevented FDA from banning saccharin, but a warning label must accompany any use.

Epidemiological studies of humans have not found an increased risk of developing bladder cancer from exposure to saccharin. It is estimated that in the United States, approximately 80 million to 100 million people consume saccharin in foods. In comparison, approximately 25,000 to 30,000 people develop bladder cancer each year in the United States. The question for society is whether the risk of developing cancer from saccharin consumption is worth the benefit of using this sweetener. In most applications aspartame can substitute for saccharin.

Nutrient Supplements

Vitamin and mineral supplements are added to foods to improve their nutritional quality, and sometimes to replace nutrients lost in processing, as in the case of enriched flour. Vitamin A is added to margarine and to some forms of milk; vitamin D is added to some dairy products. Potassium iodide is added to salt.

preservatives Compounds that extend the shelf life of foods by inhibiting microbial growth or minimizing the destructive effect of oxygen and metals.

Preservatives

There are many types of **preservatives.** Some function as antioxidants, inhibitors of microbial growth, or **sequestrants** (see later category). Sodium benzoate, sorbic acid, and calcium propionate are common preservatives. Calcium propionate is a natural part of some cheeses.

Nitrates—and the related form, nitrites—are used as preservatives, especially to prevent growth of *C. botulinum.* Sodium and potassium nitrates and nitrites are used to preserve meats such as bacon, ham, salami, and hot dogs (Figure 19-5). Nitrates and nitrites have been used for centuries—in conjunction with salt—to preserve meat. An added effect of nitrates is their reaction with myoglobin pigments in meat to form a bright pink color. This gives the characteristic appearance to ham, hot dogs, and other cured meats.

If nitrates and nitrites form chemical substances that can cause cancer, why aren't they banned? In the United States, USDA regulates the use of these chemicals in meats, and the governing laws are not part of the 1938 Federal Food, Drug, and Cosmetic Act. Therefore the Delaney clause, an amendment to the 1938 law, does not apply. Currently, USDA sees no clear threat to public safety from the regulated use of nitrates or nitrites in meats, and so no action appears warranted.

Nitrate consumption from both cured foods and natural vegetables has been associated with the synthesis of nitrosamines in the stomach. These are potent cancer-causing agents, particularly in the stomach and esophagus. However, actual risk appears to be low, except for people with low stomach acid output (some elderly people, for example). FDA also feels that consumers "take for granted" a margin of microbial safety from nitrite use in cured meats. People often serve them cold or at least underheated. Consequently government agencies have chosen not to ban nitrate or nitrite use in foods, but rather to change manufacturing practices to lower amounts of preformed nitrosamines.

The addition of vitamin C to cured meats, such as bacon, is one way to reduce the amount of nitrosamines formed in foods.[25] This is a common practice today. Other antioxidants, such as vitamin E, also reduce synthesis of nitrosamines. About 35% of the nitrite in our food supply is added in manufacturing, as is about 13% of nitrates. The rest is found naturally in foods, mostly in vegetables and baked goods.

Stabilizers and Thickeners

These give a smooth texture and uniform color and flavor to candies, ice creams and other frozen deserts, chocolate milk, and artificially sweetened beverages. Commonly used substances are pectins, vegetable gums (such as guar gum and carrageenan), gelatins, and agars. These compounds work by absorbing water. Without stabilizers and thickeners, ice crystals form in ice cream and other frozen desserts, and particles of chocolate separate from chocolate milk. These stabilizers are also used to prevent evaporation and deterioration of the volatile flavor oils used in cakes, puddings, and gelatin mixes.

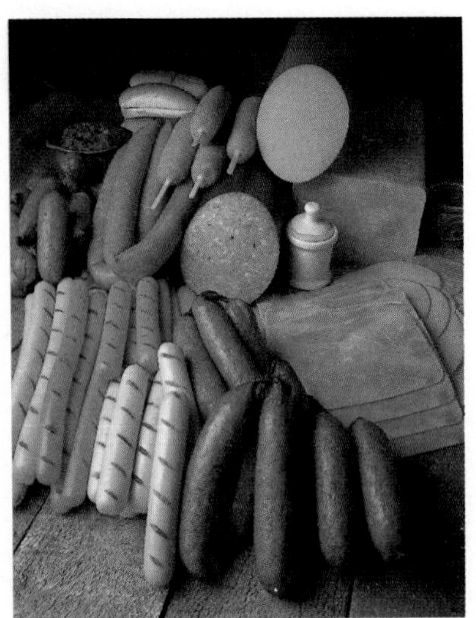

Figure 19-5 Cured meats rely on nitrates/nitrites for their pink color. The National Cancer Institute advises moderation with these foods, as they pose some cancer risk.

Sequestrants

These additives bind metal ions, such as iron and copper, that cause undesirable effects on flavor and appearance of foods. They also reduce the ability to cause rancidity in products containing fat. Examples of sequestrants include Ethylenediamine tetraacetic acid (EDTA) and citric acid.

• • •

If this list of compounds seems bewildering, you can easily avoid most of them. By emphasizing unprocessed whole foods, you can essentially eliminate most of them from your diet (Figure 19-6). However, no evidence shows that this will necessarily make you healthier. It amounts to a personal decision. Do you have enough faith in FDA and food manufacturers to protect your health and welfare, or would you like to minimize your intake of compounds not naturally found in foods? Choose the path that seems best to you.

> **CONCEPT CHECK**
>
> Food additives are used to reduce spoilage from microbial growth, oxygen, metals, and other compounds. Additives are also used to adjust pH, improve flavor and color, leaven, provide nutritional fortification, thicken, and emulsify food components. Additives are classified as intentional (direct), which are those purposefully added to foods, and incidental (indirect), which are those that turn up in foods due to environmental contamination or manufacturing practices. The addition of an additive to a food is limited to 1/100 of the highest amount that has no observable effect when fed to animals. The Delaney clause further limits intentional addition cancer-causing compounds to food in the United States. Carcinogens that incidentally enter foods have maximum levels set for their presence in foods.

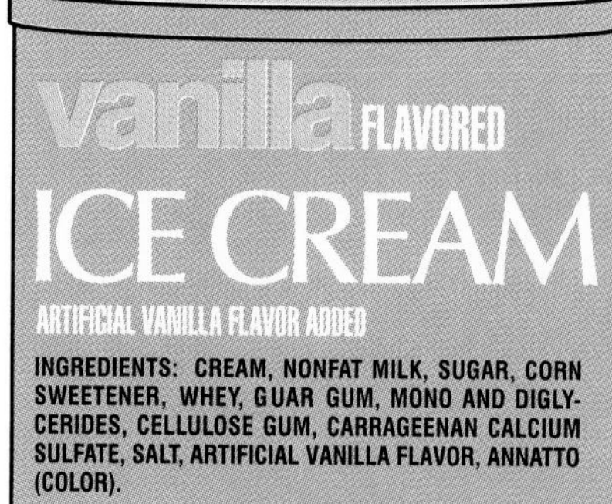
vanilla FLAVORED
ICE CREAM
ARTIFICIAL VANILLA FLAVOR ADDED
INGREDIENTS: CREAM, NONFAT MILK, SUGAR, CORN SWEETENER, WHEY, GUAR GUM, MONO AND DIGLY-CERIDES, CELLULOSE GUM, CARRAGEENAN CALCIUM SULFATE, SALT, ARTIFICIAL VANILLA FLAVOR, ANNATTO (COLOR).

Figure 19-6 Depending on our food choices, we can either eat a diet essentially devoid or full of food additives. The course each of us takes, for the most part, is a personal decision.

Naturally Occurring Substances in Foods That can Cause Illness

Foods contain a variety of naturally occurring substances that can cause illness. Following are some of the more important examples:[18]

Safrole—found in sassafras, mace, and nutmeg; causes cancer.

Solanine—found in potato shoots and green spots on potato skins; inhibits the action of neurotransmitters.

Aflatoxin—found on moldy grains (especially corn, peanuts, and wheat); causes cancer.

Avidin—found in raw egg whites; binds biotin, preventing its absorption.

Goitrogens—found in brussels sprouts, broccoli, kale, and soybeans; they inhibit thyroid hormone metabolism.

Thiaminase—found in raw clams and mussels; destroys the vitamin thiamin.

Glycyrrhizic acid—found in pure licorice extracts; causes hypertension.

Tetrodotoxin—found in puffer fish; causes respiratory paralysis.

Protease inhibitor—found in raw soybeans; inhibits digestive enzymes.

Saponins—found in alfalfa sprouts; can destroy red blood cell membranes.

Tannins—found in tea; can bind calcium and iron.

Oxalic acid—found in spinach; binds calcium.

Herbal teas—containing senna or comfrey; can cause diarrhea and liver damage.

Nitrates—found in spinach, lettuce, and beets; can be converted into the carcinogen nitrosamine.

Browning products—found in toasted grains; can cause DNA mutations.

People have coexisted for centuries with these naturally occurring substances and have learned to avoid some of them. Today they pose little health risk. Farmers know potatoes must be stored in the dark so that solanine won't be synthesized. Operators of grain elevators check grain deliveries for the presence of aflatoxins. (Aflatoxins fluoresce under ultraviolet light.) And we have naturally limited our consumption of other of these substances or developed cooking and food preparation methods to limit their potency. Nevertheless, it is important to understand that some potentially harmful chemicals in foods occur naturally.

TOXIC ENVIRONMENTAL CONTAMINANTS IN FOOD

A variety of toxic environmental contaminants may be found in foods. We mention some of them here:

Lead

This metal can cause anemia, kidney disease, and damage to the nervous system. Lead toxicity is especially a problem for children and is related to poor learning ability and decreased growth.[8] It is important not to store food in a can with a lead solder joint after the can has been opened, nor in a bread bag turned inside out (lead can be part of the ink). Contact with air speeds degradation of the solder joint and the release of lead into the food product. This is especially important for acidic food products, such as tomatoes. Many cans today are lead free if used for acidic products, like soft drinks. In addition, never store acidic products, such as fruit juice, sauerkraut, or pickled vegetables, in galvanized or other metal containers, except stainless steel. Acid can dissolve the metal, and lead will then leach into the food product. Lead can also leak out of solder joints in copper pipes, so let tap water run 2 minutes or so before drinking it or cooking with it, especially first thing in the morning.[9] Also, don't use hot tap water for cooking or preparing infant formula as lead leaches more easily into hot water.

Lead can enter the food supply via pottery glazes. Lead is no longer used in glazes on commercially produced dishes in the United States because of this hazard. However, there is no way to ensure the safety of homemade or imported pottery items. It is important not to use antiques or collectibles for food or beverage storage because of the potential presence of lead.

Dioxin

This is an abbreviated name for a complex chemical defoliant. Dioxin is believed to cause cancer and other harmful effects in animals, even in small doses, but its toxicity to humans in low doses is still under question. Our major food sources of dioxin are bottom fish from the Great Lakes—an area with a great deal of industrial activity and chemical production. Dioxin is primarily a problem for people who frequently consume fish caught locally.[3] People who eat commercial fish normally eat a variety, and even people who stick to one type of fish do not usually have a problem because fish in interstate commerce generally come from different waters, only a few of which may contain dioxin.

Mercury

FDA first limited mercury in foods in 1969 after 120 people in Japan became ill from eating fish contaminated with high amounts. Birth defects in offspring of some of those people were also blamed on the mercury poisoning. The fish most often contaminated was swordfish. Currently, swordfish shipments are automatically detained until they are shown to meet mercury standards.

Urethane in Alcoholic Beverages

This chemical forms during fermentation of alcoholic beverages. If the fermented product is heated, as in the production of sherry and bourbon, urethane levels increase even more. Although urethane causes cancer in animals, it is unclear whether it causes cancer in humans. FDA research on urethane in food products is now a high priority.

Polychlorinated Biphenyls (PCBs)

These chemicals were widely used for years in a variety of industrial products, but because they are linked to liver tumors and reproductive problems in animals, they are no longer produced. FDA had banned their use in machinery associated with food and animal feed and has established limits for PCBs in susceptible foods and in paper used for food-packaging material.

The most significant food source of PCB residues is fish, primarily freshwater fish such as Coho and Chinook salmon from the Great Lakes and bottom-feeding fresh water species from waters in other industrial areas. A key point in fish consumption is variety and moderation when local sources have the potential for contamination.

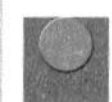

How Safe is the American Food Supply?

JOHN N. HATHCOCK, PH.D.

Today, those who take too seriously every scary headline about pesticides, food additives, and bacterial contamination are apt to feel that practically anything they eat may lead to dire consequences. On one hand, we are told to eat more fruits, vegetables, fish, and poultry, and on the other, we are warned that these foods may contain dangerous substances. Within a recent short period, we were alarmed by reports that poisons in apples, grapes, fish, poultry, and eggs could make us ill, even violently so. Often one set of claims contradicted another, leading to widespread confusion. How can we distinguish between extremist claims and the truth?

The concept of safety

What is a safe food supply? To a nutritionist, it is a food supply available in quantity and at prices allowing easy selection of a variety of diets that provide good nutrition without excessive intakes of specific food components, such as fats. To a toxicologist, it is a food supply that allows easy selection of a variety of diets that doesn't generate significant hazard because of toxic components.

Absolute safety is the total absence of hazard. Because of the logic and statistical nature of the evidence, proof of absolute safety would require proof of a negative—that something cannot occur. The science of toxicology never allows such a proof. It does provide evidence that supports the conclusion that almost all foods in the American food supply usually provide adequate safety. "Usually" and "adequately" may seem like hedge words, but really they are not; they simply recognize that proof of absolute safety is not possible and that, occasionally, some particular foods may not be adequately safe. Why don't we strive for "always" in safety? There are three reasons: (1) it's not possible; (2) there are trade-offs that make it unwise—that is, actions taken to decrease one type of risk may generate another; and (3) maximum reduction in many types of risk would be prohibitively expensive.

Trade-offs in food safety

Cooking improves food safety. Safety is improved because microbes are killed, reducing food spoilage and food-borne infections. On the other hand, cooking may produce mutagenic and carcinogenic chemicals in very small quantities, usually through heat destruction of fat or protein. Although these chemicals are produced in only trace quantities, some of them may cause more risk of cancer than the worrisome pesticides and food additives.

The safety of food additives, such as sodium nitrite, has been widely questioned in the popular press and by some scientists. Nitrite has antibacterial properties that help protect against the growth of the bacteria that cause botulism, a disease that quickly causes death. Nitrite also contributes color and flavor to some foods. No responsible scientist will tell you that the use of nitrite is perfectly safe. It can react with naturally present amines and other essential substances to produce nitrosamines. Many nitrosamines have some potential to cause cancer in experimental animals. With only this in mind, it may seem logical to avoid all nitrite-containing foods, but that is not the case. The first reason relates to the protective action of nitrite against botulism. The second is that such avoidance would have little effect on exposure to nitrite. Most nitrite in the human body does not come from food additives. Instead, nitrates normally present in vegetables are converted by bacteria in the mouth and intestine to nitrite. Vegetable sources provide most of the nitrite to which most people are exposed (approximately 75%, depending on the particular dietary pattern).

Many foods, especially those containing polyunsaturated oils, have synthetic antioxidants (such as BHA, BHT, and propyl gallate) added to prevent rancidity. Some products formed when fats undergo oxidative rancidity have toxic effects, possibly including risk of cancer and accelerated aging. The safety of these synthetic antioxidant food additives has been questioned in relation to reports that BHT can have cancer-enhancing effects under some experimental conditions. These reports indicate that bladder cancer increases but liver cancer decreases in experimental animals also treated with certain chemical carcinogens. Under other experimental conditions, treatment with synthetic antioxidants decreases the effects of chemical carcinogens. Overall, the evidence indicates that the antioxidants are more likely to decrease risk of cancer in humans than to increase it. Nevertheless, if synthetic antioxidants have any adverse effects, why not replace them with a natural antioxidant, such as vitamin E? The answer relates to comparative effectiveness and to avoidance of excessive intakes of any one substance—including vitamin E.

The replacement of all other antioxidants by vitamin E is not desirable for several reasons. Such replacement would dramatically increase intakes of vitamin E, and if intakes become high enough, questions of the safety of high intakes of vitamin E would arise. Furthermore, vitamin E as a food antioxidant is more expensive than synthetic antioxidants.

Conclusions

The familiar advice to eat a variety of foods to ensure nutritional adequacy also makes sense for avoiding excessive intakes of any particular substance. Certainly, eating a variety of foods increases the probability that a variety of contaminating chemicals will be consumed in small quantities. The common fear that such multiple exposure will dramatically enhance toxicity of those substances is not well founded. Actually, just the opposite is likely. Often one substance will enhance our ability to metabolize and detoxify others, thereby decreasing risk of toxicity rather than increasing it.

Overall, the American food supply is outstandingly safe. Occasional exceptions, such as contamination with microbes or their toxins can make certain foods unsafe. Absolute safety of food is impossible, but the greatest dietary risks are associated with too much food, too much fat, and too much sodium rather than with chemical contaminants.

Dr. Hathcock is a senior scientist with FDA. No official support or endorsement by the Food and Drug Administration is intended or should be inferred.

Table 19-4 What you can do

FDA's sampling and testing show that pesticide residues in foods do not pose a health hazard. Nevertheless, if you want to reduce dietary exposure to pesticides, follow this advice from the Environmental Protection Agency:

- Thoroughly rinse and scrub (with a brush, if possible) fruits and vegetables. Peel them, if appropriate—though some nutrients will be peeled away.
- Remove outer leaves of leafy vegetables, such as lettuce and cabbage.
- Trim fat from meat and poultry and skin (which contains most of the fat) from poultry and fish, and discard fats and oils in broths and pan drippings. Residues of some pesticides in feed concentrate in the animals' fat. Trim skin and fatty deposits from fish.
- Throw back the big fish—the little ones have less time to take up and concentrate pesticides and other harmful residues.

Adapted from: Food and Drug Administration, FDA Consumer: Safety first: protecting America's food supply, p. 26, November 1988.

PROTECTING YOURSELF FROM ENVIRONMENTAL TOXINS IN FOODS

To avoid toxins that naturally occur in food, find out which foods pose a risk. We have reviewed some of them. In addition, emphasize variety and moderation in your food selection. The presence of mercury in swordfish may concern you, but it is a health risk only if your diet is dominated by swordfish. The small amount of mercury in most swordfish is not harmful if you are exposed to it infrequently. Table 19-4 provides some other practical tips for limiting the amount of pesticides in your diet.

CONCEPT CHECK

You can avoid many food additives by consuming unprocessed foods. This is a personal choice. No evidence suggests avoidance is necessary. A general program to minimize exposure to environmental contaminants includes thoroughly rinsing and scrubbing fruits and vegetables, removing outer leaves of leafy vegetables, and trimming fat from meat and poultry, including the skin, and discarding any fat that is rendered from meat or fish during cooking.

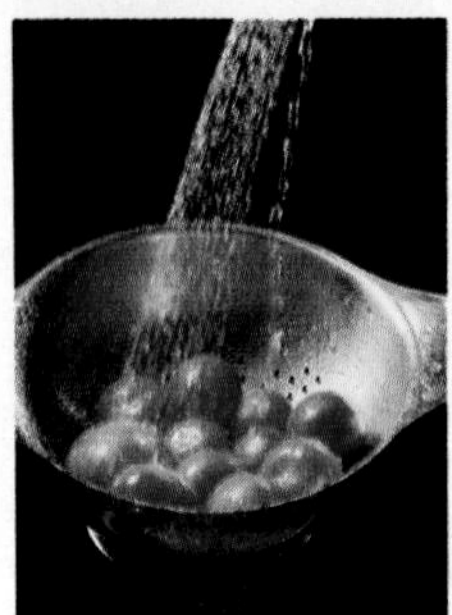

Summary

1. Bacteria and other microbes in foods pose the greatest risk for food-borne illness. In the past, salt, sugar, smoke, fermentation, and drying were used mostly to protect against food-borne illness. Today, careful cooking, pasteurization, and keeping hot foods hot and cold foods cold provide additional insurance.
2. Cross-contamination commonly causes food-borne illness. It occurs when bacteria on raw animal products contact foods that can support bacterial growth. Because of the risk of cross-contamination, no food should be kept at room temperature for more than 2 hours if there is a possibility that it has come in contact with raw animal products and can support bacterial growth.
3. Treatment for food-borne illness usually requires drinking a lot of fluids, avoiding food-handling while diarrhea is present, thorough hand washing, and bedrest. Botulism, *Vibrio vulnificus* and hepatitis A viral infections, and trichinosis represent the types of food-borne illness that require prompt medical attention.
4. The three major causes of food-borne illness today are the bacteria *Salmonella, Staphylococcus aureus,* and *Clostridium perfringens*. To protect against these bacteria that cause food-borne illness, cover cuts on the hands, do not sneeze or cough on foods, avoid contact between raw meat or poultry products and other food

products, and rapidly cool and then thoroughly reheat leftovers. Thorough cooking of foods and the use of pasteurized dairy products further protects against other bacteria and viruses that scientists are only now beginning to understand.

5. Food additives are used primarily to extend shelf life by preventing microbial growth and destruction of food components by oxygen, metals, and other substances. Food additives are classified as those intentionally added to foods and those that incidentally end up in foods. An additive to a food is limited to 1/100 to 1/1000 of the greatest amount that causes no observable symptoms in animals. In most cases, the Delaney clause bans use of any intentional food additive in the United States if it causes cancer.

6. Antioxidants, such as BHA, BHT, vitamins E and C, and sulfites, prevent oxygen and enzyme destruction of food products. Emulsifiers suspend fat in water, improving the uniformity, smoothness, and body of foods, such as ice cream. Common preservatives include sodium benzoate and sorbic acid, which prevent bacterial growth. Sequestrants bind metals, and so prevent spoilage of food from metal contamination.

7. Toxic substances occur naturally in a variety of foods, such as green potatoes, moldy grains, raw fish, raw soybeans, and raw egg whites. Cooking foods limits their toxic effects. Over the centuries, people have purposely avoided some of these foods, such as moldy grains and the green parts of potatoes.

8. A variety of environmental contaminants can be found in foods. Because most of them are fat soluble, trimming fat from meats and discarding fat that is rendered during cooking of meats, fish, and poultry are good steps to minimize exposure. In addition, washing fruits and vegetables thoroughly and discarding the outer leaves of leafy vegetables are also helpful.

Study Questions

1. Identify three major classes of microorganisms that are responsible for food-borne illness and explain how they differ in structure and biological activity.

2. Which kinds of foods are most likely to be involved in food-borne illness. Why are they targets for contamination?

3. Discuss five techniques that are important in preventing the spread of food-borne illness.

4. Define the term food additive and give examples of four intentional food additives. What are their specific functions in foods? What is their relationship to the GRAS list?

5. Discuss the federal legislation that governs the use of food additives, including the Delaney clause?

REFERENCES

1. American Dietetic Association: Food and water safety, *Journal of The American Dietetic Association* 90:111, 1990.
2. Blair D: Uncertainties in pesticide risk estimation and consumer concern, *Nutrition Today,* Nov/Dec 1989, p 13.
3. Blumenthal D: Deciding about dioxins, *FDA Consumer,* February 1990, p 10.
4. Blumenthal D: Red dye no. 3 and other colorful controversies, *FDA Consumer,* May 1990, p 18.
5. Carnevale RA, Sachs S: Counting down on residues—1990, *FSIS Food Safety Review,* Fall 1991, p 4.
6. Farley D: Food safety crucial for people with lowered immunity, FDA Consumer, July/Aug 1990, p 7.
7. Farley D: Setting safe limits on pesticide residues, *FDA Consumer,* Oct 1988, p 8.
8. Frisancho AR, Ryan AS: Decreased stature associated with moderate blood lead concentrations in Mexican-American children, *American Journal of Clinical Nutrition* 54:516, 1991.
9. Greeley A: Getting the lead out of just about everything, *FDA Consumer,* July/Aug 1991, p 27.
10. Guerrant RL, Bobak DA: Bacterial and protozoal gastroenteritis, *The New England Journal of Medicine* 325:327, 1991.
11. Hecht A: Preventing food-borne illness, *FDA Consumer* Jan/Feb 1991, p 18.
12. Herrmann JE and others: Astroviruses as a cause of gastroenteritis in children, *The New England Journal of Medicine* 324:1757, 1991.
13. Klontz KC and others: Syndromes of *Vibrio vulnificus* infections, *Annals of Internal Medicine* 109:318, 1988.
14. Leikos CW: An order of fries—hold the sulfites, FDA Consumer, p 10, March 1988.
15. Liston J and others: Seafood Safety, *Nutrition Reviews* 49:357, 1991.
16. Miller RW: Get hooked on seafood safety, *FDA Consumer,* June 1991, p 7.
17. Murray PR and others: *Medical Microbiology,* St Louis, 1990, Mosby–Yearbook.

18. Newberne PM: Naturally occurring food-borne toxicants. In Schils ME, Young VR, editors: *Modern nutrition in health and disease,* Philadelphia, 1988, Lea & Febiger.
19. Rogan A, Glaros G: Food irradiation: the process and implications for dietitians, *Journal of The American Dietetic Association* 88:833, 1988.
20. Ryser ET, Marth EH: New food-borne pathogens of public health significance, *Journal of The American Dietetic Association* 89:949, 1989.
21. Segal M: Determining risk—is it worth the worry? *FDA Consumer,* June 1990, p 7.
22. Senti FR: Food additives and contaminants. In Schils ME, Young VR, editors: *Modern nutrition in health and disease,* Philadelphia, 1988, Lea & Febiger.
23. Skinner KJ: *Listeria*—battling back against one tough bug, *FDA Consumer,* July/Aug 1988, p 13.
24. Snider S: FDA insures quality of imports, *FDA Consumer,* March 1991, p 13.
25. Tannenbaum SR, Wishnok JS, Leaf CD: Inhibition of nitrosamine formation by ascorbic acid, *American Journal of Clinical Nutrition* 53:247S, 1991.
26. Thonney PR, Bisogni CA. Residues of agricultural chemicals on fruits and vegetables, *Nutrition Today* Nov/Dec 1989, p 6.
27. Williams RD: So long, sunny side up, *FDA Consumer,* Dec 1991, p 8.
28. Wittner MW and others: Eustrongylidiasis—a parasitic infection acquired by eating sushi, *The New England Journal of Medicine* 320:1124, 1989.

SUGGESTED READINGS

An excellent source of information about food-borne illness and food additive safety is FDA Consumer. We have cited articles from this source often throughout the chapter. See the article by Guerrant and Bobak, as well as the article by Skinner to learn more about food-borne illness. The articles by Klontz and others and Ryser and Marth discuss "new" food-borne bacteria of interest, including *Vibrio vulnificus*. For a review of parasites in seafood, see the article by Wittner and others. To review the potential for food irradiation as a method of food preservation, see the article by Rogan and Glaros. These articles plus the material in this chapter will enable you to evaluate the safety of your daily food intake.

TAKE ACTION

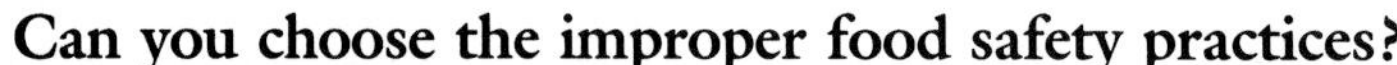

Can you choose the improper food safety practices?

In this chapter you learned the following facts: (1) 1/3 to 1/2 of all diarrhea cases in America are induced by food-borne organisms; (2) Diarrhea caused by food-borne illness hits about one of every ten to 35 Americans per year.

Carefully preparing foods to prevent food-borne illness can minimize its occurrence for most of us. Read the excerpt below and pick the food safety violations that could contribute to this risk.

A LOCAL HEALTH DEPARTMENT INSPECTOR GIVES THE FOLLOWING ACCOUNT OF HIS VISIT TO A LOCAL DINER:

Workers at the Morningside Diner try hard to give good service and provide tasty, satisfying food. As I walked through the kitchen I noticed that each food handler washed his/her hands thoroughly with hot, soapy water before handling the food, especially after handling raw meat, fish, poultry, or eggs. Before preparing raw foods they also thoroughly wash the cutting boards, dishes, and other equipment. As they use their cutting boards, after cutting food, they wipe them with a damp rag and use them again to cut more food.

When preparing fresh fruits and vegetables, they wash them but are careful to leave a little dirt on them for fear of washing important nutrients from the outside. The cooks generally cook meats to an internal temperature of 180° F (82° C). However, for pork, to preserve the flavor, it is cooked to an internal temperature of 140° F (60° C). Some cooked foods that are to be served later are cooled to 40° F (4° C) within 2 hours, and foods like beef stew are cooled in shallow pans.

To save the customer money, the management of the diner uses canned foods, even when the cans are dented. Often these can be purchased at lower prices. When leftovers are reheated, they are raised to an internal temperature of 150° F (66° C) and served immediately. Food handlers take great care to remove moldy portions of food. The cooks prepare stuffing separately from the poultry. On examining the temperature of their refrigerators, they were approximately 55° F (13° C).

1. Below, list the violations of food safety practices that could contribute to food-borne illness.

____

____

2. If you were writing a report describing ways they could correct these practices, what would you say?

____

____

NUTRITION PERSPECTIVE

Pesticides in Foods

Pesticides used in food production produce both desirable and unwanted effects. Many health authorities feel the benefits outweigh the risks. Pesticides help ensure an adequate food supply, make foods available at reasonable cost, and help ensure safety of the food supply. Alternatively, sentiment is growing nationwide that pesticides pose significant and avoidable health risks. Consumers have come to assume that "man made" is dangerous and "organic" is safe. But such is not always the case. Some researchers believe this sentiment is grounded in fear and fueled by unbalanced reports. Other researchers say concern about pesticides is valid and overdue.

The public is struggling to make sense of conflicting information. Alar in apples illustrates this point. Apple growers have routinely sprayed Alar on trees to control ripening. We now know that one component of Alar changes into a potential carcinogen when heated, as it is when apples are processed into juice. Manufacturers and apple growers have now moved quickly to eliminate the use of Alar. Still, as some school systems were taking apples off menus, the U.S. Environmental Protection Agency (EPA) stated that it is unlikely that a person would be harmed from eating apples containing Alar. The agency felt it was safer to eat apples while Alar was being phased out than it was to drive a car or live on mostly hamburgers and candy bars. Furthermore, FDA analysis of 683 samples between 1981 and March 1989 turned up no apples with amounts of Alar that even approached EPA's safe limits.

Most concern about pesticide residues in foods focuses on chronic rather than acute toxicity since the amounts of residues, if present at all, are extremely small.[2] These low concentrations found in foods are not known to produce adverse effects in the short-term, although the high levels that occasionally result from accidents or misuse have done so. For humans, pesticides pose a danger mainly in their cumulative effects. Hence, their threats to health are difficult to determine. However, growing evidence, including the problems of contamination of underground water supplies, indicates that in terms of our nation's health we would be better off if we reduced our use of pesticides.[1]

What Actually is a Pesticide?

Federal law defines a pesticide as any substance or mixture of substances intended to prevent, destroy, repel, or mitigate any pest.[26] Their built-in toxic properties lead to the possibility that other nontarget organisms, including humans, might also be harmed. The term pesticide tends to be used as a generic reference to many types of products, including insecticides, herbicides, fungicides, and rodenticides. A pesticide product may be chemical or bacterial, natural or man made. For agriculture, the EPA allows about 10,000 pesticide uses, involving some 300 active ingredients.[26] Pesticide use in general substantially contributes to the chemical load applied intentionally to the earth's surface. About 2.6 billion pounds of pesticides are used each year in the United States, 60% of which is applied to agricultural crops (Figure 19-7).[2]

Once a pesticide is applied, it can turn up in a number of unintended and unwanted places. It may be carried in the air and dust by wind currents, remain in soil attached to soil particles, be taken up by organisms in the soil, decompose to other compounds, be taken up by plant roots, or enter aquatic habitats. Each is a route to the food chain; some are more direct than others.

Why Use Pesticides?

In the United States alone, pests destroy nearly $20 billion of food crops yearly, despite extensive pesticide use. The primary reason for using pesticides is economic—use of agricultural chemicals increases production and lowers the cost of food, at

NUTRITION PERSPECTIVE

Pesticides in Foods—cont'd

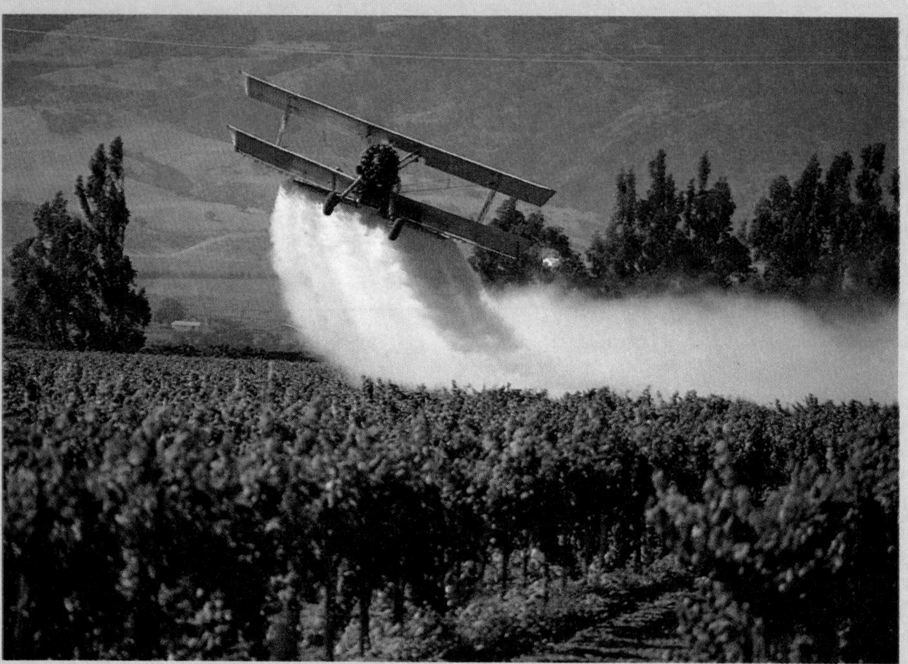

Figure 19-7 Pesticide use poses a risk verses benefit question. Each side has points we need to consider.

least in the short run. Pesticides decrease erosion by eliminating cultivation of plants otherwise needed to get rid of weeds growing by the plants. Before the 1950s crop rotation was the primary way to replenish the soil, reduce erosion, and limit pests. Unless pesticides are applied, farming must depend much more on crop rotations to limit damage from pests. U.S. government subsidies that encourage planting the same crop year after year discourage crop rotation, and so stimulate pesticide use. (See the discussion on sustainable agriculture in Chapter 20. Crop rotation is a key feature of that farming technology.)

Consumer demands have also changed over the years. At one time we would not think twice about buying an apple with a worm hole; we simply took it home, cut out the wormy part, and ate the apple. Today, consumers find worm holes less acceptable, and so farmers rely more and more on pesticides to produce cosmetically attractive fruits and vegetables.[21] On the practical side, pesticides can protect against rotting and decay of fresh fruits and vegetables. This is helpful since our food distribution system does not usually permit consumer purchase within hours of harvest. Also, food grown without pesticides can contain naturally occurring organisms that produce carcinogens at levels far above current standards for pesticide residues. For example, fungicides help prevent the potential human carcinogen aflatoxin (due to growth of a mold) from forming on some crops. So while some pesticides may improve the appearance of food products, others help keep some foods fresher and safer to eat.

Regulating Pesticides

Currently, a pesticide is exhaustively tested, perhaps over 10 years or more, before it can be used. EPA must decide both that the pesticide causes no unreasonable adverse effects to man and the environment, and that benefits outweigh the risks of using it. However, there is concern about older chemicals registered before 1970, when less stringent testing conditions were permitted.[2,26] EPA is now asking chemical companies to retest the old compounds using more rigorous tests. But inadequate funding at EPA has hampered the review of older pesticides. The slow pace for this retesting has angered the critics of pesticide use. When weighing whether to approve or cancel a pesticide, EPA considers how much more it would cost the farmer to use an alternative pesticide or process, and whether cancellation would decrease productivity.[26] After determining the dollar cost to the farmer, EPA then looks at costs to processors and consumers as well.

Once approved for use, setting limits that yield at least a 100-fold margin of safety is a standard requirement for use to minimize health effects other than cancer (such as kidney damage or birth defects). In other words, these limits set the safety standard at 100 times less than the highest dose at which the pesticide causes no ill effects in animals—or lower.[7] Note this is the same as used for food additives. If the pesticide causes cancer, its use must not incur more than one cancer case in one million people over their lifetimes.

How Safe are Pesticides?

A person's risk of poisoning from exposure to pesticides through food depends on how potent the chemical poison is, how concentrated it is in the food, how much and how frequently it's eaten, and the person's resistance or susceptibility to the substance. Pesticide use is clearly associated with impure water quality. Accumulating information also links pesticide use to increased cancer rates in farm communities. For U.S. rural counties, the incidence of lymph, genital, and digestive tract cancers increases with higher-than-average herbicide use.[2] Respiratory cancer cases increase with greater insecticide use. In tests using laboratory animals, scientists have found that some of the chemicals present in pesticide residues cause birth defects, sterility, tumors, organ damage, and injury to the central nervous system. Some pesticides persist in the environment for years.

Still, the cancer risk from pesticide residues is most likely hundreds of times less than the risk of eating substances naturally found in foods such as peanut butter, brown mustard, and basil. Plants manufacture their own toxic substances to defend themselves against insects, birds, and grazing animals (including humans). When plants are stressed or damaged, they produce even more of these toxins. Because of this, many foods contain naturally occurring chemicals considered toxic, even carcinogenic. Other scientists argue that if natural carcinogens in large numbers are already in the food supply, then we should reduce the number of added carcinogens whenever possible. In other words, we should do what we can to help the problem.

The mere presence of a pesticide in food or water at any concentration frightens some people. The levels of pesticide residues found in foods are almost always well below the tolerance levels that have been set to meet safety concerns.[7] High and obviously hazardous concentrations are very rare, usually as the result of spills or improper uses. But the major challenge for scientists and regulators goes beyond detecting and measuring pesticide residues; it is rather a question of what, if any, biological significance they have.

The Risks of Pesticides to Children

Any discussions of pesticides and associated health risks need to focus attention on children. Children face a higher risk from pesticides than adults for several reasons:[2]

1. Their exposure is greater; children eat more food in proportion to their body weight than do adults.

NUTRITION PERSPECTIVE

Pesticides in Foods—cont'd

2. Children consume more foods that are potential sources of pesticide residues, than do adults. For example, they eat more fruit.
3. Exposure at an early age carries a greater risk than exposure later in life; residues accumulate to toxic levels over a longer period. Also cancer has more time to develop.
4. Physiological susceptibility to the effects of carcinogens and neurotoxins in pesticides may be greater; the cells in children are dividing rapidly and the enzyme systems that detoxify chemicals are not fully developed.

Until recent years, EPA did not consider these factors in risk calculations. EPA now looks at age-level consumption data for approval of new pesticides. Although children are at greater risk from pesticides, the magnitude of that risk and how best to calculate it are open to debate.

Testing Levels of Pesticides in Foods

FDA tests thousands of raw products a year for pesticide residues and consistently finds 96% to 99% free of illegal residues.[5] (A pesticide is considered illegal in this case if it is not approved for use on the crop in question, or if the amount used exceeds the allowed levels.) Residues sometimes appear on the wrong crops or in excess amounts because of contamination from nearby farms via wind or water. Still, actual crop residues are usually considerably lower than the legal limits because worst-case scenarios of crop treatment and residue level are used to set the limits. In animals, when illegal residues are found, they are usually concentrated in kidney, liver, or fat, rather than muscle meat. When a problem is identified, FDA takes steps to make sure it's corrected and that the tainted food never reaches the consumer. However, of 600 pesticides available on international markets, many are not even detected by any of FDA's multiresidue tests.[2] This has raised concern by pesticide critics with regards to imported foods. Better tests that detect single residues are less frequently used because of cost.

Personal Action

We often take risks in our own lives, but we prefer to have a choice in the matter after weighing the pros and cons. For instance, we can choose not to immunize a child, but we do so with the understanding that the child might get sick. It is a personal risk that we choose to take. One can also choose to risk cancer from smoking or to avoid that risk. But with pesticides in produce, someone else is deciding what is acceptable and what is not.[26] Our only choice is whether to buy or avoid pesticide-containing foods. And, in reality, it is almost impossible to avoid pesticides entirely because all produce generally contains traces of pesticides, probably from cross-contamination from nearby farms.

Short-term studies of the effects of pesticides on laboratory animals cannot pinpoint long-term cancer risks precisely. But it should be clearly understood that the presence of minute traces of an environmental chemical in food does not mean that any adverse effect will result from consumption of that food. FDA feels the hazards are comparatively low, and in the short run are less than the hazards of food-borne illness created in our own kitchens.[7] We can't avoid the risks entirely, but we can limit pesticide exposure by carefully washing vegetables and fruits and following the other advice in Table 19-4.

In the future, we can encourage farmers to use fewer pesticides in an effort to protect our foods and water supplies, and we will have to settle for produce that isn't perfect in appearance. Are you concerned enough about pesticides on food to change your shopping habits and take more political action?

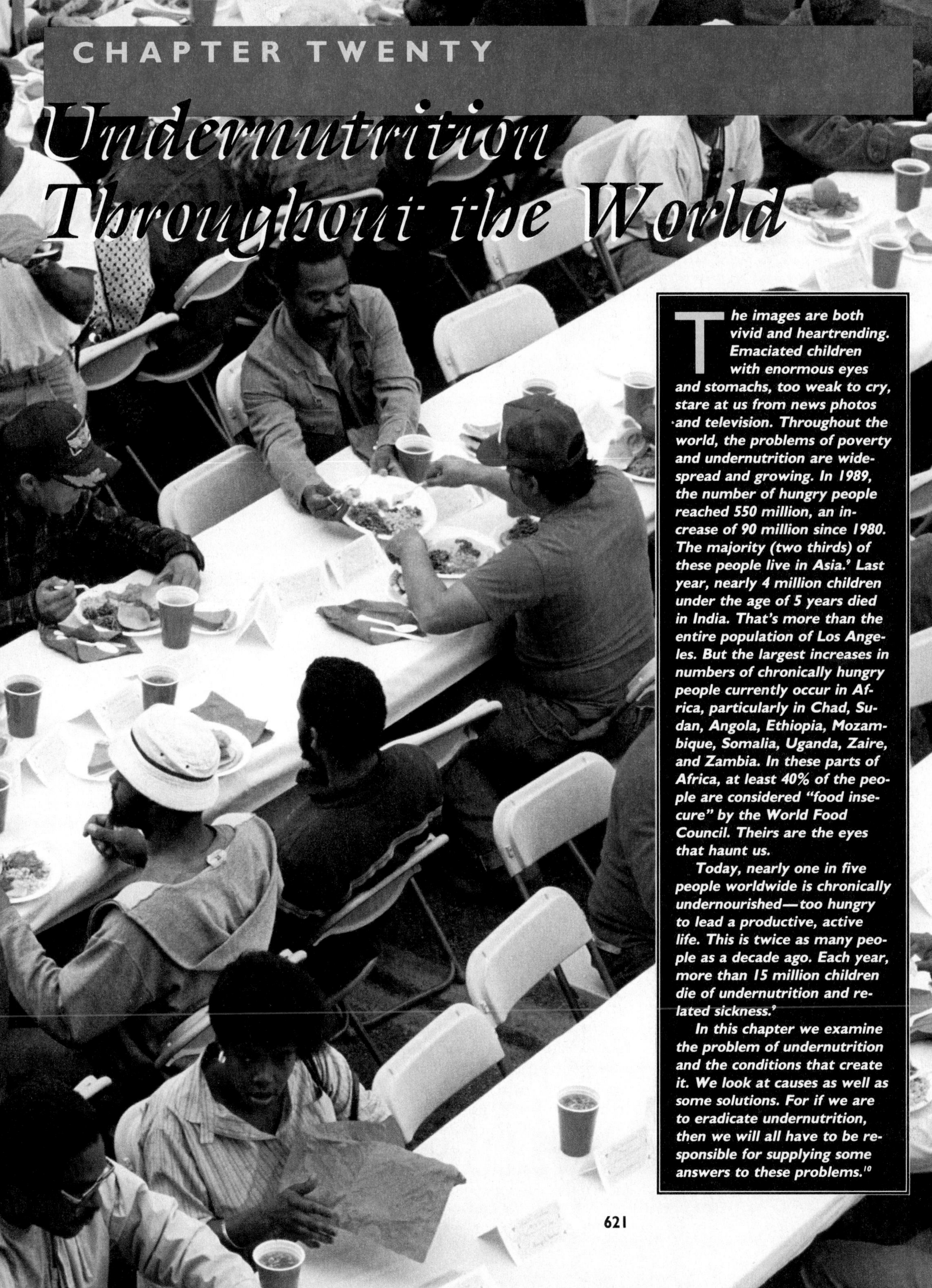

CHAPTER TWENTY

Undernutrition Throughout the World

The images are both vivid and heartrending. Emaciated children with enormous eyes and stomachs, too weak to cry, stare at us from news photos and television. Throughout the world, the problems of poverty and undernutrition are widespread and growing. In 1989, the number of hungry people reached 550 million, an increase of 90 million since 1980. The majority (two thirds) of these people live in Asia.[9] Last year, nearly 4 million children under the age of 5 years died in India. That's more than the entire population of Los Angeles. But the largest increases in numbers of chronically hungry people currently occur in Africa, particularly in Chad, Sudan, Angola, Ethiopia, Mozambique, Somalia, Uganda, Zaire, and Zambia. In these parts of Africa, at least 40% of the people are considered "food insecure" by the World Food Council. Theirs are the eyes that haunt us.

Today, nearly one in five people worldwide is chronically undernourished—too hungry to lead a productive, active life. This is twice as many people as a decade ago. Each year, more than 15 million children die of undernutrition and related sickness.[9]

In this chapter we examine the problem of undernutrition and the conditions that create it. We look at causes as well as some solutions. For if we are to eradicate undernutrition, then we will all have to be responsible for supplying some answers to these problems.[10]

NUTRITION AWARENESS INVENTORY

What have you learned from reading Chapter 20? Here are 15 statements about undernutrition in the world. Read them to test your current knowledge. If you think the statement is true or mostly true, circle T; if you think the statement is false or mostly false, circle F. Use the scoring key at the end of the book to compute your total score. To review, take this test again later, and especially before tests.

1. T F Hunger is partly the psychological state resulting when not enough food is eaten.
2. T F The primary cause of undernutrition is poverty.
3. T F Diabetes is more common when food supplies are low.
4. T F Undernutrition is the most common form of malnutrition among the poor.
5. T F The risk of dying from pregnancy-related causes highlights the gap between the developing and industrialized countries.
6. T F The greatest risk from poor nutrition during pregnancy is borne by the infant.
7. T F 9-year-old children suffering from undernutrition can look like 4-year-olds.
8. T F Marginal deficiencies of iron affect few people worldwide.
9. T F Years of undernutrition can be overcome in several weeks on a high-protein, high-carbohydrate diet.
10. T F Compared with other industrialized countries, the United States has one of the lowest infant mortality rates in the world.
11. T F Homelessness in the United States is much more evident today than in 1980.
12. T F The world population is rapidly outstripping the global food supply.
13. T F Traditionally, poorer people bear more children.
14. T F In Third World countries, the urban population consists mostly of the poor.
15. T F Wherever they live, a key factor for the health of people is a safe water supply.

World Hunger Continues to Plague Mankind

The famines that occurred in Ethiopia and Sudan in the 1980s called attention to the problem of undernutrition in the developing world. The plight of millions of starving people consolidated widespread public support for immediate aid for the victims of famine. Then from 1990 through today, hunger again was and still is frequently in the news, as evidenced by recent strife in Somalia. Continuing civil wars in Africa, coupled with drought, have brought more than 30 million people to the brink of starvation. Relief aid has been arriving, but often too little, too late. The deadly combination of war and poor weather also has led to increasing hunger recently in Bangladesh, Afghanistan, the Philippines, and Cambodia.[9] The problem of undernutrition in developing nations is ongoing, and one that requires our attention.

Undernutrition and Poverty

Let's first define some key words:

Hunger is the psychological and physiological state that results when not enough food is eaten to meet energy needs. It also describes an uneasiness, discomfort, weakness, or pain caused by lack of food. If hunger is not attended to, the resulting medical and social costs from undernutrition are high—infant prematurity and mental retardation, inadequate growth and development in childhood that contribute to poor school performance, decreased work output in adulthood, and chronic disease (Table 20-1). Symptoms of chronic hunger can be found not only in the developing world, but also in many people living at or below the poverty level in the United States and elsewhere.[9]

Table 20-1 The realities of undernutrition

- Nearly one in five people worldwide is chronically malnourished—too hungry to lead a productive, active life.
- Today, 60,000 people will die of hunger—two thirds of them children.
- Approximately half of all children who die each year in developing countries do so from causes that could be prevented at low cost.
- At least 250,000 children are permanently blinded each year simply through lack of vitamin A.
- Women in poor countries average up to four times more births than women in the United States.
- Every day, the world produces about 3000 kcalories/day for each person, well above the average need of 2300 kcalories.
- Poor women in Third World countries face a 300-fold increased risk of death in pregnancy compared to women in the United States.
- Almost half the world's people earn less than $200 a year—many use 80% to 90% of that income to obtain food.
- Of the nearly 5.4 billion people on earth, more than 1.2 billion drink contaminated water.
- In many developing countries, life expectancy of the population is one half to two thirds of that in the United States.
- 1.8 billion people in the world are without proper sanitation facilities.
- Developing countries have two thirds of the 13 million HIV infections worldwide.

The primary cause of chronic hunger is poverty. Unemployment and underemployment, homelessness, drug addiction, functional illiteracy, marital breakups leading to single parent families (often headed by a woman who has limited earning potential), wage discrimination, poor health, inadequate governmental programs, and war and civil strife all contribute to this poverty. In developing nations, poverty; the problems of lack of resources, war, and civil strife; and inadequacy of governmental programs are intensified.[9]

malnutrition Failing health that results from a long-standing dietary intake that either fails to meet or greatly exceeds nutritional needs.

Malnutrition is a condition of impaired development or function caused by a long-term deficiency or excess or imbalance of kcalories and/or nutrients. The occurrence of specific diseases of malnutrition depends mostly on the food/population ratio. When food supplies are low and the population large, undernutrition leading to nutritional deficiency diseases, such as xerophthalmia (eye and other health problems due to a poor vitamin A intake), is common. However, when the food supply is ample or overabundant, poor food choices coupled with an overgenerous intake can lead to nutrition-related chronic diseases, such as certain forms of diabetes. Note, however, pockets of undernutrition among the poor may still be found in areas where food is abundant.

Genetics plays an important role in both forms of malnutrition. Not every child in Thailand who eats mainly rice develops protein-energy malnutrition (see Chapter 5); similarly, not every adult in New York City who consumes a high-fat, high-kcalorie diet develops diabetes. Genetics influences the development of these diseases.[24,29]

undernutrition Failing health that results from a long-standing dietary intake that does not meet nutritional needs.

Undernutrition, referred to many times in this book, is the malnutrition that results from an inadequate intake, absorption, or utilization of the nutrients or kcalories needed for optimal growth, development, and body function. Worldwide, overall kcalorie intake deserves a special focus, more so than protein intake. The earliest response to undernutrition is a reduction in activity, which allows the individual to preserve energy for growth and other vital functions. With persistent undernutrition, the second sign is a reduced rate of weight gain or poor weight maintenance.[18] Later, in children, the rate of growth in height is reduced.

Undernutrition is the most common form of malnutrition among the poor in developing countries. It is also the primary cause of specific nutrient deficiencies that in turn can result in muscle wasting, blindness (from xerophthalmia), scurvy, pellagra, beriberi, anemia, rickets, goiter, and a host of other effects (Table 20-2). For example, more than 250,000 children develop blindness from xerophthalmia each year. Of the 5.3 billion people in the world, at least half a billion suffer some form of undernutrition.[3] Death and disease from infections, particularly those causing severe diarrhea, measles, and tuberculosis, are dramatically increased when the infections are superimposed on a state of chronic undernutrition.[24]

protein-energy malnutrition (PEM) This results when a person regularly consumes insufficient amounts of kcalories and protein. The deficiency eventually results in body wasting and an increased susceptibility to infections.

Protein-energy malnutrition (PEM) is a form of undernutrition caused by an extremely deficient intake of kcalories and/or protein and generally an accompanying illness. The typically dramatic results of protein-energy malnutrition—kwashiorkor and marasmus—were covered in Chapter 5. We will concentrate in this chapter on the more subtle effects of a chronic lack of food.

famine Times of massive starvation, often associated with crop failures, war, and political strife.

Famine is not the same thing as chronic hunger. Although both are results of poverty and a lack of food, famine is the extreme form of chronic hunger. Periods of famine are characterized by large-scale loss of life, social disruption, and economic chaos that slows food production. As a result of these extremes, there is a downward spiral of events, including human distress; sales of land, livestock, and other important farm assets; migration; division and impoverishment of the poorest families; crime; and the weakening of customary moral codes, as seen recently in Somalia. Antisocial behavior—hoarding, crime, etc.—increases.[12] In the midst of all this, undernutrition rates soar, infectious diseases spread, and people die in unusual numbers. Successfully halting this spiral requires more than just feeding those in need. Special efforts are needed to eradicate the fundamental causes of famine.

Because famine strikes areas that typically have high mortality rates and poor record-keeping, death counts are mostly guesswork. More than 3 million people may have perished in the great Bengal, India, famine of 1943. In 1974, another 1.5 million from that region starved in the new country of Bangladesh. China suffered an almost unbelievable famine from 1959 to 1961—estimates of mortality range from 16 to 64 million.

Causes of famine vary by region and decade, but the most common underlying cause is crop failure. The most obvious causes of crop failure are bad weather, war and civil strife, or both. War deserves a special focus: It contributes to food crisis by drawing labor from food production, disrupting the marketing of agricultural inputs and crops, destroying fields, creating refugees, and hindering relief efforts. Food relief now can even become a weapon.[9] War is linked to many famines in recent years. In fact, these types of man-made disasters absorb more than three quarters of the disaster assistance channeled through the World Food Program.

Consequences of Undernutrition—A Closer Look

Prolonged undernutrition is detrimental to health at any time throughout life, but results are more critical during some periods of growth and in the elderly years.

THE CRITICAL PERIODS

The human organism is particularly susceptible to the effects of undernutrition during periods of rapid growth, especially pregnancy, infancy, and childhood.

Pregnancy

The period of greatest health risk from undernutrition is in pregnancy. A pregnant woman needs extra nutrients to meet her own needs as well as those of her developing fetus. If the mother's nutrient intake is inadequate during pregnancy, her own health can be seriously jeopardized.[20] Stores of maternal nutrients may be depleted to provide for the baby. Maternal iron-deficiency anemia is one possible consequence.

Table 20-2 Nutrient deficiency diseases commonly seen in states of undernutrition in the world

Disease and key nutrient involved	Typical result	Excellent dietary sources for the nutrient
Xerophthalmia		
Vitamin A	Blindness, poor growth, increased infections	Liver, fortified milk, sweet potatoes, spinach, greens, carrots, cantaloupe, apricots
Rickets		
Vitamin D	Weakened bones, bow legs, fractures	Fortified milk, fish oils, (sun exposure)
Beriberi		
Thiamin	Nerve degeneration, poor muscle coordination, heart problems	Sunflower seeds, pork, whole and enriched grains, dried beans
Ariboflavinosis		
Riboflavin	Inflammation of face and oral cavity	Milk, mushrooms, spinach, liver, enriched grains
Pellagra		
Niacin	Diarrhea, skin inflammation, mental deterioration	Mushrooms, bran, tuna, chicken, beef, peanuts, whole and enriched grains
Scurvy		
Vitamin C	Poor wound healing, bleeding skin and gums	Citrus fruits, strawberries, broccoli
Iron-deficiency anemia		
Iron	Poor work output, poor growth, increased health risk in pregnancy	Meats, spinach, seafood, broccoli, peas, bran, whole-grain and enriched breads
Goiter		
Iodide	Enlarged thyroid gland, poor growth in infancy and childhood, possible mental retardation	Iodized salt, saltwater fish

Note that often two or more nutrition-deficiency diseases are found in an undernourished person in the Third World. This separate discussion of nutrients just makes it easier to see the important role of each nutrient.

Pregnancy-induced hypertension (preeclampsia), a life-threatening condition involving rapid weight gain from fluid retention and a sharp increase in blood pressure, is also thought to reflect inadequate prenatal nutrition, especially a poor calcium intake.

In Africa, women birth on average more than six live babies. Coupled with chronic undernutrition, this high birthrate creates a 1 in 20 lifetime risk of dying from pregnancy-related causes. In contrast, American women face a risk of 1 in about 6,000. No other social indicator—literacy, life expectancy, or infant mortality included—shows a wider gap between the developing world and the industrialized world.

Fetal and Infant Stages

The greatest risk from undernutrition during pregnancy actually is borne by the fetus. A growing fetus requires a rich supply of protein, vitamins, and minerals as it develops. When these needs are not met, the infant is often born before 37 weeks of gestation, whereas about 40 weeks' gestation is ideal. Results of prematurity include poor lung function and a weakened immune response.[9] These conditions lessen health and make death more likely. Long-term problems in growth and development can result if the infant survives. At the extreme, low-birth-weight babies, 2500 grams or less (about 5.5 pounds or less), face 30 to 40 times the normal risk of dying before the age of 1 year, primarily due to their poor lung development. When low birth weight is accompanied by other physical abnormalities, medical intervention in the United States costs upwards of $100,000 per baby. When severe retardation occurs, the lifetime cost of care can be over $2 million per child.

In the United States, low birth weight accounts for more than half of all infant deaths and for 75% of deaths of babies under 1 month of age. And the rate of occurrence is currently increasing. Worldwide, more than half of infant deaths stem from low birth weight.[9]

Childhood

The rapid growth years of early childhood comprise another period of high risk from undernutrition.[19] Because the human brain grows most rapidly from conception through early childhood, the brain and central nervous system are particularly vulnerable. After the preschool years, brain growth and development slow dramatically until maturity and then stop. Nutritional deprivation, especially in early infancy, can lead to permanent brain impairment. Beyond early childhood, learning may be jeopardized by a deprived environment, but the basic size and structure of the brain are set. Note that currently about 5 million children suffer from chronic hunger.

In general, poor children experience more nutritional deprivation and overall illness and are more severely affected by them than are other children. For example, iron-deficiency anemia, indicated by the presence of an abnormally low concentration of hemoglobin in the blood, is much more common among poor children than nonpoor children. This deficiency can lead to reduced stamina and learning problems.

Undernutrition in childhood also can weaken resistance to infection, as immune function decreases when other micronutrients, such as zinc, are very low in a diet or show lower bioavailability because the food sources are primarily of plant origin.[13] Poorly nourished youngsters are then at risk for more frequent colds, ear infections, and other infectious diseases.[16] Their immune systems may not even respond to vaccinations, and so the value of this form of help is reduced. In addition, in recent years the height of several groups of growth-retarded children in the United States, including Hispanic children in Colorado, has been shown to improve after zinc supplementation. Note that nearly half of all African-American children in the United States live in poverty.

Symptoms of undernutrition in children are not always obvious. Visitors to developing countries may miss undernutrition in children—children who appear to be 3 or 4 years old are actually 8 or 9 years old. Failure of children to grow is a common result of undernutrition and a warning sign that more extreme effects may follow.

The Elderly

We also need to consider one more group at risk for undernutrition—the elderly and the infirm. These people often require nutrient-dense foods, the amount depending on their state of health and levels of activity. Because many have fixed incomes and significant medical costs, food is often a low priority item. In addition, the elderly and the chronically ill are often unable to take care of their own needs, are sometimes isolated, and are more apt to be depressed—all important factors that can influence food intake (see Chapter 18).

GENERAL EFFECTS OF SEMISTARVATION

The results of undernutrition from semistarvation in their initial stages are often so mild that physical symptoms are absent, and blood tests typically do not detect the slight changes in metabolism. Even in the absence of clinical symptoms, however, undernourishment may affect reproductive capacity, resistance to or recovery from disease, activity, work output, attitudes, and behavior.[4] Recall from Chapter 2 that as tissues continue to be depleted of nutrients, blood tests eventually detect biochemical changes, such as a drop in blood hemoglobin concentration. Physical symptoms, such as body weakness, become apparent with further depletion. Finally, the full-blown symptoms of the predominating deficiency become obvious enough to be recognized, such as scurvy from a vitamin C deficiency.

In general, the occurrence of severe deficiency in a few people in a population represents the tip of the iceberg. This usually means that a much greater number have milder degrees of undernutrition. As we have noted, mild nutrient deficiencies, though perhaps not life threatening, can in certain critical combinations still cause very important practical difficulties in health, as well as in life in general. These should not, therefore, be dismissed as trivial, especially in the developing world.[4] It is becoming clear that combined deficiencies of certain vitamins and minerals (e.g., iron and zinc), although less severe than those causing overt physical symptoms, can seriously reduce work performance. **Marginal** deficiencies of iodide, iron, and zinc are known to affect hundreds of millions of people worldwide.

marginal Noticeable, but not severe.

Detailed experiments studying the effects of chronic undernutrition were performed by Dr. Ansel Keys in the 1940s. He maintained 32 men on a diet averaging about 1600 kcalories daily for 6 months. The subjects were conscientious objectors to war, who during World War II volunteered to help scientists understand the physiological responses to starvation and refeeding. These studies were undertaken to gain information deemed useful in helping victims of undernutrition from the war. During the 6 months of study the men lost an average of 24% of their body weight. After about 3 months, the subjects complained of tiredness, muscle soreness, irritability, and hunger pains. They showed a loss of ambition, poor self-discipline, and poor concentration. They were often moody and depressed. Their ability to laugh heartily and sneeze was reduced, and they became intolerant to heat. Decreases in heart rate and muscle tone were also noted.

These cumulative stresses of undernutrition, then, eventually caused emotional instability and an overall apathetic frame of mind. Persistent hunger made it difficult for the subjects to pursue cultural interests, perform manual activities, and study. This in turn produced a frustrating discrepancy between their desire and ability to pursue activities. When they were permitted to eat normally again, even after 12 weeks of rehabilitation, the desire for more food and a feeling of tiredness continued for the subjects. By 20 weeks they had largely, but not fully, recovered—that required about 33 weeks.

These same responses can be expected from undernutrition wherever it appears in the world. This state diminishes the ability of people, communities, and even whole countries to perform at peak levels of physical and mental capacity, robbing people and nations of human resources. Furthermore, the effects of undernutrition in poor countries are likely even greater than that seen by Dr. Keys because his subjects had adequate vitamin and mineral intakes. In addition, the populations in poorer countries must also contend with recurrent infections, poor sanitary conditions, extreme weather conditions, and regular exposure to very infectious diseases. Their greater nutrient needs—especially iron—to combat rampant parasitism and infection compound the problem further. Again, iron and zinc deficiency both can lead to poor immune function, and so these deficiencies increase the risk of disease due to infections, such as diarrhea, pneumonia, and dysentery.

As we mentioned earlier, a common consequence of undernutrition both in the United States and worldwide is an increased rate of infant mortality. The United States infant mortality rate is currently in twenty-fourth place worldwide.[2] Countries that fare better include Scandinavia; western European nations, such as England, France, and Germany; and Asian nations, such as Japan. We have seen a decline in the United States' position in infant mortality rates from a rank of sixth in the 1950s to its current position. The African-American infant mortality rate in the United States is 18.6 per thousand live births, a figure comparable to that of developing countries. The rate for white Americans is 8.1 per thousand. Additional data for poor whites in the United States suggest that this African-American/white ratio reflects the impact of economic and social circumstances, rather than any biological difference between racial groups.

CONCEPT CHECK

Hunger is the uneasiness and pain that results when insufficient food is eaten to meet energy needs. Chronic hunger leads to undernutrition and in turn to growth failure for children and weakness in adults. Risk of infection increases and nutrient-deficiency diseases also result. The primary cause of undernutrition is poverty. The critical periods when undernutrition most adversely influences health are pregnancy, infancy, and childhood. The effects in infancy are the most dramatic, as evidenced by infant mortality rates about twice that of healthy populations.

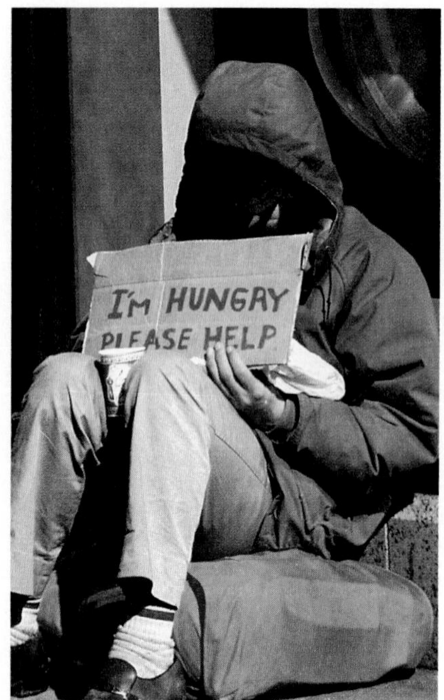

We feel food and shelter for all should be considered a right for everyone.

Undernutrition in America—How Widespread is It?

About 34 million Americans—nearly one in seven people—live at or near the poverty level. This is currently set at about $13,400 annually for a family of four. Two thirds of poor Americans experience chronic hunger; and 8 million are children—nearly 20% of all children.[2] Overall, African-Americans have the highest poverty rate of any racial group at 32%. The poverty rate for whites is 11%; Hispanics, 28%; and Asians and Pacific Islanders, 12%.

Our poor citizens generally eat enough to prevent overt emaciation, so undernutrition in the United States presents itself quite differently from that in the developing world. Kwashiorkor and marasmus, evident in the pictures of Ethiopian children in the mid 1980s, rarely occur here. Instead, undernutrition here tends to take the form the World Health Organization terms "silent undernutrition." It is reflected in the young child whose weight is several pounds below the low end of the normal range on a growth chart. The untrained eye may miss this condition, or simply see a skinny child. The trained professional will recognize that the size of the child reflects growth failure.[2]

The poor amongst us often face difficult choices: whether to buy groceries for the family or pay this month's rent; whether to have dental work done or pay the utility bill; or whether to replace clothes the children have outgrown or pay for transportation to apply for a job. Food is one of the few flexible items in a poor person's budget. Rents are fixed, utility costs aren't negotiable, the price of medical care and prescription drugs can't be bargained down, and bus drivers won't accept less than the going rate to transport riders. But a person can always eat less.[1] The short-term consequences may be less dramatic than having the utilities shut off. The long-term cumulative effects, however, are disturbing.

In sheer numbers, as well as in severity of health risks posed, undernutrition in the United States is a troubling problem. Note that in the United States the threat of hunger for most citizens was virtually eliminated in the 1970s.[2] The fact that major pockets of undernutrition reemerged and spread rapidly in the 1980s and remain in the 1990s suggests that the roots of undernutrition in the United States are mainly political and socioeconomic, rather than technical. Resources are available for feeding all citizens. In the developing world, far more factors complicate this problem, as we will discuss later.

The presence of undernutrition in the United States raises a broad question for our society at large: Where can people in such situations turn when their own resources fail? The responsibility for helping those in need could lie with the federal government, state government, local government, religious groups, charitable organizations, or perhaps with the individuals themselves. It turns out all can be part of the solution.

UNDERNUTRITION IN THE UNITED STATES IS NOT A NEW PROBLEM

The problem of undernutrition in the United States actually began when the Pilgrims landed.[21] Studies in the 1930s during the Depression documented both famine and the existence of widespread pellagra (niacin deficiency) and rickets (vitamin D deficiency). In response, the government opened soup kitchens and began distributing food commodities (Table 20-3). Congress organized school lunch programs in 1946 after testimony by the United States Surgeon General that 70% of the men who had poor nutrition during the Depression era (10 to 12 years earlier) were being rejected for physical reasons by the draft.

In the 1950s, it was assumed that all Americans had enough to eat. Nevertheless, occasional reports of undernutrition surfaced, mostly among the chronic poor: migrant workers, Native Americans, southern African-Americans, unemployed minorities, and some of the elderly.

After observing extensive hunger and poverty during his presidential campaign, President John F. Kennedy in the 1960s revitalized the food stamp program, a program begun two decades earlier, and expanded commodity distribution programs.[2] The food stamp program for low-income people, still in effect, allows recipients to use food stamps like cash to purchase food and seeds—but not tobacco, cleaning items, alcoholic beverages, or nonedible products—at stores authorized to accept them. One in ten Americans relies on this program for help (Table 20-3).

The school breakfast program won passage in 1965 as politicians began to see firsthand the number of children coming to school hungry. Both school lunch and breakfast programs still enable low-income students to receive meals at reduced cost or no cost if certain income guidelines are met. In the same year Congress funded group noon-time (congregate) meals and home-delivered meals for all senior citizens over 60 years of age. Both are still active programs serving the elderly and others.

Political and social awareness of hunger and undernutrition in the late 1960s was spurred on by the book *Hunger USA* and a resulting television documentary, *Hunger in America,* shown in May 1968. The film graphically demonstrated that hunger existed in all areas and ethnic groups in the United States. The response was dramatic.[2] Between 1969 and 1971, some already large federal food programs were expanded and others were newly created. The food stamp program served only 2 million people in 1968, but by 1971, it was serving 11 million citizens. Today it serves more than 23 million people. The school lunch program, which had served only 2 million poor children before 1970, was serving 8 million by 1971. In 1982 about 23 million children took part in the program. The school breakfast program, which was still only a pilot program for children living in poverty areas, became nationally available by 1975.[21]

In the early 1970s the Special Supplemental Feeding Program for Women, Infants, and Children (WIC) was authorized. This program provides food vouchers and nutrition education to low-income pregnant and lactating women and their young children, and currently serves 5 million Americans. WIC has repeatedly shown to be cost effective, especially in reducing the numbers of premature, low-birth-weight babies. WIC is also credited for much of the drop in iron-deficiency anemia seen in children in the last decade. Reports also show that for each dollar spent on prenatal WIC benefits, between $1.92 and $4.21 is recouped later in lower Medicaid costs for mothers and newborns. The current federal budget shortfalls over the last few years have threatened both the scope and existence of this program. "Of all the dumb ways of saving money, not feeding pregnant women and kids is the dumbest," says Dr. Jean Mayer, a leading expert on nutrition.[21]

UNDERNUTRITION IN UNITED STATES—A REEVALUATION

In 1977, a team of physicians resurveyed areas of undernutrition visited 10 years earlier. They found that the degree of poverty in regions like Appalachia and the

Table 20-3 Some federally subsidized programs that supply foods for Americans

Program	Eligibility	Description
Food stamps	Low income	Coupons are given to purchase food at grocery stores, the amount based on size of household and income.
Emergency food system	Low income	Food stamps issued on 24-hour notice for 1 month, while eligibility for further use of the program can be investigated.
Commodity supplemental food	Certain income populations, such as pregnant women, young children, and elderly	USDA surplus foods are distributed by county agencies.
Special Supplemental Food Program for Women, Infants, and Children (WIC)	Low income pregnant/lactating women, infants, children less than 5 years old at nutritional risk	Coupons are given to purchase milk, cheese, fruit juice, cereal, infant formula, and other specific food items at grocery stores.
School lunch	Low income	Free or reduced-price lunch distributed by the school. Meal follows USDA pattern based on the Guide to Daily Food Choices. Cost for the child depends on family income. In schools without a lunch program, special milk programs may be available.

slums of big cities had not changed. If anything, poverty was often worse than in 1967. Yet undernutrition had essentially disappeared as a social phenomenon. As a population, we had more food resources available to us. The large federal food programs—food stamps, the school lunch and school breakfast programs, and WIC—contributed to this difference. Politicians had responded to the demands of the American people by directing federal resources toward a massive human problem, and the effort succeeded.[2] Certainly some Americans still fell through the cracks, but a food "safety net" was catching many whose needs had not been met before.

THE 1980s

The first official recognition in 1982 that widespread hunger reappeared in the United States came from the United States Conference of Mayors. While the news media had been reporting the appearance of soup kitchens and breadlines in the

Table 20-3 Some federally subsidized programs that supply foods for Americans—cont'd

Program	Eligibility	Description
School breakfast	Low income	Free or reduced-price breakfast distributed by the school. Meal follows USDA pattern. Cost for the child depends on family income.
Special milk	Low income	Provides milk for school children.
Child and Adult Care Food	Child enrolled in organized child care program; income guidelines are the same as school lunch program. Adult guidelines are enrollment in an adult day-care program and low income	Reimbursement given for meals supplied to children or adults at the site. Meals must follow USDA guidelines, which is based on the Guide to Daily Food Choices.
Congregate Meals for the Elderly	Age 60 or over (no income guidelines)	Free noon meal is furnished at a site. Meal follows specific pattern based on one third of the RDA.
Home-delivered meals	Homebound individuals	Noon meal is delivered at no cost or for a fee, depending on income, at least 5 days a week. Sometimes other meals for later consumption are delivered at the same time. Often refered to as "Meals on Wheels."

nation's cities since the beginning of the decade, the mayors identified growing hunger as a national problem.

Why was there a sudden increase in hungry people in the United States? First, unemployment in the United States rose from 6.2% in early 1980 to 10.8% in 1983. Although it has since fallen to about 7.6%, more Americans are still unemployed today than were unemployed in 1980. Second, in every year but one since 1976, the scope of the food stamp program has been narrowed and eligibility tightened, so that participants lost 7 to 10 billion dollars worth of foods in the period from 1982 to 1985. In 1981, the school lunch program was reduced by one third. In addition, during that time funding levels for the senior citizen meal programs lagged far behind the increases in food and operating costs, as well as behind the increasing numbers of people in this age group.[2]

At the same time, many volunteer programs also reported an inability to adequately feed those in need. More than 70% of soup kitchens and food pantries said that private donations also did not meet increasing needs.

In a 1985 report, *Hunger in America: The Growing Epidemic,* a group of physicians associated the reappearance of widespread hunger in the United States with government policies and budget cutbacks. Other contemporary reports pointed out that for the majority of food programs, at least half the clients were families with children—those most at risk from undernutrition.[2]

Although cuts in the food stamp and school meal programs were made in the early 1980s, attempts to cut WIC were not successful. A bipartisan coalition in Congress protected WIC against proposed funding reductions. This coalition maintained and even increased WIC participation in the mid 1980s in the face of annual efforts to cut funds. This points to the political nature of the problems we discuss in the United States. Who went hungry depended very heavily on political decisions.

CONGRESS ACTS AGAIN

During 1986 and 1987, concern over undernutrition and associated adverse health outcomes began to take hold in Washington. Congressional leaders became more concerned. Four hundred million dollars were then added back to the food stamp and school meal programs, and Congress increased funding for WIC. These changes, however, while signaling a growing awareness of undernutrition, still fell and remain far short of the amount needed to end the problem. As a nation, in 1989 the United States was not as well off nutritionally as in the late 1970s but was much better off in 1989 than in 1985.[21]

THE 1990s

Hunger increased in the United States in 1990 and 1991. The U.S. Conference of Mayors reported that 1990 emergency food requests were up 22% and shelter requests up 24% over 1989. The Salvation Army said requests for aid increased 20% in 1990. There are currently more than 180 food banks, 23,000 food pantries, and 3300 soup kitchens trying to cope with this problem. Just over two of every three people requesting emergency food assistance in the survey cities were members of families—children and their parents. Across the nation the problem of hunger among some citizens remains.[9]

POVERTY IS ALSO AT THE HEART OF THE CURRENT PROBLEM

The root cause of hunger and undernutrition continues to be poverty. In 1992, there were more than 34 million Americans living at or below the poverty threshold. Recent increases were fueled by the unequal distribution of wealth in the 1980s. From 1980 to 1989, the richest 20% of American families received a 33% increase in after-tax income. The richest 5% of families received a 51% increase.[21] Meanwhile, the poorest 20% of families netted a 0.5% decrease in after-tax income.

Of the 13 million jobs created between 1980 and 1985, most were in a sector, such as quick-service restaurants, that offers low pay. If both parents have such full-time, low-paying jobs, the family may still operate at or below poverty level, again currently $13,400 for a family of four. Note that parents in most poor families do work—nearly two in three poor families in 1989 included at least one worker. In sum, not only have the impoverished in the United States had to exist with less federal assistance, they have also netted a dwindling amount of the national family income.

Homelessness in the United States

The economics of poverty and undernutrition have recently changed in one more very important way. Homelessness is much more evident now than in 1980. This is partly because the cost of housing has substantially increased and partly because federal support for subsidized housing was cut dramatically during the 1980s. Many working poor cannot afford any of the available rents on their minimum-wage earnings. In 1969, the average American spent about 33% of his or her income on housing. Today about 3.5 million people at or below the poverty line spend about 50% for housing.[21] The government considers housing costs, which include rent and utilities, to be affordable if they consume no more than 30% of a family's income. When so much is spent for shelter, almost every other expense is pushed aside, including enough food for children. The larger the family, the less money left to feed each child. Other important causes of homelessness include release of the mentally ill from mental institutions, employment, substance abuse, and personal crises.

An additional important variable related to nutrient intake of the poor is the availability of cooking facilities. In the absence of cooking facilities, people may buy expensive foods that require no preparation. These, typically processed snack foods, tend to provide kcalories but limited nutrients.

The stereotypical image of a homeless person is someone out of step with society who might refuse to work. However, each year, as more and more "typical Americans" find themselves on the streets, we are having to rethink this stereotype. They represent what some observers have labeled the "new homeless," reportedly the fastest-growing segment of the homeless. These citizens have suffered sudden economic difficulties, and usually remain homeless for a short time, waiting for an opportunity to propel them and their families back into mainstream society.[9]

In Columbus, Ohio during 1989, of the 10,562 people who used structures funded by the Community Shelter Board over a 9-month period, 47% had at least a high school diploma, 22% were employed, 17% had recently been employed, and 18% were children; the total included 513 families. In an affluent California community (Contra Costa County) in 1989, investigators found 48% of emergency food recipients were members of families with children. Only 2% were transient people. Forty-five percent of adult emergency food recipients were employed in low-paying jobs or had recently lost a job. Many emergency food recipients were disabled (16% of survey respondents), raising dependent children alone (27%), or were children themselves (33%). Nationwide, the composition of the homeless population is estimated to be 50% single men, 35% families with children, 12% single women and 3% unaccompanied youth. Children comprise 24% of the homeless population.[9]

Food and Shelter for All Americans

The reasons for both homelessness and undernutrition in America then are many. Still, people left behind by society do not go away, as the recent riots in Los Angeles revealed. We may deny being our brother's keeper, but we cannot avoid being his neighbor. Blaming the victims obscures the real issues. Problems surrounding poverty, hunger, and homelessness increased in the 1980s, linked to political and economic factors. Opponents of federal nutrition programs raise the issue of cost, often citing the federal deficit as a reason for limiting spending and stating much money is wasted by bureaucrats and drug-addicted recipients. This argument in our opinion does not outweigh the even greater need of society to meet nutritional needs of its citizens.[21] Consider that when money was needed for the Gulf War, it was there, and when it was needed for the Savings & Loan bailout, it was there. If we decided to do something about homelessness and poverty, it would be there, too. The approximately 1.2 trillion dollar budget of the United States allows for many choices.

Undernutrition, especially in the United States, is a condition that need not exist. Nutrition programs and community intervention, if utilized fully and effec-

EXPERT OPINION

A Call to Action on Childhood Hunger

ANN K. KITTLAUS

Millions of kids are hungry in America. But these children are often invisible. In fact, many Americans are unaware of the dimensions of the tragic but solvable problem of hunger here at home. It's time to make childhood hunger a national priority.

Extent of hunger

During the 1980s, reports from local feeding programs, state networks, and regional coalitions spoke painfully of the growing specter of hunger, especially among families with children. To document this need, a comprehensive, scientifically valid study of hunger among low-income families with children was developed by the Connecticut Association for Human Services. Replication of the survey—called the Community Childhood Hunger Identification Project, or CCHIP—is being coordinated in sites across the country by the Food Research and Action Center (FRAC).

Interviewers hired from within the community conduct door-to-door surveys among a predetermined random sample of low-income families with at least one child under age 12. CCHIP measures hunger by asking a series of questions about the resources available for a household to buy food, the adequacy of the food consumed, food shortages, and the prevalence of hunger. The CCHIP survey also collects information regarding the relationship between hunger and such factors as child health, school absenteeism, household expenses, food assistance program participation, and strategies families employ to avoid hunger.

Based on the first round of CCHIP surveys, FRAC estimates that roughly 5 million American children under 12 years of age are hungry every month and millions more are at risk of hunger.

The CCHIP findings are consistent with other recent surveys that have documented dramatic increases in demand for emergency food assistance across the country.

America's hungry children do not have the distended bellies and emaciated bodies that children in famine-stricken areas of the world display. Instead, the impact of hunger on children here often manifests itself in the lower birth weights of newborns and in many specific health problems, such as unwanted weight loss, fatigue, headaches, irritability, an inability to concentrate, and frequent colds. CCHIP has found that hungry children experience two to three times as many of these problems as do children whose families do not experience hunger. The capacity of hungry children to learn is compromised, and their physical development, stamina, and resistance to disease are impaired.

Causes of hunger

Hunger is a condition of poverty. Living below the poverty line puts tremendous strains on a household budget, adversely affecting the ability to purchase a nutritionally adequate diet. In fact, government surveys show that as income goes down, the nutritional adequacy of the diet goes down as well.

Hunger has increased in the last decade primarily due to a combination of economic factors and cuts in federal assistance programs. Despite the nation's economic expansion in the 1980s, poverty remained consistently high. As recession hit in 1990, an already high poverty rate began to grow. According to the U.S. Census Bureau, 33.6 million Americans, including one in five children, lived in poverty in 1990. These figures reflect only the early impact of the recession of the early 1990s.

tively, could go a long way toward meeting the food needs of those at highest risk.[21] More employment opportunities could then help solidify the improvements. The near elimination of large-scale undernutrition in the United States in the 1970s demonstrates that this national problem can be solved.

Private emergency food network systems also are important, but not sufficient to meet all food needs in the United States. Private donations often taper off during economic hardship in a given geographic area. In addition, much of what is donated is limited in nutritional value. Of necessity, processed and canned grocery items predominate rather than protein-rich foods or perishable items such as fresh produce and milk.[2]

During recent years, an extensive network of private agencies to feed the hungry has sprung up. There are 180 food banks around the United States in the Chicago-based Second Harvest system. These food banks distribute corporate surplus to 42,000 soup kitchens and food pantries operating out of church basements and social-service agencies.[2] Interestingly, Second Harvest officials note that left-over Gulf War food has been their largest and most diverse donation ever from a single donor, over 100 million pounds of food. Yet despite this extraordinary effort, a

EXPERT OPINION

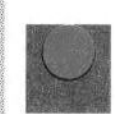

A Call to Action on Childhood Hunger—cont'd

This recession also exacerbated the lasting effects of cuts to federal "safety net" programs in the early 1980s. State and local governments and private charities, which were enlisted to fill the gap, have been increasingly unable to shoulder the burden. Without significant improvements in the economy and stronger safety-net programs, hunger will persist.

Public attitudes toward hunger

The public is very concerned about hunger. A national public-opinion poll released in April 1992 reveals that over 90% of registered voters believe that hunger in the United States is a serious and growing problem. Voters place the primary responsibility for ending hunger with government, and support for federal food assistance programs is very high. In fact, a strong majority of voters is willing to earmark $100 more in taxes annually to end hunger. The poll was released with the Medford Declaration to End Hunger in the United States, which has been endorsed by over 3000 leaders of American society and is the broadest collective statement ever made that hunger in this country can and must be ended.

What you can do to fight childhood hunger

Hunger hurts everybody. We all have a stake in preventing underweight births, in improving the performance of children at school, in ensuring the food security of families, and in preventing expensive health problems caused by hunger. Only when our children are well-nourished can they reach their full potential and become contributing members of society.

There is an urgent need to find long-term solutions to the many problems caused by poverty. But no child should have to go to bed hungry while we work to resolve these long-term problems. Effective programs exist today to alleviate hunger. They include the Special Supplemental Food Program for Women, Infants and Children; the school lunch and breakfast programs; the child and adult care food program; the summer food program for children; and the food stamp program. With sufficient funding and proper administration, these programs can dramatically improve nutritional intake and reduce childhood hunger in this nation.

The Food Research and Action Center, in partnership with a 50-state network of antihunger groups and more than 100 national organizations, has launched the **Campaign to End Childhood Hunger.** Through individual and organizational involvement at the local, state and national levels, the campaign is working to educate the public on the extent and causes of childhood hunger and is advocating immediate and long-term solutions to the problem.

If you are not hungry yourself, or living in poverty, or involved in helping those who are, it is all too easy to be ignorant of the misfortune and misery of others. And while many may avert their eyes and close their minds, the problems are real and they are severe. Unless concerted action is taken now, these problems will only increase in magnitude until the cost of attacking them becomes overwhelming and millions of children suffer needlessly. For humanitarian as well as for hard economic reasons, we must band together to promote changes both in our local communities and at the national level.

Millions of kids are hungry in America and there are solutions. ●

Ann K. Kittlaus is Communications Director for the Food Research and Action Center, 1875 Connecticut Avenue, N.W. Suite 540, Washington, D.C. 20009.

huge gap remains between overall federal (and state) aid and human need. There is no getting around the fact that federal assistance is the most effective way to help poor Americans attain adequate nutrition. When federal assistance is a priority, undernutrition can be beaten.

So while the problems of poverty and hunger are related, they are not necessarily synonymous. If hunger is instead thought of as food insecurity, the opposite then is food security, described as having two elements: the ready availability of quality foods and an assured ability to acquire personally acceptable foods.[6] Food security is in turn actually an investment. Considering the link between food and health, there is a level of nutrient intake that has clear economic benefit. Not just an issue for the poor: food security belongs to all of us.

Overall, poor Americans eventually need longer-term solutions to poverty—beginning with increased opportunities for education, jobs with adequate wages and benefits, affordable housing, and child care.[8] If this country can develop the potential of more people, it can remain the land of opportunity for all. However, providing sufficient funding and outreach for federal food assistance programs alone would eliminate much of the hunger in the United States today.

When big city mayors were recently asked what recommendations they would make to enable the nation to eliminate hunger and homelessness by the end of the century, most focused on housing and employment policies and programs. Recommended most frequently were: a substantial federal affordable housing program, job creation and expanded job training, full employment, and increases in the minimum wage. Also recommended were increases and improvements in the food stamp and WIC Programs.

As part of this discussion, we should consider the responsibility of both the well off and the poor themselves. All citizens have a responsibility to contribute answers to our economic and social problems if we are to remain a moral and just society. The government must often step in with its programs when individual members of society fail to shoulder responsibility for themselves and others around them. Is the government to blame when a father walks out on his wife and children, leaving them without adequate resources to buy food and clothing, or when an unwed 16-year-old women is pregnant with her second child? The long-term solution to these problems is partly governmental in nature, and partly social; all citizens should develop a sense of ethical responsibility. The Reverend Jesse Jackson sees this second thrust as a key goal for American society as a whole.

It is not fair to solely blame the victims of poverty. Unemployment and expensive housing are formidable foes. Even while they desire a better life, and most do, people do not strive indefinitely against circumstances sure to defeat them.[17] Many of the poor are ill equipped for the battle—the elderly, sick, handicapped, female heads of households, and young children.[9] But it is also not fair for the government to shoulder all the blame. In terms of undernutrition in America, is there so much blame that it goes around and touches almost all of us? Until the economy can accept all of us, it is important for all of society to take the initiative and reach out to others in need.

CONCEPT CHECK

Hunger and undernutrition in the United States were recognized by political leaders in the 1960s. In response, federally-subsidized food programs, such as food stamps, school lunch, and congregate meals for the elderly, were started or received substantially increased funding. This federal response greatly reduced undernutrition in the United States; but the number of at-risk people increased in the 1980s as funding for these programs was reduced and an economic recession took place. Since 1985 some funding has been restored, but elimination of undernutrition remains a challenge for the United States—government and citizens alike.

Undernutrition in the Third World

Undernutrition in the Third World is also tied to poverty. So any true solution must address this problem. However, the countries that are considered to be Third World—those that are not industrialized—have a multitude of structural problems so complex and interrelated that they cannot be treated separately. Programs that have proven immensely helpful in the United States would only be a starting point in the Third World. Systematic solutions have to consider major obstacles, such as:[9]

- extreme imbalances in the food/population ratio in different regions of a country.
- the rapid depletion of natural resources.
- cultural attitudes towards certain foods.
- poor **infrastructure**—especially poor housing; sanitation and storage facilities; and education, communication, and transportation systems.
- war and civil unrest.
- mounting external debt.

infrastructure The basic framework of a system or organization. For a society, this includes roads, bridges, telephones, and other basic technologies.

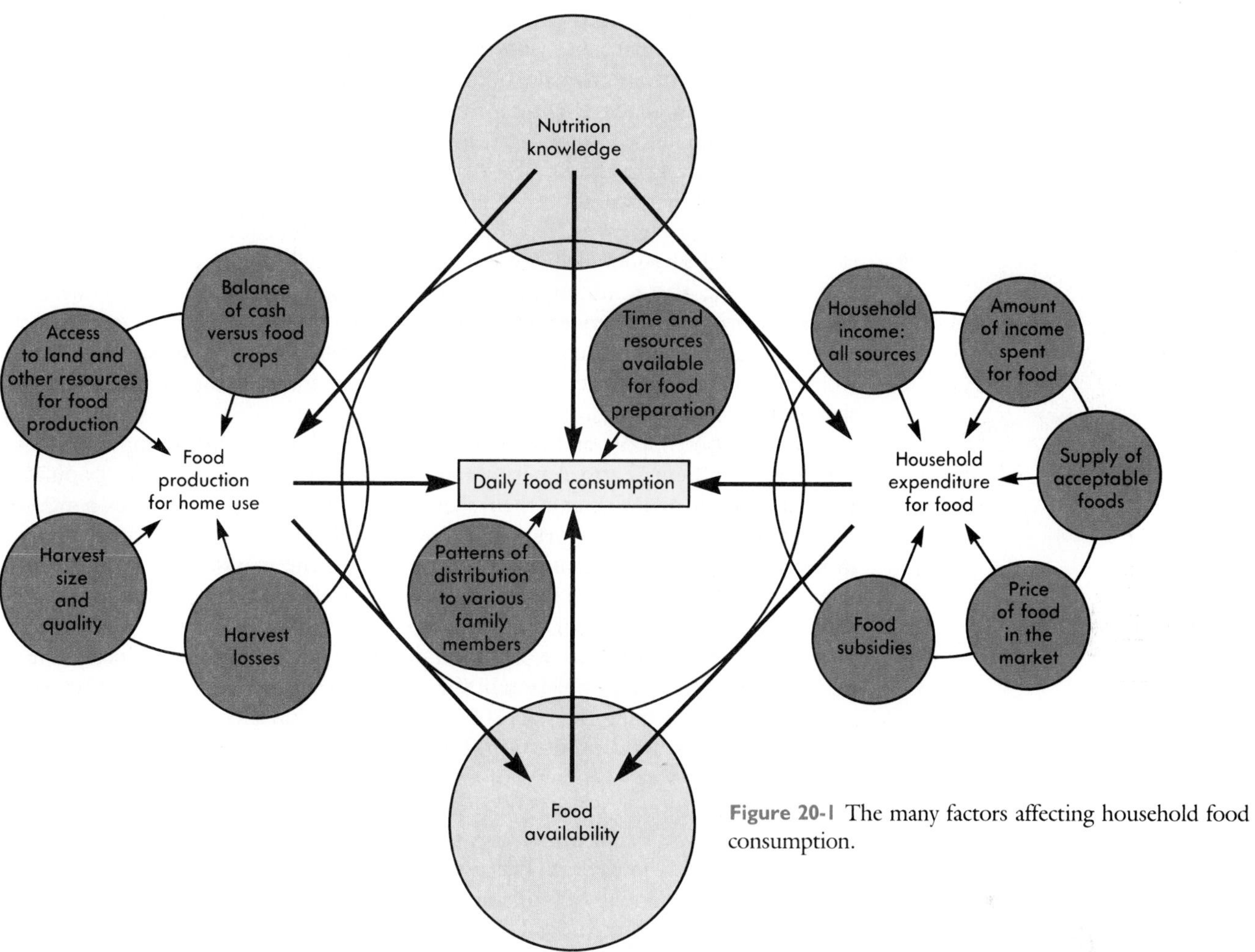

Figure 20-1 The many factors affecting household food consumption.

Let's examine each problem individually. Figure 20-1 depicts factors relating to an individual's food intake.

The Food/Population Ratio

Whether the earth can yield enough food for all has been a long-standing question. As early as 1798, the English demographer and economist, Thomas Malthus, proposed a rather pessimistic view of the prospects for humans. He said that given the passion between the sexes (which he felt was something to be counseled against) the population would always increase in a **geometric ratio**—2, 4, 8, 16, 32 and so on. Meanwhile, at best, the food supply would increase only **arithmetically**—2, 4, 6, 8, 10 and so on. This prediction means that while the food/population ratio might begin at 2/2, eventually population will grow to 32 while food supplies will only increase to feed 10.[24]

geometric ratio A group of numbers where the division of each number by the one to the left of it yields the same answer.

arithmetic ratio A group of numbers where the difference between each number is the same.

Malthus felt that in the likely absence of sexual restraint, the growing population would be subject to recurring checks imposed by famine, war, or natural catastrophe brought on by disease. His proposals became the object of intense controversy in England and elsewhere, often meeting vigorous opposition. Eminent scientists in Britain pointed out that scientific advances in agriculture would greatly increase food production. In fact, that has been true. Nevertheless, the population "explosion" is just that. Malthus was correct in his prediction of geometric growth in the world

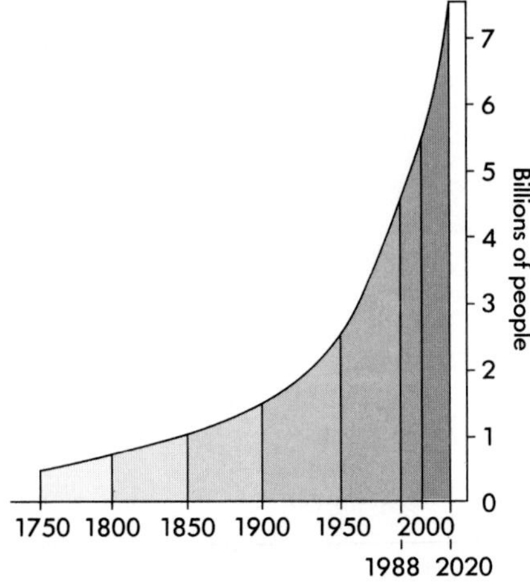

Figure 20-2 World population trends since 1750.

population. So far this growth has not been slowed significantly by either natural checks or recent human interventions, such as birth control (Figure 20-2).

Birth-control programs have been effective in developed countries, but are relatively ineffective in developing countries that could really profit from them.[11] Whereas women in the United States average 1.9 live births each, women in Rwanda (in eastern Africa) average 8.5 live births each (Figure 20-3).

At this time, there are about 5.4 billion persons in the world. About three fourths live in developing Third World countries. Many experts believe that the global supply of food would provide adequate nutrition for all 5.4 billion of us—about 3000 kcalories daily. But food supplies are not distributed equally among consumers. Gross disparities exist between developed and developing countries, among socioeconomic groups within countries, and even within families. In some instances, women and children get less to eat than men, and sometimes girl children get less than boy children.[20]

As well, food supply and population trends within the developing world itself are clearly different. Latin America and Asia both have had declining population growth rates since 1970, and their share of the world population will have risen only marginally between the years 1950 and 2025. On the other hand, the population in Africa will have more than doubled, to 19% of the world population, over the same 75-year period.[11] Here the population will likely rise from 650 million in 1992 to 900 million by the end of the century.

Economists estimate that world food production will continue to increase more rapidly than the world population in the near future, allowing the food/population ratio to increase through the year 2000. In the short run then, the primary problem appears not to be food production, but equitable distribution and utilization, especially in poverty-stricken areas of the developing nations.

Eventually, though, food production will begin to lag behind population growth.[11] And we are currently drifting in that direction. Most good farmland in the world is already in use, and because of poor farming practice or competing land-use demands, the number of farmable acres worldwide decreases annually. For many reasons, sustainable world food output—that which does *not* deplete the earth's resources—is now running well behind food consumption. This suggests that food production in less-developed countries will barely keep up with population growth, and will soon lag behind. That in turn will reduce the reserves needed to both combat and help stave off undernutrition, particularly famine, in poor countries. At present, international grain reserves are at levels barely above what is needed to fill the pipeline from field to table, and were at the lowest levels in December 1991 than at any time in the last 15 years. This is the world's main insurance against undernutrition.

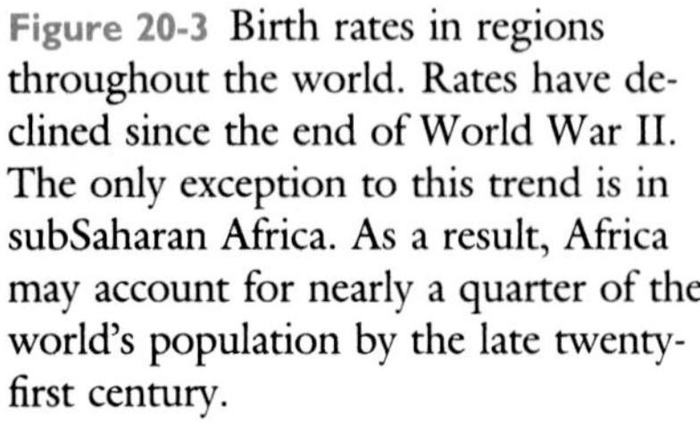

Figure 20-3 Birth rates in regions throughout the world. Rates have declined since the end of World War II. The only exception to this trend is in subSaharan Africa. As a result, Africa may account for nearly a quarter of the world's population by the late twenty-first century.

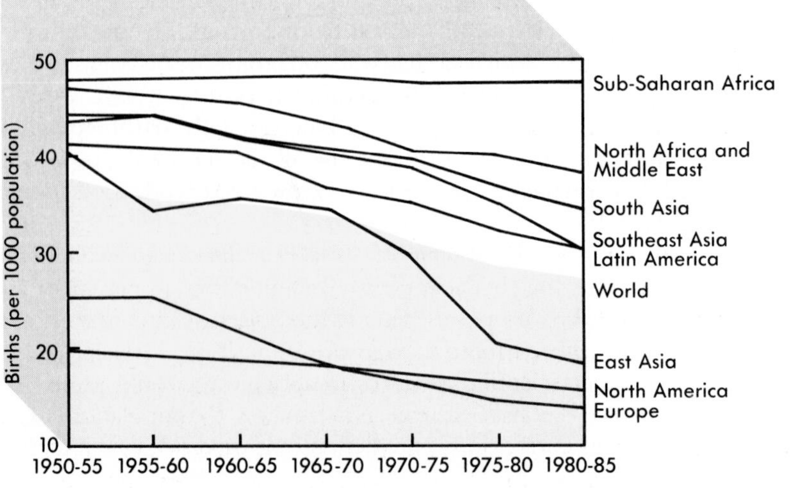

A RENEWED FOCUS ON POPULATION CONTROL

While efforts on the supply side of the food/population ratio are essential, some, but not all scientists in this area of research feel there is no substitute for reducing the demand side. They argue that the survival of our civilization depends on limiting reproduction.[11]

For millions of years, maximizing reproduction has been a measure of biological success. Because disease and difficult living conditions often claimed young lives, producing many offspring by couples was one strategy for carrying on the family. These conditions still hold in Third World countries and constitute as well a key method for providing support in old age. Contrast life expectancy at birth in the United States and Canada—about 76 years—to that in Africa—about 50 years. In the small African country of Sierra Leone life expectancy is about 34 years—a figure reduced partly by averaging in a high infant mortality rate. More children also means more helpers to farm, hunt, and prepare food. Traditionally, poorer people bear more children—unlike what you might predict.

Now, in an evolutionary blink of the eye—mere decades—poor people are being asked to change their entire attitude toward having children. It is a difficult undertaking. In 1888, 1.5 billion people inhabited the earth. Now the population exceeds 5.4 billion and is growing fast. Currently the population increases by three people every second, or about a quarter million every day. In essence, the world must accommodate a new population roughly equivalent to that of the United States and Canada every 3 years!

Even though the overall rate of growth has begun to decline, most population experts believe population size will still pass 10 billion during the next 50 years. The poorest countries are increasing the most, further straining their ability to cope. A 1988 United Nations World Food Council report concluded that earlier progress in fighting undernutrition and poverty has either come to a halt or is being reversed in many parts of the world. This is particularly evident in Africa. The pressure of more people to feed will intensify these problems.

STEMMING THE HUMAN TIDE

Attempts to implement family-planning programs in Third World nations have been met with only partial success. Some small countries, such as Singapore, Taiwan, Thailand, Columbia, Costa Rica, and several Caribbean countries have achieved substantial reductions in their birthrates. Larger countries, including India and Mexico, are struggling.[11]

China has explicitly recognized that it is already overpopulated. It has the world's most stringest family-planning program: The government allows only one child per urban couple, two at most in rural areas. Penalties for having extra children include restricted housing and employment opportunities. China's program, though successful by world standards, has encountered opposition. A new policy that allows families to earn private income, while very successful in increasing food production, has unexpectedly created an incentive to have more children to help earn the income. The overall result has been a recent surge in the birthrate, which has been countered by new efforts to impose restraints.

In the final analysis, successful birth-control programs have to recognize that only when people have enough to eat and are financially secure, will they feel safe having fewer children.[11] By providing the poor with a livelihood that allows access to food, shelter, health care, and enough money to support themselves in old age, experts believe more couples will then *choose* to have fewer children.

Promoting breast-feeding is important to family health and population control. It helps naturally space births farther apart. Solely breast-feeding an infant lessens ovulations in women, and so fertilization, for an average of about 6 months (though it cannot be relied on as a form of birth control). When childbirths are more widely spaced, the health of mother and infant are aided, and fewer total births occur. In addition, in Third World countries breast-feeding cuts infant mortality by providing some of the mother's immune factors for the infant, while also lessening the risk from water-borne diseases. Exclusive breast-feeding in early infancy improves the chance of infant survival, compared with a combination of breast-feeding and bottle-feeding. Other nutritional benefits will be discussed later.

In 1960, families in South Korea were averaging six children each. Economic policies coupled with a strong family-planning program transformed South Korea from a struggling country to an economic success. Today, Korean families average slightly fewer than two children each and the population will soon stabilize.[11] However, nations do not have to wait to become industrialized before launching population control programs. Indonesia, South Korea, and Thailand took great economic strides while at the same time controlling population growth. Still, to date, population stabilization—as in Western countries—has mainly been accompanied by relative wealth and security.

In addition to economics, another unavoidable road block to family-planning programs lies with cultural, religious, and traditional beliefs. In sub-Saharan Africa being childless not only carries an aura of evil for the woman, but also marks the end of a line of descent. The Yoruba believe, for example, that a childless woman has made a pact with evil spirits before her own birth to kill her children; then, devoid of descendants, she will return to join these evil spirits in some otherworldly sphere. Women are almost as afraid of being rendered functionally infertile by the death of all their children as they are of bearing none.[5] Thus female sterilization and even contraception are widely feared. Even women with four or five children fear, not unreasonably, that all the children may suddenly die.

In India, a rigid class structure that leaves those in the lower classes destitute and poor encourages these families to have more children for many of the economic reasons discussed above. Also, Moslem religious practices typically promote a large, abundant family as a sign of prosperity and health.

Malthus' gloomy mathematical prediction may soon become fact. If we cannot find ways of humanely controlling population growth, nature may solve the problem by killing off large portions of humanity in the ways Malthus predicted. Only the future will tell.

CONCEPT CHECK

Currently, world food production is sufficient to meet the energy needs of the world's population. Undernutrition exists, despite adequate food resources, because of poverty, politics, and unequal distribution. Projected population growth may soon overwhelm food production. Limiting population growth, especially in Third World countries where birth rates are high, is a challenging priority.

The Declining State of Agricultural Resources

Population control has become more critical lately as we quickly exhaust and, in some cases, deplete the earth's resources. The productive capacity of agriculture is approaching its limits worldwide. As we mentioned, food production, especially in parts of the Third World, is being undermined by environmentally unsustainable farming methods.

green revolution A time during the 1960s when there was much emphasis in improving strains and cultivation practices of cereal grains, such as rice, wheat, and corn.

The term **"green revolution"** describes a phenomenon starting in the 1960s where a dramatic rise in crop yields in some countries, such as the Philippines, India, and Mexico, was made possible because of increased use of fertilizers and the development of superior crops through careful plant breeding. Many of the "green revolution" technologies have now achieved most of their potential. One example is that rice yield has not increased significantly since the release of superior varieties in 1966. Wheat is another example: India more than tripled its wheat harvest between 1965 and 1983, a period when high-yielding crop strains were introduced. Since

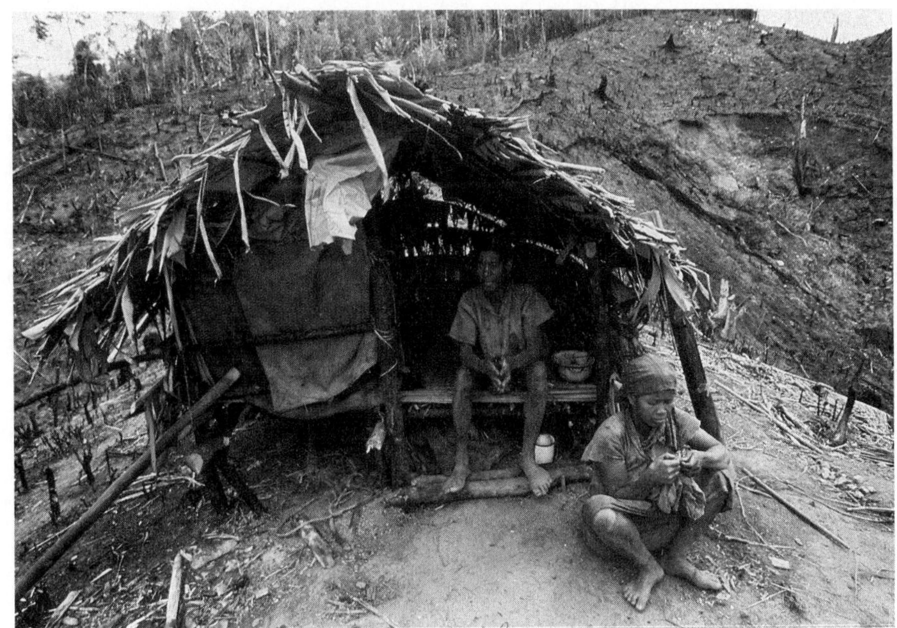

Figure 20-4 Losing ground in their effort to grow rice, farmers in Madagascar survey erosion on hills cleared of rain forest. Farming further depletes the soil, and in turn new land must be cleared. Slash-and-burn farming destroys 50 acres of rain forest an hour worldwide.

then, its grain output has not increased. Future gains in productivity may be much harder to accomplish because of the need to farm less-productive soils.[9]

Africa benefitted least from the green revolution because most farmers there do not grow wheat or rice. They produce cassava, cowpeas, millet, yams, and sorghum. Until the introduction of yet another superior wheat or rice strain, developing countries will not benefit greatly from recent more modest breakthroughs in biotechnology (see the Nutrition Issue). Actually, the green revolution was never supposed to solve the world's food problems, according to Dr Norman Borlaug, its chief architect. It was just a stopgap measure until world leaders could get population growth under control.

Areas of the world that remain uncultivated or ungrazed are mostly of poor quality: rocky, steep, infertile, too dry, too wet, or inaccessible. Much of this land is also invaluable for providing humans crucial **ecosystem** benefits. This is particularly true for humid tropical areas, such as the Amazon basin rain forests, which significantly influence the earth's climate, notably through oxygen production.[11] Some nations, such as Brazil, can still expand onto land that will sustain cultivation, but such countries are in the distinct minority. The overwhelming experience over the last few decades has been overextension of agriculture onto erodible land, followed by predictable degradation, erosion, and abandonment (Figure 20-4).[26]

ecosystem A community in nature that includes plant and animals and the environment associated with them.

The prospects of obtaining substantially more food from the oceans are also poor. Since the early 1970s, the world fish catch per person has been declining. Clearly, we can exploit the earth's resources only so far—world population cannot continue to expand as it does today without potentially invoking serious famine and death.

Attitudes Toward Certain Foods

Culture affects food use just as it does family size. In India, for example, the Hindu reverence for cattle has worsened some already significant nutrition problems. These sacred cows consume food rather than provide it; the wandering cows also considerably damage vegetation which could otherwise feed humans. Although the cows provide milk, there is no effort to improve milk production through selective breeding practices.

In certain areas of India, a child may not be fed milk curds because of a superstitious belief that these inhibit growth, nor bananas because they supposedly cause

Note in the United States many of us shun potential foods like horse meat, insects, textured soy protein, and algae.

convulsions. These are obstacles, but not roadblocks to good nutrition. Given enough food resources, a healthful diet that allows for individual food taboos and prejudices is possible.

The Effects of Poor Infrastructure on Health: Shelter and Sanitation in the Third World

When people die from undernutrition in Third World countries, other influences almost always contribute, such as inadequate shelter and sanitation. Poor sanitation raises the risk for infection, as does undernutrition. Together these represent a lethal combination (Figure 20-5). More than 1 billion people today occupy inadequate and deteriorating shelter with poor conditions. The future looks even worse. By the year 2000, Mexico City will house more than 26 million people, with Sao Paulo, Brazil, Calcutta, India and Bombay, India not far behind. Many of the 15 million child deaths each year in developing countries (half of them in children under 5 years old) could be prevented if standards of environmental hygiene were improved.

Urban populations of some developing countries are currently growing at an annual rate of 5% to 7%. This urban explosion is the result of both high birth rates and continuing migration to the cities from the countryside. It is estimated that by the year 2000 about half of the world's population will live in cities and towns. Such a skewed population distribution will result in further impoverishment. In Brazil, for example, migrants displaced by multinational land developers have flooded from the north and northeast into Rio de Janeiro and Sao Paulo, attracted by the prospect of jobs. There they have built shanty towns next to apartment towers and affluent suburbs, but the jobs do not materialize and the desperate poverty begets more poverty.[11]

In Third World countries, the poor make up most of the urban population, and their needs for housing and community services often outstrip available governmental resources. Most of these urban poor live in overcrowded, self-made shelter that is only partially served by public utilities and lacks a safe and adequate water supply. The shanty towns and ghettos of the Third World countries provide surroundings that are often worse than the rural areas that the people left behind. And because the people now need cash to purchase food, they find themselves with diets that are even more meager than their home-grown rural fare.[20] To make matters worse, makeshift shelters often lack facilities to protect food from spoilage or from the ravages of insects and rodents. In some developing countries food losses can amount to as much as 30% to 40% of the perishable foods.

A move from rural to urban life takes its greatest toll on infants and children. Infants are often weaned early from the breast, partly because the mother seeks employment and partly because she may be trying to emulate the image of sophisticated, formula-using women promoted in advertisements. Unfortunately, infant formulas are relatively expensive, and so poor parents may use too little to meet the baby's needs, or they may overdilute the mixture. Since the water supply may not be safe, the prepared formula is also likely to be grossly contaminated with bacteria. In many nations, bottle-fed infants contract far more illnesses and are as much as 25 times more likely to die in childhood than those who are exclusively breast-fed for the first 6 months of life.

Breast milk is hygienic, readily available, nutritionally sound, and again provides infants with some immune factors. And as we mentioned, breast-feeding encourages longer intervals between births for the mother. In a developing world, advantages of breast-feeding over formula-feeding can mean the difference between life and death. In spite of this, major corporations continue to heavily market infant formulas in these regions.

Overall, the most important single activity that can be undertaken for the health of people, wherever they live, is the provision of a safe and convenient water supply.[9]

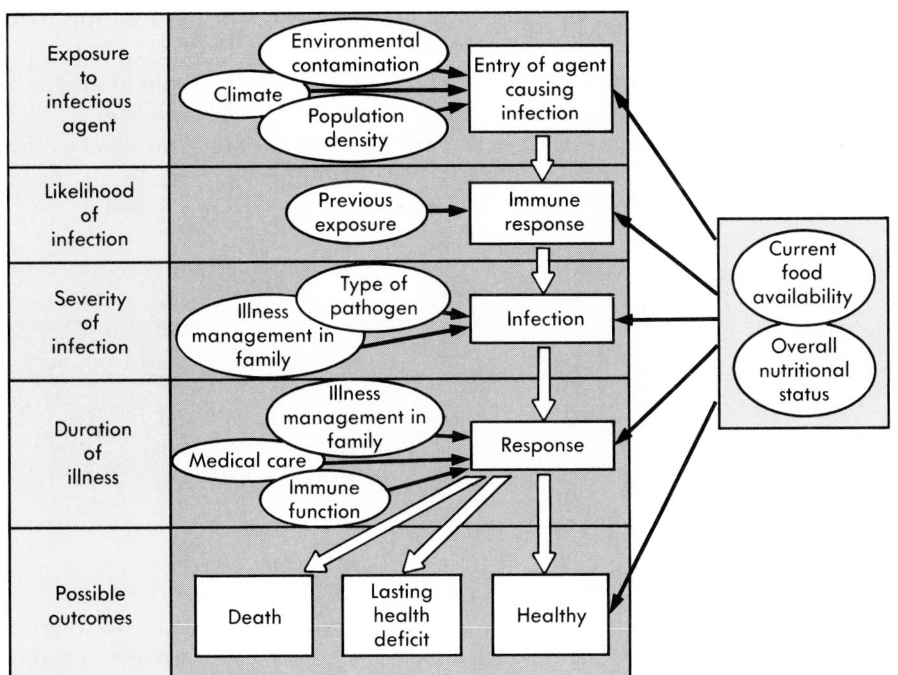

Figure 20-5 Nutrition and infection. The ultimate effect of an infection depends in part on the nutritional state of the person, as well as on many environmental influences.

The World Health Organization (WHO) estimates that 1.2 billion people, about one fifth of all people, were without a safe and adequate water supply in 1990.

Poor sanitation, another example of inadequate infrastructure in the Third World, creates a further critical public health problem. It is common to see human feces, rotting garbage, and associated insect and rodent infestations in Third World cities. Human excreta is a potent source of disease organisms, and ends up as one of the most dangerous substances with which people can come into contact. In some developing countries, diarrheal diseases account for as many as one third of all deaths in children under 5 years of age. WHO estimates that even with progress in housing, 1.8 billion people in the world are still without proper sanitation in 1990.

Health may be further jeopardized by the uncertainty and stress associated with lack of employment, threats to family welfare, effects of poor environment, such as noise and odors, the lack of efficient health care services, and generally deficient socioeconomic circumstances. This goes on to hinder education, parent-child relations, and home life, and may encourage drug and alcohol abuse. Poor living conditions today can create even poorer conditions for children of tomorrow.

To this already unbalanced equation, add the threat to health from Acquired Immune Deficiency Syndrome (AIDS). Developing countries now have two thirds of the world's approximately 13 million human immunodeficiency virus (HIV) infections, and could have 90% of the 40 million infections expected by the year 2000. The continent hardest hit is Africa; Asia follows close behind and is gaining. Note there is no cure for AIDS. AIDS-related infections already represent up to 80% of the hospital admissions in Zambia. Researchers who studied 1458 women living in Kigali, the capital of Rwanda, found an overall HIV-infection rate of 32%. It can take 10 years or longer for a person infected with the AIDS virus to develop AIDS symptoms. Most people with AIDS symptoms then die within a few years. By 2015 AIDS is likely to be the leading cause of death in African countries south of the Sahara desert, with about 70 million cases.

Because the pattern for transmission of HIV is different in most of Africa than in industrialized nations, entire families and villages are being affected. Nearly all of the spread of HIV in Africa is attributed to heterosexual contact. In the United

States, the disease is most frequent among homosexual males and IV drug users. Reuse of hypodermic needles, tainted blood supplies, transfer of the virus to the infant at birth, multiple sexual partners, and prostitution all contribute to the spread of HIV in Africa. The economic impact as more become ill will be enormous.[9] Note that since most of the AIDS-related deaths are among able-bodied men and women who are rearing families, many children are left without parents. In an already weakened economy, the long-term effects may be similar to a prolonged war.

CONCEPT CHECK

Poor housing conditions, impure water, inadequate sanitation, and high-risk AIDS-related practices worldwide increase the risk for infection and disease. Infection then combines with undernutrition to further compromise health status. A healthy diet, clean drinking water, breast-feeding infants, and sanitary handling of human waste all contribute to health—all should be the rights of every human being. Lessening the spread of AIDS must be a worldwide priority.

War and Civil Unrest

The President of Mali recently stated, "... Only by translating our sense of common destiny into action will we be able to resolve the paradox of currently spending $1 trillion each year in the production of lethal weapons, while only a fraction of that sum would make our planet a land of prosperity for millions of people who today suffer from illness, hunger, thirst and ignorance."

Worldwide military spending has doubled over the past 20 years to more than $2 million dollars a minute.[9] The amount spent on weapons every minute could feed 2000 undernourished children for 1 year. The Third World's share of the global arms budget increased from 9% to 16% from 1977 to 1987, draining resources that could be used to combat poverty and hunger. Presently, less than one half of 1% of the total world yearly production of goods and services is devoted to economic development assistance, while approximately 6% goes to military expenditures.

In the worst of cases, civil disruptions and war contribute in large measure to massive undernutrition. There are more civil conflicts being fought in Africa today than in any other region of the world. The militarization of the continent has decreased somewhat with the easing of tensions between the United States and the former Soviet Union, but military spending in Angola, Chad, Ethiopia (through the end of 1990), Uganda, and Zaire remained double the combined total of health and education outlays. The recent war in Angola left 800,000 homeless, 80,000 maimed, and cost the country $20 billion dollars.

Even when food might be available, political divisions may well impede distribution—using food as a weapon—such that undernutrition will continue to be the lot of many people for years into the future. In addition, aid programs aimed at the poor, especially during emergencies, have been undermined by poor administration, corruption, and political influence.

In the 1970s, the problem of undernutrition was perceived as a technical one—how to produce enough food for the growing world population. Today, the problem is largely a political one—a focus of which is how to achieve cooperation among and within nations.

External Debt

At a recent meeting of the United Nations, many developing countries asserted that they were on the verge of economic collapse, and felt that a major contributing factor was the $1.3 trillion external debt they collectively owed. Latin American debt represents 45% of the region's gross regional output of goods and services. Nearly 40% of total export earnings are spent in paying off this debt. One option is for Latin American nations to form a comprehensive plan aimed at renegotiating the external debt on more realistic terms. The current debt of the United States limits its ability to help correct this problem (and to help its own poor as well).

Many African nations carry large debt burdens. Still, they need to import—and pay for—machinery, concrete, trucks, and consumer goods. To make up the difference between export income and import expenses, countries have been forced to borrow billions of dollars from international banks. While the African debts are much smaller in absolute terms than the debts of Brazil, Argentina, and Mexico, for example, the actual burden is greater when national incomes and export earnings are considered. Nearly half the money African nations earn from exports goes to paying off the continent's multibillion dollar debt. As a result, African nations have had to impose austerity programs, in turn restricting imports of food, fuel, and farm machinery. The effects of wage cuts and the increased prices for food and consumer goods can push many of these poor nations over the edge into widespread undernutrition.

Possible Solutions to Undernutrition in the Third World

As you have probably guessed, eliminating undernutrition in the Third World will be complicated. It actually may likely be impossible without bold new thinking and initiatives. In the 1980s it was a common practice for the more abundant nations of the world to supply famished areas with direct food aid.[27] Though highly publicized and praised at the time, direct food aid is not a long-term solution. While reducing the number of deaths from famine, it can also reduce incentives for local production for farmers by driving down local prices. In addition, the affected countries may have little or no means of transporting the food to those who need it most. Furthermore, the donated foods may meet with little cultural acceptance.

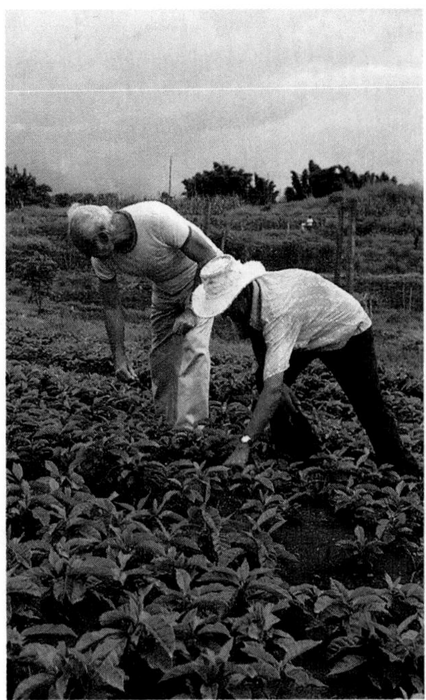

Poor people in less developed countries benefit from access to the land to help maintain food security.

In the short run, there is no choice—aid must be given because people are starving. Still, improving the infrastructure for poor people, especially rural people, needs to be the long-term focus. This is because the most significant factor affecting undernutrition of people in impoverished areas is their reliance on outside sources for basic needs. Their dependence makes them constantly vulnerable.[12]

Recall that in the last 20 years world food supplies have grown faster than population. Thus the increase in undernutrition during this time period is due mainly to an increase in the number of people cut off from their fair share of this supply. Millions of farmers are losing access to resources they need in order to be self-reliant. And the number of households with insufficient means to support themselves is growing. In response, careful small-scale, regional development is needed.[9] There is a growing realization that the rural landless will flock to the overcrowded cities unless economic opportunities can be created for them.

Small-scale rural enterprises and off-farm activities would ensure that poor people in rural areas who have no access to land or other assets can acquire "entitlement" to food. Such enterprises can be run by the people who stand to benefit, either as individuals or as members of small groups, using very limited capital. A prerequisite would be access to credit, appropriate technologies, a market, and ability to transport the product to that market. Households that presently have land could be helped in different ways so that they would be able to feed themselves.

cash crop Crops grown by countries with specific intent to export in order to gain the ability to purchase goods from other countries, rather than feed the country's citizens. Examples are coffee, tea, cocoa, and bananas.

In Africa and elsewhere in the developing world, women tend to produce most of the food crops consumed in the home, and often produce as much as half the **cash crops** sold for income. Lack of credit is a major obstacle when women take over homes and farms. Strengthening the opportunities for rural women must be seen as a goal that will benefit not only women, but all of Africa and other parts of the developing world. Women especially need access to the inputs that can allow subsistence food production to happen.[20]

For the most part, the problem is one of helping people produce much of their own needs for subsistence and directing them to resources and employment opportunities. Experience has shown that credit—along with training, food-storage facilities, and marketing—allows rural people to participate in development to their benefit and the benefit of their families and communities. Suitable technologies for processing, preserving, marketing, and distributing traditional, nutritious local staples need to be encouraged.

Land ownership brings many advantages, particularly available food. If instead food resources become concentrated in the hands of a few, as often happens in unequal land ownership, it won't be equally distributed unless efficient transportation systems are in place. Inequitable distribution then leads to problems that prove very difficult to resolve.

Raising the economic status of impoverished people by employing them turns out to be as important as expanding the food supply.[9] If an increase in food supply is achieved without an accompanying rise in employment, then there may be no long-term change in the number of undernourished people. It is possible to see food prices fall with increased mechanization, use of fertilizers, and other modern technologies. But these very same advances can displace jobs for more people. When this happens, the food that is produced will still be out of reach for those who need it most.

A shipment of high-tech tractors, for example, might put local laborers out of work. Rice might be planted more efficiently using farm machinery, but using human power eventually leaves more humans with the resources to buy food. Success in reducing undernutrition in the Third World must occur by employing more poor people in a productive manner on available land, or by providing other jobs. From a Third World point of view, it is of little consequence that these jobs are technologically primitive by Western standards.

Finally, current exploitation of Third World countries, such as the massive marketing effort of infant formula manufacturers, must be examined by the American public. Recent disturbing reports of deaths from toxic pesticides and medicines banned in the United States but sold to developing countries raises many questions. What are the roles and responsibilities of wealthier nations in our global community, and how can we direct our resources to help developing nations, rather than to reap profits from their dependence on us?

CONCLUDING THOUGHTS

It is prudent to assume that the developing world will have to rely largely on its own resources to finance development, especially in light of the current budget deficit in the United States. It is even more essential then to make full use of human resources available in the developing world itself. The "right" choice for production ends up depending on the relative need to employ people and the numbers of people available to do the work.

Overemphasizing cash crops, such as coffee, tea, rubber, and cocoa—as some developing countries have done, especially in Latin America—is not likely to solve the nutritional problems of poor people. Cash crops are usually grown at the expense of food crops on the assumption that money earned from the cash crops will be used to purchase enough food for the families of the workers. However, this is not always the case.[20] Food can be bought, but it may not be enough and it would be more expensive. In such a situation, poorer families are at greater risk than others since the money earned from cash crops is often not enough to meet other basic family needs, let alone their food needs. As with poor families in the United States, buying quality foods often takes second priority, resulting in nutritional deprivation.

The battle against world undernutrition then is twofold: to supply nutrients to the undernourished and to reduce the number of people in danger of undernutrition. The second part of this battle is a very real one. Many delegates to a recent Food and Agriculture Organization of the United Nations (FAO) conference stressed the need for strategies that could supply food to vulnerable households, subsidize basic commodities purchased by the poor, and raise the employment and income-generating capacity of the poor.

NUTRITION FOCUS

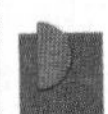

Low Input Sustainable Agriculture Is Also Needed

The Food and Agriculture Organization (FAO) of the United Nations works on this principle: "The fight to ensure that all people have enough nutritious food to eat is worthy of our greatest efforts, but it must be fought with the full recognition that it cannot be won unless agricultural, fisheries, and forestry production returns to the earth as much—or more—than it takes." These words suggest we need to take immediate steps to protect an already fragile environment from further deterioration if the world is to feed a population of 6 billion by the year 2000 (Figure 20-4).

Low input sustainable agriculture (LISA) is one method to achieve this goal. This practice seeks to reduce use of purchased inputs (chemicals, machinery, etc.), while maintaining or increasing yields and farm profits.[7] The overall objective is to reduce costs, environmental and health hazards, and natural resource degradation. Sustainable agriculture offers a system of farm production that relies chiefly on working with nature, rather than trying to conquer it. The biological and stewardship techniques employed have already demonstrated adequate agricultural returns, without locking farmers into an expensive and environmentally damaging array of new farm inputs. Pesticides, fertilizers, water, and soil erosion are all receiving special attention. The LISA concept is gaining support both in the United States and Third World countries.

Rather than resorting to **herbicide** exclusively to knock out weeds, farmers can combine timely cultivation with variations in planting dates and seeding rates to produce thicker canopies at the right time to shade out weeds. LISA is also reintroducing crop rotations—a traditional farming practice that provides effective pest control with sufficient economic returns. In many instances commercial pesticides are still the best, most cost-effective, or only means for growing a successful crop. But, LISA techniques can substantially reduce use of chemical pesticides.

Export of American-made agrichemicals to Third World countries is a time bomb in the area of worker safety. Virtually all chemical use in those countries is by hand application. Many of the extremely toxic materials, such as methyl parathion, are virtually impossible to apply safely by hand under tropical conditions. Sooner or later, political, if not moral pressure will force an industry response to this very real problem.

Today, the conventional emphasis on maximum yields relies on heavy additions of fertilizers. The LISA farm community is seeking soil nutrient management practices that focus instead on long-term soil health rather than short-term yields. This in turn allows for maximum economic return, use of the soil's internal capacity for regeneration, and minimization of damage to ground and surface water. Crop rotation is an important tool in this effort.

Although not widely recognized at this time, recent growth in world food output has been achieved in part by practicing unsustainable methods, such as plowing highly erodible land and depleting water tables through overirrigation.[11] In Africa, a land area twice the size of New Jersey is turned into unproductive desert each year because of soil erosion. Since World War II, more than 3 billion acres of agricultural land—an area larger than China and India combined—have been damaged by human actions and may prove costly or impossible to reclaim. The erosion is caused by overgrazing livestock, destructive farming techniques, and destroying mature rain forests. LISA can help stem this. Many of Africa's cash crops damage the land, draining the soil of vital nutrients. Then, when the land has been used up, farmers move on to other areas, leaving behind desolated land ripe for soil erosion. In the short run, farmers can overplow and overpump with impressive results, but in doing so they are using up the natural resources on which long-term farm productivity depends.

Nearly all available irrigation water worldwide is currently used, and groundwater supplies are becoming depleted at rapid rates in many regions. China, which has more than 20% of the world's irrigated land, is plagued with a growing scarcity of fresh water. Third World countries often overconcentrate poultry, swine, and milk production around metropolitan areas, in turn polluting and overdrafting ground water.

Today, one third of the earth's population does not receive enough food to maintain an active working life, though enough grain is still produced to supply 3000 kcalories daily for every man, woman, and child on the planet. More than half of this grain is grown in the Third World. The economic loss is staggering, and the amount of human pain and suffering is incalculable.[9] With all the international relief efforts, government assistance, and private organizations combined, we are still operating in the Dark Ages in our battle against undernutrition.

PREVENTING FAMINE

Policies to prevent famine must focus on increasing the productivity of rural people and reducing war and civil strife. Then as agricultural surpluses grow, producers can sell some, rather than consume all of their harvest. Livestock numbers will grow, absorbing surplus grain and providing animal protein. As rural wealth grows, food becomes a smaller portion of the household budget. If disaster strikes, food stocks will be adequate, livestock can be slaughtered, and price swings are more tolerable. The conditions of scarcity that characterize famine then cease to arise.[12] In the end, it is positive government action that must strengthen the rural economies, thus ending the kind of desperate poverty that links natural or man-made disasters to famine, and ultimately to widespread death. Little such preparedness planning exists in Africa today. Famine-prone African countries are very fully dependent on international sources of supply for food, medicine, transport, and famine management. However, these usually arrive on the scene after the famine has already peaked. Local remedies, such as food reserves, can be put into action much sooner. Perhaps if we rid ourselves of negative government actions worldwide, the task could become easier?

CONCEPT CHECK

War, civil strife, and external debt contribute to the difficulty of ending undernutrition in many Third World countries. Overall, the solution seems to lie in providing sufficient employment so that people can purchase the food their families need and/or providing access to land and other food production resources. Programs must be sensitive to regional conditions to ensure that new technologies introduced don't intensify existing problems for the poorest people. Simple approaches are appropriate if people using them are left with the resources needed to feed their families.

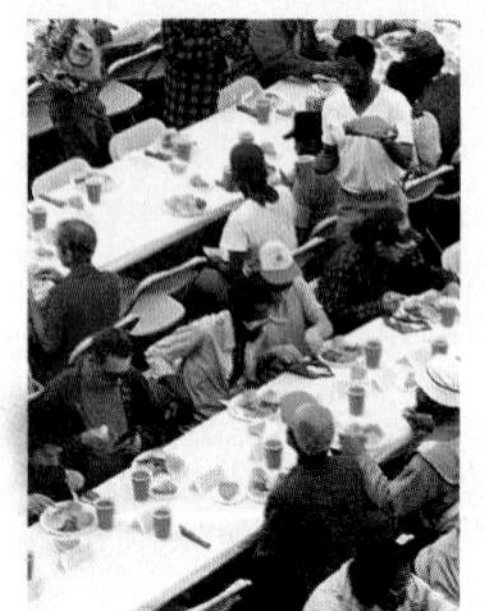

Summary

1. Poverty is a common thread wherever people show undernutrition. Malnutrition can occur when the food supply is either scarce or abundant. The resulting deficiency conditions or degenerative diseases are influenced by genetic makeup.
2. Undernutrition is the most common form of malnutrition in developing countries. It results from inadequate intake, absorption, or use of nutrients or kcalories. Many deficiency conditions then appear and infectious diseases thrive because the immune system cannot function properly.
3. The greatest risk of undernutrition occurs during critical periods of growth and development: pregnancy, infancy, and childhood. Low birth weight is a leading cause of infant deaths worldwide. Many developmental problems are caused by nutritional deprivation during critical periods of brain growth.
4. Undernutrition diminishes both physical and mental capabilities. In poor countries, this is worsened by recurrent infections, poor sanitary conditions, extreme weather, inadequate shelter, and exposure to diseases.
5. In the United States, famine has been nonexistent since the 1930s, but undernutrition is present. Soup kitchens, food stamps, school lunch and breakfast programs, and the Supplemental Feeding Program for Women, Infants, and Children (WIC) have focused on improving the nutritional health of poor and at-risk people. These programs have proven effective in reducing undernutrition, especially when adequately funded.
6. Multiple factors contribute to the problem of undernutrition in Third World countries. In densely populated countries, food resources may be inadequate and the means for distributing food may be poor. Farming methods often encourage erosion, which deprives the soil of valuable nutrients, thus defeating future efforts to grow food. Poor water availability hampers food production. Naturally occurring devastation from droughts, excessive rainfall, fire, crop infestation, and human causes, such as urbanization, civil unrest, war, debt, and poor sanitation, all contribute to the major problem of undernutrition, as well as famine.

7. Any proposed solutions to the problem of world undernutrition must consider the interaction of multiple factors, many of which are thoroughly embedded in cultural traditions. Family planning efforts, for example, may not succeed until life expectancy can be raised. Through education, efforts should be made to improve farming methods, encourage breast-feeding, and improve sanitation and hygiene. Direct food aid is only a short-term solution. In what may appear to be a step backward, a focus on subsistence-level farming, away from the specialization of cash crops, is needed in order to increase the economic status of people reliant on traditional rain-fed agriculture. Low input sustainable agriculture is one method to employ. The overall goal is to gain meaningful employment and purchasing power for vast numbers of the rural poor.

Study Questions

1. Describe in a short paragraph evidence of undernutrition that you have seen in the society around you while you were growing up. What are/were the roots of these problems?

2. Why is solving the problem of undernutrition a key factor in development of the ultimate potential of Third World countries? What basic nutrients are keys to the health and growth of these people?

3. Choose one problem that contributes to the complex picture of famine. In one page, describe the problem and discuss possible solutions.

4. What do you believe contributes to undernutrition in wealthy nations, such as the United States? What are some solutions to these problems?

5. A person you recently met asks you where to find food and shelter. Where would you first direct this person in your community for help? If you are unsure, try to find out.

REFERENCES

1. American Dietetic Association: Position of The American Dietetic Association: domestic hunger and inadequate access to food, *Journal of The American Dietetic Association* 90:1437, 1990.
2. Brown JL, Allen D: Hunger in America, *Annual Reviews of Public Health* 9:503, 1988.
3. Brown LR: The world food crisis, *USA Today,* March 1989.
4. Buzina R and others: Workshop on functional significance of mild-to-moderate malnutrition, *American Journal of Clinical Nutrition* 50:172, 1989.
5. Caldwell JC, Caldwell P: High fertility in sub-Saharan Africa, *Scientific American,* May 1990, p 118.
6. Campbell C and others: The role of nutrition professionals in the hunger debate, *Journal of the Canadian Dietetic Association* 49:230, 1988.
7. Chabot BF: Sustainable agriculture is model for extension, *Community Nutrition Institute News,* March 1990, p 4.
8. Cohen BE and others: Food sources and intake of homeless persons, *Journal of Nutrition Education* 24:45S, 1992.
9. Cohen MJ, Hoehn RA: *Hunger 1992,* Washington, D.C., 1991, Bread for the World Institute.
10. Cotugna N, Vickery CE: Nurturing social responsibility: Nutrition students volunteer in hunger projects, *Journal of The American Dietetic Association* 92:297, 1992.
11. Ehrlich PR, Ehrlich AH: Population, plenty, and poverty, *National Geographic,* December 1988, p 913.
12. Field JO: Famine: A perspective for the nutrition community, *Nutrition Reviews* 49:144, 1991.
13. Gibson RS and others: Growth in children from the Wosera subdistrict, Papua New Guinea, in relation to energy and protein intakes and zinc status, *American Journal of Clinical Nutrition* 53:782, 1991.
14. Grumbach MM and others: Bovine somatotropin and the safety of cows' milk: National Institutes of Health Technology Assessment Conference Statement, *Nutrition Reviews* 49:227, 1991.
15. Husaini MA and others: Developmental effects of short-term supplementary feeding in nutritionally-at-risk Indonesian infants, *American Journal of Clinical Nutrition* 54:799, 1991.
16. Keusch GT: Vitamin A supplements—too good not to be true, *The New England Journal of Medicine* 323:985, 1990.
17. Knapp STF: Reflections on nutrition education for the rural, low-income community, *Nutrition Today,* Nov/Dec 1991, p 32.
18. Latham MC and others: Improvements in growth following iron supplementation in young Kenyan school children, *Nutrition* 6:159, 1990.
19. Lewis S: Food security, environment, poverty, and the world's children, *Journal of Nutrition Education* 24:3S, 1992.
20. Marangu L: Food crisis in Africa, *Canadian Home Economics Journal* 39:144, 1989.
21. Mayer J: Nutritional problems in the United States: Then and now two decades later, *Nutrition Today,* Jan/Feb 1990, p 17.
22. Meyers AF: Undernutrition, hunger, and learning in children, *Nutrition News* 52:1, 1989.
23. Miller HI, Ackerman SJ: Perspective on food biotechnology, *FDA Consumer,* March 1990, p 6.
24. Olson RE: World food production and problems in human nutrition, *Nutrition Today,* Jan/Feb 1989, p 18.

25. Rivera JA and others: Effect of supplementary feeding on recovery from mild to moderate wasting in preschool children, *American Journal of Clinical Nutrition* 54:62, 1991.
26. Saran R: Food and the environment, *Food Policy,* Feb 1990, p 76.
27. Singer HW: The African food crisis and the role of food aid, *Food Policy,* Aug 1989, p 196.
28. Walker SP and others: Nutritional supplementation, psychosocial stimulation, and growth of stunted children: the Jamaican study, *American Journal of Clinical Nutrition* 54:642, 1991.
29. Zeitlin M: Nutritional resilience in a hostile environment: positive deviance in child nutrition, *Nutrition Reviews* 49:259, 1991.

SUGGESTED READINGS

The article by Brown and Allen provides a detailed review of the changing face of hunger in America. The article by Mayer asks us to take a close look at the political reasons for our current hunger crisis. Both these articles set the stage for understanding the position paper by The American Dietetic Association. The article by the Ehrlichs outlines the role of overpopulation in world hunger. These scientists have been leading advocates for population control for the last 30 years. The article by Olson further discusses world food problems in the context of population control and food production. The article by Singer discusses the dilemma faced when food aid is given during times of semistarvation. It points out that there are no simple solutions to this problem of world hunger—a theme echoed by this chapter.

TAKE ACTION

Fighting world undernutrition on a personal level

The following are suggested activities for doing something about world and domestic undernutrition. Like any change in behavior, don't try to do too many things at once. Try one or two of them, representing your personal stand against this gigantic problem.

1. Donate money, possibly $5 to $10 dollars per week, to a voluntary agency that does work in the United States and abroad such as those listed below:

   Bread for the World
802 Rhode Island Ave., N.E.
Washington, D.C. 20018

   The Hunger Project
2015 Steiner St.
San Francisco, CA 94115

   Oxfam America
115 Broadway
Boston, MA 02116

   Seeds
222 East Lake Dr.
Decatur, GA 30030

   Save the Children Federation
P.O. Box 970
Westport, CT 06881

   Institute for Food and Development Policy
1885 Mission St.
San Francisco, CA 94103

   Food Research and Action Center
1875 Connecticut Ave., N.W. #540
Washington, D.C. 20009

   Catholic Relief Services
209 W Fayette St.
Baltimore, MD 21201

   Interreligious Taskforce on U.S. Food Policy
110 Maryland Ave. NE
Washington, D.C. 20002

   CARE
660 First Ave.
New York, NY 10016

   Children's Defense Fund
122 C Street, N.W.
Washington, DC 20001

   Lutheran World Relief
390 Park Ave. S
New York, NY 10016

   Second Harvest
116 South Michigan Ave.
Suite #4
Chicago, IL 60603

2. Write a letter to one of your senators or congressmen asking what they are doing about ending domestic and world undernutrition.
3. Volunteer at a local soup kitchen or homeless shelter for a time-limited period (a few days to 1 month).
4. Call your local social service agency and ask what services are available locally to deal with hunger and undernutrition in the community. Then ask about how to donate money or volunteer your services.
5. Sponsor a child in a foreign country with monthly financial aid for food and clothing. To do this you can write:

   World Vision International
Box 0
Pasadena, CA 91109

6. Contribute to World Food Day activities each October 16th.
7. Organize students on your campus. At Miami University in Oxford, Ohio, two students saw the successful culmination of a year-long effort to provide food for the homeless in the suburban Cincinnati area by distributing excess food from the university's dining halls. Let us know about your efforts! ▲

NUTRITION PERSPECTIVE

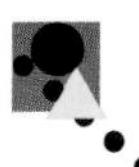

Biotechnology As An Answer to Food Shortage

The human ability to manipulate nature has enabled us to improve the production and yield of many important foods. Traditional **biotechnology** is almost as old as agriculture. The first farmer to selectively improve his stock by breeding the best bull with the best cows was implementing biotechnology in a simple sense. The first baker who used yeast to make bread rise was likewise using biotechnology to produce an improved product.

biotechnology Use of advanced scientific techniques to alter and ideally improve characteristics of animals.

By the 1930s, biotechnology made it possible to selectively breed better plant hybrids; as a result corn production in the United States quickly doubled. Through similar methods, agricultural wheat was crossed with wild grasses in order to acquire more desirable properties, such as greater yield, increased resistance to mildew and bacterial diseases, and tolerance to salt or adverse climatic conditions.

Another type of biotechnology uses hormones rather than breeding. In the last decade Canadian salmon have been treated with a hormone that allows them to mature three times faster than normal—without changing the fish in any other way.

The New Biotechnology

The "new biotechnology" that is part of agriculture today includes a number of methods that directly modify products. It differs from traditional methods because it directly changes some of the genetic material (DNA) of organisms to improve characteristics. No longer is cross-breading plants or animals the only tool.[23] The new process, called **genetic engineering,** was developed mostly in the 1970s. It now covers a wide range of cell and subcell techniques for synthesizing and then placing genetic material in organisms. This allows access to a wider gene pool, and it permits faster and more accurate production of new and more useful microbial, plant, and animal species. However, it is important to note that genetic engineering does not replace conventional breeding practices; both work together.

genetic engineering Alteration of genetic material in plants or animals with the intent of improving growth, disease resistance, or other characteristics.

Currently, genetic engineering at the farm level has led to new types of seeds, availability of new growth hormones, and application of microbial inoculants to stop pests and frost damage. Biotechnology is also being used to develop drought-tolerant crops, as well as for methods to better detect the bacteria that cause food-borne illness, such as *Listeria*. Plants are being engineered to grow without pesticides and new forms of potatoes can last without preservatives. To our eyes and palates, these first benefits of the new biotechnology may seem only subtly different, but the ultimate benefits could be substantial.

Questions surround the use of the new biotechnology. Take, for instance, research on a new tomato genetically-engineered to allow it to stay firm longer. Is it still a tomato? It looks the same, feels the same, tastes the same, and even has the identical nutritional value as that of the original product. The only change researchers have made is to counteract the action of a single gene in the DNA that makes tomatoes rot rapidly. The reversal of just one gene out of 10,000 is the only change needed to make the "biotech" tomato different from the standard garden variety.[23]

Still, ultimately the question remains: How many properties can be changed in a plant, animal, or bacteria before it becomes something else? A tomato altered in only one specific way still seems to be a tomato, but does it remain one if it is "improved" in 10 or 20 ways? Will its ability to thwart pests pose toxic risks to us as well? When traditional methods crossed a tangerine with a grapefruit, the new genetic structure was clearly something else, now commonly known as a tangelo.

Is the New Biotechnology Safe?

The above questions force the new biotechnology to continue to develop under protest. Although genetically modified organisms offer the possibility of reducing environmentally detrimental activities, such as the use of chemical pesticides, critics

NUTRITION PERSPECTIVE

Biotechnology As An Answer to Food Shortage—cont'd

point out past mistakes of releasing "foreign agents," such as insects and plants, into areas with no natural predators. While the risks may appear to be momentarily negligible, they may be cumulative, and so, dangerous in the long run.

Public opinion has long been turning against processes perceived as harmful to the environment, such as producing "unnatural" products. Since food reserves are high in the United States, Canada, and Europe, even increasing food production has been questioned. The prime example of skepticism concerning unnatural products is western Europe's ban of the growth hormone previously used in beef production there. They felt the increase in meat supply was not worth the perceived risks posed by the product. In the United States, the first genetically-engineered food product for humans, an enzyme called renin that is used in making cheese, is in wide use after FDA approval. Will a protest over use of renin arise?

Other potentially beneficial applications of the new biotechnology are currently being studied by both scientists and concerned consumer groups. Bovine somatotropin (BST), a hormone produced by cattle, has been known since the 1930s to increase milk production when injected into dairy cattle. Today an identical BST produced through genetic engineering can be used to greatly increase milk yield.[14] Because it is a protein, any BST in the milk produced would be digested and, therefore, inactivated when eaten. People even produce their own form of somatotropin, but it is structured considerably different from that in BST. Since cows produce BST naturally, it has always been present in their milk. Treating the animals with the proposed higher levels of BST won't increase the level of hormone occurring naturally in the milk, nor will it alter the milk's nutrient composition.

While FDA is still evaluating the animal and environmental safety of BST, the agency has determined that the milk from treated animals is safe for humans. One question is whether the increased milk production will stress the health of the cows themselves, leading farmers to use more antibiotics, which can show up in milk. The public already appears to oppose it, and European Economic Community has banned its use. Again, with milk surpluses in the United States and Europe, there is little to help garner public support. Furthermore, dairy farmers in Wisconsin, as well as other dairy-producing regions, are generally opposed to the introduction of the hormone because they fear negative consumer reaction will cause lower milk consumption. The industry is also concerned that a sharp increase in milk output would adversely affect prices and, in turn, harm thousands of small dairy farms facing an already precarious economic situation.

Will the New Biotechnology Help Reduce Third World Undernutrition?

Whether genetically engineered applications will help reduce Third World undernutrition remains to be seen. Unless price cuts parallel the increased production, landowners and suppliers of biotechnology will capture the benefits of biotechnology, and so its rewards will most likely remain unshared. This principle needs to be emphasized; the person who couldn't afford a tangelo yesterday probably won't be able to afford one tomorrow. The same can be said for improved tomatoes. And as with most innovations, the more successful farmers, often those with larger farms, will adopt the new biotechnology first. Because of this, the present trend to fewer, larger farms will continue in the Third World—a trend that is counterproductive in addressing the most pressing undernutrition issues there. Furthermore, biotechnology does not promise dramatic gains in grain production—the primary food resource in the world.

For the Third World, the focus needs to be on providing people with resources to produce and/or purchase their own food, rather than on simply growing more food. Biotechnology is merely a useful tool, not a panacea.

Appendices

APPENDIX A

Food Composition Tables

Baby Foods

Food Name	Portion	WT. Gm	KCAL Kc	PROT Gm	CARB Gm	FAT Gm	CHOL Mg	SAFA Gm	MUFA Gm	PUFA Gm	SOD Mg	POT Mg
BABY-CARROTS	OUNCE	28.4	8	0.2	1.7	0	0	0	0	0	11	55.6
BABY-TEETHING BISCUITS	ITEM	11	43	1.2	8.4	0.5	0	—	—	—	40	35
BABY-MIXED CEREAL/MILK	OUNCE	28.4	32	1.3	4.5	1	0	—	—	—	13.3	56
BABY-OATMEAL CEREAL/MILK	OUNCE	28.4	33	1.4	4.3	1.2	0	—	—	—	13	58
BABY-RICE CEREAL/MILK	OUNCE	28.4	33	1.1	4.7	1	0	—	—	—	13	54
BABY-BEEF LASAGNA	OUNCE	28.4	22	1.2	2.8	0.6	—	—	—	—	129	35
BABY-BEEF STEW	OUNCE	28.4	14	1.4	1.5	0.3	3.55	0.16	0.12	0.01	98	40
BABY-MIXED VEGETABLES	OUNCE	28.4	11	0.3	2.7	0.028	0	0	0	0	2	34
BABY-TURKEY & RICE	OUNCE	28.4	14	0.5	2.1	0.4	2.84	0.12	0.15	0.04	5	12
BABY-VEAL & VEGETABLES	OUNCE	28.4	20	1.7	1.7	0.8	—	—	—	—	7	43
BABY-APPLE BLUEBERRY	OUNCE	28.4	17	0.1	4.6	0.1	0	0	0	0	0	20
BABY-APPLESAUCE	OUNCE	28.4	12	0.1	3.1	0	0	0	0	0	1	20
BABY-PEACHES	OUNCE	28.4	20	0.1	5.4	0	0	0	0	0	2	46
BABY-PEARS	OUNCE	28.4	12	0.1	3.1	0	0	0	0	0	1	37
BABY-APPLE PEACH JUICE	FL OZ	31	14	0	3.6	0	0	0	0	0	1	28
BABY-APPLE PEACH JUICE	FL OZ	31	13	0	3.2	0	0	0	0	0	0.31	30
BABY-ORANGE JUICE	FL OZ	31	14	0.2	3.2	0.1	0	0	0	0	0	57
BABY-BEEF	OUNCE	28.4	30	3.9	0	1.5	—	0.73	0.62	0.06	23	62
BABY-CHICKEN	OUNCE	28.4	37	3.9	0	2.2	—	0.58	1.01	0.54	13	40
BABY-EGG YOLKS	SERVING	28.4	58	2.8	0.3	4.9	223	1.47	1.8	0.54	11	22
BABY-HAM	OUNCE	28.4	32	3.9	0	1.6	—	0.55	0.78	0.22	12	58
BABY-LAMB	OUNCE	28.4	29	4	0	1.3	0	0.66	0.53	0.06	18	58
BABY-LIVER	OUNCE	28.4	29	4.1	0.4	1.1	52	0.39	0.22	0.02	21	64
BABY-PORK	OUNCE	28.4	35	4	0	2	—	0.68	1.02	0.22	12	63
BABY-TURKEY	OUNCE	28.4	32	4	0	1.7	—	0.54	0.62	0.41	16	65
BABY-BEANS-GREEN	OUNCE	28.4	7	0.4	1.7	0	0	0	0	0	1	45
BABY-COOKIE-ARROWROOT	ITEM	6	24	0.4	4.3	0.9	0	0.2	0.539	0.05	22	9
BABY-GARDEN VEGETABLES	OUNCE	28.4	11	0.7	1.9	0.1	0	0	0	0	10	48
BABY-PEAS	OUNCE	28.4	11	1	2.3	0.1	0	0	0	0	1	32
BABY-SQUASH	OUNCE	28.4	7	0.2	1.6	0.1	0	0	0	0	1	51
BABY-SWEET POTATOES	OUNCE	28.4	16	0.3	3.7	0	0	0	0	0	6	75
BABY-PRETZELS	ITEM	6	24	0.7	4.9	0.1	0	0	0	0	16	8
BABY-ZWIEBACK	PIECE	7	30	0.7	5.2	0.7	1.46	0.28	0.24	0.05	16	21
BABY-CEREAL & EGG YOLKS	OUNCE	28.4	15	0.5	2	0.5	18	0.17	0.22	0.04	9	11
BABY-APPLE BETTY	OUNCE	28.4	20	0.1	5.6	0	0	0	0	0	3	14
BABY-BEEF & EGG NOODLES	OUNCE	28.4	15	0.6	2	0.5	—	—	—	—	8	13
BABY-BEANS-GREEN-BUTTERED	OUNCE	28.4	9	0.3	1.9	0.2	—	—	—	—	1	45
BABY-BEETS	OUNCE	28.4	10	0.4	2.2	0	0	0	0	0	24	52
BABY-CORN-CREAMED	OUNCE	28.4	16	0.4	4	0.1	0	0	0	0	12	26
BABY-PEAS-CREAMED	OUNCE	28.4	15	0.6	2.5	0.5	0	—	—	—	4	25
BABY-SPINACH-CREAMED	OUNCE	28.4	11	0.7	1.6	0.4	0	—	—	—	14	54

Beverages

Food Name	Portion	WT. Gm	KCAL Kc	PROT Gm	CARB Gm	FAT Gm	CHOL Mg	SAFA Gm	MUFA Gm	PUFA Gm	SOD Mg	POT Mg
BEER-LIGHT	FL OZ	29.5	8.26	0.059	0.384	0	0	0	0	0	0.885	5.31
BEER-REGULAR	FL OZ	29.7	12.2	0.089	1.1	0	0	0	0	0	1.49	7.43
BRANDY/COGNAC-PONY	ITEM	30	73	—	—	0	0	0	0	0	—	—
CARN INST BREAK-CHOC-ENV	ITEM	36	130	7	23	1	—	—	—	—	136	422
CHAMPAGNE-DOMESTIC-GLASS	ITEM	120	84	0.2	3	0	0	0	0	0	—	—
CHOC BEV DRINK-NO MILK-DRY	OUNCE	28.4	99.1	0.937	25.6	0.88	0	0.521	0.287	0.026	59.6	168

Key to Abbreviations

KCAL, kcalories
PROT, protein
CARB, carbohydrate
FAT, fat
CHOL, cholesterol
SAFA, saturated fat
MUFA, monounsaturated fat
PUFA, polyunsaturated fat
SOD, sodium
POT, potassium
MAG, magnesium
IRON, iron
ZINC, zinc
V-A, vitamin A
V-C, vitamin C
THIA, thiamin
RIBO, riboflavin
NIAC, niacin
V-B6, vitamin-B6
FOL, folate
VB12, vitamin-B12
CALC, calcium
PHOS, phosphorus
SEL, selenium
FIBD, dietary fiber
VE, vitamin E

MAG Mg	IRON Mg	ZINC Mg	V-A RE	V-C Mg	THIA Mg	RIBO Mg	NIAC Mg	V-B6 Mg	FOL Ug	VB12 Ug	CALC Mg	PHOS Mg	SEL Mg	FIBD Gm	V-E Mg
3	0.1	0.043	325	1.6	0.007	0.011	0.131	0.021	4.22	0	6	6	0	0.7	0.204
4	0.39	0.102	1	1	0.026	0.059	0.476	0.012	2.2	0.008	29	18	—	0.1	—
8	2.96	0.202	6	0.3	0.122	0.165	1.64	0.019	3.2	0.085	62	40	—	0.25	0.287
10	3.44	0.262	6	0.4	0.143	0.16	1.7	0.017	2.84	0.085	62	45	0.001	0.7	0.241
13	3.46	0.182	6	0.3	0.132	0.142	1.48	0.032	2.3	0.085	68	50	0.001	0.25	0.236
3	0.25	0.198	100	0.5	0.02	0.025	0.384	0.02	1.7	0.145	5	11	—	0.1	0.088
3	0.2	0.247	95	0.9	0.004	0.018	0.372	0.021	1.7	0.145	3	12	0.003	0.34	0.088
3.12	0.09	0.046	77	0.8	0.004	0.009	0.142	0.021	2.3	0	6	—	0	0.25	0.207
2.27	0.07	0.071	27	0.3	0.001	0.006	0.087	0.009	0.9	0.028	6	6	—	0	0.088
2	0.17	0.284	21	0.5	0.006	0.021	0.457	0.024	1.7	0.128	3	15	—	0.1	0.088
0.851	0.06	0.01	1	7.9	0.005	0.01	0.034	0.01	1	0	1	2	0	0.1	0.193
1	0.06	0.007	0	10.9	0.003	0.008	0.017	0.009	0.5	0	1	2	0	0.7	0.193
2	0.07	0.024	5	8.9	0.003	0.009	0.173	0.004	1.1	0	2	3	0	0.7	0.193
2	0.07	0.021	1	7	0.004	0.008	0.054	0.002	1	0	2	3	0	0.55	0.193
1	0.18	0.009	1	18	0.002	0.005	0.026	0.009	0	0	1	2	0	0.25	0.211
1	0.17	0.008	2	18.1	0.002	0.003	0.066	0.007	0.4	0	1	1	0	0.25	0.211
3	0.05	0.017	2	19.4	0.014	0.009	0.074	0.017	8.2	0	4	3	0	0.25	0.211
5	0.42	0.696	16	0.6	0.003	0.04	0.808	0.04	1.6	0.403	2	24	0.003	0	0.119
4	0.4	0.343	11	0.5	0.004	0.043	0.923	0.057	2.9	0.113	18	27	0.003	0	0.119
2	0.78	0.543	107	0.4	0.02	0.075	0.007	0.045	26.1	0.437	22	81	0.005	0	0.471
4	0.29	0.637	3	0.6	0.039	0.044	0.746	0.071	0.6	0.028	2	23	0.003	0	0.119
4	0.42	0.781	7	0.3	0.005	0.057	0.829	0.043	0.6	0.621	2	27	0.004	0	0.119
4	1.5	0.844	3247	5.5	0.014	0.514	2.36	0.097	95.7	0.612	1	58	0.007	0	0.119
3	0.28	0.644	3	0.5	0.041	0.058	0.643	0.058	0.5	0.281	1	27	0.004	0	0.119
4	0.34	0.519	48	0.6	0.005	0.059	1.04	0.051	3.2	0.284	7	36	0.003	0	0.119
7	0.21	0.058	13	1.5	0.007	0.024	0.098	0.011	9.8	0	11	6	0	0.39	0.207
1	0.18	0.032	—	0.3	0.03	0.026	0.344	0.002	0.6	0.004	2	7	—	0.1	0.014
6	0.24	0.074	172	1.6	0.017	0.02	0.221	0.028	11.4	0	8	8	0	0.7	0.207
4	0.27	0.099	16	1.9	0.023	0.017	0.289	0.02	7.4	0	6	12	0	0.7	0.207
3	0.08	0.04	57	2.2	0.003	0.016	0.1	0.018	4.4	0	7	4	0	0.7	0.207
4	0.1	0.058	183	2.8	0.008	0.009	0.101	0.026	2.8	0	4	7	0	0.7	0.207
2	0.23	0.047	0	0.2	0.028	0.021	0.214	0.005	5.67	0	1	7	—	0	0.046
1	0.04	0.038	0	0.4	0.015	0.017	0.092	0.006	1.4	0	1	4	—	0	—
1	0.13	0.081	11	0.2	0.003	0.012	0.014	0.006	0.9	0.02	7	11	—	0	0.111
0.567	0.05	0.003	0	9.8	0.004	0.01	0.013	0.003	0.1	0.011	5.39	0.851	—	0.1	0.065
2	0.12	0.106	31	0.3	0.01	0.012	0.205	0.014	1.4	0.026	3	8	0.003	0.1	0.088
—	0.36	—	13	2.3	0.005	0.03	0.096	—	8.1	—	18	—	0.17	0.7	0.207
4	0.09	0.034	1	0.7	0.003	0.012	0.037	0.007	8.7	0	4	4	—	0.4	0.207
2	0.08	0.054	2	0.6	0.004	0.013	0.145	0.012	3.2	0.005	6	9	—	0.9	0.207
4.54	0.16	0.11	2	0.5	0.025	0.016	0.23	0.013	6.4	0.023	4	9	—	0.7	0.207
16	0.18	0.088	118	2.5	0.004	0.029	0.061	0.021	17.2	0.017	25	15	—	1.12	0.207

MAG Mg	IRON Mg	ZINC Mg	V-A RE	V-C Mg	THIA Mg	RIBO Mg	NIAC Mg	V-B6 Mg	FOL Ug	VB12 Ug	CALC Mg	PHOS Mg	SEL Mg	FIBD Gm	V-E Mg
1.48	0.012	0.009	0	0	0.003	0.009	0.116	0.01	1.2	0.003	1.48	3.54	0	0	—
1.78	0.009	0.006	0	0	0.002	0.008	0.135	0.015	1.78	0.006	1.49	3.56	—	0.07	—
—	—	—	—	—	—	—	—	—	—	—	—	—	—	0	—
80	4.5	3	525	27	0.3	0.07	5	0.4	0	0.6	100	150	—	—	5
—	—	—	—	—	—	—	—	—	—	—	—	—	—	0	—
27.8	0.892	0.44	0.568	0.199	0.01	0.041	0.143	0.003	1.62	0	10.5	36.4	—	—	0.63

Continued.

Beverages—cont'd

Food Name	Portion	WT. Gm	KCAL Kc	PROT Gm	CARB Gm	FAT Gm	CHOL Mg	SAFA Gm	MUFA Gm	PUFA Gm	SOD Mg	POT Mg
CIDER-FERMENTED	FL OZ	30	11.8	—	0.3	0	0	0	0	0	0	—
CLUB SODA	FL OZ	29.6	0	0	0	0	0	0	0	0	6.22	0.592
COFFEE SUBSTITUTE-PREPARED	FL OZ	30.3	1.52	0.03	0.303	0	0	0.002	0.002	0.007	1.21	7.27
COFFEE-BREWED	FL OZ	29.6	0.592	0.03	0.118	0	0	0.001	0	0.001	0.592	16
COFFEE-INSTANT-PREPARED	CUP	239	4.78	0.239	0.956	0	0	0.005	0	0.005	7.17	86
CORDIALS/LIQUEUR-54-PROOF	FL OZ	34	97	—	11.5	0	0	0	0	0	1	1
CREAM SODA	FL OZ	30.9	15.8	0	4.1	0	0	0	0	0	3.71	0.309
FRUIT PUNCH DRINK-CAN	FL OZ	31	14.6	0	3.69	0	0	0.001	0.001	0.001	6.82	7.75
GATORADE-THIRST QUENCHER	FL OZ	30.1	7.53	0	1.9	0	0	0	0	0	12	3.31
HOT COCOA-PREP/MILK-HOME	CUP	250	218	9.1	25.8	9.05	33.3	5.61	2.65	0.33	123	480
LEMON LIME SODA-7UP	FL OZ	30.7	12.3	0	3.19	0	0	0	0	0	3.38	0.307
OVALTINE-CHOC-PREP/MILK	CUP	265	227	9.53	29.2	8.79	—	—	—	—	228	600
PERRIER-MINERAL WATER	CUP	237	0	0	0	0	0	0	0	0	2.37	0
POSTUM-INST GRAIN BEV-DRY	OUNCE	28.4	103	1.93	24.1	0.028	0	0	0	0	28.4	896
TANG-INST DRINK-ORANGE-DRY	OUNCE	28.4	104	0	26.1	0	0	0	0	0	12.8	80.9
TEA-BREWED	FL OZ	29.6	0.296	0	0.089	0	0	0.001	0	0.001	0.888	11
TEA-HERB-BREWED	FL OZ	29.6	0.296	0	0.059	0	0	0.001	0	0.001	0.296	2.66
TEA-INSTANT-PREP-SWEETENED	CUP	259	88.1	0.259	22.1	0	0	0.008	0.003	0.021	7.77	49.2
TEA-INSTANT-PREP-UNSWEET	CUP	237	2.37	0	0.474	0	0	0	0	0	7.11	47.4
TONIC WATER-QUININE SODA	FL OZ	30.5	10.4	0	2.68	0	0	0	0	0	1.22	0
WATER	CUP	237	0	0	0	0	0	0	0	0	7.11	0
WHIS/GIN/RUM/VOD-100 PROOF	FL OZ	27.8	82	0	0	0	0	0	0	0	0	0
WHIS/GIN/RUM/VOD-80 PROOF	FL OZ	27.8	64	0	0	0	0	0	0	0	0.278	0.556
WHIS/GIN/RUM/VOD-86 PROOF	FL OZ	27.8	69.5	0	0.028	0	0	0	0	0	0.278	0.556
WHIS/GIN/RUM/VOD-90 PROOF	FL OZ	27.7	72.9	0	0	0	0	0	0	0	0.554	0
WHIS/GIN/RUM/VOD-94 PROOF	FL OZ	27.8	76.5	0	0	0	0	0	0	0	0	0
WINE COOLER-WHITE WINE/7UP	SERVING	102	54.9	0.05	5.72	0	0	0	0	0	7.48	41
WINE-DESSERT	FL OZ	30	45.9	0.06	3.54	0	0	0	0	0	2.7	27.6
WINE-RED-TABLE	FL OZ	29.5	21	0.059	0.502	0	0	0	0	0	1.48	33
WINE-ROSE-TABLE	FL OZ	29.5	20.9	0.059	0.413	0	0	0	0	0	1.48	29.2
WINE-VERMOUTH-DRY-GLASS	ITEM	100	105	0	1	0	0	0	0	0	4	75
WINE-VERMOUTH-SWEET-GLASS	ITEM	100	167	0	12	0	0	0	0	0	—	—
WINE-WHITE-TABLE	FL OZ	29.5	20.1	0.03	0.236	0	0	0	0	0	1.48	23.6

Breads

Food Name	Portion	WT. Gm	KCAL Kc	PROT Gm	CARB Gm	FAT Gm	CHOL Mg	SAFA Gm	MUFA Gm	PUFA Gm	SOD Mg	POT Mg
BAGEL-EGG	ITEM	55	163	6.02	30.9	1.41	8	—	—	—	198	40.7
BAGEL-WATER	ITEM	55	163	6.02	30.9	1.41	0	0.2	0.4	0.6	198	40.7
BISCUITS-PREPARED/MIX	ITEM	28.4	104	1.63	13	5.05	1.4	3.31	1.29	0.196	221	32.8
BREAD STICK-VIENNA TYPE	ITEM	35	106	3.3	20.3	1.1	0	—	—	—	548	33
BREAD-CORN-HOME REC	SLICE	45	108	2.21	15.6	3.94	0	—	—	—	126	42.3
BREAD-CRACKED WHEAT	SLICE	25	65.5	2.32	12.5	0.868	0	0.1	0.2	0.2	108	33.3
BREAD-FRENCH-ENRICHED	SLICE	35	98	3.33	17.7	1.36	0	0.2	0.4	0.4	193	30.1
BREAD-MIXED GRAIN	SLICE	25	64.3	2.49	11.7	0.93	0	—	—	—	103	54.5
BREAD-PITA	ITEM	38	105	3.95	20.6	0.57	0	—	—	—	215	44.8
BREAD-PUMPERNICKEL	SLICE	32	81.6	2.93	15.4	1.1	0	—	—	—	173	139
BREAD-RAISIN-ENRICHED	SLICE	25	69.5	2.05	13.2	0.99	0	0.2	0.3	0.2	94	60
BREAD-RYE-AMERICAN-LIGHT	SLICE	25	65.5	2.12	12	0.913	0	—	—	—	174	51
BREAD-WHEAT-FIRM-TOASTED	SLICE	21	59	2.31	10.9	1.05	0	0.1	0.2	0.3	153	42.4
BREAD-WHITE-FIRM	SLICE	23	61.4	1.9	11.2	0.902	0	0.2	0.3	0.3	118	25.8
BREAD-WHITE-FIRM-TOASTED	SLICE	20	65	2	12	1	0	0.2	0.3	0.3	117	28
BREAD-WHOLE WHEAT-FIRM	SLICE	25	61.3	2.41	11.3	1.09	0	0.1	0.2	0.3	159	44
BREAD-WHOLE WHEAT-HOME REC	SLICE	25	66.5	2.25	11.6	1.61	0	—	—	—	89	85
BREADCRUMBS-DRY-GRATED	CUP	100	390	13	73	5	0	1	1.6	1.4	736	152
CRACKERS-ANIMAL	ITEM	1.9	8.67	0.127	1.47	0.2	0	—	—	—	7.53	1.67
CRACKERS-CHEDDAR SNACKS	ITEM	1.6	7.22	0.144	1.11	0.261	—	—	—	—	14.3	2.17
CRACKERS-CHEESE	ITEM	1	5.38	0.091	0.52	0.327	—	0.09	0.09	0.03	12	1.86
CRACKERS-GRAHAM-PLAIN	ITEM	7	27.5	0.5	5	0.5	0	0.1	0.25	0.15	33	27.5
CRACKERS-GRAHAM-SUG/HONEY	ITEM	7	30.1	0.519	5.4	0.732	0	0.1	0.4	0.1	32.9	11.7
CRACKERS-RITZ	ITEM	3.33	18	0.233	2.13	0.967	0	—	—	—	32.3	2.67
CRACKERS-RY KRISP-NATURAL	ITEM	2.1	7.5	0.25	1.67	0.033	0	0	0	0	18.5	10.2
CRACKERS-RYE WAFERS	ITEM	6.5	22.5	1	5	0	0	0	0	0	57	39

MAG Mg	IRON Mg	ZINC Mg	V-A RE	V-C Mg	THIA Mg	RIBO Mg	NIAC Mg	V-B6 Mg	FOL Ug	VB12 Ug	CALC Mg	PHOS Mg	SEL Mg	FIBD Gm	V-E Mg
—	—	—	—	—	—	—	—	—	—	—	—	—	—	0	—
0.296	0.003	0.03	0	0	0	0	0	0	0	0	1.48	0	—	0	0
1.21	0.018	0.009	0	0	0.002	0	0.065	0.003	0.091	0	0.909	2.12	—	0	—
1.48	0.015	0.006	0	0	0	0	0.066	0	0.03	0	0.592	0.296	0	0	—
9.56	0.12	0.072	0	0	0	0.003	0.676	0	0	0	7.17	7.17	0	0	—
0	0.02	0.02	—	0	—	—	—	—	—	0	0	—	0	—	
0.309	0.015	0.022	0	0	0	0	0	0	0	0	1.55	0	—	0	0
0.62	0.065	0.037	1.2	9.18	0.007	0.007	0.007	0	0.403	0	2.48	0.31	0	0	—
0.301	0.015	0.006	0	0	0.002	0	0	0	0	0	0	2.71	—	0	0
56	0.78	1.23	95.5	2.4	0.102	0.435	0.365	0.108	12.3	0.87	298	270	—	3	—
0.307	0.021	0.015	0	0	0	0	0.005	0	0	0	0.614	0	—	0	0
52	4.77	1.13	700	29	0.63	0.97	12.7	0.766	29	0.871	392	302	—	—	—
0	0	0	0	0	0	0	0	0	0	0	33.2	0	—	0	0
—	1.87	—	0	0	0.165	0.076	6.76	—	—	—	76.7	189	—	0	—
—	0.028	—	535	107	0	0	0	—	—	—	71	75.8	—	—	—
0.888	0.006	0.006	0	0	0	0.004	0	0	1.54	0	0	0.296	0	0	—
0.296	0.024	0.012	0	0	0.003	0.001	0	0	0.178	0	0.592	0	—	0	0
5	0.05	0.078	0	0	0	0.0047	0.093	0.005	9.6	0	5.18	2.59	0	0	—
4.74	0.04	0.071	0	0	0	0.005	0.088	0.005	0.711	0	4.74	2.37	0	0	—
0	0.003	0.031	0	0	0	0	0	0	0	0	0.305	0	—	0	0
2.37	0.024	0.071	0	0	0	0	0	0	0	0	4.74	0	—	0	0
0	0.01	0.01	0	0	0.002	0.001	0.004	0	0	0	0	1	—	0	0
0	0.033	0.019	0	0	0.002	0	0	0	0	0	0	1.39	0	0	0
0	0.008	0.014	0	0	0.002	0	0.014	0	0	0	0	1.39	0	0	0
0	0	0	0	0	0	0	0	0	0	0	0	0	0	0	0
0	0.01	0.01	0	0	0.002	0.001	0.004	0	0	0	0	1	—	0	0
5	0.193	0.063	—	—	0.002	0.003	0.043	0.007	0.1	0	6.11	6.95	—	0	—
2.7	0.072	0.021	0	0	0.005	0.005	0.064	0	0.12	0	2.4	2.7	—	0	—
3.84	0.127	0.027	0	0	0.001	0.008	0.024	0.01	0.59	0.003	2.36	4.13	—	0	—
2.95	0.112	0.018	0	0	0.001	0.005	0.022	0.007	0.325	0.003	2.36	4.43	—	0	—
—	—	—	—	—	0.01	0.01	0.2	—	—	—	8	—	0.005	0	—
—	—	—	—	—	—	—	—	—	—	—	—	—	—	0	—
2.95	0.09	0.02	0	0	0.001	0.001	0.02	0.004	0.059	0	2.66	4.13	—	0	—

MAG Mg	IRON Mg	ZINC Mg	V-A RE	V-C Mg	THIA Mg	RIBO Mg	NIAC Mg	V-B6 Mg	FOL Ug	VB12 Ug	CALC Mg	PHOS Mg	SEL Mg	FIBD Gm	V-E Mg
11	1.46	0.286	23.5	0	0.209	0.16	1.94	0.024	13.2	0.052	23.1	36.9	—	1.16	—
11	1.46	0.286	0	0	0.209	0.16	1.94	0.024	13.2	0	23.1	36.9	0.018	1.16	—
3.36	0.616	0.109	37	0	0.101	0.067	1.75	0.011	2.24	0.036	33.9	98.6	0.005	0.504	0.694
—	0.3	—	0	0	0.02	0.03	0.3	—	—	—	16	31	—	1.02	—
8.1	0.671	0.212	7.25	0	0.081	0.081	0.675	0.032	4.5	0.077	43.7	48.6	0.005	1.17	—
8.75	0.665	—	0	0	0.095	0.095	0.84	0.023	—	0	16.3	31.8	0.011	1.33	0.225
7	1.08	0.221	0	0	0.161	0.123	1.4	0.019	13	0	38.5	28.4	0.01	0.805	0.417
12.3	0.815	0.3	0	0	0.098	0.095	1.04	0.026	16.3	0	26	53	0.011	1.58	0.225
—	0.916	—	0	0	0.171	0.076	1.4	—	—	—	30.8	38	—	0.608	—
21.8	0.877	0.365	0	0	0.109	0.166	1.06	0.049	—	0	22.7	69.8	0.014	1.89	0.288
6.25	0.775	0.155	0	0	0.083	0.155	1.02	0.009	8.75	0	25.5	22.5	—	0.55	—
6	0.68	0.318	0	0	0.103	0.08	0.828	0.023	9.75	0	20	36.3	0.009	1.55	—
22.5	0.823	0.403	0	0	0.067	0.05	0.92	0.045	13.2	0	17.2	63	0.011	2.38	0.189
4.83	0.653	0.143	0	0	0.108	0.071	0.863	0.008	8.05	0	29	24.8	0.006	0.437	0.274
4.8	0.6	0.142	0	0	0.07	0.06	0.8	0.008	8	0	22	23	0.006	0.5	0.238
23.3	0.855	0.42	0	0	0.088	0.053	0.958	0.047	13.8	0	18	65	0.011	2.83	0.225
23.3	0.67	0.562	10.8	0	0.068	0.038	0.798	0.05	12.3	0.027	19.8	63.3	0.011	2.83	0.225
32	3.6	—	0	0	0.35	0.35	4.8	—	—	—	122	141	0.02	3.65	—
0.267	0.059	0.009	0	0	0.005	0.009	0.073	0	0.2	0.001	0.2	1.2	0	0.027	0.035
0.278	0.068	0.012	0.18	0	0.009	0.007	0.067	0.001	0.222	0.009	1.22	1.89	0.001	0.056	0.029
0.22	0.035	0.01	—	0	0.004	0.004	0.082	—	—	—	1.05	2.1	0	0.025	0.018
3.57	0.25	0.053	0	0	0.01	0.04	0.25	0.006	0.91	0	3	10.5	0.001	0.224	0.128
2.31	0.183	0.053	0	0	0.024	0.019	0.218	0.006	0.91	0	2.66	8.26	0.001	0.119	0.127
—	0.1	—	—	—	0.013	0.013	0.1	—	—	—	5	8	—	0.107	—
2.5	0.092	0.057	—	—	0.006	0.005	0.033	0.007	0.833	—	0.833	6.83	0.001	0.34	0.038
—	0.25	—	0	0	0.02	0.015	0.1	—	—	—	3.5	25	0.001	1.05	0.118

Continued.

Breads—cont'd

Food Name	Portion	WT. Gm	KCAL Kc	PROT Gm	CARB Gm	FAT Gm	CHOL Mg	SAFA Gm	MUFA Gm	PUFA Gm	SOD Mg	POT Mg
CRACKERS-SALTINES	ITEM	2.75	12.5	0.25	2	0.25	0.75	0.1	0.1	0.05	36.8	3.25
CRACKERS-TRISCUITS	ITEM	4.5	21	0.4	3.1	0.75	0	—	—	—	—	—
CRACKERS-WHEAT THINS	ITEM	1.8	9	0.125	1.25	0.35	0	—	—	—	—	—
CROISSANT-ROLL-SARA LEE	ITEM	26	109	2.3	11.2	6.1	—	—	—	—	140	40
FRENCH TOAST-HOME RECIPE	SLICE	65	153	5.67	17.2	6.73	—	—	—	—	257	85.8
MUFFIN-BLUEBERRY-HOME REC	ITEM	40	110	3	17	4	21	1.1	1.4	0.7	252	46
MUFFIN-BRAN-HOME REC	ITEM	40	112	2.96	16.7	5.08	21	1.2	1.4	0.8	168	98.8
MUFFIN-CORN-HOME REC	ITEM	40	125	3	19	4	21	1.2	1.6	0.9	192	54
MUFFIN-ENGLISH-PLAIN	ITEM	56	133	4.43	25.7	1.09	0	—	—	—	358	314
MUFFIN-ENGLISH-PLAIN-TOAST	ITEM	53	154	5.13	29.8	1.26	0	—	—	—	414	364
MUFFIN-PLAIN-HOME REC	ITEM	40	120	3	17	4	21	1	1.7	1	176	50
MUFFIN-SOY	ITEM	40	119	3.9	16.7	4.4	0	—	—	—		—
PANCAKES-BUCKWHEAT-MIX	ITEM	27	55	2	6	2	20	0.8	0.9	0.4	160	66
PANCAKES-PLAIN-HOME RECIPE	ITEM	27	60	2	9	2	20	0.5	0.8	0.5	160	33
PANCAKES-PLAIN-MIX	ITEM	27	58.9	1.85	7.87	2.17	20	0.7	0.7	0.3	160	43.2
ROLL-BROWN & SERVE-ENR	ITEM	26	85	2	14	2	0	0.4	0.7	0.5	144	25
ROLL-HAMBURGER/HOT DOG	ITEM	40	114	3.43	20.1	2.09	0	0.5	0.8	0.6	241	36.8
ROLL-HARD-ENRICHED	ITEM	50	155	5	30	2	0	0.4	0.6	0.5	312	49
ROLL-SUBMARINE/HOAGIE-ENR	ITEM	135	390	12	75	4	0	0.9	1.4	1.4	761	122
ROLL-WHOLE WHEAT-HOMEMADE	ITEM	35	90	3.5	18.3	1	0	—	—	—	197	102
WAFFLES-ENR-HOME RECIPE	ITEM	75	245	6.93	25.7	12.6	45	2.3	2.8	1.4	445	129
WAFFLES-FROZEN	ITEM	37	103	2.15	15.9	3.52	0	—	—	—	256	77.7

Breakfast Cereals

Food Name	Portion	WT. Gm	KCAL Kc	PROT Gm	CARB Gm	FAT Gm	CHOL Mg	SAFA Gm	MUFA Gm	PUFA Gm	SOD Mg	POT Mg
CEREAL-100% BRAN	CUP	66	178	8.25	48.1	3.3	0	0.587	0.574	1.87	457	824
CEREAL-ALL BRAN	CUP	85.2	212	12.2	63.4	1.53	0	—	—	—	961	1051
CEREAL-ALPHA BITS	CUP	28.4	111	2.2	24.6	0.6	0	—	—	—	219	110
CEREAL-BRAN BUDS	CUP	85.2	220	11.8	64.8	2.04	0	—	—	—	523	1425
CEREAL-BRAN CHEX	CUP	49	156	5.05	39	1.37	0	—	—	—	455	394
CEREAL-BRAN FLAKES-KELLOGG	CUP	39	127	4.91	30.5	0.741	0	0	0	0	303	248
CEREAL-C.W. POST-PLAIN	CUP	97	432	8.7	69.4	15.2	0.184	11.3	1.72	1.42	167	198
CEREAL-CHEERIOS	CUP	22.7	88.8	3.42	15.7	1.45	0	0.27	0.515	0.597	246	81
CEREAL-CORN BRAN	CUP	36	125	2.45	30.3	1.26	0	—	—	—	310	70.2
CEREAL-CORN CHEX	CUP	28.4	111	2.02	24.9	0.114	0	0	0	0	271	23
CEREAL-CORN FLAKES-KELLOGG	CUP	22.7	88.3	1.84	19.5	0.068	0	0	0	0	232	20.9
CEREAL-CORN GRITS-ENRICHED	CUP	242	145	3.39	31.5	0.484	0	0.073	0.121	0.194	0	53.2
CEREAL-CORN-SHREDDED-SUGAR	CUP	25	95	2	22	0	0	0	0	0	247	—
CEREAL-CRACKLIN BRAN	CUP	60	229	5.52	41.2	8.76	0	—	—	—	487	355
CEREAL-CREAM/WHEAT-INSTANT	CUP	241	153	4.4	31.6	0.6	0	0	0	0	6	48
CEREAL-CREAM/WHEAT-PACKET	ITEM	150	132	2.5	28.9	0.4	0	0	0	0	241	55
CEREAL-CREAM/WHEAT-REG-HOT	CUP	251	133	3.8	27.7	0.5	0	0	0	0	2	43
CEREAL-CRISPY RICE	CUP	28.4	112	1.82	25.2	0.114	0	0	0	0	208	27
CEREAL-FARINA-COOK-ENR	CUP	233	117	3.26	24.7	0.233	0	0.023	0.023	0.07	0	30.3
CEREAL-FORTIFIED OAT FLAKE	CUP	48	177	8.98	34.8	0.72	0	0	0	0	429	343
CEREAL-FROST FLAKE-KELLOGG	CUP	35	133	1.75	31.7	0.07	0	0	0	0	284	22.4
CEREAL-FROSTED MINI WHEATS	ITEM	7.1	25.5	0.731	5.86	0.071	0	0	0	0	2.06	24.2
CEREAL-GRANOLA-HOMEMADE	CUP	122	594	15	67.3	33.2	0	5.84	9.37	17.2	12.2	612
CEREAL-GRANOLA-NATURE VAL	CUP	113	503	11.5	75.5	19.6	0	13	2.93	2.75	232	389
CEREAL-GRAPE NUTS	CUP	114	407	13.3	93.5	0.456	0	0	0	0	792	381
CEREAL-GRAPE NUTS FLAKES	CUP	32.5	116	3.48	26.6	0.358	0	0	0	0	183	113
CEREAL-HEARTLAND NATURAL	CUP	115	499	11.6	78.5	17.7	0	—	—	—	293	385
CEREAL-HONEY BRAN	CUP	35	119	3.08	28.6	0.735	0	0	0	0	202	151
CEREAL-HONEY NUT CHERRIOS	CUP	33	125	3.63	26.5	0.759	0	0.132	0.31	0.304	299	115
CEREAL-LIFE-PLAIN/CINNAMON	CUP	44	162	8.1	31.5	0.836	0	0	0	0	229	197
CEREAL-LUCKY CHARMS	CUP	32	125	2.91	26.1	1.22	0	0.224	0.426	0.493	227	66.2
CEREAL-MALT O MEAL-COOK	CUP	240	122	3.6	25.9	0.24	0	0	0	0	2.4	31.2
CEREAL-MAYPO-COOK-HOT	CUP	240	170	5.8	31.8	2.4	0	—	—	—	9.6	211
CEREAL-NUTRI GRAIN-BARLEY	CUP	41	153	4.47	33.9	0.328	0	0	0	0	277	108
CEREAL-NUTRI GRAIN-CORN	CUP	42	160	3.36	35.4	0.966	0	—	—	—	276	98
CEREAL-NUTRI GRAIN-RYE	CUP	40	144	3.48	33.9	0.28	0	0	0	0	272	71.6
CEREAL-NUTRI GRAIN-WHEAT	CUP	44	158	3.83	37.2	0.44	0	0	0	0	299	120

MAG Mg	IRON Mg	ZINC Mg	V-A RE	V-C Mg	THIA Mg	RIBO Mg	NIAC Mg	V-B6 Mg	FOL Ug	VB12 Ug	CALC Mg	PHOS Mg	SEL Mg	FIBD Gm	V-E Mg
0.77	0.125	0.017	0	0	0.125	0.013	0.1	0.001	0.495	0	0.5	2.5	0.004	0.072	0.05
—	—	—	—	—	—	—	—	—	—	—	—	—	0.001	0.155	0.082
—	—	—	—	—	—	—	—	—	—	—	—	—	0	0.099	0.033
7	1.04	—	8.2	0	0.28	0.1	1.2	—	—	—	12	32	—	0.56	—
11.7	1.34	0.553	22.2	0	0.124	0.163	1.01	0.038	17.6	0.291	72.2	84.5	—	2.02	—
10	0.6	—	18	0	0.09	0.1	0.7	—	—	—	34	53	—	0.85	—
35.2	1.26	1.08	40	2.48	0.1	0.112	1.26	0.111	16.8	0.092	53.6	111	—	2.52	—
18.4	0.7	—	25	0	0.1	0.1	0.7	—	—	—	42	68	—	0.95	—
10.6	1.58	0.403	0	0	0.258	0.179	2.1	0.022	17.9	0	90.7	62.7	0.015	1.29	—
12.2	1.83	0.466	0	0	0.239	0.207	2.43	0.026	20.7	0	105	72.6	0.015	1.49	—
10.8	0.6	—	8	0	0.09	0.12	0.9	—	—	—	42	60	—	0.85	—
52	0.9	—	40	0	0.08	0.1	0.5	—	—	—	35	56	—	0.835	—
5.13	0.4	0.192	12	0	0.04	0.05	0.2	0.057	2.97	0.355	59	91	0.002	0.621	—
5.13	0.4	0.192	6	0	0.06	0.07	0.5	0.057	2.97	0.355	27	38	0.002	0.45	—
5.13	0.265	0.192	7.66	0	0.038	0.059	0.254	0.057	2.97	0.355	35.6	70.7	0.003	0.394	—
5.46	0.8	0.19	0	0	0.1	0.06	0.9	0.016	9.88	—	20	23	0.008	0.988	1.73
7.6	1.19	0.248	0	0	0.196	0.132	1.58	0.014	14.8	—	53.6	32.8	0.012	1.01	0.212
11.5	1.2	0.3	0	0	0.2	0.12	1.7	0.018	29.5	0	24	46	0.015	1.5	0.265
—	3	—	0	0	0.54	0.32	4.5	0.047	—	—	58	115	0.041	3.75	0.716
40	0.8	—	0	0	0.12	0.05	1.1	—	—	—	34	98	0.016	1.83	0.315
16.5	1.48	0.653	28	0	0.18	0.24	1.46	0.054	14.3	0.365	154	135	0.011	1.05	—
7.77	1.8	0.303	95	0	0.167	0.2	1.93	0.098	0.74	—	30	141	—	0.888	—

MAG Mg	IRON Mg	ZINC Mg	V-A RE	V-C Mg	THIA Mg	RIBO Mg	NIAC Mg	V-B6 Mg	FOL Ug	VB12 Ug	CALC Mg	PHOS Mg	SEL Mg	FIBD Gm	V-E Mg
312	8.12	5.74	0	62.7	1.58	1.78	20.9	2.11	46.9	6.27	46.2	801	0.02	19.5	—
318	13.5	11.2	1125	45.2	1.11	1.28	15	1.53	301	0	69	794	0.025	25.5	7.78
17	1.8	1.5	375	0	0.4	0.4	5	0.5	100	1.5	8	51	0.01	0.3	—
271	13.5	11.2	1125	45.2	1.11	1.28	15	1.53	301	0	57.1	740	0.025	23.6	3.45
126	7.8	2.14	11	26	0.6	0.26	8.6	0.9	173	2.6	29	327	0.01	7.9	—
71	24.8	5.15	516	0	0.507	0.585	6.86	0.702	138	2.1	19.1	192	0.004	5.5	0.823
67	15.4	1.64	1284	0	1.3	1.5	17.1	1.7	342	5.1	47	224	—	2.2	—
31.3	3.61	0.629	300	12	0.295	0.341	4	0.409	4.99	1.2	38.8	107	0.01	0.863	—
18.4	12.2	4	7.56	0	0.374	0.698	10.9	0.858	232	1.39	41.4	51.8	0.002	6.84	—
3.98	1.79	0.1	14	15.1	0.369	0.068	5	0.511	100	1.51	3.12	11.1	0.002	0.5	—
2.72	1.43	0.064	300	12	0.295	0.341	4	0.409	80.1	0	0.681	14.3	0.001	0.454	—
9.68	1.55	0.169	—	—	0.242	0.145	1.96	0.058	2.42	0	0	29	0.024	0.6	3.34
3.5	0.6	0.088	0	13	0.33	0.05	4.4	0.45	88.3	1.33	1	10	0.002	1.54	0.538
116	3.78	3.18	794	31.8	0.78	0.9	10.6	1.1	212	0	39.6	241	0.01	9.1	—
14	12	0.41	0	0	0.2	0.1	1.8	0.029	11	0	59	43	—	2.21	—
9	8.1	0.23	1250	0	0.4	0.2	5	0.5	100	0	40	20	—	2.02	1.41
10	10.3	0.33	0	0	0.251	0	1.51	0.035	10	0	50.2	42	—	1.94	—
11.9	0.71	0.471	0	1.14	0.114	0.028	2.02	0.044	3.12	0.083	5.11	31	0.004	1	—
4.66	1.17	0.163	—	—	0.186	0.117	1.28	0.023	4.66	0	4.66	28	—	3.26	2.19
57.6	13.7	1.5	636	0	0.624	0.72	8.45	0.864	169	2.54	68.2	176	0.01	1.2	—
2.8	2.21	0.049	463	18.6	0.455	0.525	6.16	0.63	124	0	1.4	25.9	—	0.77	—
5.82	0.447	0.376	94	3.76	0.092	0.107	1.25	0.128	25.1	0	2.34	18.5	—	0.54	0.153
141	4.84	4.47	10	1.22	0.732	0.305	2.14	0.428	98.8	0	75.6	494	0.023	12.8	—
116	3.78	2.19	—	—	0.39	0.19	0,83	—	85	—	71	354	0.037	4.2	—
76.4	4.95	2.51	1500	0	1.48	1.71	20.1	2.05	402	6.04	10.8	286	0.034	5.47	—
35.8	9.3	0.65	430	0	0.423	0.488	5.72	0.585	115	1.72	13	96.9	0.01	2.08	0.686
147	4.33	3.04	—	1.15	0.36	0.161	1.61	0.194	64.4	0	74.8	416	—	5.4	—
45.9	5.6	0.903	463	18.6	0.455	0.525	6.16	0.63	23.5	1.86	16.1	132	—	3.9	—
38.6	5.25	0.865	437	17.5	0.429	0.495	5.81	0.594	21.5	1.75	23.1	122	—	1.3	—
14.1	11.6	1.45	—	—	0.955	0.999	11.6	0.084	37	0	154	238	—	1.4	—
26.9	5.09	0.563	424	17	0.416	0.48	5.63	0.576	6.4	1.7	36.2	88.6	—	0.6	—
4.8	9.6	0.168	0	0	0.48	0.24	5.76	0.019	4.8	0	4.8	24	—	0.6	—
51	8.4	1.49	702	28.8	0.72	0.72	9.36	0.96	9.6	2.88	125	248	—	1.2	—
32.4	1.45	5.41	543	21.7	0.533	0.615	7.22	0.738	145	2.17	11.1	126	0.027	2.4	—
27	0.89	5.54	556	22.3	0.546	0.63	7.39	0.756	148	2.23	1.26	121	0.003	2.6	—
30.4	1.13	5.28	530	21.2	0.52	0.6	7.04	0.72	141	2.12	8.4	104	—	2.56	—
34.3	1.24	5.81	583	23.3	0.572	0.66	7.74	0.792	155	2.33	12.3	165	0.007	2.8	—

Continued.

Breakfast Cereals—cont'd

Food Name	Portion	WT. Gm	KCAL Kc	PROT Gm	CARB Gm	FAT Gm	CHOL Mg	SAFA Gm	MUFA Gm	PUFA Gm	SOD Mg	POT Mg
CEREAL-OATMEAL-INST-PACKET	ITEM	177	104	4.4	18.1	1.7	0	0.289	0.597	0.697	286	100
CEREAL-OATMEAL-RAW	CUP	81	311	13	54.2	5.1	0	0.9	1.6	1.87	3	284
CEREAL-OATS-PUFFED-SUGAR	CUP	25	100	3	19	1	0	0.185	0.075	0.465	294	—
CEREAL-PRODUCT 19	CUP	33	126	3.23	27.4	0.231	0	0	0	0	378	51.5
CEREAL-RAISIN BRAN-KELLOGG	CUP	49.2	154	5.31	37.1	0.984	0	—	—	—	359	256
CEREAL-RALSTON-COOKED	CUP	253	134	5.57	28.2	0.8	0	0	0	0	4	153
CEREAL-RICE CHEX	CUP	25.2	99.5	1.34	22.5	0.101	0	0	0	0	211	29.2
CEREAL-RICE KRISPIES	CUP	28.4	112	1.93	24.8	0.199	0	0	0	0	340	29.5
CEREAL-RICE-PUFFED-PLAIN	CUP	14	56.3	0.882	12.6	0.07	0	0	0	0	0.42	15.8
CEREAL-RICE-PUFFED-SUGAR	CUP	28.4	115	1	26	0	0	0	0	0	21	43
CEREAL-ROMAN MEAL-COOKED	CUP	241	147	6.51	33	0.964	0	—	—	—	3	302
CEREAL-SPECIAL K	CUP	21.3	83.1	4.2	16	0.085	0.028	0	0	0	199	36.8
CEREAL-SUGAR CORN POPS	CUP	28.4	108	1.42	25.7	0.085	0	0	0	0	104	17.3
CEREAL-SUGAR SMACKS	CUP	37.9	141	2.65	33	0.72	0	0	0	0	100	56.1
CEREAL-TEAM	CUP	42	164	2.69	36	0.756	0	0	0	0	259	71
CEREAL-TOASTIES	CUP	22.7	87.8	1.84	19.5	0.045	0	0	0	0	238	26.3
CEREAL-TOTAL	CUP	33	116	3.3	26	0.693	0	0.099	0.066	0.343	409	123
CEREAL-TRIX	CUP	28.4	109	1.53	25.2	0.398	0	0	0	0	181	26.7
CEREAL-WHEAT CHEX	CUP	46	169	4.55	37.8	1.15	0	—	—	—	308	173
CEREAL-WHEAT FLAKES-SUGAR	CUP	30	105	3	24	0	0	0	0	0	368	81
CEREAL-WHEAT GERM-SUGAR	CUP	113	426	24.6	68.7	9.04	0	1.57	1.31	5.49	3.39	802
CEREAL-WHEAT GERM-TOASTED	CUP	113	432	32.9	56.1	12.1	0	2.07	1.7	7.48	4.52	1070
CEREAL-WHEAT-PUFFED-PLAIN	CUP	12	43.7	1.76	9.55	0.144	0	0	0	0	0.48	41.8
CEREAL-WHEAT-PUFFED-SUGAR	SERVING	38	138	5.59	30.2	0.456	0	—	0.122	0.141	1.52	132
CEREAL-WHEAT-ROLLED-COOKED	CUP	240	180	5	41	1	0	0.182	0.07	0.475	535	202
CEREAL-WHEAT-SHRED-BISCUIT	ITEM	23.6	83	2.6	18.8	0.3	0	0	0	0	0.472	77
CEREAL-WHEAT-WHOLE MEAL	CUP	245	110	4	23	1	0	0.182	0.07	0.475	535	118
CEREAL-WHEATENA-COOKED	CUP	243	136	4.86	28.7	1.22	0	—	—	—	4.86	187
CEREAL-WHEATIES	CUP	29	101	2.8	23.1	0.5	0	0.07	0.05	0.24	276	108
CEREAL-WHOLE WHEAT NATURAL	CUP	242	150	4.84	33.2	0.968	0	—	—	—	1	171

Combination Foods

Food Name	Portion	WT. Gm	KCAL Kc	PROT Gm	CARB Gm	FAT Gm	CHOL Mg	SAFA Gm	MUFA Gm	PUFA Gm	SOD Mg	POT Mg
BEANS/PORK/FRANKFURTER-CAN	CUP	257	365	17.3	39.6	16.9	15.4	6.05	7.27	2.15	1105	604
BEANS/PORK/SWEET SAUCE-CAN	CUP	253	281	13.4	53.1	3.69	17.7	1.42	1.6	0.473	850	673
BEANS/PORK/TOM SAUCE-CAN	CUP	253	248	13.1	49.1	2.61	17	0.999	1.12	0.331	1113	759
BEEF & VEGETABLE STEW	CUP	245	220	16	15	11	72	4.9	4.5	0.5	1006	613
BEEF POTPIE-HOME RECIPE	SLICE	210	515	21	39	30	44	7.9	12.9	7.4	596	334
BEEF-RAVIOLIOS-CANNED	OUNCE	28.4	27.5	1.14	4.26	0.568	—	0.11	0.16	0.254	131	45.7
CHICKEN A LA KING-HOME REC	CUP	245	470	27	12	34	186	12.9	13.4	6.2	759	404
CHICKEN CHOW MEIN-CANNED	CUP	250	95	7	18	0	98	0	0	0	722	418
CHICKEN POTPIE-BAKED-HOME	SLICE	232	545	23	42	31	72	11	13.5	5.5	593	343
CHILI CON CARNE/BEANS-CAN	CUP	255	340	19	31	16	38	7.5	7.2	1	1354	594
CHILI WITH BEANS-CANNED	CUP	255	286	14.6	30.4	14	43.4	6	5.95	0.923	1331	931
MACARONI & CHEESE-ENR-CAN	CUP	240	230	9	26	10	42	4.2	3.1	1.4	729	139
MACARONI & CHEESE-ENR-HOME	CUP	200	430	17	40	22	42	8.9	8.8	2.9	1086	240
MEAT LOAF-CELERY/ONIONS	SERVING	87.6	213	15.8	5.23	13.9	107	5.29	5.9	0.613	103	182
PIZZA-CHEESE-BAKED	SLICE	63	140	7.68	20.5	3.21	9	1.54	0.99	0.491	336	110
PIZZA-PEPPERONI-BAKED	SLICE	71	181	10.1	19.9	6.96	14	2.24	3.14	1.17	267	153
SALAD-CARROT RAISIN-HOME	CUP	268	306	3.8	55.8	11.6	—	—	—	—	—	—
SALAD-CHEF SALAD-HAM/CHEES	SERVING	200	196	13.4	7.42	12.7	46	6.98	4.09	0.739	567	415
SALAD-CHICKEN	CUP	205	502	26	17.4	36.2	—	—	—	—	1395	521
SALAD-COLESLAW	TBSP	8	5.52	0.103	0.993	0.209	1	0.031	0.057	0.108	1.84	14.5
SALAD-FRUIT-CAN/JUICE	CUP	249	125	1.27	32.5	0.075	0	0.01	0.012	0.027	12.5	289
SALAD-GREEN SALAD-TOSSED	SERVING	207	32	2.6	6.67	0.16	0	0.021	0.008	0.07	53	356
SALAD-MACARONI	SERVING	28.4	50.7	0.7	5.3	3	—	—	—	—	148	21
SALAD-MANDARIN ORANGE GEL	SERVING	28.4	22.7	0.4	5.7	0	0	0	0	0	14	9
SALAD-POTATO	CUP	250	358	6.7	27.9	20.5	170	3.57	6.2	9.34	1323	635
SALAD-THREE BEAN-DEL MONTE	OUNCE	28.4	22.4	0.71	5.06	0.056	0	0	0	0	101	38.3
SALAD-TUNA	CUP	205	350	30	7	22	68	4.3	6.3	6.7	434	—
SAND-BAC/LET/TOM/MAYO	ITEM	148	282	6.8	28.8	15.6	—	—	—	—	—	—
SANDWICH-CLUB	ITEM	315	590	35.6	41.7	20.8	—	—	—	—	—	—

MAG Mg	IRON Mg	ZINC Mg	V-A RE	V-C Mg	THIA Mg	RIBO Mg	NIAC Mg	V-B6 Mg	FOL Ug	VB12 Ug	CALC Mg	PHOS Mg	SEL Mg	FIBD Gm	V-E Mg
42.5	6.32	0.867	455	0	0.531	0.283	5.47	0.74	150	0	163	133	0.015	1.62	2.71
120	3.41	2.48	8.2	0	0.59	0.11	0.63	0.097	26	0	42	384	0.022	4.6	—
28	4	0.693	275	13	0.33	0.38	4.4	0.45	5.5	1.33	44	102	0.006	2.65	—
12.2	21	0.495	1748	70	1.75	1.98	23.3	2.34	466	7	3.96	46.5	—	0.4	—
63.5	22.3	5.02	500	0	0.492	0.59	6.69	0.689	133	2.02	17.2	183	0.005	5.31	—
59	1.64	1.42	0	0	0.2	0.18	2.05	0.114	17.7	0.109	12.7	148	—	4.2	2.38
6.3	1.59	0.348	1.85	13.4	0.328	0.008	4.44	0.454	89	1.34	3.53	24.7	0.004	0.151	0.071
10.2	1.79	0.48	375	15.1	0.369	0.426	5	0.511	100	0	3.98	34.4	0.004	0.1	0.08
3.5	0.148	0.144	0	0	0.015	0.014	0.42	0.011	2.66	0	0.84	13.7	0.001	0.1	—
7.56	0	1.48	300	15	0	0	0	0.504	98.8	1.48	3	14	0.002	0.2	—
109	2.12	1.78	0	0	0.241	0.12	3.08	0.113	24.1	0	28.9	215	—	2.31	—
11.7	3.39	2.81	280	11.3	0.277	0.32	3.75	0.383	75.2	0.011	6.18	41.3	0.013	0.17	—
1.99	1.79	1.51	375	15.1	0.369	0.426	5	0.511	100	0	1.14	28.1	—	0.2	—
18.2	2.39	0.379	500	20.1	0.493	0.569	6.67	0.682	134	0	4.17	41.3	—	0.531	—
18.5	2.57	0.584	556	22.3	0.546	0.63	7.39	0.756	6.72	2.23	6.3	65.1	0.007	0.7	—
3.41	0.597	0.066	300	—	0.295	0.341	4	0.409	80.1	1.2	0.908	10	—	0.386	—
37	21	0.78	1748	70	1.75	1.98	23.3	2.34	466	7	282	137	—	2.4	—
6.25	4.52	0.13	371	15.1	0.369	0.426	5	0.511	2.56	1.51	5.68	19	—	0.32	—
58.4	7.31	1.23	—	24.4	0.598	0.166	8.1	0.828	162	2.44	17.9	182	—	3.4	0.971
32.7	4.8	0.669	330	16	0.4	0.45	5.3	0.54	9	1.59	12	83	0.003	2.7	0.633
271	7.71	14.1	0	—	1.41	0.7	4.73	0.829	298	0	37.3	971	—	5.7	—
362	10.3	18.8	50	7	1.89	0.93	6.31	1.11	398	0	50.9	1295	—	14.6	31.1
17.4	0.568	0.283	0	0	0.024	0.028	1.3	0.02	3.84	0	3.36	42.6	—	0.4	—
55.1	1.8	0.897	0	0	0.076	0.087	4.1	0.065	12.2	0	10.6	135	—	2.11	—
52.8	1.7	1.15	0	0	0.17	0.07	2.2	—	26.4	—	19	182	—	2.87	9.72
40.1	0.74	0.59	0	0	0.07	0.06	1.08	0.06	12	0	9.68	86	—	2.2	0.508
53.9	1.2	1.18	0	0	0.15	0.05	1.5	—	27	—	17	127	—	1.61	9.92
48.6	1.36	1.68	0	0	0.024	0.049	1.34	0.046	17	0	9.72	146	0.058	2.6	—
31.6	4.61	0.65	384	15.4	0.377	0.435	5.1	0.522	102	1.54	43.8	100	0.003	2	0.612
54	1.5	1.16	0	0	0.17	0.12	2.15	0.177	26.6	0	16.9	167	0.058	2.7	9.8

MAG Mg	IRON Mg	ZINC Mg	V-A RE	V-C Mg	THIA Mg	RIBO Mg	NIAC Mg	V-B6 Mg	FOL Ug	VB12 Ug	CALC Mg	PHOS Mg	SEL Mg	FIBD Gm	V-E Mg
72	4.45	4.81	38.6	5.91	0.149	0.144	2.32	0.118	77.1	0	123	267	—	12.8	2.75
86	4.2	3.8	27.8	7.59	0.119	0.154	0.888	0.215	94.6	0	154	266	—	14	2.75
88	8.3	14.8	62	7.8	0.132	0.116	1.26	0.175	56.9	0	141	297	—	13.8	2.75
—	2.9	—	480	17	0.15	0.17	4.7	—	—	0.002	29	184	—	3.19	1.35
—	3.8	—	344	6	0.3	0.3	5.5	—	—	—	29	149	—	3.9	—
—	0.312	—	50	0.426	0.026	0.023	0.398	—	—	—	4.54	—	—	0.23	0.136
—	2.5	—	226	12	0.1	0.42	5.4	—	—	—	127	358	—	1.2	—
—	1.3	—	30	13	0.05	0.1	1	—	—	—	45	85	—	0.9	0.125
—	3	—	618	5	0.34	0.31	5.5	—	—	—	70	232	0.032	4.2	—
—	4.3	—	30	—	0.08	0.18	3.3	0.263	—	—	82	321	—	5	—
115	8.75	5.1	86.7	4.34	0.122	0.268	0.913	0.337	57.9	0.03	120	393	—	6.93	—
—	1	—	52	0	0.12	0.24	1	—	—	—	199	182	—	1.44	—
52	1.8	—	172	0	0.2	0.4	1.8	—	—	—	362	322	0.028	1.2	—
13.6	1.91	3.08	12.3	0.725	0.052	0.148	3.16	0.162	10.9	1.52	22.8	112	0.001	0.11	0.068
16	0.58	0.82	74	1.3	0.18	0.16	2.48	0.04	59	0.33	116	113	—	1.59	—
8	0.94	0.52	54	1.7	0.14	0.23	3.05	0.05	53	0.19	65	75	—	1.48	—
—	3	—	1100	12	0.16	0.16	1	—	—	—	96	130	—	16.7	—
28.4	1.17	1.73	740	24	0.337	0.24	2.21	0.206	46	0.474	227	251	0.019	2.39	0.995
—	—	—	—	—	—	—	—	—	—	—	—	—	—	—	—
0.8	0.047	0.016	6.56	2.62	0.005	0.005	0.022	0.01	2.12	0	3.6	2.56	—	0.297	—
21	0.62	0.349	149	8.22	0.027	0.035	0.886	0.067	6.47	0	27.4	34.9	0.001	1.64	—
22	1.3	0.43	235	48	0.06	0.1	1.15	0.16	77	0	26	80	0.001	2.11	—
—	—	—	—	—	—	—	—	—	—	—	—	—	—	0.29	—
—	—	—	—	—	—	—	—	—	—	—	—	—	—	0.57	—
37.5	1.63	0.775	82.5	25	0.193	0.15	2.23	0.353	16.8	0.385	47.5	130	—	5.25	—
6.25	0.284	0.093	8	0.852	0.014	0.014	0.085	—	—	—	9.66	16.2	—	1.52	—
—	2.7	—	118	2	0.08	0.23	10.3	—	—	—	41	291	—	1.03	3.05
—	1.5	—	174	13	0.16	0.14	1.6	—	—	—	53	89	—	2.88	—
—	4.3	—	350	27	0.38	0.41	10.2	—	—	—	103	394	—	4.17	—

Continued.

Combination Foods—cont'd

Food Name	Portion	WT. Gm	KCAL Kc	PROT Gm	CARB Gm	FAT Gm	CHOL Mg	SAFA Gm	MUFA Gm	PUFA Gm	SOD Mg	POT Mg
SPAGHETTI/TOM/CHE-CAN	CUP	250	190	6	39	2	4	0.5	0.3	0.4	955	303
SPAGHETTI/TOM/CHE-HOME REC	CUP	250	260	9	37	9	4	2	5.4	0.7	955	408
SPAGHETTI/TOM/MEAT-CAN	CUP	250	260	12	29	10	39	2.2	3.3	3.9	1220	245
SPAGHETTI/TOM/MEAT-HOME	CUP	248	330	19	39	12	75	3.3	6.3	0.9	1009	665
TACO	ITEM	171	370	20.7	26.7	20.6	57	11.4	6.58	0.959	802	473
VEGETABLES-MIXED-FROZ-BOIL	CUP	182	107	5.21	23.8	0.273	0	0.056	0.018	0.132	63.7	308

Dairy Products

Food Name	Portion	WT. Gm	KCAL Kc	PROT Gm	CARB Gm	FAT Gm	CHOL Mg	SAFA Gm	MUFA Gm	PUFA Gm	SOD Mg	POT Mg
CHEESE FOOD-AMERICAN-PROC	OUNCE	28.4	93	5.56	2.07	6.97	18	4.38	2.04	0.2	337	79
CHEESE SPREAD-PROCESSED	OUNCE	28.4	82	4.65	2.48	6.02	16	3.78	1.76	0.18	381	69
CHEESE-AMERICAN-PROCESSED	OUNCE	28.4	106	6.28	0.45	8.86	27	5.58	2.54	0.28	406	46
CHEESE-BLUE	OUNCE	28.4	100	6.06	0.659	8.14	21	5.29	2.21	0.23	395	72.9
CHEESE-CAMEMBERT-WEDGE	ITEM	38	114	7.52	0.18	9.22	27	5.8	2.67	0.28	320	71
CHEESE-CHEDDAR-SHREDDED	CUP	113	455	28.1	1.45	37.5	119	23.8	10.6	1.06	701	111
CHEESE-COTTAGE-4%-LAR CURD	CUP	225	232	28.1	6.03	10.1	33.8	6.41	2.88	0.315	911	189
CHEESE-CREAM	OUNCE	28.4	100	2.17	0.759	10	31.4	6.31	2.82	0.365	85.1	34.4
CHEESE-FETA	OUNCE	28.4	75	4.03	1.16	6.03	25	4.24	1.31	0.17	316	18
CHEESE-GOUDA	OUNCE	28.4	101	7.07	0.63	7.78	32	4.99	2.2	0.19	232	34
CHEESE-LIMBURGER	OUNCE	28.4	93	5.68	0.14	7.72	26	4.75	2.44	0.14	227	36
CHEESE-MONTEREY	OUNCE	28.4	106	6.94	0.19	8.58	25.2	5.41	2.48	0.255	152	23
CHEESE-MOZZARELLA-SKIM MILK	OUNCE	28.4	72	6.88	0.78	4.51	16	2.87	1.28	0.13	132	24
CHEESE-PARMESAN-GRATED	CUP	100	456	41.6	3.74	30	79	19.1	8.73	0.66	1862	107
CHEESE-PROVOLONE	OUNCE	28.4	100	7.25	0.61	7.55	20	4.84	2.1	0.22	248	39
CHEESE-RICOTTA-SKIM MILK	CUP	246	340	28	12.6	19.5	76	12.1	5.69	0.64	307	308
CHEESE-ROMANO	OUNCE	28.4	110	9.02	1.03	7.64	29	4.85	2.22	0.168	340	24.5
CHEESE-ROQUEFORT	OUNCE	28.4	105	6.11	0.57	8.69	26	5.46	2.4	0.37	513	26
CHEESE-SWISS	OUNCE	28.4	107	8.06	0.96	7.78	26	5.04	2.06	0.28	74	31
CHEESE-SWISS-PROCESSED	OUNCE	28.4	95	7.01	0.6	7.09	24	4.55	2	0.18	388	61
CREAM-COFFEE-TABLE-LIGHT	CUP	240	469	6.48	8.78	46.3	159	28.9	13.4	1.72	95	292
CREAM-HALF & HALF-FLUID	CUP	242	315	7.16	10.4	27.8	89	17.3	8.04	1.03	98	314
CREAM-SOUR-CULTURED	CUP	230	493	7.27	9.82	48.2	102	30	13.9	1.79	123	331
CREAM-SOUR-HALF & HALF	TBSP	15	20	0.44	0.64	1.8	6	1.12	0.52	0.07	6	19
CREAM-SOUR-IMITATION	OUNCE	28.4	59	0.68	1.88	5.53	0	5.04	0.17	0.02	29	46
CREAM-WHIP-IMIT-FROZ	CUP	75	239	0.94	17.3	19	0	16.3	1.21	0.39	19	14
CREAM-WHIP-IMIT-PRESSURIZE	CUP	70	184	0.69	11.3	15.6	0	13.2	1.35	0.17	43	13
CREAM-WHIP-PRESSURIZED	CUP	60	154	1.92	7.49	13.3	46	8.3	3.85	0.5	78	88
CREAM-WHIPPING-HEAVY	CUP	238	821	4.88	6.64	88.1	326	54.8	25.4	3.27	89	179
MILK-1% FAT-LOWFAT-FLUID	CUP	244	102	8.03	11.7	2.59	10	1.61	0.75	0.1	123	381
MILK-2% FAT-LOWFAT-FLUID	CUP	244	121	8.12	11.7	4.68	18	2.92	1.35	0.17	122	377
MILK-2%-MILK SOLIDS ADDED	CUP	245	125	8.53	12.2	4.7	18	2.93	1.36	0.18	128	397
MILK-BUTTERMILK-FLUID	CUP	245	99	8.11	11.7	2.16	9	1.34	0.62	0.08	257	371
MILK-CHOCOLATE-WHOLE	CUP	250	208	7.92	25.9	8.48	30	5.26	2.48	0.31	149	417
MILK-CONDENSED-SWEET-CAN	CUP	306	982	24.2	166	26.6	104	16.8	7.43	1.03	389	1136
MILK-EGGNOG-COMMERCIAL	CUP	254	342	9.68	34.4	19	149	11.3	5.67	0.86	138	420
MILK-EVAPORATED-SKIM-CAN	CUP	255	199	19.3	28.9	0.51	10.2	0.309	0.158	0.015	293	847
MILK-EVAPORATED-WHOLE-CAN	CUP	252	338	17.2	25.3	19.1	73.1	11.6	5.9	0.605	267	764
MILK-HUMAN-WHOLE-MATURE	CUP	246	171	2.53	17	10.8	34	4.94	4.08	1.22	42	126
MILK-WHOLE-3.3% FAT-FLUID	CUP	244	150	8.03	11.4	8.15	33	5.07	2.35	0.3	120	370
MILK-WHOLE-LOW SODIUM	CUP	244	149	7.56	10.9	8.44	33	5.26	2.44	0.31	6	617
MILKSHAKE-CHOCOLATE-THICK	ITEM	300	356	9.15	63.5	8.1	32	5.04	2.34	0.3	333	672
MILKSHAKE-VANILLA-THICK	ITEM	313	350	12.1	55.6	9.48	37	5.9	2.74	0.35	299	572
YOGURT-FRUIT FLAVOR-LOWFAT	CUP	227	231	9.92	43.2	2.45	10	1.58	0.67	0.07	133	442
YOGURT-PLAIN-LOWFAT	CUP	227	144	11.9	16	3.52	14	2.27	0.97	0.1	159	531
YOGURT-PLAIN-NONFAT	CUP	227	127	13	17.4	0.41	4	0.264	0.112	0.012	174	579
YOGURT-PLAIN-WHOLE	CUP	227	139	7.88	10.6	7.38	29	4.76	2.03	0.21	105	351

MAG Mg	IRON Mg	ZINC Mg	V-A RE	V-C Mg	THIA Mg	RIBO Mg	NIAC Mg	V-B6 Mg	FOL Ug	VB12 Ug	CALC Mg	PHOS Mg	SEL Mg	FIBD Gm	V-E Mg
28	2.8	—	186	10	0.35	0.28	4.5	—	—	—	40	88	0.025	2.5	—
—	2.3	—	216	13	0.25	0.18	2.3	—	—	—	80	135	—	2.5	—
28	3.3	—	200	5	0.15	0.18	2.3	—	—	—	53	113	—	2.75	—
—	3.7	—	—	22	0.25	0.3	4	—	—	—	124	236	0.022	2.73	—
71	2.42	3.93	147	2.2	0.15	0.45	3.22	0.24	23	1.04	221	203	—	2.67	—
40	1.49	0.892	778	5.82	0.129	0.218	1.55	0.135	34.6	0	45.5	92.8	0.001	6.92	

MAG Mg	IRON Mg	ZINC Mg	V-A RE	V-C Mg	THIA Mg	RIBO Mg	NIAC Mg	V-B6 Mg	FOL Ug	VB12 Ug	CALC Mg	PHOS Mg	SEL Mg	FIBD Gm	V-E Mg
9	0.24	0.85	77.8	0	0.008	0.125	0.04	0.04	2.07	0.317	163	130	0.006	0	—
8	0.09	0.73	67	0	0.014	0.122	0.037	0.033	2	0.113	159	202	0.006	0	—
6	0.11	0.85	103	0	0.008	0.1	0.02	0.02	2	0.197	174	211	0.003	0	0.28
6.99	0.09	0.749	61.2	0	0.008	0.108	0.287	0.047	9.98	0.344	150	110	0.006	0	—
8	0.12	0.9	105	0	0.011	0.185	0.239	0.086	24	0.492	147	132	0.008	0	—
31	0.77	3.51	359	0	0.031	0.424	0.09	0.084	21	0.935	815	579	0.018	0	—
11.3	0.315	0.833	110	0	0.047	0.367	0.284	0.151	27	1.4	135	297	0.052	0	—
2.03	0.344	0.152	122	0	0.005	0.057	0.029	0.013	4.05	0.122	23.3	30.4	0.001	0	—
5	0.18	0.82	36.3	0	0.044	0.239	0.281	0.12	9.07	0.479	140	96	—	0	—
8	0.07	1.11	55	0	0.009	0.095	0.018	0.023	6	0.435	198	155	0	0	—
6	0.04	0.6	109	0	0.023	0.143	0.045	0.024	16	0.295	141	111	—	0	—
8	0.2	0.85	80.8	0	0.004	0.111	0.026	0.022	5.16	0.234	212	126	0.013	0	—
7	0.06	0.78	49.8	0	0.005	0.086	0.03	0.02	2	0.232	183	131	0.003	0	—
51	0.95	3.19	211	0	0.045	0.386	0.315	0.105	8	1.4	1376	807	0.024	0	—
8	0.15	0.92	69.4	0	0.005	0.091	0.044	0.021	3	0.415	214	141	—	0	—
36	1.08	3.3	319	0	0.052	0.455	0.192	0.049	32.2	0.716	669	449	—	0	—
11.6	0.218	0.731	48.6	0	0.01	0.105	0.022	0.024	2	0.319	302	215	—	0	—
8	0.16	0.59	89.2	0	0.011	0.166	0.208	0.035	14	0.182	188	111	—	0	—
10.1	0.05	1.11	72.1	0	0.006	0.103	0.026	0.024	2	0.475	272	171	0.002	0	0.2
8	0.17	1.02	68.8	0	0.004	0.078	0.011	0.01	1.67	0.348	219	216	0.002	0	—
21	0.1	0.65	519	1.82	0.077	0.355	0.137	0.077	6	0.528	231	192	0.001	0	1.51
25	0.17	1.23	315	2.08	0.085	0.361	0.189	0.094	6	0.796	254	230	0.001	0	1.52
26	0.14	0.62	546	1.98	0.081	0.343	0.154	0.037	25	0.69	268	195	—	0	—
2	0.01	0.08	20.4	0.13	0.005	0.022	0.01	0.002	2	0.045	16	14	—	0	—
1.81	0.111	0.335	0	0	0	0	0	0	0	0	1	13	—	0	0
1	0.09	0.02	194	0	0	0	0	0	0	0	5	6	—	0	—
1	0.01	0.01	99.4	0	0	0	0	0	0	0	4	13	—	0	—
6	0.03	0.22	165	0	0.022	0.039	0.042	0.025	1.56	0.175	61	54	—	0	—
17	0.07	0.55	1051	1.38	0.052	0.262	0.093	0.062	9	0.428	154	149	—	0	1.5
34	0.12	0.95	150	2.37	0.095	0.407	0.212	0.105	12	0.898	300	235	0.003	0	0.22
33	0.12	0.95	150	2.32	0.095	0.403	0.21	0.105	12	0.888	297	232	0.007	0	0.22
35	0.12	0.98	150	2.45	0.098	0.424	0.22	0.11	13	0.936	313	245	0.007	0	0.22
27	0.12	1.03	24.3	2.4	0.083	0.377	0.142	0.083	12.3	0.537	285	219	0.003	0	0.98
33	0.6	1.02	90.7	2.28	0.092	0.405	0.313	0.1	12	0.835	280	251	0.003	0.15	—
78	0.58	2.88	302	7.96	0.275	1.27	0.643	0.156	34	1.36	868	775	0.003	0	0.337
47	0.51	1.17	268	3.81	0.086	0.483	0.267	0.127	2	1.14	330	278	0.003	0	—
68.9	0.74	2.3	300	3.16	0.115	0.788	0.444	0.14	23	0.609	740	497	0.003	0	0.459
60.5	0.479	1.94	184	4.74	0.118	0.796	0.489	0.126	20.2	0.411	658	509	0.003	0	0.454
8	0.07	0.42	178	12.3	0.034	0.089	0.435	0.027	13	0.111	79	34	0.004	0	2.44
33	0.12	0.93	92.2	2.29	0.093	0.395	0.205	0.102	12	0.871	291	228	0.003	0	0.22
12	0.122	0.927	95.2	2.29	0.049	0.256	0.105	0.083	12.2	0.876	246	209	0.003	0	0.22
48	0.93	1.44	77.5	0	0.141	0.666	0.372	0.075	15	0.945	396	378	0.005	0.75	—
37	0.31	1.22	107	0	0.094	0.61	0.457	0.131	21	1.63	457	361	0.005	0.2	—
33	0.16	1.68	31.2	1.5	0.084	0.404	0.216	0.091	21	1.06	345	271	0.011	0.8	—
40	0.18	2.02	45	1.82	0.1	0.486	0.259	0.111	25	1.28	415	326	0.011	0	—
43	0.2	2.2	4.8	1.98	0.109	0.531	0.281	0.12	28	1.39	452	355	0.011	0	—
26	0.11	1.34	83.8	1.2	0.066	0.322	0.17	0.073	17	0.844	274	215	0.011	0	—

Desserts

Food Name	Portion	WT. Gm	KCAL Kc	PROT Gm	CARB Gm	FAT Gm	CHOL Mg	SAFA Gm	MUFA Gm	PUFA Gm	SOD Mg	POT Mg
CAKE-ANGELFOOD-MIX/PREP	SLICE	53	142	4.2	31.5	0.122	0	—	—	—	142	51.9
CAKE-CHEESECAKE-COMMERCIAL	SLICE	85	257	4.61	24.3	16.3	—	—	—	—	189	83.3
CAKE-FRUIT-DARK-HOME REC	SLICE	15	56.9	0.72	8.96	2.3	6.75	0.48	1.31	0.47	23.7	74.4
CAKE-GINGERBREAD-MIX/PREP	SLICE	63	175	2	32	4	1	1.1	1.8	1.1	90	173
CAKE-POUND-HOME RECIPE	SLICE	33	160	2	16	10	68	5.9	3	0.6	58	20
CAKE-SHEET-NO ICING-HOME	SLICE	86	315	4	48	12	1	3.3	4.9	2.6	382	68
CAKE-SPONGE-HOME RECIPE	SLICE	66	188	4.82	35.7	3.14	162	1.1	1.3	0.5	164	59.4
CAKE-STRAWBERRY SHORTCAKE	SERVING	175	344	4.8	61.2	8.9	—	—	—	—	—	—
CAKE-YELLOW/ICING-HOME REC	SLICE	69	268	2.9	40.3	11.4	36	3	3	1.4	191	72.5
COOKIE-CHOC CHIP-HOME REC	ITEM	10	46.3	0.5	6.41	2.68	5.25	0.6	1.15	0.8	20.6	20.5
COOKIE-CHOCOLATE CHIP-MIX	ITEM	10.5	50	0.5	6.96	2.42	5.52	0.7	0.9	0.6	37.8	13.5
COOKIE-MACAROON	ITEM	19	90	1	12.5	4.5	0	—	—	—	6	88
COOKIE-OATMEAL/RAISIN-MIX	ITEM	13	61.5	0.732	8.93	2.6	0	0.5	0.825	0.5	37.1	22.6
COOKIE-PEANUT BUTTER-MIX	ITEM	10	50	0.8	5.87	2.64	—	—	—	—	56.6	19.4
COOKIE-SANDWICH-CHOC/VAN	ITEM	10	50	0.5	7	2.25	0	0.55	0.975	0.55	63	3.75
COOKIE-SUGAR-MIX	ITEM	20	98.8	0.908	13.1	4.79	—	—	—	—	109	13.6
COOKIE-VANILLA WAFER	ITEM	4	18.5	0.2	3	0.6	2.5	0.1	0.2	0.1	10	2.9
CUPCAKE/CHOCOLATE ICING	ITEM	36	130	2	21	5	15	2	1.7	0.7	120	42
CUSTARD-BAKED	CUP	265	305	14	29	15	278	6.8	5.4	0.7	209	387
DANISH PASTRY-PLAIN	ITEM	65	250	4.06	29.1	13.6	0	4.7	6.1	3.2	249	60.5
DOUGHNUTS-CAKE-PLAIN	ITEM	25	104	1.28	12.2	5.77	10	1.2	1.2	2	139	27.3
DOUGHNUTS-YEAST-GLAZED	ITEM	50	205	3	22	11.2	13	3	5.8	3.3	117	34
FROZ YOGURT-FRUIT VARIETY	CUP	226	216	7	41.8	2	—	—	—	—	—	—
GRANOLA BAR	ITEM	24	109	2.35	16	4.23	—	—	—	—	66.7	78.2
ICE CREAM SUNDAE-HOT FUDGE	ITEM	165	297	5.89	49.8	9.01	21.5	5.25	2.43	0.843	190	413
ICE CREAM-VAN-HARD-10% FAT	CUP	133	269	4.8	31.7	14.3	59	8.92	4.14	0.533	116	257
ICE CREAM-VAN-SOFT SERVE	CUP	173	377	7.04	38.3	22.5	153	13.5	5.85	0.65	153	338
ICE MILK-VAN-SOFT-2.6% FAT	CUP	175	223	8.03	38.4	4.62	13	2.88	1.16	0.1	163	412
PIE-APPLE-HOME REC	SLICE	135	323	2.75	49.1	13.6	0	3.9	6.4	3.6	207	115
PIE-BANANA CREAM-HOME REC	SLICE	130	285	6	40	12	40	3.8	4.7	2.3	252	264
PIE-CHERRY-HOME REC	SLICE	135	350	4	52	15	0	4	6.4	3.6	410	142
PIE-CUSTARD-HOME REC	SLICE	130	285	8	30	14	—	4.8	5.5	2.5	373	178
PIE-LEMON MERINGUE-HOME	SLICE	120	300	3.86	47.3	11.2	0	3.7	4.8	2.3	223	52.8
PIE-MINCE-HOME REC	SLICE	135	365	3	56	16	0	4	6.6	3.6	604	240
PIE-PEACH-HOME REC	SLICE	135	345	3	52	14	0	3.5	6.2	3.6	361	21
PIE-PECAN-HOME REC	SLICE	118	495	6	61	27	0	4	14.4	6.3	260	145
PIE-PUMPKIN-HOME REC	SLICE	130	275	5	32	15	0	5.4	5.4	2.4	278	208
PIECRUST-MIX/PREP-BAKED	ITEM	160	743	10	70.5	46.5	0	11.4	19.9	11.7	1300	89.5
PUDD-CHOC-COOKED-MIX/MILK	CUP	260	320	9	59	8	32	4.3	2.6	2	335	354
PUDD-CHOC-INST-MIX/MILK	CUP	260	325	8	63	7	28	3.6	2.2	0.3	322	335
PUDD-RICE/RAISINS	CUP	265	387	9.5	70.8	8.2	—	—	—	—	188	469
PUDD-TAPIOCA CREAM-HOME	CUP	165	220	8	28	8	80	4.1	2.5	0.5	257	223
SHERBET-ORANGE-2% FAT	CUP	193	270	2.16	58.7	3.82	14	2.38	0.96	0.09	88	198
TURNOVER-APPLE	OUNCE	28.4	85.2	0.738	10.5	4.71	1.42	—	—	—	109	13.9
TWINKIE-HOSTESS	ITEM	42	143	1.25	25.6	4.2	21	—	—	—	189	—

Eggs

Food Name	Portion	WT. Gm	KCAL Kc	PROT Gm	CARB Gm	FAT Gm	CHOL Mg	SAFA Gm	MUFA Gm	PUFA Gm	SOD Mg	POT Mg
EGG-HARD-LARGE-NO SHELL	ITEM	50	77	6.29	0.56	5.3	213	1.63	2.04	0.707	62	63
EGG-POACHED-WHOLE-LARGE	ITEM	50	74	6.22	0.61	4.99	212	1.54	1.9	0.679	140	60
EGG-SUBSTITUTE-LIQUID	CUP	251	211	30.1	1.61	8.31	2.51	1.65	2.25	4.02	444	828
EGG-WHITE-RAW-LARGE	ITEM	33.4	17	3.52	0.34	0	0	0	0	0	55	48
EGG-WHOLE-RAW-LARGE	ITEM	50	75	6.25	0.61	5.01	213	1.55	1.91	0.682	63	60
EGG-YOLK-RAW-LARGE	ITEM	16.6	59	2.78	0.3	5.12	213	1.59	1.95	0.698	7	16

MAG Mg	IRON Mg	ZINC Mg	V-A RE	V-C Mg	THIA Mg	RIBO Mg	NIAC Mg	V-B6 Mg	FOL Ug	VB12 Ug	CALC Mg	PHOS Mg	SEL Mg	FIBD Gm	V-E Mg
5.83	0.451	0.106	0	0	0.064	0.122	0.594	0.007	4.77	0.015	50	63	0.003	0.037	4.5
8.5	0.408	0.357	43	4.25	0.026	0.111	0.391	0.054	15.3	0.421	47.6	74.8	—	1.79	—
—	0.42	—	3.6	0.06	0.024	0.024	0.165	—	—	—	10.8	17	—	0.313	—
14	0.9	0.284	0	0	0.09	0.11	0.8	0.048	5	0.066	57	63	0.004	1.83	—
—	0.5	—	16	0	0.05	0.06	0.4	—	1.98	—	6	24	0.002	0.08	2.8
12	0.9	0.301	30	0	0.13	0.15	1.1	0.024	6.02	0.087	55	88	0.006	0.96	7.3
7.26	1.11	0.799	25	0	0.092	0.132	0.726	0.037	14.5	0.332	25.1	65.3	0.004	0	5.6
—	2	—	86	89	0.17	0.21	1.3	—	—	—	73	84	—	2.14	—
13.1	0.787	0.338	9.5	0	0.076	0.097	0.656	0.023	5.52	0.123	57.3	60.7	0.004	0.552	5.86
3.5	0.249	0.044	1	0	0.015	0.015	0.146	0.002	0.9	0.01	3.3	8.4	0.001	0.27	0.545
2.52	0.228	0.053	6.09	0	0.014	0.022	0.195	0.002	0.945	—	2.94	7.46	0.001	0.284	0.573
—	0.15	—	0	0	0.01	0.03	0.1	—	—	—	5	16	0.001	0.437	1.04
3.64	0.285	0.085	2.08	0	0.022	0.021	0.241	0.006	1.56	—	4.42	14.4	0.001	0.351	0.708
3.9	0.19	0.75	3.04	0	0.019	0.016	0.381	0.008	2.4	—	11.5	23.5	—	0.18	0.545
5.1	0.175	0.086	0	0	0.015	0.025	0.175	0.004	0.3	0	2.5	24	0.001	0.15	0.545
1.6	0.386	0.054	2.96	0	0.036	0.024	0.466	0.011	1.8	—	20.8	37.8	0.001	0.262	1.09
0.68	0.06	—	1	0	0.01	0.009	0.08	—	—	—	1.6	2.5	0	0.01	0.218
—	0.4	—	12	0	0.05	0.06	0.4	—	—	—	47	71	0.003	0.42	0.72
—	1.1	—	87	1	0.11	0.5	0.3	—	—	—	297	310	0.003	1.02	—
9.75	1.2	0.546	11	0	0.156	0.15	1.47	—	—	—	68.9	66.3	—	0.582	—
5.75	0.365	0.128	2.2	0	0.06	0.05	0.428	0.009	2	—	11	55	0.002	0.325	1.01
9.5	0.6	—	5	0	0.1	0.1	0.8	—	11	—	16	33	0.004	1.1	2.03
24	0	—	0	0	0.01	0.26	0	—	—	—	200	200	—	—	—
—	0.763	—	—	—	0.067	0.026	—	—	—	0	14.4	66.5	—	0.96	—
34.7	0.611	0.99	46.2	2.48	0.066	0.314	1.12	0.132	9.9	0.677	216	238	—	—	—
18	0.12	1.41	133	0.7	0.052	0.329	0.134	0.061	3	0.625	176	134	0.002	0	0.466
25	0.43	1.99	199	0.92	0.08	0.448	0.178	0.095	9	0.996	236	199	0.002	0	0.606
29	0.28	0.86	44	1.17	0.117	0.541	0.184	0.133	5	1.37	274	202	0.003	0	0.61
10.8	1.22	0.23	5.1	2	0.149	0.108	1.24	0.035	6.75	0	12.2	31.1	0.015	2.16	9.84
—	1	—	66	1	0.11	0.22	1	—	—	—	86	107	0.015	1.4	—
9.45	0.9	—	118	0	0.16	0.12	1.4	—	—	0	19	34	0.015	1.08	9.84
—	1.2	—	60	0	0.11	0.27	0.8	—	—	—	125	147	0.015	2.08	9.48
7.2	0.9	0.336	33.4	3.66	0.096	0.12	0.72	0.029	10.8	0.191	15.6	48	0.013	1.44	8.75
24.3	1.9	—	0	1	0.14	0.12	1.4	—	—	—	38	51	0.015	1.96	9.84
9.45	1.2	—	198	4	0.15	0.14	2	—	—	0	14	39	0.015	1.82	9.84
—	3.7	—	40	0	0.26	0.14	1	—	—	—	55	122	0.012	4.13	—
16.9	1	—	320	0	0.11	0.18	1	—	—	—	66	90	0.015	3.51	9.48
—	3.05	—	0	0	0.535	0.395	4.95	—	—	—	65.5	136	—	4.23	1.39
—	0.8	—	68	2	0.05	0.39	0.3	—	—	—	265	247	—	0	—
—	1.3	—	68	2	0.08	0.39	0.3	—	—	—	374	237	—	0	—
—	1.1	—	35	0	0.08	0.37	0.5	—	—	—	260	249	—	1.42	—
—	0.7	—	60	2	0.07	0.3	0.2	—	—	—	173	180	—	0.56	—
15	0.31	1.33	39	3.86	0.033	0.089	0.131	0.025	14	0.158	103	74	—	0	—
2.56	0.312	0.054	2.28	0.284	0.028	0.02	0.332	0.011	1.14	0.028	3.98	11.4	—	0.21	2.07
—	0.545	—	8.1	0	0.055	0.06	0.5	—	—	—	19	—	—	—	—

MAG Mg	IRON Mg	ZINC Mg	V-A RE	V-C Mg	THIA Mg	RIBO Mg	NIAC Mg	V-B6 Mg	FOL Ug	VB12 Ug	CALC Mg	PHOS Mg	SEL Mg	FIBD Gm	V-E Mg
5	0.6	0.52	84	0	0.033	0.256	0.032	0.06	22	0.56	25	86	0.012	0	0.7
5	0.72	0.55	95.2	0	0.025	0.215	0.031	0.059	18	0.4	25	89	0.012	0	0.7
21.9	5.27	3.26	542	0	0.276	0.753	0.276	0.008	37.4	0.748	133	304	—	0	—
4	0.01	0	0	0	0.002	0.151	0.031	0.001	1	0.07	2	4	0.005	0	0
5	0.72	0.55	95.2	0	0.031	0.254	0.037	0.07	23	0.5	25	89	0.022	0	0.7
1	0.59	0.52	97	0	0.028	0.106	0.002	0.065	24	0.52	23	81	0.007	0	0.7

Fast Foods*

Food Name	Portion	WT. Gm	KCAL Kc	PROT Gm	CARB Gm	FAT Gm	CHOL Mg	SAFA Gm	MUFA Gm	PUFA Gm	SOD Mg	POT Mg
ARTHUR TREACHER-CHICK SAND	ITEM	156	413	16.2	44	19.2	—	—	—	6.7	708	279
BURGER KING-WHOP HAMBURGER	ITEM	261	630	26	50	36	104	16.5	13.8	2.22	990	520
CHURCHS CHICK-WHITE MEAT	ITEM	100	327	21	10	23	—	—	—	—	498	186
DAIRY QUEEN-BANANA SPLIT	ITEM	383	540	10	91	15	30	—	—	—	—	—
DAIRY QUEEN-CONE-REGULAR	ITEM	142	226	5.37	33.2	8.43	38.3	4.87	2.5	0.494	126	233
DAIRY QUEEN-DIP CONE-REG	ITEM	156	300	7	40	13	20	—	—	—	—	—
DAIRY QUEEN-FLOAT	ITEM	397	330	6	59	8	20	—	—	—	—	—
DAIRY QUEEN-MALT-REGULAR	ITEM	418	600	15	89	20	50	—	—	—	—	—
DIARY QUEEN-SUNDAE-REGULAR	ITEM	177	319	6.31	53.4	9.66	23	5.63	2.61	0.904	204	443
JACK/BOX-BREAK JACK SAND	ITEM	121	301	18	28	13	182	—	—	—	1037	190
JACK/BOX-JUMBO JACK HAMBUR	ITEM	246	551	28	45	29	80	11.4	12.6	2.42	1134	492
JACK/BOX-JUMBO JACK/CHEESE	ITEM	272	628	32	45	35	110	15	12.6	2.03	1666	499
JACK/BOX-MOBY JACK	ITEM	141	455	17	38	26	56	—	—	—	837	246
JACK/BOX-ONION RINGS-BAG	ITEM	83	275	3.7	31.3	15.5	14	6.95	6.65	0.665	430	129
MCDONALD-BIG MAC HAMBURGER	ITEM	215	560	25.2	42.5	32.4	103	10.1	20.1	1.5	950	237
MCDONALD-QP HAMBURGER W/CH	ITEM	194	520	28.5	35.1	29.2	118	11.2	16.5	1.51	1150	341
MCDONALDS-CHEESEBURGER	ITEM	116	310	15	31.2	13.8	53	5.17	7.66	0.93	750	223
MCDONALDS-EGG MCMUFFIN	ITEM	138	290	18.2	28.1	11.2	226	3.82	6.1	1.29	740	213
MCDONALDS-FILET O FISH	ITEM	142	440	13.8	37.9	26.1	50	5.16	10.2	10.8	1030	150
MCDONALDS-HAMBURGER	ITEM	102	260	12.3	30.6	9.5	37	3.63	5.09	0.77	500	215
MCDONALDS-QP HAMBURGER	ITEM	166	410	23.1	34	20.7	86	8.09	11.4	1.21	660	322
TACO BELL-BEAN BURRITO	ITEM	168	332	16.7	42.6	11.5	79	5.6	4.23	0.633	1030	405
TACO BELL-BEEF BURRITO	ITEM	110	262	13.3	29.3	10.4	32.5	5.23	3.7	0.427	746	370
TACO BELL-BEEFY TOSTADA	ITEM	225	334	16.1	29.7	16.9	75	11.5	3.51	0.538	870	490
TACO BELL-BURRITO SUPREME	ITEM	225	457	21	43	22	126	7.7	7.35	1.65	367	350
TACO BELL-TACO-REGULAR	ITEM	171	370	20.7	26.7	20.6	57	11.4	6.58	0.959	802	473
TACO BELL-TOSTADA-REGULAR	ITEM	144	223	9.6	26.5	9.86	30	5.37	3.05	0.749	543	403
WENDYS-DOUBLE HAMBURGER	ITEM	226	540	34.3	40.3	26.6	122	10.5	10.3	2.8	791	569
WENDYS-SINGLE HAMBURGER	ITEM	218	511	25.7	40.1	27.4	86	10.4	11.4	2.2	825	479
WENDYS-TRIPLE HAMBURGER	ITEM	259	693	50	28.6	41.5	142	15.9	18.2	2.74	713	785

*For more fast foods, see pp A-34 to A-45.

Fats Oils

Food Name	Portion	WT. Gm	KCAL Kc	PROT Gm	CARB Gm	FAT Gm	CHOL Mg	SAFA Gm	MUFA Gm	PUFA Gm	SOD Mg	POT Mg
ANIMAL FAT-COOKING-CHICKEN	TBSP	12.8	115	0	0	12.8	11	3.8	5.7	2.7	0	0
BUTTER-REGULAR-TABLESPOON	TBSP	14	100	0.119	0.008	11.4	30.7	7.07	3.28	0.421	116	3.64
BUTTER-WHIPPED-TABLESPOON	TBSP	9	64.5	0.077	0.005	7.3	19.7	4.54	2.11	0.271	74.3	2.34
MARGARINE-CORN-REG-HARD	TSP	4.7	33.8	0	0	3.8	0	0.6	2.2	0.8	44.3	1.99
MARGARINE-CORN-REG-SOFT	TSP	4.7	33.7	0	0	3.8	0	0.7	1.5	1.5	50.7	1.77
MARGARINE-DIET-MAZOLA	TBSP	14	50	0	0	5.7	0	1	2.1	2.6	130	—
MARGARINE-REG-HARD-STICK	ITEM	113	812	1.02	1.02	91	0	17.9	40.5	28.7	1066	47.9
MARGARINE-VEG SPRAY-MAZOLA	SERVING	0.72	6	0	0	0.72	0	0.08	0.17	0.4	0	—
MAYONNAISE-IMITATION-SOY	TBSP	15	34.7	0.045	2.4	2.9	3.6	0.495	0.675	1.59	74.6	1.5
MAYONNAISE-LIGHT-LOW CAL	TBSP	14	40	0	1	4	5	—	—	—	—	—
MIRACLE WHIP-LIGHT-LOW CAL	TBSP	14	45	0	2	4	5	—	—	—	95	—
SAL DRESS-BLUE CHE-LOW CAL	TBSP	16	10	0	1	1	4	0.5	0.3	0	177	5
SAL DRESS-BLUE CHEESE	TBSP	15.3	77.1	0.7	1.1	8	2.6	1.5	1.9	4.3	167	5.66
SAL DRESS-CAESAR	TBSP	15	70	0	1	7	—	—	—	—	—	—
SAL DRESS-FRENCH	TBSP	15.6	67	0.1	2.7	6.4	1.95	1.5	1.2	3.4	214	12.3
SAL DRESS-FRENCH-LOW CAL	TBSP	16.3	21.9	0.033	3.5	0.9	0.978	0.13	0.228	0.554	128	12.9
SAL DRESS-ITALIAN	TBSP	14.7	68.7	0	1.5	7.1	0	1	1.7	4.1	116	2
SAL DRESS-ITALIAN-LOW CAL	TBSP	15	15.8	0	0.7	1.5	1	0.2	0.3	0.9	118	2
SAL DRESS-MAYO-LOW CAL	TBSP	16	20	0	2	2	2	0.4	0.4	1	44	1
SAL DRESS-MAYONNAISE TYPE	TBSP	14.7	57.3	0.132	4.91	4.91	3.82	0.72	1.32	2.65	104	1.32
SAL DRESS-RANCH STYLE	TBSP	15	54	0.4	0.6	5.7	—	—	—	—	97	—
SAL DRESS-RUSSIAN	TBSP	15.3	76	0.2	1.6	7.8	0	1.1	1.8	4.5	133	24
SAL DRESS-RUSSIAN-LOW CAL	TBSP	16.3	23	0.082	4.5	0.652	1	0.1	0.2	0.4	141	26
SAL DRESS-THOU ISL-LOW CAL	TBSP	15.3	24.3	0.1	2.5	1.6	2	0.2	0.4	1	153	17
SAL DRESS-THOUSAND ISLAND	TBSP	15.6	58.9	0.14	2.4	5.6	4.9	0.9	1.3	3.1	109	18
SAL DRESS-VINEGAR/OIL-HOME	TBSP	15.6	70	0	0.39	7.81	0	1.42	2.31	3.76	0.078	1.17
SANDWICH SPREAD-COMMERCIAL	TBSP	15.3	59.5	0.1	3.4	5.2	12	0.8	1.1	3.1	153	5.36
SHORTENING-VEGETABLE-SOY	CUP	205	1812	0	0	205	0	51.2	89	52.2	—	—
VEGETABLE OIL-CORN	CUP	218	1927	0	0	218	0	27.7	52.7	128	0	0
VEGETABLE OIL-OLIVE	CUP	216	1909	0	0	216	0	29.2	159	18.2	0.08	0

MAG Mg	IRON Mg	ZINC Mg	V-A RE	V-C Mg	THIA Mg	RIBO Mg	NIAC Mg	V-B6 Mg	FOL Ug	VB12 Ug	CALC Mg	PHOS Mg	SEL Mg	FIBD Gm	V-E Mg
27	1.7	—	36.9	19	0.17	0.24	8.1	—	—	—	59	147	—	—	—
50	6	5.25	192	13	0.02	0.03	5.2	0.312	31.2	2.81	104	312	—	—	—
—	1	—	48	1	0.1	0.18	7.2	—	—	—	94	—	—	—	—
—	1.8	—	225	18	0.6	0.6	0.8	—	—	0.9	350	250	—	—	—
21.3	0.213	0.781	87.4	1.56	0.071	0.355	0.426	0.085	7.1	0.284	212	192	—	—	—
—	0.4	—	90.1	0	0.09	0.34	0	—	—	0.6	200	150	—	—	—
—	0	—	30	0	0.12	0.17	0	—	—	0.6	200	200	—	—	—
—	3.6	—	225	3.6	0.12	0.6	0.8	—	—	1.8	500	400	—	—	—
37.2	0.655	1.06	74.5	2.66	0.071	0.336	1.2	0.142	10.6	0.726	232	255	—	—	—
24	2.5	1.8	133	3	0.41	0.47	5.1	0.14	—	1.1	177	310	—	—	—
44	4.5	4.2	73.9	3.7	0.47	0.34	11.6	0.3	—	2.68	134	261	—	—	—
49	4.6	4.8	220	4.9	0.52	0.38	11.3	0.31	—	3.05	273	411	—	—	—
30	1.7	1.1	72.1	1	0.3	0.21	4.5	0.12	—	1.1	167	263	—	—	—
15	0.85	0.35	2.4	0.6	0.09	0.1	0.92	0.06	11	0.12	73	86	—	—	5.36
38	4	4.7	106	1.68	0.48	0.41	6.81	0.27	21	1.8	256	314	—	—	—
41	3.72	5.7	211	3.24	0.37	0.39	6.73	0.23	23	2.15	295	382	—	—	—
21	2.3	2.09	118	2.15	0.29	0.21	3.86	0.12	18	0.94	199	177	—	—	—
33	2.77	1.8	150	1.38	0.47	0.33	3.71	0.16	44	0.8	256	319	—	—	—
27	1.83	0.9	43.8	0.06	0.3	0.15	2.68	0.1	20	0.82	165	229	—	1.11	—
23	2.29	2.05	45.6	2.15	0.28	0.16	3.84	0.12	17	0.84	122	110	—	—	—
37	3.68	5.1	67	3.24	0.36	0.29	6.7	0.27	23	1.88	142	249	—	—	—
0.407	3.84	3.04	240	3.3	0.275	0.6	3.86	0.205	73	0.995	144	143	—	—	—
40.5	3.05	2.37	41.7	0.55	0.115	0.46	3.23	0.16	19.5	0.985	42	87.5	—	—	—
68	2.45	3.18	383	3.9	0.09	0.5	2.85	0.26	0.26	1.13	190	173	—	—	—
51.8	3.8	5.85	216	8	0.45	0.923	6.17	0.27	42.8	1.53	146	245	—	—	—
71	2.42	3.93	257	2.2	0.15	0.45	3.22	0.24	23	1.04	221	203	—	—	—
59	1.88	1.9	187	1.3	0.1	0.33	1.33	0.17	75	0.68	211	116	—	—	—
49	5.95	5.68	30.6	1.2	0.36	0.39	7.57	0.54	27	4.07	102	314	—	—	—
43	4.92	4.87	93.4	2.5	0.42	0.38	7.28	0.33	36	2.38	96	233	—	—	—
55	8.33	10.8	47.4	1.4	0.31	0.56	11	0.62	31	4.92	65	393	—	—	—

MAG Mg	IRON Mg	ZINC Mg	V-A RE	V-C Mg	THIA Mg	RIBO Mg	NIAC Mg	V-B6 Mg	FOL Ug	VB12 Ug	CALC Mg	PHOS Mg	SEL Mg	FIBD Gm	V-E Mg
0	0	0	0	0	0	0	0	0	0	0	0	0	—	0	0.3
0.28	0.022	0.007	105	0	0.001	0.005	0.006	0	0.42	0.018	3.36	3.22	0	0	0.221
0.18	0.014	0.005	67.9	0	0	0.003	0.004	0	0.27	0.011	2.16	2.07	0	0	0.142
0.12	0	—	47	0.008	0	0.002	0.001	0	0.06	0.004	1.41	1.08	0	0	2.71
0.11	0	0	47	0.007	0	0.002	0.001	0	0.05	0.004	1.25	0.95	0	0	2
—	0	—	130	0	0	0	0	—	—	—	0	—	0	0	1.35
2.94	0.068	0	338	0.181	0.011	0.042	0.026	0.01	1.34	0.108	33.8	25.9	0.002	0	65.1
—	0	—	0	0	0	0	0	—	—	—	0	0	—	0	—
0.002	0	0.017	0	0	0	0	0	0	0	0	0.002	0.008	—	0	2.7
—	—	—	—	—	—	—	—	—	—	—	—	—	—	0	8.12
—	—	—	—	—	—	—	—	—	—	—	—	—	—	0	4.2
—	0	—	9	0	0	0.01	0	—	—	—	10	8	—	0	7.6
0	0.031	0	9.5	0.3	0.002	0.02	0.015	0.006	1.24	0.042	12.4	11.3	—	0.05	7.5
—	—	—	—	—	—	—	—	—	—	—	—	—	—	0.04	7.13
0	0.1	0.01	3.12	0	0.001	0.002	0	0.002	0.654	0.022	1.7	2.2	—	0.1	7.41
0	0.1	0.03	0	0	0	0	0	0	0	0	2	2.28	—	0.09	7.75
0.094	0	0.02	3.53	0	0	0	0	0.002	0.719	0.024	1	1	—	0.05	6.99
0	0	0.017	0	0	0	0	0	0	0	0	0	1	—	0.09	7.13
—	0	—	12	—	0	0	0	—	—	—	3	4	—	0	4.8
0.29	0.029	0.026	9.6	0	0.002	0.004	0	0.002	0.923	0.031	2.06	3.82	—	0	4.41
—	—	—	—	—	—	—	—	—	—	—	—	—	—	0	4.5
0.23	0.1	0.07	31.8	1	0.01	0.01	0.1	0.005	1.59	0.046	3	6	—	0	7.27
0.075	0.098	0.016	2.61	0.978	0.001	0.002	0	0.001	0.569	0.019	3.1	6.03	—	0.2	7.74
0.107	0.1	0.024	14.8	0	0	0	0	0.002	0.854	0.028	2	3	—	0.3	6.99
0.312	0.1	0.02	15	0	0	0	0	0.003	0.98	0.032	2	3	—	0.6	7.45
0	0	0	0	0	0	0	0	0	0	0	—	—	—	0	8.05
0	0	0	0	0	0	0	0	0	0	0	0	0	—	0.02	5.28
—	—	—	—	—	—	—	—	—	—	—	—	—	—	0	197
0	0	0	0	0	0	0	0	0	0	0	0	0	—	0	181
0.02	0.83	0.13	0	0	0	0	0	0	0	0	0.38	2.63	—	0	27.3

Fish

Food Name	Portion	WT. Gm	KCAL Kc	PROT Gm	CARB Gm	FAT Gm	CHOL Mg	SAFA Gm	MUFA Gm	PUFA Gm	SOD Mg	POT Mg
FISH-ANCHOVY-FILLET-CAN	ITEM	4	8.4	1.16	0	0.388	3.4	0.088	0.151	0.102	147	21.8
FISH-BLUEFISH-BAKED/BUTTER	ITEM	155	246	40.6	0	8.1	108	1.83	1.84	3.94	161	—
FISH-CARP-COOKED-DRY HEAT	SERVING	85	138	19.4	0	6.1	71.4	1.18	2.54	1.56	54	363
FISH-CATFISH-FRIED-BREADED	SERVING	85	195	15.4	6.83	11.3	68.9	2.79	4.77	2.83	238	289
FISH-CLAM-CAN-SOLID/LIQUID	OUNCE	28.4	12.8	2.33	0.667	0.333	17.7	0.067	0	0	14.7	39.7
FISH-CLAMS-BREADED-FRIED	SERVING	85	172	12.1	8.78	8.78	51.9	2.28	3.86	2.44	309	277
FISH-CLAMS-CKD-MOIST HEAT	SERVING	85	126	21.7	4.36	1.65	57	0.16	0.146	0.469	95	534
FISH-CLAMS-RAW-MEAT ONLY	SERVING	85	62.9	10.9	2.18	0.83	28.9	0.08	0.068	0.24	47.6	267
FISH-COD-COOKED-DRY HEAT	PIECE	180	189	41.1	0	1.55	99	0.302	0.223	0.526	140	439
FISH-CRAB CAKE	ITEM	60	93	12.1	0.288	4.51	90	0.89	1.69	1.36	198	194
FISH-CRAB MEAT-KING-CAN	CUP	135	135	24	1	3.2	135	0.6	0.6	2	675	149
FISH-CRAB-IMITATION-SURIMI	SERVING	85	86.7	10.2	8.69	1.11	17	0.221	0.17	0.57	715	76.5
FISH-CRAB-STEAMED-PIECES	CUP	155	150	30	0	2.39	82.2	0.206	0.287	0.831	1662	406
FISH-CRAYFISH-CKD-MOIST	SERVING	85	96.9	20.3	0	1.15	151	0.197	0.32	0.281	57.8	298
FISH-FLATFISH-CKD-DRY HEAT	SERVING	85	99.5	20.5	0	1.3	58	0.309	0.263	0.35	89.3	292
FISH-GROUPER-CKD-DRY HEAT	SERVING	85	100	25.7	0	1.11	40	0.254	0.228	0.343	45	403
FISH-HADDOCK-COOK-DRY HEAT	SERVING	85	95.2	20.6	0	0.79	62.9	0.142	0.128	0.263	74	339
FISH-HALIBUT-BROILED-DRY	SERVING	85	119	22.7	0	2.5	34.9	0.354	0.822	0.799	58.7	490
FISH-LOBSTER-CKD-MOIST	OUNCE	28.4	27.8	5.82	0.364	0.168	20.4	0.03	0.045	0.026	108	100
FISH-MACKEREL-ATLANTIC-CAN	CUP	190	296	44.1	0	12	150	3.53	4.23	3.14	720	369
FISH-MACKEREL-CKD-DRY HEAT	SERVING	85	223	20.3	0	15.1	63.8	3.55	5.96	3.66	70.6	341
FISH-MUSSEL-BLUE-CKD-MOIST	SERVING	85	147	20.2	6.28	3.81	47.6	0.723	0.862	1.03	313	228
FISH-OCEAN PERCH-CKD-DRY	SERVING	85	103	20.3	0	1.78	45.9	0.266	0.681	0.465	82	298
FISH-OYSTER-EAST-CKD-MOIST	SERVING	85	117	12	6.65	4.21	92.7	1.07	0.425	1.26	190	389
FISH-OYSTER-EASTERN-CANNED	CUP	248	171	17.5	9.7	6.14	136	1.57	0.62	1.83	278	568
FISH-OYSTERS-PACIFIC-RAW	SERVING	85	68.9	8.03	4.21	1.96	42.5	0.434	0.304	0.76	90.1	143
FISH-OYSTERS-RAW-MEAT ONLY	CUP	248	171	17.5	9.7	6.14	136	1.56	0.62	1.83	277	568
FISH-PERCH-BREADED-FRIED	PIECE	85	195	16	6	11	32	2.7	4.4	2.3	128	242
FISH-PERCH-COOKED-DRY HEAT	SERVING	85	99.5	21.1	0	1	98	0.201	0.166	0.401	67.2	292
FISH-POLLOCK-ATLANTIC-RAW	SERVING	85	78.2	16.5	0	0.833	60.4	0.115	0.095	0.411	73.1	303
FISH-POLLOCK-CKD-DRY HEAT	SERVING	85	96.1	20	0	0.952	81.6	0.196	0.148	0.445	98.6	329
FISH-POMPANO-CKD-DRY HEAT	SERVING	85	179	20.1	0	10.3	54.4	3.82	2.82	1.24	64.6	541
FISH-RED SNAPPER-CKD-DRY	SERVING	85	109	22.4	0	1.46	40	0.31	0.274	0.5	48.5	444
FISH-ROCKFISH-CKD-DRY HEAT	SERVING	100	121	24	0	2.01	44	0.474	0.447	0.594	77	520
FISH-ROE-RAW-EGGS	OUNCE	28.4	39.4	6.34	0.426	1.82	106	0.414	0.472	0.754	25.8	62.8
FISH-SALMON-CKD-MOIST HEAT	SERVING	85	157	23.3	0	6.41	41.7	1.19	2.22	1.87	50.2	454
FISH-SALMON-PINK-CAN	SERVING	85	118	16.8	0	5.14	46.8	1.3	1.54	1.74	471	277
FISH-SALMON-SMOKED	SERVING	100	117	18.3	0	4.32	23	0.929	2.02	0.995	784	175
FISH-SARDINES-CAN/OIL	ITEM	12	25	2.95	0	1.37	17	0.184	0.464	0.618	60.5	47.6
FISH-SCALLOPS-STEAMED	OUNCE	28.4	31.8	6.59	0.511	0.398	15.1	—	—	—	75.2	135
FISH-SEA BASS-CKD-DRY HEAT	SERVING	85	105	20.1	0	2.18	45.1	0.557	0.462	0.81	74	279
FISH-SHAD-BAKE/MARG/BACON	SERVING	100	201	23.2	0	11.3	69.4	2.45	2.23	5.9	79	377
FISH-SHRIMP-CKD-MOIST HEAT	SERVING	85	84.2	17.8	0	0.918	166	0.246	0.167	0.374	190	155
FISH-SHRIMP-FRENCH FRIED	SERVING	85	206	18.2	9.75	10.4	150	1.77	3.24	4.32	292	191
FISH-SHRIMP-MEAT-CAN	CUP	128	154	29.5	1.32	2.51	221	0.477	0.375	0.966	216	269
FISH-SMELT-COOKED-DRY HEAT	SERVING	85	105	19.2	0	2.64	76.5	0.492	0.699	0.965	65.5	316
FISH-SOLE/FLOUNDER-BAKED	SERVING	127	148	30.7	0	1.94	86	0.461	0.392	0.523	133	436
FISH-SQUID-COOKED-FRIED	SERVING	85	149	15.3	6.62	6.36	221	1.6	2.34	1.82	260	237
FISH-STICK-BREAD-FROZ-COOK	OUNCE	28.4	77.2	4.44	6.75	3.47	31.8	0.894	1.44	0.899	165	74.1
FISH-SURIMI	SERVING	85	84.2	12.9	5.82	0.765	25.5	0.153	0.119	0.391	122	95.2
FISH-SWORDFISH-BROIL/MARG	SERVING	100	174	28	0	6	4	—	—	—	—	—
FISH-SWORDFISH-COOKED-DRY	SERVING	85	132	21.6	0	4.37	42.5	1.2	1.68	1.01	97.8	314
FISH-TROUT-BROOK-COOKED	SERVING	100	196	23.5	0.4	11.2	—	—	—	—	78.8	—
FISH-TROUT-RAINBOW-CKD-DRY	SERVING	85	128	22.4	0	3.66	62.1	0.707	1.13	1.31	28.9	539
FISH-TUNA-CAN/OIL-DRAINED	SERVING	85	168	24.8	0	6.98	15.3	1.3	2.51	2.45	301	176
FISH-TUNA-DIET-LOW SODIUM	OUNCE	28.4	35.5	7.67	0.011	0.54	9.94	0.09	0.163	0.199	11.4	73.8
FISH-TUNA-LIGHT-CAN/WATER	SERVING	85	111	25.1	0	0.525	15.3	0.136	0.122	0.111	303	267
FISH-TUNA-WHITE-CAN/WATER	SERVING	85	116	22.7	0	2.09	35.7	0.556	0.551	0.78	333	241
FISH-TUNA-YELLOWFIN-RAW	SERVING	85	91.8	19.9	0	0.81	38.3	0.2	0.131	0.241	31.5	377
FISH-WHITE PERCH-FRI-FILET	ITEM	65	108	12.5	0	5.3	—	—	—	—	—	—
FISH-WHITEFISH-BAKE/STUFF	SERVING	100	215	15.2	5.8	14	—	—	—	—	195	291
FISH-WHITING-CKD-DRY HEAT	SERVING	85	98	20	0	1.43	71.4	0.269	0.4	0.456	112	369

MAG Mg	IRON Mg	ZINC Mg	V-A RE	V-C Mg	THIA Mg	RIBO Mg	NIAC Mg	V-B6 Mg	FOL Ug	VB12 Ug	CALC Mg	PHOS Mg	SEL Mg	FIBD Gm	V-E Mg
2.76	0.185	0.098	0.84	0	0.003	0.015	0.796	0.008	0.5	0.035	9.28	10.1	0.002	0	—
43.3	1.1	—	24	—	0.17	0.16	2.9	—	—	1.64	44.6	445	0.047	0	—
32.3	1.35	1.62	7.65	1.36	0.119	0.06	1.79	0.186	14.7	1.25	44.2	451	0.026	0	—
23	1.22	0.731	6.8	0	0.062	0.113	1.94	0.162	14	1.62	37.4	184	—	0.8	—
—	1.17	0.347	—	—	0.003	0.03	0.3	—	—	5.4	15.7	38.7	0.046	0	—
11.9	11.8	1.24	76.5	8.5	0.085	0.207	1.75	0.051	15.5	34.2	53.6	160	—	0.32	—
16	23.8	2.32	145	18.8	0.128	0.362	2.85	0.094	—	84.1	78	287	—	0	—
7.65	11.9	1.16	76.5	11.1	0.068	0.181	1.5	0.051	13.6	42	39.1	144	0.016	0	—
76	0.882	1.04	25.2	1.8	0.158	0.142	4.52	0.509	14.6	1.89	25.2	248	0.081	0	—
19.8	0.648	2.45	48.6	1.68	0.054	0.048	1.74	0.102	24.9	3.56	63	128	0.013	0.03	—
29	1.1	5.83	—	—	0.11	0.11	2.6	—	—	13.5	61	246	0.03	0	—
36.6	0.332	0.281	17	0	0.027	0.023	0.153	0.026	1.36	1.36	11.1	240	0.019	0	—
97.7	1.18	11.8	14	11.8	0.082	0.085	2.08	0.279	79.1	17.8	91.5	434	0.034	0	1.89
26.4	2.67	1.43	8.17	2.81	0.153	0.065	2.5	0.153	2.98	2.94	25.5	281	—	0	—
49.3	0.289	0.536	9.35	0	0.068	0.097	1.85	0.204	7.82	2.13	15.3	246	—	0	—
32	0.969	0.434	42.5	0	0.069	0.005	0.324	0.298	8.67	0.588	17.9	121	—	0	—
42.5	1.15	0.408	16.2	0	0.034	0.038	3.94	0.294	11.3	1.18	35.7	205	0.025	0	1.02
91	0.91	0.45	45.9	0	0.059	0.077	6.06	0.337	11.7	1.16	51	242	0.051	0	—
9.94	0.111	0.829	7.38	0	0.002	0.019	0.304	0.022	3.15	0.883	17.3	52.5	0.023	0	—
70.3	3.88	1.94	247	1.71	0.076	0.403	11.7	0.399	9.5	13.2	458	572	0.089	0	2.52
82.5	1.33	0.799	45.9	0.34	0.135	0.35	5.82	0.391	1.28	16.2	12.8	236	0.03	0	—
32	5.71	2.27	77.4	11.6	0.255	0.357	2.55	0.085	64.3	20.4	28	242	—	0	—
33	1	0.52	11.9	0.68	0.111	0.114	2.07	0.23	8.84	0.981	116	235	0.03	0	—
92.7	11.4	155	145	7.23	0.247	0.282	2.12	0.081	15.2	32.5	75.7	236	0.051	0	—
134	16.6	226	223	12.4	0.372	0.412	3.09	0.236	22.1	47.5	112	344	0.149	0	—
18.7	4.34	14.1	68.9	6.8	0.057	0.198	1.71	0.043	8.5	13.6	6.8	138	0.056	0	—
134	16.6	226	223	12.4	0.372	0.412	3.25	0.124	24.6	47.5	112	345	0.141	0	—
—	1.1	—	—	—	0.1	0.1	1.6	—	—	0.85	28	192	0.02	0.05	—
32.3	0.986	1.21	8.5	1.45	0.068	0.102	1.62	0.119	4.93	1.87	86.7	218	0.03	0	—
57	0.391	0.4	9.01	0	0.04	0.157	2.78	0.244	2.55	2.71	51	188	—	0	—
62.1	0.238	0.51	19.6	0	0.063	0.065	1.4	0.059	3.06	3.57	5.1	410	—	0	—
26.4	0.57	0.587	30.6	0	0.578	0.128	3.23	0.196	14.7	1.02	36.6	290	—	0	—
31.5	0.204	0.374	29.8	1.36	0.045	0.003	0.294	0.391	4.93	2.98	34	171	—	0	—
34	0.53	0.53	66	0	0.044	0.084	3.92	0.27	10.4	1.2	12	228	0.039	0	—
5.68	0.17	0.284	22.4	4.54	0.068	0.21	0.511	0.045	22.7	2.84	6.25	114	0.014	0	—
31.5	0.757	0.442	15.3	0.85	0.162	0.17	7.14	0.391	3.91	3.06	39.1	248	0.026	0	—
28.9	0.714	0.782	14.5	0	0.02	0.158	5.56	0.255	13.1	3.74	181	280	0.045	0	1.54
18	0.85	0.31	26	0	0.023	0.101	4.72	0.278	1.9	3.26	11	164	0.061	0	—
4.68	0.35	0.157	8.04	0	0.01	0.027	0.63	0.02	1.42	1.07	45.8	58.8	0.006	0	—
—	0.852	—	—	—	—	—	—	—	—	—	32.7	96	0.015	0	—
45.1	0.315	0.442	54.4	0	0.111	0.128	1.62	0.391	4.93	0.255	11.1	211	—	0	—
—	0.6	—	9.01	—	0.13	0.26	8.6	—	—	—	24	313	—	0	2
28.9	2.63	1.33	56.1	1.87	0.026	0.027	2.2	0.108	2.98	1.26	33.2	116	0.054	0	—
34	1.07	1.17	47.6	1.28	0.11	0.116	2.61	0.083	6.9	1.59	57	185	0.027	0.48	—
52.5	3.5	1.61	23	2.94	0.035	0.047	3.53	0.142	2.3	1.43	75.5	298	0.041	0	—
32.3	0.978	1.8	14.5	0	0.629	0.124	1.5	0.145	3.91	3.37	65.5	251	0.105	0	—
74	0.43	0.8	14.4	—	0.102	0.145	2.77	0.305	—	3.19	23	368	0.16	0	—
32.3	0.859	1.48	9.35	3.57	0.048	0.389	2.21	0.049	4.51	1.04	33.2	213	—	0.3	—
7.1	0.21	0.187	8.8	0	0.036	0.05	0.596	0.017	5.17	0.51	5.68	51.4	0.003	0.665	—
36.6	0.221	0.281	17	0	0.017	0.018	0.187	0.026	1.36	1.36	7.65	240	—	0	—
—	1.3	—	616	—	0.04	0.05	10.9	—	—	—	—	275	0.047	0	—
28.9	0.884	1.25	34.9	0.935	0.037	0.099	10	0.324	1.96	1.72	5.1	286	—	0	—
35	1.1	—	95.8	1	0.12	0.06	2.5	—	—	—	218	272	—	0	0.2
33.2	2.07	1.18	18.7	3.15	0.072	0.191	5.87	0.391	14.7	2.98	73.1	273	—	0	—
26.4	1.18	0.765	19.6	0	0.032	0.102	10.5	0.094	4.51	1.87	11.1	264	0.061	0	—
9.09	0.341	0.142	6.91	—	0.009	0.014	3.52	0.105	0	0.398	1.42	62.5	0.033	0	0.8
24.7	2.72	0.374	19.6	0	0.034	0.102	10.5	0.321	4	1.87	10.2	158	0.061	0	—
28.9	0.51	0.4	20.4	0	0.003	0.039	4.93	0.366	3.49	1.87	3.4	227	0.061	0	—
42.5	0.62	0.442	15.3	0.85	0.369	0.04	8.33	0.765	1.62	0.442	13.6	162	0.085	0	—
—	0.7	—	0	0	0.04	0.05	2.7	—	—	—	9	113	0.016	0	—
—	0.5	—	601	0	0.11	0.11	2.3	—	—	—	—	246	—	0.58	—
23	0.357	0.45	28.9	0	0.058	0.051	1.42	0.153	12.8	2.21	52.7	242	—	0	—

Frozen Dinners

Food Name	Portion	WT. Gm	KCAL Kc	PROT Gm	CARB Gm	FAT Gm	CHOL Mg	SAFA Gm	MUFA Gm	PUFA Gm	SOD Mg	POT Mg
BEEF DINNER-SWANSON	ITEM	326	320	25	34	9	—	—	—	—	1085	—
BEEF SIRLOIN TIPS-LE MENU	ITEM	326	400	29	27	19	—	—	—	—	1100	—
BEEF/GREEN PEPPERS-STOUF	ITEM	220	225	10	18	11	—	—	—	—	960	420
CABBAGE ROLL/TOM SAUC-HORM	OUNCE	28.4	23	1.1	3.2	0.7	3	0.281	0.226	0.043	127	87
CHICKEN CACCIATORE-STOUF	ITEM	319	310	25	29	11	—	—	—	—	1135	300
CHICKEN DINNER-SWANSON	ITEM	326	660	26	64	33	—	—	—	—	1610	—
CHICKEN KIEV-LE MENU	ITEM	234	500	21	35	30	—	—	—	—	745	—
CHICKEN PARMIGIANA-LE MENU	ITEM	333	390	26	28	19	—	—	—	—	900	—
EGG ROLL-BEEF/SHRIMP-FROZ	ITEM	12	27	0.9	3.5	1	—	—	—	—	80.5	—
FETTUCINI ALFREDO-STOUFFER	ITEM	142	270	8	19	18	—	—	—	—	1195	240
FISH & CHIPS-VAN DE KAMP'S	ITEM	224	500	16	45	30	—	—	—	—	551	—
FISH DIVAN-LEAN CUISINE	ITEM	351	270	31	16	10	85	—	—	—	780	850
HAM-FROZ DIN-BANQUET	ITEM	284	369	16.8	47.7	12.2	—	—	—	—	1590	125
LASAGNA-STOUFFER	ITEM	298	385	28	36	14	—	—	—	—	1200	580
MANICOTTI-CHEESE-LE MENU	ITEM	241	310	18	29	13	—	—	—	—	840	—
MEATBALLS/NOODLES-STOUFFER	ITEM	312	475	25	33	27	—	—	—	—	1620	395
MEATLOAF-FROZ DIN-BANQUET	ITEM	312	412	20.9	29	23.7	—	—	—	—	1991	468
MEXICAN DINNER-SWANSON	ITEM	454	590	20	64	29	—	—	—	—	1865	—
SALISBURY STEAK DIN-BANQ	ITEM	312	390	18.1	24	24.6	—	—	—	—	2059	387
SOLE-LIGHT-VAN DE KAMP'S	ITEM	142	293	16	17	18	—	—	—	—	412	—
TURKEY DINNER-SWANSON	ITEM	326	340	20	42	10	—	—	—	—	1295	—
TURKEY PIE-STOUFFER	ITEM	284	460	20	35	26		—	—	—	1735	270
VEAL PARMIGIANA-FROZ DIN	ITEM	213	296	24	17	14	—	—	—	—	973	466
VEGETABLE LASAGNA-LE MENU	ITEM	312	400	15	30	24	—	—	—	—	1135	—

Fruits

Food Name	Portion	WT. Gm	KCAL Kc	PROT Gm	CARB Gm	FAT Gm	CHOL Mg	SAFA Gm	MUFA Gm	PUFA Gm	SOD Mg	POT Mg
APPLE JUICE-CANNED/BOTTLED	CUP	248	116	0.15	29	0.28	0	0.047	0.012	0.082	7	296
APPLE JUICE-FROZEN-DILUTED	CUP	239	112	0.34	27.6	0.239	0	0.043	0.005	0.074	16.7	301
APPLES-RAW-PEELED-BOILED	CUP	171	90.6	0.45	23.3	0.61	0	0.099	0.024	0.178	1.71	150
APPLES-RAW-UNPEELED	ITEM	138	81	0.262	21.1	0.497	0	0.08	0.021	0.145	1	159
APPLESAUCE-CAN-SWEETENED	CUP	255	194	0.459	50.8	0.47	0	0.077	0.018	0.138	8	156
APPLESAUCE-CAN-UNSWEETENED	CUP	244	105	0.415	27.6	0.12	0	0.02	0.005	0.034	4.88	183
APRICOT-RAW-WITHOUT PIT	ITEM	35.3	16.9	0.494	3.93	0.138	0	0.01	0.06	0.027	0.353	104
APRICOTS-CAN/JUICE	CUP	248	119	1.56	30.6	0.09	0	0.007	0.042	0.017	9	409
APRICOTS-DRIED-COOKED-UNSW	CUP	250	213	3.24	54.8	0.4	0	0.028	0.178	0.08	9	1222
APRICOTS-DRIED-UNCOOKED	CUP	130	309	4.75	80.3	0.6	0	0.042	0.26	0.117	13	1791
AVOCADO-RAW-CALIFORNIA	ITEM	173	306	3.65	12	30	0	4.48	19.4	3.53	20.8	1097
BANANAS-RAW-PEELED	ITEM	114	105	1.17	26.7	0.547	0	0.211	0.047	0.101	1.14	451
BLACKBERRIES-FROZEN-UNSW	CUP	151	96.6	1.78	23.7	0.649	0	—	—	—	1.51	211
BLACKBERRIES-RAW	CUP	144	74.9	1.04	18.4	0.562	0	0.07	0.17	0.299	0	282
BLUEBERRIES-FROZEN-UNSWEET	CUP	155	79.1	0.651	18.9	0.992	0	—	—	—	1.55	83.7
BLUEBERRIES-RAW	CUP	145	81.2	0.972	20.5	0.551	0	0.07	0.16	0.292	8.7	129
BOYSENBERRIES-FROZEN-UNSW	CUP	132	66	1.45	16.1	0.343	0	—	—	—	1.32	183
CHERRIES-SWEET-RAW	ITEM	6.8	4.9	0.082	1.13	0.065	0	0.015	0.018	0.02	0	15.2
CRANAPPLE JUICE-CAN	CUP	253	170	0.253	43.3	0	0	0	0	0	5.06	68.3
CRANBERRY SAUCE-CAN-SWEET	CUP	277	418	0.554	108	0.416	0	0.06	0.14	0.22	80.3	72
DATES-NATURAL-DRIED-CHOP	CUP	178	490	3.51	131	0.801	0	0.05	0.31	0.42	5.34	1161
FIGS-DRIED-UNCOOKED	CUP	199	507	6.07	130	2.33	0	0.466	0.513	1.11	21.9	1417
FRUIT COCKTAIL-CAN/JUICE	CUP	248	114	1.14	29.4	0.025	0	0.005	0.007	0.015	9.92	236
FRUIT ROLL UP-CHERRY	ITEM	14.4	50	0	12	1	0	—	—	—	5	45
GRAPE DRINK-CANNED	CUP	253	154	1.42	37.8	0.202	0	0.063	0.008	0.056	7.59	334
GRAPE JUICE-CAN & BOTTLE	CUP	253	154	1.42	37.8	0.202	0	0.063	0.008	0.056	7.59	334
GRAPE JUICE-FROZ-DILUTED	CUP	250	128	0.475	31.9	0.225	0	0.073	0.01	0.065	5	52.5
GRAPEFRUIT JUICE-CAN-SWEET	CUP	250	115	1.45	27.8	0.225	0	0.03	0.03	0.053	5	405
GRAPEFRUIT JUICE-CAN-UNSW	CUP	247	93.9	1.28	22.1	0.247	0	0.032	0.032	0.057	2.47	378
GRAPEFRUIT JUICE-FROZ-DILU	CUP	247	101	1.36	24	0.321	0	0.047	0.044	0.079	2.47	336
GRAPEFRUIT JUICE-RAW	CUP	247	96.3	1.24	22.7	0.247	0	0.035	0.032	0.059	2.47	400
GRAPEFRUIT-RAW-PINK & RED	ITEM	246	74	1.36	18.5	0.246	0	0.034	0.032	0.06	0	312
GRAPEFRUIT-RAW-WHITE	ITEM	236	78	1.63	19.8	0.236	0	0.033	0.03	0.057	0	349
KIWIFRUIT-RAW	ITEM	76	46.4	0.752	11.3	0.334	0	0	0	0	3.8	252
LEMON JUICE-CAN & BOTTLE	CUP	244	51.2	0.976	15.8	0.708	0	0.093	0.027	0.207	51.2	249

MAG Mg	IRON Mg	ZINC Mg	V-A RE	V-C Mg	THIA Mg	RIBO Mg	NIAC Mg	V-B6 Mg	FOL Ug	VB12 Ug	CALC Mg	PHOS Mg	SEL Mg	FIBD Gm	V-E Mg
—	—	—	—	—	—	—	—	—	—	—	—	—	—	—	—
—	—	—	—	—	—	—	—	—	—	—	—	—	—	—	—
—	2.33	—	136	0	0.078	0.155	3.88	—	—	—	0	—	—	—	—
4	0.25	0.19	—	0.18	0.76	0.02	0.29	0.03	2.9	0.1	5.9	15.7	—	—	—
—	—	—	—	—	—	—	—	—	—	—	—	—	—	—	—
—	—	—	—	—	—	—	—	—	—	—	—	—	—	—	—
—	—	—	—	—	—	—	—	—	—	—	—	—	—	—	—
—	—	—	—	—	—	—	—	—	—	—	—	—	—	—	—
—	—	—	—	—	—	—	—	—	—	—	—	—	—	0.12	—
—	—	—	—	—	—	—	—	—	—	—	—	—	—	—	—
—	—	—	—	—	—	—	—	—	—	—	—	—	—	—	—
—	—	—	—	—	—	—	—	—	—	—	—	—	—	—	—
—	2.5	—	1311	57	0.57	0.23	3.4	—	—	—	151	278	—	—	—
—	3.15	—	248	0	0.21	0.42	4.2	—	—	—	410	—	—	—	—
—	—	—	—	—	—	—	—	—	—	—	—	—	—	—	—
—	—	—	—	—	—	—	—	—	—	—	—	—	—	—	—
—	4.3	—	427	8	0.16	0.22	4.2	—	—	—	84	243	—	—	—
—	—	—	—	—	—	—	—	—	—	—	—	—	—	—	—
—	3.5	—	791	7	0.16	0.19	3.6	—	—	—	90	206	—	—	—
—	—	—	—	—	—	—	—	—	—	—	—	—	—	—	—
—	—	—	—	—	—	—	—	—	—	—	—	—	—	—	—
—	—	—	—	—	—	—	—	—	—	—	—	—	—	—	—
—	2.3	—	123	6.4	0.3	0.38	6.8	—	—	—	97	—	—	—	—
—	—	—	—	—	—	—	—	—	—	—	—	—	—	—	—

MAG Mg	IRON Mg	ZINC Mg	V-A RE	V-C Mg	THIA Mg	RIBO Mg	NIAC Mg	V-B6 Mg	FOL Ug	VB12 Ug	CALC Mg	PHOS Mg	SEL Mg	FIBD Gm	V-E Mg
8	0.92	0.07	0.2	2.3	0.052	0.042	0.248	0.074	0.248	0	17.4	18	0.002	0.52	—
12	0.621	0.09	—	1.43	0.007	0.036	0.091	0.079	0.717	0	14.3	16.7	0.002	0.55	—
5	0.32	0.068	7.5	0.342	0.027	0.021	0.162	0.075	1.03	0	8.55	13	0.001	4.1	—
6	0.25	0.05	7.4	7.8	0.023	0.019	0.106	0.066	3.9	0	10	10	0.001	3.04	0.911
7	0.89	0.102	2.8	4.34	0.033	0.071	0.479	0.066	1.53	0	10.2	17	0.001	3.06	—
7.32	0.29	0.073	7	2.93	0.032	0.061	0.459	0.063	1.46	0	7.32	17.1	0.001	3.66	—
2.82	0.191	0.092	92.2	3.53	0.011	0.014	0.212	0.019	3.04	0	4.94	6.71	0	0.67	—
24	0.74	0.27	420	12.2	0.045	0.047	0.853	0.134	4.22	0	30	50	0.001	2.81	—
42	4.17	0.66	591	4	0.015	0.075	2.36	0.285	0	0	40	104	—	19.5	—
61	6.11	0.97	941	3.12	0.01	0.196	3.9	0.203	13.4	0	59	152	—	10.1	—
70	2.04	0.727	106	13.7	0.187	0.211	3.32	0.484	113	0	19	73	—	6.13	—
33	0.35	0.182	9.2	10.4	0.051	0.114	0.616	0.659	21.8	0	6.84	22	0.001	1.82	0.365
33.2	1.21	0.378	17.2	4.68	0.044	0.069	1.82	0.092	51.3	0	43.8	45.3	0.001	7.55	—
28.8	0.821	0.39	23.7	30.2	0.043	0.058	0.576	0.084	49	0	46.1	30.2	0.001	8.93	—
7.75	0.279	0.109	12.6	3.88	0.05	0.057	0.806	0.091	10.4	0	12.4	17.1	0.001	4.94	—
7.25	0.247	0.16	14.5	18.9	0.07	0.073	0.521	0.052	9.28	0	8.7	14.5	0.001	3.34	—
21.1	1.12	0.29	8.9	4.09	0.07	0.049	1.01	0.074	83.6	0	35.6	35.6	0.001	5.15	—
0.748	0.026	0.004	1.46	0.476	0.003	0.004	0.027	0.002	0.286	0	1.02	1.29	0	0.1	—
5.06	0.152	0.101	0	81	0.013	0.051	0.152	0.053	0.506	0	17.7	7.59	0.001	0	—
8.31	0.609	0.139	5.5	11.1	0.042	0.058	0.277	0.039	—	0	11.1	16.6	0.001	3.2	—
62.3	2.05	0.516	8.9	0	0.16	0.178	3.92	0.342	22.4	0	57	71.2	—	15.5	—
117	4.44	1.01	26.4	1.59	0.141	0.175	1.38	0.446	14.9	0	287	135	—	18.5	—
17.4	0.521	0.223	75.7	6.7	0.03	0.04	0.999	0.126	6.2	0	19.8	34.7	0.001	1.51	—
—	—	—	—	—	—	—	—	—	—	—	—	—	—	—	—
25.3	0.607	0.127	2.02	0.253	0.066	0.094	0.663	0.164	6.58	0	22.8	27.8	—	0	—
25.3	0.607	0.127	2	0.253	0.066	0.094	0.663	0.164	6.58	0	22.8	27.8	0.001	0	—
10	0.25	0.1	1.9	59.8	0.038	0.065	0.31	0.105	3.25	0	10	10	0.001	0	—
25	0.9	0.15	0	67.3	0.1	0.058	0.798	0.05	26	0	20	27.5	0.001	0	0.45
24.7	0.494	0.222	1.8	72.1	0.104	0.049	0.571	0.049	25.7	0	17.3	27.2	0.001	0.442	0.445
27.2	0.346	0.124	2.2	83.2	0.101	0.054	0.536	0.109	8.89	0	19.8	34.6	0.001	0	0.44
29.6	0.494	0.124	2.47	93.9	0.099	0.049	0.494	0.109	25.2	0	22.2	37.1	0.001	0.5	0.44
20	0.3	0.18	63.7	91	0.098	0.05	0.492	0.104	23.1	0	36	22	0.001	3.2	0.627
21.2	0.142	0.165	2.4	78.6	0.087	0.047	0.634	0.102	23.6	0	28.3	18.9	0.001	2.5	0.614
22.8	0.312	—	13.3	74.5	0.015	0.038	0.38	—	—	0	19.8	30.4	—	2.58	—
19.5	0.317	0.146	3.7	60.5	0.1	0.022	0.481	0.105	24.6	0	26.8	22	0.001	0.732	—

Continued.

Fruits—cont'd

Food Name	Portion	WT. Gm	KCAL Kc	PROT Gm	CARB Gm	FAT Gm	CHOL Mg	SAFA Gm	MUFA Gm	PUFA Gm	SOD Mg	POT Mg
LEMON JUICE-RAW	CUP	244	61	0.927	21.1	0	0	0	0	0	2.44	303
LEMONADE-FROZ-DILUTED	CUP	248	105	0	28	0	0	0	0	0	0	40
LEMONS-RAW-PEELED	ITEM	58	16.8	0.638	5.41	0.174	0	0.023	0.006	0.052	1.16	80
LIME JUICE-CAN & BOTTLE	CUP	246	51.7	0.615	16.5	0.566	0	0.064	0.054	0.157	39.4	185
LIME JUICE-RAW	CUP	246	66.4	1.08	22.2	0.246	0	0.027	0.025	0.066	2.46	268
LIMES-RAW	ITEM	67	20.1	0.469	7.06	0.134	0	0.015	0.013	0.037	1.34	68.3
MELONS-CANTALOUPE-RAW	CUP	160	56	1.41	13.4	0.448	0	0	0	0	14.4	494
MELONS-CASABA-RAW	CUP	170	44.2	1.53	10.5	0.17	0	0	0	0	20.4	357
MELONS-HONEYDEW-RAW	CUP	170	59.5	0.782	15.6	0.17	0	0	0	0	17	461
NECTARINES-RAW	ITEM	136	66.6	1.28	16	0.626	0	—	—	—	0	288
ORANGE JUICE-CAN	CUP	249	104	1.47	24.5	0.349	0	0.045	0.062	0.085	4.98	436
ORANGE JUICE-FROZ-DILUTED	CUP	249	112	1.69	26.8	0.149	0	0.017	0.025	0.03	2.49	473
ORANGE JUICE-RAW	CUP	248	111	1.74	25.8	0.496	0	0.06	0.089	0.099	2.48	496
ORANGES-RAW-ALL VARIETIES	ITEM	131	61.6	1.23	15.4	0.157	0	0.02	0.03	0.033	0	237
PAPAYA NECTAR-CAN	CUP	250	143	0.425	36.3	0.375	0	0.118	0.103	0.088	12.5	77.5
PAPAYAS-RAW	CUP	140	54.6	0.854	13.7	0.196	0	0.06	0.053	0.043	4.2	359
PEACHES-CAN/WATER PACK	CUP	244	58.6	1.07	14.9	0.146	0	0.015	0.051	0.068	7.32	242
PEACHES-DRIED-COOKED-UNSW	CUP	258	199	2.99	50.8	0.645	0	0.067	0.23	0.304	5.16	826
PEACHES-DRIED-UNCOOKED	CUP	160	382	5.78	98.1	1.22	0	0.131	0.445	0.587	11.2	1594
PEACHES-FROZ-SLICED-SWEET	CUP	250	235	1.58	60	0.33	0	0.035	0.12	0.16	15	325
PEACHES-RAW-SLICED	CUP	170	73.1	1.19	18.9	0.153	0	0.017	0.058	0.077	0	335
PEACHES-RAW-WHOLE	ITEM	87	37.4	0.609	9.66	0.078	0	0.009	0.03	0.039	0	171
PEARS-CAN/JUICE	CUP	248	124	0.843	32.1	0.174	0	0.01	0.035	0.037	9.92	238
PEARS-RAW-BARTLET-UNPEELED	ITEM	166	97.9	0.647	25.1	0.664	0	0.037	0.139	0.156	0	208
PINEAPPLE JUICE-CAN	CUP	250	140	0.8	34.5	0.2	0	0.013	0.023	0.07	2.5	335
PINEAPPLE JUICE-FROZ-DILU	CUP	250	130	1	31.9	0.075	0	0.005	0.008	0.025	2.5	340
PINEAPPLE-CAN/JUICE	CUP	250	150	1.05	39.3	0.2	0	0.015	0.025	0.073	4	305
PINEAPPLE-RAW-DICED	CUP	155	76	0.605	19.2	0.667	0	0.05	0.074	0.226	1.55	175
PLUMS-RAW-PRUNE TYPE	ITEM	28.4	20	0	6	0	0	0	0	0	0	48
POMEGRANATES-RAW	ITEM	154	105	1.46	26.4	0.462	0	—	—	—	4.62	399
PRUNE JUICE-CAN & BOTTLE	CUP	256	182	1.56	44.7	0.077	0	0.008	0.054	0.018	10.2	707
PRUNES-DRIED-UNCOOKED	CUP	161	385	4.2	101	0.837	0	0.066	0.547	0.18	6.44	1199
RAISINS-SEEDLESS	CUP	145	435	4.67	115	0.667	0	0.218	0.026	0.196	17.4	1089
RAISINS-SEEDLESS-PACKET	ITEM	14	42	0.451	11.1	0.064	0	0.021	0.003	0.019	1.68	105
RASPBERRIES-RAW	CUP	123	60.3	1.12	14.2	0.677	0	0.023	0.065	0.385	0	187
RHUBARB-RAW-COOKED-SUGAR	CUP	270	380	1	97	0	0	0	0	0	5	548
STRAWBERRIES-FROZ-UNSWEET	CUP	149	52.2	0.641	13.6	0.164	0	0.009	0.022	0.08	2.98	221
STRAWBERRIES-RAW-WHOLE	CUP	149	44.7	0.909	10.5	0.551	0	0.03	0.077	0.277	1.49	247
TANGERINES-RAW-PEELED	ITEM	84	37	0.53	9.4	0.16	0	0.018	0.029	0.031	0.84	132
WATERMELON-RAW	CUP	160	51.2	0.992	11.5	0.688	0	—	—	—	3.2	186

Grains

Food Name	Portion	WT. Gm	KCAL Kc	PROT Gm	CARB Gm	FAT Gm	CHOL Mg	SAFA Gm	MUFA Gm	PUFA Gm	SOD Mg	POT Mg
BISQUICK MIX-DRY	CUP	112	480	8	76	16	—	—	—	—	1400	—
CORN CHIPS	OUNCE	28.4	155	1.7	16.9	9.14	0	1.5	3.39	4.25	164	43.3
CORNMEAL-DEGERM-ENR-COOKED	CUP	240	878	20.4	186	3.96	0	0.54	0.989	1.7	7.2	389
CROUTONS-HERB SEASONED	CUP	30	100	4.29	20	0	0	0	0	0	372	38.6
FLOUR-WHEAT-ENR-SIFTED	CUP	115	419	11.9	87.7	1.12	0	0.178	0.1	0.475	2.3	123
MACARONI-COOKED-FIRM-HOT	CUP	130	183	6.2	36.9	0.871	0	0.124	0.102	0.355	1.3	40.3
NOODLES-EGG-ENR-COOKED	CUP	160	200	7	37	2	50	—	—	—	3	70
NOODLES-RAMEN-ORIENTAL	CUP	227	207	5.9	30.7	8.6	—	—	—	—	829	—
POPCORN-POPPED-PLAIN	CUP	6	25	1	5	0	0	0	0	0	0	—
POPCORN-POPPED-SUGAR COAT	CUP	35	135	2	30	1	0	0.5	0.2	0.4	0	—
PRETZEL-THIN-STICK	ITEM	0.3	1.19	0.028	0.242	0.011	0	0	0	0	4.83	0.303
RICE CAKE-REGULAR	ITEM	9.31	35	0.7	7.6	0.28	0	—	—	—	10.8	27.2
RICE-BROWN-UNCLE BEN'S	CUP	146	220	5	46.4	1.82	0	0.462	0.425	0.616	2.4	172
RICE-SPANISH-HOME RECIPE	CUP	245	213	4.4	40.7	4.2	0	—	—	—	774	566
RICE-WHITE-INSTANT-HOT	CUP	165	162	3.4	35.1	0.264	0	0.073	0.084	0.072	4.95	6.6
RICE-WHITE-LONG GRAIN-COOK	CUP	205	264	5.51	57.2	0.574	0	0.158	0.18	0.156	4.1	80
RICE-WHITE-PARBOIL-COOKED	CUP	175	199	4.01	43.3	0.473	0	0.128	0.147	0.126	5.25	64.8
SHAKE'N BAKE	OUNCE	28.4	116	2.44	17.7	4.26	—	—	—	—	984	56.8
SPAGHETTI-COOK-TENDER-HOT	CUP	140	155	5	32	1	0	—	—	—	1	85

MAG Mg	IRON Mg	ZINC Mg	V-A RE	V-C Mg	THIA Mg	RIBO Mg	NIAC Mg	V-B6 Mg	FOL Ug	VB12 Ug	CALC Mg	PHOS Mg	SEL Mg	FIBD Gm	V-E Mg
14.6	0.073	0.122	4.9	112	0.073	0.024	0.244	0.124	31.5	0	17.1	14.6	0.001	0.732	—
—	0.1	—	1	17	0.01	0.02	0.2	—	12	—	2	3	0.001	0.56	—
4.64	0.348	0.035	1.7	30.7	0.023	0.012	0.058	0.046	6.15	0	15.1	9.28	0.001	0.58	—
17.2	0.566	0.148	4	15.7	0.081	0.007	0.401	0.066	19.4	0	29.5	24.6	0.001	0	—
14.8	0.074	0.148	2.5	72.1	0.049	0.025	0.246	0.106	20.2	0	22.1	17.2	—	0	—
4.02	0.402	0.074	0.7	19.5	0.02	0.013	0.134	0.029	5.49	0	22.1	12.1	0.001	0.353	—
17.6	0.336	0.256	516	67.5	0.058	0.034	0.918	0.184	27.2	0	17.6	27.2	0.001	1.28	0.496
13.6	0.68	—	5.1	27.2	0.102	0.034	0.68	—	—	0	8.5	11.9	0.001	2	0.527
11.9	0.119	—	6.8	42.2	0.131	0.031	1.02	0.1	—	0	10.2	17	0.001	1.53	0.527
10.9	0.204	0.122	100	7.34	0.023	0.056	1.35	0.034	5.03	0	6.8	21.8	0.001	2.18	—
27.4	1.1	0.174	43.7	85.7	0.149	0.07	0.782	0.219	45.1	0	19.9	34.9	0.001	0.26	0.498
24.9	0.249	0.125	19.4	96.9	0.197	0.045	0.503	0.11	109	0	22.4	39.8	0.001	0.498	0.498
27.3	0.496	0.124	49.6	124	0.223	0.074	0.992	0.099	75.1	0	27.3	42.2	0.001	1.98	0.496
13.1	0.131	0.09	26.9	69.7	0.114	0.052	0.369	0.079	39.7	0	52.4	18.3	0.002	3.14	0.314
7.5	0.85	0.375	27.7	7.5	0.015	0.01	0.375	0.023	5.25	0	25	0	0.001	1.2	—
14	0.14	0.098	282	86.5	0.038	0.045	0.473	0.027	53.2	0	33.6	7	0.001	1.27	—
12.2	0.781	0.22	130	7.08	0.022	0.046	1.27	0.046	8.3	0	4.88	24.4	0.001	1.08	—
33.5	3.38	0.464	50.8	9.55	0.013	0.054	3.92	0.098	0.258	0	23.2	98	0.001	6.7	—
67.2	6.5	0.912	346	7.68	0.003	0.339	7	0.107	0.48	0	44.8	190	0.001	14	—
12.5	0.925	0.125	70.9	236	0.033	0.088	1.63	0.045	8	0	7.5	27.5	0.001	5.99	—
11.9	0.187	0.238	91	11.2	0.029	0.07	1.68	0.031	5.78	0	8.5	20.4	0.001	2.72	—
6.09	0.096	0.122	46.5	5.74	0.015	0.036	0.861	0.016	2.96	0	4.35	10.4	0.001	1.39	—
17.4	0.719	0.223	1.4	3.97	0.027	0.027	0.496	0.035	2.98	0	22.3	29.8	0.001	4.71	—
9.96	0.415	0.199	3.3	6.64	0.033	0.066	0.166	0.03	12.1	0	18.3	18.3	0.001	4.32	—
32.5	0.65	0.275	1.2	26.8	0.138	0.055	0.643	0.24	57.8	0	42.5	20	0.002	0.25	—
22.5	0.75	0.275	2.5	30	0.175	0.05	0.5	0.185	26.5	0	27.5	20	0.002	0.3	—
35	0.7	0.25	9.5	23.8	0.238	0.048	0.71	0.185	12	0	35	15	0.002	1.88	0.25
21.7	0.57	0.124	3.5	23.9	0.143	0.056	0.651	0.135	16.4	0	10.9	10.9	0.001	1.86	0.155
1.96	0.1	0.028	8	1	0.01	0.01	0.1	0.023	0.616	0	3	5	0	0.588	—
4.62	0.462	—	0	9.39	0.046	0.046	0.462	0.162	—	0	4.62	12.3	0.001	1.1	—
35.8	3.02	0.538	0.9	10.5	0.041	0.179	2.01	0.558	1.02	0	30.7	64	0.001	2.56	—
72.5	3.99	0.853	320	5.31	0.13	0.261	3.16	0.425	5.96	0	82.1	127	0.001	11	—
47.9	3.02	0.392	1.1	4.79	0.226	0.128	1.19	0.361	4.79	0	71.1	141	0.001	7.69	—
4.62	0.291	0.038	0.112	0.462	0.022	0.012	0.115	0.035	0.462	0	6.86	13.6	0	0.742	—
22.1	0.701	0.566	16	30.8	0.037	0.111	1.11	0.07	32	0	27.1	14.8	0.001	5.5	—
32.4	1.6	0.216	22	16	0.05	0.14	0.8	0.054	14.3	0	211	41	0.001	5.4	—
16.4	1.12	0.194	6.6	61.4	0.033	0.055	0.688	0.042	25	0	23.8	19.4	0.001	3.9	0.596
14.9	0.566	0.194	4.1	84.5	0.03	0.098	0.343	0.088	26.4	0	20.9	28.3	0.001	3.87	0.387
10.1	0.084	0.202	77.3	25.9	0.088	0.018	0.134	0.056	17.1	0	11.8	8.4	0.001	1.68	—
17.6	0.272	0.112	58.5	15.4	0.128	0.032	0.32	0.23	3.52	0	12.8	14.4	0.001	0.64	—

MAG Mg	IRON Mg	ZINC Mg	V-A RE	V-C Mg	THIA Mg	RIBO Mg	NIAC Mg	V-B6 Mg	FOL Ug	VB12 Ug	CALC Mg	PHOS Mg	SEL Mg	FIBD Gm	V-E Mg
—	—	—	—	—	—	—	—	—	—	—	—	—	—	3.02	2.78
21.9	0.376	0.435	—	—	0.048	0.026	0.554	0.054	—	0	37.1	54.6	0.002	1.66	—
96	9.91	1.73	98.4	0	1.72	0.977	12.1	0.617	115	0	12	202	0.006	1.9	1.01
11.4	1.54	0.3	0	—	0.129	0.2	1.72	0	0	—	—	—	—	1.41	—
25.3	5.34	0.81	0	0	0.903	0.569	6.79	0.051	30.4	0	17.3	124	0.005	3.11	0.265
23.4	1.82	0.689	0	0	0.265	0.127	2.18	0.046	0.93	0	9.1	70.2	0.032	2.08	0.351
43.2	1.4	—	11	0	0.22	0.13	1.9	0.141	19.2	0	16	94	0.094	3.52	—
—	—	—	—	—	—	—	—	—	—	—	—	—	—	2.04	—
—	0.2	0.5	—	0	—	0.01	0.1	0.012	—	0	1	17	0.001	0.4	—
—	0.5	—	—	0	—	0.02	0.4	—	—	—	2	47	0.007	1.35	—
0.072	0.006	0.003	0	0	0.001	0.001	0.013	0	0.048	0	0.0078	0.273	—	—	0.002
—	—	—	—	—	—	—	—	—	—	—	—	—	—	0.158	—
—	0.9	—	0	0	0.18	0.04	4.2	—	—	—	16	222	0.057	2.48	2.98
—	1.5	—	162	37	0.1	0.07	1.7	—	—	—	34	96	—	1.83	—
8.25	1.04	0.396	0	0	0.124	0.076	1.45	0.016	6	0	13.2	23.1	0.033	1.32	0.644
26.7	2.25	0.943	0	0	0.334	0.027	3.03	0.191	6.15	0	22.6	96.4	0.041	2.13	0.8
21	1.97	0.543	0	0	0.437	0.031	2.45	0.033	6	0	33.3	73.5	0.035	0.875	0.683
—	0.71	—	62	0.284	0.162	0.184	2.19	—	—	—	13.9	43.5	—	—	—
23.8	1.3	0.7	0	0	0.2	0.11	1.5	0.09	16.8	0	11	70	0.085	2.24	1.68

Continued.

Grains—cont'd

Food Name	Portion	WT. Gm	KCAL Kc	PROT Gm	CARB Gm	FAT Gm	CHOL Mg	SAFA Gm	MUFA Gm	PUFA Gm	SOD Mg	POT Mg
STUFFING-MIX-DRY FORM	CUP	30	111	3.9	21.7	1.1	—	—	—	—	399	52
STUFFING-MIX-PREPARED	CUP	140	501	9.1	49.8	30.5	—	—	—	—	1254	126
TACO SHELLS	ITEM	11	49.8	0.967	7.24	2.15	0	—	—	—	—	—
TORTILLA CHIPS-DORITOS	OUNCE	28.4	139	2	18.6	6.6	0	1.43	3.19	1.77	180	51
TORTILLA-CORN	ITEM	30	67.2	2.15	12.8	1.14	0	—	—	—	53.4	52.2
TORTILLA-FLOUR	ITEM	30	95	2.5	17.3	1.8	0	—	—	—	—	—

Meats

Food Name	Portion	WT. Gm	KCAL Kc	PROT Gm	CARB Gm	FAT Gm	CHOL Mg	SAFA Gm	MUFA Gm	PUFA Gm	SOD Mg	POT Mg
BACON BITS	TBSP	6	26.6	1.92	1.72	1.55	0	—	—	—	165	—
BACON-PORK-BROILED/FRIED	SLICE	6.3	36.3	1.92	0.037	3.1	5.36	1.1	1.49	0.366	101	30.6
BEEF-LIVER-FRIED/MARG	SLICE	85	184	22.7	6.67	6.8	410	2.4	1.45	1.53	90.1	309
BOLOGNA-PORK	SLICE	23	56.8	3.52	0.168	4.57	13.6	1.58	2.25	0.488	272	64.6
BRAUNSCHWEIGER-SAUS-PORK	SLICE	18	64.6	2.43	0.56	5.78	28.1	1.96	2.68	0.67	206	35.8
CANADIAN BACON-PORK-GRILL	SLICE	23.3	43	5.64	0.315	1.96	13.5	0.66	0.94	0.185	360	90.5
CORNED BEEF HASH-CANNED	CUP	220	400	19	24	25	50	11.9	10.9	0.5	1188	440
DEVILED HAM-CANNED	TBSP	13	45	2	0	4	10	1.5	1.8	0.4	160	—
FRANKFURTER-HOT DOG-NO BUN	ITEM	57	183	6.43	1.46	16.6	28.5	6.13	7.79	1.56	638	95
HAM-REG-LUNCH MEAT-11% FAT	SLICE	28.4	52	4.98	0.88	3	16.2	0.962	1.41	0.344	374	94
HAM-REG-ROASTED-PORK	CUP	140	249	31.7	0	12.6	82.6	4.37	6.22	1.97	2100	573
HAMBURGER-GROUND-REG-BAKED	SERVING	85	244	19.6	0	17.8	74	6.99	7.79	0.663	51	188
HAMBURGER-GROUND-REG-FRIED	SERVING	85	260	20.3	0	19.2	75.7	7.53	8.39	0.714	71.4	255
ITALIAN SAUSAGE-PORK-LINK	ITEM	67	216	13.4	1.01	17.2	52	6.05	8.01	2.2	618	204
KIELBASA-PORK/BEEF	SLICE	26	80.6	3.45	0.56	7.06	17.4	2.58	3.36	0.8	280	70.5
KNOCKWURST-PORK/BEEF-LINK	ITEM	68	209	8.08	1.2	18.9	39.4	6.94	8.71	1.98	687	136
LAMB-CHOP-LEAN/FAT-BROILED	SERVING	85	307	18.8	0	25.2	84.2	10.8	10.3	2.02	64.6	230
LAMB-CHOP/RIB-LEAN-BROILED	SERVING	57	134	15.8	0	7.38	51.9	2.65	2.97	0.673	48.5	178
LAMB-LEG-LEAN/FAT-ROASTED	SLICE	85	219	21.7	0	14	79	5.85	5.92	1.01	56	266
LIVERWURST/LIVER SAUS-PORK	SLICE	18	59	2.54	0.4	5.14	28	1.91	2.4	0.47	215	—
MORTADELLA-PORK/BEEF	SLICE	15	46.7	2.46	0.458	3.81	8.4	1.43	1.71	0.468	187	24.5
POLISH SAUSAGE-PORK	ITEM	227	740	32	3.71	65.2	159	23.4	30.7	7	1989	538
PORK-CHOP-LEAN-BROILED	ITEM	66	169	18.4	0	10.1	63	3.48	4.53	1.23	49.5	276
PORK-CHOP-LEAN/FAT-BROILED	ITEM	82	284	19.3	0	22.3	77	8.06	10.2	2.53	54.1	288
PORK-LOIN-LEAN-ROASTED	SLICE	72	173	20.5	0	9.42	65.5	3.25	4.23	1.14	49.7	261
PORK-LOIN-LEAN/FAT-ROAST	ITEM	88	268	22.4	0	19.1	80	6.92	8.76	2.18	56.3	283
PORK-TENDERLOIN-LEAN-ROAST	OUNCE	28.4	47.1	8.18	0	1.37	26.3	0.471	0.613	0.165	19	153
POT ROAST-ARM-BEEF-COOKED	SLICE	100	231	33	0	9.98	101	3.79	4.35	0.4	66	289
ROAST BEEF-RIB-LEAN	SLICE	51	122	13.9	0	7.03	41.3	2.96	3.06	0.209	37.7	192
ROAST BEEF-RIB-LEAN/FAT	SLICE	85	308	18.3	0	25.5	73.1	10.8	11.4	0.9	52	257
SALAMI-COOKED-BEEF	SLICE	23	60.3	3.46	0.646	4.76	15	2.07	2.17	0.237	270	51.5
SALAMI-DRY OR HARD-PORK	SLICE	10	40.7	2.26	0.16	3.37	7.9	1.19	1.6	0.374	226	37.8
SAUSAGE-LINK-PORK-COOKED	ITEM	13	48	2.55	0.13	4.05	10.8	1.41	1.81	0.495	168	46.9
SAUSAGE-PATTY-PORK-COOKED	ITEM	27	100	5.31	0.28	8.41	22.4	2.92	3.75	1.03	349	97
SPARERIBS-PORK-BRAISED	OUNCE	28.4	113	8.25	0	8.61	34.4	3.34	4.02	0.997	26.4	90.9
STEAK-CHICKEN FRIED	ITEM	100	389	17.9	12.3	30	—	—	—	—	815	126
STEAK-RIB-COOKED	ITEM	100	221	28	0	11.2	80	4.75	4.91	0.34	69	394
STEAK-ROUND-LEAN/FAT	SLICE	85	179	26.2	0	7.5	72	2.8	3.09	0.33	51	365
STEAK-SIRLOIN-LEAN-BROILED	ITEM	56	116	17	0	4.89	49.8	2	2.16	0.207	37	226
STEAK-SIRLOIN-LEAN/FAT	ITEM	85	238	23.3	0	15.3	76.5	6.38	6.86	0.612	53.6	306

Food Name	Portion	WT. Gm	KCAL Kc	PROT Gm	CARB Gm	FAT Gm	CHOL Mg	SAFA Gm	MUFA Gm	PUFA Gm	SOD Mg	POT Mg
BAKING POWDER-HOME USE	TSP	3	3.87	0.003	0.936	0	0	0	0	0	329	4.5
BAKING POWDER-LOW SODIUM	TSP	4.3	7.4	0.004	1.79	0	0	0	0	0	0.258	471
BAKING SODA	TSP	3	0	0	0	0	0	0	0	0	821	—
CHEWING GUM-CANDY COATED	ITEM	1.7	5	—	1.6	—	0	0	0	0	—	—

MAG Mg	IRON Mg	ZINC Mg	V-A RE	V-C Mg	THIA Mg	RIBO Mg	NIAC Mg	V-B6 Mg	FOL Ug	VB12 Ug	CALC Mg	PHOS Mg	SEL Mg	FIBD Gm	V-E Mg
—	1	—	0	0	0.07	0.08	1	—	—	—	37	57	—	—	—
—	2.2	—	91	0	0.13	0.17	2.1	—	—	—	92	136	—	—	—
11.4	0.286	0.142	—	—	0.032	0.017	0.189	—	—	0	15.6	25.4	—	0.88	—
21	0.5	0.24	5.2	0	0.03	0.03	0.04	0.1	4	—	30	59	—	1.85	—
19.5	0.57	0.426	—	0	0.048	0.03	0.384	0.091	5.7	0	42	54.9	0.002	1.56	—
7	1.1	—	0.2	0	0.01	0.08	1	—	—	—	46	25	0.005	0.778	—

MAG Mg	IRON Mg	ZINC Mg	V-A RE	V-C Mg	THIA Mg	RIBO Mg	NIAC Mg	V-B6 Mg	FOL Ug	VB12 Ug	CALC Mg	PHOS Mg	SEL Mg	FIBD Gm	V-E Mg
—	0.3	—	0	0.18	0.025	0.018	0.138	—	—	—	8.4	18.1	—	—	—
1.51	0.101	0.205	0	2.11	0.044	0.018	0.464	0.017	0.315	0.11	0.756	21.2	0.001	0	0.037
19.6	5.34	4.63	9216	19.5	0.179	3.52	12.3	1.22	187	95	9.35	392	0.048	0	1.38
3.22	0.177	0.467	0	8.12	0.12	0.036	0.897	0.062	1.15	0.214	2.53	32	0.004	0	0.112
1.98	1.68	0.506	759	1.73	0.045	0.275	1.51	0.059	7.92	3.62	1.62	30.2	0.002	0	0.124
5	0.19	0.395	0	5	0.192	0.046	1.61	0.105	1	0.18	2.5	69	0.003	0	—
—	4.4	—	—	—	0.02	0.2	4.6	—	—	—	29	147	—	—	0.088
1.69	0.3	0.238	0	—	0.02	0.01	0.2	0.042	—	0.091	1	12	0.002	0	0.068
6	0.66	1.05	0	14.8	0.113	0.068	1.5	0.08	2	0.74	6.27	49	0.005	0	0.08
5	0.28	0.61	0	7.95	0.245	0.071	1.49	0.097	0.852	0.236	2	70	0.013	0	0.146
30.8	1.88	3.46	0	31.8	1.02	0.462	8.61	0.434	4.2	0.98	11.2	393	0.066	0	0.728
12.8	2.05	4.16	0	0	0.026	0.136	4.04	0.196	7.65	1.99	8.5	116	—	0	—
17	2.08	4.31	0	0	0.026	0.17	4.96	0.204	7.65	2.3	9.35	145	—	0	—
12.1	1.01	1.59	0	1.34	0.417	0.156	2.79	0.22	3.35	0.871	16.1	114	0.022	0	—
4.16	0.377	0.52	0	5.46	0.059	0.056	0.749	0.05	1.3	0.42	11.4	38.5	0.004	0	0.083
8	0.62	1.13	0	18.4	0.233	0.095	1.86	0.11	1.36	0.8	7.48	66.6	0.01	0	0.388
19.6	1.6	3.4	0	0	0.08	0.19	5.95	0.09	12	2.16	16.2	151	0.014	0	0.285
16.5	1.26	3	0	0	0.057	0.143	3.73	0.086	12	1.5	9.12	121	0.01	0	0.182
20	1.69	3.74	—	—	0.09	0.23	5.6	0.13	17	2.2	9	162	0.014	0	—
—	1.15	—	—	—	0.049	0.185	—	0.03	5	2.42	5	41	0.003	0	0.124
1.65	0.21	0.315	0	3.9	0.018	0.023	0.401	0.019	0.45	0.222	2.7	14.6	0.002	0	0.048
32	3.26	4.39	0	2.27	1.14	0.336	7.82	0.42	4.54	2.23	27.2	308	0.066	0	0.726
19.1	0.614	1.93	1.5	0.198	0.641	0.278	3.93	0.304	3.3	0.713	4.62	184	0.011	0	0.396
20.5	0.664	2.01	2.1	0.246	0.69	0.294	4.32	0.312	4.1	0.804	5.74	193	0.014	0	0.492
15.1	0.785	1.64	1.8	0.288	0.654	0.188	3.93	0.324	0.72	0.432	4.32	158	0.023	0	0.431
16.7	0.87	1.8	2.1	0.264	0.727	0.21	4.44	0.352	0.88	0.528	4.4	172	0.028	0	0.527
7.1	0.437	0.852	0.601	0.114	0.266	0.111	1.33	0.119	1.7	0.156	2.56	81.8	0.009	0	0.21
24	3.79	8.66	0	0	0.081	0.289	3.72	0.33	11	3.4	9	268	0.006	0	—
12.8	1.33	3.54	0	0	0.042	0.107	2.1	0.153	4.08	1.49	5.1	109	0.012	0	—
17	1.77	4.28	0	0	0.065	0.146	2.65	0.25	5.1	2.37	9.35	140	0.02	0	—
3.22	0.504	0.497	0	3.98	0.024	0.043	0.745	0.05	0.46	1.11	2.07	26	0.004	0	0.156
2	0.13	0.42	0	0	0.093	0.033	0.56	0.06	0.2	0.28	1.3	23	0.002	0	0.068
2.21	0.16	0.325	0	0.26	0.096	0.033	0.587	0.04	0.26	0.22	4.16	23.9	0.004	0	0.042
5	0.34	0.68	0	0	0.2	0.069	1.22	0.09	0.54	0.47	9	50	0.003	0	0.086
6.82	0.525	1.31	0.901	—	0.116	0.108	1.55	0.1	1.14	0.307	13.3	74.1	0.005	0	0.17
—	2.3	—	7.81	—	0.11	0.14	2.7	—	—	—	11	110	—	0	0.55
27	2.57	6.99	0	0	0.105	0.216	4.8	0.4	8	3.32	13	208	0.006	0	—
25.5	2.39	4.59	0	0	0.097	0.221	4.98	0.459	10.2	2.07	5.1	203	0.029	0	0.468
17.9	1.88	3.65	3	0	0.071	0.165	2.4	0.252	5.6	1.6	6.16	137	0.019	0	0.308
23.8	2.56	4.89	15	0	0.095	0.224	3.29	0.34	7.65	2.26	9.35	185	0.029	0	0.468

MAG Mg	IRON Mg	ZINC Mg	V-A RE	V-C Mg	THIA Mg	RIBO Mg	NIAC Mg	V-B6 Mg	FOL Ug	VB12 Ug	CALC Mg	PHOS Mg	SEL Mg	FIBD Gm	V-E Mg
—	0	—	0	0	0	0	0	—	—	—	58	87.1	—	—	—
—	0	—	0	0	0	0	0	—	—	—	207	314	—	—	—
—	—	—	0	0	0	0	0	0	0	0	—	—	—	0	0
—	—	—	—	0	0	0	0	—	—	—	—	—	—	—	—

Continued.

Miscellaneous—cont'd

Food Name	Portion	WT. Gm	KCAL Kc	PROT Gm	CARB Gm	FAT Gm	CHOL Mg	SAFA Gm	MUFA Gm	PUFA Gm	SOD Mg	POT Mg
CHEWING GUM-WRIGLEYS	ITEM	3	10	0	2.3	—	0	0	0	0	0	0
GEL-DZERT A-LOW CAL-PREP	CUP	240	16	4	0	0	0	0	0	0	—	—
GELATIN DESSERT-PREP	CUP	240	140	4	34	0	0	0	0	0	0	—
GELATIN-DRY-ENVELOPE	ITEM	7	25	6	0	0	0	0	0	0	8	180
JELLO-GEL-SUGAR FREE-PREP	CUP	240	16	2	0	0	0	0	0	0	120	—
OLIVES-GREEN-PICKLED-CAN	ITEM	4	3.75	0.1	0.1	0.5	0	0.05	0.35	0.035	80.8	1.75
OLIVES-MISSION-RIPE-CAN	ITEM	3	5	0.1	0.1	0.667	0	0.067	0.41	0.034	19.2	0.667
PICKLE RELISH-SWEET	TBSP	15	20	0	5	0	0	0	0	0	124	—
PICKLE-DILL-CUCUMBER-MED	ITEM	65	5	0	1	0	0	0	0	0	928	130
PICKLE-FRESH PACK-CUCUMBER	ITEM	7.5	5	0	1.5	0	0	0	0	0	50	—
PICKLE-SWEET/GHERKIN-SMALL	ITEM	15	20	0	5	0	0	0	0	0	128	—
PICKLE/HAMBURGER RELISH	OUNCE	28.4	30	0	7	0	0	0	0	0	325	—
PICKLE/HOT DOG RELISH	OUNCE	28.4	35	0	8	0	0	0	0	0	200	—
POPSICLE	ITEM	95	70	0	18	0	0	0	0	0	0	—
VINEGAR-CIDER	TBSP	15	0	0	1	0	0	0	0	0	0.125	15
VINEGAR-DISTILLED	CUP	240	29	0	12	0	0	0	0	0	2	36
YEAST-BAKER-DRY-ACT-PACKET	SERVING	7	20	3	3	0	0	0	0	0	1	140
YEAST-BREWERS-DRY	TBSP	8	25	3	3	0	0	0	0	0	9	152

Nuts/Seeds

Food Name	Portion	WT. Gm	KCAL Kc	PROT Gm	CARB Gm	FAT Gm	CHOL Mg	SAFA Gm	MUFA Gm	PUFA Gm	SOD Mg	POT Mg
NUT-FILBERT/HAZEL-DRI-CHOP	CUP	115	727	15	17.6	72	0	5.29	56.5	6.9	3.45	512
NUT-WALNUT-PERSIAN/ENGLISH	CUP	120	770	17.2	22	74.2	0	6.7	17	47	12	602
NUTS-ALMOND-SHELLED-SLIVER	CUP	115	677	22.9	23.5	60	0	5.69	39	12.6	12.7	842
NUTS-BRAZIL-DRIED-SHELLED	CUP	140	918	20.1	17.9	92.7	0	22.6	32.2	33.8	2.8	840
NUTS-CASHEWS-DRY ROASTED	CUP	137	786	21	44.8	63.5	0	12.5	37.4	10.7	21.9	774
NUTS-MACADAMIA-DRIED	CUP	134	941	11.1	18.4	98.8	0	14.8	77.9	1.7	6.7	493
NUTS-MIXED-DRY ROASTED	CUP	137	814	23.7	34.7	70.5	0	9.45	43	14.8	16.4	818
NUTS-MIXED-OIL ROASTED	CUP	142	876	23.8	30.4	80	0	12.4	45	18.9	15.6	825
NUTS-PEANUTS-OIL ROASTED	CUP	144	837	37.9	27.3	71	0	9.85	35.2	22.4	8.46	982
NUTS-PEANUTS-OIL-SALTED	CUP	144	837	37.9	27.3	71	0	9.85	35.2	22.4	624	982
NUTS-PEANUTS-SPANISH-DRIED	CUP	146	828	37.7	23.6	71.9	0	9.98	35.7	22.7	26.3	1029
NUTS-PECANS-DRIED-HALVES	CUP	108	720	8.37	19.7	73.1	0	5.85	45.5	18.1	1.08	423
NUTS-PECANS-OIL ROASTED	CUP	110	754	7.65	17.7	78.3	0	6.27	48.8	19.4	1.1	395
NUTS-PISTACHIO-DRIED	CUP	128	739	26.3	31.8	61.9	0	7.84	41.8	9.36	7.68	1399
NUTS-PISTACHIO-DRY ROASTED	CUP	128	776	19.1	35.2	67.6	0	8.56	45.6	10.2	8	1242
NUTS-WALNUT-BLACK-DRI-CHOP	CUP	125	759	30.4	15.1	70.7	0	4.54	15.9	46.9	2	655
PEANUT BUTTER-CHUNK STYLE	TBSP	16.1	94.8	3.87	3.48	8.04	0	1.54	3.79	2.31	78.2	121
PEANUT BUTTER-LOW SODIUM	TBSP	16	95	5	2.5	8.5	0	1.36	3.95	2.46	5	110
PEANUT BUTTER-OLD FASHION	TBSP	16	95	4.2	2.7	8.1	0	1.5	—	2.7	75	110
PEANUT BUTTER-SMOOTH TYPE	TBSP	16	94.1	3.94	3.32	8	0	1.53	3.77	2.3	76.5	115
SEEDS-PUMPKIN/SQUASH-ROAST	CUP	64	285	11.9	34.4	12.4	0	2.35	3.86	5.66	11.5	588
SEEDS-SESAME-ROASTED-WHOLE	OUNCE	28.4	161	4.82	7.31	13.6	0	1.91	5.15	5.98	3.12	135
SEEDS-SUNFLOWER-OIL ROAST	CUP	135	830	28.8	19.9	77.6	0	8.13	14.8	51.2	4.05	652

Poultry Products

Food Name	Portion	WT. Gm	KCAL Kc	PROT Gm	CARB Gm	FAT Gm	CHOL Mg	SAFA Gm	MUFA Gm	PUFA Gm	SOD Mg	POT Mg
CHICK-BREAST-NO SKIN-ROAST	ITEM	172	284	53.4	0	6.14	146	1.74	2.14	1.32	126	440
CHICK-THIGH-NO SKIN-ROAST	ITEM	52	109	13.5	0	5.66	49	1.57	2.16	1.29	46	124
CHICKEN ROLL-LIGHT	SLICE	28.4	45	5.54	0.695	2.09	14.2	0.574	0.84	0.455	166	64.5
CHICKEN SPREAD-CANNED	TBSP	13	25	2	0.7	1.52	—	—	—	—	50.2	13.8
CHICKEN-BREAST-FRI/BATTER	ITEM	280	728	69.6	25.2	36.9	238	9.86	15.3	8.62	770	564
CHICKEN-BREAST-FRIED/FLOUR	ITEM	196	436	62.4	3.22	17.4	176	4.8	6.86	3.84	150	506
CHICKEN-BREAST-NO SKIN-FRI	ITEM	172	322	57.5	0.88	8.1	156	2.22	2.96	1.84	136	474
CHICKEN-BREAST-ROASTED	ITEM	196	386	58.4	0	15.3	166	4.3	5.94	3.26	138	480
CHICKEN-BREAST-STEWED	ITEM	220	404	60.3	0	16.3	166	4.58	6.38	3.48	136	390

MAG Mg	IRON Mg	ZINC Mg	V-A RE	V-C Mg	THIA Mg	RIBO Mg	NIAC Mg	V-B6 Mg	FOL Ug	VB12 Ug	CALC Mg	PHOS Mg	SEL Mg	FIBD Gm	V-E Mg
0	0	0	0	0	0	0	0	0	0	0	3	0	—	—	0
—	—	—	—	—	—	—	—	—	—	—	—	—	—	0	—
—	—	—	—	—	—	—	—	—	—	—	—	—	0.016	0	—
—	0.4	—	—	4	0	0	0	0	—	—	0	0	0.002	0	—
—	—	—	—	—	—	—	—	—	—	—	—	—	—	0	—
—	0.05	—	1	—	—	—	—	—	0.04	0	2	0.5	0	0.104	—
—	0.033	0.01	1	—	0	0	—	0	0.033	0	3	0.333	0	0.09	—
—	0.1	0.01	—	—	—	—	—	—	—	—	3	2	0	—	—
7.8	0.7	0.176	7	4	0	0.01	0	0.005	0.65	0	17	14	0	0.78	—
—	0.15	0.02	1	0.5	0	0	0	0.001	0.075	0	2.5	2	0	0.09	—
0.15	0.2	0.02	1	1	0	0	0	0.001	0.15	0	2	2	0	0.165	—
—	0.189	—	—	—	—	—	—	—	—	—	5.67	3.78	0	—	—
—	0.189	—	—	—	—	—	—	—	—	—	5.6	3.7	0	—	—
—	0	—	0	0	0	0	0	—	—	—	0	—	—	—	—
—	0.1	0.02	—	—	—	—	—	0	—	—	1	1	0.013	0	—
0	—	—	—	—	—	—	—	—	—	—	—	—	0.074	0	—
3.78	1.1	—	0	0	0.16	0.38	2.6	0.14	286	0	3	90	0	2.21	—
18.4	1.4	—	0	0	1.25	0.34	3	0.2	313	0	17	140	0	—	—

MAG Mg	IRON Mg	ZINC Mg	V-A RE	V-C Mg	THIA Mg	RIBO Mg	NIAC Mg	V-B6 Mg	FOL Ug	VB12 Ug	CALC Mg	PHOS Mg	SEL Mg	FIBD Gm	V-E Mg
328	3.76	2.76	7.7	1.15	0.575	0.127	1.3	0.704	82.6	0	216	359	0.002	9.77	—
203	2.93	3.28	14.8	3.84	0.458	0.178	1.25	0.67	79.2	0	113	380	0.023	5.76	23.5
340	4.21	3.36	0	0.69	0.243	0.896	3.87	0.13	67.5	0	306	598	0.005	10.7	28.2
315	4.76	6.43	—	0.98	1.4	0.171	2.27	0.351	5.6	0	246	840	2.26	10.8	—
356	8.22	7.67	0	0	0.274	0.274	1.92	0.351	94.8	0	62	671	0.007	10	15
155	3.23	2.29	0	0	0.469	0.147	2.87	0.263	21	0	93.8	182	0.007	12.4	—
308	5.07	5.21	2.1	0.548	0.274	0.274	6.44	0.406	69	0	96	596	0.007	11.6	16.4
333	4.56	7.22	2.8	0.71	0.707	0.315	7.19	0.341	118	0	153	659	0.007	12.8	17
266	2.64	9.55	0	0	0.364	0.156	20.6	0.367	181	0	127	744	0.055	12.8	16.7
266	2.64	9.55	0	0	0.364	0.156	20.6	0.367	181	0	127	744	0.055	12.8	16.8
245	6.69	4.77	0	0	0.934	0.197	17.6	0.508	350	0	134	549	0.007	11.7	17.3
138	2.3	5.91	13.8	2.16	0.916	0.138	0.958	0.203	42.3	0	38.9	314	0.003	7.02	21.4
142	2.32	6.05	—	2.2	0.338	0.113	0.982	0.208	43.3	0	37.4	323	0.006	8.47	21.9
202	8.68	1.72	29.9	9.22	1.05	0.223	1.38	0.32	74.2	0	173	644	0.007	13.8	—
166	4.06	1.74	30.7	9.34	0.541	0.315	1.8	0.326	75.6	0	90	609	0.007	13.8	—
252	3.84	4.28	37	4	0.271	0.136	0.863	0.693	81.9	0	72	580	0.024	8.08	24.5
25.6	0.306	0.448	0	0	0.02	0.018	2.21	0.073	14.8	0	6.6	51.1	0.001	1.06	—
28	0.29	0.47	—	0	0.024	0.017	2.15	0.062	13.1	0	5	60	0.002	1.7	3.2
30	0.3	0.5	—	—	0.01	0.01	2.3	—	—	—	5	60	0.002	1.06	—
25.1	0.267	0.402	—	0	0.022	0.016	2.09	0.06	12.5	0	5.44	51.7	0.002	0.96	3.2
168	2.12	6.59	3.84	0.192	0.022	0.033	0.183	0.024	5.76	0	35.2	58.9	—	29.4	—
101	4.19	2.03	0.284	0	0.228	0.071	1.3	0.228	27.9	0	281	181	—	5.32	6.45
171	9.05	7.03	6.75	1.89	0.432	0.378	5.58	1.07	316	0	75.6	1538	0.104	9.18	70.4

MAG Mg	IRON Mg	ZINC Mg	V-A RE	V-C Mg	THIA Mg	RIBO Mg	NIAC Mg	V-B6 Mg	FOL Ug	VB12 Ug	CALC Mg	PHOS Mg	SEL Mg	FIBD Gm	V-E Mg
50	1.78	1.72	10.8	0	0.12	0.196	23.6	1.02	6.88	0.58	26	392	0.046	0	0.946
12	0.68	1.34	10.2	0	0.038	0.12	3.39	0.18	4	0.16	6	95	0.021	0	0.286
5	0.275	0.205	6.82	0	0.019	0.037	1.5	0.06	0.568	0.043	12	44.5	—	0	0.148
1.56	0.3	0.15	3.25	0	0.001	0.015	0.357	0.02	0.39	0.017	16.3	11.6	—	—	0.068
68	3.5	2.66	56.5	0	0.322	0.408	29.5	1.2	16	0.82	56	516	0.03	—	1.54
58	2.34	2.14	29.4	0	0.16	0.256	26.9	1.14	8	0.68	32	456	0.021	0.07	1.08
54	1.96	1.86	12	0	0.136	0.215	25.4	1.1	6.88	0.62	27.5	423	0.031	0	0.946
54	2.08	2	54.7	0	0.13	0.234	24.9	1.08	6	0.64	28	420	0.053	0	1.08
48	2.02	2.12	54.1	0	0.09	0.253	17.2	0.64	6	0.46	28	344	0.053	0	1.21

Continued.

Poultry Products—cont'd

Food Name	Portion	WT. Gm	KCAL Kc	PROT Gm	CARB Gm	FAT Gm	CHOL Mg	SAFA Gm	MUFA Gm	PUFA Gm	SOD Mg	POT Mg
CHICKEN-DRUMSTICK-FRIED	ITEM	49	120	13.2	0.8	6.72	44	1.79	2.66	1.58	44	112
CHICKEN-FRANKFURTER	ITEM	45	116	5.82	3.06	8.76	45.5	2.49	3.82	1.82	617	37.8
CHICKEN-GIBLETS-FRI/FLOUR	CUP	145	402	47.2	6.31	19.5	647	5.5	6.41	4.9	164	478
CHICKEN-GIBLETS-SIMMERED	CUP	145	228	37.5	1.37	6.92	570	2.16	1.73	1.56	84.1	229
CHICKEN-LEG-NO SKIN-ROAST	ITEM	95	182	25.7	0	8.01	89	2.18	2.9	1.87	87	230
CHICKEN-LEG-NO SKIN-STEWED	ITEM	101	187	26.5	0	8.14	90	2.22	2.95	1.9	78	192
CHICKEN-LEG-ROASTED	ITEM	114	265	29.6	0	15.4	105	4.24	5.97	3.42	99	256
CHICKEN-LIVER PATE-CAN	TBSP	13	26	1.75	0.85	1.7	—	—	—	—	50.2	12.4
CHICKEN-LIVER-SIMMERED	CUP	140	219	34.1	1.23	7.63	883	2.58	1.88	1.25	71	196
CHICKEN-THIGH-FRIED/FLOUR	ITEM	62	162	16.6	1.97	9.29	60	2.54	3.64	2.11	55	147
CHICKEN-WING-FRIED/FLOUR	ITEM	32	103	8.36	0.76	7.09	26	1.94	2.84	1.58	25	57
CHICKEN-WING-ROASTED	ITEM	34	99	9.13	0	6.62	29	1.85	2.6	1.41	28	62
CHICKEN-WING-STEWED	ITEM	40	100	9.11	0	6.73	28	1.88	2.64	1.43	27	56
DUCK-FLESH & SKIN-ROASTED	ITEM	764	2574	145	0	217	640	73.9	98.6	27.9	454	1560
DUCK-NO SKIN-ROASTED	ITEM	442	890	104	0	49.5	396	18.4	16.4	6.3	286	1114
TURK HAM-CURED THIGH MEAT	SLICE	28.4	36.5	5.37	0.105	1.44	15.9	0.483	0.327	0.43	283	92
TURK-BREAST-NO SKIN-ROAST	ITEM	612	826	184	0	4.5	508	1.47	0.796	1.22	318	1787
TURKEY LOAF-BREAST	SERVING	28.4	31.2	6.39	0	0.449	11.6	0.136	0.127	0.08	406	79
TURKEY PASTRAMI	SLICE	28.4	40	5.21	0.47	1.76	15.3	0.514	0.582	0.452	297	73.8
TURKEY ROLL-LIGHT	OUNCE	28.4	41.7	5.31	0.15	2.05	12.2	0.574	0.71	0.494	139	71.3
TURKEY-DARK MEAT-NO SKIN	CUP	140	262	40	0	10.1	119	3.39	2.3	3.02	110	406
TURKEY-LIGHT-NO SKIN-ROAST	CUP	140	219	41.9	0	4.5	97	1.44	0.784	1.2	89	426
TURKEY-LIGHT/DARK-NO SKIN	CUP	140	238	41	0	6.95	107	2.29	1.45	2	99	418

Sauces/Dips

Food Name	Portion	WT. Gm	KCAL Kc	PROT Gm	CARB Gm	FAT Gm	CHOL Mg	SAFA Gm	MUFA Gm	PUFA Gm	SOD Mg	POT Mg
DIP-FRENCH ONION-KRAFT	TBSP	15	30	0.5	1.5	2	0	—	—	—	120	—
DIP-GUACAMOLE-KRAFT	TBSP	15	25	0.5	1.5	2	0	—	—	—	108	—
GRAVY-BEEF-CANNED	CUP	233	123	8.74	11.2	5.49	6.99	2.69	2.24	0.187	1305	189
GRAVY-CHICKEN-CANNED	CUP	238	188	4.59	12.9	13.6	4.76	3.36	6.07	3.4	1373	260
GRAVY-TURKEY-CANNED	CUP	238	121	6.2	12.2	5.01	4.76	1.48	2.14	1.17	1373	259
HORSERADISH-PREPARED	TBSP	15	6	0.2	1.4	0	0	0	0	0	165	44
MUSTARD-BROWN-PREPARED	CUP	250	228	14.8	13.3	15.8	0	—	—	—	3268	325
MUSTARD-YELLOW-PREPARED	TSP	5	5	0.1	0.1	0.1	0	0	0	0	65	7
SAUCE-BARBECUE	CUP	250	188	4.5	32	4.5	0	0.675	1.93	1.7	2032	435
SAUCE-BEARNAISE-MIX/MILK	CUP	255	701	8.34	17.5	68.3	189	41.8	19.9	3.03	1265	298
SAUCE-CHEESE-MIX/MILK	CUP	279	307	16	23.2	17.1	53	9.32	5.3	1.59	1565	552
SAUCE-CHILI-BOTTLED	TBSP	15	16	0.4	3.7	0	0	0	0	0	201	56
SAUCE-CURRY-MIX/MILK	CUP	272	269	10.7	25.7	14.7	35.4	6.04	5.14	2.75	1276	495
SAUCE-HEINZ 57	TBSP	15	15	0.4	2.7	0.2	0	0	0	0	265	—
SAUCE-MARINARA-CANNED	CUP	250	170	4	25.5	8.38	0	1.2	4.28	2.3	1573	1060
SAUCE-MUSHROOM-MIX/MILK	CUP	267	227	11.3	23.8	10.3	34	5.39	3.28	1.09	1535	494
SAUCE-PICANTE-CANNED	FL OZ	16	9	0.3	1.9	0.5	0	0	0	0	218	77
SAUCE-SALSA/CHILIES-CANNED	FL OZ	16	10	0.4	2	0.7	0	0	0	0	111	87
SAUCE-SOUR CREAM-MIX/MILK	CUP	314	509	19.1	45.4	30.2	91	16.1	9.86	2.76	1005	733
SAUCE-SOY	TBSP	18	9.54	0.931	1.53	0.014	0	0.002	0.002	0.006	1029	32.4
SAUCE-SPAGHETTI-CANNED	CUP	249	271	4.53	39.7	11.9	0	1.7	6.07	3.25	1235	956
SAUCE-SWEET/SOUR-MIX/PREP	CUP	313	294	0.751	72.7	0.063	0	0	0	0	779	66
SAUCE-TABASCO	TSP	5	0	0.1	0.1	0	0	0	0	0	22	3
SAUCE-TACO-CANNED	FL OZ	16	11	0.4	2.2	0.7	0	—	—	—	128	88
SAUCE-TARTAR-REGULAR	TBSP	14	75	0	1	8	9	1.5	1.8	4.1	98	11
SAUCE-TERIYAKI-BOTTLED	TBSP	18	15.1	1.07	2.87	0	0	0	0	0	690	40.5
SAUCE-TOMATO-CAN-LOW SOD	CUP	226	90	4	18	0	0	0	0	0	65	—
SAUCE-TOMATO-CAN-SALT ADD	CUP	245	73.5	3.26	17.6	0.417	0	0.059	0.061	0.164	1482	908
SAUCE-TOMATO-SPANISH-CAN	CUP	244	80.5	3.51	17.7	0.659	0	0.092	0.098	0.264	1152	900
SAUCE-WORCESTERSHIRE	TBSP	15	12	0.3	2.7	0	0	0	0	0	147	120
TOMATO CATSUP	TBSP	15	15	0	4	0	0	0	0	0	156	54

MAG Mg	IRON Mg	ZINC Mg	V-A RE	V-C Mg	THIA Mg	RIBO Mg	NIAC Mg	V-B6 Mg	FOL Ug	VB12 Ug	CALC Mg	PHOS Mg	SEL Mg	FIBD Gm	V-E Mg
11	0.66	1.42	12.3	0	0.04	0.11	2.96	0.17	4	0.16	6	86	0.005	0	0.27
4.5	0.9	0.468	17.1	0	0.03	0.052	1.39	0.144	1.8	0.108	43	48.2	0.01	0	—
37	15	9.09	5195	12.7	0.141	2.21	15.9	0.88	550	19.3	26	414	0.025	—	2.09
29	9.34	6.63	3234	11.6	0.126	1.38	5.95	0.49	545	14.7	17.4	332	0.025	0	2.09
23	1.24	2.71	18	0	0.071	0.22	6	0.35	8	0.31	11.4	174	0.013	0	0.523
21	1.41	2.81	18	0	0.06	0.218	4.85	0.22	8	0.23	11	151	0.013	0	0.556
26	1.52	2.96	46.2	0	0.078	0.243	7.06	0.37	8	0.35	14	199	0.016	0	0.627
1.69	1.19	0.278	28.2	1.3	0.007	0.182	0.977	0.034	41.7	1.05	1.3	22.8	—	0.01	0.046
29	11.9	6.07	6886	22.2	0.214	2.45	6.23	0.82	1077	27.1	20	437	0.099	0	2.02
15	0.93	1.56	18.3	0	0.058	0.151	4.31	0.21	5	0.19	8	116	0.011	0.04	0.341
6	0.4	0.56	12	0	0.019	0.044	2.14	0.13	1	0.09	5	48	0.006	0	0.176
7	0.43	0.62	16.2	0	0.014	0.044	2.26	0.14	1	0.1	5	51	0.006	0	0.187
6	0.45	0.65	15.9	0	0.016	0.041	1.85	0.09	1	0.07	5	48	0.006	0	0.22
124	20.6	14.2	483	0	1.33	2.06	36.9	1.4	50	2.26	86	1190	—	0	5.35
88	11.9	11.5	103	0	1.15	2.08	22.5	1.1	44	1.76	52	898	—	0	3.09
4.54	0.785	0.835	0	0	0.015	0.07	1	0.068	1.7	0.068	2.5	54	—	0	—
177	9.36	10.6	0	0	0.263	0.802	45.9	3.42	36.7	2.39	73.4	1370	0.049	0	—
5.68	0.113	0.321	0	0	0.011	0.03	2.36	0.102	1.14	0.574	1.99	65	—	0	—
3.98	0.471	0.613	0	0	0.016	0.071	1	0.077	1.42	0.068	2.56	56.8	—	0	—
4.54	0.364	0.443	0	0	0.025	0.064	1.99	0.091	1.14	0.068	11.4	52	—	0	—
34	3.27	6.25	0	0	0.088	0.347	5.11	0.5	12.6	0.52	45	286	0.035	0	—
39	1.88	2.85	0	0	0.085	0.181	9.57	0.75	8	0.52	27	307	—	0	—
37	2.49	4.34	0	0	0.087	0.255	7.62	0.64	10	0.52	35	298	0.035	0	—

MAG Mg	IRON Mg	ZINC Mg	V-A RE	V-C Mg	THIA Mg	RIBO Mg	NIAC Mg	V-B6 Mg	FOL Ug	VB12 Ug	CALC Mg	PHOS Mg	SEL Mg	FIBD Gm	V-E Mg
—	—	—	—	—	—	—	—	—	—	—	—	—	—	—	—
—	—	—	—	—	—	—	—	—	—	—	—	—	—	—	—
4.66	1.63	2.33	0	0	0.075	0.084	1.54	0.023	4.66	0.23	14	69.9	—	0.093	—
4.76	1.12	1.9	264	0	0.04	0.102	1.05	0.024	4.76	0.238	47.6	69	—	—	—
4.76	1.67	1.9	0	0	0.048	0.191	3.1	0.024	4.76	0	9.52	69	—	—	—
—	0.1	—	—	—	—	—	—	—	—	—	9	5	—	—	—
—	4.5	—	—	—	—	—	—	—	—	—	310	335	—	—	10.4
2	0.1	—	—	—	—	—	—	—	—	—	4	4	0	0.06	0.208
45	2.25	0.5	218	17.5	0.075	0.05	2.25	0.188	10	0	48	50	—	2.3	—
25.5	0.255	0.765	757	1.79	0.077	0.255	0.255	0.077	10.2	0.51	230	186	—	0.09	—
47.4	0.279	0.971	117	2.23	0.148	0.564	0.318	0.14	12.6	1.12	569	438	—	0.1	—
—	0.1	—	21	2	0.01	0.01	0.2	—	—	—	3	8	0	—	—
46.2	1.09	1.09	40.8	2.72	0.109	0.544	0.544	0.109	16.3	1.09	484	280	—	0.9	—
—	—	—	—	—	—	—	—	—	—	—	—	—	0	—	—
60	2	0.675	240	32	0.113	0.148	3.98	0.62	33.8	0	45	87.5	—	—	—
37.4	0.534	1.34	93.5	1.87	0.187	0.801	4.81	0.187	40.1	0.801	302	166	—	0.5	—
—	0.25	—	23	8.8	0.02	0.01	0.22	—	—	—	3.8	8	—	—	—
—	0.28	—	39	9.1	0.02	0.01	0.29	—	—	—	4.2	9.3	—	—	—
44	0.61	1.37	144	2.51	0.126	0.704	0.556	0.126	15.7	0.942	546	—	—	—	—
6.12	0.364	0.067	0	0	0.009	0.023	0.605	0.031	2.79	0	3.06	19.8	—	—	—
59.8	1.62	0.523	306	27.9	0.137	0.147	3.75	0.879	53.8	0	69.7	89.6	—	—	—
9.39	1.62	0.091	0	0	0.009	0.097	0.939	0.313	1.88	0	40.7	—	—	—	—
—	—	—	—	—	0	0.01	0	—	—	—	—	—	—	0	—
—	0.3	—	4.4	6.2	0.02	0.01	0.27	—	—	—	5.9	9.8	—	—	—
—	0.1	—	3	0	0	0	0	—	—	—	3	4	—	—	7.21
11	0.306	0.018	0	0	0.005	0.013	0.229	0.018	3.6	0	4.5	27.7	—	—	—
—	—	—	—	—	—	—	—	—	—	—	—	—	0.002	3.39	—
46.6	1.89	0.613	240	32.1	0.162	0.142	2.82	0.38	23	0	34.3	78.4	—	3.68	—
46.4	8.49	0.83	242	21	0.181	0.151	3.15	0.432	32.9	0	41.5	117	—	3.66	—
—	0.9	—	5.1	27	0	0.03	0	—	—	—	15	9	—	—	—
3.6	0.1	0.034	21	2	0.01	0.01	0.2	0.016	0.75	0	3	8	0	—	—

Soups

Food Name	Portion	WT. Gm	KCAL Kc	PROT Gm	CARB Gm	FAT Gm	CHOL Mg	SAFA Gm	MUFA Gm	PUFA Gm	SOD Mg	POT Mg
SOUP-BEAN/BACON-CAN-WATER	CUP	253	173	7.89	22.8	5.94	2.53	1.52	2.18	1.82	952	403
SOUP-BEEF BROTH-CAN-READY	CUP	240	16.8	2.74	0.096	0.528	0	0.264	0.216	0.024	782	130
SOUP-BEEF BROTH-DEHY-CUBED	ITEM	3.6	6.12	0.62	0.58	0.14	0.144	0.072	0.06	0.006	864	14.5
SOUP-BEEF-CHUNKY-CAN	CUP	240	170	11.7	19.6	5.14	14.4	2.55	2.14	0.216	866	336
SOUP-BLACK BEAN-CAN-WATER	CUP	247	116	5.63	19.8	1.51	0	0.395	0.543	0.469	1198	274
SOUP-CHEESE-CAN-MILK	CUP	251	230	9.46	16.2	14.6	47.7	9.11	4.09	0.452	1019	341
SOUP-CHICK BROTH-CAN/WATER	CUP	244	39	4.93	0.93	1.39	0	0.39	0.586	0.268	776	210
SOUP-CHICKEN NOODLE-CAN	CUP	241	74.7	4.05	9.35	2.46	7.23	0.65	1.11	0.554	1106	55.4
SOUP-CHICKEN-CHUNKY-CAN	CUP	251	178	12.7	17.3	6.63	30.1	1.98	2.96	1.38	889	176
SOUP-CHICKEN/RICE-CAN	CUP	240	127	12.3	13	3.19	12	0.96	1.44	0.672	888	108
SOUP-CLAM-MANHATTAN-WATER	CUP	244	78.1	2.2	12.2	2.22	2.44	0.383	0.383	1.29	578	188
SOUP-CLAM-NEW ENGLAND-MILK	CUP	248	163	9.47	16.6	6.6	22.3	2.95	2.26	1.09	992	300
SOUP-CREAM/CELERY-CAN-MILK	CUP	248	164	5.68	14.5	9.7	32.2	3.94	2.46	2.65	1009	310
SOUP-CREAM/CHICK-CAN-MILK	CUP	248	191	7.46	15	11.5	27.3	4.64	4.46	1.64	1046	273
SOUP-CREAM/MUSHROOM-MILK	CUP	248	203	6.05	15	13.6	19.8	5.13	2.98	4.61	1076	270
SOUP-CREAM/POTATO-CAN-MILK	CUP	248	148	5.78	17.2	6.45	22.3	3.77	1.74	0.57	1060	323
SOUP-MINESTRONE-CAN-WATER	CUP	241	81.9	4.26	11.2	2.51	2.41	0.554	0.699	1.11	911	313
SOUP-ONION-CAN-WATER	CUP	241	57.8	3.75	8.17	1.74	0	0.265	0.747	0.651	1053	67.5
SOUP-ONION-DEHY-PACKET	SERVING	39	115	4.52	20.9	2.33	1.95	0.538	1.36	0.269	3493	260
SOUP-PEA-SPLIT-CAN-WATER	CUP	250	165	8.6	26.5	2.94	0	1.4	1	0.375	988	190
SOUP-PEA-SPLIT-CAN-WATER	CUP	253	189	10.3	28	4.4	7.59	1.77	1.8	0.633	1008	399
SOUP-TOMATO RICE-CAN-WATER	CUP	247	119	2.11	21.9	2.72	2.47	0.519	0.593	1.36	815	330
SOUP-TOMATO-CAN-MILK	CUP	248	161	6.1	22.3	6	17.4	2.9	1.61	1.12	932	449
SOUP-TOMATO-CAN-WATER	CUP	244	85.4	2.05	16.6	1.92	0	0.366	0.439	0.952	871	263
SOUP-TURKEY NOODLE-CAN	CUP	244	68.3	3.9	8.63	1.99	4.88	0.561	0.805	0.488	815	75
SOUP-TURKEY VEGETABLE-CAN	CUP	241	72.3	3.09	8.63	3.04	2.41	0.892	1.33	0.675	905	175
SOUP-TURKEY-CHUNKY-CAN	CUP	236	135	10.2	14.1	4.41	9.44	1.23	1.77	1.09	923	361
SOUP-VEGETABLE BEEF-CAN	CUP	245	78.4	5.61	10.2	1.91	4.9	0.858	0.809	0.123	960	174
SOUP-VEGETARIAN-CAN-WATER	CUP	241	72	2.1	12	1.93	0	0.289	0.819	0.723	822	209

Sugars/Sweets

Food Name	Portion	WT. Gm	KCAL Kc	PROT Gm	CARB Gm	FAT Gm	CHOL Mg	SAFA Gm	MUFA Gm	PUFA Gm	SOD Mg	POT Mg
CANDY-ALMOND JOY	OUNCE	28.4	151	1.7	18.5	7.8	—	1.74	2.47	1.72	—	—
CANDY-BIT O HONEY	OUNCE	28.4	121	0.9	21.2	3.6	—	1.65	1.63	0.188	—	—
CANDY-CARAMELS-PLAIN/CHOC	OUNCE	28.4	115	1	22	3	0	1.6	1.1	0.1	74	54
CANDY-CHOC COATED PEANUTS	OUNCE	28.4	160	5	11	12	0	4	4.7	2.1	16	143
CANDY-CHOCOLATE-SEMISWEET	CUP	170	860	7	97	61	0	36.2	19.8	1.7	3	553
CANDY-FONDANT-UNCOATED	OUNCE	28.4	105	0	25	1	0	0.1	0.3	0.1	60	1
CANDY-FUDGE-CHOC-PLAIN	OUNCE	28.4	115	1	21	3	0	1.3	1.4	0.6	54	42
CANDY-GUM DROPS	OUNCE	28.4	100	0	25	0	0	0	0	0	10	1
CANDY-HARD	OUNCE	28.4	110	0	28	0	0	0	0	0	9	1
CANDY-JELLY BEANS	ITEM	2.8	6.6	0	2.64	0	0	0	0	0	0.3	0
CANDY-KIT KAT BAR	ITEM	43	210	3	25	11	—	5.6	3.77	0.448	38	129
CANDY-LIFE SAVERS	ITEM	2	7.8	0	1.94	0.02	0	0	0	0	0.6	0
CANDY-LOLLIPOP	ITEM	28.4	108	0	28	0	0	0	0	0	—	—
CANDY-M & M'S-PACKAGE	ITEM	45	220	3	31	10	—	—	—	—	—	—
CANDY-MILK CHOC/ALMONDS	OUNCE	28.4	151	2.6	14.5	10.1	—	4.06	3.92	1.38	23	125
CANDY-MILK CHOC/PEANUTS	OUNCE	28.4	154	4	12.6	10.8	—	5.22	5.04	1.78	19	138
CANDY-MILK CHOCOLATE-PLAIN	OUNCE	28.4	145	2	16	9	0	5.5	3	0.3	28	109
CANDY-MILKY WAY BAR	ITEM	60	260	3	43	9	—	5.05	3.61	0.336	—	—
CANDY-PEANUT BRITTLE	OUNCE	28.4	123	2.4	20.4	4.4	—	1.85	1.79	0.632	9	43
CANDY-PEANUT BUTTER CUP	PIECE	17	92	2.2	8.7	5.35	2.5	2.8	1.83	0.751	54.5	68
CANDY-SNICKERS BAR	ITEM	57	270	6	33	13	—	4.73	5.03	2.04	—	—
HONEY-STRAINED/EXTRACTED	TBSP	21	65	0	17	0	0	0	0	0	1	11
ICING-CAKE-CHOC-MIX/PREP	CUP	275	1035	9	185	38	0	23.4	11.7	1	882	536
ICING-CAKE-FUDGE-MIX/WATER	CUP	245	830	7	183	16	0	5.1	6.7	3.1	568	238
ICING-CAKE-WHITE-BOILED	CUP	94	295	1	75	0	0	0	0	0	134	17
ICING-CAKE-WHITE-UNCOOKED	CUP	319	1200	2	260	21	0	12.7	5.1	0.5	156	57
ICING-CAKE-WHITE/COCO-BOIL	CUP	166	605	3	124	13	0	11	0.9	0	195	277
JAMS/PRESERVES-REGULAR	TBSP	20	55	0	14	0	0	0	0	0	2	18
MARSHMALLOWS	OUNCE	28.4	90	1	23	0	0	0	0	0	11	2
MOLASSES-CANE-BLACKSTRAP	TBSP	20	45	0	11	—	0	—	—	—	18	585

MAG Mg	IRON Mg	ZINC Mg	V-A RE	V-C Mg	THIA Mg	RIBO Mg	NIAC Mg	V-B6 Mg	FOL Ug	VB12 Ug	CALC Mg	PHOS Mg	SEL Mg	FIBD Gm	V-E Mg
45.5	2.05	1.03	89	1.6	0.089	0.033	0.567	0.04	31.9	0.051	81	132	0.008	3.2	—
4.8	0.408	0	0	0	0.005	0.05	1.87	0.024	4.8	0.168	14.4	31.2	0.008	0	—
1.8	0.08	0.008	0.54	0	0.007	0.009	0.119	0.007	1.15	0.036	2.16	8.1	0	—	—
4.8	2.33	2.64	261	7	0.058	0.151	2.71	0.132	13.4	0.61	31.2	120	0.008	—	—
42	2.15	1.41	49	0.8	0.077	0.054	0.534	0.094	24.7	0.02	44.5	106	0.008	—	—
20.1	0.803	0.688	147	1.2	0.063	0.334	0.502	0.078	10	0.44	288	251	0.008	—	—
2	0.51	0.249	0	0	0.01	0.071	3.35	0.024	4.88	0.24	9	73	0.008	0	—
4.82	0.771	0.395	72	0.2	0.053	0.06	1.39	0.027	2.17	0.145	16.9	36.2	0.008	1.45	—
7.53	1.73	1	130	1.3	0.085	0.173	4.42	0.05	4.6	0.25	24	113	0.008	—	—
9.6	1.87	0.96	586	3.84	0.024	0.098	4.1	0.048	3.84	0.312	33.6	72	0.008	1.44	—
12.2	1.63	0.976	96	3.9	0.029	0.039	0.817	0.1	9.76	4.05	26.8	41.5	0.008	—	—
22.3	1.49	0.799	40	3.47	0.067	0.236	1.03	0.126	9.67	10.2	186	156	0.008	—	—
22.3	0.694	0.196	68	1.4	0.074	0.248	0.436	0.064	8.5	0.496	186	151	0.008	0.77	—
17.4	0.675	0.675	94	1.3	0.074	0.258	0.923	0.067	7.7	0.546	181	151	0.008	0.5	—
19.8	0.59	0.64	38	2.23	0.077	0.28	0.913	0.064	9.92	0.496	178	156	0.008	—	—
17	0.54	0.675	67	1.1	0.082	0.236	0.642	0.089	9.2	0.496	166	160	0.008	—	—
7.23	0.916	0.735	234	1.21	0.053	0.043	0.942	0.099	16.1	0	34	55.4	0.008	1.9	—
2.41	0.675	0.612	0	1.21	0.034	0.024	0.6	0.048	15.2	0	26.5	12.1	0.008	—	—
25	0.58	0.231	1	0.897	0.111	0.238	1.99	0.039	6.32	0	55	126	0	2.2	—
39	1.95	1.71	20	1.7	0.108	0.068	1.24	0.053	1.8	0	27.5	124	0.008	—	—
48	2.28	1.32	44	1.52	0.147	0.076	1.48	0.068	2.53	0	22.8	213	0.008	—	—
5	0.79	0.514	76	14.8	0.062	0.049	1.06	0.077	13.6	0	22.2	33	0.008	1.7	—
22.3	1.81	0.29	108	67.7	0.134	0.248	1.52	0.164	20.9	0.44	159	149	0.008	0.8	—
8	1.76	0.244	69	66.4	0.088	0.051	1.42	0.112	14.7	0	12.2	34	0.008	0.9	—
5	0.94	0.583	29	0.244	0.073	0.063	1.4	0.037	2.2	0.146	12	48	0.008	0.7	—
4	0.771	0.612	244	0	0.029	0.039	1.01	0.048	4.82	0.17	16.9	40	0.008	0.964	—
23.6	1.91	2.12	716	6.4	0.035	0.106	3.59	0.307	11.1	2.12	50	104	0.008	2.5	—
4.9	1.13	1.55	189	2.45	0.037	0.049	1.03	0.076	10.5	0.31	17.2	41.7	0.008	0.98	—
7	1.08	0.46	300	1.45	0.053	0.046	0.916	0.055	10.6	0	21.7	35	0.008	1.21	—

MAG Mg	IRON Mg	ZINC Mg	V-A RE	V-C Mg	THIA Mg	RIBO Mg	NIAC Mg	V-B6 Mg	FOL Ug	VB12 Ug	CALC Mg	PHOS Mg	SEL Mg	FIBD Gm	V-E Mg
—	—	—	—	—	—	—	—	—	—	—	—	—	0.001	—	1.18
—	0.25	—	—	—	0	0.13	1.4	—	—	—	13	—	0.001	—	—
1	0.4	—	0	0	0.01	0.05	0.1	—	—	—	42	35	0.001	0.784	—
—	0.4	—	0	0	0.1	0.05	2.1	—	—	—	33	84	0.001	—	—
—	4.4	—	9	0	0.02	0.14	0.9	—	—	—	51	255	0.006	—	—
—	0.3	—	0	0	0	0	0	—	—	—	4	2	0.001	0	—
12.6	0.3	—	0	0	0.01	0.03	0.1	—	—	—	22	24	0.001	—	—
—	0.1	—	0	0	0	0	0	—	—	—	2	0	0.001	0	—
—	0.5	—	0	0	0	0	0	—	—	—	6	2	0.001	0	—
—	0.03	—	0	0	0	—	—	—	—	—	0.3	0.1	0	0	—
19	0.56	0.43	9	—	0.03	0.11	0.1	—	—	—	65	78	0.002	—	—
—	0.04	—	0	0	0	0	0	—	—	—	0.4	0.2	0	0	—
—	0	—	0	0	0	0	0	—	—	—	0	0	0.001	0	—
—	—	—	—	—	—	—	—	—	—	—	—	—	0.002	—	1.89
—	0.5	—	21	0	0.02	0.12	0.2	—	—	—	65	77	0.001	—	1.18
—	0.4	—	15	0	0.07	0.07	1.4	—	—	—	49	83	0.001	—	1.18
16	0.3	—	24	0	0.02	0.1	0.1	—	1.96	—	65	65	0.001	—	1.57
—	—	—	—	—	—	—	—	—	—	—	—	—	0.002	—	2.52
—	0.56	—	2.4	0	0.02	0.01	1.3	—	—	—	11	35	0.001	—	—
14.5	0.24	0.24	1	—	0.05	0.03	0.8	—	—	—	14.5	41	0.001	—	0.714
—	—	—	—	—	—	—	—	—	—	—	—	—	0.002	—	2.39
0.63	0.1	0.02	0	0	0	0.01	0.1	0.004	—	0	1	1	0.001	0.06	—
—	3.3	—	174	1	0.06	0.28	0.6	—	—	—	165	305	0.003	—	—
—	2.7	—	0	0	0.05	0.2	0.7	—	—	—	96	218	0.003	—	—
—	0	—	0	0	0	0.03	0	—	—	—	2	2	0.001	0	—
—	0	—	258	0	0	0.06	0	—	—	—	48	38	0.003	0	—
—	0.8	—	0	0	0.02	0.07	0.3	—	—	—	10	50	0.002	—	—
—	0.2	—	0	0	0	0.01	0	0.004	1.6	0	4	2	0	0.2	—
—	0.5	0.01	0	0	0	0	0	—	—	—	5	2	0	0	—
—	3.2	—	—	—	0.02	0.04	0.4	0.004	—	0	137	17	0.013	0	—

Continued.

Sugars/Sweets—cont'd

Food Name	Portion	WT. Gm	KCAL Kc	PROT Gm	CARB Gm	FAT Gm	CHOL Mg	SAFA Gm	MUFA Gm	PUFA Gm	SOD Mg	POT Mg
MOLASSES-CANE-LIGHT	TBSP	20	50	0	13	—	0	—	—	—	3	183
NUTS-COCONUT CREAM-RAW	CUP	240	792	8.7	16	83.2	0	73.8	3.54	0.91	10	781
NUTS-COCONUT-DRI-FLAKE-CAN	CUP	77	341	2.58	31.5	24.4	0	21.6	1.04	0.267	15.4	249
NUTS-COCONUT-DRIED-SHRED	CUP	93	466	2.68	44.3	33	0	29.3	1.4	0.361	244	313
SUGAR-BROWN-PRESSED DOWN	CUP	220	820	0	212	0	0	0	0	0	66	757
SUGAR-EQUAL-PACKET	ITEM	1	4	0	1	0	0	0	0	0	0	0
SUGAR-SWEET & LOW-PACKET	ITEM	1	4	—	0.9	—	0	—	—	—	4	3
SUGAR-WHITE-GRANULATED	TBSP	12	45	0	12	0	0	0	0	0	0.12	0
SUGAR-WHITE-POWDER-SIFTED	CUP	100	385	0	100	0	0	0	0	0	0.83	3

Vegetables

Food Name	Portion	WT. Gm	KCAL Kc	PROT Gm	CARB Gm	FAT Gm	CHOL Mg	SAFA Gm	MUFA Gm	PUFA Gm	SOD Mg	POT Mg
ALFALFA SEEDS-SPROUTED-RAW	CUP	33	9.57	1.32	1.25	0.228	0	0.023	0.018	0.135	1.98	26.1
ARTICHOKES-BOIL-DRAIN	ITEM	120	60	4.18	13.4	0.192	0	0.044	0.006	0.081	114	425
ASPARAGUS-FROZ-BOIL-SPEARS	CUP	180	50.4	5.31	8.77	0.756	0	0.171	0.023	0.331	7.2	392
BEANS-BAKED BEANS-CANNED	CUP	254	236	12.2	52.1	1.14	0	0.295	0.099	0.493	1008	752
BEANS-GARBANZO-CAN	SERVING	28.4	27.8	1.31	4.66	0.511	0	0.07	0.17	0.26	113	54.8
BEANS-GREEN-FROZ-FRENCH	CUP	135	35.1	1.84	8.26	0.189	0	0.041	0.007	0.093	17.6	151
BEANS-LIMA-CAN	CUP	248	186	11.3	34.4	0.744	0	0.168	0.042	0.357	618	667
BEANS-LIMA-FROZ-BOIL-DRAIN	CUP	170	170	10.3	32	0.578	0	0.131	0.034	0.277	90.1	694
BEANS-MUNG-SPROUTED-BOIL	CUP	125	26.3	2.54	5.24	0.113	0	0.031	0.015	0.04	12.5	126
BEANS-NAVY PEA-DRY-COOKED	CUP	190	225	15	40	1	0	—	—	—	13	790
BEANS-PINTO-FROZ-BOIL	OUNCE	28.4	46	2.64	8.77	0.136	0	0.016	0.01	0.078	23.6	183
BEANS-RED KIDNEY-CAN	CUP	255	230	15	42	1	0	—	—	—	833	673
BEANS-REFRIED BEANS	CUP	253	271	15.8	46.8	2.7	0	1.04	1.17	0.347	1073	994
BEANS-SHELLIE-CAN	CUP	245	73.5	4.31	15.2	0.466	0	0.056	0.034	0.27	818	267
BEANS-SNAP-GREEN-CAN-CUTS	CUP	135	27	1.55	6.08	0.135	0	0.03	0.005	0.069	339	147
BEANS-SNAP-GREEN-RAW-BOIL	CUP	125	43.8	2.36	9.86	0.35	0	0.08	0.014	0.181	3.75	374
BEANS-SNAP-WAX-RAW-BOIL	CUP	125	43.8	2.36	9.86	0.35	0	0.08	0.014	0.181	3.75	374
BEANS-SNAP-YELLOW/WAX-CAN	CUP	136	27.2	1.56	6.12	0.136	0	0.03	0.005	0.069	341	148
BEETS-CAN-SLICED-DRAIN	CUP	170	52.7	1.55	12.2	0.238	0	0.039	0.048	0.086	466	252
BROCCOLI-FROZ-BOIL-DRAIN	CUP	185	51.8	5.74	9.85	0.21	0	0.033	0.015	0.102	44.4	333
BROCCOLI-RAW	CUP	88	24.6	2.62	4.61	0.308	0	0.048	0.021	0.147	23.8	286
BROCCOLI-RAW-BOIL-DRAIN	CUP	155	43.4	4.62	7.84	0.543	0	0.084	0.037	0.259	40.3	453
CABBAGE-CELERY-RAW	CUP	76	12.2	0.912	2.45	0.152	0	0.033	0.017	0.055	6.84	181
CABBAGE-COMMON-BOIL-DRAIN	CUP	145	30.5	1.39	6.92	0.363	0	0.046	0.026	0.173	27.6	297
CABBAGE-COMMON-RAW-SHRED	CUP	90	21.6	1.09	4.83	0.162	0	0.021	0.012	0.078	16.2	221
CABBAGE-RED-RAW-SHREDDED	CUP	70	18.9	0.973	4.28	0.182	0	0.024	0.013	0.088	7.7	144
CABBAGE-WHITE MUSTARD-BOIL	CUP	170	20.4	2.65	3.03	0.272	0	0.036	0.02	0.131	57.8	631
CABBAGE-WHITE MUSTARD-RAW	CUP	70	9.1	1.05	1.53	0.14	0	0.018	0.011	0.067	45.5	176
CARROT-RAW-SHRED-SCRAPED	CUP	110	47.3	1.13	11.2	0.209	0	0.033	0.008	0.084	38.5	355
CARROT-RAW-WHOLE-SCRAPED	ITEM	72	31	0.74	7.3	0.137	0	0.022	0.006	0.055	25.2	233
CARROTS-BOIL-DRAIN-SLICED	CUP	156	70.2	1.7	16.3	0.28	0	0.053	0.014	0.138	103	354
CARROTS-CAN-SLICED-DRAIN	CUP	146	33.6	0.934	8.08	0.277	0	0.052	0.013	0.134	352	261
CARROTS-FROZEN-BOIL-DRAIN	CUP	146	52.6	1.74	12	0.161	0	0.031	0.007	0.077	86.1	231
CAULIFLOWER-FROZ-BOIL	CUP	180	34.2	2.9	6.75	0.396	0	0.059	0.027	0.185	32.4	250
CAULIFLOWER-RAW-BOIL-DRAIN	CUP	124	30	2.32	5.74	0.22	0	0.046	0.022	0.144	8	400
CAULIFLOWER-RAW-CHOPPED	CUP	100	24	1.99	4.92	0.18	0	0.027	0.012	0.083	15	355
CELERY-PASCAL-RAW-DICED	CUP	120	19.2	0.9	4.38	0.168	0	0.044	0.032	0.082	104	344
CELERY-PASCAL-RAW-STALK	ITEM	40	6.4	0.3	1.46	0.056	0	0.015	0.011	0.027	34.8	115
CHIVES-RAW-CHOPPED	TBSP	3	0.75	0.084	0.114	0.018	0	0.003	0.003	0.008	0.18	7.5
COLLARDS-FROZEN-BOIL-DRAIN	CUP	170	61.2	5.05	12.1	0.697	0	—	—	—	85	427
COLLARDS-RAW-BOIL-DRAIN	CUP	128	34.6	1.73	7.85	0.243	0	—	—	—	20.5	168
CORN-FROZ-BOIL-KERNELS	CUP	165	134	4.98	33.9	0.116	0	0.018	0.035	0.056	8.25	229
CORN-KERNELS FROM 1 EAR	ITEM	77	83.2	2.56	19.3	0.986	0	0.152	0.288	0.464	13.1	192
CORN-KERNELS&COB-FROZ-BOIL	ITEM	126	117	3.92	28.1	0.932	0	0.144	0.272	0.438	5.04	316
CORN-SWEET-CAN-DRAINED	CUP	165	134	4.32	30.7	1.65	0	0.254	0.482	0.777	533	322
CORN-SWEET-CREAM STYLE-CAN	CUP	256	184	4.45	46.4	1.08	0	0.166	0.315	0.507	730	343
COWPEAS-BLACKEYE-FROZ-BOIL	CUP	170	224	14.4	40.4	1.12	0	0.298	0.102	0.476	8.5	638
COWPEAS-BLACKEYE-RAW-BOIL	CUP	165	160	5.23	33.5	0.627	0	0.158	0.056	0.266	6.6	690
CUCUMBER-RAW-SLICED	CUP	104	13.5	0.562	3.03	0.135	0	0.034	0.003	0.053	2.08	155
EGGPLANT-BOILED-DRAINED	CUP	96	26.9	0.8	6.37	0.221	0	0.042	0.019	0.089	2.88	238

MAG Mg	IRON Mg	ZINC Mg	V-A RE	V-C Mg	THIA Mg	RIBO Mg	NIAC Mg	V-B6 Mg	FOL Ug	VB12 Ug	CALC Mg	PHOS Mg	SEL Mg	FIBD Gm	V-E Mg
—	0.9	—	—	—	0.01	0.01	0	0.04	—	0	33	9	0.013	0	—
—	5.47	2.3	0	6.7	0.072	0	2.14	—	—	0	26	293	—	1.6	—
37.7	1.42	1.22	0	0	0.023	0.015	0.235	0.182	5.47	0	10.8	79.3	—	4.4	—
46.5	1.79	1.69	0	0.651	0.029	0.019	0.441	0.252	7.53	0	14	99.5	0.016	39	—
—	7.5	—	0	0	0.02	0.07	0.4	—	—	—	187	42	0.003	0	—
0	0	0	0	0	0	0	0	0	0	0	0	0	0	—	0
—	—	—	—	—	—	—	—	—	—	—	—	—	0	—	—
—	0	0.006	0	0	0	0	0	—	—	—	0	0	0	0	—
—	0.1	—	0	0	0	0	0	—	—	—	0	0	0.001	0	—

MAG Mg	IRON Mg	ZINC Mg	V-A RE	V-C Mg	THIA Mg	RIBO Mg	NIAC Mg	V-B6 Mg	FOL Ug	VB12 Ug	CALC Mg	PHOS Mg	SEL Mg	FIBD Gm	V-E Mg
8.91	0.32	0.304	5.28	2.7	0.025	0.042	0.159	0.011	11.9	0	10.6	23.1	—	0.726	—
72	1.55	0.59	21.6	12	0.078	0.08	1.2	0.133	61.2	0	54	103	—	4	—
23.4	1.15	1	148	43.9	0.117	0.185	1.87	0.036	242	0	41.4	99	0.007	2.16	2.86
81.3	0.737	3.56	43.2	7.87	0.389	0.152	1.09	0.34	60.7	0	127	264	—	19.6	—
9.37	0.71	0.264	0.568	1.42	0.003	0.011	0.085	—	—	—	11.1	30.1	—	1.4	0.871
28.4	1.11	0.837	71.6	11.1	0.065	0.1	0.563	0.076	11.1	0	61	32.4	0.001	2.16	0.325
84.3	3.94	1.59	42.2	21.6	0.072	0.106	1.32	0.154	39.7	0	69.4	176	0.004	10.4	—
57.8	2.31	0.748	32.3	21.8	0.126	0.104	1.8	0.207	36	0	37.4	107	0.001	8.33	13
17.5	0.813	0.588	1.25	14.3	0.062	0.126	1.01	0.068	36.6	0	15	35	—	2.7	2.46
—	5.1	1.8	0	0	0.27	0.13	1.3	1.06	66.5	0	95	281	0.021	9.31	4.29
15.3	0.77	0.196	0	0.199	0.078	0.031	0.18	0.055	9.51	0	14.8	28.4	—	1.39	—
9.94	4.6	1.91	1	7.65	0.13	0.1	1.5	1.12	35.7	0	74	278	0.009	12.5	0.128
98.7	4.48	3.47	0	15.2	0.124	0.139	1.23	0.253	211	0	116	213	—	11.6	—
36.8	2.43	0.662	56.4	7.6	0.078	0.132	0.502	0.12	44.1	0	71.1	73.5	—	12	—
17.6	1.22	0.392	47.3	6.48	0.02	0.075	0.27	0.05	42.9	0	35.1	25.7	0.001	1.76	0.068
31.3	1.6	0.45	83.8	12.1	0.093	0.121	0.768	0.07	41.6	0	57.5	48.8	0.001	2.25	0.138
31.3	1.6	0.45	83.8	12.1	0.093	0.121	0.768	0.07	41.6	0	57.5	48	0.001	2.25	—
17.7	1.22	0.394	47.6	6.53	0.02	0.076	0.274	0.05	43.2	0	35.4	25.8	0.001	1.77	—
28.9	3.09	0.357	1.7	6.97	0.017	0.068	0.267	0.097	51.3	0	25.5	28.9	0.001	2.89	—
37	1.13	0.555	350	74.2	0.101	0.15	0.843	0.241	104	0	94.4	102	0.003	7.3	1.18
22	0.774	0.352	136	82	0.057	0.105	0.561	0.14	62.5	0	42.2	58.1	0.001	2.46	0.563
37.2	1.3	0.589	215	116	0.085	0.175	0.89	0.222	77.5	0	71.3	91.5	0.003	4.03	0.992
9.88	0.236	0.175	91.2	20.5	0.03	0.038	0.304	0.176	59.8	0	58.5	22	0.002	0.76	0.098
21.8	0.566	0.232	13.1	35.2	0.083	0.08	0.33	0.093	29.4	0	47.9	36.3	0.003	4	2.42
13.5	0.504	0.162	11.7	42.6	0.045	0.027	0.27	0.086	51	0	42.3	20.7	0.002	1.8	1.5
10.5	0.343	0.147	2.8	39.9	0.035	0.021	0.21	0.147	14.5	0	35.7	29.4	0.002	1.4	0.14
18.7	1.77	0.289	437	44.2	0.054	0.107	0.728	0.282	69	0	158	49.3	0.004	2.72	1.19
13.3	0.56	0.133	210	31.5	0.028	0.049	0.35	0.136	46	0	73.5	25.9	0.002	0.7	0.091
16.5	0.55	0.22	3094	10.2	0.106	0.064	1.02	0.162	15.4	0	29.7	48.4	0.002	3.52	0.561
10.8	0.36	0.144	2025	6.7	0.07	0.042	0.668	0.106	10.1	0	19.4	31.7	0.002	2.3	0.367
20.3	0.967	0.468	3830	3.59	0.053	0.087	0.789	0.384	21.7	0	48.4	46.8	0.002	5.77	0.713
11.7	0.934	0.38	2010	3.94	0.026	0.044	0.806	0.164	13.4	0	36.5	35	0.002	2.19	0.672
14.6	0.686	0.35	2584	4.09	0.039	0.054	0.639	0.188	15.8	0	40.9	38	0.003	5.4	0.672
16.2	0.738	0.234	3.6	56.3	0.066	0.096	0.558	0.158	73.8	0	30.6	43.2	0.001	3.24	0.162
14	0.52	0.3	1.8	68.6	0.078	0.064	0.684	0.25	63.4	0	34	44	0.001	2.73	0.113
14	0.58	0.18	2	71.5	0.076	0.057	0.633	0.231	66.1	0	29	46	0.001	2.4	0.09
13.2	0.48	0.156	15.6	8.4	0.055	0.054	0.388	0.104	33.6	0	48	30	0	1.92	0.876
4.4	0.16	0.052	5.2	2.8	0.018	0.018	0.129	0.035	11.2	0	16	10	0	0.64	0.292
1.65	0.048	0.013	19.2	2.37	0.003	0.005	0.021	0.005	0.405	0	2.43	1.53	—	0.096	—
51	1.9	0.459	1017	44.9	0.08	0.196	1.08	0.194	129	0	357	45.9	0.001	5.2	—
8.96	0.205	0.141	349	15.5	0.027	0.067	0.371	0.067	7.68	0	29.4	10.2	0.001	2.1	—
29.7	0.495	0.578	41.3	4.29	0.114	0.12	2.1	0.165	37.6	0	3.3	77.6	0.001	3.47	1.06
24.6	0.47	0.37	16.9	4.77	0.166	0.055	1.24	0.046	35.7	0	1.54	79.3	0.001	2.85	0.868
36.5	0.769	0.794	26.5	6.05	0.219	0.086	1.91	0.282	38.4	0	3.78	94.5	0.001	2.65	1.47
33	1.42	0.644	26.4	14	0.054	0.129	1.98	0.078	80.2	0	8.25	107	0.001	2.31	1.02
43.5	0.973	1.36	25.6	11.8	0.064	0.136	2.46	0.161	115	0	7.68	131	0.001	3.07	1.59
85	3.6	2.42	13.6	4.42	0.442	0.109	1.24	0.162	240	0	39.1	207	—	9.8	1.11
85.8	1.85	1.7	130	3.63	0.166	0.244	2.32	0.107	210	0	211	84.2	—	11	4.47
11.4	0.291	0.239	5.2	4.89	0.031	0.02	0.312	0.054	14.5	0	14.6	17.7	0.001	1.04	0.322
12.5	0.336	0.144	5.76	1.25	0.073	0.019	0.576	0.083	13.8	0	5.76	21.1	—	2.69	—

Continued.

Vegetables—cont'd

Food Name	Portion	WT. Gm	KCAL Kc	PROT Gm	CARB Gm	FAT Gm	CHOL Mg	SAFA Gm	MUFA Gm	PUFA Gm	SOD Mg	POT Mg
ENDIVE-RAW-CHOPPED	CUP	50	8.5	0.625	1.68	0.1	0	0.024	0.002	0.044	11	157
GARLIC-RAW-CLOVE	ITEM	3	4.47	0.191	0.992	0.015	0	0.003	0	0.007	0.51	12
LEEKS-BOIL-DRAIN	ITEM	124	38.4	1.01	9.45	0.248	0	0.033	0.004	0.138	12.4	108
LETTUCE-BUTTERHEAD-LEAVES	SLICE	15	1.95	0.194	0.348	0.03	0	0.004	0.001	0.018	0.75	38.6
LETTUCE-ICEBERG-RAW-CHOP	CUP	55	7.15	0.556	1.15	0.105	0	0.014	0.003	0.055	4.95	86.9
LETTUCE-ICEBERG-RAW-LEAVES	PIECE	20	2.61	0.202	0.418	0.038	0	0.005	0.001	0.02	1.81	31.6
LETTUCE-LOOSELEAF-RAW	CUP	55	9.9	0.715	1.93	0.165	0	0.022	0.006	0.09	4.95	145
LETTUCE-ROMAINE-RAW-SHRED	CUP	56	8.96	0.9	1.33	0.112	0	0.014	0.004	0.059	4.48	162
MISO-FERMENTED SOYBEANS	CUP	275	567	32.5	76.9	16.7	0	2.41	3.69	9.43	10030	451
MUSHROOMS-BOIL-DRAIN	ITEM	12	3.24	0.26	0.617	0.056	0	0.007	0.001	0.022	0.24	42.7
MUSHROOMS-CAN-DRAIN	ITEM	12	2.88	0.224	0.595	0.035	0	0.005	0.001	0.014	51	15.5
MUSHROOMS-RAW-CHOPPED	CUP	70	17.5	1.46	3.26	0.294	0	0.039	0.005	0.119	2.8	259
NUTS-CHESTNUTS-ROASTED	OUNCE	28.4	67.9	1.27	14.9	0.34	0	0.05	0.176	0.087	1.14	135
ONION RINGS-FROZ-PREP-HEAT	ITEM	10	40.7	0.534	3.82	2.67	0	0.858	1.09	0.511	37.5	12.9
ONIONS-MATURE-BOIL-DRAIN	CUP	210	92.4	2.86	21.3	0.399	0	0.065	0.056	0.153	6.3	349
ONIONS-MATURE-RAW-CHOPPED	CUP	160	60.8	1.86	13.8	0.256	0	0.042	0.037	0.099	4.8	251
ONIONS-YOUNG GREEN	ITEM	5	1.25	0.087	0.278	0.007	0	0.001	0	0	0.2	12.8
PARSLEY-RAW-CHOPPED	TBSP	4	1.32	0.088	0.276	0.03	0	0.005	0.012	0.005	1.56	21.4
PEAS-GREEN-CAN-DRAINED	CUP	170	117	7.51	21.4	0.595	0	0.105	0.053	0.277	372	294
PEAS-GREEN-FROZ-BOIL-DRAIN	CUP	160	125	8.24	22.8	0.432	0	0.078	0.038	0.206	139	269
PEAS-SPLIT-DRY-COOKED	CUP	200	230	16	42	1	0	—	—	—	8	592
PEPPERS-HOT-RED-DRIED	TSP	2	5	0	1	0	0	0	0	0	20	20
PEPPERS-JALAPENO-CAN-CHOP	CUP	136	32.6	1.09	0.664	0.816	0	0.084	0.046	0.445	1990	185
POTATO CHIPS-SALT ADDED	ITEM	2	10.5	0.128	1.04	0.708	0	0.181	0.125	0.36	9.38	26
POTATO PANCAKES-HOME REC	ITEM	76	495	4.63	26.4	12.6	93.5	3.42	5.35	2.54	388	538
POTATO SKIN-BAKED	ITEM	58	115	2.49	26.7	0.058	0	0.015	0.001	0.025	12.2	332
POTATO-AU GRATIN-HOME REC	CUP	245	323	12.4	27.6	18.6	56.4	11.6	5.27	0.676	1061	970
POTATO-FRENCH FRIED-FROZ	ITEM	5	11.1	0.173	1.7	0.438	0	0.208	0.178	0.033	1.55	22.9
POTATO-FRENCH FRIED-RAW	ITEM	5	13.5	0.2	1.8	0.7	0	0.17	0.178	0.033	11.1	42.7
POTATO-HASH BROWN-PREP-RAW	CUP	156	239	3.77	11.6	21.7	—	8.48	9.69	2.5	37.4	501
POTATO-HASHED BROWN-FROZ	CUP	156	340	4.93	43.8	17.9	0	7.01	8.01	2.07	53	680
POTATO-MASHED-DEHY-PREP	CUP	210	166	4.2	27.5	4.62	4	1.43	1.35	1.33	491	704
POTATO-MASHED-MILK/BUTTER	CUP	210	223	3.95	35.1	8.88	4.2	2.17	3.72	2.54	620	607
POTATO-SCALLOP-HOME REC	CUP	245	211	7.03	26.4	9.02	29.4	5.52	2.55	0.407	821	926
POTATO-SCALLOP-MIX-PREP	OUNCE	28.4	26.4	0.602	3.63	1.22	—	0.748	0.344	0.055	96.8	57.7
PUMPKIN PIE MIX-CAN	CUP	270	281	2.94	71.3	0.351	0	0.176	0.043	0.019	562	373
RADISHES-RAW	ITEM	4.5	0.765	0.027	0.162	0.024	0	0.001	0.001	0.002	1.08	10.4
RUTABAGAS-BOIL-DRAIN	CUP	170	57.8	1.87	13.2	0.323	0	0.042	0.041	0.143	30.6	488
SAUERKRAUT-CANNED	CUP	236	44.8	2.15	10.1	0.33	0	0.083	0.031	0.144	1560	401
SEAWEED-WAKAME-RAW	OUNCE	28.4	12.8	0.861	2.6	0.182	0	0.037	0.016	0.062	248	14.2
SOYBEAN-DRY-COOKED	CUP	180	234	19.8	19.4	10.3	0	—	—	—	4	972
SPINACH-CAN-SOLIDS/LIQUIDS	CUP	234	44.5	4.94	6.83	0.866	0	0.14	0.023	0.363	746	538
SPINACH-FROZ-BOIL-CHOPPED	CUP	205	57.4	6.44	10.9	0.431	0	0.068	0.012	0.176	176	611
SPINACH-RAW-BOIL-DRAIN	CUP	180	41.4	5.35	6.75	0.468	0	0.076	0.013	0.194	126	839
SPINACH-RAW-CHOPPED	CUP	56	12.3	1.6	1.96	0.196	0	0.032	0.006	0.082	44.2	312
SQUASH-ACORN-BAKED	CUP	205	115	2.29	29.9	0.287	0	0.059	0.021	0.121	8.2	896
SQUASH-BUTTERNUT-BAKED	CUP	205	82	1.84	21.5	0.185	0	0.039	0.014	0.078	8.2	582
SQUASH-HUBBARD-BOIL-MASH	CUP	236	70.8	3.49	15.2	0.873	0	0.179	0.066	0.368	11.8	505
SQUASH-SUMMER-BOIL-SLICED	CUP	180	36	1.64	7.76	0.558	0	0.115	0.041	0.236	2	346
SQUASH-WINTER-BAKE-MASH	CUP	205	80	1.82	17.9	1.29	0	0.267	0.096	0.543	2.05	896
SQUASH-ZUCCHINI-FROZ-BOIL	CUP	223	37.9	2.56	7.94	0.29	0	0.06	0.022	0.123	4.46	433
SQUASH-ZUCCHINI-ITALIA-CAN	CUP	227	65.8	2.34	15.5	0.25	0	0.052	0.018	0.107	850	622
SQUASH-ZUCCHINI-RAW-BOIL	CUP	180	28.8	1.15	7.07	0.09	0	0.018	0.007	0.038	5.4	455
SQUASH-ZUCCHINI-RAW-SLICED	CUP	130	18.2	1.51	3.77	0.182	0	0.038	0.014	0.078	3.9	322
SUCCOTASH-BOIL-DRAIN	CUP	192	221	9.73	46.8	1.54	0	0.284	0.298	0.732	32.6	787
SWEET POTATO-BAKE-PEEL	ITEM	114	117	1.96	27.7	0.125	0	0.027	0.005	0.056	11.4	397
SWEET POTATO-BOIL-MASHED	CUP	328	344	5.41	79.6	0.984	0	0.21	0.036	0.433	42.6	604
SWEET POTATO-CAN-MASHED	CUP	255	258	5.05	59.2	0.51	0	0.11	0.02	0.227	191	536
SWEET POTATO-CANDIED	PIECE	105	144	0.914	29.3	3.41	0	1.42	0.658	0.154	73.5	198
TOFU-SOYBEAN CURD	PIECE	120	86	9.4	2.9	5	0	—	—	—	8	50
TOMATO JUICE-CAN	CUP	244	41.5	1.85	10.3	0.146	0	0.02	0.022	0.058	881	537
TOMATO JUICE-LOW SODIUM	CUP	244	41.5	1.85	10.3	0.146	0	0.02	0.022	0.059	24.4	537
TOMATO PASTE-CAN-LOW SOD	CUP	262	220	9.9	49.3	2.33	0	0.333	0.351	0.948	170	2442
TOMATO PASTE-CAN-SALT ADD	CUP	262	220	9.9	49.3	2.33	0	0.332	0.351	0.948	2070	2442
TOMATO POWDER	OUNCE	28.4	85.8	3.67	21.2	0.125	0	0.018	0.019	0.05	38.1	547
TOMATO PUREE-CAN-LOW SOD	CUP	250	103	4.18	25.1	0.3	0	0.04	0.043	0.118	50	1050
TOMATO PUREE-CAN-SALT ADD	CUP	250	103	4.18	25.1	0.3	0	0.04	0.043	0.118	998	1050
TOMATO-CAN-LOW SODIUM-DIET	CUP	240	48	2.23	10.3	0.576	0	0.084	0.089	0.238	31.2	530

MAG Mg	IRON Mg	ZINC Mg	V-A RE	V-C Mg	THIA Mg	RIBO Mg	NIAC Mg	V-B6 Mg	FOL Ug	VB12 Ug	CALC Mg	PHOS Mg	SEL Mg	FIBD Gm	V-E Mg
7.5	0.415	0.395	103	3.25	0.04	0.038	0.2	0.01	71	0	26	14	—	—	—
0.75	0.051	0.035	0	0.936	0.006	0.003	0.021	0.037	0.093	0	5.43	4.59	0	—	—
17.4	1.36	0.074	5.7	5.2	0.032	0.025	0.248	0.14	30.1	0	37.2	21.1	0	3.97	—
1.95	0.045	0.026	14.6	1.2	0.009	0.009	0.045	0.008	11	0	4.8	3.45	0	0.15	0.113
4.95	0.275	0.121	18.2	2.15	0.025	0.017	0.103	0.022	30.8	0	10.5	11	0	0.55	0.413
1.81	0.1	0.044	6.61	0.78	0.009	0.006	0.037	0.008	11.2	0	3.81	4	0	0.2	0.15
6.05	0.77	0.16	105	9.9	0.028	0.044	0.224	0.03	27.4	0	37.4	13.8	0	0.76	0.413
3.36	0.616	0.14	146	13.4	0.056	0.056	0.28	0.026	76	0	20.2	25.2	0	0.952	0.42
116	7.54	9.13	24.8	0	0.267	0.688	2.37	0.591	90.8	0	182	421	—	9.9	—
1.44	0.209	0.104	0	0.48	0.009	0.036	0.535	0.011	2.18	0	0.72	10.4	0.001	0.264	0.035
1.8	0.095	0.086	0	0	0.01	0.003	0.191	0.007	1.48	0	1.32	7.92	0.005	0.216	0.035
7	0.868	0.511	0	2.45	0.072	0.314	2.88	0.068	14.8	0	3.5	72.8	0.009	0.91	0.203
25.6	0.426	0.264	0.1	10.9	0.043	0.026	0.426	0.124	20.5	0	5.4	29	0.002	2.19	—
1.9	0.169	0.042	2.3	0.14	0.14	0.014	0.361	0.008	1.3	0	3.1	8.1	—	0.382	—
23.1	0.504	0.441	0	10.9	0.088	0.048	0.346	0.271	31.5	0	46.2	73.5	0.007	1.68	0.651
16	0.352	0.304	0	10.2	0.067	0.032	0.236	0.186	30.4	0	32	52.8	0.003	2.56	0.496
1	0.095	0.022	25	2.25	0.004	0.007	0.001	—	0.685	0	3	1.65	0	0.12	0.016
1.76	0.248	0.029	20.8	3.6	0.003	0.004	0.052	0.004	7.32	0	5.2	1.64	0	0.176	0.101
28.9	1.62	1.21	131	16.3	0.206	0.132	1.24	0.109	75.3	0	34	114	0.001	5.78	4.47
46.4	2.51	1.5	107	15.8	0.452	0.16	2.37	0.18	93.8	0	38.4	144	0.001	6.08	1.04
—	3.4	2.1	8	—	0.3	0.18	1.8	—	—	—	22	178	0.003	10.5	4.54
3.4	0.3	0.054	130	0	0	0.02	0.2	—	—	0	5	4	0	0.685	—
16.3	3.81	0.258	231	17.7	0.041	0.068	0.68	0.28	18.4	0	35.4	23.1	0	—	—
1.18	0.024	0.021	0	0.832	0.003	0	0.084	0.01	0.904	0	0.48	3.06	0	0.029	0.146
24	1.21	0.68	26.6	0.456	0.104	0.095	1.61	0.29	21.5	0.217	21	78	—	—	—
24.9	4.08	0.284	0	7.8	0.071	0.061	1.78	0.356	12.5	0	19.7	58.6	—	3.02	—
49	1.57	1.69	93.1	24.3	0.157	0.284	2.43	0.426	19.9	0.492	292	277	—	4.41	—
1.1	0.067	0.021	0	0.545	0.006	0.002	0.115	0.012	0.825	0	0.45	4.3	0	0.16	—
—	0.07	—	0	1.1	0.007	0.004	0.16	0.009	1.1	0	0.8	5.6	0	0.16	—
31.2	1.26	0.468	0	8.89	0.115	0.031	3.12	0.434	12	0	12.5	65.5	—	3.12	—
26.5	2.36	0.499	0	9.83	0.173	0.031	3.78	0.196	38.8	0	23.4	112	0.001	1.5	—
33.6	1.26	0.525	27.3	6.3	0.063	0.105	1.68	0.422	14.9	0	65.1	92.4	0.001	1.2	—
37.8	0.546	0.567	42	12.8	0.176	0.084	2.27	0.47	16.7	0	54.6	96.6	0.001	3.15	0.126
46.6	1.4	0.98	46.6	26	0.169	0.225	2.58	0.436	21.3	0	140	154	—	4.41	—
3.98	0.108	0.071	5.96	0.937	0.005	0.016	0.292	0.012	2.7	0	10.2	15.9	—	0.54	—
43.2	2.86	0.729	2241	9.45	0.043	0.319	1.01	0.429	94.5	0	99.9	122	—	—	—
0.405	0.013	0.014	0.045	1.03	0	0.002	0.014	0.003	1.22	0	0.945	0.81	0	0.1	—
35.7	0.799	0.51	0	37.2	0.122	0.062	1.07	0.153	26.4	0	71.4	83.3	—	2.5	—
30.7	3.47	0.448	4.72	34.7	0.05	0.052	0.337	0.307	55.9	0	70.8	47.2	0.024	6.06	—
30.4	0.619	0.108	10.2	0.852	0.017	0.065	0.454	0.001	55.5	0	42.6	22.7	0.001	1.2	—
—	4.9	—	5	0	0.38	0.16	1.1	—	—	—	131	322	—	—	—
131	3.7	0.983	1505	31.6	0.042	0.248	0.634	0.187	136	0	194	74.9	0.003	5.08	0.14
141	3.12	1.44	1595	25.2	0.123	0.344	0.859	0.299	220	0	299	98.4	0.002	4.51	6.15
157	6.43	1.37	1474	17.7	0.171	0.425	0.882	0.436	262	0	245	101	0.002	3.96	5.4
44.2	1.52	0.297	376	15.7	0.044	0.106	0.406	0.11	108	0	55.4	27.4	0.001	1.46	1.65
88.2	1.91	0.349	88.2	22.1	0.342	0.027	1.81	0.398	38.4	0	90.2	92.3	0.002	4.3	—
59.5	1.23	0.267	1435	30.9	0.148	0.035	1.99	0.254	39.4	0	84.1	55.4	0.002	3.5	—
32	0.67	0.236	946	15.3	0.099	0.066	0.788	0.243	22.9	0	23.6	33	0.002	4.2	—
44	0.648	0.71	52.2	9.9	0.079	0.074	0.923	0.117	36.2	0	48.6	69	0.006	2.52	—
16.4	0.677	0.533	730	19.7	0.174	0.049	1.44	0.148	57.4	0	28.7	41	0.006	5.74	—
29	1.07	0.446	95.9	8.25	0.091	0.089	0.861	0.1	17.4	0	37.9	55.8	0.007	3.23	—
31	1.54	0.59	123	5.2	0.095	0.091	1.2	0.345	68.6	0	38.6	66	—	7.02	—
39.6	0.63	0.324	43.2	8.28	0.074	0.074	0.77	0.14	30.2	0	23.4	72	0.006	2.3	—
28.6	0.546	0.26	44.2	11.7	0.091	0.039	0.52	0.116	28.7	0	19.5	41.6	0.004	2	—
102	2.92	1.22	55.7	15.7	0.323	0.184	2.55	0.223	63	0	32.6	225	—	14	—
22.8	0.513	0.33	2487	28	0.083	0.145	0.689	0.275	25.8	0	31.9	62.7	0.001	3.42	5.24
32.8	1.84	0.886	5592	56.1	0.174	0.459	2.1	0.8	36.4	0	68.9	88.6	0.002	9.84	15.1
61.2	3.39	0.54	3858	13.3	0.069	0.23	2.44	0.599	27.3	0	76.5	133	0.002	4.59	—
11.6	1.19	0.158	440	7.04	0.019	0.044	0.414	0.043	12	0	27.3	27.3	0.001	1.1	—
—	2.3	—	0	0	0.07	0.04	0.1	—	—	—	154	151	0.002	1.44	—
26.8	1.42	0.342	137	44.7	0.114	0.076	1.64	0.271	48.6	0	22	46.4	0.001	2.9	1.73
26.8	1.42	0.342	137	44.7	0.114	0.076	1.64	0.271	48.6	0	22	46.4	0.001	2.8	1.73
134	7.83	2.1	647	111	0.406	0.498	8.44	0.996	58.7	0	91.7	207	0.003	11.3	—
134	7.83	2.1	647	111	0.406	0.498	8.44	0.996	—	0	91.7	207	0.003	11.3	—
50.6	1.3	0.486	490	33.1	0.259	0.216	2.59	0.13	34.1	0	47.1	83.8	—	—	—
60	2.33	0.55	340	88.3	0.178	0.135	4.29	0.38	27.5	0	37.5	100	0.003	5.75	1.78
60	2.33	0.55	340	88.3	0.178	0.135	4.29	0.38	27.5	0	37.5	100	0.003	5.75	1.78
28.8	1.46	0.384	144	36.3	0.108	0.074	1.76	0.216	18.7	0	62.4	45.6	0.002	1.69	—

Continued.

Vegetables—cont'd

Food Name	Portion	WT. Gm	KCAL Kc	PROT Gm	CARB Gm	FAT Gm	CHOL Mg	SAFA Gm	MUFA Gm	PUFA Gm	SOD Mg	POT Mg
TOMATO-RAW-RED-RIPE	ITEM	123	25.8	1.05	5.71	0.406	0	0.056	0.062	0.166	11.1	273
TOMATO-RED-CAN-STEWED	CUP	255	66.3	2.37	16.5	0.357	0	0.051	0.054	0.148	648	609
TOMATO-RED-CAN-WHOLE	CUP	240	48	2.23	10.3	0.576	0	0.084	0.089	0.238	391	530
TOMATO-RED-RAW-BOIL	CUP	240	64.8	2.57	14	0.984	0	0.137	0.151	0.407	26.4	670
TOMATO-STEW-COOK-HOME REC	CUP	101	79.8	1.98	13.2	2.71	0	0.526	1.06	0.886	460	249
V-8 VEG JUICE-LOW SODIUM	CUP	243	51	0	9.72	0	0	0	0	0	58.3	571
VEGETABLE JUICE-CAN	CUP	242	46	1.52	11	0.218	0	0.032	0.034	0.092	883	467

Fast Foods—cont'd

Food Name	Portion	WT. Gm	KCAL Kc	PROT Gm	CARB Gm	FAT Gm	CHOL Mg	SAFA Gm	MUFA Gm	PUFA Gm	SOD Mg	POT Mg
ARBY'S-BEEF AND CHEESE SANDWICH	ITEM	176	402	32.2	27.1	18	77	9.03	3.66	3.51	1634	345
ARBY'S-CHICKEN BREAST SANDWICH	ITEM	184	493	23	47.9	25	91	5.1	9.6	10.3	1019	330
ARBY'S-CLUB SANDWICH	ITEM	252	560	30	43	30	100	11.6	9.28	8.4	1610	466
ARBY'S-HAM AND CHEESE SANDWICH	ITEM	146	353	20.7	33.4	15.5	58	6.44	6.74	1.38	772	290
ARBY'S-ROAST BEEF SANDWICH	ITEM	139	346	21.5	33.5	13.8	52	3.61	6.8	1.71	792	316
ARBY'S-SUPER ROAST BEEF SANDWICH	ITEM	234	501	25.1	50.4	22.1	40	8.5	8.2	5.4	798	503
ARBY'S-TURKEY DELUXE	ITEM	236	510	28	46	24	70	—	—	—	1220	—
ARBYS-SOUP-BOSTON CLAM CHOWDER	SERVING	227	207	10	18	11	28	4	5	2	1157	319
ARBYS-SOUP-CREAM OF BROCCOLI	SERVING	227	180	9	19	8	3	5	2	1	1113	455
ARBYS-SOUP-FRENCH ONION	SERVING	227	67	2	7	3	0	1	2	1	1248	106
ARBYS-SOUP-LUMBERJACK MIXED VEGETABLE	SERVING	227	89	2	13	4	4	2	1	1	1075	268
ARBYS-SOUP-OLD FASHIONED CHICKEN NOODLE	SERVING	227	99	6	15	2	25	1	1	1	929	78
ARBYS-SOUP-PILGRIM CLAM CHOWDER	SERVING	227	193	10	18	11	28	4	5	2	1157	379
ARBYS-SOUP-ROAST BEEF AND VEGETABLE	SERVING	227	96	5	14	3	10	1	1	1	996	211
ARBYS-SOUP-SPLIT PEA AND HAM	SERVING	227	200	8	21	10	30	5	1	1	1029	272
ARBYS-SOUP-TOMATO FLORENTINE	SERVING	227	84	3	15	2	2	1	1	1	910	221
ARBYS-SOUP-WISCONSIN CHEESE	SERVING	227	287	9	19	19	31	8	8	3	1129	441
BEEF BURGER-FAST FOOD	OUNCE	28.3	72.3	4.99	7.26	2.58	—	—	—	—	54.7	45.9
BUN-HAMBURGER/HOTDOG-FAST FOOD	OUNCE	28.3	97.8	2.66	16.3	2.41	—	—	—	—	22.1	31.2
BURGER KING-BACON DOUBLE CHEESE-DELUXE	SERVING	195	592	33	28	39	111	16	14	6	804	463
BURGER KING-BARBECUE BACON DOUBLE CHEESE	ITEM	174	536	32	31	31	105	14	13	2	795	429
BURGER KING-BK BROILER	ITEM	168	379	24	31	18	53	3	7.96	3.84	764	324
BURGER KING-BK BROILER SAUCE	SERVING	14	90	0	0	10	7	1	2	5	95	—
BURGER KING-CHICKEN TENDERS	PIECE	90	39.3	2.67	2.33	2.17	7.67	0.5	0.833	0.5	90.2	249
BURGER KING-CROISSANT-EGG AND CHEESE	ITEM	127	369	12.8	24.3	24.7	216	14.1	7.54	1.37	551	174
BURGER KING-CROISSANT-EGG/CHEESE/HAM	ITEM	152	475	18.9	24.2	33.6	213	17.5	11.4	2.36	1080	272
BURGER KING-DOUBLE CHEESEBURGER	ITEM	172	483	30	29	27	100	13	11	2	851	344
BURGER KING-FISH TENDERS	SERVING	99	267	12	18	16	28	3	7	4	870	176
BURGER KING-MUSHROOM SWISS DOUBLE CHEESE	ITEM	176	473	31	27	27	95	12	11	2	746	—
BURGER KING-RANCH DIP SAUCE	SERVING	28	171	0	2	18	0	3	4	10	208	—
BURGER KING-SWEET & SOUR SAUCE	SERVING	28	45	0	11	0	0	0	0	0	52	9.14
BURGER KING-TARTAR DIP SAUCE	SERVING	28	174	0	3	18	16	3	4	11	302	13.8
BURGER KING-TATER TENDERS	SERVING	71	213	2	25	12	3	3	6	3	318	—

MAG Mg	IRON Mg	ZINC Mg	V-A RE	V-C Mg	THIA Mg	RIBO Mg	NIAC Mg	V-B6 Mg	FOL Ug	VB12 Ug	CALC Mg	PHOS Mg	SEL Mg	FIBD Gm	V-E Mg
13.5	0.554	0.11	76.3	23.5	0.073	0.059	0.772	0.098	18.5	0	6.15	29.5	0.001	1.6	0.603
30.6	1.86	0.434	140	33.9	0.117	0.089	1.82	0.043	13.8	0	84.2	51	0.002	2.04	1.81
28.8	1.46	0.384	144	36.3	0.108	0.074	1.76	0.216	18.7	0	62.4	45.6	0.002	1.93	—
33.6	1.34	0.264	178	54.7	0.168	0.138	1.8	0.228	31.2	0	14.4	74.4	0.001	2.1	1.18
15.2	1.07	0.182	67.7	18.4	0.109	0.081	1.12	0.087	11.1	0	26.3	38.4	0.001	1.04	0.495
—	1.46	—	437	53	0.049	0.073	1.94	—	—	—	38.9	—	0.001	2.7	—
26.6	1.02	0.484	283	67	0.104	0.068	1.76	0.339	51.1	0	26.6	41.1	0.001	2.7	—

MAG Mg	IRON Mg	ZINC Mg	V-A RE	V-C Mg	THIA Mg	RIBO Mg	NIAC Mg	V-B6 Mg	FOL Ug	VB12 Ug	CALC Mg	PHOS Mg	SEL Mg	FIBD Gm	V-E Mg
40	5.05	5.37	58	0	0.38	0.46	5.9	0.34	41	2.05	183	401	—	1.06	0.484
45.8	3.45	1.66	15.3	0	0.447	0.388	14.8	0.65	32.3	0.339	111	290	—	1.56	3.1
46.2	3.6	3.13	127	28.3	0.68	0.43	7	0.396	43.6	0.937	200	433	—	2.27	3.92
16	3.25	1.38	95.8	2.7	0.31	0.49	2.69	0.2	71	0.54	130	152	—	1.04	1.36
31	4.23	3.39	63.1	2.1	0.38	0.31	5.86	0.27	40	1.22	54	239	—	0.974	0.257
58.3	6.38	10.7	0	0	0.526	0.601	9.44	0.484	41.1	4.29	115	402	—	1.64	0.432
—	2.7	—	—	—	0.45	0.34	8	—	—	—	80	—	—	—	—
20.4	1.36	0.731	100	3.6	0.061	0.216	0.944	0.116	8.85	9.38	170	143	—	1.36	0.163
54.8	0.792	0.738	50	9	0.113	0.422	0.751	0.175	45.5	0.588	237	193	—	1.75	1.7
2.27	0.636	0.577	10	2.4	0.032	0.023	0.565	0.045	14.3	0	25	11.4	—	0.908	0.326
5.68	1.87	2.72	250	9	0.061	0.102	1.85	0.152	14.2	0.295	40.9	90.8	—	1.25	0.436
4.54	0.726	0.372	200	1.2	0.05	0.057	1.31	0.025	2.04	0.136	15.9	34	—	0.681	0.079
19.2	1.95	1.06	350	3.6	0.061	0.163	1.34	0.148	9.36	9.67	134	126	—	1.92	0.275
4.54	1.04	1.44	300	4.8	0.034	0.045	0.96	0.07	9.76	0.295	15.9	38.6	—	0.454	0.354
36.3	2.02	2.95	300	1.2	0.109	0.089	2.38	0.204	4.31	0.227	31.8	168	—	3.86	0.163
10.2	1.64	0.236	100	12	0.091	0.093	1.34	0.116	15	0.102	44.8	57.9	—	0.454	2.8
6.81	1.32	1.13	90.1	2.4	0.03	0.238	0.704	0.045	6.81	0	252	241	—	1.82	0.436
—	0.255	—	8.22	0.17	0.017	0.037	0.822	—	—	—	3.4	24.9	—	0.028	—
—	0.227	—	0	0.142	0.071	0.023	0.397	—	—	—	9.36	13	—	0	—
37.5	3.95	6.36	71.4	7.59	0.298	0.392	8.12	0.365	31.4	3.24	156	373	—	1.06	1.78
36.1	3.96	6.52	48.7	4.42	0.294	0.393	8.25	0.348	27.1	3.34	158	379	—	0.799	0.758
29.1	3.23	3.17	43.7	6.22	0.274	0.262	5.21	0.242	37.5	1.52	73.7	153	—	1.8	3.1
—	—	—	—	—	—	—	—	—	—	—	—	—	—	0	—
21.6	1.03	0.738	25.2	0	0.135	0.117	6.21	0.315	9	0.297	9	234	—	0.27	0.362
22	2.2	1.76	300	0.2	0.19	0.38	1.51	0.1	36	0.78	244	349	—	2.05	0.83
26	2.13	2.17	135	11.4	0.52	0.3	3.19	0.23	36	1.01	144	336	—	—	—
30.6	2.95	3.95	100	5.84	0.215	0.308	4.94	0.237	31.4	1.81	189	305	—	1.44	2.12
33.1	1.7	0.589	19.6	0.005	0.232	0.167	2.29	0.055	22.7	1.05	60	191	—	1.12	1.55
—	4.14	—	—	—	—	—	—	—	—	—	—	—	—	—	—
—	—	—	—	—	—	—	—	—	—	—	—	—	—	—	—
2.09	0.1	0.013	0	0	0.001	0.003	0.059	0.003	0.301	0	1.02	2.65	—	0.014	—
1.01	0.255	0.053	25.5	0.248	0.002	0.005	0.013	0.076	2.17	0.059	6.99	7.81	—	0.042	4.67
—	—	—	—	—	—	—	—	—	—	—	—	—	—	—	—

Continued

Fast Foods—cont'd

Food Name	Portion	WT. Gm	KCAL Kc	PROT Gm	CARB Gm	FAT Gm	CHOL Mg	SAFA Gm	MUFA Gm	PUFA Gm	SOD Mg	POT Mg
CHEESE BURGER-FAST FOOD	OUNCE	28.3	78	5.61	6.55	3.26	12.3	1.73	1.65	0.241	198	68
CHICKEN-BREAST AND WING-BREADED-FRIED	SERVING	163	494	35.7	19.6	29.5	149	7.84	12.2	6.79	975	566
CHICKEN-BREAST-FAST FOOD	OUNCE	28.3	73.1	7.65	2.61	3.57	23.6	0.616	0.852	0.467	142	85
CHICKEN-DRUMSTICK & THIGH-BREADED-FRIED	SERVING	148	430	30.1	15.7	26.7	165	7.05	10.9	6.32	756	446
CHICKEN-DRUMSTICK-FAST FOOD	OUNCE	28.3	59	7.03	4.2	1.56	25.6	0.858	1.2	0.703	133	73.7
CHICKEN-FRIED-FAST FOOD-VARIOUS PORTIONS	OUNCE	28.3	82.2	4.71	5.67	4.51	25.4	1.14	1.66	0.958	153	70.9
CHICKEN-MEAT-SHAPED-FRIED-FAST FOOD	OUNCE	28.3	81.6	4.85	4.65	4.85	—	—	—	—	141	39.7
CHICKEN-SHOULDER-FAST FOOD	OUNCE	28.3	92.4	5.33	3.18	6.49	—	—	—	—	150	73.7
CHICKEN-THIGH-FAST FOOD	OUNCE	28.3	104	7.26	2.75	7.14	26.2	1.22	1.73	0.962	139	68
CHICKEN-WING-FAST FOOD	OUNCE	28.3	91.9	7.85	2.78	5.47	—	—	—	—	198	53.9
COLESLAW-FAST FOOD	OUNCE	28.3	23.8	0.68	2.75	1.13	1.07	0.206	0.374	0.759	76.5	45.4
DOUBLE CHEESE BURGER-FAST FOOD	OUNCE	28.3	66.3	4.2	6.63	2.55	16.6	2.2	1.94	0.238	49.9	85.3
FAST FOOD-PIZZA WITH CHEESE	OUNCE	28.4	63.2	3.46	9.23	1.45	4.25	0.693	0.445	0.221	151	49.3
FAST FOOD-PIZZA WITH PEPPERONI	OUNCE	28.4	72.3	4.04	7.93	2.78	5.67	0.893	1.25	0.465	107	61
FISH CAKE-FRIED-WITH BUN-FAST FOOD	OUNCE	28.3	84.5	2.72	7.63	4.79	19.7	0.388	0.761	0.455	167	51.6
FRANKFURTER-CONEY DOG-FAST FOOD	OUNCE	28.3	69.2	3.12	6.95	3.2	14.7	3.09	3.99	0.81	242	48.8
FRANKFURTER-HOT DOG-FAST FOOD	OUNCE	28.3	77.7	3.12	7.37	3.97	14.7	3.09	3.99	0.81	219	48.2
HAMBURGER-DOUBLE PATTY-EVERYTHING ON IT	OUNCE	28.4	67.8	4.3	5.05	3.33	15.3	1.32	1.3	0.351	99.2	71.4
HARDEE-BACON AND EGG BISCUIT	SERVING	124	410	15	35	24	155	5	14	5	990	180
HARDEE-BACON EGG AND CHEESE BISCUIT	SERVING	137	460	17	35	28	165	8	15	5	1220	200
HARDEE-BIG COUNTRY BREAKFAST-COUNTRY HAM	SERVING	254	670	29	52	38	345	9	21	8	2870	710
HARDEE-BIG COUNTRY BREAKFAST-SAUSAGE	SERVING	274	850	33	51	57	340	16	31	11	1980	670
HARDEE-BIG COUNTRY BREAKFAST-WITH BACON	SERVING	217	660	24	51	40	305	10	22	8	1540	530
HARDEE-BIG COUNTRY BREAKFAST-WITH HAM	SERVING	251	620	28	51	33	325	7	19	8	1780	620
HARDEE-BIG ROAST BEEF SANDWICH	SERVING	134	300	18	32	11	45	5	5	2	880	320
HARDEE-BIG TWIN HAMBURGER	SERVING	173	450	23	34	25	55	11	9	5	580	280
HARDEE-BISCUIT N GRAVY	SERVING	221	440	9	45	24	15	6	14	5	1250	210
HARDEE-CHICKEN N PASTA SALAD	SERVING	414	230	27	23	3	55	1	1	1	380	620
HARDEE-CRISPY CURLS	SERVING	85	300	4	36	16	0	3	8	5	840	370
HARDEE-GRILLED CHICKEN SANDWICH	SERVING	192	310	24	34	9	60	1	3	5	890	410
HARDEE-HAM & EGG BISCUIT	SERVING	138	370	15	35	19	160	4	12	4	1050	210
HARDEE-HAM EGG & CHEESE BISCUIT	SERVING	151	420	18	35	23	170	6	13	4	1270	230
HARDEE-MUSHROOM N SWISS HAMBURGER	SERVING	186	490	30	33	27	70	13	12	2	940	370
HARDEE-REGULAR ROAST BEEF SANDWICH	SERVING	114	260	15	31	9	35	4	4	2	730	260
HARDEE-THE LEAN ONE SANDWICH	ITEM	220	420	27	37	18	85	8	8	2	760	510
HARDEE-THREE PANCAKES	SERVING	137	280	8	56	2	15	1	1	1	890	240
KFC-CHICKEN HOT WINGS	PIECE	119	62.6	3.66	2.99	3.99	24.6	0.832	10.3	0.666	113	218
KFC-CHICKEN SANDWICH	SERVING	166	482	21	39	27	47	6	3.91	9	1060	297
KFC-CRISPY CHICKEN-BREAST	PIECE	135	342	33	12	20	114	5	4.7	2	790	347
KFC-CRISPY CHICKEN-DRUMSTICK	PIECE	69	204	14	6	14	71	3	3.72	2	324	157
KFC-CRISPY CHICKEN-THIGH	PIECE	119	406	20	14	30	129	8	6.95	4	688	280
KFC-CRISPY CHICKEN-WING	PIECE	65	254	12	9	19	67	4	5.74	3	422	115
LONG JOHN SILVER-BATTERED SHRIMP-9 PIECE	PIECE	357	95.4	2.66	9.76	4.99	13.9	1.11	3.22	0.555	163	94.3

MAG Mg	IRON Mg	ZINC Mg	V-A RE	V-C Mg	THIA Mg	RIBO Mg	NIAC Mg	V-B6 Mg	FOL Ug	VB12 Ug	CALC Mg	PHOS Mg	SEL Mg	FIBD Gm	V-E Mg
5.88	0.567	0.722	9.36	0.283	0.023	0.048	0.624	0.038	6.79	0.311	25.2	33.2	—	0.057	0.142
38	1.49	1.55	57.7	0	0.14	0.3	12	0.57	9	0.67	60	307	—	0.261	1.18
7.6	0.17	0.287	9.36	0.68	0.02	0.048	1.98	0.158	1.13	0.09	3.97	51.9	—	0	0.089
37	1.6	3.24	66.7	0	0.14	0.43	7.21	0.33	10	0.83	36	240	—	0.237	1.58
6.47	0.312	0.807	6.52	0.425	0.02	0.062	1.42	0.096	2.25	0.09	4.25	41.1	—	0	0.089
7.05	0.283	0.575	6.52	0.454	0.02	0.051	1.62	0.116	1.76	0.087	4.25	38.6	—	0	0.212
—	0.312	—	5.95	0.425	0.009	0.006	0.794	—	—	—	3.97	33.5	—	0	—
—	0.142	—	4.25	0.34	0.02	0.037	1.87	—	—	—	3.69	31.8	—	0	—
6.19	0.085	0.664	6.24	0.283	0.023	0.068	1.42	0.087	1.97	0.082	4.25	36.9	—	0	0.089
—	0.227	—	6.52	0.624	0.017	0.043	1.47	—	—	—	5.1	31.2	—	0	—
3.81	0.51	0.045	7.65	0.425	0.009	0.003	0.028	0.022	8.87	0.008	9.92	9.07	—	0	0.498
5.86	0.624	0.906	7.94	0.057	0.02	0.04	0.765	0.045	5.39	0.422	3.4	30.9	—	0.142	0.139
7.09	0.261	0.366	33.2	0.567	0.082	0.074	1.12	0.02	26.4	0.15	52.4	50.7	—	0.576	0.386
3.4	0.374	0.207	21.8	0.652	0.054	0.094	1.22	0.023	21	0.074	25.8	30.1	—	0.576	—
7.98	0.482	0.682	5.67	0.113	0.017	0.043	1.39	0.033	11.8	0.845	13.9	34.3	—	0	0.389
2.86	0.964	0.554	7.37	0.51	0.065	0.068	1.08	0.031	1.02	0.333	12.2	30.3	—	0	0.08
2.86	0.567	0.554	4.54	0.454	0.011	0.006	0.567	0.031	1.02	0.333	5.67	33.2	—	0	0.08
6.24	0.734	0.712	1.42	0.142	0.045	0.048	0.95	0.068	5.84	0.51	12.8	39.4	—	0.285	0.172
24.8	2.18	1.37	116	2.92	0.331	0.445	3.01	0.136	13.9	0.467	253	358	—	0.625	1.45
27.4	2.41	1.52	129	3.23	0.366	0.492	3.32	0.151	15.4	0.516	279	396	—	0.69	1.61
—	—	—	—	—	—	—	—	—	—	—	—	—	—	—	—
—	—	—	—	—	—	—	—	—	—	—	—	—	—	—	—
23.4	2.46	2.54	333	0	0.312	0.796	1.84	0.343	52.8	1.5	77.5	347	—	0	5.69
—	—	—	—	—	—	—	—	—	—	—	—	—	—	—	—
33.4	3.65	6.14	0	0	0.301	0.344	5.41	0.277	23.5	2.45	66	230	—	0.939	0.247
34.9	4	4.57	16.7	3.26	0.277	0.306	6.72	0.27	33.9	2.27	79.6	197	—	1.74	1.05
—	—	—	—	—	—	—	—	—	—	—	—	—	—	—	—
—	9	—	—	—	—	—	—	—	—	—	—	—	—	—	—
—	—	—	—	—	—	—	—	—	—	—	—	—	—	—	—
44.1	3	2.66	413	0.033	0.43	0.593	4.17	0.1	31	0.472	542	611	—	2.21	4.09
25.5	2.75	1.62	127	8.73	0.56	0.535	3.87	0.207	39.3	0.73	94.9	234	—	1.06	2.33
30.2	2.65	1.67	142	3.56	0.403	0.542	3.66	0.166	16.9	0.569	308	436	—	0.761	1.78
—	—	—	—	—	—	—	—	—	—	—	—	—	—	—	—
28.4	3.11	5.22	0	0	0.257	0.293	4.6	0.236	20	2.09	56.1	196	—	0.799	0.211
—	—	—	—	—	—	—	—	—	—	—	—	—	—	—	—
25.4	1.86	0.914	63.2	0.719	0.215	0.388	1.39	0.099	13.5	0.415	341	411	—	1.35	1.86
22.3	1.48	2.1	63.4	0.206	0.05	0.149	7.65	0.491	3.69	0.333	17.9	175	—	0.061	1.05
41.4	3.11	1.5	13.8	0	0.403	0.35	13.4	0.586	29.1	0.305	99.9	261	—	1.41	2.8
40.2	1.61	1.47	20	0	0.113	0.171	18.4	0.771	5.38	0.459	21.4	312	—	0.08	0.742
16	0.92	1.98	17.4	0	0.057	0.155	4.14	0.238	5.54	0.217	8.42	120	—	0.041	0.637
28.8	1.77	2.97	35.2	0	0.108	0.293	8.22	0.395	9.75	0.362	16	221	—	0.136	0.668
12.4	0.81	1.14	24.5	0	0.038	0.089	4.33	0.265	2.33	0.18	9.87	97.2	—	0.056	0.72
132	10.3	4.23	242	4.89	0.3	0.496	9.86	0.364	33.5	3.4	214	764	—	1.77	16.9

Continued

Fast Foods—cont'd

Food Name	Portion	WT. Gm	KCAL Kc	PROT Gm	CARB Gm	FAT Gm	CHOL Mg	SAFA Gm	MUFA Gm	PUFA Gm	SOD Mg	POT Mg
LONG JOHN SILVER-BREADED SHRIMP	PIECE	420	51	1.19	6.19	2.43	5.95	0.524	1.57	0.286	85.2	41
LONG JOHN SILVER-CATFISH FILLET	SERVING	373	860	28	90	42	65	10	26	6	990	1180
LONG JOHN SILVER-CHICKEN PLANK-4 PIECE	SERVING	415	940	39	94	44	70	10	29	5	1660	1320
LONG JOHN SILVER-CHICKEN-LIGHT HERB	SERVING	498	630	35	85	17	85	3	5	7	2170	790
LONG JOHN SILVER-CLAM CHOWDER WITH COD	SERVING	198	140	11	10	6	20	2	3	2	590	380
LONG JOHN SILVER-CLAM DINNER	SERVING	363	980	21	122	45	15	10	30	6	1200	870
LONG JOHN SILVER-COLE SLAW	SERVING	98	140	1	20	6	15	1	2	4	260	190
LONG JOHN SILVER-FISH & CHICKEN ENTREE	SERVING	398	870	35	91	40	70	9	26	5	1520	1290
LONG JOHN SILVER-FISH & MORE ENTREE	SERVING	381	800	31	88	37	70	8	23	5	1390	1260
LONG JOHN SILVER-FISH AND FRYES-3 PIECE	SERVING	358	810	42	77	38	85	9	27	2	1630	1340
LONG JOHN SILVER-FISH SAND-WICH PLATTER	SERVING	379	870	26	108	38	55	8	22	7	1110	1050
LONG JOHN SILVER-FRIES	SERVING	85	220	3	30	10	5	3	7	1	60	390
LONG JOHN SILVER-GARDEN SALAD	SERVING	246	170	9	13	9	5	0.846	1	0.777	380	20
LONG JOHN SILVER-GUMBO-COD & SHRIMP BOBS	SERVING	198	120	9	4	8	25	2	3	3	740	310
LONG JOHN SILVER-HOMESTYLE FISH SANDWICH	SERVING	196	510	22	58	22	45	5	13	3	780	470
LONG JOHN SILVER-HOMESTYLE FISH-3 PIECE	SERVING	456	960	43	97	44	100	10	29	5	1890	1540
LONG JOHN SILVER-HOMESTYLE FISH-6 PIECE	SERVING	513	1260	49	124	64	130	14	43	6	1590	1660
LONG JOHN SILVER-HUSH-PUPPIES	PIECE	24	70	2	10	2	5	1	1	1	25	65
LONG JOHN SILVER-LIGHT FISH-LEMON	SERVING	291	320	24	49	4	75	1	1	1	900	470
LONG JOHN SILVER-LIGHT FISH-PAPRIKA	SERVING	284	300	24	45	2	70	1	1	1	650	460
LONG JOHN SILVER-MIXED VEGE-TABLES	SERVING	113	60	2	9	2	0	1	1	1	330	120
LONG JOHN SILVER-OCEAN CHEF SALAD	SERVING	321	250	24	19	9	80	2	2	2	1340	160
LONG JOHN SILVER-RICE PILAF	SERVING	142	210	5	43	2	0	1	1	1	570	140
LONG JOHN SILVER-SEAFOOD PLATTER	SERVING	400	970	30	109	46	70	10	30	6	1540	1100
LONG JOHN SILVER-SEAFOOD SALAD	SERVING	337	270	16	36	7	90	1	2	3	670	100
LONG JOHN SILVER-SEAFOOD SALAD-SCOOP	SERVING	142	210	14	26	5	90	1	2	3	570	100
LONG JOHN SILVER-SHRIMP & FISH DINNER	SERVING	348	770	25	85	37	80	8	23	5	1250	1030
LONG JOHN SILVER-SHRIMP FISH & CHICKEN	SERVING	380	840	31	89	40	80	9	26	5	1450	1170
LONG JOHN SILVER-SHRIMP SCAMPI	SERVING	529	610	25	87	18	220	3	6	7	2120	560
MCDONALDS-APPLE BRAN MUFFIN	SERVING	85	190	5	46	0	0	0	0	0	230	202
MCDONALDS-APPLE DANISH	SLICE	115	390	5.8	51.2	17.9	25.7	3.49	10.8	1.96	370	68.6
MCDONALDS-APPLE PIE	SERVING	83	260	2.2	30	14.8	0	4.83	9.11	0.87	240	49.5
MCDONALDS-BACON AND EGG BISCUIT	SERVING	156	440	17.5	33.3	26.4	253	8.22	16.1	2.01	1230	237
MCDONALDS-BACON BITS	SERVING	3	16	1.3	0.1	1.19	0	0	1.19	0	95	4.35
MCDONALDS-BARBEQUE (BARBE-CUE) SAUCE	SERVING	32	50	0.3	12.1	0.5	0	0.06	0.19	0.22	340	55.7
MCDONALDS-BISCUIT WITH SPREAD	SERVING	75	260	4.6	31.9	12.7	1	3.39	8.64	0.64	730	99.5
MCDONALDS-CHEF SALAD	SERVING	283	230	20.5	7.5	13.3	128	5.91	6.52	0.91	490	—
MCDONALDS-CHICKEN MCNUG-GETS-6 PIECE	SERVING	113	290	19	16.5	16.3	65	4.1	10.4	1.78	520	—

MAG Mg	IRON Mg	ZINC Mg	V-A RE	V-C Mg	THIA Mg	RIBO Mg	NIAC Mg	V-B6 Mg	FOL Ug	VB12 Ug	CALC Mg	PHOS Mg	SEL Mg	FIBD Gm	V-E Mg
156	12.1	4.97	285	5.75	0.353	0.584	11.6	0.428	39.4	3.99	252	899	—	2.08	19.9
121	4.63	3.43	317	11	0.201	0.489	9.69	0.869	67.4	9.41	200	1017	—	0.071	6.85
—	—	—	—	—	—	—	—	—	—	—	—	—	—	—	—
94.6	4.83	3.59	120	0	0.324	0.647	26.3	1.05	9.96	0.747	214	782	—	0	1.58
16.7	1.7	0.923	73.9	4.21	0.053	0.143	1.17	0.129	8.17	8.44	117	110	—	1.67	0.24
40.6	56.7	6.18	365	46.9	0.341	0.911	7.17	0.258	54.1	201	209	572	—	0	5.41
13.1	0.5	0.149	225	29.8	0.039	0.026	0.256	0.127	36.8	0.032	36.1	23.1	—	2.33	5.28
—	—	—	—	—	—	—	—	—	—	—	—	—	—	—	—
131	3.25	2.14	71.2	5	0.392	0.495	12.3	0.724	46.4	5.17	133	769	—	1.69	9.28
—	—	—	—	—	—	—	—	—	—	—	—	—	—	—	—
93.7	6.39	2.25	64.6	2.14	0.872	0.648	11.1	0.421	89.1	2.29	238	488	—	4.06	6.82
28.9	0.646	0.323	0	8.76	0.15	0.024	2.76	0.201	24.6	0	16.1	79.1	—	2.93	0.209
40	1.73	1.1	239	25.6	0.14	0.15	11.4	0.561	65.7	0.268	42	217	—	2.07	1.12
41.1	2.28	0.776	300	21.4	0.117	0.079	1.98	0.168	46.5	0.24	100	105	—	3.02	2.09
48.4	18	1.16	33.4	1.11	0.451	0.335	5.73	0.218	46.1	1.19	123	252	—	2.1	3.53
157	3.89	2.56	85.3	5.99	0.47	0.593	14.7	0.866	55.5	6.19	159	920	—	2.02	11.1
177	4.38	2.88	95.9	6.74	0.528	0.667	16.6	0.975	62.4	6.97	179	1035	—	2.27	12.5
—	—	—	—	—	—	—	—	—	—	—	—	—	—	—	—
56.1	2.29	1.39	79.7	10.2	0.291	0.146	3.38	0.335	46.1	0.576	40.4	238	—	2.43	3.66
97.7	2.43	1.6	53.1	3.73	0.293	0.369	9.18	0.54	34.6	3.86	99	573	—	1.26	6.91
24.1	0.899	0.536	75	3.5	0.078	0.132	0.931	0.081	20.8	0.003	28.5	56.4	—	5.9	0.935
—	—	—	—	—	—	—	—	—	—	—	—	—	—	—	—
16.6	1.77	0.618	59.5	0.565	0.148	0.016	1.51	0.082	5.32	0.006	16.9	44.6	—	0.778	0.936
114	4.13	2.2	59	13.4	0.42	0.368	8.22	0.876	36.9	1.68	109	484	—	5.33	5.2
86	3.22	5.2	129	19.9	0.128	0.158	3.72	0.27	46.7	2.89	148	444	—	1.33	8.9
36.2	1.36	2.19	250	8.38	0.054	0.067	1.57	0.114	19.7	1.22	62.5	187	—	0.562	3.76
81.7	3.45	1.55	27.5	16.5	0.372	0.212	6.64	0.64	35	1.06	54.1	422	—	7.33	5.29
—	—	—	—	—	—	—	—	—	—	—	—	—	—	—	—
203	13.6	6.22	364	11.3	0.132	0.196	13.6	0.55	9.89	5.57	299	1156	—	0	15.5
54.8	0.6	1.23	1	0.7	0.02	0.08	0.4	0.374	76.8	0.784	31	178	—	4.47	0.454
8.09	1.37	0.232	34.5	16.1	0.28	0.2	2.2	0.026	3.42	0	14	30.7	—	1.57	4.51
5.84	0.71	0.168	0	11.4	0.06	0.02	0.32	0.019	2.47	0	10.7	22.1	—	1.13	3.25
31.2	2.56	1.73	160	0	0.36	0.33	2.47	0.172	17.5	0.588	185	451	—	0.786	1.82
2.85	0	0.056	0	0	0	0	0	0.002	3.81	0.036	0	6.51	—	0	0.248
5.76	0.31	0.064	30	2.34	0.01	0.01	0.17	0.024	1.28	0	12.8	6.4	—	1.89	2.1
14.1	1.31	0.704	0	0	0.23	0.11	1.65	0.028	5.95	0.102	75	168	—	0.977	2.14
—	1.51	—	411	13.6	0.31	0.29	3.6	—	—	—	256	—	—	—	—
—	1	—	0	0	0.11	0.12	8.97	—	—	—	12.8	—	—	—	—

Continued

Fast Foods—cont'd

Food Name	Portion	WT. Gm	KCAL Kc	PROT Gm	CARB Gm	FAT Gm	CHOL Mg	SAFA Gm	MUFA Gm	PUFA Gm	SOD Mg	POT Mg
MCDONALDS-CHOCOLATE MILK-SHAKE-LOWFAT	SERVING	293	320	11.6	66	1.7	10	0.76	0.92	0.05	240	—
MCDONALDS-CHUNKY CHICKEN SALAD	SERVING	250	140	23.1	5.3	3.4	78	0.94	1.99	0.52	230	436
MCDONALDS-CINNAMON AND RAISIN DANISH	ITEM	110	440	6.4	57.5	21	34.7	4.2	13	1.6	430	—
MCDONALDS-COOKIE-CHOCOLATY	SERVING	56	330	4.2	41.9	15.6	4	5.04	10.2	0.39	280	71.7
MCDONALDS-COOKIE-MCDONALD-LAND	SERVING	56	290	4.2	47.1	9.2	0	1.85	6.8	0.52	300	37.5
MCDONALDS-CROUTONS	SERVING	11	50	1.39	6.8	2.17	0	0.45	1.32	0.11	140	19.9
MCDONALDS-ENGLISH MUFFIN	SERVING	59	170	5.4	26.7	4.6	9	2.38	1.68	0.5	270	74.3
MCDONALDS-FRENCH FRIES-LARGE	SERVING	122	400	5.61	45.9	21.6	16	9.06	11.6	0.89	200	866
MCDONALDS-FRENCH FRIES-MEDIUM	SERVING	97	320	4.44	36.3	17.1	12	7.17	9.21	0.7	150	692
MCDONALDS-FRENCH FRIES-REGULAR ORDER	SERVING	68	220	3.13	25.6	12	9	5.05	6.49	0.5	110	484
MCDONALDS-GARDEN SALAD	SERVING	213	110	7.1	6.2	6.6	83	2.9	3.16	0.53	160	450
MCDONALDS-HASHBROWN POTATO	SERVING	55	130	1.4	14.9	7.3	9	3.24	3.66	0.37	330	238
MCDONALDS-HONEY SAUCE	SERVING	14	45	0	11.5	0	0	0	0	0	0	—
MCDONALDS-HOT CAKES WITH SYRUP	SERVING	176	410	8.2	74.4	9.2	21	3.66	3.09	2.46	640	187
MCDONALDS-HOT CARAMEL SUNDAE	SERVING	174	270	6.6	59.3	2.8	13	1.51	1.22	0.09	180	414
MCDONALDS-HOT FUDGE SUNDAE	SERVING	169	240	7.3	50.5	3.2	6	2.35	0.76	0.05	170	274
MCDONALDS-HOT MUSTARD SAUCE	SERVING	30	70	0.5	8.2	3.6	5	0.51	1.23	1.86	250	25.6
MCDONALDS-ICED CHEESE DANISH	SERVING	110	390	7.4	42.3	21.8	47	5.95	12.1	1.77	420	—
MCDONALDS-McCHICKEN SAND-WICH	SERVING	190	490	19.2	39.8	28.6	42.6	5.4	11.5	11.6	780	340
MCDONALDS-McDLT HAMBURGER	ITEM	234	580	26.3	36	36.8	109	11.5	16.7	8.5	990	—
MCDONALDS-MCLEAN DELUXE HAMBURGER	SERVING	206	320	22	35	10	60	4	5	1	670	290
MCDONALDS-MILKSHAKE-CHOCO-LATE-LOWFAT	SERVING	293	320	12	66	2	10	1	1	0	240	—
MCDONALDS-MILKSHAKE-STRAW-BERRY-LOWFAT	SERVING	293	320	11	67	1	10	1	1	0	170	—
MCDONALDS-MILKSHAKE-VA-NILLA-LOWFAT	SERVING	293	290	11	60	1	10	1	1	0	170	643
MCDONALDS-PORK SAUSAGE	SERVING	48	180	8.4	0	16.3	48	5.88	8.51	1.9	350	—
MCDONALDS-RASPBERRY DANISH	ITEM	117	410	6.1	61.5	15.9	26	3.11	10.2	1.1	310	—
MCDONALDS-SALAD DRESSING-PEPPERCORN	OUNCE	28.4	160	0	2	18	14	2	4	10	170	22.4
MCDONALDS-SALAD DRESSING-RED FRENCH	OUNCE	28.4	80	0	10	4	0	0	2	2	220	22.4
MCDONALDS-SAUSAGE AND EGG BISCUIT	ITEM	180	520	19.9	32.6	34.5	275	11.2	20	2.54	1250	319
MCDONALDS-SAUSAGE BISCUIT	ITEM	123	440	13	31.9	29	49	9.27	17.2	2.54	1080	196
MCDONALDS-SAUSAGE MCMUFFIN	ITEM	117	370	16.5	27.3	21.9	64	7.79	11.7	2.43	830	179
MCDONALDS-SAUSAGE MCMUFFIN WITH EGG	ITEM	167	440	22.6	27.9	26.8	263	9.45	14.2	3.15	980	255
MCDONALDS-SCRAMBLED EGGS	SERVING	98	140	12.4	1.2	9.8	399	3.33	5.03	1.44	290	102
MCDONALDS-SIDE SALAD	SERVING	115	60	3.7	3.3	3.3	41	1.45	1.59	0.27	85	219
MCDONALDS-STRAWBERRY MILK-SHAKE-LOWFAT	SERVING	293	320	10.7	67	1.3	10	0.63	0.64	0.05	170	—
MCDONALDS-STRAWBERRY SUNDAE	SERVING	171	210	5.7	49.2	1.1	5	0.63	0.39	0.04	95	263
MCDONALDS-SWEET AND SOUR SAUCE	SERVING	32	60	0.2	13.8	0.2	0	0.03	0.1	0.1	190	10.4
MCDONALDS-VANILLA MILK-SHAKE-LOWFAT	SERVING	293	290	10.8	60	1.3	10	0.63	0.67	0.05	170	—
MCDONALDS-VANILLA-FROZEN YOGURT	SERVING	80	100	4	22	0.75	3	0.41	0.28	0.06	80	—
PIZZA-BEEF/CHICKEN/ONION	OUNCE	28.3	72.6	5.53	7.23	2.38	—	—	—	—	267	49
PIZZA-BEEF/ONION	OUNCE	28.3	72.9	4.34	7.88	2.66	—	—	—	—	132	49.9
PIZZA-CHICKEN CURRY/PEAS	OUNCE	28.3	81.6	3.74	9.41	3.23	—	—	—	—	146	44.5
PIZZA-CHICKEN/MUSHROOM/TOMATO	OUNCE	28.3	60.7	4.9	7.31	1.3	—	—	—	—	167	44.2

MAG Mg	IRON Mg	ZINC Mg	V-A RE	V-C Mg	THIA Mg	RIBO Mg	NIAC Mg	V-B6 Mg	FOL Ug	VB12 Ug	CALC Mg	PHOS Mg	SEL Mg	FIBD Gm	V-E Mg
—	0.84	—	91.9	0	0.13	0.5	0.4	—	—	—	332	—	—	—	—
36.6	1.02	2.94	366	19.9	0.22	0.17	8.5	0.6	26.6	0.63	33.8	257	—	0.955	13
—	1.81	—	33	3.2	0.32	0.24	2.8	—	—	—	35.1	—	—	—	—
20.2	2.18	0.515	0	0	0.18	0.21	2.47	0.028	5.04	0.073	23.9	71.1	—	1.12	1.73
12.9	2.07	0.325	0	0	0.25	0.18	2.54	0.028	3.92	0.067	8.91	91.3	—	0.56	1.73
4.62	0.35	0.103	0	0.14	0.05	0.03	0.42	0.007	3.41	0	6.48	15.4	—	0.517	0.114
12.2	1.61	0.396	36.6	0	0.33	0.14	2.47	0.097	51.1	0.001	151	59.8	—	1.56	0.16
40.1	0.93	0.633	0	14.6	0.24	0	3.29	0.317	40.1	0.147	17.8	162	—	4.21	0.3
32	0.73	0.506	0	11.6	0.19	0	2.6	0.253	32	0.117	14.1	129	—	3.35	0.239
22.4	0.52	0.354	0	8.16	0.14	0	1.84	0.177	22.4	0.082	9.93	90.4	—	—	—
34.7	1.26	0.956	391	13.5	0.1	0.16	0.59	0.486	56.9	0.232	149	188	—	1.8	0.974
9.3	0.27	0.175	0	1.59	0.06	0.02	0.85	0.069	3.55	0	5.58	39.4	—	1.09	0.125
—	0.07	—	0	0.14	0	0.01	0.04	—	—	—	—	—	—	—	—
25	2.08	0.6	52	4.71	0.32	0.33	2.82	0.12	9	0.19	114	501	—	—	—
50.5	0.08	1.1	87.4	0	0.08	0.35	0.26	0.383	19.1	0.661	222	198	—	1.04	1.38
32	0.48	1.29	64.3	0	0.08	0.35	0.3	0.074	7.23	0.597	235	178	—	1.25	1.36
5.47	0.22	0.094	1.6	0.45	0.01	0.01	0.15	0.01	1.27	0	15	7.3	—	0.252	1.45
—	1.42	—	37.6	1.1	0.29	0.23	2.1	—	—	—	32.9	—	—	—	—
47.3	2.61	1.72	31.2	2.42	0.96	0.21	8.92	0.671	33.3	0.35	143	299	—	1.61	3.19
—	3.91	—	226	7.38	0.39	0.36	6.87	—	—	—	225	—	—	—	—
34.8	3.78	3.24	66.6	9.74	0.354	0.311	5.81	0.257	47.7	1.48	92.5	170	—	2.4	3.2
—	—	—	—	—	—	—	—	—	—	—	332	—	—	—	—
—	—	—	—	—	—	—	—	—	—	—	327	—	—	—	—
48.1	0.205	2.43	38.1	2.2	0.123	0.589	0.314	0.132	30.8	1.54	327	394	—	0	0.12
—	0.67	—	0	0	0.27	0.1	2.31	—	—	—	8.24	—	—	0	—
—	1.47	—	35.1	3.2	0.33	0.21	2.1	—	—	—	14.2	—	—	—	—
0	0.114	0.023	5.68	0	0.002	0.005	0.001	0.003	1.19	0.039	3.12	3.98	—	0	2.87
0	0.114	0.023	5.68	0	0.002	0.005	0.001	0.003	1.19	0.039	3.12	3.98	—	0	2.87
25	3.16	2.16	88.3	0.1	0.53	0.35	3.99	0.2	40	1.37	116	490	—	—	—
19.8	1.98	1.54	0	0	0.49	0.21	3.96	0.114	8.73	0.504	83.2	443	—	1.35	3.66
20	2.3	1.67	72.1	1.27	0.6	0.29	4.8	0.133	47.7	0.503	235	273	—	1.1	1.94
28.6	3.34	2.39	150	0	0.64	0.42	4.82	0.19	68.1	0.718	263	390	—	1.56	2.77
10.2	2.08	1.09	156	1.18	0.07	0.26	0.05	0.075	27.2	1.68	57	136	—	0	3.44
12.4	0.67	0.252	217	7.4	0.05	0.08	0.32	0.059	40.3	0	763	25.5	—	1.23	0.469
—	0.09	—	91.9	0	0.13	0.48	0.31	—	—	—	327	—	—	—	—
19	0.16	1.17	64.3	1.3	0.07	0.29	0.25	0.067	8.77	0.54	190	127	—	0.687	0.754
2.38	0.17	0.014	64.8	0.64	0	0.01	0.08	0.004	0.344	0	10.9	3.03	—	0.016	—
—	0.1	—	91.9	0	0.13	0.48	0.31	—	—	—	327	—	—	—	—
—	0.23	—	38.4	0	0.04	0.18	0.37	—	—	—	112	—	—	—	—
—	0.709	—	23.2	1.25	0.026	0.023	1.25	—	—	—	72.9	53	—	0.028	—
—	0.17	—	23.2	0.227	0.011	0.017	0.879	—	—	—	21.3	35.7	—	0.113	—
—	0.17	—	29.8	0.198	0.02	0.026	1.73	—	—	—	19.3	36.6	—	0.198	—
—	0.198	—	22.7	0.312	0.009	0.011	0.765	—	—	—	24.1	36.6	—	0.085	—

Continued

Fast Foods—cont'd

Food Name	Portion	WT. Gm	KCAL Kc	PROT Gm	CARB Gm	FAT Gm	CHOL Mg	SAFA Gm	MUFA Gm	PUFA Gm	SOD Mg	POT Mg
PIZZA-CHICKEN/PINEAPPLE	OUNCE	28.3	80.5	4.22	6.32	4.25	—	—	—	—	267	37.4
PIZZA-COMBINATION SUPREME	OUNCE	28.3	50.5	4.14	7.09	0.624	5.66	1.33	1.47	0.408	165	45.1
PIZZA-CURRY BEEF/PEAS	OUNCE	28.3	70.6	4.51	7.31	2.58	8.33	0.856	1.62	1.01	130	47.3
PIZZA-ONION/TOMATO/GREEN PEPPER/MUSHROOM	OUNCE	28.3	45.4	3.49	6.58	0.567	—	—	—	—	136	42.8
PIZZA-PEPPERONI/BEEF/SALAMI/ MUSHROOM/ETC	OUNCE	28.3	83.3	5.07	4.56	4.96	—	—	—	—	367	61.2
PIZZA-SHRIMP/CUCUMBER	OUNCE	28.3	68.6	4.45	6.83	2.61	—	—	—	—	143	46.2
PIZZA-SHRIMP/SQUID/MUSH-ROOM	OUNCE	28.3	70.3	4.96	7.43	2.3	—	—	—	—	160	33.2
POTATOES-FRENCH FRIED-FAST FOOD	OUNCE	28.3	91.3	1.08	10.3	5.07	2.76	1.8	1.93	0.755	17	130
POTATOES-MASHED-FAST FOOD	OUNCE	28.3	26.4	0.624	5.44	0.227	0.544	0.284	0.481	0.328	82.2	48.2
RAX-GRILLED CHICKEN SAND-WICH	ITEM	190	440	24	36	19	87.9	2.92	4.48	5.37	1050	340
SALAD-FAST FOOD	OUNCE	28.3	33.5	0.454	3.29	2.04	—	—	—	—	128	39.7
SPAGHETTI-VEGETABLES/ SAUCE/CHEESE	OUNCE	28.3	28.3	3.8	3.01	0.113	—	—	—	—	83.6	52.4
SUBWAY SANDWICH-HAM AND CHEESE-ON WHEAT	ITEM	194	673	39	86	22	73	7	8	4	2508	918
SUBWAY-BMT SANDWICH-ON HONEY WHEAT ROLL	ITEM	220	1011	45	88	57	133	20	25	7	3199	1002
SUBWAY-BMT SANDWICH-ON ITALIAN ROLL	ITEM	213	982	44	83	55	133	20	24	7	3139	917
SUBWAY-CLUB SANDWICH-ON HONEY WHEAT	ITEM	220	722	47	89	23	84	7	9	4	2777	1055
SUBWAY-CLUB SANDWICH-ON ITALIAN ROLL	ITEM	213	693	46	83	22	84	7	8	4	2717	971
SUBWAY-COLD CUT COMBO SAND-WICH-ITALIAN	ITEM	184	853	46	83	40	166	12	15	10	2218	876
SUBWAY-COLD CUT COMBO SAND-WICH-ON WHEAT	ITEM	191	883	48	88	41	166	12	15	10	2278	1010
SUBWAY-HAM & CHEESE SAND-WICH-ON ITALIAN	ITEM	184	643	38	81	18	73	7	8	4	1710	834
SUBWAY-MEATBALL SANDWICH-ON ITALIAN ROLL	ITEM	215	918	42	96	44	88	17	17	4	2022	1210
SUBWAY-MEATBALL-ON HONEY WHEAT ROLL	ITEM	224	947	44	101	45	88	17	18	4	2082	1498
SUBWAY-ROAST BEEF SANDWICH-ITALIAN ROLL	ITEM	184	689	42	84	23	83.3	8	9	4	2288	910
SUBWAY-ROAST BEEF SANDWICH-ON WHEAT ROLL	ITEM	189	717	41	89	24	75	8	9	4	2348	994
SUBWAY-SALAD DRESSING-BUTTERMILK RANCH	SERVING	56.7	348	1	2	37	6	5	7	24	492	17
SUBWAY-SALAD DRESSING-LITE ITALIAN	SERVING	56.7	23	1	4	1	0	3.97	6.35	15.9	952	13
SUBWAY-SEAFOOD/CRAB SAND-WICH-ON ITALIAN	ITEM	210	986	29	94	57	56	11	15	28	1967	557
SUBWAY-SEAFOOD/CRAB SAND-WICH-ON WHEAT	ITEM	219	1015	31	100	58	56	11	16	28	2027	641
SUBWAY-SPICY ITALIAN SAND-WICH-ON ITALIAN	ITEM	213	1043	42	83	63	137	23	28	7	2282	880
SUBWAY-STEAK & CHEESE SAND-WICH-ITALIAN	ITEM	213	765	43	83	32	82	12	12	4	1556	909
SUBWAY-TURKEY BREAST SAND-WICH-WHEAT ROLL	ITEM	192	674	42	88	20	67	6	7	7	2520	605
TACO BELL-DOUBLE BEEF BURRITO SUPREME	ITEM	255	457	23.6	41.7	21.8	56.8	10.1	15.4	2.09	1053	431
TACO BELL-ENCHIRITO	ITEM	213	382	19.8	30.9	19.7	54.2	9.32	—	1.51	1243	—
TACO BELL-MEXICAN PIZZA	SERVING	223	575	21.3	39.7	36.8	52	11.4	8.16	9.74	1031	408
TACO BELL-NACHOS	SERVING	106	346	7.49	37.5	18.5	8.82	5.74	9.96	1.55	399	159
TACO BELL-NACHOS BELL-GRANDE	SERVING	287	649	21.6	60.6	35.3	36.3	12.3	—	2.61	997	674
TACO BELL-PINTOS & CHEESE	SERVING	128	190	8.97	19	8.72	16.2	3.6	4.92	0.814	642	399
TACO BELL-SOFT TACO	ITEM	92.1	228	11.8	17.9	11.8	31.8	5.37	3.71	1.21	516	178
TACO BELL-TACO BELLGRANDE	ITEM	163	355	18.3	17.7	23.1	55.9	10.9	6.57	1.32	472	334
TACO BELL-TACO LIGHT	ITEM	170	410	19	18.1	28.8	55.6	11.6	—	5.36	594	316
TACO BELL-TACO SALAD WITH SALSA/NO SHELL	SERVING	530	520	30.6	30	31.4	79.8	14.4	19.2	1.7	1431	1151

MAG Mg	IRON Mg	ZINC Mg	V-A RE	V-C Mg	THIA Mg	RIBO Mg	NIAC Mg	V-B6 Mg	FOL Ug	VB12 Ug	CALC Mg	PHOS Mg	SEL Mg	FIBD Gm	V-E Mg
—	0.397	—	25.2	0.879	0.026	0.026	2.13	—	—	—	85.9	114	—	0.057	—
6.45	0.227	0.343	9.64	0.624	0.017	0.017	1.81	0.038	6.9	0.084	26.6	39.4	—	0.17	0.348
7.03	0.17	0.725	28.6	0.879	0.02	0.023	3.57	0.058	2.45	0.366	23.8	37.7	—	0.17	0.784
—	0.227	—	9.07	0.425	0.014	0.023	1.64	—	—	—	24.7	32.9	—	0.227	—
—	0.227	—	21.5	0.198	0.02	0.003	3.06	—	—	—	76.3	58.7	—	0.085	—
—	0.198	—	11.9	0.397	0.009	0.011	2.32	—	—	—	24.7	48.2	—	0.142	—
—	0.17	—	13	0.369	0.009	0.014	0.936	—	—	—	22.4	37.7	—	0.142	—
9.62	0.595	0.108	6.24	0.312	0.023	0.011	0.369	0.067	8.21	0	2.27	20.1	—	0	0.07
5.15	0.765	0.077	14.7	0.227	0.017	0.011	0.198	0.063	2.25	0.016	3.12	14.2	—	0	0.208
47.3	3.56	1.72	15.8	0	0.462	0.401	15.3	0.671	33.3	0.35	114	299	—	1.61	3.19
—	0.652	—	4.25	0.85	0.017	0.006	0.028	—	—	—	5.39	14.2	—	0	—
—	0.312	—	3.97	0.085	0.011	0.011	0.227	—	—	—	3.97	9.64	—	0.34	—
—	—	—	—	—	—	—	—	—	—	—	—	—	—	6	—
—	—	—	—	—	—	—	—	—	—	—	—	—	—	6	—
66.1	4.26	6.08	66.5	5.4	0.271	0.341	5.06	0.481	62.6	2.33	63.6	308	—	5	6.1
39.7	3.18	1.39	83	15.1	0.486	0.348	9.3	0.455	43.1	0.44	96.3	247	—	6	5.04
65.6	3.09	2.5	74	20.2	0.477	0.334	12.5	0.581	47	0.946	57.5	384	—	5	1.61
27.5	2.86	2.73	87	17.3	0.359	0.333	3.8	0.201	39	1.23	227	315	—	5	1.08
28.5	2.97	2.83	90.3	18	0.372	0.346	3.94	0.208	40.5	1.28	23.5	327	—	6	1.13
49.6	2.17	2.8	174	16.8	0.528	0.388	3.56	0.335	45.1	0.756	304	527	—	5	4.6
47.1	4.97	6.2	71.9	18.7	0.333	0.391	9.36	0.4	34.9	3.21	77.6	263	—	3.02	1.18
—	—	—	—	—	—	—	—	—	—	—	—	—	—	—	—
57.1	3.68	5.26	57.5	4.67	0.234	0.294	4.37	0.416	54.1	2.01	54.9	266	—	5	5.26
58.6	3.78	5.4	59	4.79	0.24	0.302	4.49	0.427	55.6	2.07	56.4	273	—	6	5.4
1.13	0.113	0.102	47.6	0	0.007	0.014	0.002	0.01	3.56	0.118	7.94	14.7	—	0	2.72
0.363	0.113	0.062	13.6	0	0.006	0.011	0.002	0.007	2.77	0.092	5.67	2.84	—	0	5.86
—	—	—	—	—	—	—	—	—	—	—	—	—	—	—	—
61.7	4.41	5.28	107	5.49	0.51	0.383	6.95	0.258	91.3	6.54	230	336	—	2.49	3.01
—	—	—	—	—	—	—	—	—	—	—	—	—	—	5	—
43.1	4.22	6.78	119	5.82	0.33	0.464	5.06	0.381	36.4	2.54	231	456	—	6	1.01
—	—	—	—	—	—	—	—	—	—	—	—	—	—	7	—
87.2	3.95	5.93	286	8.68	0.427	2.19	3.68	0.354	132	2.18	145	548	—	5.68	2.78
—	2.84	—	290	28.1	0.256	0.418	2.32	—	—	—	269	—	—	—	—
62.9	3.74	2.32	295	30.9	0.319	0.326	2.96	0.274	113	0.198	257	360	—	5.75	3.02
42.8	0.934	2.58	169	1.88	0.006	0.163	0.679	0.122	15.7	0.615	191	439	—	1.39	3.36
—	3.48	—	341	57.8	0.104	0.339	2.17	—	—	—	297	—	—	—	—
49.8	1.42	1.08	132	51.4	0.05	0.146	0.396	0.192	98.1	0.076	156	175	—	4.87	1.68
30.6	2.27	1.36	64	1.22	0.387	0.224	2.74	0.159	40.3	0.31	116	132	—	2.56	1.1
54.1	1.92	2.4	254	5.48	0.107	0.291	2.02	0.282	71.3	0.549	182	234	—	4.54	1.94
—	2.44	—	199	4.7	0.199	0.325	2.51	—	—	—	155	—	—	—	—
111	5.14	9.14	908	76.1	0.264	0.64	3.17	0.779	98.8	4.29	367	567	—	7.04	7.25

Continued

Fast Foods—cont'd

Food Name	Portion	WT. Gm	KCAL Kc	PROT Gm	CARB Gm	FAT Gm	CHOL Mg	SAFA Gm	MUFA Gm	PUFA Gm	SOD Mg	POT Mg
TACO BELL-TACO SALAD WITH SALSA/SHELL	SERVING	595	941	36	63.1	61.3	80.4	18.7	21.6	12.1	1662	1212
TACO BELL-TACO SALAD-NO SALSA-NO SHELL	SERVING	530	502	29.5	26.3	31.3	79.8	14.4	19.2	1.7	1056	988
WENDYS-BACON AND CHEESE POTATO	SERVING	347	450	15	57	18	10	37.1	38.2	14.1	1125	1580
WENDYS-BIG CLASSIC-QUARTER POUND BURGER	SERVING	277	570	27	46	33	85	15.9	14.8	4.26	1075	590
WENDYS-BROCCOLI AND CHEESE POTATO	SERVING	377	400	9	59	16	0	—	—	—	470	1555
WENDYS-CHEESE POTATO	SERVING	348	470	13	57	21	0	12.1	9.26	4	580	1435
WENDYS-CHEESE SAUCE	SERVING	56	40	1	5	2	0	1.87	1.06	0.319	300	70
WENDYS-CHEESE TORTELLINI/ SPAGHETTI SAUCE	SERVING	112	120	4	24	1	5	2.8	2.15	0.888	280	110
WENDYS-CHICKEN CLUB SAND-WICH	SERVING	231	500	30	42	24	75	5.45	8.46	8.02	950	515
WENDYS-CHICKEN SALAD	SERVING	56	120	7	4	8	0	3	2.81	3	215	60
WENDYS-CHILI	SERVING	255	220	21	23	7	45	3	5.66	1.05	750	495
WENDYS-FRENCH FRIES-REGULAR SIZE	SERVING	134	440	5	53	23	25	8.51	9.13	3.58	265	855
WENDYS-KIDS MEAL HAMBURGER	SERVING	104	260	14	30	9	35	3.5	4.75	0.768	545	205
WENDYS-REFRIED BEANS	SERVING	56	70	4	10	3	0	1	2.21	1	215	210
WENDYS-SEAFOOD SALAD	SERVING	56	110	4	7	7	0	1	4.46	4	455	40
WENDYS-SINGLE CHEESEBURGER/ EVERYTHING	SERVING	252	490	29	35	27	90	10.8	11.2	4.58	1155	495
WENDYS-SINGLE HAMBURGER/ EVERYTHING	SERVING	234	420	25	35	21	70	6.72	9.4	4.43	865	495
WENDYS-SPANISH RICE	SERVING	56	70	2	13	1	0	0.121	0.298	1	440	130
WENDYS-TACO SALAD WITH TACO CHIPS	SERVING	791	660	40	46	37	35	28.8	28.7	15.4	1110	1330
WENDYS-TUNA SALAD	SERVING	56	100	8	4	6	0	1	0.796	3	290	90

MAG Mg	IRON Mg	ZINC Mg	V-A RE	V-C Mg	THIA Mg	RIBO Mg	NIAC Mg	V-B6 Mg	FOL Ug	VB12 Ug	CALC Mg	PHOS Mg	SEL Mg	FIBD Gm	V-E Mg
125	7.1	10.3	888	77	0.508	0.753	4.78	0.875	111	4.82	398	637	—	7.91	8.14
111	4.54	9.14	572	74.3	0.246	0.498	3.17	0.779	98.8	4.29	331	567	—	7.04	7.25
167	15.3	6.99	266	76.5	1.04	0.805	14.5	1.94	75.4	2.26	713	1015	—	9.85	5.83
49.2	4.75	6.36	162	9.41	0.346	0.496	7.95	0.382	50.5	2.92	304	491	—	2.32	3.42
—	—	—	—	—	—	—	—	—	—	—	—	—	—	—	—
71.9	2.25	2.43	288	33.9	0.223	0.425	3.47	0.574	30.6	0.299	417	398	—	3.59	2.75
9.52	0.056	0.195	23.5	0.448	0.03	0.113	0.064	0.028	2.52	0.224	114	87.9	—	0.168	0.08
14.3	1.34	0.643	110	4.24	0.12	0.175	1.21	0.085	12.2	0.17	74.5	92.3	—	1.01	1.14
41.7	14.4	1.46	87.1	15.8	0.511	0.365	16	0.478	45.3	0.462	101	259	—	2.3	5.29
8.2	0.5	0.659	21.5	1.08	0.022	0.077	1.79	0.134	5.96	0.141	12.8	57.5	—	0.214	2.89
53.2	6.3	4.12	146	18.9	0.158	0.258	4.81	0.232	41.3	1.46	55.2	228	—	6	2.11
45.6	1.02	0.509	0	13.8	0.237	0.038	4.36	0.316	38.9	0	25.5	125	—	4.62	0.33
21.6	2.47	2.22	7.3	1.43	0.226	0.198	3.82	0.135	24.9	0.998	62.6	110	—	1.32	0.641
24.7	1.16	0.493	0	1.68	0.082	0.039	0.177	0.087	71.1	0	24.6	72.3	—	3	0.566
14.3	0.535	0.865	21.4	3.3	0.021	0.026	0.619	0.045	7.76	0.481	24.7	73.7	—	0.222	1.48
43.7	4.31	4.27	136	10.9	0.403	0.423	6.52	0.302	55.1	1.8	234	348	—	2.69	3.8
39.5	4.29	3.69	75.6	11.1	0.402	0.353	6.6	0.292	54.2	1.68	105	193	—	2.73	3.64
8.92	0.692	0.196	23.9	9.2	0.046	0.017	0.586	0.057	3.6	0	15.3	17.4	—	0.744	0.36
166	9.23	13.6	1478	67.4	0.396	0.925	15.2	1.16	147	6.41	532	847	—	10.5	10.8
10.3	0.557	0.176	14.9	1.23	0.018	0.041	3.75	0.045	3.9	0.679	9.25	61.9	—	0.312	0.638

APPENDIX B

Chemistry: A Tool for Understanding Nutrition

BY DR. ALLAN BURKITT, PROFESSOR OF CHEMISTRY, DILLARD UNIVERSITY

An understanding of basic chemistry can make the study of nutrition easier and more interesting. It helps to connect nutrient characteristics with the structural and chemical characteristics of the individual compounds.

You have already taken at least one basic college course in chemistry; consequently this appendix serves only to review key chemical points that arise in the study of nutrition. One concept to keep firmly in mind is that the physical and chemical properties of almost anything are intimately related to its structure. This is true of atoms, molecules, organisms—anything composed of matter. A basic knowledge of chemical structures can help you visualize important concepts in nutrition.

Let's briefly review those aspects of chemistry closely related to nutrition. We hope that this overview will make it easier to see what nutrition is all about.

Matter and Mass

All living and nonliving things are composed of matter. Two characteristics of matter are its mass and its volume. Mass is related to the amount of force it takes to move the object—it takes less force to move a paper clip than a car, therefore the clip has a less mass. Volume is related to the amount of space an object occupies—a pint of water occupies less space than a gallon, therefore a pint has the smaller volume. Both of these properties depend on how much of the substance you have. A lake has a larger volume and a larger mass than a puddle of water.

A more fundamental property of matter is its density, which is defined to be the mass of an object divided by its volume (d = Mass/Volume). Density is a more fundamental property because it is independent of how much matter is available. The density of water in the lake and in the puddle is about 1.0 gram per milliliter. The units of density are usually reported in units of g mL^{-1} for solids and liquids and g L^{-1} for gases.

The density of pure water is 1.0 gram per milliliter; lean body tissue has a density of about 1.1 grams per milliliter; and that of body fat is about 0.9 gram per milliliter. Substances with a density less than that of water are buoyant (they tend to float), while substances with a density greater than water tend to sink. The more fat people contain, the more buoyant they are when placed in water. This physical property—tendency to float or sink in water—is used to determine the amount of body fat stored in a person (see Chapter 8).

Elements and Atoms

Most matter is composed of atoms. Atoms are substances that cannot be broken down into simpler forms by ordinary chemical means. An **element** is composed of atoms of only one kind. For example, the element carbon is composed of only carbon atoms, and the element oxygen is composed of only oxygen atoms. There are more than 100 elements, such as hydrogen, oxygen, carbon, iron, and nitrogen. Many of these elements can be found in molecules found in nutrition.

Each element (atom) is identified by its atomic number. For example, the atom containing 6 protons (atomic number = 6) is called carbon (C). Overall, then, elements are identified by the number of protons they contain. A periodic table lists the atomic number for each element (Table B-1).

Atomic Structure

Atoms are composed of protons (possessing a unit positive charge), neutrons (zero charge) and electrons (unit negative charge). All atoms are spherically shaped. At the center of the sphere is the nucleus containing all the protons and neutrons. The nucleus is surrounded by an electron cloud. The volume occupied by the electron cloud is about 10,000 times greater than the volume occupied by the nucleus. Consequently the volume of the electron cloud defines the atomic volume.

Protons and neutrons have about the same mass and that mass is 2000 times larger than the mass of the electron. Essentially, all the mass of the atom is located within the nucleus. The structure of an atom can therefore be pictured as a very tiny, highly dense nuclear core surrounded by a cloud of electrons.

Electrons surrounding the nucleus have a somewhat peculiar nonintuitive behavior. For instance, its impossible to know precisely where any given electron is located at any particular moment. In is only possible to define a volume of space where the electron is most likely to be found. This volume has a specific size and shape and is called an orbital. Any orbital can contain up to two electrons.

Different orbitals have different energies. Orbitals of similar energy are grouped together into electron shells. A shell can contain either 1, 4, 9, or 16 different orbitals. Therefore shells can hold a maximum of 2, 8, 18, or 32 electrons depending on the number of orbitals in the shell. Any shell can hold less than the maximum number of electrons. Most atoms have electrons occupying more than one shell. Carbon has two shells, the first holding two electrons (the maximum number) and the second holding six electrons (two less than the maximum number of eight). Shells themselves are always spherical, and this gives rise to the spherical shape of the atoms. The outermost shell in an atom is called the valence shell. The number of electrons in the valence shell and the energy of those electrons determine chemical behavior. Since these are unique for each element, each element has a unique chemistry.

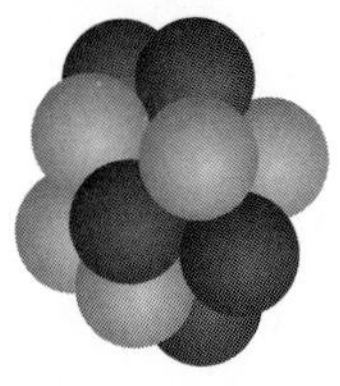

Carbon 14
6 Protons
8 Neutrons
6 Electrons

Atoms that have not undergone chemical change are electrically neutral. This means that the number of protons equals the number of electrons in these atoms. Each element has a unique number of protons in its atoms. All neutral atoms of carbon, for example, contain six protons and six electrons, although the number of neutrons may vary (see the next section). The number of protons an atom of an element contains is defined as the atomic number. Each element has a unique atomic number. The atomic number of each element and its symbol are given (among other things) in the periodic table.

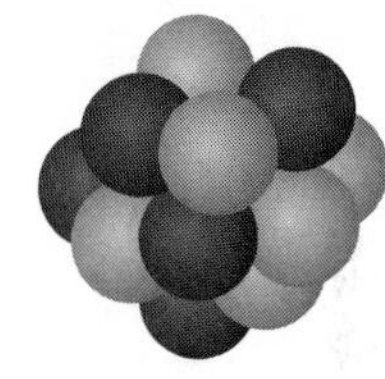

Carbon 12
6 Protons
6 Neutrons
6 Electrons

Isotopes

In the previous section it was pointed out that all the atoms of a given element contain the same number of protons, but that the number of neutrons in the nucleus may vary. Carbon nuclei, for example can contain 6, 7, or 8 neutrons. Atoms with identical numbers of electrons and different numbers of neutrons are called **isotopes.** Scientists distinguish between isotopes by adding the number of protons and neutrons together and writing the resultant sum as a superscript to the left of the elemental symbol. For example, consider carbon with its six protons. The predominant isotope of carbon contains six neutrons and is written as ^{12}C. The isotope containing seven neutrons is labeled ^{13}C, and the isotope containing eight neutrons is labeled ^{14}C. Note that having 6 protons means that all the atoms are carbon, but since they differ in the number of neutrons, they represent the isotopes of carbon. The isotopes of carbon are shown in the margin.

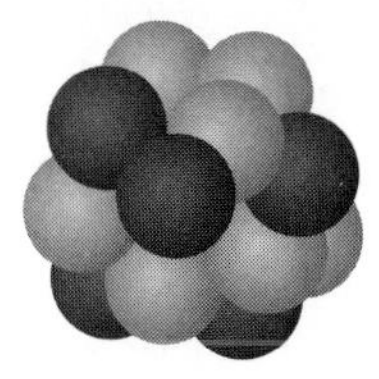

Carbon 13
6 Protons
7 Neutrons
6 Electrons

Table B-1 Periodic table of the elements

1 H 1.00794	Atomic number Symbol Atomic weight

Main-group elements (groups 1–2, 13–18); Transition metals (groups 3–12)

Period	1 IA	2 IIA	3 IIIB	4 IVB	5 VB	6 VIB	7 VIIB	8	9 VIIIB	10	11 IB	12 IIB	13 IIIA	14 IVA	15 VA	16 VIA	17 VIIA	18 VIIIA
1	1 H 1.00794																	2 He 4.002602
2	3 Li 6.941	4 Be 9.012182											5 B 10.811	6 C 12.011	7 N 14.00674	8 O 15.9994	9 F 18.9984032	10 Ne 20.1797
3	11 Na 22.989768	12 Mg 24.3050											13 Al 26.981539	14 Si 28.0855	15 P 30.973762	16 S 32.066	17 Cl 35.4527	18 Ar 39.948
4	19 K 39.0983	20 Ca 40.078	21 Sc 44.955910	22 Ti 47.88	23 V 50.9415	24 Cr 51.9961	25 Mn 54.93805	26 Fe 55.847	27 Co 58.93320	28 Ni 58.69	29 Cu 63.546	30 Zn 65.39	31 Ga 69.723	32 Ge 72.61	33 As 74.92159	34 Se 78.96	35 Br 79.904	36 Kr 83.80
5	37 Rb 85.4678	38 Sr 87.62	39 Y 88.90585	40 Zr 91.224	41 Nb 92.90638	42 Mo 95.94	43 Tc (98)	44 Ru 101.07	45 Rh 102.90550	46 Pd 106.42	47 Ag 107.8682	48 Cd 112.411	49 In 114.82	50 Sn 118.710	51 Sb 121.75	52 Te 127.60	53 I 126.90447	54 Xe 131.29
6	55 Cs 132.90543	56 Ba 137.327	57 La* 138.9055	72 Hf 178.49	73 Ta 180.9479	74 W 183.85	75 Re 186.207	76 Os 190.2	77 Ir 192.22	78 Pt 195.08	79 Au 196.96654	80 Hg 200.59	81 Tl 204.3833	82 Pb 207.2	83 Bi 208.98037	84 Po (209)	85 At (210)	86 Rn (222)
7	87 Fr (223)	88 Ra (226)	89 Ac** (227)	104 Unq (261)	105 Unp (262)	106 Unh (263)	107 Uns (262)	108 Uno (265)	109 Une (267)									

Inner-Transition Metals

*Lanthanides	58 Ce 140.115	59 Pr 140.90765	60 Nd 144.24	61 Pm (145)	62 Sm 150.36	63 Eu 151.965	64 Gd 157.25	65 Tb 158.92534	66 Dy 162.50	67 Ho 164.93032	68 Er 167.266	69 Tm 168.93421	70 Yb 173.04	71 Lu 174.967
**Actinides	90 Th 232.0381	91 Pa (231)	92 U 238.0289	93 Np (237)	94 Pu (244)	95 Am (243)	96 Cm (247)	97 Bk (247)	98 Cf (251)	99 Es (252)	100 Fm (257)	101 Md (258)	102 No (259)	103 Lr (262)

Metal

Metalloid

Nonmetal

Key to abbreviations

Name	Symbol	Name	Symbol	Name	Symbol	Name	Symbol
Key to abbreviations							
Actinium	Ac	Erbium	Er	Molybdenum	Mo	Samarium	Sm
Aluminum	Al	Europium	Eu	Neodymium	Nd	Scandium	Sc
Americium	Am	Fermium	Fm	Neon	Ne	Selenium	Se
Antimony	Sb	Fluorine	F	Neptunium	Np	Silicon	Si
Argon	Ar	Francium	Fr	Nickel	Ni	Silver	Ag
Arsenic	As	Gadolinium	Gd	Niobium	Nb	Sodium	Na
Astatine	At	Gallium	Ga	Nitrogen	N	Strontium	Sr
Barium	Ba	Germanium	Ge	Nobelium	No	Sulfur	S
Berkelium	Bk	Gold	Au	Osmium	Os	Tantalum	Ta
Beryllium	Be	Hafnium	Hf	Oxygen	O	Technetium	Tc
Bismuth	Bi	Helium	He	Palladium	Pd	Tellurium	Te
Boron	B	Homium	Ho	Phosphorus	P	Terbium	Tb
Bromine	Br	Hydrogen	H	Platinum	Pt	Thallium	Tl
Cadmium	Cd	Indium	In	Plutonium	Pu	Thorium	Th
Calcium	Ca	Iodine	I	Polonium	Po	Thulium	Tm
Californium	Cf	Iridium	Ir	Potassium	K	Tin	Sn
Carbon	C	Iron	Fe	Praseodymium	Pr	Titanium	Ti
Cerium	Ce	Krypton	Kr	Promethium	Pm	Tungsten	W
Cesium	Cs	Lanthanum	La	Protactinium	Pa	Uranium	U
Chlorine	Cl	Lead	Pb	Radium	Ra	Vanadium	V
Chromium	Cr	Lithium	Li	Radon	Rn	Xenon	Xe
Cobalt	Co	Lutetium	Lu	Rhenium	Re	Ytterbium	Yb
Copper	Cu	Magnesium	Mg	Rhodium	Rh	Yttrium	Y
Curium	Cm	Manganese	Mn	Rubidium	Rb	Zinc	Zn
Dysprosium	Dy	Mendelevium	Md	Ruthenium	Ru	Zirconium	Zr
Einsteinium	Es	Mercury	Hg				

While the ordinary chemical behavior of different isotopes of the same element are virtually identical, the *radiochemical* behavior is sometimes different. These radioactive isotopes are frequently important in nutrition. The element phosphorus has radioactive isotopes, such as ^{48}P. These isotopes emit radiation that can be detected and measured by instruments designed for that purpose. Other isotopes are not radioactive but still can be traced in body fluids or tissues, again using instruments designed for that purpose. Examples include ^{13}C and ^{15}N.

Isotope "markers" such as ^{48}P and ^{13}C can be used to trace nutrients as they follow the chemical pathways in which they are metabolized. For example, you could "mark" a glucose molecule with a radioactive carbon atom (^{14}C). This allows you to see where the glucose ends up in your body and also helps inform you what chemical transformations glucose undergoes when metabolized. Such studies have demonstrated that glucose can become part of the fat stored in adipose cells or form CO_2 (detected as $^{14}CO_2$) that is exhaled in the breath. Isotope techniques are widely used in nutrition.

Atomic and Molar Mass

The atomic masses that appear on the periodic table are obtained by measuring the mass of each element relative to the mass of the ^{12}C isotope. The units are called Daltons and one ^{12}C atom has the arbitrarily assigned mass of 12.000 Daltons. This unit is useful for expressing the mass of individual atoms and molecules, but is inconveniently sized to be generally useful. One carbon atom also has a mass 1.993×10^{-23} grams; grams being a much more familiar unit than Daltons.

In nature, however, not all the atoms of a given element have the same mass. For example, naturally occurring carbon is 98.90% ^{12}C and 1.10% ^{13}C. (The ^{14}C used in the experiments involving glucose described above is man made). These masses are averaged ($12 \text{ Daltons} \times 0.989 + 13 \text{ Daltons} \times 0.110 = 12.011$ Daltons) to give the average mass of the isotopes that occur in nature. It is the average masses that appear on the periodic table. So, for example, if you look up the mass of carbon on the periodic table you will find 12.011 and not 12.000.

A mole is defined to be the number of "things" equal to the number of atoms in 12 grams of ^{12}C. The number of atoms in 12 grams of ^{12}C is:

$$12\text{g C} \times \frac{1 \text{ atom}}{1.993 \times 10^{-23} \text{ gC}} = 6.023 \times 10^{23} \text{ atoms}$$

Therefore the number of "objects" in a mole is 6.02×10^{23}, which is frequently called Avogadro's number. The point is that one ^{12}C atom has a mass of 12 Daltons and one mole of ^{12}C atoms has a mass of 12 grams.

This concept can be extended directly. One mole of naturally occurring carbon (containing ^{12}C and ^{13}C) has a mass of 12.011 grams (from the periodic table), and one mole of naturally occurring hydrogen has a mass of 1.00795 grams, etc.

Ions

Atoms are electrically neutral because they have identical numbers of positively charged protons and negatively charged electrons. The electrons in metal atoms (those elements that have luster and conduct electricity) are not tightly bound to the nucleus, so when metals undergo chemical transformations they frequently lose one or more electrons. This results in a metallic species containing more protons than electrons, and therefore possesses a net positive charge. Species with a net positive charge are called cations.

$$Na \rightarrow Na^{+} + e^{-}$$ **(a sodium metal atoms loses an electron forming a cation.)**

In nonmetallic elements, the electrons are very tightly held by the nucleus and cations are formed rarely and then only under forcing conditions. Instead nonmetallic

Table B-2 Important ions in the human body

Common ions	Symbol	Function
Calcium	Ca^{2+}	Component of bones and teeth, necessary for blood clotting and muscle contraction
Sodium	Na^{+}	Helps maintain membrane potentials (electrical charge differences across a membrane) and water balance
Potassium	K^{+}	Helps maintain membrane potentials
Hydrogen	H^{+}	Helps maintain acid-base balance
Hydroxide	OH^{-}	Helps maintain acid-base balance
Chloride	Cl^{-}	Helps maintain acid-base balance
Bicarbonate	HCO_3^{-}	Helps maintain acid-base balance
Ammonium	NH_4^{+}	Helps maintain acid-base balance
Phosphate	PO_4^{3-}	Component of bone and teeth, involved in energy exchange and acid-base balance
Iron	Fe^{2+}	Necessary for red blood cell formation and function
Magnesium	Mg^{2+}	Necessary for enzymes

elements can readily accept additional electrons. This results in a species with a net negative charge, called anions.

$Cl + e^{-} \rightarrow Cl^{-}$ (a nonmetallic chlorine atom gains an electron to form an anion)

These charged atoms—where electron(s) have been added or removed—are collectively known as **ions.** Sodium (Na^{+}), potassium (K^{+}), and calcium (Ca^{+2}) are found in the body as cations. Chlorine (Cl^{-}) is a common anion in the body. A more complete list of common ions found in the body is given in Table B-2.

Salts

Salts are substances composed of cations and anions. Table salt ($Na^{+}\ Cl^{-}$ or simply NaCl) is a good example. Salts can be formed by the interaction of acids and bases, and in that case they are one product of the neutralization reaction that took place (water is other product). The hydrogen ions of the acid are exchanged by the positive ions of the base, and a salt forms (see a later description of acids and bases if these are unfamiliar terms). For example, when hydrochloric acid reacts with sodium hydroxide (NaOH), table salt is produced.

$$HCl + NaOH \rightarrow NaCl + H_2O$$

The formula for salts can be misleading. For example, NaCl can suggest that table salt exists as discrete entities containing one sodium ion and one chloride ion. An inspection of the structure of table salt, however, shows that table salt is actually a three-dimensional stack of layers—much like having a ream of paper with all the pages glued together. In each layer, the sodium ions are surrounded by four chloride ions and vice versa. The layers are stacked on top each other so that a chloride ion is below a sodium ion on the layer above and above the sodium ion on the layer beneath. The point of all this is that no sodium ion is "attached" to a single chloride ion; it can be thought of as being associated with **all** the neighboring chloride ions. Distinct NaCl molecules are not observed except under special laboratory situations and in the gas phase.

Salts dissociate—separate—to form positively and negatively charged ions when dissolved in water. Substances that dissolve in water and conduct electricity are called electrolytes. Sodium, potassium, calcium, and chloride are important electrolytes in the body.

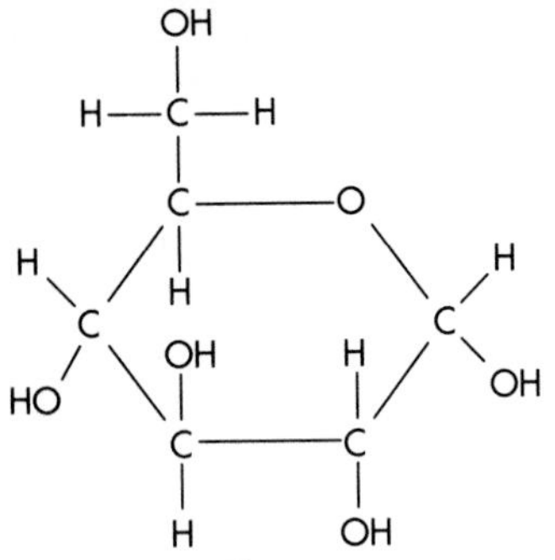

Molecules

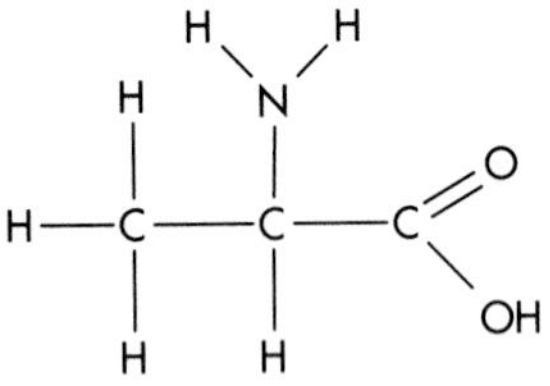

Molecules form when atoms combine with each other in associated groups. You know many examples—H_2O, N_2, O_2, H_2SO_4 are all molecules with which you are familiar. The term compound refers to molecules composed of more than one element, H_2O for example. Each compound possesses its own properties, such as color, taste, density, etc. Some complex molecules that are useful in nutrition are given in the margin.

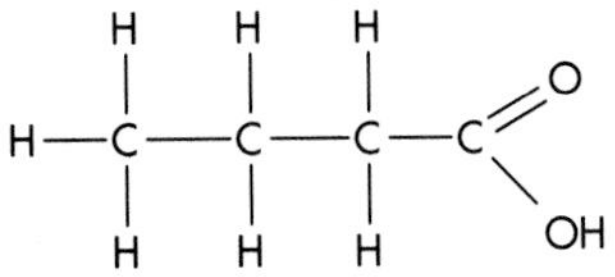

Glucose

Alanine

Butyric acid

A molecular formula gives the elemental composition of a molecule. This consists of the symbols of the atoms in the molecule plus a subscript denoting the number of each type of atom. If no subscript appears, then only one atom of that element is in the molecule. The molecular formula for ethanol (alcohol) is C_2H_6O, indicating that ethanol has two carbons, six hydrogens, and one oxygen atom in each molecule. A structural formula shows how the atoms are arranged with respect to each other. Molecular and ball-and-stick models approximate the shape of the molecule (Figure B-1).

When molecules recombine with each other atoms are conserved. This means that all the atoms present in the starting materials **must** be present in the products. For example, when glucose is combined with oxygen in the presence of a suitable catalyst, carbon dioxide (CO_2) and water (H_2O) are formed.

$$\underset{\text{Glucose}}{C_6H_{12}O_6} + 6\,O_2 \xrightarrow{\text{Catalyst}} 6\,CO_2 + 6\,H_2O$$

Notice that all six carbon atoms originally in glucose are present in carbon dioxide at the end of the transformation. Similar observations can be made about the total distribution of hydrogen and oxygen atoms between the molecules on both sides of the arrow.

The products, then, are simply different combinations of the same atoms found in the original glucose and O_2. The overall process exhibits conservation of mass.

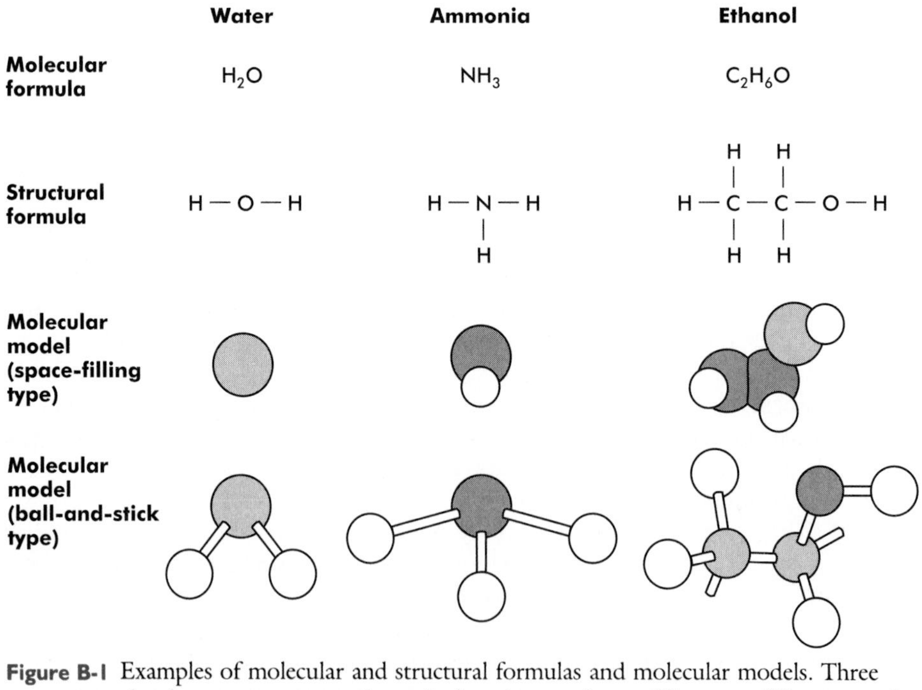

	Water	**Ammonia**	**Ethanol**
Molecular formula	H_2O	NH_3	C_2H_6O
Structural formula	H—O—H	H—N—H (with H below N)	H—C—C—O—H (each C with H above and below)
Molecular model (space-filling type)			
Molecular model (ball-and-stick type)			

Figure B-1 Examples of molecular and structural formulas and molecular models. Three common molecules—water, ammonia, and ethanol—are shown. The space-filling type of model gives a more realistic feeling of the space occupied by the atoms. On the other hand, the ball-and-stick type shows the bonds and bond angles more clearly.

Chemical Bonding

Why do atoms combine to form molecules? The key lies in the structure of the atom. You know that the atom consists of a nucleus surrounded by a cloud of electrons. The nucleus is very dense and has a positive charge. The positive charge on the nucleus attracts the electrons in the atom, but it also attracts electrons in the valence shells of other atoms. When two atoms come in close proximity, each nuclei attracts the electrons in the valence shell of the other. This can result in each atom sharing electrons with the other atom. When this occurs a **covalent bond** is formed. Specifically, when this type of bonding occurs, the atoms share valence electrons (up to six) with each other.

For example, consider a simple description of how methane (CH_4) is formed. Hydrogen has one electron in its valence shell, and that valence shell can hold a maximum of two electrons. Carbon has four electrons in its valence shell, and that shell can hold a maximum of eight electrons. Both carbon and hydrogen fill their valence shells to the maximum by sharing electrons with each other. This is illustrated in the margin. Notice that each hydrogen in methane contains two electrons and that the carbon atom has eight electrons in its valence shell. A good way to look at this is that the hydrogen atoms share one pair of electrons, while the carbon atom shares four pair of electrons.

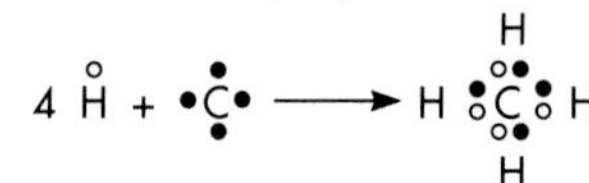

∘ Hydrogren electrons

• Carbon electrons

There are some guidelines that govern this behavior:

1. There must be room in the valence shell of each element to accommodate additional electrons.
2. Second row nonmetallic elements of the periodic table (e.g., carbon, nitrogen, oxygen) and hydrogen typically fill their valence shells by sharing the necessary number of electrons with another element.
3. Third row nonmetals and beyond the periodic table (e.g., phosphorus, sulfur, chloride) frequently make fewer covalent bonds than is necessary to fill the valence shell. Sulfur, for example, typically makes two bonds instead of six.

A single bond exists when two atoms share one electron pair. A double bond forms when two atoms share two electron pairs. For example, fatty acids commonly have a few carbon-carbon double bonds, as shown below for oleic acid. This is found in large amounts in olive oil and canola oil. Double covalent bonds are indicated by a double line between the atoms (e.g., —C = C—).

```
H  H  H  H  H  H  H  H  H  H  H  H  H  H  H  H  H  O
|  |  |  |  |  |  |  |        |  |  |  |  |  |  |  ||
C—C—C—C—C—C—C—C—C=C—C—C—C—C—C—C—C—C—OH
|  |  |  |  |  |  |  |        |  |  |  |  |  |  |
H  H  H  H  H  H  H  H        H  H  H  H  H  H  H
```

The stability associated with completed electron shells for second row elements and hydrogen is one reason why carbon is almost always found forming four bonds. For the same reason nitrogen tends to make three bonds and oxygen two. As noted above, sulfur forms two bonds. Phosphorus often forms five bonds.

The backbone of large molecules consists of a chain of carbon atoms bound together (occasionally the chain contains an atom other than carbon). Variations in the length of the chains and their atomic combinations allow the formation of a wide variety of molecules. For example, some starches have thousands of carbons bound by covalent bonds to one another. Protein typically contains many atoms, such as carbon, nitrogen, sulfur, hydrogen, and oxygen. Without the ability of atoms to form covalent bonds, the complex molecules that are common to living organisms could not exist.

When two different atoms form a covalent bond, the bonding electrons are never shared equally. Consider the H—O bond in water. It is unreasonable to expect that the hydrogen nucleus (containing one proton) and the oxygen nucleus (containing eight protons) have identical forces of attraction for the shared electron pair. In addition other factors come into play—such has how many shells each atom has,

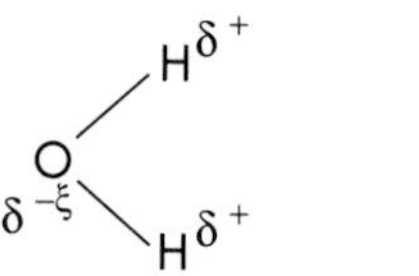

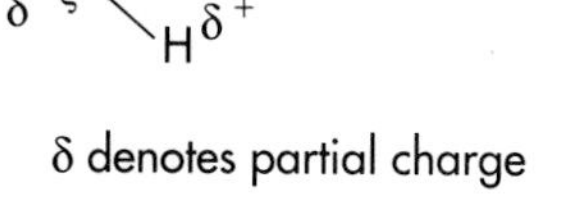
δ denotes partial charge

how many electrons are in the shells, and the distance the shared electrons are from each nucleus. All of these suggest an unequal sharing of electrons in a covalent bond made between different atoms.

The ability of an atom to attract electrons toward itself is called electronegativity. It is highest toward the top right corner of the periodic table and lowest toward the bottom left. Metals have low electronegativity, nonmetals have relatively high electronegativities. Oxygen and nitrogen have the highest electronegativities of the elements typically found in compounds important to nutrition.

In a water molecule, the electrons tend to be associated more closely with the more electronegative oxygen atom than with the hydrogen atoms. This unequal sharing of electrons can result in one end (an electrical pole) of the molecule having a charge opposite to that of the other end. The end containing the more electronegative element is the negative end of the molecule. This results in a polar molecule, meaning that the molecule itself has a net polarity.

While all bonds formed between two different atoms are polar, not all molecules containing such bonds are polar. The distinction between bond polarity and molecular polarity is important. The figure in the margin shows that water with two H—O bonds is polar. However CO_2 containing two polar CO bonds is not polar as shown below.

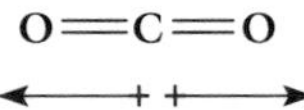

Although each CO bond in carbon dioxide is polar, the molecule itself has zero polarity because the electrical vectors (to the left and right in the figure) are equal in magnitude and opposite in direction.

Polar molecules are weakly attracted both to ions and to other polar molecules. The positive end of the molecule can align itself with an anion or with the negative end of another molecule. These attractive forces, called respectively ion-dipole and dipole-dipole forces, are much weaker than covalent bonds individually, but there can be so many of them that they make a significant contribution to the total energy of a collection of some molecules. Water has a much higher boiling point than expected because the molecules are "glued" together by such forces.

In fact water and most other molecules containing a O—H or N—H bond have a particularly strong dipole-dipole interaction called hydrogen bonding. Hydrogen bonds play an important role in determining the shape and stability of complex molecules, such as large proteins, because the hydrogen bonds between different parts of that molecule hold the molecule together.

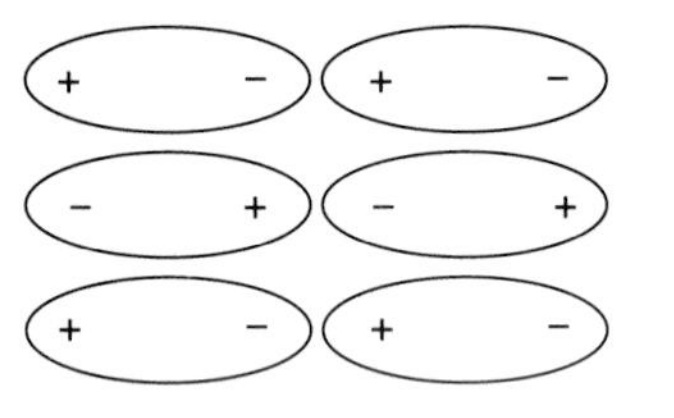
dipole-dipole

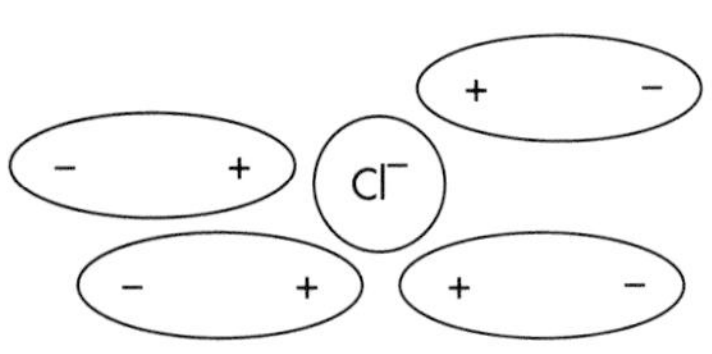

ion-dipole

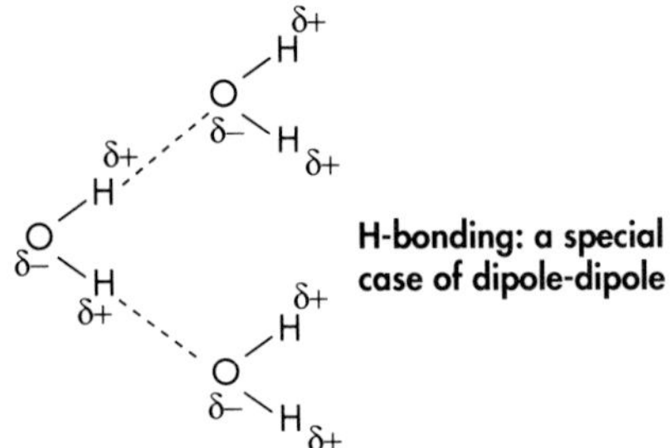
H-bonding: a special case of dipole-dipole

Acids and Bases

Many molecules are classified as acids or bases. For most purposes an acid is defined as a proton donor. Because a hydrogen atom without its electron is a proton (H^+), any substance that releases hydrogen ions when in water is an acid. For example, hydrogen chloride (HCl) forms hydrogen and chloride ions (H^+ and Cl^-) in solution and therefore is an acid.

$$HCl \rightarrow H^+ + Cl^-$$

A base is defined as a proton acceptor, and so any substance that can form accepts hydrogen ions while in water is a base. Many bases can function as proton acceptors by releasing hydroxide ions (OH^-) when dissolved in water. For example, the base sodium hydroxide (NaOH) dissolves in water to form sodium and hydroxide ions:

$$NaOH \rightarrow Na^+ + OH^-$$

The hydroxide ions are proton acceptors as they go on to combine with hydrogen ions to form water:

$$OH^- + H^+ \rightarrow H_2O$$

Acids and bases are classified as strong or weak. Strong acids and bases dissociate completely when dissolved in water. Consequently, they release all of their hydrogen ions or hydroxide ions when dissolved. In general, the more completely the acid or base dissociates the stronger it is. Hydrochloric acid, for example, is a strong acid because it completely dissociates in water.

Weak acids only partically dissociate in water. Consequently, they only release some of their acidic hydrogens. For example, when acetic acid ($CH_3\overset{\displaystyle O}{\overset{\|}{C}}-OH$, the principle component of vinegar) is dissolved in water, the acetic acid only partially dissociates.

$$CH_3\overset{O}{\overset{\|}{C}}-OH \rightleftharpoons CH_3\overset{O}{\overset{\|}{C}}-O^- + H^+$$

The equilibrium lies far to the left so that only a small fraction of the acetic acid in a bottle of vinegar has dissociated.

Most weak bases release hydroxide into solution by reacting with the water itself. For example ammonia (NH_3) reacts with water to form NH_4^+ and OH^-.

$$NH_3 + H_2O \rightleftharpoons NH_4^+ + OH^-$$

pH

The term pH describes the hydrogen ion (H^+) concentration of a solution. Specifically, pH is equal to the negative logarithm of the hydrogen ion concentration ($pH = {}^-Log_{10}[H^+]$). As the hydrogen ion concentration increases, the pH decreases. Because of the exponential relationship, a one unit change in pH represents a tenfold change in hydrogen ion concentration.

Keep in mind that a neutral pH is 7, an acid pH lies between 0 and 7, and an alkaline or basic pH lies between 7 and 14.

The stomach has a pH of 1 to 2 and is very acidic. Since pH is based on an exponent, the stomach doesn't have merely seven times more hydrogen ions than the blood, it actually has one million times more hydrogen ions. Other acidic solutions include coffee at pH 5, orange juice at pH 4, and vinegar at pH 3.

In a basic solution, hydroxide ions (OH^-) are in greater amounts than hydrogen ions. Basic solutions include household ammonia at pH 11 and concentrated lye (sodium hydroxide) at pH 14 (Figure B-2).

Free Radicals

We saw in a previous section that atoms tend to share electron pairs when forming chemical bonds, and there is a tendency to share enough electrons to completely fill the valence shell. A consequence is that atoms or elements are rarely found with an odd number of electrons. A molecule with an odd number of electrons is called a **free radical.** Free radicals are reactive, primarily because they contain unpaired electrons (shown as a dot). They can be formed when a molecule is exposed to an energy source such as sunlight or heat, or by collisions with other free radicals.

The formation of radicals occurs when a bond breaks and each atom or molecular fragment recovers the electron originally used to make the chemical bond.

$$A-B + \text{energy} \rightarrow A\cdot + B\cdot$$

Being reactive, free radicals sometime cause reactions that do not occur normally. Free radicals are believed to promote the development of some cancers (skin and lung cancers for example). However, some normal physiological functions in the body, such as in respiration, also are linked to free radical formation.

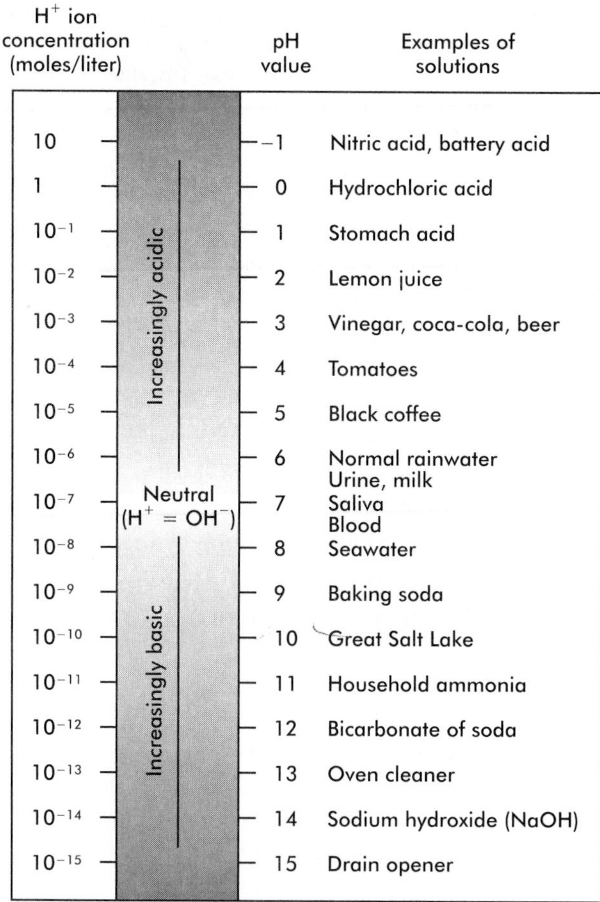

Figure B-2 The pH values of common substances. Note that "acid" tomatoes aren't really that acidic.

Some molecules, called antioxidants, are used extensively in the food industry to trap or prevent the formation of free radicals. This increases the storage time of food by decreasing chemical breakdown. They are part of the class of food additives called preservatives.

Isomerism

Compounds that have *identical* chemical formulas and *different* structures are called isomers. A simple example of this are two compounds with the formula C_2H_6O.

ethanol	**methyl ether**
CH_3CH_2OH	CH_3-O-CH_3

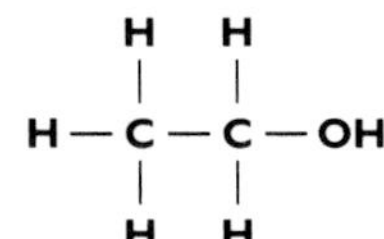

Ethanol is imbibed by millions of people daily. Methyl ether is a foul tasting poisonous substance that has little practical utility.

An important point about isomers is that since isomers have different structures they *must* have different properties. The difference in properties between two isomers can be large (as in the example above) or very subtle, but the differences are there and detectable. There are different types of isomerism and we will briefly review two of the more common types.

STRUCTURAL ISOMERS

H H
H—C—O—C—H
H H

Isomers in which the number and kinds of bonds differ are called structural **isomers.** Look at the ethanol and methyl ether whose structures are given in the margin. Ethanol has five C—H bonds, one O—H bond, and one C—C bond. Methyl ether has six C—H bonds and two C—O bonds. This analysis demonstrates that these two C_2H_6O compounds are structural isomers.

Compounds containing chains of carbon atoms typically have many structural isomers. Any variation in the way the chain is branched gives rise to an new isomer. For example, pentane C_5H_{12} has three isomers as shown below:

Pentane $CH_3—CH_2—CH_2—CH_2—CH_3$

Neopentane $CH_3—CH_2—CH(CH_3)—CH_3$

Isopentane $CH_3—C(CH_3)_2—CH_3$

STEREOISOMERS

Stereoisomers have the same number and types of bonds but different spacial arrangements (different configurations in space). The point is that the only difference between stereoisomers are the way the atoms are arranged in space.

A good way to illustrate this is to look at molecules containing double bonds. Because there is restricted rotation about a C = C bond, molecules containing double bonds frequently exhibit stereoisomerism. (C = C single bonds are easily rotated, like a pin wheel; if you put a second pin in the pinwheel forming a "double bond" you won't be able to spin it.) For example, in the relatively simple molecule two-butene ($CH_3CH = CHCH_3$) the methyl groups ($-CH_3$) can be located on the same side of the double bond (cis isomer) or on opposite sides of the double bond (trans isomer). This is illustrated below.

$(H_3C)(H)C=C(CH_3)(H)$ **_cis_-2-butene; the methyl groups are on the same side of the double bond**

$(H)(H_3C)C=C(CH_3)(H)$ **_trans_-2-butene; the methyl groups are on opposite sides of the double bond**

You will note that both isomers have one C = C bond, two C—C bonds, and eight C—H bonds. The only difference between the two isomers is the position of the methyl groups. Another example involving a larger molecule, oleic acid and its isomer elaidic acid, is given in Figure B-3, *A*. Oleic acid is a *cis* isomer. In making margarine some of the *trans* isomer forms, which is called elaidic acid. Collectively, these isomer types are sometimes called **geometric isomers.**

Another type of stereoisomerism occurs in molecules that cannot be superimposed on their mirror images—just like a right hand glove cannot be superimposed on a left hand glove. This type of isomerism occurs very frequently in biological molecules, and they are referred to as **optical isomers** for historical reasons. In simple systems the isomers are distinguished by calling one isomer the D-form and the other one the L-form.

Just as a right hand glove and a left hand glove are mirror images, they cannot be superimposed on each other. Also note that the three dimensional model of D-alanine is a nonsuperimposible mirror image of its L-isomer (Figure B-3, *B*). This nonsuperimposibility on the mirror image is the only criterion used to determine the existence of optical isomers.

The differences between the D and L isomers is very subtle. For example the chemistry of D-alanine is identical to the chemistry of L-alanine except when they

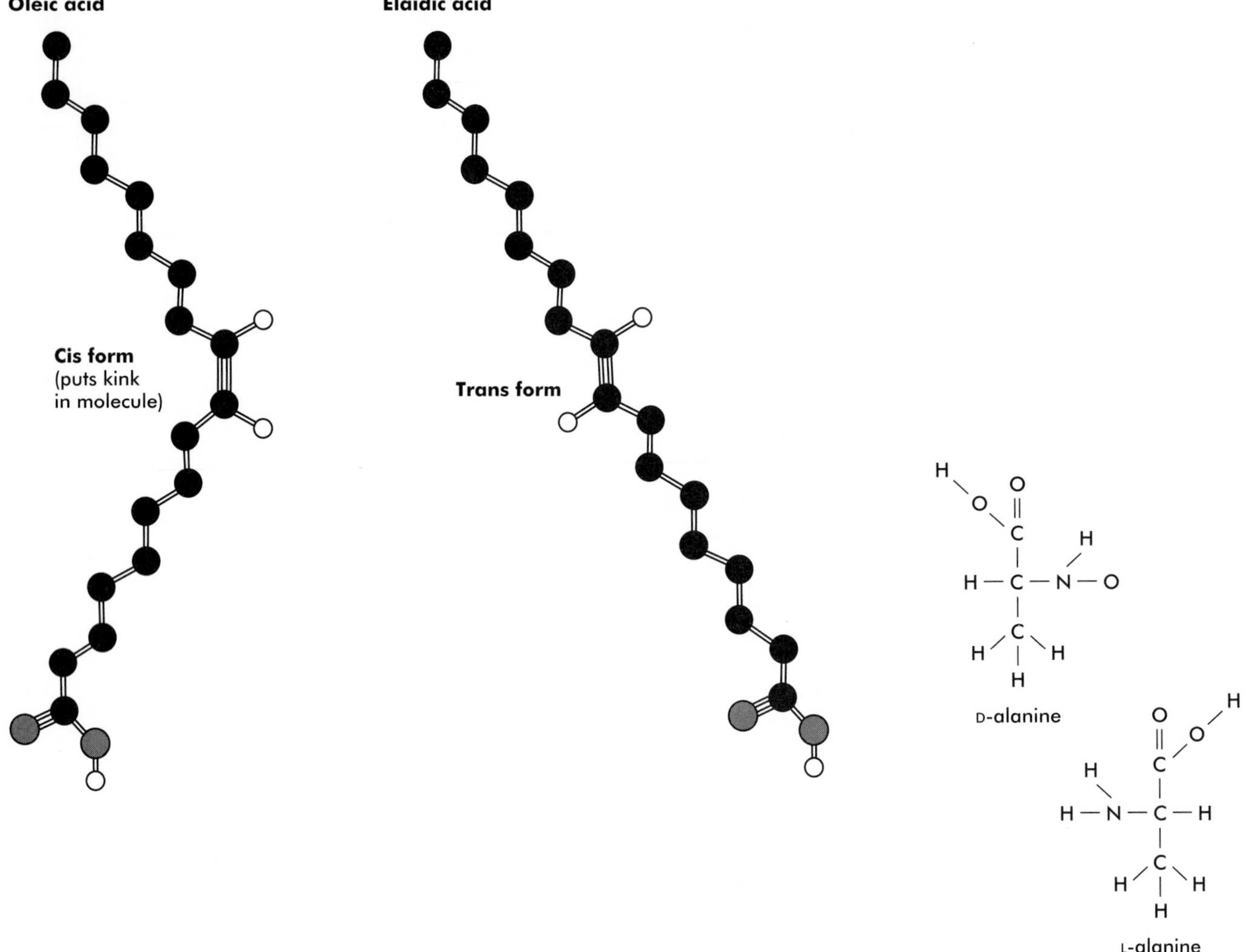

Figure B-3 Cis and trans isomers of fatty acids. Cis forms are the most common forms in unprocessed foods.

react with other optical isomers; then the chemistry can be profoundly different. This is similar to trying to use the right-hand glove on the left hand—the glove doesn't interact act well with the wrong hand. Since most biological molecules are one unique optical isomers, this chemical difference that arises from isomerism can be very profound in biological systems. For example, L-alanine can be used by the body to make proteins, but not the D-form.

Chemical Reactions

One of the most important properties of chemical compounds is the reactions they undergo. It is chemical reactions that ultimately allow you to see, walk, and think.

In a chemical reaction, a compound or several compounds (the reactants) is converted into another compound or set of compounds (the products) accompanied by the absorption or release of energy (heat in most biological processes). In effect the reactants simply reshuffle their atoms to form products. Clearly then, chemical reactions create and break down molecules. It is important to recognize that no atoms lose their identity during a chemical reaction, and no atoms are gained, lost, or converted to other atoms during the course of a normal chemical reaction.

Chemists have grouped reactions according to their similarities in chemical behavior. Body cells undergo some of these reactions over and over. What follows is a brief overview of some of these important reaction types.

CONDENSATION REACTIONS

A condensation reaction occurs when two molecules join together to form a larger molecule and a small molecule (usually water). The two compounds typically each contain a hydroxyl group, meaning you have two —OH groups. A simple example is the condensation of ethanol to make ethyl ether and water:

$$\underset{\text{ethanol}}{CH_3CH_2OH} + \underset{\text{ethanol}}{CH_3CH_2OH} \rightarrow \underset{\text{ethyl ether}}{CH_3CH_2{-}O{-}CH_2CH_3} + H_2O$$

While this reaction does not occur in the body it illustrates the essential features of condensation reactions. One OH group gains a proton and forms a water molecule. The other OH group loses a proton and forms a bond with the other molecule—in exactly the same place as the water molecule leaves. Note this is an overall description of what happens, not how it happens. The exact details of how some condensation reactions occur can be quite complex and are beyond the scope of this appendix.

A condensation reaction that occurs in the body is the formation of maltose from two glucose molecules as shown in Figure B-4.

While it is typical for both molecules to contain an OH group in a condensation reaction, it is not a requirement for the reaction. Figure B-4, *A* illustrates a condensation reaction where only one of the reactants contains an OH group.

HYDROLYSIS REACTIONS

Hydrolysis reactions are reactions that occur when water is added to a compound. In biological systems hydrolysis reactions are very frequently the reverse of condensation reactions. That is, water is added to a large molecule, which results in the formation of two smaller molecules. This can be illustrated by adding water to ethyl ether to form ethanol—the reverse of a reaction discussed above.

$$CH_3CH_2{-}O{-}CH_2CH_3 + H_2O \rightarrow 2\ CH_3CH_2\text{-}OH$$

In fact, this reaction is reversible and can be run in either direction depending on conditions. Another example is given in Figure B-4, *B*; notice this is simply the reverse of the reaction shown in Figure B-4, *A*.

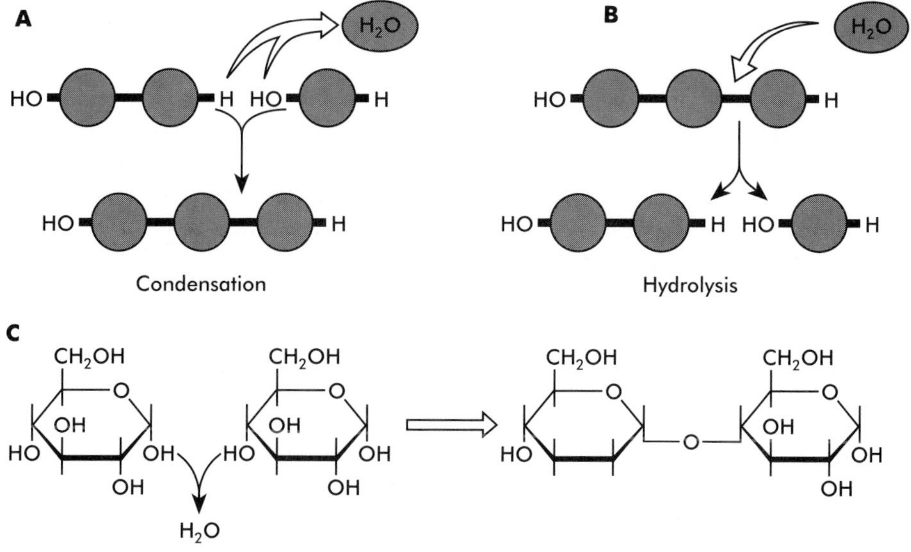

Figure B-4 Making (and breaking) molecules. Biological molecules are formed by linking subunits together. The covalent bond between the subunits is often formed in a condensation reaction, in which a water molecule is eliminated. Breaking such a bond requires adding a water molecule, a hydrolysis reaction.

All of this is quite important in body chemistry. As molecules are formed in cells, condensation reactions take place. As compounds are broken down into smaller fragments, hydrolysis reactions take place. When the body breaks down foodstuffs during digestion to absorb them, such as the sugar maltose, it uses a hydrolysis reaction. When the body makes protein for muscles, carbohydrates for storage in muscles, or fat to fuel muscles, it uses condensation reactions (Figure B-4, *C*).

OXIDATION AND REDUCTION REACTIONS

The formal meaning of oxidation and reduction can be summarized as:

A species is oxidized when it loses one or more electrons.

A species is reduced when it gains one or more electrons.

Clearly, then, it is electron flow that governs oxidation-reduction processes. It is important to note that if one species loses electrons (is oxidized) another species *must* gain electrons (is reduced). The two processes go together; you cannot have one without the other. By way of illustration, consider the reaction between zinc and Cu^{2+} ion.

$$\mathbf{Zn + Cu^{2+} \rightarrow Zn^{2+} + Cu}$$

Here Zn is oxidized by losing two electrons ($Zn \rightarrow Zn^{2+} + 2\ e^-$) and copper is reduced by gaining two electrons ($Cu^{2+} + 2e^- \rightarrow Cu$).

The body undergoes many oxidation-reduction reactions. For example, the iron in hemoglobin is oxidized to Fe^{3+} and reduced to Fe^{2+} during the transport of oxygen to the body cells.

Oxidation-reduction reactions involving carbon-containing compounds is somewhat more difficult to visualize. A simple rule has been developed to determine oxidation-reduction in these compounds.

> If the compound gains oxygen or loses hydrogen it is oxidized; if it loses oxygen or gains hydrogen the compound is reduced.

The processes illustrated below exemplify this definition.

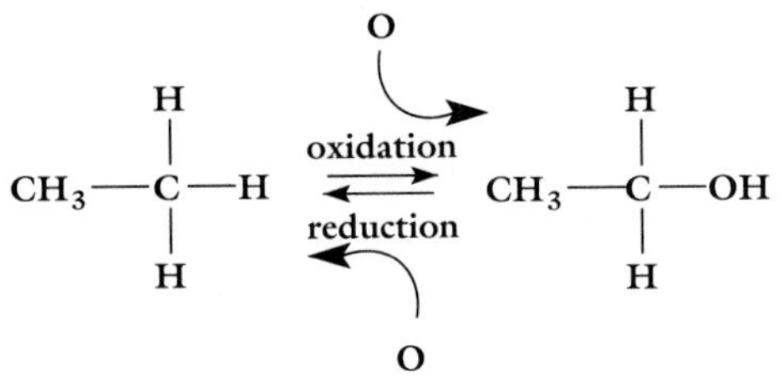

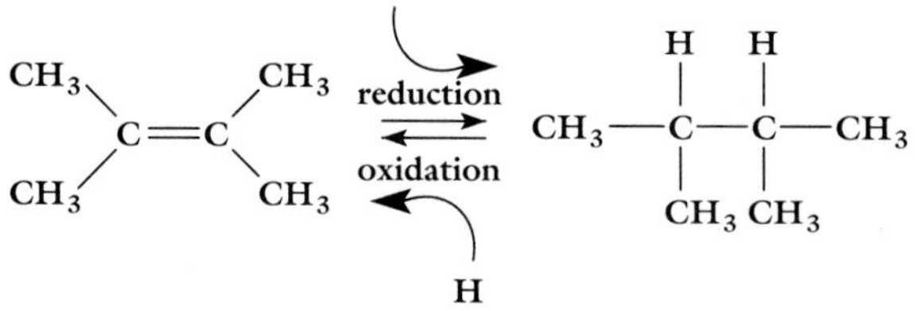

$$CH_3\text{—}CH_2\text{—}H \;\underset{\text{reduction }(-\mathrm{O})}{\overset{\text{oxidation }(+\mathrm{O})}{\rightleftharpoons}}\; CH_3\text{—}CH_2\text{—}OH$$

$$(CH_3)_2C{=}C(CH_3)_2 \;\underset{\text{oxidation }(-\mathrm{H})}{\overset{\text{reduction }(+\mathrm{H})}{\rightleftharpoons}}\; CH_3\text{—}CH(CH_3)\text{—}CH(CH_3)\text{—}CH_3$$

This method of determining oxidation and reduction is extensively used in fields related to organic chemistry, namely biology and biochemistry. For example, pyruvic acid (made from glucose) is reduced to form lactic acid by gaining two hydrogens. This happens during intense exercise (see Chapter 10). Lactic acid is oxidized back to pyruvic acid by losing two hydrogens.

Common Chemical Structures

As we saw earlier, carbon can form four bonds, nitrogen three, oxygen two, sulfur two, and hydrogen one. Most compounds in the body are made up carbons, hy-

Functional group	Name	Typically found in	Example
—OH	hydroxide	alcohols	CH_3—OH
—C=O | H	aldehyde	aldehydes	CH_3C=O | H
C—C=O | C	ketone	ketones	CH_3C=O | CH_3
—C=O | OH	carboxyl	carboxylic acids	CH_3C=O | OH
—S—S—	disulfide	disulfides	CH_3—S—S—CH_3
—C=O |	carbonyl	aldehydes, ketones, carboxylic acids, amides	$(CH_3)_2$C=O
—C—NH_2 |	amine	amines	CH_3—NH_2
—C=O | NH_2	amide	amides	CH_3C=O | NH_2
OH | HO—P=O | OH	phosphate	phosphates	OH | CH_3—O—P=O | O—CH_3
—C=O | O—C	ester	esters	CH_3—C=O | CH_3CH_2—O

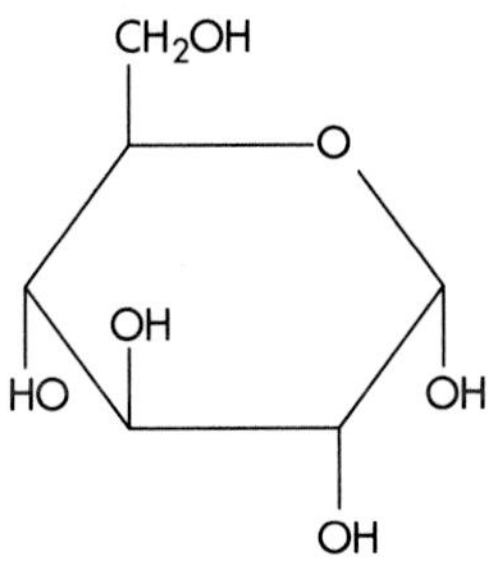

Glucose

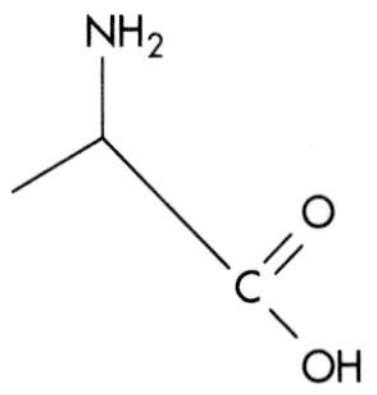

Alanine

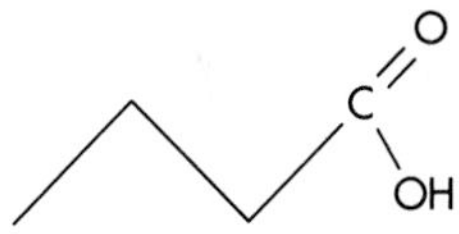

Butyric acid

drogen, oxygen, sulfur, and other elements, with carbon often being the predominant element. Some very commonly encountered combinations of atoms, called functional groups, have been given specific names because these appear in many compounds. You need to be familiar with them for they are some of the most important features that differentiate compounds. These are summarized in the box below. Study them because the names and structures of these groups appear frequently throughout the book.

Drawing Chemical Structures

Chemists have developed a short hand notation for writing chemical formulas called stick structures. In stick structures neither carbon atoms nor the hydrogens bonded to the carbon atoms are expressly shown. What is shown is the bonds between the carbon atoms (the structure) and the position of all non carbon and hydrogen atoms. The thing to keep in mind is that there are carbon atoms at the apices of every angle in the structure (with the appropriate number of hydrogens connected to the carbon) **and** at the terminal ends of the sticks. By way of illustration, look at a stick structure of propane ($CH_3CH_2CH_3$):

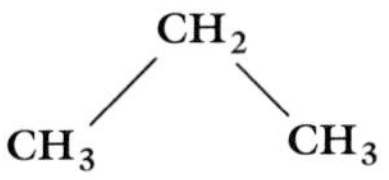

CH_2

CH_3 CH_3

Propane

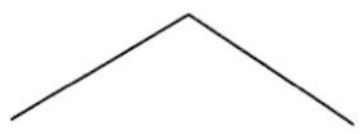

Stick structure of propane

The big advantage of using stick structures is that it allows for a clear representation of complex molecules without "cluttering up the picture." This notation will be used throughout the text so you should become familiar with it. It becomes handy when large structures such as those encountered in the body have to be represented.

• • •

This is a brief review of basic principles of chemistry. Ideally it has reinforced earlier coursework. If these ideas are mostly new to you and you are confused, perhaps you have a classmate who can help you understand these key chemistry principles?

APPENDIX C

Clinical and Biochemical Measures of Nutritional Status

Clinical Signs and Symptoms of Various Nutrient Deficiencies

Area of examination	Sign/symptom	Potential nutrient deficiency
Hair	Loss	Zinc, essential fatty acids
	Easy pluckability	Protein, essential fatty acids
	Lackluster	Protein, zinc
	"Corkscrew" hair	Vitamin C, vitamin A
	Decreased pigmentation	Protein, copper
Eyes	Xerosis of conjunctiva	Vitamin A
	Corneal vascularization	Riboflavin
	Xerophthalmia	Vitamin A
	Bitot's spots	Vitamin A
GI tract	Nausea, vomiting	Pyridoxine
	Diarrhea	Zinc, niacin
	Mouth inflammation	Pyridoxine, riboflavin, iron
	Cheilosis	Pyridoxine, iron
	Tongue inflammation	Pyridoxine, zinc, niacin, folate, vitamin B-12
	Magenta tongue	Riboflavin
	Swollen, bleeding gums	Vitamin C
	Fissured tongue	Niacin
	Enlarged liver	Protein
Skin	Dry and scaling	Vitamin A, essential fatty acids, zinc
	Petechiae/ecchymoses (small hemorrhages)	Vitamin C, vitamin K
Skin	Follicular hyperkeratosis	Vitamin A, essential fatty acids
	Nose-lip dryness	Niacin, pyridoxine, riboflavin
	Bilateral dermatitis	Niacin, zinc
Extremities	Subcutaneous fat loss	Kcalories
	Muscle wastage	Kcalories, protein
	Edema	Protein
	Osteomalacia, bone pain, rickets	Vitamin D
	Bone pain	Vitamin C
Hematologic	Anemia	Vitamin B-12, iron, folate, copper, vitamin E, vitamin K
	Low white cell count	Copper
	Low prothrombin, prolonged clotting time	Vitamin K
Neurologic	Disorientation	Niacin, thiamin
	Confabulation	Thiamin
	Nerve degeneration	Thiamin, pyridoxine, chromium
	Poor coordination, feeling	Thiamin, pyridoxine, vitamin B-12
Cardiovascular	Congestive heart failure, cardiomegaly, tachycardia	Thiamin
	Heart degeneration	Selenium

From Ross Laboratories.

Biochemical indicators of good nutrition status

Nutrient or measurement	Test		Normal or acceptable levels	
			Men	**Women**
Iron	Hemoglobin (g/100 ml)		≥14.0	≥12.0
		Infants (under 2 years)	≥10.0	≥10.0
		Children (6-12 years)	≥11.5	≥11.5
		Pregnancy (2nd trimester)		≥11.0
		(3rd trimester)		≥10.5
Protein	Serum albumin (g/100 ml)		≥3.5	≥3.5
Normal lipid metabolism	Serum cholesterol (mg/100 ml)		<200	<200
	Serum triglyceride (mg/100 ml)		<150	<150
Normal carbohydrate metabolism	Serum glucose (mg/100 ml)		75-110	75-110
Sodium	Serum sodium (mEq/l)		130-150	130-155
Potassium	Serum potassium (mEq/l)		3.5-5.3	3.5-5.3
Vitamin A	Plasma vitamin A (μg/100 ml)		>20	>20
Vitamin C	Serum vitamin C (mg/100 ml)		≥0.3	≥0.3
Riboflavin	Erythrocyte glutathione peroxidase (% stimulation of activity by added riboflavin cofactor)		<20	<20
Vitamin B-6	Trytophan load test—increase in excretion of xanthurenic acid (mg/day)		<25	<25
Folate	Serum folate (nanogram/ml)		>6.0	>6.0
Thiamin	Urinary thiamin (μg/g creatinine)		>65	>65
Zinc	Plasma zinc (μg/100 ml)		80-115	80-115

Some information obtained from: Roe DA: *Drug-induced nutritional deficiencies,* AVI Press, Westport, Conn, 1976, and Sauberlich HE, Skala HH, and Dowdy RP: *Laboratory tests for the assessment of nutritional status,* CRC Press, Inc, Cleveland, 1974.

APPENDIX D

Nutrient Recommendations for Canadians

Summary examples of recommended nutrient intake based on age and body weight expressed as daily rates

Age	Sex	Weight kg	Protein g	Vit. A RE*	Vit. D ug	Vit. E mg	Vit. C mg	Folate ug	Vit. B_{12} ug	Calcium mg	Phosphorus mg	Magnesium mg	Iron mg	Iodine ug	Zinc mg
Months															
0-4	Both	6.0	12⁺	400	10	3	20	25	0.3	250†	150	20	0.3§	30	2§
5-12	Both	9.0	12	400	10	3	20	40	0.4	400	200	32	7	40	3
Years															
1	Both	11	13	400	10	3	20	40	0.5	500	300	40	6	55	4
2-3	Both	14	16	400	5	4	20	50	0.6	550	350	50	6	65	4
4-6	Both	18	19	500	5	5	25	70	0.8	600	400	65	8	85	5
7-9	M	25	26	700	2.5	7	25	90	1.0	700	500	100	8	110	7
	F	25	26	700	2.5	6	25	90	1.0	700	500	100	8	95	7
10-12	M	34	34	800	2.5	8	25	120	1.0	900	700	130	8	125	9
	F	36	36	800	2.5	7	25	130	1.0	1100	800	135	8	110	9
13-15	M	50	49	900	2.5	9	30	175	1.0	1100	900	185	10	160	12
	F	48	46	800	2.5	7	30	170	1.0	1000	850	180	13	160	9
16-18	M	62	58	1000	2.5	10	40‖	220	1.0	900	1000	230	10	160	12
	F	53	47	800	2.5	7	30‖	190	1.0	700	850	200	12	160	9
19-24	M	71	61	1000	2.5	10	40‖	220	1.0	800	1000	240	9	160	12
	F	58	50	800	2.5	7	30‖	180	1.0	700	850	200	13	160	9
25-49	M	74	64	1000	2.5	9	40‖	230	1.0	800	1000	250	9	160	12
	F	59	51	800	2.5	6	30‖	185	1.0	700	850	200	13	160	9
50-74	M	73	63	1000	5	7	40‖	230	1.0	800	1000	250	9	160	12
	F	63	54	800	5	6	30‖	195	1.0	800	850	210	8	160	9
75 +	M	69	59	1000	5	6	40‖	215	1.0	800	1000	230	9	160	12
	F	64	55	800	5	5	30‖	200	1.0	800	850	210	8	160	9
Pregnancy (additional)															
1st Trimester			5	0	2.5	2	0	200	1.2	500	200	15	0	25	6
2nd Trimester			20	0	2.5	2	10	200	1.2	500	200	45	5	25	6
3rd Trimester			24	0	2.5	2	10	200	1.2	500	200	45	10	25	6
Lactation (additional)			20	400	2.5	3	25	100	0.2	500	200	65	0	50	6

* Retinol Equivalents.
⁺Protein is assumed to be from breast milk and must be adjusted for infant formula.
† Infant formula with high phosphorus should contain 375 mg calcium.
§ Breast milk is assumed to be the source of the mineral.
‖ Smokers should increase vitamin C by 50%.
From Scientific Review Committee: *Nutrition Recommendations,* Ottawa, Canada, 1990, Health and Welfare.

Summary of examples of recommended nutrients based on energy expressed as daily rates

Age	Sex	Energy kcal	Thiamin mg	Riboflavin mg	Niacin Ne⁺	n-3 PUFA* g	n-6 PUFA g
Months							
0-4	Both	600	0.3	0.3	4	0.5	3
5-12	Both	900	0.4	0.5	7	0.5	3
Years							
1	Both	1100	0.5	0.6	8	0.6	4
2-3	Both	1300	0.6	0.7	9	0.7	4
4-6	Both	1800	0.7	0.9	13	1.0	6
7-9	M	2200	0.9	1.1	16	1.2	7
	F	1900	0.8	1.0	14	1.0	6
10-12	M	2500	1.0	1.3	18	1.4	8
	F	2200	0.9	1.1	16	1.2	7
13-15	M	2800	1.1	1.4	20	1.5	9
	F	2200	0.9	1.1	16	1.2	7
16-18	M	3200	1.3	1.6	23	1.8	11
	F	2100	0.8	1.1	15	1.2	7
19-24	M	3000	1.2	1.5	22	1.6	10
	F	2100	0.8	1.1	15	1.2	7
25-49	M	2700	1.1	1.4	19	1.5	9
	F	1900	0.8	1.0	14	1.1	7
50-74	M	2300	0.9	1.2	16	1.3	8
	F	1800	0.8†	1.0†	14†	1.1†	7†
75 +	M	2000	0.8	1.0	14	1.1	7
	F§	1700	0.8†	1.0†	14†	1.1†	7†
Pregnancy (additional)							
1st Trimester		100	0.1	0.1	1	0.05	0.3
2nd Trimester		300	0.1	0.3	2	0.16	0.9
3rd Trimester		300	0.1	0.3	2	0.16	0.9
Lactation (additional)		450	0.2	0.4	3	0.25	1.5

* PUFA, polyunsaturated fatty acids.
⁺Niacin equivalents.
† Level below which intake should not fall.
§ Assumes moderate physical activity.
From Scientific Review Committee: *Nutrition Recommendation*, Ottawa, Canada, 1990, Health and Welfare.

APPENDIX E

Dietary Intake Assessment

Though it may seem overwhelming at first, it is actually very easy to track the foods you eat. One tip is to record foods and beverages consumed as close as possible to the actual time of consumption.

Fill in the food record form that follows. We supply a blank copy on the next page. Then, to estimate the nutrient values of the foods you are eating, consult food labels and the food composition table in Appendix A or use your Mosby nutrition software package. If these resources do not have the serving size you need, adjust the value. If you drink ½ cup of orange juice, for example, but a table has values for only 1 cup, halve all values before you record them. Consider pooling all the same food to save time; if you drink a cup of 1% milk three times throughout the day, enter your milk consumption only once as 3 cups. As you record your intake for use on the nutrient analysis form consider the following tips:

- Measure and record the amounts of food eaten in portion sizes of cups, teaspoons, tablespoons, ounces, slices, or inches (or convert metric units to these units).
- Record brand names of all food products, such as "Quick Quaker Oats."
- Measure and record all those little extras, such as gravies, salad dressings, taco sauces, pickles, jelly, sugar, ketchup, and margarines.
- For beverages
  - —List the type of milk, such as whole, skim, 2%, evaporated, chocolate, or reconstituted dry.
  - —Indicate whether fruit juice is fresh, frozen, or canned.
  - —Indicate type for other beverages, such as fruit drink, fruit-flavored drink, Kool-Aid, and hot chocolate made with water or milk.
- For fruits
  - —Indicate whether fresh, frozen, dried, or canned.
  - —If whole, record as number eaten and size with approximate measurements (such as 1 apple—3 inches in diameter).
  - —Indicate whether processed in water, light syrup, heavy syrup, or other medium.
- For vegetables
  - —Indicate fresh, frozen, canned, dried.
  - —Record as portion of cup, teaspoon, or tablespoon or as pieces (such as 2 carrot sticks—4 inches long, ½ inch thick).
  - —Record preparation method.
- For cereals
  - —Record cooked cereals in portions of tablespoon or cup, (a level measurement after cooking).
  - —Record dry cereal in level portions of cup or tablespoons.
  - —If margarine, milk, sugar, fruit, or something else is added, then measure and record amount and type.
- For breads
  - —Indicate whether whole wheat, rye, white, and so on.
  - —Measure and record number and size of portion (biscuit—2 inches across,

1 inch thick; slice of homemade rye bread—3 inches by 4 inches, ¼ inch thick.
- —Sandwiches: list ALL ingredients (lettuce, mayonnaise, tomato, and so on) with amounts.

- For meats, fish, poultry, cheese
  - —Give size (length, width, thickness) in inches or weight in ounces after cooking for meats, fish, and poultry (such as cooked hamburger patty—3 inches across, ½ inch thick).
  - —Give size (length, width, thickness) in inches or weight in ounces for cheese.
  - —Record measurements only on the cooked edible part—without bone or fat that is left on the plate.
  - —Describe how meat was prepared.
- For eggs
  - —Record as soft or hard cooked, fried, scrambled, poached, or omelet.
  - —If milk, butter, or drippings are used, specify kinds and amount.
- For desserts
  - —List commercial brand or "homemade" or "bakery" under brand.
  - —Purchased candies, cookies, and cakes: Specify kind and size.
  - —Measure and record portion size of cakes, pies, and cookies by specifying thickness, diameter, and width or length, depending on the item.

Time	Minutes Spent Eating	M or S*	H⁺	Activity While Eating	Place of Eating	Food and Quantity	Others Present	Reason for Food Choice

M or S; meal or snack
⁺Hunger (0 none; 3 maximum)

Now complete the nutrient analysis form as shown using your food record. A blank copy of this form also follows for your use.

Nutrient Analysis Form (Sample)

Quantity	Name	Kcalories	Protein (grams)	Carbohydrate (grams)	Fat-total (grams)	Cholesterol (milligrams)	Saturated fat (grams)	Monounsaturated fat (grams)	Polyunsaturated fat (grams)	Sodium (milligrams)	Potassium (milligrams)	Magnesium (milligrams)
1 ea.	Egg bagel-3.5 inch diam.	180	7.45	34.7	1.00	44.0	0.171	0.286	0.400	300	65.0	18.0
1 Tbs.	Jelly	49.0	0.018	12.7	0.018	—	0.005	0.005	0.005	4.00	16.0	0.720
1.5 cup	Orange juice-prep fr/frzn	165	2.52	40.2	0.210	—	0.025	0.037	0.045	3.00	711	36.0
2 ea.	Cheeseburger-McD	636	30.2	57.0	32.0	80.0	13.3	12.2	2.18	1460	314	45.8
1 ea.	Serving-French fries-McD	220	3.00	26.1	11.5	8.57	4.61	4.37	0.570	109	564	26.7
1.5 cup	Cola beverage-regular	151	—	38.5	—	—	—	—	—	15.0	4.00	3.00
4 oz.	Pork loin chop-brld-lean	261	36.2	—	11.9	112	4.09	5.35	1.43	88.2	476	34.0
1 ea.	Baked potato with skin	220	4.65	51.0	0.200	—	0.052	0.004	0.087	16.0	844	55.0
.5 cup	Peas-frozen-cooked	63.0	4.12	11.4	0.220	—	0.039	0.019	0.103	70.0	134	23.0
20 gr.	Margarine-reg/soft-80% fat	143	0.160	0.100	16.1	—	2.76	5.70	6.92	216	7.54	0.467
2 cup	Iceberg lettuce-chopped	14.6	1.13	2.34	0.212	—	0.028	0.008	0.112	10.1	177	10.1
2 oz.	French dressing	300	0.318	3.63	32.0	—	4.94	14.2	12.4	666	7.03	5.81
1 cup	2% lowfat milk	121	8.12	11.7	4.78	22.0	2.92	1.35	0.170	122	377	33.0
2 ea.	Graham crackers	60.0	1.04	10.8	1.46	—	0.400	0.600	0.400	86.0	36.0	6.00
	Totals:	2584	99.0	300	112	266	33.4	44.1	24.8	3165	3732	298
RDA or minimum requirement*		2900	58							500	2000	350
% of RDA or minimum requirement		89	170							633	187	85

*Values from inside cover of textbook. The values listed are for a male age 19 to 24 years. Note that kcalories are just rough estimates. It is better to base energy needs on actual energy output.

Iron (milligrams)	Zinc (milligrams)	Vitamin A (RE)	Vitamin C (milligrams)	Thiamin (milligrams)	Riboflavin (milligrams)	Niacin (milligrams)	Vitamin B-6 (milligrams)	Folate (micrograms)	Vitamin B-12 (micrograms)	Calcium (milligrams)	Phosphorus (milligrams)	Selenium (micrograms)	Dietary Fiber (grams)	Vitamin E (milligrams)
2.10	0.612	7.00	—	2.58	0.197	2.40	0.030	16.3	0.065	20.0	61.0	5.00	0.748	1.80
0.120	—	0.200	0.710	0.002	0.005	0.036	0.005	2.00	—	2.00	1.00	0.360	—	0.016
0.411	0.192	28.5	145	0.300	0.060	0.750	0.165	163	—	33.0	60.0	0.735	1.49	0.714
5.68	5.20	134	4.10	0.600	0.480	8.66	0.230	42.0	1.82	338	410	58.0	0.460	0.560
0.605	0.320	5.00	12.5	0.122	0.020	2.26	0.218	19.0	0.027	9.10	101	0.600	4.19	0.203
0.120	0.049	—	—	—	—	—	—	—	—	9.00	46.0	—	—	—
1.04	2.54	3.15	0.454	1.30	0.350	6.28	0.535	6.77	0.839	5.67	277	20.6	—	0.405
2.75	0.650	—	26.1	0.216	0.067	3.32	0.701	22.2	—	20.0	115	1.80	3.90	0.100
1.25	0.750	53.4	7.90	0.226	0.140	1.18	0.090	46.9	—	19.0	72.0	3.20	3.61	0.400
—	0.041	199	0.028	0.002	0.006	0.004	2.19	0.211	0.017	5.29	4.06	0.199	—	0.028
0.560	0.246	37.0	4.36	0.052	0.034	0.210	0.044	62.8	—	21.2	22.4	0.448	1.68	0.120
0.227	0.045	0.023		—	—	—	0.006	—	—	7.10	3.63		0.431	15.9
0.120	0.963	140	2.32	0.095	0.403	0.210	0.105	12.0	0.888	297	232	5.66	—	0.080
0.367	0.113	—	—	0.020	0.030	0.600	0.011	1.80	—	6.00	20.0	1.54	1.40	
15.4	11.7	607	204	5.52	1.79	25.9	2.14	395	3.65	792	1425	98.2	17.9	22.5
10	15	1000	60	1.5	1.7	19	2	200	2	1200	1200	70	—	10
54	78	61	340	368	105	132	107	198	180	66	118	140	—	225

Nutrient Analysis Form (Sample)

Quantity	Name	Kcalories	Protein (grams)	Carbohydrate (grams)	Fat-total (grams)	Cholesterol (milligrams)	Saturated fat (grams)	Monounsaturated fat (grams)	Polyunsaturated fat (grams)	Sodium (milligrams)	Potassium (milligrams)	Magnesium (milligrams)
Totals:												
RDA or minimum requirement*												
% of RDA or minimum requirement												

*Values from inside cover of textbook. The values listed are for a male age 19 to 24 years. Note that kcalories are just rough estimates. It is better to base energy needs on actual energy output.

Iron (milligrams)	**Zinc (milligrams)**	**Vitamin A (RE)**	**Vitamin C (milligrams)**	**Thiamin (milligrams)**	**Riboflavin (milligrams)**	**Niacin (milligrams)**	**Vitamin B-6 (milligrams)**	**Folate (micrograms)**	**Vitamin B-12 (micrograms)**	**Calcium (milligrams)**	**Phosphorus (milligrams)**	**Selenium (micrograms)**	**Dietary Fiber (grams)**	**Vitamin E**

Complete the following Table as you summarize your dietary intake.

Percentage of kcalories from protein, fat, carbohydrate, and alcohol

Intake				
Protein (P):	____ g/day × 4 kcal/g	=	(P)______	kcal/day.
Fat (F):	____ g/day × 9 kcal/g	=	(F)______	kcal/day.
Carbohydrate (C):	____ g/day × 4 kcal/g	=	(C)______	dcal/day.
Alcohol (A):			(A)______	kcal/day.*
	Total kcal (T)/day	=	(T)______	kcal/day.

Percentage of kcalories from protein:

$\frac{(P)}{(T)} \times 100 =$ ____ % of total kcalories.

Percentage of kcalories from fat:

$\frac{(F)}{(T)} \times 100 =$ ____ % of total kcalories.

Percentage of kcalories from carbohydrate:

$\frac{(C)}{(T)} \times 100 =$ ____ % of total kcalories.

Percentage of kcalories from alcohol:

$\frac{(A)}{(T)} \times 100 =$ ____ % of total kcalories.

Note: The four percentages can total 99, 100, or 101, depending on the way in which figures were rounded off earlier.

*To find out how many kcalories in a beverage are from alcohol, look up the beverage in Appendix A. Figure out how many kcalories are from carbohydrate (multiply carbohydrate grams times 4), fat (fat grams times 9), and protein (protein grams times 4). The remaining kcalories are from alcohol.

For this same day you keep your food record, also keep a 24-hour record of your activities. Include sleeping, sitting, and walking, as well as the obvious forms of exercise. Calculate your kcalorie expenditure for these activities using Appendix M. Try to substitute a similar activity if your particular activity is not listed in Appendix M. Calculate the total kcalories you used for the day (total for column 3). Here is an example of an activity record. A blank form follows for your use.

Weight (lb or kg):		**Gender (M or F)**		
		Energy cost		
Activity	**Time (minutes); convert to hours;**	**Column 1 kcal/hr (from table)**	**Column 2 time (hr)**	**Column 3 (kcal) (Column 1 × Column 2)**
Example for 150-lb man: Brisk walking	0.5 hr (30 min)	299	0.5	150

Weight (lb or kg):		**Gender (M or F)**		
		Energy cost		
Activity	**Time (minutes); convert to hours;**	**Column 1 kcal/hr (from table)**	**Column 2 time (hr)**	**Column 3 (kcal) (Column 1 × Column 2)**
Total kcalories used (from adding all of column 3)				

This Appendix is now completed. See if your instructor wants you to complete more work before turning in this assignment.

APPENDIX F

U.S. RDA, RDI and DRV

U.S. recommended daily allowances (U.S. RDA)

Vitamins and minerals	Unit of measurement	Adults and children 4 or more years of age*	Infants	Children under 4 years of age	Pregnant or lactating women
Protein	Grams	65†	25†	28	‡
Vitamin A	International Units	5000	1500	2500	8000
Vitamin D	"	400	400	400	400
Vitamin E	"	30	5.0	10	30
Vitamin C	Milligrams	60	35	40	60
Folic Acid	"	0.4	0.1	0.2	0.8
Thiamin	"	1.5	0.5	0.7	1.7
Riboflavin	"	1.7	0.6	0.8	2.0
Niacin	"	20	8.0	9.0	20
Vitamin B-6	"	2.0	0.4	0.7	2.5
Vitamin B-12	Micrograms	6.0	2.0	3.0	8.0
Biotin	Milligrams	0.3	0.05	0.15	0.3
Pantothenic Acid	"	10	3.0	5.0	10
Calcium	Grams	1.0	0.6	0.8	1.3
Phosphorus	"	1.0	0.5	0.8	1.3
Iodine	Micrograms	150	45	70	150
Iron	Milligrams	18	15	10	18
Magnesium	"	400	70	200	450
Copper	"	2.0	0.6	1.0	2.0
Zinc	"	15	5.0	8.0	15

*These U.S. RDA values are on most nutrition labels.

†If the protein efficiency ratio of the food protein in question is equal to or better than that of casein, U.S. RDA is 45 g for adults, 20 g for children under 4 yrs, and 18 g for infants (see Chapter 8)

‡Not specified because this U.S. RDA is used only in vitamin and mineral supplements for pregnant or lactating females.

(Proposed) Reference Daily Intakes (RDIs)*,†
(to replace the U.S. RDAs)

Nutrient	Unit of measurement	Adults and children 4 or more years of age	Children less than 4 years of age†	Infants‡	Pregnant women	Lactating women
Vitamin A	Retinol equivalents§	875	400	375	800	1300
Vitamin C	Milligrams	60	40	33	70	95
Calcium	Milligrams	900	800	500	1200	1200
Iron	Milligrams	12	10	8.0	30	15
Vitamin D	Micrograms‖	6.5	10	9.0	10	10
Vitamin E	*alpha*-Tocopherol equivalents§	9.0	6.0	3.5	10	12
Vitamin K	Micrograms	65	15	7.5	65	65
Thiamin	Milligrams	1.2	0.7	0.4	1.5	1.6
Riboflavin	Milligrams	1.4	0.8	0.5	1.6	1.8
Niacin	Niacin equivalents§	16	9.0	5.5	17	20
Vitamin B_6	Milligrams	1.5	1.0	0.5	2.2	2.1
Folate	Micrograms	180	50	30	400	280
Vitamin B_{12}	Micrograms	2.0	0.7	0.4	2.2	2.6
Biotin	Micrograms	60	20	13	65	65
Pantothenic acid	Milligrams	5.5	3.0	2.5	5.5	5.5
Phosphorus	Milligrams	900	800	400	1200	1200
Magnesium	Milligrams	300	80	50	320	355
Zinc	Milligrams	13	10	5.0	15	19
Iodine	Micrograms	150	70	45	175	200
Selenium	Micrograms	55	20	13	65	75
Copper	Milligrams	2.0	0.9	0.6	2.5	2.5
Manganese	Milligrams	3.5	1.3	0.6	3.5	3.5
Fluoride	Milligrams	2.5	1.0	0.5	3.0	3.0
Chromium	Micrograms	120	50	33	13	130
Molybdenum	Micrograms	150	38	26	160	160
Chloride	Milligrams	3150	1000	650	3400	3400

*The following abbreviations are allowed: "mg" for "milligrams"; "mcg" for "micrograms"; "mcg RE" for "retinol equivalents"; "mg *a*-TE" for *alpha*-tocopherol equivalents"; "mg NE" for "niacin equivalents."
†The term "children less than 4 years of age" means persons 13 through 47 months of age.
‡The term "infants" means persons not more than 12 months of age.
§1 retinol equivalent = 1 microgram retinol or 6 micrograms *beta*-carotene; 1 *alpha*-tocopherol equivalent = 1 milligram *d-alpha*-tocopherol; 1 niacin equivalent = 1 milligram niacin or 60 milligrams of dietary tryptophan.
‖As cholecalciferol.

(Proposed) Daily Reference Values (DRVs)†‡
(to provide intake guidelines for substances not included in the 1989 RDAs)

Food component	Unit of measurement*	DRV
Fat	Grams	75
Saturated fatty acids	Grams	25
Unsaturated fatty acids	Grams	50
Cholesterol	Milligrams	300
Carbohydrate	Grams	325
Fiber	Grams	25
Sodium	Milligrams	2400
Potassium	Milligrams	3500

*The following abbreviations are allowed: "g" for "grams" and "mg" for "milligrams."
†From *The Federal Register,* July 19, 1990, pp. 29485-29486.
‡Written comments on these proposals were accepted until November 11, 1990. Many comments were received; therefore changes are possible. After the problems identified in the comments are resolved, final rules will be published. The RDIs and DRVs will each become effective one year after publication of their final rules.

APPENDIX G

Exchange System Lists

Milk Exchange List

Skim milk (12 grams carbohydrate, 8 grams protein, 0 grams fat, 90 kcalories)

1 cup	skim or nonfat milk (½% and 1%)
⅓ cup	powdered (nonfat dry, before adding liquid)
½ cup	canned, evaporated skim milk
1 cup	buttermilk made from skim milk
1 cup	yogurt made from skim milk (plain, unflavored)

Low-fat milk (12 grams carbohydrate, 8 grams protein, 5 grams fat, 120 kcalories)

1 cup	2% fat milk
1 cup	plain nonfat yogurt (added milk solids)

Whole milk (12 grams carbohydrate, 8 grams protein, 8 grams fat, 150 kcalories)

1 cup	whole milk
1 cup	custard-style yogurt made from whole milk (plain, unflavored)

Vegetable Exchange List

(5 grams carbohydrate, 2 grams protein protein, 0 grams fat, 25 kcalories) 1 exchange equals:

½ cup cooked vegetables or vegetable juice
1 cup raw vegetables

artichoke (½ medium)
asparagus
beans (green, wax, Italian)
bean sprouts
beets
broccoli
brussels sprouts
cabbage, cooked
carrots
cauliflower
eggplant
green pepper
greens
mushrooms (cooked)
onions
pea pods
sauerkraut
spinach (cooked)
squash, summer, zucchini
string beans (green, yellow)
tomato
tomato juice
turnips
vegetable juice
zucchini (cooked)

Fruit Exchange List

(15 grams carbohydrate, 0 grams protein, 0 grams fat, 60 kcalories) 1 fruit exchange equals:

1	apple (2 inches in diameter)
4 rings	dried apple
½ cup	apple juice
½ cup	applesauce (unsweetened)

Fruit Exchange List—cont'd

4	apricots, fresh
½ cup	apricots, canned
7 halves	apricots, dried
½	banana, 9 inches
¾ cup	blackberries
¾ cup	blueberries
1 cup	raspberries
1¼ cup	strawberries
⅓ melon	cantaloupe (5 inches in diameter)
12	cherries (large, raw)
½ cup	cherries, canned
½ cup	cider
⅓ cup	cranberry juice cocktail
2½ medium	dates
2	figs, fresh (2 inches in diameter)
1½	figs, dried
½	grapefruit
½ cup	grapefruit juice
15	grapes
⅓ cup	grape juice
⅛ melon	honeydew melon (7 inches in diameter; cubes = 1 cup)
1	kiwi (large)
¾ cup	mandarin oranges
½ small	mango
1 small	nectarine (1½ inches in diameter)
1 small	orange (2½ inches in diameter)
½ cup	orange juice
1 medium or ¾ cup	peach, fresh (2¾ inches in diameter)
½ cup or 2 halves	peach, canned
1 small or ½ large	pear, fresh
½ cup or 2 halves	pear, canned
¾ cup	pineapple, raw
⅓ cup	pineapple, canned
½ cup	pineapple juice
2	plums (2 inches in diameter)
3	prunes, dried
⅓ cup	prune juice
2 tablespoons	raisins
2	tangerine (2½ inches in diameter)
1¼ cups	watermelon (cubes)

Starch/Bread Exchange List

(15 grams carbohydrate, 3 grams protein, 0 grams fat, 80 kcalories)

1 starch/bread exchange equals:

Bread

1 slice	white (including French and Italian)
1 slice	whole wheat
1 slice	rye or pumpernickel
1 slice	raisin (unfrosted)
2 (⅔ ounces)	bread sticks (crisp, 4 inches long, ½ inch wide)
½ (1 ounce)	bagel, small
½	English muffin
1 (small)	plain roll
½ (1 ounce)	frankfurter bun
½ (1 ounce)	hamburger bun

3 tablespoons	dried bread crumbs
1	tortilla (6 inches in diameter)
½	pita (6 inches in diameter)

Cereal/Grains/Pasta

½ cup	bran flakes
¾ cup	other ready-to-eat unsweetened cereal
1½ cups	puffed cereal (unfrosted)
½ cup	cereal (cooked)
⅓ cup	rice or barley (cooked)
3 tablespoons	grapenuts
½ cup	shredded wheat
3 tablespoons	wheat germ
½ cup	pasta (cooked spaghetti, noodles, macaroni)
2½ tablespoons	cornmeal (dry)
2½ tablespoons	flour (dry)

Crackers/Snacks

3	graham (2½ inch square)
¾ ounce	matzoh (4 inches × 6 inches)
24	oyster
4	rye crisp (2 inches × 3½ inches)
6	saltines
8	animal
5 slices	melba toast
3 cups	popcorn (popped with no added fat)
¾ ounce	pretzels

Dried Beans/Peas/Lentils

⅓ cup	dried beans, such as kidney, white, split, blackeye (cooked)
⅓ cup	lentils (cooked)
¼ cup	baked beans

Starchy Vegetables

½ cup	corn
1	corn on the cob (6 inches)
½ cup	lima beans
½ cup	peas, green (canned or frozen)
1 small	potato, white (3 ounces baked)
½ cup	potato, mashed
1 cup	winter squash, acorn or butternut
⅓ cup	yam or sweet potato

Starch Group (With Fat)

1 starch/bread exchange
1 fat exchange

1	biscuit (2½ inches across)
1 (2 ounce)	corn bread (2-inch cube)
6	cracker, round butter type
10 (1½ ounce)	french fries (2 inches to 3½ inches)
1	muffin, plain, small
2	pancake (4 inches in diameter)
¼ cup	stuffing, bread (prepared)
2	taco shell (6 inches across)
1	waffle (4½ inches square)
4-6 (1 ounce)	whole-wheat crackers (such as Triscuits)

Meat Exchange List

Lean (0 grams carbohydrate, 7 grams protein, 3 grams fat, 55 kcalories)

Beef	1 ounce	baby beef (lean), chipped beef, chuck, flank steak, tenderloin, plate ribs, round (bottom, top), all cuts rump, spare ribs, tripe
Pork	1 ounce	leg (whole rump, center shank), ham (center slices), USDA good or choice grades such as round, sirloin, flank, and tenderloin
	1½ ounce	95% fat-free luncheon meat
Veal	1 ounce	leg, loin, rib, shank, shoulder, chops, roasts, all cuts except cutlets (ground or cubed)
Poultry	1 ounce	chicken, turkey, cornish hen (without skin)
	3 (½ cup)	egg whites, egg substitutes
Fish	2 ounces	fresh or frozen, any type canned salmon, tuna, mackerel, crab, or lobster
	1 ounce	clams, oysters, scallops, shrimp
	3 ounces	sardines, drained
Cheeses	1 ounce	cottage, farmer's, or pot (low-fat), grated parmesan

Medium fat (0 grams carbohydrate, 7 grams protein, 5 grams fat, 75 calories)

Beef	1 ounce	all ground beef, roast (rib, chuck, rump), steak (cubed, porterhouse, T-bone), meat loaf
Lamb	1 ounce	leg, rib, sirloin, loin (roast and chops), shank, shoulder
Pork	1 ounce	loin (all cuts tenderloin), chops, roast, Boston butt, cutlets
Poultry	1 ounce	capon, duck (domestic), goose, ground turkey, chicken with skin
Veal	1 ounce	cutlets
Organ meats	1 ounce	all types
Fish	¼ cup	tuna (canned in oil); salmon (canned)
Cheeses	¼ cup or 1 ounce	cottage (creamed), mozzarella (made with skim milk), ricotta, Neufchatel
Egg	1	egg
Other	4 ounces	tofu

High fat (0 grams carbohydrate, 7 grams protein, 8 grams fat, 100 kcalories)

Beef	1 ounce	brisket, corned beef (commercial), chuck (ground commercial), roasts (rib), steaks (club and rib); most USDA prime cuts of beef
Lamb	1 ounce	patties (ground lamb)
Pork	1 ounce	spare ribs, loin (back ribs), pork (ground), country-style ham, deviled ham, pork sausage
Cheeses	1 ounce	all regular cheeses (American, blue, brick, Camembert, cheddar, Gouda, Limburger, Muenster, Swiss, Monterey), all processed cheeses
Cold cuts	1 ounce	bologna, salami, pimento loaf
Frankfurter	1 ounce	(turkey or chicken)
Peanut butter	1 tablespoon	
Sausage	1 ounce	(Polish, Italian)

Fat Exchange List

(0 grams carbohydrate, 0 grams protein, 5 grams fat, 45 kcalories)

1/8 medium	avocado
1 strip	bacon, crisp
1 teaspoon	butter, margarine
2 tablespoons	cream, light
2 tablespoons	cream, sour
1 tablespoon	cream, heavy
1 tablespoon	cream cheese
Dressing	
2 teaspoons	all varieties
	mayonnaise type
1 tablespoon	reduced calorie
1 tablespoon	gravy, meat
Olives	
10 small or 5 large	

Nuts, 6	almonds, whole, dry roasted
2 large	pecans, whole
20 small or 10 large	peanuts, Spanish, whole
10	peanuts, Virginia, whole
2 whole	walnuts
1 tablespoon	cashews, dry roasted
1 tablespoon	seeds (pine, sunflower)
2 teaspoons	pumpkin seeds
1 tablespoon	other
Oil	
1 teaspoon	corn, cottonseed, safflower, soy, sunflower, olive, peanut, canola

Free Foods

A free food is any food or drink that contains less than 20 kcalories per serving. You can eat as much as you want of those items that have no serving size specified. You may eat two or three servings per day of those items that have a specific serving size. Be sure to spread them out through the day.

Drinks:
- Bouillon or broth without fat
- Bouillon, low-sodium
- Carbonated drinks, sugar-free
- Carbonated water
- Club soda
- Cocoa powder, unsweetened (1 tablespoon)
- Coffee/Tea
- Drink mixes, sugar-free
- Tonic water, sugar-free

Nonstick pan spray

Fruit:
- Cranberries, unsweetened (½ cup)
- Rhubarb, unsweetened (½ cup)

Vegetables:
(raw, 1 cup)
- Cabbage
- Celery
- Chinese cabbage
- Cucumber
- Green onion
- Hot peppers
- Mushrooms (fresh)
- Radishes
- Zucchini

Salad greens:
- Endive
- Escarole
- Lettuce
- Romaine
- Spinach

Sweet Substitutes:
- Candy, hard, sugar-free
- Gelatin, sugar-free
- Gum, sugar-free
- Jam/Jelly, sugar-free (2 teaspoons)
- Pancake syrup, sugar-free (1-2 tablespoons)
- Sugar substitutes (saccharin, aspartame)
- Whipped topping (2 tablespoons)

Condiments:
- Catsup (1 tablespoon)
- Horseradish
- Mustard
- Pickles, dill, unsweetened
- Salad dressing, low-calorie (2 tablespoons)
- Taco sauce (3 tablespoons)
- Vinegar

Seasonings:
- Basil (fresh)
- Celery seeds
- Cinnamon
- Chili powder
- Chives
- Curry
- Dill
- Flavoring extracts (vanilla, almond, walnut, peppermint, butter, lemon, etc.)
- Garlic
- Garlic powder
- Herbs
- Hot pepper sauce
- Lemon
- Lemon juice
- Lemon pepper
- Lime
- Lime juice
- Mint
- Onion powder
- Oregano
- Paprika
- Pepper
- Pimento
- Spices
- Soy sauce
- Soy sauce, low-sodium (lite)
- Wine, used in cooking (¼ cup)
- Worcestershire sauce

APPENDIX H

Fatty Acids, Including Omega-3 Fatty Acids in Foods

Chain length and number of double bonds for common fatty acids

Common name of fatty acids	Number of carbon atoms and site of double bond counting from methyl end ($—CH_3$)
Saturated fatty acids	
Formic	1
Acetic	2:0
Propionic	3:0
Butyric	4:0
Valeric	5:0
Caproic	6:0
Caprylic	8:0
Capric	10:0
Lauric	12:0
Myristic	14:0
Palmitic	16:0
Stearic	18:0
Unsaturated fatty acids	
Oleic	18:1 (9-10) w-9
Linoleic	18:2 (6-7, 9-10) w-6
alpha-Linolenic	18:3 (3-4, 6-7, 9-10) w-3
Arachidonic	20:4 (6-7, 9-10, 12-13, 15-16) w-6
Eicosapentaenoic	20:5 (3-4, 6-7, 9-10, 12-13, 15-16) w-3
Docosahexaenoic	22:6 (3-4, 6-7, 9-10, 12-13, 15-16, 18-19) w-3

Fatty acids composition of selected foods*

Food item	Fatty acid†									
	<C12:0	C12:0	14:0	C16:0	C18:0	C18:1 w-9	C18:2 w-6	C18:3 w-3	C20:5 w-3	C22:6 w-3
Fats and oils		Lauric acid	Mysistic acid	Palmitic acid	Stearic acid	Oleic acid	Linoleic acid	Alpha linolenic acid	EP-A‡	DHA‡
Beef tallow	—	0.9	3.7	24.9	18.9	36.0	3.1	0.6	—	—
Butter	7.0	2.3	8.2	21.3	9.8	20.4	1.8	1.2	—	—
Cocoa butter	—	—	0.1	25.4	33.2	32.6	2.8	0.1	—	—
Corn oil	—	—	—	12.0	2.0	25.0	60.0	0.5	—	—
Cottonseed oil	—	—	0.8	22.7	2.3	17.0	51.5	0.2	—	—
Lard	0.1	0.2	1.3	23.8	13.5	41.2	10.2	1.0	—	—
Olive oil	—	—	—	13.0	2.5	74.0	9.0	0.5	—	—
Palm kernel oil	7.2	47.0	16.4	8.1	2.8	11.4	1.6	—	—	—
Palm oil	—	0.1	1.0	43.5	4.0	36.6	9.1	0.2	—	—
Safflower oil	—	—	—	6.5	2.5	11.5	79.0	0.5	—	—
Shortening§	0.2	0.4	0.4	19.3	9.9	50.6	13.5	0.6	—	—
Margarine, stick	2	1	10	23	9	31	7	1	—	—
Margarine, tub	1	1	1	12	8	22	52	1	—	—
Canola oil	—	—	—	5	1	62	22	9	—	—
Soybean oil	—	—	—	10	4	24	53	7	—	—
Coconut oil	14	45	17	8	3	6	2	—	—	—
Meat, fish, and poultry										
Beef, lean only, uncooked	—	—	0.17	1.4	0.74	2.4	0.2	0.01	—	—
Chicken, white meat, uncooked	—	—	0.01	0.3	0.1	0.4	0.2	0.01	—	—
Salmon, coho, raw	—	—	0.3	0.6	0.2	1.2	0.3	0.2	0.3	0.5
Tuna, light, canned in oil	—	—	0.03	1.4	0.1	2.8	2.7	0.07	0.03	0.1

*Only major fatty acids are presented.
†Values represent %/100 edible portion.
‡EPA eicosapentaenoic acid, DHA docosahexaenoic acid } fish oil fatty acids
§Soybean and palm oils, hydrogenated.
From USDA Agriculture Handbook No. 8-4 (28).

Omega-3 fatty acids in foods

Food item	Edible portion, raw (grams/100 grams)
Fish oils	
Cod liver oil	19.2
Herring oil	12.0
Menhaden oil	21.7
Salmon oil	20.9
Finned fish	
Anchovy, European	1.4
Bluefish	1.2
Dogfish, spiny	1.9
Carp	0.6
Catfish	0.3
Cod	0.3
Flounder	0.2
Halibut	0.9
Herring, Atlantic	1.7
Herring, Pacific	1.8
Mackerel, Atlantic	2.6
Mackerel, king	2.2
Mullet, unspecified	1.1
Perch	0.4
Sablefish	1.5
Salmon, Atlantic	1.4
Salmon, Chinook	1.5
Scad, Muroaji	2.1
Shark	0.5
Smelt	0.7
Sprat	1.3
Sturgeon, Atlantic	1.5
Swordfish	0.2
Trout, lake	2.0
Tuna, albaccore	1.5
Tuna, bluefin	1.6
Whitefish, lake	1.3
Fats and oils	
Butter	1.2
Butter oil	1.5
Chicken fat	1.0
Duck fat	1.0
Lard	1.0
Linseed oil	53.3
Margarine, hard, soybean	1.5
Margarine, hard, soybean oil and hydrogenated soybean oil	1.9
Margarine, hard, hydrogenated soybean oil and palm oil	2.3
Margarine, hard, hydrogenated soybean oil and cottonseed oil	2.8
Margarine, hard, hydrogenated palm oil	3.0
Margarine, liquid, hydrogenated soybean oil, soybean oil and cottonseed oil	2.4
Fats and oils—cont'd	
Margarine, soft, hydrogenated soybean oil and cottonseed oil	1.6
Margarine, soft, hydrogenated soybean oil and palm oil	1.9
Margarine, soft, soybean oil, hydrogenated soybean oil and hydrogenated cottonseed oil	2.8
Rapeseed oil (canola)	11.1
Rice bran oil	1.6
Salad dressing, commercial, blue cheese, regular	3.7
Salad dressing, commercial, Italian, regular	3.3
Salad dressing, commercial, mayonnaise (imitation), soybean, without cholesterol	4.6
Salad dressing, commercial, mayonnaise, safflower and soybean	3.0
Salad dressing, commercial, mayonnaise, soybean	4.2
Salad dressing, commercial, mayonnaise-type	2.0
Salad dressing, commercial, Thousand Island, regular	2.5
Salad dressing, home recipe, French	1.9
Salad dressing, home recipe, vinegar and soybean oil	1.4
Shortening, special purpose, for bread, soybean (hydrogenated) and cottonseed	4.0
Shortening, special purpose, heavy-duty, frying, soybean (hydrogenated)	2.4
Soybean lecithin	5.1
Soybean oil	6.8
Walnut oil	10.4
Legumes	
Soybeans, dry	1.6
Nuts and seeds	
Beechnuts, dried	1.7
Butternuts, dried	1.7
Butternuts, dried	8.7
Chia seeds, dried	3.9
Walnuts, black	3.3
Walnuts, English/Persian	6.8
Vegetables	
Soybeans, green, raw	3.2
Soybeans, mature seeds, sprouted cooked	2.1

From U.S. Department of Agriculture Human Nutrition Information Service: *Provisional tables on the content of omega-3 fatty acids and other fat components of selected foods,* HNIS/PT-103, 1988.

APPENDIX I

U.S. dietary goals 2nd edition, 1977

1. To avoid overweight, consume only as much energy (calories) as is expended; if overweight, decrease energy intake and increase energy expenditure.
2. Increase the consumption of complex carbohydrates and "naturally occurring" sugars from about 28% of energy intake to about 48% of energy intake.
3. Reduce the consumption of refined and processed sugars by about 45% to account for about 10% of total energy intake.
4. Reduce overall fat consumption from approximately 40% to about 30% of energy intake.
5. Reduce saturated fat consumption to account for about 10% of total energy intake; and balance that with polyunsaturated and monounsaturated fats, which should account for about 10% of energy intake each.
6. Reduce cholesterol consumption to about 300 mg a day.
7. Limit the intake of sodium by reducing the intake of salt to about 5 g a day.

The Goals Suggest the Following Changes in Food Selection and Preparation:

1. Increase consumption of fruits and vegetables and whole grains.
2. Decrease consumption of refined and other processed sugars and foods high in such sugars.
3. Decrease consumption of foods high in total fat, and partially replace saturated fats, whether obtained from animal or vegetable sources, with polyunsaturated fats.
4. Decrease consumption of animal fat, and choose meats, poultry and fish which will reduce saturated fat intake.
5. Except for young children, substitute low-fat and non-fat milk for whole milk, and low-fat dairy products for high fat dairy products.
6. Decrease consumption of butterfat, eggs and other high cholesterol sources. Some consideration should be given to easing the cholesterol goal for premenopausal women, young children and the elderly in order to obtain the nutritional benefits of eggs in the diet.
7. Decrease consumption of salt and foods high in salt content.

US Senate Select Committee on Nutrition and Human Needs: *Dietary Goals for the United States,* ed 2, 1977.

APPENDIX J

Estimating Energy Needs and Additional Height-Weight Tables

Estimates of Resting Energy Needs

Harris-Benedict equations

Women:

655 + [9.56 × weight (in kilograms)] + [1.85 × height (in centimeters)] − [4.68 × age (in years)]

Men:

66.5 + [13.8 × weight (in kilograms)] + [5 × height (in centimeters)] − [6.76 × age (in years)]

Owen equations

Women:

795 + [7.18 × weight (in kilograms)]

Men:

879 + [10.2 × weight (in kilograms)]

Boothby and Berkson nomogram for estimation of caloric requirements

Food nomogram

Directions for Estimating Caloric Requirement: To determine the desired allowance of calories, proceed as follows: 1. Locate the ideal weight on Column 1 by means of a common pin. 2. Bring edge of one end of a 12- or 15-inch ruler against the pin. 3. Swing the other end of the ruler to the patient's height on Column II. 4. Transfer the pin to the point where the ruler crosses Column III. 5. Hold the ruler against the pin in Column III. 6. Swing the left hand end of the ruler to the patient's sex and age (measured from last birthday) given in Column IV (these positions correspond to the Mayo Clinic's metabolism standards for age and sex). 7. Transfer the pin to the point where the ruler crosses Column V. This gives the basal caloric requirement (basal calories) of the patient for 24 hours and represents the calories required by the fasting patient when resting in bed. 8. To provide the extra calories for activity and work, the basal calories are increased by a percentage. To the basal calories for adults add: 50 to 80 percent for manual laborers, 30 to 40 percent for light work or 10 to 20 percent for restricted activity such as resting in a room or in bed. To the basal calories for children add 50 to 100 percent for children ages 5 to 15 years. This computation may be done by simple arithmetic or by the use of Columns VI and VII. If the latter method is chosen, locate the "percent above or below basal" desired in Column VI. By means of the ruler connect this point with the pin on Column V. Transfer the pin to the point where the ruler crosses Column VII. This represents the calories estimated to be required by the patient.

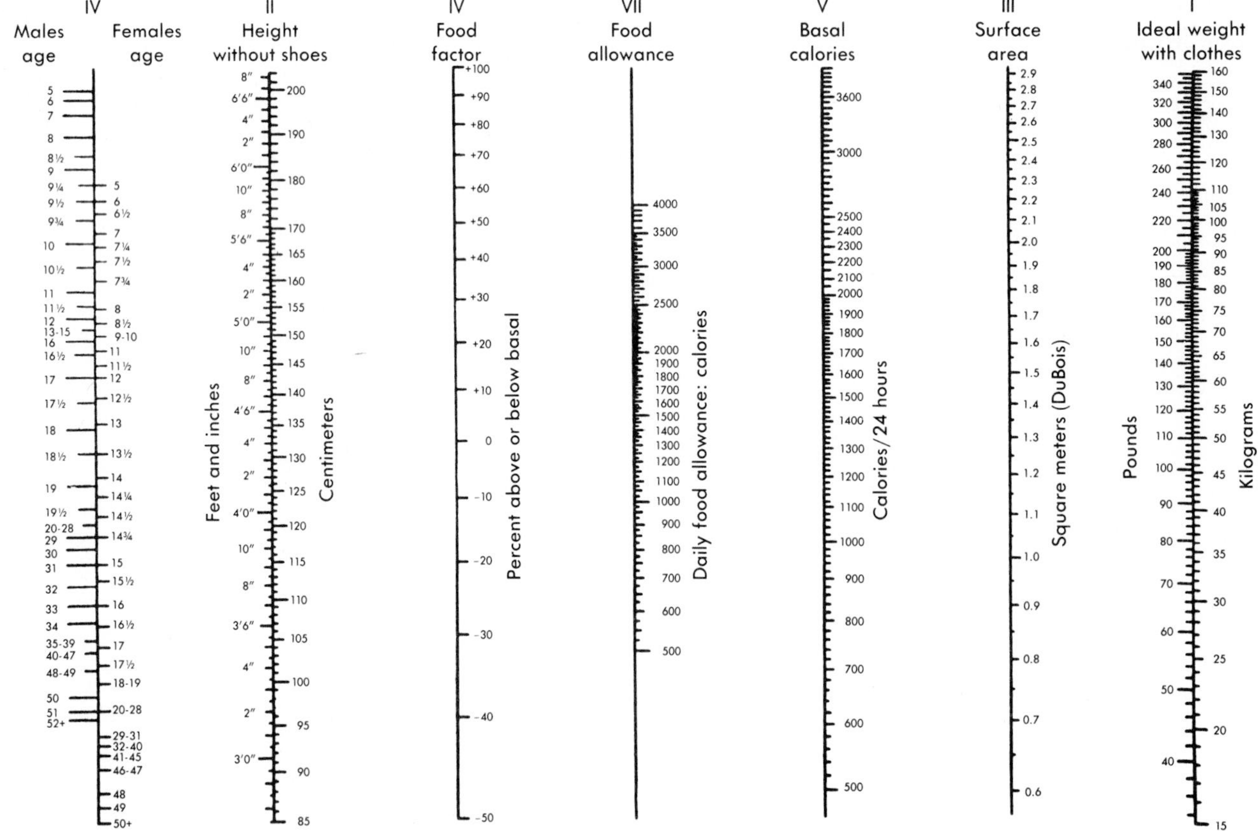

Height-Weight Tables

1983 Metropolitan Life Insurance Company height-weight table in metric units

	Males				Females		
Height (cm)	Small frame (kg)	Medium frame (kg)	Large frame (kg)	Height (cm)	Small frame (kg)	Medium frame (kg)	Large frame (kg)
157.5	58.2–60.9	59.4–64.1	62.7–68.2	147.5	46.4–50.5	49.5–55.0	53.6–59.5
160	59.1–61.8	60.5–65.0	63.6–69.5	150	46.8–51.4	50.5–55.9	54.5–60.9
162.5	60.0–62.7	61.4–65.9	64.5–70.9	152.5	47.3–52.3	51.4–57.3	55.5–62.3
165	60.9–63.7	62.3–67.3	65.5–72.7	155	48.2–53.6	52.3–58.6	56.8–63.6
167.5	61.8–64.5	63.2–68.6	66.4–74.5	157.5	49.1–55.0	53.6–60.0	58.2–65.0
170	62.7–65.9	64.5–70.0	67.7–76.4	160	50.5–56.4	55.0–61.4	59.5–66.8
173	63.6–67.3	65.9–71.4	69.1–78.2	162.5	51.8–57.7	56.4–62.7	60.9–68.6
175	64.5–68.6	67.3–72.7	70.5–80.0	165	53.2–59.1	57.7–64.1	62.3–70.5
178	65.4–70.0	68.6–74.1	71.8–81.8	167.5	54.5–60.5	59.1–65.5	63.6–72.3
180	66.4–71.4	70.0–75.5	73.2–83.6	170	55.9–61.8	60.5–66.8	65.0–74.1
183	67.7–72.7	71.4–77.3	74.5–85.6	173	57.3–63.2	61.8–68.2	66.4–75.9
185.5	69.1–74.5	72.7–79.1	76.4–87.3	175	58.6–64.5	63.2–69.5	67.7–77.3
188	70.5–76.4	74.5–80.9	78.2–89.5	178	60.0–65.9	64.5–70.9	69.1–78.6
190.5	71.8–78.2	75.9–82.7	80.0–91.8	180	61.4–67.3	65.9–72.3	70.5–80.0
193	73.6–80.0	77.7–85.0	82.3–94.1	183	62.3–68.6	67.3–73.6	71.8–81.4

Andres table for adults and the elderly—age-specific weight-for-height tables* (Gerontology Research Center)

Height	Weight range for men and women by age (years) in pounds†				
	25	35	45	55	65
ft-in					
4–10	84–111	92–119	99–127	107–135	115–142
4–11	87–115	95–123	103–131	111–139	119–147
5–0	90–119	98–127	106–135	114–143	123–152
5–1	93–123	101–131	110–140	118–148	127–157
5–2	96–127	105–136	113–144	122–153	131–163
5–3	99–131	108–140	117–149	126–158	135–168
5–4	102–135	112–145	121–154	130–163	140–173
5–5	106–140	115–149	125–159	134–168	144–179
5–6	109–144	119–154	129–164	138–174	148–184
5–7	112–148	122–159	133–169	143–179	153–190
5–8	116–153	126–163	137–174	147–184	158–196
5–9	119–157	130–168	141–179	151–190	162–201
5–10	122–162	134–173	145–184	156–195	167–207
5–11	126–167	137–178	149–190	160–201	172–213
6–0	129–171	141–183	153–195	165–207	177–219
6–1	133–176	145–188	157–200	169–213	182–225
6–2	137–181	149–194	162–206	174–219	187–232
6–3	141–186	153–199	166–212	179–225	192–238
6–4	144–191	157–205	171–218	184–231	197–244

*Values in this table are in pounds for height without shoes and weight without clothes. To convert inches to centimeters, multiply by 2.54; to convert pounds to kilograms, multiply by 0.455. †Data from Andres R: Gerontology Research Center, National Institute of Aging, Baltimore, Md.

Desireable weights* for men and women aged 20 to 74 years by height: United States, 1971-74, HANES, 1979

Height (inches)†	Weight (pounds)	
	Men	Women
57	—	113
58	—	117
59	—	120
60	—	123
61	—	127
62	136	130
63	140	134
64	145	137
65	150	140
66	155	144
67	159	147
68	163	151
69	168	154
70	173	158
71	178	—
72	182	—
73	187	—
74	192	—

*Based on average weights estimated from regression equation of weight on height for men and women aged 20 to 29 years. †Height measured without shoes. Clothing ranged from 0.20 to 0.62 pounds, which was not deducted from weight shown.

Nomogram for determining waist-to-hip ratio (WHR). To use this nomogram, place a straightedge between your waist circumference on the left and your hip circumference on the right. The point at which the line crosses the center column is your WHR. (From Bray GA and Gray DS: Obesity, Pt I, Pathogenesis, *Western Journal of Medicine* 149:429-441, 1988)

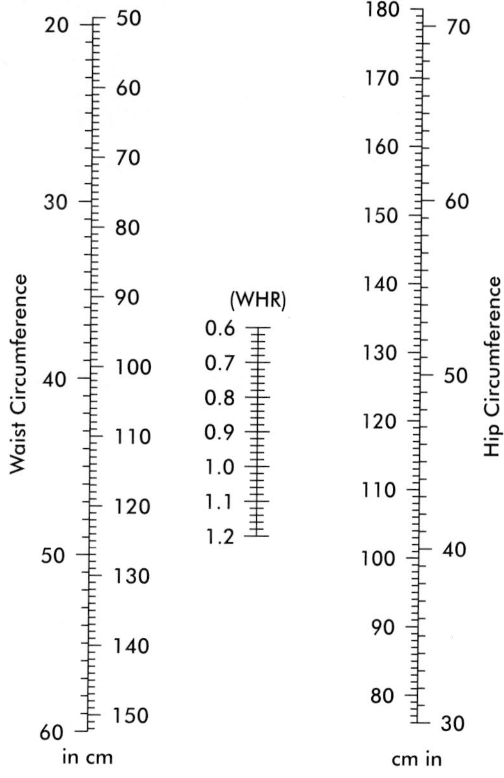

APPENDIX K

Determination of Frame Size

Determination of frame size

Method 1

Height is recorded without shoes.

Wrist circumference is measured just beyond the bony (styloid) process at the wrist joint on the right arm using a tape measure.

The following formula is used:

$$r = \frac{\text{height (cm)}}{\text{wrist circumference (cm)}}$$

Frame size can be determined as follows:

Males	Females
$r > 10.4$ small	$r > 11.0$ small
$r = 9.6\text{-}10.4$ medium	$r = 10.1\text{-}11.0$ medium
$r < 9.6$ large	$r < 10.1$ large

From Grant JP: *Handbook of Total Parenteral Nutrition*, Philadelphia, 1980, WB Saunders.

Method 2

The patient's right arm is extended forward perpendicular to the body, with the arm bent so the angle at the elbow forms 90 degrees with the fingers pointing up and the palm turned away from the body. The greatest breadth across the elbow joint is measured with a sliding caliper along the axis of the upper arm, on the two prominent bones on either side of the elbow. This is recorded as the elbow breadth. The following tables give the elbow breadth measurements for medium-framed men and women of various heights. Measurements lower than those listed indicate a small frame size; higher measurements indicate a large frame size.

Men		Women	
Height in 1″ heels	**Elbow breadth**	**Height in 1″ heels**	**Elbow breadth**
5′2″-5′3″	2½-2⅞	4′10″-4′11″	2¼-2½
5′4″-5′7″	2⅝-2⅞	5′0″-5′3″	2¼-2½
5′8″-5′11″	2¾-3	5′4″-5′7″	2⅜-2⅝
6′0″-6′3″	2¾-3⅛	5′8″-5′11″	2⅜-2⅝
6′4″ and over	2⅞-3¼	6′0″ and over	2½-2¾

From Metropolitan Life Insurance Co, 1983.

APPENDIX L

Energy Cost of Various Activities

Activity	Body weight		
	120 Pounds (54 Kilograms) Kcal/Hour	150 Pounds (68 Kilograms) Kcal/Hour	180 Pounds (82 Kilograms) Kcal/Hour
Aerobics—heavy	435	544	653
Aerobics—light	163	204	244
Aerobics—medium	272	340	408
Back-packing	489	612	734
Badminton	277	346	416
Ballroom dancing	166	208	249
Basketball—vigorous	544	680	816
Bicycling (5.5 MPH)	163	204	244
Billiards	108	136	163
Bowling	212	265	318
Calisthenics—heavy	435	544	653
Calisthenics—light	217	272	326
Canoeing (2.5 MPH)	179	224	269
Carpentry—general	272	340	408
Circuit training	604	755	906
Cleaning (F)	202	253	303
Cleaning (M)	189	236	284
Climbing (100 FT/HR)	391	489	587
Cooking (F)	146	183	220
Cooking (M)	156	195	235
Cycling (13 MPH)	527	659	791
Disco dancing	326	408	489
Ditch digging—hand	315	394	473
Dressing/showering	85	106	128
Driving	93	117	140
Eating (sitting)	75	93	112
Fencing	239	299	359
Food shopping (F)	202	253	303
Food shopping (M)	189	236	284
Football—touch	380	476	571
Gardening	174	217	261
Gardening—digging	411	514	617
Gardening—raking	176	220	264
Golf	195	244	293
Horseback riding—trotting	277	346	416
Housework—cleaning	217	272	326
Ice skating (10 MPH)	315	394	473
Jazzercize—heavy	435	544	653

Activity	Body weight 120 Pounds (54 Kilograms) Kcal/Hour	150 Pounds (68 Kilograms) Kcal/Hour	180 Pounds (82 Kilograms) Kcal/Hour
Jazzercize—light	163	204	244
Jazzercize—medium	272	340	408
Jogging—medium	489	612	734
Jogging—slow	380	476	571
Judo	636	795	955
Lawn mowing (hand)	212	265	318
Lawn mowing (power)	195	244	293
Lying—at ease	71	89	107
Piano playing	130	163	195
Racquetball—social	435	544	653
Roller skating	277	346	416
Rowboating (2.5 MPH)	239	299	359
Running or jogging (10 MPH)	718	897	1077
Scull rowing (race)	669	836	1004
Sewing—hand	104	130	156
Shuffleboard/skeet	163	204	244
Sitting quietly	68	85	102
Skiing (10 MPH)	478	598	718
Sleeping	64	80	97
Square dancing	277	346	416
Squash or handball	478	598	718
Swimming (.25 MPH)	239	299	359
Table tennis	282	353	424
Tennis	331	414	497
Volleyball	277	346	416
Walking (2.5 MPH)	163	204	244
Walking (3.75 MPH)	239	299	359
Water skiing	380	476	571
Weight lifting—heavy	489	612	734
Weight lifting—light	217	272	326
Window cleaning (F)	192	240	288
Window cleaning (M)	189	236	284
Wood chopping/sawing	315	394	473
Writing (sitting)	94	118	142

From *Nutritionist 3 software,* Salem, Ore, N-Squared Computing.

APPENDIX M

Infant and Child Growth Charts

Girls: Birth to 36 Months Physical Growth NCHS Percentiles*

Name ____________________ Record # __________

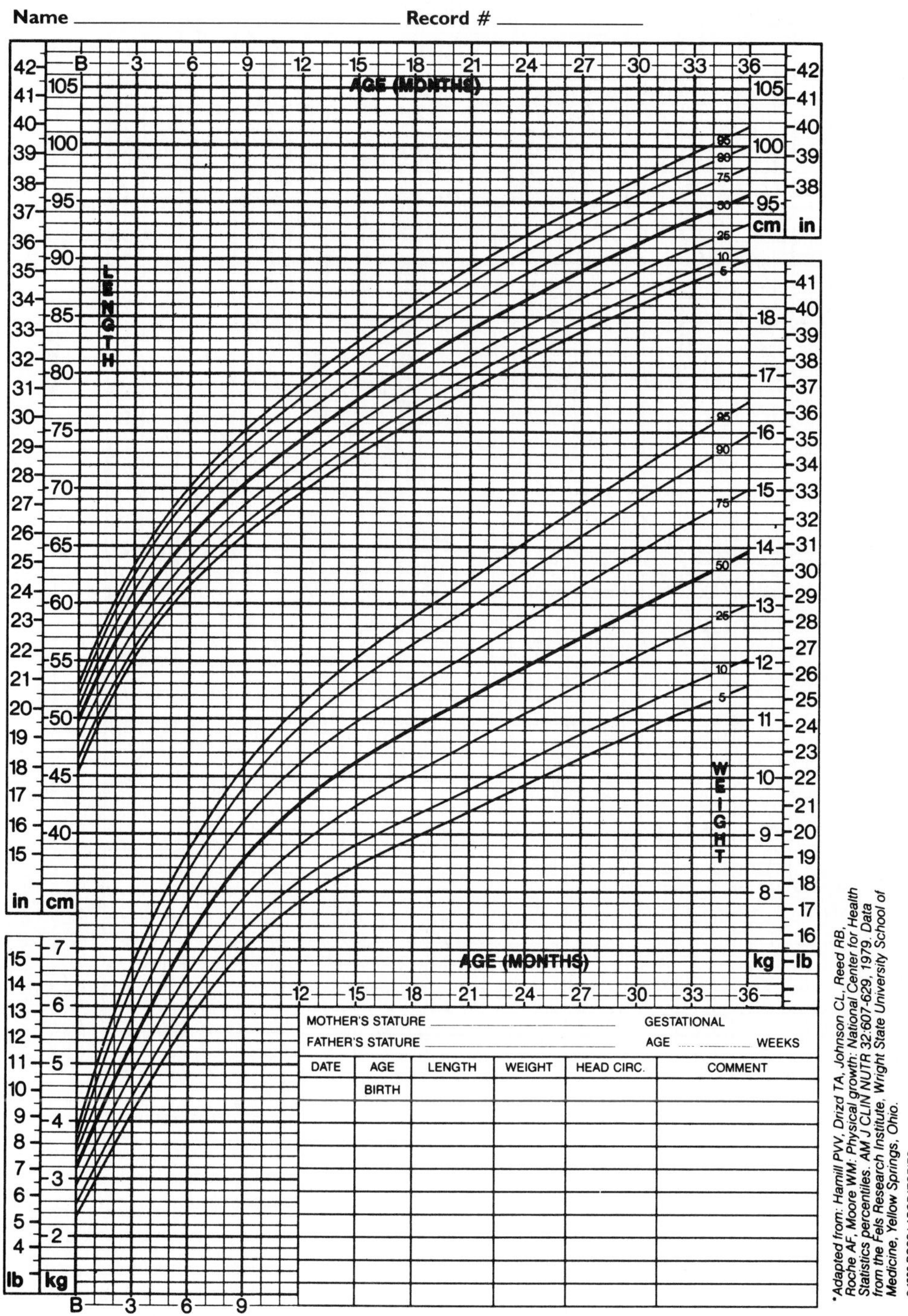

*Adapted from: Hamill PVV, Drizd TA, Johnson CL, Reed RB, Roche AF, Moore WM: Physical growth: National Center for Health Statistics percentiles. AM J CLIN NUTR 32:607-629, 1979. Data from the Fels Research Institute, Wright State University School of Medicine, Yellow Springs, Ohio.

Boys: Birth to 36 Months Physical Growth NCHS Percentiles*

Name ______________________ **Record #** ____________

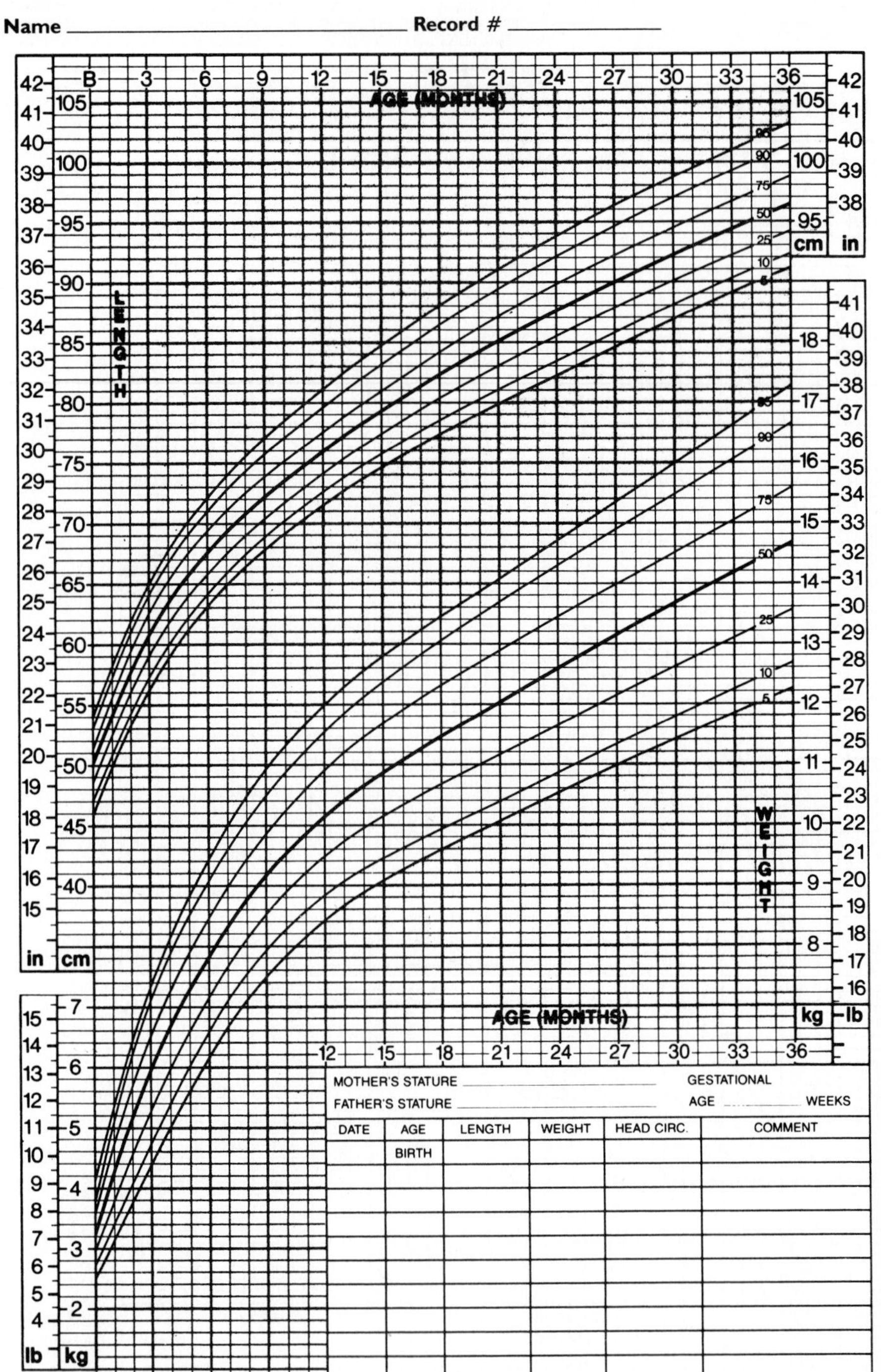

*Adapted from: Hamill PVV, Drizd TA, Johnson CL, Reed RB, Roche AF, Moore WM: Physical growth: National Center for Health Statistics percentiles. AM J CLIN NUTR 32:607-629, 1979. Data from the Fels Research Institute, Wright State University School of Medicine, Yellow Springs, Ohio.

Girls: Birth to 36 Months Physical Growth NCHS Percentiles*

Name ______________________ Record # __________

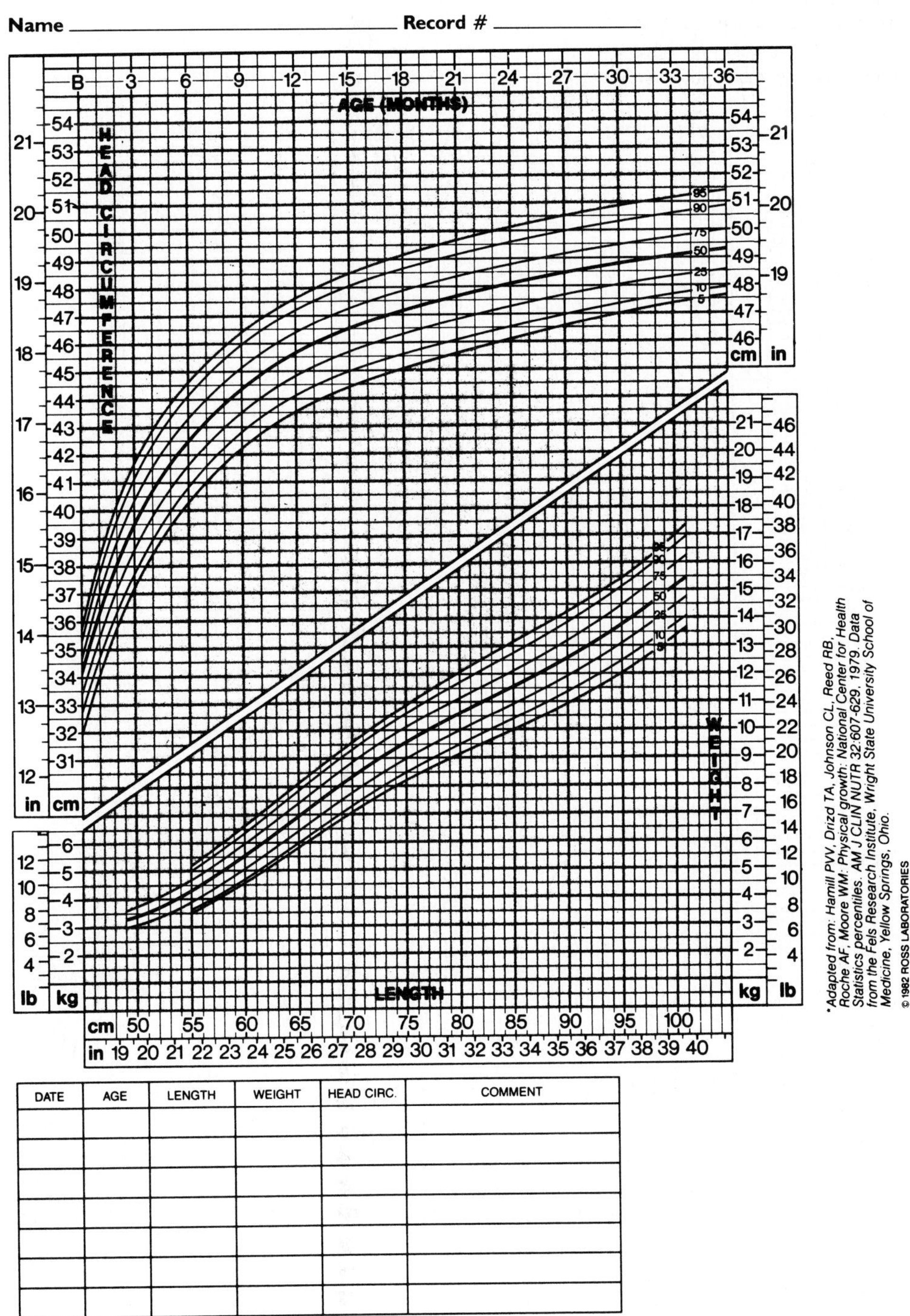

DATE	AGE	LENGTH	WEIGHT	HEAD CIRC.	COMMENT

*Adapted from: Hamill PVV, Drizd TA, Johnson CL, Reed RB, Roche AF, Moore WM: Physical growth: National Center for Health Statistics percentiles. AM J CLIN NUTR 32:607-629, 1979. Data from the Fels Research Institute, Wright State University School of Medicine, Yellow Springs, Ohio.

Boys: Birth to 36 Months Physical Growth NCHS Percentiles*

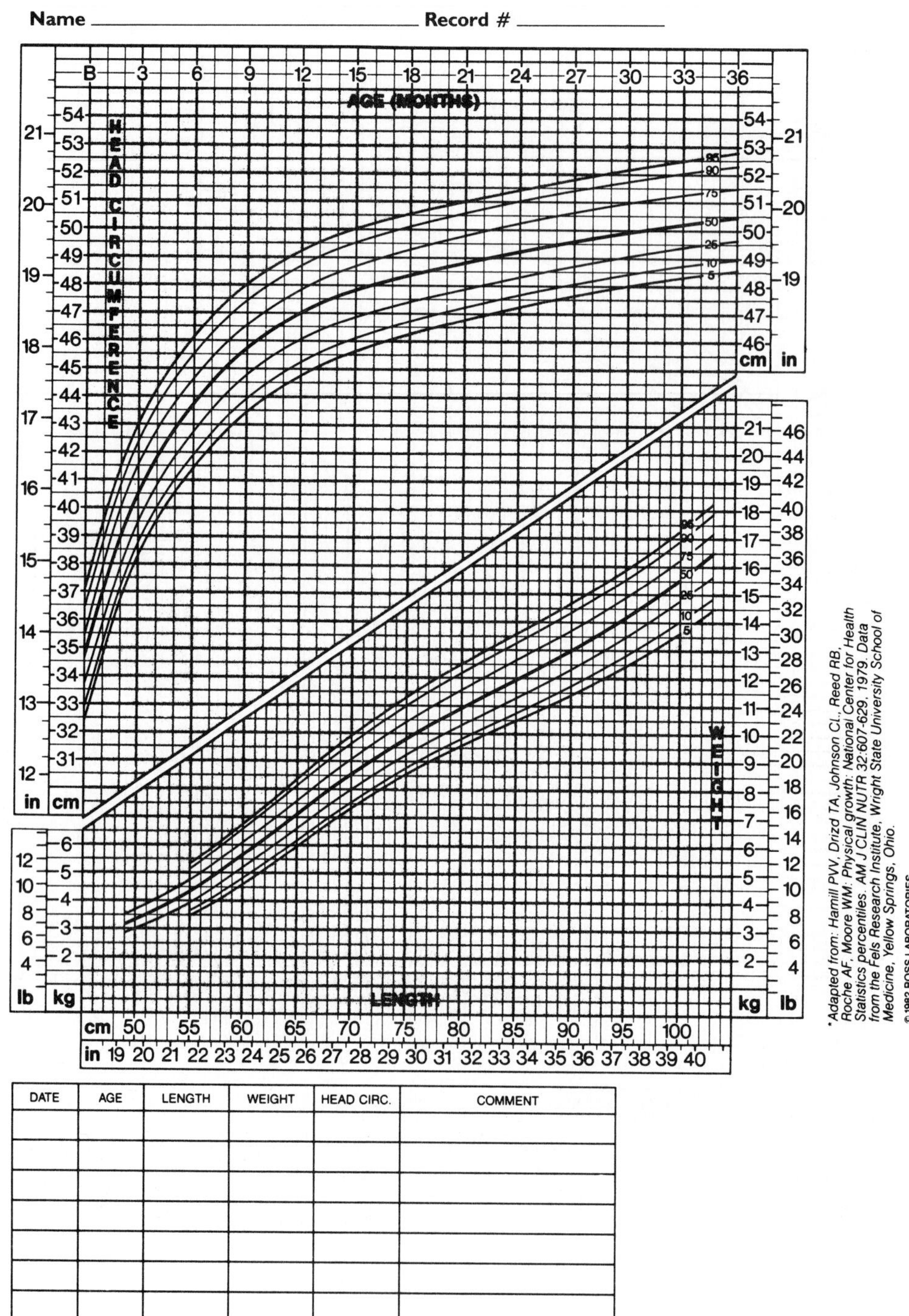

DATE	AGE	LENGTH	WEIGHT	HEAD CIRC.	COMMENT

*Adapted from: Hamill PVV, Drizd TA, Johnson CL, Reed RB, Roche AF, Moore WM: Physical growth: National Center for Health Statistics percentiles. AM J CLIN NUTR 32:607-629, 1979. Data from the Fels Research Institute, Wright State University School of Medicine, Yellow Springs, Ohio.

Boys: Prepubescent Physical Growth NCHS Percentiles*

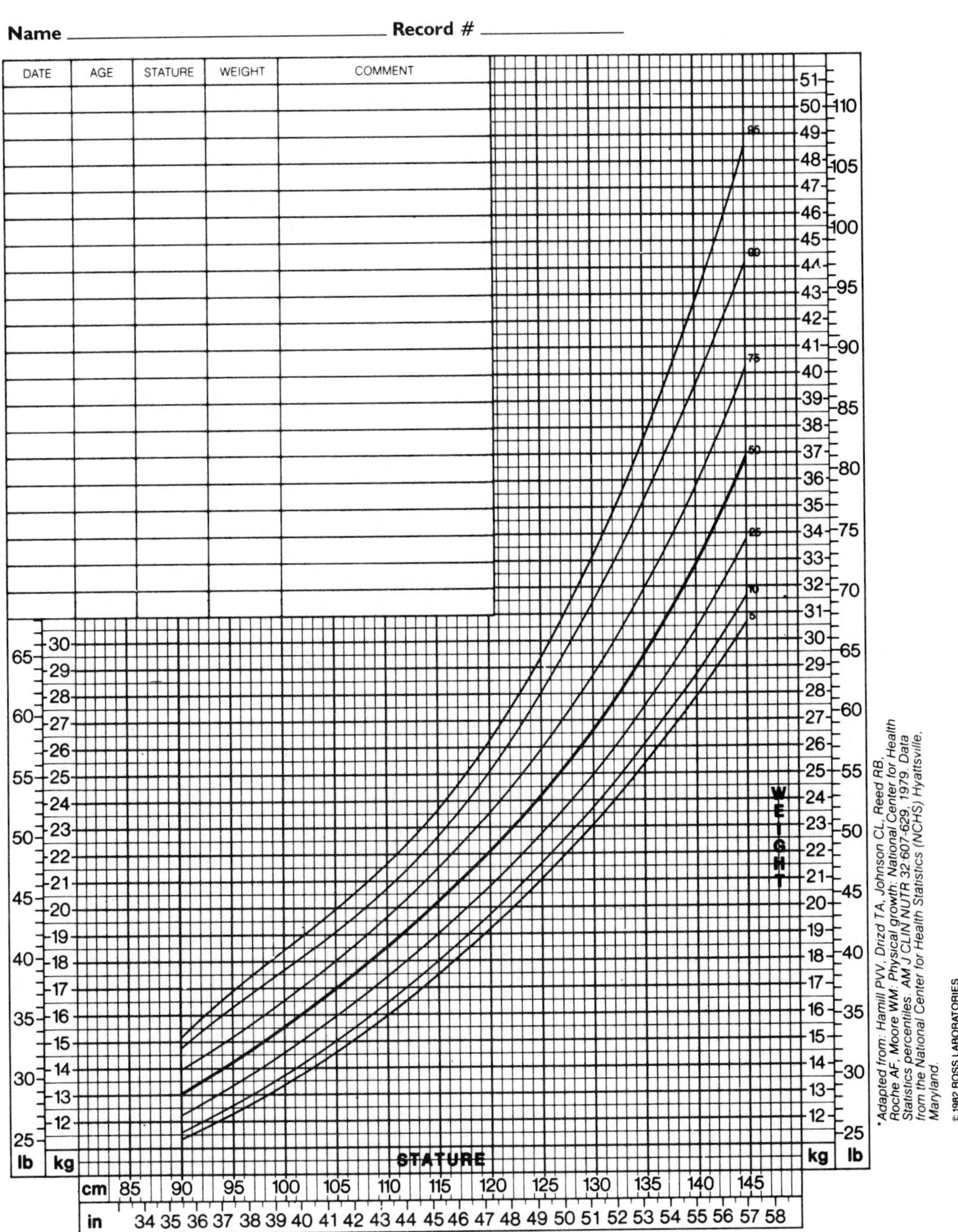

*Adapted from: Hamill PVV, Drizd TA, Johnson CL, Reed RB, Roche AF, Moore WM: Physical growth: National Center for Health Statistics percentiles. AM J CLIN NUTR 32:607-629, 1979. Data from the National Center for Health Statistics (NCHS) Hyattsville, Maryland.

Girls: Prepubescent Physical Growth NCHS Percentiles*

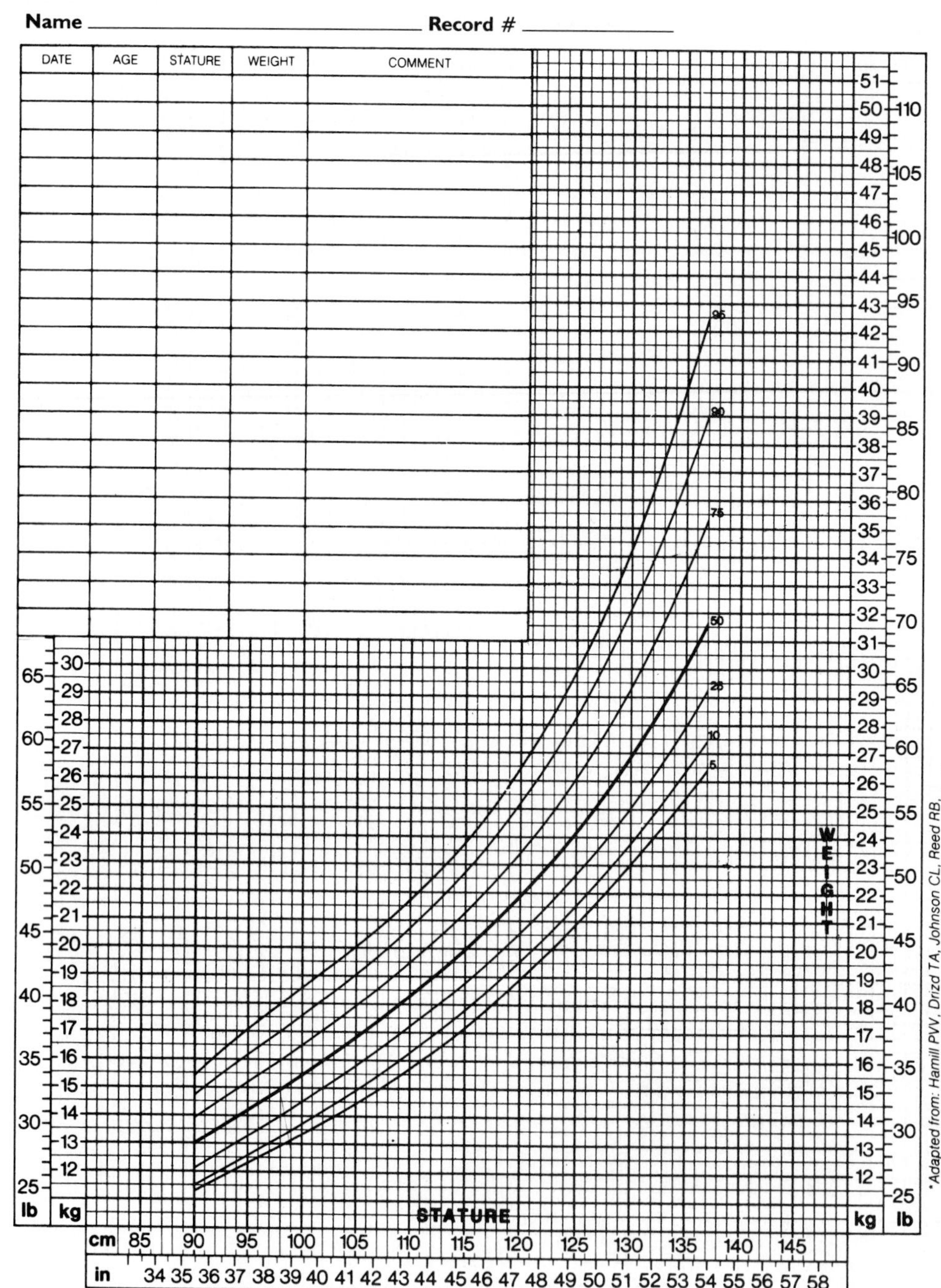

Girls: 2 to 18 Years Physical Growth NCHS Percentiles*

Name ______________________ **Record #** ______________

MOTHER'S STATURE ____________ FATHER'S STATURE ____________

DATE	AGE	STATURE	WEIGHT	COMMENT

AGE (YEARS)

STATURE

WEIGHT

*Adapted from: Hamill PVV, Drizd TA, Johnson CL, Reed RB, Roche AF, Moore WM: Physical growth: National Center for Health Statistics percentiles. AM J CLIN NUTR 32:607-629, 1979. Data from the National Center for Health Statistics (NCHS) Hyattsville, Maryland.

Boys: 2 to 18 Years Physical Growth NCHS Percentiles*

Name ______________________ **Record #** ____________

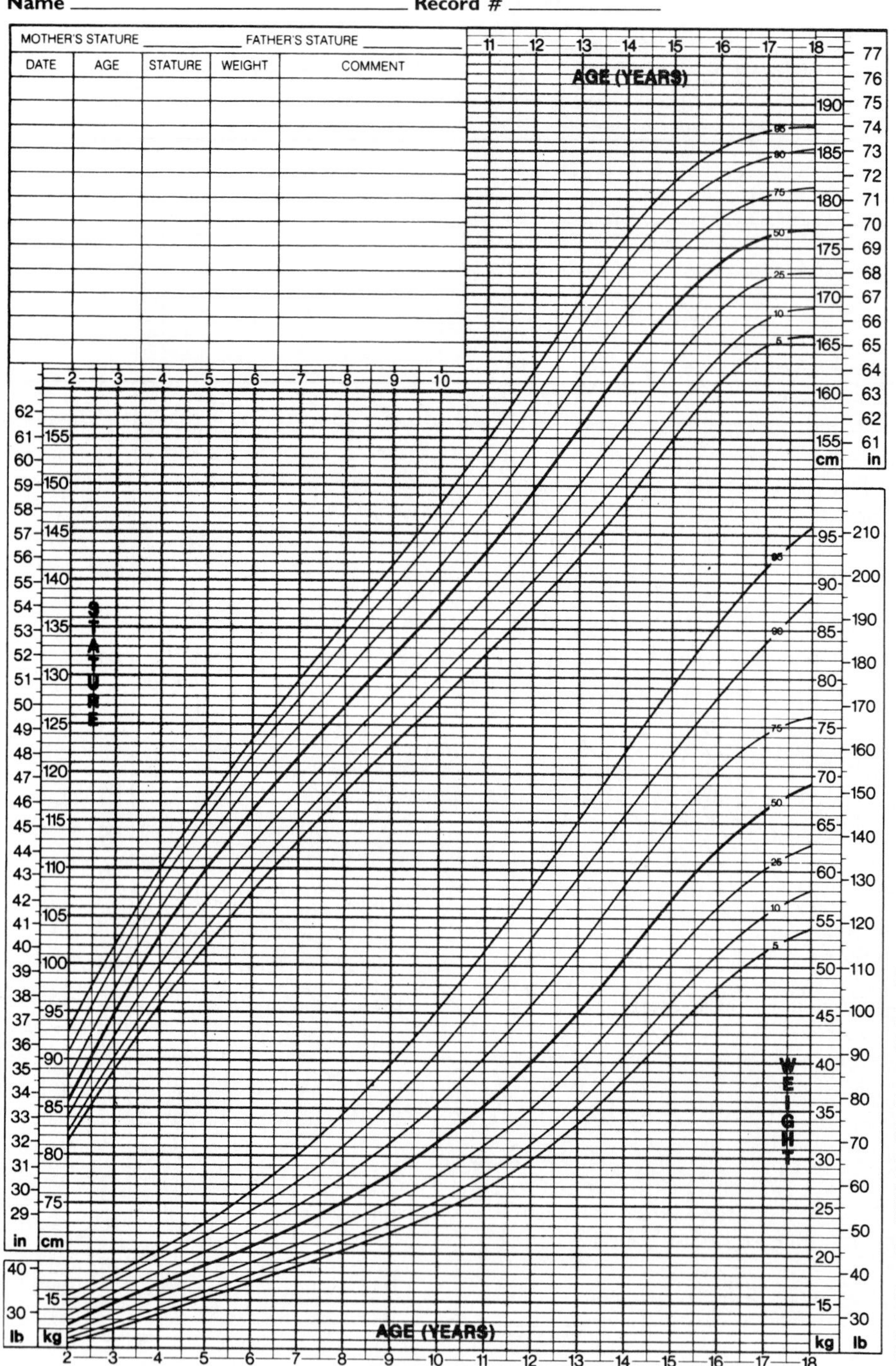

*Adapted from: Hamill PVV, Drizd TA, Johnson CL, Reed RB, Roche AF, Moore WM: Physical growth: National Center for Health Statistics percentiles. AM J CLIN NUTR 32:607-629, 1979. Data from the National Center for Health Statistics (NCHS) Hyattsville, Maryland.

Glossary

absorptive cells (ab-SORP-tiv) A class of cells that line the villi, fingerlike projections in the small intestine that participate in nutrient absorption.

acesulfame (ay-see-SUL-fame) An alternate sweetener that yields no energy to the body; it is 200 times sweeter than sucrose.

achlorhydria (ay-clor-HIGH-dre-ah) A state of reduced acid production by the stomach, primarily resulting from loss of the acid-producing cells in the stomach associated with aging.

acid ash Acid compounds that form from the residue of metabolized sulfur- and phosphorus-containing foods, such as protein foods.

acid pH A pH less than 7. Lemon juice has an acid pH.

active absorption Absorption in which a carrier is used and ATP energy is expended. In this way, the absorptive cell can absorb nutrients, such as glucose, against a concentration gradient.

adaptive thermogenesis Adaptive energy expended, resulting in the heat production, due to exposure to cold environmental conditions or overfeeding.

adenosine triphosphate (ATP) (ah-DEN-o-sin try-FOS-fate) The main energy currency for cells. ATP energy is used to promote ion pumping, enzyme activity, and muscular contraction.

adipose (fat) cells (ADD-ih-pos) Fat-storing cells.

adipsin (ah-DIP-sin) A protein that appears to be made by adipose cells and acts as a communication link between adipose cells and the brain.

adult-onset obesity Obesity that develops in adulthood; characterized by a normal number of adipose cells, but each cell is enlarged because of fat storage.

aerobic (air-ROW-bic) Requiring oxygen; aerobic activities use large muscle groups at moderate intensities. This permits the body to use oxygen to supply energy and to maintain a steady rate for more than a few minutes.

alcohol Ethyl alcohol or ethanol, CH_3CH_2OH.

alcohol dehydrogenase (dee-high-DRO-jen-ase) The enzyme used in alcohol (ethanol) breakdown; the major enzyme used in the liver when alcohol is in low concentrations.

aldosterone (al-DOS-ter-own) A powerful hormone produced by the adrenal glands that acts on the kidney to cause sodium reabsorption and, in turn, water conservation.

alimentary canal (al-ih-MEN-tah-ree) Gastrointestinal tract.

alkaline ash (AL-kah-line) Alkaline compounds that form in the body from residue of metabolized potassium- and sodium-containing foods, such as fruits and vegetables.

alkaline (basic) pH (Al-kah-line) A pH greater than 7. Baking soda in water yields an alkaline pH.

allergy (AL-ler-jee) An immune response when antibodies react with a foreign substance (antigen).

alpha bond (AL-fa) A type of carbohydrate bond that can be digested by human intestinal enzymes.

alpha-linolenic acid (AL-fah-lin-oh-LE-nik) An essential acid with 18 carbon atoms and 3 double bonds (omega-3).

alveoli (al-VE-o-lye) Small air sacs of the lung.

amino acid (ah-MEE-noh AH-sid) The building block for proteins containing a central carbon atom with a nitrogen atom and other atoms attached.

amniotic fluid (am-nee-OTT-ik) The fluid that surrounds and protects the fetus in the uterus.

amylase (AM-uh-lace) Starch-digesting enzymes from the salivary glands or pancreas.

amylopectin (am-ih-low-PEK-tin) A digestible branched-chain polysaccharide made of glucose units.

amylose (AM-uh-los) A digestible straight-chain digestible polysaccharide made of glucose units.

anabolic In a state of anabolism.

anabolism (an-AH-bol-iz-um) The process of building compounds.

anaerobic (AN-ah-ROW-bic) Not requiring oxygen; anaerobic sports activities use muscle groups at high intensities that exceed the body's capacity to supply energy using only oxygen-requiring pathways.

anaphylactic shock (an-ah-fih-LAK-tic) A severe allergic response that results in greatly lowered blood pressure, as well as respiratory and gastrointestinal distress.

androgen (AN-dro-jen) A general term for hormones that stimulate development in male sex organs; for example, testosterone.

android obesity (AN-droyd) Obesity in which fat storage is located primarily in the abdominal area; defined as a waist-to-hip circumference ratio greater than 0.9 in men and 0.8 in women. Android obesity is closely associated with a high risk of heart disease, hypertension, and diabetes.

anergy (AN-er-jee) Lack of an immune response to foreign compounds entering the body.

angiotensin I (an-jee-oh-TEN-sin) An intermediary compound produced during the body's attempt to conserve water and sodium; it is converted to angiotensin II.

angiotensin II A compound, produced in response to low blood pressure, that increases blood vessel constriction and triggers production of the hormone aldosterone.

animal model Study of disease in animals that duplicates human disease. This can be used to understand more about the human disease.

anorexia nervosa (an-oh-REX-ee-uh ner-VOH-sah) An eating disorder involving a psychological loss of appetite and self-starvation, resulting in part from a distorted body image and various social pressures associated with puberty.

anthropometry (an-throw-po-MEH-tree) The measurement of weight, lengths, circumferences, and thicknesses of the body.

antibody (AN-tih-bod-ee) Blood proteins that inactivate foreign proteins found in the body. This helps prevent infections.

antidiuretic hormone (ADH) (an-tie-dye-URET-ik) A hormone, secreted by the pituitary gland, that acts on the kidney to cause a decrease in water excretion.

antioxidant A compound that prevents the oxidation of substances in food or the body, particularly lipids. Antioxidants are especially important in preventing the oxidation of polyunsaturated lipids in the membranes of cells. An antioxidant is able to donate electrons to electron-seeking compounds. This in turn reduces electron capture and thus breakdown of unsaturated fatty acids and other cell components by oxidizing agents.

apoferritin (ape-oh-FERR-ih-tin) A protein in the intestinal cell that binds with the ferric form of iron (Fe^{+3}) to form ferritin.

apolipoproteins (APE-oh-lip-oh-PRO-teens) Proteins inbedded in the outer shell of lipoproteins. They help other enzymes function, act as a lipid transfer protein, or help bind to a receptor.

appetite (AP-peh-tight) The external (psychological) influences that encourage us to find and eat food, often in the absence of obvious hunger.

arachidonic acid (ar-a-kih-DON-ik) A fatty acid with 20 carbon atoms and four double bonds (omega-6).

areola (ah-REE-oh-lah) The circular dark area of skin at the center of the breast.

ariboflavinosis (aH-rih-bo-flay-vih-NOH-sis) A condition resulting from a lack of riboflavin. The "a" stands for "without", and the "osis" stands for "a condition of".

arithmetic ratio A group of numbers in which the difference between each number is the same.

aseptic processing (ah-SEP-tik) A method by which food and container are simultaneously sterilized. It allows manufacturers to produce boxes of milk that can be stored at room temperature. Variations of this process are also known as ultra high temperature (UHT) packaging.

aspartame (AH-spar-tame) A sweetener made of two amino acids and methanol; it is 200 times sweeter than sucrose.

atherosclerosis (ath-e-roh-scle-ROH-sis) A buildup of fatty material in the arteries, including those surrounding the heart.

atom Smallest combining unit of an element.

autodigestion Literally, self-digestion. The stomach limits autodigestion by covering itself with a thick layer of mucous and producing enzymes and acid only when needed for digestion of foodstuffs.

autoimmune Immune reactions against normal body cells; self against self.

avidin (AV-ih-din) A protein found in raw egg whites that can bind biotin and inhibit its absorption. Avidin is destroyed by cooking.

baryophobia (bear-ee-oh-FO-bee-ah) A disorder associated with a poor rate of growth in children because the parents underfeed them in an attempt to prevent development of obesity and/or heart disease.

basal metabolism (BAY-sal) The minimum energy the body requires to support itself when resting and awake. To have basal metabolic rate (BMR) measured, a person must not have eaten in the previous 12 hours and be maintained in a warm, quiet environment during the measurement. It amounts to roughly 1 kilocalorie per minute, or about 1400 kcalories per day.

beriberi (BEAR-ee-BEAR-ee) The thiamin deficiency disorder characterized by muscle weakness, loss of appetite, nerve degeneration, and sometimes edema.

beta bond (BAY-tuh) A type of carbohydrate bond that is not digested by human intestinal enzymes when it is part of a long chain of monosaccharides.

beta-oxidation The breakdown of a fatty acid into numerous acetyl-CoA molecules

BHA and BHT (Butylated hydroxyanisole and butylated hydroxytoluene) Two common synthetic antioxidants added to foods.

bile A substance made in the liver and stored in the gallbladder; it is released into the small intestine to aid fat absorption by emulsifying it into micelles.

bile acids Emulsifiers synthesized by the liver and released by the gallbladder during digestion to aid in fat digestion.

bioavailability The degree to which the amount of an ingested nutrient actually gets absorbed and so is available to the body.

biochemical lesion (LEE-zhun) Nutritional deficiency symptoms observed in the blood or urine, such as low levels of nutrient byproducts or low enzyme activities, indicating reduced body function.

bioelectrical impedance (im-PEE-dance) A method to estimate total body fat that uses a low-energy electrical current. The more fat storage a person has, the more impedance (resistance) to electrical flow will be exhibited.

biological value (BV) of a protein The body's ability to retain protein absorbed from a food.

biotechnology The use of advanced scientific techniques to alter and, ideally, improve characteristics of animals and plants.

blood doping A technique by which an athlete's red blood cell count is increased. Blood is taken from the athlete, and the red blood cells are concentrated and then later reintroduced into the athlete.

B-lymphocytes (LIM-fo-site) White blood cells synthesized by lymph tissues and responsible for antibody production.

body mass index Weight (in kilograms) divided by height squared (in meters). A value of 30 or greater shows obesity-related health risks.

bomb calorimeter (kal-oh-RIM-eh-ter) An instrument used to determine the kcalorie content of a food.

bond A sharing of electrons, charges, or attractions. This links two atoms.

bound water Water that is attached to organic substances. This is not available for microbial use.

brown adipose tissue (ADD-ih-pos) A specialized form of adipose tissue that produces large amounts of heat by metabolizing energy-yielding nutrients without synthesizing much ATP. The energy released simply forms heat.

buffer Compounds that can take up or release hydrogen ions to maintain a certain pH value in a solution.

bulimia (boo-LEEM-ee-uh) An eating disorder in which large quantities of food are eaten at one time (bingeing) and then purged from the body by vomiting, use of laxatives, or other means.

cafeteria-fed animal A laboratory animal that is fed a high-fat, high-sugar diet to encourage it to overeat and become obese.

calcitriol (kal-sih-TRIH-ol) The active hormone form of vitamin D (1,25-dihydroxy–vitamin D). It contains a derivative of cholesterol as part of its structure.

calmodulin (kal-MOD-you-lin) A cell protein that, once it binds calcium, can influence the activity of certain enzymes in the cell.

cancer A condition characterized by uncontrolled growth of abnormal body cells.

carbohydrate (kar-bow-HIGH-drate) A compound containing carbon, hydrogen, and oxygen atoms; most are known as sugars, starches, and dietary fibers.

carbohydrate-loading A process in which a 600-gram carbohydrate intake (or 70% of total energy, whichever is larger) is consumed for 6 to 7 days before an athletic event in an attempt to increase muscle glycogen stores.

cardiac output (CARD-ee-ack) Amount of blood pumped by the heart.
cardiovasculer Referring to the heart and blood vessels.
cariogenic (CARE-ee-oh-jen-ik) A substance, often carbohydrate-rich (such as caramels), that promotes dental caries.
carnitine (CAR-nih-teen) A compound used to shuttle fatty acids from the cytosol of the cell into mitochrondria.
carotenes (CARE-oh-teens) Pigment substances in plants that can often form vitamin A. Beta-carotene is the most active form.
carpal tunnel syndrome (CAR-pull) (SIN-drom) A disease where nerves that travel to the wrist are pinched as they pass through a narrow opening in a bone in the wrist.
casein (KAY-seen) Proteins in milk that form hard curds. These are difficult for infants to digest.
cash crops Crops grown by a country specifically for export rather than to feed the country's citizens (e.g., coffee, tea, cocoa, and bananas).
catalyst (CAT-ul-ist) A compound that speeds reaction rates but is not altered by the reaction.
catabolic/catabolism (cat-ah-BOL-ik) Breaking down compounds.
celiac disease Also known as gluten-induced enteropathy. It is caused by an allergy to protein found in wheat, rye, oats, and barley. If untreated, it causes a severe flattening of the villi in the intestine, leading to severe malabsorption of nutrients.
cell (SELL) A minute structure, the living basis of plant and animal organization. In animals it is bounded by a cell membrane. Cells contain both genetic material and systems for synthesizing energy-yielding compounds. Cells have the ability to both take up compounds from and excrete compounds into their surroundings.
cellulose (SELL-you-los) A straight-chain polysaccharide of glucose molecules that is undigestible because of the presence of beta carbohydrate bonds.
Celsius A centigrade measure of temperature. For conversion:
(degrees in Fahrenheit $-$ 32) $\times$ 5/9 $=$ °C
(degrees in centigrade $\times$ 9/5) $+$ 32 $=$ °F.
cerebrovascular accident (CVA) (se-REE-bro-VAS-cue-lar) Death of part of the brain tissue due to a blood clot.
ceruloplasmin (se-RUE-low-PLAS-min) A blue, copper-containing protein component of plasma that changes iron to Fe^{+3} (ferric form) so it can bind with apoferritin.
chain-breaking Breaking the link between two or more behaviors that encourage problem behaviors, such as snacking while watching television.
chemical reaction An interaction between two chemicals that changes both participants.
chemical score A ratio comparing the essential amino acid content of the protein in a food with the essential amino acid content in a reference protein, such as one established by the Food and Agriculture Organization. The lowest ratio for an essential amino acid is the chemical score.
cholecystokinin (CCK) (ko-la-sis-toe-KY-nin) A hormone that stimulates enzyme release from the pancreas and bile release from the gallbladder.
cholesterol (ko-LES-te-rol) A waxy lipid, it has a structure containing multiple chemical rings.
chronic (KRON-ik) Long-standing, developing over time; slow to develop or resolve. When referring to disease, this indicates that the disease progress, once developed, is slow and tends to remain; a good example is coronary heart disease.
chylomicrons (kye-lo-MY-krons) Dietary fat surrounded by a shell of cholesterol, phospholipids, and protein. These are made in the intestine after fat absorption and travel through the lymphatic system to the bloodstream.
chyme (KIME) A mixture of stomach secretions and partially digested food.
cirrhosis (see-ROH-sis) A loss of functioning liver cells, which are replaced by nonfunctioning connective tissue. Any substance that poisons liver cells can lead to cirrhosis. The most common cause is a long-standing, excessive alcohol intake.
cis isomer (sis-I-so-mer) An isomer form seen in compounds with double bonds, such as fat, where the hydrogens on both ends of the double bond lie on the same side of that bond.
citric acid cycle (SIT-rik) A pathway that breaks down acetyl-CoA, yielding carbon dioxide, $FADH_2$, NADH, and GTP. The pathway can also be used to synthesize compounds.
clinical lesion (LEE-zhun) Nutritional deficiency sign seen on physical examination.
clostridium botulinum (klo-STRID-ee-um BOT-you-LY-num) A bacterium that can cause a fatal type of food poisoning.
cognitive restructuring Changing negative, self-defeating, or pessimistic thoughts that undermine weight control efforts to those that are positive, optimistic, and supportive of weight control.
colic (KOL-ik) Periodic crying in a healthy infant, apparently resulting from gastrointestinal gas build-up.
colostrum (ko-LAHS-trum) The first fluid secreted by the breast during late pregnancy and the first days after birth. This thick fluid is rich in immune factors and protein.
complement A group of serum proteins involved in immune responses, such as phagocytosis and the destruction of bacteria.
complementarity of proteins The ability of two food protein sources to make up for each other's insufficient contribution of specific essential amino acids, such that together they yield a high-quality protein diet.
complete proteins Proteins that contain ample amounts of all nine essential amino acids.
compound A group of different types of atoms bonded together in definite proportion (see **molecule**)
compression of morbidity Using good health practices to delay the onset of disabilities caused by chronic disease.
condensation reaction A reaction that forms a bond between two compounds by removing a water molecule.
conditioning The process through which an originally neutral stimulus repeatedly paired with a reinforcing agent elicits a predictable response.
conjugase (KON-ju-gase) Enzyme systems in the intestine that enhance folate absorption; they remove glutamate molecules from polyglutamate forms.
connective tissue Protein tissue that holds different structures in the body together.
contingency management Forming a plan of action for responding to an environment in which overeating is likely, such as when snacks are within easy reach at a party.
control group Participants in an experiment whose habits are not altered.
cortical bone (KORT-ih-kal) Dense, compact bone that comprises the outer surface and shafts of bone.
cortisol (KORT-ih-sol) A hormone made by the adrenal gland that, among other functions, stimulates the production of glucose from amino acids.
covalent bond (ko-VAY-lent) A union of two atoms formed by the sharing of electrons.
cretinsim (KREET-in-ism) Stunting of body growth and poor mental development in an infant that results from inadequate maternal intake of iodine during pregnancy.

Crohn's disease (Krown) A disease of unknown cause in which the small intestine becomes severly inflamed and its absorptive capacity limited.
crude fiber What remains of dietary fiber after acid and alkaline treatment. This consists of primarily cellulose and lignin.
cystic fibrosis (SIS-tik-figh-BRO-sis) A disease that often leads to overproduction of mucus. Mucus can invade the pancreas, decreasing enzyme output. The lack of lipase enzyme output then contributes to severe fat malabsorption.
cytochromes (SITE-o-krome) Electron-transfer agents that participate in the electron transport chain.
cytotoxic test (SITE-o-TOX-ik) An unreliable test to diagnose food allergies that involves mixing whole blood with food proteins.
Daily Reference Values (DRV) Standards of intake for certain parts of a diet, such as carbohydrate, fat, saturated fat, cholesterol, sodium, potassium, and dietary fiber, set by FDA for which no U.S. RDA exist. These values are intended to be used for comparing intakes of these factors to desirable (or maximum) levels of intake.
deamination (dee-am-ih-NA-shun) The removal of an amine group from an amino acid.
Delaney clause This clause to the 1958 Food Additives Amendment of the Pure Food and Drug Act prevents the intentional (direct) addition to foods of a compound that has been shown to cause cancer in animals or man.
denature (dee-NAY-ture) Alteration of the tertiary structure of a protein, usually as a result of treatment by heat, acid, base, or agitation.
dental caries (KARE-ees) Erosions in the surface of a tooth caused by acids made by bacteria as they metabolize sugars.
depolarize To create a neutral or uncharged condition.
dextrin Partial breakdown products of starch that contain few to many glucose molecules. These appear while starch is being digested into many units of maltose.
diabetes mellitus (DYE-uh-BEET-eez MELL-uh-tus) A disease characterized by high blood sugar levels (hyperglycemia), resulting from either an insufficient insulin release by the pancreas or a general inability for insulin to act on certain body cells, such as adipose cells (see **insulin-dependent diabetes mellitus** and **noninsulin-dependent diabetes mellitus**).
diastolic blood pressure (dye-ah-STOL-ik) The pressure in the bloodstream found when the heart is between beats.
dietary fiber Substances in food (essentially from plants) that are not digested by the processes present in the stomach and small intestine.
dietary goals Specific goals for nutrient intakes set in 1977 by a Committee of the U.S. Senate.
dietary guidelines General goals for nutrient intake and diet composition set by government agencies—USDA and DHHS.
dietitian See **registered dietitian.**
digestibility (dye-JES-tih-bil-it-ee) The proportion of food substances eaten that can be broken down in the intestinal tract and absorbed into the bloodstream.
diphosphoglycerate (dye-foss-foe-gliss-er-ate) A compound used in the red blood cells that is involved in the release of oxygen from hemoglobin.
direct calorimetry (kal-oh-RIM-eh-tree) A method to determine energy use by the body by measuring heat that emanates from the body, usually using an insulated chamber.
disaccharides (dye-SACK-uh-rides) Class of sugars formed by the chemical bonding of two monosaccharides.
diuretic (dye-URET-ik) A substance that, when ingested, increases the flow of urine.
diverticula (DYE-ver-TIK-you-luh) Pouches that protrude through the wall of the large intestine to the outside of the intestine.
diverticulitis (DYE-ver-tik-you-LITE-us) An inflammation of the diverticula caused by acids produced by bacterial metabolism inside the diverticula.
diverticulosis (DYE-ver-tik-you-LOH-sis) The condition of having many diverticula in the colon.
docosahexaenoic acid (DHA) An omega-3 fatty acid with 22 carbons and six carbon-carbon double bonds. DHA is also present in fish oils and also may be synthesized from alpha-linolenic acid.
double-blind study An experiment in which the subjects and researchers are unaware of the subjects assignment (test or placebo) nor the outcome of the study until it is completed. An independent third party holds the code and the data until the study is completed.
duodenum (doo-oh-DEE-num, or doo-ODD-num) The first 12 inches (30 centimeters) of the small intestine.
ecosystem A "community" in nature that includes plants and animals and the environment associated with them.
ectomorph (EK-tuh-morf) A body type associated with very long, thin bones and very long, thin fingers.
edema (uh-DEE-muh) The build-up of fluid in extracellular spaces.
eicosanoids (eye-KOH-san-oyds) Hormonelike compounds synthesized from polyunsaturated fatty acids. Within this class of compounds are prostaglandins, thromboxanes, and leukotrienes.
eicosapentaenoic acid (EPA) (eye-KOH-sah-pen-tah-NO-ik) An omega-3 fatty acid with 20 carbon atoms and five double bonds; present in fish oils and may be synthesized from alpha-linolenic acid.
electrolytes (ih-LEK-tro-lites) Substances that break down into ions in water and, in turn, are able to conduct an electrical current. These include sodium, chloride, and potassium.
electron A part of an atom that is negatively charged. Electrons orbit the nucleus.
electron transport chain A series of reactions using oxygen that convert NADH and $FADH_2$ into free NAD and FAD, yielding water and ATP.
elements Substances that cannot be broken down further by using ordinary chemical procedures.
elimination diet A restrictive diet that systematically tests foods that may cause an allergic response by first eliminating suspected foods and then adding them back, one at a time.
embryo (Em-bree-oh) In humans the developing infant during the second to eighth week after conception.
emulsify (ee-MULL-sih-fye) To suspend fat in water by isolating individual fat drops using sheets of water molecules or other substances to prevent the fat from coalescing.
endocrine-onset obesity (EN-doh-krin) Obesity caused by rare hormonal abnormalities or rare genetic disorders. This is the cause of less than 10% of obesity in America.
endometrium (en-doh-ME-tree-um) A layer of cells that line the wall of the uterus.
endomorph (En-doh-morf) A body type characterized by short, stubby bones, a short trunk, and short fingers.
endorphins (en-DOR-fins) Natural body tranquilizers that may be involved in the feeding response and function in pain reduction.

endotoxin A toxin made by bacteria that is released by bacteria as they die and their cell walls are broken.

enriched A term generally meaning that the vitamins thiamin, niacin, and riboflavin and the mineral iron have been added to a grain product to improve nutritional quality.

enterohepatic circulation (EN-ter-oh-heh-PAT-ik) Recycling of compounds between the small intestine circulation and the liver over and over again, as happens with bile acids.

enzyme (EN-zime) A compound that speeds the rate of a chemical reaction but is not altered by the chemical reaction. Almost all enzymes are proteins.

epidemiology (ep-uh-dee-me-OLL-uh-gee) The study of how disease rates vary between different population groups, such as the rate of stomach cancer in Japan compared with that in Canada.

epigenetic carcinogens (promoters) (ep-ih-je-NET-ik car-SIN-oh-jens) Compounds that increase cell division and thereby increase the chance that a cell with altered DNA will develop into cancer.

epinephrine (ep-ih-NEE-rin) Also known as adrenaline. This hormone is released by the adrenal gland and various nerve endings in the body. It acts to increase glycogen breakdown in the liver, among other functions.

epithelial cells (ep-ih-THEE-lee-ul) The surface cells that line the outside of the body and all external passages within it.

equilibrium (ee-kwih-LIB-ree-um) In nutrition, a state in which nutrient intake equals nutrient losses. Thus the body maintains a stable condition.

ergogenic (ur-go-jen-ic) Work producing.

erythropoietin (eh-REE-throw-POY-eh-tin) A protein secreted by the kidneys that enhances red blood cell synthesis and stimulates red blood cell release from bone marrow.

essential (indespensible) amino acids Amino acids not efficiently synthesized by humans that must therefore be included in the diet. There are nine essential amino acids.

essential fatty acids Fatty acids that must be present in the diet to maintain health. These are linoleic acid and alpha-linolenic acid.

essential nutrient In nutritional terms, this represents a substance that, when left out of a diet, leads to signs of poor health. Then, if added back to a diet before permanent damage occurs the aspects of health affected are restored.

esterification (e-ster-ih-fih-KAY-shun) With regard to fats, the process of attaching fatty acids to a glycerol molecule, creating an ester bond. Removing a fatty acid is called deesterification; reattaching a fatty acid is called reesterification.

estimated safe and adequate daily dietary intake (ESADDI) Nutrient intake recommendations by the Food and Nutrition Board. A range for intake of some nutrients is given as not enough information is available to set a more specific RDA.

eustachian tubes (you-STAY-shun) Thin tubes connected to the middle ear that open into the throat.

exchange The serving size of a food within a specific exchange system group.

exchange system A grouping of foods into six lists. When the proper serving size for any food in a list is consumed, all foods within the list yield a similar amount of carbohydrate, fat, protein, and energy.

exotoxin A toxin made by bacteria that is excreted into its surrounding medium as the toxin is made.

experiment A test made to examine the validity of a hypothesis.

extracellular fluid Fluid present outside the cells; this includes intravascular and interstitial fluids.

extracellular space The space between cells.

facilitated absorption Absorption where a carrier is used to shuttle substances into the absorptive cells, but no energy is expended. A concentration gradient higher in the intestinal contents than in the absorptive cell drives the absorption.

failure to thrive Inadequate gains in height and weight in infancy, often due to an inadequate food intake.

famine A time of massive starvation, often associated with crop failures, war, and political strife.

fasting hypoglycemia (HIGH-po-gligh-SEE-me-uh) Low blood sugar that follows a day or so of fasting.

fatty acids Acids found in lipids, composed of carbon atoms and hydrogen atoms with an acid group

$$(-\overset{\overset{\displaystyle O}{\|}}{C}-OH)$$

at one end and a methyl group ($-CH_3$) at the other.

feeding center A group of cells in the hypothalamus that, when stimulated, causes hunger. These cells are also known as the lateral feeding centers.

ferritin (FERR-ih-tin) A protein compound that serves as the storage form of iron in the blood and tissues.

fetal alcohol syndrome (FAS) (FEET-al) A group of physical and mental abnormalities in the infant that result from the mother consuming alcohol during pregnancy.

fetus (FEET-us) The developing life form from 8 weeks until birth.

flavin adenine dinucleotide (FAD) (FLAY-vin ADD-eh-neen dye-NUK-lee-oh-tide) A hydrogen carrier in the cell; synthesized from the vitamin riboflavin.

fluoroapatite (fleur-oh-APP-uh-tite) Tooth crystals containing fluoride ions that are relatively acid resistant.

food-borne illness Sickness caused by ingestion of foods containing toxic substances produced by microorganisms.

food intolerance An adverse reaction to food that does not involve an immune response.

food sensitivity A mild reaction to a substance in a food that might be expressed as slight itching or redness of the skin.

fore milk (FOR) The first breast milk delivered in the nursing session.

fortified A term generally meaning that vitamins, minerals, or both have been added to a food product in excess of what was originally found in the product.

fraternal twins Fetuses that develop from two separate ova and sperm and therefore have separate genetic identities, although they develop simultaneously in the mother.

free erythrocyte protoporphyrins (FEP) (eh-RITH-row-sight pro-tow-POR-fy-rins) Immature forms of red blood cells released from the bone marrow. An increased serum level of FEP reflects a decreased ability to make red blood cells and suggests iron-deficiency anemia. Lead poisoning also raises blood FEP levels.

free radical Short-lived form of compounds that exist with an unpaired electron in their outer electron shell. This causes it to have an electron-seeking nature, which can be very destructive to electron-dense areas of a cell, such as DNA and cell membranes.

free water The water not bound to the components in a food. This is available for microbial use.

fructose (FROOK-tose) A monosaccharide with six carbons that form a five-membered ring with oxygen in the ring; found in fruits and honey.

fruitarian (froot-AIR-een-un) A person who eats primarily fruits, nuts, honey, and vegetable oils.
galactose (gah-LAK-tose) A six-carbon monosaccharide; an isomer of glucose.
galactosemia (gah-LAK-toh-SEE-mee-ah) A disease characterized by the buildup of the monosaccharide galactose in the bloodstream resulting from the inability of the liver to metabolize it. If present at birth and left untreated, this disease causes severe growth and mental retardation in the infant.
gastric balloon (GAS-trik) A balloon about the size of a soft drink can that is inserted surgically into the upper part of the stomach to stimulate feelings of satiety.
gastric inhibitory peptide (GAS-trik in-HIB-ih-tor-ee-PEP-tide) A hormone that slows gastric motility and stimulates insulin release from the pancreas.
gastrin (GAS-trin) A hormone that stimulates enzyme and acid secretion in the stomach.
gastrointentional distention Expansion of the walls of the stomach or intestines due to pressure caused by the presence of gases, food, drink, or other factors.
gastrointestinal (GI) tract (GAS-troh-in-TES-tin-al) The main sites in the body used for digestion and absorption of nutrients. It consists of the mouth, esophagus, stomach, small intestine, large intestine, rectum, and anus.
gastroplasty (GAS-troh-plas-tee) Surgery performed on the stomach to limit its volume to approximately 50 milliliters, the size of a shot glass.
gene (JEAN) The genetic material on chromosomes that provides the blueprint for the production of cell proteins.
generally recognized as safe (GRAS) A group of food additives that in 1958 were considered safe, therefore allowing manufacturers to use them thereafter when needed in food products. The FDA bears responsibility for proving they are not safe and can remove unsafe products.
genetic engineering Alteration of genetic material in plants or animals with the intent of improving growth, disease resistance, or other characteristics.
genotoxic carcinogen (initiator) (JEH-no-TOK-sik car-SIN-oh-jen) A compound that alters DNA in a cell, in turn providing the potential for cancer to develop.
geometric ratio A group of numbers in which the division of each number by the one to the left of it yields the same answer.
gestation (jes-TAY-shun) The time between conception and birth of the fetus.
gestational diabetes (jes-TAY-shun-al) A high blood glucose level that develops during pregnancy but returns to normal after birth. One cause is production of hormones by the placenta that antagonize the action of the hormone insulin.
glucagon (GLOO-kuh-gon) A hormone made by the pancreas that stimulates the breakdown of glycogen in the liver into glucose; this raises the blood glucose level. Glucagon also performs other functions.
gluconeogenesis (gloo-ko-nee-oh-JEN-uh-sis) The production of new glucose molecules by metabolic pathways in the cell. The source of the carbon atoms for these new glucose molecules is usually amino acids.
glucose (GLOO-kos) A six-carbon atom carbohydrate found in blood and in table sugar bound to fructose; also known as dextrose, it is one of the simple sugars.
glucose polymer A carbohydrate source used in some sports drinks that consists of bonding of a few glucose molecules together.
glutathione peroxidase (gloo-tah-THIGH-own per-OX-ih-dase) A selenium-containing enzyme that can break down peroxides. It acts in conjunction with vitamin E to stabilize free radicals.
glycemic index (gligh-SEE-mik) A ratio used to measure the relative ability of a carbohydrate to raise blood glucose levels as opposed to the ability of white bread (or glucose) to raise blood glucose levels.
glycerol (GLISS-er-ol) An alcohol containing three hydroxyl groups (—OH); used to help form triglyceride molecules.
glycogen (GLIGH-ko-jen) A carbohydrate made of multiple units of glucose; exhibits a highly branched structure; the storage form of carbohydrate for muscle and liver; sometimes known as animal starch.
glycolysis (gligh-COLL-ih-sis) The pathway that results in the breakdown of glucose into two pyruvate (lactate) molecules.
glycosidic bond (gligh-coh-SID-ik) The covalent bond formed between two monosaccharides when a water molecule is lost.
goiter (GOY-ter) An enlargement of the thyroid gland often caused by a lack of iodide in the diet.
goitregens (GOY-troh-jens) Substances in food that interfere with thyroid hormone metabolism and so may cause goiter if consumed in large amounts.
gram Measure of weight in the metric system. One gram equals 1/28 of an ounce.
green revolution A period in the 1960s when much emphasis was placed on improving strains and cultivation practices of cereal grains, such as rice, wheat, and corn.
growth hormone A pituitary hormone that produces body growth and the release of fat from storage, among other effects.
gum A dietary fiber containing chains of galactose, glucuronic acid, and other monosaccharides; characteristically found in exudates from plant stems.
gynecoid obesity (GIGH-nih-coyd) Obesity in which fat storage is located primarily in the buttocks and thigh area.
H_2 blockers Medications, such as cimetidine, that block the stimulation of stomach acid production caused by histamine.
Harris-Benedict equation An equation that predicts resting metabolic rate based on a person's weight, height, and age.
heartburn A pain emanating from the esophagus, caused by stomach acid backing up into the esophagus and irritating the esophageal tissue.
heart disease Disease usually caused by the deposition of fatty material in the blood vessels in the heart. This in turn reduces blood flow to the heart, thereby reducing heart function.
heat-labile (LAY-bile) A structure or activity that is changed by heating.
hematocrit (hee-MAT-oh-krit) The percentage of total blood volume occupied by red blood cells.
heme iron (HEEM) Iron provided from animal tissues as products of hemoglobin and myoglobin. Appoximately 40% of the iron in meat is heme iron. This is readily absorbed.
hemicellulose (hem-ih-SELL-you-los) A dietary fiber containing xylose, galactose, glucose, and other monosaccharides bonded together.
hemochromatosis (heem-oh-krom-ah-TOS-sis) A disorder of iron metabolism characterized by increased iron absorption, increased saturation of iron-binding proteins, and deposition of hemosiderin in the liver tissue.
hemoglobin (HEEM-oh-glow-bin) The iron-containing protein in the red blood cell that carries oxygen to the cells and carbon dioxide away from the cells. It is also responsible for the red color of blood.
hemolysis (hee-MOL-ih-sis) A breakdown of red blood cells caused by the destruction of the red blood cell membranes.

hemorrhoids (HEM-or-oyds) A pronounced swelling in a large vein, particularly veins found in the anal region.

hemosiderin (heem-oh-SID-er-in) An insoluble iron-protein compound found in the liver. Hemosiderin stores increase as the amount of iron in the liver exceeds the storage capacity of ferritin.

herbicide (erb-ih-side) A compound that reduces the growth and reproduction of plants.

hexose (HEK-sos) A general term describing a carbohydrate containing six carbon atoms.

high-density lipoprotein (HDL) The lipoprotein synthesized by the liver and intestine that picks up cholesterol from dying cells and other sources and transfers it to the other lipoproteins in the bloodstream. A low HDL level increases the risk for heart disease.

high-fructose corn syrup A corn syrup that has been manufactured to contain between 40% and 90% fructose.

high-quality proteins Proteins that contain ample amounts of all nine essential amino acids.

hind milk (HYND) The milk secreted at the end of a nursing session; it is higher in fat than fore milk.

histamine (HISS-tuh-meen) A breakdown product of the amino acid histidine that stimulates acid secretion by the stomach and other effects on the body, such as contraction of smooth muscles, increased nasal secretions, relaxation of blood vessels, and changes in relaxation of airways.

homeostasis A series of adjustments that act to prevent change in the internal environment in the body.

hormone A compound secreted into the bloodstream that acts to control the function of target organ cells. Hormones can be either proteinlike or fatlike, such as insulin or estrogen.

hunger The internal or physiological drive to find and eat food.

hydrogenation (high-dro-jen-AY-shun) The addition of hydrogen atoms to the double bonds of polyunsaturated and monounsaturated fatty acids to reduce the extent of unsaturation. This process turns liquid vegetable oils into solid fats.

hydroloysis reaction (high-DROL-ih-sis) A reaction in which a compound is split into parts, releasing water in the process.

hydrophilic (high-dro-FILL-ik) Attracts water (literally, "water loving").

hydrophobic (high-dro-FO-bik) Repels water (literally, "water fearing").

hydroxyapatite (high-drox-ee-APP-uh-tite) A compound composed of calcium and phosphate that is deposited into the bone protein matrix to give bone strength and rigidity.

hyperactivity A poorly defined term generally used to label inattention, irritability, and excessively active behavior in children.

hypercalcemia (high-per-kal-SEE-mee-ah) A high level of calcium in the bloodstream. This can lead to loss of appetite, calcium deposits in organs, and other health problems.

hypercarotenemia (high-per-car-oh-teh-NEEM-ee-ah) High level of carotene in the bloodstream, usually caused by a diet high in carrots or other yellow/orange vegetables.

hyperglycemia (HIGH-per-gligh-SEE-me-uh) High blood glucose levels, above 140 milligrams per 100 milliliters of blood.

hyperplasia (high-per-PLAY-zee-uh) An increase in cell number.

hypertension (high-per-TEN-shun) A condition in which blood pressure remains persistently elevated, especially when the heart is between beats.

hypertrophy (high-PURR-tro-fee) An increase in cell size.

hypochromic (high-po-KROME-ik) Pale red blood cells lacking sufficient hemoglobin (often caused by an iron deficiency); these have reduced oxygen-carrying ability.

hypoglycemia (HIGH-po-gligh-SEE-mee-uh) Low blood glucose levels, below 40 to 50 milligrams per 100 milliliters of blood.

hypothalamus (high-po-THALL-uh-mus) A part of the brain that contains cells that play a role in the regulation of hunger, respiration, body temperature, and other body functions.

hypothesis (high-POTH-eh-sis) An "educated guess" by a scientist to explain a phenomenon.

identical twins Two fetuses that develop from a single ovum and sperm and, consequently, have the same genetic makeup.

ileum (ILL-ee-um) The terminal segment of the small intestine.

incidental food additives Additives that gain access to food products indirectly from environmental contamination of food ingredients or during the manufacturing process.

incomplete (low-quality) proteins Food protein that lacks ample amount of one or more of the essential amino acids needed to support human protein needs.

indirect calorimetry (kal-oh-RIM-eh-tree) A method to measure the energy output by the body by measuring oxygen uptake and/or carbon dioxide output. Formulas are then used to convert these gas exchange values into kcalorie use.

infectious disease (in-FEK-shus) Any disease caused by an invasion of the body by microorganisms, such as bacteria, fungi, or viruses.

infrastructure The basic framework of a system or organization. For society, this includes roads, bridges, telephones, and other basic technologies.

inorganic Free of carbon atoms bonded to hydrogen atoms.

insensible losses Fluid losses that are not perceptible to the senses, such as losses through lungs, feces, and skin (an exception is heavy perspiration).

insoluble fibers (in-sol-you-bul) Fibers that, for the most part, do not dissolve in water nor are digested by bacteria in the large intestine. These include cellulose, some hemicelluloses, and lignin.

insulin (IN-suh-lin) A hormone produced by the beta cells of the pancreas. Insulin increases the synthesis of glycogen in the liver and the movement of glucose from the bloodstream into muscle and adipose cells, among other processes.

insulin-dependent diabetes mellitus A form of diabetes prone to ketosis and that requires insulin therapy.

intentional food additives Additives knowingly (directly) incorporated into food products by manufacturers.

intermediate density lipoprotein (IDL) (lip-oh-PRO-teen) The product formed after a very low density lipoprotein (VLDL) has most of its triglyceride removed.

international unit (IU) A crude measure of vitamin activity, often based on the growth rate of animals. Today these units have been replaced by more precise microgram quantities.

interstitial fluid (in-ter-STISH-ul) Fluid between cells.

intestinal bypass A surgical procedure that causes intentional malabsorption of food by shortening the length of the intestine by about 12 of its normal 15 feet. This procedure is no longer used to treat obesity because of the many medical problems that result.

intracellular fluid Fluid contained within a cell.

intravascular fluid Fluid within the bloodstream (that is, in the arteries, veins, and capillaries).

intraveneous (in-tra-VEEN-us) Introduced directly into the bloodstream.
intrinsic factor A proteinlike compound produced by the stomach that enhances vitamin B-12 absorption.
in utero (in YOU-ter-oh) "In the uterus" or, in other words, during pregnancy.
ion An atom with an unequal number of electrons and protons. If the number of electrons exceeds the number of protons, the ion is negative. If the number of protons exceeds the number of electrons, the ion is positive.
ionic bond (eye-OH-ik) A union between two atoms formed by an attraction of a positive ion to a negative ion, as seen in table salt (Na^+Cl^-).
irradiation (ir-RAY-dee-AY-shun) A process in which radiation energy is applied to foods. This then creates compounds (free radicals) in the food that destroy cell membranes, break down DNA, link proteins together, limit enzyme activity, and alter a variety of other proteins and cell functions that can lead to food spoilage. The net result is less food spoilage.
isomer (EYE-so-mer) Different chemical structures for compounds that share the same chemical formula.
isotope (EYE-so-towp) An alternate form of a chemical element. It differs from other atoms of the same element in the number of neutrons in its nucleus.
jaundice (JAWN-diss) A yellow staining of the skin and sclera (white of the eye) resulting from a buildup of bile pigments in the bloodstream. Liver or gallbladder disease is often the cause.
jejunem (je-JOON-um) The first half of the small intestine (minus the first 12 inches, which is the duodenum).
juvenile-onset obesity Obesity that develops in childhood; often characterized by an excess number of adipose cells that are also very large because of abundant fat storage.
kcalories (kay-KAL-oh-rees) The heat needed to raise the temperature of 1000 grams (1 liter) of water 1 degree Celsius.
ketone (kee-tone) Incomplete breakdown products of fat containing three or four carbons. These contain a ketone chemical group, hence, the name. An example is acetoacetic acid.
ketone bodies (KEE-tone) Products of acetyl-CoA (fat) metabolism containing three to four carbon atoms: acetoacetic acid, beta-hydroxybutyric acid, and acetone. These contain a ketone group, hence, the name.
ketogenic A name often given to diets that lead to the abundant production of ketones by the liver. This can be caused by a low carbohydrate intake.
ketosis (kee-TOE-sis) The condition of having high levels of ketones in the bloodstream.
kidney nephrons (NEF-rons) Cells of the kidney that filter waste out of the blood.
kjoule (KAY-jool) A measure of work in which one kjoule equals the work needed to move 1 kilogram a distance of 1 meter with the force of one newton. One kcalorie equals 4.18 kjoules.
kwashiorkor (kwash-ee-OR-core) A disease seen primarily in young children who have an existing disease and who consume a marginal amount of kcalories and considerably insufficient protein in the face of high needs. The child will suffer from infections and exhibit edema, poor growth, weakness, and an increased susceptibility to further illness.
lactic acid (LAK-tik AS-id) A three-carbon acid; also called lactate, formed during anaerobic cell metabolism; a partial breakdown product of glucose.
lactobacillus bifidus factor (lak-toe-bah-SIL-us BIFF-id-us) A protective factor secreted in human milk that encourages growth of beneficial bacteria in the intestine of the infant.
lacto-ovo vegetarian A person who consumes only plant products, dairy products, and eggs.
lacto-ovo-pesco vegetarian A person who consumes only plant products, dairy products, eggs, and fish.
lactose (lak-tose) A sugar made up of glucose linked to another sugar, called galactose.
lactose intolerance (primary and secondary) Primary lactose intolerance takes place when lactase production declines for no apparent reason. Secondary lactose intolerance takes place when a specific cause, like long-standing diarrhea, results in a decline in lactase production.
lactovegetarian (lak-toe vej-eh-TEAR-ree-an) A person who consumes only plant products and dairy products.
lanugo (lah-NEW-go) Downlike hair that appears after one has lost much body fat during semistarvation. The hair stands erect and traps air, which acts as insulation to the body, replacing that usually supplied by body fat. Fetuses also show lanugo.
larvae (LAR-vee) An early developmental stage in the life history of some microorganisms, such as parasites.
laxative A medication or other substance that stimulates evacuation of the intestinal tract.
lean body mass The part of the human body that is free of all but essential body fat. About 2% of body weight as fat is essential to retain. The rest of the fat in the body represents storage and so is not part of lean body mass. Lean body mass includes muscle, bone, organs, connective tissue, skin, and other body parts.
lecithin (less-uh-thin) A group of phospholipids containing two fatty acids, a phosphate group, and a choline molecule.
"let-down reflex" A reflex stimulated by infant suckling that causes the release (ejection) of milk from milk ducts in the mother's breasts.
leukotriene An important mediator of many diseases involving inflammatory or hypersensitivity reactions, such as asthma.
life expectancy Average length of life for a given group of people.
life span Potential oldest age to which a person can survive.
lignin (LIG-nin) An insoluble fiber made up of a multiringed alcohol (noncarbohydrate) structure.
limiting amino acid The essential amino acid in the lowest concentration in a food in comparison with the body's need.
linoleic acid (lin-oh-LEE-ik) An essential fatty acid with 18 carbon atoms and two double bonds; omega-6.
lipase (LYE-pase) Fat digesting enzymes; linguinal lipase is produced by the tongue, gastric lipase by the stomach, and pancreatic lipase by the pancreas.
lipid (LIP-id) A compound containing much carbon and hydrogen, little oxygen, and sometimes other atoms. Lipids dissolve in ether or benzene and include fats, oils, and cholesterol.
lipofuscin (ceroid pigments) (lip-oh-FEW-shun SER-oyd) Signs of accumulation of lipid breakdown products, often seen as brown spots on the skin.
lipogenesis (lye-poh-JEN-eh-sis) The building of fatty acids using derivatives of acetyl-CoA molecules.
lipogenic (lye-poh-JEN-ik) Means creating lipid. The liver is the major lipogenic organ in the human body.
lipolysis (lye-POL-ih-sis) The breakdown of lipid.
lipoprotein (lye-poh-PRO-teen) A compound found in the bloodstream containing a core of lipids with a shell of protein, phospholipid, and cholesterol.

lipoprotein lipase (lye-poh-PRO-teen LYE-pase) An enzyme attached to the outsides of some cells that line the bloodstream; it breaks down triglycerides into free fatty acids and glycerol.

liter (LEE-ter) A measure of volume in the metric system. One liter equals 0.96 quarts.

lobules (LOB-you-els) Saclike structures in the breast that store milk.

long-chain fatty acids Fatty acids that contain more than 12 carbon atoms.

low birth weight (LBW) Infant weight at birth of less than 2500 grams (5.5 pounds); caused by either premature birth or growth retardation during pregnancy.

low-density lipoprotein (LDL) The product of the intermediate density lipoprotein (IDL) containing primarily cholesterol. An elevated level is strongly linked to heart disease risk.

low input sustainable agriculture (LISA) A form of farming that attempts to limit use of purchased materials, such as manufactured fertilizers and pesticides. Use of manure and crop rotation are typical substitutes.

low-quality (incomplete) proteins Food proteins that lack an ample amount of one or more amino acids essential for human protein needs.

lumen (LOO-men) The inside cavity of a tube, such as the GI tract.

lymphatic system (lim-FAT-ick) A system of vessels in the body that can convey lymph particles, such as chylomicrons, from tissues into the bloodstream.

lysosome (LYE-so-som) A cellular organelle that contains digestive enzymes for use inside the cell for turnover of cell parts.

lysozyme (LYE-so-zime) A substance produced by a variety of cells in the body that can destroy bacteria.

macrocyte (MAC-row-site) A greatly enlarged mature red blood cell having a short lifespan.

major mineral A mineral vital to health that is required in the diet in amounts greater than 100 milligrams per day.

malnutrition Failing health that results from a long-standing dietary intake that fails to match nutritional needs.

maltose (MAWL-tose) Glucose bonded to glucose; a simple sugar.

mannitol (MAN-it-tol) An alcohol derivative of fructose.

marasmus (mah-RAZ-mus) Results from a person consuming insufficient protein and kcalories; usually seen in infancy. It is the equivalent of protein-energy malnutrition in adults. The person will have little or no fat stores and show muscle wasting.

marginal Noticeable but not severe.

mass movement A peristaltic wave that simultaneously coordinates contraction over a large area of the colon. Mass movements move material from one portion of the colon to another and from the colon into the rectum.

mast cells Cells in the body that contain histamine and are responsible for some aspects of allergic and inflammatory reactions.

maximum volume of oxygen consumption (Vo_2 max) The maximum amount of oxygen consumption a person can achieve during exercise, such as when riding a bicycle or running on a treadmill.

meconium (mee-KOH-nee-um) The first thick, mucousy stool passed after birth.

medium-chain fatty acids Fatty acids that contain 8 to 10 carbon atoms.

megaloblast (MEG-ah-low-blast) A large, immature red blood cell that results from an inability for cell division during red blood cell development.

menaquinones (men-AH-kwih-nones) Forms of vitamin K that come from animal food sources or bacterial synthesis.

menarche (men-AR-kee) Onset of menses in women, usually between ages 10 to 13 years.

menopause (MEN-oh-paws) The cessation of menses in women, usually beginning at about 50 years of age.

mesomorph (mez-oh-morf) A body type associated with average bone size, trunk size, and finger length.

metabolism (meh-TAB-oh-lizm) Chemical reactions that occur in the body, enabling cells to release energy from foods, convert one substance into another, and prepare end products for excretion.

metallothionein (meh-TAL-oh-THIGH-oh-neen) Protein that binds and regulates the release of zinc and copper (and other positive ions) in intestinal and liver cells.

meter (MEET-er) A measure of length in the metric system. One meter equals 39.4 inches.

micelles (MY-sells) An emulsification product in which individual emulsifiers organize with their hydrophobic parts to the center of the micelle and their hydrophilic parts to the outside. Lipids are attracted to the center area and water is attracted to the outside periphery.

microcytic (my-kro-SIT-ik) Literally, "small cell." Red blood cells that are smaller than normal.

microfractures Small fractures, undetectable by x-rays or other bone scans, that may occur frequently in bones.

microsomol ethanol oxidizing system (my-kro-SO-mol ETH-an-ol) An alternative pathway for alcohol metabolism when alcohol is in high concentrations in the liver; uses rather than yields energy.

minerals Elements used in the body to promote chemical reactions and help form body structures.

miscarriage Termination of pregnancy that occurs before the fetus can survive; also called spontaneous abortion.

mitochondria Organelles inside most cells, including muscle cells. These are the main sites of energy production in a cell. Mitochondria also contain the pathway for burning fat for fuel, among other metabolic pathways.

modified food starch Starch molecules that have been chemically linked together to increase stability.

molecule A group of like or unlike atoms chemically combined (see **compound**).

monoglyceride (mon-oh-GLIS-er-ide) A breakdown product of a triglyceride consisting of one fatty acid bonded to a glycerol backbone.

monosaccharide (mon-oh-SACK-uh-ride) A single sugar, such as glucose, that is not broken down further during digestion.

monounsaturated fatty acid A fatty acid containing one $C = C$ double bond.

mortality Death rate. The term morbidity refers to the amount of sickness present.

mottling (MOT-ling) Discoloration or marking of the surface of teeth caused by a high fluoride content.

mucilage (MYOO-sih-laj) A dietary fiber consisting of chains of galactose, mannose, and other monosaccharides; characteristically found in seaweed.

mucopolysaccharides (MYOO-ko-POL-ee-SAK-ah-rides) Substances containing protein and carbohydrate parts; found in bone and other organs.

mucus (MYOO-cuss) A thick fluid secreted by glands throughout the body. It contains a compound that has both carbohydrate and protein parts (glycoprotein). It acts as a lubricant and means of protection for cells.

mycotoxins (MY-ko-tok-sins) A group of toxic compounds produced by molds, such as aflatoxin B-1 found on moldy grains.

myocardial infarction (MY-oh-CARD-ee-ahl in-FARK-shun) Death of part of the heart muscle.

myoglobin (my-oh-GLOW-bin) Iron-containing compound that binds oxygen (O_2) in muscle.

net protein utilization Biological value of a protein multiplied by digestibility of that protein.

neutron (NEW-tron) The part of an atom that has no charge.

neutrophil (NEW-tro-fil) The major form of white blood cells, comprising 55% to 65% of the total.

nicotinamide adenine dinucleotide (NAD) (nik-oh-TIN-ah-mide AD-en-een dye-NUK-lee-oh-tide) A hydrogen carrier that represents a potential form of energy; made from the vitamin niacin.

nonessential (dispensible) amino acids Amino acids that can be readily made by the body. There are 11 nonessential amino acids found in foods.

nonheme iron Iron provided from plant sources and animal tissues other than part of hemoglobin and myoglobin. Nonheme iron needs to be changed to Fe^{+2} before absorption; less efficiently absorbed than heme iron.

noninsulin-dependent diabetes mellitus A form of diabetes in which ketosis is not commonly seen. Insulin therapy can be used, but often is not required.

nonpolar A compound with no charges present; no positive or negative poles present.

no observable effect level (NOEL) The highest dose of an additive that, when fed, produces no deleterious health effect in animals.

nucleus (NEW-klee-us) In chemistry, the core of an atom; it consists of protons and neutrons.

nutrient density The ratio formed by dividing a food's contribution to the needs for a nutrient by its contribution to kcalorie needs. When the contribution to nutrient needs exceeds that of kcalorie needs, the food is considered to have a favorable nutrient density for that nutrient.

nutrients Chemical substances in food that nourish the body by providing energy, building materials, and factors to regulate needed chemical reactions in the body.

nutrition The Council on Food and Nutrition of the American Medical Association defines nutrition as "the science of food; the nutrients and the substances therein; their action, interaction, and balance in relation to health and disease;" and the process by which the organism (i.e., body) ingests, digests, absorbs, transports, utilizes, and excretes food substances."

nutrition label A label format that must be included on foods under certain circumstances, such as when nutrients are added to foods or when a nutritional claim is made for the food. The nutrition label follows specific guidelines set by the FDA. New labeling laws are likely to alter the current format.

nutritional status The nutritional health of a person as determined by **a**nthropometric measures (height, weight, circumferences, and so on), **b**iochemical measures of nutrients or their by-products in blood and urine, a **c**linical (physical) examination, and a **d**ietary analysis (ABCD).

nutritionist A person who advises about nutrition and/or works in the field of food and nutrition. In many states in the United States a person does not need formal training to use this title. Some states reserve this title for Registered Dietitians.

obesity (oh-BEES-ih-tee) A condition characterized by excess body fat, usually defined as 20% above desirable weight.

oleic acid A fatty acid with 18 carbons and one carbon-carbon double bond; omega-9.

oligosaccharides (ol-ih-go-SAK-ah-rides) Carbohydrates containing three to ten monosaccharide units.

omega-3 (ω-3) fatty acid A fatty acid with its first double bond first appearing at the third carbon atom from the methyl end ($—CH_3$).

omega-6 (ω-6) fatty acid A fatty acid with its first double bonds first appearing at the sixth carbon atom from the methyl end ($—CH_3$).

omnivore (ahm-nih-voor) A person who consumes foods from both plants and animals.

oncogenes (ahn-ko-jeens) Genes that code for proteins that in turn cause growth.

oncotic force (ahn-KAH-tik) The osmotic potential exerted by proteins in the bloodstream.

organ A group of tissues designed to perform a specific function; for example, the heart. It contains muscle tissue, nerve tissue, and so on.

organic A compound that contains carbon atoms bonded to hydrogen atoms.

organism A living thing. The human body is an organism consisting of many organs that act in a coordinated manner to support life.

osmotic potential (oz-MOT-ik) The tendency to attract water across a semipermeable membrane, usually to dilute some constituent in a fluid.

osmotic pressure The pressure needed to be exerted to keep particles in a solution from drawing liquid across a semipermeable membrane.

osteomalacia (OS-tee-oh-mal-AY-shuh) Adult rickets. A vitamin D deficiency disease that causes weak bones and increases fracture risk.

osteopenia (os-tee-oh-PEE-nee-ah) Decreased bone mass, resulting from cancer, hyperthyroidism, or other causes.

osteoporosis (os-tee-oh-po-ROH-sis) A bone disease that develops primarily after menopause in women and is characterized by a decrease in bone density.

ostomy (OSS-toh-mee) A surgically created short circuit in intestinal flow where the exit point is usually through the abdomen, rather than at the anus.

outpatient A person treated by medical personnel outside the hospital setting; for example, in a clinic or a physician's office.

overnutrition A state in which nutritional intake exceeds the body's needs.

oxidize (OX-ih-dize) To lose an electron or gain an oxygen atom.

oxidizing agent In one sense, a substance capable of capturing an electron from another compound.

palatable (PAL-it-ah-bull) Pleasing to taste.

passive absorption Absorption that uses no energy. It requires permeability for the substance through the wall of the intestine and a concentration gradient higher in the lumen of the intestine than in the absorptive cell.

pasteurization (pas-tur-eye-ZAY-shun) The process of heating food products to kill pathogenic microorganisms. One method heats milk at 161° F for at least 20 seconds.

pathway A metabolic progression of individual steps from starting materials to ending products, like $C_6H_{12}O_6$ (glucose) + $O_2 \rightarrow\rightarrow\rightarrow CO_2 + H_2O$.

pectin (PEK-tin) A dietary fiber containing chains of galacturonic acid and other monosaccharides; characteristically found between plant cell walls.

peer-reviewed journal A journal that publishes research only after two or three scientists, who were not part of the study, agree it was well conducted and the results are fairly represented. Thus the research has been approved by peers of the research team.

pellagra (peh-LAHG-rah) A disease characterized by inflammation of the skin, diarrhea, and eventual mental incapacity resulting from the lack of the vitamin niacin in the diet.

pepsin (PEP-sin) A protein-digesting enzyme produced by the stomach.

peptide bond A bond formed by the reaction of an amine group with an acid group while splitting off a water molecule. This is the main bond that links amino acids in a protein.

peptides A few amino acids bonded together; often two to four.

peptones A partial breakdown product of proteins.

percentile Classification of a measurement of a unit into divisions of 100 units.

peristalsis (per-ih-STALL-sis) A coordinated muscular contraction that is used to propel food down the gastrointestinal tract.

pernicious anemia (per-NISH-us ah-NEE-mee-ah) The anemia that results from a lack of vitamin B-12 absorption. It is pernicious (deadly) because of the associated nerve degeneration that can result in eventual paralysis and death.

pH measure of the hydrogen ion concentration in a solution.

phagocytosis/pinocytosis (FAG-oh-sigh-TOW-sis/PIN-oh-sigh-TOW-sis) A form of active absorption in which the absorptive cell forms an indentation, and particles or fluids entering the indentation are then engulfed by the cell.

phenylalanine An amino acid.

phenylketonuria (PKU) (fen-ihl-kee-toh-NEW-ree-ah) A disease caused by a defect in the ability of the person's liver to metabolize the amino acid phenylalanine into the amino acid tyrosine.

phenylpropanolamine (fen-ihl-pro-pan-OL-ah-meen) An over-the-counter decongestant that has a mild appetite-reducing effect.

phosphocreatine (PCr) A high-energy compound that can be used to reform adenosine triphosphate (ATP) from adenosine diphosphate (ADP).

photosynthesis (foto-sin-tha-sis) The process by which plants use energy from the sun to produce energy-yielding compounds, such as glucose.

phylloquinone (fil-oh-KWIN-own) A form of vitamin K that comes from plants.

physiological The normal increase in blood volume in pregnancy that ends up diluting the quantity of red blood cells, resulting in anemia; also called hemodilution.

phytic acid (phytate) (FY-tick, FY-tate) A constituent of plant fibers that binds positive ions to its multiple phosphate groups.

phytobezoars (fy-tow-BEE-zors) A pellet of fiber characteristically found in the stomach.

pica (PIE-kah) The practice of eating nonfood items such as dirt, laundry starch, or clay.

placebo (plah-SEE-bo) A fake medicine used to disguise the roles of participants in an experiment; if fake surgery is performed, that is called a sham operation.

placenta (plah-SEN-tah) An organ formed only during pregnancy that secretes hormones and makes possible the transfer of oxygen and nutrients from the mother's blood to the fetus and the removal of fetal wastes.

plaque (PLACK) In terms of heart disease, a cholesterol-rich substance deposited in the blood vessels. It also contains various white blood cells and other lipids.

polar A compound with distinct positive and negative charges (poles) on it. These charges act like poles on a magnet.

polyglutamate form (POL-ee-GLOO-tah-mate) Folate with more than one glutamate molecule attached.

polypeptide (POL-ee-PEP-tide) Fifty to 100 amino acids bonded together.

polysaccharides (POL-ee-SACK-uh-rides) Carbohydrates containing many glucose units, up to 3000 or more.

polyunsaturated fatty acid A fatty acid containing two or more $C=C$ double bonds.

pool The amount of a nutrient residing within the cell (body) that can be readily mobilized when needed.

portal vein A large vein that distributes blood from the intestine to the liver through capillaries.

positive balance A state in which a nutrient intake exceeds losses. This causes a net gain of the nutrient in the body, such as when tissue protein is gained during growth. The opposite of this would be negative balance, where losses exceed intake, as in cases of starvation.

precursor A compound that comes before; to precede.

pregnancy-induced hypertension A serious disorder that can involve high blood pressure, kidney failure, convulsion, and even death of the mother and the fetus. Although the exact cause is not known, good nutrition and prenatal care can prevent or limit its severity. Protein in the urine is an early sign; also known as pre-eclampsia.

premature An infant born before 38 weeks of gestation.

premenstrual syndrome A disorder (also referred to as PMS) found in some women a few days before the onset of menses and characterized by depression, headache, bloating, and mood swings.

preservatives Compounds that extend the shelf life of foods by inhibiting microbial growth or minimizing the destructive effect of oxygen and metals.

primary disease A disease process that is not caused by another disease process.

primary structure of a protein The order of amino acids in the protein molecule.

progestins (pro-JES-tins) Hormones including progesterone, that are necessary for pregnancy and lactation.

prognosis (prog-NO-sis) A forecast of the probable course of a disease.

prolactin (pro-LACK-tin) A hormone secreted by the mother that stimulates the synthesis of milk.

prostacyclin A prostaglandin that is a potent inhibitor of blood clotting made by the blood vessel walls.

prostaglandin I_2 (pros-tah-GLAN-din) An inhbitor of blood clotting made by blood vessel cells.

prostate A gland located near the urinary tract in males that produces a fluid used for the discharge of semen.

protein Compounds made of amino acids; contain carbon, hydrogen, oxygen, nitrogen, and sometimes other atoms, in a specific configuration.

protein efficiency ratio (PER) A measure of protein quality determined by the ability of a protein to support the growth of a young animal.

protein-energy malnutrition (PEM) This results when a person regularly consumes insufficient amounts of kcalories and protein. The deficiency eventually results in body wasting and an increased susceptibility to infections.

prothrombin (pro-THROM-bin) A blood protein needed for blood clotting that requires vitamin K for its synthesis.

proton (PRO-ton) The part of an atom that is positively charged.

proto-oncogenes (PRO-tow-ahn-ko-jeens) Growth-promoting genes found naturally in human cells.

psyllium (sil-see-um) A mostly soluble type of dietary fiber found in the seeds of the plantain plant.

raffinose (RAF-ih-nos) An indigestible oligosaccharide containing three monosaccharide units.

rancid (RAN-sid) Containing products of decomposed fatty acids; these yield off-flavors and odors.

reactive hypoglycemia (HIGH-po-gligh-SEE-mee-uh) Low blood sugar that follows a meal high in simple sugars, with corresponding symptoms of irritability, headache, nervousness, and sweating.

receptive framework for learning The process by which a person opens oneself to learning more about a problem; it usually involves seeking more information about the issue from books and people. In the case of seeking behavior changes, it involves examining one's own background experiences to evaluate whether a behavior change is feasible.

receptor A site in a cell at which compounds (such as hormones) bind. Cells that contain receptors for a specific compound are partially controlled by that compound.

receptor pathway for cholesterol uptake A process by which LDL molecules (cholesterol-containing) are bound by cell receptors, with the incorporation of the LDL molecule into the cell.

Recommended Dietary Intake (RDI) Recommendations from the original tenth edition RDA Committee that were published in 1987 in the American Journal of Clinical Nutrition after the National Academy of Sciences refused to publish the original tenth edition of the RDA.

Recommended Nutritient Intakes (RNI) The Canadian version of RDA.

reducing agent In one sense, a compound capable of donating electrons (also hydrogen ions) to another compound.

reduction To gain an electron or hydrogen atom.

Reference Daily Intakes (RDI) Standards of expressing nutrient content on nutrition labels. RDI figures are based on average 1989 RDA values set for a nutrient that span a particular age range, such as children over 4 years through adults. RDI soon should replace U.S. RDA.

Registered Dietitian (RD) (dye-eh-TISH-shun) A person who has completed both a baccalaureate degree program approved by The American Dietetic Association, performed at least 900 hours of supervised professional practice, and passed a registration examination.

relapse prevention A set of strategies used by people to help prevent and cope with weight control lapses.

requirement The amount of a nutrient required by one person to maintain health. This varies between individuals. We do not know our individual requirements for each nutrient.

renin (REN-in) An enzyme formed in the kidney in response to low blood pressure; it acts on a blood protein to produce angiotensin I.

reserve capacity The extent to which an organ can preserve essentially normal function despite the loss of cells or reduction in cell activity.

resting metabolic rate The number of kcalories used during rest, without stringently controlling recent physical activity. Essentially the same as the basal metabolic rate, but the subject does not need to meet the strict conditions used for a basal metabolic rate determination. Today, both terms are often used interchangeably.

restraint A feeling that occurs as a result of restricted food intake, often associated with the belief that there are good and bad foods.

retinoids (RET-ih-noyds) Forms of preformed vitamin A; one source is animal foods, like liver.

reverse transport of cholesterol The process by which cholesterol is picked up by HDL molecules and transferred to other lipoproteins that can dispose of it in the liver.

rhodopsin (row-DOP-sin) A protein involved in vision; it is made in the eye and incorporates a protein called opsin and a form of vitamin A; especially important in night vision.

ribose (RIGH-bos) A five-carbon sugar found in genetic material, specifically RNA.

rickets A disease characterized by softening of the bones because of poor calcium deposition. This deficiency disease arises from lack of vitamin D activity in the body.

risk factor A characteristic or a behavior that contributes to the chances of developing an illness.

R-protein A protein produced by the salivary glands that enhances vitamin B-12 absorption.

runner's anemia (ah-NEE-mee-ah) A decrease in the blood's ability to carry oxygen that may be caused by iron loss through perspiration, red blood cell destruction resulting from the impact of exercise, or increased blood volume; found in athletes.

saccharin (SACK-ah-rin) An alternate sweetener that yields no energy to the body; it is 500 times sweeter than sucrose.

saliva (sah-LIGH-vah) A watery fluid produced by the salivary glands in the mouth that contains lubricants, enzymes, and other substances.

salt Generally refers to a mixture of sodium and chloride in a 40:60 ratio.

satiety (suh-TIE-uh-tee) A state in which there is no longer a desire to eat.

satiety center A group of cells in the hypothalamus that, when stimulated, causes satiety. These cells are also known as the ventromedial satiety center.

saturated fatty acid A fatty acid containing no C = C double bonds.

scavenger pathway for cholesterol uptake A process by which LDL molecules (cholesterol-containing) are taken up by scavenger cells imbedded in the blood vessels.

scurvy (SKER-vee) The deficiency disease that results after a few weeks of consuming a diet free of vitamin C; pinpoint hemorrhages on the skin are an early sign.

sebaceous glands (seh-BAY-shus) Glands surrounding hair follicles on the face, back, and elsewhere that secrete fatty substances.

sebum (SEE-bum) Secretion of the sebaceous glands, consisting of lipids, waxes, and other triglycerides.

secondary deficiency A deficiency caused not by lack of the nutrient in question, but by lack of a substance that is needed for that nutrient to function.

secondary disease A disease process that develops as a result of another disease.

secondary structure of a protein The interactions (bonds) formed between amino acids placed close together in the primary structure.

secretin (SEE-kreh-tin) A hormone that causes bicarbonate ion release from the pancreas.

self-monitoring A process of tracking foods eaten and conditions affecting eating; actions are usually recorded in a diary, along with location, time, and state of mind. This is a tool to help a person understand more about his or her eating habits.

semi essential amino acids Amino acids that, when consumed, spare the need to use an essential amino acids for their synthesis. Tyrosine in the diet, for example, spares the need to use phenylalanine for its synthesis.

sequesterants (see-KWES-ter-ants) Compounds that bind free metal ions. By so doing, they reduce the ability of ions to cause rancidity in compounds containing fat.

serotonin (ser-oh-TONE-in) A neurotransmitter synthesized from the amino acid tryptophan that appears to both decrease the desire to eat carbohydrates and induce sleep.

set point Often refers to the close regulation of body weight. It is not known what cells control this set point nor how it actually functions in weight regulation. There is no doubt, however, that there are mechanisms that help regulate weight.

short-chain fatty acids Fatty acids that contain fewer than eight carbon atoms.

sickle cell anemia An anemia that results from a malformation of the red blood cell because of an incorrect primary structure in part of its hemoglobin protein chains. The disease can lead to episodes of severe bone and joint pain, abdominal pain, headache, convulsions, paralysis, and even death.

sign A change in health status that is apparent on physical examination.

small-for-gestational age (SGA) (jes-TAY-shun-al) Infants born after normal gestation time (38 weeks), but weighing less than 2500 grams (about 5.5 pounds).

sodium bicarbonate An alkaline substance made basically of sodium and carbon dioxide ($NaHCO_3$).

soluble fibers (SOL-you-bull) Fibers that either dissolve or swell when put into water or are metabolized (fermented) by bacteria in the large intestine. These include pectins, gums, mucilages, and some hemicelluloses.

solvent A substance that other substances dissolve in.

sorbitol (SOR-bih-tol) An alcohol derivative of glucose.

sphincter (SFINK-ter) A muscular valve that controls flow of foodstuffs in the GI tract.

stable isotope (I-so-tope) An isotope form of an element that does not emit radiation.

stachyose (STAK-ee-os) An indigestible oligosaccharide with four monosaccharide units.

Standard of Identity If a food is produced according to a specific recipe on file with the FDA, the label does not have to list its ingredients. In that case, the manufacturer is using its Standard of Identity to avoid disclosing its ingredients.

starch A carbohydrate made of multiple units of glucose attached together in a form the body can digest; also known as complex carbohydrate.

steroids (stare-oydes) A group of hormones and related compounds that are derivatives of cholesterol.

stimulus control Altering the environment to minimize the stimuli for eating; for example, removing foods from sight and storing them in kitchen cabinets.

stress fracture A fracture that occurs from repeated jarring of a bone. Common sites include bones of the foot.

stroke The loss of body function that results from a blood clot in the brain, which in turn causes the death of brain tissue.

subclinical Not seen on a clinical (physical) examination.

subclinical disease Disease or disorder that is present but not severe enough to produce symptoms that can be detected or diagnosed.

subjects Participants in an experiment.

sucrose (SOO-kros) Fructose bonded to glucose; table sugar.

sugar Simple carbohydrate forms with a chemical composition of (CH_2O). Most sugars form ringed structures when in solution.

superoxide dismutase (soo-per-OX-ide DISS-myoo-tase) An enzyme that can neutralize a superoxide free radical.

sympathetic nervous system Part of the nervous system that regulates involuntary vital functions, including the activity of the heart, smooth muscles, and glands. The sympathetic nervous system specifically accelerates heart rate, constricts blood vessels, and raises blood pressure. The parasympathetic nervous system slows heart rate, increases intestinal peristalsis and gland activity, and relaxes sphincters.

symptom A change in health status noted by the person with the problem, such as a stomach pain.

synapse Spaces between nerve cells. One nerve cell stimulates other nearby cells, including other nerve cells, by releasing chemicals that cross the synapse. These chemicals are what excites neighboring cells.

systolic blood pressure (sis-TOL-lik) The pressure in the arteries associated with the pumping of blood from the heart.

teratogen (ter-a-toe-jen) An agent that causes physical defects in a developing fetus.

tertiary structure of a protein (TER-she-air-ee) The three-dimensional structure of a protein, formed by interactions of amino acids placed far apart in the primary structure.

tetany (TET-ah-nee) A syndrome marked by sharp contraction of muscles with failure to relax afterward; usually caused by abnormal calcium metabolism.

theory An explanation for a phenomenon that has numerous lines of evidence to support it.

thermic effect of food The increase in kcalorie use that occurs during the digestion, absorption, and metabolism of energy-yielding nutrients.

"thrifty" metabolism A metabolism that characteristically uses less kcalories than normal, such that the risk of weight gain and obesity is enhanced.

thromboxane (throm-BOX-ane) A stimulus for blood clotting made by particles (platelets) in the bloodstream.

thyroid-stimulating hormone A hormone that regulates the uptake of iodide by the thyroid gland and is secreted in response to low levels of circulating thyroid hormone.

tissue A group of cells designed to perform a specific function; nerve tissue is an example.

t-lymphocyte (tee-LYMF-oh-site) White blood cells processed by the thymus gland and responsible for recognition of foreign substances (for example, bacterial cells) in the body.

tocopherols (tuh-KOFF-er-alls) The chemical name for some forms of vitamin E.

trabecular bone (trah-BEK-you-lar) The spongy, inner matrix of bone, found primarily in the spine, pelvis, and ends of bones.

trace mineral A mineral vital to health that is required in the diet in amounts less than 100 milligrams per day.

transamination (trans-am-ih-NAT-shun) The transfer of an amine group from an amino acid to a carbon skeleton to form a new amino acid.

trans isomer (EYE-so-mer) An isomer form found in compounds with double bonds, such as fatty acids, where the hydrogens of both carbon atoms forming the double bond lie on opposite sides of that bond.

triglyceride (try-GLISS-uh-ride) The major form of lipid in food. It is composed of three fatty acids bonded to glycerol, an alcohol.

trimester The normal pregnancy of 38 to 42 weeks is divided into three 13 to 14 week periods called trimesters.

trypsin (TRIP-sin) A protein-digesting enzyme secreted by the pancreas (in a zymogen form) that acts in the small intestine.

ulcer (UL-sir) Erosion of the tissue lining usually in the stomach or the upper small intestine. These are generally referred to as peptic ulcers.

uncoupling The dissociation between the liberation of energy from energy-yielding substances and the formation of ATP.

undernutrition Failing health that results from a longstanding dietary intake that regularly fails to meet nutritional needs.

underwater weighing A method to estimate total body fat by weighing individuals under water; the more fat a person has the less they will weigh under water.

U.S. Recommended Daily Allowances (U.S. RDA) Standards established by the FDA for use on nutrition labels. For the most part, the four existing versions use the highest nutrient recommendation in the appropriate age and gender category from the 1968 publication of the RDA. The version that includes children over 4 years of age and adults is most commonly seen on nutrition labels.
variability In a nutritional sense, the variation one would expect to see for nutrient requirements in a group of individuals.
vegan (VEE-gun) A person who eats only plant foods.
very low calorie diet (VLCD) Known also as protein-sparing, modified fast (PSMF), this diet allows a person 400 to 700 kcalories per day, often in liquid form. Of this, 30 to 120 grams are carbohydrate; the rest is high biological value protein.
very low density lipoprotein (VLDL) The lipoprotein that intitially leaves the liver. It carries both the cholesterol and lipid newly synthesized by the liver.
villi (VIL-eye) Fingerlike protrusions into the small intestine that participate in digestion and absorption of foodstuffs.
vitamins Organic compounds needed in very small amounts in the diet to help regulate and support chemical reactions in the body.
VO_2 max Maximum volume of oxygen consumed per unit of time during exercise.
water activity A measure of the amount of free water in a food. Most bacteria need a water activity greater than 0.9 to grow, while molds can grow in water activity as low as 0.6.
whey (WAY) Proteins, such as lactalbumin, that are found in great amounts in human milk and are easy to digest.
whole grains Grains containing the entire seed of the plant, including the bran, germ, and endosperm (starchy interior).
xanthinine dehydrogenase (ZAN-thin-een dh-HY-droj-eh-nase) An enzyme, containing molydenum and iron, that functions in the formation of uric acid and the mobilization of iron from liver ferritin stores.
xerophthalmia (zer-op-THAL-mee-uh) A cause of blindness that results from infection of the eye secondary to a vitamin A deficiency. The specific cause is a lack of mucus production by the eye, which then leaves it more vulnerable to surface dirt and bacterial infections.
xylitol (ZIGH-lih-tol) An alcohol derivative of the five-carbon monosaccharide, xylose.
yo-yo dieting The practice of losing weight and then regaining it, only to lose it and regain it again.
zymogen (zigh-MO-gin) An inactive form of an enzyme.

Answers to Nutrition Awareness Inventory

CHAPTER 1

1. *True.* Water is a large component of many foods, even meats.

2. *False.* Minerals cannot be further broken down or converted into other substances by ordinary chemical means.

3. *False.* Kcalories (kilocalories) are 1000-calorie units. Although most people talk about energy units as calories, what they really mean is kilocalories. As a nutrition student, you need to be aware of the proper term.

4. *True.* One gram of protein yields 4 kcalories, 1 gram of carbohydrate 4 kcalories, 1 gram of fat 9 kcalories, and 1 gram of alcohol 7 kcalories.

5. *False.* Vitamins have no caloric value in and of themselves. They merely aid in certain energy-yielding reactions.

6. *True.* When nutrient intake does not meet nutrient needs, your nutrient stores can be used, like calcium found in bones. However, as these stores are depleted, serious health problems may result.

7. *False.* Many minerals, such as calcium and magnesium, are required in larger amounts than vitamins.

8. *False.* Water has no capacity to yield a metabolizable energy source in the body. Do not confuse this fact with the definition of the heat measurement unit, the kcalorie, which uses water.

9. *False.* Organic refers to carbon atoms bonded to hydrogen atoms. The term has nothing to do with organic gardening.

10. *False.* Malnutrition represents a poor nutrition state due to either an excess or insufficient nutrient intake. Undernutrition refers to an insufficient nutrient intake.

11. *True.* In a person severely deficient in iron, weakness is common and temperature control may be altered, causing the person to feel cold.

12. *True.* Five of the ten leading causes of death in America display strong links to overnutrition.

13. *False.* Vitamins A and D and minerals such as iron and selenium can even be harmful if taken in large amounts for long periods of time.

14. *True.* Alcoholic beverages are the third leading contributor to energy intakes in the United States.

15. *False.* Food choices are most often determined by taste and habit. Nutrition knowledge is not scarce, but it sometimes seems it is in everyday life!

CHAPTER 2

1. *True.* These are the substances provided by foods that are necessary for life.

2. *False.* Children need to be in positive protein balance, where intake exceeds output, in order to grow.

3. *False.* Few healthy people need vitamin and mineral supplements in order meet their nutrient needs (see Chapter 12).

4. *False.* A cup of water equals about 250 milliliters, or ¼ liter.

5. *False.* One pound equals about 454 grams.

6. *False.* RDA is the abbreviation for recommended dietary allowances.

7. *False.* No nutrient is absolutely required daily. You can maintain health for about 4 days on a diet free of water and about 10 days on a diet free of the vitamin thiamin.

8. *True.* While nutrient recommendations are often similar, groups of scientists from different countries may disagree with each other. In addition, the type of diet consumed influences nutrient needs.

9. *False.* The RDAs form a recommendation only for group needs. It does not provide personal nutrient requirements.

10. *False.* Active people are likely to require closer to 2200 to 2800 kcalories or more to meet energy needs.

11. *True.* Potatoes and bread have very similar carbohydrate : protein : fat ratios.

12. *True.* The exchange system relieves us of having to memorize the composition of all foods: rather, it is a powerful tool for quickly and conveniently estimating the energy, protein, carbohydrate, and fat contents of a food or meal.

13. *True.* Nutrient density is an important concept, especially for people on a low-kcalorie diet. It refers to the ratio of a food's nutrients to its kcalorie content.

14. *True.* The term kilocalories, or kcalories, is used to measure food energy. Nutritionists often use the term calories when speaking, but the written word should be kcalories.

15. *True.* No one food contains all the nutrients needed to maintain good health. Milk, for example is low in iron, while eggs are low in calcium.

CHAPTER 3

1. *True.* Glucose combined with fructose forms sucrose, or table sugar.

2. *True.* Starch is the storage form of carbohydrates in plants. Glycogen is the storage form of carbohydrates in animals. The amount of glycogen present in meat that comes to the table is so small that it should not be considered a food source of carbohydrates.

3. *False.* Fat contains more kcalories per gram than carbohydrates (9 versus 4 kcalories per gram).

4. *True.* Carbohydrates are important energy-supplying nutrients.

5. *True.* Fiber is referred to as bulk, but dietary fiber is the preferred term.

6. *False.* Although there is no RDA for carbohydrates, at least 50 to 100 grams per day will prevent the body from breaking down its own protein to make glucose. About 55% of kcalories should come from carbohydrates.

7. *False.* Fiber mostly improves the health of the large intestine.

8. *True.* The frequency and form of the sugars eaten are more important than the total amount of sugars consumed.

9. *True.* When eaten in excess of energy needs, carbohydrates are stored as glycogen and to some extent fat.

10. *False.* Most all bread, including white bread, contains wheat flour. It is whole wheat flour that includes the fiber portion of the grain.

11. *True.* The American food supply yields about 125 pounds of simple sugars annually for each of us. Many nutritionists believe that consumption of sugars is too high. Only 10% or so of kcalories should be from sugar. This allows for more healthful foods in the diet.

12. *True.* Honey may contain bacteria spores that grow and become fatal to infants because their stomachs have yet to develop the strong acidic environment that adult stomachs have. Acid reduces the harmful bacterium's growth.

13. *False.* Diabetes is a disorder of high blood glucose levels.

14. *False.* There is scant corroborating evidence for these theories. Sugars have a low nutrient density, and kcalories from these may replace foods that contain essential nutrients. This is the main problem with food containing sugars in our diets.

15. *True.* This was observed by Dr. Denis Burkitt, who attributes this phenomenon to the high dietary fiber intakes of Africans as compared with North Americans.

CHAPTER 4

1. *True.* Polyunsaturated fats are liquid at room temperature. Thus, vegetable oils are liquid at room temperature.

2. *True.* Fats yield 9 kcalories per gram, while carbohydrates and proteins yield 4 kcalories per gram.

3. *False.* While one's blood cholesterol helps predict the risk of cardiovascular disease, knowing the LDL cholesterol level and the ratio of total cholesterol to HDL cholesterol is more important.

4. *True.* But don't be misled by advertisers who state certain products are "cholesterol-free." The product may still contain saturated fat, which is a more important determinant of one's blood cholesterol level.

5. *True.* Animal fats are often rich in saturated fat.

6. *True.* Triglyceride is the primary form of lipid in both foods and the body.

7. *False.* Fat is absolutely necessary for life because it supplies essential fatty acids used to make vital body compounds.

8. *True.* In some cases this process makes food production easier; hydrogenation prevents the oils in many foods from turning rancid in transit and storage. In addition a hydrogenated oil may give a product the consistency that the consumer expects.

9. *True.* Most fruits and vegetables contain only traces of fat. Avocados and olives are exceptions.

10. *True.* BHA and BHT are examples of antioxidants found in salad dressings.

11. *True.* Vitamins A, E, D, and K are fat soluble, and their absorption is enhanced by dietary fat.

12. *False.* Everyone age 20 years or more should monitor and track his or her blood cholesterol levels. (Some groups recommend that anyone over 2 years old who has a family history of early heart disease should do the same.) Certain elevated blood lipoprotein levels are risk factors for cardiovascular disease.

13. *True.* Butter, however, contains more saturated fats than margarine.

14. *True.* Studies with both animals and humans have shown fish oils can positively affect a number of aspects of health. However, high doses of fish oil should be used only in experimental conditions, under supervision of a physician experienced in this area.

15. *False.* Nondairy creamers often contain coconut oil, which is very high in saturated fat.

CHAPTER 5

1. *False.* Most of us eat such a varied assortment of food that if enough kcalories are consumed, it would be difficult not to have a high-quality protein diet; one that contains enough of all nine essential amino acids.

2. *True.* Protein is particularly important for building new tissue during periods of rapid growth.

3. *True.* Only a few enzymes are composed of other compounds.

4. *True.* Insulin, as an example, contains only amino acids.

5. *True.* Biological value represents the body's ability to retain the protein absorbed.

6. *True.* Milk proteins provide one of the highest possible biological values from foods. An egg white has the very best biological value.

7. *False.* More protein per weight is required during periods of growth.

8. *False.* All of us, including athletes, can meet our protein needs with basic foods, and rarely is an intake greater than twice the RDA necessary.

9. *True.* For this reason trimming meats of fat and broiling them is a good idea. Vegetable sources, such as legumes, provide protein without fat, unless of course it is added during preparation.

10. *True.* Although a lack of energy can be caused by other things, it is a symptom of severe protein deficiency.

11. *False.* Gelatin is a low-quality protein; it lacks several of the essential amino acids.

12. *True.* Starvation in infancy leads to marasmus, which means "to waste away."

13. *False.* Plant proteins contain much fiber and magnesium; in comparison, animal proteins supply the most absorbable form of iron.

14. *True.* It is 85% protein.

15. *True.* Fruits contain mostly carbohydrate and water.

CHAPTER 6

1. *False.* For many foods some digestion actually begins during cooking when protein structures unfold, starch granules swell, and tough vegetable fibers are softened.

2. *True.* Water-soluble nutrients use a special portal vein that connects the intestinal tract to the liver. Many nutrients can enter the bloodstream only after passing through the liver.

3. *True.* A living person's small intestine is approximately 10 feet long; at autopsy it is approximately 23 feet long.

4. *False.* It is the acid produced by the stomach that is responsible for killing most of the bacteria that enter the stomach.

5. *True.* The term colon also refers to the large intestine.

6. *False.* The digestive enzymes work efficiently no matter what combination of foods is eaten.

7. *True.* Stomach enzymes require an acid pH for maximum activity, whereas the small intestine has a more neutral pH.

8. *False.* The cells that line the walls of the small intestine would be unable to effectively absorb nutrients through a thick mucus layer (like that of the stomach). The mechanism by which the small intestine is protected is the presence of a sphincter (the pyloric sphincter) that regulates the influx of stomach contents to the intestine. In addition, the pancreas secretes bicarbonate, a substance by which the stomach acids entering the small intestine may be neutralized.

9. *True.* Although bile is not required for the digestion of proteins and starches, it is absolutely essential for the digestion, emulsification, and absorption of fats (especially long-chain fatty acids).

10. *False.* The liver, the pancreas, and the gallbladder all play key roles in digestion, but they are not part of the direct path taken by nutrients through the body.

11. *False.* The overwhelming amount of absorption (nearly 95%) takes place in the small intestine. The large intestine serves in only limited absorption of minerals, water and the bacterial by-products, such as vitamin K, the vitamin biotin, and short-chain fatty acids.

12. *True.* The sugar glucose is absorbed from the small intestine into the bloodstream against a concentration gradient. Much glucose from the bloodstream is present in the cells of the intestine. So energy must be expanded if more glucose in the intestinal tract is to enter the intestinal cells. Conversely, the concentration of fat in the intestinal cells is low, allowing fat to be passively absorbed into them.

13. *True.* The peristaltic waves that propel food down the intestinal tract require a coordination of both longitudinal muscles (which lie lengthwise down the intestinal tract) and circular muscles (which surround the intestinal tract).

14. *True.* Many undigested foods that enter the colon are nutrient sources for bacteria found there. The bacteria then make a variety of products, including various gases.

15. *False.* In the stomach, bacterial growth is hampered by the gastric acids. The valve (ileocecal sphincter) that regulates the influx of contents from the small intestine into the colon also serves to prevent the prominent bacterial growth within the colon from moving into the small intestine. If these bacteria were able to get within the small intestine they would compete for the nutrients and create problems with fat digestion.

CHAPTER 7

1. *True.* Carbohydrates provide both energy for the body and carbons that can be synthesized into fat.

2. *True.* Fat can be stored in adipose tissue for future needs or used for energy by cells, such as muscle cells.

3. *False.* The carbons in protein can become the carbons of fat; high-protein diets can be fattening.

4. *True.* The brain uses glucose primarily for energy. Ketone bodies can be used under special circumstances, such as in cases of semi-starvation.

5. *True.* Ketone body levels in the bloodstream rise during fasting, partly because the liver is engaged in gluconeogenesis and is prevented from metabolizing fat efficiently. Ketone bodies are then synthesized from breakdown products of fatty acids.

6. *False.* The carbons in alcohol can become the carbons of fat.

7. *True.* These form coenzymes used in metabolism, such as NAD and FAD.

8. *True.* The removal of amino groups from amino acids (deamination) requires vitamin B-6.

9. *True.* Both iron and copper participate in the election transport chain. This is where most ATP is made in a cell.

10. *False.* Carnitine is used to shuttle fatty acids into a cell's mitochondria for energy metabolism.

11. *False.* Ketones are primarily formed from acetyl-coA, a breakdown product of fatty acids. Glycerol can form acetyl-CoA, but there is not enough glycerol in our diets to be of nutritional importance.

12. *True.* Mitochondria are the major sites of ATP production in the cell.

13. *True.* Carbons of carbohydrate, fat, protein, and alcohol molecules can all become the carbons of acetyl-coA. This compound then has a pivotal role in energy metabolism. In essence, all roads lead to acetyl-CoA.

14. *True.* Using photosynthesis, plants trap solar energy and store it in the chemical bonds of glucose and other organic compounds.

15. *True.* When liver and muscle glycogen stores are depleted, body proteins are degraded to provide building blocks for glucose. The glycerol portion of the fat molecule also can be used in gluconeogenesis, but it represents only a small amount of glucose produced.

CHAPTER 8

1. *True.* When the brain receives signals that the liver is metabolizing absorbed nutrients, it then signals satiety in the brain.

2. *False.* Adipose cell size may be involved with the regulation of eating week to week and month to month. It is involved in long-term hunger regulation.

3. *False.* The RDA represents an average energy need for a person performing light activity. The range given may or may not accurately estimate a person's energy needs.

4. *True.* To keep a resting body alive, there is need to maintain heart rate, respiration, body temperature, and other functions. The energy used represents basal or resting metabolism, depending on the conditions in which it was measured.

5. *False.* Brown adipose tissue mostly disappears between infancy and adulthood. Its role in the average adult is unclear, but is likely of minor importance.

6. *False.* In general, obesity increases risk for health problems and reduces life expectancy. The greater the obesity, the greater the effect it has on life expectancy. Occasionally a person may escape the health problems associated with obesity, but most people do not.

7. *True.* Your body weight may be greater than a desirable figure, as predicted from the Metropolitan Life Insurance Table, but excess weight yields a health risk only if it is from excess body fat. Extra muscle mass poses no risk.

8. *False.* Women tend to store fat in the hip and thigh areas, whereas men tend to store fat in the abdominal area.

9. *True.* Health problems usually begin when a person exceeds desirable weight by more than 20%; the greater the difference, the greater the health risk.

10. *True.* Muscle tissue metabolizes energy at a high rate and thus has a great influence on basal metabolism.

11. *True.* The extra weight carried by an obese person raises the kcalorie cost of physical activity.

12. *False.* There is little evidence that adult obesity in men is related to childhood obesity; however, there is a strong relationship between childhood and adult obesity in women.

13. *False.* Probably less than 10% of all cases of obesity in the United States arise from diagnosed problems in thyroid or other hormone levels in the bloodstream.

14. *False.* Consuming no more than a few hundred extra kcalories daily for a few years can create an obese state. Once an obese state is achieved, it takes very few extra kcalories to maintain it.

15. *True.* At the beginning of a meal, people usually choose a variety of foods. At the end of a meal, choices narrow and sweet food choices often predominate.

CHAPTER 9

1. *False.* Although physical activity is helpful, a low-kcalorie diet is equally important.

2. *True.* Diet relapse is a critical issue that is just now receiving focused attention.

3. *True.* A diet with fewer than 1000 kcalories is likely to cause hunger and fatigue.

4. *False.* Most people regain the weight they lost within 1 year.

5. *True.* It is impractical to lose fat tissue rapidly because of the high-kcalorie deficit required.

6. *True.* Changes in behavior are likely to reduce the tendency to relapse into bad habits.

7. *False.* There is no evidence that eating one affects the body's use of the other.

8. *True.* High-carbohydrate foods generally contain fewer kcalories than high-fat foods.

9. *False.* Recent studies show that a low-fat diet is practical and can have significant satiety if high in dietary fiber.

10. *True.* People who can change their habits are able to have more control over their food choices and behavior.

11. *True.* An example might be to avoid a candy machine that is on the way to class.

12. *False.* You must burn about 3000 extra kcalories to lose 1 pound.

13. *True.* More than 70% of obese children become obese adults.

14. *True.* Brisk walking burns about 5 kcalories per minute.

15. *True.* Weighing twice one's desirable body weight is another measure of morbid obesity.

CHAPTER 10

1. *False.* A cell must first convert the energy stored in carbohydrate to ATP energy.

2. *False.* Carbohydrates and fats both provide energy for the body.

3. *False.* Only initial stages do not require oxygen to function. Ultimate burning to carbon dioxide and water does require oxygen input.

4. *True.* Complete burning of all body fuels yields carbon dioxide as one of the by-products.

5. *False.* No evidence supports this assertion.

6. *False.* Rapid weight loss, such as seen in wrestlers, can weaken the body. Long-term weight loss can reduce muscle mass and make it hard to keep glycogen stores adequate.

7. *False.* Given high kcalorie intakes of athletes, protein needs are easily met from typical food choices. No supplements are needed.

8. *True.* This is the key recommendation for carbohydrate-loading strategies.

9. *True.* The carbohydrate present can reduce glycogen use and the electrolytes can help maintain blood volume.

10. *True.* Caffeine can enhance fat use by muscles, which may improve athletic performance in some endurance events.

11. *False.* The target heart rate range to promote general aerobic conditioning is 60% to 85% of maximum heart rate.

12. *False.* Cool-down exercises are just as important—if not more—as warm-up exercises.

13. *False.* Thirst is not a good indication for fluid replacement needs. A much better guide is weight loss: 2 cups (½ liter) of water should eventually be consumed for every pound (½ kilogram) lost while exercising.

14. *False.* Loading up on carbohydrate will not be beneficial for short, sprint-type exercise; it benefits exercise lasting longer than 1.5 to 2 hours.

15. *True.* Anabolic steroids are illegal substances. They are also unsafe to use.

CHAPTER 11

1. *True.* Some cultures use certain foods as ceremonial foods. In the United States waffles are a breakfast food, while in England they are dessert.

2. *True.* About 5% of young women suffer from an eating disorder.

3. *False.* They have an intense fear of gaining weight.

4. *True.* This is referred to as purging.

5. *True.* People with anorexia nervosa tend to be extremely competitive.

6. *True.* People with anorexia nervosa see themselves as fat, even when they are thin.

7. *True.* But they don't like to admit it.

8. *False.* People with bulimia are extremely secretive.

9. *True.* This attitude is reflected in advertisements.

10. *True.* Most people with eating disorders see themselves as inadequate.

11. *True.* People with eating disorders are often obsessively neat and highly aware of imperfections.

12. *True.* The damaging effects of late stages of these conditions increase the risk of permanent injury.

13. *True.* Bingeing and purging characterize bulimia.

14. *False.* Treatment should emphasize choice as opposed to restriction.

15. *True.* This should be suspected in children who exhibit poor growth rates.

CHAPTER 12

1. *False.* No vitamin missing from a diet for less than a week leads to deficiency symptoms. Earliest signs of deficiency appear with a thiamin-free diet after about 10 days. The first symptoms of a vitamin C deficiency are seen after about 20 to 40 days.

2. *False.* Of the fat-soluble vitamins, vitamin K is more readily excreted from the body.

3. *True.* Mineral oil is not absorbed by the intestine. During its passage, mineral oil can dissolve fat-soluble vitamins and pull them into the colon for eventual elimination.

4. *False.* Because fat-soluble vitamins do not dissolve rapidly in boiling water, they are not leached out of foods during cooking to the same extent as most water-soluble vitamins.

5. *False.* There is a slight chance that one more vitamin remains to be discovered, but for the most part nutrition scientists feel they have isolated all the vitamins necessary for human health.

6. *True.* When in the active form, vitamin D, through a variety of mechanisms, can improve calcium absorption from the small intestine.

7. *True.* Vitamin A enhances night vision by participating in the formation of the compound rhodopsin.

8. *True.* Vitamin A has a high potential for causing toxicity, especially in pregnant women and children.

9. *True.* Aided by the action of sunlight, the skin produces vitamin D, which can then be metabolized by the liver and kidneys to form the active vitamin D hormone. By definition this compound is a hormone since it is made in one part of the body and acts in another.

10. *False.* The skin (as an organ) is capable of using sunlight to produce inactive vitamin D. Foods in general are not capable of performing this process; vitamin D itself added to foods will supplement the product.

11. *False.* Instead, vitamin E stabilizes free radical compounds by donating an electron. This decreases the tendency for free radicals to steal electrons from fatty acids and other electron-dense compounds.

12. *True.* Vitamin K is able to add carbon dioxide molecules to one type of amino acid, glutamate, in turn imparting calcium-binding properties to the proteins containing that amino acid.

13. *True.* Antibiotics can reduce the growth of bacteria in the small intestine and colon. These bacteria synthesize a form of vitamin K that we absorb and use.

14. *True.* Vegetables are a good source of vitamin K. This is another reason why we should "eat our vegetables."

15. *True.* The American Medical Association recently recommended that a reasonable nutrient supplement dosage is generally 50% to 150% of the U.S. RDA for most vitamins.

CHAPTER 13

1. *False.* Thiamin needs are more closely tied to carbohydrate intake because the conversion of pyruvate to acetyl-CoA requires thiamin. Carbohydrate foods generate pyruvate.

2. *True.* Pork is an excellent source of thiamin, along with sunflower seeds and dried beans.

3. *False.* Normally, highly processed grains like white rice are stripped of much of their vitamin value. However, in the United States, grains are usually enriched and thus contain extra niacin, thiamin, riboflavin, and iron. Thus, enriched white rice is a good source of niacin.

4. *True.* Milk is the best source of riboflavin in the American diet.

5. *True.* A deficiency in a major B vitamin, such as riboflavin, suggests other B vitamins will also be deficient, since most are found in similar foods.

6. *True.* In the elderly years, cells in the stomach commonly decrease the synthesis of a factor that is vital for vitamin B-12 absorption. The treatment is usually monthly injections of vitamin B-12.

7. *True.* The amino acid tryptophan is converted into niacin in the body. Niacin needs then are met by consuming both niacin-containing foods and protein in the diet.

8. *True.* A niacin deficiency causes severe dermatitis and skin redness, especially where the sun strikes, as well as diarrhea and dementia.

9. *True.* Nicotinic acid in pharmacological (high) doses can lower serum cholesterol levels. At the same time, it often causes redness of the skin and itching.

10. *True.* Alcohol decreases the absorption of vitamin B-6, thiamin, and folate. Alcoholism is a major cause of B vitamin deficiencies.

11. *False.* Excessive supplementation of folate may mask a B-12 deficiency. One of the early warning signs of the onset of a severe B-12 deficiency is an impaired ability to recycle folate. If excessive amounts of folate are available, this sign will not be readily apparent and may escape the eye of a physician.

12. *True.* Vitamin B-12 is not found in plants unless its presence is due to fermentation or contamination of the product from bits of soil or insects.

13. *True.* Pinpoint hemorrhages in the skin near hair follicles is an early sign of scurvy. These occur after about 20 to 40 days of no vitamin C intake.

14. *True.* Vitamin C converts iron into a form that is absorbed more readily.

15. *False.* High doses of vitamin C may moderately reduce the symptoms and duration of a cold; no food or medication can prevent colds.

CHAPTER 14

1. *False.* An electrolyte is a substance that dissociates into ions and so is able to conduct electricity. Although, in a water molecule, the hydrogen atoms are slightly positive and the oxygen atom negative, each water molecule does not break down into individual ions.

2. *False.* The terms major and trace are not designations of nutritional importance. They are classifications referring only to the amount needed for daily functioning.

3. *True.* For example, the coenzyme for the vitamin thiamin requires magnesium to function efficiently.

4. *False.* Animal foods are often the best mineral sources, since animals concentrate the minerals they consume from plants. The exception is magnesium, which is plentiful in green plants.

5. *True.* The body can conserve water, but some must be lost every day. Thus after only a few days, severe dehydration and death can result from lack of water intake. Death from starvation can take as long as 50 or more days in an adult.

6. *True.* Water evaporation from the skin requires heat energy. So when perspiration evaporates, heat energy is taken from the skin, leaving you feeling cooler.

7. *True.* This simple method of estimation yields results similar to those derived by totaling all typical water losses via lungs, skin, feces, and urine.

8. *False.* In cases of some mental disorders, such as schizophrenia, people may drink tremendous amounts of water in a short time. This can overwhelm the kidneys' excretion capacity and lead to headaches, blurred vision, and cramps.

9. *True.* About one half of the sodium consumed by Americans is supplied by processed foods. Sodium is prevalent in foods such as frozen dinners, canned soups, and convenience entrees.

10. *False.* Many substances commonly found in dietary fiber, such as phytate in grain fibers, as well as oxalic acid in spinach and other vegetables, can actually bind minerals, inhibiting their absorption.
11. *True.* Although part of our preference for salt is related to the sodium receptors on the tongue, habit also has a role. If you grow up consuming salty foods, you are more likely to prefer salty foods. Preferences can be relearned by gradually decreasing added salt.
12. *False.* Cheese has added salt unless it is a "low salt" cheese. Milk does not have added salt and so is lower in sodium per kcalorie.
13. *True.* Perspiration on the skin tastes salty, not because it has a higher sodium concentration than blood, but because once the water evaporates, concentrated sodium is left behind.
14. *False.* The effectiveness of dietary calcium in entirely preventing bone loss has been disproved, but adequate dietary amounts can slow some bone loss in old age.
15. *False.* It is estimated that only 10% to 15% of the population is at risk for developing hypertension from excess sodium intake. These people can benefit from restricting sodium. No data verify the need for consuming a low-sodium diet if blood pressure is normal, but many scientists feel this is a prudent course to take to prevent future hypertension.

CHAPTER 15

1. *True.* The small amounts needed by the body make trace mineral deficiencies difficult to detect in humans. Laboratory techniques are not even available to adequately measure some trace elements in tissues, and there are gaps in our knowledge about metabolism and storage of many minerals. This hampers interpretation of laboratory results.
2. *True.* Trace minerals that have the same charge and are chemically similar or use the same carrier proteins often compete with each other during absorption and metabolism. This must be considered when setting the RDA for a trace mineral and when using mineral supplements.
3. *True.* Eating a variety of foods will ensure an intake from a variety of soil conditions and help maximize the chances of consuming an adequate amount of trace minerals.
4. *True.* The refinement process strips a food, such as flour, of many minerals. The enrichment process only replaces one: iron.
5. *True.* Women in their childbearing years have a greater need for iron due to their greater iron loss during menstruation.
6. *False.* The body has no efficient mechanism for eliminating excess iron. Excess iron intake can be very damaging. In response, iron absorption is very carefully regulated in an attempt to prevent excess absorption.
7. *True.* A main function of zinc is promoting growth and development. A zinc deficiency can cause poor growth in children, whereas a zinc supplement can help increase appetite and the rate of weight gain in children recovering from undernutrition.
8. *False.* Hair analysis is not a reliable method at this time. Too many contaminating substances, such as shampoos, invalidate the results.
9. *True.* Taking zinc supplements often disrupts the natural nutrient balance found in a good diet and so can do more harm than good.
10. *True.* Copper is a component of the protein ceruloplasmin. This compound converts Fe^{+2} into Fe^{+3}, the form in which iron can leave the mucosal cell and storage sites in the liver to bind with transferrin in the blood.
11. *True.* Copper and zinc compete with each other for absorption.
12. *False.* Most iodide in our diets comes from iodized salt added to foods during processing, cooking, or at the table.
13. *True.* Fluoride prevents caries in two ways. It inhibits the growth of bacteria on teeth, and it makes teeth resistant to acid during tooth development.
14. *False.* We know little about chromium metabolism, and it is likely that, as happens with other trace minerals, it is quite toxic even at moderate doses.
15. *False.* A prolonged iron deficiency can eventually lead to iron-deficiency anemia, but most people with poor iron intakes take years to develop symptoms if they remain untreated. In addition, some types of anemia are caused by conditions other than an iron deficiency.

CHAPTER 16

1. *True.* Infants weighing less than 5.5 pounds (2.5 kilograms) at birth are considered to have low birth weight. The risk of sickness and death in the early months of life is much greater for these infants.
2. *False.* During the first trimester (13 weeks), when organs and body parts are forming, the potential for birth defects is greatest.
3. *True.* The quality of the mother's diet and the amount of weight she gains during pregnancy are more important than genetic background in determining birth weight.
4. *True.* During pregnancy, an average increase of 300 kcalories per day is needed. Energy demands are greatest during the second and third trimesters.
5. *True.* This range of weight gain normally allows optimal development of the fetus without an excessive increase of fat stores in the mother.
6. *True.* Gaining excessive weight from eating too many kcalories is a problem for many pregnant women.
7. *False.* Eating a healthful diet requires learning wise food choices.
8. *True.* Many mineral needs, but particularly those for iron, calcium and zinc, are increased. Iron requirements usually necessitate taking supplements in addition to changing the diet.
9. *True.* Symptoms of gestational diabetes will first occur during pregnancy and then disappear after birth. This happens more frequently in women who have a family history of diabetes.
10. *True.* Immune factors passed from mother to infant via breast milk reduce the number of respiratory and intestinal infections.
11. *True.* Almost all women are capable of breast-feeding; the size of the breasts, and even the presence of twins, pose no major barrier.
12. *True.* Many substances ingested by the mother, including medicines, are secreted into the milk.
13. *True.* The placenta is a specialized organ of pregnancy that both secretes hormones and allows for the transfer of oxygen, nutrients, and wastes between mother and fetus.
14. *True.* This means good nutrition and health habits should be started early, ideally before pregnancy begins.
15. *False.* Unaltered cow's milk is too difficult for an infant to digest and fully metabolize until approximately 6 to 12 months of age.

CHAPTER 17

1. *True.* Although all nutrients and an adequate kcalorie intake are needed for growth, protein is particularly important for reaching one's genetic potential.
2. *True.* Infancy is a period of very rapid growth.
3. *False.* Brain growth rate is maximal at birth and continues through 12 to 15 months of age.
4. *False.* No evidence strongly links infant obesity to obesity in childhood or adulthood.
5. *False.* Infant energy needs are higher per pound.
6. *False.* Infants need relatively high-fat diets to support brain growth and supply enough energy for other growth with a small volume of food.
7. *False.* Infants are not usually developmentally or nutritionally ready for solid food until 4 to 6 months of age.
8. *True.* It is not necessary to add salt, sugar, or spices to infant foods.
9. *True.* However, little besides patience helps a parent deal with colic.
10. *True.* Cow's milk should not be fed to a child until about 6 months of age at the earliest, and preferably not until 12 months of age.
11. *True.* Cow's milk is low in iron, and the protein is more difficult to digest than that in human milk. This may cause intestinal irritation that contributes to iron losses.
12. *False.* What is eaten is most important—not when.
13. *True.* Anemia and obesity are the nutritional problems clinicians need to focus on.
14. *False.* Parents should control what food is available, but let children decide the amount to eat. With good foods available, children can reliably decide on serving size.

15. *False.* Scientific studies have never shown a very strong link between any dietary factor and acne.

CHAPTER 18

1. *False.* The average length of time Americans live has increased during the last century, but not the age of the oldest people.

2. *True.* This amount of exercise is thought to adequately stimulate the cardiovascular system and help reduce stress and obesity.

3. *True.* Drug-nutrient interactions can be a problem at any age, but because the elderly generally take more and different combinations of drugs over a long period, nutritional status is more likely to be affected.

4. *True.* Being overweight contributes to almost all the chronic diseases common in our society.

5. *True.* In addition, because the elderly population is rapidly growing, society will need to continue dealing with this concern.

6.. *False.* Good nutrition can delay some symptoms of aging, but no diet can magically prevent aging; aging probably begins at conception.

7. *False.* The senses of smell and taste tend to decrease with age. Adding seasonings can enhance food appeal.

8. *True.* The sense of thirst may diminish with age, but not the need for fluids.

9. *True.* Stomach secretions that promote absorption of vitamin B-12 decrease with age.

10. *True.* Increasing fiber and fluid intakes can help reduce constipation.

11. *True.* Excessive intake of vitamin A supplements results in many toxicity problems. These are only a few examples (see Chapter 12).

12. *True.* Be aware of these nutrients if you are involved in the care of elderly people or have the chance to advise elderly relatives.

13. *True.* Exercise is an important part of body maintenance.

14. *False.* People differ in genetic backgrounds, abilities to regulate cholesterol metabolism, and responsiveness to diets aimed at lowering blood cholesterol. There is, however, no way to know how much a diet will help until a person tries it.

15. *False.* This age-group varies more in physical ability than any other.

CHAPTER 19

1. *True.* We often do not realize food-borne illness is so common because the symptoms mimic other disorders, such as flu.

2. *False.* Foods having the potential to cause food-borne illness often show no signs of it in taste, smell, or appearance.

3. *False.* Imported foods, such as soft cheeses from Mexico, have been implicated in food-borne illness. While foods are inspected when they enter from foreign countries, there is not enough manpower to inspect all foods carefully.

4. *False.* Chemical structure—not origin—is the key to evaluating chemicals: Whether a chemical is made in a laboratory or found in nature is irrelevant to its harmfulness to humans. Some naturally occurring toxins in foods, such as solanine in green potatoes, are much more toxic than synthetic food additives.

5. *True.* When the pulp of an apple is exposed to oxygen, it turns brown. Antioxidants, such as vitamin C found in lemon and orange juice, can prevent this browning.

6. *True.* The growth of bacteria and fungi in foods requires sufficient free water, that is, water not bound by other food compounds. If the water content of a food is reduced considerably, the lack of free water curtails growth of bacteria and fungi.

7. *False.* Only a few of the many bacteria, fungi, viruses, and other earthly microbes are known to cause food-borne illness.

8. *True.* And for this reason, foods generally should be kept cold (below 40° F or 4° C) or hot (above 140° F or 60° C).

9. *True.* The symptoms of food-borne illness are abdominal bloating, gas, diarrhea, vomiting, and headache, all of which are also symptoms of flu.

10. *False.* One incident of food-borne illness provides no immunity against future attacks.

11. *True.* *Salmonella* bacteria are commonly associated with chickens, especially raw chicken carcasses. Raw chicken should be handled very carefully so that juices do not contaminate other foods, thereby spreading *Salmonella* bacteria to other foods.

12. *True.* The bacterium that produces the very deadly botulism toxin is present in all soil.

13. *True.* *Clostridium botulinum* grows only in the absence of air. Thus it may be found in improperly canned foods and in thick foods where air is excluded from the center. Chili is an example.

14. *True.* Many viruses and parasites that may be present in raw fish are destroyed by cooking. Consuming raw fish poses a significant health risk for hepatitis, parasite infections, and other health problems.

15. *False.* Aside from the alcohol present in high amounts (which over time can lead to cirrhosis of the liver), alcoholic beverages contain urethanes, which FDA is now studying carefully to assess the degree of health risk these agents pose.

CHAPTER 20

1. *True.* But hunger is also physiological as well, and can be described as an uneasiness, discomfort, weakness, or pain caused by lack of food.

2. *True.* And this poverty can be caused by unemployment, homelessness, illiteracy, poor health, and other factors.

3. *False.* Diabetes is more common when food supplies are abundant.

4. *True.* Undernutrition is also the primary cause of many nutrient deficiency diseases, such as scurvy, pellagra, anemia, and many others.

5. *True.* No other social indicator shows a wider gap between the developing and industrialized world.

6. *True.* The growing fetus needs a diet rich in vitamins, protein, and minerals.

7. *True.* Failure of children to grow is a common result of undernutrition.

8. *False.* Marginal iron deficiencies affect hundreds of millions of people worldwide.

9. *False.* Full recovery may never happen, and if it does, it is likely to take months to years.

10. *False.* The United States is in twenty-second place.

11. *True.* This is partly because the cost of housing has substantially increased, and partly because federal support for subsidized housing was cut during the 1980s.

12. *False.* Economists estimate that world food production will continue to increase more rapidly than the world population in the near future, allowing the food/population ratio to increase through the year 2000.

13. *True.* There are many reasons for this. Among them is an economic imperative to have large families. Experts believe couples will choose to have fewer children once each couple experiences an increased livelihood.

14. *True.* Most of these urban poor live in overcrowded, self-made shelter with inadequate public utilities.

15. *True.* WHO estimates that more than one billion people are without a safe and adequate water supply.

Credits

Front matter p. iii, Photo Researchers; p. iv, The Stock Market; p. v, The Stock Market; p. vi, Ron Rovtar, FPG International; p. vii, Margaret Miller, Photo Researchers; p. vii, Eleanor Thompson, The Stock Market.

Chapter 1 p. 3, Daniel Hunnel, The Image Bank; p. 10 (left), Janeart Ltd., Image Bank; (right) John Kelly, The Image Bank; p. 15, Superstock; p. 18, Patrick La Croix, The Image Bank; p. 20, Ray Block, H. Armstrong Roberts; p. 23, Tom Ebenhoh, Photographic Resources; p. 25, Daniel Hunnel, The Image Bank.

Chapter 2 p. 33, Susan Kinast, WAK Pictures, Inc.; p. 36, courtesy of Laura Edwards; p. 41, Donald O'Connor Gaphic Studios; p. 45, U.S. Department of Agriculture; p. 52-54, International Diabetes Center, Minneapolis, Minn; p. 56, Susan Kinast, WAK Pictures, Inc.; p. 61, Chick Harrity, *U.S. News and World Report.*

Chapter 3 p. 67, Superstock; p. 69, Wolff Communications; p. 70, Cathy Lander-Golberg, Lander Photographics; p. 74, Jeffry W. Myers, Stock Boston; p. 90, courtesy of the Rice Council; p. 94, Superstock; p. 99, Richard H. Smith, FPG International.

Chapter 4 p. 101, Superstock; p. 106, from Deitel, M: *Nutrition in clinical surgery,* ed 2, Baltimore, 1985, Williams & Wilkins; p. 108, Wolff Communications; p. 110, Superstock; p. 122, courtesy of the National Livestock and Meat Board; p. 128, Superstock.

Chapter 5 p. 138, Michael Pruzan, The Stock Market; p. 140, Wolff Communications; p. 146 (left), Bill Longcore, Science Source; (right), Omikron/Science Source; p. 150, Lennart Nilsson, Boehringer Ingelheim International GmbH; p. 151, Cathy Lander-Goldberg, Lander Photographics; p. 159, Superstock FourByFive; p. 163, FPG International; p. 164, Michael Pruzan, The Stock Market.

Chapter 6 p. 172, Cathy Lander-Goldberg, Lander Photographics; p. 177 (top left), H. Armstrong Roberts; (middle right), Ed Reschke; (bottom), Science Photo Library, Photo Researchers; p. 178, International Diabetes Center, Minneapolis, Minn; p. 182, Superstock; p. 190, art by Christy Krames, from Raven PH, Johnson GB: *Understanding biology,* ed 2, St Louis, 1991, Mosby–Year Book; p. 196, Cathy Lander-Goldberg; p. 199, Wolff Communications.

Chapter 7 p. 205, Louis Goldman, FPG International; p. 207, K.G. Multi/Visuals Unlimited, from Raven PH, Johnson GB: *Understanding biology,* ed 1, Times Mirror Mosby College Publishing; p. 222, Nik Kleinberg, Stock Boston; p. 223, John Coletti, Stock Boston; p. 228, Louis Goldman, FPG International.

Chapter 8 p. 233, Elizabeth Hathon, The Stock Market; p. 235 (bottom), O'Connor Graphic Studio; p. 245, Medical Graphics Corporation, St. Paul, Minn; p. 248, Diana Linsley, from Payne WA, Hahn DB: *Understanding your health,* ed 2, Times Mirror Mosby College Publishing; p. 257, Bob Daemmrich, Stock Boston; p. 258, Wasye Szkodzinsky, Photo Researchers; p. 259, Elizabeth Hathon, The Stock Market.

Chapter 9 p. 264, Cathy Lander-Goldberg, Lander Photographics; p. 271, James Schnepf, Woodfin Camp and Associates; p. 282, W. Metzen, H. Armstrong Roberts; p. 292, Linsley Photographics; p. 293, Cathy Lander-Goldberg, Lander Photographics.

Chapter 10 p. 299, Charles Gupton, The Stock Market; p. 309, Cathy Lander-Goldberg, Lander Photographics; p. 311, Superstock, FourByFive; p. 318, Wide World Photos, Inc; p. 319, Charles Gupton, The Stock Market.

Chapter 11 p. 323, Cathy Lander-Goldberg, Lander Photographics; p. 326, Paul Buddle, H. Armstrong Roberts; p. 327, Wolff Communications; p. 332, Cathy Lander-Goldberg, Lander Photographics; p. 333, courtesy of Paul S. Casamassimo, D.D.S., M.S.; p. 335, Cathy Lander-Goldberg, Lander Photographics; p. 338, Cathy Lander-Goldberg, Lander Photographics; p. 343, **A,** Culver Pictures, Inc, **B,** Kobal Collection, Superstock, **C,** Caron/Gamma Liason, **D,** Linsley Photographics.

Chapter 12 p. 347, S. Feld, H. Armstrong Roberts; p. 353, from McLaran DS: *A colour atlas of nutritional disorders,* ed 1, 1981, Wolfe Medical Publications; p. 356, Friend Denny, Stock Shop; p. 358, Wally McNamee, Woodfin Camp and Associates, Inc; p. 360, from McLaran DS: *A colour atlas of nutritional disorders,* ed 1, 1981, Wolfe Medical Publications, Ltd; p. 362, George Obrenski, The Image Bank; p. 366 (left), Bill Longcore, Science Source; p. 368, R.J. Bennett, H. Armstrong Roberts; p. 371, Al Assid, The Stock Market; p. 373, S. Feld, H. Armstrong Roberts.

Chapter 13 p. 380, H. Armstrong Roberts; p. 384, International Diabetes Center, Minneapolis, Minn; p. 385, from McLaran DS: *A colour atlas of nutritional disorders,* ed 1, 1981, Wolfe Medical Publicatons, Ltd; p. 386, George Obresnki, The Image Bank; p. 387, from McLaran S: A *colour atlas of nutritional disorders,* ed 1, 1981, Wolfe Medical Publications, Ltd; p. 391, Michael Gadomski, Photo Researchers; p. 400, Mike Yamashita, The Stock Shop; p. 403, from McLaran DS: *A colour atlas of nutritional disorders,* ed 1, 1981, Wolfe Medical Publications, Ltd; p. 404, Peter Vandermark, Stock Boston; p. 410, H. Armstrong Roberts.

Chapter 14 p. 421, Jeffrey MacMillan, *U.S. News and World Report;* p. 424, Gerald Vendystadt, Photo Researchers; p. 431, Plessner International, The Stock Shop; p. 435, J. Villegiep, Photo Researchers; p. 446, FPG International; p. 449, courtesy of National Cancer Institute; p. 452, Jeffrey MacMillan, *U.S. News and World Report.*

Chapter 15 p. 458, Superstock; p. 461, Norm Thomas, Photo Researchers; p. 462, courtesy of the National Cancer Institute; p. 464 (left), CNRI, Science Photo Library, Photo Researchers; p. 466, from Powers LW: *Diagnostic hematology;* 1989, The CV Mosby Co; p. 468, Frank Oberle, Photographic Resources; p. 471, Anada S. Prasad, M.D., Ph.D., *American Journal of Medicine,* 31:532-546, 1961; p. 477, from McLaran DS: *A colour atlas of nutritional disorders,* ed 1, 1981, Wolfe Medical Publications, Ltd; p. 482, Day Williams, Photo Researchers; p. 483, Superstock; p. 488, B. Zak Photography.

Chapter 16 p. 491, Lennart Nilsson: *A child is born,* Dell Publishing Company; p. 496, Gabe Palmer, The Stock Market; p. 509, William Hubbel, Woodfin Camp and Associates; p. 511, art by Kevin Sommerville for Seeley RR, Stephens TD, Tate P: *Anatomy and Physiology,* ed 2, 1992, Mosby–Year Book; p. 514, Peter Menzel, Stock Boston; p. 516, Lennart Nilsson: *A child is born,* Dell Publishing Company; p. 519 (right), George Steinmetz.

Chapter 17 p. 521, Superstock; p. 525, Peter Pearson, H. Armstrong Roberts; p. 526, David de Lossy, The Image Bank; p. 533, FourByFive; p. 535, Nick Pavloff, The Image Bank; p. 541, John Coletti, Stock Boston; p. 543, H. Armstrong Roberts; p. 544, Jeffrey Myers, West Stock; p. 547, Superstock.

Chapter 18 p. 554, K. Reno, H. Armstrong Roberts; p. 556, George Obremski, The Image Bank; p. 567, Will and Deri McIntyre, Photo Researchers; p. 571, Sandy King, The Image Bank; p. 577, K. Reno, H. Armstrong Roberts.

Chapter 19 p. 589, Jose Luis Banus, FPG International; p. 591, Wolff Communications; p. 592 Wolff Communications; p. 593, George Contorakes, The Stock Market; p. 598 (top), Stacey Pick, Stock Boston; (bottom), Eleanor Thompson, The Stock Market; p. 608, J. Barry O'Rourke, The Stock Market; p. 610, Zanetti, The Stock Market; p. 614, Jose Luis Banus, FPG International; p. 618, Superstock, FourByFive.

Chapter 20 p. 621, Joe Sohm/Chromosom, The Stock Market; p. 628, Roy Morsch, The Stock Market; p. 641, Frans Lanting, Minden Pictures; p. 645, Suzanne L. Murphy, FPG International; p. 648, Joe Sohm/Chromosom, The Stock Market.

Index

B

W

MEDIAN HEIGHTS AND WEIGHTS AND RECOMMENDED ENERGY INTAKE 10TH EDITION RDA

Category	Age (years) or Condition	Weight (kg)	Weight (lb)	Height (cm)	Height (in)	REE[a] (kcal/day)	Average Energy Allowance (kcal): Multiples of REE	Average Energy Allowance (kcal): Per kg	Average Energy Allowance (kcal): Per day[b]
Infants	0.0-0.5	6	13	60	24	320		108	650
	0.5-1.0	9	20	71	28	500		98	850
Children	1-3	13	29	90	56	740		102	1,300
	4-6	20	44	112	44	950		90	1,800
	7-10	28	62	132	52	1,130		70	2,000
Males	11-14	45	99	157	62	1,440	1.70	55	2,500
	15-18	66	145	176	69	1,760	1.67	45	3,000
	19-24	72	160	177	70	1,780	1.67	40	2,900
	25-50	79	174	176	70	1,800	1.60	37	2,900
	51+	77	170	173	68	1,530	1.50	30	2,300
Females	11-14	46	101	157	62	1,310	1.67	47	2,200
	15-18	55	120	163	64	1,370	1.60	40	2,200
	19-24	58	128	164	65	1,350	1.60	38	2,200
	25-50	63	138	163	64	1,380	1.55	36	2,200
	51+	65	143	160	63	1,280	1.50	30	1,900
Pregnant	1st Trimester								+0
	2nd Trimester								+300
	3rd Trimester								+300
Lactating	1st 6 months								+500
	2nd 6 months								+500

[a] Resting energy expenditure (REE); calculation based on FAO equations, then rounded. This is the same as RMR.
[b] Figure is rounded.

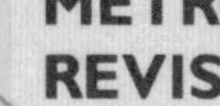

METROPOLITAN LIFE INSURANCE COMPANY HEIGHT-WEIGHT DATA, REVISED 1983

Height-Weight Tables for Adults (1983)

Height: Ft	Height: In	WOMEN Frame*: Small	WOMEN Frame*: Medium	WOMEN Frame*: Large	Height Ft	Height In	MEN Frame*: Small	MEN Frame*: Medium	MEN Frame*: Large
4	10	102-111	109-121	118-131	5	2	128-134	131-141	138-150
4	11	103-113	111-123	120-134	5	3	130-136	133-143	140-153
5	0	104-115	113-126	122-137	5	4	132-138	135-145	142-156
5	1	106-118	115-129	125-140	5	5	134-140	137-148	144-160
5	2	108-121	118-132	128-143	5	6	136-142	139-151	146-164
5	3	111-124	121-135	131-147	5	7	138-145	142-154	149-168
5	4	114-127	124-138	134-151	5	8	140-148	145-157	152-172
5	5	117-130	127-141	137-155	5	9	142-151	148-160	155-176
5	6	120-133	130-144	140-159	5	10	144-154	151-163	158-180
5	7	113-136	133-147	143-163	5	11	146-157	154-166	161-184
5	8	126-139	136-150	146-167	6	0	149-160	157-170	164-188
5	9	129-142	139-153	149-170	6	1	152-164	160-174	168-192
5	10	132-145	142-156	152-173	6	2	155-168	164-178	172-197
5	11	135-148	156-159	155-176	6	3	158-172	167-182	176-202
6	0	138-151	148-162	158-179	6	4	162-176	171-187	181-207

Based on a weight-height mortality study conducted by the Society of Actuaries and the Association of Life Insurance Medical Directors of America, Metropolitan Life Insurance Company, revised 1983.

*Weights at ages 25 to 59 based on lowest mortality. Height includes 1-in heel. Weight for women includes 3 lb. for indoor clothing. Weight for men includes 5 lb. for indoor clothing. (see p. 347 for controversy surrounding the use and abuse of these tables over the years and Appendix K for determination of frame size.)

W9-CSI-053

The Brothers Karamazov

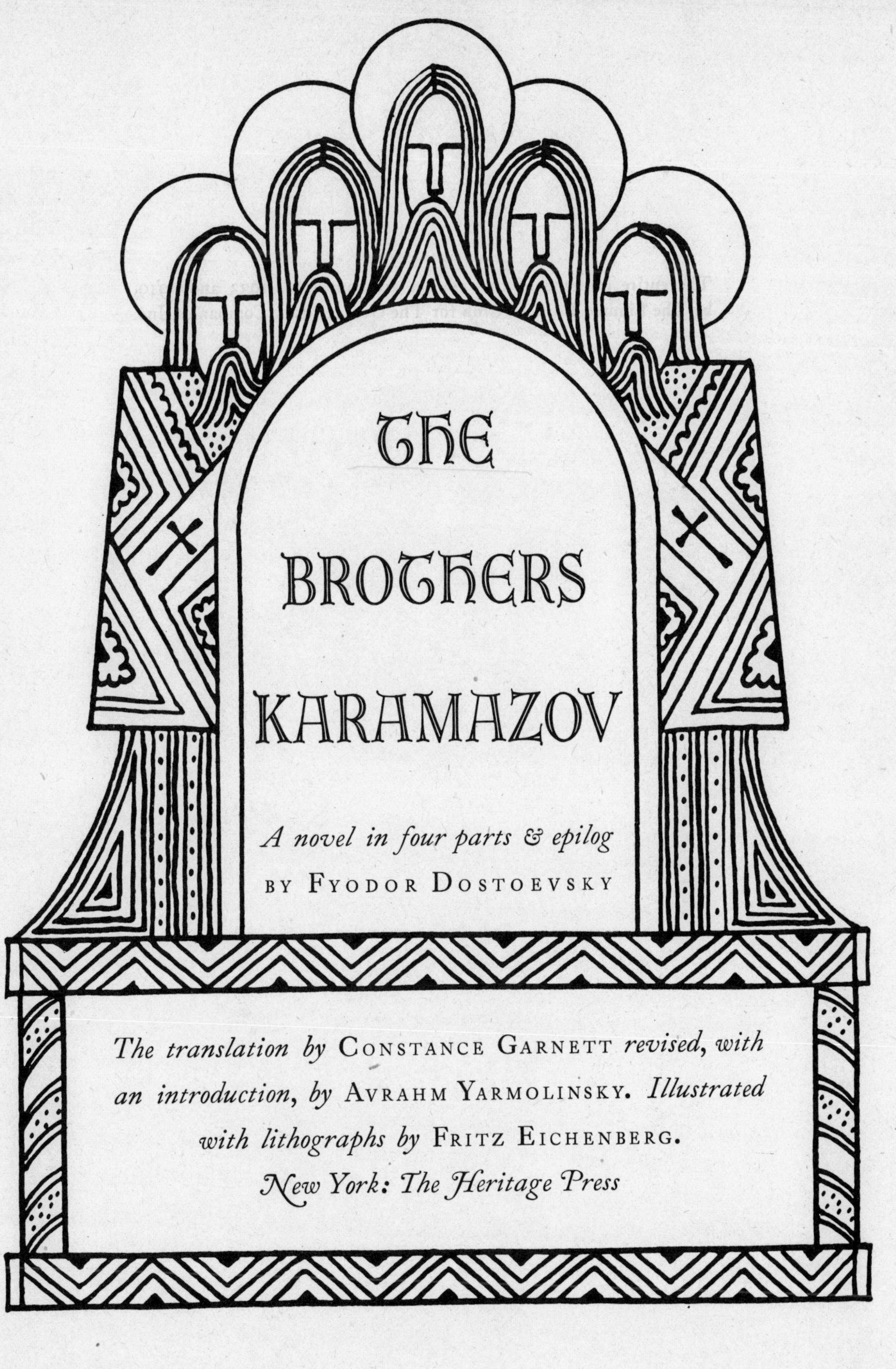

THE BROTHERS KARAMAZOV

A novel in four parts & epilog

BY FYODOR DOSTOEVSKY

The translation by CONSTANCE GARNETT *revised, with an introduction, by* AVRAHM YARMOLINSKY. *Illustrated with lithographs by* FRITZ EICHENBERG.

New York: The Heritage Press

INTRODUCTION

Of the nineteenth century novelists, none have worn so well as the Russians, but whereas the passage of time has given Turgenev a slightly old-fashioned air, and has neither subtracted from nor yet added to the excellences of Tolstoy, it has only served to bring out the profundity and imaginative power of Dostoevsky's work. Within the last two or three decades his reputation has climbed to dizzying heights. For one thing, the malaise through which our civilization is passing has brought us closer to a man who, we must admit, foresaw pretty clearly the progress of our spiritual disease, even though he would have medicined us with a religion which we cannot swallow. Further, a better and more widely diffused knowledge of mental processes has made this generation more appreciative of the first novelist to have such an astonishing insight into human motives and into all the contradictions and confusions of the mind. His present extraordinary vogue may suffer an eclipse abroad, for causes not necessarily the same as those that have weakened his influence at home, where both his convictions and his perplexities are out of harmony with the practical temper of the times. Yet his greatness as a novelist is one of the few certainties in an uncertain world.

Dostoevsky's crowning achievement was "The Brothers Karamazov." Few novels of any time and any country have been so heartily praised in our own day, and by connoisseurs so diverse. Marcel Proust, himself a master builder in the field of fiction, allowed it a mysterious beauty, a sculptural grandeur. Arnold Bennett classed it as "one of the supreme marvels of the world." Sigmund Freud, who brings to his judgment of literature the acumen of a pioneer psychologist, does not hesitate to call it "the most magnificent novel ever written." Translated into practically every civilized language, broadcast in inexpensive editions, the book is finding its way to a widening circle of readers. And yet, though it carries the thrills of a detective story, the elementary interest of melodrama and romance, the persuasiveness of realistic fiction, it will always be, to some degree, caviar to the general. Its psychological subtleties, its passionate philosophizing, will inevitably limit its deepest appeal to the mature and the discriminating.

"The Brothers Karamazov" was at once the culmination and the close of Dostoevsky's career: when he put finis to it, in November, 1880, he had only two months to live. He had been occupied with the actual writing of it for three years, but some of its elements had been present in his mind before he set pen to paper, and indeed are discoverable in his earliest writings. As though he feared that the sands were running out for him, he gave more of himself to the book than to any previous work. He put into it the affirmation which was the difficult yield of so many doubts; he put into it the doubts, too, along with his understanding of character, his intimate knowledge of the obscure ways of the human soul, his sense of life, with its burden of mystery, terror and pity, and its core of pure joy. The book bears witness to the strength of a creative power miraculously preserved in a body racked by disease and distress, by the accumulated fatigues of nearly sixty lacerating years.

It is far from obvious precisely how Dostoevsky's personal fortunes shaped his novels, and particularly "The Brothers Karamazov," yet a glance at the more significant among the author's experiences and private opinions, and at the influences that worked upon him, may contribute something to the appreciation of the book.

Fyodor Dostoevsky was born in 1821, in the pious old city of Moscow, where he spent his childhood and early youth. He was the son of an army doctor, a stern, moody, irascible man, who belonged to the gentry, and the growing family led a shabby-genteel existence in a corner of the charity hospital where he served. A religious atmosphere prevailed in the home, and the memory of childhood pilgrimages to a neighboring monastery must have fed the imagination of the man who wrote the scenes from monastic life in "The Brothers Karamazov." From the first, Dostoevsky's taste for reading was encouraged by his parents, who were not without literary interests, and who were at pains to give him a good schooling. As a boy he spent several summers on his father's modest property in the provinces, but the spacious manorial setting in which Turgenev and Tolstoy, his two famous contemporaries, grew up, was alien to him. His mind was at home in the city, and practically all his characters have the urban stamp upon them.

His mother died just before he left Moscow, at the age of sixteen, to attend a military engineering school in what was then St. Petersburg. There, his unaccustomed surroundings, the severity of the discipline, the roughness and vulgarity of his schoolmates, the uncongenial character of his studies, his humiliating poverty (his tuition had been paid by a well-to-do relative), combined to make a brooding solitary of the proud, dreamy, high-strung boy. He was in his second year at school when news reached him that his father had been murdered. The doctor had retired to his country place and given himself up to drink, and the killing was no doubt an act of vengeance on a brutal master perpetrated by his own serfs. The psychoanalytic view of the matter is that the effect of the tragedy on Dostoevsky, who allegedly harbored a strong unconscious death-wish against his father, was a shattering one, and indeed, brought out his latent tendency to epilepsy. Posthumous psychoanalysis is admittedly guess-work, but it is at least noteworthy that Dostoevsky's last and greatest novel revolves around the murder of a repulsive old sot by his servant, who is also his bastard, while two other sons of his commit the crime of parricide in their minds, and that one of the major themes is the problem of moral responsibility for a crime which is a wish rather than an act.

The profession of engineering held no attractions for the young man, and within a year of graduation he retired from the service, determined to make his living by his pen, even if he had to starve for it. From then on almost to the end of his days he lived in the grip of crushing poverty, enduring for a while a kind of literary peonage, and always writing desperately against time. He broke into print at the age of twenty-four with "Poor Folk," a short novel, which had an immediate and dazzling success. He followed it up with a story called "The Double," a striking and penetrating study of the split personality, a theme which was to haunt his mind and to recur again in his last work. He was hailed as a prodigy by Belinsky, and was welcomed into the circle over which this influential critic presided. Here Dostoevsky was exposed to liberal and even radical views, and more particularly to the ideas of the Westernists, who wished to see Russia follow the lead of Europe. A break soon took place between him and his newfound friends, partly owing to his touchiness and arrogance — his success had gone to his head — and partly to intellectual incompatibility. His fame seemed to be withering as rapidly as it had bloomed, the stories he was now writing being coldly received; his earnings were of the meagrest; and to add to his harassments, he was ill: he had various nervous symptoms and seems to have already become subject to epileptic seizures.

Although living under the iron rule of a paternalistic autocrat, a handful of young Russian intellectuals were sensitive to the movement that prepared the revolutions of 1848 abroad. Dostoevsky was one of these young men: he followed eagerly the events in Europe, he read the books of the French socialists, and he attended Friday night gatherings at which opinions directed against church and state were aired. At the same time, paradoxically enough, he seems to have entertained some nationalistic and pietistic notions which were then being popularized by the Slavophils. At all events, it is highly doubtful whether he subscribed to the more subversive views of his companions; he was certainly no atheist, and a socialist of only the mildest variety; if he uttered some wild words it was because he was carried away by a generous impulse toward social justice. The result of it all was that on the morning of Holy Saturday in 1849 he, as well as dozens of other young men who had attended the Fridays, was arrested and thrust into prison. Charged with having attended the meetings and with having read aloud a seditious letter, he was condemned, and sentenced to four years of hard labor in Siberia, to be followed by service in the ranks. But together with the other prisoners, he was taken to a public square, where a sentence of capital punishment was read aloud, and the preliminaries to execution by shooting were carried out. For some interminable minutes Dostoevsky believed that he was about to die. Suddenly, in accordance with the grim comedy prearranged by the czar, who had a taste for theatricals, the true sentence was announced.

Dostoevsky endured four years of penal servitude in a foul prison, shaven and fettered like the common criminals who were his constant companions, without the merest decencies of existence, without privacy, without any book but the New Testament, without a word from home. Furthermore, he now came to recognize for the first time that he was an epileptic. On his release he became a private in a Siberian regiment largely recruited from ex-convicts and stationed in a miserable frontier town thousands of miles from civilization. He accepted his punishment as though he deserved it, and did not shrink from his brutish fellows. He was later to assert that his intimate contact with the common people had opened his eyes to the ancient treasure of the Russian folk: their Orthodox faith and their childlike confidence in the czar. His experiences no doubt helped to stimulate his preoccupation with crime, which was to him a token of man's spiritual nature. His exile lasted ten years in all, and when he returned to Petersburg in 1859, he was not only toughened in soul and body, but a firmer adherent of the Russian Christ and a loyal subject of his emperor. He was moreover a married man, having allied himself with a widow, a delicate and destitute gentlewoman, for whom he had conceived a passion not unmixed with pity.

Dostoevsky, now approaching forty, had to start again at the bottom. He had brought from Siberia two rather mediocre tales, which he had difficulty in placing. The problem of how to earn enough to support himself, his wife, and his stepson was acute. The rôle of a publicist had always fascinated him, and now, with the quickening of Russia's intellectual and political life, prior to the great reforms of the sixties, it seemed more attractive than ever. Although he knew that fiction was his métier, he had a strong impulse to make his influence felt in a more direct fashion. With his brother Mikhail, who was himself something of a littérateur and who had besides a head for business, he launched a monthly review. It was a conservative periodical waging war against the nihilists, and just tinged with liberalism to suit the times. Through a misunderstanding it was suppressed in 1863, and was resumed shortly under another name. It was to these magazines that Dostoevsky contributed, besides some miscellaneous papers, an inferior novel, and a remarkable chronicle of his prison days, as well as "Notes From the Underground," that disturbing mixture of controversy and confession which, both in its probing of a sick soul and its implied aspiration toward spiritual health, is the true preamble to his great novels.

During these years his personal life was an agitated one. There was a peaceful interval when he fulfilled his long cherished dream of visiting Western Europe. The trip confirmed him in the prejudices he took with him against the West and also in his faith in Russia's manifest destiny. He went abroad unaccompanied by his wife. His marriage had turned out badly. The two seem to have been bound to each other by the double ties of love and hate, which he was to represent in his novels so often as the basis of the passional relation. His devotion to her did not prevent him from having a brief liaison with a young student, who took the initiative in terminating their intimacy. In 1863, while his wife lay desperately ill with consumption, he went abroad for the second time, ostensibly to be treated for epilepsy, actually to be with his fickle mistress, and it was on this trip that he contracted the gambling fever which was to be the curse of his existence for years. The following spring his wife died, and a few months later his brother Mikhail, too, passed away suddenly, leaving a mass of debts incurred in connection with the magazine, and a family without visible means of support. Dostoevsky took over the magazine, sank in it his share of his aunt's fortune, only to see the review fail within a few months, and to find himself, an ailing, middle-aged man, deep in debt, with his own stepson and his brother's family on his hands, and no one and nothing to live for.

And yet he sometimes felt, strangely enough, that his life was just beginning, and indeed, his best work was still to come. One evening in Wiesbaden, in September, 1865, after he had lost everything at roulette, the main outline of his first important novel, "Crime and Punishment," suddenly crystallized in his brain. In this "psychological account of a crime," as Dostoevsky himself described his superb work, the author expresses his fascinated horror at a mind which allows itself to be guided by reason alone, and which in its aberration dares to set itself beyond good and evil. Ideas of this order recur.

He was forced to interrupt the writing of the novel and to dash off another story in order to fulfill an onerous contract into which he had entered in a moment of utter penury. In this short novel, "The Gambler," he drew upon his experiences at the tables and also upon his unhappy liaison. He had to work at record speed and so resorted to the services of a stenographer, probably an unprecedented occurrence in the history of Russian letters. The girl — she was only twenty — was not the first to whom he proposed after becoming a widower, but she was the first to accept him. His marriage, early in 1867, to this steadfast, brave, humdrum young person, won him a loving wife, a devoted helpmate, and a capable manager of his affairs. A few weeks after the wedding the couple went abroad, partly to escape creditors, but more particularly to save their union, seemingly so incongruous, from the attacks upon it made by his relatives.

The couple stayed abroad, chiefly in Germany, four years, and at times this second exile seemed to him worse than his Siberian captivity. They were constantly in want, often not knowing where the next meal was to come from, and reduced to pawning even their necessaries. His periodic and disastrous gambling fits contributed not a little to their misery. Two children were born to them here, but the parents knew the sorrow of leaving their firstborn in a foreign cemetery. Dostoevsky's seizures, though less frequent, persisted. His homesickness was made acute by his hatred of the alien scene, but more by the feeling that he was losing touch with his country and so with the source of his art and the springs of life itself. Under these harassing circumstances, Dostoevsky wrote "The Idiot," a work of great originality and power, in which for the first time he made the attempt, repeated in "The Brothers Karamazov," to depict the perfect Christian confronting the world, the flesh, and the devil. He also began "The Possessed," a huge novel which savagely attacks the revolutionary movement, then still in its infancy, and which is further concerned with the tragedy of a rootless soul, unable to lay hold of anything on earth or in heaven which gives validity to life, — another motif which Dostoevsky resumes in his last novel.

"The Possessed" was finished in 1872, when he was again settled in Petersburg. In his last decade his life was uneventful and less irregular than it had ever been before. There were still creditors to satisfy, his health was worse, and what with the needs of a growing family, he had to drive his pen harder and faster than ever, but thanks to the business sense of his energetic wife, toward the end he knew relative security and ease. The winters were spent in the capital and the summers in a provincial town, which Dostoevsky used as the setting for "The Brothers Karamazov." The great sorrow of these latter years was the loss of his youngest child, Alyosha — only two of his four children survived — and there are echoes of it in that moving passage of his last novel in which the peasant woman bereaved of her child pours out her heart to the elder Zosima.

He occupied himself alternately with journalism and fiction, giving almost equal time to each. For a while he edited a conservative weekly, to which he contributed, besides comment on foreign politics, informal miscellaneous feuilletons dealing with matters of current interest, which he called "A Writer's Diary." He gave up the burdensome editorial task to write "A Raw Youth," which first appeared in 1875, serially, like all his novels. This sprawling narrative, which is the least integrated of Dostoevsky's works, has for one of its dominant themes the father-son relation which is touched upon again in "The Brothers Karamazov." Both the assent to life arrived at by the adolescent hero, who had been possessed by a withering cerebral dream, and the inner peace found by his father, the divided soul, announce Dostoevsky's final work. Having completed "A Raw Youth," he resumed his "Writer's Diary," this time as a monthly miscellany, of which he was the publisher and to which he was the sole contributor. He made this the vehicle for the expression of his belief in the messianic destiny of his country, and of other views as vehement as they were contradictory. His forensic writings, added to his novels, won him a wide reputation even among those who were hostile to his nationalistic and pietistic opinions, and he was looked to for spiritual guidance by many, so that the speech which he delivered at the unveiling of a statue of Pushkin in Moscow was the occasion of a public ovation approximating that tendered the aged Voltaire on his final visit to Paris. The Pushkin festival occurred in the summer of 1880.

The most obvious claim that this book makes upon the reader's attention is its excellence as a crime novel. Dostoevsky was not averse to using the tricks of his trade, and in this story of parricide he contrived suspense and surprise with extraordinary skill. It owes much of its effectiveness to its dramatic quality. It exhibits the tempo and tension of high tragedy: there are prolixities and interpolations, but the main action is crowded into a few days; the protagonists are observed not in the sober light of common day but in the flash of the thunderbolt; a sense of impending catastrophe broods over the scenes.

The characters — there are some fifty men and women in the book — are drawn with that understanding of emotional ambivalence and the rôle of the unconscious which distinguishes Dostoevsky's art. They are not transcripts of ordinary humanity. Their ecstasies and agonies are too intense, their soul-searchings too keen, their tossings between good and evil, between love and hatred, too abrupt, their impulses too perverse. Yet they have a compelling reality. The inwardness and authority with which Dostoevsky portrayed the Karamazovs may be due to the fact that they are projections of the several elements at war within his own breast. They are creatures of flesh and blood, endowed with a distinct life of their own, but they may also be taken as symbols. The old man Karamazov seems to be the pattern of the sensualist in all his unredeemable animalism; his bastard, Smerdyakov, the moral idiot, being the evil growth of his blind lust. It is with the three legitimate sons that we reach the human plane, and the violent Dmitri, the subtle Ivan, the gentle Alyosha, appear respectively as the body, the mind, and the spiritual member. It belongs to the substance of Dostoevsky's thinking that he should represent the body as striving toward union with the spirit, the intellect as cruelly divided against itself and fundamentally inimical to life.

The book derives further significance from the fact that it is concerned with ideas. The crime novel is also a philosophical novel, but that does not mean that the author engages in dry abstract disquisitions. With Dostoevsky, intellection has the force and heat of emotion. The ideas either grow naturally out of the situations, or are formulated in the course of those absorbing arguments which are among the high points of the narrative. They revolve around the whole complex of problems that cluster about morality and religion. "The Brothers Karamazov" may be viewed as a vast parable, or, better still, as a religious disputation, such as is carried on, with a difference, in the Book of Job. Ivan, the dialectician, upholds the negative: if God can allow the suffering of the innocent, of children, above all, even though this be the price of some future beatitude, then the world is meaningless and unacceptable. His blasphemies go further. In his fantasy, "The Grand Inquisitor," he shows the Catholic Church at the height of its power serving not Christ, but the Evil One who tempted Him in the desert; the church is using the means that Christ had spurned, in order to make men happy and save them from His terrible gift of freedom. It is Ivan's tragedy that he cannot wholeheartedly side with Christ against Satan and the Grand Inquisitor. To understand Dostoevsky's intention here one must remember that among his favorite ideas was the dubious notion that Catholicism, in arrogating to itself temporal power, had betrayed Christ, and so become the mother of socialism. The latter Dostoevsky abhorred as a crass destructive doctrine which set the nourishment of man's body above the well-being of his soul, and which would result in the establishment of a sane, safe, social order, orphaned of God. Ivan's own fate, no less than Dmitri's regeneration, the serene faith which guides Alyosha, and the saintly life and Orthodox teachings of his master, Zosima, all indirectly refute Ivan's argument and proclaim a religious acceptance of life. The reader must decide for himself who wins the debate. As for Dostoevsky, he was, consciously at least, on the side of the angels, as the final scene emphatically attests.

Often after completing a novel, Dostoevsky was left with a feeling of the inadequacy of what he had set down. Some such feeling must have haunted him when he finished his last work, for the end of the book was by no means the end of the story of the Karamazovs. Indeed, the novel closes before he has fairly launched the youngest brother, the novice, on his career in the world. As is indicated in the author's foreword, which the present edition offers for the first time in English, "The Brothers Karamazov" was to have had a second part, with Alyosha as the hero. Dostoevsky did not live to write it, so that, in a sense, the novel is a torso, not unlike that other Russian masterpiece, Gogol's "Dead Souls." Little is known of the author's plans for the sequel. It is said that Alyosha was to have become involved with revolutionists and to have committed a political crime, — it will be recalled that during Dostoevsky's last years the terrorists were increasingly active and, indeed, his own death antedated by one month the assassination of the czar. The possibilities of such a novel as this projected sequel fairly dazzle the imagination. But there is no need to speak of might-have-beens. The work as it stands is sufficient to engage profoundly the mind and the emotions of the reader, and to leave him shaken by a sense of the large potentialities of the soul.

Avrahm Yarmolinsky

Verily, verily, I say unto you, Except a corn of wheat fall into the ground and die, it abideth alone: but if it die, it bringeth forth much fruit. JOHN XII. 24.

THE TABLE OF CONTENTS

THE TABLE OF CONTENTS

A LIST OF THE LITHOGRAPHS

The Brothers Karamazov

AUTHOR'S FOREWORD

In commencing the life-story of my hero, Alexey Fyodorovich Karamazov, I find myself somewhat perplexed: although I call Alexey Fyodorovich my hero, nevertheless I myself know that he is by no means a great man, and hence I foresee that there will inevitably arise such questions as these: "What is so remarkable about your Alexey Fyodorovich, that you have chosen him as your hero? What has he accomplished? For what is he known, and by whom? Why should a reader like myself spend time over the facts of his life?"

The last question is the most embarrassing one, for I can answer it only by saying: "Perhaps you will see for yourself from the novel." And what if you do read it, and fail to see, and so do not agree that my Alexey Fyodorovich is remarkable? I say this because unhappily I anticipate such an eventuality. To my mind he is remarkable, but I doubt very much if I shall succeed in proving it to the reader. The fact is that he is perhaps a leader, but a leader in the making, still unformed. Indeed, it would be strange to require in an age like ours that a man should have a clearly defined viewpoint. One thing perhaps is plain: he is a queer character, indeed an original. But queerness and oddity are more apt to repel than to command attention, especially at a time when all are striving to eliminate differences and to find some unifying principle in the general confusion. But an original is in most cases the very essence of what is particular and apart from the commonalty. Isn't that so?

Should you disagree with this notion and answer: "No, it isn't so," or "It isn't always so," then I might feel more encouraged about the significance of my hero, Alexey Fyodorovich. For not only is an original "not always particular and apart from the commonalty," but, on the contrary, it happens sometimes that such a person is near the very heart of the commonalty, and the rest of the men of his age have temporarily been swept away from it, as by a gust of wind. . . .

I should not have entered into these uninteresting and vague explanations and should have begun simply without any introduction, saying to myself: "If they like it, they will read it," but the trouble is that while there is one life-story, there are two tales here. The main narrative is the second one, — it has to do with the activity of my hero in our own day, precisely at the present moment. As for the first tale, it deals with events of thirteen years ago, and properly speaking, it is not an entire novel, but only the description of one episode in my hero's early youth. I cannot do without this first tale, because much in the second tale would become unintelligible without it. But in this way my original embarrassment is rendered even greater: if I, that is, the biographer himself, find that my immature and modest hero seems not to deserve even one tale, why appear with two, and how can I justify such presumption?

At a loss as to how to answer these questions, I choose to evade them. Of course, the perspicuous reader has long since guessed that such was my intention from the first, and was only vexed with me for wasting words and time. To this, here is my direct reply: I was wasting words and time, first, out of courtesy, second, out of shrewdness: at least I gave my readers fair warning. Besides, I am even glad that my book has of itself split into two narratives, without injury, however, to its essential unity: having perused the first tale, the reader will decide for himself whether it is worth his while to attempt the second. Of course, there is no obligation in the matter, — you may throw the book aside after the first two pages and never open it again. But there are readers so conscientious that they will certainly wish to read the book to the end, so as to form a judicious estimate of it. Such, for instance, are all the Russian critics. It is by this type of reader that I feel I have done my duty. I have given these scrupulous and conscientious folk a legitimate pretext for tossing the book aside at the outset. Well, here is my whole foreword. I fully agree that it is altogether useless, but as it has been written, let it stand. And now to business.

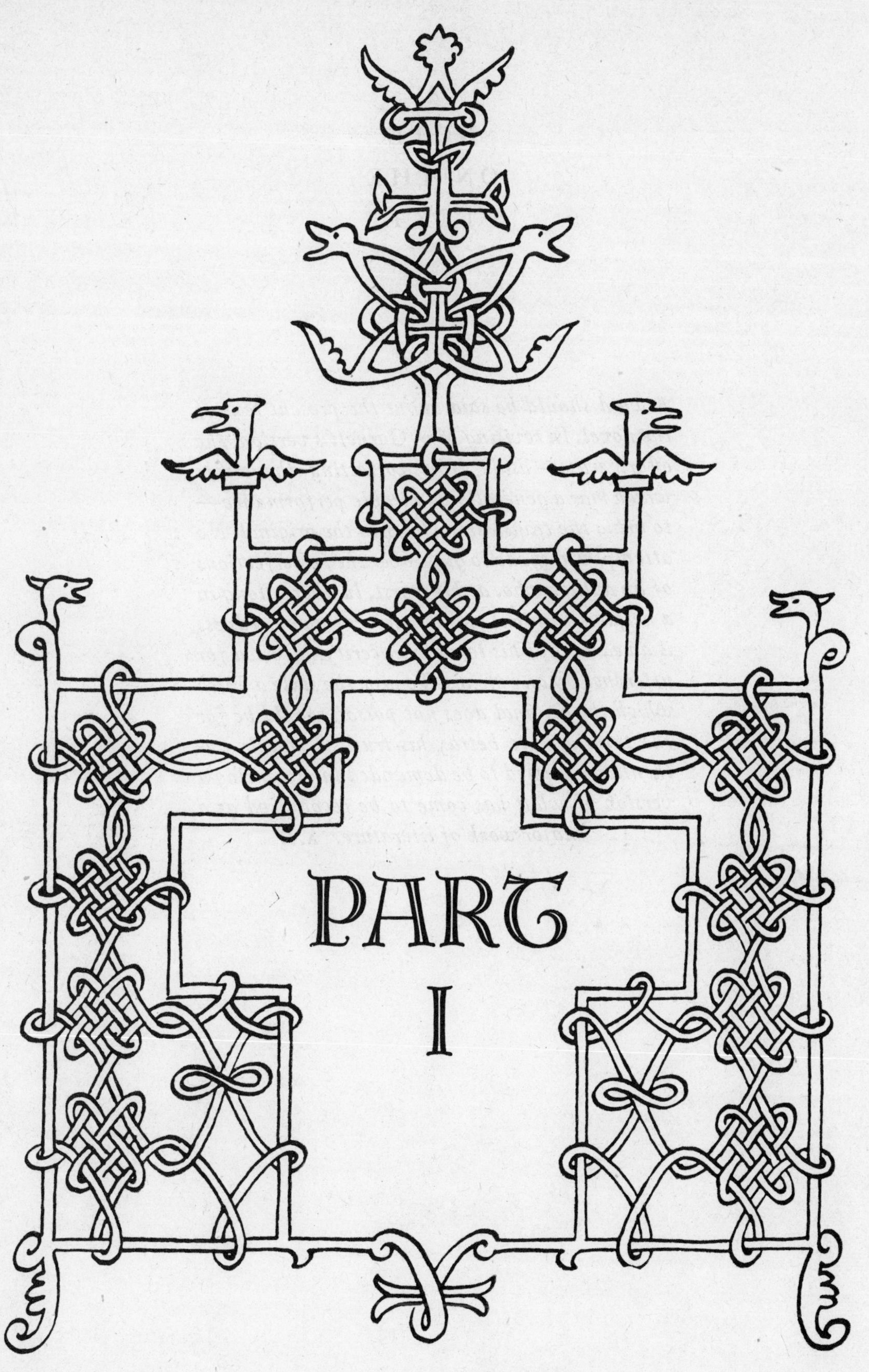
PART
I

A NOTE ON THE TEXT

A word should be said about the present text of the novel. In revising Mrs. Garnett's version, the effort was — aside from correcting the errors which mar a generally admirable performance — to bring the translation closer to the original. No attempt was made to gloss over the imperfections of an author who, at his worst, lumbers along in a helpless fashion, and whose very awkwardness is an earnest of his terrible sincerity, his need for utterance by any means. To give the style a finish which the original does not possess would be for the translator to betray his trust. Certainly authenticity seemed to be demanded in presenting a version of what has come to be recognized as a major work of literature. A.Y.

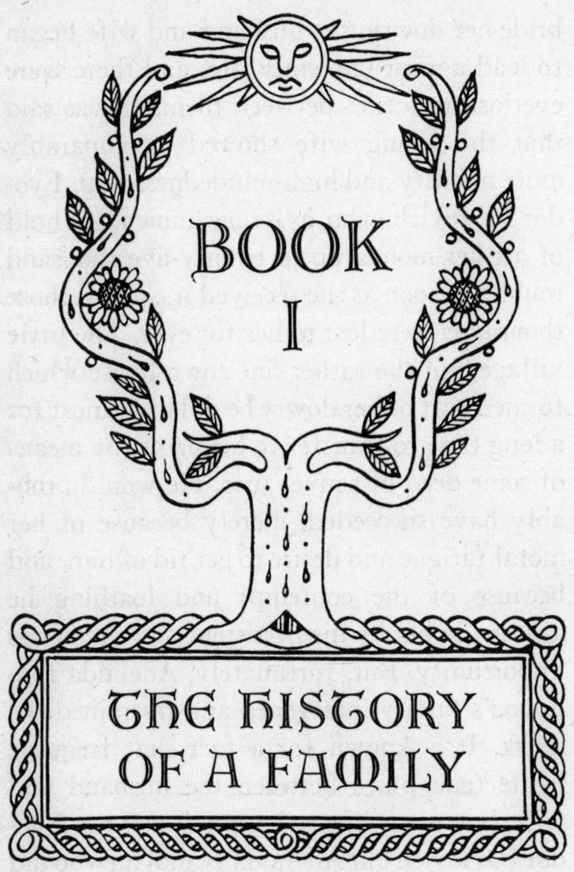

CHAPTER I

FYODOR PAVLOVICH KARAMAZOV

ALEXEY FYODOROVICH KARAMAZOV was the third son of Fyodor Pavlovich Karamazov, a landowner well known in our district in his own day, and still remembered among us owing to his tragic and obscure death, which happened just thirteen years ago, and of which I shall speak in its proper place. For the present I will only say that this "landowner"—for so we used to call him, although he hardly spent a day of his life on his estate—was a strange sort, yet one pretty frequently to be met with, a worthless and dissolute and at the same time senseless type of man. But he was one of those senseless persons who are very well able to look after their worldly affairs, and, apparently, after nothing else. Fyodor Pavlovich, for instance, began with next to nothing; his estate was of the smallest; he ran to dine at other men's tables, and was on the look-out for a chance to become a hanger-on, yet at his death it appeared that he had a hundred thousand roubles in hard cash. At the same time, he was all his life one of the most senseless eccentrics in the whole district. I repeat, it was not stupidity—the majority of these eccentrics are shrewd and intelligent enough—but just senselessness, and a peculiar national form of it.

He was married twice, and had three sons, the eldest, Dmitri, by his first wife, and two, Ivan and Alexey, by his second. Fyodor Pavlovich's first spouse, Adelaïda Ivanovna, belonged to the gentry, coming of a fairly rich and distinguished family, also landowners in our district, the Miüsovs. How it came to pass that a girl with a dowry, who was also a beauty, and moreover one of those lively, intelligent girls, so common in this generation, but sometimes also to be found in the last, could have married such a seedy nonentity, as everybody called him then, I won't attempt to explain. I knew a young lady of the last "romantic" generation who after some years of an enigmatic passion for a gentleman, whom she might quite easily have married at any moment, invented insuperable obstacles to their union, and ended by throwing herself one stormy night into a rather deep and rapid river from a high bank, almost a precipice, and so perished, entirely to satisfy her own caprice, and to be like Shakespeare's Ophelia. Indeed, if this precipice, a chosen and favourite spot of hers, had been less picturesque, if there had been a prosaic flat bank in its place, most likely the suicide would never have occurred. This is a fact, and probably there have been not a few similar instances in Russia in the last two or three generations. Adelaïda Ivanovna Miüsov's action was likewise, no doubt, an echo of other people's ideas, and was due to the "chafing of imprisoned thought." She wanted, perhaps, to show her feminine independence, to defy social conventions and the despotism of her family. And a pliable imagination persuaded her, we must suppose, for a brief moment, that Fyodor Pavlovich, in spite of his parasitic position, was one of the bold and ironical spirits of that progressive epoch, though he was, in fact, an ill-natured buffoon and nothing more. What gave the marriage piquancy was that it was preceded by an elopement, and this greatly captivated Adelaïda Ivanovna's fancy. Fyodor Pavlovich's position at the time made him specially eager for any such enterprise, for he was passionately anxious to make a career in one way or another. To attach himself to a good family and obtain a dowry was an alluring prospect. As for love, apparently the bride felt none for the groom, nor, in spite of Adelaïda Ivanovna's beauty, he any for her. This was, perhaps, a unique case in the life of Fyodor Pavlovich, who was always of a sensuous temperament, and ready to run after any petticoat on the slightest encouragement. She seems to have been the only woman who made no particular appeal to his senses.

Immediately after the elopement Adelaïda Ivanovna discerned in a flash that she had no feeling for her husband but contempt. The marriage accordingly showed itself in its true colours with extraordinary rapidity. Although the family became reconciled to the event pretty quickly and apportioned the runaway bride her dowry, the husband and wife began to lead a most unseemly life, and there were everlasting scenes between them. It was said that the young wife showed incomparably more nobility and high-mindedness than Fyodor Pavlovich, who, as is now known, got hold of all her money up to twenty-five thousand roubles as soon as she received it, so that those thousands were lost to her for ever. The little village and the rather fine town house which formed part of her dowry he did his utmost for a long time to transfer to his name, by means of some deed of conveyance. He would probably have succeeded, merely because of her moral fatigue and desire to get rid of him, and because of the contempt and loathing he aroused in her by his persistent and shameless importunity. But, fortunately, Adelaïda Ivanovna's family intervened and restrained the shark. It is known for a fact that frequent fights took place between the husband and wife, but, according to legend, it was not Fyodor Pavlovich but Adelaïda Ivanovna who did the beating, for she was a hot-tempered, bold, dark-browed, impatient woman, possessed of remarkable physical strength. Finally, she left the house and ran away from Fyodor Pavlovich with a destitute divinity student, leaving Mitya, a child three years old, on her husband's hands. Immediately Fyodor Pavlovich introduced a regular harem into the house, and abandoned himself to orgies of drunkenness. In the intervals he used to drive all over the province, complaining tearfully to each and all of Adelaïda Ivanovna's having left him, going into details too disgraceful for a husband to mention in regard to his own married life. What seemed to gratify him most and flatter him was to play the ridiculous part of the injured husband, and to parade his woes.

"One would think that you'd got a promotion, Fyodor Pavlovich, you seem so pleased in spite of your sorrow," scoffers said to him.

Many added that he was glad of a new comic part in which to play the buffoon, and that it was simply to make it funnier that he pretended to be unaware of his ludicrous position. But, who knows, it may indeed have been simplicity. At last he succeeded in getting on the track of his runaway wife. The poor woman turned out to be in Petersburg, where she had gone with her divinity student, and where she had thrown herself into a life of complete emancipation. Fyodor Pavlovich at once began bustling about, making preparations to go to Petersburg, with what object he could not himself have said. He would perhaps really have gone; but having determined to do so he felt at once entitled to fortify himself for the journey by another bout of reckless drinking. And just at that time his wife's family received the news of her death in Petersburg. She had died quite suddenly in a garret, according to one story, of typhus, or, as another version had it, of starvation. Fyodor Pavlovich was drunk when he heard of his wife's death, and the story is that he ran out into the street and began shouting with joy, raising his hands to heaven: "Lord, now lettest Thou Thy servant depart in peace," but others say he wept without restraint like a little child, so much so that people were sorry for him, in spite of the disgust he inspired. It is quite possible that both versions were true, that he rejoiced at his release, and at the same time wept for her who released him. As a general rule, people, even the wicked, are much more naïve and simple-hearted than we suppose. And we ourselves are, too.

CHAPTER II

HE GETS RID OF HIS ELDEST SON

YOU can easily imagine what a father such a man could be and how he would bring up his children. His behaviour as a father was exactly what might be expected. He completely abandoned the child of his marriage with Adelaïda Ivanovna, not from malice, nor because of his grievances as a husband, but simply because he forgot him altogether. While he was wearying every one with his tears and complaints, and turning his house into a sink of debauchery, a faithful servant of the family, Grigory, took the three-year-old Mitya into his care. If he hadn't looked after him there would have been no one even to change the child's little shirt.

It happened moreover that the child's relations on his mother's side also forgot him at first. His grandfather was no longer living, the widow, Mitya's grandmother, had moved to Moscow, and was seriously ill, while his aunts were married, so that Mitya remained for almost a whole year in old Grigory's charge and lived with him in the servant's cottage. But even if his father had remembered him (he could not, indeed, have been altogether unaware of his existence), he would have sent him back to the cottage, as the child would only have been in the way of his debaucheries. But a cousin of Mitya's mother, Pyotr Alexandrovich Miüsov, happened to return from Paris. He was afterwards to reside abroad for many years, and at that time, still quite a young man, he was distinguished among the Miüsovs as a person of enlightened ideas of European culture, who had lived in the capitals and abroad. Towards the end of his life he became a Liberal of the type common in the forties and fifties. In the course of his career he had come into contact with many of the most liberal men of his epoch, both in Russia and abroad. He had known Proudhon and Bakunin personally, and in his declining years was very fond of describing the three days of the Paris Revolution of February 1848, hinting that he himself had almost taken part in the fighting on the barricades. This was one of the most grateful recollections of his youth. He had an independent property of about a thousand souls, to reckon in the old style. His splendid estate lay on the outskirts of our little town and bordered on the lands of our famous monastery, with which Pyotr Alexandrovich began an endless lawsuit, almost as soon as he came into the estate, concerning the rights of fishing in the river or wood-cutting in the forest, I don't know exactly which. He regarded it as his duty as a citizen and a man of culture to bring an action against the "clericals." Hearing all about Adelaïda Ivanovna, whom he, of course, remembered, and in whom he had at one time been interested, and learning of the existence of Mitya, he intervened, in spite of all his youthful indignation and his contempt for Fyodor Pavlovich. It was then that he made the latter's acquaintance for the first time, and told him directly that he wished to undertake the child's education. He used long afterwards to tell, as a characteristic touch, that when he began to speak of Mitya, Fyodor Pavlovich looked for some time as though he did not understand what child he was talking about, and even as though he was surprised to hear that he had a little son in the house. The story may have been exaggerated, yet it must have been something like the truth. But Fyodor Pavlovich was all his life fond of acting, of suddenly playing an unexpected part, sometimes without any motive for doing so, and even to his own direct disadvantage, as, for instance, in the present case. This habit, however, is characteristic of a very great number of people, some of them very clever ones, not like Fyodor Pavlovich.

Pyotr Alexandrovich carried the business through vigorously, and was appointed, with Fyodor Pavlovich, joint guardian of the child, because, after all, he had a small property, a house and land, left him by his mother. Mitya did, in fact, pass into this cousin's keeping, but as the latter had no family of his own, and after securing the revenues of his estates was in haste to return at once to Paris, he left the boy in charge of one of his cousins, a lady living in Moscow. It came to pass that, settling permanently in Paris, he, too, forgot the child, especially when the February revolution broke out, making an impression on his mind that he remembered all the rest of his life. The Moscow lady died, and Mitya passed into the care of one of her married daughters. I believe he changed his home a fourth time later on. I won't enlarge upon that now, as I shall have much to tell later of Fyodor Pavlovich's firstborn, and must confine myself now to the most essential facts about him, without which I could not begin my story.

In the first place, this Mitya, or rather Dmitri Fyodorovich, was the only one of Fyodor Pavlovich's three sons who grew up in the belief that he had property, and that he would be independent on coming of age. He spent an irregular boyhood and youth. He did not finish his studies at the gymnasium, got into a military school, then went to the Caucasus, was promoted, fought a duel, and was degraded to the ranks, earned promotion again, led a wild life, and spent a good deal of money.

He did not begin to receive any income from Fyodor Pavlovich until he came of age, and until then kept getting into debt. He saw and got to know his father, Fyodor Pavlovich, for the first time on coming of age, when he visited our neighbourhood on purpose to settle with him about his property. Even then he seems not to have liked his father. He did not stay long with him, and made haste to get away, having only succeeded in obtaining a certain sum of money, and entering into an agreement for future payments from the estate, of the revenues and value of which he was unable (a fact worthy of note), upon this occasion, to get a statement from his father. Fyodor Pavlovich remarked for the first time then (this, too, should be noted) that Mitya had an exaggerated and mistaken idea of his property. Fyodor Pavlovich was very well satisfied with this, as it fell in with his own designs. He gathered that the young man was frivolous, unruly, of violent passions, impatient, and dissipated, and that if he could only obtain ready money he would be satisfied, although only, of course, for a short time. So Fyodor Pavlovich began to take advantage of this, sending him from time to time small doles, irregular remittances. In the end, when, four years later, Mitya, losing patience, came a second time to our little town to settle up once for all with his father, it suddenly turned out to his amazement that he had nothing, that it was even difficult to get an account, that he had received the whole value of his property in sums of money from Fyodor Pavlovich, and was perhaps even in debt to him, that by various agreements into which he had, of his own desire, entered at various previous dates, he had no right to demand anything more, and so on, and so on. The young man was overwhelmed, suspected dishonesty and cheating, was almost beside himself, and, as it were, lost his head. It was indeed this circumstance that led to the catastrophe, the account of which forms the subject of my first introductory story, or rather the external side of it. But before I pass to that story I must tell about Fyodor Pavlovich's other two sons, and of their origin.

CHAPTER III

THE SECOND MARRIAGE AND THE SECOND FAMILY

VERY shortly after getting the four-year-old Mitya off his hands Fyodor Pavlovich married a second time. His second marriage lasted eight years. He took this second wife, Sofya Ivanovna, also a very young girl, from another province, where he had gone upon some small piece of business in company with a Jew. Though Fyodor Pavlovich was a drunkard and a lecher he never neglected investing his capital, and managed his business affairs very successfully, though, no doubt, not over-scrupulously. Sofya Ivanovna was the daughter of an obscure deacon, and was left from childhood an orphan without relations. She grew up in the house of a wealthy old lady, General Vorohov's widow, who was at once her benefactress and tormentor. I do not know the details, but I have only heard that the orphan girl, a meek, gentle, long-suffering creature, was once cut down from a halter in which she was hanging from a nail in the lumber-room, so terrible were her sufferings from the crotchets and everlasting nagging of this old woman, who was apparently not bad-hearted but had become an insufferable tyrant through idleness.

Fyodor Pavlovich offered her his hand; inquiries were made about him and he was sent packing. But again, as in his first marriage, he proposed an elopement to the orphan. There is very little doubt that she would not on any account have married him if she had learned a little more about him in time. But he came from another province; besides, what could a little girl of sixteen know about it, except that she would be better off at the bottom of the river than remaining with her benefactress. So the poor child exchanged a benefactress for a benefactor. Fyodor Pavlovich did not get a penny this time, for the general's widow was furious. She gave them nothing and cursed them both into the bargain. But this time he had not even reckoned on a dowry; what allured him was the remarkable beauty of the innocent girl, above all her innocent appearance, which made a deep impression on a vicious sensualist who had hitherto admired only the coarser types of feminine beauty.

"Those innocent eyes slit my soul up like a razor," he used to say afterwards, with his loathsome snigger. In a man so depraved this might, of course, mean no more than sensual attraction. As he had received no dowry with his wife, and had, so to speak, taken her "from the halter," he did not stand on ceremony with her. Making her feel that she had "wronged" him, he took advantage of her phenomenal meekness and submissiveness to trample on the elementary decencies of marriage. He gathered loose women into his house, and carried on orgies of debauchery in his wife's presence. To show what a pass things had come to, I may mention that Grigory, the gloomy, stupid, obstinate, argumentative servant, who had hated his first mistress, Adelaïda Ivanovna, took the side of his new mistress. He championed her cause, abusing Fyodor Pavlovich in a manner little befitting a servant, and on one occasion broke up the revels and drove all the disorderly women out of the house by main force. In the end this unhappy young woman, kept in terror since childhood, fell a victim to that kind of nervous disease which is most frequently found in peasant women who are said to be possessed by devils. At times, after terrible fits of hysterics, she even lost her reason. Yet she bore Fyodor Pavlovich two sons, Ivan and Alexey, the elder in the first year of marriage and the second three years later. When she died, little Alexey was in his fourth year, and, strange as it seems, I know that he remembered his mother all his life, like a dream, of course. At her death almost exactly the same thing happened to the two little boys as to their elder brother, Mitya. They were completely forgotten and abandoned by their father. They were looked after by the same Grigory and lived in his cottage, where they were found by the tyrannical old lady who had brought up their mother. She was still alive, and had not, all those eight years, forgotten the insult done her. All that time she had been getting exact information as to her Sofya's manner of life, and hearing of her illness and hideous surroundings she declared aloud two or three times to her retainers:

"It serves her right. God has punished her for her ingratitude."

Exactly three months after Sofya Ivanovna's death the general's widow suddenly appeared in our town, and went straight to Fyodor Pavlovich's house. She spent only half an hour in the town but she accomplished a great deal. It was evening. Fyodor Pavlovich, whom she had not seen for those eight years, came in to her tipsy. The story is that instantly upon seeing him, without any sort of explanation,

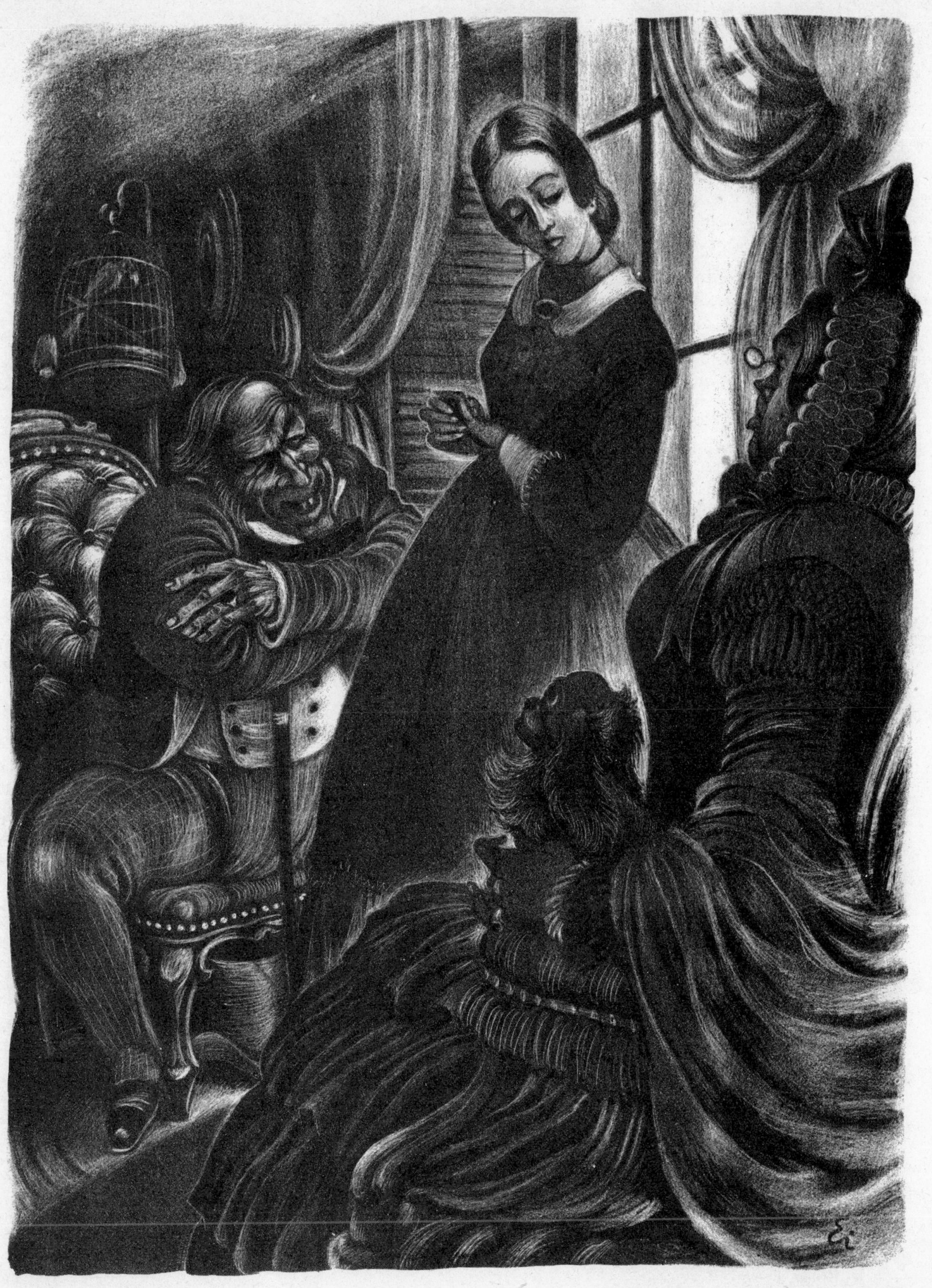

FYODOR'S SECOND MARRIAGE

she gave him two good, resounding slaps in the face, seized him by a tuft of hair, and shook him three times up and down. Then, without a word, she went straight to the cottage to the two boys. Seeing, at the first glance, that they were unwashed and in dirty linen, she promptly gave Grigory, too, a slap in the face, and announcing that she would carry off both the children she wrapped them just as they were in a plaid, put them in the carriage, and drove off to her own town. Grigory accepted the blow like a devoted slave, without a rude word, and when he escorted the old lady to her carriage he made her a low bow and pronounced impressively that, "God would repay her for the orphans." "You are a blockhead all the same," the old lady shouted to him as she drove away.

Fyodor Pavlovich, thinking it over, decided that it was a good thing and did not refuse his formal consent to having his children brought up by the general's widow. As for the slaps she had given him, he drove all over town telling the story.

It happened that the old lady died soon after this, but she left the boys in her will a thousand roubles each "for their instruction, and so that all be spent on them without fail, with the condition that it be so portioned out as to last till they are of age, for even a pittance of this sort is sufficient for such children, and if other people wish to open up their purses, let them." I have not read the will myself, but I heard that it did contain something queer of the sort, very whimsically expressed. The old woman's principal heir, Yefim Petrovich Polenov, the Marshal of Nobility of the province, turned out, however, to be an honest man. Having communicated with Fyodor Pavlovich, and discerning at once that he could extract nothing from him for his children's education (though the latter never directly refused but only procrastinated as he always did in such cases, and was, indeed, at times effusively sentimental), Yefim Petrovich took a personal interest in the orphans. He became especially fond of the younger, Alexey, who lived for a long while as one of his family. I beg the reader to note this from the beginning. And to Yefim Petrovich, a man of a nobility and kindness rarely to be met with, the young men were more indebted for their education and bringing up than to any one. He kept the two thousand roubles left to them by the general's widow intact, so that by the time they came of age their portions had been doubled by the accumulation of interest. He educated them both at his own expense, and certainly spent far more than a thousand roubles upon each of them. I won't enter into a detailed account of their boyhood and youth, but will only mention a few of the most important circumstances. Of the elder, Ivan, I will only say that he grew into a somewhat morose and reserved, though far from timid, boy. At ten years old he had realised that they were living not in their own home but on other people's charity, and that their father was a man of whom it was disgraceful to speak. This boy began very early, almost in his infancy (so they say at least), to show a brilliant and unusual aptitude for learning. I don't know precisely why, but he left the family of Yefim Petrovich when he was hardly thirteen, entering a Moscow gymnasium, and boarding with an experienced and celebrated teacher, an old friend of Yefim Petrovich. Ivan used to declare afterwards that this was all due to the "ardour for good works" of Yefim Petrovich, who was captivated by the idea that a boy of genius should be trained by a teacher of genius. But neither Yefim Petrovich nor this teacher was living when the young man graduated from the gymnasium and entered the university. As Yefim Petrovich had made no provision for the payment of the tyrannical old lady's legacy, which had grown from one thousand to two, it was delayed, owing to formalities inevitable in Russia, and the young man was in great straits for the first two years at the university, as he was forced to keep himself all the time he was studying. It must be noted that he did not even attempt to communicate with his father, perhaps from pride, from contempt for him, or perhaps because of his cool common sense, which told him that from such a father he would get no assistance worth mentioning. However that may have been, the young man was by no means despondent and succeeded in getting work, at first doing miserably paid tutoring and afterwards getting paragraphs on street incidents into the newspapers under the signature of "Eye-Witness." These paragraphs, it was said, were so interesting and piquant that they were snapped up. This alone showed the young man's practical and intellectual superiority over the masses of needy and unfortunate students of both sexes who hang about the offices of the newspapers and magazines, from morning till night, unable to think of anything better than everlasting entreaties for copying and translations from the French. Having once got into touch with the editors Ivan Fyodorovich always kept up his connection with them, and in his latter years at the university he published brilliant reviews of books upon various special subjects, so that he became well known in literary circles. But only in his last year he suddenly succeeded in attracting the attention of a far wider circle of readers, so that a great many people noticed and remembered him. It was rather a curious incident. When he had just left the university and was preparing to go abroad upon his two thousand roubles, Ivan Fyodorovich published in one of the larger newspapers a strange article, which attracted general notice, on a subject of which he might have been supposed to know nothing, as he was a student of natural science. The article dealt with a subject which was being debated everywhere at the time — the question of the ecclesiastical courts. After discussing several opinions on the subject he went on to explain his own view. What was most striking about the article was its tone, and its unexpected conclusion. Many of the Church party regarded him as decidedly on their side. And yet not only the anti-clericals but even atheists joined them in their applause. Finally some sagacious persons opined that the article was nothing but an impudent satirical burlesque. I mention this incident particularly because in due time this article reached the famous monastery in our neighbourhood, where the brethren, being particularly interested in the question of the ecclesiastical courts, were completely bewildered by it. Learning the author's name, they were interested in his being a native of the town and the son of "that Fyodor Pavlovich." And just then it was that the author himself made his appearance among us.

Why Ivan Fyodorovich had come amongst us I remember asking myself at the time with a certain uneasiness. This fateful visit, which was the first step leading to so many consequences, I never fully explained to myself. It seemed strange on the face of it that a young man so learned, so proud, and apparently so cautious, should suddenly visit such an infamous house and a father who had ignored him all his life, hardly knew him, did not remember him, and would not under any circumstances have given him money, though he was always afraid that his sons Ivan and Alexey would come to ask him for it. And here the young man was staying in the house of such a father, had been living with him for two months, and they were on the best possible terms. This last fact was a special cause of wonder to many others as well as to me. Pyotr Alexandrovich Miüsov, of whom I have spoken already, the cousin of Fyodor Pavlovich's first wife, happened to be in the neighbourhood again on a visit to his estate. He had come from Paris, which was his permanent home. I remember that he was more surprised than any one when he made the acquaintance of the young man, who interested him extremely, and with whom he sometimes argued and not without an inner pang compared himself in acquirements.

"He is proud," he said to us at the time, "he will never be in want of money; he has got enough to go abroad now. What does he want here? Every one can see that he hasn't come for money, for his father would never give him any. He has no taste for drink and dissipation, and yet his father can't do without him. They get on so famously together!"

That was the truth; the young man had an unmistakable influence over the old man, who, though often extremely and even spitefully perverse, positively appeared to be behaving more decently and even seemed at times ready to obey his son.

It was only later that we learned that Ivan had come partly at the request of, and in the interests of, his elder brother, Dmitri, whom he saw for the first time on this very visit, though before leaving Moscow he had been in correspondence with him about an important matter of more concern to Dmitri than to himself.

What that business was the reader will learn fully in due time. Yet even when I did know of this special circumstance I still felt Ivan Fyodorovich to be an enigmatic figure, and thought his visit rather puzzling.

I may add that Ivan appeared at the time in the light of a mediator between his father and his elder brother Dmitri, who was in open quarrel with his father and even planning to bring an action against him.

The little family, I repeat, was now united for the first time, and some of its members met for the first time in their lives. The younger brother, Alexey, had already been a year among us, having been the first of the three to arrive. It is of that brother Alexey I find it most difficult to speak in this introduction before I have brought him on the scene. Yet I must give some preliminary account of him, if only to explain one queer fact, which is that I have to introduce my future hero to the reader wearing the cassock of a novice. Yes, he had been for the last year in our monastery, and seemed willing to be cloistered there for the rest of his life.

CHAPTER IV

THE THIRD SON, ALYOSHA

He was only twenty, his brother Ivan was in his twenty-fourth year at the time, while their elder brother Dmitri was in his twenty-eighth year. First of all, I must explain that this young man, Alyosha, was not a fanatic, and, in my opinion, at least, was not even a mystic. I may as well state my full opinion from the beginning. He was simply an early lover of humanity, and if he adopted the monastic way of life it was simply because at that time it struck him, so to say, as the ideal escape for his soul struggling as it was from the darkness of worldly wickedness to the light of love. And the reason this way of life struck him thus was that he found here at that time an extraordinary being, as he thought, our celebrated elder, Zosima, to whom he became attached with all the first ardour of his unappeasable heart. But I do not dispute that he was very strange even at that time, and had been so indeed from his cradle. I have mentioned already, by the way, that though he lost his mother in his fourth year he remembered her all his life — her face, her caresses, "as though she stood living before me." Such memories may persist, as every one knows, from an even earlier age, even from two years old, but only standing out through a whole lifetime like spots of light out of darkness, like a corner torn out of a huge picture, which has all faded and vanished except that fragment. That is how it was with him. He remembered one still summer evening, an open window, the slanting rays of the setting sun (that he recalled most vividly of all); in a corner of the room the holy image, before it a lighted lamp, and on her knees before the image his mother, sobbing hysterically with shrieks and moans, snatching him up in both arms, squeezing him close till it hurt, and praying for him to the Mother of God, holding him out in both arms to the image as though to put him under the Mother's protection . . . and suddenly a nurse runs in and snatches him from her in terror. That was the picture! And Alyosha remembered his mother's face at that minute. He used to say that it was frenzied but beautiful, as he remembered. But he rarely cared to speak of this memory to any one. In his childhood and youth he was by no means expansive, and talked little indeed, but not from distrust or shyness or a sullen unsociability; quite the contrary, from something different, from a sort of inner preoccupation entirely personal and unconcerned with other people, but so important to him that he seemed, as it were, to forget others on account of it. But he was fond of people: he seemed throughout his life to put implicit trust in people: yet no one ever looked on him as a simpleton or a naïve person. There was something about him which made one feel at once (and it was so all his life afterwards) that he did not care to be a judge of others — that he would never take it upon himself to criticise and would never condemn any one for anything. He seemed, indeed, to accept everything without the least condemnation, though often grieving bitterly: and this was so much so that no one could surprise or frighten him even in his earliest youth. Coming at twenty to his father's house, which was a very sink of filthy debauchery, he, chaste and pure as he was, simply withdrew in silence when to look on was unbearable, but without the slightest sign of contempt or condemnation. His father, who had once been in a dependent position, and so was sensitive and ready to take offence, met him at first with distrust and sullenness. "He does not say much," he used to grumble, "and thinks the more." But soon, within a fortnight indeed, he took to embracing him and kissing him terribly often, with drunken tears, with sottish sentimentality, yet he evidently felt a real and deep affection for him, such as he had never been capable of feeling for any one before.

Every one, indeed, loved this young man wherever he went, and it was so from his earliest childhood. When he entered the household of his patron and benefactor, Yefim Petrovich Polenov, he gained the hearts of all the family, so that they looked on him quite as their own child. Yet he entered the house at such a tender age that he could not have acted from design or artfulness in winning affection. So that the gift of making himself loved directly and naturally was inherent in him, in his very being so to speak. It was the same at school, though he seemed to be just one of those children who are distrusted, sometimes ridiculed, and even hated by their schoolfellows. He was dreamy, for instance, and rather solitary. From his earliest childhood he was fond of creeping into a corner to read, and yet he was a general favourite all the while he was at school. He was rarely playful or merry, but any one could see at the first glance that this was not from any sullenness. On the contrary, he was serene and even-tempered. He never tried to show off before his schoolfellows. Perhaps because of this, he was never afraid of any one, yet the boys immediately understood that he was not proud of his fearlessness and seemed to be unaware that he was brave and fearless. He never bore a grudge. It would happen that an hour after the offence he would address the offender or answer some question with as trustful and open an expression as though nothing had happened between them. And it was not that he seemed to have forgotten or intentionally forgiven the affront, but simply that he did not regard it as an affront, and this completely conquered and captivated the boys. He had one characteristic which made all his schoolfellows from the bottom class to the top want to make fun of him, not from malice but because it amused them. This characteristic was a wild frantic bashfulness and chastity. He could not bear to hear certain words and certain conversations about women. It is unfortunately impossible to eradicate these words and conversations in schools. Boys pure in mind and heart, almost children, are fond of talking in school among themselves, and even aloud, of things, pictures, and images of which even soldiers would sometimes hesitate to speak. More than that, much that soldiers have no knowledge or conception of is familiar to quite young children of our intellectual and higher classes. There is no moral depravity, no real corrupt inner cynicism in it, but there is the appearance of it, and it is often looked upon among them as something refined, subtle, smart, and worthy of imitation. Seeing that Alyosha Karamazov put his fingers in his ears when they talked of "that," they used sometimes to crowd round him, pull his hands away, and shout nastiness into both ears, while he struggled, slipped to the floor, tried to hide himself without uttering one word of abuse, enduring their insults in silence. But at last they left him alone and gave up taunting him with being a "regular girl," and what's more they looked upon it with compassion. And by the way, he was always one of the best in the class but was never first.

After Yefim Petrovich's death, Alyosha spent two more years at the provincial gymnasium. Almost immediately after the man's decease the inconsolable widow went for a long visit to Italy with her whole family, which consisted only of persons of the female sex. Alyosha found himself in the house of two distant relations of Yefim Petrovich, ladies whom he had never seen before. On what terms he lived with them he did not know himself. It was very characteristic of him, indeed, that he never cared at whose expense he was living. In that respect he was a striking contrast to his elder brother Ivan, who struggled with poverty for his first two years in the university, maintained himself by his own efforts, and had from childhood been bitterly conscious of living at the expense of his benefactor. But this strange trait in Alyosha's character must not, I think, be condemned too severely, for at the slightest acquaintance with him any one would have perceived that Alyosha was one of those youths, verging on the "fool in Christ" type, who, if they were suddenly to come into possession of a large fortune, would not hesitate to give it away for the asking, either for good works or perhaps to a clever rogue. In general he seemed scarcely to know the value of money, not, of course, in a literal sense. When he was given pocket-money, which he never asked for, he was either terribly careless of it so that it was gone in a moment, or he kept it for weeks together, not knowing what to do with it.

In later years Pyotr Alexandrovich Miüsov, a man very sensitive on the score of money and bourgeois honesty, pronounced the following judgment, after getting to know Alyosha:

"Here is perhaps the one man in the world whom you might leave alone without a penny, in the centre of an unknown town of a million inhabitants, and he would not come to harm, he would not die of cold and hunger, for he would be fed and sheltered at once; and if he were not, he would find a shelter for himself, and it would cost him no effort or humiliation. And to shelter him would be no burden, but, on the contrary, would probably be looked on as a pleasure."

He did not finish his studies at the gymnasium. A year before the end of the course he suddenly announced to the ladies that he was going to see his father about a plan which had occurred to him. They were sorry and unwilling to let him go. The journey was not an expensive one, and the ladies would not let him pawn his watch, a parting present from his benefactor's family. They provided him liberally with money and even fitted him out with new clothes and linen. But he returned half the money they gave him, saying that he intended to go third class. On his arrival in the town he made no answer to his father's first inquiry why he had come before completing his studies, and seemed, so they say, unusually pensive. It soon became known that he was looking for his mother's grave. He practically acknowledged at the time that that was the only object of his visit. But it can hardly have been the whole reason for it. It is more probable that he himself did not understand and could not explain what had suddenly arisen in his soul and drawn him irresistibly into a new, unknown, but inevitable path. Fyodor Pavlovich could not show him where his second wife was buried, for he had never visited her grave since her coffin had been covered with earth, and in the course of years had entirely forgotten where she was buried.

Fyodor Pavlovich, by the way, for some time previously had not been living in our town. Three or four years after his wife's death he had gone to the south of Russia and finally turned up in Odessa, where he spent several years. He made the acquaintance at first, in his own words, "of a lot of low Jews, Jewesses, and Jewkins," and ended by being received by "Jews high and low alike." It may be presumed that at this period he developed a peculiar faculty for making and squeezing out money. He finally returned to our town

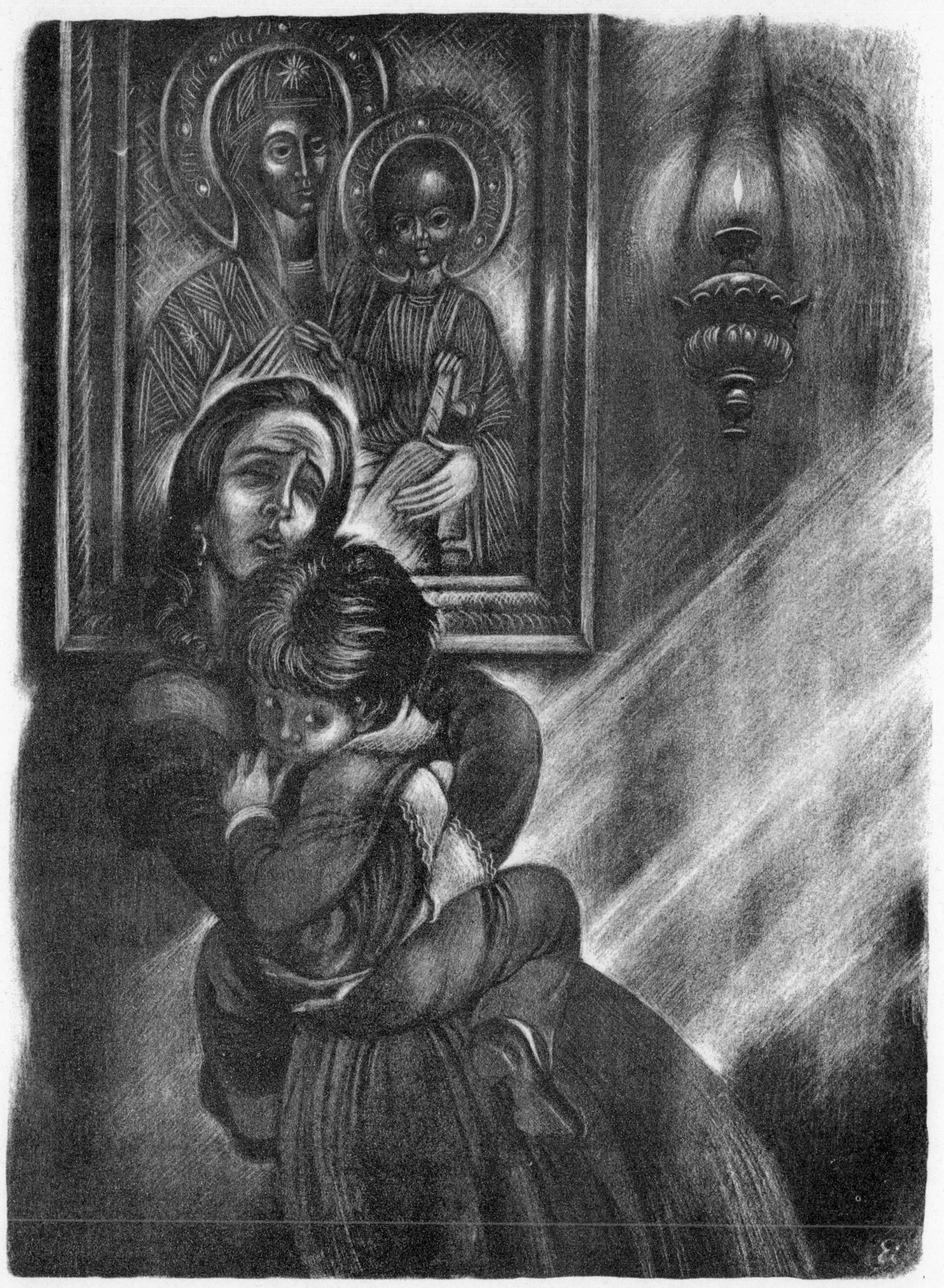

ALYOSHA THE BOY

only three years before Alyosha's arrival. His former acquaintances found him looking terribly aged, although he was by no means an old man. He behaved not exactly with more dignity but with more effrontery. The former buffoon showed an insolent propensity for making buffoons of others. His vile behaviour with women was not simply what it used to be, but even more revolting. In a short time he opened a great number of new pot-houses in the district. It was evident that he was worth perhaps a hundred thousand roubles or not much less. Many of the inhabitants of the town and district were soon in his debt, and, of course, had given good security. Of late, too, he looked somehow bloated and seemed more irresponsible, more uneven, had sunk into a sort of incoherence, used to begin one thing and end with another, as though he were falling to pieces. He was more and more frequently drunk, and, if it had not been for the same servant Grigory, who by that time had aged considerably, too, and used to look after him sometimes almost like a nurse, Fyodor Pavlovich might have got into terrible scrapes. Alyosha's arrival seemed to affect him even morally, as though something had awakened in this prematurely old man which had long been dead in his soul.

"Do you know," he used often to say, looking at Alyosha, "that you are like her, 'the possessed woman' " — that was what he used to call his dead wife, Alyosha's mother. Grigory it was who pointed out the "possessed woman's" grave to Alyosha. He took him to our town cemetery and showed him in a remote corner a cast-iron tombstone, cheap but decently kept, on which were inscribed the name and age of the deceased and the date of her death, and below something by way of a funerary quatrain, such as are commonly used on old-fashioned middle-class tombs. To Alyosha's amazement this tombstone turned out to be Grigory's doing. He had put it up on the poor "possessed woman's" grave at his own expense, after Fyodor Pavlovich, whom he had often pestered about the grave, had gone to Odessa, abandoning the grave and all his memories. Alyosha showed no particular emotion at the sight of his mother's grave. He only listened to Grigory's sententious and solemn account of the erection of the tombstone; he stood with bowed head and walked away without uttering a word. It was perhaps a year before he visited the cemetery again. But this little episode was not without an influence upon Fyodor Pavlovich — and a very peculiar one. He suddenly took a thousand roubles to our monastery to pay for requiems for the soul of his wife; but not for the second, Alyosha's mother, the "possessed woman," but for the first, Adelaïda Ivanovna, who used to thrash him. In the evening of the same day he got drunk and abused the monks to Alyosha. He himself was far from being religious; he had probably never put a five-copeck candle before the image of a saint. Strange impulses of sudden feeling and sudden thought are common in men of that sort.

I have mentioned already that he had come to look bloated. His countenance at this time testified unmistakably to the character of the life he had led. Besides the long fleshy bags under his little eyes, always full of insolence, suspicion, and mockery; besides the multitude of deep wrinkles in his small fat face, below his sharp chin the Adam's apple hung fleshy and long, like a purse, which gave him a peculiar, repulsive, sensual appearance; add to that a voluptuary's wide mouth with full lips, between which could be seen little stumps of black decayed teeth. He slobbered every time he began to speak. He was fond indeed of making fun of his own face, though, I believe, he was well satisfied with it. He used particularly to point to his nose, which was not very large, but very delicate and conspicuously aquiline. "A regular Roman nose," he used to say; "with my Adam's apple I've quite the countenance of an ancient Roman patrician of the decadent period." He seemed proud of it.

Not long after visiting his mother's grave Alyosha suddenly announced to him that he wanted to enter the monastery, and that the monks were willing to receive him as a novice. He explained that this was his strong desire, and that he was solemnly asking his consent as a father. The old man knew that the elder Zosima, who was living in the monastery hermitage, had made a special impression upon his "gentle boy."

"That is the most honest monk among them, of course," he observed, after listening in thoughtful silence to Alyosha, and seeming scarcely surprised at his request. "H'm! . . . So that's where you want to go, my gentle boy?"

He was half drunk, and suddenly he grinned his slow half-drunken grin, which was not without a certain cunning and tipsy slyness. "H'm! . . . I had a presentiment that you would end in something like this. Would you believe it? You were making straight for it. Well, to be sure you have your own two thousand. That's a dowry for you. And I'll never desert you, my angel. And I'll pay what's wanted for you there, if they ask for it. But, of course, if they don't ask, why should we worry them? What do you say? You know, you spend money like a canary, two grains a week. H'm! . . . Do you know that near one monastery there's a place outside the town where every baby knows there are none but 'the monks' wives' living, as they are called. Thirty women, I believe. I have been there myself. You know, it's interesting in its own way, of course, for a change. The worst of it is, it's awfully Russian. There are no French women there. Of course they could be gotten, there is plenty of money there. If they get to hear of it they'll come along. Well, there's nothing of that sort here, no 'monks' wives,' and two hundred monks. They're honest. They keep the fasts. I admit it. . . . H'm. . . . So you want to be a monk? And do you know I'm sorry to lose you, Alyosha; would you be lieve it, I've really grown fond of you? Well, it's a good opportunity. You'll pray for us sinners; we have sinned too much here. I've always been thinking who would pray for me, and whether there's any one in the world to do it. My dear boy, I'm awfully stupid about that. You wouldn't believe it. Awfully. You see, however stupid I am about it, I keep thinking, I keep thinking—from time to time, of course, not all the while. It's impossible, I think, for the devils to forget to drag me down to hell with their hooks when I die. Then I wonder — hooks? Where would they get them? What of? Iron hooks? Where do they forge them? Have they a factory there of some sort? The monks in the monastery probably believe that there's a ceiling in hell, for instance. Now I'm ready to believe in hell, but without a ceiling. It makes it more refined, more enlightened, more Lutheran that is. And, after all, what does it matter whether it has a ceiling or not? But, do you know, there's a damnable question involved in it? If there's no ceiling there can be no hooks, and if there are no hooks it all breaks down, which is unlikely again, for then there would be none to drag me down to hell, and if they don't drag me down what justice is there in the world? *Il faudrait les inventer*, those hooks, on purpose for me alone, for, if you only knew, Alyosha, what a loose fish I am."

"There are no hooks there," said Alyosha, looking gently and seriously at his father.

"Yes, yes, only the shadows of hooks. I know, I know. That's how a Frenchman described hell: '*J'ai vu l'ombre d'un cocher qui avec l'ombre d'une brosse frottait l'ombre d'une carosse.*' How do you know there are no hooks, darling? When you've lived with the monks you'll sing a different tune. But go and get at the truth there, and then come and tell me. Anyway it's easier going to the other world if one knows for a fact what there is there. Besides, it will be more seemly for you with the monks than here with me, with a drunken old man and his wenches . . . though you're like an angel, nothing touches you. And I dare say nothing will touch you there. That's why I give you my permission, because I hope it will be so. You've got all your wits about you. Go ahead and get over it; you will be cured and come back again. And I will wait for you. I feel that you're the only creature in the world who has not condemned me. My dear boy, I feel it, you know. I can't help feeling it."

And he even began blubbering. He was sentimental. He was vicious and sentimental.

CHAPTER V

ELDERS

SOME of my readers may imagine that my young man was a sickly, ecstatic, poorly developed creature, a pale dreamer, a feeble, consumptive little fellow. On the contrary, Alyosha was at this time a well-grown, red-cheeked, clear-eyed lad of nineteen, radiant with health. He was very handsome, too, graceful, moderately tall, with hair of a dark brown, with a regular, rather long, oval-shaped face, and wide-set dark grey, shining eyes; he was very thoughtful, and apparently very serene. I shall be told, perhaps, that red cheeks are not incompatible with fanaticism and mysticism; but I fancy that Alyosha was more of a realist than any one. Oh! no doubt, in the monastery he fully believed in miracles, but, to my thinking, miracles are never a stumbling-block to the realist. It is not miracles that dispose realists to belief. The true realist, if he is an unbeliever, will always find strength and ability to disbelieve in an actual miracle, and if he is confronted with a miracle as an irrefutable fact he would rather disbelieve his own senses than admit the fact. Even if he admits it, he admits it as a natural phenomenon till then unknown to him. Faith does not, in the realist, spring from the miracle but the miracle from faith. If the realist once believes, then he is bound by his very realism to admit the miraculous also. The Apostle Thomas said that he would not believe till he saw, but when he did see he said, "My Lord and my God!" Was it the miracle forced him to believe? Most likely not, but he believed solely because he desired to believe and possibly he fully believed in his secret heart even when he said, "I do not believe till I see."

I shall be told, perhaps, that Alyosha was stupid, undeveloped, had not finished his studies, and so on. That he did not finish his studies is true, but to say that he was stupid or foolish would be a great injustice. I'll simply repeat what I have said above. He entered upon this path only because, at that time, it alone struck his imagination and presented itself to him as offering an ideal means of escape for his soul from darkness to light. Add to that that he was to some extent a youth of our own time — that is, honest in nature, demanding the truth, seeking it and believing in it, and seeking to serve it at once with all the strength of his soul, demanding immediate action, and ready to sacrifice everything, life itself, for it. Though these young men unhappily fail to understand that the sacrifice of life is, in many cases, the easiest of all sacrifices, and that to sacrifice, for instance, five or six years of their seething youth to hard and tedious study, if only to multiply ten-fold their powers of serving the truth and the cause they have set before them as their goal — such a sacrifice is utterly beyond the strength of many of them. The path Alyosha chose was a path going in the opposite direction, but he chose it with the same thirst for swift and noble action. As soon as he reflected seriously he was convinced of the existence of God and immortality, and at once he naturally said to himself: "I want to live for immortality, and I will accept no compromise." In the same way, if he had decided that God and immortality did not exist, he would at once have become an atheist and a socialist. For socialism is not merely the labour question, or the question of the so-called fourth estate, it is above all things the atheistic question, the question of the form taken by atheism to-day, the question of the tower of Babel built without God, not to mount to heaven from earth but to bring heaven down to earth. Alyosha found it strange and impossible to go on living as before. It is written: "Give all that thou hast to the poor and follow Me, if thou wouldst be perfect." Alyosha said to himself: "I can't give two roubles instead of 'all,' and only go to mass instead of 'following Him.' " Perhaps his memories of childhood brought back our monastery, to which his mother may have taken him to mass. Perhaps the slanting sunlight and the holy image to which his poor "possessed" mother had held him up still acted upon his imagination. Brooding on these things, he may have come to us perhaps only to see whether here he could sacrifice all or only "two roubles," and in the monastery he met this elder. . . .

This elder was, as I have already explained, elder Zosima. I must digress to say a few words about what an "elder" is in Russian monasteries, and I am sorry that I do not feel very competent to do so. I will try, however, to give a superficial account of it in a few words. Authorities on the subject assert that the institution of "elders" is of recent date, not more than a hundred years old in our monasteries, though in the orthodox East, especially at Sinai and Athos, it has existed over a thousand years. It is maintained that the institution existed in ancient times in Russia also, but owing to the calamities which befell Russia — the Tatars, civil war, the interruption of relations with the East after the destruction of Constantinople — it fell into oblivion and "elders" disappeared. It was revived among us towards the end of the last century by one of the great "ascetics," as they called him, Païssy Velichkovsky, and his disciples. But to-day, even after a hundred years, it exists in a few monasteries only, and has sometimes been almost persecuted as an innovation unheard of in Russia. It flourished especially in the celebrated Kozelski Optin Monastery. When and how it was introduced into our monastery I cannot say. There had already been three such elders and Zosima was the last of them. But he was almost dying of weakness and disease, and they had no one to take his place. The question for our monastery was an important one, for it had not been distinguished by anything in particular till then: they had neither relics of saints, nor wonder-working ikons, nor glorious traditions, nor historical exploits in the service of the country. It had flourished and been glorious all over Russia through its elders, to see and hear whom pilgrims had flocked for thousands of miles from all parts.

What then is an elder? An elder is one who takes your soul, your will, into his soul and his will. When you choose an elder, you renounce your own will and yield it to him in complete submission, complete self-abnegation. This novitiate, this terrible discipline, is undertaken voluntarily, in the hope of self-conquest, of self-mastery, in order, after a life of obedience, to attain perfect freedom, that is, from self; to escape the lot of those who have lived their whole lives without finding their true selves in themselves. This institution of elders is not founded on theory, but was derived in the East from the practice of a thousand years. The obligations due to an elder are not the ordinary "obedience" which has always existed in our Russian monasteries. What is involved here is continual confession to the elder by all who have submitted themselves to him, and an indissoluble bond between him and them.

The story is told, for instance, that in the early days of Christianity one such novice, failing to fulfil some command laid upon him by his elder, left his monastery in Syria and went to Egypt. There, after great exploits, he was found worthy at last to suffer torture and a martyr's death for the faith. When the Church, regarding him as a saint, was burying him, suddenly, at the deacon's exhortation, "Depart all ye unbaptized," the coffin containing the martyr's body left its place and was cast forth from the church, and this took place three times. And only at last they learnt that this holy man had broken his vow of obedience and left his elder, and, therefore, could not be forgiven without the elder's absolution in spite of his great deeds. Only after this could the funeral take place. This, of course, is only an old legend. But here is a recent and true occurrence.

In our own day a monk who was dwelling at Athos was suddenly commanded by his elder to quit the place, which he loved as a sacred and tranquil haven of refuge, and to go, first to Jerusalem to do homage to the Holy Places and thence north to Siberia: "There is the place for thee and not here." The monk, overwhelmed with sorrow, went to the Œcumenical Patriarch at Constantinople and besought him to release him from his vow of obedience. But the Patriarch replied that not only was he unable to release him, but there was not and could not be on earth a power which could release him except the elder who had himself laid that vow upon him. In this way the elders are endowed in certain cases with unbounded and unfathomable authority. That is why in many of our monasteries the institution at first met with extreme hostility. Meantime the elders gained high respect among the masses. Simple people as well as men of the highest station flocked, for instance, to the elders of our monastery to confess their doubts, their sins, and their sufferings, and ask for counsel and admonition. Seeing this, the opponents of the elders added to other accusations this, that the sacrament of confession was being arbitrarily and frivolously degraded, though the continual opening of the heart to the elder by the novice or the layman had nothing of the character of the sacrament. In the end, however, the institution of elders has been retained and is gradually becoming established in Russian monasteries. It is true, perhaps, that this tried and tested thousand-year-old instrument for the emancipation of man from slavery and his moral regeneration may become a two-edged tool and it may lead some not to humility and complete self-control but to the most satanic pride, that is, to bondage and not to freedom.

The elder Zosima was about sixty-five. He came of a family of landowners, had been in the army in his early youth, and served in the Caucasus as an officer. He had, no doubt, struck Alyosha by some peculiar quality of his soul. Alyosha lived in the cell of the elder, who grew very fond of him and made him his intimate. It must be noted that at that time Alyosha was not as yet bound by any obligation and could go where he pleased and be absent for whole days. If he wore the monastic dress it was voluntarily, so as not to be different from the other inhabitants of the monastery. No doubt he liked it, too. Possibly his youthful imagination was deeply stirred by the power and fame of his elder. It was commonly said that so many people had for years past come to open their hearts to Father Zosima and to entreat him for words of advice and healing, he had taken into his soul so many revelations and confessions, so much contrition, that he had acquired the keenest intuition and could tell from a stranger's face what he wanted, and what pain was tearing at his conscience. He sometimes astounded and almost alarmed his visitors by his knowledge of their secrets before they had spoken a word.

Alyosha noticed that many, almost all, went in to the elder for the first time with apprehension and uneasiness, but came out with bright and happy faces. Alyosha was particularly struck by the fact that Father Zosima was not at all stern. On the contrary, he was always almost gay in his dealings with people. The monks said that he was drawn precisely to those who were more sinful, and the greater the sinner the more he loved him. There were, no doubt, up to the end of his life, among the monks some who hated and envied him, but they were becoming fewer and they held their peace, though among them were several of high standing in the monastery, for instance, one of the oldest monks distinguished for his long periods of silence and strict fasting. But the majority were on Father Zosima's side and very many of them loved him with all their hearts, warmly and sincerely. Some were almost fanatically devoted to him, and declared, though not quite aloud, that he was a saint, beyond any doubt, and, seeing that his end was near, they anticipated miracles and great glory to the monastery in the immediate future from his relics. Alyosha believed unquestioningly in the miraculous power of the elder, just as he had unquestioning faith in the story of the coffin that flew out of the church. He saw many who came with sick children or relatives and besought the elder to lay hands on them and to pray over them, return shortly after — some the next day — and, falling in tears at the elder's feet, thank him for healing their sick.

Whether they had really been healed or were simply better in the natural course of the disease was a question which did not exist for Alyosha, for he fully believed in the spiritual power of his master and rejoiced in his fame, in his glory, as though it were his own triumph.

His heart beat loudest, and he beamed, as it were, all over when the elder came out to the gates of the hermitage into the waiting crowd of pilgrims of the humbler class who had flocked from all parts of Russia to see the elder and obtain his blessing. They fell down before him, wept, kissed his feet, kissed the earth on which he stood, and wailed, while the women held up their children to him and brought him the sick "possessed of devils." The elder spoke to them, read a brief prayer over them, blessed them, and dismissed them. Of late he had been so weakened by attacks of illness that he was sometimes unable to leave his cell, and the pilgrims waited several days for him to come out. Alyosha did not wonder why they loved him so, why they fell down before him and wept with emotion merely at seeing his face. Oh! he understood that for the humble soul of the Russian commoner, worn out by grief and toil, and still more by the everlasting injustice and everlasting sin, his own and the world's, it was the greatest need and comfort to find some one or something holy to fall down before and worship: "Among us there is sin, unrighteousness, and temptation, but yet, somewhere on earth there is some one holy and exalted. He possesses righteousness; he knows what righteousness is; so it is not dead upon the earth; so it will come one day to us, too, and rule over all the earth according to the promise."

Alyosha knew that this was just how the people felt and even reasoned. He understood it, but that the elder Zosima was this saint and custodian of God's justice — of that he had no more doubt than the weeping peasants and the sick women who held out their children to the elder. The conviction that after his death the elder would bring extraordinary glory to the monastery was even stronger in Alyosha than in any one there, and, of late, a kind of deep burning inner ecstasy flamed ever higher in his heart. He was not at all troubled at this elder's standing as a solitary example before him.

"No matter. He is holy. He carries in his heart the secret of renewal for all: that power which will, at last, establish righteousness on earth, and all men will be holy and love one another, and there will be neither rich nor poor, neither exalted nor humbled, but all will be as the children of God, and the true Kingdom of Christ will come." That was the dream in Alyosha's heart.

The arrival of his two brothers, whom he had not known till then, seemed to make a great impression on Alyosha. He more quickly made friends with his half-brother Dmitri (though he arrived later) than with his own brother Ivan. He was extremely interested in his brother Ivan, but when the latter had been two months in the town, though they had met fairly often, they were still not intimate. Alyosha was naturally reserved, and he seemed to be expecting something, ashamed of something, while his brother Ivan, though Alyosha noticed at first that he looked long and curiously at him, seemed soon to have left off thinking about him. Alyosha noticed it with some embarrassment. He ascribed his brother's indifference at first to the disparity of their age and education. But he also wondered whether the absence of interest and sympathy in Ivan might be due to some other cause entirely unknown to him. He kept fancying that Ivan was absorbed in something — something inward and important — that he was striving towards some goal, perhaps very hard to attain, and that that was why he had no thought for him. Alyosha wondered, too, whether there was not some contempt on the part of the learned atheist for him — a silly novice. He knew for certain that his brother was an atheist. He could not take offence at this contempt, if it existed; yet, with an uneasy embarrassment which he did not himself understand, he waited for his brother to come nearer to him. Dmitri used to speak of Ivan with the deepest respect and with a peculiar emotion. From him Alyosha learnt all the details of the important affair which had of late formed such a close and remarkable bond between the two elder brothers. Dmitri's enthusiastic references to Ivan were the more striking in Alyosha's eyes since Dmitri was, compared with Ivan, almost uneducated, and the two brothers were such a contrast in personality and character that it would be difficult to find two men more unlike.

It was at this time that the meeting, or rather gathering, of the members of this ill-assorted family took place in the cell of the elder who had such an extraordinary influence on Alyosha. The pretext for this gathering was really a false one. It was at this time that the difference between Dmitri and his father with regard to money matters seemed at its acutest stage and their relations had become insufferably strained. Fyodor Pavlovich seems to have been the first to suggest, apparently in jest, that they should all meet in Father Zosima's cell, and that, without resorting directly to his mediation, they might more decently come to an understanding under the conciliating influence of the elder's presence. Dmitri, who had never seen the elder, naturally supposed that his father was trying to intimidate him, but, as he secretly blamed himself for his outbursts of temper with his father on several recent occasions, he accepted the challenge. It must be noted that he was not, like Ivan, staying with his father, but living apart at the other end of the town. It happened that Pyotr Alexandrovich Miüsov, who was staying in the district at the time, caught eagerly at the idea. A Liberal of the forties and fifties, a free-thinker and an atheist, he may have been led on to take a hand in the affair by boredom or the hope of frivolous diversion. He was suddenly seized with the desire to see the monastery and the holy man. As his lawsuit with the monastery still dragged on, he made a pretended attempt to settle it amicably the pretext for seeing the Father Superior. A visitor coming with such laudable intentions might be received with more attention and consideration than if he came from simple curiosity. Pressure from within the monastery was brought to bear on the ailing elder, who of late had scarcely left his cell, and had been forced by illness to deny even his ordinary visitors. In the end he consented to see them, and the day was fixed. "Who has made me a judge over them?" was all he said, smilingly, to Alyosha.

Alyosha was much perturbed when he heard of the proposed visit. Of all the wrangling, quarrelsome party, Dmitri was the only one who could regard the interview seriously. All the others would come from frivolous motives, perhaps insulting to the elder. Alyosha was well aware of that. Ivan and Miüsov would come from curiosity, perhaps of the coarsest kind, while his father might be contemplating some piece of buffoonery. Though he said nothing, Alyosha thoroughly understood his father. The boy, I repeat, was far from being as simple as every one thought him. He awaited the day with a heavy heart. No doubt he was always deeply worried in his heart as to how the family discord could be ended. But his chief anxiety concerned the elder. He trembled for him, for his reputation, and dreaded any affront to him, especially the refined, courteous irony of Miüsov and the supercilious half utterances of the highly educated Ivan. He even wanted to venture on warning the elder, telling him something about them, but, on second thoughts, said nothing. He only sent word the day before, through a friend, to his brother Dmitri, that he loved him and expected him to keep his promise. Dmitri wondered, for he could not remember what he had promised, but he answered by letter that he would do his utmost not to let himself be provoked "by vileness," but that, although he had a deep respect for the elder and for his brother Ivan, he was convinced that the meeting was either a trap for him or an unworthy farce. "Nevertheless I would rather swallow my tongue than be lacking in respect to the sainted man whom you reverence so highly," he wrote. Alyosha was not greatly cheered by the letter.

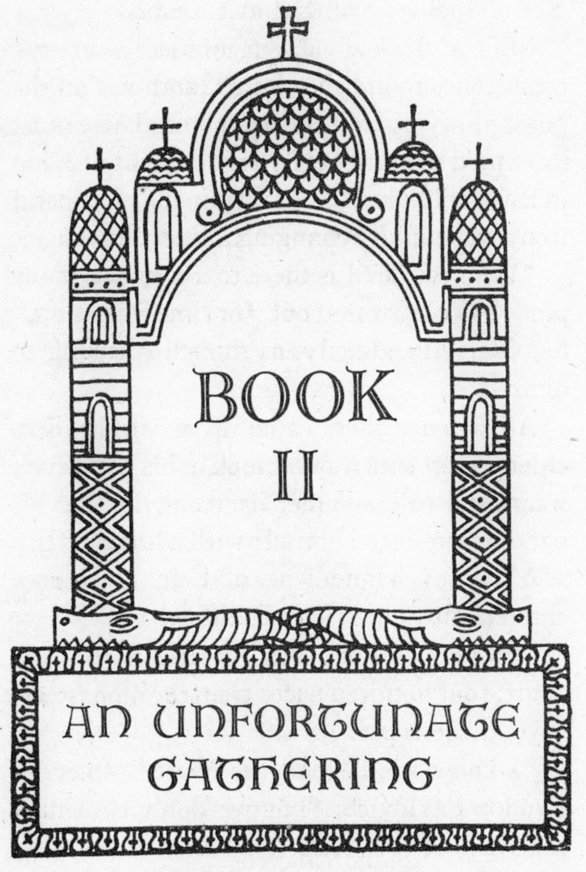

BOOK II

AN UNFORTUNATE GATHERING

CHAPTER I

THEY ARRIVE AT THE MONASTERY

It was a warm, bright day at the end of August. The interview with the elder had been fixed for half-past eleven, immediately after late mass. Our visitors were not present at the service, but arrived just as it was over. First an elegant open carriage, drawn by two valuable horses, drove up with Miüsov and a distant relative of his, a young man of twenty, called Pyotr Fomich Kalganov. This young man was preparing to enter the university. Miüsov, with whom he was staying for the time, was trying to persuade him to go abroad to the university of Zürich or Jena. The young man was still undecided. He was thoughtful and absent-minded, as it were. He had a pleasant face, was strongly built, and rather tall. There was a strange fixity in his gaze at times. Like all very absent-minded people he would sometimes stare at a person for quite a while without seeing him. He was silent and rather awkward, but sometimes, when he was alone with some one, he became very talkative in a spasmodic fashion, and would laugh at anything or nothing. But his animation vanished as quickly as it appeared. He was always well and even elegantly dressed; he had already some independent fortune and expectations of much more. He was a friend of Alyosha's.

In an ancient, creaking, but roomy, hired carriage, with a pair of old pinkish-grey horses, a long way behind Miüsov's carriage, came Fyodor Pavlovich, with his son Ivan. Dmitri was late, though he had been informed of the time the evening before. The visitors left their carriage at the hostelry, outside the precincts, and entered the gates of the monastery on foot. Except Fyodor Pavlovich, none of the party had ever seen the monastery, and Miüsov had probably not even been to church for some thirty years. He looked about him with curiosity, and with assumed ease. But, aside from the church and the living quarters, though these too were ordinary enough, he found nothing of interest in the interior of the monastery. The last of the worshippers were coming out of the church, bareheaded and crossing themselves. Among the humbler people were a few of higher rank — two or three ladies and a very old general. They were all staying at the hostelry. Our visitors were at once surrounded by beggars, but none of them gave them anything, except young Kalganov, who took a ten-copeck piece out of his purse, and, nervous and embarrassed — God knows why! — hurriedly gave it to an old woman, saying: "Divide it equally." None of his companions made any remark upon it, so that he had no reason to be embarrassed; but, perceiving this, he was even more overcome.

It was strange that their arrival did not seem expected, and that they were not received with special honour, though one of them had recently made a donation of a thousand roubles, while another was a very wealthy and highly cultured landowner, upon whom the monastery might become dependent for its fishing-rights if the lawsuit took a certain turn. Yet no monastic official met them.

Miüsov looked absent-mindedly at the tombstones round the church, and was on the point of saying that the dead buried here must have paid a pretty penny for the right of lying in this "holy place," but refrained. His liberal irony was rapidly changing almost into anger.

"Who the devil is there to ask in this crazy place? We must find out, for time is passing," he observed suddenly, as though speaking to himself.

All at once there came up a bald-headed, elderly man with a sweet look in his little eyes, wearing a full, summer overcoat. Lifting his hat, he introduced himself with a honeyed lisp as Maximov, a landowner of Tula. He at once entered into our visitors' difficulty.

"Father Zosima lives in the hermitage, apart, four hundred paces from the monastery, beyond the copse."

"I know it's beyond the copse," observed Fyodor Pavlovich, "but we don't remember the way. It is a long time since we've been here."

"This way, through this gate, and straight across the copse . . . the copse. Come with me, won't you? I'll show you. I have to go . . . I am going myself. This way, this way."

They came out of the gate and turned towards the copse. Maximov, a man of sixty, ran rather than walked, turning sideways to stare at them all, with an incredible degree of nervous curiosity. His eyes bulged.

"You see, we have come to the elder upon business of our own," observed Miüsov severely. "That personage has granted us an audience so to speak, and so, though we thank you for showing us the way, we cannot ask you to accompany us."

"I've been there. I've been already; *un chevalier parfait*," and Maximov snapped his fingers in the air.

"Who is a *chevalier?*" asked Miüsov.

"The elder, the splendid elder, the elder! The honour and glory of the monastery, Zosima. Such an elder!"

But his incoherent talk was cut short by a very pale, wan-looking monk of medium height, wearing a monk's hood, who overtook them. Fyodor Pavlovich and Miüsov stopped.

The monk, with an extremely courteous, profound bow, announced:

"The Father Superior invites all of you gentlemen to dine with him after your visit to the hermitage. At one o'clock, not later. And you also," he added, addressing Maximov.

"That I certainly will, without fail," cried Fyodor Pavlovich, hugely delighted at the invitation. "And, believe me, we've all given our word to behave properly here. . . . And you, Pyotr Alexandrovich, will you go, too?"

"Yes, of course. What have I come for but to study all the customs here? The only thing that embarrasses me is your company. . . ."

"Yes, Dmitri Fyodorovich isn't here yet."

"It would be a capital thing if he didn't turn up. Do you suppose I like all this business, and in your company, too? So we will come to dinner. Thank the Father Superior," he said, turning to the monk.

"No, it is my duty now to conduct you to the elder," answered the monk.

"If so I'll go straight to the Father Superior — to the Father Superior," chirped Maximov.

"The Father Superior is engaged just now. But as you please——" the monk hesitated.

"A most annoying old man!" Miüsov observed aloud, while Maximov ran back to the monastery.

"He's like von Sohn," Fyodor Pavlovich said suddenly.

"Is that all you can think of? . . . In what way is he like von Sohn? Have you ever seen von Sohn?"

"I've seen his portrait. It's not the features, but something indefinable. He's a second von Sohn. I can always tell from the physiognomy."

"Ah, I dare say you are a connoisseur in that. But, look here, Fyodor Pavlovich, you said just now that we had given our word to behave properly. Remember it. I advise you to control yourself. But if you begin to play the buffoon I don't intend to be associated with you here. . . . You see what a man he is" — he turned to the monk — "I'm afraid to go among decent people with him." A thin, subtle smile, not without a certain slyness, came to the pale, bloodless lips of the monk, but he made no reply, and it was evident that he held his peace from a sense of his own dignity. Miüsov frowned more than ever.

"Oh, devil take them all! It's just surface polish kept up for centuries, and nothing but charlatanism and nonsense underneath," flashed through Miüsov's mind.

"Here's the hermitage. We've arrived,"

cried Fyodor Pavlovich. "The gates are shut."

And he began ostentatiously to make the sign of the cross before the saints painted above and on the sides of the gates.

"In Rome do as the Romans do. Here in this hermitage there are twenty-five saints being saved. They look at one another, and eat cabbage. And not one woman goes in at this gate. That's what is remarkable. And that really is so. But I did hear that the elder receives ladies," he remarked suddenly to the monk.

"Women of the people are here, too, now, lying in the portico there waiting. But for ladies of rank two rooms have been built adjoining the portico, but outside the precincts — you can see the windows — and the elder goes out to them by an inner passage when he is well enough. They are always outside the precincts. There is a Harkov lady, Madame Hohlakov, waiting there now with her ailing daughter. Probably he has promised to come out to her, though of late he has been so weak that he has hardly shown himself even to the people."

"So then there are loopholes, after all, to creep out of the hermitage to the ladies. Don't suppose, holy father, that I mean any harm. But do you know that at Athos not only the visits of women are prohibited, but no creature of the female sex is allowed — no hens, nor turkey-hens, nor young cows."

"Fyodor Pavlovich, I warn you I shall go back and leave you here. They'll turn you out when I'm gone."

"But I'm not interfering with you, Pyotr Alexandrovich. Look," he cried suddenly, stepping within the precincts, "what a vale of roses they live in!"

Though there were no roses now, there were numbers of rare and beautiful autumn flowers growing wherever there was space for them, and evidently tended by a skilful hand; there were flower-beds round the church, and between the tombs; and the one-storeyed wooden house where the elder lived was also surrounded with flowers.

"And was it like this in the time of the last elder, Varsonofy? That one didn't care for such elegance. They say he used to jump up and thrash even ladies with a stick," observed Fyodor Pavlovich, as he went up the steps.

"The elder Varsonofy did sometimes act rather queerly, but a great deal that's told is foolishness. He never thrashed any one," answered the monk. "Now, gentlemen, if you will wait a minute I will announce you."

"Fyodor Pavlovich, for the last time, remember our agreement, do you hear? Behave properly or I will pay you out!" Miüsov had time to mutter again.

"I can't think why you are so agitated," Fyodor Pavlovich observed sarcastically. "Are you uneasy about your sins? They say he can tell by one's eyes what one has come about. And what a lot you think of their opinion! you, a Parisian, and so advanced. I'm surprised at you."

But Miüsov had no time to reply to this sarcasm. They were asked to come in. He walked in, somewhat annoyed.

"Now, I know myself, I am irritated, I shall lose my temper and begin to argue — and lower myself and my ideas," he reflected.

CHAPTER II

THE OLD BUFFOON

They entered the room almost at the same moment that the elder came in from his bedroom. There were already in the cell, awaiting the elder, two monks of the hermitage, one the

Father Librarian, and the other Father Païssy, a very learned man, so they said, in delicate health, though not old. There was also a tall young fellow, who looked about two and twenty, standing in the corner throughout the interview. He had a broad, fresh face, and clever, observant, narrow brown eyes, and was wearing ordinary dress. He was a divinity student, and a future theologian, who was for some reason befriended by the monks. His expression was one of unquestioning, but self-respecting, reverence. Being in a subordinate and dependent position, and so not on an equality with the guests, he did not greet them with a bow.

Father Zosima was accompanied by a novice, and by Alyosha. The two monks rose and greeted him with a very deep bow, touching the ground with their fingers; then kissed his hand, asking his benediction. Blessing them, the elder replied with as deep a reverence to them, and asked the blessing of each of them. The whole ceremony was performed very gravely, not as though it were an everyday rite, but with some emotion. But Miüsov fancied that it was all done with intentional impressiveness. He stood in front of the other visitors. He ought — he had reflected upon it the evening before — from simple politeness, since it was the custom here, to have gone up to receive the elder's blessing, even if he did not kiss his hand. But when he saw all this bowing and kissing on the part of the monks he instantly changed his mind. With dignified gravity he made a rather deep, conventional bow, and moved away to a chair. Fyodor Pavlovich did the same, mimicking Miüsov like an ape. Ivan bowed with great dignity and courtesy, but he too kept his hands at his sides, while Kalganov was so confused that he did not bow at all. The elder let fall the hand raised to bless them, and, bowing to them again, asked them all to sit down. The blood rushed to Alyosha's cheeks. He was ashamed. His forebodings were coming true.

Father Zosima sat down on a very old-fashioned mahogany sofa, upholstered in leather, and made his visitors sit down in a row along the opposite wall on four mahogany chairs, covered with shabby black leather. The monks sat, one at the door and the other at the window. The divinity student, the novice, and Alyosha remained standing. The cell was by no means spacious and had a faded look. It contained nothing but the most necessary furniture, of coarse and poor quality. There were two pots of flowers in the window, and a number of ikons in the corner. Before one huge ancient ikon of the Virgin a lamp was burning. Near it were two other holy pictures in shining settings, and, next them, carved cherubim, china eggs, a Catholic cross of ivory with a Mater Dolorosa embracing it, and several foreign engravings of the works of the great Italian artists of past centuries. Next to these costly and artistic engravings were several of the crudest Russian lithographs of saints and martyrs, such as are sold for a few copecks at all the fairs. On the other walls were portraits of Russian bishops, past and present.

Miüsov cast a cursory glance at all these "conventional" ornaments and bent an intent look upon the elder. He had a high opinion of his own insight, a weakness excusable in him, as he was fifty, an age at which a clever man of the world of established position can hardly help taking himself rather seriously. At the first moment he did not like the elder. There was, indeed, something in the elder's face which many people besides Miüsov might not have liked. Zosima was a short, bent, little man, with very weak legs, and, though he was only sixty-five, he looked at least ten years older. His face was very thin and covered with a network of fine wrinkles, particularly numerous about his eyes, which were small, light-coloured, quick, and shining like two bright points. He had a sprinkling of grey hair about his temples. His pointed beard was small and scanty, and his lips, which smiled frequently, were as thin as two threads. His nose was not long, but sharp, like a bird's beak.

"To all appearances a malicious, small soul, full of petty pride," thought Miüsov. He felt altogether dissatisfied with himself.

A cheap little clock on the wall struck twelve hurriedly, and helped to start the conversation.

"Precisely the hour," cried Fyodor Pavlovich, "but no sign of my son, Dmitri. I apologise for him, sacred elder!" (Alyosha shuddered all over at "sacred elder.") "I am always punctual myself, to the minute, remembering that punctuality is the courtesy of kings . . ."

"But you are no king, anyway," Miüsov muttered, losing his self-restraint at once.

"Yes; that's true. I'm not a king, and, would you believe it, Pyotr Alexandrovich, I was aware of that myself. But, there! I always say the wrong thing. Your reverence," he cried, with sudden pathos, "you behold before you a buffoon, a buffoon in good sooth! I introduce myself as such. It's an old habit, alas! And if I sometimes talk nonsense out of place it's with an object, with the object of amusing people and making myself agreeable. One must be agreeable, mustn't one? I was seven years ago in a little town where I had business, and I made friends with some merchants there. We went to the *ispravnik* [captain of police] because we had to ask a favour of him, and to invite him to dine with us. He was a tall, fat, fair, sullen man, the most dangerous type in such cases. It's their liver. I went straight up to him, and with the ease of a man of the world, you know, 'Mr. Ispravnik,' said I, 'be our Napravnik, so to speak.' 'What do you mean by Napravnik?' said he. I saw, at the first half-second, that it had missed fire. He stood there so glum. 'I wanted to make a joke,' said I, 'for the general diversion, as Mr. Napravnik is our well-known Russian orchestra conductor and what we need for the harmony of our undertaking is some one of that sort.' And I explained my comparison very sensibly, didn't I? 'Excuse me,' said he, 'I am an *ispravnik*, and I do not allow puns to be made on my calling.' He turned and walked away. I followed him, shouting, 'Yes, yes, you are an *ispravnik*, not a Napravnik.' 'No,' he said, 'since you called me a Napravnik I am one.' And would you believe it, it ruined our business! And I'm always like that, always like that. Always injuring myself with my amiability. Once, many years ago, I said to an influential, you might say, person: 'Your wife is a ticklish lady,' in an honourable sense, of the moral qualities, so to speak. And what do you suppose he asked me, 'Why, have you tickled her?' I thought I'd be polite, so I couldn't help saying, 'Yes, I have,' and he gave me a fine tickling on the spot. Only that happened long ago, so I'm not ashamed to tell the story. I'm always injuring myself like that."

"You're doing it now, too," muttered Miüsov, with disgust.

Father Zosima scrutinised them both in silence.

"Am I? Would you believe it, I was aware

of that, too, Pyotr Alexandrovich, and let me tell you, indeed, I foresaw I should as soon as I began to speak. And do you know I foresaw, too, that you'd be the first to remark on it. The minute I see my joke isn't coming off, your reverence, both my cheeks feel as though they were cleaving to the lower jaw and there is almost a spasm in them. That's been so since I was young, when I used to be a hanger-on, and made my living that way in the houses of the gentry. I am an inveterate buffoon, and from my birth, your reverence, there's been a crazy streak in me. I do not deny that there may be an unclean spirit in me. But only a little one. A more important one would have chosen another lodging. But not your soul, Pyotr Alexandrovich; you're not a lodging worth having either. But I do believe — I believe in God, it's only of late that I have had doubts. But now I sit and await words of wisdom. I'm like the philosopher, Diderot, your reverence. Did you ever hear, most holy father, how Diderot went to see the Metropolitan Platon, in the time of the Empress Catherine? He went in and said straight out, 'There is no God.' Whereat the exalted and holy dignitary lifted up his finger and answered, 'The fool hath said in his heart there is no God.' The philosopher fell down at his feet on the spot. 'I believe,' he cried, 'and will be christened.' And so he was. Princess Dashkov was his godmother, and Potyomkin his godfather."

"Fyodor Pavlovich, this is unbearable! You know you're telling lies and that that stupid anecdote isn't true. Why are you playing the fool?" cried Miüsov in a shaking voice, quite unable to control himself.

"I suspected all my life that it wasn't true," Fyodor Pavlovich cried with conviction. "But I'll tell you the whole truth, gentlemen. Great elder! Forgive me, the last thing about Diderot's christening I made up just now. I never thought of it before. I made it up to add piquancy. I play the fool, Pyotr Alexandrovich, to make myself agreeable. Though I really don't know myself, sometimes, what I do it for. And as for Diderot, I heard as far as 'the fool hath said in his heart' twenty times from the gentry about here when I was young. Among others I heard your aunt tell the story, Pyotr Alexandrovich. They all believe to this day that the infidel Diderot came to dispute about God with the Metropolitan Platon. . . ."

Miüsov got to his feet, so thoroughly out of patience that he forgot himself. He was furious, and conscious that as a result he was ridiculous himself.

What was taking place in the cell was really incredible. For forty or fifty years past, since the times of former elders, no visitors had entered that cell without feelings of the profoundest veneration. Almost every one admitted to the cell felt that a great favour was being shown him. Many remained kneeling during the whole visit. Of those visitors, many had been men of high rank and learning, some even free-thinkers, attracted by curiosity, but all without exception, whether coming singly or in groups, felt called upon to show the profoundest reverence and delicacy, all the more so since here there was no question of money, but only, on the one side, love and grace, and on the other penitence and eager desire to resolve some spiritual problem or crisis. So that Fyodor Pavlovich's buffoonery amazed and bewildered the spectators, or at least some of them. The monks, with unchanged countenances, waited, with earnest attention, to hear what the elder would say, but seemed on the point of getting up, like Miüsov. Alyosha stood, with hanging head, on the verge of tears. What seemed to him strangest of all was that his brother Ivan, on whom alone he had rested his hopes, and who alone had such influence on his father that he could have stopped him, sat now quite unmoved, with downcast eyes, apparently waiting with interest to see how it would end, as though he were altogether an outsider. Alyosha did not even dare to look at Rakitin, the divinity student, whom he also knew very well, indeed, almost intimately. For he knew Rakitin's thoughts — he was the only one in the monastery who did.

"Forgive me," began Miüsov, addressing Father Zosima, "for perhaps I seem to be taking part in this unworthy foolery. I made a mistake in believing that even a man like Fyodor Pavlovich would understand what was due on a visit to a person so highly esteemed. I did not suppose I should have to apologise simply for having come with him. . . ."

Pyotr Alexandrovich could say no more, and was about to leave the room, overwhelmed with confusion.

"Don't distress yourself, I beg." The elder suddenly got on to his feeble legs, and taking Pyotr Alexandrovich by both hands made him sit down again. "I beg you not to disturb yourself. I particularly beg you to be my guest." And with a bow he went back and sat down again on his little sofa.

"Great elder, speak out! Do I annoy you by my vivacity or not?" Fyodor Pavlovich cried suddenly, clutching the arms of his chair in both hands, as though ready to leap up from it if the answer were unfavourable.

"I earnestly beg you, too, not to disturb yourself, but to be at your ease," the elder said impressively. "Be at your ease. Make yourself quite at home. And, above all, do not be so ashamed of yourself, for that is at the root of it all."

"Quite at home? To be my natural self? Oh, that is much too much, but I accept it with feeling. Do you know, blessed father, you'd better not invite me to be my natural self. Don't risk it. . . . I will not go so far as that myself. I warn you for your own sake. Well, the rest is still wrapped in the mists of uncertainty, though there are people who'd be pleased to give you a complete picture of me. I mean that for you, Pyotr Alexandrovich. But as for you, most holy one, let me tell you, I am brimming over with ecstasy."

He started to get up and, lifting his hands, declaimed, "Blessed be the womb that bare thee, and the paps that gave thee suck — the paps especially. When you said just now, 'Don't be so ashamed of yourself for that is at the root of it all,' you pierced right through me with that remark, and read me to the core. Indeed, I always feel when I meet people that I am lower than all, and that they all take me for a buffoon. So I say, 'Let me really play the buffoon. I am not afraid of your opinion, for you are every one of you worse than I am.' That is why I am a buffoon. It is from shame, great elder, from shame; it's simply over-sensitiveness that I run riot. If I were only sure that every one would accept me as the kindest and wisest of men, oh, Lord, what a good man I should be then! Master!" he fell suddenly on his knees, "what shall I do to inherit eternal life?"

It was difficult even now to decide whether he was joking or really moved.

Father Zosima, lifting his eyes, looked at him, and said with a smile:

"You have known for a long time what you

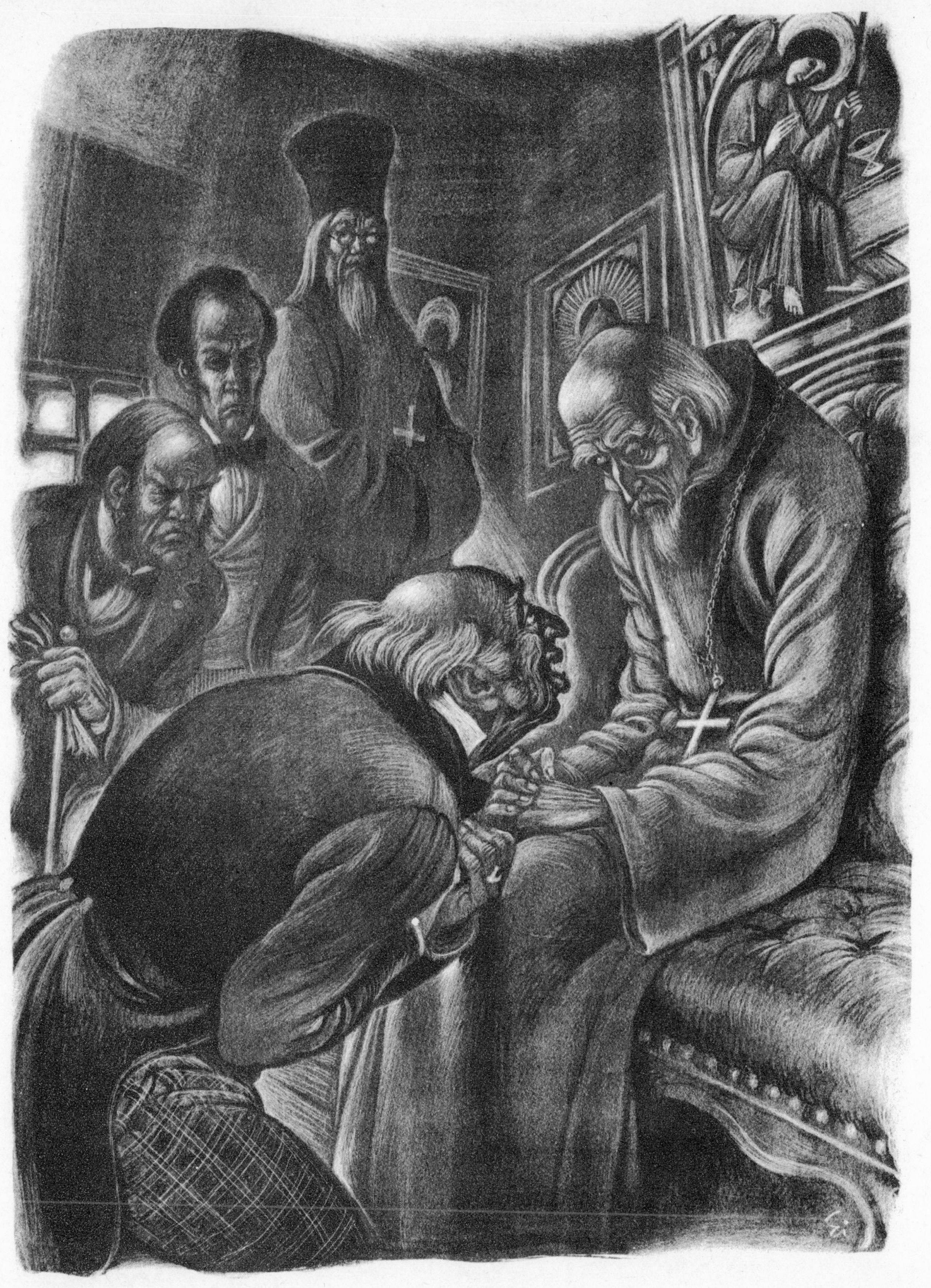

THE OLD BUFFOON

must do. You have sense enough: don't give way to drunkenness and incontinence of speech; don't give way to sensual lust; and, above all, to the love of money. And close your pot-houses. If you can't close all, at least two or three. And, above all — don't lie."

"You mean about Diderot?"

"No, not about Diderot. Above all, don't lie to yourself. The man who lies to himself and listens to his own lie comes to such a pass that he cannot distinguish the truth within him, or around him, and so loses all respect for himself and for others. And having no respect he ceases to love, and in order to occupy and distract himself without love he gives way to passions and coarse pleasures, and sinks to bestiality in his vices, all from continual lying to other men and to himself. The man who lies to himself can be more easily offended than any one. You know it is sometimes very pleasant to take offence, isn't it? A man may know that nobody has insulted him, but that he has invented the insult for himself, has lied and exaggerated to make it picturesque, has caught at a word and made a mountain out of a molehill — he knows that himself, yet he will be the first to take offence, and will revel in his resentment till he feels great pleasure in it, and so pass to genuine vindictiveness. But get off your knees, sit down, I beg you. All this, too, is deceitful posturing . . ."

"Blessed man! Give me your dear hand to kiss."

Fyodor Pavlovich skipped up, and imprinted a rapid kiss on the elder's thin hand. "It is, it is pleasant to take offence. You said that so well, as I never heard it before. Yes, I have been all my life taking offence, to please myself, taking offence on æsthetic grounds, for to be insulted is not only a matter of pleasure, but sometimes a matter of beauty — that you had forgotten, great elder, of beauty! I shall make a note of that. But I have been lying, lying positively my whole life long, every day and hour of it. Truly, I am a lie, and the father of lies. Though I believe I am not the father of lies. I am getting mixed in my texts. Say, the son of lies, and that will be enough. Only . . . my angel . . . I may sometimes talk about Diderot! Diderot will do no harm, though sometimes a word will do harm. Great elder, by the way, I was forgetting, though I had been meaning for the last two years to come here on purpose to ask and to find out something. Only do tell Pyotr Alexandrovich not to interrupt me. Here is my question: Is it true, great father, that the story is told somewhere in the 'Lives of the Saints' of a holy miracle-worker martyred for his faith who, when his head was cut off at last, stood up, picked up his head, and 'fondly kissed it'? He walked a long way, carrying it in his hands, and kissing it. Is that true or not, honoured fathers?"

"No, it is untrue," said the elder.

"There is nothing of the kind in all the lives of the saints. What saint do you say the story is told of?" asked the Father Librarian.

"I do not know what saint. I do not know, and can't tell. I was deceived. That was the way I was told the story. I had heard it, and do you know who told it? Pyotr Alexandrovich Miüsov here, who was so angry just now about Diderot. It was he who told the story."

"I have never told it you, I never speak to you at all."

"It is true you did not tell me, but you told it when I was present. It was three years ago. I mentioned it because by that ridiculous story you shook my faith, Pyotr Alexandrovich.

You knew nothing of it, but I went home with my faith shaken, and I have been getting more and more shaken ever since. Yes, Pyotr Alexandrovich, you were the cause of a great fall. That was worse than Diderot!"

Fyodor Pavlovich got excited and pathetic, though it was perfectly clear to every one by now that he was playing a part again. Yet Miüsov was stung to the quick by his words.

"What nonsense, and it is all nonsense," he muttered. "I may really have told it, some time or other . . . but not to you. I was told it myself. I heard it in Paris from a Frenchman. He told me it was read at our mass from the 'Lives of the Saints' . . . he was a very learned man who had made a special study of Russian statistics and had lived a long time in Russia. . . . I have not read the 'Lives of the Saints' myself, and I am not going to read them . . . all sorts of things are said at dinner — we were dining then."

"Yes, you were dining then, and so I lost my faith!" said Fyodor Pavlovich, teasing him.

"What do I care for your faith?" Miüsov was on the point of shouting, but he suddenly checked himself, and said with contempt, "You literally defile everything you touch."

The elder suddenly rose from his seat. "Excuse me, gentlemen, for leaving you a few minutes," he said, addressing all his guests. "I have visitors awaiting me who arrived before you. But don't you tell lies all the same," he added, turning to Fyodor Pavlovich with a good-humoured face. He went out of the cell. Alyosha and the novice flew to escort him down the steps. Alyosha was breathless: he was glad to get away, but he was glad, too, that the elder was good-humoured and not offended. Father Zosima was going towards the portico to bless the people waiting for him there. But Fyodor Pavlovich persisted in stopping him at the door of the cell.

"Most blessed man!" he cried, with feeling. "Allow me to kiss your dear hand once more. Yes, with you I could still talk, I could still get on. Do you think I always lie and play the fool like this? Believe me, I have been acting like this all the time on purpose to try you. I have been testing you all the time to see whether I could get on with you. Is there room for my humility beside your pride? I am ready to give you a testimonial that one can get on with you! But now, I'll be quiet; I will keep quiet all the time. I'll sit in a chair and hold my tongue. Now it is for you to speak, Pyotr Alexandrovich. You are the principal person left now — for ten minutes."

CHAPTER III

PEASANT WOMEN WHO HAVE FAITH

NEAR the wooden portico below, built on to the outer wall of the precinct, there was a crowd of about twenty peasant women. They had been told that the elder was at last coming out, and they had gathered together in anticipation. Two ladies, Madame Hohlakov and her daughter, had also come out into the portico to wait for the elder, but in a separate part of it set aside for ladies of rank.

Madame Hohlakov was wealthy, still young and attractive, and always dressed with taste. She was rather pale, and had lively black eyes. She was not more than thirty-three, and had been five years a widow. Her daughter, a girl of fourteen, was partially paralysed. The poor child had not been able to walk for the last six months, and was wheeled about in a chair. She had a charming little face, rather thin from illness, but full of gaiety. There was a gleam of mischief in her big dark eyes with their long lashes. Her mother had been intending to take her abroad ever since the spring, but they had been detained all summer by business connected with their estate. They had been staying a week in our town, where they had come more for purposes of business than devotion, but had visited Father Zosima once already, three days before. Though they knew that the elder saw scarcely any one, they had now suddenly turned up again, and urgently entreated "the happiness of looking once again on the great healer."

The mother was sitting on a chair by the side of her daughter's wheel-chair, and two paces from her stood an old monk, not of our monastery, but a visitor from an obscure religious house in the far north. He, too, sought the elder's blessing.

But Father Zosima, on entering the portico, went first straight to the peasant women who were crowded at the foot of the three steps that led up into the portico. Father Zosima stood on the top step, put on his stole, and began blessing the women who thronged about him. One "possessed" woman was led up to him. As soon as she caught sight of the elder she began shrieking, hiccuping, and writhing in convulsions. Laying the stole on her forehead, he read a short prayer over her, and she was at once soothed and quieted.

I do not know how it may be now, but in my childhood I often happened to see and hear these "possessed" women in the villages and monasteries. They used to be brought to mass; they would squeal and bark like a dog so that they were heard all over the church. But when the sacrament was carried in and they were led up to it, at once the "possession" ceased, and the sick women were always soothed for a time. I was greatly impressed and amazed at this as a child; but then I heard from country neighbours and from my town teachers that the whole illness was simulated to avoid work, and that it could always be cured by suitable severity; various anecdotes were told to confirm this. But later on I learnt with astonishment from medical specialists that there is no pretence about it, that it is a terrible illness to which women are subject, specially prevalent among us in Russia, and that it is due to the hard lot of the peasant women. It is a disease, I was told, arising from exhausting toil too soon after hard, abnormal, and unassisted labour in childbirth, and from the hopeless misery, from beatings, and so on, which some women were not able to endure like others. The strange and instant healing of the frantic and struggling woman as soon as she was led up to the holy sacrament, which had been explained to me as due to malingering and the trickery of the "clericals," arose probably in the most natural manner. Both the women who supported her and the invalid herself fully believed as truth beyond question that the evil spirit in possession of her could not hold out if the sick woman were brought to the sacrament and made to bow down before it. And so, with a nervous and psychically deranged woman, a sort of convulsion of the whole organism always took place, and was bound to take place, at the moment of bowing down to the sacrament, a convulsion aroused by the expectation of the miracle of healing and the implicit belief that it would come to pass; and it did come to pass, though only for a moment. It was exactly the same now as soon as the elder touched the sick woman with the stole.

Many of the women in the crowd were moved to tears of ecstasy by the effect of the moment; some strove to kiss the hem of his garment; others wailed in sing-song voices.

He blessed them all and talked with some of them. The "possessed" woman he knew already. She came from a village only six versts from the monastery, and had been brought to him before.

"But here is one from afar." He pointed to a woman by no means old but very thin and wasted, with a face not merely sunburnt but almost blackened by exposure. She was kneeling and gazing with a fixed stare at the elder; there was something almost frenzied in her eyes.

"From afar off, father, afar off! Two hundred miles from here. From afar off, father, from afar off!" the woman began in a sing-song voice as though she were chanting a dirge, swaying her head from side to side with her cheek resting in her hand.

There is among the masses silent and long-suffering sorrow. It withdraws into itself and is quiet. But there is a grief that breaks out in tears and from then on finds vent in wailing. This is particularly common with women. But it is no lighter a grief than the silent kind. Lamentation comforts only by lacerating the heart still more. Such grief does not desire consolation. It feeds on the sense of its hopelessness. Lamentation springs only from the constant craving to keep the wound green.

"You are of the townspeople?" said Father Zosima, looking curiously at her.

"Townfolk we are, father, townfolk. We work the land though we live in the town. I have come to see you, oh, father! We heard of you, father, we heard of you. I have buried my little son, and I have come to pray to God. I have been in three monasteries on my pilgrimage, but they told me, 'Go, Nastasya, go to this place' — that is to you, little dove, to you. I have come; I was yesterday at the service, and to-day I have come to you."

"What are you weeping for?"

"It's my little son I'm grieving for, father. He was three years old — three years all but three months. For my little boy, father, I'm in anguish, for my little boy. He was the last one left. We had four, my Nikita and I, but we don't keep our children, my dear, we don't keep them. I buried the first three without grieving overmuch, and now I have buried the last I can't forget him. It's as though he were standing before me. He doesn't leave me. He has dried up my heart. I look at his little clothes, his little shirt, his little boots, and I cry. I lay out all that is left of him, all his little things. I look at them and cry. I say to Nikita, my husband, let me go on a pilgrimage, master. He is a driver. We're not poor people, father, not poor; we are independent. It's all our own, the horses and the carriage. And what good is it all to us now? My Nikita has begun drinking while I am away. I'm sure of it. It used to be so before. As soon as I turn my back he gives way to it. But now I don't think about him either. It's three months since I left home. I've forgotten him. I've forgotten everything. I don't want to remember. And what would our life together be now? I've done with him, I've done. I've done with them all. I don't care to look upon my house and my goods. I don't care to see anything at all!"

"Listen, mother," said the elder. "Once in olden times a great saint saw in church a mother like you weeping for her little one, her only one, whom God had called to him. 'Knowest thou not,' said the saint to her, 'how bold these little ones are before the throne of God? Verily there are none bolder than they in the Kingdom of Heaven. "Thou didst give us life, O Lord," they say, "and scarcely had we looked upon it when Thou didst take it back again." And so boldly they ask and ask again that God gives them at once the rank of angels. Therefore,' said the saint, 'thou, too, woman, rejoice and weep not, for thy little one is now with the Lord in the host of his angels.' That's what the saint said to the weeping mother of old. He was a great saint and he could not have spoken falsely. Therefore you, too, mother, know that your little one is surely before the throne of God, is rejoicing and happy, and praying to God for you. Therefore do you also weep, but rejoice." The woman listened to him with downcast eyes, leaning her cheek on her hand. She sighed deeply.

"My Nikita tried to comfort me with the same words as you. 'Foolish one,' he said, 'why weep? Our son is no doubt chanting with the angels before God.' He says that to me, but he weeps himself. I see that he cries like me. 'I know, Nikita,' said I. 'Where could he be if not with the Lord God? Only, he is not here with us, sitting beside us as he used to before.' And if only I could look upon him one little time, if only I could peep at him just once, without going up to him, without speaking, if I could hide myself in a corner and only see him for one little minute, hear him playing in the yard. He used to come and call in his little voice, 'Mammy, where are you?' If only I could hear him just once, only once, pattering about the room on his little feet, pit-a-pat, with his little feet, so quick, quick; I remember how he used to run to me and shout and laugh, if only I could hear his little feet, hear them, recognise them! But he's gone, father, he's gone, and I shall never hear him again. Here's his little sash, but he isn't here, him I shall never see or hear now."

She drew out of her bosom her boy's little sash, with braid on it, and as soon as she looked at it she began shaking with sobs, hiding her eyes with her fingers through which the tears flowed in a sudden stream.

"It is Rachel of old," said the elder, "weeping for her children, and will not be comforted because they are not. Such is the lot set on earth for you mothers. Be not comforted. Consolation is not what you need. Weep and be not consoled, but weep. Only every time that you weep be sure to remember that your little son is one of the angels of God, that he looks down from there at you and sees you, and rejoices at your tears, and points at them to the Lord God; and a long while yet will you keep that great mother's grief. But it will turn in the end into quiet joy, and your bitter tears will be only tears of tender sorrow that purifies the heart and delivers it from sin. And I shall pray for the peace of your child's soul. What was his name?"

"Alexey, father."

"A sweet name. After Alexey, the man of God?"

"Yes, father."

"What a saint he was! I will remember him in my prayers, mother, and your grief, and I will pray for your husband's health. It is a sin for you to leave him. Your little one will see from heaven that you have forsaken his father, and will weep over you. Why do you trouble his happiness? He is living, for the soul lives for ever, and though he is not in the house he is near you, unseen. How can he go into the house when you say that the house is hateful to you? To whom is he to go if he find you not together, his father and mother? He comes to you in dreams now, and you are tormented. But then he will send you gentle dreams. Go to your husband, mother; go this very day."

"I will go, father, at your word. I will go. You've touched my heart. Nikita, my Nikita, you are waiting for me," the woman began in a sing-song voice; but the elder had already turned away to a very old woman, dressed like a townswoman, not like a pilgrim. Her eyes showed that she had come with an object, and in order to ask a question. She said she was the widow of a non-commissioned officer, and lived close by in the town. Her son Vasenka was in the commissariat service, and had gone to Irkutsk in Siberia. He had written twice from there, but now a year had passed since he had written.

She did inquire about him, but she did not know whether she had inquired in the proper place.

"Only the other day Stepanida Ilyinishna Bedryagin — she's a rich merchant's wife — said to me, 'You go, Prohorovna, and put your son's name down for prayer in the church, that they may pray for the peace of his soul as though he were dead. His soul will be troubled,' she said, 'and he will write you a letter.' And Stepanida Ilyinishna told me it was a certain thing and well-tried. Only I am in doubt. . . . Oh, light of our lives! is it true or isn't it, and would it be right?"

"Don't think of it. It's shameful to ask the question. How is it possible to pray for the peace of a living soul as though for the dead? And his own mother, too! It's a great sin, akin to sorcery. Only for your ignorance it is forgiven you. Better pray to the Queen of Heaven, our swift defence and help, for his good health, and that she may forgive you for your erring thought. And another thing I will tell you, Prohorovna. Either he will soon come back to you, your son, or he will be sure to send a letter. Go, and henceforward be in peace. Your son is alive, I tell you."

"God reward you, dear father, our benefactor, who prays for all of us and for our sins!"

But the elder had already noticed in the crowd two burning eyes fixed upon him. An exhausted, consumptive-looking peasant woman, still young, was looking at him in silence. Her eyes besought him, but she seemed afraid to approach.

"What is it, my child?"

"Absolve my soul, father," she articulated softly and slowly, sank on her knees and bowed down at his feet. "I have sinned, father. I fear my sin."

The elder sat down on the lower step. The woman crept closer to him, still on her knees.

"I am a widow these three years," she began in a half-whisper, with a sort of shudder. "I had a hard life with my husband. He was an old man. He used to beat me cruelly. He lay ill; I thought looking at him, if he were to get well, if he were to get up again, what then? And then the thought came to me — "

"Stay!" said the elder, and he put his ear close to her lips.

The woman went on in a low whisper, so that it was almost impossible to catch anything. She had soon done.

"Three years ago?" asked the elder.

"Three years. At first I didn't think about it, but now I've been taken ill, and the thought never leaves me."

"Have you come a distance?"

"Over three hundred miles."

"Have you told it in confession?"

"I have confessed it. Twice I have confessed it."

"Have you been admitted to Communion?"

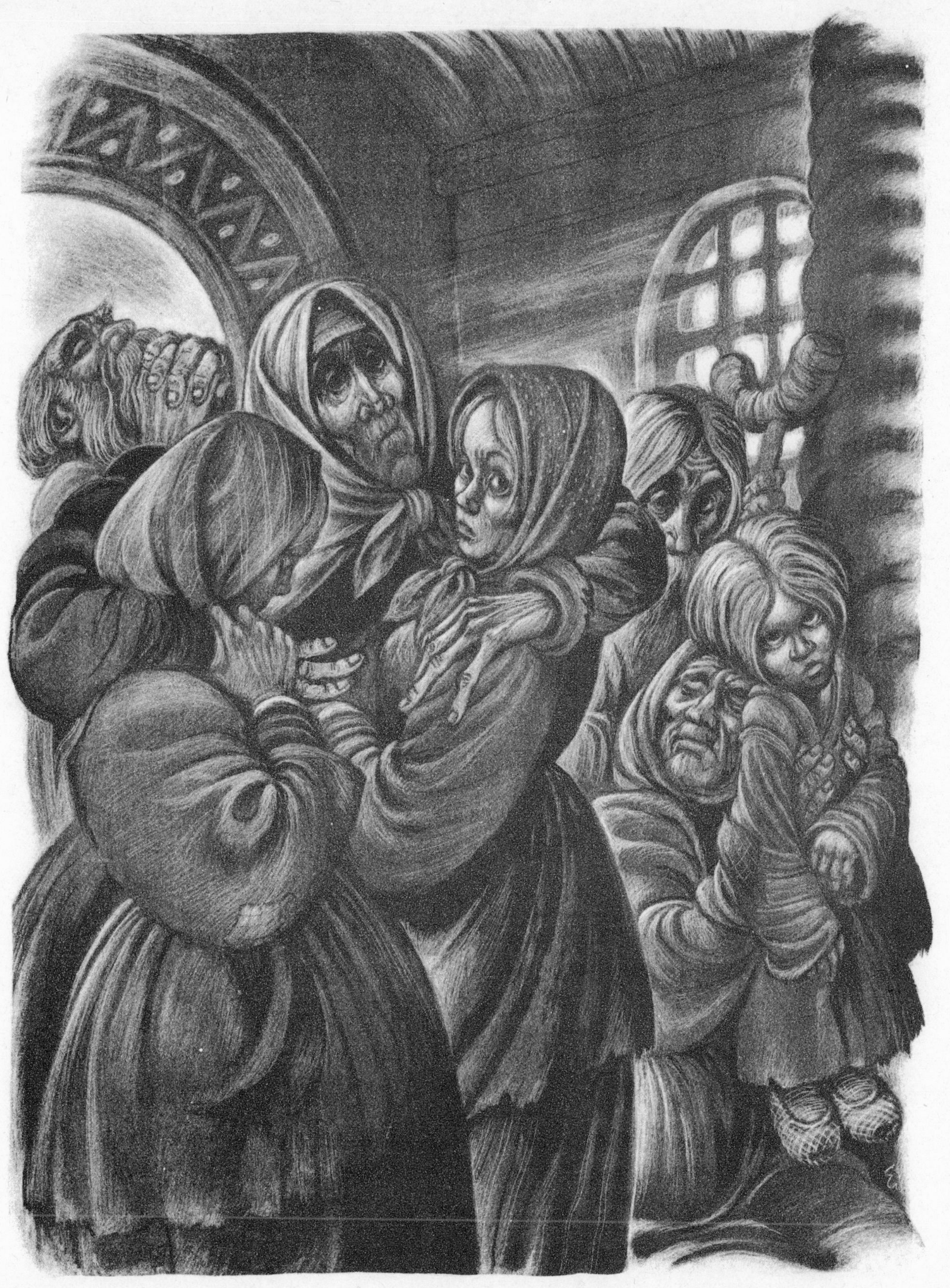

WOMEN OF GREAT FAITH

"Yes. I am afraid. I am afraid to die."

"Fear nothing and never be afraid; and don't fret. If only your penitence fail not, God will forgive all. There is no sin, and there can be no sin on earth, which the Lord will not forgive to the truly repentant! Man cannot commit a sin so great as to exhaust the infinite love of God. Can there be a sin which could exceed the love of God? Think only of repentance, continual repentance, but dimiss fear altogether. Believe that God loves you inconceivably; that He loves you with your sin, in your sin. It has been said of old that over one repentant sinner there is more joy in heaven than over ten righteous men. Go, and fear not. Be not bitter against men, be not angry if you are wronged. Forgive the dead man in your heart what wrong he did you. Be reconciled with him in truth. If you are penitent, you love. And if you love you belong to God. All things are redeemed, all things are saved by love. If I, a sinner, even as you are, am tender with you and have pity on you, how much more will God. Love is such a priceless treasure that you can purchase the whole world with it, and expiate not only your own sins but the sins of others. Go, and do not fear."

He signed her three times with the sign of the cross, took from his own neck a little ikon and put it upon her. Without a word, she bowed down to the earth before him.

He got up and looked cheerfully at a healthy peasant woman with a tiny baby in her arms.

"From Vyshegorye, dear father."

"Five miles you have dragged yourself with the baby. What do you want?"

"I've come to look at you. I have been to you before — or have you forgotten? You've no great memory if you've forgotten me. They told us you were ill. Thinks I, I'll go and see him for myself. Now I see you, and you're not ill! You'll live another twenty years. God bless you! There are plenty to pray for you; how should you be ill?"

"I thank you for all, daughter."

"By the way, I have a thing to ask, not a great one. Here are sixty copecks. Give them, dear father, to some one poorer than me. I thought as I came along, better give through him. He'll know whom to give to."

"Thanks, my dear, thanks! You are a good woman. I love you. I will do so certainly. Is that your little girl?"

"My little girl, father, Lizaveta."

"May the Lord bless you both, you and your babe Lizaveta! You have gladdened my heart, mother. Farewell, dear children, farewell, dear ones."

He blessed them all and bowed low to them.

CHAPTER IV

A LADY OF LITTLE FAITH

A LADY, watching the scene between the elder and the peasant women and his blessing them, shed silent tears and wiped them away with a dainty handkerchief. She was a sentimental society lady with a disposition genuinely good in many respects. When the elder went up to her at last she met him enthusiastically.

"Ah, what I have been feeling, as I watched this touching scene! . . . " She could not go on for emotion. "Oh, I understand the people's love for you. I love the people myself. I want to love them. And who could help loving them, our splendid Russian people, so simple in their greatness!"

"How is your daughter's health? You wanted to talk to me again?"

"Oh, I have been urgently begging for it,

I have prayed for it! I was ready to fall on my knees and remain kneeling for three days at your windows until you let me in. We have come, great healer, to express our ardent gratitude. You have healed my Lise, healed her completely, merely by praying over her last Thursday and laying your hands upon her. We have hastened here to kiss those hands, to pour out our feelings and our homage."

"What do you mean by healed? But she is still lying in her chair."

"But her night fevers have entirely ceased ever since Thursday," said the lady with nervous haste. "And that's not all. Her legs are stronger. This morning she got up well; she had slept all night. Look at her rosy cheeks, her bright eyes! She used to be always crying, but now she laughs and is gay and happy. This morning she insisted on my letting her stand up, and she stood up for a whole minute without any support. She wagers that in a fortnight she'll be dancing a quadrille. I've called in Dr. Herzenstube. He shrugged his shoulders and said, 'I am amazed; I can make nothing of it.' And would you have us not disturb you, not fly here to thank you? Lise, thank him — thank him!"

Lise's pretty little laughing face became suddenly serious. She rose in her chair as far as she could and, looking at the elder, clasped her hands before him, but could not restrain herself and broke into laughter.

"It's at him," she said, pointing to Alyosha, with childish vexation at herself for not being able to repress her mirth.

If any one had looked at Alyosha standing a step behind the elder, he would have caught a quick flush mantling his cheeks in an instant. His eyes flashed and fell.

"She has a message for you, Alexey Fyodorovich. How are you?" the mother went on, holding out her exquisitely gloved hand to Alyosha.

The elder turned round and all at once looked attentively at Alyosha. The latter approached Lise and, smiling in a strangely awkward way, held out his hand to her, too. Lise assumed an important air.

"Katerina Ivanovna has sent you this through me." She handed him a little note. "She particularly begs you to go and see her as soon as possible; that you will not fail her, but will be sure to come."

"She asks me to go and see her? Me? What for?" Alyosha muttered in great astonishment. His face at once looked anxious.

"Oh, it all has to do with Dmitri Fyodorovich and — with what has happened lately," the mother explained hurriedly. "Katerina Ivanovna has made up her mind, but she must see you about it without fail. . . . Why? Of course, I can't say. But she asks you to come as soon as possible. And you will do it, you will surely do it. Your feelings as a Christian will make you."

"I have only seen her once," Alyosha protested with the same perplexity.

"Oh, she is such a noble, exalted creature! Her sufferings alone . . . Think what she has gone through, what she is enduring now! Think what awaits her! It's all terrible, terrible!"

"Very well, I will come," Alyosha decided, after rapidly scanning the brief, enigmatic note, which consisted of an urgent entreaty that he would come, without any sort of explanation.

"Oh, how sweet and how splendid that would be of you!" cried Lise with sudden animation. "And I told mamma: he is sure not to go, he is saving his soul. How splendid you are! I've always thought you were splendid. How glad I am to tell you so now!"

"Lise!" said her mother impressively, but at once broke into a smile.

"You have quite forgotten us, Alexey Fyodorovich," she said; "you never come to see us. Yet Lise has told me twice that she is never happy except with you."

Alyosha raised his downcast eyes and again flushed, and again smiled without knowing why. But the elder was no longer watching him. He had engaged in conversation a monk who, as mentioned before, had been awaiting his entrance by Lise's chair. He was evidently a monk of the humblest, that is of the peasant, class, of a narrow outlook, but a true believer, and, in his own way, a stubborn one. He announced that he had come from the far north, from Obdorsk, from St. Sylvester, and was a member of a poor monastery, consisting of only nine monks. The elder gave him his blessing and invited him to come to his cell whenever he liked.

"How can you presume to do such deeds?" the monk asked suddenly, pointing solemnly and significantly at Lise. He was hinting at her "cure."

"It's too early, of course, to speak of that. Relief is not complete cure, and may proceed from other causes. But if there has been any healing, it is by no power but God's will. It's all from God. Visit me, father," he added to the monk. "It's not always I can see visitors. I am ill, and I know that my days are numbered."

"Oh, no, no! God will not take you from us. You will live a long, long time yet," cried the lady. "And in what way are you ill? You look so well, so gay and happy."

"I am extraordinarily better to-day. But I know that it's only for a moment. I understand my disease now thoroughly. If you say that I seem so cheerful to you, you could never tell me anything that would please me more. For men are made for happiness, and any one who is completely happy has a right to say to himself, 'I have done God's will on earth.' All the righteous, all the saints, all the holy martyrs were happy."

"Oh, how you speak! What bold and lofty words!" cried the lady. "You seem to pierce with your words. And yet — happiness, happiness — where is it? Who can say of himself that he is happy? Oh, since you have been so good as to let us see you once more to-day, let me tell you what I could not utter last time, what I dared not say, all I am suffering and have been for so long! I am suffering! Forgive me! I am suffering!"

And in a rush of fervent feeling she clasped her hands before him.

"From what specially?"

"I suffer . . . from lack of faith."

"Lack of faith in God?"

"Oh, no, no! I dare not even think of that. But the future life — it is such an enigma! And no one, no one can solve it. Listen! You are a healer, you are deeply versed in the human soul, and of course I dare not expect you to believe me entirely, but I assure you on my word of honour that I am not speaking lightly now. The thought of the life beyond the grave agitates me to the point of suffering, of fright, of terror. And I don't know to whom to appeal, and have not dared to all my life. And now I am so bold as to ask you. Oh, God! What will you think of me now?"

She struck her hands together.

"Don't distress yourself about my opinion

of you," said the elder. "I quite believe in the sincerity of your anguish."

"Oh, how thankful I am to you! You see, I shut my eyes and ask myself: if every one has faith, where did it come from? They say that it all comes from terror at the menacing phenomena of nature, and that none of it's real. And I say to myself, 'I've been believing all my life, and what if, when I come to die, there's nothing but burdocks growing on the grave? — as I read in some book.' It's awful! How — how can I get back my faith? But really I only believed when I was a little child, mechanically, without thinking of anything. How, how is one to prove it? I have come now to lay my soul before you and to ask you about it. If I let this chance slip, no one all my life will answer me. How can one prove it? How can one convince oneself? Oh, how unhappy I am! I stand and look about me and see that scarcely any one else cares; no one troubles his head about it, and I'm the only one who can't stand it. It's deadly — deadly!"

"No doubt. But there's no proving it, though you can be convinced of it."

"How?"

"By the experience of active love. Strive to love your neighbour actively and tirelessly. In so far as you advance in love you will grow surer of the reality of God and of the immortality of your soul. If you attain to perfect self-forgetfulness in the love of your neighbour, then you will believe without doubt, and no doubt can possibly enter your soul. This has been tried. This is certain."

"In active love? There's another question — and such a question! You see, I so love humanity that — would you believe it? — I often dream of forsaking all that I have, leaving Lise, and becoming a sister of mercy. I close my eyes and think and dream, and at that moment I feel full of strength to overcome all obstacles. No wounds, no festering sores could at that moment frighten me. I would bind them up and wash them with my own hands. I would nurse the afflicted. I would be ready to kiss such wounds."

"It is much, and well that your mind is full of such dreams and not others. Sometime, unawares, you may do a good deed in reality."

"Yes. But could I endure such a life for long?" the lady went on fervently, almost frantically. "That's the chief question — that's my most agonising question. I shut my eyes and ask myself, 'Would you persevere long on that path? And if the patient whose wounds you are washing did not meet you with gratitude, but worried you with his whims, without valuing or remarking your charitable services, began abusing you and rudely commanding you, and complaining to the superior authorities of you (which often happens when people are in great suffering) — what then? Would you persevere in your love, or not?' And do you know, I came with horror to the conclusion that, if anything could dissipate my active love for humanity, it would be ingratitude. In short, I am a hired servant, I expect my payment at once — that is, praise, and the repayment of love with love. Otherwise I am incapable of loving any one."

She was in a very paroxysm of self-castigation, and, concluding, she looked with defiant resolution at the elder.

"It's just the same story as a doctor once told me," observed the elder. "He was a man getting on in years, and undoubtedly clever. He spoke as frankly as you, though in jest, in sorrowful jest. 'I love humanity,' he said, 'but I wonder at myself. The more I love humanity in general, the less I love man in particular, that is, as separate individuals. In my dreams,' he said, 'I have often come to making enthusiastic schemes for the service of humanity, and perhaps I might actually have faced crucifixion if it had been suddenly necessary; and yet I am incapable of living in the same room with any one for two days together, as I know by experience. As soon as any one is near me, his personality disturbs my self-importance and restricts my freedom. In twenty-four hours I begin to hate the best of men: one because he's too long over his dinner; another because he has a cold and keeps on blowing his nose. I become hostile to people the moment they come close to me. But it has always happened that the more I detest men individually the more ardent becomes my love for humanity in general."

"But what's to be done? What can one do in such a case? Must one despair?"

"No. It is enough that you are distressed by it. Do what you can, and it will be reckoned unto you. Much is done already in you since you can so deeply and sincerely know yourself. If you have been talking to me so sincerely, simply to gain approbation for your frankness, as you did from me just now, then of course you will not attain to anything in the achievement of real love; it will all get no further than dreams, and your whole life will slip away like a phantom. In that case you will naturally cease to think of the future life, too, and will of yourself grow calmer after a fashion in the end."

"You have crushed me! Only now, as you speak, I understand that I was really only seeking your approbation for my sincerity when I told you I could not endure ingratitude. You have revealed me to myself. You have seen through me and explained me to myself!"

"Are you speaking the truth? Well, now, after such a confession, I believe that you are sincere and good at heart. If you do not attain happiness, always remember that you are on the right road, and try not to leave it. Above all, avoid falsehood, every kind of falsehood, especially lying to yourself. Watch over your own deceitfulness and look into it every hour, every minute. Avoid also being scornful, both of others and of yourself. What seems to you abominable within you is purified by the very fact of your observing it in yourself. Avoid fear, too, though fear is only the consequence of every sort of falsehood. Never be frightened at your own faint-heartedness in the attainment of love. Don't be frightened overmuch even at your evil actions. I am sorry I can say nothing more consoling to you, for love in action is a harsh and dreadful thing compared with love in dreams. Love in dreams thirsts for immediate action, rapidly performed and in the sight of all. Men will even give their lives if only the ordeal does not last long but is soon over, with all looking on and applauding as though on the stage. But active love is labour and fortitude, and for some people, too, perhaps, a whole science. But I predict that just when you see with horror that in spite of all your efforts you are getting further from your goal instead of nearer to it — at that very moment I predict that you will reach it and behold clearly the miraculous power of the Lord who has been all the time loving and mysteriously guiding you. Forgive me for not being able to stay longer with you. They are waiting for me. Good-bye."

The lady was weeping.

"Lise, Lise! Bless her — bless her!" she cried, starting up suddenly.

"She does not deserve to be loved. I have seen her naughtiness all along," the elder said jestingly. "Why have you been laughing at Alexey?"

Lise had in fact been occupied in mocking at him all the time. She had noticed before that Alyosha was shy and tried not to look at her, and she found this extremely amusing. She waited intently to catch his eye. Alyosha, unable to endure her persistent stare, was irresistibly and suddenly drawn to glance at her, and at once she smiled triumphantly in his face. Alyosha was even more disconcerted and vexed. At last he turned away from her altogether and hid behind the elder's back. After a few minutes, drawn by the same irresistible force, he turned again to see whether he was being looked at or not, and found Lise almost hanging out of her chair to peep sideways at him, eagerly waiting for him to look. Catching his eye, she laughed so that the elder could not help saying, "Why do you tease him like that, naughty girl?"

Lise suddenly and quite unexpectedly blushed. Her eyes flashed and her face became terribly serious. She began speaking quickly and nervously in a warm and resentful voice:

"Why has he forgotten everything, then? He used to carry me about when I was little. We used to play together. He used to come to teach me to read, do you know it? Two years ago, when he went away, he said that he would never forget me, that we were friends for ever, for ever, for ever! And now he's afraid of me all at once. Am I going to eat him? Why doesn't he want to come near me? Why doesn't he talk? Why won't he come and see us? It's not that you won't let him. We know that he goes everywhere. It's not good manners for me to invite him. He ought to have thought of it first, if he hasn't forgotten me. No, now he's saving his soul! Why have you put that long gown on him? If he runs he'll fall."

And suddenly she hid her face in her hand and went off into irresistible, prolonged, nervous, inaudible laughter, that fairly shook her. The elder listened to her with a smile, and blessed her tenderly. As she kissed his hand she suddenly pressed it to her eyes and began crying.

"Don't be angry with me. I'm silly and good for nothing . . . and perhaps Alyosha's right, quite right, in not wanting to come and see such a ridiculous girl."

"I will send him without fail," said the elder.

CHAPTER V

SO BE IT! SO BE IT!

The elder's absence from his cell had lasted for about twenty-five minutes. It was more than half-past twelve, but Dmitri, on whose account they had all met there, had still not appeared. But he seemed almost to be forgotten, and when the elder entered the cell again, he found his guests engaged in eager conversation. Ivan and the two monks took the leading share in it. Miüsov, too, was trying to take a part, and apparently very eagerly, in the conversation. But he was unsuccessful in this also. He was evidently in the background, and his remarks were treated with neglect, which increased his irritability. He had had intellectual encounters with Ivan before and he could not endure with equanimity a certain carelessness Ivan showed him.

"Hitherto at least I have stood in the front ranks of all that is progressive in Europe, and here the new generation positively ignores us," he thought.

Fyodor Pavlovich, who had given his word to sit still and be quiet, had actually been quiet for some time, but he watched his neighbour Miüsov with an ironical little smile, obviously enjoying his discomfiture. He had been waiting for some time to pay off old scores, and now he could not let the opportunity slip. Bending over his shoulder, he began teasing him again in a whisper.

"Why didn't you go away just now, after the 'fondly kissing'? Why did you consent to remain in such unseemly company? It was because you felt insulted and injured, and you remained to vindicate yourself by showing off your intelligence. Now you won't go till you've displayed your intellect to them."

"You again? . . . On the contrary, I'm just going."

"You'll be the last, the last of all to go!" Fyodor Pavlovich delivered him another thrust. At that moment Father Zosima returned.

The discussion died down for a moment, but the elder, seating himself in his former place, looked at them all as though cordially inviting them to go on. Alyosha, who knew every expression of his face, saw that he was fearfully exhausted and forcing himself to keep up. Of late he had been liable to fainting fits from exhaustion. His face had the pallor that was common before such attacks, and his lips were white. But he evidently did not want to break up the gathering. He seemed to have some special object of his own in acting thus. What object? Alyosha watched him intently.

"We are discussing this gentleman's most interesting article," said Father Iosif, the librarian, addressing the elder, and pointing to Ivan. "He brings forward much that is new, but I think the argument cuts both ways. It is an article written in answer to a book by an ecclesiastical authority on the question of the ecclesiastical jurisdiction and its scope."

"I'm sorry I have not read your article, but I've heard of it," said the elder, looking keenly and intently at Ivan.

"He takes a most interesting position," continued the Father Librarian. "As far as Church jurisdiction is concerned he is apparently quite opposed to the separation of Church from State."

"That's interesting. But in what sense?" Father Zosima asked Ivan. The latter, at last, answered him, not condescendingly, as Alyosha had feared, but with modesty and reserve, with evident goodwill and apparently without the slightest mental reservation.

"I start from the thesis that this confusion of elements, that is, of the essential principles of Church and State, taken separately, will, of course, go on for ever, in spite of the fact that it is impossible, and that the confusion of these elements cannot be reduced to any order or harmony, for there is falsity at the very root of the thing. Compromise between Church and State in such questions as, for instance, jurisdiction, is, to my thinking, impossible in any real sense. My clerical opponent maintains that the Church holds a precise and definite position in the State. I argued, on the contrary, that the Church ought to contain within itself the whole State, and not simply occupy a corner in it, and, if this is, for some reason, impossible at present, then it ought, in reality, to be set up as the direct and chief goal of the future development of Christian society!"

"Perfectly true," Father Païssy, the silent and learned monk, assented nervously but firmly. "The purest Ultramontanism!" cried Miüsov, impatiently crossing his legs.

"Oh, but we have no mountains," cried Father Iosif, and turning to the elder he continued: "the gentleman replies to the following 'fundamental and essential' propositions of his opponent, who is, you must note, an ecclesiastic. First, that 'no social organisation can or ought to arrogate to itself power to dispose of the civil and political rights of its members.' Secondly, that 'criminal and civil jurisdiction ought not to belong to the Church, and is inconsistent with its nature, both as a divine institution and as a union of men for religious purposes,' and, finally, in the third place, 'the Church is a kingdom not of this world.' "

"A most unworthy play upon words for an ecclesiastic!" Father Païssy could not refrain from breaking in again. "I have read the book to which you made reply," he added, addressing Ivan, "and was astounded at the words 'the Church is a kingdom not of this world.' If it is not of this world, then it cannot exist on earth at all. In the Gospel, the words 'not of this world' are not used in that sense. To play with such words is indefensible. Our Lord Jesus Christ came precisely to set up the Church upon earth. The Kingdom of Heaven, of course, is not of this world, but in heaven; but it is entered only through the Church which has been founded and established upon earth. And so a frivolous play upon words in such a connection is unpardonable and improper. The Church is, in truth, a kingdom and is ordained to rule, and in the end must undoubtedly become the kingdom embracing all the earth. For that we have divine promise."

He ceased speaking suddenly, as though checking himself.

After listening to him attentively and respectfully, Ivan went on, addressing the elder with perfect composure but as before with ready cordiality:

"The whole point of my article is that during the first three centuries Christianity existed on earth only in the Church and was nothing but the Church. When the pagan Roman State desired to become Christian, it inevitably happened that, by becoming Christian, it merely included the Church within it, but remained a pagan State in very many of its functions. In the nature of things, this was bound to happen. But Rome as a State retained too much of the pagan civilisation and culture, as, for example, the very objects and fundamental principles of the State. As for the Christian Church, on entering into the State it could, of course, surrender no part of its fundamental principles — the rock on which it stood — and could pursue no aims but its own, those which have been ordained and revealed by God Himself, and among them that of transforming the whole world, and therefore the ancient pagan State itself, into the Church. In that way (that is, with a view to the future) it is not the Church that should seek a definite position in the State, like 'every social organisation,' or as 'a union of men for religious purposes' (as my opponent calls the Church), but, on the contrary, every earthly State should be, in the end, completely transformed into the Church and should become nothing else but a Church, rejecting every purpose incongruous with the aims of the Church. All this will not degrade it in any way or take from its honour and glory as a great State, nor from the glory of its rulers, but only turns it from a false, still pagan, and mistaken path to the true and rightful path, which alone leads to the eternal goal. This is why the author of the book 'On the Foundations of Church Jurisdiction' would have judged correctly if, in seeking and laying down those foundations, he had looked upon them as only a temporary compromise inevitable in our sinful and imperfect days. But as soon as the author ventures to declare that the foundations which he predicates now, part of which Father Iosif just enumerated, are the unshakable, primal, and eternal foundations, he is going directly against the Church and its sacred, eternal, and unshakable destiny. That is the gist of my article."

"That is, in brief," Father Païssy began again, laying stress on each word, "according to certain theories only too clearly formulated in the nineteenth century, the Church ought to be transformed into the State, as though this would be an advance from a lower to a higher form, so as subsequently to disappear into it, making way for science, for the spirit of the age, and civilisation. And if the Church resists and is unwilling, some corner is set apart for her in the State, and even that under surveillance — and this is so everywhere in all modern European countries. But Russian thinking, Russian hopes and conceptions demand not that the Church should pass as from a lower into a higher type into the State, but, on the contrary, that the State should end by being worthy to become only the Church and nothing else. So be it! So be it!"

"Well, I confess you've reassured me somewhat," Miüsov said smiling, again crossing his legs. "So far as I understand then, the realisation of such an ideal is infinitely remote, and will take place only at the second coming of Christ. That's as you please. It's a beautiful Utopian dream of the disappearance of war, diplomacy, banks, and so on — something after the fashion of socialism, indeed. But I imagined that it was all meant seriously, and that the Church might be *now* going to try criminals, and sentence them to beating, prison, and even death."

"But if there were even now none but the ecclesiastical court, the Church would not sentence a criminal to prison or to death. Crime and the way of regarding it would inevitably change, not all at once of course, but fairly soon," Ivan replied calmly, without flinching.

"Are you serious?" Miüsov glanced keenly at him.

"If everything became the Church, the Church would excommunicate all the criminal and disobedient, and would not cut off their heads," Ivan went on. "I ask you, what would become of the excommunicated? He would be cut off then not only from men, as now, but from Christ. By his crime he would have transgressed not only against men but against the Church of Christ. This is so even now, of course, strictly speaking, but it is not clearly enunciated, and very, very often the criminal of to-day compromises with his conscience: 'I steal,' he says, 'but I don't go against the Church, I'm not an enemy of Christ.' That's what the criminal of to-day is continually saying to himself, but when the Church takes the place of the State it will be difficult for him, in opposition to the Church all over the world, to say: 'All men are mistaken, all in error, all mankind are the false Church. I, a thief and a murderer, am the only true Christian Church.' It will be very difficult to say this to himself; it requires a rare combination of unusual circumstances. Now, on the other hand, take the Church's own view of crime: is it not bound to renounce the present almost pagan attitude, and instead of mechanically cutting off its tainted member for the preservation of society, as at present, to adopt completely and honestly the idea of the regeneration of the man, of his resurrection and salvation?"

"What do you mean? I fail to understand again," Miüsov interrupted. "Some sort of dream again. Something shapeless and even incomprehensible. What do you mean by excommunication? What sort of excommunication? I suspect you are simply amusing yourself, Ivan Fyodorovich."

"Yes, but you know, in reality it is so now," said the elder suddenly, and all turned to him at once. "If there were no Church of Christ now, there would be nothing to restrain the criminal from evil doing, no real chastisement for it afterwards; none, that is, but the mechanical punishment spoken of just now, which in the majority of cases only embitters the heart; and not the real punishment, the only effectual one, the only deterrent and softening one, which lies in the recognition of sin by one's own conscience."

"How is that, may one inquire?" asked Miüsov, with lively curiosity.

"Why," began the elder, "all these punishments, — hard labour, and formerly flogging also, reform no one, and what's more, deter hardly a single criminal, and the number of crimes does not diminish but is continually on the increase. You must admit that. Consequently the security of society is not preserved, for, although the obnoxious member is mechanically cut off and sent far away out of sight, another criminal always comes to take his place at once, and perhaps two of them. If anything does preserve society, even in our time, and does regenerate and transform the criminal, it is only the law of Christ speaking with the voice of his conscience. It is only by recognising his guilt as a member of Christ's society — that is, of the Church — that he recognises his guilt before society — that is, before the Church. Thus, the criminal of today can recognise his guilt only before the Church, and not before the State. Now, if jurisdiction belonged to society as a Church, then it would know whom to recall from exclusion and bring back into the fold. But at present the Church, having no active jurisdiction, but only the power of moral condemnation, refrains of her own accord from imposing active punishment on the criminal. She does not excommunicate him but merely does not deprive him of fatherly exhortation. What is more, the Church even tries to preserve all Christian communion with the criminal. She admits him to church services, to the holy sacrament, gives him alms, and treats him more as a captive than as a convict. And what would become of the criminal, O Lord, if the Christian society too — that is, the Church — were to reject him even as the civil law rejects him and cuts him off? What would become of him if the Church, too, punished him with her excommunication as the immediate and automatic consequence of the punishment inflicted by secular law? There could be no more terrible despair, at least for a Russian criminal, for Russian criminals still have faith. Though, who knows, perhaps then a fearful thing would happen, perhaps the despairing heart of the criminal would lose its faith and then what would become of him? But the Church, like a tender, loving mother, refrains from active punishment herself, as the sinner is too severely punished already by the State court, and there must be some one to have pity on him. The Church holds aloof, above all, because its judgment is the only one that contains the truth, and therefore cannot either from a practical or a moral standpoint ally itself with any other judgment even as a temporary compromise. No compact is possible here. The foreign criminal, they say, rarely repents, for the very doctrines of to-day confirm him in the idea that his crime is not a crime, but only a rebellion against an unjustly oppressive force. Society cuts him off completely by a force that triumphs over him mechanically and (so at least they say of themselves in Europe) accompanies this exclusion with hatred, forgetfulness, and the most profound indifference as to the ultimate fate of the erring brother. In this way, it all takes place without the compassionate intervention of the Church, for in many cases there are no churches there at all, for though ecclesiastics and splendid church buildings remain, the churches themselves have long ago striven to pass from Church into State and to disappear in it completely. So it seems at least in Lutheran countries. As for Rome, it was proclaimed a State instead of a Church a thousand years ago. And so the criminal is no longer conscious of being a member of the Church and, having been excommunicated, sinks into despair. If he returns to society, often it is with such hatred that he, as it were, cuts himself off from society. You can judge for yourself how it must end. In many cases it would seem to be the same with us, but the difference is that besides the established law courts we have the Church, too, which always keeps up relations with the criminal as a dear and still precious son. And besides that, there is still preserved, though only in thought, the judgment of the Church, which though at present in a state of suspension is still living as a dream for the future, and is, no doubt, instinctively recognised by the criminal in his soul. What was said here just now is true, too, that is, that if the jurisdiction of the Church were introduced in practice in its full force, that is, the whole of society were turned into the Church, not only the judgment of the Church would have influence on the reformation of the criminal such as it never has now, but possibly also the crimes themselves would be incredibly diminished. And there can be no doubt that the Church would look upon the criminal and the crime of the future in many cases quite differently and would succeed in restoring the excluded, in restraining those who plan evil, and in regenerating the fallen. It is true," said Father Zosima, with a smile, "Christian society now is not ripe and is only resting on some seven righteous men, but as they are never lacking, it will continue still unshaken in expectation of its complete transformation from a society almost heathen in character into a single universal and regnant Church. So be it, so be it. Even though at the end of the ages, for it is ordained to come to pass! And there is no need to be troubled about times and seasons, for the secret of the times and seasons is in the wisdom of God, in His foresight, and His love. And what in human reckoning seems still afar off, may by the Divine ordinance already be, on the eve of its appearance, standing at the gates. And so be it, so be it!"

"So be it, so be it!" Father Païssy repeated austerely and reverently.

"Strange, extremely strange!" Miüsov pronounced it, not so much with heat as with latent indignation.

"What strikes you as so strange?" Father Iosif inquired cautiously.

"Why, it's beyond anything!" cried Miüsov, suddenly breaking out, "the State is eliminated and the Church is raised to the position of the State. It's not simply Ultramontanism, it's arch-ultramontanism! It's beyond the dreams of Pope Gregory the Seventh!"

"You are completely misunderstanding it," said Father Païssy sternly; "understand the Church is not to be transformed into the State. That is Rome and its dream. That is the third temptation of the devil. On the contrary, the State is transformed into the Church, ascends to the Church and becomes a Church over the whole world — which is the complete opposite of Ultramontanism and Rome, and your interpretation, and is only the glorious destiny ordained for the Orthodox Church. This star will arise in the east!"

Miüsov was significantly silent. His whole figure expressed extraordinary personal dignity. A supercilious and condescending smile played on his lips. Alyosha watched it all with a throbbing heart. The whole conversation stirred him profoundly. He glanced casually at Rakitin, who was standing immovable in his place by the door listening and watching intently though with downcast eyes. But from the colour in his cheeks Alyosha guessed that Rakitin was probably no less excited, and he knew what caused his excitement.

"Allow me to tell you one little anecdote, gentlemen," Miüsov said impressively, with a peculiarly important air. "Some years ago, soon after the *coup d'état* of December, I happened to be calling in Paris on an extremely influential personage in the Government, and I met a very interesting man in his house. This individual was not precisely a detective but was a sort of superintendent of a whole regiment of political detectives — a rather powerful position in its own way. I was prompted by curiosity to seize the opportunity of conversation with him. And as he had not come as a visitor but as a subordinate official coming to present a report, and as he saw the reception given me by his chief, he deigned to speak with some openness, to a certain extent only, of course. He was rather courteous than open, as Frenchmen know how to be courteous, especially to a foreigner. But I thoroughly understood him. The subject of our talk was the socialist revolutionaries who were at that time persecuted. I will quote only one most curious remark dropped by this person. 'We are not particularly afraid,' said he, 'of all these socialists, anarchists, infidels, and revolutionists; we keep watch on them and know all their moves. But there are a few peculiar men among them who believe in God and are Christians, but at the same time are socialists. Those are the people we are most afraid of. They are terrible people! The socialist who is a Christian is more to be dreaded than a socialist who is an atheist.' The words struck me at the time, and now they have suddenly come back to me here, gentlemen."

"You apply them to us, and look upon us as socialists?" Father Païssy asked directly, without beating about the bush.

But before Pyotr Alexandrovich could think what to answer, the door opened, and the guest so long expected, Dmitri Fyodorovich, came in. They had, in fact, given up expecting him, and his sudden appearance caused some surprise for a moment.

CHAPTER VI

WHY IS SUCH A MAN ALIVE?

DMITRI FYODOROVICH, a young man of eight and twenty, of medium height and agreeable countenance, looked much older than his years. He was muscular, and showed signs of considerable physical strength. Yet there was something almost sickly in his face. It was rather thin, his cheeks were hollow, and there was an unhealthy sallowness in their colour. His rather large, prominent, dark eyes had an expression of firm determination, and yet there was a vague look in them, too. Even when he was excited and spoke irritably, his eyes somehow did not obey his mood, but expressed something else, sometimes quite incongruous with what was passing. "It's hard to tell what he's thinking," those who talked to him sometimes declared. People who saw something pensive and sullen in his eyes were startled by his sudden laugh, which bore witness to mirthful and light-hearted thoughts at the very time when his expression was so gloomy. A certain unhealthy look in his face was easy to understand at this moment. Every one knew or had heard of the extremely restless and dissipated life which he had been leading of late, as well as of the violent anger to which he had been roused in his quarrels with his father about money. There were several stories current in the town about it. It is true that he was irritable by nature, "of an unstable and faulty mind," as our justice of the peace, Semyon Ivanovich Kachalnikov, happily described him at a gathering.

He was dressed stylishly and irreproachably in a carefully buttoned frock-coat. He wore black gloves and carried a top hat. Having only lately left the army, he still had moustaches and no beard. His dark brown hair was cropped short, and combed forward on his temples. He had the long determined stride of a military man. He stood still for a moment on the threshold, and glancing at the whole party went straight up to the elder, guessing him to be their host. He made him a low bow, and asked his blessing. Father Zosima, rising in his chair, blessed him. Dmitri kissed his hand respectfully, and with intense agitation, almost anger, he said:

"Be so generous as to forgive me for having kept you waiting so long, but Smerdyakov, my father's valet, in reply to my insistent inquiry, told me twice over that the appointment was for one o'clock. Now I suddenly learn — "

"Don't be upset," interposed the elder. "No matter. You are a little late. It's of no consequence. . . ."

"I'm extremely obliged to you, and expected no less from your kindness."

Dmitri spoke curtly and bowed once more. Then, turning suddenly towards his father, made him, too, a similarly low and respectful bow. He had evidently decided upon it beforehand, and made this bow in all sincerity, thinking it his duty to show his respect and good intentions.

Although Fyodor Pavlovich was taken unawares, he was equal to the occasion. In response to Dmitri's bow he jumped up from his chair and made his son a bow as low in return. His face was suddenly solemn and impressive, which gave him, however, a positively malignant look. Dmitri then bowed to all present, and without a word walked to the window with his long, resolute stride, sat down on the only empty chair, near Father Païssy, and, bending forward, prepared to listen to the conversation he had interrupted.

Dmitri's entrance had taken no more than two minutes, and the conversation was resumed. But this time Miüsov thought it unnecessary to reply to Father Païssy's persistent and almost irritable question.

"Allow me to withdraw from this discussion," he observed with a certain well-bred nonchalance. "It's a subtle question, too. Here Ivan Fyodorovich is smiling at us. He must have something interesting to say about that also. Ask him."

"Nothing special, except one little remark," Ivan replied at once. "European Liberals in general, and even our liberal dilettanti, often mix up the final results of socialism with those of Christianity. This absurd conclusion is, of course, a characteristic feature. But it's not only Liberals and dilettanti who confuse socialism and Christianity, but, in many cases, it appears, the police, too — that is, the foreign police, of course. Your Paris anecdote is rather to the point, Pyotr Alexandrovich."

"I ask your permission to drop this subject altogether," Miüsov repeated. "I will tell you instead, gentlemen, another interesting and rather characteristic anecdote about Ivan Fyodorovich himself. Only five days ago, at a gathering here, principally of ladies, he solemnly declared in argument that there was nothing in the whole world to make men love their neighbours. That there was no law of nature that man should love mankind, and that, if there had been any love on earth hitherto, it was not owing to a natural law, but simply because men have believed in their immortality. Ivan Fyodorovich added in parenthesis that the whole natural law lies in that faith, and that if you were to destroy in mankind the belief in immortality, not only love but every living force maintaining the life of the world would at once be dried up. Moreover, nothing then would be immoral, everything would be permitted, even cannibalism. That's not all. He ended by asserting that for every individual, like ourselves, who does not believe in God or immortality, the moral law of nature must immediately be changed into the exact contrary of the former religious law, and that egoism, even to the point of crime, must become, not only permissible but even recognised as the inevitable, the most rational, all but honourable outcome of his position. From this paradox, gentlemen, you can judge the rest of the theories which our eccentric and paradoxical friend, Ivan Fyodorovich, has set forth or intends to offer."

"Excuse me," Dmitri cried suddenly, "if I've heard aright: crime must not only be permitted but even recognised as the inevitable and the most logical outcome of his position for every atheist! Is that so or not?"

"Quite so," said Father Païssy.

"I'll remember it."

Having said this, Dmitri ceased speaking as suddenly as he had flung himself into the conversation. Every one looked at him with curiosity.

"Is that really your conviction as to the consequences of the disappearance of the belief in immortality?" the elder asked Ivan suddenly.

"Yes. That was my contention. There is no virtue if there is no immortality."

"You are blessed in believing that, or else most unhappy."

"Why unhappy?" Ivan asked smiling.

"Because in all probability you don't believe yourself in the immortality of your soul, nor in what you have written in your article on the Church and on the Church question."

"Perhaps you are right! . . . But I wasn't altogether joking," Ivan suddenly and strangely confessed, flushing quickly.

"You were not altogether joking. That's true. The question is not settled and is still fretting your heart. But even the martyr likes sometimes to divert himself with his despair, as it were driven to it by despair itself. Meanwhile, in your despair, you, too, divert yourself with magazine articles, and drawing-room discussions, though you don't believe your own arguments, and with an aching heart mock at them inwardly. . . . That question you have not settled, and it is your great grief, for it clamours for an answer."

"But can it be answered by me? Answered in the affirmative?" Ivan went on asking strangely, still looking at the elder with the same inexplicable smile.

"If it can't be decided in the affirmative, it will never be decided in the negative. You know that that is the peculiarity of your heart, and all its suffering is due to it. But thank the Creator who has given you a lofty heart capable of such suffering; of thinking and seeking higher things, for our dwelling is in the heavens. God grant that your heart will attain the answer on earth, and may God bless your ways."

The elder raised his hand and would have made the sign of the cross over Ivan from where he stood. But the latter rose from his seat, went up to him, received his blessing, and kissing his hand went back to his place in silence. His expression was firm and earnest. This action and all the preceding conversation with the elder, which was so surprising coming from Ivan, impressed every one by its strangeness and a certain solemnity, so that all were silent for a moment, and there was a look almost of apprehension in Alyosha's face. But Miüsov suddenly shrugged his shoulders. And at the same moment Fyodor Pavlovich jumped up from his seat.

"Divine and most holy elder," he cried, pointing to Ivan, "that is my son, flesh of my flesh, the dearest of my flesh! He is my most dutiful Karl Moor, so to speak, while this son who has just come in, Dmitri, against whom I am seeking a judgment from you, is the undutiful Franz Moor — they are both out of Schiller's *Robbers*, and so I am no less than *regierender* Graf von Moor! Judge and save us! We need not only your prayers but your prophecies!"

"Speak without buffoonery, and don't begin by insulting the members of your family," answered the elder, in a faint, exhausted voice. He was obviously getting more and more fatigued, and his strength was visibly failing.

"An unseemly farce which I foresaw when I came here!" cried Dmitri indignantly. He leapt up. "Forgive it, reverend father," he added, addressing the elder. "I am not a cultivated man, and I don't even know how to address you properly, but you have been deceived and you have been too good-natured in letting us meet here. All my father wants is a scandal. Why he wants it only he can tell. He always has some motive. But I believe I know why ——"

"They all blame me, all of them!" cried Fyodor Pavlovich in his turn. "Pyotr Alexandrovich here blames me, too. You have been blaming me, Pyotr Alexandrovich, you have!" he turned suddenly to Miüsov, although the latter was not dreaming of interrupting him. "They all accuse me of having hidden the children's money in my boots, and cheated them, but allow me, isn't there a court of law? There they will reckon out for you, Dmitri Fyodorovich, from your receipts, your letters, and your agreements, how much money you had, how much you have spent, and how much you have left. Why does Pyotr Alexandrovich refuse to pass judgment? Dmitri is not a stranger to him. Because they are all against me, while Dmitri Fyodorovich is in debt to me, and not a little, but some thousands, of which I have documentary proof. The whole town is ringing with his debaucheries. And where he was stationed before, he would spend a thousand or two to seduce some respectable girl; we know all about that, Dmitri Fyodorovich, the most secret details of it. I'll prove it. . . . Would you believe it, holy father, he has captivated the heart of the most honourable of young ladies of good family and fortune, the daughter of a gallant and distinguished colonel, formerly his superior officer, who had been decorated with the Order of Anna. He promised to marry the girl and now she is here, an orphan; she is betrothed to him, yet before her very eyes he is paying court to a certain local enchantress. And although this enchantress has lived in, so to speak, civil marriage with a respectable man, yet she is of an independent character, an impregnable fortress, so to speak, for everybody, just like a lawful wife — for she is virtuous, yes, holy fathers, she is virtuous. And Dmitri Fyodorovich wants to open this fortress with a golden key, and that's why he is insolent to me now, trying to get money from me, though he has wasted thousands on this enchantress already. He's continually borrowing money for the purpose. From whom do you think? Shall I say, Mitya?"

"Hold your tongue!" cried Dmitri; "wait till I'm gone. Don't dare in my presence to asperse the good name of a most honourable girl! That you should utter a word about her is an outrage, and I won't permit it!"

He was choking.

"Mitya! Mitya!" cried Fyodor Pavlovich nervously, squeezing out a tear. "And is your father's blessing nothing to you? If I curse you, what then?"

"Shameless hypocrite!" growled Dmitri furiously.

"He says that to his father! his father! What would he do to others? Gentlemen, only fancy; there's a poor but honourable man living here, burdened with a numerous family, a captain who got into trouble and was discharged from the army, but not publicly, not by court-martial, with no slur on his honour. And three weeks ago, Dmitri seized him by the beard in a tavern, dragged him out into the street and beat him publicly, and all because he is an agent, on the quiet, in a little business of mine."

"It's all a lie! Outwardly it's the truth, inwardly it's a lie!" Dmitri was trembling with rage. "Father, I don't justify my action. Yes, I confess it publicly, I behaved like a brute to that captain, and I regret it now, and I'm disgusted with myself for my brutal rage. But this captain, this agent of yours, went to that lady whom you call an enchantress, and suggested to her from you that she should take IOU's of mine which were in your possession, and should sue me for the money so as to get me into prison by means of them, if I persisted in claiming an account of my property from you. Now you reproach me for having a weakness for that lady when you yourself incited her to captivate me! She told me so to my face. . . . She told me the story and laughed at you. . . . You want to put me in prison only because you are jealous of me on her account, because you'd begun to force your attentions upon her; and I know all about that, too; she laughed at you for that as well — you hear — she laughed at you as she described it. So here, holy fathers, you have this man, this father who reproaches his profligate son! Gentlemen, forgive my anger, but I foresaw that this crafty old man had only brought you together to create a scandal. I had come to forgive him if he held out his hand; to forgive him, and ask forgiveness! But as he has just this minute insulted not only me, but an honourable young lady for whom I feel such reverence that I dare not take her name in vain, I have made up my mind to show up his game, though he is my father. . . . "

He could not go on. His eyes were glittering and he breathed with difficulty. But every one in the cell was stirred, too. All except Father Zosima rose in alarm from their seats. The monks looked austere but waited for the elder to make his will known. He sat still, very pale, not from excitement but from the weakness of disease. An imploring smile lighted up his face; from time to time he raised his hand, as though to check the storm, and, of course, a gesture from him would have been enough to end the scene; but he seemed to be waiting for something and watched them intently as though trying to make out something which was not perfectly clear to him. At last Miüsov felt completely humiliated and disgraced.

"We are all to blame for this scandalous scene," he said hotly. "But I did not foresee it when I came, though I knew with whom I had to deal. This must be stopped at once! Believe me, your reverence, I had no precise knowledge of the details that have just come to light, I was unwilling to believe them, and I learn for the first time. . . . A father is jealous of his son's relations with a woman of loose behaviour and intrigues with the creature to get his son into prison! This is the company in which I have been forced to appear here! I was deceived. I declare to you all that I was as much deceived as any one."

"Dmitri Fyodorovich," yelled Fyodor Pavlovich suddenly, in an unnatural voice, "if you were not my son I would challenge you this instant to a duel . . . with pistols, at three paces . . . across a handkerchief, across a handkerchief," he ended, stamping with both feet.

With old liars who have been acting all their lives there are moments when they enter so completely into their part that they tremble or shed tears of emotion in earnest, although at that very moment, or a second later, they are able to whisper to themselves, "You know you are lying, you shameless old sinner! You're play-acting now, in spite of your 'holy' wrath."

Dmitri frowned terribly, and looked with unutterable contempt at his father.

"I thought . . . I thought," he said, in a soft and, as it were, controlled voice, "that I was coming to my native place with the angel of my heart, my betrothed, to cherish his old age, and I find nothing but a depraved sensualist, a despicable clown!"

"A duel!" yelled the old wretch again, breathless and spluttering at each syllable. "And you, Pyotr Alexandrovich Miüsov, let me tell you that there has never been in all your family a loftier, and more honest — you hear — more honest woman than this 'creature,' as you have dared to call her! And you,

Dmitri Fyodorovich, have given up your betrothed for that 'creature,' so you must yourself have thought that your betrothed wasn't worth her little finger. That's the woman called a 'creature'!"

"Shameful!" broke from Father Iosif.

"Shameful and disgraceful!" Kalganov, flushing crimson, cried in a boyish voice, trembling with emotion. He had been silent till that moment.

"Why is such a man alive?" Dmitri, beside himself with rage, growled in a muffled voice, hunching up his shoulders till he looked almost deformed. "No, but tell me, should he be allowed to go on defiling the earth?" He looked round at every one and pointed at the old man. He spoke evenly and deliberately.

"Listen, listen, monks, to the parricide!" cried Fyodor Pavlovich, rushing up to Father Iosif. "That's the answer to your 'shameful'! What is shameful? That 'creature,' that 'woman of loose behaviour' is perhaps holier than you are yourselves, you monks who are seeking salvation! She fell perhaps in her youth, ruined by her environment. But she loved much, and Christ himself forgave the woman 'who loved much.' "

"It was not for such love Christ forgave her," broke impatiently from the gentle Father Iosif.

"Yes, it was for such, monks, it was! You save your souls here, eating cabbage, and think you are the righteous. You eat gudgeons, a gudgeon a day, and you think you bribe God with gudgeon."

"This is unendurable!" was heard on all sides in the cell.

But this unseemly scene was cut short in a most unexpected way. Father Zosima rose suddenly from his seat. Almost distracted with anxiety for the elder and every one else, Alyosha succeeded, however, in supporting him by the arm. Father Zosima moved towards Dmitri and reaching him sank on his knees before him. Alyosha thought that he had fallen from weakness, but this was not so. Having knelt, the elder distinctly and deliberately bowed down at Dmitri's feet till his forehead touched the floor. Alyosha was so astounded that he failed to assist him when he got up again. There was a faint smile on the elder's lips.

"Farewell! Forgive me, all of you!" he said, bowing on all sides to his guests.

Dmitri stood for a few moments in amazement. Bowing down to him — what did it mean? Suddenly he cried aloud, "Oh, God!" hid his face in his hands, and rushed out of the room. All the guests flocked out after him, in their confusion not saying good-bye, or bowing to their host. Only the monks went up to him again for a blessing.

"What did it mean, falling at his feet like that? Was it symbolic or what?" said Fyodor Pavlovich, suddenly quieted and trying to reopen conversation without daring to address anybody in particular. They were all passing out of the precincts of the hermitage at the moment.

"I can't answer for a madhouse and for madmen," Miüsov answered at once ill-humouredly, "but I will spare myself your company, Fyodor Pavlovich, and, trust me, for ever. Where's that monk?"

"That monk," that is, the monk who had invited them to dine with the Superior, did not keep them waiting. He met them as soon as they came down the steps from the elder's cell, as though he had been waiting for them all the time.

"Reverend father, kindly do me a favour. Convey my deepest respects to the Father Superior, apologise for me, Miüsov, personally, to his reverence, telling him that I deeply regret that owing to unforeseen circumstances I am unable to have the honour of being present at his table, greatly as I should desire to do so," Miüsov said irritably to the monk.

"And that unforeseen circumstance, of course, is myself," Fyodor Pavlovich cut in immediately. "Do you hear, father; this gentleman doesn't want to remain in my company or else he'd come at once. And you shall go, Pyotr Alexandrovich, pray go to the Father Superior and good appetite to you. I will decline, and not you. Home, home, I'll eat at home, I don't feel equal to it here, Pyotr Alexandrovich, my amiable relative."

"I am not your relative and never have been, you contemptible man!"

"I said it on purpose to madden you, because you always disclaim the relationship, though you really are a relation in spite of your shuffling. I'll prove it by the church calendar. As for you, Ivan, stay if you like. I'll send the horses for you later. Propriety requires you to go to the Father Superior, Pyotr Alexandrovich, to apologise for the disturbance we've been making. . . ."

"Is it true that you are going home? Aren't you lying?"

"Pyotr Alexandrovich! How could I dare after what's happened! Forgive me, gentlemen, I was carried away! And upset besides! And, indeed, I am ashamed. Gentlemen, one man has the heart of Alexander of Macedon and another the heart of the little dog Fido. Mine is that of the little dog Fido. I am abashed! After such an escapade how can I go to dinner, to gobble up the monastery's sauces? I am ashamed, I can't. You must excuse me!"

"The devil only knows, what if he deceives us," thought Miüsov, still hesitating, and watching the retreating buffoon with distrustful eyes. The latter turned round and, noticing that Miüsov was watching him, waved him a kiss.

"Well, are you coming to the Superior?" Miüsov asked Ivan abruptly.

"Why not? I was especially invited yesterday."

"Unfortunately I feel myself compelled to go to this confounded dinner," said Miüsov with the same irritability, regardless of the fact that the monk was listening. "We ought, at least, to apologise for the disturbance, and explain that it was not our doing. What do you think?"

"Yes, we must explain that it wasn't our doing. Besides, Father won't be there," observed Ivan.

"Well, I should hope not! Confound this dinner!"

They all walked on, however. The monk listened in silence. On the road through the copse he made one observation however — that the Father Superior had been waiting a long time, and that they were more than half an hour late. He received no answer. Miüsov looked with hatred at Ivan. "Here he is, going to the dinner as though nothing had happened," he thought. "A brazen face, and the conscience of a Karamazov!"

CHAPTER VII

A DIVINITY STUDENT BENT ON A CAREER

ALYOSHA helped his elder to his bedroom and seated him on his bed. It was a little room furnished with the bare necessities. There was a narrow iron bedstead, with a strip of felt for a mattress. In the corner, under the ikons, was a reading-desk with a cross and the Gospel lying on it. The elder sank exhausted on the bed. His eyes glittered and he breathed hard. He looked intently at Alyosha, as though considering something.

"Go, my dear boy, go. Porfiry is enough for me. Make haste, you are needed there, go and wait on the Father Superior's table."

"Allow me to stay here," Alyosha entreated.

"You are more needed there. There is no peace there. You will wait on them, and be of service. If evil spirits rise up, repeat a prayer. And remember, my boy (the elder liked to call him that), this is not the place for you in the future. When it is God's will to call me, leave the monastery. Go away for good."

Alyosha started.

"What is it? This is not your place for the time being. I consecrate you to a great novitiate in the world. Yours will be a long pilgrimage. And you will have to take a wife, too, you must. You will have to bear *all* before you come back. There will be much to do. But I don't doubt of you, and so I send you forth. Christ is with you. Do not abandon Him and He will not abandon you. You will see great sorrow, and in that sorrow you will be happy. This is my last message to you: in sorrow seek happiness. Work, work unceasingly. Remember my words, for although I shall talk with you again, not only my days but my hours are numbered."

Alyosha's face again betrayed strong emotion. The corners of his mouth quivered.

"What is it again?" Father Zosima asked, smiling gently. "The worldly may follow their dead with tears, but here we rejoice over the father who is departing. We rejoice and pray for him. Leave me, I must pray. Go and make haste. Be with your brothers. And not with one only, but with both."

Father Zosima raised his hand to bless him. It was impossible to protest, though Alyosha had a great longing to remain. He longed, moreover, to ask what was the significance of this bow to Dmitri; indeed, the question was on the tip of his tongue, but he dared not ask it. He knew that the elder would have explained it unasked if he had thought fit. But evidently such was not his pleasure. That gesture had made a terrible impression on Alyosha; he believed blindly that it had a mysterious significance. Mysterious, and perhaps dreadful.

As he hastened out of the hermitage precincts to reach the monastery in time to wait on the Father Superior's table, he felt a sudden pang at his heart, and stopped short. He seemed to hear again Father Zosima's words, foretelling his approaching end. What he had foretold so exactly must infallibly come to pass. Alyosha believed that implicitly. But how could he be left without him? How could he live without seeing and hearing him? Where should he go? He had told him not to weep, and to leave the monastery. Good God! It was long since Alyosha had known such anguish. He hurried through the copse that divided the hermitage from the monastery and, unable to bear the burden of his thoughts, he gazed at the ancient pines beside the path. He had not far to go — about five hundred paces. He expected to meet no one at that hour, but at the first turn of the path he noticed Rakitin. He was waiting for some one.

"Are you waiting for me?" asked Alyosha, overtaking him.

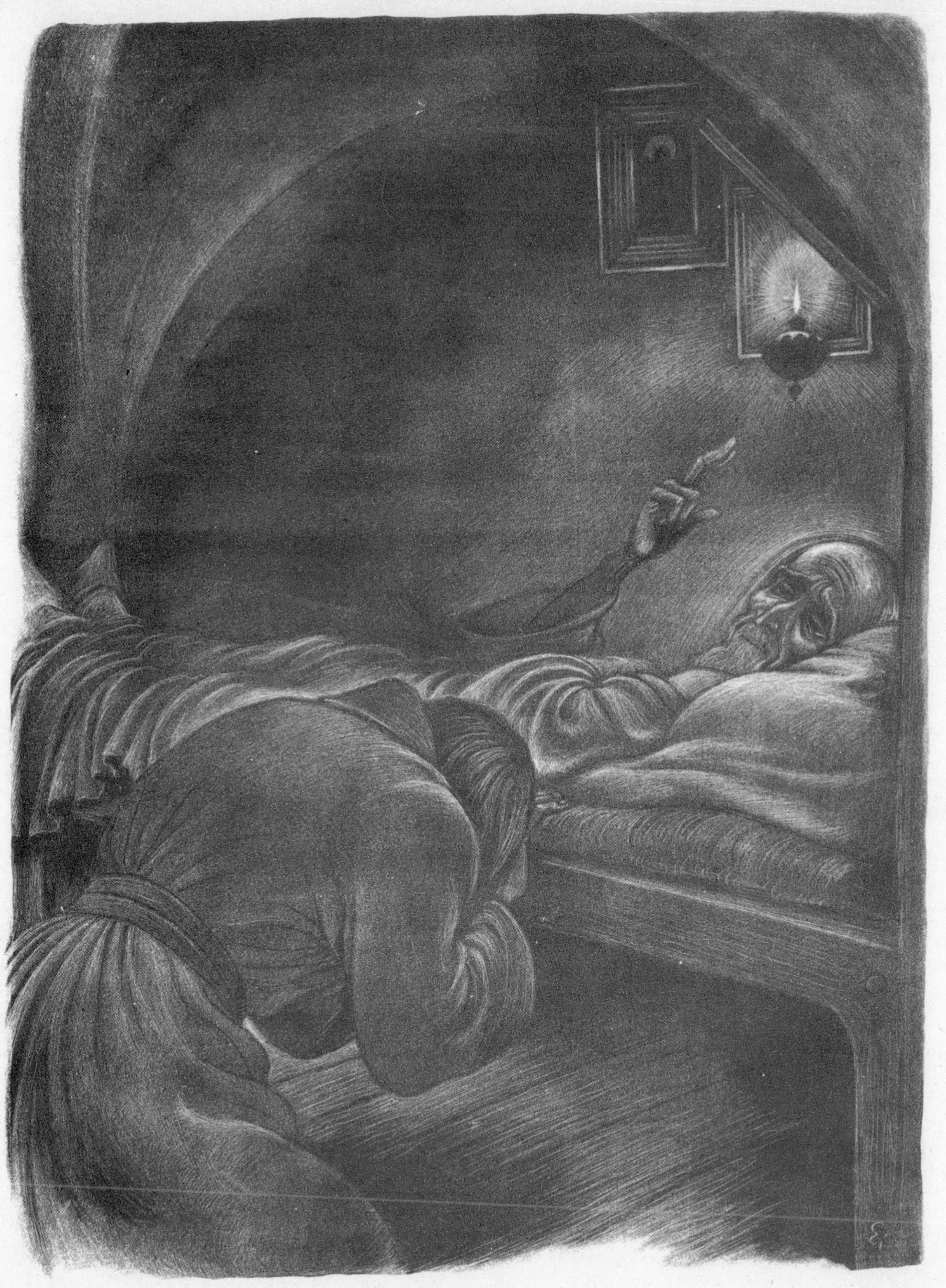

THE BLESSING OF FATHER ZOSIMA

"Yes," grinned Rakitin. "You are hurrying to the Father Superior, I know; he has a banquet. There's not been such a banquet since the Superior entertained the Bishop and General Pahatov, do you remember? I shan't be there, but you go and hand the sauces. Tell me one thing, Alexey, what does that dream mean? That's what I want to ask you."

"What dream?"

"That bowing to your brother, Dmitri. And didn't he tap the ground with his forehead, too!"

"You speak of Father Zósima?"

"Yes, of Father Zosima."

"Tapped the ground?"

"Ah, I have expressed myself irreverently? Well, what of it? Anyway, what does that dream mean?"

"I don't know what it means, Misha."

"I knew he wouldn't explain it to you! There's nothing wonderful about it, of course, only the usual holy mummery. But the hocus-pocus was not without a purpose. All the bigots in the town will talk about it and spread the story through the province, wondering what it meant. To my thinking the old man really has a keen nose; he sniffed a crime. Your house stinks."

"What crime?"

Rakitin evidently had something he was eager to speak of.

"It'll be in your family, this crime. Between your brothers and your rich old father. So Father Zosima flopped down to be ready for what may turn up. If something happens later on, it'll be: 'Ah, the holy man foresaw it, prophesied it!' though it's a poor sort of prophecy, flopping like that. 'Ah, but it was symbolic,' they'll say, 'an allegory,' and the devil knows what all! It'll be remembered to his glory: 'He predicted the crime and marked the criminal!' That's always the way with these pious ecstatics; they cross themselves at the pot-house and throw stones at the church. Your elder's that sort: he takes a stick to a just man and falls at the feet of a murderer."

"What crime? What murderer? What do you mean?"

Alyosha stopped dead. Rakitin stopped, too.

"What murderer? As though you didn't know! I'll bet you've thought of it before. That's interesting, too, by the way. Listen, Alyosha, you always speak the truth, though you're always between two stools. Have you thought of it or not? Answer."

"I have," answered Alyosha in a low voice. Even Rakitin was taken aback.

"What? Have you really?" he cried.

"I . . . I've not exactly thought of it," muttered Alyosha, "but directly you began speaking so strangely, I fancied I had thought of it myself."

"You see (and how well you expressed it!), you see? Looking at your father and your brother Mitya to-day you thought of a crime. Then I'm not mistaken?"

"But wait, wait a minute," Alyosha broke in uneasily; "what has led you to see all this? Why does it interest you? That's the first question."

"Two questions, disconnected, but natural. I'll deal with them separately. What led me to see it? I shouldn't have seen it, if I hadn't suddenly understood your brother Dmitri, seen right into the very heart of him all at once. I caught the whole man from one trait. These very honest but passionate people draw a line which mustn't be crossed. If it were, he'd stick a knife even into his father. But his father's a drunken and abandoned old sinner, who has never known how to restrain himself — they'll both let themselves go, and they'll come to grief."

"No, Misha, no. If that's all, you've reassured me! It won't come to that."

"But why are you trembling all over? Let me tell you; he may be honest — your Mitya (he is stupid, but honest), but he's — a sensualist. That's the very definition and inner essence of him. It's your father has handed him on his low sensuality. Do you know, I simply wonder at you, Alyosha, how you can have kept your purity. You're a Karamazov, too, you know! In your family sensuality is carried to a disease. But now, these three sensualists are watching one another, with their knives in their boots. The three of them are knocking their heads together, and you may be the fourth."

"You are mistaken about that woman. Dmitri — despises her," said Alyosha, with a sort of shudder.

"Grushenka? No, brother, he doesn't despise her. Since he has openly given up his betrothed for her, he doesn't despise her. There's something here, my dear boy, that you don't understand yet. A man will fall in love with some beauty, with a woman's body, or even with a part of a woman's body (a sensualist can understand that), and he'll surrender his own children for her, sell his father and mother, and his country, Russia, too. If he's honest, he'll steal; if he's humane, he'll murder; if he's faithful, he'll deceive. Pushkin, the poet of women's feet, sang of their feet in his verse. Others don't sing their praises, but they can't look at women's feet without a thrill — and it's not only their feet. Contempt's no help here, brother, even if he did despise Grushenka. He does, but he can't tear himself away."

"I understand that," Alyosha jerked out suddenly.

"Really? Well, I dare say you do understand, since you blurt it out at the first word," said Rakitin, malignantly.

"That escaped you unawares, and the confession's the more precious. So it's a familiar subject; you've thought about it already, about sensuality, I mean! Oh, you virgin soul! You're a quiet one, Alyosha, you're a saint, I know, but the devil only knows what you've thought about, and what you know already! You are pure, but you've been down into the depths. . . . I've been watching you a long time. You're a Karamazov yourself; you're a thorough Karamazov — no doubt birth and selection have something to answer for. You're a sensualist through your father, a saintly fool through your mother. Why do you tremble? Is it true, then? Do you know, Grushenka has been begging me to bring you along; 'I'll pull off his cassock,' she says. You can't think how she keeps begging me to bring you. I wondered why she took such an interest in you. Do you know, she's an extraordinary woman, too!"

"Thank her and say I'm not coming," said Alyosha, with a crooked smile. "Finish what you were saying, Misha. I'll tell you my idea after."

"There's nothing to finish. It's all clear. It's the same old tune, brother. If even you are a sensualist at heart, what of your brother Ivan? He's a Karamazov, too. What is at the root of all you Karamazovs is that you're all grasping sensualists and saintly fools! Your brother Ivan writes theological articles in jest, for some idiotic, unknown reason of his own, though he's an atheist, and he admits it's a fraud himself — that's your brother Ivan. Besides, he's trying to get Mitya's betrothed for himself, and I fancy he'll succeed, too. And what's more it's with Mitya's consent. For Mitya will surrender his betrothed to him to be rid of her, the sooner to run to Grushenka. And he's ready to do that in spite of all his nobility and disinterestedness. Observe that. Those are the most fatal people! Who the devil can make you out? He recognises his vileness and goes on with it! Let me tell you, too, the old man, your father, is now crossing Mitya's path. He has suddenly gone crazy over Grushenka. His mouth waters at the sight of her. It's simply on her account he made that scene in the cell just now, simply because Miüsov called her an 'abandoned creature.' He's worse than a tom cat in love. At first she was only employed by him in connection with his pot-houses and in some other shady business, but now he has suddenly realised all she is and has gone wild about her. He keeps pestering her with his offers, not honourable ones, of course. And they'll clash, the precious father and son, on that path! But Grushenka favours neither of them, she's still playing with them, and teasing them both, considering which she can get most out of. For though she could filch a lot of money from the papa he wouldn't marry her, and maybe he'll turn stingy in the end and pull his purse-strings tight. That's where Mitya's value comes in, he has no money, but he's ready to marry her. Yes, ready to marry her! to abandon his betrothed, a rare beauty, Katerina Ivanovna, who's rich, and the daughter of a colonel, and to marry Grushenka, the former kept woman of a dissolute old merchant, Samsonov, a coarse, uneducated, provincial mayor. Some murderous conflict may well come to pass from all this, and that's what your brother Ivan is waiting for. It would suit him down to the ground. He'll carry off Katerina Ivanovna, for whom he is languishing, and pocket her dowry of sixty thousand. That's very alluring to start with, for a man of no consequence and a beggar. And, take note, he won't be wronging Mitya, but doing him the greatest service. For I know for a fact that Mitya, only last week, when he was with some gipsy girls drunk in a tavern, shouted that he was unworthy of his betrothed, Katya, but that his brother Ivan, he was the man who deserved her. And Katerina Ivanovna will not in the end refuse such a fascinating man as Ivan. She's hesitating between the two of them already. And how has that Ivan won you all, so that you all worship him? He is laughing at you, and enjoying himself at your expense."

"How do you know? How can you speak so confidently?" Alyosha asked sharply, frowning.

"Why do you ask, and why are you frightened at my answer in advance? It shows that you know I'm speaking the truth."

"You don't like Ivan. Ivan wouldn't be tempted by money."

"Really? And the beauty of Katerina Ivanovna? It's not only the money, though a fortune of sixty thousand is an attraction."

"Ivan is above that. He wouldn't be tempted by thousands. It is not money, it's not comfort Ivan is seeking. Perhaps it's suffering he is seeking?"

"What wild dream now? Oh, you — aristocrats!"

"Ah, Misha, he has a stormy spirit. His mind is in bondage. He is haunted by a great, unresolved idea. He is one of those who don't want millions, but an answer to their questions."

"That's plagiarism, Alyosha. You're paraphrasing your elder. Ah, Ivan has set you a riddle!" cried Rakitin, with undisguised malice. He even changed colour, and his lips twitched. "And the riddle's a stupid one. It isn't worth guessing at it. Think a bit — and you'll see through it. His article is absurd and ridiculous. And did you hear his stupid theory just now: if there's no immortality of the soul, then there's no virtue, and everything is permissible. (And by the way, do you remember how your brother Mitya cried out: 'I will remember!') An attractive theory for scoundrels! — (I'm being abusive, that's stupid.) Not for scoundrels, but for sophomoric poseurs, 'haunted by profound, unsolvable problems.' He's showing off, and what it all comes to is, 'on the one hand we cannot but admit' and 'on the other, it must be confessed'! His whole theory is vile! Humanity will find in itself the power to live for virtue even without believing in immortality. It will find it in the love of freedom, of equality, of fraternity."

Rakitin could hardly restrain himself in his heat, but, suddenly, as though remembering something, he stopped short.

"Well, that's enough," he said, with a still more crooked smile. "Why are you laughing? Do you think I'm a vulgarian?"

"No, I never dreamed of thinking you a vulgarian. You are clever but . . . never mind, I was silly to smile. I understand your getting hot about it, Misha. I guess from your warmth that you are not indifferent to Katerina Ivanovna yourself; I've suspected that for a long time, brother, that's why you don't like my brother Ivan. Are you jealous of him?"

"And jealous of her money, too? Won't you add that?"

"I'll say nothing about money. I am not going to insult you."

"I believe it, since you say so, but confound you, and your brother Ivan with you. Don't you understand that one might very well dislike him, apart from Katerina Ivanovna? And why the devil should I like him? He condescends to abuse me, you know. Why haven't I a right to abuse him?"

"I never heard of his saying anything about you, good or bad. He doesn't speak of you."

"And I heard that the day before yesterday at Katerina Ivanovna's he was abusing me for all he was worth — you see what an interest he takes in your humble servant. And which is the jealous one after that, brother, I can't say. He was so good as to express the opinion that, if I don't go in for the career of an archimandrite in the immediate future and don't take orders, I shall be sure to go to Petersburg and get on to some solid magazine as a critic, that I shall write for the next ten years, and in the end become the owner of the magazine. Then, he said, I'll go on editing it, in a liberal and atheistic spirit, with a socialistic tinge, with a tiny gloss of socialism, but keeping a sharp look-out all the time, that is, keeping in with both sides and hoodwinking the fools. According to your brother's account, the tinge of socialism won't hinder me from laying by the proceeds and investing them under the guidance of some Jew, till at the end of my career I build a large house in Petersburg and move my publishing offices to it, and let out the rest to lodgers. He has even chosen the place for it, near the new stone bridge which they say is to be built across the Neva at Liteinaya Street."

"Ah, Misha, perhaps that's just what will really happen, every word of it," cried Alyosha, unable to restrain a good-humoured smile.

"You are pleased to be sarcastic, too, Alexey Fyodorovich."

"No, no, I'm joking, forgive me. I've something quite different in my mind. But, excuse me, who can have told you all this? You can't have been at Katerina Ivanovna's yourself when he was talking about you?"

"I wasn't there, but Dmitri Fyodorovich was; and I heard him tell it with my own ears; if you want to know, he didn't tell me, but I overheard him, unintentionally, of course, for I was sitting in Grushenka's bedroom and I couldn't go away because Dmitri Fyodorovich was in the next room."

"Oh, yes, I'd forgotten she was a relation of yours."

"A relation! That Grushenka a relation of mine!" cried Rakitin, turning crimson. "Are you mad? You're out of your mind!"

"Why, isn't she a relation of yours? I heard so."

"Where can you have heard it? You Karamazovs brag of being an ancient, noble family, though your father used to run about playing the buffoon at other men's tables, and was only admitted to the kitchen as a favour. I may be only a priest's son, and dirt in the eyes of gentlemen like you, but don't insult me so lightly and wantonly. I have a sense of honour, too, Alexey Fyodorovich, I couldn't be a relation of Grushenka, a common wench. I beg you to understand that!"

Rakitin was intensely irritated.

"Forgive me, for goodness' sake, I had no idea . . . besides . . . how can you call her that? Is she . . . that sort of woman?" Alyosha flushed suddenly. "I tell you again, I heard that she was a relation of yours. You often go to see her, and you told me yourself you're not having a love affair with her. I never dreamed that you of all people had such contempt for her! Does she really deserve it?"

"I may have reasons of my own for visiting her. That's not your business. But as for relationship, your brother, or even your father is more likely to make her yours, than mine. Well, here we are. You'd better go to the kitchen. Hullo! what's wrong, what is it? Are we late? They can't have finished dinner so soon! Have the Karamazovs been making trouble again? No doubt they have. Here's your father and your brother Ivan after him. They've broken away from the Father Superior's party. And look, Father Isidor's shouting after them from the steps. And your father's shouting and waving his arms. I expect he's swearing. Bah, and there goes Miüsov driving away in his carriage. You see, he's going. And there's old Maximov running! —but this is a scandal! There can't have been any dinner. Have they beaten up the Father Superior? Or have they, perhaps, been beaten up? It would serve them right!"

There was reason for Rakitin's exclamations. Indeed, there had been an unprecedented and unheard-of scandal. It had all happened on the spur of the moment.

CHAPTER VIII

THE SCANDALOUS SCENE

Miüsov, as a man of breeding and delicacy, could not but feel some inward qualms, when he reached the Father Superior's quarters with Ivan: he felt ashamed of having lost his temper. He felt that he ought to have disdained that despicable wretch, Fyodor Pavlovich, too much to have been upset by him in Father Zosima's cell, and so to have forgotten himself. "The monks were not to blame, in any case," he decided, on the steps. "And if they're decent people here, too (and the Father Superior, I understand, is of the gentry), why not be courteous and friendly with them? I won't argue, I'll fall in with everything, I'll win them by politeness, and . . . and . . . show them that I've nothing to do with that Æsop, that buffoon, that Pierrot, and have merely been taken in over this affair, just as they have."

He determined to drop his litigation with the monastery, and relinquish his claims to the wood-cutting and fishery rights once and for all that very day. He was the more ready to do this because the rights had become much less valuable, and he had indeed the vaguest idea where the wood and river in question were.

These excellent intentions were strengthened when they entered the Father Superior's dining-room, though, strictly speaking, it was not a dining-room, for the Father Superior had only two rooms altogether; they were, however, much larger and more comfortable than Father Zosima's. But there was no great luxury about the furnishing of these rooms either. The furniture was of mahogany, upholstered in leather, in the old-fashioned style of the twenties; the floor was not even stained, but everything was shining with cleanliness, and there were many choice flowers in the windows; the most sumptuous thing in the room at the moment was, of course, the luxuriously appointed table. The cloth was clean, the service shone; there were three kinds of well-baked bread, two bottles of wine, two of excellent mead, and a large glass jug of kvass — both the latter made in the monastery, and famous in the neighbourhood. There was no vodka. Rakitin related afterwards that the dinner included five courses: fish soup made of sterlets, served with little fish patties; delicious boiled fish served in a special way; salmon cutlets; ice cream and compote; and finally, blanc-mange. Rakitin nosed out all these good things, for he could not resist peeping into the kitchen, where he already had connections. He had connections everywhere, and got information about everything. He had a restless and envious heart. He was well aware of his own considerable abilities, but nervously exaggerated them in his self-conceit. He knew he would play a prominent part of some sort, but Alyosha, who was strongly attached to him, was distressed to see that his friend Rakitin was dishonourable, and quite unconscious of being so, considering, on the contrary, that because he would not steal money left on the table he was a man of the highest integrity. Neither Alyosha nor any one else could have done anything about that.

Rakitin, of course, was a person of too little consequence to be asked to the dinner, to which Father Iosif, Father Païssy, and only one other monk had been invited. They were already waiting in the dining-room when Miüsov, Kalganov, and Ivan Fyodorovich arrived. The other guest, Maximov, stood a little aside, waiting also. The Father Superior stepped into the middle of the room to receive his guests. He was a tall, thin, but still vigorous old man, with black hair streaked with grey, and a long, grave, ascetic face. He bowed to his guests in silence. But this time they approached to receive his blessing. Miüsov even tried to kiss his hand, but the Father Superior drew it back in time to avoid the salute. But Ivan Fyodorovich and Kalganov went through the ceremony in the most simple-hearted and complete manner, kissing his hand as peasants do.

"We must apologise most humbly, your reverence," began Miüsov, simpering affably, and yet speaking in a dignified and respectful tone. "Pardon us for having come alone without the other gentleman you invited, Fyodor Pavlovich. He felt obliged to decline the honour of your hospitality, and not without reason. In the reverend Father Zosima's cell he was carried away by the unhappy dissension with his son, and let fall words which were quite out of keeping . . . in fact, quite unseemly . . . as" (he glanced at the monks) "your reverence is, no doubt, already aware. And therefore, recognising that he had been to blame, he felt sincere regret and shame, and begged me, and his son Ivan Fyodorovich, to convey to you his apologies, regrets, and contrition. In brief, he hopes and desires to make amends later. For the present, he asks your blessing, and begs you to forget what has taken place."

As he uttered the last word of his tirade, Miüsov completely recovered his self-complacency, and all traces of his former irritation disappeared. He fully and sincerely loved humanity again.

The Father Superior listened to him with dignity, and, with a slight bend of the head, replied:

"I sincerely deplore his absence. Perhaps at our table he might have learnt to like us, and we him. Pray join us in our repast, gentlemen."

He stood before the holy image, and began to say grace, aloud. All bent their heads reverently, and Maximov stepped forward, clasping his hands before him, with peculiar fervour.

It was at this moment that Fyodor Pavlovich played his last prank. It must be noted that he really had meant to go home, and really had felt the impossibility of going to dine with the Father Superior as though nothing had happened, after his disgraceful behaviour in the elder's cell. Not that he was so very much ashamed of himself or that he felt himself much at fault — quite the contrary perhaps. But still he felt it would be unseemly to go to dinner. Yet his creaking carriage had hardly been brought to the steps of the hostelry, and he had hardly got into it, when he suddenly stopped short. He remembered his own words at the elder's: "I always feel when I meet people that I am lower than all, and that they all take me for a buffoon; so I say let me play the buffoon, for you are, every one of you, stupider and lower than I." He had the sudden desire to revenge himself on every one for his own vileness. He suddenly recalled how he had once in the past been asked, "Why do you hate so and so, so much?" And he had answered them, in a fit of clownish impudence, "I'll tell you. He has done me no harm. But I played him a dirty trick, and ever since I have hated him."

Remembering that now, he smiled quietly and malignantly, hesitating for a moment. His eyes flashed, and his lips positively began to quiver. "Well, since I have begun, I may as well finish," he decided suddenly. His inmost thought at that moment might be expressed in the following words, "Well, there is no clearing myself now. So I'll go the limit. I will show them I have no shame before them — that's all!"

He told the coachman to wait, while with rapid steps he returned to the monastery and went straight to the Father Superior's quarters. He had no clear idea what he would do, but he knew that he was no longer in control of himself, and that a touch might drive him to the utmost limits of obscenity, but only to obscenity, to nothing criminal, nothing for which he could be legally punished. In the last resort, he could always restrain himself, and indeed had marvelled at himself, on that score, sometimes. He appeared in the Father Superior's dining-room, just at the moment when the prayer was over, and all were moving to the table. Standing in the doorway, he scanned the company and, with a prolonged, impudent, malicious chuckle, looked them all boldly in the face. "They thought I had gone, and here I am again," he shouted so that the room rang.

For one moment every one stared at him without a word; and at once every one felt that something revolting, grotesque, positively scandalous, was about to happen. Miüsov passed immediately from the most benevolent frame of mind to the most savage. All the feelings that had subsided and died down in his heart revived instantly.

"No! this I cannot endure!" he cried. "I absolutely cannot! and . . . I certainly cannot!" The blood rushed to his head. He positively stammered, but he was beyond thinking of style; and he seized his hat.

"What is it he cannot?" cried Fyodor Pavlovich, "that he absolutely cannot and certainly cannot? Your reverence, am I to come in or not? Will you receive me as your guest?"

"You are heartily welcome," answered the Superior. "Gentlemen!" he added, "may I venture to beg you most earnestly to lay aside your dissensions, and to be united in love and family harmony — with prayer to the Lord — at our humble table."

"No, no, it is impossible!" cried Miüsov, beside himself.

"Well, if it is impossible for Pyotr Alexandrovich, it is impossible for me, and I won't stop. That is why I came. I will stay with Pyotr Alexandrovich everywhere now. If you will go away, Pyotr Alexandrovich, I will go away, too; if you remain, I will remain. You stung him by what you said about family harmony, Father Superior, he does not admit he is my relation. That's right, isn't it, von Sohn? Here's von Sohn. How are you, von Sohn?"

"Do you mean me?" muttered Maximov, puzzled.

"Of course I mean you," cried Fyodor Pavlovich. "Who else? The Father Superior could not be von Sohn."

"But I am not von Sohn either. I am Maximov."

"No, you are von Sohn. Your reverence, do you know who von Sohn was? It was a famous murder case. He was killed in a house of harlotry — I believe that is what such places are called among you — he was killed and robbed, and in spite of his venerable age, he was nailed up in a box and sent from Petersburg to Moscow in the luggage van. And while they were nailing him up, the harlots sang songs and played the harp, that is to say, the piano. So this is that very von Sohn. He has risen from the dead, haven't you, von Sohn?"

"What can this mean? What is this?" voices were heard in the group of monks.

"Let us go," cried Miüsov, addressing Kalganov.

"No, permit me," Fyodor Pavlovich broke in shrilly, taking another step into the room. "Allow me to finish. There in the cell I was blamed for behaving disrespectfully just because I mentioned gudgeon. Pyotr Alexandrovich Miüsov, my relation, prefers to have *plus de noblesse que de sincérité* in his words, but I prefer in mine *plus de sincérité que de noblesse*, and — damn the noblesse! That's right, isn't it, von Sohn? Allow me, Father Superior, though I am a buffoon and play the buffoon, yet I am the soul of honour, and I want to speak my mind. Yes, I am the soul of honour, while in Pyotr Alexandrovich there is wounded vanity and nothing else. I had come perhaps to have a look round and speak my mind. My son, Alexey, is here, saving his soul. I am a father; I care for his welfare, and it is my duty to care. While I've been playing the fool, I have been listening and having a look on the sly; and now I want to give you the last act of the performance. You know how things are with us? As a thing falls, so it lies. As a thing once has fallen, so it must lie for ever. Not a bit of it! I want to get up again. Holy fathers, you revolt me. Confession is a great sacrament, before which I am ready to bow down reverently; but there in the cell, they all kneel down and confess aloud. Can it be right to confess aloud? The holy fathers ordained that confession should be whispered into the ear: only then your confession will be a sacrament, and so it has been since olden times. But this way how can I explain to him before every one that I did this and that, for instance. . . . I mean, this and that, you understand? Sometimes it would not be proper to talk about it — why, it's a scandal! No, fathers, this way lies sectarian heresy, I dare say. . . . At the first opportunity I shall write to the Synod, and I shall take my son, Alexey, home."

We must note here that Fyodor Pavlovich knew where to look for the weak spot. There had been at one time malicious gossip which had even reached the Archbishop (not only regarding our monastery, but also others where the institution of elders existed) that too much respect was paid to the elders, even to the detriment of the authority of the Superior, that the elders abused the sacrament of confession, and so on and so on — absurd charges which had died away of themselves everywhere. But the spirit of devilish folly, which had caught up Fyodor Pavlovich, and was spurring him on in his wrongheadedness to lower and lower depths of ignominy, prompted him with this old slander. Fyodor Pavlovich did not understand a word of it, and he could not even put it sensibly, for on this occasion no one had been kneeling and confessing aloud in the elder's cell, so that he could not have seen anything of the kind. He was only speaking from confused memory of old slanders. But as soon as he had uttered his foolish tirade, he felt he had been talking absurd nonsense, and at once longed to prove to his audience, and above all to himself, that he had not been talking nonsense. And, though he knew perfectly well that with each word he would be adding more and more absurdity, he could not restrain himself, and plunged forward blindly.

"How abominable!" cried Pyotr Alexandrovich.

"Pardon me!" said the Father Superior. "It was said of old, 'Many have begun to speak against me and have uttered wicked words. And hearing it I have said within me: it is the medicine of the Christ, and He has sent it to heal my vainglorious soul.' And so we humbly thank you, precious guest!" and he made Fyodor Pavlovich a low bow.

"Tut-tut-tut! Bigotry and stock phrases! Stock phrases and stock gestures. The old lies and formal prostrations. We know all about them. A kiss on the lips and a dagger in the heart, as in Schiller's *Robbers*. I don't like sham, fathers, I want the truth. But the truth is not to be found in gudgeon, and that I proclaim aloud! Father monks, why do you fast? Why do you expect reward in heaven for that? Why, for reward like that I will come and fast, too! No, saintly monk, you try being virtuous in the world, be useful to society, without shutting yourself up in a monastery at other people's expense, and without expecting a reward up aloft for it — you'll find that a bit harder. I can talk sense, too, Father Superior. What have they got here?" He went up to the table. "Old port wine, mead brewed by the Eliseyev Brothers. Fie, fie, fathers! That's better than gudgeon. Look at the bottles the fathers have brought out, he! he! he! And who has provided it all? The Russian peasant, the toiler, brings here the groat earned by his horny hand, wringing it from his family and the tax-gatherer! You bleed the people, you know, holy fathers."

"This is altogether disgraceful, coming from you," said Father Iosif.

Father Païssy kept obstinately silent. Miüsov rushed from the room, and Kalganov after him.

"Well, father, I will follow Pyotr Alexandrovich! I am not coming to see you again. You may beg me on your knees, I shan't come. I sent you a thousand roubles, so you're casting sheep's-eyes at me again. He, he, he! No, you won't get any more from me. I am taking my revenge for my youth, for all the humiliation I endured." He thumped the table with his fist in a paroxysm of simulated feeling. "This monastery has played a great part in my life! It has cost me many bitter tears. You used to set my wife, the possessed one, against me. You cursed me with bell and book, you spread stories about me all over the place. Enough, fathers! This is the age of Liberalism, the age of steamers and railways. Neither a thousand, nor a hundred roubles, no, nor a hundred copecks will you get out of me!"

It must be noted again that our monastery had never played any great part in his life, and he had never shed a bitter tear because of it. But he was so carried away by his simulated emotion that for one moment he almost believed it himself. He almost wept with emotion. But at that very instant, he felt that it was time to draw back.

The Father Superior bowed his head at his malicious lie, and again spoke impressively:

"It is written again, 'Bear circumspectly and gladly dishonour that cometh upon thee by no act of thine own, be not confounded and hate not him who hath dishonoured thee.' And so will we."

"Tut-tut-tut! Church lingo and all that rigmarole. Farewell, fathers, I am going. But I will take my son, Alexey, away from here for ever, on my parental authority. Ivan Fyodorovich, my most dutiful son, permit me to order you to follow me. Von Sohn, what are you staying here for? Come to my place now. It is fun there. It is only one short verst; instead of lenten oil, I will give you sucking-pig and kasha. We will have dinner with French brandy and liqueurs. I've cloudberry wine. . . . Hey, von Sohn, don't lose your chance." He went out, shouting and gesticulating.

It was at that moment Rakitin saw him and pointed him out to Alyosha.

"Alexey!" his father shouted, from far off, catching sight of him. "You come home to me to-day, for good, and bring your pillow and mattress, and leave no trace behind."

Alyosha stood rooted to the spot, watching the scene in silence. Meanwhile, Fyodor Pavlovich had got into the carriage, and Ivan was about to follow him in grim silence without even turning to say good-bye to Alyosha. But at this point another almost incredible scene of grotesque buffoonery gave the finishing touch to the episode. Suddenly, beside the footboard of the carriage, Maximov appeared. He ran up, panting, afraid of being too late. Rakitin and Alyosha saw him running. He was in such a hurry that in his impatience he put his foot on the step on which Ivan's left foot was still resting, and clutching the carriage he kept trying to jump in. "I am going with you!" he kept shouting, laughing a thin mirthful laugh with a look of reckless glee in his face. "Take me, too."

"There!" cried Fyodor Pavlovich, delighted. "Did I not say he was von Sohn? It is von Sohn himself, risen from the dead. Why, how did you tear yourself away? What were you *vonsohning* in there? And how could you get away from the dinner? You must really be brazen-faced! I am that myself, but I am surprised at you, brother! Jump in, jump in! Let him in, Ivan. It will be fun. He can lie somewhere at our feet. Will you, von Sohn? Or perch on the box with the coachman. Skip onto the box, von Sohn!"

But Ivan, who had by now taken his seat, without a word gave Maximov a violent punch in the breast and sent him flying. It was pure luck that he did not fall. "Drive on!" Ivan shouted angrily to the coachman.

"Why, what are you doing, what are you about? Why did you do that?" Fyodor Pavlovich protested.

But the carriage had already driven away. Ivan made no reply.

"Well, you are a fellow," Fyodor Pavlovich said again.

After a pause of two minutes, looking askance at his son, "Why, it was you got up all this monastery business. You put me up to it, you approved of it. Why are you angry now?"

"You've talked rot enough. You might rest a bit now," Ivan snapped sullenly.

Fyodor Pavlovich was silent again for two minutes.

"A drop of brandy now would go to the right spot," he observed sententiously, but Ivan made no response.

"You shall have some, too, when we get home."

Ivan was still silent. Fyodor Pavlovich waited another two minutes.

"But I will take Alyosha away from the monastery, though you will dislike it so much, most respectful Karl von Moor."

Ivan shrugged his shoulders contemptuously, and turning away stared at the road. And they did not speak again all the way home.

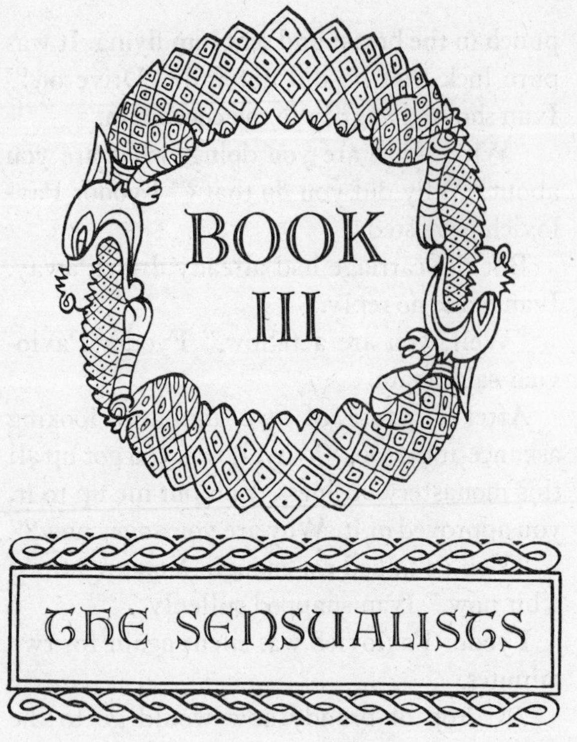

BOOK III

THE SENSUALISTS

CHAPTER I

IN THE SERVANTS' QUARTERS

THE Karamazov house was far from being in the centre of the town, but neither was it on the outskirts. It was a pleasant-looking old house of two storeys, painted grey, with a red iron roof. It was roomy and snug, and might still last many years. There were all sorts of unexpected little cupboards and closets and staircases. There were rats in it, but Fyodor Pavlovich did not altogether dislike them. "One doesn't feel so lonesome when one's left alone in the evening," he used to say. It was his habit to send the servants away to the lodge for the night and to lock himself up alone. The lodge was a spacious and solid building in the yard. Fyodor Pavlovich used to have the cooking done there, although there was a kitchen in the house; he did not like the smell of cooking, and, winter and summer alike, the dishes were carried in across the courtyard. The house was built for a large family; there was room for five times as many, with their servants. But at the time of our story there was no one living in the house but Fyodor Pavlovich and his son Ivan. And in the lodge there were only three servants: old Grigory, his old wife Marfa, and the servant Smerdyakov, still a young man. Of these three we must say a few words. Of Grigory Vasilyevich Kutuzov we have said something already. He was firm and determined and went stubbornly and undeviatingly towards his goal, if once he had been brought by any reasons (and they were often amazingly illogical ones) to believe that it was the right one. He was honest and incorruptible. His wife, Marfa Ignatyevna, had obeyed her husband's will implicitly all her life, yet she had pestered him terriby after the emancipation of the serfs. She was set on leaving Fyodor Pavlovich and opening a little shop in Moscow with their small savings. But Grigory decided then, once for all, that "the woman's talking nonsense, for every woman is without honour," and that they ought not to leave their old master, whatever he might be, "for that was now their duty."

"Do you understand what duty is?" he asked Marfa Ignatyevna.

"I know about duty, Grigory Vasilyevich, but why it's our duty to stay here, that I can't understand," Marfa answered firmly.

"Well, don't understand then. But so it shall be. And you hold your tongue."

And so it was. They did not go away, and Fyodor Pavlovich named a sum, a small one, as wages, and paid it regularly. Grigory knew, too, that he had an indisputable influence over his master. It was true, and he was aware of it. Fyodor Pavlovich was an obstinate and cunning buffoon, yet, though his will was strong enough "in some of the affairs of life," as he expressed it, he found himself, to his surprise, of a somewhat weak character when it came to certain other emergencies. He knew his weaknesses and was afraid of them. There are positions in which one has to keep a sharp look-out. And that's not easy without a trustworthy man, and Grigory was a most trustworthy man. Many times in the course of his life Fyodor Pavlovich had only just escaped a sound thrashing through Grigory's intervention, and on each occasion the old servant gave him a lecture. But it wasn't only thrashings that Fyodor Pavlovich was afraid of. There were graver situations, and very subtle and complicated ones, in which Fyodor Pavlovich felt an inexplicable and extraordinary craving for some one faithful and devoted, which sometimes unaccountably came upon him all in a moment. It was almost a morbid condition. Dissolute and often cruel in his lust, like some noxious insect, Fyodor Pavlovich was sometimes, in moments of drunkenness, overcome by a spiritual terror and a moral convulsion which took an almost physical form. "My soul's simply quaking in my throat at such times," he used to say. At such moments he liked to feel that there was near at hand, in the lodge if not in the room, a steady, devoted soul, a man untainted by vice, and indeed, totally unlike himself, one who had seen all his debauchery and knew all his secrets, but was ready in his devotion to overlook all that, not to oppose him, above all, not to reproach him or threaten him with anything, either in this world or in the next, and, in case of need, to defend him — from whom? From somebody unknown, but terrible and dangerous. What he needed was to feel that there was *another* human being, an old and tried friend, that he might call him in his sick moments merely to look at his face, or, perhaps, exchange some quite irrelevant words with him. And if this person were not angry, he felt comforted, and if he were angry, he was more dejected. It happened even (very rarely however) that Fyodor Pavlovich went at night to the lodge to wake Grigory and fetch him for a moment. When the old man came, Fyodor Pavlovich would begin talking about the most trivial matters, and would soon dismiss him, sometimes even with mockery and a jest. And then Fyodor Pavlovich would spit, get into bed, and sleep the sleep of the just. Something of the same sort had happened to Fyodor Pavlovich on Alyosha's arrival. Alyosha "pierced his heart" by "living with him, seeing everything and condemning nothing." Moreover, Alyosha brought with him something his father had never known before: a complete absence of contempt for him and an invariable kindness, a perfectly natural unaffected devotion to the old man who deserved it so little. All this was a complete surprise to the old lecher, who had been leading a bachelor's life. It was a new and startling experience for him, who had till then loved nothing but "evil." When Alyosha had left him, he confessed to himself that he had learnt something he had not till then been willing to learn.

I mentioned already at the beginning of my tale that Grigory had detested Adelaïda Ivanovna, the first wife of Fyodor Pavlovich and the mother of Dmitri, and that he had, on the contrary, protected Sofya Ivanovna, the poor "possessed woman," against his master and any one who chanced to speak ill or lightly of her. His sympathy for this unhappy woman had become something sacred to him, so that even now, twenty years after, he could not bear a slighting allusion to her from any one, and would at once check the offender. Externally, Grigory was a cold, dignified, and reserved man, whose words, when he did speak, were weighty and grave. It was impossible to tell at first blush whether he loved his meek, obedient wife; but he really did love her, and she knew it.

Marfa Ignatyevna was by no means stupid; indeed, she was probably cleverer than her spouse, or, at least, more prudent than he in worldly affairs, and yet she had given in to him in everything without question or complaint ever since her marriage, and respected him for his spiritual superiority. It was remarkable how little they spoke to one another in the course of their lives, and only of the most necessary daily affairs. Grave and dignified, Grigory thought over all his affairs and troubles alone, so that Marfa Ignatyevna had long grown used to knowing that he did not need her advice. She felt that her husband prized her silence, and took it as a sign of her good sense. He had never beaten her but once, and then only slightly. Once during the year after Fyodor Pavlovich's marriage to Adelaïda Ivanovna, the village girls and women — at that time serfs — were called together before the house to sing and dance. They were beginning "In the Green Meadows," when Marfa, at that time a young woman, skipped forward and danced "the Russian Dance," not in the village fashion, but as she had danced it when she was a servant in the service of the rich Miüsov family, in their private theatre, where the actors were taught to dance by a dancing master from Moscow. Grigory saw how his wife danced, and, an hour later, at home in their cottage he gave her a lesson, pulling her hair a little. But there it ended: the beating was never repeated, and Marfa Ignatyevna gave up dancing.

God had not blessed them with children. One child was born but it died. Grigory was fond of children, and was not ashamed of showing it. When Adelaïda Ivanovna had run away, Grigory took Dmitri, then a child of three, combed his hair and washed him in a tub with his own hands, and looked after him for almost a year. Afterwards he had looked after Ivan and Alyosha for which the general's widow had rewarded him with a slap in the face; but I have already related all that. The only happiness his own child had brought him had been in the anticipation of its birth. When it was born, his heart was stricken with grief and horror. The baby had six fingers. Grigory was so crushed by this that he was not only silent till the day of the christening, but kept away in the garden. It was spring, and he spent three days digging the kitchen garden. The third day was fixed for christening the baby: meantime Grigory had reached a conclusion. Going into the cottage where the clergy were assembled and the visitors had arrived, including Fyodor Pavlovich, who was to stand godfather, he suddenly announced that the baby "ought not to be christened at all." He announced this quietly, briefly, speaking through his teeth, and gazing with dull intentness at the priest.

"Why not?" asked the priest with good-humoured surprise.

"Because it's a dragon," muttered Grigory.

"A dragon? What dragon?"

Grigory did not speak for some time. "It's a confusion of nature," he muttered vaguely, but firmly, obviously unwilling to say more.

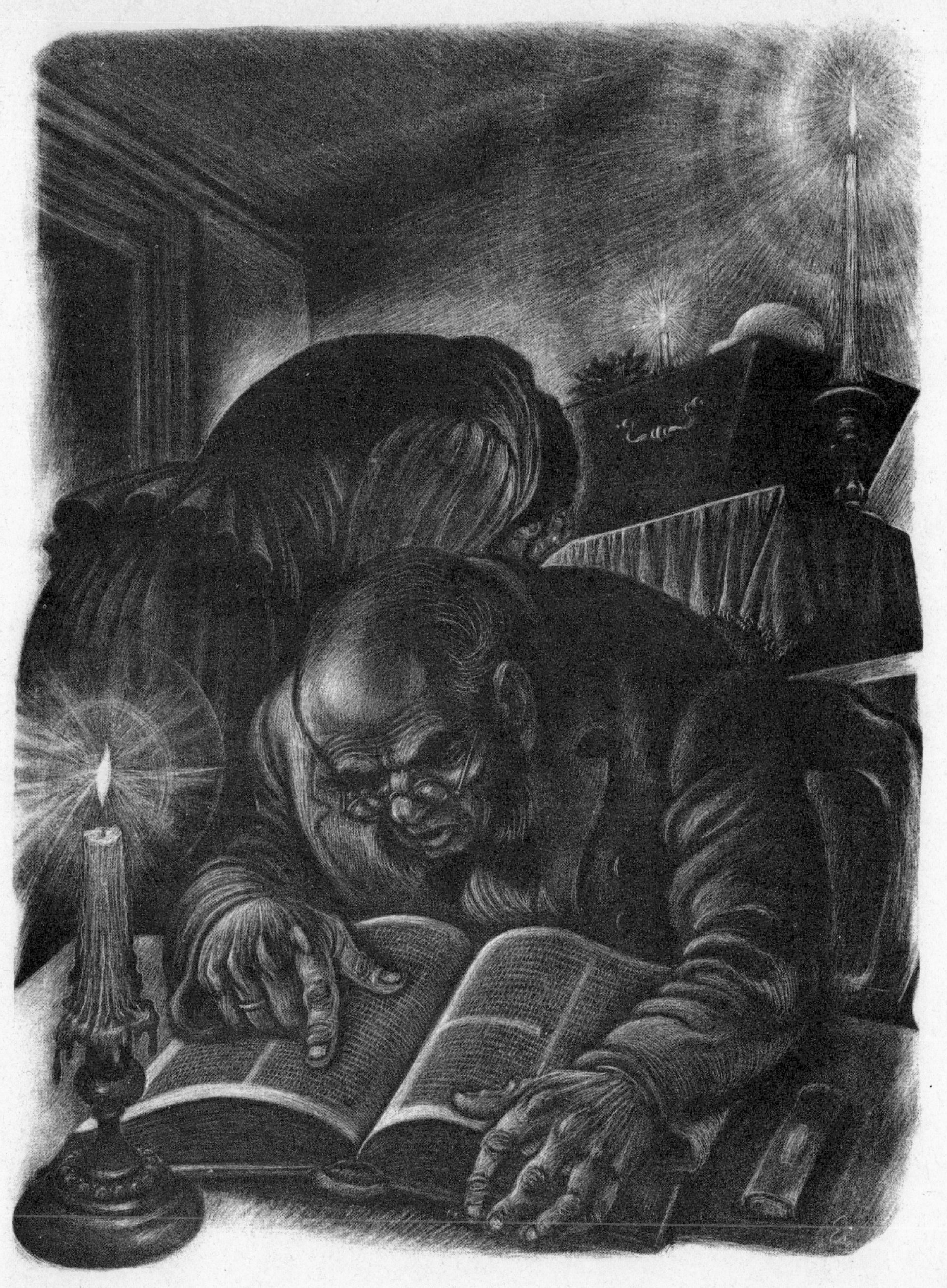

GRIGORY AND THE CHILD

They laughed, and of course christened the poor baby. Grigory prayed earnestly at the font, but his opinion of the new-born child remained unchanged. Yet he did not interfere in any way. As long as the sickly infant lived he scarcely looked at it, tried indeed not to notice it, and for the most part kept out of the cottage. But when, at the end of a fortnight, the baby died of thrush, he himself laid the child in its little coffin, looked at it in profound grief, and when they were filling up the shallow little grave he fell on his knees and bowed down to the earth. He did not for years afterwards mention his child, nor did Marfa speak of the baby before him, and, even if Grigory were not present, she never spoke of it above a whisper. Marfa observed that, from the day of the burial, he devoted himself to "religion" and took to reading the "Lives of the Saints," for the most part sitting alone and in silence, and always putting on his big, round, silver-rimmed spectacles. He rarely read aloud, only perhaps during Lent. He was fond of the book of Job, and had somehow got hold of a copy of the discourses and sermons of "our godly Father Isaac the Syrian," which he read persistently for years together, understanding practically nothing of it, but perhaps prizing and loving it the more for that. Of late he had begun to listen to the doctrines of the sect of Flagellants settled in the neighbourhood. He was evidently shaken by them, but judged it unfitting to go over to the new faith. His habit of edifying reading gave him an expression of still greater gravity.

He was perhaps predisposed to mysticism. And the birth of his deformed child, and its death, had, as though by special design been accompanied by another strange and marvellous event, which, as he said later, had left an "imprint" upon his soul. It happened that, on the very night after the burial of his child, Marfa was awakened by the wail of a new-born baby. She was frightened and waked her husband. He listened and said he thought it was more like some one groaning, "it might be a woman." He got up and dressed. It was a rather warm night in May. As he went down the steps, he distinctly heard groans coming from the garden. But the gate from the yard into the garden was locked at night, and there was no other way of entering it, for it was enclosed all round by a strong, high fence. Going back into the house, Grigory lighted a lantern, took the garden key, and taking no notice of the hysterical terror of his wife, who was still persuaded that she heard a child crying, and that it was her own baby crying and calling for her, went into the garden in silence. There he heard at once that the groans came from the bath-house that stood near the garden gate, and that they were the groans of a woman. Opening the door of the bath-house, he saw a sight which petrified him. An idiot girl, who wandered about the streets and was known to the whole town by the nickname of Lizaveta Smerdyashchaya (Stinking Lizaveta), had got into the bath-house and had just given birth to a child. She lay dying with the baby beside her. She said nothing, for she had never been able to speak. But her story needs a chapter to itself.

CHAPTER II

LIZAVETA

THERE was one circumstance which struck Grigory particularly, and confirmed a very unpleasant and revolting suspicion. This Lizaveta was a dwarfish creature, "not five foot within a wee bit," as many of the pious old women said pathetically about her, after her death. The broad, healthy, red face of the twenty-year old girl had a look of blank idiocy and the fixed stare in her eyes was unpleasant, in spite of their meek expression. She wandered about, summer and winter alike, barefooted, wearing nothing but a hempen smock. Her coarse, almost black hair curled like lamb's wool, and formed a sort of huge cap on her head. It was always crusted with mud, and had leaves, bits of stick, and shavings clinging to it, as she always slept on the ground and in the dirt. Her father, a homeless, sickly drunkard, called Ilya, had lost everything and lived many years as a workman with some well-to-do tradespeople. Her mother had long been dead. Spiteful and ailing, Ilya used to beat Lizaveta inhumanly whenever she returned to him. But she rarely did so, for every one in the town was ready to look after her as being an idiot, and so specially dear to God. Ilya's employers, and many others in the town, especially of the tradespeople, tried to clothe her better, and always rigged her out with high boots and a sheepskin coat for the winter. But, although she allowed them to dress her up without resisting, she usually went away, preferably to the cathedral porch, and taking off all that had been given her — kerchief, sheepskin, skirt, or boots — she left them there and walked away barefoot in her smock as before. It happened on one occasion that a new governor of the province, making a tour of inspection in our town, saw Lizaveta, and was wounded in his tenderest feelings. And though he was told she was an idiot, he pronounced that for a young woman of twenty to wander about in nothing but a smock was a breach of the proprieties, and must not occur again. But the governor went his way, and Lizaveta was left as she was. At last her father died, which endeared her, being thus orphaned, even more to the pious people of the town. In fact, every one seemed to love her; even the boys did not tease her, and the boys of our town, especially the schoolboys, are a mischievous set. She would walk into strange houses and no one drove her away. On the contrary, every one was kind to her and gave her a groat. If she were given a copper, she would take it, and at once drop it in the alms-jug of the church or the prison. If she were given a roll or a bun in the market, she would hand it to the first child she met. Sometimes she would stop one of the richest ladies in the town and give it to her, and the lady would be pleased to take it. She herself never tasted anything but black bread and water. If she went into a fine shop, where there were costly goods or money lying about, no one kept watch on her, for they knew that if she saw thousands of roubles overlooked by them, she would not have touched a groat. She scarcely ever went to church. She slept either on a church porch or, having climbed over a hurdle (to this day there are many hurdles instead of fences in our town), in a kitchen garden. She used at least once a week to turn up "at home," that is at the house of her father's former employers, and in the winter went there every night, and slept either in the passage or the cowhouse. People were amazed that she could stand such a life, but she was accustomed to it, and, although she was so tiny, she was of a robust constitution. Some of the townspeople declared that she did all this only from pride, but that is hardly credible. She could hardly speak, and only from time to time uttered an inarticulate grunt. How could she have been proud?

Now it happened one clear, warm, moonlight night in September (a long time ago) that five or six drunken revellers were returning from the club at a very late hour, according to our provincial notions. They passed through the "back-way," which led between the back gardens of the houses, with hurdles on either side. This way leads out on to the bridge over the long, stinking pool which we were accustomed to call a river. Among the nettles and burdocks beside the hurdle our revellers saw Lizaveta asleep. They stopped to look at her, laughing, and began jesting with unbridled licentiousness. It occurred to one young gentleman to make the whimsical inquiry whether any one could possibly look upon such an animal as a woman, and so forth. . . . They all pronounced with lofty repugnance that it was impossible. But Fyodor Pavlovich, who was of the company, thrust himself forward and declared that it was by no means impossible, and that, indeed, there was a certain piquancy about it, and so on. . . . It is true that at that time he was overdoing his part as a buffoon. He liked to put himself forward and entertain the company, ostensibly on equal terms, of course, though in reality he was on a servile footing with them. It was just at the time when he had received the news of his first wife's death in Petersburg, and, with crape upon his hat, was drinking and behaving so shamelessly that even the most reckless among us were shocked at the sight of him. The revellers, of course, laughed at this unexpected opinion; and one of them even began encouraging him to act upon it. The others repelled the idea even more emphatically, although still with the utmost hilarity, and at last they went on their way. Later on, Fyodor Pavlovich swore that he had gone with them, and perhaps it was so, no one knows for certain, and no one ever knew. But five or six months later, all the town was talking, with intense and sincere indignation, of Lizaveta's condition, and trying to find out who was the miscreant who had wronged her. Then suddenly a terrible rumour was all over the town that this miscreant was no other than Fyodor Pavlovich. Who set the rumour going? Of that drunken band five had left the town and the only one still among us was an elderly and estimable civil councillor, the father of grown-up daughters, who could hardly have spread the tale, even if there had been any foundation for it. But rumour pointed straight at Fyodor Pavlovich, and persisted in pointing at him. Of course this was no great grievance to him: he would not have troubled to contradict a set of tradespeople. In those days he was proud, and did not condescend to talk except in his own circle of officials and gentlemen, whom he entertained so well.

At the time, Grigory stood up for his master vigorously. He provoked quarrels and altercations in defence of him and succeeded in bringing some people round to his side. "It's the wench's own fault," he asserted, and the culprit, according to him, was none but "Karp with the Screw," a dangerous convict, who had escaped from prison and who had hidden in our town. This conjecture sounded plausible, for it was remembered that Karp had been in the neighbourhood just at that time in the autumn, and had robbed three people. But this affair and all the talk about it did not estrange popular sympathy from the poor idiot. She was better looked after than ever. A well-to-do merchant's widow named Kondratyeva arranged to take her into her house at the end of April, meaning not to let her go out until after the confinement. They kept a constant watch over her, but in spite of their vigilance she escaped on the very last day, and made her way into Fyodor Pavlovich's garden. How, in her condition, she managed to climb over the high, strong fence, remained a mystery. Some maintained that she must have been lifted over by somebody; others hinted at something more uncanny. The most likely explanation is that it happened naturally — that Lizaveta, accustomed to clambering over hurdles to sleep in gardens, had somehow managed to climb this fence, in spite of her condition, and had leapt down, injuring herself.

Grigory rushed to Marfa and sent her to Lizaveta, while he ran to fetch an old midwife who lived close by. They saved the baby, but Lizaveta died at dawn. Grigory took the baby, brought it home, and making his wife sit down, put it on her lap. "A child of God, an orphan, is akin to all," he said, "and to us above others. Our little lost one has sent us this infant who has sprung from the devil's son and a holy innocent. Nurse him and weep no more."

So Marfa brought up the child. He was christened Pavel, to which people were not slow in adding Fyodorovich (son of Fyodor). Fyodor Pavlovich did not object to any of this, and thought it amusing, though he persisted vigorously in denying his responsibility. The townspeople were pleased at his adopting the foundling.

Later on, Fyodor Pavlovich invented a surname for the child, calling him Smerdyakov, after his mother's nickname.

So this Smerdyakov became Fyodor Pavlovich's second servant, and was living in the lodge with Grigory and Marfa at the time our story begins. He was employed as cook. I ought to say something of this Smerdyakov, but I am ashamed of keeping my readers' attention so long occupied with these common menials, and I will go back to my story, hoping to say more of Smerdyakov in the course of it.

CHAPTER III

THE CONFESSION OF AN ARDENT HEART — IN VERSE

ALYOSHA remained for some time irresolute after hearing the command his father shouted to him from the carriage. But in spite of his uneasiness he did not stand still. That was not his way. He went at once to the kitchen to find out what mischief his father had been doing upstairs. Then he set off, trusting that on the way to town he would find some answer to the question tormenting him. I hasten to add that his father's shouts, commanding him to return home "with his mattress and pillow," did not frighten him in the least. He understood perfectly that those peremptory shouts were merely "a flourish" to produce an effect. In the same way a tradesman in our town who was celebrating his name-day with a party of friends, getting angry at being refused more vodka, smashed up his own crockery and furniture and tore his own and his wife's clothes, and finally broke his windows, all for the sake of effect. Next day, of course, when he was sober, he regretted the broken cups and saucers. Alyosha knew that his father would let him go back to the monastery next day, possibly even that evening. Moreover, he was fully persuaded that his father might injure any one else, but would not injure him. Alyosha was certain that no one in the whole world ever would want to injure him, and, what is more, he knew that no one could injure him. This was for him an axiom, assumed once for all without question, and he went his way without hesitation, relying on it.

But at that moment a fear of a different sort disturbed him, and worried him the more because he could not define it. It was the fear of a woman, of Katerina Ivanovna, who had so urgently entreated him in the note handed to him by Madame Hohlakov to come and see her about something. This request and the necessity of going had at once aroused an uneasy feeling in his heart, and this feeling had grown more and more painful as the morning wore on, in spite of the scenes at the hermitage and at the Father Superior's. He was not uneasy because he did not know what she would say and what he would answer. And he was not afraid of her simply as a woman. Though he knew little of women, he had spent his life, from early childhood till he entered the monastery, entirely with women. He was afraid of that particular woman, Katerina Ivanovna. He had been afraid of her from the first time he saw her. He had only seen her two or three times, and had only chanced to say a few words to her. He remembered her as a beautiful, proud, imperious girl. It was not her beauty which troubled him, but something else. And the vagueness of his apprehension increased the apprehension itself. The girl's aims were of the noblest, he knew that. She was trying to save his brother Dmitri simply through generosity, though he had already behaved badly to her. Yet, although Alyosha recognised and did justice to all these fine and generous sentiments, a shiver began to run down his back when he drew near her house.

He reflected that he would not find Ivan, who was so intimate a friend, with her, for Ivan was certainly now with his father. Dmitri he was even more certain not to find there, and he had a foreboding of the reason. And so his conversation would be with her alone. He had a great longing to run and see his brother Dmitri before that fateful interview. Without showing him the letter, he could have a talk with him. But Dmitri lived a long way off, and he was sure to be away from home, too. Standing still for a minute, he reached a final decision. Crossing himself with a rapid and accustomed gesture, and at once smiling, he turned resolutely in the direction of his terrible lady.

He knew her house. If he went by Bolshaya Street and then across the market-place, it would be a long way round. Though our town is small, the houses are far apart, and the distances are rather great. And meanwhile his father was expecting him, and perhaps had not yet forgotten his command. He might be unreasonable, and so he had to make haste to get there and back. So he decided to take a short cut by the back-way, for he knew every inch of the ground. This meant skirting fences, climbing over hurdles, and crossing other people's back-yards, where every one he met knew him and greeted him. In this way he could reach Bolshaya Street in half the time.

He had to pass the garden adjoining his father's, and belonging to a little tumbledown house with four windows. The owner of this house, as Alyosha knew, was a bedridden old woman, living with her daughter, who had been a genteel maid-servant in generals' families in Petersburg. Now she had been at home a year, looking after her sick mother. She always dressed up in fine clothes, though her old mother and she had sunk into such poverty that they went every day to Fyodor Pavlovich's kitchen for soup and bread, which Marfa gave readily. Yet, though the young woman came for soup, she had never sold any of her dresses, and one of these even had a long train — a fact which Alyosha had learned from Rakitin, who always knew everything that was going on in the town. He had forgotten it as soon as he had heard it, but now, on reaching the garden, he remembered the dress with the train, raised his head, which had been bowed in thought, and came upon something quite unexpected.

Over the hurdle in the garden, Dmitri, mounted on something, was leaning forward, gesticulating violently, beckoning to him, obviously afraid to utter a word for fear of being overheard. Alyosha ran up to the hurdle.

"It's a good thing you looked up. I nearly shouted to you," Mitya said in a joyful, hurried whisper. "Climb in here quickly! How splendid that you've come! I was just thinking of you!"

Alyosha was delighted, too, but he did not know how to get over the hurdle. Mitya put his powerful hand under his elbow to help him jump. Tucking up his cassock, Alyosha leapt over the hurdle with the agility of a barelegged street urchin.

"Well done! Now come along," said Mitya in an enthusiastic whisper.

"Where?" whispered Alyosha, looking about him and finding himself in a deserted garden with no one in it but themselves. The garden was small, but the house was at least fifty paces away.

"There's no one here. Why do you whisper?" asked Alyosha.

"Why do I whisper? Deuce take it!" cried Dmitri at the top of his voice. "Why, indeed? You see what silly tricks nature plays one. I am here in secret, and on the watch. I'll explain later on, but, knowing it's a secret, I began whispering like a fool, when there's no need. Let us go. Over there. Till then be quiet. I want to kiss you.

Glory be to God in heaven,
Glory be to God in me . . .

I was just repeating that, sitting here, before you came."

The garden was about three acres in extent, and planted with trees along the fence on all four sides. There were apple-trees, maples, limes, and birch-trees. The middle of the garden was a bare grass-plot, which yielded several loads of hay in the summer. The garden was leased in the spring for a few roubles. There were also patches of raspberries and currants and gooseberries along the fences; a kitchen garden had been planted lately near the house.

Dmitri led his brother to the most secluded corner of the garden. There, in a thicket of lime-trees and old bushes of black currant, elder, snowball-tree, and lilac, there stood a tumbledown green summer-house, blackened with age. Its walls were of lattice-work, but there was still a roof which could give shelter. God knows when this summer-house was built. There was a tradition that it had been put up some fifty years before by a retired colonel called von Schmidt, who owned the house at that time. It was all in decay, the floor was rotting, the planks were loose, the wood smelled musty. In the summer-house there was a green wooden table fixed in the ground, and round it were some green benches upon which it was still possible to sit. Alyosha had at once observed his brother's exalted condition, and on entering the arbour he saw half a bottle of cognac and a wineglass on the table.

"That's cognac," Mitya laughed. "I see

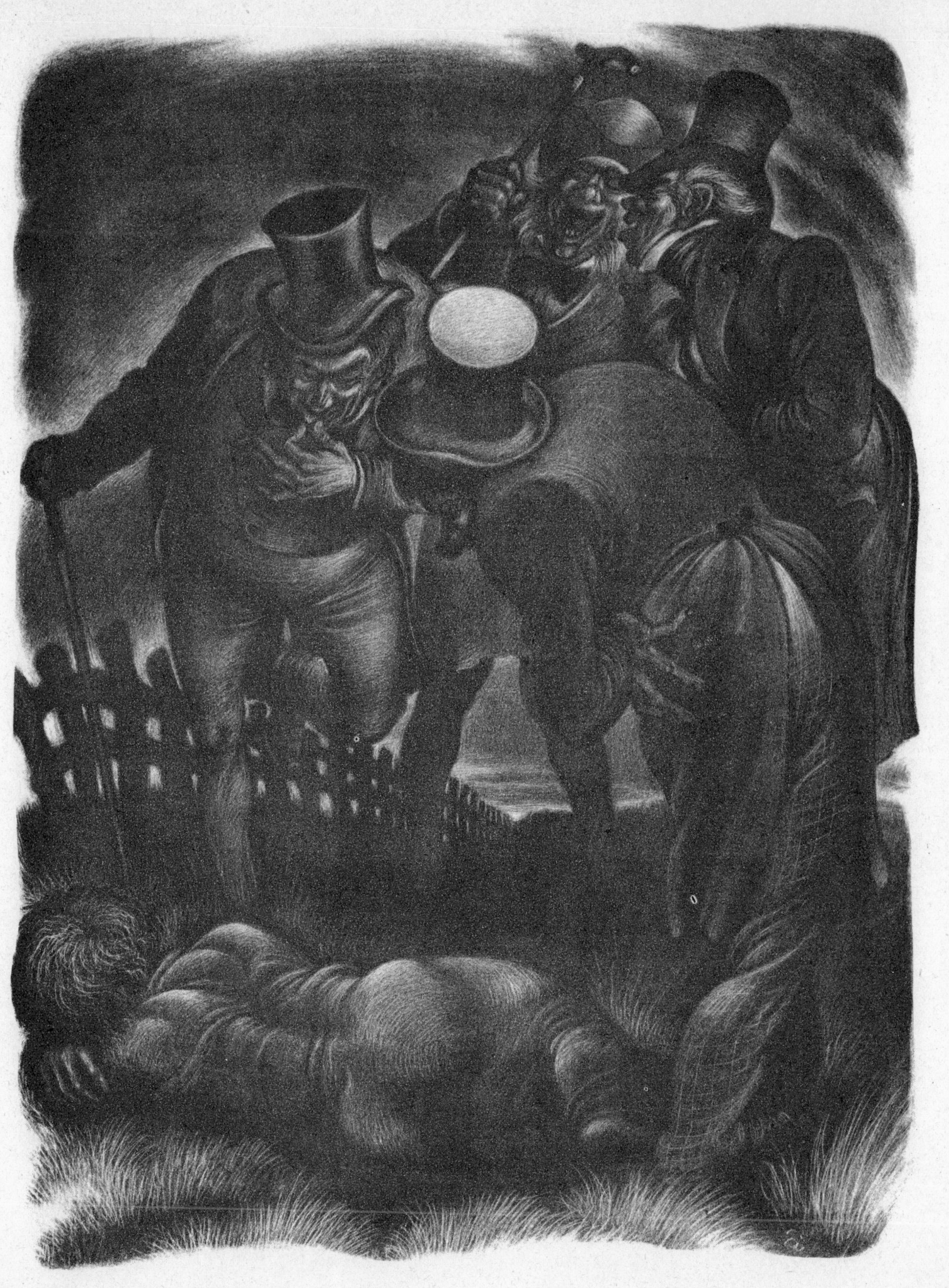

THE FINDING OF LIZAVETA

your look: 'He's drinking again!' Distrust the phantom.

Distrust the vapid, lying crowd,
And lay aside thy doubts.

I'm not drinking, I'm only 'indulging,' as that pig, your Rakitin, says. He'll be a councillor of state one day, but he'll always talk about 'indulging.' Sit down. I could take you in my arms, Alyosha, and press you to my bosom till I crushed you, for in the whole world — really — re-al-ly (can you take it in?) — I love no one but you!"

He uttered the last words in a sort of ecstasy.

"No one but you and one 'jade' I have fallen in love with, to my ruin. But being in love doesn't mean loving. You may be in love with a woman and yet hate her. Remember that! I can still talk about it cheerfully. Sit down here at the table and I'll sit beside you and look at you, and go on talking. You shall keep quiet and I'll go on talking, for the time has come. But on reflection, you know, I'd better speak quietly, for here — here — you can never tell what ears are listening. I will explain everything, as they say, 'to be continued.' Why have I been longing for you? Why have I been thirsting for you all these days, and just now? (It's five days since I've cast anchor here.) Because it's only to you I can tell everything; because I must, because I need you, because to-morrow I shall fly from the clouds, because to-morrow life will end and begin. Have you ever experienced, have you ever dreamt of falling down a precipice into a pit? That's just what I'm doing now, but not in a dream. And I'm not afraid, and don't you be afraid. At least, I am afraid, but it's sweet. It's not pleasure though, but ecstasy. Damn it all, whatever it is! A strong spirit, a weak spirit, a womanish spirit — whatever it is! Let us praise nature: look at all the sunshine, how clear the sky is, the leaves are all green, it's still summer; four o'clock in the afternoon, and the stillness! Where were you going?"

"I was going to see father, but I meant to go to Katerina Ivanovna's first."

"To her, and to father! Oo! what a coincidence! Why was I waiting for you? Hungering and thirsting for you in every cranny of my soul and even in my ribs? Why, to send you to father and to her, Katerina Ivanovna, so as to have done with her and with father. To send an angel. I might have sent any one, but I wanted to send an angel. And here you are on your way to see father and her."

"Did you really mean to send me?" cried Alyosha with a pained expression.

"Stay! You knew it! And I see that you have understood it all at once. But be quiet, be quiet for a time. Don't be sorry, and don't cry."

Dmitri stood up, thought a moment, and put his finger to his forehead.

"She's asked you, written you a letter or something, that's why you're going to her? You wouldn't be going except for that?"

"Here is her note." Alyosha took it out of his pocket. Mitya glanced through it quickly.

"And you were going the back-way! Oh, gods, I thank you for sending him by the back-way, and he got into my hands like the golden fish to the silly old fisherman in the fairy-tale. Listen, Alyosha, listen, brother! Now I mean to tell you everything, for I must tell some one. An angel in heaven I've told already; but I want to tell an angel on earth. You are an angel on earth. You will hear and judge and forgive. And that's what I need, that some one above me should forgive. Listen! If two people break away from everything on earth and fly off into the unknown, or at least one of them, and before flying off or going to ruin he comes to some one else and says, 'Do this for me'—some favour never asked before that could only be asked on one's deathbed—would that other refuse, if he were a friend or a brother?"

"I will do it, but tell me what it is, and make haste," said Alyosha.

"Make haste! H'm! . . . Don't be in a hurry, Alyosha, you hurry and worry yourself. There's no need to hurry now. Now the world has turned a corner. Ah, Alyosha, what a pity you can't understand ecstasy. But what am I saying to him? As though you didn't understand it. What an ass I am, what am I saying: 'Be noble, oh, man!' Whose verse is that?"

Alyosha made up his mind to wait. He felt that, perhaps, indeed, his work lay here. Mitya sank into thought for a moment, with his elbow on the table and his head in his hand. Both were silent.

"Alyosha," said Mitya, "you're the only one who won't laugh. I should like to begin—my confession—with Schiller's 'Hymn to Joy,' *An die Freude!* I don't know any German, I only know it's called that. Don't think I'm talking nonsense because I'm drunk. I'm not a bit drunk. Brandy's all very well, but I need two bottles to make me drunk:

Silenus with his rosy phiz
Upon his stumbling ass.

But I've not drunk even a quarter of a bottle, and I'm not Silenus. I'm not Silenus, but I am strong,* for I've made a decision once for all.

*In Russian, "silen."

Forgive me the pun; you'll have to forgive me a lot more than puns to-day. Don't be uneasy. I'm not spinning it out. I'm talking sense, and I'll come to the point in a minute. I won't keep you in suspense. Stay, how does it go?"

He raised his head, thought a minute, and began ecstatically:

"In the craggy clefts deep-hidden
Crouched the fearful troglodyte;
And the nomad left but barren
Traces, in his desert flight.
Savage spear and keen-tipped arrow
Through the woods the hunter bore;
Woe unto the wave-tossed stranger
Flung upon the luckless shore!

"On her way sad Ceres greeted
Mournfully a coast so bare,
Seeking still her daughter's footsteps,
Where was nothing green or fair!
Not an omen there of comfort,
Not a welcome where she trod,
Not one temple's shining columns
Spoke of reverence due a god.

"There no fruit of sweetest harvest
Bade her share the meal serene;
On the horrid altars smoking
Human sacrifice was seen.
Yea, as far as she might wander
Only misery met her gaze,
Deep within her mighty spirit
She bewailed man's fallen ways."

Mitya sobbed and seized Alyosha's hand. "My dear, my dear, in degradation, in degradation now, too. There's a terrible amount of suffering for man on earth, a terrible lot of grief. Don't think I'm only a brute in an officer's uniform, who swills cognac and wallows in debauchery. I hardly think of anything but of that degraded man — if only I'm not lying. God keep me from lying and boasting. I think about that man because I am such a man.

That man's soul might rise from vileness,
And attain to light and worth,
He did frame a pact eternal
With primeval Mother Earth.

Only here is the difficulty: how am I to frame an eternal pact with Mother Earth? I don't kiss her. I don't cleave to her bosom. Am I to become a peasant or a shepherd? I go ahead and I don't know whether I'm on my way to stench and shame or to light and joy. That's the trouble, for everything in the world is a riddle! And whenever I've happened to sink to the lowest depths of depravity (and that's all I've been doing) I always read that poem about Ceres and man. Has it reformed me? Never! For I'm a Karamazov. For when I do leap into the abyss I pitch in head foremost and heels up, and am positively pleased to be falling in that degrading attitude, and pride myself upon it. And in the very depths of that degradation I suddenly begin a hymn. Let me be accursed. Let me be vile and base, but let me, too, kiss the hem of the garment in which my God is clothed. Though I may be following the devil, I am Thy son, O Lord, and I love Thee, and I feel the joy without which the world cannot exist and have its being.

Joy, each blade of grass announces,
Nature's precept to rehearse,
Joy, 'tis joy that turns the wheeling
Watchworks of the universe.
Flowers from the bud she beckons,
Stars and suns she brings to pass,
Filling space with worlds undreamed of,
Hidden from the seer's glass.
Joy all creatures drink unstinting
From great Nature's bounteous breast,
All the virtuous, all the wicked,
Seek her rosy path with zest.
Wine and kisses both she gave us,
Friendship, faithful to its trust;
To the cherub, sight of Godhead,
To the insect — sensual lust.

But enough poetry! I am in tears; let me cry. It may be foolishness that every one would laugh at. But you won't laugh. Your eyes are shining, too. Enough poetry. I want to tell you now about the insects to whom God gave 'sensual lust.'

To the insect — sensual lust.

I am that insect, brother, and the words are said of me specially. And all of us Karamazovs are the same kind, and, angel as you are, that insect lives in you, too, and stirs up tempests in your blood. Tempests, because sensual lust is a tempest — worse than a tempest! Beauty is a terrible and awful thing! It is terrible because unfathomable; and it cannot be fathomed, because God sets us nothing but riddles. Here the boundaries meet and all contradictions dwell together. I am not a cultivated man, brother, but I've thought a lot about this. What a terrible lot of mysteries there are! Too many riddles weigh men down on earth. We must solve them as best we can, and try to keep a dry skin in the water. Beauty! I can't endure the thought that a man of lofty mind and heart begins with the ideal of the Madonna and ends with the ideal of Sodom. What's still more dreadful is that a man with the ideal of Sodom in his soul does not renounce the ideal of the Madonna, and his heart is on fire with that ideal, genuinely on fire, just as in the days of his youth and innocence. Yes, man is broad, too broad, indeed. I'd have him narrower. The devil only knows what to make of it! What seems disgraceful to the mind is beauty and nothing else to the heart. Is there beauty in Sodom? Believe me, that the overwhelming majority of mankind find beauty in Sodom. Did you know that secret? The awful thing is that beauty is not only a terrible but a mysterious thing. God and the devil are fighting there and the battlefield is the heart of man. But a man talks of what ails him. Listen, now to come to the facts."

CHAPTER IV

THE CONFESSION OF AN ARDENT HEART — IN ANECDOTE

"I WAS leading a wild life there. Father said just now that I spent several thousand roubles in seducing girls. That's a swinish invention, and there was nothing of the sort. And if there was, I didn't need money simply for *that*. With me money is an accessory, the overflow of my heart, the background. To-day she would be my lady, to-morrow a wench out of the streets in her place. I entertained them both. I threw away money by the handful on music, rioting, gipsies. Sometimes I gave it to the women, too, for they'll take it greedily, that must be admitted, and be pleased and thankful for it. Ladies used to be fond of me: not all of them, but it happened, it happened. But I always liked side-paths, little dark back-alleys behind the square — there one finds adventures and surprises, and gold in the dirt. I am speaking figuratively, brother. In the town I was in, there were no such back-alleys in the literal sense, but morally there were. If you were like me, you'd know what that means. I loved vice, I loved the ignominy of vice. I loved cruelty; am I not a bug, am I not a noxious insect? In fine, a Karamazov! Once we went, a whole lot of us, for a picnic, in seven sledges. It was dark, it was winter, and I began squeezing a girl's hand, and forced her to kiss me. She was the daughter of an official, a sweet, gentle, submissive creature. She allowed me, she allowed me much in the dark. She thought, poor thing, that I would come next day to make her an offer (I was looked upon as a good match, too). But I didn't say a word to her for five months. I used to see her in a corner at dances (we were always having dances), her eyes watching me. I saw how they glowed with fire — a fire of gentle indignation. This game only tickled that insect lust I cherished in my soul. Five months later she married an official and left the town, still angry, and still, perhaps, in love with me. Now they live happily. Observe that I told no one. I didn't boast of it. Though I'm full of low desires, and love what's low, I'm not dishonourable. You're blushing; your eyes flashed. Enough of this filth for you. And all this was nothing much — wayside blossoms *à la* Paul de Kock — though the cruel insect was growing stronger in my soul. I've a perfect album of reminiscences, brother. God bless them, the darlings. I tried to break it off without quarreling. And I never gave them away. I never bragged of one of them. But that's enough. You can't suppose I brought you here simply to talk of such dirt. No, I'm going to tell you something more curious; and don't be surprised that I'm glad to tell you, instead of being ashamed."

"You say that because I blushed," Alyosha said suddenly. "I wasn't blushing at what you were saying or at what you've done. I blushed because I am the same as you are."

"You? Come, that's going a little too far!"

"No, it's not going too far," said Alyosha

warmly (obviously the idea was not a new one). "It's like the rungs of the same ladder. I'm on the bottom rung, and you're above, somewhere about the thirteenth. That's how I see it. But it's all the same. Absolutely the same in kind. Any one on the bottom step is bound to go up to the top one."

"Then one ought not to step on at all."

"Any one who can help it had better not."

"But can you?"

"I think not."

"Hush, Alyosha, hush, darling! I could kiss your hand, you touch me so. That hussy, Grushenka, is a judge of men. She told me once that she'd devour you one day. There, there, I won't! From this field of corruption, this place fouled by flies, let's pass to my tragedy, also befouled by flies, that is by every sort of vileness. Although the old man told lies abut my seducing innocence, there really was something of the sort in my tragedy, though it was only once, and then it did not come off. The old man who has reproached me with what never happened does not even know of this fact; I never told any one about it. You're the first, except Ivan, of course — Ivan knows everything. He knew about it long before you. But Ivan's a tomb."

"Ivan's a tomb?"

"Yes."

Alyosha listened with great attention.

"I was lieutenant in a line regiment, but still I was under surveillance, like a kind of exile. Yet I was awfully well received in the little town. I spent money right and left. I was thought to be rich; I thought so myself. But I must have pleased them in other ways as well. Although they shook their heads over me, they liked me. My colonel, who was an old man, took a sudden dislike to me. He was always down on me, but I had powerful friends, and, moreover, all the town was on my side, so he couldn't get me into trouble. I was at fault myself for refusing to treat him with proper respect. I was proud. This obstinate old fellow, who was really a very good sort, kind-hearted and hospitable, had had two wives, both dead. His first wife, who was of a humble family, left a daughter as unpretentious as herself. She was a young woman of four and twenty when I was there, and was living with her father and an aunt, her mother's sister. The aunt was a simple, silent woman; the niece was simple, too, but lively. When I look back, I like to say a good word about people. I never knew a woman of more charming character than Agafya — fancy, her name was Agafya Ivanovna! And she wasn't bad-looking either, in the Russian style: tall, stout, with a full figure, and beautiful eyes, though a rather coarse face. She had not married, although she had had two suitors. She refused them, but was as cheerful as ever. I was intimate with her, not in 'that' way, it was pure friendship. I have often been friendly with women quite innocently. I used to talk to her with shocking frankness, and she only laughed. Many women like such freedom, and she was a girl, too, which made it very amusing. Another thing, one could never think of her as a young lady. She and her aunt lived in her father's house with a sort of voluntary humility, not putting themselves on an equal footing with other people. She was a general favourite, and of use to every one, for she was a clever dressmaker. She had a talent for it. She gave her services freely without asking for payment, but if any one offered her payment, she didn't refuse. The lieutenant-colonel, of course, was a very different matter. He was one of the chief personages in the district. He kept open house, entertained the whole town, gave suppers and dances. At the time I arrived and joined the battalion, all the town was talking of the expected return of the lieutenant-colonel's second daughter, a great beauty, who had just left a fashionable school in the capital. This second daughter is this very Katerina Ivanovna, and she was the child of the colonel's second wife, who belonged to a distinguished family, being the daughter of a general; although, as I learnt on good authority, she brought the lieutenant-colonel no money. She had connections, and that was all. There may have been expectations, but they had come to nothing.

"Yet, when the young lady came from boarding-school on a visit, the whole town revived. Our most distinguished ladies — two 'Excellencies' and a colonel's wife — and all the rest following their lead, at once took her up and gave entertainments in her honour. She was the belle of the balls and picnics, and they got up *tableaux vivants* in aid of distressed governesses. As for me, I took no notice, I went on as wildly as before, and one of my exploits at the time set all the town talking. I saw her eyes taking my measure one evening at the battery commander's, but I didn't go up to her, as though I disdained her acquaintance. I did go up and speak to her at an evening party not long after. She scarcely looked at me, and compressed her lips scornfully. 'Wait a bit. I'll have my revenge,' thought I. I behaved like an awful rowdy on many occasions at that time, and I was conscious of it myself. The main thing was that I felt that 'Katenka' was not an innocent boarding-school miss, but a person of character, proud and really high-principled; above all, she had education and intellect, and I had neither. You think I meant to make her an offer? No, I simply wanted to revenge myself, because I was such a capital fellow and she didn't seem to notice it.

"Meanwhile, I spent my time in drink and riot, till the lieutenant-colonel put me under arrest for three days. Just at that time father sent me six thousand roubles in return for my sending him a deed giving up all claims upon him — settling our accounts, so to speak, and saying that I wouldn't demand anything more. I didn't understand a word of it at the time. Until I came here, Alyosha, till the last few days, indeed, perhaps even now, I haven't been able to make head or tail of my money affairs with father. But let all that go to the deuce, we'll talk of it later.

"Just as I received the money, I got a letter from a friend telling me something that interested me immensely. The authorities, I learnt, were dissatisfied with our lieutenant-colonel. He was suspected of irregularities; in fact, his enemies were preparing a surprise for him. And then the commander of the division arrived, and kicked up the devil of a shindy. Shortly afterwards he was ordered to retire. I won't tell you how it all happened. He had enemies certainly. Suddenly there was a marked coolness in the town towards him and all his family. His friends all turned their backs on him. Then I took my first step. I met Agafya Ivanovna, with whom I'd always kept up a friendship, and said, 'Do you know there's a deficit of 4,500 roubles of government money in your father's accounts?'

" 'What do you mean? What makes you say so? The general was here not long ago, and everything was all right.'

" 'Then it was, but now it isn't.'

"She was terribly scared.

" 'Don't frighten me!' she said. 'Who told you so?'

" 'Don't be uneasy,' I said, 'I won't tell any one. You know I'm as silent as the grave. I only wanted, in view of "possibilities," to add, that when they demand that 4,500 roubles from your father, and he can't produce it, he'll be tried, and demoted to the ranks in his old age. But you just send me your boarding-school miss secretly. I've received some money lately. I'll give her four thousand, maybe, and keep the secret religiously.'

" 'Ah, you scoundrel!' that's what she said. 'You vicious scoundrel! How dare you!'

"She went away furiously indignant, while I shouted after her once more that the secret should be kept sacred. Those two simple creatures, Agafya and her aunt, I may as well say at once, behaved like innocent angels all through this business. They genuinely adored their 'Katya,' thought her far above them, and waited on her, hand and foot. But Agafya told her of our conversation. I found that out afterwards. She didn't keep it back, and of course that was just what I wanted.

"Suddenly the new major arrived to take command of the battalion. The old lieutenant-colonel was taken ill at once, couldn't leave his room for two days, and didn't hand over the government money. Dr. Kravchenko declared that he really was ill. But I knew for a fact, and had known for a long time, that for the last four years the money had never been in his hands except when the Commander made his visits of inspection. He used to lend it to a trustworthy person, a merchant of our town called Trifonov, an old widower, with a big beard and gold-rimmed spectacles. He used to go to the fair, do a profitable business with the money, and return the whole sum to the colonel, bringing with it a present from the fair, as well as interest on the loan. But this time (I heard all about it quite by chance from Trifonov's son and heir, a drivelling youth and one of the most vicious in the world)—this time, I say, Trifonov brought nothing back from the fair. The lieutenant-colonel flew to him. 'I've never received any money from you, and couldn't possibly have received any.' That was all the answer he got. So now our lieutenant-colonel is confined to the house, with a towel round his head, while they're all three busy putting ice on it. All at once an orderly arrives on the scene with a book and an order to 'hand over the government money immediately, within two hours.' He signed his name in the book (I saw the signature in the book afterwards), stood up, saying he would put on his uniform, ran to his bedroom, loaded his double-barrelled gun with a service bullet, took the boot off his right foot, fixed the gun against his chest, and began feeling for the trigger with his foot. But Agafya, remembering what I had told her, had her suspicions. She stole up and peeped into the room just in time. She rushed in, flung herself upon him from behind, threw her arms round him, and the gun went off, but the bullet hit the ceiling, and hurt no one. The others ran in, took away the gun, and held him by the arms. I heard all about this afterwards. I was at home, it was getting dusk, and I was just preparing to go out. I had dressed, brushed my hair, scented my handkerchief, and taken up my cap, when suddenly the door opened, and there in my lodging facing me stood Katerina Ivanovna.

"It's strange how things happen sometimes. No one had seen her in the street, so that no one knew of it in the town. I lodged with two decrepit old ladies, who looked after me. They were most obliging old things, ready to do anything for me, and at my request were as silent afterwards as two cast-iron posts. Of course I grasped the situation at once. She walked in and looked straight at me, her dark eyes determined, even defiant, but on her lips and round her mouth there was an expression of uncertainty.

" 'My sister told me,' she began, 'that you would give me 4,500 roubles if I came to you for it — myself. I have come . . . give me the money!'

"She couldn't keep it up. She choked, frightened, her voice failed her, and the corners of her mouth and the lines round it quivered. Alyosha, are you listening, or are you asleep?"

"Mitya, I know you will tell the whole truth," said Alyosha in agitation.

"I am telling it. If I tell the whole truth just as it happened I shan't spare myself. My first thought was a — Karamazov one. Once I was bitten by a centipede, brother, and laid up for a fortnight with fever from it. Well, I felt as though a centipede stung my heart then — a noxious insect, you understand? I looked her up and down. You've seen her? She's a beauty. But she was beautiful in another way then. At that moment she was beautiful because she was noble, and I was a scoundrel; she in all the grandeur of her generosity and sacrifice for her father, and I — a bug! And, scoundrel and bug that I was, she was altogether at my mercy, body and soul. She was hemmed in. I tell you frankly, that thought, that venomous thought, so possessed my heart that it almost swooned. It seemed as if there could be no resisting it; that I would act like a bug, like a venomous spider, without a spark of pity. My breath failed me. Understand, I should have gone next day to ask for her hand, so that it might end honourably, so to speak, and that nobody would or could know. For though I'm a man of base desires, I'm honest. And at that very second some voice seemed to whisper in my ear, 'But when you come tomorrow to make your proposal, that girl won't even see you; she'll order her coachman to kick you out of the yard. "Publish it through all the town," she would say, "I'm not afraid of you." ' I looked at the young lady, my voice had not deceived me. That is how it would be, not a doubt of it. I could see from her face now that I should be turned out of the house. My spite was roused. I longed to play her the nastiest swinish cad's trick: to look at her with a sneer, and on the spot where she stood before me to stun her with a tone of voice that only a shopman could use.

" 'Four thousand! What do you mean? I was joking. You've been reckoning without your host, madam. Two hundred, perhaps, yes, with pleasure. But four thousand is not a sum to throw away on such frivolity. You've put yourself out to no purpose.'

"I should have lost the game, of course. She'd have run away. But it would have been an infernal revenge. It would have been worth it all. I'd have howled with regret all the rest of my life, only to have played that trick. Would you believe it, it has never happened to me with any other woman, not one, to look at her at such a moment with hatred. But, on my oath, I looked at her for three seconds, or five perhaps, with fearful hatred — that hate which is only a hair's-breadth from love, from the maddest love!

"I went to the window, put my forehead

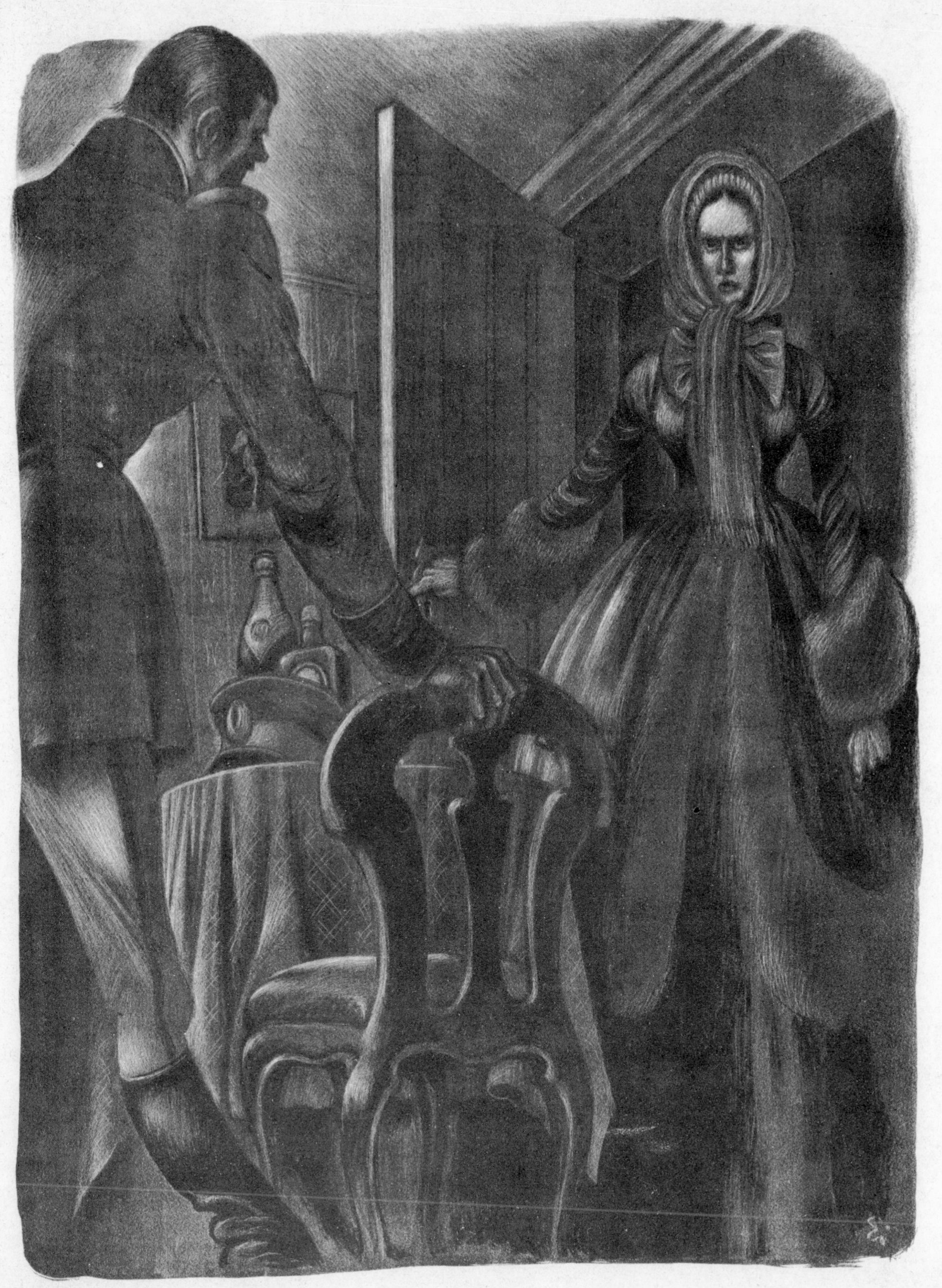

THE ARDENT HEART

against the frozen pane, and I remember the ice burnt my forehead like fire. I did not keep her long, don't be afraid. I turned round, went up to the table, opened the drawer and took out a bank-note for five thousand roubles (it was lying in a French dictionary). Then I showed it her in silence, folded it, handed it to her, opened the door into the passage, and, stepping back, made her a deep bow, a most respectful, a most impressive bow, believe me! She shuddered all over, gazed at me for a second, turned horribly pale — white as a sheet, in fact — and all at once, also without a word, not impetuously but softly, gently, bowed down to my feet — not a boarding-school curtsey, but a Russian bow, with her forehead to the floor. She jumped up and ran away. I was wearing my sword. I drew it and nearly stabbed myself with it on the spot; why, I don't know. It would have been frightfully stupid, of course. I suppose it was out of ecstasy. Can you understand that one might kill oneself out of ecstasy? But I didn't stab myself. I only kissed my sword and put it back in the scabbard — which there was no need to have told you, by the way. And I fancy that in telling you about my inner conflict I have laid it on rather thick to glorify myself. But let it pass, and to hell with all who pry into the human heart! Well, so much for that 'adventure' with Katerina Ivanovna. So now Ivan knows of it, and you — no one else."

Dmitri got up, took a step or two in his excitement, pulled out his handkerchief and mopped his forehead, then sat down again, not in the same place as before, but on the opposite side, so that Alyosha had to turn quite round to face him.

CHAPTER V

THE CONFESSION OF AN ARDENT HEART — "HEELS UP"

"Now," said Alyosha, "I understand the first half."

"You understand the first half. That half is a drama, and it was played out there. The second half is a tragedy, and it will be enacted here."

"And I understand nothing of that second half so far," said Alyosha.

"And I? Do you suppose I understand it?"

"Stop, Dmitri. There's one important question. Tell me, you were betrothed, you are betrothed still?"

"We weren't betrothed at once, not for three months after that adventure. The next day I told myself that the incident was closed, concluded, and that there would be no sequel. It seemed to me caddish to make her an offer. On her side she gave no sign of life for the six weeks that she remained in the town; except, indeed, for one action. The day after her visit the maid-servant slipped round with an envelope addressed to me. I tore it open; it contained the change out of the bank-note. Only 4,500 was needed, but there was a discount of about 200 on changing it. She only sent me about 260 roubles, I don't remember exactly, but not a note, not a word of explanation. I searched the packet for a pencil mark — n-nothing! Well, I spent the rest of the money on such an orgy that the new major was obliged to reprimand me.

"Well, the lieutenant-colonel produced the government money, to the astonishment of every one, for nobody believed that he had the money intact. He'd no sooner paid it than he fell ill, took to his bed, and, three weeks later, softening of the brain set in, and he died five days afterwards. He was buried with military honours, for he had not had time to receive his discharge. Ten days after his funeral, Katerina Ivanovna, with her aunt and sister, went to Moscow. And, behold, on the very day they went away (I hadn't seen them, didn't see them off or take leave) I received a tiny note, a sheet of blue lace-edged paper, and on it only one line in pencil: 'I will write to you. Wait. K.' And that was all.

"I'll explain the rest now, in two words. In Moscow their fortunes changed with the swiftness of lightning and the unexpectedness of an Arabian fairy-tale. That general's widow, their nearest relation, suddenly lost the two nieces who were her heiresses and next-of-kin — both died in the same week of small-pox. The old lady, prostrated with grief, welcomed Katya as a daughter, as her one hope, pounced upon her, altered her will in Katya's favour. But that concerned the future. Meanwhile she gave her, for present use, eighty thousand roubles, as a marriage portion, to do what she liked with. She was an hysterical woman. I saw something of her in Moscow, later.

"Well, suddenly I received by post four thousand five hundred roubles. I was speechless with surprise, as you may suppose. Three days later came the promised letter. I have it with me now. I always keep it, and shall keep it till I die. Shall I show you? You must read it. She offers to be my wife, offers herself to me. 'I love you madly,' she says, 'even if you don't love me, never mind. Be my husband. Don't be afraid. I won't hamper you in any way. I will be your chattel. I will be the carpet under your feet. I want to love you for ever. I want to save you from yourself.' Alyosha, I am not worthy to repeat those lines in my vile words and in my vile tone, my everlastingly vile tone, that I can never cure myself of. That letter stabs me even now. Do you think I don't mind — that I don't mind even now? I wrote her an answer at once, as it was impossible for me to go to Moscow. I wrote to her with tears. One thing I shall be ashamed of for ever. I referred to her being rich and having a dowry while I was only a stuck-up beggar! I mentioned money! I ought to have borne it in silence, but it slipped from my pen. Then I wrote at once to Ivan, and told him all I could about it in a letter of six pages, and sent him to her. Why do you look like that? Why are you staring at me? Yes, Ivan fell in love with her; he's in love with her still. I know that. I did a stupid thing, in the world's opinion; but perhaps that one stupid thing may be the saving of us all now. Oo! Don't you see what a lot she thinks of Ivan, how she respects him? When she compares us, do you suppose she can love a man like me, especially after all that has happened here?"

"But I'm convinced that she does love a man like you, and not a man like him."

"She loves her own *virtue*, not me." The words broke involuntarily, and almost maliciously, from Dmitri. He laughed, but a minute later his eyes flashed, he flushed crimson and struck the table violently with his fist.

"I swear, Alyosha," he cried, with intense and genuine anger at himself; "you may not believe me, but as God is holy, and as Christ is our Lord, I swear that though I mocked at her lofty sentiments just now, I know that I am a million times baser in soul than she, and that these lofty sentiments of hers are as sincere as a heavenly angel's. That's the tragedy of it — that I know that for certain. What if one does show off a bit? Don't I do it myself?

And yet I'm sincere, sincere. As for Ivan, don't I understand how he must be cursing Fate now — with his intellect, too! To see the preference given — to whom, to what? To a monster who, though he is betrothed and all eyes are fixed on him, can't restrain himself from debauchery — and before the very eyes of his betrothed! And a man like me is preferred, while he is rejected. And why? Because a girl wants to ruin her life and future out of gratitude. Absurd! I've never said a word of this to Ivan, and Ivan of course has never dropped a hint of the sort to me. But destiny will take its course, and the worthy man will come into his own, while the undeserving one will vanish into his back-alley for ever — his filthy back-alley, his beloved back-alley where he is at home, and there in filth and stench he will perish, of his own free will and with joy. I've been talking foolishly. I've worn out all my words. I use them at random, but it will be as I have said. I shall drown in the back-alley, and she will marry Ivan."

"Stop, brother," Alyosha interrupted again with great anxiety. "There's one thing you haven't made clear yet: you are still betrothed all the same, aren't you? How can you break off the engagement if she, your betrothed, doesn't want to?"

"Yes, formally and solemnly betrothed. It was all done on my arrival in Moscow, with great ceremony, with ikons, all in fine style. The general's widow blessed us, and — would you believe it? — congratulated Katya. 'You've made a good choice,' she said, 'I see right through him.' And, would you believe it, she didn't like Ivan, and hardly greeted him? I had a lot of talk with Katya in Moscow. I told her about myself — sincerely, honourably. She listened to everything.

There was sweet confusion,
There were tender words.

Though there were proud words, too. She wrung out of me a mighty promise to reform. I gave my promise, and here ——"

"What?"

"Why, I called to you and brought you out here to-day, this very day — remember it — to send you — this very day again — to Katerina Ivanovna, and ——"

"What?"

"To tell her that I shall never come to see her again, and that I send her my compliments."

"But is that possible?"

"That's just the reason I'm sending you in my place, because it's impossible. How could I tell her myself?"

"And where will you go?"

"To the back-alley."

"To Grushenka then!" Alyosha exclaimed sorrowfully, striking his hands together. "Can Rakitin really have told the truth? I thought that you had just visited her, and that was all."

"Can a betrothed man pay such visits? Is such a thing possible and with such a betrothed, and before the eyes of all the world? Confound it, I have some honour! As soon as I began visiting Grushenka, I ceased to be betrothed, and to be an honest man. I understand that. Why do you look at me? You see, I went in the first place to give her a beating. I had heard, and I know for a fact now, that that captain, father's agent, had handed Grushenka an IOU of mine for her to sue me for payment, so as to put a spoke in my wheels. They wanted to scare me. I set out to thrash Grushenka. I had had a glimpse of her before.

She doesn't strike one at first sight. I knew about her old merchant, who's lying ill now, paralysed; but he will leave her a decent little sum, anyhow. I knew, too, that she was fond of money, that she hoarded it, and lent it at a wicked rate of interest, that she's a merciless cheat and swindler. I went to thrash her, and I stayed. A storm broke, — a plague struck me. I'm plague-stricken still, and I know that everything is over, that there will never be anything more for me. The cycle of time is accomplished. That's my position. And though I'm a beggar, as fate would have it, I had three thousand just then in my pocket. I drove with Grushenka to Mokroye, a place twenty-five versts from here. I got gipsies there and champagne and made all the peasants there drunk on it, and all the women and girls. I sent the thousands flying. In three days' time I was stripped bare, but a hero. Do you suppose the hero had gained his end? Nothing of the sort. I tell you: it's a curve. That hussy, Grushenka, has a certain curve to her body. You can see it even in her little foot, even in the little toe of her left foot. I saw it, and kissed it, but that was all, I swear! 'I'll marry you, if you like,' she said, 'you're a beggar, you know. Say that you won't beat me, and will let me do anything I choose, and perhaps I will marry you.' She laughed, and she's laughing still!"

Dmitri leapt up in a sort of fury. It seemed all at once as though he were drunk. His eyes became suddenly bloodshot.

"And do you really mean to marry her?"

"At once, if she is willing. And if she isn't, I shall stay all the same. I'll be the porter at her gate, Alyosha!" he cried. He stopped short before him, and taking him by the shoulders began shaking him violently. "Do you know, you innocent boy, that this is all delirium, senseless delirium, for there's a tragedy here. Let me tell you, Alexey, that I may be a low man, with low and degraded passions, but a thief, a pickpocket, a housebreaker, Dmitri Karamazov can never be. Well, then; let me tell you that I am a thief and a pickpocket. That very morning, just before I went to thrash Grushenka, Katerina Ivanovna sent for me, and in strict secrecy (why I don't know, I suppose she had some reason) asked me to go to the city and to post three thousand roubles to Agafya Ivanovna in Moscow, so that nothing should be known of it in the town here. So I had that three thousand roubles in my pocket when I went to see Grushenka, and it was that money we spent at Mokroye. Afterwards I pretended I had been to the city, but did not show her the post office receipt. I said I had sent the money and would bring the receipt, and so far I haven't brought it. I've forgotten it. Now what do you think you'll answer her to-day when you say: 'He sends his compliments,' and she asks you, 'What about the money?' You could still have said to her, 'He's a degraded sensualist, and a low creature, with uncontrollable passions. He didn't send your money then, but embezzled it, because, like a low brute, he couldn't restrain himself.' But still you might have added, 'He isn't a thief though. Here is your three thousand; he sends it back. Send it yourself to Agafya Ivanovna. But he told me to say "he sends his compliments."' But, as it is, she will ask, 'But where is the money?'"

"Mitya, you are unhappy, yes! But not as unhappy as you think. Don't kill yourself with despair, don't."

"What, do you suppose I'd shoot myself because I can't get three thousand to pay back? That's just it. I shan't shoot myself. I haven't the strength now. Afterwards, perhaps. But now I'm going to Grushenka. The hell with it."

"And what will you do there?"

"I'll be her husband if she deigns to have me, and when her lover comes, I'll go into the next room. I'll clean her friends' goloshes, fan the coals for the samovar, run errands."

"Katerina Ivanovna will understand it all," Alyosha said solemnly. "She'll understand the depth of your sorrow and will forgive you. She has a lofty mind, and no one could be more unhappy than you. She'll see that for herself."

"She won't be reconciled to everything," said Dmitri, with a grin. "There's something in it, brother, that no woman could reconcile herself to. Do you know what would be the best thing to do?"

"What?"

"Pay back the three thousand."

"Where can we get it from? I say, I have two thousand. Ivan will give you another thousand — that makes three. Take it and pay it back."

"And when would you get it, your three thousand? You're not of age, besides, and you must — you absolutely must — convey my farewell to her to-day, with the money or without it, for I can't drag on any longer, things have come to such a pass. To-morrow is too late. I shall send you to father."

"To father?"

"Yes, to father first. Ask him for three thousand."

"But, Mitya, he won't give it."

"As though he would! I know he won't. Do you know the meaning of despair, Alexey?"

"Yes."

"Listen. Legally he owes me nothing. I've had it all from him, I know that. But morally he owes me something, doesn't he? You know he started with twenty-eight thousand of my mother's money and made a hundred thousand with it. Let him give me back only three out of the twenty-eight thousand, and he'll draw my soul out of hell, and it will atone for many of his sins. With that three thousand — I give you my solemn word — I'll make an end of everything, and he shall hear nothing more of me. For the last time I give him the chance to be a father. Tell him God Himself sends him this chance."

"Mitya, he won't give it for anything."

"I know he won't. I know it perfectly well. Now, especially. That's not all. I know something more. Now, only a few days ago, perhaps only yesterday, he found out for the first time *in earnest* (underline *in earnest*) that Grushenka is perhaps really not joking, and may indeed leap into marriage with me. He knows her character; he knows the cat. And do you suppose he's going to give me money to help to bring that about when he's crazy about her himself? And that's not all, either. I can tell you more than that. I know that for the last five days he has had three thousand drawn out of the bank, changed into notes of a hundred roubles, packed into a large envelope, sealed with five seals, and tied across with red tape. You see how well I know all about it! On the envelope is written: 'For my angel, Grushenka, if she will come to me.' He scrawled it himself in silence and in secret, and no one knows that the money's there except the valet, Smerdyakov, whom he trusts like himself. So now he has been expecting Grushenka for the last three or four days; he hopes she'll come for the money. He has sent her word of it, and she has sent him word that perhaps she'll come. And if she does go to the old man, can I marry her after that? You understand now why I'm here in secret and what I'm on the watch for."

"For her?"

"Yes, for her. Foma has a room in the house of these sluts here. Foma comes from our parts; he was a soldier in our regiment. He does jobs for them. He's watchman at night and goes grouse shooting in the day-time; and that's how he lives. I've established myself in his place. Neither he nor the women of the house know the secret — that is, that I am on the watch here."

"No one but Smerdyakov knows, then?"

"No one else. He will let me know if she goes to the old man."

"It was he told you about the money, then?"

"Yes. It's a dead secret. Even Ivan doesn't know about the money, or anything. The old man is sending Ivan to Chermashnya for a stay of two or three days. A purchaser has turned up for the copse: he'll give eight thousand for the timber. So the old man keeps asking Ivan to help him by going there to arrange it. It will take him two or three days. That's what the old man wants, so that Grushenka can come while he's away."

"Then he's expecting Grushenka to-day?"

"No, she won't come to-day; there are signs. She's certain not to come," cried Mitya suddenly. "Smerdyakov thinks so, too. Father's drinking now. He's sitting at table with Ivan. Go to him, Alyosha, and ask for the three thousand."

"Mitya, dear, what's the matter with you?" cried Alyosha, jumping up from his place, and looking keenly at his brother's frenzied face. For one moment the thought struck him that Dmitri had gone mad.

"What is it? I'm not insane," said Dmitri, looking intently and earnestly at him. "No fear. I am sending you to father, and I know what I'm saying. I believe in miracles."

"In miracles?"

"In a miracle of Divine Providence. God knows my heart. He sees my despair. He sees the whole picture. Surely He won't let something awful happen. Alyosha, I believe in miracles. Go!"

"I am going. Tell me, will you wait for me here?"

"Yes. I know it will take some time. You can't go at him point blank. He's drunk now. I'll wait three hours — four, five, six, seven. Only remember you must go to Katerina Ivanovna to-day, if it has to be at midnight, *with the money or without the money*, and say, 'He sends his compliments to you.' I want you to say that line to her: 'He sends his compliments to you.' "

"Mitya! And what if Grushenka comes to-day — if not to-day, to-morrow, or the next day?"

"Grushenka? I shall see her. I will rush out and prevent it."

"And if ——?"

"If there's an if, it will be murder. I couldn't endure it."

"Who will be murdered?"

"The old man. I shan't kill her."

"Brother, what are you saying?"

"Oh, I don't know. . . . I don't know. Perhaps I shan't kill him, and perhaps I shall. I'm afraid that his face will suddenly become so loathsome to me at that moment. I hate his throat, his nose, his eyes, his shameless snigger. I feel a physical repulsion. That's what I'm afraid of. That's what may be too much for me."

"I'll go, Mitya. I believe that God will order things for the best, that nothing awful may happen."

"And I will sit and wait for the miracle. And if it doesn't come to pass ——"

Alyosha went thoughtfully towards his father's house.

CHAPTER VI

SMERDYAKOV

HE did in fact find his father still at table. Though there was a dining-room in the house, the table was laid as usual in the drawing-room, which was the largest room, and furnished with old-fashioned ostentation. The furniture was white and very old, upholstered in worn red silky material. In the spaces between the windows there were mirrors in elaborate white and gilt frames, with old-fashioned carving. On the walls, covered with a white paper, which was cracked in many places, there hung two large portraits — one of some prince who had been governor of the district thirty years before, and the other of a bishop, also long since deceased. In the right-hand corner there were several ikons, before which a lamp was lighted at nightfall . . . not so much for devotional purposes as to light the room. Fyodor Pavlovich used to go to bed very late, at three or four o'clock in the morning, and would wander about the room at night or sit in an armchair, thinking. This had become a habit with him. He often slept quite alone in the house, sending his servants to the lodge; but usually Smerdyakov remained, sleeping on a bench in the hall.

When Alyosha came in, dinner was over, but coffee and preserves had been served. Fyodor Pavlovich liked sweet things with cognac after dinner. Ivan was also at table, having coffee. The servants, Grigory and Smerdyakov, were standing by. Both the gentlemen and the servants seemed in singularly good spirits. Fyodor Pavlovich was roaring with laughter. Before he entered the room, Alyosha heard the shrill laugh he knew so well, and could tell from the sound of it that his father had reached only the good-humoured stage, and was far from being completely drunk.

"Here he is! Here he is!" yelled Fyodor Pavlovich, highly delighted at seeing Alyosha. "Join us. Sit down. Coffee is a lenten dish, but it's hot and good. I don't offer you cognac, you're keeping the fast. But would you like some? No; I'd better give you some liqueur, — it's fine. Smerdyakov, go to the cupboard, the second shelf on the right. Here are the keys. Look sharp!"

Alyosha refused the liqueur.

"Never mind. If you won't have it, we will," said Fyodor Pavlovich, beaming. "But hold on — have you dined?"

"Yes," answered Alyosha, who had in truth eaten only a piece of bread and drunk a glass of kvass in the Father Superior's kitchen. "Though I should like to have some hot coffee."

"Bravo, my darling! He'll have some coffee. Does it want warming? No, it's boiling. It's capital coffee: Smerdyakov's making. My Smerdyakov's an artist at coffee and at fish patties, and at fish soup, too. You must come one day and have some fish soup. Let me know beforehand. . . . But hold on, hold on; didn't I tell you this morning to come home with your mattress and pillow and all? Have you brought your mattress? He, he, he!"

"No, I haven't," said Alyosha, smiling, too.

"Ah, but you were frightened, you were frightened this morning, weren't you? There, my darling, would I do anything to vex you? Do you know, Ivan, I can't resist the way he looks one straight in the face and laughs. I can't. It makes me shake with laughter. I just love him. Alyosha, let me give you my paternal blessing."

Alyosha rose, but Fyodor Pavlovich had already changed his mind.

"No, no," he said, "I'll just make the sign of the cross over you, now. Sit still. Now we've a treat for you, in your own line, too. It'll make you laugh. Balaam's ass has begun talking here — and how he talks! How he talks!"

Balaam's ass, it appeared, was the valet, Smerdyakov. He was a young man of about four and twenty, terribly unsociable and taciturn. Not that he was shy or bashful. On the contrary, he was conceited and seemed to despise everybody.

We must say a few words about him now. He was brought up by Grigory and Marfa, but the boy grew up "with no sense of gratitude," as Grigory expressed it; he was an unfriendly boy, and seemed to look at the world distrustfully. In his childhood he was very fond of hanging cats, and burying them with great ceremony. He used to dress up in a sheet as though it were a surplice, and sang, and waved some object over the dead cat as though it were a censer. All this he did on the sly, with the greatest secrecy. Grigory caught him once at this diversion and gave him a sound beating. He shrank into a corner and sulked there for a week. "He doesn't care for you or me, the monster," Grigory used to say to Marfa, "and he doesn't care for any one. Are you a human being?" he said, addressing the boy directly. "You're not a human being. You grew from bath-house slime. That's what you are." Smerdyakov, it appeared afterwards, could never forgive him those words. Grigory taught him to read and write, and when he was twelve years old began teaching him the Scriptures. But this teaching came to nothing. At the second or third lesson the boy suddenly grinned.

"What's the matter?" asked Grigory, looking at him threateningly over his spectacles.

"Oh, nothing. God created light on the first day, and the sun, moon, and stars on the fourth day. Where did the light come from on the first day?"

Grigory was thunderstruck. The boy looked sarcastically at his teacher. There was something positively haughty in his expression. Grigory could not restrain himself. "I'll show you where!" he cried, and gave the boy a violent slap on the cheek. The boy took the slap without a word, but withdrew into his corner again for some days. A week later he had his first attack of the disease to which he was subject all the rest of his life — epilepsy. When Fyodor Pavlovich heard of it, his attitude to the boy seemed changed at once. Till then he had taken no notice of him, though he never scolded him, and always gave him a copeck when he met him. Sometimes, when he was in good humour, he would send the boy something sweet from his table. But as soon as he heard of his illness, he showed an active interest in him, sent for a doctor, and tried remedies, but the disease turned out to be incurable. The fits occurred, on an average, once a month, but at various intervals. The fits varied, too, in violence: some were light and some were very severe. Fyodor Pavlovich strictly forbade Grigory to use corporal punishment on the boy, and began allowing him to come upstairs to him. He forbade him to be taught anything whatever for a time, too. One day when the boy was about fifteen, Fyodor Pavlovich noticed him lingering by the bookcase, and reading the titles through the glass. Fyodor Pavlovich had a fair number of books — over a hundred — but no one ever saw him reading. He at once gave Smerdyakov the key to the bookcase. "Come, read. You shall be my librarian. It'll be better for you to sit reading than to wander about the courtyard. Come, read this," and Fyodor Pavlovich gave him "Evenings in a Cottage near Dikanka."

He read a little, but didn't like it. He did not smile once, and ended by frowning.

"Why? Isn't it funny?" asked Fyodor Pavlovich.

Smerdyakov did not speak.

"Answer, stupid!"

"It's all untrue," mumbled the boy, with a grin.

"Then go to the devil! You have the soul of a lackey. Stay, here's Smaragdov's 'Universal History.' That's all true. Read that."

But Smerdyakov did not get through ten pages of Smaragdov. He thought it dull. So the bookcase was closed again.

Shortly afterwards Marfa and Grigory reported to Fyodor Pavlovich that Smerdyakov was gradually beginning to show an extraordinary fastidiousness. He would sit before his soup, take up his spoon and look into the soup, bend over it, examine it, take a spoonful and hold it to the light.

"What is it? A beetle?" Grigory would ask.

"A fly, perhaps," observed Marfa.

The squeamish youth never answered, but he did the same with his bread, his meat, and everything he ate. He would hold a piece on his fork to the light, scrutinise it as through a microscope, and only after long deliberation decide to put it in his mouth.

"Ach! What fine gentlemen's airs!" Grigory muttered, looking at him.

When Fyodor Pavlovich heard of this development in Smerdyakov he determined to make him his cook, and apprenticed him to a chef in Moscow. The apprenticeship lasted several years and he came back remarkably changed in appearance. He looked extraordinarily old for his age. His face had grown wrinkled, yellow, and he resembled a eunuch. In character he seemed almost exactly the same as before he went away. He was just as unsociable, and showed not the slightest inclination for any companionship. In Moscow, too, as we heard afterwards, he had always been silent. Moscow itself had little interest for him; he saw very little there, and took scarcely any notice of anything. He went once to the theatre, but returned silent and displeased with it. On the other hand, he came back to us from Moscow well dressed, in a clean coat and clean linen. He invariably brushed his clothes most scrupulously twice a day, and was very fond of cleaning his smart calf boots with a special English polish, so that they shone like a mirror. He turned out a first-rate cook. Fyodor Pavlovich paid him a salary, almost the whole of which Smerdyakov spent on clothes, pomade, perfumes, and such things. But he seemed to have as much contempt for the female sex as for men; he was sedate, almost unapproachable, with them. Fyodor Pavlovich began to regard him rather differently. His fits were becoming more frequent, and on the days he was ill Marfa cooked, which did not suit Fyodor Pavlovich at all.

"Why are your fits getting worse?" Fyodor Pavlovich would ask, looking askance at his new cook. "Would you like to get married? Shall I find you a wife?"

But Smerdyakov would turn pale with vexation, and make no reply. Fyodor Pavlovich would leave him with a gesture of surrender. The great thing was that he had absolute confidence in his honesty. It happened once, when Fyodor Pavlovich was drunk, that he dropped in the muddy courtyard three hundred-rouble notes which he had only just received. He missed them only the next day, and was just hastening to search his pockets when he saw the notes lying on the table. Where had they come from? Smerdyakov had picked them up and brought them in the day before.

"Well, my lad, I've never met any one like you," Fyodor Pavlovich said shortly, and gave him ten roubles. We may add that he not only believed in his honesty, but had, for some reason, a liking for him, although the young man looked as morosely at him as at every one and was always silent. He rarely spoke. If it had occurred to any one to wonder at the time what the young man was interested in, and what was in his mind, it would have been impossible to tell by looking at him. Yet he used sometimes to stop suddenly in the house, or even in the yard or street, and stand still for ten minutes, lost in thought. A physiognomist studying his face would have said that there was no thought in it, no reflection, but only a sort of contemplative look. There is a remarkable picture by the painter Kramskoy, called "Contemplation." It shows a forest in winter, and on a roadway through the forest, in absolute solitude, stands a peasant in a torn kaftan and bast shoes. He stands, as it were, lost in thought. Yet he is not thinking; he is "contemplating." If one touched him he would start and look at one as though awakening but bewildered. It's true he would come to himself immediately; but if he were asked what he had been thinking about, he would remember nothing. Yet probably he has hidden within himself the impression which had dominated him during the period of contemplation. Those impressions are dear to him and no doubt he hoards them imperceptibly, and even unconsciously. How and why, of course, he does not know either. He may suddenly, having accumulated impressions for many years, abandon everything and go off to Jerusalem on a pilgrimage for his soul's salvation, or perhaps he will suddenly set fire to his native village, or perhaps do both. There are a good many "contemplatives" among the peasantry. Well, Smerdyakov was probably one of them, and he probably was greedily hoarding up his impressions, hardly knowing why.

CHAPTER VII

CONTROVERSY

But Balaam's ass had suddenly spoken. The subject was a strange one. Grigory had gone in the morning to make purchases, and had heard from the shopkeeper Lukyanov the story of a Russian soldier which had appeared in the newspaper that day. This soldier had been taken prisoner in some remote part of Asia, and was threatened with an immediate agonising death if he did not renounce Christianity and embrace Islam. He refused to deny his faith, and was tortured, flayed alive, and died, praising and glorifying Christ. Grigory had related the story at table. Fyodor Pavlovich always liked, over the dessert after dinner, to laugh and talk, if only with Grigory. This afternoon he was in a particularly good-humoured and expansive mood. Sipping his cognac and listening to the story, he observed that a soldier like that should be immediately canonised and his skin dispatched to some monastery. "That would bring the crowds and the money."

Grigory frowned, seeing that Fyodor Pavlovich was by no means touched, but, as usual, was beginning to blaspheme. At that moment, Smerdyakov, who was standing by the door, grinned. Smerdyakov often waited at table towards the end of dinner, and since Ivan's arrival in our town he had done so every day.

"What are you grinning at?" asked Fyodor Pavlovich, catching the smile instantly, and knowing that it referred to Grigory.

"Well, my opinion is, sir," Smerdyakov began suddenly and unexpectedly in a loud voice, "that if that soldier's praiseworthy exploit was so very great there would have been, to my thinking, no sin in it if he had in such an emergency renounced, so to speak, the name of Christ and his own christening, to save by that same his life, for good deeds, by which, in the course of years to expiate his cowardice."

"How could it not be a sin? You're talking nonsense. For that you'll go straight to hell and be roasted there like mutton," put in Fyodor Pavlovich.

It was at this point that Alyosha came in, and Fyodor Pavlovich, as we have seen, was highly delighted at his appearance.

"We're on your subject, your subject," he chuckled gleefully, making Alyosha sit down to listen.

"As for mutton, sir, that's not so, and there'll be no punishment there for this, and there shouldn't be either, in all justice, sir," Smerdyakov maintained sedately.

"How do you mean 'in all justice'?" Fyodor Pavlovich cried still more gaily, nudging Alyosha with his knee.

"He's a rascal, that's what he is!" burst from Grigory. He looked Smerdyakov wrathfully in the face.

"As for being a rascal, wait a little, Grigory Vasilyevich," answered Smerdyakov with perfect composure. "You'd better consider yourself that, once I am taken prisoner by the enemies of the Christian race, and they demand that I curse the name of God and renounce my holy baptism, I am fully empowered by my own reason to do so, for there would be no sin in it."

"But you've said that before. Don't waste words. Prove it," cried Fyodor Pavlovich.

"Bouillon-maker!" muttered Grigory contemptuously.

"As for being a bouillon-maker, wait a bit, too, and consider for yourself, Grigory Vasilyevich, without abusing me. For as soon as I say to those torturers, 'No, I'm not a Christian, and I curse my true God,' then at once, by God's high judgment, I become immediately and specially anathema accursed, and am cut off from the Holy Church, exactly as though I were a heathen, so that at that very instant, not only when I say it aloud, but when I think of saying it, before a quarter of a second has passed, I am cut off. Is that so or not, Grigory Vasilyevich?"

He addressed Grigory with obvious satisfaction, though he was really answering Fyodor Pavlovich's questions, and was well aware of it, and intentionally pretending that the questions had come from Grigory.

"Ivan," cried Fyodor Pavlovich suddenly, "stoop down, I must whisper something to you. He's got this all up for your benefit. He wants you to compliment him. Compliment him."

Ivan listened with perfect seriousness to his father's excited whisper.

"Wait, Smerdyakov, be quiet a minute," cried Fyodor Pavlovich once more. "Ivan, your ear again."

Ivan bent down again with a perfectly grave face.

"I love you as I do Alyosha. Don't think I don't love you. Some cognac?"

"Yes." But you're rather drunk yourself, thought Ivan, looking steadily at his father.

He was watching Smerdyakov with great curiosity.

"You're anathema accursed, as it is," Grigory suddenly burst out, "and how dare you argue, you rascal, after that, if . . ."

"Don't scold him, Grigory, don't scold him," Fyodor Pavlovich cut him short.

"You should wait, Grigory Vasilyevich, if only a short time, and listen, for I haven't finished all I had to say. For at the very moment I become accursed of God, at that same highest moment, I become exactly like a heathen, and my baptism is removed and becomes of no avail. Isn't that so?"

"Make haste and finish, my boy," Fyodor Pavlovich urged him, sipping from his wineglass with relish.

"And if I've ceased to be a Christian, then I told no lie to the torturers when they asked whether I was a Christian or not a Christian, seeing I had already been relieved by God Himself of my Christianity by reason of the thought alone, before I had time to utter a word to the torturers. And if I have already been demoted, in what manner and with what sort of justice can I be held responsible as a Christian in the other world for having denied Christ, when, through the very thought alone, before denying Him I had been relieved of my baptism? If I'm no longer a Christian, then I can't renounce Christ, for I've nothing then to renounce. Who will hold an unclean Tatar responsible, Grigory Vasilyevich, even in heaven, for not having been born a Christian? And who would punish him for that, considering that you can't take two skins off one ox? For God Almighty Himself, even if He did make the Tatar responsible, when he dies would give him the smallest possible punishment, I imagine (since he must be punished), judging that he is not to blame if he has come into the world an unclean heathen, from heathen parents. The Lord God can't surely take a Tatar and say he was a Christian? That would mean that the Almighty would tell a real untruth. And can the Lord of heaven and earth tell a lie, even in one word?"

Grigory was thunderstruck and looked at the orator, his eyes nearly starting out of his head. Though he did not clearly understand what was said, he had caught something in this rigmarole, and stood, looking like a man who has just hit his head against a wall. Fyodor Pavlovich emptied his glass and went off into his shrill laugh.

"Alyosha! Alyosha! What do you say to that! Ah, you casuist! He must have been with the Jesuits somewhere, Ivan. Oh, you stinking Jesuit, who taught you? But you're talking nonsense, you casuist, nonsense, nonsense, nonsense. Don't cry, Grigory, we'll reduce him to smoke and ashes in a moment. Tell me this, oh, ass; you may be right before your torturers, but you have renounced your faith all the same in your own heart, and you say yourself that in that very hour you became anathema accursed. And if once you're anathema they won't pat you on the head for it in hell. What do you say to that, my fine Jesuit?"

"There is no doubt, sir, that I have renounced it in my own heart, sir, but there was no special sin in that. Or if there was sin, sir, it was of the most ordinary kind."

"How's that, the most ordinary kind?"

"You lie, accursed one!" hissed Grigory.

"Consider yourself, Grigory Vasilyevich," Smerdyakov went on, staid and unruffled, conscious of his triumph, but, as it were, generous to the vanquished foe. "Consider yourself, Grigory Vasilyevich; it is said in Scripture that if you have faith, even as a mustard seed, and bid a mountain move into the sea, it will move without the least delay at your bidding. Well, Grigory Vasilyevich, if I'm without faith and you have so great a faith that you are continually swearing at me, you try yourself telling this mountain, not to move into the sea, for that's a long way off, but even to our stinking little river which runs beyond our garden. You'll see for yourself that it won't budge, but will remain just where it is however much you shout at it, and that shows, Grigory Vasilyevich, that you haven't faith in the proper manner, and only abuse others about it. Again, taking into consideration that no one in our day, not only you, but actually no one, from the highest person to the lowest peasant, can shove mountains into the sea — except perhaps some one man in the world, or, at most, two, and they most likely are saving their souls in secret somewhere in the Egyptian desert, so you wouldn't find them — if so it be, if all the rest have no faith, will God curse all the rest? that is, the population of the whole earth, except about two hermits in the desert, and in His well-known mercy will He not forgive one of them? And so I trust that though I may once have doubted I shall be forgiven if I shed tears of repentance."

"Wait!" cried Fyodor Pavlovich, in a transport of delight. "So you do suppose there are two who can move mountains, that they do exist? Ivan, make a note of it, write it down. There you have the Russian all over!"

"You're quite right in saying it's characteristic of the people's faith," Ivan assented, with an approving smile.

"You agree. Then it must be so, if you agree. It's true, isn't it, Alyosha? That's the Russian faith all over, isn't it?"

"No, Smerdyakov has not the Russian faith at all," said Alyosha firmly and gravely.

"I'm not talking about his faith. I mean those two in the desert, only that idea. Surely that's Russian, isn't it?"

"Yes, that's purely Russian," said Alyosha, smiling.

"Your words are worth a gold piece, oh, ass, and I'll give it to you to-day. But as for the rest, you talk nonsense, nonsense, nonsense. Let me tell you, stupid, that we here are all of little faith, only from carelessness, because we haven't time; in the first place, things are too much for us, and, in the second place, the Lord God has given us so little time, only twenty-four hours in the day, so that one hasn't even time to get sleep enough, much less to repent of one's sins. But you there, you denied your faith to your torturers when you'd nothing else to think about but your faith and nothing else to do but show your faith. So I consider, brother, that it constitutes a sin."

"Constitute a sin it may, but consider yourself, Grigory Vasilyevich, that it only extenuates it, if it does constitute it. If I had believed then in very truth, as I ought to have believed, then it really would have been sinful if I had not faced tortures for my faith, and had gone over to the filthy Mohammedan faith. But, of course, it wouldn't have come to torture then, because I should only have had to say at that instant to the mountain, 'Move and crush the tormentor,' and it would have moved and at the very instant have crushed him like a black-beetle, and I should have walked away as though nothing had happened, praising and glorifying God. But, suppose at that very moment I had tried all that, and cried to that mountain, 'Crush these tormentors,' and it hadn't crushed them, how could I have helped doubting, pray, at such a time, and at such a dread hour of mortal terror? And apart from that, I should know already that I could not attain to the fulness of the Kingdom of Heaven (for since the mountain had not moved at my word, they could not think very much of my faith up aloft, and there could be no very great reward awaiting me in the world to come). So why should I let them flay the skin off me as well, and to no good purpose? For, even though they had flayed my skin half off my back, even then the mountain would not have moved at my word or at my cry. And at such a moment not only doubt might come over one, but one might lose one's reason from fear, so that one would not be able to think at all. And, therefore, how should I be particularly to blame, if, not seeing my advantage or reward there or here, I should, at least, save my skin? And so trusting fully in the grace of the Lord I should cherish the hope that I might be altogether forgiven, sir."

CHAPTER VIII

OVER THE COGNAC

THE controversy was over. But strange to say Fyodor Pavlovich, who had been so gay, suddenly began frowning. He frowned and gulped some cognac, and it was already a glass too much.

"Get along with you, Jesuits!" he cried to the servants. "Get out, Smerdyakov. I'll send you the gold piece I promised you to-day, but be off! Don't cry, Grigory. Go to Marfa. She'll comfort you and put you to bed. The rascals won't let me sit in peace after dinner," he snapped peevishly, as the servants promptly withdrew at his word.

"Smerdyakov always pokes himself in now, after dinner. It's you he's so interested in. What have you done to fascinate him?" he added to Ivan.

"Nothing whatever," answered Ivan. "He's pleased to have a high opinion of me; he's a lackey and a mean soul. Worms'-meat of progress, however, when the time comes."

"Of progress?"

"There will be others and better ones. But there will be some like him as well. His kind will come first, and better ones after."

"And when will the time come?"

"The rocket will go off and fizzle out, perhaps. The people are not very fond of listening to these bouillon-makers, so far."

"Ah, brother, but a Balaam's ass like that thinks and thinks, and the devil knows where he'll end."

"He's storing up ideas," said Ivan, smiling.

"You see, I know he can't bear me, nor any one else, even you, though you fancy that he has a high opinion of you. Worse still with Alyosha, he despises Alyosha. But he doesn't steal, that's one thing, and he's not a gossip, he holds his tongue, and doesn't wash our dirty linen in public. He makes capital fish patties, too. But, damn him, is he worth talking about so much?"

"Of course he isn't."

"And as for the ideas he may be hatching, the Russian peasant, generally speaking, needs flogging. That I've always maintained. Our peasant is a swindler, and doesn't deserve to be pitied, and it's a good thing he's still thrashed sometimes. Russia's strength is in the birch. If they destroy the forests, Russia will perish. I stand up for the clever people. We've left off thrashing the peasants, we've grown so clever, but they go on thrashing themselves. And a good thing, too. 'For with what measure ye mete it shall be measured to you again,' or how does it go? Anyhow, it will be measured out. But Russia's all swinishness. My dear, if you only knew how I hate Russia. . . . That is, not Russia, but all this vice! But maybe I mean Russia. *Tout cela c'est de la cochonnerie.* . . . Do you know what I like? I like wit."

"You've had another glass. That's enough."

"Wait. I'll have one more, and then another, and then I'll stop. No, stop, you interrupted me. At Mokroye I was talking to an old peasant, and he told me: 'There's nothing we like so much as sentencing girls to be thrashed, and we always give the lads the job of thrashing them. And the girl he has thrashed to-day, the young man will ask in marriage to-morrow. So it quite suits the girls, too,' he said. There's a set of de Sades for you! But it's clever, anyway. Shall we go over and have a look at it, eh? Alyosha, are you blushing? Don't be bashful, child. I'm sorry I didn't stay to dinner at the Father Superior's and tell the monks about the girls at Mokroye. Alyosha, don't be angry that I offended your Superior this morning. I lost my temper. If there is a God, if He exists, then, of course, I'm to blame, and I shall have to answer for it. But if there isn't a God at all, don't they deserve worse, your fathers? It's not enough to cut their heads off, for they keep back progress. Would you believe it, Ivan, that this hurts my feelings? No, you don't believe it, as I see from your eyes. You believe what people say, that I'm nothing but a buffoon. Alyosha, do you believe that I'm nothing but a buffoon?"

"No, I don't believe it."

"And I believe you don't, and that you speak the truth. You look sincere and you speak sincerely. But not Ivan. Ivan's supercilious. . . . I'd make an end of your monastery, though, all the same. I'd take all that mystic stuff and suppress it, once for all, all over Russia, so as to bring all the fools to reason. And the gold and the silver that would flow into the mint!"

"But why suppress it?" asked Ivan.

"That Truth may prevail the sooner."

"Well, if Truth were to prevail, you know, you'd be the first to be robbed and . . . suppressed."

"Bah! I dare say you're right. Ah, I'm an ass!" burst out Fyodor Pavlovich, striking himself lightly on the forehead.

"Well, your monastery may stand then, Alyosha, if that's how it is. And we clever people will sit snug and enjoy our cognac. You know, Ivan, it must have been so ordained by the Almighty Himself. Ivan, speak, is there a God or not? Wait: speak the truth, speak seriously. Why are you laughing again?"

"I'm laughing because you made a clever remark just now about Smerdyakov's belief in the existence of two saints who could move mountains."

"Why, am I like him now, then?"

"Very much."

"Well, that shows I'm a Russian, too, and I have a Russian trait. And you may be caught in the same way, though you are a philosopher. Shall I catch you? What do you bet that I'll catch you to-morrow. Speak, all the same, is there a God, or not? Only, be serious. I want you to be serious now."

"No, there is no God."

"Alyosha, is there a God?"

"There is."

"Ivan, and is there immortality, some sort of immortality, just a little, just a tiny bit?"

"There is no immortality either."

"None at all?"

"None at all."

"There's absolute nothingness then. Perhaps there is just something? Not altogether nothing!"

"Absolute nothingness."

"Alyosha, is there immortality?"

"There is."

"God and immortality?"

"God and immortality. In God is immortality."

"H'm! It's more likely Ivan's right. Good Lord! to think what faith, what force of all kinds, man has lavished for nothing, on that dream, and for how many thousand years. Who is it that is making a mock of man this way? Ivan! For the last time, once for all, is there a God or not? I ask for the last time!"

"And for the last time, there is not."

"Who is laughing at man, then, Ivan?"

"The devil, perhaps," said Ivan, smiling.

"And the devil? Does he exist?"

"No, he doesn't."

"It's a pity. Damn it all, what wouldn't I do to the man who first invented God! Hanging on a bitter aspen tree would be too good for him."

"There would have been no civilisation if they hadn't invented God."

"Wouldn't there have been? Without God?"

"No. And there would have been no cognac either. But I must take your cognac away from you, anyway."

"Stop, stop, stop, dear boy, one more little glass. I've hurt Alyosha's feelings. You're not angry with me, Alyosha? My dear little Alexey!"

"No, I am not angry. I know your thoughts. Your heart is better than your head."

"My heart better than my head, is it? Oh, Lord! And that from you. Ivan, do you love Alyosha?"

"I do."

"You must love him." (Fyodor Pavlovich was getting very drunk.) "Listen, Alyosha, I was rude to your elder this morning. But I was excited. But there's wit in that elder, don't you think, Ivan?"

"Very likely."

"There is, there is. *Il y a du Piron là dedans*. He's a Jesuit, a Russian one, that is. As he's an honourable person there's a hidden indignation boiling within him at having to pretend and affect holiness."

"But, of course, he believes in God."

"Not a bit of it. Didn't you know? Why, he tells every one so, himself. That is, not every one, but all the clever people who come to him. He said straight out to Governor Schultz not long ago: '*Credo*, but I don't know in what.' "

"Really?"

"He really did. But I respect him. There's something of Mephistopheles about him, or rather of 'The hero of our time.' . . . Arbenin, or what's his name? . . . You see, he's a sensualist. He's such a sensualist that I should be afraid for my daughter or my wife if she went to confess to him. You know, when he begins telling stories . . . The year before last he invited us to tea, tea with liqueur (the ladies send him liqueur), and began telling us about old times till we nearly split our sides. . . . Especially how he once cured a paralysed woman. 'If my legs were not bad I know a dance I could dance you,' he said. What do you say to that? 'I've played plenty of tricks in my time,' said he. He did Demidov, the merchant, out of sixty thousand."

"What, he stole it?"

"He brought him the money as a man he could trust, saying, 'Take care of it for me, brother, the police will be searching my place to-morrow.' And he kept it. 'You have given it to the Church,' he declared. I said to him: 'You're a scoundrel,' I said. 'No,' said he, 'I'm not a scoundrel, but I'm broad-minded.' But that wasn't he, that was some one else. I've muddled him with some one else . . . without noticing it. Come, another glass and that's enough. Take away the bottle, Ivan. I've been telling lies. Why didn't you stop me, Ivan, and tell me I was lying?"

"I knew you'd stop of yourself."

"That's a lie. You did it from spite, from simple spite against me. You despise me. You have come to me and you despise me in my own house."

"Well, I'll leave. It's the cognac working in you."

"I've begged you for Christ's sake to go to Chermashnya for a day or two, and you don't go."

"I'll go to-morrow if you're so set up on it."

"You won't go. You want to keep an eye on me. That's what you want, you spiteful soul. That's why you won't go."

The old man persisted. He had reached that state of drunkenness when the drunkard who has till then been inoffensive tries to pick a quarrel and to assert himself.

"Why are you looking at me? Why do you look like that? Your eyes look at me and say, 'The drunken mug!' Your eyes are suspicious, they're contemptuous. . . . You've come here with some design. Alyosha, here, looks at me and his eyes shine. Alyosha doesn't despise me. Alexey, you mustn't love Ivan."

"Don't be cross with my brother. Leave off insulting him," Alyosha said suddenly and with emphasis.

"Oh, all right. Ugh, my head aches. Take away the cognac, Ivan. It's the third time I've told you."

He mused, and suddenly a slow, cunning grin spread over his face.

"Don't be angry with a feeble old man, Ivan. I know you don't love me, but don't be angry all the same. There's nothing to love me for. You go to Chermashnya. I'll come to you myself and bring you a present. I'll show you a little wench there. I've had my eye on her a long time. She's still running about barefoot. Don't be afraid of bare-footed wenches — don't despise them — they're pearls!"

And he kissed his hand with a smack.

"To me . . ." he revived at once, seeming to grow sober the instant he touched on his favourite topic. "To me . . . Ah, you boys! You children, little sucking pigs, to me . . . all my life a woman has never seemed ugly — that's been my rule! Can you understand that? How could you understand it? You've still milk in your veins, not blood. You're not hatched yet. My rule has been that you can always find something devilishly interesting in every woman that you wouldn't find in any other. Only, one must know how to find it, that's the point! That's a talent! To my mind there are no homely women. The very fact that she is a woman is half the battle . . . but how could you understand that? Even in *vieilles filles*, even in them you may discover something that makes you simply wonder that men have been such fools as to let them grow old without noticing them. Bare-footed girls or unattractive ones, you must take by surprise. Didn't you know that? You must astound them till they're fascinated, pierced, ashamed that such a gentleman should fall in love with such a little slut. It's a jolly good thing that there always are and always will be masters and slaves in the world, so there always will be a little maid-of-all-work and her master, and you know, that's all that's needed for happiness. Wait . . . listen, Alyosha, I always used to astonish your late mother, but in a different way. I used to neglect her completely, but all at once, when the moment came, I'd be all devotion to her, crawl on my knees, kiss her feet, and I always, always — I remember it as though it were to-day — reduced her to that tinkling, quiet, nervous, queer little laugh. It was peculiar to her. I knew her attacks always used to begin like that, the next day she would begin shrieking hysterically, and this little laugh was not a sign of delight, but it made a very good counterfeit. That's what it means to be able to find the right thing in every one. Once Belyavsky — he was a handsome fellow, and rich — he courted her and made a habit of coming here — suddenly gave me a slap in the face in my own house and in her presence. And she — such a sheep — why, I thought she would have knocked me down for that blow. How she set on me! 'You're beaten, beaten now,' she said. 'You've taken a blow from him. You have been trying to sell me to him,' she said. . . . 'And how dared he strike you in my presence! Don't dare come near me again, never, never! Run at once, challenge him to a duel!' . . . I took her to the monastery then to bring her to her senses. The holy fathers prayed over her. But I swear, by God, Alyosha, I never harmed my poor possessed girl! Only once, perhaps, in the first year; she was already very fond of praying. She used to keep the feasts of Our Lady particularly and used to turn me out of her room then. I'll knock that mysticism out of her, thought I! 'Here,' said I, 'you see your holy image. Here it is. Here I take it down. You believe it's a miracle-working ikon, but here, I'll spit on it directly and nothing will happen to me for it!' . . . When she saw it, good Lord! I thought she would kill me. But she only jumped up, struck her hands together, then suddenly hid her face in them, began trembling all over and fell on the floor . . . fell all of a heap. Alyosha, Alyosha, what's the matter?"

The old man jumped up in alarm. From the time he had begun speaking about his mother, a change had gradually come over Alyosha's face. He flushed crimson, his eyes glowed, his lips quivered. The old sot had gone spluttering on, noticing nothing, till the moment when something very strange happened to Alyosha. Precisely what he was describing in the possessed woman was suddenly repeated in Alyosha. He jumped up from his seat exactly as his mother was said to have done, struck his hands together, hid his face in them, and dropped into the chair, shaking all over in an hysterical paroxysm of sudden, violent, silent weeping. His extraordinary resemblance to his mother particularly startled the old man.

"Ivan, Ivan! Water, quickly! It's like her, exactly as she used to be then, his mother. Spurt some water on him from your mouth, that's what I used to do to her. He's upset about his mother, his mother," he muttered to Ivan.

"But she was my mother, too, I believe, his mother. Was she not?" said Ivan, with uncontrolled anger and contempt. The old man shrank before his flashing eyes. But something very strange had happened, though only for a second; it seemed really to have escaped the old man's mind that Alyosha's mother actually was Ivan's mother, too.

"Your mother?" he muttered, not understanding. "What do you mean? What mother are you talking about? Was she? . . . Why, damn it! of course she was yours, too! Damn it! My mind's gone back on me, that never happened to me before. Excuse me, why, I was thinking, Ivan . . . He, he, he!" He stopped. A broad, drunken, half senseless grin overspread his face.

At that moment a fearful noise and clamour was heard in the hall, there were violent shouts, the door was flung open, and Dmitri burst into the room. The old man rushed to Ivan in terror.

"He'll kill me! He'll kill me! Don't let him get at me!" he screamed, clinging to the skirt of Ivan's coat.

CHAPTER IX

THE SENSUALISTS

GRIGORY and Smerdyakov ran into the room right after Dmitri. They had been struggling with him in the passage, refusing to admit him, acting on instructions given them by Fyodor Pavlovich some days before. Taking advantage of the fact that Dmitri stopped a moment on entering the room to look about him, Grigory ran round the table, closed the double doors on the opposite side of the room leading to the inner apartments, and stood before the closed doors, stretching wide his arms, prepared to defend the entrance, so to speak, with the last drop of his blood. Seeing this, Dmitri uttered a scream rather than a shout and rushed at Grigory.

"Then she's there! She's hidden there! Out of the way, scoundrel!"

He tried to pull Grigory away, but the old servant pushed him back. Beside himself with fury, Dmitri struck out, and hit Grigory with all his might. The old man fell like a log, and Dmitri, leaping over him, broke in the door. Smerdyakov remained pale and trembling at the other end of the room, huddling close to Fyodor Pavlovich.

"She's here!" shouted Dmitri. "I saw her turn towards the house just now, but I couldn't catch her. Where is she? Where is she?"

That shout, "She's here!" produced an indescribable effect on Fyodor Pavlovich. All his fright left him.

"Hold him! Hold him!" he cried, and dashed after Dmitri. Meanwhile Grigory had got up from the floor, but still seemed stunned. Ivan and Alyosha ran after their father. In the third room something was heard to fall on the floor with a ringing crash: it was a large glass vase — not an expensive one — on a marble pedestal which Dmitri had brushed against as he ran past it.

"At him!" shouted the old man. "Help!"

Ivan and Alyosha caught the old man and were forcibly bringing him back.

"Why do you run after him? He'll murder you outright," Ivan cried wrathfully at his father.

"Ivan! Alyosha! She must be here. Grushenka's here. He said he saw her himself, running."

He was choking. He was not expecting

Grushenka at the time, and the sudden news that she was there overwhelmed him. He was trembling all over. He seemed frantic.

"But you've seen for yourself that she hasn't come," cried Ivan.

"But she may have come by that other entrance."

"You know that entrance is locked, and you have the key."

Dmitri suddenly reappeared in the drawing-room. He had, of course, found the other entrance locked, and the key actually was in Fyodor Pavlovich's pocket. The windows of all the rooms were closed, too, so that Grushenka could not have come in anywhere nor have run out anywhere.

"Hold him!" shrieked Fyodor Pavlovich, as soon as he saw him again. "He's been stealing money in my bedroom." And tearing himself from Ivan he rushed again at Dmitri. But Dmitri threw up both hands and suddenly clutched the old man by the two tufts of hair that remained on his temples, tugged at them, and flung him with a crash on the floor. He kicked him two or three times in the face with his heel. The old man moaned shrilly. Ivan, though not so strong as Dmitri, threw his arms round him, and with all his might pulled him away. Alyosha helped him with his slender strength, holding Dmitri in front.

"Madman! You've killed him!" cried Ivan.

"Serve him right!" shouted Dmitri breathlessly. "If I haven't killed him, I'll come again and kill him. You can't protect him!"

"Dmitri! Go away at once!" cried Alyosha commandingly.

"Alexey! You tell me. It's only you I can believe; was she here just now, or not? I saw her myself creeping this way by the fence from the lane. I shouted, she ran away."

"I swear she's not been here, and no one expected her."

"But I saw her. . . . So she must . . . I'll find out at once where she is. . . . Good-bye, Alexey! Not a word to Æsop about the money now. But go to Katerina Ivanovna at once and be sure to say, 'He sends his compliments to you!' Compliments, his compliments! Just compliments and farewell! Describe the scene to her."

Meanwhile Ivan and Grigory had lifted up the old man and seated him in an armchair. His face was covered with blood, but he was conscious and listened greedily to Dmitri's cries. He was still fancying that Grushenka really was somewhere in the house. Dmitri looked at him with hatred as he went out.

"I don't repent shedding your blood!" he cried. "Beware, old man, beware of your dream, for I have my dream, too. I curse you, and disown you altogether."

He ran out of the room.

"She's here. She must be here. Smerdyakov! Smerdyakov!" the old man wheezed, almost inaudibly, beckoning to him with his finger.

"No, she's not here, you old lunatic!" Ivan shouted at him angrily. "Here, he's fainting! Water! A towel! Hurry, Smerdyakov!"

Smerdyakov ran for water. At last they got the old man undressed, and put him to bed. They wrapped a wet towel round his head. Exhausted by the cognac, by his violent emotion, and the blows he had received, he shut his eyes and fell asleep as soon as his head touched the pillow. Ivan and Alyosha went back to the drawing-room. Smerdyakov removed the fragments of the broken vase, while Grigory stood by the table looking gloomily at the floor.

"Shouldn't you put a wet bandage on your head and go to bed, too?" Alyosha said to him.

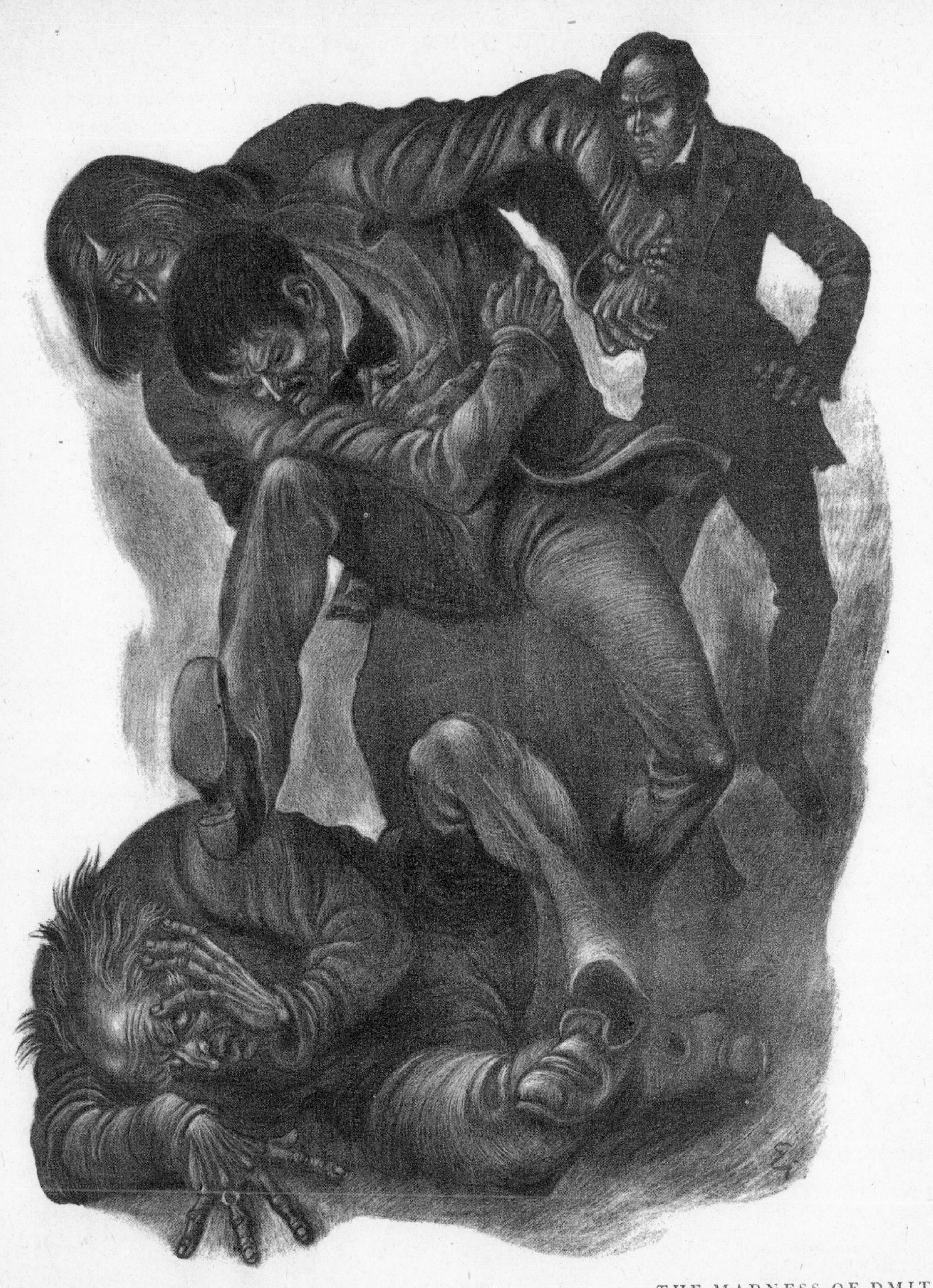

THE MADNESS OF DMITRI

"We'll look after him. My brother gave you a terrible blow — on the head."

"He's insulted me!" Grigory articulated gloomily and distinctly.

"He's 'insulted' his father, not only you," observed Ivan with a forced smile.

"I used to wash him in his tub. He's insulted me," repeated Grigory.

"Damn it all, if I hadn't pulled him away perhaps he'd have murdered him. It wouldn't take much to do for Æsop, would it?" whispered Ivan to Alyosha.

"God forbid!" cried Alyosha.

"Why should He forbid?" Ivan went on in the same whisper, with a malignant grimace. "One reptile will devour the other. And serve them both right, too."

Alyosha shuddered.

"Of course I won't allow the murder to take place any more than I did just now. Stay here, Alyosha, I'll go for a turn in the yard. My head's begun to ache."

Alyosha went to his father's bedroom and sat by his bedside behind the screen for about an hour. The old man suddenly opened his eyes and gazed for a long while at Alyosha, evidently remembering and thinking. All at once his face betrayed extraordinary excitement. "Alyosha," he whispered apprehensively, "where's Ivan?"

"In the yard. He's got a headache. He's on the watch."

"Give me that looking-glass. It stands over there. Give it me."

Alyosha gave him a little round folding looking-glass which stood on the chest of drawers. The old man looked at himself in it; his nose was considerably swollen, and on the left side of his forehead there was a rather large crimson bruise.

"What does Ivan say? Alyosha, my dear, my only son, I'm afraid of Ivan. I'm more afraid of Ivan than of the other. You're the only one I'm not afraid of. . . ."

"Don't be afraid of Ivan either. He is angry, but he'll defend you."

"Alyosha, and what of the other? He's run to Grushenka. My angel, tell me the truth, was she here just now or not?"

"No one has seen her. It was a mistake. She has not been here."

"You know Mitya wants to marry her, to marry her."

"She won't marry him."

"She won't. She won't. She won't. She won't on any account!"

The old man fairly fluttered with joy, as though nothing more comforting could have been said to him. In his delight he seized Alyosha's hand and pressed it warmly to his heart. Tears positively glittered in his eyes.

"That image of the Mother of God of which I was telling you just now," he said. "Take it home and keep it for yourself. And I give you permission to go back to the monastery. . . . I was joking this morning, don't be angry with me. My head aches, Alyosha. . . . Alyosha, comfort my heart. Be an angel and tell me the truth!"

"You're still asking whether she has been here or not?" Alyosha said sorrowfully.

"No, no, no. I believe you. I'll tell you what it is: you go to Grushenka yourself, or see her somehow; make haste and ask her; see for yourself, which she means to choose, him or me? Eh? What? Can you, or can't you?"

"If I see her I'll ask her," Alyosha muttered, embarrassed.

"No, she won't tell you," the old man interrupted, "she's a minx. She'll begin kissing you and say that it's you she wants. She's a deceitful, shameless hussy. You mustn't go to her, you mustn't!"

"No, father, and it wouldn't be suitable, it wouldn't be right at all."

"Where was he sending you just now? He shouted 'Go' as he ran away."

"To Katerina Ivanovna."

"For money? To ask her for money?"

"No. Not for money."

"He's no money; not a bit. I'll settle down for the night, and think things over, and you can go. Perhaps you'll meet her. . . . Only be sure to come to me to-morrow in the morning. Be sure to. I have a word to say to you to-morrow. Will you come?"

"Yes."

"When you come, pretend you've come of your own accord to ask after me. Don't tell any one I told you to. Don't say a word to Ivan."

"Very well."

"Good-bye, my angel. You stood up for me, just now. I shall never forget it. I've a word to say to you to-morrow — but I must think about it."

"And how do you feel now?"

"I shall get up to-morrow and go out, perfectly well, perfectly well!"

Crossing the yard, Alyosha found Ivan sitting on the bench at the gateway. He was sitting writing something in pencil in his notebook. Alyosha told Ivan that their father had waked up, was conscious, and had let him go back to sleep at the monastery.

"Alyosha, I should be very glad to meet you to-morrow morning," said Ivan cordially, standing up. His cordiality was a complete surprise to Alyosha.

"I shall be at the Hohlakovs' to-morrow," answered Alyosha, "I may be at Katerina Ivanovna's, too, if I don't find her now."

"But you're going to her now, anyway? For that 'compliments and farewell,'" said Ivan, smiling. Alyosha was disconcerted.

"I think I quite understand his exclamations just now, and part of what went before. Dmitri has asked you to go to her and say that he — well, in fact — takes his leave of her?"

"Brother, how will all this horror end between father and Dmitri?" exclaimed Alyosha.

"One can't tell for certain. Perhaps in nothing: it may all fizzle out. That woman is a beast. In any case we must keep the old man indoors and not let Dmitri into the house."

"Brother, let me ask one thing more: has any man a right to look at other men and decide who is worthy to live and who isn't?"

"Why bring in the question of worth? The matter is most often decided in men's hearts on other grounds much more natural. And as for rights — who has not the right to wish?"

"Not for another man's death?"

"What even if for another man's death? Why lie to oneself, since all men live so and perhaps cannot help living so. Are you referring to what I said just now — that one reptile will devour the other? In that case let me ask you, do you think me, like Dmitri, capable of shedding Æsop's blood, murdering him?"

"What are you saying, Ivan? Such an idea never crossed my mind. I don't think Dmitri is capable of it, either."

"Thanks, if only for that," smiled Ivan. "Be sure, I should always defend him. But in my wishes I reserve myself full latitude in this case. Good-bye till to-morrow. Don't condemn me, and don't look on me as a villain," he added with a smile.

They shook hands warmly as they had never done before. Alyosha felt that his brother had taken the first step towards him, and that he had certainly done this with some definite purpose.

CHAPTER X

BOTH TOGETHER

ALYOSHA left his father's house feeling even more broken and dejected in spirit than when he had entered it. His mind, too, seemed crushed and scattered, as it were, while he felt that he was afraid to put together the disjointed fragments and form a general idea from all the agonising and conflicting experiences of the day. He felt something bordering upon despair, which he had never known till then. Towering like a mountain above all the rest stood the fatal insoluble question: How would things end between his father and his brother Dmitri with this terrible woman? Now he had himself been a witness of it, he had been present and seen them face to face. Yet only his brother Dmitri could be made unhappy, terribly, completely unhappy: there was trouble awaiting him. It appeared, too, that there were other people concerned, far more so than Alyosha could have supposed before. There was something positively mysterious in it, too. Ivan had made a step towards him, which was what Alyosha had long been desiring. Yet now he felt for some reason that he was frightened by this advance. And these women? Strange to say, that morning he had set out for Katerina Ivanovna's in the greatest embarrassment; now he felt nothing of the kind. On the contrary, he was hastening there as though expecting to find guidance from her. Yet to give her this message was obviously more difficult than before. The matter of the three thousand was decided irrevocably, and Dmitri, feeling himself dishonoured and losing his last hope, might sink to any depth. He had, moreover, told him to describe to Katerina Ivanovna the scene which had just taken place with his father.

It was by now seven o'clock, and it was getting dark as Alyosha entered the very spacious and comfortable house on Bolshaya Street occupied by Katerina Ivanovna. Alyosha knew that she lived with two aunts. One of them, a silent woman, was that aunt of her half-sister Agafya Ivanovna who had looked after her in her father's house when she came from boarding-school. The other aunt was a Moscow lady of style and consequence, though in straitened circumstances. It was said that they both gave way in everything to Katerina Ivanovna, and that she kept them with her only for the sake of the proprieties. Katerina Ivanovna herself heeded no one but her benefactress, the general's widow, who had been kept by illness in Moscow, and to whom she was obliged to write twice a week a full account of all her doings.

When Alyosha entered the hall and asked the maid who opened the door to announce him, it was evident that they were already aware of his arrival. Possibly he had been noticed from the window. At least, Alyosha heard a noise, caught the sound of flying footsteps and rustling skirts. Two or three women perhaps had run out of the room.

Alyosha thought it strange that his arrival should cause such excitement. But he was conducted to the drawing-room at once. It was a large room, elegantly and amply furnished, not at all in provincial style. There were many sofas, lounges, settees, big and little tables. There were pictures on the walls, vases and lamps on the tables, masses of flowers, and even an aquarium by the window. It was twilight and rather dark. Alyosha made out a silk mantle thrown down on the sofa, where people had evidently just been sitting; and on a table in front of the sofa were two unfinished cups of chocolate, biscuits, a crystal dish with blue raisins, and another with sweetmeats. Alyosha saw that he had interrupted visitors, and frowned. But at that instant the portière was raised, and with rapid, hurrying footsteps Katerina Ivanovna came in, holding out both hands to Alyosha with a radiant smile of delight. At the same instant a servant brought in two lighted candles and set them on the table.

"Thank God! At last you have come, too! I've been simply praying for you all day! Sit down."

Alyosha had been struck by Katerina Ivanovna's beauty when, three weeks before, Dmitri had first brought him, at Katerina Ivanovna's special request, to be introduced to her. There had been no conversation between them at that interview, however. Supposing Alyosha to be very shy, Katerina Ivanovna had talked all the time to Dmitri to spare him. Alyosha had been silent, but he had seen a great deal very clearly. He was struck by the imperiousness, proud ease, and self-confidence of the haughty girl. And all that was certain, Alyosha felt that he was not exaggerating it. He thought her great glowing black eyes were very fine, especially with her pale, even rather sallow, longish face. But in those eyes and in the lines of her exquisite lips there was something with which his brother might well be passionately in love, but which perhaps could not be loved for long. He expressed this thought almost plainly to Dmitri when, after the visit, his brother besought and insisted that he should not conceal the impressions his betrothed made on him.

"You'll be happy with her, but perhaps — not tranquilly happy."

"Quite so, brother. Such people remain always the same. They don't yield to fate. So you think I shan't love her for ever."

"No; perhaps you will love her for ever. But perhaps you won't always be happy with her."

Alyosha had given his opinion at the time, blushing, and angry with himself for having yielded to his brother's entreaties and put such "foolish" ideas into words. For his opinion had struck him as awfully foolish immediately after he had uttered it. He felt ashamed, too, of having given so confident an opinion about a woman. It was with the more amazement that he felt now, at the first glance at Katerina Ivanovna as she ran in to him, that he had perhaps been utterly mistaken. This time her face was beaming with unfeigned good-natured kindliness, and direct warm-hearted sincerity. The "pride and haughtiness," which had struck Alyosha so much before, were betrayed now only in a frank, generous energy and a sort of bright strong faith in herself. Alyosha realised at the first glance, at the first word, that all the tragedy of her position in relation to the man she loved so dearly was no secret to her; that she perhaps already knew everything, positively everything. And yet, in spite of that, there was such brightness in her face, such faith in the future. Alyosha felt at once that he had gravely wronged her in his thoughts. He was conquered and captivated immediately. Besides all this, he noticed at her first words that she was in great excitement, an excitement perhaps quite exceptional and almost approaching ecstasy. "I was so eager to see you, because I can learn from you the whole truth — from you and no one else."

"I have come," muttered Alyosha confusedly, "I — he sent me."

"Ah, he sent you! I foresaw that. Now I know everything — everything!" cried Katerina Ivanovna, her eyes flashing. "Wait a moment, Alexey Fyodorovich, I'll tell you why I've been so longing to see you. You see, I know perhaps far more than you do yourself, and I don't need any news from you. I'll tell you what I want from you. I want to know your own last impression of him. I want you to tell me most directly, plainly, coarsely even (oh, as coarsely as you like!), what you thought of him just now and of his position after your meeting with him to-day. That will perhaps be better than if I had a personal explanation with him, as he does not want to come to me. Do you understand what I want from you? Now, tell me simply, tell me every word of the message he sent you with (I knew he would send you)."

"He told me to give you his compliments — and to say that he would never come again — but to give you his compliments."

"His compliments? Was that what he said — his own expression?"

"Yes."

"Accidentally perhaps he made a mistake in the word, perhaps he did not use the right word?"

"No; he told me precisely to repeat that word. He begged me two or three times not to forget to say so."

Katerina Ivanovna flushed hotly.

"Help me now, Alexey Fyodorovich. Now I really need your help. I'll tell you what I think, and you must simply say whether it's right or not. Listen! If he had sent me his compliments in passing, without insisting on your repeating the words, without emphasising them, that would be the end of everything! But if he particularly insisted on those words, if he particularly told you not to forget to repeat them to me, then perhaps he was in excitement, beside himself. He had made his decision and was frightened by it. He wasn't walking away from me with a resolute step, but leaping headlong. The emphasis on that phrase may have been simply bravado."

"Yes, yes!" cried Alyosha warmly. "I believe that is it."

"And, if so, he's not altogether lost. He's only in despair, but I can still save him. Wait! Did he not tell you anything about money — about three thousand roubles?"

"He did speak about it, and it's that more than anything that's crushing him. He said he had lost his honour and that nothing mattered now," Alyosha answered warmly, feeling a rush of hope in his heart and believing that there really might be a way of escape and salvation for his brother. "But do you know about the money?" he added, and suddenly broke off.

"I've known of it a long time; I telegraphed to Moscow to inquire, and heard long ago that the money had not arrived. He hadn't sent the money, but I said nothing. Last week I learnt that he was still in need of money. My only object in all this was that he should know to whom to return, and who was his true friend. No, he doesn't wish to believe that I am his truest friend; he won't know me, and looks on me merely as a woman. I've been tormented all week, trying to think how to prevent him from being ashamed to face me because he spent that three thousand. That is, let him feel ashamed of himself, let him be ashamed before other people, but not before me. He can tell God everything without shame. Why is it he still does not understand how much I am ready to bear for his sake? Why, why doesn't he know me? How dare he not know me after all that has happened? I want to save him for ever. Let him forget me as his betrothed. And here he fears that he is dishonoured in my eyes. Why, he wasn't afraid to be open with you, Alexey Fyodorovich. How is it that I don't deserve the same?"

The last words she uttered in tears. Tears gushed from her eyes.

"I must tell you," Alyosha began, his voice trembling, too, "what happened just now between him and my father."

And he described the whole scene, how Dmitri had sent him to get the money, how he had broken in, knocked his father down, and after that had again specially and emphatically begged him to take his compliments and farewells.

"He went to that woman," Alyosha added softly.

"And do you suppose that I can't put up with that woman? Does he think I can't? But he won't marry her," she suddenly laughed nervously. "Could such a passion last for ever in a Karamazov? It's passion, not love. He won't marry her because she won't marry him." Again Katerina Ivanovna laughed strangely.

"He may marry her," said Alyosha mournfully, looking down.

"He won't marry her, I tell you. That girl is an angel. Do you know that? Do you know that?" Katerina Ivanovna exclaimed suddenly with extraordinary heat. "She is one of the most fantastic of fantastic creatures. I know how bewitching she is, but I know, too, that she is kind, firm, and noble. Why do you look at me like that, Alexey Fyodorovich? Perhaps you are wondering at my words, perhaps you don't believe me? Agrafena Alexandrovna, my angel!" she cried suddenly to some one, peeping into the next room, "come in to us. This is a friend. This is Alyosha. He knows all about our affairs. Show yourself to him."

"I've only been waiting behind the curtain for you to call me," said a soft, one might even say sugary, feminine voice.

The portière was raised and Grushenka herself, smiling and beaming, came up to the table. A violent revulsion passed over Alyosha. He fixed his eyes on her and could not take them off. Here she was, that awful woman, the "beast," as Ivan had called her half an hour before. And yet one would have thought the creature standing before him most simple and ordinary, a good-natured, kind woman, handsome certainly, but so like other handsome ordinary women! It is true she was very, very good-looking with that Russian beauty so passionately loved by many men. She was a rather tall woman, though a little shorter than Katerina Ivanovna, who was exceptionally tall. She had a full figure, and moved softly, noiselessly, as it were, her movements having a peculiar soft and cloying quality, like her voice. She moved, not like Katerina Ivanovna, with a vigorous, bold step, but silently. Her feet made absolutely no sound on the floor. She sank softly into an armchair, softly rustling her sumptuous black silk dress, and delicately wrapping her milk-white neck and broad shoulders in a costly black cashmere shawl. She was twenty-two years old, and her face looked exactly that age. She was very white in the face, with a pale pink tint on her cheeks. Her face might be said to be too broad, and the lower jaw was set a trifle forward. Her upper lip was thin, but the slightly prominent lower lip was at least twice as full, and looked slightly swollen, as it were. But her magnificent, abundant dark brown hair, her fine brown eyebrows and charming grey-blue eyes with their long lashes, would have made the most indifferent person, meeting her casually in a crowd in the street, stop at the sight of her face and remember it long after. What struck Alyosha most in that face was its expression of childlike good-nature. There was a childlike look in her eyes, a look of childish delight. She came up to the table, beaming with delight and seeming to expect something with childish, impatient, and confiding curiosity. The light in her eyes gladdened the soul — Alyosha felt that. There was something else in her which he could not understand, or would not have been able to define, and which yet perhaps unconsciously affected him. It was that softness, that voluptuousness of her bodily movements, that catlike noiselessness. Yet it was a vigorous, ample body. Under the shawl could be guessed full broad shoulders, a high, still quite girlish bosom. Her figure suggested the lines of the Venus of Milo, though already in somewhat exaggerated proportions. That could be divined. Connoisseurs of Russian beauty could have foretold with certainty, looking at Grushenka, that this fresh, still youthful, beauty would lose its perfection when she reached thirty, would "spread"; that the face would become puffy, and that wrinkles would very soon appear upon her forehead and round the eyes; the complexion would grow coarse and red perhaps — in fact, that it was a momentary beauty, the fleeting beauty which is so often met with in Russian women. Alyosha, of course, did not think of this; but though he was fascinated, yet he wondered with an unpleasant sensation, and as it were regretfully, why she drawled in that way and could not speak naturally. She did so evidently feeling there was a charm in the exaggerated, honeyed modulation of the syllables. It was, of course, only a bad, underbred habit that showed lack of education and a false idea of good manners. And yet this intonation and manner of speaking impressed Alyosha as almost incredibly incongruous with the childishly simple and happy expression of her face, the soft, babyish radiance in her eyes. Katerina Ivanovna at once made her sit down in an armchair facing Alyosha, and ecstatically kissed her several times on her smiling lips. She seemed quite in love with her.

"This is the first time we've met, Alexey Fyodorovich," she said rapturously. "I wanted to know her, to see her. I wanted to go to her, but I'd no sooner expressed the wish than she came to me. I knew we should settle everything together — everything. My heart told me so — I was begged not to take the step, but I foresaw it would be a way out of the difficulty, and I was not mistaken. Grushenka has explained everything to me, told me all she means to do. She flew here like an angel of goodness and brought us peace and joy."

"You did not disdain me, sweet, excellent young lady," drawled Grushenka in her singsong voice, still with the same charming smile of delight.

"Don't dare to speak to me like that, you sorceress, you witch! Disdain you! Here I must kiss your lower lip once more. It looks as though it were swollen, and now it will be more so, and more and more. Look how she laughs, Alexey Fyodorovich! It does one's heart good to see the angel."

Alyosha flushed, and faint, imperceptible shivers ran through him.

"You make so much of me, dear young lady, and perhaps I am not at all worthy of your kindness."

"Not worthy! She's not worthy of it!" Katerina Ivanovna cried again with the same heat. "You know, Alexey Fyodorovich, we're fanciful, we're self-willed, but proudest of the proud in our little heart. We're noble, we're generous, Alexey Fyodorovich, let me tell you. We have only been unfortunate. We were too ready to make every sacrifice for an unworthy, perhaps, or fickle man. There was one man — one, an officer too, we loved him, we sacrificed everything to him. That was long ago, five years ago, and he has forgotten us, he has married. Now he is a widower, he has written, he is coming here, and, do you know, we've loved him, none but him, all this time, and we've loved him all our life! He will come, and Grushenka will be happy again. For the last five years she's been wretched. But who can reproach her, who can boast of her favour? Only that bedridden old merchant, but he is more like her father, her friend, her protector. He found her then in despair, in agony, deserted by the man she loved. She was ready to drown herself then, but the old merchant saved her — saved her!"

"You defend me very kindly, dear young lady. You are in a great hurry about everything," Grushenka drawled again.

"Defend you! Is it for me to defend you? Should I dare to defend you? Grushenka, angel, give me your hand. Look at that charming soft little hand, Alexey Fyodorovich! Look at it! It has brought me happiness and has lifted me up, and I'm going to kiss it, outside and inside, here, here, here!"

And three times she kissed the certainly charming, though rather plump, hand of Grushenka in a sort of rapture. She held out her hand with a charming, musical, nervous little laugh, watched the "sweet young lady," and obviously liked having her hand kissed.

"Perhaps there's rather too much rapture," thought Alyosha. He blushed. His heart was peculiarly uneasy the whole time.

"You won't make me blush, dear young lady, kissing my hand like this before Alexey Fyodorovich."

"Do you think I meant to make you blush?" said Katerina Ivanovna, somewhat surprised. "Ah, my dear, how little you understand me!"

"Yes, and you, too, perhaps quite misunderstand me, dear young lady. Maybe I'm not so good as I seem to you. I've a bad heart; I will have my own way. I fascinated poor Dmitri Fyodorovich that day simply for fun."

"But now you'll save him. You've given me your word. You'll explain it all to him. You'll break it to him that you have long loved another man, who is now offering you his hand."

"Oh, no! I didn't give you my word to do that. It was you kept talking about that. I didn't give you my word."

"Then I didn't quite understand you," said Katerina Ivanovna slowly, turning a little pale. "You promised . . ."

"Oh, no, angel lady, I've promised nothing," Grushenka interrupted softly and evenly, still with the same gay and simple expression. "You see at once, dear young lady,

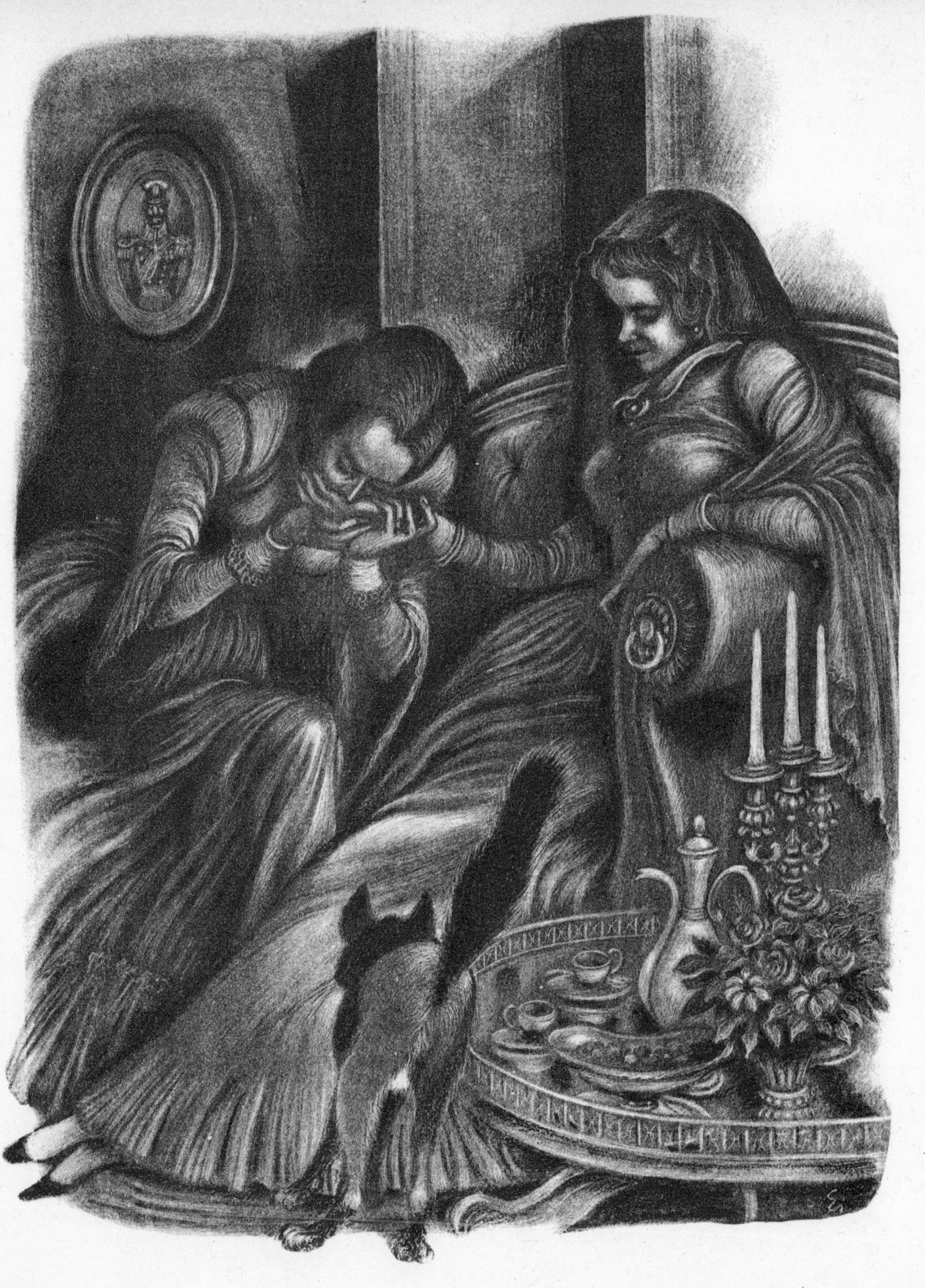

KATERINA KISSES GRUSHENKA'S HAND

what a wilful wretch I am compared with you. I do what I feel like doing. I may have made you some promise just now. But now again I'm thinking: I may take to Mitya again. I liked him very much once — liked him for almost a whole hour. Now maybe I shall go and tell him to stay with me from this day forward. You see, I'm so changeable."

"Just now you said — something quite different," Katerina Ivanovna whispered faintly.

"Ah, just now! But, you know, I'm such a soft-hearted, silly creature. Only think what he's gone through on my account! What if when I go home I feel sorry for him? What then?"

"I never expected ——"

"Ah, young lady, how good and generous you are compared with me! Now perhaps you won't care for a silly creature like me, now you know my character. Give me your sweet little hand, angelic lady," she said tenderly, and with a sort of reverence took Katerina Ivanovna's hand.

"Here, dear young lady, I'll take your hand and kiss it as you did mine. You kissed mine three times, but I ought to kiss yours three hundred times to be even with you. Well, but let that pass. And then it shall be as God wills. Perhaps I shall be your slave entirely and want to do your bidding like a slave. Let it be as God wills, without any agreements or promises. What a sweet hand — what a sweet hand you have! You sweet young lady, you incredible beauty!"

She slowly raised the hand to her lips, with the strange object indeed of "being even" with her in kisses.

Katerina Ivanovna did not take her hand away. She listened with timid hope to the last words, though Grushenka's promise to do her bidding like a slave was very strangely expressed. She looked intently into her eyes; she still saw in those eyes the same simple-hearted, confiding expression, the same serene gaiety.

"She's perhaps too naïve," thought Katerina Ivanovna, with a gleam of hope.

Grushenka meanwhile seemed enthusiastic over the "sweet hand." She raised it slowly to her lips. But as it reached her lips, she suddenly held it there for two or three moments, as though reconsidering something.

"Do you know, angel lady," she suddenly drawled in an even more soft and sugary voice, "do you know, after all, I think I won't kiss your hand?" And she laughed a little merry laugh.

"As you please. What's the matter with you?" said Katerina Ivanovna, starting suddenly.

"So that you may be left to remember that you kissed my hand, but I didn't kiss yours."

There was a sudden flash in her eyes. She looked with awful intentness at Katerina Ivanovna.

"Insolent creature!" cried Katerina Ivanovna, as though suddenly grasping something. She flushed all over and leapt up from her seat.

Grushenka too got up, but without haste.

"So I shall tell Mitya how you kissed my hand, but I didn't kiss yours at all. And how he will laugh!"

"Vile slut! Out with you!"

"Ah, for shame, young lady! Ah, for shame! That's unbecoming, dear young lady, a word like that from you."

"Out with you! You're a creature for sale!" screamed Katerina Ivanovna. Every feature was working now in her utterly distorted face.

"For sale indeed! You used to visit gentlemen in the dusk for money once; you brought your beauty for sale. You see, I know."

Katerina Ivanovna shrieked, and would have rushed at her, but Alyosha held her with all his strength.

"Not a step, not a word! Don't speak, don't answer her. She'll go away — she'll go at once."

At that instant Katerina Ivanovna's two aunts ran in at her cry, and with them a maid-servant. All hurried to her.

"I will go away," said Grushenka, taking up her mantle from the sofa. "Alyosha, darling, see me home!"

"Go away — go away, make haste!" cried Alyosha, clasping his hands imploringly.

"Dear little Alyosha, see me home! I've got a pretty little story to tell you on the way. I got up this scene for your benefit, Alyosha. See me home, darling, you'll be glad of it afterwards."

Alyosha turned away, wringing his hands. Grushenka ran out of the house, laughing musically.

Katerina Ivanovna went into a fit of hysterics. She sobbed, and was shaken with convulsions. Every one fussed round her.

"I warned you," said the elder of her aunts. "I tried to prevent your doing this. You're too impulsive. How could you do such a thing? You don't know these creatures, and they say she's worse than any of them. You are too self-willed."

"She's a tigress!" yelled Katerina Ivanovna. "Why did you hold me, Alexey Fyodorovich? I'd have beaten her — beaten her!"

She could not control herself before Alyosha; perhaps, indeed, she did not care to.

"She ought to be flogged in public on a scaffold!"

Alyosha withdrew towards the door.

"But, my God!" cried Katerina Ivanovna, striking her hands together. "He! He! He could be so dishonourable, so inhuman! Why, he told that creature what happened on that fatal, accursed day! 'You brought your beauty for sale, dear young lady.' She knows it! Your brother's a scoundrel, Alexey Fyodorovich."

Alyosha wanted to say something, but he couldn't find a word. His heart ached.

"Go away, Alexey Fyodorovich! It's shameful, it's awful for me! To-morrow, I beg you on my knees, come to-morrow. Don't condemn me. Forgive me. I don't know what I shall do with myself now!"

Alyosha walked out into the street reeling. He could have wept as she did. Suddenly he was overtaken by the maid.

"The young lady forgot to give you this letter from Madame Hohlakov; it's been left with us since dinner-time." Alyosha took the little pink envelope mechanically and put it, almost unconsciously, into his pocket.

CHAPTER XI

ANOTHER REPUTATION RUINED

It was not much more than three-quarters of a mile from the town to the monastery. Alyosha walked quickly along the road, at that hour deserted. It was almost night, and too dark to see anything clearly at thirty paces ahead. Half-way there his road was crossed by another. A figure came into sight under a solitary willow at the cross-roads. As soon as Alyosha reached the cross-roads the figure tore from its place and rushed at him, shouting savagely: "Your money or your life!"

"So it's you, Mitya," cried Alyosha, in surprise, violently startled however.

"Ha, ha, ha! You didn't expect me? I wondered where to wait for you. Near her house? There are three roads leading from it, and I might have missed you. At last I thought of waiting here, for you had to pass here, there's no other way to the monastery. Come, tell me the truth. Crush me like a beetle. But what's the matter?"

"Nothing, brother — it's the fright you gave me. Oh, Dmitri! A while ago — that blood!" (Alyosha began to cry; he had been on the verge of tears for a long time, and now something seemed to snap in his soul.) "You almost killed father — cursed him — and now — here — you're playing practical jokes — 'Your money or your life!' "

"Well, what of that? It's not proper — is that it? Not suitable in my position?"

"No — I only ——"

"Stop. Look at the night. You see what a dark night, what clouds, what a wind has risen. I hid here under the willow waiting for you. And as God's above, I suddenly thought, why go on in misery any longer, what is there to wait for? Here I have a willow, a handkerchief, a shirt, I can twist them into a rope in a minute, and braces besides, and why go on burdening the earth, dishonouring it with my vile presence. And then I heard you coming — Heavens, it was as though something flew down to me suddenly. So there is a man, then, whom I love. Here he is, that man, my dear little brother, whom I love more than any one in the world, the only one I love in the world. And I loved you so much, so much at that moment that I thought, 'I'll fall on his neck at once.' Then a stupid idea struck me: 'I'll joke with him, I'll scare him.' I shouted, like a fool, 'Your money!' Forgive my foolery — it was only nonsense, and there's nothing unseemly in my soul. . . . Damn it all, tell me what's happened. What did she say? Strike me, crush me, don't spare me! Was she furious?"

"No, not that. . . . There was nothing like that, Mitya. There — I found them both there."

"Both? Whom?"

"Grushenka at Katerina Ivanovna's."

Dmitri was struck dumb.

"Impossible!" he cried. "You're raving! Grushenka with her?"

Alyosha described all that had happened from the moment he went in to Katerina Ivanovna's. He was ten minutes telling his story. He can't be said to have told it fluently and consecutively, but he seemed to make it clear, not omitting any word or action of significance, and vividly describing, often in one word, his own sensations. Dmitri listened in silence, gazing at him with a terrible fixed stare, but it was clear to Alyosha that he understood it all, and had grasped every point. But as the story went on, his face became not merely gloomy, but menacing. He scowled, he clenched his teeth, and his fixed stare became still more rigid, more concentrated, more terrible, when suddenly, with incredible rapidity, his wrathful, savage face changed, his tightly compressed lips parted, and Dmitri Fyodorovich broke into uncontrolled, spontaneous laughter. He literally shook with laughter. For a long time he could not speak.

"So she wouldn't kiss her hand! So she didn't kiss it; so she ran away!" he kept exclaiming with hysterical rapture; insolent rapture it might have been called, if it had not been so spontaneous. "So the other one called her a tigress! And a tigress she is! So she ought to be flogged on a scaffold? Yes, yes, so she ought. That's just what I think; she ought to have been long ago. It's like this, brother, let her be punished, but I must recover first. I understand the queen of impudence. That's her all over! You saw her all over in that hand-kissing, the she-devil! She's the queen of all the infernal women you can imagine in the world! She's magnificent in her own line! So she ran home? I'll go — ah — I'll run to her! Alyosha, don't blame me, I agree that strangling is too good for her."

"But Katerina Ivanovna!" exclaimed Alyosha sorrowfully.

"I see her, too! I see right through her, as I've never done before! It's like a discovery of the four continents of the world, that is, of the five! What a thing to do! That's just like Katya, who was not afraid to face a coarse, unmannerly officer and risk a deadly insult on a generous impulse to save her father! But the pride, the recklessness, the defiance of fate, the unbounded defiance! You say that aunt tried to stop her? That aunt, you know, is an overbearing woman, herself. She's the sister of the general's widow in Moscow, and even more stuck-up than she. But her husband was caught stealing government money. He lost everything, his estate and all, and the proud wife had to lower her colours, and hasn't raised them since. So she tried to hold Katya back, but she wouldn't listen to her! She thinks she can overcome everything, that everything will give way before her. She thought she could bewitch Grushenka if she liked, and she believed it herself; she plays a part to herself, and whose fault is it? Do you think she kissed Grushenka's hand first, on purpose, with a sly design? No, she really, really fell in love with Grushenka, that's to say, not with Grushenka, but with her own dream, her own delusion — because it was *her* dream, *her* delusion! Alyosha, darling, how did you escape from them, those women? Did you pick up your cassock and run? Ha, ha!"

"Brother, you don't seem to have noticed how you've insulted Katerina Ivanovna by telling Grushenka about that day. And she flung it in her face just now that she had gone to gentlemen in secret to sell her beauty! Brother, what could be worse than that insult?" What worried Alyosha more than anything was that, incredible as it seemed, his brother appeared pleased at Katerina Ivanovna's humiliation.

"Bah!" Dmitri frowned fiercely, and struck his forehead with his palm. He only now realised it, though Alyosha had just told him of the insult, and Katerina Ivanovna's cry: "Your brother is a scoundrel!"

"Yes, perhaps, I really did tell Grushenka about that 'fatal day,' as Katya calls it. Yes, I did tell her, I remember! It was that time at Mokroye. I was drunk, the gipsies were singing. . . . But I was sobbing. I was sobbing then, kneeling and praying to Katya's image, and Grushenka understood it. She understood it all then. I remember, she cried herself. . . . Damn it all! But it was bound to turn out this way. Then she cried, but now 'thrust the dagger into the heart'! That's how women are."

He looked down and sank into thought.

"Yes, I am a scoundrel, a thorough scoundrel!" he said suddenly, in a gloomy voice. "It doesn't matter whether I cried or not, I'm a scoundrel! Tell her I accept the name, if that's any comfort. Come, that's enough. Good-bye. It's no use talking! It's not amusing. You go your way and I mine. And I don't want to see you again until perhaps the very last moment. Good-bye, Alexey!" He warmly pressed Alyosha's hand, and still looking down, without raising his head, as though tearing himself away, turned rapidly towards the town.

Alyosha looked after him, unable to believe he would go away so abruptly.

"Wait, Alexey, one more confession to you alone!" cried Dmitri, suddenly turning back. "Look at me. Look at me well. You see here, here — there's terrible disgrace in store for me." (As he said "here," Dmitri struck his chest with his fist with a strange air, as though the dishonour lay precisely on his chest, and was hidden in some spot there, in a pocket, perhaps, or hanging round his neck.) "You know me now, a scoundrel, an avowed scoundrel, but let me tell you that I've never done anything before and never shall again, anything that can compare in baseness with the dishonour which I bear now at this very minute on my breast, here, here, which will come to pass, though I'm perfectly free to stop it. I can stop it or carry it through, note that. Well, let me tell you, I shall carry it through. I shan't stop it. I told you everything just now, but I didn't tell you this, because even I had not brass enough for it. I can still stop; if I do, I can give back the full half of my lost honour to-morrow. But I shan't pull up. I shall carry out my base plan, and you can bear witness that I told you so beforehand. Darkness and ruin! No need to explain. You'll find out in due time. The filthy back-alley and the she-devil. Good-bye. Don't pray for me, I'm not worth it. And there's no need, no need at all. . . . I don't need it! Away!"

And he suddenly retreated, this time finally. Alyosha went towards the monastery.

"What? I shall never see him again! What is he saying?" he wondered wildly. "Why, I shall certainly see him to-morrow. I shall look him up. I shall make a point of it. What does he mean?"

He went round the monastery, and crossing the pine-wood went straight to the hermitage. The door was opened to him, though no one was admitted at that hour. There was a tremor in his heart as he went into Father Zosima's cell.

Why, why, had he gone forth? Why had his elder sent him into the world? Here was peace. Here was holiness. But there was confusion, there was darkness in which one lost one's way and went astray at once. . . .

In the cell he found the novice Porfiry and Father Païssy, who came every hour to inquire after Father Zosima. Alyosha learnt with alarm that he was getting worse and worse. Even his usual evening discourse with the brothers could not take place that day. As a rule every evening after service the monks flocked into Father Zosima's cell, and all confessed aloud their sins of the day, their sinful thoughts and temptations; even their disputes, if there had been any. Some confessed kneeling. The elder absolved, reconciled, exhorted, imposed penance, blessed, and dismissed them. It was against this general "confession" that the opponents of "elders" protested, maintaining that it was a profanation of the sacrament of confession, almost a sacrilege, though this was quite a different thing. They even represented to the diocesan authorities that such confessions attained no good object, but actually to a large extent led to sin and temptation. Many of the brothers disliked going to the elder, and went against their own will because every one went, and for fear they should be accused of pride and rebellious ideas. People said that some of the monks agreed beforehand, saying, "I'll confess I lost my temper with you this morning, and you confirm it," simply in order to have something to say. Alyosha knew that this actually happened sometimes. He knew, too, that there were among the monks some who deeply resented the fact that letters from relations were habitually taken to the elder, to be opened and read by him before those to whom they were addressed.

It was assumed, of course, that all this was done freely, and in good faith, by way of voluntary submission and salutary edification. But, in fact, there was sometimes no little insincerity, and much that was false and strained in this practice. Yet the older and more experienced of the monks adhered to their opinion, arguing that "for those who have come within these walls sincerely seeking salvation, such obedience and sacrifice will certainly be salutary and of great benefit; those, on the other hand, who find it irksome, and murmur against it, are no true monks, and have made a mistake in entering the monastery — their proper place is in the world. Even in church one cannot be safe from sin and the devil. So it was no good being too lenient."

"He is weaker, a drowsiness has come over him," Father Païssy whispered to Alyosha, as he blessed him. "It's difficult to rouse him. And he must not be roused. He waked up for five minutes, sent his blessing to the brothers, and begged their prayers for him at night. He intends to take the sacrament again in the morning. He remembered you, Alexey. He asked whether you had gone away, and was told that you were in the town. 'I blessed him for that work,' he said, 'his place is there, not here, for awhile.' Those were his words about you. He remembered you lovingly, with anxiety; do you understand how he honoured you? But how is it that he has decided that you shall spend some time in the world? He must have foreseen something in your destiny! Understand, Alexey, that if you return to the world, it must be to do the duty laid upon you by your elder, and not for frivolous vanity and worldly pleasures."

Father Païssy went out. Alyosha had no doubt that Father Zosima was dying, though he might live another day or two. Alyosha firmly and ardently resolved that in spite of his promises to his father, the Hohlakovs, and Katerina Ivanovna, he would not leave the monastery next day, but would remain with his elder to the end. His heart glowed with love, and he reproached himself bitterly for having been able for one instant to forget him whom he had left in the monastery on his death-bed, and whom he honoured above every one in the world. He went into Father Zosima's bedroom, knelt down, and bowed to the ground before the elder, who slept quietly without stirring, with regular, hardly audible breathing and a peaceful face.

Alyosha returned to the other room, where Father Zosima had received his guests in the morning. Taking off his boots, he lay down on the hard, narrow, leathern sofa, which he had long used as a bed, bringing nothing but a pillow. The mattress, about which his father had shouted to him that morning, he had long forgotten to place there. He took off his cassock, which he used as a covering. But before going to bed, he fell on his knees and prayed a long time. In his fervent prayer he did not beseech God to lighten his darkness but only thirsted for the joyous emotion which always visited his soul after the praise and adoration of which his evening prayer usually consisted. That joy always brought him light untroubled sleep. As he was praying, he suddenly felt in his pocket the little pink note the servant had handed him as he left Katerina Ivanovna's. He was disturbed, but finished his prayer. Then, after some hesitation, he opened the envelope. In it was a note to him, signed by Lise, the young daughter of Madame Hohlakov, who had laughed at him before the elder in the morning.

"Alexey Fyodorovich," she wrote, "I am writing to you without any one's knowledge, even mamma's, and I know how wrong it is. But I cannot live without telling you the feeling that has sprung up in my heart, and this no one but we two must know for a time. But how am I to say what I want so much to tell you? Paper, they say, does not blush, but I assure you it's not true and that it's blushing just as I am now, all over. Dear Alyosha, I love you, I've loved you from my childhood on, since our Moscow days, when you were very different from what you are now, and I shall love you all my life. My heart has chosen you, to unite our lives, and pass them together till our old age. Of course, on condition that you will leave the monastery. As for our age, we will wait for the time fixed by the law. By that time I shall certainly be quite strong, I shall be walking and dancing. There can be no doubt of that.

"You see how I've thought of everything. There's only one thing I can't imagine: what you'll think of me when you read this? I'm always laughing and being naughty. I made you angry this morning, but I assure you before I took up my pen, I prayed before the Image of the Mother of God, and now I'm praying, and almost crying.

"My secret is in your hands. When you come to-morrow, I don't know how I shall look at you. Ah, Alexey Fyodorovich, what if I can't restrain myself like a silly and laugh when I look at you as I did to-day? You'll think I'm a nasty girl making fun of you, and you won't believe my letter. And so I beg you, dear one, if you've any pity for me, when you come to-morrow, don't look me straight in the face, for if I meet your eyes, it will be sure to make me laugh, especially as you'll be in that long gown. I feel cold all over when I think of it, so when you come, don't look at me at all for a time, look at mamma or at the window. . . .

"Here I've written you a love-letter. Oh, God, what have I done? Alyosha, don't despise me, and if I've done something very horrid and wounded you, forgive me. Now the secret of my reputation, ruined perhaps for ever, is in your hands.

"I shall certainly cry to-day. Good-bye till our meeting, our *awful* meeting. Lise.

"P.S. Alyosha! You must, must, must come! Lise."

Alyosha read the note in amazement, read it through twice, thought a little, and suddenly laughed a soft, sweet laugh. He started. That laugh seemed to him sinful. But a minute later he laughed again just as softly and happily. He slowly replaced the note in the envelope, crossed himself and lay down. The agitation in his heart passed at once. "God have mercy upon all of them, have all these unhappy and turbulent souls in Thy keeping, and set them in the right path. All ways are Thine. Save them according to Thy wisdom. Thou art love. Thou wilt send joy to all!" Alyosha murmured, crossing himself, and falling into peaceful sleep.

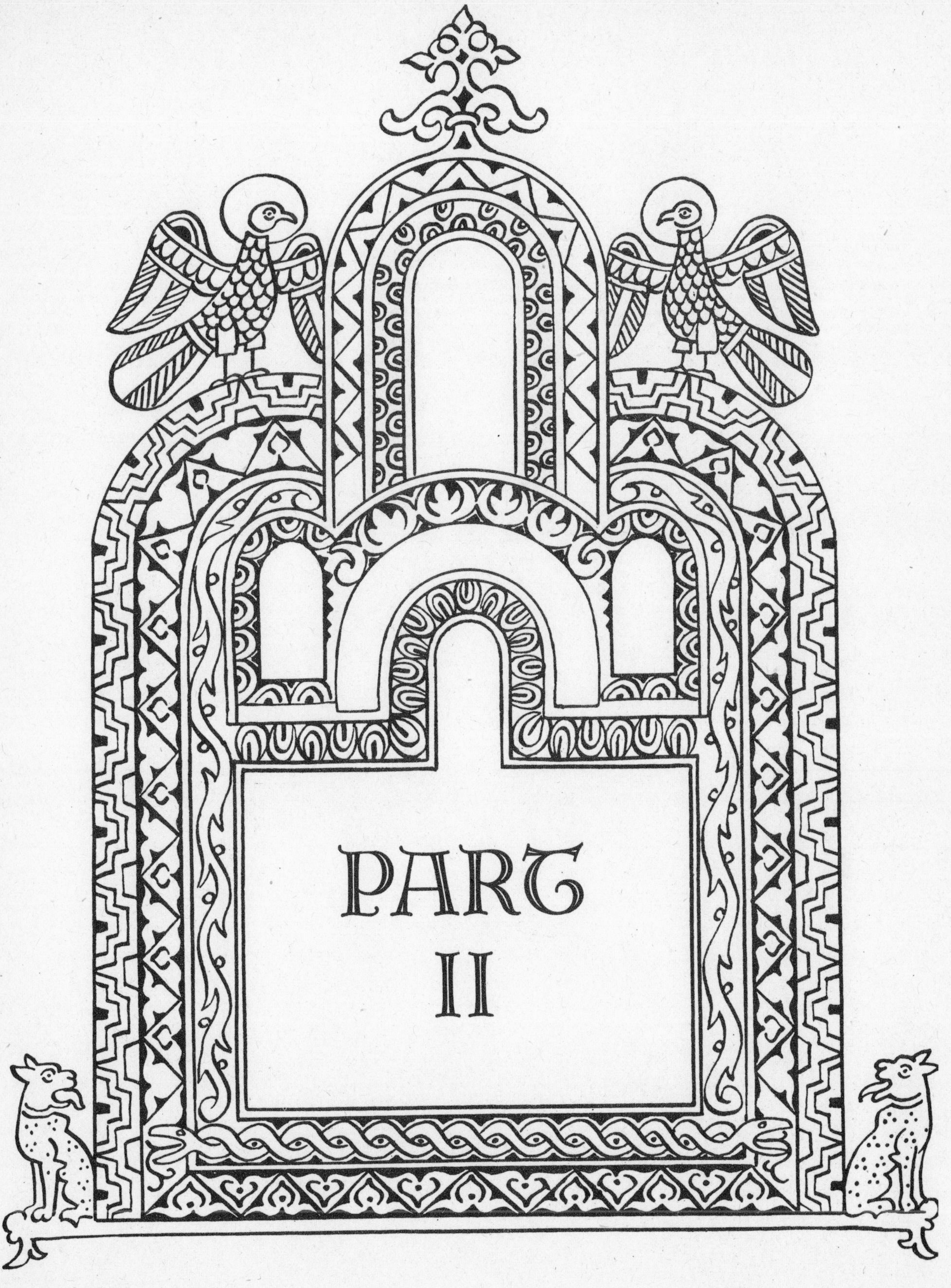
PART
II

CHAPTER I

FATHER FERAPONT

Alyosha was roused early, before daybreak. Father Zosima woke up feeling very weak, though he wanted to get out of bed and sit up in a chair. His mind was quite clear; his face looked very tired, yet serene and almost joyful. It wore an expression of gaiety, kindness, and cordiality. "May be I shall not live through the day," he said to Alyosha. Then he desired to confess and take the sacrament at once. His confessor was always Father Païssy. After the communion, came the service of extreme unction. The monks assembled and the cell was gradually filled up by the inmates of the hermitage. Meantime it grew light. People began coming from the monastery, too. After the service was over the elder desired to take leave of every one, and kissed them all. As the cell was so small the earlier visitors withdrew to make room for others. Alyosha stood beside the elder, who was seated again in his armchair. He talked and preached as much as he could. Though his voice was weak, it was fairly steady.

"I've been teaching you so many years, and therefore I've been talking aloud so long, that I've got into the habit of talking, and so much so that it's almost more difficult for me to hold my tongue than to talk, even now, in spite of my weakness, dear fathers and brethren," he jested, looking with emotion at the group crowding round him.

Alyosha remembered afterwards something of what he said to them. But though he spoke out distinctly and his voice was fairly steady, his speech was somewhat disconnected. He spoke of many things, he seemed anxious before the moment of death to say everything he had not said in his life, and not simply for the sake of edifying them, but as though thirsting to share with all men and all creation his joy and ecstasy, and once more in his life to open his whole heart.

"Love one another, fathers," said the elder, as far as Alyosha could remember afterwards. "Love God's people. Because we have come here and shut ourselves within these walls, we are no holier than those who are outside, but on the contrary, from the very fact of coming here, each of us has confessed to himself that he is worse than the laity, than all men on earth. . . . And the longer the monk lives in his seclusion, the more keenly he must recognise that. Else he would have had no reason to come here. When he realises that he is not only worse than others, but that he is responsible to all men for all and everything, for all human sins, communal and individual, only then the aim of our seclusion is attained. For know, dear ones, that every one of us is undoubtedly responsible for everything and shares the guilt of all men on earth, not merely through the general universal guilt, but each one is personally responsible for all mankind and every individual man. This knowledge is the crown of the monastic way of life and of every man on earth. For monks are not a special sort of men, but only what all men on earth ought to be. Only then our heart would grow soft with infinite, universal, unquenchable love. Then every one of you will have the power to win over the whole world by love and to wash away the sins of the world with your tears. . . . Each of you keep watch over your heart and confess your sins to yourself unceasingly. Be not afraid of your sins, even when perceiving them, if only there be penitence, but make no conditions with God. Again I say, Be not proud. Be proud neither before the little nor before the great. Hate not those who reject you, who disgrace you, who abuse and slander you. Hate not the atheists, the teachers of evil, the materialists — and I mean not only the good ones — for there are many good ones among them, especially in our day — hate not even the wicked ones. Remember them in your prayers thus: Save, O Lord, all those who have none to pray for them, save all those who will not pray. And add: it is not in pride that I make this prayer, O Lord, for I am more abominable than all men. . . . Love God's people, let not strangers ravish the flock, for if you slumber in your slothfulness and squeamish pride, or worse still, in covetousness, they will come from all sides and ravish your flock. Expound the Gospel to the people unceasingly . . . be not extortionate. . . . Do not love gold and silver, do not hoard them. . . . Have faith. Cling to the banner and raise it on high."

But the elder spoke more disconnectedly than Alyosha reported his words afterwards. Sometimes he broke off altogether, as though to take breath and recover his strength, but he was in a sort of ecstasy. They heard him with emotion, though many wondered at his words and found them obscure. . . . Afterwards all these words were remembered.

When Alyosha happened for a moment to leave the cell, he was struck by the general excitement and suspense that swayed the monks who were crowding about it. Some were alarmed, others were solemn, but all were expecting that some great miracle would happen immediately after the elder's disease. Their expectation was, in a sense, almost frivolous, but even the most austere of the monks were affected by it. The most austere of all was the countenance of Father Païssy.

Alyosha had absented himself from the cell only because he had been mysteriously summoned by a monk to see Rakitin, who had arrived from town with a singular letter for him from Madame Hohlakov. In it she informed Alyosha of a curious and very appropriate incident. It appeared that among the women who had come on the previous day to receive Father Zosima's blessing there had been an old woman from the town, a sergeant's widow, called Prohorovna. She had inquired whether she might pray for the rest of the soul of her son, Vasenka, who had gone to Irkutsk, and had sent her no news for over a year. To which Father Zosima had answered sternly, forbidding her to do so, and saying that to pray for the living as though they were dead was a kind of sorcery. He afterwards forgave her on account of her ignorance, and added "as though reading the book of the future" (this was Madame Hohlakov's expression) words of comfort: "that her son Vassya was certainly alive and he would either come himself very shortly or send a letter, and that she was to go home and wait for him." And "would you believe it," exclaimed Madame Hohlakov enthusiastically, "the prophecy has been fulfilled literally indeed, and more than that." Scarcely had the old woman reached home when they gave her a letter from Siberia which had been awaiting her. But that was not all; in the letter written on the road from Ekaterinburg, Vassya informed his mother that he was returning to Russia with an official, and that three weeks after her receiving the letter he hoped "to embrace his mother."

Madame Hohlakov warmly entreated Alyosha to report this new "miracle of prediction" to the Superior and all the brotherhood. "All, all, ought to know of it!" she concluded. The letter had been written in haste, the excitement of the writer was apparent in every line of it. But Alyosha had no need to tell the monks, for all knew of it already. Rakitin had commissioned the monk who brought his message "to inform most respectfully his reverence Father Païssy, that he, Rakitin, must speak with him on a matter of such gravity that he dare not defer it for a moment, and humbly begs forgiveness for his presumption." As the monk had given the message to Father Païssy before delivering the note to Alyosha, the latter found after reading it that there was nothing left for him to do but to hand it to Father Païssy in confirmation of the story.

And even that austere and cautious man, though he frowned as he read the news of the "miracle," could not completely restrain some inner emotion. His eyes flashed, and a grave and solemn smile came to his lips. "We shall see greater things!" broke from him.

"We shall see greater things, greater things yet!" the monks around repeated.

But Father Païssy, frowning again, begged all of them, at least for a time, not to speak of the matter "till it be more fully confirmed, seeing there is so much credulity among the worldlings, and indeed this might well have chanced naturally," he added, prudently, as it were to satisfy his conscience, though scarcely believing his own disavowal, a fact his listeners very clearly perceived.

Within the hour the "miracle" was of course known to the whole monastery, and to many outsiders who had come for the mass. No one seemed more impressed by it than the monk who had come the day before from St. Sylvester, from the little monastery of Obdorsk in the far North. It was he who had been standing near Madame Hohlakov the previous day and had asked Father Zosima with great earnestness, referring to the "healing" of the lady's daughter, "How can you presume to do such things?"

He was now somewhat puzzled and did not know what to believe. The evening before he had visited Father Ferapont in his cell apart, behind the apiary, and had been greatly impressed and overawed by the visit. This Father Ferapont was that aged monk so devout in fasting and observing silence, who has been mentioned already as antagonistic to Father Zosima and the whole institution of "elders," which he regarded as a pernicious and frivolous innovation. He was a very formidable opponent, in spite of the fact that because of his practice of silence he scarcely spoke a word to any one. What made him formidable was that a number of monks fully shared his feeling, and many of the visitors looked upon him as a great saint and ascetic, although they had no doubt that he was a fool in Christ. But it was just this that attracted them.

Father Ferapont never went to see the elder. Though he lived in the hermitage, they did not insist on his keeping its regulations, and this, too, because he behaved as though he were out of his mind. He was seventy-five or more, and he lived in a corner beyond the apiary in an old decaying wooden cell which had been built long ago for another great ascetic, Father Iona, who had lived to be a hundred and five, and of whose saintly doings many curious stories were still current in the monastery and the neighbourhood.

Father Ferapont had succeeded in getting himself installed in this same solitary cell seven years previously. It was simply a peasant hut, though it looked like a chapel, for it contained an extraordinary number of ikons with lamps perpetually burning before them — which had been brought as offerings. It was as though Father Ferapont had been appointed to look after them and keep the lamps burning. It was said (and indeed it was true) that he ate only two pounds of bread in three days. The beekeeper, who lived close by the apiary, used to bring him the bread every three days, and even to this man who waited upon him Father Ferapont rarely uttered a word. The four pounds of bread, together with the sacrament bread, regularly sent him on Sundays after the late mass by the Father Superior, made up his weekly ration. The water in his jug was changed every day. He rarely appeared at mass. Visitors who came to do him homage saw him sometimes kneeling all day long at prayer without looking round. If he addressed them, he was brief, abrupt, strange, and almost always rude. On very rare occasions, however, he would strike up a conversation with visitors, but for the most part he would utter some one strange saying which was a complete riddle, and no entreaties would induce him to pronounce a word in explanation. He was not a priest, but a simple monk. There was a strange rumour, chiefly current, however, among the most ignorant, that Father Ferapont had communication with heavenly spirits and conversed only with them, and so was silent with men.

The monk from Obdorsk, having been directed to the apiary by the beekeeper, who was also a very silent and surly monk, went to the corner where Father Ferapont's cell stood. "Maybe he will speak as you are a stranger and maybe you'll get nothing out of him," the beekeeper had warned him. The monk, as he related afterwards, approached with the utmost awe. It was rather late in the evening. Father Ferapont was sitting at the door of his cell on a low bench. A huge old elm was lightly rustling overhead. There was an evening freshness in the air. The monk from Obdorsk bowed down before the saint and asked his blessing.

"Do you want me to bow down to you, monk?" said Father Ferapont. "Rise!"

The monk got up.

"Blessing, be blessed! Sit beside me. Whence do you come?"

What most struck the poor monk was the fact that in spite of his strict fasting and great age, Father Ferapont still looked a vigorous old man. He was tall, held himself erect, and had a thin, but fresh and healthy face. There was no doubt he still had considerable strength. He was of athletic build. In spite of his great age he was not even quite grey, and still had very thick hair and a full beard, both

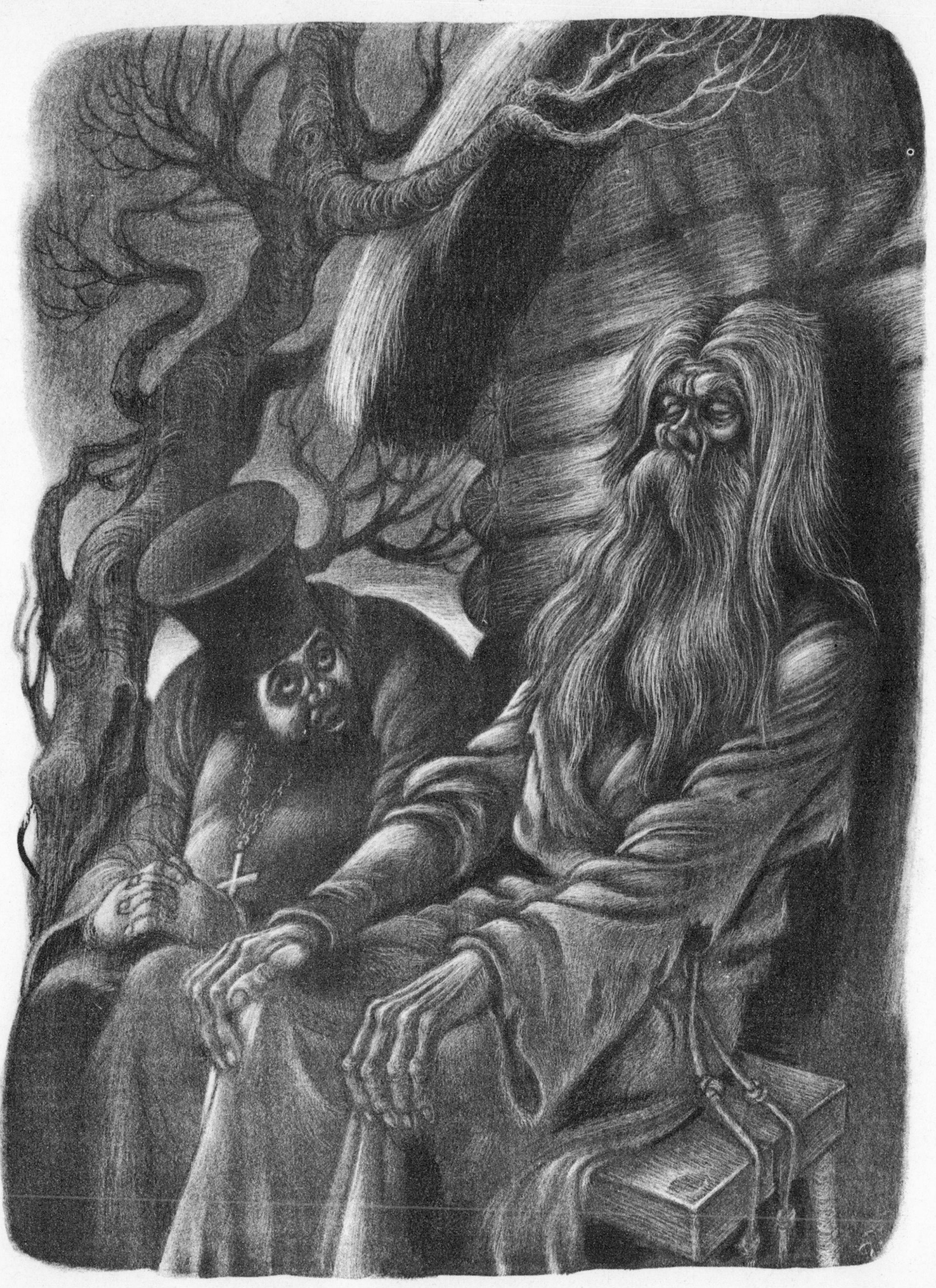

FATHER FERAPONT

of which had once been black. His eyes were grey, large and luminous, but strikingly prominent. He spoke with a broad accent. He was dressed in a peasant's long reddish coat of coarse convict cloth (as it used to be called) and had a stout rope round his waist. His throat and chest were bare. Beneath his coat, his shirt of the coarsest linen showed almost black with dirt, not having been changed for months.

They said that he wore irons weighing thirty pounds under his coat. His stockingless feet were thrust into old slippers almost dropping to pieces.

"From the little Obdorsk monastery, from St. Sylvester," the monk answered humbly, whilst his keen and inquisitive, but rather frightened little eyes kept watch on the hermit.

"I have been at your Sylvester's. I used to stay there. Is Sylvester well?"

The monk hesitated.

"You are a senseless lot! How do you keep the fasts?"

"Our dietary is according to the ancient conventual rules. During Lent there are no meals provided Mondays, Wednesdays, and Fridays. On Tuesday and Thursday we have white bread, stewed fruit with honey, wild berries, or salt cabbage and oatmeal stirabout. On Saturday white cabbage soup, noodles with peas, kasha, all with hemp oil. On weekdays we have dried fish and kasha with the cabbage soup. From Monday till Saturday evening, six days in Holy Week, we have only bread and water and uncooked vegetables, and that sparingly; if possible we do not take food every day, just as in the first week in Lent. On Good Friday nothing is eaten. In the same way on Saturday of Holy Week we have to fast till three o'clock, and then take a little bread and water and drink a single cup of wine. On Holy Thursday we drink wine and have something cooked without oil or not cooked at all. Inasmuch as the Laodicean council lays down for Holy Thursday: 'It is unseemly to break the fast on the Holy Thursday and dishonour the whole of Lent!' This is how we keep the fast. But what is that compared with you, holy father," added the monk, growing more confident, "for all the year round, even at Easter, you take nothing but bread and water, and what we should eat in two days lasts you full seven. It's truly marvellous — your great abstinence."

"And mushrooms?" asked Father Ferapont, suddenly.

"Mushrooms?" repeated the surprised monk.

"Yes. I can give up their bread, not needing it at all, and go away into the forest and live there on the mushrooms or the berries, but they can't give up their bread here, wherefore they are in bondage to the devil. Nowadays the unclean deny that there is need of such fasting. Haughty and unclean is their judgment."

"Och, true," sighed the monk.

"And have you seen devils among them?" asked Ferapont.

"Among them? Among whom?" asked the monk timidly.

"I went to the Father Superior on Trinity Sunday last year, I haven't been since. I saw a devil sitting on one man's chest hiding under his cassock, only his horns poked out; another had one peeping out of his pocket with such sharp eyes, he was afraid of me; another settled in the unclean belly of one, another was hanging round a man's neck, and so he was carrying him about without seeing him."

"You—can see spirits?" the monk inquired.

"I tell you I can see, I can see through them. When I was coming out from the Superior's I saw one hiding from me behind the door, and a husky one, a yard and a half or more high, with a thick long grey tail, and the tip of his tail was in the crack of the door and I was quick and slammed the door, pinching his tail in it. He squealed and began to struggle, and I made the sign of the cross over him three times. And he croaked on the spot like a crushed spider. He must have rotted there in the corner and be stinking, but they don't see, they don't smell it. It's a year since I have been there. I reveal it to you, as you are a stranger."

"Your words are fearful! But, holy and blessed father," said the monk, growing bolder and bolder, "is it true, as they noise abroad even to distant lands about you, that you are in continual communication with the Holy Ghost?"

"He does fly down at times. It happens."

"How does he fly down? In what form?"

"As a bird."

"The Holy Ghost in the form of a Dove?"

"There's the Holy Ghost and there's the Holy Spirit. The Holy Spirit can appear as other birds—sometimes as a swallow, sometimes a goldfinch and sometimes as a bluetit."

"How do you know him from an ordinary tit?"

"He speaks."

"How does he speak, in what language?"

"Human language."

"And what does he tell you?"

"Why, to-day he told me that a fool would visit me and would ask unseemly questions. You want to know too much, monk."

"Fearful are your words, most holy and blessed father," the monk shook his head. But there was a doubtful look in his frightened little eyes.

"Do you see this tree?" asked Father Ferapont, after a pause.

"I do, blessed father."

"You think it's an elm, but to me it looks otherwise."

"How does it look?" inquired the monk, after a pause of vain expectation.

"It happens at night. You see those two branches? In the night it is Christ holding out His arms to me and seeking me with those arms, I see it clearly and tremble. Oh, terror, terror!"

"What is terrible about it, if it's Christ Himself?"

"Why, He'll seize me and carry me aloft."

"Alive?"

"In the spirit and glory of Elijah, haven't you heard? He will take me in His arms and bear me away."

Although after this talk the monk returned to the cell he was sharing with one of the brothers, in considerable perplexity of mind, he was undoubtedly drawn towards Father Ferapont rather than towards Father Zosima. The monk from Obdorsk stood for fasting, above all, and it was not strange that one who kept so rigid a fast as Father Ferapont should "see marvels." His words certainly seemed queer, but only the Lord knew what was hidden in those words, and were not worse words and acts usual with those who renounced their intellects for the sake of Christ? The pinching of the devil's tail he was ready and eager to believe, and not only in the figurative sense. Besides he had, before visiting the monastery, a strong prejudice against the institution of "elders," which he only knew of by hearsay and believed to be a pernicious innovation. Before he had been long at the monastery, he had detected the secret murmurings of some frivolous brothers who disliked the institution. He was, besides, a meddlesome, inquisitive man, who poked his nose into everything. This was why the news of the fresh "miracle" performed by Father Zosima reduced him to extreme perplexity. Alyosha remembered afterwards how their inquisitive guest from Obdorsk had been continually flitting to and fro from one group to another, listening and asking questions among the monks who were crowding within and without the elder's cell. But he did not pay much attention to him at the time, and only recollected it afterwards.

He had no thought to spare for it indeed, for when Father Zosima, feeling tired again, had gone back to bed, he thought of Alyosha as he was closing his eyes, and sent for him. Alyosha ran at once. There was no one else in the cell but Father Païssy, Father Iosif, and Porfiry, a novice. The elder, opening his weary eyes and looking intently at Alyosha, asked him suddenly:

"Are your people expecting you, my son?"

Alyosha hesitated.

"Haven't they need of you? Didn't you promise some one yesterday to see them today?"

"I did promise—to my father—my brothers—others, too."

"You see. Go without fail. Don't grieve. Be sure I shall not die without your being by to hear my last word. To you I will say that word, my son, it will be my legacy to you. To you, dear son, because you love me. But now go to keep your promise."

Alyosha immediately obeyed, though it was hard to go. But the promise that he should hear his last word on earth, and above all that it would be bequeathed to him, Alyosha, sent a thrill of rapture through his soul. He made haste that he might finish what he had to do in the town and return quickly. Father Païssy, too, uttered some words of exhortation which moved and surprised him greatly. He spoke as they left the cell together.

"Remember, young man, constantly," Father Païssy began, without preface, "that the science of this world, which has become a great power, has, especially in the last century, analysed everything divine handed down to us in the holy books. After this cruel analysis, the learned of this world have nothing left of all that was sacred of old. But they have only analysed the parts and overlooked the whole, and indeed their blindness is astounding. Yet the whole still stands steadfast before their eyes, and the gates of hell shall not prevail against it. Has it not lasted nineteen centuries, is it not still a living, a moving power in the individual soul and among the masses of the people? It dwells as unshakably as before in the souls of the very atheists, who have destroyed everything! For even those who have renounced Christianity and rebel against it, in their inmost being still follow the Christian ideal, for hitherto neither their subtlety nor the ardour of their hearts has been able to create a higher image of man and of virtue than the image manifested by Christ of old. When it has been attempted, the result has been only grotesque. Remember this especially, young man, since you are being sent into the world by your departing elder. Maybe, remembering this great day, you will not forget my words, uttered from the heart for your guidance, seeing you are young, and the temptations of the world are great and beyond your strength to endure. Well, now go, my orphan."

With these words Father Païssy blessed him. As Alyosha left the monastery and thought them over, he suddenly realised that he had met a new and unexpected friend, a warmly loving teacher, in this austere monk who had hitherto treated him sternly. It was as though Father Zosima had bequeathed him to him at his death, and "perhaps that's just what had passed between them," Alyosha thought suddenly. The philosophic reflections he had just heard so unexpectedly testified to the ardour of Father Païssy's heart. He was in haste to arm the boy's mind for battle with temptation and to guard the young soul left in his charge with the strongest defence he could imagine.

CHAPTER II
AT HIS FATHER'S

FIRST of all, Alyosha went to his father. As he approached the house he recalled that his father had insisted the day before that he should come without his brother Ivan seeing him. "Why so?" Alyosha wondered suddenly. "Even if my father has something to say to me alone, why should I go in unseen? Most likely in his excitement yesterday he meant to say something different," he decided. Yet he was very glad when Marfa Ignatyevna, who opened the garden gate to him (Grigory, it appeared, was ill in bed in the lodge), told him in answer to his question that Ivan Fyodorovich had gone out two hours ago.

"And my father?"

"He is up, taking his coffee," Marfa answered somewhat drily.

Alyosha went in. The old man was sitting alone at the table, wearing slippers and an old dressing-gown. He was amusing himself by looking through some accounts, rather inattentively however. He was quite alone in the house, for Smerdyakov, too, had gone out, marketing. Though he had got up early and was trying to put a bold face on it, he looked tired and weak. His forehead, upon which huge purple bruises had come out during the night, was bandaged with a red handkerchief; his nose had swollen terribly in the night, and some smaller bruises covered it in patches, giving his whole face a peculiarly spiteful and irritable look. The old man was aware of this, and turned a hostile glance on Alyosha as he came in.

"The coffee is cold," he cried harshly; "I won't offer you any. I've ordered nothing but a lenten fish soup to-day, and I don't invite any one to share it. Why have you come?"

"To find out how you are," said Alyosha.

"Yes. Besides, I told you to come yesterday. It's all of no consequence. You need not have troubled. But I knew you'd drag yourself here directly."

He said this with the most hostile feeling. At the same time he got up and looked anxiously in the looking-glass (perhaps for the fortieth time that morning) at his nose. He began, too, adjusting the red handkerchief on his forehead more becomingly.

"Red's better. It's just like the hospital in a white one," he observed sententiously. "Well, how are things over there? How is your elder?"

"He is very ill; he may die to-day," answered Alyosha. But his father had not listened, and had forgotten his own question at once.

"Ivan's gone out," he said suddenly. "He

is doing his utmost to carry off Mitya's fiancée. That's what he is staying here for," he added maliciously, and, twisting his mouth, looked at Alyosha.

"Surely he did not tell you so?" asked Alyosha.

"Yes, he did, long ago. Would you believe it, he told me three weeks ago? You don't suppose he, too, came to murder me, do you? He must have had some object in coming."

"What do you mean? Why do you say such things?" said Alyosha, troubled.

"He doesn't ask for money, it's true, but yet he won't get a groat from me. I intend living as long as possible, you may as well know, my dear Alexey Fyodorovich, and so I need every copeck, and the longer I live, the more I shall need it," he continued, pacing from one corner of the room to the other, keeping his hands in the pockets of his loose greasy dressing-gown, which was made of yellow cotton material. "Now I am still a man, I am only fifty-five, but I want to remain something of a man for another twenty years yet. As I get older, you know, I'll become disgusting. The wenches won't come to me of their own accord, so I shall need my money. So I am saving up more and more, simply for myself, my dear son Alexey Fyodorovich. You may as well know. For I mean to wallow in my filth to the end, let me tell you. For filth is sweet; all abuse it, but all men live in it, only others do it on the sly, and I openly. And so all the other dirty ones fall upon me for being so simple. And your paradise, Alexey Fyodorovich, is not to my taste, let me tell you that; and it's not the proper place for a gentleman, your paradise, even if it exists. I believe that I fall asleep and don't wake up again, and that's all. You can pray for my soul if you like. And if you don't want to, don't, damn you! That's my philosophy. Ivan talked well here yesterday, though we were all drunk. Ivan is a conceited coxcomb, but he has no particular learning . . . nor education either. He sits silent and smiles at one without speaking —that's what pulls him through."

Alyosha listened to him in silence.

"Why won't he talk to me? If he does speak, he gives himself airs. Your Ivan is a scoundrel! And I'll marry Grushenka in a minute if I want to. For if you've money, Alexey Fyodorovich, you have only to want a thing and you can have it. That's what Ivan is afraid of, he is on the watch to prevent me getting married and that's why he is egging on Mitya to marry Grushenka himself. He hopes to keep me from Grushenka by that (as though I should leave him my money if I don't marry her!). Besides if Mitya marries Grushenka, Ivan will carry off his rich fiancée, that's what he's reckoning on! He is a scoundrel, your Ivan!"

"How cross you are. It's because of yesterday; you had better lie down," said Alyosha.

"There! you say that," the old man observed suddenly, as though it had struck him for the first time, "and I am not angry with you. But if Ivan said it, I should be angry with him. It is only with you I have good moments, otherwise you know I am an ill-natured man."

"You are not an ill-natured man, but a warped one," said Alyosha with a smile.

"Listen. I meant this morning to get that ruffian Mitya locked up and even now I don't know what I shall decide about it. Of course in these fashionable days fathers and mothers are looked upon as a prejudice, but even now the law does not allow you to drag your old father about by the hair, to kick him in the face with your heels in his own house, and brag of murdering him outright — all in the presence of witnesses. If I liked, I could nab him and have him locked up at once for what he did yesterday."

"Then you don't mean to lodge a complaint?"

"Ivan has dissuaded me. I shouldn't care about Ivan, but there's another thing."

And bending down to Alyosha, he went on in a confidential half-whisper.

"If I send the ruffian to prison, she'll hear of it and run to see him at once. But if she hears that he has beaten me, a weak old man, within an inch of my life, she may give him up and come to me. . . . For that's her way, everything by contraries. I know her through and through! Won't you have a drop of cognac? Take some cold coffee and I'll pour a quarter of a glass into it, it's delicious, my boy."

"No, thank you. I'll take that roll with me if I may," said Alyosha, and taking a three-copeck French roll he put it in the pocket of his cassock. "And you'd better not have cognac, either," he suggested apprehensively, looking into the old man's face.

"You are quite right, it irritates my nerves instead of soothing them. Only one little glass. I'll get it out of the cupboard."

He unlocked the cupboard, poured out a glass, drank it, then locked the cupboard and put the key back in his pocket.

"That's enough. One glass won't kill me."

"You see you are in a better humour now," said Alyosha, smiling.

"Um! I love you even without the cognac, but with scoundrels I am a scoundrel. Ivan is not going to Chermashnya — why is that? He is bent on spying, he wants to know how much I give Grushenka if she comes. They are all scoundrels! But I don't recognise Ivan, I don't know him at all. Where does he come from? He is not one of us in soul. As though I'd leave him anything! I shan't leave a will at all, you may as well know. And I'll crush Mitya like a beetle. I squash black beetles at night with my slipper; they squelch when you tread on them. And your Mitya will squelch, too. *Your* Mitya, for you love him. Yes, you love him and I am not afraid of your loving him. But if Ivan loved him I should be afraid for myself at his loving him. But Ivan loves nobody. Ivan is not one of us. People like Ivan are not our sort, my boy. They are like a cloud of dust. When the wind blows, the dust will be gone. . . . I had a silly idea in my head when I told you to come to-day; I wanted to find out from you about Mitya. If I were to hand him over a thousand or maybe two now, would the beggarly wretch agree to take himself off altogether for five years or, better still, thirty-five, and without Grushenka, and give her up once for all, eh?"

"I — I'll ask him," muttered Alyosha. "If you would give him three thousand, perhaps he ——"

"That's nonsense! You needn't ask him now, no need! I've changed my mind. It was a nonsensical idea of mine. I won't give him anything, not a penny, I want my money myself," cried the old man, waving his hand. "I'll crush him like a beetle without it. Don't say anything to him or else he will begin hoping. There's nothing for you to do here, you needn't stay. Is that fiancée of his, Katerina Ivanovna, whom he has kept so carefully hidden from me all this time, going to marry him or not? You went to see her yesterday, I believe?"

"Nothing will induce her to leave him."

"There you see how dearly these fine young ladies love a rake and a scoundrel. They are trash, I tell you, those pale young ladies, very different from . . . Ah, if I had his youth and the looks I had then (for I was better-looking than he at eight and twenty) I'd have been a conquering hero just as he is. He is a low cad! But he shan't have Grushenka, anyway, he shan't! I'll wipe the floor with him!"

His anger had returned with the last words.

"You can go. There's nothing for you to do here to-day," he snapped harshly.

Alyosha went up to say good-bye to him, and kissed him on the shoulder.

"What's that for?" the old man was a little surprised. "We shall see each other again, or do you think we shan't?"

"Not at all, I didn't mean anything."

"Nor did I, I did not mean anything," said the old man, looking at him. "Listen, listen," he shouted after him, "make haste and come again and I'll have a fish soup for you, a fine one, not like to-day. Be sure to come! Come to-morrow, do you hear, to-morrow!"

And as soon as Alyosha had gone out the door, he went to the cupboard again and gulped down another half-glass.

"That's enough!" he muttered, clearing his throat, and again he locked the cupboard and put the key in his pocket. Then he went into his bedroom, lay down on the bed, exhausted, and in one minute he was asleep.

CHAPTER III

A MEETING WITH SCHOOLBOYS

"THANK goodness he did not ask me about Grushenka," thought Alyosha, as he left his father's house and turned towards Madame Hohlakov's, "or I might have had to tell him of my meeting with Grushenka yesterday."

Alyosha felt painfully that since yesterday both combatants had renewed their energies, and that their hearts had grown hard again. "Father is spiteful and angry, he's made some plan and will stick to it. And what of Dmitri? He, too, will be harder than yesterday, he, too, must be spiteful and angry, and he, too, no doubt, has made some plan. Oh, I must succeed in finding him to-day, whatever happens."

But Alyosha had not long to meditate. An incident occurred on the road, which, though apparently of little consequence, made a great impression on him. Just after he had crossed the square and turned into an alley in order to reach Mihailovsky Street, which is divided by a small ditch from Bolshaya Street (our whole town is intersected by ditches), he saw a group of schoolboys between the ages of nine and twelve, at the bridge. They were going home from school, some with their bags on their shoulders, others with leather satchels slung across them, some in short jackets, others in little overcoats. Some even had those high boots with pleats round the ankles, such as little boys spoilt by rich fathers love to wear. The whole group was talking eagerly about something, apparently holding a council. Since his Moscow days Alyosha had never been able to pass children without taking notice of them, and although he was particularly fond of children of three or thereabouts, he liked schoolboys of ten and eleven, too. And so, anxious as he was to-day, he wanted at once to turn aside to talk to them. He looked into their excited rosy faces, and noticed at once that all the boys had stones in their hands. Beyond the ditch some thirty paces away, there was another schoolboy standing by a fence. He, too, had a satchel at his side. He was about ten years old, pale, delicate-looking, and with sparkling black eyes. He kept an attentive and anxious watch on the other six, obviously his schoolfellows with whom he had just come out of school, but with whom he evidently had a feud.

Alyosha went up and addressing a fair, curly-headed, rosy boy in a black jacket observed:

"When I had a satchel like yours, I always used to carry it on my left side, so as to have my right hand free, but you've got yours on your right side. So it will be awkward for you to get at it."

It was without premeditated artfulness that Alyosha began with this practical remark. But it is the only way for a grown-up person to get at once into confidential relations with a child, or still more with a group of children. One must begin in a serious businesslike way so as to be on a perfectly equal footing. Alyosha understood this by instinct.

"But he is left-handed," another, a fine healthy-looking boy of eleven, answered promptly. All the others stared at Alyosha.

"He even throws stones with his left hand," observed a third.

At that instant a stone flew into the group, but only just grazed the left-handed boy, though it was well and vigorously thrown by the boy standing on the other side of the ditch.

"Give it him, hit him back, Smurov," they all shouted. But Smurov, the left-handed boy, needed no telling, and at once revenged himself; he threw a stone, but it missed the boy and hit the ground. The boy on the other side of the ditch, the pocket of whose coat was visibly bulging with stones, flung another stone at the group; this time it flew straight at Alyosha and hit him rather painfully on the shoulder.

"He aimed it at you, he meant it for you. You are Karamazov, Karamazov!" the boys shouted, laughing. "Come, let's all go for him at once, go!" and six stones flew at the boy. One struck the boy on the head and he fell down, but at once leapt up and began ferociously returning their fire. Both sides threw stones incessantly. Many of the group had their pockets full, too.

"What are you about! Aren't you ashamed? Six against one! Why, you'll kill him," cried Alyosha.

He ran forward and met the flying stones to screen the solitary boy. Three or four ceased throwing for a minute.

"He began first!" cried a boy in a red shirt in an angry childish voice. "He is a beast, he stabbed Krasotkin in class the other day with a penknife. It bled. Krasotkin wouldn't tell tales, but he must be thrashed."

"But what for? I suppose you tease him."

"There, he sent a stone at your back again, he knows you," cried the children. "It's you he is aiming at now, not us. Come, all of you, at him again, don't miss, Smurov!" and again a fire of stones, and a very vicious one, began. The boy on the other side of the ditch was hit in the chest; he screamed, began to cry, and ran away uphill towards Mihailovsky Street. They all shouted: "Aha, he is funking, he is running away. Bath-mop!"

"You don't know what a beast he is, Karamazov, killing is too good for him," said the boy in the jacket, with flashing eyes. He seemed to be the eldest.

"What's wrong with him?" asked Alyosha, "is he a tell-tale or what?"

The boys looked at one another as though derisively.

"Are you going that way, to Mihailovsky?" the same boy went on. "Catch up with him. . . . You see he's stopped again, he is waiting and looking at you."

"He is looking at you," the other boys chimed in.

"You ask him, if he likes a ragged bath-mop. Do you hear, ask him that!"

There was a general burst of laughter. Alyosha looked at them, and they at him.

"Don't go near him, he'll hurt you," cried Smurov in a warning voice.

"I shan't ask him about the bath-mop, for I expect you tease him with that question somehow. But I'll find out from him why you hate him so."

"Find out then, find out," cried the boys, laughing.

Alyosha crossed the bridge and walked uphill by the fence, straight towards the boy.

"You'd better look out," the boys called after him; "he won't be afraid of you. He will stab you in a minute, on the sly, as he did Krasotkin."

The boy waited for him without budging. Coming up to him, Alyosha saw facing him a child about nine years old. He was an undersized weakly boy with a thin long pale face, with large dark eyes that gazed at him vindictively. He was dressed in a rather shabby old overcoat, which he had monstrously outgrown. His bare arms stuck out of his sleeves. There was a large patch on the right knee of his trousers, and in his right boot just at the toe there was a big hole in the leather, carefully blackened with ink. Both the pockets of his overcoat were weighed down with stones. Alyosha stopped two steps in front of him, looking inquiringly at him. The boy, seeing at once from Alyosha's eyes that he wouldn't beat him, became less defiant, and addressed him first.

"I am alone, and there are six of them. I'll beat them all, alone!" he said suddenly, with flashing eyes.

"I think one of the stones must have hurt you badly," observed Alyosha.

"But I hit Smurov on the head!" cried the boy.

"They told me that you know me, and that you threw a stone at me on purpose," said Alyosha.

The boy looked darkly at him.

"I don't know you. Do you know me?" Alyosha continued.

"Let me alone!" the boy cried irritably; but he did not move, as though he were expecting something, and again there was a vindictive light in his eyes.

"Very well, I am going," said Alyosha; "only I don't know you and I don't tease you. They told me how they tease you, but I don't want to tease you. Good-bye!"

"Monk in silk trousers!" cried the boy, following Alyosha with the same vindictive and defiant expression, and he threw himself into an attitude of defence, feeling sure that now Alyosha would fall upon him; but Alyosha turned, looked at him, and walked away. He had not gone three steps before the biggest stone the boy had in his pocket hit him a painful blow in the back.

"So you'll hit a man from behind! They tell the truth, then, when they say that you attack on the sly," said Alyosha, turning round again. This time the boy threw a stone savagely right into Alyosha's face; but Alyosha just had time to guard himself, and the stone struck him on the elbow.

"Aren't you ashamed? What have I done to you?" he cried.

The boy waited in silent defiance, certain that now Alyosha would attack him. Seeing that even now he would not, his rage was like a little wild beast's; he flew at Alyosha himself, and before Alyosha had time to move, the spiteful child had seized his left hand with both of his and bitten his middle finger. He fixed his teeth in it and it was ten seconds before he let go. Alyosha cried out with pain and pulled his finger away with all his might. The child let go at last and retreated to his former distance. Alyosha's finger had been badly bitten to the bone, close to the nail; it began to bleed.

Alyosha took out his handkerchief and bound it tightly round his injured hand. He was a full minute bandaging it. The boy stood waiting all the time.

At last Alyosha raised his gentle eyes and looked at him.

"Very well," he said, "you see how badly you've bitten me. That's enough, isn't it? Now tell me, what have I done to you?"

The boy stared in amazement.

"Though I don't know you and it's the first time I've seen you," Alyosha went on with the same serenity, "yet I must have done something to you — you wouldn't have hurt me like this for nothing. So what have I done? How have I wronged you, tell me?"

Instead of answering, the boy broke into a loud tearful wail and ran away. Alyosha walked slowly after him towards Mihailovsky Street, and for a long time he saw the child running in the distance as fast as ever, not turning his head, and no doubt still keeping up his tearful wail. He made up his mind to find him out as soon as he had time, and to solve this mystery. Just now he had not the time.

CHAPTER IV

AT THE HOHLAKOVS'

ALYOSHA soon reached Madame Hohlakov's house, a handsome stone house of two storeys, one of the finest in our town. Though Madame Hohlakov spent most of her time in another province where she had an estate, or in Moscow, where she had a house of her own, yet she had a house in our town, too, inherited from her forefathers. The estate in our district was the largest of her three estates, yet she had been very little in our province before this time. She ran out to Alyosha in the hall.

"Did you get my letter about the new miracle?" She spoke rapidly and nervously.

"Yes."

"Did you show it to every one? He restored the son to his mother!"

"He will die to-day," said Alyosha.

"I have heard, I know, oh, how I long to talk to you, to you, or some one about all this. No, to you, to you! And how sorry I am I can't see him! The whole town is in excitement, they are all suspense. But now — do you know Katerina Ivanovna is here now?"

"Ah, that's lucky," cried Alyosha. "Then I shall see her here. She told me yesterday to be sure to come and see her to-day."

"I know, I know all. I've heard exactly what happened yesterday — and the atrocious behaviour of that — creature. *C'est tragique*, and if I'd been in her place I don't know what I should have done. And your brother Dmitri Fyodorovich, what do you think of him? — my goodness! Alexey Fyodorovich, I am wandering, only fancy; your brother is in there with her, not that dreadful brother who was so shocking yesterday, but the other, Ivan Fyodorovich, he is sitting with her talking;

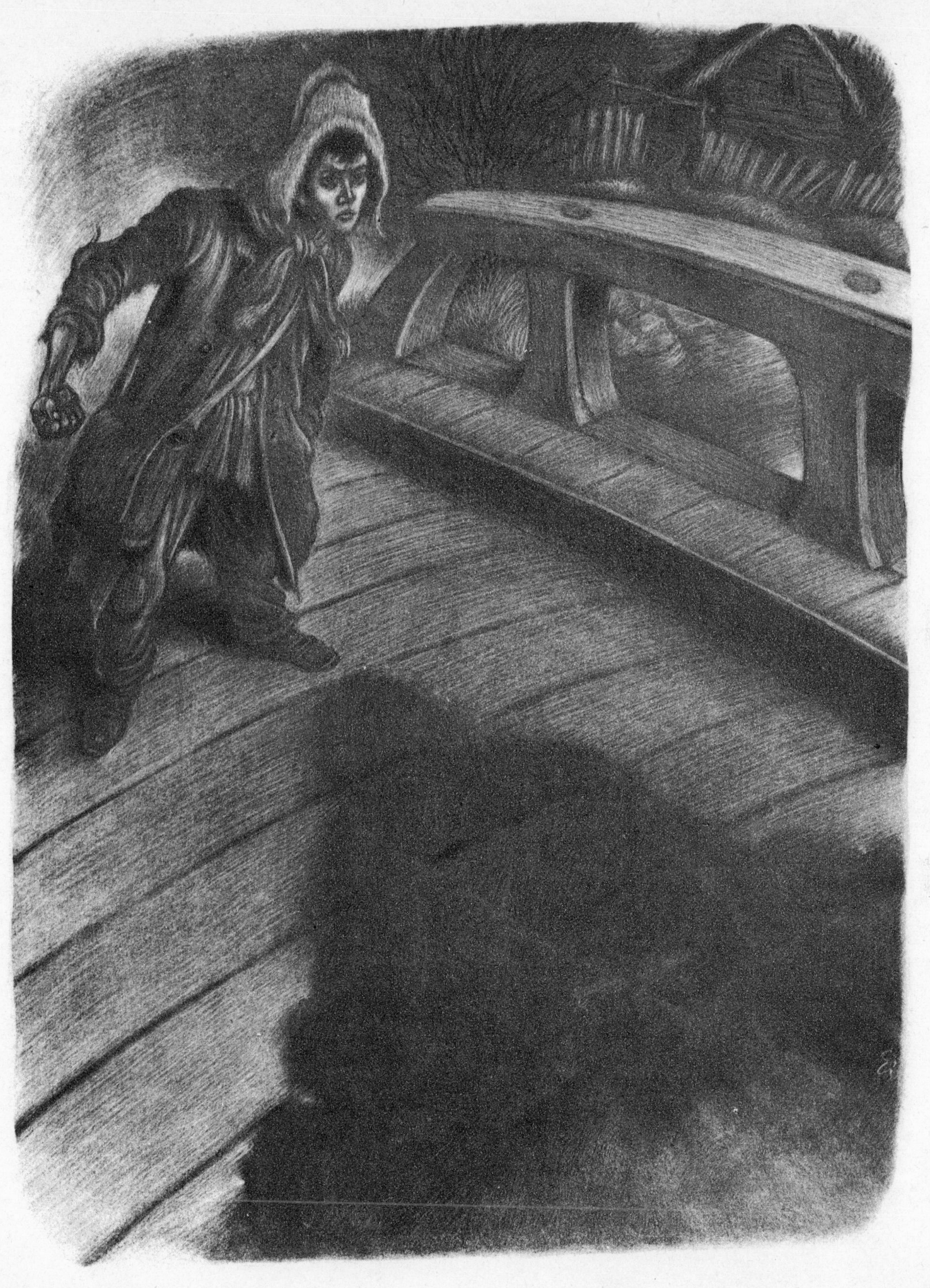

THE BOY WHO THREW THE STONE

they are having a serious conversation. If you could only imagine what's passing between them now — it's awful, I tell you, it's lacerating, it's like some incredible tale of horror. They are ruining themselves for no reason any one can see. They both recognize this and revel in it. I've been waiting for you! I've been thirsting for you! It's too much for me, that's the worst of it. I'll tell you all about it presently, but now I must speak of something else, the most important thing — I had quite forgotten what's most important. Tell me, why has Lise been in hysterics? As soon as she heard you were here, she threw a fit!"

"*Maman*, it's you who are hysterical now, not I." Lise's voice chirped through a tiny crack of the door leading into an inner room. Her voice sounded as though she wanted to laugh, but was doing her utmost to control it. Alyosha at once noticed the crack, and no doubt Lise was peeping through it, but that he could not see.

"And no wonder, Lise, no wonder . . . your caprices will make me hysterical, too. But she is so ill, Alexey Fyodorovich, she has been so ill all night, feverish and moaning! I could hardly wait for the morning and for Herzenstube to come. He says that he can make nothing of it, that we must wait. Herzenstube always comes and says that he can make nothing of it. As soon as you approached the house, she screamed, went into hysterics, and insisted on being wheeled back into her old room here."

"Mamma, I didn't know he had come. It wasn't on his account I wanted to be wheeled into this room."

"That's not true, Lise, Yulia ran to tell you that Alexey Fyodorovich was coming. She was on the look-out for you."

"My darling mamma, it's not at all clever of you. But if you want to make up for it and say something very clever, dear mamma, you'd better tell our honoured visitor, Alexey Fyodorovich, that he has shown his want of wit by venturing to come to us after what happened yesterday and although every one is laughing at him."

"Lise, you go too far. I declare I shall have to be severe. Who laughs at him? I am so glad he has come, I need him, I can't do without him. Oh, Alexey Fyodorovich, I am exceedingly unhappy!"

"But what's the matter with you, mamma, darling?"

"Ah, your caprices, Lise, your fidgetiness, your illness, that awful night of fever, that awful everlasting Herzenstube, everlasting, everlasting, that's the worst of it! Everything, in fact, everything. . . . Even that miracle, too! Oh, how it has upset me, how it has struck me, that miracle, dear Alexey Fyodorovich! And that tragedy in the drawing-room there, it's more than I can bear, I warn you. I can't bear it. A comedy, perhaps, not a tragedy. Tell me, will Father Zosima live till to-morrow, will he? Oh, my God! What is happening to me? Every minute I close my eyes and see that it's all nonsense, all nonsense."

"I should be very grateful," Alyosha interrupted suddenly, "if you could give me a clean rag to bind up my finger with. I have hurt it, and it's very painful."

Alyosha unbound his bitten finger. The handkerchief was soaked with blood. Madame Hohlakov screamed and shut her eyes.

"Good heavens, what a wound, how awful!"

But as soon as Lise saw Alyosha's finger through the crack, she flung the door open.

"Come, come here," she cried imperiously. "No nonsense now! Good heavens, why did you stand there saying nothing about it all this time? He might have bled to death, mamma! How did you do it? Water, water! You must wash it first of all, simply hold it in cold water to stop the pain, and keep it there, keep it there. . . . Make haste, mamma, some water in a slop basin. But do make haste," she finished nervously. She was quite frightened at the sight of Alyosha's wound.

"Shouldn't we send for Herzenstube?" cried Madame Hohlakov.

"Mamma, you'll be the death of me. Your Herzenstube will come and say that he can make nothing of it! Water, water! Mamma, for goodness' sake go yourself and hurry Yulia, she is such a slowcoach and never can come quickly! Make haste, mamma, or I shall die."

"Why, it's a trifle," cried Alyosha, frightened by this alarm.

Yulia ran in with water and Alyosha put his finger in it.

"Some lint, mamma, for mercy's sake, bring some lint and that muddy caustic lotion for cuts, what's it called? We've got some, we have. You know where the bottle is, mamma; it's in your bedroom in the right-hand cupboard, there's a big bottle of it there with the lint."

"I'll bring everything in a minute, Lise, only don't scream and don't fuss. You see how bravely Alexey Fyodorovich bears it. Where did you get such a dreadful wound, Alexey Fyodorovich?"

Madame Hohlakov hastened away. This was all Lise was waiting for.

"First of all, answer the question, where did you get hurt like this?" she asked Alyosha quickly. "And then I'll talk to you about something quite different. Well?"

Instinctively feeling that the time of her mother's absence was precious to her, Alyosha hastened to tell her of his enigmatic meeting with the schoolboys in the fewest words possible. Lise struck her hands together at his story.

"How can you, and in that dress too, get mixed up with schoolboys!" she cried angrily, as though she had rights over him. "You are nothing but a boy yourself if you can do that, a little boy! But you must find out for me about that horrid boy and tell me all about it, for there's some mystery in it. Now for the second thing, but first a question: can you, Alexey Fyodorovich, in spite of the pain, talk about the merest trifles, but talk sensibly?"

"Of course, and I don't feel much pain now."

"That's because your finger is in the water. It must be changed directly for it will get warm in a minute. Yulia, bring some ice from the cellar and another basin of water. Now she is gone, I can speak; will you give me the letter I sent you yesterday, dear Alexey Fyodorovich — be quick for mamma will be back in a minute and I don't want ——"

"I haven't got the letter."

"That's not true, you have. I knew you would say that. You've got it in that pocket. I've been regretting that foolish joke all night. Give me back the letter at once, give it me."

"I've left it at home."

"But you can't consider me as a child, a little girl, after that silly joke! I beg your pardon for that silliness, but you must bring me the letter, if you really haven't got it — bring it to-day, you must, you must."

"To-day I can't possibly, for I am going

back to the monastery and I shan't come and see you for the next two days — three or four perhaps — for Father Zosima ——"

"Four days, what nonsense! Listen. Did you laugh at me very much?"

"I didn't laugh a bit."

"Why not?"

"Because I believed all you said."

"You are insulting me!"

"Not at all. As soon as I read it, I thought that all that would come to pass, for as soon as Father Zosima dies, I am to leave the monastery. Then I shall go back and finish my studies, and when you reach the legal age we will be married. I shall love you. Though I haven't had time to think about it, I believe I couldn't find a better wife than you, and Father Zosima tells me I must marry."

"But I am a cripple, wheeled about in a chair," laughed Lise, flushing crimson.

"I'll wheel you about myself, but I'm sure you'll get well by then."

"But you are mad," said Lise, nervously, "to turn a joke into all this nonsense! Here's mamma, very conveniently, perhaps. Mamma, you are always late, how can you be so long! And here's Yulia with the ice!"

"Oh, Lise, don't scream, above all things don't scream. That scream drives me . . . How can I help it when you stuck the lint in another place. I've been hunting and hunting — I do believe you did it on purpose."

"But I couldn't tell that he would come with a bad finger, or else perhaps I might have done it on purpose. Angel mamma, you begin to say really witty things."

"Never mind my being witty, but I must say you show nice feeling for Alexey Fyodorovich's sufferings! Oh, my dear Alexey Fyodorovich, what's killing me is no one thing in particular, not Herzenstube, but everything together, that's what is too much for me."

"That's enough, mamma, enough about Herzenstube," Lise laughed gaily. "Hurry up with the lint and the lotion, mamma. That's simply Goulard water, Alexey Fyodorovich, I remember the name now, but it's a splendid lotion. Would you believe it, mamma, on the way here he had a fight with the boys in the street, and it was a boy bit his finger; isn't he a child, a child himself? Is he fit to be married after that? For only fancy, he wants to be married, mamma. Just think of him married, isn't it funny, isn't it awful?"

And Lise kept laughing her thin hysterical giggle, looking slyly at Alyosha.

"But why married, Lise? What makes you talk of such a thing? It's quite out of place — and perhaps the boy was rabid."

"Why, mamma! As though there were rabid boys!"

"Why not, Lise, as though I had said something stupid! Your boy might have been bitten by a mad dog and he would become mad and bite any one near him. How well she has bandaged it, Alexey Fyodorovich. I couldn't have done it. Do you still feel the pain?"

"It's nothing much now."

"You don't feel afraid of water?" asked Lise.

"Come, that's enough, Lise, perhaps I really was rather too quick talking of the boy being rabid, and you pounced upon it at once. Katerina Ivanovna has only just heard that you are here, Alexey Fyodorovich, she simply rushed at me, she's dying to see you, dying!"

"Ach, mamma, go to them yourself. He can't go just now, he is in too much pain."

"Not at all, I can go quite well," said Alyosha.

"What! You are going away? Is that what you say?"

"Well, when I've seen them, I'll come back here and we can talk as much as you like. But I should like to see Katerina Ivanovna at once, for I am very anxious to be back at the monastery as soon as I can."

"Mamma, take him away quickly. Alexey Fyodorovich, don't trouble to come and see me afterwards, but go straight back to your monastery — and a good riddance. I want to sleep, I didn't sleep all night."

"Ah, Lise, you are only making fun, but how I wish you would sleep!" cried Madame Hohlakov.

"I don't know what I've done. . . . I'll stay another three minutes, five if you like," muttered Alyosha.

"Even five! Do take him away quickly, mamma, he is a monster."

"Lise, you are crazy. Let us go, Alexey Fyodorovich, she is too capricious to-day. I am afraid to cross her. Oh, the trouble one has with nervous girls! Perhaps she really will be able to sleep after seeing you. How quickly you have made her sleepy, and how fortunate it is."

"Ah, mamma, how sweetly you talk. I must kiss you for it, mamma."

"And I kiss you, too, Lise. Listen, Alexey Fyodorovich," Madame Hohlakov began mysteriously and importantly, speaking in a rapid whisper. "I don't want to suggest anything, I don't want to lift the veil, you will see for yourself what's going on. It's appalling. It's the most fantastic farce. She loves your brother Ivan, and she is doing her utmost to persuade herself she loves your brother Dmitri. It's appalling! I'll go in with you, and if they don't turn me out, I'll stay to the end."

CHAPTER V

LACERATION IN THE DRAWING-ROOM

But in the drawing-room the conversation was already over. Katerina Ivanovna was greatly excited, though she looked resolute. At the moment Alyosha and Madame Hohlakov entered, Ivan Fyodorovich stood up to take leave. His face was rather pale, and Alyosha looked at him anxiously. The fact is, that at that moment a doubt, a harassing enigma, which had for some time haunted Alyosha, was being cleared up for him. During the preceding month it had been several times suggested to him that his brother Ivan was in love with Katerina Ivanovna, and, what was more, that he meant "to snatch her away" from Dmitri. Until quite lately the idea had seemed monstrous to Alyosha, though it worried him extremely. He loved both his brothers, and dreaded such rivalry between them. Meantime, Dmitri had said outright on the previous day that he was glad that Ivan was his rival, and that it was a great assistance to him, Dmitri. In what way would it help him? Would it enable him to marry Grushenka? But that Alyosha considered the worst thing possible. Besides all this, Alyosha had implicitly believed till the evening before that Katerina Ivanovna had a steadfast and passionate love for Dmitri; but he had only believed it till the evening before. He had fancied, too, that she was incapable of loving a man like Ivan, and that she did love Dmitri, and loved him just as he was, in spite of the monstrosity of such a passion.

But during yesterday's scene with Grushenka another idea had vaguely suggested itself to him. The word "lacerating," which Madame Hohlakov had just uttered, almost made him start, because half waking up towards daybreak that night he had cried out, "Laceration, laceration," probably in response to a dream of his. He had been dreaming all night of the previous day's scene at Katerina Ivanovna's. And now Alyosha was struck by Madame Hohlakov's blunt and persistent assertion that Katerina Ivanovna was in love with Ivan, and was only deceiving herself through some sort of pose, from "self-laceration," and was torturing herself with her pretended love for Dmitri out of some fancied sense of duty. "Yes," he thought, "perhaps the whole truth lies in those words." But in that case what was Ivan's position? Alyosha felt instinctively that a character like Katerina Ivanovna's must dominate, and she could only dominate some one like Dmitri, and never a man like Ivan. For Dmitri might at last submit to her domination "and be happy" (which was what Alyosha would have desired), but Ivan — no, Ivan could not submit to her, and such submission would not give him happiness. That was the notion that for some reason Alyosha had formed in his mind about Ivan. And now all these doubts and reflections flitted through his mind as he entered the drawing-room. Another idea, too, suddenly and irresistibly took hold of him: "What if she loved neither of them — neither Ivan nor Dmitri?"

I must note that Alyosha felt as it were ashamed of his own thoughts and had reproached himself when they kept recurring to him during the last month. "What do I know about love and women and how can I decide such questions?" he thought self-reproachfully, after each such thought or conjecture. And yet it was impossible not to think about it. He felt instinctively that this rivalry was of immense importance in his brothers' lives and that a great deal depended upon it.

"One reptile will devour the other," Ivan had pronounced the day before, speaking in anger of his father and Dmitri. So Ivan looked upon Dmitri as a reptile, and perhaps had long done so. Was it perhaps since he had known Katerina Ivanovna? That phrase had, of course, escaped Ivan unawares yesterday, but that only made it more important. If he felt like that, what chance was there of peace? Were there not, on the contrary, new grounds for hatred and hostility in their family? And with which of them was Alyosha to sympathise? And what was he to wish for each of them? He loved them both, but what could he desire for each in the midst of such terrible conflicts? He might go quite astray in this maze, and Alyosha's heart could not endure uncertainty, because his love was always of an active character. He was incapable of passive love. If he loved any one, he set to work at once to help him. And to do so he must know what he was aiming at; he must know for certain what was best for each, and having ascertained this it was natural for him to help them both.

But instead of a definite aim, he found nothing but uncertainty and perplexity on all sides. "It was lacerating," as was said just now. But what could he understand even in this "laceration"? He did not understand the first word in this perplexing maze.

Seeing Alyosha, Katerina Ivanovna said quickly and joyfully to Ivan, who had already got up to go: "One minute! Stay another minute! I want to hear the opinion of this person here whom I trust absolutely. Don't go away," she added, addressing Madame Hohlakov. She made Alyosha sit down beside her, and Madame Hohlakov sat opposite, beside Ivan.

"You are all my friends here, all I have in the world, my dear friends," she began ardently, in a voice which quivered with tears of genuine suffering, and again Alyosha's heart turned to her at once. "You, Alexey Fyodorovich, were a witness yesterday of that terrible scene, and saw how I acted. You did not see it, Ivan Fyodorovich, he did. What he thought of me yesterday I don't know. I only know one thing, that if it were repeated to-day, this minute, I should have the same feelings again as yesterday — have the same feelings, speak the same words, make the same gestures. You remember my actions, Alexey Fyodorovich; you checked me in one of them . . . (as she said that, she flushed and her eyes gleamed). I must tell you that I can't get reconciled to anything. Listen, Alexey Fyodorovich. I don't even know whether I still love *him*. I feel *pity* for him, and that is a poor sign of love. If I loved him, if I still loved him, perhaps I shouldn't pity him now, but should hate him."

Her voice quivered, and tears glittered on her eyelashes. Alyosha shuddered inwardly. "That girl is truthful and sincere," he thought, "and she does not love Dmitri any more."

"That's true, that's true," cried Madame. "Wait, dear. I haven't told you the chief, the final decision I came to during the night. I feel that perhaps my decision is a terrible one — for me, but I foresee that nothing will induce me to change it — nothing. It will be so all my life. My dear, kind, ever-faithful and generous adviser, the one friend I have in the world, Ivan Fyodorovich, with his deep insight into the heart, approves and commends my decision. He knows it."

"Yes, I approve of it," Ivan assented, in a subdued but firm voice.

"But I should like Alyosha, too (Ah! Alexey Fyodorovich, forgive my calling you simply Alyosha), I should like Alexey Fyodorovich, too, to tell me before my two friends whether I am right. I feel instinctively that you, Alyosha, my dear brother (for you are a dear brother to me)," she said again ecstatically, taking his cold hand in her hot one, "I foresee that your decision, your approval, will bring me peace, in spite of all my sufferings, for, after your words, I shall be calm and submit — I feel that."

"I don't know what you are asking me," said Alyosha, flushing. "I only know that I love you and at this moment wish for your happiness more than my own! . . . But I know nothing about such affairs," something impelled him to add hurriedly.

"In such affairs, Alexey Fyodorovich, in such affairs, the chief thing is honour and duty and something higher — I don't know what — but higher perhaps even than duty. I am conscious of this irresistible feeling in my heart, and it compels me irresistibly. But it may all be put in two words. I've already decided, even if he marries that — creature (she began solemnly), whom I never, never can forgive, *even then I will not abandon him*. Henceforward I will never, never abandon him!" she cried, torn by a sort of pale, forced ecstasy. "Not that I would tag after him continually, get in his way and worry him. Oh, no! I will go away to another town — wherever you please — but I will watch over him all my life — I will watch over him all my life untiringly. When he becomes unhappy with that woman, and that is bound to happen quite soon, let him come to me and he will find a friend, a sister. . . . Only a sister, of course, and so for ever; but he will learn at least that that sister is really his sister, who loves him and has sacrificed all her life to him. I will gain my point. I will insist on his finally getting to know me and confiding entirely in me, without reserve," she cried, in a sort of frenzy. "I will be his god, to whom he will pray — and that, at least, he owes me for his treachery and for what I suffered yesterday through him. And let him see that all my life I will be true to him and the promise I gave him, in spite of his being untrue and betraying me. I will — I will become nothing but a means for his happiness, or — how shall I say? — an instrument, a machine for his happiness, and this all my life, all my life, and he will see this all his life! That's my decision. Ivan Fyodorovich fully approves of me."

She was breathless. She had perhaps intended to express her thought in a more dignified, graceful, and natural way, but it was expressed too hastily and crudely. Her manner was full of youthful impulsiveness, it betrayed that she was still smarting from yesterday's insult, and that her pride craved satisfaction. She felt this herself. Her face suddenly darkened, an unpleasant look came into her eyes. Alyosha at once saw it and felt a pang of sympathy. His brother Ivan made it worse by putting in:

"I've only expressed my own view. Coming from any one else," he said, "this would have been affected and overstrained, but from you — no. Any other woman would have been wrong, but you are right. I don't know how to explain it, but I see that you are absolutely sincere and, therefore, you are right."

"But that's only for the moment. And what does this moment mean? Nothing but yesterday's insult." Madame Hohlakov obviously had not intended to interfere, but she could not refrain from this very just comment.

"Quite so, quite so," cried Ivan, with peculiar eagerness, obviously annoyed at being interrupted, "in any one else this moment would be due only to yesterday's impression and would be only a moment. But with Katerina Ivanovna's character, that moment will last all her life. What for any one else would be only a promise is for her an everlasting, burdensome, grim, perhaps, but unremitting duty. And she will be sustained by the sense of having fulfilled this duty. Your life, Katerina Ivanovna, will henceforth be spent in painful contemplation of your own feelings, your own heroism, and your own sorrow; but in the end that suffering will be softened and your life will turn into sweet contemplation of a bold and proud design which has been carried out. Yes, proud it certainly is, and desperate in any case, but a triumph for you. And the consciousness of it will in the end be a source of complete satisfaction and will reconcile you to everything else."

This was unmistakably said with some malice and obviously with intention; even perhaps with no desire to conceal that he spoke ironically and mockingly.

"Oh, dear, how wrong it all is!" Madame Hohlakov cried again.

"Alexey Fyodorovich, you speak. I want dreadfully to know what you will say!" cried Katerina Ivanovna, and suddenly burst into tears. Alyosha got up from the sofa.

"It's nothing, nothing!" she went on through her tears. "I'm upset, I didn't sleep last night. But by the side of two such friends as you and your brother I still feel strong — for I know — you two will never desert me."

"Unluckily I may be obliged to return to Moscow — to-morrow — and to leave you for a long time — And, unluckily, it's unavoidable," Ivan said suddenly.

"To-morrow — to Moscow!" her face was suddenly contorted; "but — but, dear me, how fortunate," she cried in a voice suddenly changed. In one instant there was no trace left of her tears. She underwent an instantaneous transformation, which amazed Alyosha. Instead of a poor, insulted girl, weeping in a sort of emotional "laceration," he saw a woman completely self-possessed and even exceedingly pleased, as though something agreeable had just happened.

"Oh, not fortunate that I am losing you, of course not," she corrected herself suddenly, with the charming smile of a woman of the world. "Such a friend as you are could not suppose that. I am only too unhappy at losing you." She rushed impulsively at Ivan, and seizing both his hands, pressed them ardently. "But what is fortunate is that in Moscow you will be able to see auntie and Agafya and to tell them all the horror of my present position. You can speak with complete openness to Agafya, but spare dear auntie. You will know how to do that. You can't think how wretched I was yesterday and this morning, wondering how I could write them that dreadful letter — for one can never tell such things in a letter. . . . Now it will be easy for me to write, for you will see them and explain everything. Oh, how glad I am! But I am only glad of that, believe me. Of course, no one can take your place. . . . I will run at once to write the letter," she finished suddenly, and took a step as though to leave the room.

"And what about Alyosha and his opinion, which you were so desperately anxious to hear?" cried Madame Hohlakov. There was a sarcastic, angry note in her voice.

"I had not forgotten that," cried Katerina Ivanovna, coming to a sudden standstill, "and why are you so antagonistic at such a moment?" she added, with warm and bitter reproachfulness. "What I said, I repeat. I must have his opinion. More than that, I must have his decision! As he says, so it shall be. You see how anxious I am for your words, Alexey Fyodorovich. . . . But what's the matter?"

"I couldn't have believed it. I can't understand it!" Alyosha cried suddenly in distress.

"What? what?"

"He is going to Moscow, and you cry out that you are glad. You said that on purpose! And you begin explaining that you are not glad of that but sorry to be — losing a friend. But that was acting, too — you were playing a part — as in a theatre!"

"In a theatre? What? What do you mean?" exclaimed Katerina Ivanovna, profoundly astonished, flushing crimson, and frowning.

"Though you assure him you are sorry to lose a friend in him, you persist in telling him to his face that it's fortunate he is going," said Alyosha breathlessly. He was standing at the table and did not sit down.

"What are you talking about? I don't understand . . ."

"I don't understand myself. . . . It's like a sudden illumination . . . I know I am not saying it properly, but I'll say it all the same," Alyosha went on in the same shaking and broken voice. "What I see is that perhaps you don't love Dmitri at all . . . and never have, from the beginning. . . . And Dmitri, too, has never loved you . . . and only esteems you. . . . I really don't know how I dare to say all this, but somebody must tell the truth . . . for nobody here wishes to tell the truth."

"What truth?" cried Katerina Ivanovna, and there was an hysterical note in her voice.

"I'll tell you," Alyosha went on with desperate haste, as though he were leaping headlong from a house-top. "Call Dmitri; I will fetch him — and let him come here and take your hand and take Ivan's and join your hands. For you're torturing Ivan, simply because you love him — and torturing him, because you love Dmitri through 'self-laceration' — with an unreal love — because you've persuaded yourself to."

Alyosha broke off and was silent.

"You . . . you . . . you are a little religious idiot — that's what you are!" Katerina Ivanovna snapped. Her face was white and her lips were contorted with anger.

Ivan suddenly laughed and got up. His hat was in his hand.

"You are mistaken, my good Alyosha," he said, with an expression Alyosha had never seen in his face before — an expression of youthful sincerity and strong, irresistibly frank feeling. "Katerina Ivanovna has never cared for me! She has known all the time that I cared for her — though I never said a word of my love to her — she knew, but she didn't care for me. I have never been her friend either, not for one moment; she is too proud to need my friendship. She kept me at her side as a means of revenge. She revenged herself through me and on me for all the insults which she has been continually receiving from Dmitri ever since their first meeting. For even that first meeting has rankled in her heart as an insult — that's what her heart is like! All the time I did nothing but listen to her speak of her love for him. I am going now; but, believe me, Katerina Ivanovna, you really love only him. And the more he insults you, the more you love him — that's your 'laceration.' You love him just as he is; you love him for insulting you. If he reformed, you'd give him up at once and cease to love him. But you need him so as to contemplate continually your heroic fidelity and to reproach him for infidelity. And it all comes from your pride. Oh, there's a great deal of humiliation and self-abasement about it, but it all comes from pride. . . . I am too young and I've loved you too much. I know that I ought not to say this, that it would be more dignified on my part simply to leave you, and it would be less offensive for you. But I am going far away, and shall never come back. . . . It is for ever. I don't want to sit beside a 'laceration.' . . . But I don't know how to speak now. I've said everything. . . . Good-bye, Katerina Ivanovna; you can't be angry with me, for I am a hundred times more severely punished than you, if only by the fact that I shall never see you again. Good-bye! I don't want your hand. You have tortured me too deliberately for me to be able to forgive you at this moment. I shall forgive you later, but now I don't want your hand. '*Den Dank, Dame, begehr ich nicht,*' " he added, with a crooked smile, showing, however, that he had read Schiller, and read him, indeed, till he knew him by heart — which Alyosha would never have believed. He went out of the room without saying good-bye even to his hostess, Madame Hohlakov. Alyosha struck his hands together.

"Ivan!" he cried desperately after him. "Come back, Ivan! No, nothing will induce him to come back now!" he cried again, with sorrowful understanding; "but it's my fault, my fault. I began it! Ivan spoke angrily, wrongly. Unjustly and angrily. He must come back here, come back," Alyosha kept exclaiming frantically.

Katerina Ivanovna went suddenly into the next room.

"You have done no harm. You behaved beautifully, like an angel," Madame Hohlakov whispered rapidly and ecstatically to Alyosha. "I will do my utmost to prevent Ivan Fyodorovich from going."

Her face beamed with delight, to the great distress of Alyosha, but Katerina Ivanovna suddenly returned. She had two hundred-rouble notes in her hand.

"I have a great favour to ask of you, Alexey Fyodorovich," she began, addressing Alyosha with an apparently calm and even voice, as though nothing had happened. "A week — yes, I think it was a week ago — Dmitri Fyodorovich was guilty of a hasty and unjust action — a very ugly action. There is a low tavern here and in it he met that discharged officer, that captain, whom your father used to employ in some business. Dmitri Fyodorovich somehow lost his temper with this captain, seized him by the beard and dragged him out into the street and along it for some distance, in that insulting fashion. And I am told that his son, a boy, still a child, who is at school here, saw it and ran beside them crying and begging for his father, appealing to every one to defend him, but every one laughed. You must forgive me, Alexey Fyodorovich, I cannot think without indignation of that disgraceful action of *his* . . . one of those actions of which only Dmitri Fyodorovich would be capable in his anger . . . and his passions! I can't speak of it even. . . . I can't find words. I've made inquiries about his victim, and find he is a very poor man. His name is Snegiryov. He did something wrong in the army and was discharged. I can't tell you what. And now he has sunk into terrible destitution, with his family — a miserable family of sick children, and, I believe, an insane wife. He has been living here a long time; he used to work as a copying clerk, but now he is getting nothing. I thought if you . . . that is I thought . . . I don't know. I am so confused. You see, I wanted to ask you, my dear Alexey Fyodorovich, to go to him, to find some excuse to go to them — I mean to that captain — oh, goodness, how badly I explain it! — and delicately, carefully, as only you know how to (Alyosha blushed), manage to give him this assistance, these two hundred roubles. He will be sure to take it. . . . I mean, persuade him to take it. . . . Or, rather, what do I mean? You see it's not by way of compensation to prevent him from taking proceedings (for I believe he meant to), but simply a token of sympathy, of a desire to assist him, from me, Dmitri Fyodorovich's betrothed, not from himself. . . . But you know. . . . I would go myself, but you'll know how to do it ever so much better. He lives in Ozyornaya Street, in the house of a woman called Kalmikov. . . . For God's sake, Alexey Fyodorovich, do it for me, and now . . . now I am rather . . . tired. Good-bye!"

She turned so quickly and disappeared behind the portière that Alyosha had not time to utter a word, though he wanted to speak. He longed to beg her pardon, to blame himself, to say something, for his heart was full and he could not bear to go out of the room without doing so. But Madame Hohlakov took him by the hand and drew him along with her. In the hall she stopped him again as before.

"She is proud, she is struggling with herself; but kind, charming, generous," she exclaimed, in a half-whisper. "Oh, how I love her, especially sometimes, and how glad I am again of everything! Dear Alexey Fyodorovich, you didn't know, but I must tell you, that we all, all — both her aunts, I and all of us, Lise, even — have been hoping and praying for nothing for the last month but that she may give up your favourite Dmitri, who takes no notice of her and does not care for her, and marry Ivan Fyodorovich — such an excellent and cultivated young man, who loves her more than anything in the world. We are in a regular plot to bring it about, and I am even staying on here perhaps on that account."

"But she has been crying — she has been wounded again," cried Alyosha.

"Never trust a woman's tears, Alexey Fyodorovich. I am never for the women in such cases. I am always on the side of the men."

"Mamma, you are spoiling and ruining him," Lise's thin voice cried from behind the door.

"No, it was all my fault. I am horribly to blame," Alyosha repeated unconsoled, hiding his face in his hands in an agony of remorse for his indiscretion.

"Quite the contrary; you behaved like an angel, like an angel. I am ready to say so a thousand times over."

"Mamma, how has he behaved like an angel?" Lise's voice was heard again.

"I somehow fancied all at once," Alyosha went on as though he had not heard Lise, "that she loved Ivan, and so I said that stupid thing. . . . What will happen now?"

"To whom, to whom?" cried Lise. "Mamma, you really want to be the death of me. I ask you and you don't answer."

At the moment the maid ran in.

"Katerina Ivanovna is ill. . . . She is crying, struggling . . . in hysterics."

"What is the matter?" cried Lise, in a tone of real anxiety. "Mamma, I shall be having hysterics, and not she!"

"Lise, for mercy's sake, don't scream, don't kill me. At your age one can't know everything that grown-up people know. I'll come and tell you everything you ought to know. Oh, mercy on us! I am coming, I am coming. . . . Hysterics is a good sign, Alexey Fyodorovich; it's an excellent thing that she is hysterical. That's just as it ought to be. In such cases I am always against the woman, against all these feminine tears and hysterics. Run and say, Yulia, that I'll fly to her. As for Ivan Fyodorovich's going away like that, it's her own fault. But he won't go away. Lise, for mercy's sake, don't scream! Oh, yes; you are not screaming. It's I am screaming. Forgive your mamma; but I am delighted, delighted, delighted! Did you notice, Alexey Fyodorovich, how young, how young Ivan Fyodorovich was just now when he went out, when he said all that and went out? I thought he was so learned, such a *savant*, and all of a sudden he behaved so warmly, openly, and youthfully, with such youthful inexperience, and it was all so fine, like you. . . . And the way he repeated that German verse, it was just like you! But I must fly, I must fly! Alexey Fyodorovich, make haste to carry out her commission, and then make haste back. Lise, do you want anything now? For mercy's sake, don't keep Alexey Fyodorovich a minute. He will come back to you at once."

Madame Hohlakov at last ran off. Before leaving, Alyosha would have opened the door to see Lise.

"On no account," cried Lise. "On no account now. Speak through the door. How have you come to be an angel? That's the only thing I want to know."

"For an awful piece of stupidity, Lise! Good-bye!"

"Don't dare to go away like that!" Lise was beginning.

"Lise, I have a real sorrow! I'll be back directly, but I have a great, great sorrow!"

And he ran out of the room.

CHAPTER VI

LACERATION IN THE COTTAGE

HE was really grieved in a way he had seldom been before. He had rushed in like a fool, and meddled in what? In a love-affair. "But what do I know about it? What can I tell about such things?" he repeated to himself for the hundredth time, flushing crimson. "Oh, being ashamed would be nothing; shame is but the punishment I deserve. The trouble is I shall certainly have caused more unhappiness. . . . And Father Zosima sent me to reconcile and unite. Is this the way to bring people together?" Then he suddenly remembered how he had tried to join their hands, and he felt fearfully ashamed again. "Though I acted quite sincerely, I must be more sensible in the future," he concluded suddenly, and did not even smile at his conclusion.

Katerina Ivanovna's commission took him to Ozyornaya Street, and his brother Dmitri lived close by, in a lane. Alyosha decided to go to him in any case before going to the captain, though he had a presentiment that he would not find his brother. He suspected that he would intentionally keep out of his way now, but he must find him anyhow. Time was passing: the thought of his dying elder had not left Alyosha for one minute from the time he set off from the monastery.

There was one point which interested him particularly about Katerina Ivanovna's commission: when she had mentioned the captain's son, the little schoolboy who had run beside his father crying, the idea had at once struck Alyosha that this must be the schoolboy who had bitten his finger when he, Alyosha, asked him what he had done to hurt him. Now Alyosha felt practically certain of this, though he could not have said why. Thinking of another subject was a relief, and he resolved to think no more about the "mischief" he had done, and not to torture himself with remorse, but to do what he had to do, let come what would. At that thought he was completely comforted. Turning to the street where Dmitri lodged, he felt hungry, and taking out of his pocket the roll he had brought from his father's, he ate it. It made him feel stronger.

Dmitri was not at home. The people of the house, an old cabinet-maker, his son, and his old wife, looked with positive suspicion at Alyosha. "He hasn't slept here for the last three nights. Maybe he has gone away," the old man said in answer to Alyosha's persistent inquiries. Alyosha saw that he was answering in accordance with instructions. When he asked whether he were not at Grushenka's or in hiding at Foma's (Alyosha spoke so freely on purpose), all three looked at him in alarm. "They are fond of him, they are doing their best for him," thought Alyosha. "That's good."

At last he found the house in Ozyornaya Street. It was a decrepit little house, leaning to one side, with three windows looking into the street, and with a muddy yard, in the middle of which stood a solitary cow. He crossed the yard and found the door opening into the passage. On the left of the passage lived the old woman of the house with her old daughter. Both seemed to be deaf. In answer to his repeated inquiry for the captain, one of them at last understood that he was asking for their lodgers, and pointed to a door across the passage. The captain's lodging turned out to be a simple cottage room. Alyosha had his hand on the iron latch to open the door, when he was struck by the strange hush within. Yet he knew from Katerina Ivanovna's words that the man had a family. "Either they are all asleep or perhaps they have heard me coming and are waiting for me to open the door. I'd better knock first," and he knocked. An answer came, but not at once, after an interval of perhaps ten seconds.

"Who's there?" shouted some one in a loud and very angry voice.

Then Alyosha opened the door and crossed the threshold. He found himself in a regular peasant's room. Though it was large, it was cumbered up with domestic belongings of all sorts, and there were several people in it. On the left was a large Russian stove. From the stove to the window on the left a rope was strung across the room, and there were rags hanging on it. There was a bedstead against the wall on each side, right and left, covered with knitted quilts. On the one on the left was a pyramid of four print-covered pillows, each smaller than the one beneath. On the other there was only one very small pillow. The opposite corner was screened off by a curtain or a sheet hung on a string. Behind this curtain could be seen a bed made up on a bench and a chair. The rough square table of plain wood had been moved against the middle window. The three windows, which consisted each of four tiny greenish mouldy panes, gave little light, and were close shut, so that the room was not very light and rather stuffy. On the table was a frying-pan with the remains of some fried eggs, a half-eaten piece of bread, and a small bottle with a few drops of vodka.

A woman of genteel appearance, wearing a cotton gown, was sitting on a chair by the bed on the left. Her face was thin and yellow, and her sunken cheeks betrayed at the first glance that she was ill. But what struck Alyosha most was the expression in the poor woman's eyes — a look of surprised inquiry and yet of haughty pride. And while he was talking to her husband, her big brown eyes moved from one speaker to the other with the same haughty and questioning expression. Beside her at the window stood a young girl, rather plain, with scanty reddish hair, poorly but very neatly dressed. She looked disdainfully at Alyosha as he came in. Beside the other bed was sitting another female figure. She was a very pathetic creature, a young girl of about twenty, but hunchbacked and crippled, "with withered legs," as Alyosha was told afterwards. Her crutches stood in the corner close by. The strikingly beautiful and gentle eyes of this poor girl looked with mild serenity at Alyosha. A man of forty-five was sitting at the table, finishing the fried eggs. He was spare, small, and weakly built. He had reddish hair and a scanty light-coloured beard, very much like a ragged bath-mop (this comparison and the phrase "bath-mop" flashed at once into Alyosha's mind for some reason, he remembered it afterwards). It was obviously this gentleman who had shouted to him, as there was no other man in the room. But when Alyosha went in, he leapt up from the bench on which he was sitting, and, hastily wiping his mouth with a ragged napkin, darted up to Alyosha.

"It's a monk come to beg for the monastery. A nice place to come to!" the girl standing in the corner on the left said aloud. The man spun round towards her instantly and answered her in an excited and breaking voice.

"No, Varvara, you are wrong. Allow me to ask, sir," he turned again to Alyosha, "what has brought you to — our retreat?"

Alyosha looked attentively at him. It was the first time he had seen him. There was something angular, flurried, and irritable about him. Though he had obviously just been drinking, he was not drunk. There was extraordinary impudence in his expression, and yet, strange to say, at the same time there was obvious cowardice. He looked like a man who had long been kept in subjection and had submitted to it, and now had suddenly turned and was trying to assert himself. Or, better still, like a man who wants dreadfully to hit you but is horribly afraid you will hit him. In his words and in the intonation of his shrill voice there was a sort of crazy humour, at times spiteful and at times cringing, and continually shifting from one tone to another. The question about "our retreat" he had asked as it were quivering all over, rolling his eyes, and skipping up so close to Alyosha that he instinctively drew back a step. He was dressed in a very shabby dark cotton coat, patched and spotted. He wore checked trousers of an extremely light colour, long out of fashion, and of very thin material. They were so crumpled and so short that he looked as though he had grown out of them like a boy.

"I am Alexey Karamazov," Alyosha began in reply.

"I quite understand that, sir," the gentleman snapped out at once to assure him that he knew who he was already. "I am Captain Snegiryov, sir, but I am still desirous to know precisely what has led you ——"

"Oh, I've come for nothing special. I wanted to have a word with you — if only you allow me."

"In that case, here is a chair, sir; kindly take a seat, sir. That's what they used to say in the old comedies, 'kindly take a seat,' " and with a rapid gesture he seized an empty chair (it was a rough wooden chair, not upholstered) and set it for him almost in the middle of the room; then, taking another similar chair for himself, he sat down facing Alyosha, so close to him that their knees almost touched.

"Nikolay Ilyich Snegiryov, sir, formerly a captain in the Russian infantry, put to shame for his vices, but still a captain. Though I don't talk like one now; it's in the last half of my life that I've learnt to say 'sir.' It's a word you use when you've come down in the world."

"That's very true," smiled Alyosha. "But is it used involuntarily or on purpose?"

"As God's above, it's involuntary, and I usen't to use it! I didn't use the word 'sir' all my life, but as soon as I sank into the depths I began to say 'sir.' It's the work of a higher power. I see you are interested in contemporary questions, but how can I have excited your curiosity, living as I do in surroundings impossible for the exercise of hospitality?"

"I've come — about that business."

"About what business?" the captain interrupted impatiently.

"About your meeting with my brother Dmitri Fyodorovich," Alyosha blurted out awkwardly.

"What meeting, sir? You don't mean that meeting? About my 'bath-mop,' then?" He moved closer so that his knees positively knocked against Alyosha.

His lips were strangely compressed to a thread.

"What mop?" muttered Alyosha.

"He is come to complain of me, father!" cried a voice familiar to Alyosha — the voice of the schoolboy — from behind the curtain. "I bit his finger just now." The curtain jerked back, and Alyosha saw his assailant lying on a little bed made up on the bench and the chair in the corner under the ikons. The boy lay covered by his coat and an old wadded quilt. He was evidently unwell, and, judging by his glittering eyes, he was in a fever. He looked at Alyosha without fear, as though he felt he was at home and could not be touched.

"What! Did he bite your finger?" The captain jumped up from his chair. "Was it your finger he bit?"

"Yes. He was throwing stones at schoolboys who were stoning him. There were six of them against him alone. I went up to him, and he threw a stone at me and then another at my head. I asked him what I had done to him. And then he rushed at me and bit my finger badly, I don't know why."

"I'll thrash him, sir, at once — this minute!" The captain jumped up from his seat.

"But I am not complaining at all, I am simply telling you. . . . I don't want him to be thrashed. Besides, he seems to be ill."

"And do you suppose I'd thrash him? That I'd take my Ilusha and thrash him before you for your satisfaction? Would you like it done at once, sir?" said the captain, suddenly turning to Alyosha, as though he were going to attack him. "I am sorry about your finger, sir; but instead of thrashing Ilusha, would you like me to chop off my four fingers with this knife here before your eyes to satisfy your just wrath? I should think four fingers would be enough to satisfy your thirst for vengeance. You won't ask for the fifth one, too?" He stopped short with a catch in his throat. Every feature in his face was twitching and working; he looked extremely defiant. He was in a sort of frenzy.

"I think I understand it all now," said Alyosha gently and sorrowfully, still keeping his seat. "So your boy is a good boy, he loves his father, and he attacked me as the brother of your assailant. . . . Now I understand it," he repeated thoughtfully. "But my brother Dmitri Fyodorovich regrets his action, I know that, and if only it is possible for him to come to you, or better still, to meet you in that same place, he will ask your forgiveness before every one — if you wish it."

"After pulling out my beard, you mean, he will ask my forgiveness? And he thinks that will be a satisfactory finish, doesn't he?"

"Oh, no! On the contrary, he will do anything you like and in any way you like."

"So if I were to ask his Excellency to go down on his knees before me in that very tavern — 'The Metropolis' it's called — or in the market-place, he would do it?"

"Yes, he would even go down on his knees."

"You've pierced me to the heart, sir. Touched me to tears and pierced me to the heart, sir. I am only too sensible of your brother's generosity. Allow me to introduce my family, my two daughters and my son — my litter. If I die, who will care for them, sir, and while I live who but they will care for a wretch like me? That's a great thing the Lord has ordained for every man of my sort, sir. For there must be some one able to love even a man like me."

"Ah, that's perfectly true!" exclaimed Alyosha.

"Oh, do leave off playing the buffoon! Some fool comes in, and you put us to shame!" cried the girl by the window, suddenly turning to her father with a scornful and contemptuous air.

"Wait a little, Varvara! Permit me to sustain my tone," cried her father, speaking peremptorily but looking at her quite approvingly. "That's her character," he said, addressing Alyosha again.

And in all nature there was naught
Whereon he let his blessing fall . . .

or rather in the feminine: whereon she let her blessing fall. But now let me present you to my spouse, Arina Petrovna. She is crippled, sir, she is forty-three; she can move, but very little, sir. She is of humble origin. Arina Petrovna, compose your countenance. This is Alexey Fyodorovich Karamazov. Get up, Alexey Fyodorovich." He took him by the hand and with unexpected force pulled him up. "You must stand up to be introduced to a lady. It's not the Karamazov, mamma, who . . . h'm . . . et cetera, but his brother, radiant with modest virtues. Come, Arina Petrovna, come, mamma, first your hand to be kissed."

And he kissed his wife's hand respectfully and even tenderly. The girl at the window turned her back indignantly on the scene; an expression of extraordinary cordiality came over the haughtily inquiring face of the woman.

"Good morning! Sit down, Mr. Chernomazov," she said.

"Karamazov, mamma, Karamazov (we are of humble origin)," he whispered again.

"Well, Karamazov, or whatever it is, but I always think of Chernomazov. . . . Sit down. Why has he pulled you up? He calls me crippled but I am not, only my legs are swollen like barrels, and I am shrivelled up myself. Once I used to be so fat, but now it's as though I had swallowed a needle."

"We are of humble origin, sir," the captain muttered again.

"Oh, father, father!" the hunchback girl, who had till then been silent on her chair, said suddenly, and she hid her eyes in her handkerchief.

"Clown!" blurted out the girl at the window.

"Have you heard our news?" said the mother, pointing at her daughters. "It's like clouds blowing over; the clouds pass and we have music again. When we were with the army, we used to have many such guests. I don't mean to make any comparisons, young man; every one to his taste. The deacon's wife used to come then and say, 'Alexander Alexandrovich is a man of the noblest heart, but Nastasya Petrovna,' she would say, 'is a child of hell.' 'Well,' I said, 'that's a matter of taste; but you are a small one, but a skunk.' 'And you want keeping in your place,' says she. 'You black sword,' said I, 'who asked you to teach me?' 'But my breath,' says she, 'is clean, and yours is unclean.' 'You ask all the officers whether my breath is unclean,' and ever since then I had it in my mind. Not long ago I was sitting here as I am now, when I saw that very general come in who came here at Easter, and I asked him: 'Your Excellency,' said I, 'could a noble lady let in fresh air?' 'Yes,' he answered; 'you ought to open a window or open the door, for the air is not fresh here.' And they all go on like that! And what is my breath to them? The dead smell worse still! 'I won't spoil the air,' said I, 'I'll order shoes and go away.' My darlings, don't reproach your own mother! Nikolay Ilyich, how is it I can't please you? There's only Ilusha who comes home from school and loves me. Yesterday he brought me an apple. Forgive your own mother — forgive a poor lonely creature! Why has my breath become unpleasant to you?" And the poor mad woman broke into sobs, and tears streamed down her cheeks. The captain rushed up to her.

"Mamma, mamma, my dear, give over! You are not lonely. Every one loves you, every one adores you." He began kissing both her hands again and tenderly stroking her face; taking the napkin, he began wiping away her tears. Alyosha fancied that he, too, had tears in his eyes. "There, you see, you hear?" he turned with a sort of fury to Alyosha, pointing to the poor imbecile.

"I see and hear," muttered Alyosha.

"Father, father, how can you — with him! Let him alone!" cried the boy, sitting up in his bed and gazing at his father with glowing eyes.

"Do give over clowning, stop your silly antics which never lead to anything!" shouted Varvara, stamping her foot with passion.

"Your anger is quite just this time, Varvara, and I'll make haste to satisfy you. Come, put on your cap, Alexey Fyodorovich, and I'll put on mine. We will go out. I have a word to say to you in earnest, but not within these walls. This girl sitting here is my daughter Nina; I forgot to introduce her to you. She is a heavenly angel incarnate . . . who has flown down to us mortals . . . if you can understand."

"There he is shaking all over, as though he were in convulsions!" Varvara went on indignantly.

"And she there stamping her foot at me and calling me a clown just now, she is a heavenly angel incarnate, too, and she has good reason to call me so. Come along, Alexey Fyodorovich, we must make an end."

And, snatching Alyosha's hand, he drew him out of the room into the street.

CHAPTER VII

AND IN THE OPEN AIR

"The air is fresh, but in my mansion it is not so in any sense of the word. Let us walk slowly, sir. I should like very much to engage your interest, sir."

"I, too, have something important to say to you," observed Alyosha, "only I don't know how to begin."

"To be sure you must have business with me. You would never have looked in upon me without some object. Unless you come simply to complain of the boy, and that's hardly likely. And, by the way, sir, about the boy: I could not explain to you in there, but here I will describe that scene to you. You see, sir, my mop was thicker a week ago — I mean my beard. That's the nickname they have given my beard, the schoolboys most of all, sir. Well, your brother Dmitri Fyodorovich was pulling me by the beard — he dragged me out of the tavern into the square; at that moment the boys were coming out of school, and with them Ilusha. As soon as he saw me in such a state, sir, he rushed up to me. 'Papa,' he cried, 'papa!' He caught hold of me, hugged me, tried to pull me away, crying to my assailant, 'Let go, let go, it's my father, forgive him!' — yes, he actually cried, 'forgive him.' He clutched at that hand, that very hand, sir, with his little hands and kissed it, sir. . . . I remember his little face at that moment, I haven't forgotten it, sir, and I never shall!"

"I swear," cried Alyosha, "that my brother will express his most deep and sincere regret, even if he has to go down on his knees in that same square. . . . I'll make him or he is no brother of mine!"

"Aha, then it's only your idea! And it does not come directly from him but simply from the generosity of your own ardent heart. You should have said so, sir. No, in that case allow me to finish telling you of your brother's highly chivalrous, soldierly high-mindedness, for he did give expression to it at the time, sir. He left off dragging me by the beard and released me: 'You are an officer,' he said, 'and I am an officer, if you can find a decent man to be your second, send me your challenge. I will give you satisfaction, though you are a scoundrel.' That's what he said, sir. A chivalrous spirit indeed! I retired with Ilusha, and that scene is a family record imprinted for ever on Ilusha's soul, sir. No, it's not for us to claim the privileges of the gentry, sir. Judge for yourself. You've just been in our mansion, what did you see there? Three ladies, one a cripple and weak-minded, another a cripple and hunchback, and the third not crippled but far too clever. She is a student, dying to get back to Petersburg, to work for the emancipation of the Russian woman on the banks of the Neva. I won't speak of Ilusha, sir, he is only nine. He is alone in the world, for if I die, what will become of all of them, I simply ask you that, sir. And if I challenge him and he kills me on the spot, what then? What will become of them all? And worse still, if he doesn't kill me but only cripples me: I couldn't work, but I should still be a mouth to feed. Who would feed it, sir, and who would feed them all? Must I take Ilusha from school and send him to beg in the streets? That's what it means for me to challenge him to a duel, sir. It's silly talk and nothing else."

"He will beg your forgiveness, he will bow down at your feet in the middle of the square," cried Alyosha again, with glowing eyes.

"I did think of prosecuting him," the captain went on, "but look in our code, sir, could I get much compensation for a personal injury? And then Agrafena Alexandrovna* sent for me and shouted at me: 'Don't dare to dream of it! If you proceed against him, I'll publish it to all the world that he beat you for your dishonesty, and then you will be prosecuted.' I call God to witness whose was the dishonesty and on whose instructions I acted, I, a mere pawn — wasn't it by her own and Fyodor Pavlovich's? 'And what's more,' she went on, 'I'll dismiss you for good and you'll never earn another penny from me. I'll speak to my merchant, too (that's what she calls her old man), and he, too, will chase you out!' And if he dismisses me, how can I earn anything? Those two are all I have to look to, for your father has not only given over employing me, for another reason, but he means to make use of papers I've signed to drag me to court. And so I kept quiet, and you have seen my family, sir. But now let me ask you: did Ilusha bite your finger badly? I didn't like to go into it in our mansion before him."

"Yes, very badly, and he was greatly irritated. He was avenging you on me as a Karamazov, I see that now. But if only you had seen how he was throwing stones at his schoolfellows! It's very dangerous. They might kill him. They are children and stupid. A stone may be thrown and break somebody's head."

"That's just what has happened. He has

* Grushenka.

been bruised by a stone to-day, sir. Not on the head but on the chest, just above the heart. He came home crying and groaning and now he is ill."

"And you know he attacks them first. He is bitter against them on your account. They say he stabbed a boy called Krasotkin with a penknife not long ago."

"I've heard about that, too, it's dangerous, sir. Krasotkin is an official here, we may hear more about it."

"I would advise you," Alyosha went on warmly, "not to send him to school at all for a time till he is calmer . . . and his anger has subsided."

"Anger!" the captain repeated, "anger indeed, sir. In a small creature, a mighty anger. You don't know all, sir. Let me tell you more. Since that incident all the boys have been teasing him about the 'bath-mop.' Schoolboys are a merciless crew; individually they are angels, but together, especially at school, they are often merciless. They began to tease him and a gallant spirit arose in Ilusha. An ordinary boy, a weak son, would have submitted, would have felt ashamed of his father, sir, but he stood up for his father against them all. For his father and for truth and justice, sir. For what he suffered when he kissed your brother's hand and cried to him, 'forgive father, forgive him' — that only God knows — and I, sir. For our children — not your children, but ours — the children of the poor gentlemen looked down upon by every one — know what justice means, sir, even at nine years old. How should the rich know? They don't explore such depths once in their lives. But at that moment in the square when he kissed his hand, at that moment my Ilusha had grasped all that justice means. That truth entered into him and crushed him for ever, sir," the captain said hotly again with a sort of frenzy, and he struck his right fist against his left palm as though he wanted to show how "the truth" had crushed Ilusha. "That very day, sir, he fell ill with fever and was delirious all night. All that day he hardly said a word to me, but I noticed he kept watching me from the corner, though he turned to the window and pretended to be learning his lessons. But I could see his mind was not on his lessons. Next day I got drunk to forget my troubles, sinful man that I am, sir, and I don't remember much, sir. Mamma began crying, too — I am very fond of mamma — well, I spent my last penny drowning my troubles. Don't despise me for that, sir, in Russia men who drink are the best. The best men amongst us are the greatest drunkards. I lay down and I don't remember about Ilusha, though all that day the boys had been jeering at him at school. 'Bath-mop,' they shouted, 'your father was pulled out of the tavern by his ragged mop, you ran by and begged forgiveness.'

"On the third day when he came back from school, I saw he looked pale and wretched. 'What is it?' I asked. He wouldn't answer. Well, there's no talking in our mansion without mamma and the girls taking part in it. What's more, the girls had heard about it the very first day. Varvara had begun snarling. 'You fools and buffoons, can you ever do anything sensible?' 'Quite so,' I said, 'can we ever do anything sensible?' for the time I turned it off like that. So in the evening I took the boy out for a walk, sir, for you must know we go for a walk every evening, always the same way, along which we are going now — from our gate to that great stone which lies alone in the road under the hurdle, which marks the beginning of the town pasture. A beautiful and lonely spot, sir. Ilusha and I walked along hand in hand as usual. He has a little hand, his fingers are thin and cold — he has trouble with his chest, you know. 'Father,' says he, 'father!' 'Well?' say I. I saw his eyes flashing. 'Father, what he did to you then!' 'It can't be helped, Ilusha,' I say. 'Don't make up with him, father, don't make up with him! At school they say that he has paid you ten roubles for it.' 'No, Ilusha,' say I, 'I would not take money from him for anything.' Then he began trembling all over, took my hand in both his and kissed it again. 'Father,' he says, 'father, challenge him to a duel, at school they say you are a coward and won't challenge him, and that you'll accept ten roubles from him.' 'I can't challenge him to a duel, Ilusha,' I answered. And I told him briefly what I've just told you. He listened. 'Father,' he said, 'anyway don't make up with him. When I grow up I'll call him out myself and kill him.' His eyes flashed and burned. Well, of course I am his father, and I had to tell him what's right: 'It's a sin to kill,' I said, 'even in a duel.' 'Father,' he said, 'when I grow up, I'll knock him down, knock the sword out of his hand with my own sword, I'll fall on him, wave my sword over him and say: "I could kill you, but I forgive you, so there!"' You see what the workings of his little mind have been during these two days; he must have been planning that vengeance all day, and raving about it at night.

"But he began to come home from school badly beaten, I found out about it the day before yesterday, and you are right, I won't send him to that school any more, sir. I heard that he was standing up alone against all the class and defying them all, that his heart was full of resentment, of bitterness — I was alarmed about him. We went for a walk again. 'Father,' he asked, 'are the rich people stronger than any one else on earth?' 'Yes, Ilusha,' I said, 'there are no people on earth stronger than the rich.' 'Father,' he said, 'I will get rich, I will become an officer and conquer everybody. The Tsar will reward me, I will come back here and then no one will dare . . .' Then he was silent and his lips still kept trembling. 'Father,' he said, 'what a horrid town this is.' 'Yes, Ilusha,' I said, 'it isn't a very nice town.' 'Father, let us move into another town, a nice one,' he said, 'where people don't know about us.' 'We will move, we will, Ilusha,' said I, 'only I must save up for it.' I was glad to be able to turn his mind from painful thoughts, and we began to dream of how we would move to another town, how we would buy a horse and cart. 'We will put mamma and your sisters inside, we will cover them up and we'll walk, you shall have a lift now and then, and I'll walk beside, for we must spare our horse, we can't all ride. That's how we'll go.' He was enchanted at that, most of all at the thought of having a horse and driving him. For of course a Russian boy is born with the idea of a horse. We chatted a long while. Thank God, I thought, I have diverted his mind and comforted him.

"That was the day before yesterday, in the evening, but last night everything was changed. He had gone to school in the morning, he came back depressed, terribly depressed. In the evening I took him by the hand and we went for a walk; he would not talk. There was a wind blowing and no sun, and a feeling of autumn; twilight was coming on. We walked along, both of us depressed. 'Well, my boy,' said I, 'how about our setting off on our travels?' I thought I might bring him back

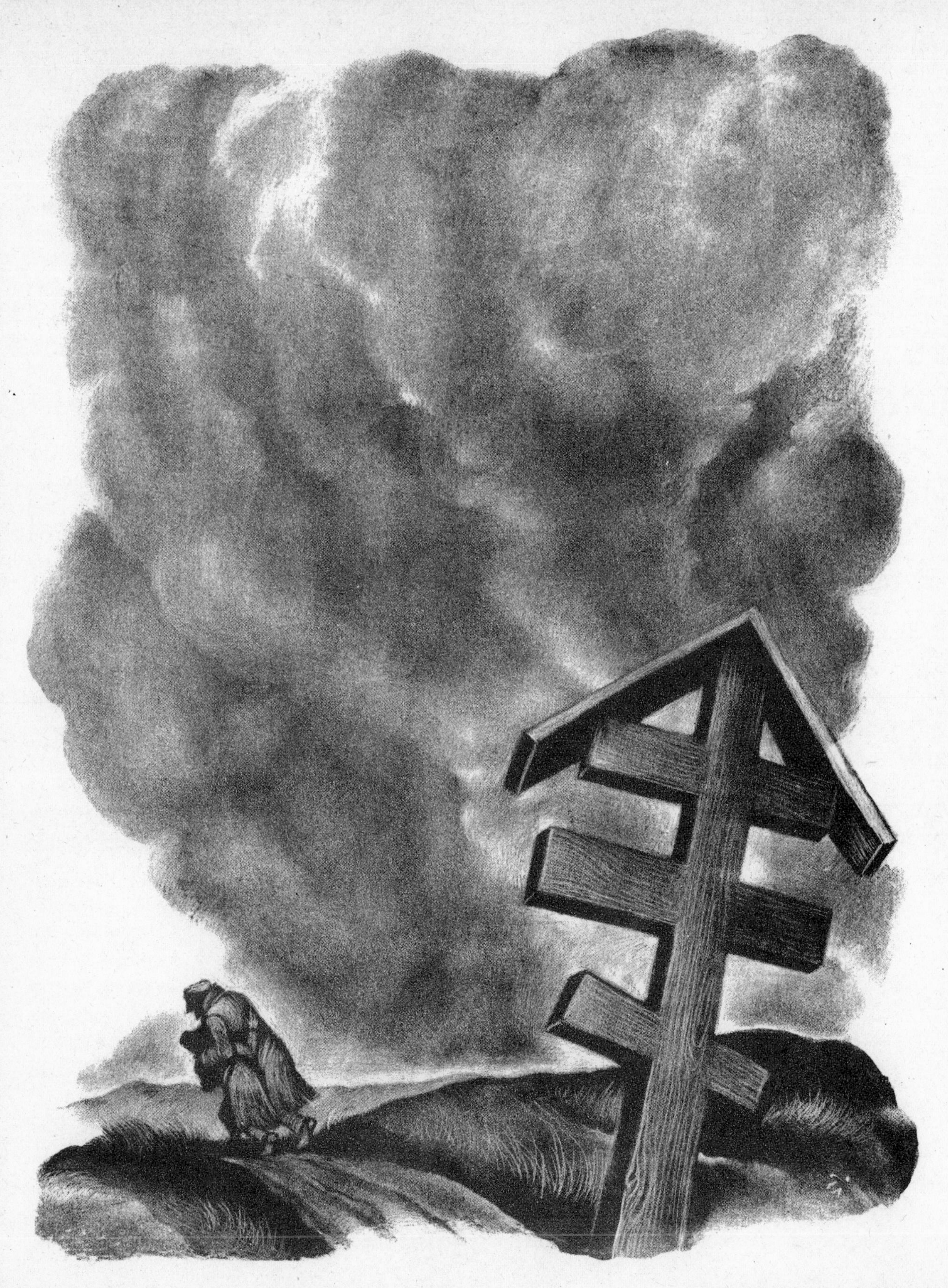

"AND IN THE OPEN AIR"

to our talk of the day before. He didn't answer, but I felt his fingers trembling in my hand. Ah, I thought, it's a bad job; there's something new. We had reached the stone where we are now. I sat down on the stone. And in the air there were lots of kites flapping and whirling. There were as many as thirty in sight. Of course, it's just the season for the kites. 'Look, Ilusha,' said I, 'it's time we got out our last year's kite again. I'll mend it, where have you put it away?' My boy made no answer. He looked away and turned sideways to me. And then a gust of wind blew up the sand. He suddenly fell on me, threw both his little arms round my neck and held me tight. You know, when children are silent and proud, and try to keep back their tears when they are in great trouble and suddenly break down, their tears flow in streams. With those warm streams of tears, he suddenly wetted my face. He sobbed and shook as though he were in convulsions, and squeezed up against me as I sat on the stone. 'Father,' he kept crying, 'dear father, how he insulted you!' And I sobbed, too. We sat shaking in each other's arms. 'Ilusha,' I said to him, 'Ilusha darling.' No one saw us then. God alone saw us, I hope he will record it to my credit, sir. You must thank your brother, Alexey Fyodorovich. No, sir, I won't thrash my boy for your satisfaction."

He had gone back to his original tone of resentful buffoonery. Alyosha felt, though, that he trusted him, and that if there had been some one else in his, Alyosha's, place, the man would not have spoken so openly and would not have told what he had just told. This encouraged Alyosha, whose heart was trembling with inward tears.

"Ah, how I would like to make friends with your boy!" he cried. "If you could arrange it —— "

"Certainly, sir," muttered the captain.

"But now listen to something quite different!" Alyosha went on. "I have a message for you. That same brother of mine, Dmitri, has insulted his betrothed, too, a noble-hearted girl of whom you have probably heard. I have a right to tell you of her wrong; I ought to do so, in fact, for hearing of the insult done to you and learning all about your unfortunate position, she commissioned me at once — just now — to bring you this help from her — but only from her alone, not from Dmitri, who has abandoned her. Nor from me, his brother, nor from any one else, but from her, only from her! She entreats you to accept her help. . . . You have both been insulted by the same man. She thought of you only when she had just received a similar insult from him — similar in its cruelty, I mean. She comes like a sister to help a brother in misfortune. . . . She told me to persuade you to take these two hundred roubles from her, as from a sister, knowing that you are in such need. No one will know of it, it can give rise to no unjust slander. There are the two hundred roubles, and I swear you must take them unless — unless all men are to be enemies on earth! But there are brothers even on earth. . . . You have a generous heart . . . you must see that, you must," and Alyosha held out two new rainbow-coloured hundred-rouble notes.

They were both standing at the time by the great stone close to the fence, and there was no one near. The notes seemed to produce a tremendous impression on the captain. He started, but at first only from astonishment. Such an outcome of their conversation was the last thing he had expected. Nothing could have been further from his dreams than help from any one — and such a sum!

He took the notes, and for a minute he was almost unable to answer, quite a new expression came into his face.

"That for me? So much money — two hundred roubles! Good heavens! Why, I haven't seen so much money for the last four years! Mercy on us! And she says she is a sister . . . And is that the truth?"

"I swear that all I told you is the truth," cried Alyosha.

The captain flushed red.

"Listen, my dear, listen. If I take it, I shan't be behaving like a scoundrel? In your eyes, Alexey Fyodorovich, I shan't be a scoundrel? No, Alexey Fyodorovich, listen, listen," he said hurriedly, touching Alyosha with both his hands. "You are persuading me to take it, saying that it's a sister sends it, but inwardly, in your heart won't you feel contempt for me if I take it, eh?"

"No, no, on my salvation I swear I shan't! And no one will ever know but me — I, you, and she, and one other lady, her great friend."

"Never mind the lady! Listen, Alexey Fyodorovich, at a moment like this you must listen, for you can't understand what these two hundred roubles mean to me now." The poor fellow went on rising gradually into a sort of incoherent, almost wild enthusiasm. He was thrown off his balance and talked extremely fast, as though afraid he would not be allowed to say all he had to say.

"Besides it's being honestly acquired from a 'sister,' so highly respected and revered, do you know that now I can look after mamma and Nina, my hunchback angel daughter? Dr. Herzenstube came to me in the kindness of his heart and was examining them both for a whole hour. 'I can make nothing of it,' said he, but he prescribed a mineral water which is to be had at a chemist's here. He said it would be sure to do her good, and he ordered foot-baths, too, with some medicine in them. The mineral water costs thirty copecks, and she'd need to drink forty bottles perhaps; so I took the prescription and laid it on the shelf under the ikons, and there it lies. And he ordered hot baths for Nina with something dissolved in them, morning and evening. But how can we carry out such a cure in our mansion, without servants, without help, without a tub, and without water? Nina is rheumatic all over, I don't think I told you that. All her right side aches at night, she is in agony, and, would you believe it, the angel bears it without groaning for fear of waking us. We eat what we can get, and she'll only take the leavings, what you'd scarcely give to a dog. 'I am not worth it, I am taking it from you, I am a burden on you,' that's what her angel eyes try to express. We wait on her, but she doesn't like it. 'I am a useless cripple, no good to any one.' As though she were not worth it, when she is the salvation of all of us with her angelic sweetness. Without her, without her gentle word it would be hell among us! She softens even Varvara. And don't judge Varvara harshly either, she is an angel, too; she, too, has suffered wrong. She came to us for the summer, and she brought sixteen roubles she had earned by lessons and saved up, to go back with to Petersburg in September, that is now. But we took her money and ate it up, so now she has nothing to go back with. Though indeed she couldn't go back, for she has to work for us like a slave. She is like an overdriven horse with all of us on her back. She waits on us all, mends and washes, sweeps the floor, puts mamma to bed. And mamma is capricious and tearful and insane! And now I can get a servant with this money, you understand, Alexey Fyodorovich, I can get medicines for the dear creatures, I can send my student to Petersburg, I can buy beef, I can feed them properly. Good Lord, but it's a dream!"

Alyosha was delighted that he had brought him such happiness and that the poor fellow had consented to be made happy.

"Wait, Alexey Fyodorovich, wait," the captain began to talk with frenzied rapidity carried away by a new daydream. "Do you know that Ilusha and I will perhaps really carry out our dream. We will buy a horse and cart, a black horse, he insists on its being black, and we will set off as we pretended the other day. I have an old friend, a lawyer in K. province, and I heard through a trustworthy man that if I were to go he'd give me a place as clerk in his office, so, who knows, maybe he would. So I'd just put mamma and Nina in the cart, and Ilusha could drive, and I'd walk, I'd walk. . . . Why, if I only succeed in getting one debt paid that's owing me, I should have perhaps enough for that, too!"

"There would be enough!" cried Alyosha. "Katerina Ivanovna will send you as much more as you need, and you know I have money, too; take what you want, as you would from a brother, from a friend, you can give it back later. . . . (You'll get rich, you'll get rich!) And you know you couldn't have a better idea than to move to another province! It would be the saving of you, especially of your boy — and you ought to go quickly, before the winter, before the cold. You must write to us when you are there, and we will always be brothers. . . . No, it's not a dream!"

Alyosha was about to hug him, he was so pleased. But glancing at him he stopped short. The man was standing with his neck outstretched and his lips protruding, with a pale and frenzied face. His lips were moving as though trying to articulate something; no sound came, but still his lips moved. It was uncanny.

"What is it?" asked Alyosha, startled.

"Alexey Fyodorovich . . . I . . . you," muttered the captain, faltering, looking at him with a strange, wild, fixed stare, and an air of desperate resolution. At the same time there was a sort of grin on his lips. "I, sir . . . you, sir . . . wouldn't you like me to show you a little trick I know?" he murmured, suddenly, in a firm rapid whisper, his voice no longer faltering.

"What trick?"

"A pretty trick, a bit of hocus-pocus," whispered the captain. His mouth was twisted on the left side, his left eye was screwed up. He still stared at Alyosha.

"What is the matter, what trick?" Alyosha cried, now thoroughly alarmed.

"Why, look," squealed the captain suddenly, and showing him the two notes which he had been holding by one corner between his thumb and forefinger during the conversation, he crumpled them up savagely and squeezed them tight in his right hand. "Do you see, do you see?" he shrieked, pale and infuriated. And suddenly flinging up his hand, he threw the crumpled notes on the sand. "Do you see?" he shrieked again, pointing to them. "Look there!"

And with wild fury he began trampling them under his heel, gasping and exclaiming as he did so: "Here's your money, sir! Here's your money, sir! Here's your money, sir! Here's your money, sir!"

Suddenly he darted back and drew himself up before Alyosha, and his whole figure expressed unutterable pride.

"Tell those who sent you that the bath-mop does not sell his honour," he cried, raising his arm in the air. Then he turned quickly and began to run; but he had not run five steps before he turned completely round and kissed his hand to Alyosha. He ran another five paces and then turned round for the last time. This time his face was not contorted with laughter, but quivering all over with tears. In a tearful, faltering, sobbing voice he cried:

"What should I say to my boy if I took money from you for our shame?"

And then he ran on without turning. Alyosha looked after him, inexpressibly grieved. Oh, he saw that till the very last moment the man had not known he would crumple up and fling away the notes. He did not turn back. Alyosha knew he would not. He would not follow him and call him back, he knew why. When he was out of sight, Alyosha picked up the two notes. They were very much crushed and crumpled, and had been pressed into the sand, but were uninjured and even rustled like new ones when Alyosha unfolded them and smoothed them out. After smoothing them out, he folded them up, put them in his pocket and went to Katerina Ivanovna to report on the success of her commission.

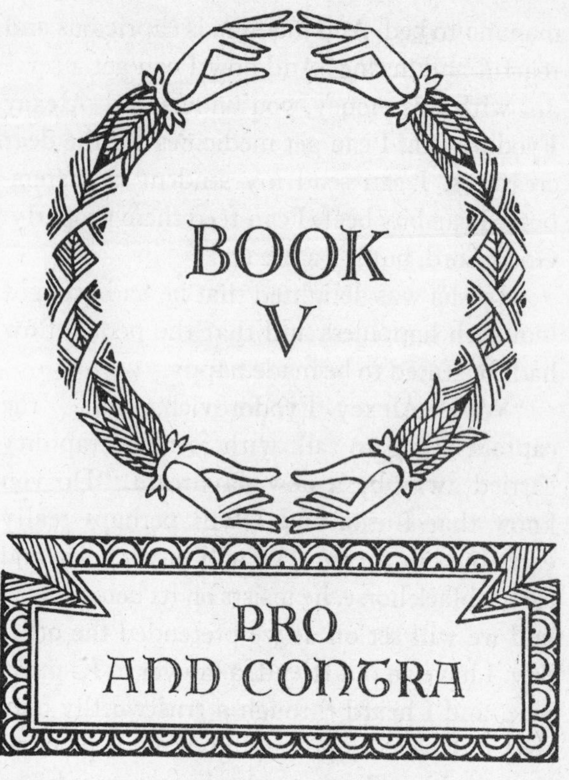

CHAPTER I

THE ENGAGEMENT

Madame Hohlakov was again the first to meet Alyosha. She was flustered; something important had happened. Katerina Ivanovna's hysterics had ended in a fainting fit, and then "a terrible, awful weakness had followed, she lay with her eyes turned up and was delirious. Now she was in a fever. They had sent for Herzenstube; they had sent for the aunts. The aunts were already here, but Herzenstube had not yet come. They were all sitting in her room, waiting. She was unconscious now, and what if it turned out to be brain fever!"

Madame Hohlakov looked gravely alarmed. "This is serious, serious," she added at every word, as though nothing that had happened to her before had been serious. Alyosha listened with distress, and began to describe his adventures, but she interrupted him at the first words. She had not time to listen. She begged him to sit with Lise and wait for her there.

"Lise," she whispered almost in his ear, "Lise has greatly surprised me just now, dear Alexey Fyodorovich. She touched me, too, and so my heart forgives her everything. Only fancy, as soon as you had gone, she began to be sincerely remorseful for having laughed at you to-day and yesterday, though she was not laughing at you, but only joking. But she was seriously sorry for it, almost ready to cry, so that I was quite surprised. She has never been really sorry for laughing at me, but has only made a joke of it. And you know she is laughing at me every minute. But this time she was in earnest. Now she is in earnest about everything. She thinks a great deal of your opinion, Alexey Fyodorovich, and don't take offence or be wounded by her if you can help it. For my part, I am always lenient towards her, for she's such a clever little thing— would you believe it? She said just now that you were a friend of her childhood, 'the greatest friend of her childhood' — just think of that — 'greatest friend' — and what about me? In that respect, she has very strong feelings and memories, and, what's more, she has these phrases, most unexpected words, which come out all of a sudden when you least expect them. She spoke lately about a pine-tree, for instance: there used to be a pine-tree in our garden in her early childhood. Very likely it's standing there still; so there's no need to speak in the past tense. Pine-trees are not like people, Alexey Fyodorovich, they don't change quickly. 'Mamma,' she said, 'I remember this pine-tree as in a dream,' only she said something so original about it that I can't repeat it. Besides, I've forgotten it. Well, goodbye! I am so worried I feel I shall go out of my mind. Ah! Alexey Fyodorovich, I've been out of my mind twice in my life, and I was being treated for it. Go to Lise, cheer her up, as you always can so charmingly. Lise," she cried, going to her door, "here I've brought you Alexey Fyodorovich, whom you insulted so. He is not at all angry, I assure you; on the contrary, he is surprised that you could imagine it."

"*Merci, maman.* Come in, Alexey Fyodorovich."

Alyosha went in. Lise looked rather embarrassed, and at once flushed crimson. She was evidently ashamed of something, and, as people always do in such cases, she began immediately talking of other things, as though they alone were of absorbing interest to her at the moment.

"Mamma has just told me all about the two hundred roubles, Alexey Fyodorovich, and your taking them to that poor officer . . . and she told me the whole awful story of how he had been insulted . . . and you know, although mamma muddles things . . . she always rushes from one thing to another . . . I cried listening to it. Well, did you give him the money and how is that poor man getting on?"

"The fact is I didn't give it to him, and it's a long story," answered Alyosha, as though he, too, could think of nothing but his regret at having failed, yet Lise saw perfectly well that he, too, looked away, and that he, too, was trying to talk of other things.

Alyosha sat down at the table and began to tell his story, but at the first words he lost his embarrassment and gained Lise's complete attention as well. He spoke with deep feeling, under the influence of the strong impression he had just received, and he succeeded in telling his story well and circumstantially. In the old days in Moscow, when Lise was a child, he had been fond of coming to Lise and describing to her what had just happened to him, what he had read, or what he remembered of his childhood. Sometimes they had made day-dreams and woven whole romances together — generally cheerful and amusing ones. Now they both felt suddenly transported to the old days in Moscow, two years before. Lise was deeply touched by his story. Alyosha, mastered by his emotion, succeeded in bringing the image of Ilusha clearly before her. When he finished describing the scene in which the luckless man trampled on the money, Lise could not help striking her hands together and crying out:

"So you didn't give him the money! So you let him run away! Oh, dear, you ought to have run after him!"

"No, Lise; it's better I didn't run after him," said Alyosha, getting up from his chair and walking across the room with a careworn look.

"How so? How is it better? Now they are without food and they will perish."

"They will not perish, for the two hundred roubles will come to them yet. He'll take the money to-morrow. To-morrow he will be sure to take it," said Alyosha, pacing up and down, pondering. "You see, Lise," he went on, stopping suddenly before her, "I made one blunder, but that, even that, is all for the best."

"What blunder, and why is it for the best?"

"I'll tell you. He is a man of weak and cowardly character; he has suffered so much and is very good-natured. I keep wondering why he took offence so suddenly, and trampled on the notes, for I assure you, up to the last minute, he did not know that he was going to trample on the money. And I think now that there was a great deal to offend him . . . and it could not have been otherwise in his position. . . . To begin with, he was vexed at having shown himself so overjoyed by the money in my presence and not having concealed it from me. If he had been pleased, but not so much; if he had not shown it; if he had begun affecting scruples and making difficulties, as other people do when they take money, he might still have endured taking it. But he was too genuinely delighted, and that was mortifying. Ah, Lise, he is a good and truthful man — that's the worst of the whole business in such cases. All the while he talked his voice was so weak, so broken, he talked so fast, so fast, he kept tittering so, or else he was crying — yes, I am sure he was crying, he was in such transports — and he talked about his daughters — and about the position he could get in another town. . . . And when he had poured out his heart, he felt ashamed at having shown me his inmost soul like that. So he began to hate me at once. He is one of those awfully sensitive poor people. What had made him feel most ashamed was that he had given in too soon and accepted me as a friend, you see. At first he had almost flown at me and tried to intimidate me, but as soon as he saw the money he began embracing me; he kept touching me with his hands. This must have been how he came to feel so humiliated by it all, and then I made that blunder, a very grave one. I suddenly said to him that if he had not money enough to move to another town, we would give it to him, and, indeed, I myself would give him as much as he wanted out of my own money. That struck him all at once. Why, he thought, did I put myself forward to help him? You know, Lise, it's awfully hard for a man who has suffered insults, when other people look at him as though they were his benefactors. . . . I've heard that; Father Zosima told me so. I don't know how to put it, but I have often seen it myself. And I feel like that myself, too. And the worst of it was that though he did not know, up to the very last minute, that he would trample on the notes, he had a kind of presentiment of it, I am sure of that. That's just what made him so ecstatic, that he had that presentiment. . . . And though it's so dreadful, it's all for the best. In fact, I believe nothing better could have happened."

"Why, why could nothing better have happened?" cried Lise, looking with great surprise at Alyosha.

"Because if he had taken the money, an hour after getting home, he would be crying with mortification, that's just what would have happened. And most likely he would have come to me early to-morrow, and perhaps have flung the notes at me and trampled upon them as he did just now. But now he has gone home awfully proud and triumphant, though he knows he has 'ruined himself.' So now nothing could be easier than to make him accept the two hundred roubles by to-morrow, for he has already vindicated his honour, tossed away the money, and trampled it under foot. . . . He couldn't know when he did it that I should bring it to him again to-morrow, and yet he is in terrible need of that money. Though he is proud of himself now, yet even to-day he'll be thinking what a help he has lost. He will think of it more than ever at night, will dream of it, and by to-morrow morning he may be ready to run to me to ask forgiveness. It's just then that I'll appear. 'Here, you are a proud man,' I shall say: 'you have proved it; but now take the money and forgive us!' And then he will take it!"

Alyosha was carried away with joy as he uttered the last words. "And then he will take it!" Lise clapped her hands.

"Ah, that's true! I understand that perfectly now. Ah, Alyosha, how do you know all this? So young and yet he knows what's in the heart. . . . I should never have worked it out."

"The great thing now is to persuade him that he is on an equal footing with us, in spite of his taking money from us," Alyosha went on in his excitement, "and not only on an equal, but even on a higher footing."

"On a higher footing is charming, Alexey Fyodorovich; but go on, go on!"

"You mean there isn't such an expression as 'on a higher footing'; but that doesn't matter because ——"

"Oh, no, of course it doesn't matter. Forgive me, Alyosha, dear. . . . You know, I scarcely respected you till now — that is, I respected you but on an equal footing; but now I shall begin to respect you on a higher footing. Don't be angry, dear, at my joking," she put in at once, with strong feeling. "I am ridiculous and small, but you, you! Listen, Alexey Fyodorovich. Isn't there in all our analysis — I mean your analysis . . . no, better call it ours — aren't we showing contempt for him, for that poor man — in analysing his soul like this, as it were, from above, eh? In deciding so certainly that he will take the money?"

"No, Lise, it's not contempt," Alyosha answered, as though he had prepared himself for the question. "I was thinking of that on the way here. How can it be contempt when we are all like him, when we are all just the same as he is. For you know we are just the same, no better. And if we were better, we should still have been just the same in his place. . . . I don't know about you, Lise, but I consider that I have a petty soul in many ways, and his soul is not petty; on the contrary, full of fine feeling. . . . No, Lise, I have no contempt for him. Do you know, Lise, my elder once said: one must take care of most people exactly as one would of children, and of some of them as one would of the sick in hospitals."

"Ah, Alexey Fyodorovich, dear, let us take care of people as we would of the sick!"

"Let us, Lise; I am ready. Though I am not really ready. I am sometimes very impatient and at other times I don't see things. It's different with you."

"Ah, I don't believe it! Alexey Fyodorovich, how happy I am."

"I am so glad you say so, Lise."

"Alexey Fyodorovich, you are wonderfully good, but you are sometimes a kind of pedant. . . . And yet you are not really a pedant at all. Go to the door, open it gently, and see whether mamma is eavesdropping," said Lise, in a nervous, hurried whisper.

Alyosha went, opened the door, and reported that no one was listening.

"Come here, Alexey Fyodorovich," Lise went on, flushing redder and redder. "Give me your hand — so. I have to make a great confession, I didn't write to you yesterday in jest, but in earnest," and she hid her eyes with her hand. It was evident that she was greatly ashamed of the confession.

Suddenly she snatched his hand and impulsively kissed it three times.

"Ah, Lise, what a fine thing!" cried Alyosha joyfully. "You know, I was perfectly sure you were in earnest."

"Sure? Upon my word!" She put aside his hand, but did not let go of it, blushing hotly, and laughing a little happy laugh. "I kiss his hand and he says, 'What a fine thing.' "

But her reproach was undeserved, Alyosha, too, was in great confusion.

"I should like to please you always, Lise, but I don't know how to do it," he muttered, blushing too.

"Alyosha, dear, you are cold and rude. Do you see? He has chosen me as his wife and is quite settled about it. He is sure that I wrote in earnest. What a thing to say! Why, that's impertinence — that's what it is."

"Why, was it wrong of me to feel sure?" Alyosha asked, laughing suddenly.

"Ah, Alyosha, on the contrary, it was altogether right," cried Lise, looking tenderly and happily at him.

Alyosha stood still, holding her hand in his. Suddenly he stooped down and kissed her on her lips.

"What's that you're doing? What is it?" cried Lise. Alyosha was terribly abashed.

"Oh, forgive me if I shouldn't. . . . Perhaps I'm awfully stupid. . . . You said I was cold, so I kissed you. . . . But I see it was stupid."

Lise laughed, and hid her face in her hands. "And in that costume!" she ejaculated in the midst of her mirth. But she suddenly ceased laughing and became serious, almost stern.

"Alyosha, we must put off kissing, because neither of us knows how, and we shall have a long time to wait," she ended suddenly. "Tell me rather why you who are so clever, so intellectual, so observant, choose a little idiot, an invalid like me? Ah, Alyosha, I am awfully happy for I don't deserve you a bit."

"You do, Lise. I shall be leaving the monastery altogether in a few days. If I go into the world, I must marry. I know that. *He* told me to marry, too. Whom could I marry better than you — and who would have me except you? I have been thinking it over. In the first place, you've known me from childhood on; and in the second place, you've a great many qualities I haven't. You have a more joyous soul than I; above all, you are more innocent than I am. I have been brought into contact with many, many things already. . . . Ah, you don't know, but I, too, am a Karamazov. What does it matter if you do laugh and make jokes, and at me, too? Go on laughing. I am so glad you do. You laugh like a little child, but in your heart you think like a martyr."

"Like a martyr? How?"

"Yes, Lise, your question just now: whether we weren't showing contempt for that poor man by dissecting his soul — that was the question of a sufferer. . . . You see, I don't know how to express it, but any one who thinks of such questions is capable of suffering. Sitting in your invalid chair you must have thought over many things already."

"Alyosha, give me your hand. Why are you taking it away?" murmered Lise in a failing voice, weak with happiness. "Listen, Alyosha. What will you wear when you come out of the monastery? What sort of suit? Don't laugh, don't be angry, it's very, very important to me."

"I haven't thought about the suit, Lise; but I'll wear whatever you like."

"I should like you to have a dark blue velvet coat, a white piqué waistcoat, and a soft grey felt hat. . . . Tell me, did you believe that I didn't care for you when I said I didn't mean what I wrote?"

"No, I didn't believe it."

"Oh, you intolerable person, you are incorrigible."

"You see, I knew that you — perhaps cared for me, but I pretended to believe that you didn't care for me to make it — easier for you."

"That makes it worse! Worse and better than all! Alyosha, I love you awfully. Just before you came this morning, I tried my fortune. I decided I would ask you for my letter, and if you brought it out calmly and gave it to me (as might have been expected from you) it would mean that you did not love me at all, that you felt nothing, and were simply a stupid worthless boy, and that I was ruined. But you left the letter at home and that cheered me. You left it behind on purpose, so as not to give it back, because you knew I would ask for it? That was it, wasn't it?"

"Ah, Lise, it was not so at all. The letter is with me now, and it was this morning, in this pocket. Here it is."

Alyosha pulled the letter out, laughing, and showed it to her at a distance.

"But I am not going to give it to you. Look at it from here."

"Why, then you told a lie? You, a monk, told a lie!"

"I told a lie if you like." Alyosha laughed, too. "I told a lie so as not to give you back the letter. It's very precious to me," he added suddenly, with strong feeling, and again he flushed. "It always will be, and I won't give it up to any one!"

Lise looked at him ecstatically. "Alyosha," she lisped again, "look at the door. Isn't mamma eavesdropping?"

"Very well, Lise, I'll look; but wouldn't it be better not to look? Why suspect your mother of such meanness?"

"What meanness? As for her spying on her daughter, it's her right, it's not meanness!" cried Lise, firing up. "You may be sure, Alexey Fyodorovich, that when I am a mother, if I have a daughter like myself I shall certainly spy on her!"

"Really, Lise? That's not right."

"Oh, my goodness! What has meanness to do with it? If it were ordinary drawing-room talk, and I were eavesdropping, it would be meanness, but when your own daughter is locked up with a young man . . . Listen, Alyosha, do you know I shall spy upon you as soon as we are married, and let me tell you I shall open all your letters and read them, so you may as well be prepared."

"Yes, of course, if that's what you mean —" muttered Alyosha, "only it's not right."

"Ah, what contempt! Alyosha, dear, let's not quarrel the very first day. I'd better tell you the whole truth. Of course, it's very wrong to eavesdrop, and, of course, I am not right and you are, only I shall eavesdrop all the same."

"Do, then; you won't find out anything," laughed Alyosha.

"And Alyosha, will you give in to me? We must decide that, too."

"I shall be delighted to, Lise, and certain to, only not in the most important things. Even if you don't agree with me, I shall do my duty in the most important things."

"That's right; but let me tell you I am ready to give in to you not only in the most important matters, but in everything. And I am ready to swear to do so now — in everything, and for all my life!" cried Lise fervently, "and I'll do it gladly, gladly! What's more I'll swear never to spy on you, never once, never to read one of your letters. For you are right and I am not. And though I shall be awfully tempted to eavesdrop, I know that I won't do it since you consider it dishonourable. You are my Providence now. . . . Listen, Alexey Fyodorovich, why have you been so sad lately — both yesterday and today? I know you have a lot of anxiety and trouble, but I see you have some special grief besides, some secret one, perhaps?"

"Yes, Lise, I have a secret one, too," answered Alyosha sadly. "I see you love me, since you guessed that."

"What grief? What about? Can you tell me?" asked Lise with timid entreaty.

"I'll tell you later, Lise — afterwards," said Alyosha, confused. "Now you wouldn't understand it perhaps — and perhaps I couldn't explain it."

"I know your brothers and your father are worrying you, too?"

"Yes, my brothers, too," murmured Alyosha, pondering.

"I don't like your brother Ivan, Alyosha," said Lise suddenly.

He noticed this remark with some surprise, but did not answer it.

"My brothers are ruining themselves," he went on, "my father, too. And they are ruining others with them. It's 'the primitive Karamazov force,' as Father Païssy said the other day, an earthy, frenzied, uncouth force. Does the spirit of God move above that force? Even that I don't know. I only know that I, too, am a Karamazov. . . . I, a monk, a monk? Am I a monk, Lise? You said just now that I was."

"Yes, I did."

"And perhaps I don't even believe in God."

"You don't believe? What is the matter?" said Lise quietly and gently. But Alyosha did not answer. There was something too mysterious, too personal in these last words of his, perhaps obscure to himself, but yet torturing him.

"And now on top of it all, my friend is leaving, the best man in the world is quitting the earth! If you knew, Lise, how bound up in soul I am with him, how welded to him! And then I shall be left alone. . . . I shall come to you, Lise. . . . In the future we will be together."

"Yes, together, together! Henceforward we shall be always together, all our lives! Listen, kiss me, I allow you."

Alyosha kissed her.

"Well, now go. Christ be with you!" and she made the sign of the cross over him. "Hurry back to *him* while he is alive. I see I've kept you cruelly. I'll pray to-day for him and you. Alyosha, we shall be happy! Shall we be happy, shall we?"

"I believe we shall, Lise."

Alyosha thought it better not to go in to Madame Hohlakov and was going out of the house without saying good-bye to her. But no sooner had he opened the door than he found Madame Hohlakov standing before him. From the first word Alyosha guessed that she had been waiting on purpose to meet him.

"Alexey Fyodorovich, this is awful. This is all childish nonsense and ridiculous. I trust you won't dream . . . It's foolishness, nothing but foolishness!" she said, attacking him at once.

"Only don't tell her that," said Alyosha, "or she will be upset, and that's bad for her now."

"Sensible advice from a sensible young man. Am I to understand that you only agreed with her from compassion for her invalid state, because you didn't want to irritate her by contradiction?"

"Oh, no, not at all. I was quite serious in what I said," Alyosha declared stoutly.

"To be serious about it is impossible, unthinkable, and in the first place I shall never be at home to you again, and I shall take her away, you may be sure of that."

"But why?" asked Alyosha. "It's all so far off. We may have to wait another year and a half."

"Ah, Alexey Fyodorovich, that's true, of course, and you'll have time to quarrel and separate a thousand times in a year and a half. But I am so unhappy! Though it's such nonsense, it's a great blow to me. I feel like Famusov in the last scene of *Sorrow from Wit*. You are Chatsky and she is Sofya, and, only fancy, I've run down to meet you on the stairs, and in the play too the fatal scene takes place on the staircase. I heard it all; I almost dropped. So this is the explanation of her dreadful night and her hysterics of late! It means love to the daughter but death to the mother. I might as well be in my grave at once. And a more serious matter still, what is this letter she has written? Show it me at once, at once!"

"No, there's no need. Tell me, how is Katerina Ivanovna now? I must know."

"She is still delirious; she has not regained consciousness. Her aunts are here; but they do nothing but sigh and give themselves airs. Herzenstube came, and he was so alarmed that I didn't know what to do for him. I nearly sent for a doctor to look after him. He was driven home in my carriage. And on top of it all, you and this letter! It's true nothing can happen for a year and a half. In the name of all that's great and holy, in the name of your dying elder, show me that letter, Alexey Fyodorovich. I'm her mother. Hold it in your hand, if you like, and I will read it so."

"No, I won't show it to you. Even if she sanctioned it, I wouldn't. I am coming tomorrow, and if you like, we can talk over many things, but now good-bye!"

And Alyosha ran downstairs and into the street.

CHAPTER II

SMERDYAKOV WITH A GUITAR

He had no time to lose indeed. Even while he was saying good-bye to Lise, the thought had struck him that he must at once attempt some stratagem to catch his brother Dmitri, who was evidently hiding from him. It was getting late, nearly three o'clock. Alyosha's whole soul turned to the monastery, to his dying saint, but the necessity of seeing Dmitri outweighed everything. The conviction that a great inevitable catastrophe was about to happen grew stronger in Alyosha's mind with every hour. What that catastrophe was, and what he wished to say at this moment to his brother, he could perhaps not have said definitely.

"Even if my benefactor must die without me, anyway I won't have to reproach myself all my life with the thought that I might have prevented something and did not, but passed by and hastened home. If I do this, I shall be following his great precept."

His plan was to catch his brother Dmitri unaware, namely, to climb over the fence, as he had the day before, get into the garden and take up his post in the summer-house. If Dmitri were not there, thought Alyosha, he would not announce himself to Foma or the women of the house, but would remain hidden in the summer-house, even if he had to wait there till evening. If, as before, Dmitri were lying in wait for Grushenka to come, he would be very likely to come to the summer-house. Alyosha did not, however, give much thought to the details of his plan, but resolved to act upon it, even if it meant not getting back to the monastery that day.

Everything happened without hindrance, he climbed over the hurdle almost at the same spot as the day before, and stole into the summer-house unseen. He did not want to be noticed. The women of the house and Foma, too, if he were there, might be loyal to his brother and obey his instructions, and so refuse to let Alyosha come into the garden, or might warn Dmitri that he was being sought and inquired for.

There was no one in the summer-house. Alyosha sat down and began to wait. He looked round the summer-house, which somehow struck him as a great deal more dilapidated than before. Though the day was just as fine as yesterday, it seemed a wretched little place this time. There was a circle on the green table, left no doubt from the glass of cognac spilt the day before. Foolish and irrelevant ideas strayed into his mind, as they always do in a time of tedious waiting. He wondered, for instance, why he had sat down precisely in the same place as the previous day, why not elsewhere. In the end he felt very depressed — depressed by suspense and uncertainty. But he had not sat there more than a quarter of an hour, when he suddenly heard the thrum of a guitar somewhere quite close. People were sitting, or had only just sat down, somewhere in the bushes not more than twenty paces away.

Alyosha suddenly recollected that on coming out of the summer-house the day before, he had caught a glimse of an old low green garden-seat among the bushes on the left, by the fence. The newcomers must have seated themselves on it now.

Who were they?

A man's voice suddenly began singing in a sugary falsetto, accompanying himself on the guitar:

> *"By impregnable ties*
> *I am bound to my dear.*
> *Oh, Lord, have mercy*
> *On her and on me!*
> *On her and on me!*
> *On her and on me!"*

The voice ceased. It was a lackey's tenor and somehow a lackey's song. Another voice, a woman's, suddenly asked ingratiatingly and bashfully, as it were, though with a great deal of mincing affectation:

"Why haven't you been to see us for so long, Pavel Fyodorovich? Why do you always look down upon us?"

"Not at all," answered a man's voice politely, but with firm and emphatic dignity. It was clear that the man had the best of the situation, and that the woman was making advances.

"I believe the man must be Smerdyakov," thought Alyosha, "to judge by his voice. And the lady must be the daughter of the house here, who has come from Moscow, the one who wears the dress with a train and goes to Marfa for soup."

"I am awfully fond of verses of all kinds, if they rhyme," the woman's voice continued. "Why don't you go on?"

The man sang again:

> *"What do I care for royal wealth*
> *If but my dear one be in health?*
> *Lord have mercy*
> *On her and on me!*
> *On her and on me!*
> *On her and on me!"*

"It was even better last time," observed the woman's voice. "You sang 'If my darling be in health'; it sounded more tender. I suppose you've forgotten to-day."

"Verse is rubbish!" said Smerdyakov curtly.

"Oh, no! I am very fond of verse."

"So far as it's verse, it's fundamentally rubbish. Consider for yourself: who ever talks in rhyme? And if we were all to talk in rhyme, even if it were decreed by the authorities, we shouldn't say much, should we? Poetry is no good, Marya Kondratyevna."

"How clever you are! How is it you've gone so deep into everything?" The woman's voice was more and more ingratiating.

"I could have done better than that. I could have learnt more than that, if it had not been for my lot from my childhood up. I would have shot a man in a duel if he called me names because I am descended from a filthy beggar and have no father. And they used to throw it in my teeth in Moscow, too. It had reached them from here, thanks to Grigory Vasilyevich. Grigory Vasilyevich blames me for rebelling against my birth: 'You,' he says, 'came forth from her womb.' Call it 'womb' if you please, but I would have allowed them to kill me before I was born so that I might not have come into the world at all. They used to say in the market-place, and your mamma, too, with great lack of delicacy, set off telling me, that her hair was like a mat on her head, and that she was short of five foot by a wee bit. Why talk of a wee bit while she might have said 'a little bit,' like every one else? She wanted to make it sound pitiful, but that's a yokel's pity, a regular peasant's feeling. Can a Russian peasant have the refined feelings of an educated man? He can't be said to have feeling at all, in his ignorance. From my childhood up when I hear 'a wee bit,' I am ready to run riot. I hate all Russia, Marya Kondratyevna."

"If you'd been a cadet in the army, or a young hussar, you wouldn't have talked like that, but would have drawn your sabre to defend all Russia."

"I don't want to be a hussar, Marya Kondratyevna, and, what's more, I should like to abolish all soldiers."

"And when an enemy comes, who is going to defend us?"

"There's no need of defence. In 1812 there was a great invasion of Russia by Napoleon, first Emperor of the French, father of the present one, and it would have been a good thing if they had conquered us. A clever nation would have conquered a very stupid one and annexed it. We should have had quite a different order of things."

"Are they so much better in their country than we are? I wouldn't change a Russian dandy for three young Englishmen," observed Marya Kondratyevna tenderly, doubtless accompanying her words with a most languishing glance.

"That depends, ma'am, on what you idolise."

"But you are just like a foreigner yourself — just like a most refined foreigner. I tell you that, though it makes me blush."

"If you care to know, when it comes to debauchery, the foreigners and our own people are all alike. They are rascals, only there the scoundrel wears patent leather boots while here he is wretchedly poor and stinking and sees no harm in it. The Russian people want thrashing, as Fyodor Pavlovich said properly yesterday, though he is crazy, and all his children, too."

"You said yourself though, you had such respect for Ivan Fyodorovich."

"But he said I was a stinking lackey. The gentleman thinks that I might get out of hand. He is mistaken there. If I had a certain sum in my pocket, I would have left here long ago. Dmitri Fyodorovich is worse than any lackey in his behaviour, in his mind, and in his poverty. He doesn't know how to do anything, and yet he is respected by every one. I may be only a bouillon-maker, but with luck I could open a café restaurant in the Petrovka section of Moscow, for my cookery is something special, and there's no one in Moscow, except the foreigners, whose cookery is anything special. Dmitri Fyodorovich is a beggar, but if he were to challenge the son of the first count in the country, he'd fight him. Though in what way is he better than I am? For he is ever so much stupider than I am. Look at the money he has wasted to no purpose!"

"It must be lovely, a duel," Marya Kondratyevna observed suddenly.

"How so?"

"It must be so frightful and so brave, especially when young officers with pistols in their hands pop at one another for the sake of some lady. A perfect picture! Ah, if only girls were allowed to look on, I'd give anything to see one!"

"It's all very well when you are firing at some one, but when he is firing straight in your mug, you must feel pretty silly. You'd be glad to run away, Marya Kondratyevna."

"You don't mean you would run away?" But Smerdyakov did not deign to reply. After a moment's silence the guitar tinkled again, and he sang again in the same falsetto:

"*Whatever you may say,*
I shall go far away.
Life will be bright and gay
In the city far away.
I shall not grieve,
I shall not grieve at all,
I don't intend to grieve at all."

Then something unexpected happened. Alyosha suddenly sneezed. They were silent. Alyosha got up and walked towards them. It was indeed Smerdyakov dressed up and wearing patent leather boots, his hair pomaded, and perhaps curled. The guitar lay on the garden-seat. His companion was the daughter of the house. She was wearing a light blue dress with a train two yards long. She was young and would not have been bad-looking, but that her face was so round and terribly freckled.

"Will my brother Dmitri soon be back?" asked Alyosha with as much composure as he could muster.

Smerdyakov got up slowly; Marya Kondratyevna rose, too.

"How am I to know about Dmitri Fyodorovich? It's not as if I were his keeper," answered Smerdyakov quietly, distinctly, and superciliously.

"But I simply asked whether you do know?" Alyosha explained.

"I know nothing of his whereabouts and don't want to."

"But my brother told me that you let him know all that goes on in the house, and promised to let him know when Agrafena Alexandrovna comes."

Smerdyakov turned a deliberate, unmoved look upon him.

"And how did you get in this time, since the gate was bolted an hour ago?" he asked, looking at Alyosha.

"I came in from the lane, over the fence, and went straight to the summer-house. I hope you'll excuse me," he added, addressing Marya Kondratyevna. "I was in a hurry to find my brother."

"Ach, as though we could take it amiss in you!" drawled Marya Kondratyevna, flattered by Alyosha's apology. "For Dmitri Fyodorovich often goes to the summer-house in that way. We don't know he is here and he is sitting in the summer-house."

"I am very anxious to find him, or to learn from you where he is now. Believe me, it's on business of great importance to him."

"He never tells us," lisped Marya Kondratyevna.

"Though I used to come here as an acquaintance," Smerdyakov began again, "Dmitri Fyodorovich has pestered me in a merciless way even here by his incessant questions about the master. 'What news?' he'll ask. 'What's going on in there now? Who's coming and going?' and can't I tell him something more. Twice already he's threatened me with death."

"With death?" Alyosha exclaimed in surprise.

"Do you suppose he'd think much of that, sir, with his temper, which you had a chance of observing yourself yesterday? He says if I let Agrafena Alexandrovna in and she spends the night there, I'll be the first he'll kill. I am terribly afraid of him, sir, and if I were not even more afraid of what that might mean, I ought to let the police know. God only knows, sir, what he might not do!"

"Dmitri Fyodorovich said to him the other day, 'I'll pound you in a mortar!'" added Marya Kondratyevna.

"Oh, if it's pounding in a mortar, it may be only talk," observed Alyosha. "If I could meet him, I might speak to him about that, too."

"Well, the only thing I can tell you is this," said Smerdyakov, as though thinking better of it; "I come here as a neighbour, an old acquaintance, and why shouldn't I come? On the other hand, Ivan Fyodorovich sent me first thing this morning to your brother's lodging in Ozyornaya Street, without a letter, but with a message to Dmitri Fyodorovich to come and dine with him at the restaurant here, in the market-place. I went, but didn't find Dmitri Fyodorovich at home, though it was eight o'clock. 'He's been here, but he is gone for good,' those were the very words of his landlady. It's as though there was a conspiracy between them. Perhaps at this moment he is in the restaurant with Ivan Fyodorovich, for Ivan Fyodorovich has not been home to dinner and Fyodor Pavlovich dined alone an hour ago, and is now taking a nap. But I beg you, sir, most particularly not to speak of me and of what I have told you, for he'd kill me, sir, for nothing at all."

"Brother Ivan invited Dmitri to the restaurant to-day?" repeated Alyosha quickly.

"That is correct, sir."

"The 'Metropolis,' in the square?"

"The very same."

"That's quite likely," cried Alyosha, much excited. "Thank you, Smerdyakov; that's important. I'll go there at once."

"Don't betray me, sir," Smerdyakov called after him.

"Oh, no, I'll step into the tavern as though by chance. Don't be anxious."

"But wait a minute, I'll open the gate for you," cried Marya Kondratyevna.

"No; this is nearer, I'll climb the fence again."

The news threw Alyosha into great agitation. He ran to the tavern. It was improper for him to go into the tavern in his monastic dress, but he could inquire at the entrance for his brothers and call them out. But just as he reached the tavern, a window was flung open, and his brother Ivan called down to him from it.

"Alyosha, can't you come up here to me? I shall be awfully obliged."

"To be sure I can, only I don't quite know whether in this dress . . ."

"But I am in a private room. Come up the steps; I'll run down to meet you."

A minute later Alyosha was sitting beside his brother. Ivan was alone, dining.

CHAPTER III

THE BROTHERS GET ACQUAINTED

Ivan was not, however, in a private room. It was only a place by the window shut off by a screen, so that those sitting there could not be seen by other people in the room. It was the first room from the entrance with a buffet along the wall. Waiters were continually darting to and fro. The only customer in the room was an old retired military man drinking tea in a corner. But there was the usual bustle going on in the other rooms of the tavern; there were shouts for the waiters, the sound of popping corks, the click of billiard balls, the drone of the organ. Alyosha knew that Ivan did not usually visit this tavern and disliked taverns in general. So he must have come here, he reflected, simply to meet Dmitri by arrangement. Yet Dmitri was not there.

"Shall I order you fish soup or anything, you don't live on tea alone, I suppose," cried Ivan, apparently delighted at having got hold of Alyosha. For his own part, he had finished dinner and was taking tea.

"Let me have soup, and tea afterwards, I am hungry," said Alyosha gaily.

"And cherry jam? They have it here. You remember how you used to love cherry jam when you were little?"

"You remember that? Let me have jam, too, I like it still."

Ivan rang for the waiter and ordered soup, tea, and jam.

"I remember everything, Alyosha, I remember you till you were eleven, I was nearly fifteen. There's such a difference between fifteen and eleven that brothers are never companions at those ages. I don't know whether I was fond of you even. When I went away to Moscow for the first few years I never thought of you at all. Then, when you came to Moscow yourself, we only met once somewhere, I believe. And now I've been here more than three months, and so far we have scarcely said a word to each other. To-morrow I am going away, and I was just thinking as I sat here how I could see you to say good-bye and just then you passed."

"Were you very anxious to see me then?"

"Very, I want to get to know you once for all, and I want you to know me. And then to say good-bye. I believe it's always best to get to know people just before parting from them. I've noticed how you've been looking at me these three months. There has been a continual look of expectation in your eyes, and I can't endure that. That's why I've kept away from you. But in the end I have learnt to respect you. The little man stands firm, I thought. Though I am laughing, I am serious. You do stand firm, don't you? I like people who are firm like that whatever it is they stand on, even if they are such little boys as you. Your expectant look ceased to annoy me, I grew fond of it in the end that expectant look. You seem to love me for some reason, Alyosha?"

"I do love you, Ivan. Dmitri says of you — Ivan is a tomb! I say of you, Ivan is a riddle. You are a riddle to me even now. But I come to understand something in you, and that only happened this morning."

"What's that?" laughed Ivan.

"You won't be angry?" Alyosha laughed, too.

"Well?"

"That you are just as young as other young men of three and twenty, that you are just a young, fresh, charming boy, unfledged in fact! Now, have I insulted you dreadfully?"

"On the contrary, I am struck by a coincidence," cried Ivan, warmly and good-humouredly. "Would you believe it that ever since that scene with her, I have thought of nothing else but what a green youth I am, and just as though you guessed that, you begin about it. Do you know I've been sitting here thinking to myself: that if I didn't believe in life, if I lost faith in the woman I love, lost faith in the order of things, were convinced in fact that everything is a disorderly, damnable, and perhaps devilish chaos, if I were struck by every horror of man's disillusionment — still I should want to live and, having once tasted of the cup, I would not turn away from it till I had drained it! At thirty, though, I shall be sure to drop the cup, even if I've not emptied it, and turn away — where I don't know. But till I am thirty, I know that my youth will triumph over everything — every disillusionment, every disgust with life. I've asked myself many times whether there is in the world any despair that would overcome this frantic and perhaps unseemly thirst for life in me, and I've come to the conclusion that there isn't, that is till I am thirty, and then I shall lose it of myself, I fancy. Some drivelling consumptive moralists — and poets especially — often call that thirst for life base. It's a feature of the Karamazovs, it's true, that thirst for life regardless of everything; you have it no doubt, too, but why is it base? The centripetal force on our planet is still fearfully strong, Alyosha. I have a longing for life, and I go on living even in spite of logic. Though I may not believe in the order of the universe, yet the sticky little leaves as they open in spring are precious to me. The blue sky is precious to me, sometimes a person is dear to me — you know, one loves people sometimes without knowing why. Some great deeds done by men are precious to me, though I've long ceased perhaps to have faith in them, yet from old habit one's heart honours them. Here they have brought the fish soup for you, eat it, and good health to you. It's first-rate soup, they know how to make it here. I want to go to Europe, Alyosha, I shall set off from here. And yet I know that I am only going to a graveyard, but it's a most precious graveyard, that's what it is! Precious are the dead that lie there, every stone over them speaks of such burning life gone by, of such passionate faith in their work, their truth, their struggle, and their science, that I know I shall fall on the ground and kiss those stones and weep over them; though I'm convinced in my heart that it's long been nothing but a graveyard. And I shall not weep out of despair, but simply because I shall be happy in my tears, I shall get drunk on my own emotion. I love the sticky leaves of spring, the blue sky — that's what it is. It's not a matter of intellect or logic, you love with your insides, with your belly. You love the first strength of your youth. Do you understand anything of my twaddle, Alyosha?" Ivan laughed suddenly.

"I understand too well, Ivan. One longs to love with one's insides, with one's belly. You said that so well and I am awfully glad that you have such a strong will to live," cried Alyosha. "I think every one should love life above every thing in the world."

"Love life more than the meaning of it?"

"Certainly, love it, regardless of logic as you say, it must be regardless of logic, and it's only then that one will understand the meaning of it, too. I have had this feeling a long time. Half your work is done, Ivan, you love life; now you've only to try to do the second half and you are saved."

"Here you are trying to save me, but perhaps I am not lost! And what does your second half mean?"

"Why, one has to raise up your dead, who perhaps have not died after all. Come, let me have tea. I am so glad of our talk, Ivan."

"I see you are in an exalted mood. I am awfully fond of such *professions de foi* from such — novices. You are a steadfast person, Alexey. Is it true that you mean to leave the monastery?"

"Yes, my elder sends me out into the world."

"We shall see each other then in the world.

We shall meet before I am thirty, when I shall begin to turn aside from the cup. Father doesn't want to turn aside from his cup till he is seventy, he dreams of hanging on till he's eighty in fact, so he says. He means it only too seriously, though he is a clown. He stands on his sensuality as on a rock — though, indeed, after we are thirty there may be nothing else to stand on. . . . But to hang on till seventy is nasty, better only until thirty; one might retain 'a shadow of nobility' by deceiving oneself. Have you seen Dmitri to-day?"

"No, but I saw Smerdyakov," and Alyosha rapidly, though minutely, described his meeting with Smerdyakov. Ivan began listening anxiously and even questioned him on some points.

"But he begged me not to tell Dmitri that he had told me about him," added Alyosha. Ivan frowned and grew thoughtful.

"Are you frowning on Smerdyakov's account?" asked Alyosha.

"Yes, on his account. Damn him, I certainly did want to see Dmitri, but now there's no need," said Ivan reluctantly.

"But are you really leaving so soon, brother?"

"Yes."

"What of Dmitri and father? how will it end?" asked Alyosha anxiously.

"You are always harping on it! What have I to do with it? Am I my brother Dmitri's keeper?" Ivan snapped irritably, but then he suddenly smiled bitterly. "Cain's answer about his murdered brother, wasn't it? Perhaps that's what you're thinking at this moment? Well, damn it all, I can't stay here to be their keeper, can I? I've finished what I had to do, and I am going. Do you imagine I am jealous of Dmitri, that I've been trying to steal his beautiful Katerina Ivanovna for the last three months? Nonsense, I had business of my own. I finished it. I am going. I finished it just now, you were witness."

"At Katerina Ivanovna's?"

"Yes, and I've released myself once for all. And after all, what have I to do with Dmitri? Dmitri doesn't come in. I had my own business to settle with Katerina Ivanovna. You know yourself, on the contrary, that Dmitri behaved as though there was an understanding between us. I didn't ask him to do it, but he solemnly handed her over to me and gave us his blessing. It's all too funny. Ah, Alyosha, if you only knew how light my heart is now! Would you believe it, I sat here eating my dinner and was nearly ordering champagne to celebrate my first hour of freedom. Phew! It's been going on nearly six months, and all at once I've thrown it off. I could never have guessed even yesterday, how easy it would be to put an end to it if I wanted."

"You are speaking of your love, Ivan?"

"Of my love, if you like. I fell in love with the young lady, the finishing-school miss, I worried myself over her and she tormented me. I hung around her . . . and all at once it's over! I spoke this morning with inspiration, but I went away and roared with laughter. Would you believe it? Yes, it's the truth."

"You seem very merry about it now," observed Alyosha, looking into his face, which had all at once really grown brighter.

"But how could I tell that I didn't care for her a bit! Ha-ha! It appears after all I didn't. And yet how she attracted me! How attractive she was just now when I made my speech! And do you know she attracts me awfully even now, yet how easy it is to leave her. Do you think I am putting it on?"

"No, only perhaps it wasn't love."

"Alyosha," laughed Ivan, "don't get into discussions about love, it doesn't become you. How you rushed into the conversation this morning! I've forgotten to kiss you for it. . . . But how she tormented me! It certainly was sitting by a 'laceration.' Ah, she knew how I loved her! She loved me and not Dmitri," Ivan insisted gaily. "Her feeling for Dmitri was simply a self-laceration. All I told her then was perfectly true, but the worst of it is, it may take her fifteen or twenty years to find out that she doesn't care for Dmitri, and loves me whom she torments, and perhaps she may never find it out at all, in spite of to-day's lesson. Well, it's better so; I just up and went, for good. By the way, how is she now? What happened after I left?"

Alyosha told him she had been hysterical, and that she was now, he heard, unconscious and delirious.

"Isn't Madame Hohlakov laying it on?"

"I think not."

"I must find out. Nobody dies of hysterics though. Well, let it be hysterics. God gave woman hysterics out of kindness. I won't go there at all. Why push myself forward again?"

"But you told her that she had never cared for you."

"I did that on purpose. Alyosha, shall I call for some champagne? Let us drink to my freedom. Ah, if only you knew how glad I am!"

"No, brother, we had better not drink," said Alyosha suddenly. "Besides I feel somehow depressed."

"Yes, you've been depressed a long time, I've noticed it."

"Have you decided on going to-morrow morning then?"

"Morning? I didn't say I should go in the morning. . . . But perhaps it may be the morning. Would you believe it, I dined here to-day only to avoid dining with the old man, I loathe him so. I should have left long ago, just to get away from him. But why are you so worried about my going away? We've plenty of time before I go, a whole eternity of it!"

"If you are going away to-morrow, what do you mean by an eternity?"

"But what does it matter to us?" laughed Ivan, "we'll have time enough for our talk, for what brought us here. Why do you look so surprised? Answer: why have we met here? To talk of my love for Katerina Ivanovna, of the old man and Dmitri? of foreign travel? of the fatal position of Russia? of the Emperor Napoleon? Is that it?"

"No."

"Then you know what for. It's different for other people; but we in our green youth have to settle the eternal questions first of all. That's what we care about. Young Russia is talking about nothing but the eternal questions now. Just when the old folks are all taken up with practical questions. Why have you been looking at me in expectation for the last three months? To ask me: 'what do you believe, or don't you believe at all?' That's what your look has been meaning for these three months, hasn't it?"

"Perhaps so," smiled Alyosha. "You are not laughing at me, now, Ivan?"

"I, laughing! I don't want to hurt my little brother who has been watching me with such expectation for three months. Alyosha, look straight at me! Of course I am just such a little boy as you are, only not a novice. And what have Russian boys been doing up till now, some of them, I mean? In this stinking tavern here, for instance, they meet and sit down in a corner. They've never met in their lives before and, when they go out of the tavern, they won't meet again for forty years. And what will they talk about during that momentary encounter in the tavern? Of the eternal questions, nothing else: is there a God, is there immortality? And those who do not believe in God will talk of socialism or anarchism, of the transformation of all humanity on a new pattern, which all comes to the same thing, they're the same questions turned inside out. And in our time numbers, numbers of the most original Russian boys do nothing but talk of the eternal questions! Isn't it so?"

"Yes, for real Russians the questions of God's existence and of immortality, or, as you say, the same questions turned inside out, come first and foremost, of course, and so they should," said Alyosha, still watching his brother with the same gentle and inquiring smile.

"Well, Alyosha, it's sometimes far from intelligent to be a Russian at all, but anything stupider than the way Russian boys spend their time nowadays one can hardly imagine. But there's one Russian boy called Alyosha I am awfully fond of."

"How nicely you put that in!" Alyosha laughed suddenly.

"Well, tell me where to begin, give your orders. The existence of God, eh?"

"Begin where you like, even from the wrong end. You declared yesterday at father's that there was no God." Alyosha looked searchingly at his brother.

"I said that yesterday at dinner on purpose to tease you and I saw how your eyes began to flash. But now I've no objection to talking things over with you, and I say so very seriously. I want to be friends with you, Alyosha, for I have no friends and want to try it. Well, only fancy, perhaps I, too, accept God," laughed Ivan, "that's a surprise for you, isn't it?"

"Yes, of course, if you are not joking now."

"Joking? I was told at the elder's yesterday that I was joking. You know, dear boy, there was an old sinner in the eighteenth century who declared that, if there were no God, he would have to be invented. *S'il n'existait pas Dieu, il faudrait l'inventer.* And man has actually invented God. And what's strange, what would be marvellous, is not that God should really exist; the marvel is that such an idea, the idea of the necessity of God, could enter the head of such a savage, vicious beast as man. So holy it is, so touching, so wise, and so great a credit it does to man. As for me, I've long resolved not to wonder whether man created God or God man. And I won't go through all the axioms laid down by Russian boys on that subject, all derived from European hypotheses; for what's a hypothesis there, is an axiom with the Russian boy, and not only with the boys but with their teachers, too, for our Russian professors are often just the same boys themselves. And so I omit all the hypotheses. For what are we aiming at now? I am trying to explain as quickly as possible my essential nature, that is, what manner of man I am, what I believe in, and what I hope for, that's it, isn't it? And therefore I tell you that I accept God simply and directly. But you must note this: if God exists and if He really did create the earth, then, as we all know, He created it according to Euclidean geometry, and the human mind has the conception of only three dimensions in space. Yet there have been and still are geometricians and philosophers, and even some of the most distinguished, who doubt whether the whole universe, or to speak more widely the whole of being, was only created according to Euclid's geometry; they even dare to dream that two parallel lines, which according to Euclid can never meet on earth, may meet somewhere in infinity. I have come to the conclusion that, since I can't understand even that, I can't expect to understand about God. I acknowledge humbly that I have no faculty for settling such questions, I have a Euclidean earthly mind, and how could I solve problems that are not of this world? And I advise you never to think about it either, my dear Alyosha, especially about God, whether He exists or not. All such questions are utterly inappropriate to a mind created with a concept of only three dimensions. And so I accept God and am glad to, and what's more I accept His wisdom, His purpose — which are utterly beyond our ken; I believe in the underlying order and the meaning of life; I believe in the eternal harmony in which they say we shall one day be blended. I believe in the Word to Which the universe is striving, and Which Itself was 'with God,' and Which Itself is God and so on, and so on, to infinity. There are all sorts of phrases for it. I seem to be on the right path, don't I? Yet would you believe it, in the last account I don't accept this world of God's, and, although I know it exists, I don't admit it at all. It's not that I don't accept God, you must understand, it's the world created by Him, it's God's world that I don't and cannot accept. Let me make it plain. I believe like a child that suffering will be healed and made up for, that all the humiliating comedy of human contradictions will vanish like a pitiful mirage, like the despicable fabrication of the impotent and infinitely small Euclidean mind of man, finally, that in the cosmic *dénouement*, at the moment of eternal harmony, something so precious will come to pass that it will suffice for all hearts, for the assuagement of all indignation, for the redemption of all the crimes of humanity, of all the blood they've shed; that it will make it not only possible to forgive but to justify all that has happened to men — but though all that may come to pass, I don't accept it. I won't accept it. Even if parallel lines do meet and I see it myself, I shall see it and say that they've met, but still I won't accept it. That's what's at the root of me, Alyosha; that's my creed. I am in earnest in what I say. I began our talk as foolishly as I could on purpose, but I've led up to my confession, for that's all you want. You didn't want to hear about God, but only to know what the brother you love lives by. And so I've told you."

Ivan concluded his long tirade with marked and unexpected feeling.

"And why did you begin 'as foolishly as you could'?" asked Alyosha, looking dreamily at him.

"To begin with, for the sake of the Russian style. Russian conversations on such subjects are always carried on as foolishly as possible. And secondly, the more foolish, the nearer to the point. The more foolish one is, the clearer one is. Foolishness is short and artless, while intelligence wriggles and hides itself. Intelligence is a knave, but foolishness is honest and straight. I've led the conversation to my despair, and the more foolishly I have presented it, the better for me."

"Will you explain why you don't accept the world?" said Alyosha.

"To be sure I will, it's not a secret, that's

what I've been leading up to. Dear little brother, I don't want to corrupt you or to push you off your rock, perhaps I want to be healed by you." Ivan smiled suddenly quite like a little gentle child. Alyosha had never seen such a smile on his face before.

CHAPTER IV

REBELLION

"I MUST make you one confession," Ivan began. "I could never understand how one can love one's neighbours. It's just one's neighbours, to my mind, that one can't love, though one might love those far away. I once read somewhere of John the Merciful, a saint, that when a hungry, frozen beggar came to him, asking for warmth, he took him into his bed, held him in his arms, and began breathing into his mouth, which was putrid and loathsome from some dreadful disease. I am convinced that he did that out of 'self-laceration,' out of the self-laceration of hypocrisy, for the sake of a dutiful charity, as a self-imposed penance. For any one to love a man, he must be hidden, for as soon as he shows his face, love is gone."

"Father Zosima has talked of that more than once," observed Alyosha, "he, too, said that the face of a man often hinders many people not practised in love, from loving him. But yet there's a great deal of love in mankind, and almost Christlike love. I know that myself, Ivan."

"Well, I know nothing of it so far, and can't understand it, and the innumerable mass of mankind are with me there. The question is, whether that's due to men's bad qualities or whether it's inherent in their nature. To my thinking, Christlike love for men is a miracle impossible on earth. True, He was God. But we, we are not gods. Suppose I, for instance, suffer intensely. Another can never know how much I suffer, because he is another and not I. And what's more, a man is rarely ready to admit another's suffering (as though it were a distinction). Why won't he admit it, do you think? Because I smell bad, because I have a stupid face, because I once trod on his foot. Besides there is suffering and suffering; degrading, humiliating suffering such as humbles me — hunger, for instance — my benefactor will perhaps allow me; but when you come to higher suffering — for an idea, for instance — he will very rarely admit that, perhaps because my face strikes him as not at all what he fancies a man should have who suffers for an idea. And so he deprives me instantly of his favour, and not at all because of an evil heart. Beggars, especially genteel beggars, ought never to show themselves, but to ask for charity through the newspapers. One can love one's neighbours in the abstract, and sometimes even at a distance, but at close quarters it's almost impossible. If it were as on the stage, in the ballet, where, if beggars come in, they wear silken rags and tattered lace and beg for alms dancing gracefully, then one might like looking at them. Like looking at them, but not love them. But enough of that. I simply wanted to show you my point of view. I meant to speak of the suffering of mankind generally, but we had better confine ourselves to the sufferings of children. That reduces the scope of my argument to a tenth of what it would be. Still we'd better keep just to the children, though it does weaken my case. But, in the first place, children can be loved even at close quarters, even when they are dirty, even when they are ugly (I fancy, though, children never are ugly). In the second place, I won't speak of grown-up people because, besides being disgusting and unworthy of love, they have a compensation — they've eaten the apple and know good and evil, and they have become 'like gods.' They go on eating it still. But the children haven't eaten of it, and are so far innocent. Are you fond of children, Alyosha? I know you are, and you will understand why I prefer to speak of them. If they, too, suffer horribly on earth, they suffer for their fathers' sins, they are punished for their fathers, who have eaten the apple; but that reasoning is of another world and is incomprehensible to the heart of man here on earth. The innocent must not suffer for another's sins, and especially such innocents! You may be surprised at me, Alyosha, but I am awfully fond of children, too. And observe, cruel people, the passionate, the carnal, the Karamazovs, are sometimes very fond of children. Children while they are quite little — up to seven, for instance — are so remote from grown-up people; they are different creatures, as it were, of a different species. I knew a criminal in prison who had, in the course of his career as a robber, murdered whole families, including several children. But when he was in prison, he had a strange affection for them. He spent all his time at his window, watching the children playing in the prison yard. He trained one little boy to come up to his window and made great friends with him. . . . You don't know why I am telling you all this, Alyosha? My head aches and I am sad."

"You speak with a strange air," observed Alyosha uneasily, "as though you were out of your mind, almost."

"By the way, a Bulgarian I met lately in Moscow," Ivan went on, seeming not to hear his brother's words, "told me about the crimes committed by Turks and Circassians in all parts of Bulgaria through fear of a general rising of the Slavs. They burn villages, murder, outrage women and children, they nail their prisoners by the ears to the fences, leave them so till morning, and in the morning they hang them — all sorts of things you can't imagine. People talk sometimes of bestial cruelty, but that's a great injustice and insult to the beasts; a beast can never be so cruel as a man, so artistically cruel. The tiger only tears and gnaws, that's all he can do. He would never think of nailing people by the ears overnight, even if he were able to do it. These Turks took a pleasure in torturing children, too; cutting the unborn child from the mother's womb, and tossing babies up in the air and catching them on the points of their bayonets before their mother's eyes. Doing it before the mother's eyes was what gave zest to the amusement. Here is another scene that I thought very interesting. Imagine a trembling mother with her baby in her arms, a circle of invading Turks around her. They've planned a diversion: they pet the baby, laugh to make it laugh. They succeed, the baby laughs. At that moment a Turk points a pistol four inches from the baby's face. The baby laughs with glee, holds out its little hands to the pistol, and suddenly the artist pulls the trigger in the baby's face and blows out its brains. Artistic, wasn't it? By the way, Turks are particularly fond of sweet things, they say."

"Brother, what are you driving at?" asked Alyosha.

"I think if the devil doesn't exist, but man has created him, he has created him in his own image and likeness."

"Just as he did God, then?" observed Alyosha.

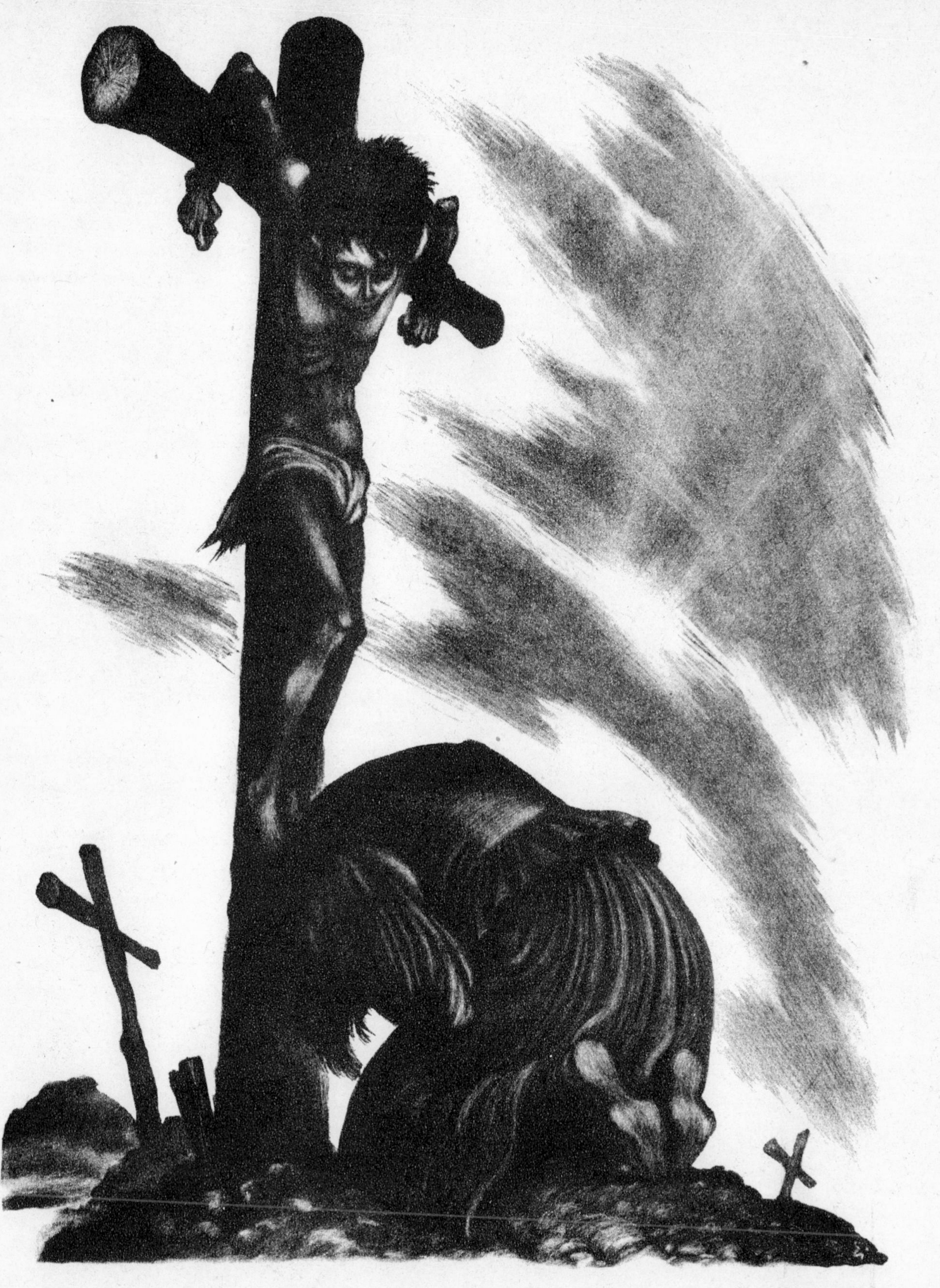

"THAT'S REBELLION"

" 'It's wonderful how you can turn words,' as Polonius says in *Hamlet*," laughed Ivan. "You turn my words against me. Well, I am glad. Yours must be a fine God, if man created Him in his image and likeness. You asked just now what I was driving at. You see, I am a connoisseur and collector of certain facts, and, would you believe, I even copy anecdotes of a certain sort from newspapers and books, and I've already got a fine collection. The Turks, of course, have gone into it, but they are foreigners. I have specimens from home that are even better than the Turks. You know we prefer beating — rods and scourges — that's our national institution. Nailing ears is unthinkable for us, for we are, after all, Europeans. But the rod and the scourge we have always with us and they cannot be taken from us. Abroad now they scarcely do any beating. Manners are more humane, or laws have been passed, so that they don't dare to flog men now. But they make up for it in another way just as national as ours. And so national that it would be practically impossible among us, though I believe we are being inoculated with it, since the religious movement began in our aristocracy. I have a charming pamphlet, translated from the French, describing how, quite recently, five years ago, a murderer, Richard, was executed — a young man, I believe, of three and twenty, who repented and was converted to the Christian faith at the very scaffold. This Richard was an illegitimate child who at the age of six was donated by his parents to some shepherds on the Swiss mountains. They brought him up to work for them. He grew up like a little wild beast among them. The shepherds taught him nothing, and scarcely fed or clothed him, but sent him out at seven to herd the flock in cold and wet, and no one hesitated or scrupled to treat him so. Quite the contrary, they thought they had every right, for Richard had been given to them as a chattel, and they did not even see the necessity of feeding him. Richard himself testifies how in those years, like the Prodigal Son in the Gospel, he longed to eat of the mash given to the pigs, which were fattened for sale. But they wouldn't even give him that, and beat him when he stole from the pigs. And that was how he spent all his childhood and his youth, till he grew up and was strong enough to go away and be a thief. The savage began to earn his living as a day labourer in Geneva. He drank what he earned, he lived like a brute, and finished by killing and robbing an old man. He was caught, tried, and condemned to death. They are not sentimentalists there. And in prison he was immediately surrounded by pastors, members of Christian brotherhoods, philanthropic ladies, and the like. They taught him to read and write in prison, and expounded the Gospel to him. They exhorted him, worked upon him, drummed at him incessantly, till at last he solemnly confessed his crime. He was converted. He wrote to the court himself that he was a monster, but that in the end God had vouchsafed him light and sent him grace. All Geneva was in excitement about him — all philanthropic and religious Geneva. All the prominent and well-bred people of the town rush to the prison, kiss Richard and embrace him: 'You are our brother, you have been visited with grace.' And Richard does nothing but weep with emotion, 'Yes, I've been visited with grace! All my childhood and youth I was glad of pigs' food, but now even I have been visited with grace. I am dying in the Lord.' 'Yes, Richard, die in the Lord; you have shed blood and must die. Though it's not your fault that you knew not the Lord, when you coveted the pigs' food and were beaten for stealing it (which was very wrong of you, for stealing is forbidden); but you've shed blood and you must die.' And on the last day, Richard, perfectly limp, did nothing but cry and repeat every minute: 'This is my happiest day. I am going to the Lord.' 'Yes,' cry the pastors and the judges and the philanthropic ladies. 'This is the happiest day of your life, for you are going to the Lord!' They all walk or drive to the scaffold in procession behind the prison van. At the scaffold they call to Richard: 'Die, brother, die in the Lord, for even you have been visited with grace!' And so, covered with his brothers' kisses, Richard is dragged on to the scaffold, and led to the guillotine. And they chopped off his head in brotherly fashion, because he, too, had been visited with grace. Yes, that's characteristic. That pamphlet has been translated into Russian by some Russian philanthropists of aristocratic rank and evangelical aspirations, and has been distributed gratis for the enlightenment of the people. The case of Richard is interesting because it's national. Though to us it's absurd to cut off a man's head, because he has become our brother and has been visited with grace, yet we have our own speciality, which is all but worse. Our own historic immediate and dearest delight lies in torture by beating. There are lines in Nekrasov describing how a peasant lashes a horse across the eyes, 'the meek eyes.' Every one has seen it, it's a peculiarly Russian trait. He describes how a feeble little nag has foundered under too heavy a load and cannot move. The peasant beats it, beats it savagely, beats it at last not knowing what he is doing in the intoxication of cruelty, thrashes it mercilessly over and over again. 'You may be on your last legs, but you must pull, if you die for it.' The nag strains, and then he begins lashing the poor defenceless creature on its weeping, on its 'meek eyes.' The frantic beast tugs and draws the load, trembling all over, gasping for breath, moving sideways, with a sort of unnatural spasmodic leaping motion — it's awful in Nekrasov. But that's only a horse, and God has given us horses to beat. So the Tatars have taught us, and they left us the knout as a remembrance. But men, too, can be beaten. A well-educated, cultured gentleman and his wife beat their own child with a birch-rod, a girl of seven. I have an exact account of it. The papa was glad that the birch was covered with twigs. 'It stings more,' said he, and so he began to do in his own daughter. I know for a fact there are people who at every blow are worked up to sensuality, to literal sensuality, which increases progressively at every blow they inflict. They beat for a minute, for five minutes, for ten minutes, more rapidly and more savagely. The child screams. At last the child cannot scream, it gasps, 'Daddy! daddy!' By some diabolical unseemly chance the case was brought into court. A counsel is engaged. The Russian people have long called a barrister 'a conscience for hire.' The counsel protests in his client's defence. 'It's such a simple thing,' he says, 'an everyday domestic event. A father corrects his child. To our shame be it said, it is brought into court.' The jury, convinced by him, retire and bring in a favourable verdict. The public roars with delight that the torturer is acquitted. Ah, a pity I wasn't there! I would have proposed establishing a scholarship fund in the torturer's name! . . . Charming pictures.

"But I've still better things about children. I've collected a great, great deal about Russian children, Alyosha. There was a little girl of five who was hated by her father and mother, 'most worthy and respectable people, of good education and breeding.' You see, I must repeat again, it is a peculiar characteristic of many people, this love of torturing children, and children only. To all other types of humanity these torturers behave mildly and benevolently, like cultivated and humane Europeans; but they are very fond of tormenting children, even fond of children themselves in that sense. It's just their defencelessness that tempts the tormentor, just the angelic confidence of the child who has no refuge and no appeal, that sets his vile blood on fire. In every man, of course, a beast lies hidden — the beast of rage, the beast of lust roused by the screams of the tortured victim, the beast of unchained lawlessness, the beast of diseases that follow on vice — gout, kidney disease, and so on.

"This poor child of five was subjected to every possible torture by those cultivated parents. They beat her, thrashed her, kicked her for no reason till her body was one bruise. Then, they went to greater refinements of cruelty — shut her up all night in the cold and frost in a privy, and because she didn't ask to be taken up at night (as though a child of five sleeping its angelic, sound sleep could be trained to wake and ask), they smeared her face with excrement and forced her to eat it, and it was her mother, her mother did this. And that mother could sleep, hearing the groans of the poor child locked up in that vile place at night! A little creature, who can't even understand what's done to her, in the dark and cold of that vile place, beats her little aching breast with her tiny fist and weeps her bloody meek unresentful tears begging dear, kind God to protect her! Do you understand this rot, friend and brother, you God-fearing and humble novice? Do you understand why this infamy is necessary and why it has come about? Without it, I am told, man could not have existed on earth, for he could not have known good and evil. But why know that devilish good and evil when it costs so much? Why, the whole world of knowledge is not worth that child's tears! I say nothing of the sufferings of grown-up people, they have eaten the apple, damn them, and the devil take them all! But these little ones! I am making you suffer, Alyosha, you are not yourself. I'll leave off if you like."

"Never mind. I, too, want to suffer," muttered Alyosha.

"One picture, only one more, because it's so curious, so characteristic, and I have only just read it in some collection of Russian antiquities. I've forgotten the name. I must look it up. It was in the darkest days of serfdom at the beginning of the century, and long live the Liberator of the People! There was in those days a general with high connections, and a very wealthy landowner, one of those men — somewhat rare, I believe, by then — who, retiring from the service to a life of leisure, were convinced that they had earned absolute power over the lives of their subjects. There were such men then. So our general, settled on his property to which his two thousand souls were attached, lives in pomp, and lords it over his poor neighbours as though they were dependents and clowns. He has kennels of hundreds of hounds and nearly a hundred whips — all mounted, and in uniform. One day a serf boy, a little child of eight, threw a stone in play and hurt the paw of the general's favourite hound. 'Why is my favourite dog lame?' He is told that the boy threw a stone that hurt the dog's paw. 'So you did it.' The general looked the child up and down. 'Take him.' He was taken — taken from his mother and kept shut up all night. Early that morning the general comes out on horseback, with the hounds, his dependents, whips, and huntsmen, all mounted, in full hunting parade, around him. The servants are summoned for their edification, and in front of them all stands the mother of the child. The child is brought from the lock-up. It's a gloomy, cold, foggy autumn day, a capital day for hunting. The general orders the child to be undressed; the child is stripped naked. He shivers, numb with terror, not daring to peep. . . . 'Make him run,' commands the general. 'Run! run!' shout the outriders. The boy runs. . . . 'At him!' yells the general, and he sets the whole pack of hounds on the child. The hounds catch him, and tear him to pieces before his mother's eyes! . . . I believe the general was afterwards declared incapable of administering his estates. Well — what did he deserve? To be shot? To be shot for the satisfaction of our moral feelings? Speak, Alyosha!"

"To be shot," murmured Alyosha, lifting his eyes to Ivan with a pale, twisted smile.

"Bravo!" cried Ivan, delighted. "If even you say so . . . You're a pretty monk! So there is a little devil sitting in your heart, Alyosha Karamazov!"

"What I said was absurd, but —— "

"That's just the point, that 'but'!" cried Ivan. "Let me tell you, novice, that the absurd is only too necessary on earth. The world stands on absurdities, and perhaps nothing would have come to pass in it without them. We know what we know!"

"What do you know?"

"I understand nothing," Ivan went on, as though in delirium. "I don't want to understand anything now. I want to stick to the fact. I made up my mind long ago not to understand. If I try to understand anything, I shall be false to the fact and I have determined to stick to the fact."

"Why are you trying me?" Alyosha cried, with sudden distress. "Will you say what you mean at last?"

"Of course, I will; that's what I've been leading up to. You are dear to me, I don't want to let you go, and I won't give you up to your Zosima."

Ivan for a minute was silent, all at once his face became very sad.

"Listen! I confined myself to children only to make my case clearer. Of the other human tears with which the earth is soaked from its crust to its centre, I will say nothing. I have narrowed my subject on purpose. I am a bug, and I recognise in all humility that I cannot understand why the world is arranged as it is. Men are themselves to blame, I suppose; they were given paradise, they wanted freedom, and stole fire from heaven, though they knew they would become unhappy, so there is no need to pity them. All that my pitiful, earthly, Euclidean understanding tells me is that there is suffering and that there are none guilty; that cause follows effect, simply and directly; that everything flows and finds its level — but that's only Euclidean nonsense, I know that, and I can't consent to live by it! What comfort is it to me that there are none guilty and that cause follows effect simply and directly, and that I know it — I must have retribution, or I will destroy myself. And not retribution in some remote infinite time and space, but here on earth, and that I see it myself. I have believed in it. I want to see it myself, and if I am dead by then, let them raise me from the dead, for if it all happens without me, it will be too great an outrage. Surely I haven't suffered, simply that I, my crimes and my sufferings, may manure the soil for future harmony for somebody else. I want to see with my own eyes the hind lie down with the lion and the victim rise up and embrace his murderer. I want to be there when every one suddenly learns what it has all been for. All the religions of the world are built on this longing, and I am a believer. But then there are the children, and what am I to do about them? That's a question I can't answer. For the hundredth time I repeat, there are numbers of questions, but I've taken only the children, because in their case what I mean is so unanswerably clear. Listen! If all must suffer to pay for the eternal harmony, what have children to do with it, tell me, please? It's beyond all comprehension why they should suffer, and why they should pay for the harmony. Why should they, too, furnish material to enrich the soil for the harmony of the future? I understand solidarity in sin among men. I understand solidarity in retribution, too; but there can be no such solidarity with children. And if it is really true that they must share responsibility for all their fathers' crimes, such a truth is not of this world and is beyond my comprehension. Some jester will say, perhaps, that the child would have grown up and have sinned, but you see he didn't grow up, he was torn to pieces by the dogs, when he was eight years old. Oh, Alyosha, I am not blaspheming! I understand, of course, how the universe will be shaken to its core, when everything in heaven and earth blends in one hymn of praise and everything that lives and has lived cries aloud: 'Thou art just, O Lord, for Thy ways are revealed.' When the mother embraces the fiend who threw her child to the dogs, and all three cry aloud with tears, 'Thou art just, O Lord!' then, of course, the crown of knowledge will be reached and all will be made clear. But what pulls me up here is that I can't accept that harmony. And while I am on earth, I make haste to take my own measures. You see, Alyosha, perhaps it really may happen that if I live to that moment, or rise again to see it, I, too, perhaps, may cry aloud with the rest, looking at the mother embracing the child's torturer, 'Thou art just, O Lord!' but I don't want to cry aloud then. While there is still time, I hasten to protect myself, and so I renounce the higher harmony altogether. It's not worth the tears of that one tortured child who beat itself on the breast with its little fist and prayed in its stinking outhouse, with its unexpiated tears to 'dear, kind God'! It's not worth it, because those tears are unatoned for. They must be atoned for, or there can be no harmony. But how? How are you going to atone for them? Is it possible? By their being avenged? But what do I care for avenging them? What do I care for a hell for oppressors? What good can hell do, since those children have already been tortured? And what becomes of harmony, if there is hell? I want to forgive. I want to embrace. I don't want more suffering. And if the sufferings of children go to swell the sum of sufferings which was necessary to pay for truth, then I assert in advance that the truth is not worth such a price. I don't want the mother to embrace the oppressor who threw her son to the dogs! She dare not forgive him! Let her forgive him for herself, if she will, let her forgive the torturer for the immeasurable suffering of her mother's heart. But the sufferings of her tortured child she has no right to forgive; she dare not forgive the torturer, even if the child were to forgive him! And if that is so, if they dare not forgive, what becomes of the harmony? Is there in the whole world a being who would have the right to forgive and could forgive? I don't want harmony. Out of love for humanity I don't want it. I would rather be left with the unavenged suffering. I would rather remain with my unavenged suffering and unassuaged indignation, *even if I were wrong*. Besides, too high a price is asked for harmony; it's beyond our means to pay so much for admission. And so I hasten to give back my ticket, and if I am an honest man I am bound to give it back as soon as possible. And that I am doing. It's not God that I don't accept, Alyosha, only I most respectfully return Him the ticket."

"That's rebellion," said Alyosha gently, looking down.

"Rebellion? I am sorry you call it that," said Ivan earnestly. "One can hardly live by rebellion, and I want to live. Tell me yourself, I challenge you — answer. Imagine that you are erecting the edifice of human destiny with the object of making men happy at last, giving them peace and rest at last, but that to this end it was essential and inevitable to torture to death only one tiny creature — that baby beating its breast with its fist, for instance — and to found that edifice on its unavenged tears, would you consent to be the architect on those conditions? Tell me, and do not lie."

"No, I wouldn't consent," said Alyosha softly.

"And can you admit the idea that men, for whom you are building it, would agree to accept a happiness based upon the unexpiated blood of a little victim? And accepting it would remain happy for ever?"

"No, I can't admit it. Brother," said Alyosha suddenly, with flashing eyes, "you said just now, is there a being in the whole world who would have the right to forgive and could forgive? But there is a Being and He can forgive everything, all and for all, because He gave His innocent blood for all and everything.

"You have forgotten Him, and on Him is built the edifice, and it is to Him they will cry aloud, 'Thou art just, O Lord, for Thy ways are revealed!' "

"Ah! the One without sin and His blood! No, I have not forgotten Him; on the contrary, I've been wondering all the time how it was you did not bring Him in before, for usually in argument those like you put Him in the foreground.

"Do you know, Alyosha — don't laugh! I made up a poem once, about a year ago. If you can waste another ten minutes on me, I'll tell it to you."

"You wrote a poem?"

"Oh, no, I didn't write it," laughed Ivan, "and I've never written two lines of poetry in my life. But I made up this poem and I remembered it. I was carried away when I made it up. You will be my first reader — that is, listener. Why should an author forego even one listener?" smiled Ivan. "Shall I tell it to you?"

"I am all attention," said Alyosha.

"My poem is called 'The Grand Inquisitor'; it's an absurd thing, but I want to tell it to you."

CHAPTER V

THE GRAND INQUISITOR

"Even this must have a preface — that is, a literary preface," laughed Ivan, "and what kind of *littérateur* am I? You see, the action takes place in the sixteenth century, and at that time, as you probably learnt at school, it was customary in poetry to bring down heavenly powers on earth. Not to speak of Dante, in France, court clerks, as well as the monks in the monasteries, used to give regular performances in which the Madonna, the saints, the angels, Christ, and God Himself were brought on the stage. In those days it was done in all simplicity. In Victor Hugo's 'Notre Dame de Paris' an edifying and gratuitous spectacle was provided for the people in the Hôtel de Ville of Paris in the reign of Louis XI in honour of the birth of the dauphin. It was called *Le bon jugement de la très sainte et gracieuse Vierge Marie*, and she appears in person on the stage and pronounces her *bon jugement*. Similar plays, chiefly from the Old Testament, were occasionally performed in Moscow, too, up to the time of Peter the Great. But besides dramatic spectacles there were current in the world all sorts of tales and songs, in which the holy angels and all the powers of heaven took part when required. In our monasteries the monks busied themselves in translating, copying, and even composing such poems — and as far back as the time of the Tatars. There is, for instance, one monastic poem (of course, from the Greek), 'The Wanderings of Our Lady through Hell,' with descriptions as bold as Dante's. Our Lady visits hell, and the Archangel Michael guides her through the torments. She sees the sinners and their tortures. There is there among others one very entertaining set of sinners in a burning lake; some of them sink so deep in the lake that they can't swim out, and 'these God forgets' — an expression of extraordinary depth and force. And so Our Lady, overcome and weeping, falls before the throne of God and begs for mercy for all in hell — for all she has seen there, indiscriminately. Her conversation with God is immensely interesting. She beseeches Him, she will not desist, and when God points to the hands and feet of her Son, nailed to the Cross, and asks, 'How can I forgive His tormentors?' she bids all the saints, all the martyrs, all the angels and archangels to kneel down with her and pray for mercy on all without distinction. It ends by her winning from God a respite from suffering every year from Good Friday till Trinity day, and the sinners at once raise a cry of gratitude from hell, chanting, 'Thou art just, O Lord, in this judgment.' Well, my poem would have been of the same sort if it had appeared at that time. In my poem He comes on the scene, but He says nothing, only appears and passes on. Fifteen centuries have passed since He promised to come in His glory, fifteen centuries since His prophet wrote, 'Behold, I come quickly'; 'Of that day and that hour knoweth no man, neither the Son, but the Father,' as He Himself said on earth. But humanity awaits him with the same faith and with the same emotion. Oh, with greater faith, for it is fifteen centuries since man has ceased to see signs from Heaven.

Believe but what the heart doth say
No signs from Heaven come to-day.

There was nothing left but faith in what the heart doth say. It is true there were many miracles in those days. There were saints who performed miraculous cures; some holy people, according to their 'Lives,' were visited by the Queen of Heaven herself. But the devil does not slumber, and doubts were already arising among men regarding the truth of these miracles. And just then there appeared in the north, in Germany, a terrible new heresy. 'A great star like unto a torch' (that is, a church) 'fell upon the fountains of the waters and they were made bitter.' These heretics began blasphemously denying miracles. But those who remained faithful were all the more ardent in their faith. Humanity poured out its tears to Him as before, awaited His coming, loved Him, hoped for Him, yearned to suffer and die for Him as before. And so many ages mankind had prayed with faith and fervour, 'O Lord our God, hasten Thy coming,' so many ages called upon Him, that in His infinite mercy He conceived the desire to descend to His worshippers. Before that day He had come down, He had visited some holy men, martyrs and hermits, as is written in their 'Lives.' Among us, Tyutchev, with absolute faith in the truth of his words, bore witness that

Bearing the Cross, in slavish dress
Weary and worn, the Heavenly King
Our mother, Russia, came to bless,
And through our land went wandering.

And that certainly was so, I assure you.

"And behold, He desired to appear, if only for a moment, to the people, to the tortured, suffering people, sunk in foul iniquity, but loving Him like children. My story is laid in Spain, in Seville, in the most terrible time of the Inquisition, when fires were lighted every day to the glory of God, and 'in magnificent *autos-da-fé* the wicked heretics were burnt.' Oh, of course, this was not the coming in which He will appear according to His promise at the end of time in all His heavenly glory, and which will be sudden 'as lightning flashing from east to west.' No, He desired to visit His children only for a moment, and just there where the flames were crackling round the heretics. In His infinite mercy He walks once more among men in that human shape in which He walked among men for three years fifteen centuries ago. He descends upon the 'torrid plazas' of the southern town in which on the day before almost a hundred heretics had, *ad majorem gloriam Dei*, been burnt by monseigneur, the Grand Inquisitor, in a magnificent *auto-da-fé*, in the presence of the king, the court, the knights, the cardinals, the most charming ladies of the court, and the whole population of Seville.

"He came softly, unobserved, and yet, strange to say, every one recognised Him. That might be one of the best passages in the poem. I mean, why they recognised Him. The people are irresistibly drawn to Him, they surround Him, they flock about Him, follow Him. He moves silently in their midst with a gentle smile of infinite compassion. The sun of love burns in His heart, light and power shine from His eyes, and their radiance, shed on the people, stirs their hearts with responsive love. He stretches out His hands to them, blesses them, and a healing virtue comes from contact with Him, even with His garments. An old man in the crowd, blind since childhood, cries out, 'O Lord, heal me and I shall see Thee!' and, as it were, scales fall from his eyes and the blind man sees Him. The crowd weeps and kisses the earth under His feet. Children throw flowers before Him, sing, and cry hosannah.

'It is He — it is He!' all repeat. 'It must be He, it can be no one but He!' He stops at the steps of the Seville cathedral at the moment when the weeping mourners are bringing in a little open white coffin. In it lies a child of seven, the only daughter of a prominent citizen. The dead child lies covered with flowers. 'He will raise your child,' people in the crowd shout to the weeping mother. The priest, coming to meet the coffin, looks perplexed, and frowns, but the mother of the dead child throws herself at His feet with a wail. 'If it be Thou, raise my child!' she cries, stretching out her hands to Him. The procession halts, the coffin is laid on the steps at His feet. He looks with compassion, and His lips once more softly pronounce, '*Talitha cumi!*' — 'and the damsel rose up.'

"The little girl sits up in the coffin and looks round, smiling with wide-open wondering eyes, holding a bunch of white roses they had put in her hand.

"There are cries, sobs, confusion among the people, and at that moment the monseigneur himself, the Grand Inquisitor, passes by the cathedral. He is an old man, almost ninety, tall and erect, with a withered face and sunken eyes, in which there is still a gleam of light. He is not dressed in the gorgeous pontifical robes, which he had flaunted before the people the previous day, when the enemies of the Roman Church were being burned — no, at this moment he is wearing his coarse, old, monk's cassock. At a distance behind him come his gloomy assistants and his slaves and the 'sacred guard.' He stops at the sight of the crowd and watches it from a distance. He had seen everything; he had seen them set the coffin down at His feet, seen the child rise up. His face darkens. He knits his thick grey brows and his eyes gleam with a sinister fire. He holds out his finger and bids the guards take Him. And such is his power, so completely are the people cowed into submission and trembling obedience to him, that the crowd immediately makes way for the guards, and in the midst of deathlike silence they lay hands on Him and lead Him away. The crowd instantly bows down to the earth, like one man, before the old Inquisitor. He blesses the people in silence and passes on. The guards lead their Prisoner to the close, gloomy, vaulted prison in the ancient palace of the Holy Inquisition and shut Him in it. The day passes and is followed by the black, hot, 'breathless' night of Seville. The air is 'fragrant with laurel and lemon.' In the pitch darkness the iron door of the prison is suddenly opened and the Grand Inquisitor himself comes in with a lantern in his hand. He is alone; the door is closed at once behind him. He stands in the doorway and for a minute or two gazes into His face. At last he goes up slowly, sets the lantern on the table and speaks.

" 'Is it Thou? Thou?' but receiving no answer, he adds at once. 'Don't answer, be silent. What canst Thou say, indeed? I know too well what Thou wouldst say. And Thou hast no right to add anything to what Thou didst say of old. Why, then, art Thou come to hinder us? For Thou hast come to hinder us, and Thou knowest that. But dost Thou know what will be to-morrow? I know not who Thou art and care not to know whether it is Thou or only a semblance of Thee, but to-morrow I shall condemn Thee and burn Thee at the stake as the worst of heretics. And the very people who have to-day kissed Thy feet, to-morrow at the faintest sign from me will rush to heap up the embers of Thy fire. Knowest

Thou that? Yes, maybe Thou knowest it,' he added with thoughtful penetration, never for a moment taking his eyes off the Prisoner."

"I don't quite understand, Ivan. What does it mean?" Alyosha, who had been listening in silence, said with a smile. "Is it simply a wild fantasy, or a mistake on the part of the old man — some impossible *qui pro quo?*"

"Take it as the last," said Ivan, laughing, "if you are so corrupted by modern realism and can't stand anything fantastic. If you like it to be a case of mistaken identity, let it be so. It is true," he went on, laughing, "the old man was ninety, and he may well have gone crazy over his set idea. He might have been struck by the appearance of the Prisoner. It might, in fact, be simply his ravings, the delusion of an old man of ninety, over-excited by the *auto-da-fé* of a hundred heretics the day before. But does it matter to us after all whether it was a mistake of identity or a wild fantasy? All that matters is that the old man should speak out, should speak openly of what he has thought in silence for ninety years."

"And the Prisoner, too, is silent? Does He look at him and not say a word?"

"That's inevitable in any case." Ivan laughed again. "The old man has told Him He hasn't the right to add anything to what He has said of old. One may say it is the most fundamental feature of Roman Catholicism, in my opinion at least. 'All has been transmitted by Thee to the Pope,' they say, 'and all, therefore, is now in the Pope's hands, and there is no need for Thee to come now at all. Thou must not meddle for the time, at least.' That's how they speak and write too — the Jesuits, at any rate. I have read it myself in the works of their theologians. 'Hast Thou the right to reveal to us one of the mysteries of that world from which Thou hast come?' my old man asks Him, and answers the question for Him. 'No, Thou hast not; that Thou mayest not add to what has been said of old, and mayest not take from men the freedom which Thou didst uphold when Thou wast on earth. Whatsoever Thou revealest anew will encroach on men's freedom of faith; for it will be manifest as a miracle, and the freedom of their faith was dearer to Thee than anything in those days fifteen hundred years ago. Didst Thou not often say then, "I would make you free"? But now Thou hast seen these "free" men,' the old man adds suddenly, with pensive irony. 'Yes, we've paid dearly for it,' he goes on, looking sternly at Him, 'but at last we have completed that work in Thy name. For fifteen centuries we have been wrestling with Thy freedom, but now it is ended and over for good. Dost Thou not believe that it's over for good? Thou lookest meekly at me and deignest not even to be wroth with me. But let me tell Thee that now, to-day, people are more convinced than ever that they have perfect freedom, yet they have brought their freedom to us and laid it humbly at our feet. But that has been our doing. Was this what Thou didst desire? Was this Thy freedom?' "

"I don't understand again," Alyosha broke in. "Is he ironical, is he jesting?"

"Not a bit of it! He claims it as a merit for himself and his Church that at last they have vanquished freedom and have done so to make men happy. 'For now' (he is speaking of the Inquisition, of course) 'for the first time it has become possible to think of the happiness of men. Man was created a rebel; and how can rebels be happy? Thou wast warned,' he says to Him. 'Thou hast had no lack of signs and warnings, but Thou didst not listen to those

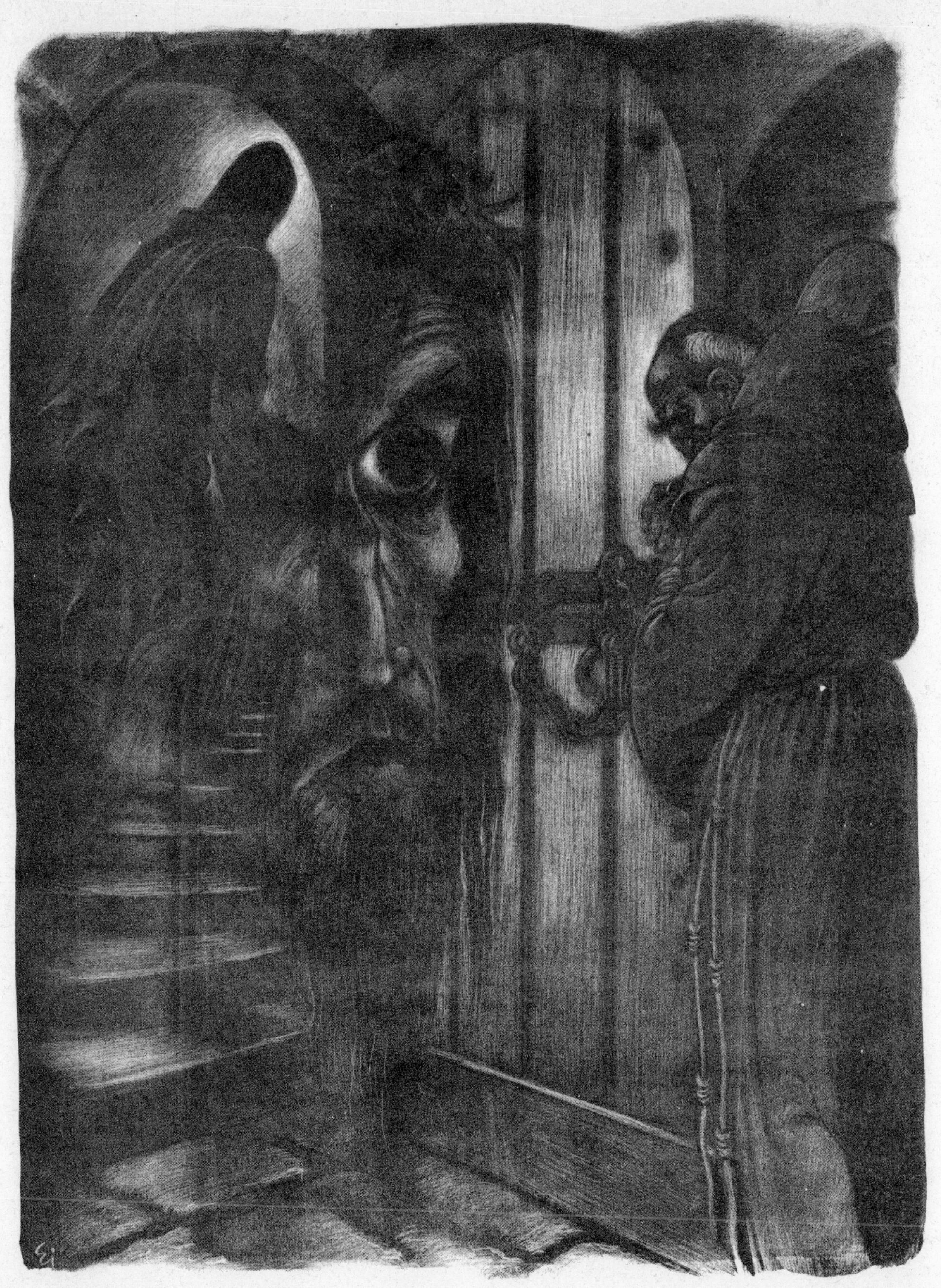

THE GRAND INQUISITOR

warnings; Thou didst reject the only way by which men might be made happy. But, fortunately, departing, Thou didst hand on the work to us. Thou hast promised, Thou hast established by Thy word, Thou hast given to us the right to bind and to unbind, and now, of course, Thou canst not think of taking it away. Why, then, hast Thou come to hinder us?' "

"And what's the meaning of 'no lack of signs and warnings'?" asked Alyosha.

"Why, that's the chief part of what the old man must say.

" 'The wise and dread spirit, the spirit of self-destruction and non-existence,' the old man goes on, 'the great spirit talked with Thee in the wilderness, and we are told in the books that he "tempted" Thee. Is that so? And could anything truer be said than what he revealed to Thee in three questions and what Thou didst reject, and what in the books is called "the temptation"? And yet if there has ever been on earth a real stupendous miracle, it took place on that day, on the day of the three temptations. The statement of those three questions was itself the miracle. If it were possible to imagine simply for the sake of argument that those three questions of the dread spirit had perished utterly from the books, and that we had to restore them and to invent them anew, in order to restore them to the books, and to do so had gathered together all the wise men of the earth — rulers, chief priests, learned men, philosophers, poets — and had set them the task of inventing three questions, such as would not only fit the occasion, but express in three words, three human phrases, the whole future history of the world and of humanity — dost Thou believe that all the combined wisdom of the earth could have invented anything in depth and force equal to the three questions which were actually put to Thee then by the wise and mighty spirit in the wilderness? From those questions alone, from the miracle of their statement, we can see that we have here to do not with the fleeting human intelligence, but with the absolute and eternal. For in those three questions the whole subsequent history of mankind is, as it were, brought together into one whole, and foretold, and in them are united all the unsolved historical contradictions of human nature. At the time it could not be so clear, since the future was unknown; but now that fifteen hundred years have passed, we see that everything in those three questions was so justly divined and foretold, and has been so truly fulfilled, that nothing can be added to them or taken from them.

" 'Judge Thyself who was right — Thou or he who questioned Thee then? Remember the first question; its meaning, though not its letter, was this: "Thou wouldst go into the world, and art going with empty hands, with some promise of freedom which men in their simplicity and their native unruliness cannot even understand, which they fear and dread — for nothing has ever been more insupportable for man and human society than freedom. But seest Thou these stones in this parched and barren wilderness? Turn them into bread, and mankind will run after Thee like a flock of sheep, grateful and obedient, though for ever trembling, lest Thou withdraw Thy hand and deny them Thy bread." But Thou didst not will to deprive man of freedom and didst reject the offer, thinking, what is that freedom worth, if obedience is bought with bread? Thou didst reply that man lives not by bread alone. But dost Thou know that for the sake of that earthly bread the spirit of the earth will rise up against Thee and will strive with Thee and overcome Thee and all will follow him, crying, "Who is like unto this beast? He has given us fire from heaven!" Dost Thou know that ages will pass, and humanity will proclaim by the lips of their sages and men of science that there is no crime, and therefore no sin; there is only hunger? "Feed men, and then ask of them virtue!" that's what they'll write on the banner, which they will raise against Thee, and with which Thy temple will be destroyed. Where Thy temple stood will rise a new building; the terrible tower of Babel will be built again, and though, like the one of old, it will not be finished, yet Thou mightest have prevented that new tower and have cut short the sufferings of men by a thousand years; for they will come back to us after a thousand years of agony with their tower. They will seek us again, hidden underground in the catacombs, for we shall be again persecuted and tortured. They will find us and cry to us, "Feed us, for those who have promised us fire from heaven haven't given it!" And then we shall finish building their tower, for he will finish the building who will feed them. And we alone shall feed them in Thy name, declaring falsely that it is in Thy name. Oh, never, never can they feed themselves without us! No science will give them bread so long as they remain free. In the end they will lay their freedom at our feet, and say to us, "Make us your slaves, but feed us." They will understand themselves, at last, that freedom and bread enough for all are inconceivable together, for never, never will they be able to share between them! They will be convinced, too, that they can never be free, for they are weak, vicious, worthless, and rebellious. Thou didst promise them the bread of Heaven, but, I repeat again, can it compare with earthly bread in the eyes of the weak, ever sinful and ignoble race of man? And if for the sake of the bread of Heaven thousands and tens of thousands shall follow Thee, what is to become of the millions and tens of thousands of millions of creatures who will not have the strength to forego the earthly bread for the sake of the heavenly? Or dost Thou care only for the tens of thousands of the great and strong, while the millions, numerous as the sands of the sea, who are weak but love Thee, must exist only to serve as raw material for the great and strong? No, we cherish the weak, too. They are sinful and rebellious, but in the end they, too, will become obedient. They will marvel at us and look on us as gods, because we are ready to endure the freedom which they have found so dreadful and to rule over them — so awful will they find it in the end to be free. But we shall tell them that we obey Thee and rule in Thy name. We shall deceive them again, for we will not let Thee come to us again. That deception will be our suffering, for we shall be forced to lie.

" 'This is the meaning of the first question in the wilderness, and this is what Thou hast rejected in the name of that freedom which Thou hast exalted above everything. Yet in this question lay hid the great mystery of this world. Choosing "bread," Thou wouldst have satisfied the universal and everlasting craving of each man and of humanity as a whole — to find some one to bow down to. Having remained free, man strives for nothing so incessantly and so painfully as to find some one to bow down to. But man seeks to bow down to what is established beyond dispute, so that all men would agree at once to bow down to it. For these pitiful creatures are concerned not only to find what one or the other can bow down to, but to find something that all would believe in and bow down to; and it is essential that they all do it *together*. This craving for *community* of worship is the chief torment of every man individually and of all humanity from the beginning of time. For the sake of common worship they've slain each other with the sword. They have set up gods and challenged one another, "Put away your gods and come and worship ours, or we will kill you and your gods!" And so it will be to the end of the world, even when gods disappear from the earth; they will fall down before idols just the same. Thou didst know, Thou couldst not but have known, this fundamental secret of human nature, but Thou didst reject the one infallible banner which was offered Thee to make all men bow down to Thee alone — the banner of earthly bread; and Thou hast rejected it for the sake of freedom and the bread of Heaven. Behold what Thou didst further. And all again in the name of freedom! I tell Thee that man is tormented by no greater anxiety than to find some one quickly to whom he can hand over that gift of freedom with which the ill-fated creature is born. But only he will take possession of their freedom who can appease their conscience. In bread there was offered Thee an infallible token; give bread, and man will worship thee, for nothing is more certain than bread. But if some one else, apart from Thee, will gain possession of his conscience — oh! then he will cast away Thy bread and follow after him who has ensnared his conscience. In that Thou wast right. For the secret of man's being is not only to live but to have something to live for. Without a stable conception of the object of life, man would not consent to go on living, and would rather destroy himself than remain on earth, though he had bread in abundance. That is true. But what happened? Instead of taking men's freedom from them, Thou didst make it greater than ever! Didst Thou forget that man prefers peace, and even death, to freedom of choice in the knowledge of good and evil? Nothing is more seductive for man than his freedom of conscience, but nothing is more painful. And behold, instead of furnishing a firm foundation for setting the conscience of man at rest for ever, Thou didst choose all that is extraordinary, vague, and conjectural; Thou didst choose what was utterly beyond the strength of men, acting as though Thou didst not love them at all — Thou who didst come to give Thy life for them! Instead of taking possession of men's freedom, Thou didst increase it, and burdened the spiritual kingdom of mankind with its sufferings for ever. Thou didst desire man's free love, that he should follow Thee freely, enticed and captivated by Thee. In place of the firm ancient law, man must hereafter with free heart decide for himself what is good and what is evil, having only Thy image before him as his guide. But did it not occur to Thee that he would at last question and indeed reject even Thy image and Thy truth, if he were weighed down with such a fearful burden as freedom of choice? They will cry aloud at last that the truth is not in Thee, for they could not have been left in greater confusion and suffering than Thou hast caused, laying upon them so many cares and insoluble problems.

" 'So that, in truth, Thou didst Thyself lay the foundation for the destruction of Thy kingdom, and no one is more to blame for it.

And yet was that what was offered Thee? There are three powers on earth, three powers alone, able to conquer and to hold captive for ever the conscience of these impotent rebels for their happiness — those powers are miracle, mystery, and authority. Thou hast rejected all three and hast set the example for doing so. When the wise and dread spirit set Thee on the pinnacle of the temple and said to Thee, "If Thou wouldst know whether Thou art the Son of God, cast Thyself down from hence, for it is written: the angels shall bear him up lest haply he dash his foot against a stone, and Thou shalt know then whether Thou art the Son of God and shalt prove then how great is Thy faith in Thy Father." But Thou didst refuse and wouldst not cast Thyself down. Oh! of course, Thou didst proudly and splendidly, like God; but the weak, unruly race of men, are they gods? Oh, Thou didst know then that in taking one step, in making one movement to cast Thyself down, Thou wouldst be tempting God and wouldst have lost all Thy faith in Him, and wouldst have been dashed to pieces against that earth which Thou didst come to save. And the wise spirit that tempted Thee would have rejoiced. But I ask again, are there many like Thee? And couldst Thou believe for one moment that men, too, could face such a temptation? Is the nature of men such, that they can reject miracle, and at the great moments of life, the moments of their deepest, most agonising spiritual difficulties, cling only to the free verdict of the heart? Oh, Thou didst know that Thy deed would be recorded in the books, would be handed down to remote times and reach the utmost ends of the earth, and Thou didst hope that man, following Thee, would cling to God without needing a miracle. But Thou didst not know that when man rejects miracle he rejects God, too; for man seeks not so much God as miracles. And as man cannot bear to be without the miracle, he will create new miracles of his own for himself, and will worship deeds of sorcery and witchcraft, though he might be a hundred times over a rebel, a heretic, and an atheist. Thou didst not come down from the Cross when they shouted to Thee, mocking and reviling Thee, "Come down from the cross and we will believe that Thou art He." Thou didst not come down, for again Thou wouldst not enslave man by a miracle, and didst crave faith given freely, not based on miracle. Thou didst crave free love and not the base raptures of the slave before the might that has overawed him for ever. But Thou didst think too highly of men therein, for they are slaves, of course, though rebellious by nature. Look round and judge; fifteen centuries have passed, look upon them. Whom hast Thou raised up to Thyself? I swear, man is weaker and baser by nature than Thou hast believed him! Can he, can he do what Thou didst? By showing him so much respect, Thou didst, as it were, cease to compassionate him, for Thou didst ask far too much from him — Thou who hast loved him more than Thyself! Respecting him less, Thou wouldst have asked less of him. That would have been more like love, for his burden would have been lighter. He is weak and vile. What though he is everywhere now rebelling against our power, and proud of his rebellion? It is the pride of a child and a school-boy. They are little children rioting and barring out the teacher at school. But their childish delight will end; it will cost them dear. They will cast down temples and drench the earth with blood. But they will see at last, the foolish children, that, though they are rebels, they are impotent rebels, unable to keep up their own rebellion. Bathed in their foolish tears, they will recognise at last that He who created them rebels must have meant to mock at them. They will say this in despair, and their utterance will be a blasphemy which will make them more unhappy still, for man's nature cannot bear blasphemy, and in the end always avenges it on itself. And so unrest, confusion, and unhappiness — that is the present lot of men after Thou didst suffer so much for their freedom! Thy great prophet tells in vision and in allegory, that he saw all those who took part in the first resurrection and that there were of each tribe twelve thousand. But if there were so many of them, they must have been not men but gods. They had borne Thy cross, they had endured scores of years in the barren, hungry wilderness, living upon locusts and roots — and Thou mayest indeed point with pride at those children of freedom, of free love, of free and splendid sacrifice in Thy name. But remember that they were only some thousands; and what of the rest? And how are the other weak ones to blame, because they could not endure what the strong have endured? How is the weak soul to blame that it is unable to receive such terrible gifts? Canst Thou have simply come to the elect and for the elect? But if so, it is a mystery and we cannot understand it. And if it is a mystery, we, too, have a right to preach a mystery, and to teach them that it's not the free judgment of their hearts, not love that matters, but a mystery which they must follow blindly, even against their conscience. So we have done. We have corrected Thy work and have founded it upon *miracle*, *mystery*, and *authority*. And men rejoiced that they were again led like sheep, and that the terrible gift that had brought them such suffering was, at last, lifted from their hearts. Were we right teaching them this? Speak! Did we not love mankind, so meekly acknowledging their feebleness, lovingly lightening their burden, and permitting their weak nature even sin with our sanction? Why hast Thou come now to hinder us? And why dost Thou look silently and searchingly at me with Thy meek eyes? Show anger. I don't want Thy love, for I love Thee not. And what use is it for me to hide anything from Thee? Don't I know to Whom I am speaking? All that I can say is known to Thee already, I read it in Thy eyes. And is it for me to conceal from Thee our secret? Perhaps it is Thy will to hear it from my lips. Listen, then. We are not with Thee, but with *him* — that is our secret. It's a long time — eight centuries — since we have been not with Thee but with *him*. Just eight centuries ago, we took from him what Thou didst reject with scorn, that last gift he offered Thee, showing Thee all the kingdoms of the earth. We took from him Rome and the sword of Cæsar, and proclaimed ourselves sole rulers of the earth, though hitherto we have not been able to bring our work to full completion. But whose fault is that? Oh, the work is only beginning, but it has begun. We have long to wait for completion and the earth has yet much to suffer, but we shall triumph and shall be Cæsars, and then we shall plan the universal happiness of man. But Thou mightest have taken even then the sword of Cæsar. Why didst Thou reject that last gift? Hadst Thou accepted that last counsel of the mighty spirit, Thou wouldst have accomplished all that man seeks on earth — that is, some one to bow down to, some one to hand his conscience to, and some means of uniting all in one unanimous and harmonious ant-heap, for the craving for universal unity is the third and last anguish of men. Mankind as a whole has always striven to organise a universal state. There have been many great nations with great histories, but the more highly they were developed the more unhappy they were, for they felt more acutely than other people the craving for world-wide union. The great conquerors, Timours and Genghis-Khans, whirled like hurricanes over the face of the earth striving to conquer the universe, but even they, though unconsciously, expressed the same great craving of mankind for universal unity. Hadst Thou taken the world and Cæsar's purple, Thou wouldst have founded the universal state and have given universal peace. For who can rule men if not he who holds their conscience and their bread in his hands. We have taken the sword of Cæsar, and in taking it, of course, have rejected Thee and followed *him*. Oh, there will yet be ages of the confusion of free thought, ages of their science and cannibalism. For having begun to build their tower of Babel without us, they will end, of course, with cannibalism. But then the beast will crawl to us and lick our feet and spatter them with tears of blood. And we shall sit upon the beast and raise the cup, and on it will be written, "Mystery." But then, and only then, the reign of peace and happiness will come for men. Thou art proud of Thine elect, but Thou hast only the elect, while we shall give rest to all. And besides, how many of those elect, those mighty ones who could become elect, have grown weary waiting for Thee, and have carried and will carry the powers of their spirit and the ardour of their heart to the other camp, and will end by raising their *free* banner against Thee. Thou didst Thyself lift up that banner. But with us all will be happy and will neither rebel nor destroy one another any more as under Thy freedom. Oh, we shall persuade them that they will become free only when they renounce their freedom in our favour and submit to us. And shall we be right or shall we be lying? They will be convinced that we are right, for they will remember the horrors of slavery and confusion to which Thy freedom brought them. Freedom, free thought and science, will lead them into such straits and will bring them face to face with such marvels and insoluble mysteries, that some of them, the fierce and rebellious, will destroy themselves, others, rebellious but weak, will destroy one another, while the rest, weak and unhappy, will crawl fawning to our feet and cry to us: "Yes, you were right, you alone possess His mystery, and we come back to you: save us from ourselves!"

" 'Receiving bread from us, they will see clearly that we take the bread made by their hands from them, to give it to them, without any miracle. They will see that we do not change the stones to bread, but in truth they will be more thankful for taking it from our hands than for the bread itself! For they will remember only too well that in old days, without our help, even the bread they made turned to stones in their hands, while since they have come back to us, the very stones have turned to bread in their hands. Too, too well will they know the value of complete submission! And until men know that, they will be unhappy. Who is most to blame for their not knowing it? Speak! Who scattered the flock and sent it astray on unknown paths? But the flock will come together again and will submit once more, and then it will be for all time.

Then we shall give them the quiet humble happiness of weak creatures such as they are by nature. Oh, we shall persuade them at last not to be proud, for Thou didst lift them up and thereby taught them pride. We shall show them that they are weak, that they are only pitiful children, but that childlike happiness is the sweetest of all. They will become timid and will look to us and huddle close to us in fear, as chicks to the hen. They will marvel at us and will be awe-stricken before us, and will be proud of our being so powerful and clever that we have been able to subdue such a turbulent flock of thousands of millions. They will tremble impotently before our wrath, their minds will grow timid, they will become as tearful as women and children, but they will be just as ready at a sign from us to pass to laughter and rejoicing, to happy mirth and childish song. Yes, we shall set them to work, but in their leisure hours we shall make their life like a child's game, with children's songs and innocent dances. Oh, we shall allow them even sin, they are weak and helpless, and they will love us like children because we allow them to sin. We shall tell them that every sin will be expiated, if it is committed with our permission, that we allow them to sin because we love them, and the punishment for these sins we take upon ourselves. And we shall take it upon ourselves, and they will adore us as their saviours who have taken on themselves their sins before God. And they will have no secrets from us. We shall allow or forbid them to live with their wives and mistresses, to have or not to have children — according to whether they have been obedient or disobedient — and they will submit to us gladly and cheerfully. The most painful secrets of their conscience, all, all they will bring to us, and we shall absolve all. And they will be glad to accept our absolution, for it will save them from the great anxiety and terrible agony they endure at present in making a free decision for themselves. And all will be happy, all the millions of creatures except the hundred thousand who rule over them. For only we, we who guard the mystery, shall be unhappy. There will be thousands of millions of happy babes, and a hundred thousand sufferers who have taken upon themselves the curse of the knowledge of good and evil. Peacefully they will die, peacefully they will expire in Thy name, and beyond the grave they will find nothing but death. But we shall keep the secret, and for their happiness we shall allure them with the reward of heaven and eternity. For if there were anything in the other world, it certainly would not be for such as they. It is prophesied that Thou wilt come again victorious, Thou wilt come with Thy chosen, the proud and strong, but we will say that they have only saved themselves, but we have saved all. We are told that the harlot who sits upon the beast, and holds in her hands *mystery*, shall be put to shame, that the weak will rise up again, and will rend her royal purple and will strip naked her loathsome body. But I will then stand up and point out to Thee the thousand millions of happy babes who knew no sin. And we who have taken their sins upon us for the sake of their happiness will stand up before Thee and say: "Judge us if Thou canst and darest." Know that I fear Thee not. Know that I, too, have been in the wilderness, I, too, have lived on roots and locusts, I, too, prized the freedom with which Thou hast blessed men, and I, too, was striving to stand among Thy elect, among the strong and powerful, thirsting "to complete the number." But I awakened and would not serve madness. I turned back and joined the ranks of those *who have corrected Thy work.* I left the proud and went back to the humble, for the happiness of the humble. What I say to Thee will come to pass, and our Kingdom will be built. I repeat, to-morrow Thou shalt see that obedient flock who at a sign from me will hasten to heap up the hot embers about the pile on which I shall burn Thee for coming to hinder us. For if there ever was one who more than all others deserved our fires, it is Thou. To-morrow I shall burn Thee. *Dixi.*' "

Ivan stopped. He was carried away as he talked and spoke with excitement; when he had finished, he suddenly smiled.

Alyosha, who had listened in silence, towards the end was greatly moved and seemed several times on the point of interrupting, but restrained himself. Now his words came with a rush.

"But . . . that's absurd!" he cried, flushing. "Your poem is in praise of Jesus, it does not blame Him — as you meant it to do. And who will believe you about freedom? Is that the way to understand it? That's not the idea of it in the Orthodox Church. . . . That's Rome, and not even the whole of Rome, it's false — those are the worst of the Catholics, the Inquisitors, the Jesuits! . . . And there could not be such a fantastic creature as your Inquisitor. What are these sins of mankind they take on themselves? Who are these keepers of the mystery who have taken some curse upon themselves for the happiness of mankind? When have they ever been seen? We know the Jesuits, they are spoken ill of, but are they really what you describe? They are not that at all, not at all. . . . They are simply the Romish army of the future universal earthly kingdom, with the Pontiff of Rome for Emperor . . . that's their ideal, but there's no sort of mystery or lofty melancholy about it. . . . It's simple lust for power, for filthy earthly goods, for domination — something like a universal serfdom with them as masters — that's all they stand for. They don't even believe in God perhaps. Your suffering Inquisitor is a mere fantasy."

"Stop, stop," laughed Ivan, "how hot you are! A fantasy you say, let it be so! Of course it's a fantasy. But allow me to say: do you really think that the Roman Catholic movement of the last centuries is actually nothing but the lust for power, for filthy goods? Is that what Father Païssy teaches you?"

"No, no, on the contrary, Father Païssy did once say something rather like what you said . . . but of course it's not that, not that at all," Alyosha hastily corrected himself.

"A precious admission, in spite of your 'not that at all.' I ask you why your Jesuits and Inquisitors have united simply for vile material gain? Why can there not be among them one martyr oppressed by great sorrow and loving humanity? You see, only suppose that there was one such man among all those who desire nothing but filthy material goods — if there's only one like my old Inquisitor, who had himself eaten roots in the desert and made frenzied efforts to subdue his flesh to make himself free and perfect. But yet all his life he loved humanity, and suddenly his eyes were opened, and he saw that it is no great moral blessedness to attain perfection and freedom, if at the same time one gains the conviction that millions of God's creatures have remained a mockery, that they will never be capable of using their freedom, that these poor rebels can never turn into giants to complete the tower, that it was not for such geese that the great idealist dreamt his dream of harmony. Seeing all that he turned back and joined — the clever people. Surely that could have happened?"

"Joined whom, what clever people?" cried Alyosha, almost in a frenzy. "They have no such great cleverness and no mysteries and secrets. . . . Perhaps nothing but atheism, that's all their secret. Your Inquisitor does not believe in God, that's his whole secret!"

"What if it is so! At last you have guessed it. It's perfectly true, it's true that that's the whole secret, but isn't that suffering, at least for a man like that, who has wasted his whole life in the desert and yet could not shake off his incurable love of humanity? In his declining days he reaches the clear conviction that nothing but what the great dread spirit advised could make any tolerable sort of life for the feeble, unruly, 'incomplete, experimental creatures fashioned in jest.' And so, convinced of this, he sees that he must follow the counsel of the wise spirit, the dread spirit of death and destruction, and therefore accept falsehood and deception, and lead men consciously to death and destruction, and yet deceive them all the way so that they may not notice where they are being led, that the poor blind creatures may at least on the way think themselves happy. And note, the deception is in the name of Him in Whose ideal the old man had so fervently believed all his life long. Isn't that a misfortune? And if only one such found himself at the head of the whole army 'filled with the lust for power only for the sake of filthy goods' — would not one such be enough to make a tragedy? More than that, one such standing at the head is enough to create the actual leading idea of the Roman Church with all its armies and Jesuits, its highest idea. I tell you frankly that I firmly believe that there has always been such a man among those who stood at the head of the movement. Who knows, there may have been some such even among the Roman Popes. Who knows, perhaps the spirit of that accursed old man who loves mankind so obstinately in his own way is to be found even now in a whole multitude of such old men, existing not by chance but by agreement, as a secret league formed long ago for the guarding of the mystery, to keep it from the weak and the unhappy, so as to make them happy. No doubt it is so, and so it must be indeed. I fancy that even among the Masons there's something of the same mystery at the bottom, and that that's why the Catholics so detest the Masons as their rivals breaking up the unity of the idea, while it is so essential that there should be one flock and one shepherd. . . . But from the way I defend my idea I might be an author impatient of your criticism. Enough of it."

"You are perhaps a Mason yourself!" broke suddenly from Alyosha. "You don't believe in God," he added, speaking this time very sorrowfully. He fancied besides that his brother was looking at him ironically. "How does your poem end?" he asked, suddenly looking down. "Or was it the end?"

"I meant to end it like this. When the Inquisitor ceased speaking he waited some time for his Prisoner to answer him. The Prisoner's silence weighs down upon him. He saw that the Prisoner had listened intently all the time, looking gently in his eyes and evidently not wishing to reply. The old man longs for Him to say something, however bitter and terrible. But He suddenly approaches the old man in silence and gently kisses him on his bloodless aged lips. That is his whole answer. The old man shudders. The corners of his lips tremble. He goes to the door, opens it, and says to Him: 'Go, and come no more . . . come not at all, never, never!' And he lets Him out into the dark streets of the town. The Prisoner goes away."

"And the old man?"

"The kiss burns in his heart, but the old man adheres to his idea."

"And you with him, you too?" cried Alyosha mournfully.

Ivan laughed.

"Why, it's all nonsense, Alyosha. It's only a silly poem by a silly student, who could never write two lines of verse. Why do you take it so seriously? Surely you don't suppose I am going straight off to the Jesuits, to join the men who are correcting His work? Good Lord, it's no business of mine. I told you, all I want is to live on till I'm thirty, and then . . . dash the cup to the ground!"

"But the little sticky leaves, and the precious graves, and the blue sky, and the woman you love! How will you live, how will you love them?" Alyosha cried sorrowfully. "With such a hell in your heart and your head, how can you? No, that's just what you are going away for, to join them . . . if not, you will kill yourself, you can't endure it!"

"There is a strength to endure everything," Ivan said with a cold smile.

"What strength?"

"The strength of the Karamazovs — the strength of the Karamazov baseness."

"To sink into debauchery, to stifle your soul with corruption, yes?"

"Possibly even that . . . only perhaps till I am thirty I shall escape it, and then . . ."

"How will you escape it? By what means will you escape it? That's impossible with your ideas."

"In the Karamazov way, again."

"'Everything is permitted,' you mean? Everything is permitted, is that it?"

Ivan scowled, and all at once turned strangely pale.

"Ah, you've caught up yesterday's phrase, which so offended Miüsov — and which Dmitri pounced upon so naïvely and paraphrased!" he smiled queerly. "Yes, if you like, 'everything is lawful' since the word has been said. I won't deny it. And Mitya's version isn't bad."

Alyosha looked at him in silence.

"I thought that going away from here I have you at least," Ivan said suddenly, with unexpected feeling; "but now I see that there is no place for me even in your heart, my dear hermit. The formula, 'everything is permitted,' I won't renounce — will you renounce me for that, yes?"

Alyosha got up, went to him and gently kissed him on the lips.

"That's plagiarism," cried Ivan, highly delighted. "You stole that from my poem. Thank you though. Get up, Alyosha, it's time we were going, both of us."

They went out, but stopped when they reached the entrance of the restaurant.

"Listen, Alyosha," Ivan began in a resolute voice, "if I am really able to care for the sticky little leaves I shall only love them, remembering you. It's enough for me that you are somewhere here, and I shan't lose my desire for life yet. Is that enough for you? Take it as a declaration of love if you like. And now you go to the right and I to the left. And it's enough, do you hear, enough. I mean even if I don't go away to-morrow (I think I certainly shall go) and we meet again, don't say a word more on these subjects. I beg that particularly. And about Dmitri, too, I ask you specially never speak to me again," he added, with sudden irritation; "it's all done with, it has all been said over and over again, hasn't it? And I'll make you one promise in return for it. When, at thirty, I am ready to 'dash the cup to the ground,' wherever I may be I'll come to have one more talk with you, even though it were from America, you may be sure of that. I'll come on purpose. It will be very interesting to have a look at you, to see what you'll be by that time. It's rather a solemn promise, you see. And we really may be parting for seven years or ten. Come, go now to your Pater Seraphicus, he is dying. If he dies without you, you will be angry with me for having kept you. Good-bye, kiss me once more; that's right, now go."

Ivan turned suddenly and went his way without looking back. It was just as Dmitri had left Alyosha the day before, though the parting had been very different. The strange thought flashed like an arrow through Alyosha's mind in the distress and dejection of that moment. He waited a little, looking after his brother. He suddenly noticed that Ivan swayed as he walked and that his right shoulder looked lower than his left. He had never noticed it before. But all at once he turned, too, and almost ran to the monastery. It was nearly dark, and he felt almost frightened; something new was growing up in him for which he could not account. The wind had risen again as on the previous evening, and the ancient pines murmured gloomily about him when he entered the hermitage copse. He almost ran. "Pater Seraphicus — he got that name from somewhere — where from?" Alyosha wondered. "Ivan, poor Ivan, and when shall I see you again? . . . Here is the hermitage. Yes, yes, that he is, Pater Seraphicus, he will save me — from him and for ever!"

Several times afterwards he wondered how on leaving Ivan he could so completely forget his brother Dmitri, though he had that morning, only a few hours before, so firmly resolved to find him and not to give up the hunt for him, even should he be unable to return to the monastery that night.

CHAPTER VI

FOR AWHILE A FAR FROM CLEAR ONE

Ivan, on parting from Alyosha, went home to Fyodor Pavlovich's house. But, strange to say, he was overcome by insufferable depression, which grew greater at every step he took towards the house. There was nothing strange in his being depressed; what was strange was that Ivan could not have said what the cause of it was. He had often been depressed before, and there was nothing surprising in his feeling so at such a moment, when he had broken off with everything that had brought him here, and was preparing that day to make a new start and enter upon a new, unknown path. He would again be as solitary as ever, and though he had great hopes, and great — too great — expectations from life, he could not have given any definite account of his hopes, his expectations, or even his desires.

Yet at that moment, though the apprehension of the new and unknown was certainly in his heart, what worried him was something quite different. "Is it loathing for my father's house?" he wondered. "Quite likely; I am so sick of it; and though it's the last time I shall cross its hateful threshold, still I loathe it. . . . No, it's not that either. Is it the parting with Alyosha and the conversation I had with him? For so many years I've been silent with the whole world and not deigned to speak, and all of a sudden I reel off a rigmarole like that." It certainly might have been the youthful vexation of youthful inexperience and vanity — vexation at having failed to express himself, especially before such a being as Alyosha, upon whom he had certainly been reckoning in his heart. No doubt that came in, that vexation, it must have indeed; but yet that was not it, that was not it either. "I feel sick with depression and yet I can't tell what I want. Better not think, perhaps."

Ivan tried "not to think," but that, too, was no use. What made his depression so vexatious and irritating was that it had a kind of casual, external character — he felt that. Some person or thing seemed to be standing out somewhere, just as something will sometimes obtrude itself upon the eye, and though one may be so busy with work or conversation that for a long time one does not notice it, yet it irritates and almost torments one till at last one realises, and removes the offending object, often quite a trifling and ridiculous one — some article left about in the wrong place, a handkerchief on the floor, a book not replaced on the shelf, and so on.

At last, feeling very cross and ill-humoured, Ivan arrived home, and suddenly, about fifteen paces from the garden gate, he guessed what was fretting and worrying him.

On a bench in the gateway the valet Smerdyakov was sitting, enjoying the coolness of the evening, and at the first glance at him Ivan knew that the valet Smerdyakov was on his mind, and that it was this man that his soul loathed. It all dawned upon him suddenly and became clear. A while ago, when Alyosha had been telling him of his meeting with Smerdyakov, he had felt a sudden twinge of gloom and loathing, which had immediately stirred responsive anger in his heart. Afterwards, as he talked, Smerdyakov had been forgotten for the time being; but still he had remained in his mind, and as soon as Ivan parted from Alyosha and was walking home alone, the forgotten sensation began to obtrude itself again. "Is it possible that this contemptible wretch can worry me so much?" he wondered, with insufferable irritation.

Indeed, Ivan had come of late to feel an intense dislike for the man, especially during the last few days. He had even begun to notice in himself a growing feeling that was almost one of hatred for the creature. Perhaps this hatred was accentuated by the fact that when Ivan first came to the neighbourhood he had felt quite differently. Then he had taken a marked interest in Smerdyakov, and had even thought him very original. He had encouraged him to talk, although he had always wondered at a certain incoherence in the man, or rather intellectual restlessness in him, and could not understand what it was that so continually and insistently worked upon the brain of "the contemplative." They discussed philosophical questions and even how there could have been light on the first day when the sun, moon, and stars were created only on the fourth day, and how that should be interpreted. But Ivan soon saw that, though the sun, moon, and stars might be an interesting subject, yet that it was quite secondary to Smerdyakov, and that he was looking for something altogether different. In one way and another, he began to betray a boundless vanity, and a wounded vanity, at that. Ivan disliked this very much. That was how his aversion arose. Later on, there had been trouble in the house. Grushenka had come on the scene, and there had been the scandals with his brother Dmitri — they discussed that, too. But though Smerdyakov always talked of that with great excitement, it was impossible to discover what his own desire in the matter was. There was, in fact, something surprising in the illogical and incoherent character of some of his desires, which came out involuntarily, yet always remained vague. Smerdyakov was always inquisitive, asking certain indirect but obviously premeditated questions, but what his object was he did not explain, and usually at the most important moment he would break off and relapse into silence or change the subject. But what finally irritated Ivan most and roused his disgust was the peculiar, revolting familiarity which Smerdyakov began to show more and more markedly. Not that he forgot himself and was rude; on the contrary, he always spoke very respectfully, yet he had obviously begun to consider — goodness knows why! — that there was some sort of understanding between him and Ivan Fyodorovich. He always spoke in a tone that suggested that those two had some kind of compact, some secret between them, that had at some time been expressed on both sides, known only to them and beyond the comprehension of those around them. But for a long while Ivan did not recognise the real cause of his growing disgust and he had only lately realised what was at the root of it.

With a feeling of disgust and irritation he tried to pass in at the gate without speaking to or looking at Smerdyakov. But Smerdyakov rose from the bench, and from that action alone Ivan knew instantly that he wanted to talk to him on a particular subject. Ivan looked at him and stopped, and the fact that he did stop, instead of passing by, as he had meant to the minute before, drove him to fury. With anger and repulsion he looked at Smerdyakov's sickly eunuch's face, with the little curls combed over the temples and a tuft of hair above the brow. His left eye, slightly screwed up, winked as though to say, "Where are you going? You won't pass by; you see that we two clever people have something to say to each other."

Ivan shook. "Get away, you blackguard; what kind of companion am I for you, you fool!" was on the tip of his tongue, but to his profound astonishment he heard himself say something entirely different: "Is my father still asleep, or has he waked?"

He asked the question softly and meekly, to his own surprise, and at once, again to his own surprise, sat down on the bench. For an instant he felt almost frightened; he remembered it afterwards. Smerdyakov stood facing him, his hands behind his back, looking at him with assurance and almost with severity.

"Still asleep, sir," he articulated deliberately. ("You were the first to speak, not I," he seemed to say.) "I am surprised at you, sir," he added, after a pause, dropping his eyes affectedly, setting his right foot forward, and playing with the tip of his polished boot.

"Why are you surprised at me?" Ivan asked abruptly and sternly, doing his utmost to restrain himself, and suddenly realising, with disgust, that he was feeling intense curiosity and would not, on any account, go away without satisfying it.

"Why don't you go to Chermashnya, sir?" Smerdyakov suddenly raised his eyes and smiled familiarly. "Why I smile you must understand of yourself, if you are a clever man," his screwed-up left eye seemed to say.

"Why should I go to Chermashnya?" Ivan Fyodorovich asked in surprise.

Smerdyakov was silent again.

"Fyodor Pavlovich himself has so earnestly begged you to, sir," he said at last, slowly and apparently attaching no significance to his answer. "I put you off with a minor reason," he seemed to suggest, "simply to say something."

"Damn you! Say outright what you want!" Ivan cried angrily at last, passing from meekness to violence.

Smerdyakov drew his right foot up to his left, pulled himself up, but went on looking at him with the same serenity and the same little smile.

"Substantially nothing — but just by way of conversation."

Another silence followed. They did not speak for nearly a minute. Ivan knew that he ought to get up and show anger, and Smerdyakov stood before him and seemed to be waiting as though to see whether he would be angry or not. So at least it seemed to Ivan. At last he moved to get up. Smerdyakov seemed to seize the moment.

"I'm in an awful position, Ivan Fyodorovich. I don't know how to help myself," he said all at once resolutely and distinctly, and at his last word he sighed. Ivan Fyodorovich sat down again.

"They are both utterly unhinged, they are no better than little children, sir," Smerdyakov went on. "I am speaking of your parent and your brother Dmitri Fyodorovich, sir. Here Fyodor Pavlovich will get up directly and begin worrying me every minute, 'Has she come? Why hasn't she come?' and so on up till midnight and even after midnight. And if Agrafena Alexandrovna doesn't come (for very likely she does not mean to come at all), then he will be at me again to-morrow morning, 'Why hasn't she come? When will she come?' — as though I were to blame for it. On the other side it's no better, sir. As soon as it gets dark, or even before, your brother will appear hereabouts with a gun in his hands: 'Look out, you rogue, you bouillon-maker. If you miss her and don't let me know she's come — I'll kill you before any one.' When the night's over, in the morning, he, too, like Fyodor Pavlovich, begins worrying me to death. 'Why hasn't she come? Will she come soon?' And he, too, thinks I am to blame because his lady hasn't come. And every day and every hour they get angrier and angrier, so that I sometimes think, sir, I shall take my own life in fright. I can't depend upon them, sir."

"And why did you stick your nose in? Why did you begin to spy for Dmitri Fyodorovich?" said Ivan irritably.

"How could I help it? Though, indeed, I haven't meddled at all, if you want to know the truth of the matter. I kept quiet from the very beginning, not daring to argue; but he appointed me to be his personal servant. He has had only one thing to say since: 'I'll kill you, you scoundrel, if you miss her.' I feel certain, sir, that I shall have a long fit to-morrow."

"What do you mean by 'a long fit'?"

"A long fit, lasting a long time — several hours, or perhaps a day or two. Once it went on for three days. I fell from the garret that time. The convulsions ceased and then began again, and for three days I couldn't come back to my senses. Fyodor Pavlovich sent for Her-

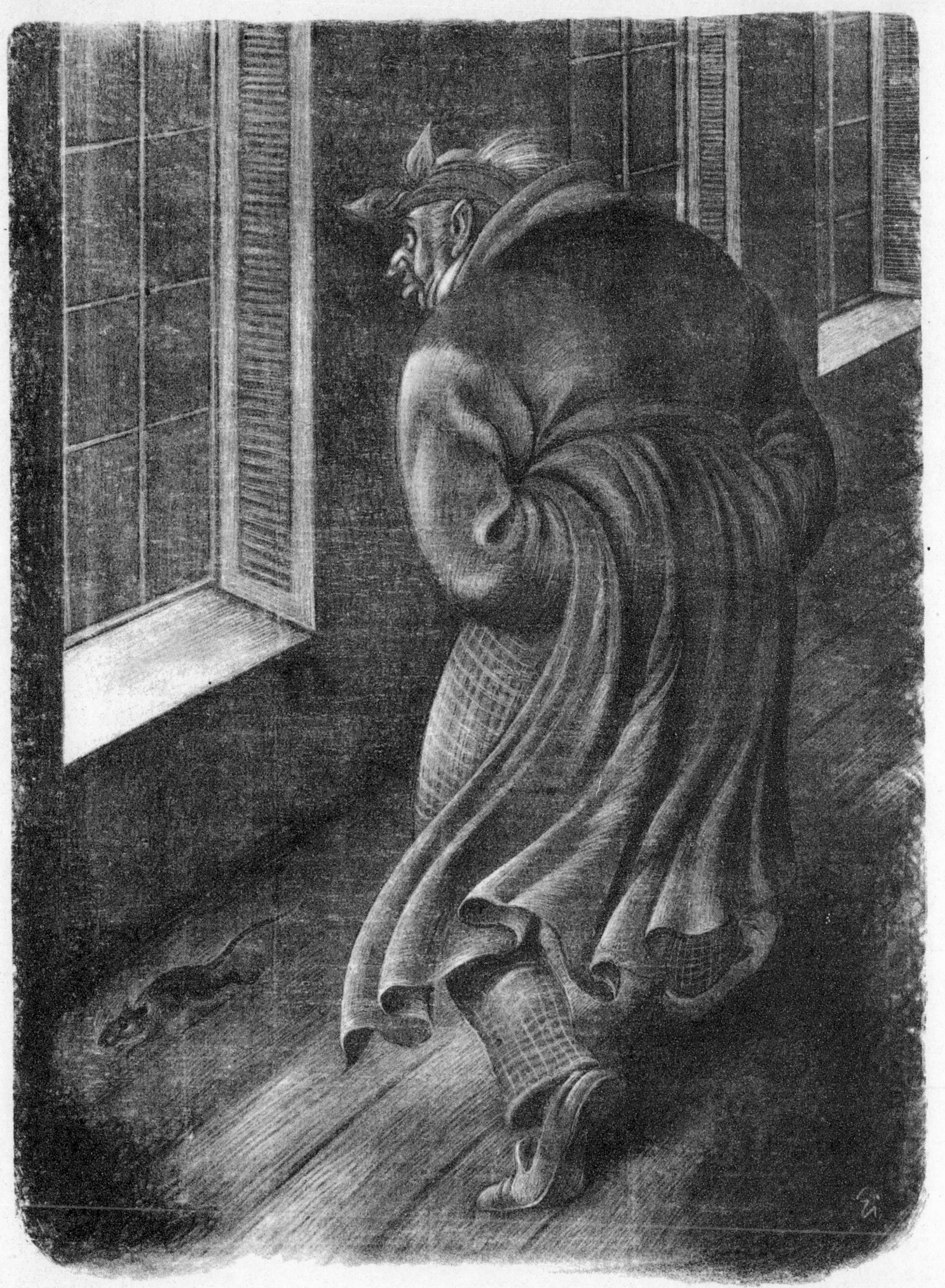

THE CRAZY OLD MAN

zenstube, the doctor here, and he put ice on my head and tried another remedy, too. . . . I might have died, sir."

"But they say one can't tell with epilepsy when a fit is coming. What makes you say you will have one to-morrow?" Ivan inquired, with a peculiar, irritable curiosity.

"That's just so. You can't tell beforehand."

"Besides you fell from the garret then."

"I climb up to the garret every day. I might fall from the garret again to-morrow. And, if not, I might fall down the cellar steps. I have to go into the cellar every day, too."

Ivan took a long look at him.

"You are talking nonsense, I see, and I don't quite understand you," he said softly, but with a sort of menace. "Do you mean to pretend to be ill for three days, beginning to-morrow, eh?"

Smerdyakov, who was looking at the ground again, and playing with the toe of his right foot, set the foot down, moved the left one forward, raised his head and, grinning, articulated:

"If I were able to play such a trick, that is, pretend to have a fit — and it would not be difficult for a man accustomed to them — I should have a perfect right to use such a means to save myself from death. For even if Agrafena Alexandrovna comes to see his father while I am ill in bed, Dmitri Fyodorovich, sir, can't blame a sick man for not telling him. He'd be ashamed to."

"Hang it all!" Ivan cried, his face working with anger. "Why are you always in such a funk over your life? All my brother Dmitri's threats are only hasty words and mean nothing. He won't kill you; it's not you he'll kill!"

"He'd kill me first of all, like a fly. But even more than that, I am afraid I shall be taken for an accomplice of his when he does something absurd to his father."

"Why should you be taken for an accomplice?"

"They'll think I am an accomplice, because I let him know the signals as a great secret."

"What signals? Whom did you tell?"

"I'm bound to admit the fact," Smerdyakov drawled with pedantic composure, "that Fyodor Pavlovich and I have a secret together in this business. As you know yourself (if only you do know it) he has for several days past locked himself in as soon as night or even evening comes on. Of late you've been going upstairs to your room early every evening, and yesterday you did not go out at all, and so perhaps you don't know how carefully he has begun to lock himself in at night, and even if Grigory Vasilyevich himself comes to the door he won't open to him till he hears his voice. But Grigory Vasilyevich does not come, sir, because I wait upon him alone in his rooms now. That's the arrangement he made himself ever since this to-do with Agrafena Alexandrovna began. But at night, by his orders, I go away to the lodge, so that I don't get to sleep till midnight, sir, but am on the watch, getting up and walking about the yard, waiting for Agrafena Alexandrovna to come, sir. For the last few days he's been perfectly frantic expecting her. What he argues is, she is afraid of him, that is, of Dmitri Fyodorovich (Mitya, as he calls him), 'and so,' says he, 'she'll come the back-way, late at night, to me. You look out for her,' says he, 'till midnight and later; and if she does come, you run up and knock at my door or at the window opening on the garden. Knock at first twice, rather slowly, and then three times more quickly, then,' says he, 'I shall understand at once that she has come, and will open the door to you quietly.' Another signal he gave me in case anything unexpected happens. At first, two knocks, and then, after an interval, another much louder. Then he will understand that something has happened suddenly and that I must see him, and he will open to me so that I can go and speak to him. That's all in case Agrafena Alexandrovna can't come herself, but sends a message. Besides, Dmitri Fyodorovich might come, too, so I must let him know he is near. Your father is awfully afraid of Dmitri Fyodorovich, so that even if Agrafena Alexandrovna had come and were locked in with him, and Dmitri Fyodorovich were to turn up anywhere near at the time, I should be bound to let him know at once, knocking three times. So that the first signal of five knocks means Agrafena Alexandrovna has come, while the second signal of three knocks means 'something important to tell you.' Your father has rehearsed them with me several times and explained them to me. And as in the whole universe no one knows of these signals but myself and your father, sir, he'd open the door without the slightest hesitation and without calling out (he is awfully afraid of calling out aloud). Well, those signals have now become known to Dmitri Fyodorovich, too."

"How are they known? Did you tell him? How dared you tell him?"

"It was out of fear I did it, sir. How could I dare to keep it back from him, sir? Dmitri Fyodorovich kept persisting every day, 'You are deceiving me, you are hiding something from me! I'll break both your legs for you.' So I told him those secret signals that he might see my slavish devotion, and might be satisfied that I was not deceiving him, but was telling him all I could."

"If you think that he'll make use of those signals and try to get in, don't let him in."

"But if I should be laid up with a fit, how can I prevent him coming in then, even if I dared to hold him back, knowing how desperate he is?"

"Hang it! How can you be so sure you are going to have a fit, confound you? Are you laughing at me?"

"How could I dare laugh at you? — and I am in no laughing humour with this fear on me. I feel I am going to have a fit. I have a presentiment. Fright alone will bring it on."

"Confound it! If you are laid up, Grigory will be on the watch. Let Grigory know beforehand; he will be sure not to let him in."

"I should never dare to tell Grigory Vasilyevich about the signals without orders from my master. And as for Grigory Vasilyevich hearing him and not admitting him, he has been ill ever since yesterday, and Marfa Ignatyevna intends to give him medicine to-morrow. They've just arranged it. It's a very curious remedy they have. Marfa Ignatyevna knows of a decoction and always keeps it on hand. It's a strong thing made from some herb. She has the secret of it, and she gives it to Grigory Vasilyevich about three times a year when his lumbago's so bad he is almost paralysed by it. Then she takes a towel, sir, wets it with the stuff, and rubs his whole back for half an hour till it's quite red and swollen, and what's left in the bottle she gives him to drink with a special prayer; but not quite all, for on such occasions she leaves some for herself, and drinks it herself. And as they never take strong drink, I assure you, sir, they both drop asleep at once and sleep soundly a very long time. And when Grigory Vasilyevich wakes up, sir, he is perfectly well after it, but Marfa Ignatyevna always has a headache from it. So, if Marfa Ignatyevna carries out her intention to-morrow, sir, they won't hear anything and won't hinder Dmitri Fyodorovich. They'll be asleep, sir."

"What a rigmarole! And it all seems to happen at once, as though it were planned. You'll have a fit and they'll both be dead to the world," cried Ivan. "But aren't you perhaps trying to arrange it this way?" broke from him suddenly, and he frowned threateningly.

"How could I, sir? . . . And why should I, when it all depends on Dmitri Fyodorovich and his designs? . . . If he means to do anything, he'll do it, sir; but if not, surely I shan't be the one to thrust him upon his father."

"And why should he go to father, especially on the sly, if, as you say yourself, Agrafena Alexandrovna won't come at all?" Ivan went on, turning white with anger. "You say that yourself, and all the while I've been here, I've felt sure it was all the old man's fancy, and the slut won't come to him. Why should Dmitri break in on him if she doesn't come? Speak, I want to know what you are thinking!"

"You know yourself why he'll come. What does it matter what I think? He will come simply because he is in a rage or suspicious on account of my illness perhaps, and he'll dash in, as he did yesterday through impatience to search the rooms, to see whether she hasn't slipped in on the sly. He is perfectly well aware, too, that Fyodor Pavlovich has a big envelope with three thousand roubles in it, tied up with ribbon and sealed with three seals. On it is written in his own hand, 'To my angel Grushenka, if she will wish to come,' to which he added three days later, 'and for my little chick.' That is what it is, sir."

"Nonsense!" cried Ivan, almost beside himself. "Dmitri isn't the one to commit robbery and kill his father while he's at it. He might have killed him yesterday on account of Grushenka, like the frantic, savage fool he is, but he won't steal."

"He is in great need of money just now — very great need, Ivan Fyodorovich. You don't know how badly he needs it, sir," Smerdyakov explained, with perfect composure and remarkable distinctness. "Besides, he looks on that three thousand as his own. He said so to me himself, sir. 'My father still owes me just three thousand,' he said. And besides that, consider, Ivan Fyodorovich, this other point: it's as good as certain, so to say, that Agrafena Alexandrovna will force him, if only she cares to, to marry her — the master himself, I mean, Fyodor Pavlovich — if only she cares to, and of course she may care to, sir. I was only talking when I said that she wouldn't come, but maybe she's looking for more than that — I mean, to be mistress here. I know myself that Samsonov, her merchant, was laughing with her about it, telling her quite openly that it would not be at all a foolish thing to do. And she's got plenty of sense, sir. She wouldn't marry a beggar like Dmitri Fyodorovich, not she, sir. So, taking that into consideration, Ivan Fyodorovich, reflect that then neither Dmitri Fyodorovich nor yourself and your brother, Alexey Fyodorovich, would get anything after the master's death, not a rouble, for Agrafena Alexandrovna would marry him simply to get hold of it all, all the money there is. But if your father were to die now, there'd surely be some forty thousand for each one of you, even for Dmitri Fyodorovich whom the master hates so, for he's made no will. . . . Dmitri Fyodorovich knows all that very well." A sort of shudder passed over Ivan's face. He suddenly flushed.

"Then why on earth," he suddenly interrupted Smerdyakov, "do you advise me to go to Chermashnya? What did you mean by that? If I go away, you see what will happen here." Ivan drew his breath with difficulty.

"Precisely so, sir," said Smerdyakov, softly and reasonably, watching Ivan intently.

"What do you mean by 'precisely so'?" Ivan questioned him, with a menacing light in his eyes, restraining himself with difficulty.

"I spoke because I felt sorry for you. If I were you I should simply throw it all up . . . rather than have anything to do with such a mess," answered Smerdyakov, with the most candid air, looking at Ivan's flashing eyes. They were both silent.

"You seem to be a confounded idiot, and what's more . . . an awful scoundrel, too." Ivan rose suddenly from the bench. He was about to pass straight through the gate, but he stopped short and turned to Smerdyakov. Something strange happened. Ivan, in a sudden paroxysm, bit his lip, clenched his fists, and, in another minute, would have flung himself on Smerdyakov. The latter, anyway, noticed it at the same moment, started, and shrank back. But the moment passed without mischief to Smerdyakov, and Ivan turned in silence, as it seemed in perplexity, to the gate.

"I am going away to Moscow to-morrow, if you care to know — early to-morrow morning. That's all!" he suddenly said aloud angrily, and wondered himself afterwards what need there was to say this then to Smerdyakov.

"That's the best thing you can do, sir," he responded, as though he had expected to hear it; "except that you may be disturbed in Moscow by a telegram, sir, if anything should happen here."

Ivan stopped again, and again turned quickly to Smerdyakov. But a change had passed over him, too. All his familiarity and carelessness had completely disappeared. His face expressed attention and expectation, intense but timid and cringing.

"Haven't you something more to say — something to add?" could be read in the intent gaze he fixed on Ivan.

"And couldn't I be sent for from Chermashnya, too — in case anything happened?" Ivan shouted suddenly, for some unknown reason raising his voice.

"From Chermashnya, too . . . you could be sent for, sir," Smerdyakov muttered, almost in a whisper, looking disconcerted, but gazing intently into Ivan's eyes.

"Only Moscow is further and Chermashnya is nearer. Is it to save my fare, or to save my going so far out of my way, that you insist on Chermashnya?"

"Precisely so, sir . . ." muttered Smerdyakov, with a breaking voice. He looked at Ivan with a revolting smile, and again made ready to draw back. But to his astonishment Ivan broke into a laugh, and went through the gate still laughing. Any one who had seen his face at that moment would have known that he was not laughing from lightness of heart, and he could not have explained himself what he was feeling at that instant. His movements had the involuntary character of convulsions.

CHAPTER VII

"A CLEVER MAN IS WORTH TALKING TO"

HIS speech, too, had the same impulsive character. Meeting Fyodor Pavlovich in the drawing-room directly he entered, he suddenly shouted to him, waving his hands, "I am going upstairs to my room, not in to you. Good-bye!" and passed by, trying not even to look at his father. Very possibly the old man was too hateful to him at that moment; but such an unceremonious display of hostility was a surprise even to Fyodor Pavlovich. And the old man evidently wanted to tell him something at once and had come to meet him in the drawing-room on purpose. Receiving this amiable greeting, he stood still in silence and with an ironical air watched his son going upstairs, till he passed out of sight.

"What's the matter with him?" he promptly asked Smerdyakov, who had followed Ivan.

"Angry about something, sir. Who can tell?" the valet muttered evasively.

"Confound him! Let him be angry then. Bring in the samovar, and get along with you. Look sharp! No news?"

Then followed a series of questions such as Smerdyakov had just complained of to Ivan, all relating to his expected visitor, and these questions we will omit. Half an hour later the house was locked, and the crazy old man paced alone through the rooms in excited expectation of hearing every minute the five knocks agreed upon. Now and then he peered out into the darkness, seeing nothing.

It was very late, but Ivan was still awake and reflecting. He went to bed late that night, about two o'clock. But we will not trouble to give an account of his thoughts, and this is not the time to look into that soul — its turn will come. And even if one tried, it would be very hard to give an account of them, for there were no thoughts in his brain, but something very vague, and, above all, intense excitement. He felt himself that he had lost his bearings. He was fretted, too, by all sorts of strange and almost surprising desires; for instance, after midnight he suddenly had an intense irresistible inclination to go down, open the door, go to the lodge and beat up Smerdyakov. But if he had been asked why, he could not have given any exact reason, except perhaps that he loathed the valet as one who had insulted him more gravely than any one in the world. On the other hand, he was more than once that night overcome by a sort of inexplicable humiliating fear, which, he felt, positively paralysed his physical powers. His head ached and he was dizzy. A feeling of hatred was rankling in his heart, as though he meant to avenge himself on some one. He even hated Alyosha, recalling the conversation he had just had with him. At moments he hated himself intensely. Of Katerina Ivanovna he almost forgot to think, and wondered greatly at this afterwards, especially as he remembered perfectly that when he had protested so valiantly to Katerina Ivanovna that he would go away next day to Moscow, something had whispered in his heart, "That's nonsense, you are not going, and it won't be so easy to tear yourself away as you are now so boastfully pretending."

Remembering that night long afterwards, Ivan recalled with peculiar repulsion how he would suddenly get up from the sofa and stealthily, as though he were afraid of being watched, open the door, go out on the staircase and listen to Fyodor Pavlovich stirring down below, listen a long while — some five minutes at a stretch — with a sort of strange curiosity, holding his breath while his heart throbbed. And why he did all this, why he was listening, he could not have said. That "action" all his life afterwards he called "infamous," and at the bottom of his heart, he thought of it as the basest action of his life. For Fyodor Pavlovich himself he felt no hatred in those moments, but was simply intensely curious to know how he was walking down there below and what he must be doing now. He wondered and imagined how he must be peeping out of the dark windows and stopping in the middle of the room, listening, listening — for some one to knock. Ivan went out onto the stairs twice to listen like this.

About two o'clock when everything was quiet, and even Fyodor Pavlovich had gone to bed, Ivan, too, had got into bed, firmly resolved to fall asleep at once, as he felt fearfully exhausted. And he did fall asleep at once, and slept soundly without dreams, but waked early, at seven o'clock, when it was broad daylight. Opening his eyes, he was surprised to feel himself extraordinarily vigorous. He jumped up at once and dressed quickly; then pulled out his trunk and began packing hastily. His linen had come back from the laundress the previous morning. Ivan positively smiled at the thought that everything was helping his sudden departure. And his departure certainly was sudden. Though Ivan had said the day before (to Katerina Ivanovna, to Alyosha, and to Smerdyakov) that he was leaving next day, yet he remembered that he had had no thought of departure when he went to bed, or, at least, had not thought for a moment that his first act in the morning would be to pack his trunk. At last his trunk and bag were ready. It was about nine o'clock when Marfa Ignatyevna came in with her usual inquiry, "Where will you take your tea, sir, in your own room or downstairs?" Ivan Fyodorovich went downstairs. He looked almost cheerful, but there was about him, about his words and gestures, something hurried and scattered. Greeting his father affably, and even inquiring specially after his health, though he did not wait to hear his answer to the end, he announced that he was starting off in an hour to return to Moscow for good, and begged him to send for the horses. His father heard this announcement with no sign of surprise, and forgot in an unmannerly way to show regret at his departure. Instead of doing so, he flew into a great flutter at the recollection of some important business of his own.

"What a fellow you are! Not to tell me yesterday! Never mind; we'll manage it all the same. Do me a great service, my dear boy. Stop at Chermashnya on the way. It only means turning to the left from the station at Volovya, only another twelve versts, and there is Chermashnya."

"I'm sorry, I can't. It's eighty versts to the railway and the train starts for Moscow at seven o'clock to-night. I can only just catch it."

"You'll catch it to-morrow or the day after, but to-day turn off to Chermashnya. It won't put you out much to humour your father! If my affairs hadn't kept me here, I would have run over myself long ago, for I've some urgent and important business there. But here I . . . it's not the time for me to go now. . . . You see, I've two pieces of woodland there, one at Begichevo and one at Dyachkino. The Maslovs, father and son, will give eight thousand for the timber. But last year I just missed a purchaser who would have given twelve. There's no getting any one about here to buy it. The Maslovs have it all in their fist. One has to take what they'll give, for no one here dare bid against them. The priest at Ilyinskoe wrote to me last Thursday that a merchant called Gorstkin, a man I know, had turned up. What makes him valuable is that he is not from these parts, so he is not afraid of the Maslovs. He says he will give me eleven thousand for the copse. Do you hear? But he'll only be here, the priest writes, for a week altogether, so you must go at once and come to terms with him."

"Well, you write to the priest; he'll make the bargain."

"He can't do it. He has no eye for business. He is a perfect treasure, I'd give him twenty thousand to keep for me without a receipt; but he has no eye for business, he is a perfect child, a crow could cheat him. And yet he is a learned man, would you believe it? This Gorstkin looks like a peasant, he wears a blue kaftan, but he is a thorough scamp. That's the common complaint. He is a liar, that's what. Sometimes he tells such lies that you wonder why he is doing it. He told me the year before last that his wife was dead and that he had married again, and would you believe it, there was not a word of truth in it? His wife never died at all, she is alive to this day and gives him a beating twice a week. So what you have to find out is whether he is lying or speaking the truth, when he says he wants to buy it and would give eleven thousand."

"I shall be no use in such a business. I have no eye either."

"Stop, wait a bit! You will be of use, for I will tell you the signs by which you can judge about Gorstkin. I've done business with him a long time. You see, you must watch his beard; he has a nasty, thin, red beard. If his beard shakes when he talks and he gets cross, it's all right, he means what he says, he wants to do business. But if he strokes his beard with his left hand and grins — he is trying to cheat you. Don't watch his eyes, you won't find out anything from his eyes, he is a deep one, a scamp — but watch his beard! I'll give you a note and you show it to him. He's called Gorstkin, though his real name is Lyagavy;* but don't call him so, he will be offended. If you come to an understanding with him, and see it's all right, write here at once. You need only write: 'He's not lying.' Stand out for eleven thousand; one thousand you can knock off, but not more. Just think! there's a difference between eight thousand and eleven thousand. It's as good as finding three thousand; it's not so easy to get a purchaser, and I'm in desperate need of money. Only let me know it's serious, and I'll run over and fix it up. I'll snatch the time somehow. But what's the good of my galloping over, if it's all a notion of the priest's? Come, will you go?"

"Oh, I can't spare the time. You must excuse me."

"Come, you might oblige your father. I shan't forget it. You've no heart, any of you — that's what it is! What's a day or two to you? Where are you going now — to Venice? Your Venice will keep another two days. I would have sent Alyosha, but what use is Alyosha in a thing like that? I send you just because you are a clever fellow. Do you suppose I don't see that? You know nothing about timber, but you've got an eye. All that is wanted is to see whether the man is in earnest. I tell you, watch his beard — if his beard shakes, you know he is in earnest."

"You force me to go to that damned Chermashnya yourself, then?" cried Ivan, with a malignant smile.

Fyodor Pavlovich did not catch, or would

* *i.e.*, setter dog.

not catch, the malignancy, but he caught the smile.

"Then you'll go, you'll go? I'll scribble the note for you at once."

"I don't know whether I shall go. I don't know. I'll decide on the way."

"Nonsense! Decide at once. My dear fellow, decide! If you settle the matter, write me a line; give it to the priest and he'll send it on to me at once. And I won't delay you longer than that. You can go to Venice. The priest will give you horses back to Volovya station."

The old man was simply in transports. He wrote the note, and sent for the horses. A light lunch was brought in, with cognac. When Fyodor Pavlovich was pleased, he usually became expansive, but this time he seemed to restrain himself. Of Dmitri, for instance, he did not say a word. He was quite unmoved by the parting, and seemed, in fact, at a loss for something to say. Ivan noticed this particularly. "He must be bored with me," he thought. Only when seeing his son off on the steps, the old man began fussing a bit, and was evidently ready to go through the ceremony of kissing. But Ivan made haste to hold out his hand, obviously avoiding the kisses. His father saw it at once, and instantly pulled himself up.

"Well, God bless you, God bless you!" he repeated from the steps. "You'll come again some time or other? Mind you do come. I shall always be glad. Well, Christ be with you!"

Ivan got into the carriage.

"Good-bye, Ivan! Don't be too hard on me!" the father called for the last time.

The whole household came out to take leave — Smerdyakov, Marfa, and Grigory. Ivan gave them ten roubles each. When he had seated himself in the carriage, Smerdyakov jumped up to arrange the rug. "You see . . . I am going to Chermashnya," broke suddenly from Ivan.

Again, as on the day before, the words seemed to drop of themselves, and he laughed, too, a peculiar, nervous laugh. He remembered it long after.

"It's a true saying then, that 'a clever man is worth talking to,'" answered Smerdyakov firmly, looking significantly at Ivan.

The carriage rolled away. Nothing was clear in the traveller's soul, but he looked eagerly around him at the fields, at the hills, at the trees, at a flock of geese flying high overhead in the bright sky. And all of a sudden he felt very happy. He tried to talk to the driver, and he felt intensely interested in an answer the peasant made him; but a minute later he realised that he was not hearing anything, and that he had not really even taken in the peasant's answer. He was silent, and it was pleasant even so. The air was fresh, pure and cool, the sky bright. The images of Alyosha and Katerina Ivanovna floated into his mind. But he smiled softly, blew gently on the friendly phantoms, and they flew away. "Their time will come," he thought. They reached the station quickly, changed horses, and galloped to Volovya. "Why is it worth while talking to a clever man? What did he mean by that?" The thought seemed suddenly to choke off his breath. "And why did I report to him that I was going to Chermashnya?" They reached Volovya station. Ivan got out of the carriage, and the drivers stood round him bargaining over the journey of twelve versts to Chermashnya. He told them to harness the horses. He went into the station, looked round, glanced at the station-master's wife, and suddenly went out again.

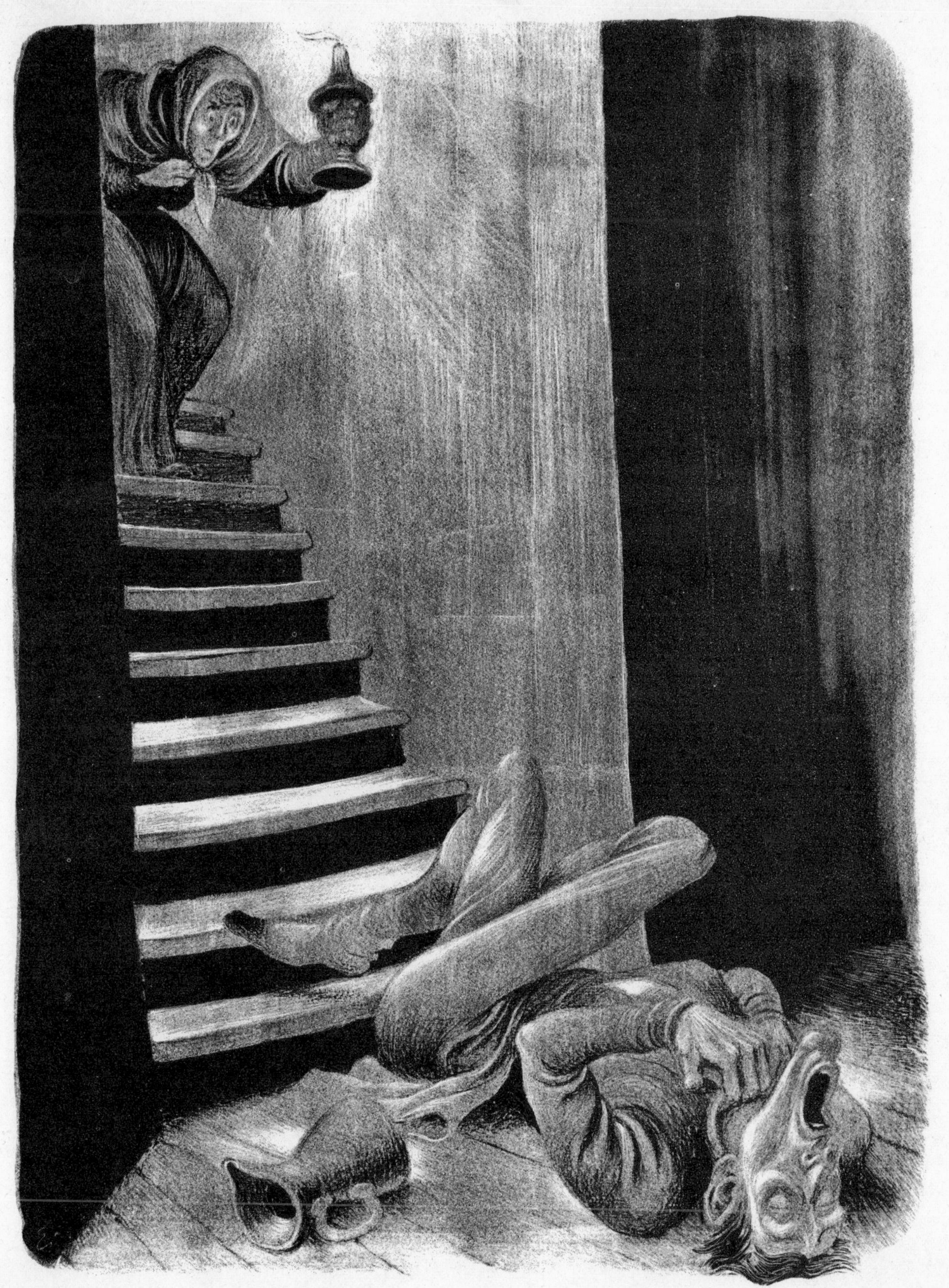

THE SCREAM OF THE EPILEPTIC

"I won't go to Chermashnya. Am I too late to reach the railway by seven, brothers?"

"We shall just do it. Shall we hitch up?"

"At once. Will any one of you be going to town to-morrow?"

"To be sure. Mitri here will."

"Can you do me a service, Mitri? Go to my father's, to Fyodor Pavlovich Karamazov, and tell him I haven't gone to Chermashnya. Can you?"

"Of course I can. I've known Fyodor Pavlovich a long time."

"And here's something for you, for I dare say he won't give you anything," said Ivan, laughing gaily.

"You may depend on it he won't." Mitri laughed, too. "Thank you, sir. I'll be sure to do it."

At seven o'clock Ivan got into the train and set off for Moscow. "Away with the past. I've done with the old world for ever, and may I have no news, no echo, from it. To a new life, new places, and no looking back!" But instead of delight his soul was filled with such gloom, and his heart ached with such anguish, as he had never known in his life before. He spent the night in thought. The train flew on, and only at daybreak, when he was approaching Moscow, he suddenly roused himself from his meditation.

"I am a scoundrel," he whispered to himself.

Meanwhile, Fyodor Pavlovich, having seen his son off, remained well satisfied. For two hours afterwards he felt almost happy, and sat sipping cognac. But suddenly something happened which was very annoying and unpleasant for every one in the house, and completely upset Fyodor Pavlovich's equanimity at once. Smerdyakov went to the cellar for something and fell down from the top of the steps. Fortunately, Marfa Ignatyevna was in the yard and heard him in time. She did not see the fall, but heard his scream — the strange, peculiar scream, long familiar to her — the scream of the epileptic falling in a fit. It was impossible to tell whether the fit had come on him at the moment he was descending the steps, so that he must have fallen while unconscious, or whether it was the fall and the shock that had caused the fit in Smerdyakov, who was known to be an epileptic. He was found at the bottom of the cellar steps, writhing in convulsions and foaming at the mouth. It was thought at first that he must have broken something — an arm or a leg — and hurt himself, but "God had preserved him," as Marfa Ignatyevna expressed it — nothing of the kind had happened. But it was difficult to get him out of the cellar. They asked the neighbours to help and managed it somehow. Fyodor Pavlovich himself was present at the whole ceremony. He helped, evidently alarmed and upset. The sick man did not, however, regain consciousness; the convulsions ceased for a time, but then began again, and every one concluded that the same thing would happen as had happened a year before, when he accidentally fell from the garret. They remembered that ice had been put on his head then. There was still ice in the cellar, and Marfa Ignatyevna had some brought up. In the evening, Fyodor Pavlovich sent for Dr. Herzenstube, who arrived at once. He was a most estimable old man, and the most careful and conscientious doctor in the province. After careful examination, he concluded that the fit was a very violent one and might have serious consequences; that meanwhile he, Herzenstube, did not fully understand it, but that by to-morrow morning, if the present remedies were unavailing, he would venture to try something else. The patient was taken to the lodge, to a room next to Grigory's and Marfa Ignatyevna's.

After that Fyodor Pavlovich had to put up with one misfortune after another. Marfa Ignatyevna cooked the dinner, and the soup, compared with Smerdyakov's, was no "better than dish water," and the fowl was so dried up that it was impossible to chew it. To her master's bitter, though deserved, reproaches, Marfa Ignatyevna replied that the fowl was a very old one to begin with, and that she had never been trained as a cook. In the evening there was another trouble in store for Fyodor Pavlovich; he was informed that Grigory, who had not been well for the last three days, was completely laid up by his lumbago. Fyodor Pavlovich finished his tea as early as possible and locked himself up alone in the house. He was in terrible excitement and suspense. That evening he reckoned on Grushenka's coming almost as a certainty. He had received from Smerdyakov that morning an assurance "that she had promised to come without fail." The irrepressible old man's heart throbbed with excitement; he paced up and down his empty rooms listening. He had to be on the alert. Dmitri might be on the watch for her somewhere, and when she knocked on the window (Smerdyakov had informed him two days before that he had told her where and how to knock) the door must be opened at once. She must not be a second in the passage, for fear — God forbid! — that she might be frightened and run away.

Fyodor Pavlovich had much to think of, but never had his heart bathed in sweeter hopes. This time he could say almost certainly that she would come!

CHAPTER I

FATHER ZOSIMA AND HIS VISITORS

WHEN with an anxious and aching heart Alyosha went into his elder's cell, he stood still almost astonished. Instead of a sick man at his last gasp, perhaps unconscious, as he had feared to find him, he suddenly saw him sitting up in his chair and, though weak and exhausted, his face was bright and cheerful, he was surrounded by visitors and engaged in a quiet and joyful conversation with them. But he had only got up from his bed a quarter of an hour before Alyosha's arrival; his visitors had gathered together in his cell earlier, waiting for him to wake, having received a most confident assurance from Father Païssy that "the teacher would get up, and, as he had himself promised in the morning, converse once more with those dear to his heart." This promise and indeed every word of the dying elder's Father Païssy believed implicitly. If he had seen him unconscious, if he had seen him breathe his last, and yet had his promise that he would rise up and take leave of him, he would not have credited perhaps his very death, but would still have expected the dead man to recover and fulfil his promise. In the morning as he lay down to sleep, Father Zosima had told him positively: "I shall not die ere I have delighted in another conversation with all of you, beloved of my heart. I shall look once more on your dear faces and pour out my heart to you once again." The monks, who had gathered for what was probably to be their last conversation with Father Zosima, had all been his devoted friends for many years. There were four of them: Father Iosif and Father Païssy, Father Mihail, the abbot of the hermitage, a man not very old and far from learned. He was of humble origin, of strong will and steadfast faith, of austere appearance, but of deep tenderness, though he seemed to conceal it as though he were almost ashamed of it. The fourth, Father Anfim, was a very old and humble little monk of the poorest peasant class. He was almost illiterate, and very quiet, scarcely speaking to any one. He was the humblest of the humble, and looked as though he had been permanently frightened by something great and dreadful beyond the scope of his intelligence. Father Zosima had a great affection for this, as it were, quaking man, and always treated him with marked respect, though perhaps there was no one he had known to whom he had said less, in spite of the fact that he had spent years wandering about holy Russia with him. That was very long ago, forty years before, when Father Zosima first began his life as a monk in a poor, little known monastery at Kostroma, and when, shortly after, he had accompanied Father Anfim on his pilgrimage to collect alms for their poor monastery.

The whole company was in the elder's bedroom which, as we mentioned before, was very small, so that there was scarcely room for the four of them (in addition to Porfiry, the novice, who was on his feet) to sit round Father Zosima on chairs brought from the living-room. It was already beginning to get dark, the room was lighted up by the lamps and wax tapers before the ikons.

Seeing Alyosha standing embarrassed in the doorway, Father Zosima smiled at him joyfully and held out his hand.

"Welcome, my quiet one, welcome, my dear, here you are, too. I knew you would come."

Alyosha went up to him, bowed down before him to the ground and wept. Something surged up from his heart, his soul was quivering, he wanted to sob.

"Come, don't mourn me yet," Father Zosima smiled, laying his right hand on his head. "You see I am sitting up talking; maybe I shall live another twenty years yet, as that dear good woman from Vyshegorye, with her little Lizaveta in her arms, wished me yesterday. God bless the mother and the little girl Lizaveta," he crossed himself. "Porfiry, did you take her offering where I told you?"

He meant the sixty copecks brought him the day before by his jolly admirer, to be given "to some one poorer than me." Such offerings, always of money gained by personal toil, are made by way of penance voluntarily undertaken. The elder had sent Porfiry the evening before to a widow, whose house had been burnt down lately, and who after the fire had gone with her children begging alms. Porfiry hastened to reply that he had given the money, as he had been instructed, "from an unknown benefactress."

"Get up, my dear boy," the elder went on, addressing Alyosha. "Let me look at you. Have you been home and seen your brother?" It seemed strange to Alyosha that he asked so confidently and precisely, about one of his brothers only — but which one? Then perhaps he had sent him out both yesterday and to-day for the sake of that brother. "I have seen one of my brothers," answered Alyosha. "I mean the elder one, to whom I bowed down."

"I only saw him yesterday and could not find him to-day," said Alyosha.

"Make haste to find him, go again to-morrow and make haste, leave everything and make haste. Perhaps you may still have time to prevent something terrible. I bowed down yesterday to the great suffering in store for him." He was suddenly silent and seemed to be pondering. The words were strange. Father Iosif, who had witnessed the scene yesterday, exchanged glances with Father Païssy. Alyosha could not resist asking a question.

"Father and teacher," he began with extreme emotion, "your words are too obscure. . . . What is this suffering in store for him?"

"Do not be curious. I seemed to see something terrible yesterday . . . as though his whole future were expressed in his eyes. A look came into his eyes — so that my heart was instantly stricken with horror at what that man is preparing for himself. Once or twice in my life I've seen such a look in a man's face . . . reflecting as it were his future fate, and that fate, alas, came to pass. I sent you to him, Alexey, for I thought your brotherly countenance would help him. But everything and all our destinies are from the Lord. 'Except a corn of wheat fall into the ground and die, it abideth alone; but if it die, it bringeth forth much fruit.' Remember that. You, Alexey, I've many times silently blessed for your countenance, know that," added the elder with a gentle smile. "This is what I think of you, you will go forth from these walls, but will live like a monk in the world. You will have many antagonists, but your very foes will love you. Life will bring you many misfortunes, but it is precisely in them you will find your happiness, and you will bless life and will make others bless it — which is what matters most. Well, that is what you are like. Fathers and teachers," he addressed his friends with a tender smile, "I have never till to-day told even him why the countenance of this youth is so dear to me. Now I will tell you. His countenance has been as it were a remembrance and a prophecy for me. At the dawn of my life when I was a child I had an elder brother who died before my eyes at seventeen. And later on in the course of my life I gradually became convinced that that brother had been for a guidance and a sign from on high for me. For had he not come into my life, I should never perhaps, so I fancy at least, have become a monk and entered on this precious path. He appeared first to me in my childhood, and here at the end of my journey he seems to have come to me over again. It is marvellous, fathers and teachers, that Alexey, who bears him some, though not great, resemblance in features, has seemed to me so like him spiritually, that many times I have taken him for that youth, my brother, mysteriously come back to me at the end of my journey, as a reminder and an inspiration. So that I positively marvelled at my having so strange a fancy. Do you hear this, Porfiry?" He turned to the novice who waited on him. "Many times I've seen in your face as it were a look of mortification because I love Alexey more than you. Now you know why that was so, but I love you, too, know that, and many times I grieved at your mortification. I should like to tell you, dear friends, of that youth, my brother, for there has been no presence in my life more precious, more prophetic and touching. My heart is full of emotion, and I look at my whole life at this moment as though living through it again."

Here I must observe that this last talk of Father Zosima with the friends who visited him on the last day of his life has been partly preserved in writing. Alexey Fyodorovich Karamazov wrote it down for remembrance, a short time after the elder's death. But whether this was only the conversation that took place then, or whether in his memoir he added parts of former conversations with his teacher, I cannot determine. In his account, Father Zosima's talk goes on without interruption, as though he told his life to his friends in the form of a story, though there is no doubt, from other accounts of it, that the conversation that evening was general. Though the visitors did not interrupt Father Zosima much, yet they, too, talked, perhaps even told something themselves. Besides, Father Zosima could not have carried on an uninterrupted narrative, for he was sometimes gasping for breath, his voice failed him, and he even lay down to rest on his bed, though he did not fall asleep and his visitors did not leave their seats. Once or twice the conversation was interrupted by Father Païssy's reading the Gospel. It is worthy of note, too, that no one of them supposed that he would die that night, for on that last evening of his life after his deep sleep during the day he seemed suddenly to have found new strength, which kept him up through this long conversation with his friends. It was like a last effort of love which was the source of incredible animation; only for a little time, however, for his life was cut short immediately. . . . But of that later. I will only state that I have preferred to confine myself to the account written down by Alexey Fyodorovich Karamazov, without going into the details of the conversation. It will be shorter and not so fatiguing, though of course, as I must repeat, Alyosha took a great deal from previous conversations, combining the parts into a whole.

CHAPTER II

NOTES ON THE LIFE OF THE ELDER ZOSIMA, PRIEST AND MONK, WHO DIED IN THE LORD; COUCHED IN HIS OWN WORDS, AND COMPILED BY ALEXEY FYODOROVICH KARAMAZOV

BIOGRAPHICAL INFORMATION

(*a*) *Concerning the youth who was the elder Zosima's brother*

BELOVED fathers and teachers, I was born in a distant northern province, in the town of V. My father was a gentleman by birth, but of no great consequence or rank. He died when I was only two years old, and I don't remember him at all. He left my mother a small frame-house, and a fortune, not large, but sufficient to keep her and her children in comfort. There were two of us, my elder brother Markel and I. He was eight years older than I was, with a hasty irritable temper, but kind-hearted and never ironical. He was remarkably silent, especially at home with me, his mother, and the servants. He did well at school, but did not get on with his schoolfellows, though he never quarrelled, at least so my mother has told me. Six months before his death, when he was past seventeen, he made friends with a political exile who had been banished from Moscow to our town for freethinking, and led a solitary existence there. The exile was a man of learning who had gained distinction in philosophy at the university. Something made him take a fancy to Markel, and he made him welcome. The young man would spend whole evenings with him during that winter, till the exile was summoned to Petersburg to take up his post again at his own request, as he had powerful friends.

It was the beginning of Lent, and Markel would not fast, he was rude and laughed at it. "That's all silly twaddle and there is no God," he said, horrifying my mother, the servants, and me, too. For though I was only nine, I, too, was aghast at hearing such words. We had four servants, all serfs, bought in the name of a landowner of our acquaintance. I remember my mother selling one of the four, the cook Afimya, who was lame and elderly, for sixty paper roubles, and hiring a free servant to take her place.

Well, in the sixth week in Lent, my brother, who was never strong and had a tendency to consumption, was taken ill. He was tall but thin and delicate-looking, and with very pleasing features. I suppose he caught cold, anyway the doctor who came soon whispered to my mother that it was galloping consumption, that he would not live through the spring. My mother began weeping, and careful not to alarm my brother, she entreated him to go to church, to confess and take the sacrament, as he was still able to move about. This made him angry, and he said something profane about the church. He grew thoughtful, however; he guessed at once that he was seriously ill, and that that was why his mother was begging him to confess and take the sacrament while he still had his strength. He had been aware, indeed, for a long time past, that he was far from well, and had a year before coolly observed at dinner to our mother and me, "I shan't be with you long, I may not live another year," which seemed now like a prophecy.

Three days passed and Holy Week had come. And on Tuesday morning my brother began going to church. "I am doing this simply for your sake, mother, to please and comfort you," he said. My mother wept with joy and grief, "his end must be near," she thought, "if there's such a change in him." But he was not able to go to church long, he took to his bed, so he had to confess and take the sacrament at home.

It was a late Easter, and the days were bright, clear, and fragrant. I remember he used to cough all night and sleep badly, but in the morning he dressed and tried to sit up in an armchair. That's how I remember him, sitting there, sweet and gentle, smiling, his face bright and joyous, in spite of his illness. A marvellous change came over him, his spirit seemed transformed. The old nurse would come in and say, "Let me light the lamp before the holy image, my dear." Formerly he would not have allowed it and would have blown it out.

"Light it, light it, dear, I was a monster to have prevented you doing it. You are praying when you light the lamp, and I pray rejoicing at you. So we are praying to the same God."

Those words seemed strange to us, and mother would go to her room and weep, but when she went in to him she wiped her eyes and looked cheerful. "Mother, don't cry, darling," he would say, "I've long to live yet, long to rejoice with you, and life is glad and joyful."

"Ah, dear boy, how can you talk of joy when you lie feverish at night, coughing as though your chest were being torn to pieces."

"Don't cry, mother," he would answer, "life is paradise, and we are all in paradise, but we won't see it; if we would, we should have heaven on earth the next day."

Every one wondered at his words, he spoke so strangely and firmly; we were all touched and wept. Friends came to see us. "Dear ones," he would say to them, "what have I done that you should love me so, how can you love any one like me, and how was it I did not know, I did not appreciate it before?"

When the servants came in to him he would say continually, "Dear, kind people, why are you doing so much for me, do I deserve to be waited on? If it were God's will for me to live, I would wait on you, for all men should wait on one another."

Mother shook her head as she listened. "My darling, it's your illness makes you talk like that."

"Mother, my joy," he would say, "there must be servants and masters, but if so I will be the servant of my servants, the same as they are to me. And another thing, mother, every one of us is guilty towards all men, of all sins, and I more than any."

Mother positively smiled at that, smiled through her tears. "Why, how could you be guilty towards all, more than anybody else? There are robbers and murderers, but what sin have you committed yet, that you blame yourself more than all?"

"Mother, my darling little life," he said (he had begun using such strange caressing words at that time), "my darling little life, my joy, believe me, every one is really responsible to all men for all and everything. I don't know how to explain it to you, but I feel it is so, painfully even. And how is it we went on living before, getting angry and not understanding anything?"

So he would get up every day, more and more sweet and joyous and full of love. When the doctor, an old German called Eisenschmidt, came: "Well, doctor, have I another day in this world?" he would ask, joking.

"You'll live many days yet," the doctor would answer, "and months and years, too."

"Months and years!" he would exclaim. "Why reckon the days? One day is enough for a man to know all happiness. My dear ones, why do we quarrel, try to outshine each other and bear grudges against each other? Let's go straight into the garden, walk and play there, love, appreciate, and kiss each other, and bless our life."

"Your son cannot last long," the doctor told my mother, as she accompanied him to the door. "The disease is affecting his mind."

The windows of his room looked out into the garden, and our garden was a shady one, with old trees in it which were coming into bud. The first birds of spring were flitting in the branches, chirruping and singing at his windows. And looking at them and admiring them, he began suddenly begging their forgiveness, too, "Birds of heaven, happy birds, forgive me, for I have sinned against you, too." That none of us could understand at the time, but he shed tears of joy. "Yes," he said, "there was God's glory all about me; birds, trees, meadows, sky, I alone lived in shame and dishonoured it all and did not notice the beauty and glory."

"You take too many sins on yourself," mother used to say, weeping.

"Mother, darling, it's for joy, not for grief I am crying. Though I can't explain it to you, I myself like to feel guilty towards them, for I don't know how to love them enough. If I have sinned against every one, yet all forgive me, too, and that's heaven. Am I not in heaven now?"

And there was a great deal more I don't remember. I remember I once went into his room when there was no one else there. It was a bright evening, the sun was setting, and the whole room was lighted up with oblique sunrays. He beckoned me, and I went up to him. He put his hands on my shoulders and looked into my face tenderly, lovingly; he said nothing for a minute, only looked at me like that.

"Well," he said, "run and play now, live for me, too."

I went out then and ran to play. And many times in my life afterwards I remembered even with tears how he told me to live for him, too. There were many other marvellous and beautiful sayings of his, though we did not understand them at the time. He died the third week after Easter. He was fully conscious though he could not talk; up to his last hour he did not change. He looked happy, his eyes beamed and sought us, he smiled at us, beckoned us. There was a great deal of talk even in the town about his end. I was impressed by all this at the time, but not too much so, though I cried a great deal at his funeral. I was young then, a child, but a lasting impression, a secret feeling about it all, remained in my heart, ready to rise up and respond when the time came. So indeed it happened.

(b) Concerning the Holy Scriptures in the life of Father Zosima

I was left alone with my mother. Her friends began advising her to send me to Petersburg as other parents did. "You have only one son now," they said, "and have a fair income, and you will perhaps be depriving him of a brilliant career if you keep him here." They suggested that mother send me to Petersburg to the Cadet Corps, that I might afterwards enter the Imperial Guard. My mother hesitated for a long time; it was awful to part with her only child, but she made up her mind to do it at last, though not without many tears, believing she was acting for my happiness. She took me to Petersburg and put me into the Cadet Corps, and I never saw her again. For she, too, died three years afterwards. She spent those three years mourning and grieving for both of us.

From the house of my childhood I have brought nothing but precious memories, for there are no memories more precious than those of early childhood in one's first home. And that is almost always so if there is any love and harmony in the family at all. Indeed, precious memories may remain even of a bad home, if only the heart knows how to find what is precious. With my memories of home I count, too, my memories of the Bible, which, child as I was, in my parents' house, I was very eager to know. I had a book of sacred history then with excellent pictures, called "A Hundred and Four Sacred Stories from the Old and New Testament," and I learnt to read from it. I have it lying on my shelf now, I keep it as a precious memento of the past. But even before I learnt to read, I remember first being visited by a kind of spiritual feeling when I was only eight years old. My mother took me alone to mass (I don't remember where my brother was at the time) on the Monday before Easter. It was a clear day, and recalling it now, it is as though I see before me the incense as it rose from the censer and softly floated upwards in rising waves, and, overhead in the cupola, melted in the rays of the sunlight that streamed in at the little window. I was stirred by the sight, and for the first time in my life I consciously received the seed of God's word into my soul. A youth came out into the middle of the church carrying a large book, so large that at the time I fancied he could scarcely carry it. He laid it on the lectern, opened it, and began reading, and suddenly for the first time I understood something read in the church of God. In the land of Uz, there lived a man, righteous and God-fearing, and he had great wealth, so many camels, so many sheep and asses, and his children feasted, and he loved them very much and prayed for them. "It may be that my sons have sinned in their feasting." And behold, the devil came before the Lord together with the sons of God, and said to the Lord that he had gone up and down the earth and under the earth. "And hast thou considered my servant Job?" God asked of him. And God boasted to the devil, pointing to his great and holy servant. And the devil laughed at God's words. "Give him over to me and Thou wilt see that Thy servant will murmur against Thee and curse Thy name." And God gave up the just man He so loved, to the devil. And the devil smote his children and his cattle and scattered his wealth, all of a sudden like a thunderbolt from heaven. And Job rent his mantle and fell down upon the ground and cried aloud, "Naked came I out of my mother's womb, and naked shall I return into the earth; the Lord gave and the Lord hath taken away. Blessed be the name of the Lord for ever and ever."

Fathers and teachers, forgive my tears now, for all my childhood rises up again before me, and I breathe now as I breathed then, with the breast of a little child of eight, and I feel as I did then, awe and wonder and gladness. The camels at that time caught my imagination, and Satan, who talked like that with God, and God who gave His servant up to destruction, and His servant crying out: "Blessed be Thy name although Thou dost punish me," and then the soft and sweet singing in the church: "Let my prayer rise up before Thee," and again incense from the priest's censer and the kneeling and the prayer. Ever since then — only yesterday I took it up — I've never been able to read that sacred tale without tears. And how much that is great, mysterious and unfathomable there is in it! Afterwards I heard the words of mockers and blasphemers, proud words, "How could God give up the most loved of His saints for the diversion of the devil, take from him his children, smite him with sore boils so that he cleansed the corruption from his sores with a potsherd — and for no object except to boast to the devil! 'See what My saint can suffer for My sake.' " But the greatness of it lies just in the fact that it is a mystery — that the transient earthly show and the eternal verity touch here. In the face of the earthly truth, the eternal truth is enacted. The Creator, just as on the first days of creation He ended each day with praise: "that is good that I have created," looks upon Job and again boasts of His creation. And Job praising the Lord, serves not only Him but all His creation for generations and generations, and for ever and ever, since for that he was ordained. Good heavens, what a book it is, and what lessons there are in it! What a book the Bible is, what a miracle, what strength is given with it to man. It is like a mould cast of the world and man and human nature, everything is named there, and indicated for all time. And what mysteries are solved and revealed; God raises Job again, gives him wealth again. Many years pass by, and he has other children and loves them. But how could he love those new ones when those first children are no more, when he has lost them? Remembering them, how could he be fully happy with those new ones, however dear to him the new ones might be? But he could, he could. It's the great mystery of human life that old grief passes gradually into quiet tender joy. The mild serenity of age takes the place of the riotous blood of youth. I bless the rising sun each day, and, as before, my heart sings to it, but now I love even more its setting, its long slanting rays and the soft tender gentle memories that come with them, the dear images from the whole of my long blessed life — and over all the Divine Truth, softening, reconciling, forgiving! My life is ending, I know that well, but every day that is left me I feel how my earthly life touches a new, infinite, unknown, but imminent life, the presentiment of which sets my soul quivering with rapture, my mind glowing and my heart weeping with joy.

Friends and teachers, I have heard more than once, and of late one may hear it more often, that the priests, and above all the village priests, are complaining on all sides of their miserable income and their humiliating lot. They plainly state, even in print — I've read it myself — that they are unable to teach the Scriptures to the people because of the smallness of their means, and if Lutherans and heretics come and lead the flock astray, they show no resistance because they have so little to live upon. May the Lord increase the sustenance that is so precious to them, for their complaint is just, too. But of a truth I say, if any one is to blame in the matter, half the fault is ours. For he may be short of time, he may say truly that he is oppressed all the time with chores and duties, but still it's not all the time, even he has an hour a week to remember God. And he does not work the whole year round. Let him gather round him once a week, some hour in the evening, if only the children at first — the fathers will hear of it and they, too, will begin to come. There's no need to build mansions for this, let him take them into his own cottage. They won't spoil his cottage, they would be there only one hour. Let him open that book and begin reading it without grand words or superciliousness, without condescension to them, but gently and kindly, being glad that he is reading to them and that they are listening with attention, loving the words himself, only stopping from time to time to explain words that are not understood by the peasants. Don't be anxious, they will understand everything, the orthodox heart will understand all! Let him read them about Abraham and Sarah, about Isaac and Rebecca, of how Jacob went to Laban and wrestled with the Lord in his dream and said, "This place is holy" — and he will impress the devout mind of the plain man. Let him read, especially to the children, how the brothers sold Joseph, the tender boy, the dreamer and prophet, into bondage, and told their father that a wild beast had devoured him, and showed him his blood-stained clothes. Let him read them how the brothers afterwards journeyed into Egypt for corn, and Joseph, already a great courtier, unrecognised by them, tormented them, accused them, kept his brothei Benjamin, and all through love: "I love you, and loving you I torment you." For he remembered all his life how they had sold him to the merchants there in the burning desert by the well, and how, wringing his hands, he had wept and besought his brothers not to sell him as a slave into a strange land. And how, seeing them again after many years, he loved them beyond measure, but he harassed and tormented them out of love. He left them at last not able to bear the suffering of his heart, flung himself on his bed and wept. Then, wiping his tears away, he went out to them joyful and told them, "Brothers, I am your brother Joseph!" Let him read them further how happy old Jacob was on learning that his darling boy was still alive, and how he journeyed to Egypt leaving his native land, and died in a strange country, uttering in his testament the great prophecy that had lain mysteriously hidden in his meek and timid heart all his life, to the effect that from his offspring, from Judah, would come the great hope of the world, its Messiah and Saviour.

Fathers and teachers, forgive me and don't be angry, because like a little child I've been babbling of what you have known for a long time, and can teach me a hundred times more skilfully. I only speak from rapture, and forgive my tears, for I love the Bible. Let him too weep, the priest of God, and be sure that the hearts of his listeners will throb in response. Only a little tiny seed is needed — drop it into the heart of the peasant and it won't die, it will live in his soul all his life, it will be hidden in the midst of his darkness and sin, like a bright spot, like a great reminder. And there's no need of much teaching or explanation, he will understand it all simply. Do you suppose that the peasants don't understand? Try reading them the touching story of the fair Esther and the haughty Vashti; or the miraculous story of Jonah in the whale. Don't forget either the parables of Our Lord, choose especially from the Gospel of St. Luke (that is what I did) and then from the Acts of the Apostles the conversion of Saul (that you mustn't leave out on any account), and from the "Lives of the Saints," for instance, the life of Alexey, the man of God and, greatest among the great, the joyful martyr, the seer of God and Christ-bearer, Mother Mary of Egypt — and you will pierce their hearts with these simple tales. Give one hour a week to it in spite of your poverty, only one little hour. And you will see for yourself that our people are gracious and grateful, and will repay you a hundredfold. Mindful of the kindness of their priest and the moving words they have heard from him, they will of their own accord help him in his fields and in his house, and will treat him with more respect than before — so that it will even increase his worldly well-being, too. The thing is so simple that sometimes one is even afraid to put it into words, for fear of being laughed at, and yet how true it is! One who does not believe in God will not believe in God's people. He who believes in God's people will see His Holiness, even though he had not believed in it till then. Only the people and their future spiritual power will convert our atheists, who have torn themselves away from their native soil.

And what good is Christ's word, unless we set an example? The masses are lost without the word of God, for their souls are athirst for the Word and for all that is beautiful.

In my youth, long ago, nearly forty years ago, I travelled all over Russia with Father Anfim, collecting alms for our monastery, and once we were benighted on the bank of a great navigable river and stayed with some fishermen there. And we were joined by a fine peasant lad, of about eighteen; he had to hurry off to work next morning, to tow a merchant's barge up the river. I noticed him looking straight before him with clear and loving eyes. It was a bright, warm, still July night, a cool mist rose from the broad river, we could hear the plash of a fish, the birds were still, all was hushed and beautiful, everything praying to God. Only we two were not sleeping, the lad and I, and we fell to talking of the beauty of this world of God's and of its great mystery. Every blade of grass, every insect, ant, and golden bee, all so marvellously know their path, though they have not intelligence, they bear witness to the mystery of God and continually accomplish it themselves. I saw the dear lad's heart was aflame. He told me that he loved the forest and the forest birds. He was a bird-catcher, knew the note of each of them, could call each bird. "I know nothing better than to be in the forest," said he, "though all things are good."

"Truly," I answered him, "all things are good and fair, because all is truth. Look," said I, "at the horse, that great beast that is so near to man; or the lowly, pensive ox, which feeds him and works for him; look at their faces, what meekness, what devotion to man, who often beats them mercilessly. What gentleness, what confidence and what beauty in its countenance! It's touching to know that there's no sin in them, for all, all except man, are sinless, and Christ has been with them before us."

"Why," asked the boy, "is Christ with them, too?"

"It cannot but be so," said I, "since the Word is for all. All creation and all creatures, every leaf is striving towards the Word, singing glory to God, crying to Christ, unwittingly accomplishing this by the mystery of their sinless life. Yonder," said I, "in the forest wanders the dread bear, fierce and menacing, and yet innocent in it. And I told him how once a bear came to a great saint who was saving his soul in a tiny cell in the wood. And the great saint felt tenderness towards him, went up to him without fear and gave him a piece of bread. "Go along," said he, "Christ be with you," and the savage beast walked away meekly and obediently, having done no harm. And the lad was touched to hear that the bear had walked away without hurting the saint, and that Christ was with him, too. "Ah," said he, "how good that is, how good and beautiful is all God's work!" He sat musing softly and sweetly. I saw he understood. And he slept beside me a light and sinless sleep. May God bless youth! And I prayed for him as I went to sleep. Lord, send peace and light to Thy people!

(c) Recollections of Father Zosima's youth before he became a monk. The duel

I spent a long time, almost eight years, in the Cadet Corps at Petersburg, and in the novelty of my surroundings there many of my childish impressions grew dimmer, though I forgot nothing. I picked up so many new habits and opinions that I was transformed into a cruel, absurd, almost savage creature. A surface polish of courtesy and society manners I did acquire, together with the French language, but we all, myself included, looked upon the soldiers in our service as the merest cattle. I was perhaps worse than the rest in that respect, for I was so much more impressionable than my companions. By the time we left the school as officers, we were ready to shed our blood for the honour of the regiment, but no one of us had any knowledge of the real meaning of honour, and if any one had come to know it, he would have been the first to ridicule it. Drunkenness, debauchery, and devilry were what we almost prided ourselves on. I don't say that we were bad by nature, all these young men were good fellows, but they behaved badly, and I worst of all. The main thing was that I found myself with money, and so I flung myself into a life of pleasure, and plunged into it headlong with all the recklessness of youth.

I was then fond of reading, yet, strange to say, the Bible was the one book I never opened at that time, though I always carried it about with me, and I was never separated from it; in very truth I was saving that book "for the day and the hour, for the month and the year," though I knew it not.

I had been in the service about four years when I chanced to be in the town of K., where our regiment was stationed at the time. The local society was varied, well-to-do, hospitable, and fond of entertainments. I met with a cordial reception everywhere, as I was of a lively temperament and was known to be well off, which always goes a long way in the world. And then a circumstance happened which was the beginning of it all.

I formed an attachment to a beautiful and intelligent young lady of serene nature and lofty character, the daughter of highly respected people. They were well-to-do people of influence and position. They always gave me a cordial and friendly reception. Well, I fancied that the young lady looked on me with favour and my heart was aflame at such an idea. Later on I saw and fully realised that I was perhaps not so passionately in love with her at all, but only respected her mind and lofty character, which I could not indeed have helped doing. I was prevented, however, from making her an offer at the time by my selfishness; I was loth to part with the allurements of my free and licentious bachelor life in the heyday of my youth, and with money in my pockets. I did drop some hint as to my feelings, however, though I put off taking any decisive step for a time. Then, all of a sudden, we were ordered off to another district.

On my return two months later, I found the young lady already married to a rich neighbouring landowner, a very amiable man, still young though older than I was, connected with the best Petersburg society, which I was not, and of excellent education, which I also lacked. I was so overwhelmed at this unexpected circumstance that my mind was positively clouded. The worst of it all was that, as I learnt then, the young landowner had been a long while betrothed to her, and I had met him indeed many times in her house, but blinded by my conceit I had noticed nothing. And this particularly mortified me; almost everybody had known all about it, while I knew nothing. I was filled with sudden irrepressible fury. With flushed face I began recalling how often I had been on the point of declaring my love to her, and as she had not attempted to stop me or to warn me, she must, I concluded, have been laughing at me all the time. Later on, of course, I reflected and remembered that she had been very far from laughing at me; on the contrary, she used to turn off any love-making on my part with a jest and begin talking of other subjects; but at that moment I was incapable of reflecting and was all eagerness for revenge. I remember with surprise that my wrath and revengeful feelings were extremely repugnant to my own nature, for being of an easy temper, I found it difficult to be angry with any one for long, and so I had to work myself up artificially and became at last revolting and absurd.

I bided my time and succeeded in insulting my "rival" at a large gathering on a perfectly extraneous pretext, jeering at his opinion upon an important public event — it was in the year 1826* — and my jibe was, so people said, clever and effective. Then I forced him to ask for an explanation, and behaved so rudely that he accepted my challenge in spite of the vast difference between us, as I was younger, a person of no consequence, and of inferior rank. I learnt afterwards for a fact that it was from a jealous feeling on his side also that he accepted my challenge; he had been rather jealous of me on his wife's account before their marriage; he fancied now that if he submitted to be insulted by me and refused to accept my challenge, and if she heard of it, she might begin to despise him and waver in her love for him. I soon found a second in a comrade, an ensign of our regiment. In those days though duels were severely punished, yet duelling was a kind of fashion among the officers — so strong and deeply rooted will a brutal prejudice sometimes be.

It was the end of June, and our meeting was to take place at seven o'clock in the morning the next day on the outskirts of the town — and then something happened that in very truth was the turning-point of my life. In the evening, returning home in a savage and brutal humour, I flew into a rage with my orderly Afanasy, and gave him two blows in the face with all my might, so that it bled. He had not been long in my service and I had struck him before, but never with such ferocious cruelty. And, believe me, though it's forty years ago, I recall it now with shame and pain. I went to bed and slept for about three hours; when I waked the day was breaking. I got up — I did not want to sleep any more — I went to the window — opened it, it looked out upon the garden; I saw the sun rising; it was warm and beautiful, the birds were trilling.

What's the meaning of it, I thought, why do I feel in my heart something vile and shameful, as it were? Is it because I am going to shed blood? No, I thought, I feel it's not that. Can it be that I am afraid of death, afraid of being killed? No, that's not it, that's not it at all. . . . And all at once I knew what it was: it was because I had struck Afanasy the evening before! It all rose before my mind, it all was, as it were, repeated over again; he stood before me and I was striking him straight on the face and he was holding his arms stiffly down, his head erect, his eyes fixed upon me as though on parade. He flinched at every blow and did not even dare to raise his hands to protect himself. That is what a man has been brought to, and that was a man beating a fellow creature! What a crime! It was as though a sharp needle had pierced me right through. I stood as if I were struck dumb, while the sun was shining, the leaves were

* The public event referred to was probably the conspiracy of December, 1825, in which many distinguished men were involved. *Translator's note.*

sparkling and rejoicing and the birds were praising God. . . . I hid my face in my hands, fell on my bed and broke into a storm of tears. And then I remembered my brother Markel and what he said on his deathbed to his servants: "My dear ones, why do you wait on me, why do you love me, am I worth your waiting on me?"

Yes, am I worth it? flashed through my mind. After all, what am I worth, that another man, a fellow creature, made in the likeness and image of God, should serve me? For the first time in my life this question forced itself upon me. He had said, "Mother, my darling little life, in truth we are each responsible to all for all, it's only that men don't know this. If they knew it, the world would be a paradise at once."

"God, can that too be false?" I thought as I wept; "in truth perhaps, I am more than all others responsible for all, a greater sinner than all men in the world." And all at once the whole truth in its full light appeared to me: what was I going to do? I was about to kill a good, intelligent, high-minded man, who had done me no wrong, and thus deprive his wife of happiness for ever, and torture and kill her, too. I lay thus in my bed with my face in the pillow, heedless how the time was passing. Suddenly my second, the ensign, came in with the pistols to fetch me.

"Ah," said he, "it's a good thing you are up already, it's time we were off, come along!"

I did not know what to do and flung myself this way and that undecided; we went out to the carriage, however.

"Wait here a minute," I said to him. "I'll be back directly, I have forgotten my purse."

And I ran back alone, straight to Afanasy's cubicle. "Afanasy," I said, "I struck you twice on the face yesterday. Forgive me," I begged.

He started as though he were frightened, and looked at me; and I saw that it was not enough, and on the spot, in my full regalia, I dropped at his feet and bowed my head to the ground. "Forgive me," I said.

Then he was completely aghast.

"Your honour . . . sir, what are you doing? Am I worth it?"

And he burst out crying as I had done before, hid his face in his hands, turned to the window and shook all over with his sobs. I flew out to my comrade and jumped into the carriage.

"Ready," I cried. "Have you ever seen a conqueror?" I asked him. "Here is one before you." I was in ecstasy, laughing and talking all the way, I don't remember what I said.

He looked at me. "Well, brother, you are a plucky fellow, you'll keep up the honour of the uniform, I can see."

So we reached the place and found them there, waiting for us. We were placed twelve paces apart; he had the first shot. I stood gaily, looking him full in the face; I did not twitch an eyelash, I looked lovingly at him, for I knew what I would do. His shot just grazed my cheek and ear.

"Thank God," I cried, "no man has been killed," and I seized my pistol, turned back and flung it far away into the wood. "That's the place for you," I cried.

I turned to my adversary.

"Forgive me, young fool that I am, sir," I said, "for my unprovoked insult to you and for forcing you to fire at me. I am ten times worse than you and more, may be. Tell that to the person whom you hold dearest in the world." I had no sooner said this than they all three shouted at me.

"Upon my word," cried my adversary, annoyed, "if you did not want to fight, why did you bother me?"

"Yesterday I was a fool, to-day I know better," I answered him gaily.

"As to yesterday, I believe you, but as for to-day, it is difficult to agree with your opinion," said he.

"Bravo," I cried, clapping my hands. "I agree with you there, too. I have deserved it!"

"Will you shoot, sir, or not?"

"No, I won't," I said, "if you like, fire at me again, but it would be better for you not to fire."

The seconds, especially mine, were shouting, too: "Can you disgrace the regiment like this, facing your antagonist and begging his forgiveness! If I'd only known this!"

I stood facing them all, not laughing now.

"Gentlemen," I said, "is it really so wonderful in these days to find a man who can repent of his stupidity and publicly confess his wrongdoing?"

"But not at the barrier," cried my second.

"That's what's so strange," I said. "For I ought to have owned my fault as soon as I got here, before he had fired a shot, before leading him into a great and deadly sin; but we have made our life so grotesque, that to act in that way would have been almost impossible, for only after I have faced his shot at the distance of twelve paces could my words have any significance for him, and if I had spoken before, he would have said, 'He is a coward, the sight of the pistols frightened him, no use listening to him.' Gentlemen," I cried suddenly, speaking straight from my heart, "look around you at the gifts of God, the clear sky, the pure air, the tender grass, the birds; nature is beautiful and sinless, and we, only we, are godless and foolish, and we don't understand that life is paradise, for we have only to understand that and it will at once be fulfilled in all its beauty, we shall embrace each other and weep."

I would have said more but I could not; my breath failed me with the sweetness and youthful gladness of it, and there was such bliss in my heart as I had never known before in my life.

"All this is sensible and edifying," said my antagonist, "and in any case you are an odd fellow."

"You may laugh," I said to him, laughing too, "but afterwards you will approve of me."

"Oh, I am ready to approve of you now," said he; "I will give you my hand, for I believe you are genuinely sincere."

"No," I said, "not now, later on when I have grown worthier and deserve your esteem, then give me your hand and you will do well."

We went home, my second upbraiding me all the way, while I kissed him. All my comrades heard of the affair at once and gathered together to pass judgment on me the same day.

"He has disgraced the uniform," they said; "let him tender his resignation."

Some stood up for me: "He faced the shot," they said.

"Yes, but he was afraid of the other shots and begged forgiveness at the barrier."

"If he had been afraid of shots, he would have fired his own pistol first before asking forgiveness, while instead he flung it loaded into the forest. No, there's something else in this, something original."

I enjoyed listening to and looking at them. "My dear friends and comrades," said I, "don't worry about my resigning my commission, for I have done so already. I have sent in my papers this morning and as soon as I get my discharge I shall go into a monastery — it's with that object I am leaving the regiment." When I had said this every one of them burst out laughing.

"You should have told us of that first, that explains everything, we can't try a monk."

They laughed and could not stop themselves, and not scornfully, but kindly and merrily. They all felt friendly to me at once, even those who had been sternest in their censure, and all the following month, until my discharge came, they could not make enough of me. "Ah, you monk," they would say. And every one said something kind to me, they began trying to dissuade me, even to pity me: "What are you doing to yourself?" "No," they would say, "he is a brave fellow, he faced the bullet and could have fired his own pistol, too, but he had a dream the night before that he should become a monk, that's why he did it."

Local society took it the same way. Till then I had been kindly received, but had not been the object of special attention, and now all took notice of me at once and extended invitations to me; they laughed at me, but they loved me. I may mention that although everybody talked openly of our duel, the authorities took no notice of it, because my antagonist was a near relation of our general, and as there had been no bloodshed and no serious consequences, and as I resigned my commission, they took it as a joke. And I began then to speak aloud and fearlessly, regardless of their laughter, for it was always kindly and not spiteful laughter. These conversations took place mostly in the evening, in the company of ladies; women particularly liked listening to me then and they made the men listen.

"But how can I possibly be responsible for all?" every one would laugh in my face. "Can I, for instance, be responsible for you?"

"You may well not know it," I would answer, "since the whole world has long been following a different road and since we consider the veriest lies as truth and demand the same lies from others. Here I have for once in my life acted sincerely and, well, you all look upon me as a saintly fool. Though you have come to love me, yet, you all laugh at me."

"But how can we help loving you?" said my hostess, laughing. The room was full of people. All of a sudden I saw arise the very young lady on whose account the duel had been fought and whom only lately I had intended to ask to be my wife. I had not noticed her coming into the room. She got up, came to me and held out her hand.

"Allow me to tell you," she said, "that I am the first who does not laugh at you, but on the contrary I thank you, with tears, and wish to say that I respect you for your action then."

Her husband, too, came up and then they all approached me and almost kissed me. My heart was filled with joy, but my attention was particularly attracted by a middle-aged man who came up to me with the others. I knew him by name already, but had never made his acquaintance nor exchanged a word with him till that evening.

(*d*) *The mysterious visitor*

He had long been an official in the town; he was wealthy, in a prominent position, respected by all, and had a reputation for benevolence. He subscribed considerable sums to the almshouse and the orphan asylum; he performed many acts of charity, too, in secret, a fact which became known only after his death. He was a man of about fifty, almost stern in appearance and not much given to conversation. He had been married about ten years and his wife, who was still young, had borne him three children. Well, I was sitting alone in my room the following evening, when my door suddenly opened and this gentleman walked in.

I must mention, by the way, that I was no longer living in my former quarters. As soon as I resigned my commission, I took rooms with an old lady, the widow of a government clerk. My landlady's servant waited upon me, for I had moved into her rooms simply because on my return from the duel I had sent Afanasy back to the regiment, as I felt ashamed to look him in the face after my last interview with him. So prone is the man of the world to be ashamed of any righteous action.

"I have listened to you," said my visitor, "with great interest when you were speaking in different houses the last few days, and I wanted at last to make your acquaintance personally so as to talk to you more fully. Can you, dear sir, grant me this favour?"

"I can, with the greatest pleasure, and I shall consider it a signal honour." I said this, though I felt almost dismayed, so greatly was I impressed from the first moment by the appearance of this man. For though other people had listened to me with interest and attention, no one had come to me before with such a serious, stern, and concentrated expression. And now he had come to see me in my own rooms. He sat down.

"You are, I see, a man of great strength of character," he said; "as you have dared to serve the truth, even when by doing so you risked incurring the contempt of all."

"Your praise is, perhaps, excessive."

"No, it's not excessive," he answered; "believe me, such a course of action is far more difficult than you think. It is that which has impressed me, and it is only on that account that I have come to you," he continued. "Tell me, please, that is if you are not annoyed by my perhaps unseemly curiosity, what were your exact sensations, if you can recall them, at the moment when you made up your mind to ask forgiveness at the duel. Do not think my question frivolous; on the contrary, in asking the question I have a secret motive of my own, which I will perhaps explain to you later on, if it is God's will that we should become more intimately acquainted."

All the while he was speaking, I was looking him straight in the face and I felt all at once a complete trust in him and great curiosity on my side also, for I felt that he was carrying some secret in his soul.

"You ask what were my exact sensations at the moment when I asked my opponent's forgiveness," I answered; "but I had better tell you from the beginning what I have not yet told any one else." And I described all that had passed between Afanasy and me, and how I had bowed down to the ground before him. "From that you can see for yourself," I concluded, "that at the time of the duel it was easier for me, for I had made a beginning already at home, and when once I had started on that road, to go further along it was far from being difficult, but became a source of joy and happiness."

I liked the way he looked at me as he listened. "All that," he said, "is exceedingly interesting, I will come to see you again and again."

And from that time forth he came to see me nearly every evening. And we should have become greater friends, if only he had talked of himself, too. But about himself he scarcely ever said a word, though he continued to question me about myself. In spite of that I became very fond of him and spoke with perfect frankness to him about all my feelings; for, thought I, what need have I to know his secrets, since I can see without that that he is a righteous man. Moreover, though he is such a serious man and my senior, he comes to see a youngster like me and doesn't look down on me. And I learnt many useful things from him, for he was a man of lofty mind.

"That life is paradise," he said to me suddenly, "I have been thinking for a long time"; and all at once he added, "indeed, I think of nothing else." He looked at me and smiled. "I am more convinced of it than you are, I will tell you later why."

I listened to him and thought that he evidently wanted to confide something to me.

"Paradise," he went on, "lies hidden within all of us — here it lies hidden in me now, and if I desire it, it will become a reality for me tomorrow and remain with me the rest of my life." I looked at him; he was speaking with great emotion and looking mysteriously at me, as if he were questioning me.

"And that each of us is responsible for all men and all things, apart from his own sins, you were quite right in thinking that, and it is wonderful how you could suddenly comprehend this thought in all its fulness. And in very truth, as soon as men understand this thought, the Kingdom of Heaven will be theirs, not in fancy, but in reality."

"And when," I cried out to him bitterly, "when will that come to pass? and will it ever come to pass? Is it not simply a dream of ours?"

"Look, already you don't believe it," he said. "You preach it and don't believe it yourself. Believe me, this dream, as you call it, will come true, without doubt; it will come true, but not now, for every process has its law. It's a matter of the soul, a psychological thing. To make the world over anew, men must turn into another path psychologically. Until you have become, in actual fact, a brother to every one, brotherhood will not come to pass. No sort of science, no kind of self-interest, will ever enable men to share their property and their rights with equal consideration for all. Every one will think his share too small and they will be always envying, complaining, and destroying one another. You ask when it will come to pass; it will come to pass, but first the period of human *isolation* must be concluded."

"What do you mean by isolation?" I asked him.

"Why, the isolation that prevails everywhere, above all in our age — it has not fully developed, it has not reached its limit yet. For nowadays every one strives to keep his individuality as distinct as possible, wishes to secure the greatest possible fulness of life for himself; but meantime all his efforts result not in fulness of life but in utter self-destruction, for instead of self-realisation he arrives at complete isolation. For in our age all mankind has split up into units, each withdraws into his own hole; each one holds aloof, hides himself and hides what he has, from the rest, and he ends by repelling others and being repelled by them. He heaps up riches in solitude and thinks, 'How strong I am now and how secure,' and in his folly he does not understand that the more he heaps up, the more he sinks into self-destructive impotence. For he is accustomed to rely upon himself alone and to cut himself off from the whole; he has trained his soul not to believe in the help of others, in men and in humanity, and only trembles for fear he should lose his money and the rights that he has won for himself. Everywhere in these days men have ceased to understand that the true security is to be found in social solidarity rather than in isolated individual effort. But this dreadful isolation must inevitably come to an end, and all will suddenly understand how unnaturally they are separated from one another. It will be the spirit of the time, and people will marvel that they have sat so long in darkness and did not see the light. And then the sign of the Son of Man will be seen in the heavens. . . . But, until then, we must guard the banner, and from time to time a man must set an example, even if it's only an isolated case, and so draw men's souls out of their solitude, and spur them to some act of brotherly communion, though it may be at the risk of appearing a saintly fool, and this to the end that the great idea may not die."

It was in such stirring and fervent talk that we spent our evenings, one after another. I gave up society and visited my friends much less frequently. Besides, my vogue was somewhat over. I say this, not in blame, for they still loved me and treated me good-humouredly, but there's no denying that fashion is a great power in society. I began to regard my mysterious visitor with deep admiration, for besides enjoying his intelligence, I began to perceive that he was brooding over some plan in his heart, and was preparing himself perhaps for a great deed. Perhaps he liked my not showing curiosity about his secret, not seeking to discover it by direct question nor by hints. But I noticed at last that he was himself fretted by the desire to open his heart to me. This had become quite evident, indeed, about a month after he first began to visit me.

"Do you know," he said to me once, "that people are very curious about us in the town and wonder why I come to see you so often. But let them wonder, for *soon all will be explained*."

Sometimes an extraordinary agitation would come over him, and almost always on such occasions he would get up and go away. Sometimes he would fix a long piercing look upon me, and I thought "He will say something directly now." But he would suddenly change the subject and speak of something ordinary and familiar. He often complained of headache, too.

One day, quite unexpectedly indeed, after he had been talking with great fervour a long time, I saw him suddenly turn pale, and his face worked convulsively, while he stared persistently at me.

"What's the matter?" I said; "do you feel ill?"—he had just been complaining of headache.

"I . . . do you know . . . I killed a human being."

He said this and smiled with a face as white as chalk. "Why is it he is smiling?" The thought flashed through my mind before I realised anything else. I, too, turned pale.

"What are you saying?" I cried.

"You see," he said, with a pale smile, "how much it has cost me to say the first word. Now I have said it, I feel I've taken the first step and shall go on."

For a long while I could not believe him, and I did not believe him at that time, but only after he had been to see me three days running and told me about it in detail. I thought he was mad, but ended by being convinced, to my great grief and amazement. His crime was a great and terrible one.

Fourteen years before, he had murdered the widow of a landowner, a wealthy and handsome young woman who had a house in our town. He had fallen passionately in love with her, declared himself and tried to persuade her to marry him. But she had already given her heart to another, a military man of noble birth and high rank in the service, who was at that time away at the front, and whom she expected to return soon. She refused his offer and asked him to stop calling on her. After he had ceased to visit her, he took advantage of his knowledge of the house to enter at night through the garden by the roof, with extreme boldness at the risk of being discovered. But as often happens, crimes committed with extraordinary audacity are the ones to be carried out successfully.

Entering the garret through the dormer window, he went down the ladder, knowing that the door at the bottom of it was sometimes, through the negligence of the servants, left unlocked. He hoped to find it so, and so it was. He made his way in the dark to her bedroom, where a light was burning before an ikon. As though on purpose, both her maids had gone off to a birthday-party in the neighbourhood, without asking leave. The other servants slept in the servants' quarters and in the kitchen on the ground-floor. His passion flamed up at the sight of her asleep, and then vindictive, jealous anger took possession of his heart, and like a drunken man, beside himself, he thrust a knife into her heart, so that she did not even cry out. Then with devilish and criminal cunning he contrived that suspicion should fall on the servants. He did not disdain to take her purse, to open her chest with keys which he drew from under her pillow, and to take some things from it, doing it all as it might have been done by an ignorant servant, that is, he left valuable papers and took only money, carried off some of the larger gold things, but left smaller articles that were ten times as valuable. He took with him, too, some things for himself as remembrances, but of that later. Having done this awful deed, he returned by the way he had come.

Neither the next day, when the alarm was raised, nor at any time after in his life, did any one dream of suspecting that he was the criminal. No one indeed knew of his love for her, for he was always reserved and uncommunicative and had no friend to whom he would have opened his heart. He was looked upon simply as an acquaintance, and not a very intimate one, of the murdered woman, all the more so since he had not even visited her during the fortnight before the murder. A serf of hers called Pyotr was at once suspected, and every circumstance confirmed the suspicion. The man knew — indeed his mistress had not concealed the fact — that having to send one of her serfs as a recruit she had decided to send him, as he had no family and, furthermore, his conduct was unsatisfactory. People had heard him angrily threatening to murder her when he was drunk in a pot-house. Two days before her death, he had run away, staying no one knew where in the town. The day after the murder, he was found on the road leading out of the town, dead drunk, with a knife in his pocket and his right hand happened to be stained with blood. He declared that his nose had been bleeding, but no one believed him. The maids confessed that they had gone to a party and that the street-door had been left open till they returned. And a number of similar details came to light, throwing suspicion on the innocent servant.

They arrested him, and he was tried for the murder; but a week after the arrest, the prisoner fell sick of a fever and died unconscious in the hospital. There the matter ended and was left to the will of God, while the judges and the authorities and every one in the town remained convinced that the crime had been committed by no one but the servant who had died in the hospital. And after that the punishment began for the real criminal.

My mysterious visitor, now my friend, told me that at first he was not in the least troubled by pangs of conscience. He was miserable a long time, but not for that reason; only from regret that he had killed the woman he loved, that she was no more, that in killing her he had killed his love, while the fire of passion was still in his veins. But of the innocent blood he had shed, of the murder of a fellow creature, he scarcely thought. The thought that his victim might have become the wife of another man was insupportable to him, and so, for a long time, he was convinced in his conscience that he could not have acted otherwise.

At first he was worried at the arrest of the servant, but his illness and death soon set his mind at rest, for the man's death was apparently (so he reflected at the time) not owing to his arrest or his fright, but to a chill he had taken on the day he ran away, when he had lain all night dead drunk on the damp ground. The theft of the money and other things troubled him little, for he argued that the theft had not been committed for gain but to avert suspicion. The sum stolen was small, and he shortly afterwards subscribed the whole of it, and much more, towards the funds for maintaining an almshouse in the town. He did this on purpose to set his conscience at rest about the theft, and it's a remarkable fact that for a long time he really was at peace — he told me this himself. He entered then upon a career of great activity in the service, volunteered for a difficult and laborious task, which occupied him two years, and being a man of strong will almost forgot the past. Whenever he recalled it, he tried not to think of it at all. He became active in philanthropy, too, founded and helped maintain many institutions in the town, did a good deal in the two capitals, and in both Moscow and Petersburg was elected a member of charitable societies.

At last, however, he began brooding over the past, and the strain of it was too much for him. Then he was attracted by a fine and intelligent girl and soon after married her, hoping that marriage would dispel his loneliness and depression, and that by entering on a new life and scrupulously doing his duty towards his wife and children, he would escape from old memories altogether. But the very opposite of what he expected happened. He began, even in the first month of his marriage, to be continually fretted by the thought, "My wife loves me — but what if she knew?" When she became pregnant with their first child, and told him of it, he was troubled: "I am giving life, but I have taken life." Children came. "How dare I love them, teach and educate them, how can I talk to them of virtue? I have shed blood." They were splendid children, he longed to caress them; "and I can't look at their innocent candid faces, I am unworthy."

At last he began to be bitterly and ominously haunted by the blood of his murdered victim, by the young life he had destroyed, by the blood that cried out for vengeance. He had begun to have terrifying dreams. But, being a man of fortitude, he bore his suffering a long time, thinking: "I shall expiate everything by this secret agony of mine." But that hope, too, was vain; the longer it went on, the more intense was his suffering.

He was respected in society for his active benevolence, though every one feared him because of his stern and gloomy character. But the more he was respected, the more intolerable it was for him. He confessed to me that he had had thoughts of killing himself. But he began to be haunted by another idea — an idea which he had at first regarded as impossible and insane, but at last it got such a hold on his heart that he could not shake it off. He dreamed of rising up, going out and confessing in the face of all men that he had committed murder. For three years this dream had pursued him, haunting him in different forms. At last he believed with his whole heart that if he confessed his crime, he would cure his soul and would be at peace for ever. But this belief filled his heart with terror, for how could he carry it out? And then suddenly came my duel. "With your example before me, I have now made up my mind."

I looked at him.

"Is it possible," I cried, striking my hands together, "that such a trivial incident should move you to such a resolution?"

"My resolution took three years to mature," he answered, "and your act only gave the last touch to it. Looking at you, I reproached myself and envied you." He said this to me almost sullenly.

"But you won't be believed," I observed; "fourteen years have elapsed."

"I have proofs, great proofs. I shall submit them." Then I cried and kissed him.

"Tell me one thing, one thing," he said (as though it all depended upon me), "my wife, my children! My wife may die of grief, and though my children won't lose their rank and property, they'll be a convict's children, and for ever! And what a memory, what a memory of me I shall leave in their hearts!"

I said nothing.

"And to part from them, to leave them for ever? It's for ever, you know, for ever!"

I sat still and repeated a silent prayer. I got up at last, I felt afraid.

"Well?" He looked at me.

"Go!" said I, "confess. Everything passes, only the truth remains. Your children will understand, when they grow up, the nobility of your great resolution."

He left me that time as though he had made up his mind. Yet for more than a fortnight afterwards, he came to me every evening, still preparing himself, still unable to bring himself to the point. He made my heart ache. One day he would come in a determined mood and say fervently:

"I know it will be heaven for me, heaven, the moment I confess. Fourteen years I've been in hell. I want to suffer. I will accept my suffering and begin to live. You can travel to the end of the world on lies, but they won't carry you back again. Now I dare not love my neighbour nor even my own children. Good God, my children will understand, perhaps, what my suffering was and will not condemn me! God is not in might but in truth."

"All will understand your high deed," I said to him, "if not at once, they will understand later; for you have served truth, the higher truth, not of this earth."

And he would go away seeming comforted, but next day he would come again, bitter, pale, sarcastic.

"Every time I come to you, you look at me so inquisitively, as though to say, 'He has still not confessed!' Wait a bit, don't despise me too much. It's not such an easy thing to do, as you would think. Perhaps I shall not do it at all. You won't go and inform against me then, will you?"

And far from looking at him with indiscreet curiosity, I was afraid to look at him at all. I was quite ill with it all, and my heart was full of tears. I could not sleep at night.

"I have just come from my wife," he went on. "Do you understand what the word 'wife' means? When I went out, the children called to me, 'Good-bye, father, make haste back to read "The Children's Magazine" with us.' No, you don't understand that! No one grows wise through another man's woe."

His eyes were glittering, his lips were twitching. Suddenly he struck the table with his fist so that everything on it danced — it was the first time he had done such a thing, he was such a mild man.

"But need I?" he exclaimed, "must I? No one has been condemned, no one has been sent to Siberia in my place, the man died of fever. And I've been punished by my sufferings for the blood I shed. And I shan't be believed, they won't believe my proofs. Need I confess, need I? I am ready to go on suffering all my life for the blood I have shed, if only my wife and children may be spared. Will it be just to ruin them with me? Aren't we making a mistake? What is right in this case? And will people recognise it, will they appreciate it, will they respect it?"

"Good Lord!" I thought to myself, "he is thinking of other people's respect at such a moment!" And I felt so sorry for him then, that I believe I would have shared his fate if it could have comforted him. I saw he was beside himself. I was aghast, realising with my heart as well as my mind what such a resolution meant.

"Decide my fate!" he exclaimed again.

"Go and confess," I whispered to him. My voice failed me, but I whispered it firmly. I took up the New Testament from the table, the Russian translation, and showed him the Gospel of St. John, ch. xii. verse 24:

"Verily, verily, I say unto you, except a corn of wheat fall into the ground and die, it abideth alone: but if it die, it bringeth forth much fruit." I had just been reading that verse when he came in. He read it.

"That's true," he said, but he smiled bitterly. "It's terrible the things you find in those books," he said, after a pause. "It's easy enough to thrust them upon one. And who wrote them? Can they have been written by men?"

"The Holy Ghost wrote them," said I.

"It's easy for you to prate." He smiled again, this time almost with hatred.

I took the book again, opened it in another place and showed him the Epistle to the Hebrews, ch. x. verse 31. He read:

"It is a fearful thing to fall into the hands of the living God."

He read it and simply flung down the book. He was trembling all over.

"A terrible text," he said. "There's no denying you've picked out fitting ones." He rose from the chair. "Well!" he said, "good-bye, perhaps I shan't come again . . . we shall meet in heaven. So I have been for fourteen years 'in the hands of the living God,' that's how one must think of those fourteen years. To-morrow I will beseech those hands to let me go." I wanted to take him in my arms and kiss him, but I did not dare — his face was contorted and sombre. He went away.

"Good God," I thought, "what has he gone to face!" I fell on my knees before the ikon and wept for him before the Holy Mother of God, our swift defender and helper. I was half an hour praying in tears, and it was late, about midnight. Suddenly I saw the door open and he came in again. I was surprised.

"Where have you been?" I asked him.

"I think," he said, "I've forgotten something . . . my handkerchief, I think. . . . Well, even if I've not forgotten anything, let me stay a little."

He sat down. I stood over him.

"You sit down, too," said he.

I sat down. We sat still for two minutes; he looked intently at me and suddenly smiled — I remember that — then he got up, embraced me warmly and kissed me.

"Remember," he said, "how I came to you a second time. Do you hear, remember it!"

And he went out.

"To-morrow," I thought.

And so it was. I did not know that evening that the next day was his birthday. I had not been out for the last few days so I had no chance of hearing it from any one. On that day he always had a great gathering, every one in the town went to it. It was the same this time. After dinner he walked into the middle of the room, with a paper in his hand — a formal declaration to his superior, who was present. This declaration he read aloud to the whole assembly. It contained a full account of the crime, with every detail.

"I cut myself off from men as a monster. God has visited me," he said in conclusion. "I want to suffer for my sin!"

Then he brought out and laid on the table all the things he had been keeping for fourteen years, that he thought would prove his crime, the jewels belonging to the murdered woman which he had stolen to divert suspicion, a cross and a locket taken from her neck with a portrait of her betrothed in the locket, her notebook and two letters; one from her betrothed, telling her that he would soon be with her, and her unfinished answer left on the table to be sent off next day. He had carried off these two letters — what for? Why had he kept them for fourteen years afterwards instead of destroying them as evidence against him?

And this is what happened: every one was amazed and horrified, every one refused to believe it and thought that he was deranged, though all listened with intense curiosity. A few days later it was fully decided and agreed upon in every house that the unhappy man had lost his mind. The legal authorities could not refuse to take up the case, but they, too, dropped it. Though the trinkets and letters made them ponder, they decided that even if they did turn out to be authentic, no final conviction could be obtained on the basis of this evidence alone. Besides, she might have given him those things for safe-keeping as a friend. I heard afterwards, however, that the genuineness of the things was proved by the friends and relations of the murdered woman, and that there was no doubt about them. Yet nothing was destined to come of it, after all.

Five days later, all had heard that he was ill and that his life was in danger. The nature of his illness I can't explain, they said it was an affection of the heart. But it became known that the doctors had been induced by his wife to investigate his mental condition also, and had come to the conclusion that it was a case of insanity. I betrayed nothing, though people ran to question me. But when I wanted to visit him, I was for a long while forbidden to do so, above all by his wife.

"It's you who have caused his illness," she said to me; "he was always gloomy, but for the last year people noticed that he was peculiarly excited and did strange things, and now you have been the ruin of him. Your preaching has brought him to this; for the last month he was always with you."

Indeed, not only his wife but the whole town were down upon me and blamed me. "It's all your doing," they said. I was silent and indeed rejoiced at heart, for I saw plainly God's mercy to the man who had turned against himself and punished himself. I could not believe in his insanity.

They let me see him at last, he insisted upon saying good-bye to me. I went in to him and saw at once that not only his days, but his hours were numbered. He was weak, yellow, his hands trembled, he gasped for breath, but his face was full of tender and happy feeling.

"It is done!" he said. "I've long been yearning to see you, why didn't you come?"

I did not tell him that they would not let me see him.

"God has had pity on me and is calling me to Himself. I know I am dying, but I feel joy and peace for the first time after so many years. There was heaven in my heart from the moment I had done what I had to do. Now I dare to love my children and to kiss them. Neither my wife nor the judges, nor any one has believed it. My children will never believe it either. I see in that God's mercy to them. I shall die, and my name will be without a stain for them. And now I feel God near, my heart rejoices as in heaven. . . . I have done my duty."

He could not speak, he gasped for breath, he pressed my hand warmly, looking fervently at me. We did not talk long, his wife kept peeping in at us. But he had time to whisper to me:

"Do you remember how I came back to you that second time, at midnight? I told you to remember it. You know what I came back for? I came to kill you!"

I started.

"I went out from you then into the darkness, I wandered about the streets, struggling with myself. And suddenly I hated you so that I could hardly bear it. Now, I thought, he is all that binds me, and he is my judge. I can't refuse to face my punishment to-morrow, for he knows all. It was not that I was afraid you would betray me (I never even thought of that) but I thought, 'How can I look him in the face if I don't confess?' And if you had been at the other end of the earth, but alive, it would have been all the same, the thought was unendurable that you were alive knowing everything and condemning me. I hated you as though you were the cause, as though you were to blame for everything. I came back to you then, remembering that you had a dagger lying on your table. I sat down and asked you to sit down, and for a whole minute I pondered. If I had killed you, I should have been ruined by that murder even if I had not confessed the other. But I didn't think that at all, and I didn't want to think of it at that moment. I only hated you and longed to revenge myself on you for everything. But the Lord vanquished the devil in my heart. But let me tell you, you were never nearer death."

A week later he died. The whole town followed him to the grave. The chief priest made a speech full of feeling. All lamented the terrible illness that had cut short his days. But all the town was up in arms against me after the funeral, and people even forbade me the house. Some, at first a few and afterwards more, began indeed to believe in the truth of his story, and they visited me and questioned me with great interest and eagerness, for man loves to see the downfall and disgrace of the righteous.

But I held my tongue, and very shortly after, I left the town, and five months later by God's grace I entered upon the safe and blessed path, praising the unseen finger which had guided me so clearly to it. But I remember in my prayer to this day the servant of God, Mihail, who suffered so greatly.

CHAPTER III

FROM THE CONVERSATIONS AND EXHORTATIONS OF FATHER ZOSIMA

(e) Concerning the Russian monk and his possible significance

FATHERS and teachers, what is a monk? In the cultivated world the word is nowadays pronounced by some people with a jeer, and by others it is used as a term of abuse, and this contempt for the monk is growing. It is true, alas, it is true, that there are many idlers, gluttons, lechers, and insolent beggars among monks. Men of the world point to these: "You are idlers, useless members of society, you live on the labour of others, you are shameless beggars."

And yet how many there are among the monks who are meek and humble, and who yearn for solitude and fervent prayer in peace. These are less noticed, or passed over in silence. And how surprised men would be if I were to say that from these meek monks, who yearn for solitary prayer, the salvation of Russia will come perhaps once more. For they are in truth prepared in peace and quiet "for the day and the hour, the month and the year." Meanwhile, in their solitude, they keep the image of Christ fair and undefiled, in the purity of God's truth, from the times of the Fathers of old, the Apostles and the martyrs. And when the time comes they will show it to the tottering truth of the world. That is a great thought. That star will shine forth out of the East.

That is my view of the monk, and is it false? is it too haughty? Look at the worldly and all who set themselves up above the people of God, has not God's image and His truth been distorted in them? They have science; but in science there is nothing but what is subject to the senses. The spiritual world, the higher part of man's being, is rejected altogether, banished with a sort of triumph, even with hatred. The world has proclaimed freedom, especially of late, but what do we see in this freedom of theirs? Nothing but slavery and self-destruction! For the world says: "You have wants and so satisfy them, for you have the same rights as the most rich and powerful. Don't be afraid of satisfying them and even multiply your wants." That is the modern doctrine of the world. In that they see freedom. And what follows from this right of multiplication of wants? In the rich, isolation and spiritual suicide; in the poor, envy and murder; for they have been given rights, but have not been shown the means of satisfying their wants. It is maintained that the world is becoming more and more united, more and more bound together in brotherly community, as it overcomes distance and transmits thoughts through the air.

Alas, put no faith in such a way of uniting

men. Interpreting freedom as the multiplication and rapid satisfaction of desires, men distort their own nature, for they thus engender in themselves many senseless and foolish desires and habits and most absurd fancies. They live only for mutual envy, for the lusts of the flesh and ostentation. To have dinners, visits, carriages, rank, and slaves to wait on one is looked upon as a necessity, for which life, honour, and human feeling are sacrificed, and men even commit suicide if they are unable to satisfy this craving. We see the same thing among those who are not rich, while the poor drown their unsatisfied wants and their envy in drink. But soon they will drink blood instead of wine, they are being led on to it. I ask you is such a man free? I knew one "champion of ideas" who told me himself that, when he was deprived of tobacco in prison, he was made so wretched by the privation that he almost went and betrayed his cause for the sake of getting tobacco again! And such a man says, "I am fighting in the cause of humanity."

How can such a one fight, what is he fit for? He is capable perhaps of some rash action, but he has no endurance. And it's no wonder that instead of gaining freedom they have sunk into slavery, and instead of serving the cause of brotherly love and the union of men have fallen, on the contrary, into disunion and isolation, as my mysterious visitor and teacher said to me in my youth. And therefore the idea of the service of humanity, of brotherly love and the solidarity of mankind, is more and more dying out in the world, and indeed this idea is sometimes treated with derision. For how can a man shake off his habits, whither shall this slave go, if he is so habituated to satisfying the innumerable wants which he has himself invented? He is isolated, and what concern has he with the rest of humanity? They have managed to accumulate a greater number of things, but the joy in the world has grown less.

The monastic way is very different. Obedience, fasting, and prayer are laughed at, yet only through them lies the way to real, true freedom. I cut off my superfluous and unnecessary wants, I subdue my proud and wanton will and chastise it with obedience, and with God's help I attain freedom of spirit and therewith spiritual joy. Which of the two is more capable of conceiving a great idea and serving it — the rich man in his isolation or the man who has freed himself from the tyranny of material things and habits? The monk is reproached for his solitude, "You have secluded yourself within the walls of the monastery for your own salvation, and have forgotten the brotherly service of humanity!" But we shall see which will be most zealous in the cause of brotherly love. For it is not we, but they, who are in isolation, though they don't see that. Even in the olden days, leaders of the people came from among us, and why should they not again? The same meek and humble ascetics will rise up and go out to work for the great cause. From the people comes the salvation of Russia. And the Russian monastery has always been on the side of the people. We are isolated only if the people are isolated. The people believe as we do, and an unbelieving reformer will never do anything in Russia, even if he is sincere in heart and a genius. Remember that! The people will meet the atheist and overcome him, and Russia will be one and orthodox. Take care of the peasant and guard his heart. Educate him quietly. That's your duty as monks, for this is a God-bearing people.

(*f*) *Of masters and servants, and of whether it is possible for them to be brothers in the spirit*

Of course, I don't deny that there is sin in the people, too. And the fire of corruption is spreading visibly, hourly, working from above downwards. The spirit of isolation is coming upon the people, too. Exploiters and oppressors are rising up. Already the merchant grows more and more eager for honours, and strives to show himself cultured though he has not a trace of culture, and to this end meanly despises his old traditions, and is even ashamed of the faith of his fathers. He visits princes, though he is only a peasant, spoiled. The people are rotting with drunkenness and cannot shake off the habit. And what cruelty to their wives, to their children even! All because of drunkenness! I've seen in the factories children nine years old, frail, rickety, bent, and already depraved. The stuffy work-room, the din of machinery, work all day long, the vile language and the drink, the drink — is that what a little child's heart needs? He needs sunshine, childish play, good examples all about him, and at least a little love. There must be no more of this, monks, no more torturing of children, rise up and preach that, make haste, make haste!

But God will save Russia, for though the masses are corrupted and cannot renounce their filthy sin, yet they know it is cursed by God and that they do wrong in sinning. So that our people still believe in righteousness, have faith in God and weep tears of devotion.

It is different with the upper classes. They, following science, want to base a just social order on reason alone, without the help of Christ, as before, and they have already proclaimed that there is no crime, that there is no sin. And that's consistent, for if you have no God, what is the meaning of crime? In Europe the people are already rising up against the rich with violence, and the leaders of the masses are everywhere leading them to bloodshed, and teaching them that their wrath is righteous. But their "wrath is accursed, for it is cruel." But God will save Russia as He has saved her many times. Salvation will come from the people, from their faith and their meekness.

Fathers and teachers, watch over the people's faith and this is not a vain dream. I've been struck all my life by the dignity, the true and seemly dignity, of our great people. I've seen it myself, I can testify to it, I've seen it and marvelled at it, I've seen it in spite of the degraded sins and poverty-stricken appearance of our peasantry. They are not servile, and even after two centuries of serfdom, they are free in manner and bearing, yet without insolence, and not revengeful and not envious. "You are rich and noble, you are clever and talented, well, be so, God bless you. I honour you, but I know that I, too, am a man. By the very fact that I honour you without envy I prove my dignity as a man."

In truth if they don't say this (for they don't know how to say this yet) that is how they act. I have seen it myself, I have experienced it myself, and, would you believe it, the poorer our Russian peasant is, the more noticeable is his seemliness and dignity, for the rich exploiters among them are for the most part corrupted already, and much of that is due to our carelessness and indifference. But God will save His people, for Russia is great in her humility. I dream of seeing, and seem to see clearly already, our future. It will come to pass that even the most corrupt of our rich will end by being ashamed of his riches before the poor, and the poor, seeing his humility, will understand and give way before him, will respond joyfully and kindly to his seemly shame. Believe me that it will end in that; things are moving in that direction. Equality is to be found only in the spiritual dignity of man, and that will only be understood among us. If we were brothers, there would be fraternity, but before that, they will never agree about the division of wealth.

We preserve the image of Christ, and it will shine forth like a precious diamond to the whole world. So be it, so be it!

Fathers and teachers, I had a touching experience once. In my wanderings I met in the city of K. my old orderly, Afanasy. It was eight years since I had parted from him. He chanced to see me in the market-place, recognised me, ran up to me, and how delighted he was, he simply rushed at me: "Master, father, is it you? is it really you I see?" He took me home with him.

He was no longer in the army, he was married and already had two little children. He and his wife earned their living as costermongers in the market-place. His room was poor, but bright and clean.

He made me sit down, set the samovar, sent for his wife, as though my appearance were a festival for them. He brought me his children; "Bless them, father."

"Is it for me to bless them, I say, I am only a simple, humble monk. I will pray to God for them. And for you, Afanasy Pavlovich, I have prayed every day since that day, for it all began with you," said I. And I explained that to him as well as I could. And what do you think? The man kept gazing at me and could not believe that I, his former master, an officer, was now before him in such a guise and garb; it made him weep.

"Why are you weeping?" said I, "better rejoice over me, dear friend, whom I can never forget, for my path is a glad and joyful one."

He did not say much, but kept sighing and shaking his head over me tenderly.

"What has become of your fortune?"

"I gave it to the monastery," I answered; "we live in common."

After tea I began saying good-bye, and suddenly he brought out half a rouble as an offering to the monastery, and another half-rouble I saw him thrusting hurriedly into my hand: "That's for you in your wanderings, it may be of use to you, father."

I took his half-rouble, bowed to him and his wife, and went out rejoicing. And on my way I thought: "Here we are both now, he at home and I on the road, sighing and shaking our heads, no doubt, and yet smiling joyfully in the gladness of our hearts, remembering how God brought about our meeting."

I have never seen him again since then. I had been his master and he my servant, but now when we kissed each other, lovingly and with spiritual emotion, a great human bond sprang up between us. I have thought a great deal about that, and now what I think is this: is it so inconceivable that that grand and simple-hearted unity might in due time become universal among the Russian people? I believe that it will come to pass and that the time is at hand.

And of servants I will add this, in former days when I was young I was often angry with servants: "the cook had served something too hot, the orderly had not brushed my clothes properly." But what enlightened me then was a thought of my dear brother's, which I had heard from him in childhood: "Am I worth it, that another should serve me and be ordered about by me because of his poverty and ignorance?" And I wondered at the time that such simple and self-evident ideas should be so slow to occur to our minds.

It is impossible that there should be no servants in the world, but act so that your servant may be freer in spirit than if he were not a servant. And why cannot I be a servant to my servant, and even let him see it, and that without any pride on my part or any mistrust on his? Why should not my servant be like my own kindred, so that I may take him into my family and rejoice in doing so? Even now this can be done, but it will lead to the magnificent union of men in the future, when a man will not seek servants for himself, or desire to turn his fellow creatures into servants as he does now, but, on the contrary, will long with his whole heart to be the servant of all, as the Gospel teaches.

And can it be a dream, that in the end man will find his joy only in deeds of enlightenment and mercy, and not in cruel pleasures as now, in gluttony, fornication, ostentation, boasting, and envious vying of one with the other? I firmly believe that it is not, and that the time is at hand. People laugh and ask: "When will that time come, and does it look as though it were coming?" I believe that with Christ's help we shall accomplish this great task. And how many ideas there have been on earth in the history of man which were unthinkable ten years before they appeared! Yet when their destined hour arrived, they came forth and spread over the whole earth. So it will be with us, and our people will shine forth in the world, and all men will say:

"The stone which the builders rejected has become the corner-stone of the building."

And we may ask the scornful themselves: if our hope is a dream, when will you build up your edifice and order things justly by your intellect alone, without Christ? If they declare that it is they who are advancing towards union, only the most simple-hearted among them believe it, so that one may positively marvel at such simplicity. Of a truth, their dreams are more fantastic than ours. They aim at a just order, but, having rejected Christ, they will end by flooding the earth with blood, for blood cries out for blood, and he that taketh the sword shall perish with the sword. And if it were not for Christ's promise, they would slaughter one another down to the last two men on earth. And those two last men would not be able to restrain each other in their pride, and the one would slay the other and then himself. And that would come to pass, were it not for the promise of Christ that for the sake of the humble and meek the time shall be shortened.

While I was still wearing an officer's uniform after my duel, I talked about servants in society, and I remember every one was amazed at me: "What!" they asked, "are we to make our servants sit down on the sofa and offer them tea?" And I answered them: "Why not, sometimes at least." Every one laughed. Their question was frivolous and my answer was not clear; but I believe there was some truth in it.

(g) *Of prayer, of love, and of contact with other worlds*

Young man, be not forgetful of prayer. Every time you pray, if your prayer is sincere, there will be new feeling and new meaning in it, which will give you fresh courage, and you will understand that prayer is an education.

Remember, too, every day, and whenever you can, repeat to yourself, "Lord, have mercy on all who have appeared before Thee to-day." For every hour and every moment thousands of men leave life on this earth, and their souls appear before the Lord. And how many of them depart in solitude, unknown, sad, dejected, because no one mourns for them or even knows whether they have lived or not. And behold, from the other end of the earth perhaps, your prayer for their rest will rise up to God though you knew them not nor they you. How touching it must be to a soul standing in dread before the Lord to feel at that instant that, for him, too, there is one to pray, that there is a fellow creature left on earth to love him, too. And God will look on you both more graciously, for if you have had so much pity on him, how much more will He have pity Who is infinitely more loving and merciful than you. And He will forgive him for your sake.

Brothers, have no fear of men's sin. Love a man even in his sin, for that is the semblance of Divine Love and is the highest love on earth. Love all God's creation, the whole and every grain of sand in it. Love every leaf, every ray of God's light. Love the animals, love the plants, love everything. If you love everything, you will perceive the divine mystery in things. Once you perceive it, you will begin to comprehend it better every day. And you will come at last to love the whole world with an all-embracing universal love. Love the animals: God has given them the rudiments of thought and unclouded joy. Do not trouble it, don't harass them, don't deprive them of their happiness, don't work against God's intent. Man, do not consider yourself superior to the animals; they are without sin, and you, with your greatness, defile the earth by your appearance on it, and leave the traces of your foulness after you — alas, it is true of almost every one of us! Love children especially, for they, too, are sinless, like the angels; they live to soften and purify our hearts and as it were to guide us. Woe to him who offends a child! Father Anfim taught me to love children. The kind, silent man used often on our wanderings to spend the farthings given us on sweets and cakes for the children. He could not pass by a child without emotion, that was the nature of the man.

At some thoughts one stands perplexed, especially at the sight of men's sin, and wonders whether one should use force or humble love. Always decide to use humble love. If you resolve on that once for all, you may subdue the whole world. Loving humility is a mighty force, the strongest of all things and there is nothing else like it.

Every day and every hour, every minute, walk round yourself and watch yourself, and see that your image be seemly. You pass by a little child, you pass by, spiteful, with ugly words, with wrathful heart; you may not have noticed the child, but he has seen you, and your image, unseemly and impious, may remain in his defenceless heart. You don't know it, but you may have sown an evil seed in him and it may grow, and all because you were not careful before the child, because you did not foster in yourself a circumspect, actively benevolent love. Brothers, love is a teacher; but one must know how to acquire it, for it is hard to acquire, it is dearly bought, it is won slowly by long labour. For we must love not only occasionally, for a moment, but for all time. Every one can love occasionally, even the wicked can.

My brother used to ask the birds to forgive him; that sounds senseless, but it is right; for all is like the ocean, all things flow and touch each other; a disturbance in one place is felt at the other end of the world. It may be folly to beg forgiveness of the birds, but birds would be happier at your side — a little happier, anyway — and children and all animals, if you yourself were nobler than you are now. It's all like an ocean, I tell you. Then you would pray to the birds, too, consumed by an all-embracing love, in a sort of transport, and pray that they will forgive you your sin. Prize this ecstasy, however senseless it may seem to men.

My friends, pray to God for gladness. Be merry as children, as the birds of heaven. And let not the sin of men confound you in your doings. Fear not that it will erase your work and hinder its being accomplished. Do not say, "Sin is mighty, wickedness is mighty, evil environment is mighty, and we are lonely and helpless, evil environment will overwhelm us and hinder our good work from being done." Fly from that dejection, children! There is only one means of salvation, then take yourself in hand and make yourself responsible for all men's sins; that is the truth, you know, friends, for as soon as you sincerely make yourself responsible for everything and for all men, you will see at once that it is really so, and that you are to blame for every one and for all things. But throwing your own indolence and impotence on others you will end by sharing the pride of Satan and murmuring against God.

Of the pride of Satan what I think is this: it is hard for us on earth to comprehend it, and therefore it is so easy to fall into error and to share it, even imagining that we are doing something great and splendid. Indeed many of the strongest feelings and movements of our nature we on earth still cannot comprehend. Do not let this tempt you, and think not that it may serve as a justification to you for anything. For the Eternal Judge will hold you responsible for what you can comprehend and not for what you cannot. You will know that yourself hereafter, for you will behold all things truly then and will not dispute them. On earth, indeed, we are as it were astray, and if it were not for the precious image of Christ before us, we should perish and be altogether lost, as was the human race before the flood. Much on earth is hidden from us, but to make up for that we have been given a precious sense of our living bond with the other world, with the higher heavenly world, and the roots of our thoughts and feelings are not here but in other worlds. That is why the philosophers say that we cannot apprehend the essence of things on earth.

God took seeds from other worlds and sowed them on this earth, and planted a garden, and everything came up that could come up, but what He grew lives and is alive only through the feeling of its contact with other mysterious worlds. If that feeling grows weak or is destroyed in you, the heavenly growth will die away in you. Then you will be indifferent to life and even grow to hate it. That's what I think.

(*h*) *Can a man judge his fellow creatures? Concerning faith to the end*

Remember particularly that you cannot be a judge of any one. For no one on earth can judge a criminal, until he recognises that he is just such a criminal as the man standing before him, and that he perhaps is more than all men to blame for that crime. When he understands that, he will be able to be a judge. Though outwardly that is absurd, it is true. For if I had been righteous myself, perhaps there would have been no criminal standing before me. If you can take upon yourself the crime of the criminal your heart is judging, take it at once, suffer for him yourself, and let him go without reproach. And even if the law itself sets you up as his judge, act in the same spirit so far as possible, for he will go away and condemn himself more bitterly than you have done. But if, after your kiss, he goes away unmoved, mocking at you, do not let that be a stumbling-block to you either. It shows his time has not yet come, but it will come in due course. And if it come not, no matter; if not he, then another in his place will understand and suffer, and judge and condemn himself, and the truth will be fulfilled. Believe that, believe it without doubt; for in that lies all the hope and faith of the saints.

Work without ceasing. If you remember in the night as you go to sleep, "I have not done what I ought to have done," rise up at once and do it. If the people around you are spiteful and callous and will not hear you, fall down before them and beg their forgiveness; for in truth you are to blame for their not wanting to heed you. And if you cannot speak to them in their bitterness, serve them in silence and in humility, never losing hope. If all men abandon you and even drive you away by force, then when you are left alone fall on the earth and kiss it, water it with your tears and it will bring forth fruit even though no one has seen or heard you in your loneliness. Believe to the end, even if all men went astray and you were left the only faithful one; bring your offering even then and praise God though you be the only one remaining. And if two of you are gathered together — then there is a whole world, a world of living love. Embrace each other tenderly and praise God, for if only in you two His truth has been fulfilled.

If you sin yourself and grieve even unto death for your sins or for your sudden sin, then rejoice for others, rejoice for the righteous man, rejoice that if you have sinned, he is righteous and has not sinned.

If the evil doing of men moves you to indignation and overwhelming distress, even to a desire for vengeance on the evil-doers, shun above all things that feeling. Go at once and seek suffering for yourself, as though you were yourself guilty of that wrong. Accept that suffering and bear it and your heart will find comfort, and you will understand that you, too, are guilty, for you might have been a light to the evil-doers, even as the one man sinless, and you were not a light to them. If you had been a light, you would have lightened the path for others, too, and the evil-doer might perhaps have been saved by your light from his sin. And even though you were a light, but you see that men were not saved by it, hold firm and doubt not the power of the heavenly light. Believe that if they were not saved now, they will be saved hereafter. And if they are not saved hereafter, then their sons will be saved, for your light will not die even when you are dead. The righteous man passes, but his light remains. Men are always saved after the death of the deliverer. Men reject their prophets and slay them, but they love their martyrs and honour those whom they have slain. You are working for the whole, you are acting for the future. Seek no reward, for great is your reward on this earth: the spiritual joy which is vouchsafed only to the righteous man. Fear not the great nor the mighty, but be wise and ever serene. Know the measure, know the times, study that. When you are left alone, pray. Love to throw yourself on the earth and kiss it. Kiss the earth and love it with an unceasing, consuming love. Love all men, love everything. Seek that rapture and ecstasy. Water the earth with the tears of your joy and love those tears. Don't be ashamed of that ecstasy, prize it, for it is a gift of God and a great one; it is not given to many but only to the elect.

(*i*) *Of hell and hell-fire: a mystic reflection*

Fathers and teachers, I ponder "What is hell?" I maintain that it is the suffering of being no longer able to love. Once in infinite existence, immeasurable in time and space, a spiritual creature was given, on his coming to earth, the power of saying to itself, "I am and I love."

Once, only once, there was given him a moment of active *living* love and for that was earthly life given him, and with it times and seasons. And what happened? — That fortunate creature rejected the priceless gift, prized it and loved it not, scorned it and remained callous. Such a one, having left the earth, sees Abraham's bosom and talks with Abraham as we are told in the parable of the rich man and Lazarus, and beholds paradise and can go up to the Lord. But that is just his torment, to rise up to the Lord without ever having loved, to be brought close to those who have loved when he has despised their love. For he sees clearly and says to himself, "Now I have understanding and though I now thirst to love, there will be nothing great, no sacrifice in my love, for my earthly life is over, and Abraham will not come even with a drop of living water (that is the gift of earthly, active life) to cool the fiery thirst of spiritual love which burns in me now, though I disdained it on earth; there is no more life for me and time will be no more! Even though I would gladly give my life for others, it can never be, for that life is passed which can be sacrificed for love, and now there is a gulf fixed between that life and this existence."

They talk of hell-fire in the material sense. I don't go into that mystery and I dread it. But I think if there were fire in the material sense, they would be glad of it, for, I imagine, that in material agony their still greater spiritual agony would be forgotten for a moment. Moreover, that spiritual agony cannot be taken from them, for that suffering is not external but within them. And if it could be taken from them, I think it would be bitterer still for the unhappy creatures. For even if the righteous in paradise forgave them, beholding their torments, and called them up to heaven in their infinite love, they would only multiply their torments, for they would arouse in them still more keenly a flaming thirst for responsive, active, and grateful love which is now impossible. In the timidity of my heart I imagine, however, that the very recognition of this impossibility would serve at last to console them. For accepting the love of the righteous together with the impossibility of repaying it, by this submissiveness and the effect of this humility, they will attain at last, as it were, to a certain semblance of that active love which they scorned on earth, to something like its outward expression. . . . I regret, friends and brothers, that I cannot express this clearly. But woe to those who have destroyed themselves on earth, woe to the suicides! I believe that there can be none more miserable than they. They tell us that it is a sin to pray for them and outwardly the Church, as it were, rejects them, but in my secret heart I believe that we may pray even for them. Love can never be an offence to Christ. For such as those I have prayed inwardly all my life, I confess it, fathers and teachers, and even now I pray for them every day.

Oh, there are some who remain proud and fierce even in hell, in spite of their certain knowledge and contemplation of the absolute truth; there are some terrible ones who have given themselves over to Satan and his proud spirit entirely. For such, hell is voluntary and unappeasable; they are tortured by their own choice. For they have cursed themselves, cursing God and life. They live upon their vindictive pride like a starving man in the desert sucking blood out of his own body. But they are never satisfied, and they refuse forgiveness, they curse God Who summons them. They cannot behold the living God without hatred, and they demand that there be no God of life, that God should destroy Himself and His own creation. And they will burn in the fire of their own wrath for ever and yearn for death and annihilation. But they will not attain to death. . . .

Here Alexey Fyodorovich Karamazov's manuscript ends. I repeat, it is incomplete and fragmentary. Biographical details, for instance, cover only the elder's earliest youth. His exhortations and opinions have been assembled to form a whole, although they were evidently uttered at different times and on different occasions. His utterances during the last few hours have not been kept separate from the rest, but their general character can be gathered from what we have in this manuscript.

The elder's death came in the end quite unexpectedly. For although those who were gathered about him that last evening realised fully that his death was approaching, yet it was difficult to imagine that it would come so suddenly. On the contrary, his friends, as I observed already, seeing him that night apparently so cheerful and talkative, were convinced that there was at least a temporary change for the better in his condition. Even five minutes before his death, they said afterwards wonderingly, it was impossible to foresee it. He seemed suddenly to feel an acute pain in his chest, he turned pale and pressed his hands to his heart. All rose from their seats and hastened to him. But though suffering, he still looked at them with a smile, sank slowly from his chair on to his knees, then bowed his face to the ground, stretched out his arms and as though in joyful ecstasy, praying and kissing the earth (as he had himself taught), quietly and joyfully gave up his soul to God.

The news of his death spread at once through the hermitage and reached the monastery. The nearest friends of the deceased and those whose position made it their duty began to lay out the body according to the ancient ritual, and all the monks gathered together in the church. And before dawn the news of the death reached the town. By morning all the town was talking of the event, and crowds were flocking from the town to the monastery. But of this we shall speak in the next book; I will only add here that before a day had passed something happened so unexpected, so strange, upsetting, and bewildering in its effect on the monks and the townspeople, that after all these years the most vivid memory of that agitating day is still preserved in our town.

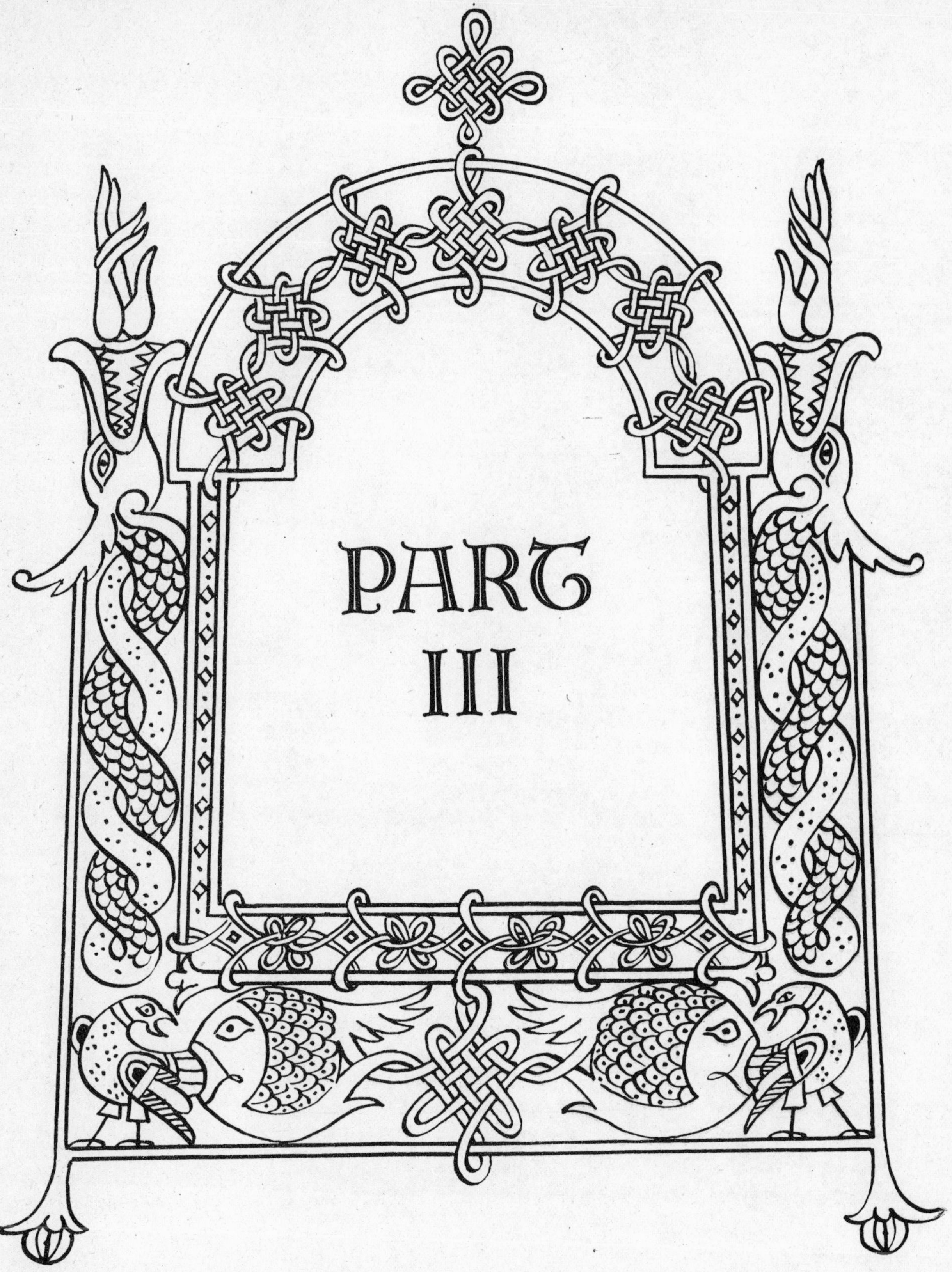
PART
III

CHAPTER I

THE BREATH OF CORRUPTION

THE body of the deceased monk, Father Zosima, was prepared for burial according to the established ritual. As is known, the bodies of dead monks and hermits are not washed. In the words of the Church Manual: "If any one of the monks depart to the Lord, the monk designated (that is, whose office it is) shall wipe the body with warm water, making first the sign of the cross with a sponge on the forehead of the deceased, on the breast, on the hands and feet and on the knees, and naught more." All this was done by Father Païssy, who then clothed the deceased in his monastic garb and wrapped him in his cloak, which was, according to custom, somewhat slit to allow of its being folded about him in the form of a cross. On his head he put a hood with an eight-cornered cross. The hood was left open and the dead man's face was covered with black cloth. In his hands was put an ikon of the Saviour. Towards morning he was put in the coffin which had been made ready long before. It was decided to leave the coffin all day in the cell, in the larger room in which the elder used to receive his visitors and fellow monks. As the deceased was a priest and monk, the Gospel, not the Psalter, had to be read over his body by ordained monks and deacons. The reading was begun by Father Iosif immediately after the requiem service. Father Païssy desired to read the Gospel later on all day and all night over his dead friend, but for the present he, as well as the Father Superior of the hermitage, was very busy and worried, for something extraordinary, an unheard of, even "unseemly" excitement and impatient expectation began to be apparent in the monks, and in the visitors arriving from the monastery hostelries, and the crowds of people flocking from the town. And as time went on, this grew more and more marked. Both the Superior and Father Païssy did their utmost to calm the general bustle and agitation.

When it was full daylight, some people began bringing their sick, in most cases children, with them from the town — as though they had been waiting expressly for this moment to do so, evidently persuaded that the dead elder's remains had a power of healing, which would be immediately made manifest in accordance with their faith. It was only then apparent how unquestionably every one in our town had accepted Father Zosima during his lifetime as a great saint. And those who came were far from being all of the humbler classes.

This intense expectation on the part of the

believers, displayed with such haste, so nakedly, even impatiently and almost demandingly, appeared to Father Païssy as a snare. Though he had long foreseen something of the sort, the actual manifestation of the feeling was beyond anything he had looked for. When he came across any of the monks who displayed this excitement, Father Païssy began to reprove them. "Such immediate expectation of something extraordinary," he said, "shows a levity, possible to worldly people but unseemly in us."

But little attention was paid him and Father Païssy noticed this with uneasiness. Yet he himself (if the whole truth must be told), secretly, at the bottom of his heart, cherished almost the same hopes and could not but be aware of it, though he was indignant at the too eager expectation around him, and saw in it light-mindedness and vanity. Nevertheless, it was particularly unpleasant to him to meet certain persons, whose presence seemed to him to bode ill. In the crowd that filled the dead man's cell he noticed with inward aversion (for which he immediately reproached himself) the presence of Rakitin and of the monk from Obdorsk, who was still staying in the monastery. Of both of them Father Païssy felt for some reason suddenly suspicious — though, indeed, he might well have felt the same about others.

The monk from Obdorsk was conspicuous as the most fussy in the excited crowd. He was to be seen everywhere; everywhere he was asking questions, everywhere he was listening, on all sides he was whispering with a peculiar, mysterious air. His expression showed the greatest impatience and even a sort of irritation because what he expected was so long in coming. As for Rakitin, he, as appeared later, had come so early to the hermitage at the special request of Madame Hohlakov. As soon as that good-hearted but weak-minded woman, who could not herself have been admitted to the hermitage, waked and heard of the death of Father Zosima, she was overtaken with such intense curiosity that she promptly despatched Rakitin to the hermitage, with instructions to keep a careful look-out and report to her by letter every half-hour or so "*everything that takes place.*" She regarded Rakitin as a most religious and devout young man. He was particularly clever in getting round people and assuming whatever part he thought most to their taste, if he detected the slightest advantage to himself in doing so.

It was a bright, clear day and many of the visitors were thronging about the tombs, which were particularly numerous round the church and scattered here and there about the hermitage. As he walked round the hermitage, Father Païssy suddenly remembered Alyosha and that he had not seen him for some time, not since the night before. And he had no sooner thought of him than he at once noticed him in the most remote corner of the hermitage garden, sitting on the tombstone of a monk who had been famous long ago for his saintliness. He sat with his back to the hermitage and his face to the wall, and seemed to be hiding behind the tombstone. Going up to him, Father Païssy saw that he was weeping quietly but bitterly, with his face hidden in his hands, and that his whole frame was shaking with sobs. Father Païssy stood over him for a little.

"Enough, dear son, enough, dear," he pronounced with feeling at last. "Why do you weep? Rejoice and weep not. Don't you know that this is the greatest of his days? Think only where he is now, at this moment!"

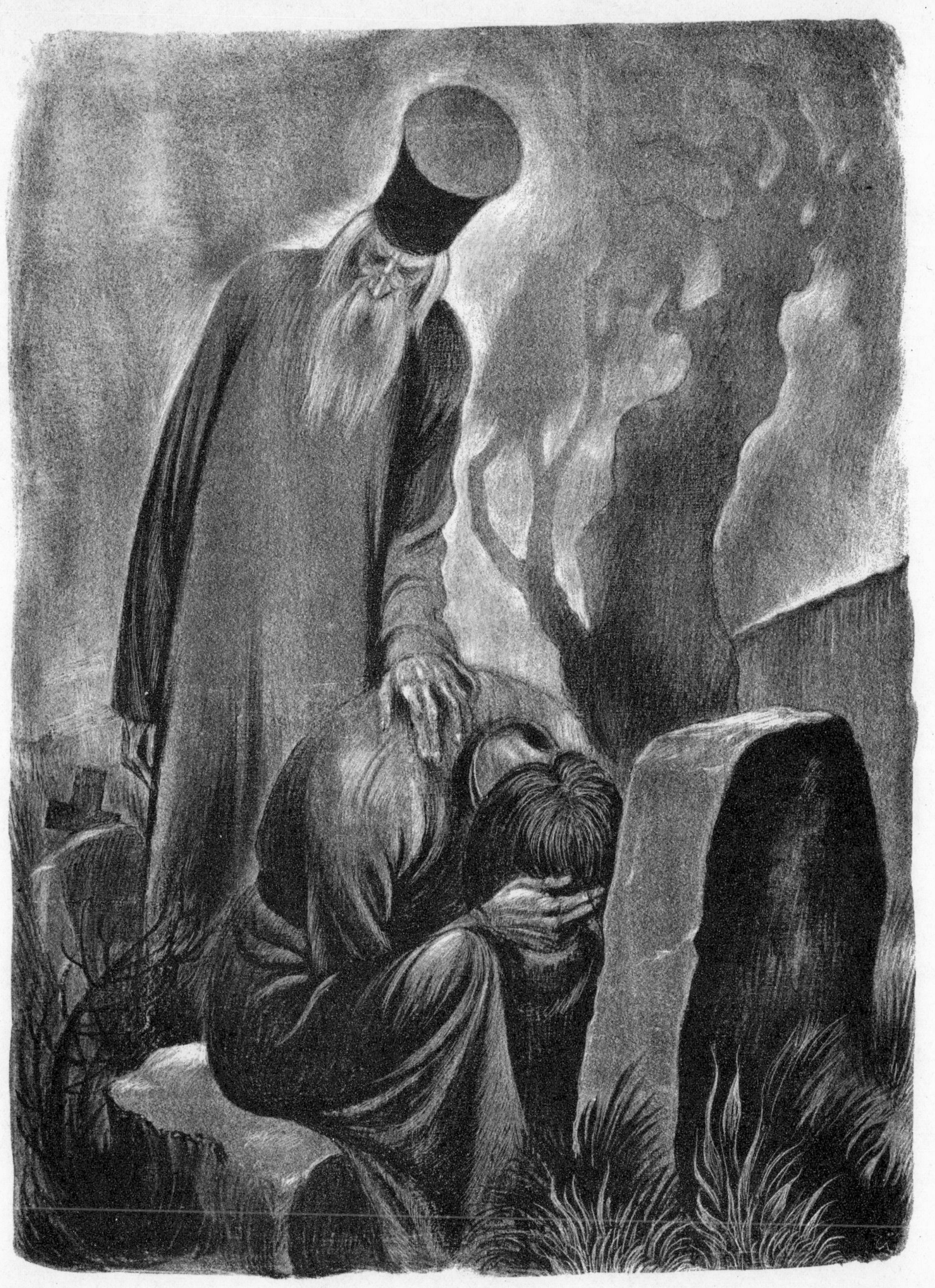

ALYOSHA AMONG THE TOMBS

Alyosha glanced at him, uncovering his face, which was swollen with crying like a child's, but turned away at once without uttering a word and hid his face in his hands again.

"May be it is well," said Father Païssy thoughtfully; "weep if you must, Christ has sent you those tears."

"Your touching tears are but a relief to your spirit and will serve to gladden your dear heart," he added to himself, walking away from Alyosha, and thinking lovingly of him. He moved away quickly, however, for he felt that he, too, might weep looking at him.

Meanwhile the time was passing; the monastery services and the requiems for the dead followed in their due course. Father Païssy again took Father Iosif's place by the coffin and began reading the Gospel. But before three o'clock in the afternoon there occurred that to which I alluded at the end of the last book, a thing so unexpected by all of us and so contrary to the general hope that, I repeat, a detailed account of this matter is remembered to this day in our town and all the surrounding neighborhood. I may add here, for myself personally, that it is almost repulsive to me to recall that event which caused such frivolous agitation and was such a stumbling-block to many, though in reality it was the most natural and trivial matter. I should, of course, have omitted all mention of it in my story, if it had not exerted a very strong influence on the heart and soul of the chief, *though future*, hero of my story, Alyosha, forming a crisis and turning-point, as it were, in his spiritual development, giving a shock to his intellect, which finally strengthened it for the rest of his life and gave it a definite aim.

And so, to return to our story. When before dawn they laid Father Zosima's body in the coffin and brought it into the front room, the question of opening the windows was raised among those who were around the coffin. But this suggestion made casually by some one was unanswered and almost unnoticed. Some of those present may perhaps have inwardly noticed it, only to reflect that the anticipation of decay and corruption from the body of such a saint was an actual absurdity, meriting compassion (if not a smile) for the lack of faith and the frivolity it implied. For they expected something quite different.

And, behold, soon after midday something began, which was at first only noted in silence by those who came in and out and each of whom was evidently afraid to communicate the thought vaguely in his mind. But by three o'clock the thing had become so clear and unmistakable that the news swiftly reached all the monks and visitors in the hermitage, promptly penetrated to the monastery, throwing all the monks into amazement, and finally, in the shortest possible time, spread to the town, exciting every one in it, believers and unbelievers alike. The unbelievers rejoiced, and as for the believers, some of them rejoiced even more than the unbelievers, for "men love the downfall and disgrace of the righteous," as the deceased elder had said in one of his exhortations.

The fact is that the breath of corruption began to come from the coffin, growing gradually more marked, and by three o'clock it was quite unmistakable. In all the past history of our monastery, no such scandal could be recalled, and in no other circumstances could such a scandal have been possible, as showed itself in unseemly disorder immediately after this discovery among the very monks themselves. Afterwards, even many years afterwards, some sensible monks, when they recalled that day, were amazed and horrified that the scandal could have reached such proportions. For in the past, monks of very holy life had died, God-fearing old men, whose saintliness was acknowledged by all, yet from their humble coffins, too, the breath of corruption had come, naturally, as from all dead bodies, but that had caused no scandal nor even the slightest excitement. Of course there had been, in former times, saints in the monastery whose memory was carefully preserved and whose relics, according to tradition, showed no signs of corruption. This fact was regarded by the monks as touching and mysterious, and the tradition of it was cherished as something seemly and miraculous, and as a promise, by God's grace, of still greater glory from their tombs in the future.

One such, whose memory was particularly cherished, was Father Job, who had died half a century earlier, at the great age of a hundred and five. He had been a celebrated ascetic, rigid in fasting and silence, and his tomb was pointed out to all visitors on their arrival with peculiar respect and mysterious hints of great hopes connected with it. (That was the very tomb on which Father Païssy had found Alyosha sitting in the morning.) Another memory cherished in the monastery was that of the famous Father Varsonofy, only recently deceased, who had preceded Father Zosima as elder, and who during his lifetime was revered as a saintly fool by all the pilgrims to the monastery. There was a tradition that both of these had lain in their coffins as though alive, that they had shown no signs of corruption when they were buried and that there had been a holy light in their countenances when they were in their coffins. And some people even insisted that a sweet fragrance came from their bodies.

Yet, in spite of these edifying precedents, it would be difficult to explain the direct cause of the frivolity, absurdity, and malice that were manifested beside the coffin of Father Zosima. It is my private opinion that several different causes were simultaneously at work, one of which was the deeply rooted hostility to the institution of elders as a pernicious innovation, an antipathy hidden deep in the hearts of many of the monks. Even more powerful was jealousy of the dead man's saintliness, so firmly established during his lifetime that it was almost a forbidden thing to question it. For though the late elder had won over many hearts, more by love than by miracles, and had gathered round him a whole world of loving adherents, none the less, in fact, rather the more on that account, he had awakened jealousy and so had come to have bitter enemies, secret and open, not only in the monastery but even among the laity. He did no one any harm, but "Why do they think him so saintly?" And that question alone gradually repeated gave rise at last to an intense, insatiable hatred of him. That I believe was why many people were extremely delighted at the smell of corruption which came so quickly, for not a day had passed since his death. At the same time there were some among those who had been hitherto reverently devoted to the elder, who were almost mortified and personally affronted by this incident. This is the way in which it all happened.

As soon as signs of decomposition had begun to appear, the whole aspect of the monks betrayed their secret motives in entering the cell. They went in, stayed a little while, and hastened out to confirm the news to the crowd of other monks waiting outside. Some of the latter shook their heads mournfully, but others did not even care to conceal the delight which gleamed unmistakably in their malicious eyes. And now no one reproached them for it, no one raised his voice in protest, which was strange, for the majority of the monks had been devoted to the dead elder. But it seemed as though God had in this case let the minority get the upper hand for a time.

Visitors from outside, particularly of the educated class, soon went into the cell, too, with the same spying intent. Of the peasantry few went into the cell, though there were crowds of them at the gates of the hermitage. After three o'clock the rush of worldly visitors was greatly increased and this was no doubt owing to the scandalous news. People were attracted who would not otherwise have come on that day and had not intended to come, and among them were some personages of high rank. But external decorum was still preserved and Father Païssy, with a stern face, continued firmly and distinctly reading aloud the Gospel, apparently not noticing what was taking place around him, though he had, in fact, observed something unusual long before. But at last the murmurs, first subdued but gradually louder and more confident, reached even him. "It shows God's judgment is not as man's," Father Païssy heard suddenly. The first to give utterance to this sentiment was a layman, an elderly official from the town, known to be a man of great piety. But he only repeated aloud what the monks had long been whispering to each other. They had long before formulated this damning conclusion, and the worst of it was that a sort of triumphant satisfaction at that conclusion became more and more apparent every moment. Soon even external decorum began to be violated and presently all almost seemed to feel they had a sort of right to violate it.

"And for what reason can *this* have happened," some of the monks said, at first with a show of regret; "he had a small frame and his flesh was dried up on his bones, why the breath?" "It must be a sign from heaven," others hastened to add, and this opinion was adopted at once without protest. For it was pointed out, too, that if the decomposition had been natural, as in the case of every dead sinner, it would have been apparent later, after a lapse of at least twenty-four hours, but this premature corruption "was in excess of nature," and so the finger of God was evident. It was meant for a sign. This conclusion seemed irresistible.

Gentle Father Iosif, the librarian, a great favourite of the dead man's, tried to reply to some of those who spoke evil that "this is not held everywhere alike," and that the incorruptibility of the bodies of the just was not a dogma of the Orthodox Church, but only an opinion, and that even in the most Orthodox regions, at Athos for instance, they were not greatly confounded by the smell of corruption, and there the chief sign of the glorification of the saved was not bodily incorruptibility, but the colour of the bones when the bodies had lain many years in the earth and had decayed in it. "And if the bones are yellow as wax, that is the great sign that the Lord has glorified the deceased saint; if they are not yellow but black, it shows that God has not deemed him worthy of such glory — that is the belief at Athos, a saintly place, where the Orthodox faith has been preserved from of old, unbroken and in the greatest purity," said Father Iosif in conclusion. But the meek father's words had little effect and even provoked a mocking retort. "That's all pedantry and innovation, no use listening to it," the monks decided. "We stick to the old doctrine; there are all sorts of innovations nowadays, are we to follow them all?" added others. "We have had as many holy fathers as they had. There they are subjects of the Turk, they have forgotten everything. Orthodoxy among them has long been impure, and they have no bells even," the greatest scoffers added.

Father Iosif walked away grieving the more since he had put forward his own opinion with little confidence as though scarcely believing in it himself. He foresaw with distress that something very unseemly was beginning and that arrant disobedience was raising its head. Little by little, all the sensible monks were reduced to silence like Father Iosif. And so it came to pass that all who loved the deceased elder and had accepted with devout obedience the institution of elders were all at once terribly cast down and glanced timidly in one another's faces when they met. Those who were hostile to the institution, as an innovation, held up their heads proudly. "There was no smell of corruption from the late elder Varsonofy, but a sweet fragrance," they recalled maliciously. "But he earned that glory not because he was an elder, but because he was a holy man."

And this was followed by a shower of criticism and even blame of Father Zosima. "His teaching was false; he taught that life is a great joy and not a vale of tears," said some of the more unreasonable. "He followed the fashionable belief, he did not recognise material fire in hell," others, still more unreasonable, added. "He was not strict in fasting, allowed himself sweet things, ate cherry jam with his tea, ladies used to send it to him. Is it right for a monk of strict rule to drink tea?" could be heard among some of the envious. "He sat in pride," the most malicious declared vindictively; "he considered himself a saint and he took it as his due when people knelt before him." "He abused the sacrament of confession," the fiercest opponents of the institution of elders added in a malicious whisper. And among these were some of the oldest monks, strictest in their devotion, genuine ascetics, who had kept silent during the life of the deceased elder, but now suddenly unsealed their lips. And this was terrible, for their words had great influence on young monks who were not yet firm in their convictions. The monk from Obdorsk heard all this attentively, heaving deep sighs and nodding his head. "Yes, clearly Father Ferapont was right in his judgment yesterday," he thought to himself, and at that moment Father Ferapont himself made his appearance, as though on purpose to increase the confusion.

I have mentioned already that he rarely left his wooden cell close by the apiary. He was seldom seen even at church and this was forgiven him on the ground of his being a saintly fool, and he was not held to rules that were binding on all the rest. But if the whole truth is to be told, he was granted these privileges out of necessity, as it were. For it would have been disgraceful to insist on burdening with the common regulations so great an ascetic, who prayed day and night (he even dropped asleep on his knees). If they had insisted, the monks would have said, "He is holier than all of us and he follows a rule harder than ours. And if he does not go to church, it's because he knows when he ought to; he has his own rule." It was to avoid the chance of such murmur and scandal that Father Ferapont was left in peace.

As every one was aware, Father Ferapont particularly disliked Father Zosima. And now the news had reached him in his hut that "God's judgment is not the same as man's," and that something had happened which was "in excess of nature." It may well be supposed that among the first to run to him with the news was the monk from Obdorsk, who had visited him the evening before and left his cell terror-stricken.

I have mentioned above, that though Father Païssy, standing firm and immovable reading the Gospel over the coffin, could not hear nor see what was passing outside the cell, he gauged most of it correctly in his heart, for he knew the men surrounding him, well. He was not confused, but awaited what would come next without fear, watching with a penetrating eye for the outcome of the general excitement which was already present to his mind.

Suddenly an extraordinary uproar in the passage in open defiance of decorum burst on his ears. The door was flung open and Father Ferapont appeared in the doorway. Behind him there could be seen a crowd of monks, together with many people from the town. They did not, however, enter the cell, but stood at the bottom of the steps, waiting to see what Father Ferapont would say and do. For they felt with a certain awe, in spite of their audacity, that he had not come for nothing. Standing in the doorway, Father Ferapont raised his arms, and under his right arm the keen inquisitive little eyes of the monk from Obdorsk peeped out. He alone, in his intense curiosity, could not resist running up the steps after Father Ferapont. The others, on the contrary, pressed further back in sudden alarm when the door was noisily flung open. Holding his hands aloft, Father Ferapont suddenly roared:

"I will cast thee out!" and, turning about, he began at once making the sign of the cross over each of the four walls and four corners of the cell in succession. All who accompanied Father Ferapont immediately understood his action. For they knew he always did this wherever he went, and that he would not sit down or say a word till he had driven out the evil spirits. "Satan, go hence! Satan, go hence!" he repeated at each sign of the cross. "I will cast thee out," he roared again.

He was wearing his coarse gown girt with a rope. His bare chest, covered with grey hair, could be seen under his hempen shirt. His feet were bare. As soon as he began waving his arms, the cruel irons he wore under his gown could be heard clanking.

Father Païssy paused in his reading, stepped forward and stood before him waiting.

"What have you come for, worthy father? Why do you offend against good order? Why do you stir up the humble flock?" he said at last, looking sternly at him.

"What have you come for? Why are you asking? What is your faith?" shouted Father Ferapont, acting like the saintly fool that he was. "I've come here to drive out your guests, the filthy devils. I've come to see how many have gathered here while I have been away. I want to sweep them out with a birch broom."

"You cast out the evil spirit, but perhaps you are serving him yourself," Father Païssy went on fearlessly. "And who can say of himself 'I am holy.' Can you, father?"

"I am unclean, not holy. I would not sit in an armchair and would not have them bow down to me as an idol," thundered Father Ferapont. "Nowadays folk destroy the true faith. The dead man, your saint," he turned to the crowd, pointing with his finger to the coffin, "did not believe in devils. He gave medicine to keep off the devils. And so they have become as common as spiders in the corners. And now he is stinking himself. In that we see a great sign from God."

The incident he referred to was this. One of the monks was haunted in his dreams and, later on, while awake, by visions of evil spirits. When in the utmost terror he confided this to Father Zosima, the elder had advised continual prayer and rigid fasting. But when that was of no use, he advised him, while persisting in prayer and fasting, to take a certain medicine.

Many persons were scandalised at the time and wagged their heads as they talked it over — and most of all Father Ferapont, to whom some of the censorious had hastened to report this "extraordinary" counsel on the part of the elder.

"Go hence, father!" said Father Païssy, in a commanding voice, "it's not for man to judge, but for God. Perhaps we see here a 'sign' which neither you, nor I, nor any one of us is able to comprehend. Go, father, and do not stir up the flock!" he repeated insistently.

"He did not keep the fasts according to the rule and therefore the sign has come. That is clear and it's a sin to hide it." The fanatic, carried away by a zeal that outstripped his reason, would not be quieted. "He was seduced by sweetmeats, ladies brought them to him in their pockets, he sipped tea, he worshipped his belly, filling it with sweet things and his mind with haughty thoughts. . . . And for this he is put to shame. . . ."

"You speak frivolously, father." Father Païssy, too, raised his voice. "I admire your fasting and severities, but you speak lightly like some frivolous youth, fickle and childish. Go hence, father, I command you!" Father Païssy thundered in conclusion.

"I will go," said Father Ferapont, seeming somewhat taken aback, but still as bitter. "You learned men! You are so clever you look down upon my humbleness. I came hither with little learning and here I have forgotten what I did know, the Lord God himself has preserved me, little as I am, from your subtlety."

Father Païssy stood over him, waiting resolutely. Father Ferapont paused and, suddenly leaning his cheek on his hand despondently, pronounced in a sing-song voice, looking at the coffin of the deceased elder:

"To-morrow they will sing over him 'Our Helper and Defender' — a splendid anthem — and over me when I croak all they'll sing will be 'What earthly joy' — a little canticle,"* he added with tearful regret. "They are proud and puffed up, this is an empty place!" he shouted suddenly like a madman, and with a wave of his hand he turned sharply and quickly descended the steps. The crowd awaiting him below wavered; some followed him at once and some lingered, for the cell was still open, and Father Païssy, following Father Ferapont on to the steps, stood watching him. But the excited old fanatic was not completely silenced. Walking twenty steps

* When a monk's body is carried out from the cell to the church and from the church to the graveyard, the canticle "What earthly joy" is sung. If the deceased was a priest as well as a monk the canticle "Our Helper and Defender" is sung instead.

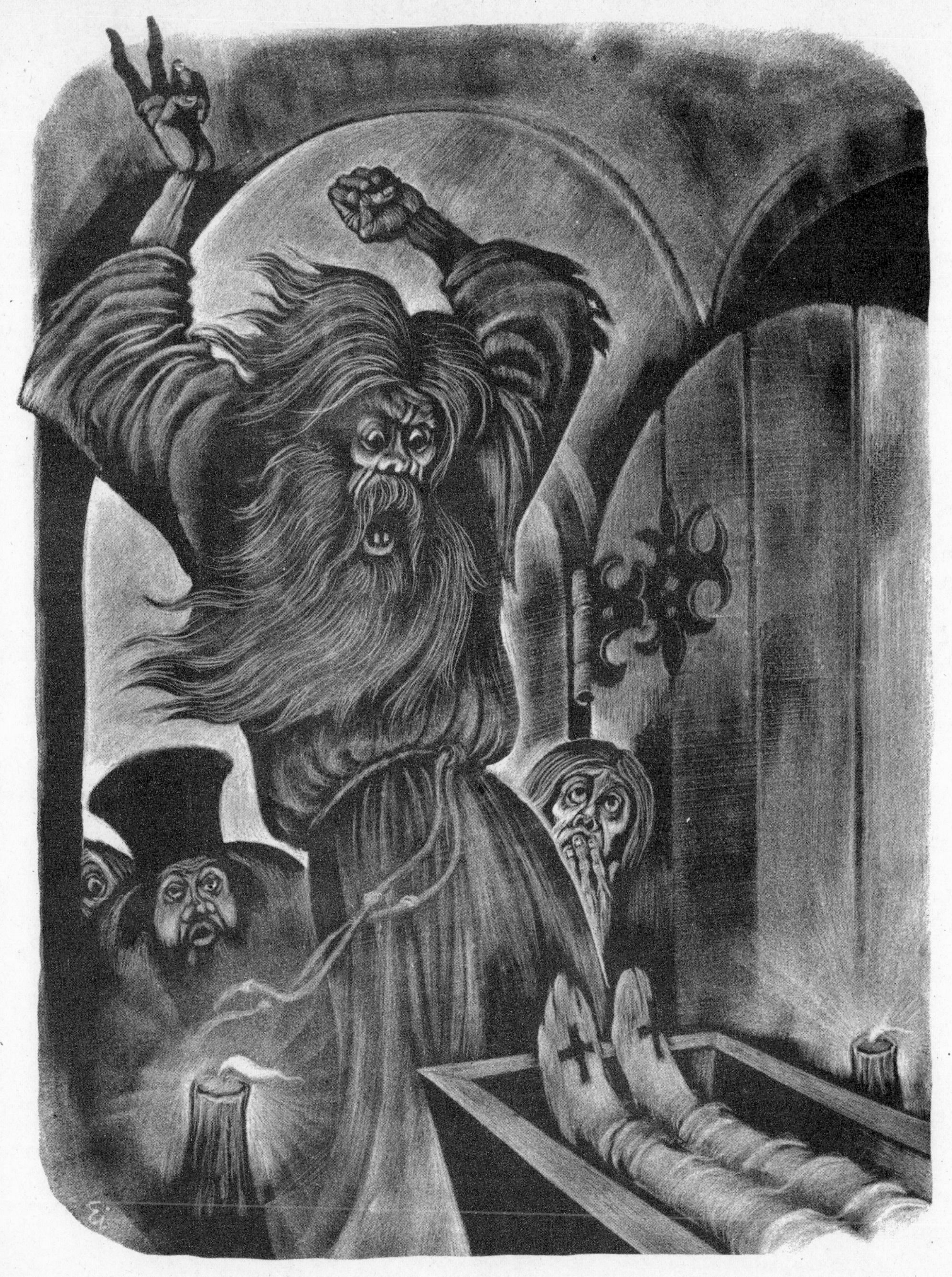

"SATAN, GO HENCE!"

away, he suddenly turned towards the setting sun, raised both his arms and, as though some one had cut him down, fell to the ground with a loud shout.

"My Lord has conquered! Christ has conquered the setting sun!" he shouted frantically, stretching up his hands to the sun, and falling face downwards on the ground, he sobbed like a little child, shaken by his tears and spreading out his arms on the ground. Then all rushed up to him; there were exclamations and sympathetic sobs . . . a kind of frenzy seemed to take possession of them all.

"This is the one who is a saint! This is the one who is a holy man!" some cried aloud, losing their fear. "This is he who should be an elder," others added maliciously.

"He wouldn't be an elder . . . he would refuse . . . he wouldn't foster the cursed innovation . . . he wouldn't imitate their foolery," other voices chimed in at once. And it is hard to say how far they might have gone, but at that moment the bell rang summoning them to service. All began crossing themselves at once. Father Ferapont, too, got up and crossing himself went back to his cell without looking round, still uttering exclamations which were utterly incoherent. A few followed him, but the greater number dispersed, hastening to service. Father Païssy let Father Iosif read in his place and went down. The frantic outcries of bigots could not shake him, but his heart was suddenly filled with sadness and began to ache strangely. He stood still and suddenly asked himself, "Why am I sad even to dejection?" and immediately grasped with surprise that his sudden sadness was due to a very small and special cause. In the crowd thronging the entrance to the cell he had noticed Alyosha and he remembered that he had felt at once a pang at heart on seeing him. "Can that boy mean so much to me now?" he asked himself, wondering.

At that moment Alyosha passed him, hurrying away, but not in the direction of the church. Their eyes met. Alyosha quickly turned away his eyes and dropped them to the ground, and from the boy's look alone Father Païssy guessed what a great change was taking place in him at that moment.

"Have you, too, fallen into temptation?" cried Father Païssy. "Can you be with those of little faith?" he added mournfully.

Alyosha stood still and gazed vaguely at Father Païssy, but quickly turned his eyes away again and again looked at the ground. He stood sideways and did not turn his face to Father Païssy, who watched him attentively.

"Where are you hastening? The bell calls to service," he said again, but again Alyosha made no answer. "Are you leaving the hermitage? What, without asking leave, without asking a blessing?"

Alyosha suddenly gave a wry smile, cast a strange, very strange, look at the father to whom his former guide, the former sovereign of his heart and mind, his beloved elder, had confided him as he lay dying. And suddenly, still without speaking, waved his hand, as though not caring even to be respectful, and with rapid steps walked towards the gates away from the hermitage.

"You will come back again!" murmured Father Païssy, looking after him with sorrowful surprise.

CHAPTER II

THE PSYCHOLOGICAL MOMENT

Father Païssy, of course, was not wrong when he decided that his "dear boy" would come back again. Perhaps indeed, to some extent, he had a penetrating insight into the true meaning of Alyosha's spiritual condition. Yet I must frankly own that it would be very difficult for me to give a clear account of that strange, vague moment in the life of my young and dearly beloved hero. To Father Païssy's sorrowful question, "are you, too, with those of little faith?" I could of course confidently answer for Alyosha, no, he is not with those of little faith. Quite the contrary. Indeed, all his distress was due precisely to the fact that he was of great faith. But still the distress was there and was so agonising that even long afterwards Alyosha thought of that sorrowful day as one of the bitterest and most fateful days of his life. If the question is asked: "Could all his grief and disturbance have been due only to the fact that his elder's body had shown signs of premature decomposition instead of at once working miraculous cures?" I must answer without beating about the bush, "Yes, it certainly was." I would only beg the reader not to be in too great a hurry to laugh at my young hero's pure heart. I am far from intending to apologise for him or to justify his innocent faith on the ground of his youth, or the little progress he had made in his studies, or any such reason. I must declare, on the contrary, that I have genuine respect for the qualities of his heart. No doubt a youth whose heart received impressions cautiously, whose love was lukewarm, and whose mind, though keen, was too prudent for his age and so worthless, such a young man might, I admit, have avoided what happened to my hero. But in some cases it is really more creditable to be carried away by an emotion, however unreasonable, which springs from a great love, than to resist such an emotion. And this is even truer of youth, for a young man who is always sensible is suspect and is of little worth — that's my opinion!

"But," sensible people will exclaim perhaps, "every young man cannot be swayed by such a superstition and your hero is no model for others." To this I reply again, yes! my hero had faith, a faith holy and steadfast, but still I am not going to apologise for him.

You see, though I declared above, and perhaps too hastily, that I would not make explanations, apologise, and justify my hero, I see that some explanation is necessary for the understanding of the rest of my story. Let me say then, it was not a question of miracles. There was no frivolous and impatient expectation of miracles in his mind. And Alyosha needed no miracles at the time, for the triumph of his convictions, for the triumph of some preconceived idea — oh, no, not at all — what he saw above all was a countenance — the countenance of his beloved elder, the countenance of that holy man whom he revered with such adoration. The fact is that all the love that lay concealed in his pure young heart for every one and everything had, for the past year, been concentrated — and perhaps wrongly so — on one being, his beloved elder. It is true that being had for so long been accepted by him as his unquestioned ideal, that all his young strength and yearning could not but turn towards that ideal, even to the forgetting at the moment of "every one and everything." He remembered afterwards how, on that terrible day, he had entirely forgotten his brother Dmitri, about whom he had been so anxious and troubled the day before; he had forgotten, too, to take the two hundred roubles to Ilusha's father, though he had so heartily intended to do so the preceding evening. But again it was not miracles he needed but only "the higher justice" which had been in his belief outraged by the blow that had so suddenly and cruelly wounded his heart. And what does it signify that this "justice" looked for by Alyosha inevitably took the shape of miracles to be wrought immediately by the remains of his adored mentor? Why, every one in the monastery cherished the same thought and the same hope, even those whose intellects Alyosha revered, Father Païssy himself, for instance. And so Alyosha, untroubled by doubts, clothed his dreams, too, in the same form as all the rest. And a whole year of life in the monastery had formed the habit of this expectation in his heart. But it was justice, justice, he thirsted for, not simply miracles.

And now the man who should, he believed, have been exalted above every one in the whole world, that man, instead of receiving the glory that was his due, was suddenly cast down and dishonoured! What for? Who had judged him? Who could have decreed this? Those were the questions that wrung his inexperienced and virginal heart. He could not endure without a sense of insult, without bitter resentment even, that the most righteous of the righteous should have been exposed to the jeering and spiteful mockery of the frivolous crowd so inferior to him. Even had there been no miracles, had there been nothing marvellous to justify his hopes, why this indignity, why this disgrace, why this premature decay, "in excess of nature," as the spiteful monks said? Why this "sign from heaven," which they so triumphantly acclaimed in company with Father Ferapont, and why did they believe they had won the right to acclaim it? Where is the finger of Providence? Why did Providence hide its face "at the most critical moment" (so Alyosha thought), as though voluntarily submitting to the blind, dumb, pitiless laws of nature?

That was why Alyosha's heart was bleeding, and, of course, as I have said already, the sting of it all was that the man he loved above everything on earth should be put to shame and disgraced! This murmuring may have been frivolous and unreasonable in my hero, but I repeat again for the third time — and am prepared to admit that it might be difficult to defend my feeling — I am glad that my hero showed himself not too reasonable at that moment, for any man of sense will always come back to reason in time, but, if love does not gain the upper hand in a boy's heart at such an exceptional moment, when will it? I will not, however, omit to mention something strange, which came for a time to the surface of Alyosha's mind at this fateful and subversive moment. This new something was the harassing impression left by the conversation with Ivan, which now persistently haunted Alyosha's mind. At this moment it haunted him. Oh, it was not that something of the fundamental, elemental, so to speak, faith of his soul had been shaken. He loved his God and believed in Him steadfastly, though he was suddenly murmuring against Him. Yet a vague but tormenting and evil impression left by his conversation with Ivan the day before, suddenly revived again now in his soul and seemed forcing its way to the surface of his consciousness.

It had begun to get dusk when Rakitin, crossing the pine copse from the hermitage to the monastery, suddenly noticed Alyosha, lying face downwards on the ground under a tree, motionless and apparently asleep. He went up and called him by his name.

"You here, Alexey? Can you have . . ." he began wondering but broke off. He had meant to say, "Can you have come to this?"

Alyosha did not look at him, but from a slight movement Rakitin at once saw that he heard and understood him.

"What's the matter?" he went on; but the surprise in his face gradually passed into a smile that became more and more ironical.

"I say, I've been looking for you for the last two hours. You suddenly disappeared. What are you about? What foolery is this? You might just look at me. . . ."

Alyosha raised his head, sat up and leaned his back against the tree. He was not crying, but there was a look of suffering and irritability in his face. He did not look at Rakitin, however, but looked away to one side of him.

"Do you know your face is quite changed? There's none of your famous meekness to be seen in it. Are you angry with some one? Have you been ill-treated?"

"Let me alone," said Alyosha suddenly, with a weary gesture of his hand, still looking away from him.

"Oho! So that's how we are feeling! So you can shout at people like other mortals. This is a come-down for an angel. I say, Alyosha, you have amazed me, do you hear? I mean it. It's long since I've been surprised at anything here. Still, I always took you for an educated man . . ." Alyosha at last looked at him, but absently, as it were, as though scarcely understanding what he said.

"Can you really be so upset simply because your old man has begun to stink? You don't mean to say you seriously believed that he was going to turn out miracles?" exclaimed Rakitin, genuinely surprised again.

"I believed, I believe, I want to believe, and I will believe, what more do you want?" cried Alyosha irritably.

"Nothing at all, darling. Damn it all, why, no schoolboy of thirteen believes in that now. But there . . . So now you are in a temper with your God, you are rebelling against Him; promotion has been withheld, the order of merit hasn't been bestowed! Eh, you are a set!"

Alyosha gazed a long while with his eyes half closed at Rakitin, and there was a sudden gleam in his eyes . . . but not of anger with Rakitin.

"I am not rebelling against my God; I simply 'don't accept His world.'" Alyosha suddenly smiled a crooked smile.

"How do you mean, you don't accept the world?" Rakitin thought a moment over his answer. "What idiocy is this?"

Alyosha did not answer.

"Come, enough nonsense, now to business. Have you had anything to eat to-day?"

"I don't remember. . . . I think I have."

"You need a bite, to judge by your looks. It makes one's heart ache to look at you. You didn't sleep all night either, I hear, you had a meeting in there. And then all this bobbery afterwards. Most likely you've had nothing to chew but a mouthful of holy bread. I've got some sausage in my pocket; I've brought it from the town in case of need, only you won't eat sausage. . ."

"Give me some."

"I say! You are going it! Why, it's a regular mutiny, with barricades! Well, my boy, we must make the most of it. Come to my place. . . . I shouldn't mind a drop of vodka myself, I am tired to death. Vodka is going too far for you, I suppose . . . or would you like some?"

"Give me some vodka, too."

"Hullo! You amaze me, brother!" Rakitin looked at him in astonishment. "Well, one way or another, vodka or sausage, this is a jolly fine chance and mustn't be missed. Come along."

Alyosha got up in silence and followed Rakitin.

"If your little brother Ivan could see this — wouldn't he be surprised! By the way, your brother Ivan set off for Moscow this morning, did you know?"

"Yes," answered Alyosha listlessly, and suddenly the image of his brother Dmitri rose before his mind. But only for a minute, and though it reminded him of something that must not be put off for a moment, some duty, some terrible obligation, even that reminder made no impression on him, did not reach his heart and instantly faded out of his mind and was forgotten. But, a long while afterwards, Alyosha remembered this.

"Your brother Ivan declared once that I was a 'liberal booby with no talents whatever.' Once you, too, could not resist letting me know I was 'dishonourable.' Well! I should like to see what your talents and sense of honour will do for you now." This phrase Rakitin finished to himself in a whisper.

"Pooh! Listen!" he said aloud, "let's take the path clear of the monastery straight to the town. H'm! I ought to go to Madame Hohlakov's by the way. Only fancy, I've written to tell her everything that happened, and would you believe it, she answered me instantly in pencil (the lady has a passion for writing notes) that 'she would never have expected *such conduct* from such an estimable elder as Father Zosima.' That was her very word: 'conduct.' She, too, is angry. Eh, you are a set! Stay!" he cried suddenly again. He stopped abruptly and taking Alyosha by the shoulder made him stop, too.

"Do you know, Alyosha" — he peeped inquisitively into his eyes, absorbed in a sudden new thought which had dawned on him, and though he was laughing outwardly he was evidently afraid to utter that new idea aloud, so difficult he still found it to believe in the strange and unexpected mood in which he now saw Alyosha. "Alyosha, do you know where we had better go now?" he brought out at last timidly, and pleadingly.

"I don't care . . . where you like."

"Let's go to Grushenka, eh? Will you come?" pronounced Rakitin at last, trembling with timid suspense.

"Let's go to Grushenka," Alyosha answered calmly, at once, and this prompt and calm agreement was such a surprise to Rakitin that he almost jumped back.

"Well! I say!" he cried in amazement, but seizing Alyosha firmly by the arm he led him along the path, still dreading that he would change his mind.

They walked along in silence, Rakitin was positively afraid to talk.

"And how glad she will be, how delighted," he muttered, but lapsed into silence again. And indeed it was not to please Grushenka that he was taking Alyosha to her. He was a practical person and never undertook anything without a prospect of gain for himself. His object in this case was two-fold, first a revengeful desire to see "the disgrace of the righteous," and Alyosha's fall "from saintliness to sin," over which he was already gloating in his imagination, and in the second place he had in view a certain material gain for himself, of which more will be said later.

"Well, this is the psychological moment," he thought to himself with spiteful glee, "and we shall catch it by the collar, for it's just what we want."

CHAPTER III

AN ONION

Grushenka lived in the busiest part of the town, near the cathedral square, renting a wooden lodge close by the house of her landlady, the widow of a merchant by the name of Morozov. The house was a large stone building of two storeys, old and of a very unprepossessing appearance. The widow, an old woman, led a secluded life there with her two unmarried nieces, who were elderly spinsters. She had no need to let her lodge, but every one knew that she had taken in Grushenka as a lodger, four years before, solely to please her kinsman, the merchant Samsonov, who was publicly known to be the girl's protector. It was said that the jealous old man's object in placing his "favourite" with the widow Morozov was that the old woman should keep a sharp eye on her new lodger's conduct. But this sharp eye soon proved to be unnecessary, and in the end the widow Morozov seldom met Grushenka and did not worry her by looking after her in any way. It is true that four years had passed since the old man had brought the slim, delicate, shy, timid, dreamy, and sad girl of eighteen from the chief town of the province, and much water had flowed under the bridges since then. Little was known of the girl's history in the town and that little was vague. Nothing more had been learnt more recently, even after many people had become interested in the great beauty that Agrafena Alexandrovna had meanwhile become. There were rumours that at seventeen she had been deceived by some one, some sort of officer, and immediately afterwards abandoned by him. The officer had gone away and afterwards married, while Grushenka had been left in destitution and disgrace. It was said, however, that though Grushenka had been actually saved from destitution by the old man, Samsonov, she came of a respectable family belonging to the clergy, that she was the daughter of a supernumerary deacon or something of the sort.

And now after four years the sensitive, injured, and pathetic little orphan had become a plump, rosy beauty of the Russian type, a woman of bold and determined character, proud and insolent. She had a good head for business, was acquisitive, saving, and careful, and by fair means or foul had succeeded, it was said, in amassing a little fortune of her own. There was only one point on which all were agreed. Grushenka was not easy of access, and except her aged protector there had not been one man who could boast of her favours during those four years. It was a positive fact, for there had been a good many, especially during the last two years, who had attempted to obtain those favours. But all their efforts had been in vain and some of these suitors had been forced to beat an undignified and even comic retreat, owing to the firm and ironical resistance they met from the strong-willed young person. It was known, too, that the young person had, especially of late, been engaging in what is called "business," and that she had shown marked abilities in that direction, so that many people called her a regular Jewess. It was not that she lent money at interest, but it was known, for instance, that she had for some time past, in partnership with old Karamazov, actually invested in the purchase of bad debts for a trifle, a tenth of their nominal value, and afterwards had made out of them ten times what they were worth.

The old widower Samsonov, a man of large fortune, was stingy and merciless. He tyrannised over his grown-up sons, but, for the last year, during which he had been ill and lost the use of his swollen legs, he had fallen greatly under the influence of his protégée, whom he had at first kept strictly and on short rations, "on lenten fare" as the wits said at the time. But Grushenka had succeeded in emancipating herself, while she established in him a boundless belief in her fidelity. The old man, now long since dead, had had a large business in his day and was also a noteworthy character, miserly and hard as flint. Though Grushenka's hold upon him was so strong that he could not live without her (it had been so especially for the last two years), he did not settle any considerable fortune on her and would not have been moved to do so, even if she had threatened to leave him. But he had presented her with a small sum, and even that was a surprise to every one when it became known.

"You are a wench with brains," he said to her, when he gave her eight thousand roubles, "and you must look after yourself, but let me tell you that except your yearly allowance as before, you'll get nothing more from me to the day of my death, and I'll leave you nothing in my will either."

And he kept his word; he died and left everything to his sons, whom, with their wives and children, he had treated all his life as servants. Grushenka was not even mentioned in his will. All this became known afterwards. He did, however, offer Grushenka advice as to how to manage her affairs, and put business in her way.

When Fyodor Pavlovich, who first came into contact with Grushenka over a matter of business, ended to his own surprise by falling madly in love with her, old Samsonov, gravely ill as he was, was immensely amused. It is remarkable that throughout their whole acquaintance Grushenka was absolutely and spontaneously open with the old man, and he seems to have been the only person in the world with whom she was on such terms. Of late, when Dmitri, too, had come on the scene with his love, the old man left off laughing. On the contrary, he once gave Grushenka a stern and earnest piece of advice.

"If you have to choose between the two, father and son, you'd better choose the old man, if only you make sure the old scoundrel will marry you and settle some money on you beforehand. But don't get mixed up with the captain, no good will come of that."

These were the very words of the old sensualist, who felt already that his death was not far off and who actually died five months later.

I will note, too, in passing, that although many in our town knew of the grotesque and monstrous rivalry of the Karamazovs, father and son, the object of which was Grushenka, scarcely any one understood what really underlay her attitude to both of them. Even Grushenka's two servants (after the catastrophe of which we will speak later) testified in court that she received Dmitri Fyodorovich simply out of fear because "he threatened to murder her." These servants were an old cook, something of an invalid and almost deaf, who came from Grushenka's old home, and her grand-daughter, a smart young girl of twenty, who performed the duties of a maid. Grushenka lived very economically and her surroundings were anything but luxurious. Her lodge consisted of three rooms containing mahogany furniture in the fashion of 1820, belonging to her landlady.

It was quite dark when Rakitin and Alyosha entered her rooms, yet they were not lighted up. Grushenka was lying down in her drawing-room on the big, hard, clumsy sofa with a mahogany back. The sofa was covered with shabby and ragged leather. Under her head she had two white down pillows taken from her bed. She was lying stretched out motionless on her back with her hands behind her head. She was dressed as though expecting some one, in a black silk dress, with a dainty lace fichu on her head, which was very becoming. Over her shoulders was thrown a lace shawl pinned with a massive gold brooch. She certainly was expecting some one. She lay as though impatient and weary, her face rather pale and her lips and eyes hot, restlessly tapping the arm of the sofa with the tip of her right foot. The appearance of Rakitin and Alyosha caused a slight excitement. From the hall they could hear Grushenka leap up from the sofa and cry out in a frightened voice, "Who's there?" But the maid met the visitors and at once called back to her mistress.

"It's not he, it's nothing, only other visitors."

"What can be the matter?" muttered Rakitin, leading Alyosha into the drawing-room.

Grushenka was standing by the sofa as though still alarmed. A thick coil of her dark brown hair escaped from its lace covering and fell on her right shoulder, but she did not notice it and did not put it back till she had scrutinised her visitors and recognised them.

"Ah, it's you, Rakitin? You quite frightened me. Whom have you brought? Who is this with you? Good heavens, you have brought him!" she exclaimed, recognising Alyosha.

"Do send for candles!" said Rakitin, with the free-and-easy air of a most intimate friend, who is privileged to give orders in the house.

"Candles . . . of course, candles. . . . Fenya, fetch him a candle. . . . Well, you have chosen a moment to bring him!" she exclaimed again, nodding towards Alyosha, and turning to the looking-glass she began quickly fastening up her hair with both hands. She seemed annoyed.

"Have I displeased you?" asked Rakitin, instantly almost offended.

"You frightened me, Rakitin, that's what it is." Grushenka turned with a smile to Alyosha. "Don't be afraid of me, my dear Alyosha, you can't think how glad I am to see you, my unexpected visitor. But you frightened me, Rakitin, I thought it was Mitya breaking in. You see, I deceived him just now, I made him promise to believe me but I told him a lie. I told him that I was going to spend the evening with my old man Kuzma Kuzmich, and should be there till late counting money. I always spend one whole evening a week with him making up his accounts. We lock ourselves in and he counts on the abacus while I sit and put things down in the book. I am the only person he trusts. Mitya believes that I am there, but I came back and have been sitting locked in here, expecting some news. How was it Fenya let you in? Fenya, Fenya, run out to the gate, open it and find out whether the captain is to be seen! Perhaps he is hiding and spying, I am dreadfully frightened."

"There's no one there, Agrafena Alexandrovna, I've just looked out; I keep running to peep through the crack, I am in fear and trembling myself."

"Are the shutters fastened, Fenya? And we must draw the curtains — that's better!" She drew the heavy curtains herself. "He'd rush in at once if he saw a light. I am afraid of your brother Mitya to-day, Alyosha."

Grushenka spoke aloud, and, though she was alarmed, she seemed to be elated over something.

"Why are you so afraid of Mitya to-day?" inquired Rakitin. "I should have thought you were not timid with him, he dances to your piping."

"I tell you, I am expecting news, priceless news, so I don't want Mitya at all now. And he didn't believe, I feel he didn't, that I would stay at Kuzma Kuzmich's. He must be in ambush now, in the back of his father's garden, watching for me. And if he's there, he won't come here, so much the better! But I really have been to Kuzma Kuzmich's, Mitya escorted me there. I told him I should stay there till midnight, and I asked him to be sure to come at midnight to fetch me home. He went away and I sat ten minutes with Kuzma Kuzmich and came back here again. Ugh, I was afraid, I ran for fear of meeting him."

"And why are you so dressed up? What a curious cap you've got on!"

"How curious you are yourself, Rakitin! I tell you, I am expecting a message. If the message comes, I shall fly, I shall gallop away and you will see no more of me. That's why I am dressed up, so as to be ready."

"And where are you flying to?"

"If you know too much, you'll get old too soon."

"Upon my word! You are all aflutter . . . I've never seen you like this before. You are dressed up as if you were going to a ball." Rakitin looked her up and down.

"Much you know about balls."

"And do you know much about them?"

"I have seen a ball. The year before last, Kuzma Kuzmich's son was married and I looked on from the gallery. Do you suppose I want to be talking to you, Rakitin, while a prince like this is standing here? Such a visitor! Alyosha, my dear boy, I look at you and can't believe my eyes. Good heavens, can you have come here to see me! To tell you the truth I never had a thought of seeing you and I didn't dream that you would ever come and see me. Though this is not the proper moment now, I am awfully glad to see you. Sit down on the sofa, here, that's right, my bright young moon. I really can't take it in even now. . . . Eh, Rakitin, if only you had brought him yesterday or the day before! But I am glad as it is! Perhaps it's better he has come now, at such a moment, and not the day before yesterday."

She gaily sat down beside Alyosha on the sofa, looking at him with positive delight. And she really was glad, she was not lying when she said so. Her eyes glowed, her lips laughed, but it was a good-natured merry laugh. Alyosha had not expected to see such a kind expression in her face. . . . He had hardly met her till the day before, he had formed an alarming idea of her, and had been horribly distressed the day before by the spiteful and treacherous trick she had played on Katerina Ivanovna. He was greatly surprised to find her now altogether different from what he had expected. And, crushed as he was by his own sorrow, his eyes involuntarily rested on her with attention. Her whole manner seemed changed for the better since yesterday, there was scarcely any trace of that mawkish sweetness in her speech, of that voluptuous softness in her movements. Everything was simple and good-natured, her gestures were rapid, direct, confiding, but she was greatly excited.

"Dear me, how everything comes together to-day," she chattered on again. "And why I am so glad to see you, Alyosha, I couldn't say myself! If you asked me, I couldn't tell you."

"Come, don't you know why you're glad?" said Rakitin, grinning. "You used to be always pestering me to bring him, you'd some object, I suppose."

"I had a different object once, but now that's over, this is not the moment. I say, I want to serve you something nice. I am good-natured now. You sit down, too, Rakitin, why are you standing? You've sat down already? There's no fear of Rakitin's forgetting to look after himself. Look, Alyosha, he's sitting there opposite us, so offended that I didn't ask him to sit down before you. Ugh, Rakitin is such a one to take offence!" laughed Grushenka. "Don't be angry, Rakitin, I'm kind today. Why are you so depressed, Alyosha, are you afraid of me?" She peeped into his eyes with merry mockery.

"He's sad. There's been no promotion," boomed Rakitin.

"What promotion?"

"His elder started to smell."

"What? You are talking some nonsense, you want to say something nasty. Be quiet, you stupid! Will you let me sit on your knee, Alyosha, like this?" She suddenly skipped forward and jumped, laughing, on his knee, like a nestling kitten, placing her right arm tenderly around his neck. "I'll cheer you up, my pious boy. Yes, really, will you let me sit on your knee, you won't be angry? If you tell me, I'll hop off."

Alyosha did not speak. He sat afraid to stir, he heard her words, "If you tell me, I'll hop off," but he did not answer, it was as though he couldn't move. But there was nothing in his heart such as Rakitin, for instance, watching him from his corner with a leer, might have expected or fancied. The great grief in his heart swallowed up every sensation that might have been aroused in him, and, if only he could have thought clearly at that moment, he would have realised that he had now the strongest armour to protect him from every snare and temptation. Yet in spite of the confusion of his spiritual condition and the sorrow that overwhelmed him, he could not help wondering at a new and strange sensation that was rising in his heart. This woman, this "dreadful" woman, had no terror for him now, none of that terror that had stirred in his soul at any passing thought of woman. On the contrary, this woman, dreaded above all women, sitting now on his knee, holding him in her arms, aroused in him now a quite different, unexpected, peculiar feeling, a feeling of the intensest and purest interest without a trace of fear, of his former terror. That was what instinctively surprised him.

"You've talked nonsense enough," cried Rakitin, "you'd much better serve us some champagne. You owe it me, you know!"

"Yes, I really do. Do you know, Alyosha, I promised him champagne on top of everything, if he'd bring you? I'll have some, too! Fenya, Fenya, bring us the bottle Mitya left! Look sharp! Though I am so stingy, I'll stand a bottle, not for you, Rakitin, you're a toadstool, but he is a lord! And though my heart is full of something very different, so be it, I'll drink with you. I long for some dissipation."

"But what is this 'moment' you're talking about? And what is this news, may I ask, or is it a secret?" Rakitin put in inquisitively, doing his best to pretend not to notice the snubs that were being continually aimed at him.

"Ah, it's not a secret, and you know it, too," Grushenka said, in a voice suddenly anxious, turning her head towards Rakitin, and drawing a little away from Alyosha, though she still sat on his knee with her arm round his neck. "My officer is coming, Rakitin, my officer is coming."

"I heard he was coming, but is he so near?"

"He is at Mokroye now, he'll send a message from there, so he wrote, I got a letter from him to-day. I am expecting the message every minute."

"You don't say so! Why at Mokroye?"

"That's a long story, I've told you enough."

"Mitya'll be up to something now — I say! Does he know or doesn't he?"

"He know! Of course he doesn't. If he knew, there would be murder. But I am not afraid of that now, I am not afraid of his knife. Be quiet, Rakitin, don't remind me of Dmitri Fyodorovich, he has bruised my heart. And I don't want to think of that at this moment. I can think of Alyosha here, I can look at Alyosha . . . smile at me, darling, cheer up, smile at my foolishness, at my pleasure. . . . Ah, he's smiling, he's smiling! How kindly he looks at me! And you know, Alyosha, I've been thinking all this time you were angry with me, because of the day before yesterday, because of that young lady. I was a cur, that's the truth. . . . But it's a good thing it happened so. It was a horrid thing, but a good thing, too." Grushenka smiled pensively and a little cruel line showed in her smile. "Mitya told me that she screamed out that I 'ought to be flogged.' I did insult her dreadfully. She sent for me, she wanted to make a conquest of me, to win me over with her chocolate. . . . No, it's a good thing it did end like that." She smiled again. "But I am still afraid of your being angry."

"Yes, that's really true," Rakitin put in suddenly with genuine surprise. "Alyosha, she is really afraid of a chicken like you."

"He is a chicken to you, Rakitin . . . because you've no conscience, that's what it is! You see, I love him with all my soul, that's how it is! Alyosha, do you believe I love you with all my soul?"

"Ah, you shameless woman! She is making you a declaration, Alexey!"

"Well, what of it, I love him!"

"And what about your officer? And the priceless message from Mokroye?"

"That is quite different."

"That's a woman's way of looking at it!"

"Don't you make me angry, Rakitin." Grushenka caught him up hotly. "This is quite different. I love Alyosha in a different way. It's true, Alyosha, I had sly designs on you before. For I am a horrid, violent creature. But at other times I've looked upon you, Alyosha, as my conscience. I've kept thinking 'how any one like that must despise a nasty thing like me.' I thought that the day before yesterday, as I ran home from the young lady's. I have thought of you a long time in that way, Alyosha, and Mitya knows, I've talked to him about it. Mitya understands. Would you believe it, I sometimes look at you and feel ashamed, utterly ashamed of myself. . . . And how, and since when, I began to think about you like that, I can't say, I don't remember. . . ."

Fenya came in and put a tray with an uncorked bottle and three glasses of champagne on the table.

"Here's the champagne!" cried Rakitin. "You're excited, Agrafena Alexandrovna, and not yourself. When you've had a glass of champagne, you'll be ready to dance. Eh, they can't even do that properly," he added, looking at the bottle. "The old woman's poured it out in the kitchen and the bottle's been brought in warm and without a cork. Well, let me have some, anyway."

He went up to the table, took a glass, emptied it at one gulp and poured himself out another.

"One doesn't often stumble upon champagne," he said, licking his lips. "Now, Alyosha, take a glass, show what you can do! What shall we drink to? The gates of paradise? Take a glass, Grushenka, you drink to the gates of paradise, too."

"What gates of paradise?"

She took a glass, Alyosha took his, tasted it and put it back.

"No, I'd better not," he smiled gently.

"And you bragged!" cried Rakitin.

"Well, if so, I won't either," chimed in Grushenka, "I really don't want any. You can drink the whole bottle alone, Rakitin. If Alyosha has some, I will."

"What calf-like sentimentality!" said Rakitin tauntingly, "and she's sitting on his knee, too! He's got something to grieve over, but what's the matter with you? He was rebelling against his God and was ready to eat sausage . . ."

"How so?"

"His elder died to-day, Father Zosima, the saint."

"So Father Zosima is dead," cried Grushenka. "Good God, I did not know!" She crossed herself devoutly. "Goodness, what have I been doing, sitting on his knee like this at such a time!" She started up as though in dismay, instantly slipped off his knee and sat down on the sofa.

Alyosha bent a long wondering look upon her and a light seemed to dawn in his face.

"Rakitin," he said suddenly, in a firm and loud voice, "don't taunt me with having rebelled against God. I don't want to feel angry with you, so you must be kinder, too. I've lost a treasure such as you have never had, and you cannot judge me now. You had much better look at her — do you see how she spared me? I came here to find a wicked soul — I felt drawn to evil because I was base and evil myself, and I've found a true sister, I have found a treasure — a loving heart. She spared me just now. . . . Agrafena Alexandrovna, I am speaking of you. You've restored my soul just now."

Alyosha's lips were quivering and he caught his breath.

"She has saved you, it seems," laughed Rakitin spitefully. "And she meant to swallow you, do you realise that?"

"Stay, Rakitin." Grushenka jumped up. "Hush, both of you. Now I'll tell you all about it. Hush, Alyosha, your words make me ashamed, for I am bad and not good — that's

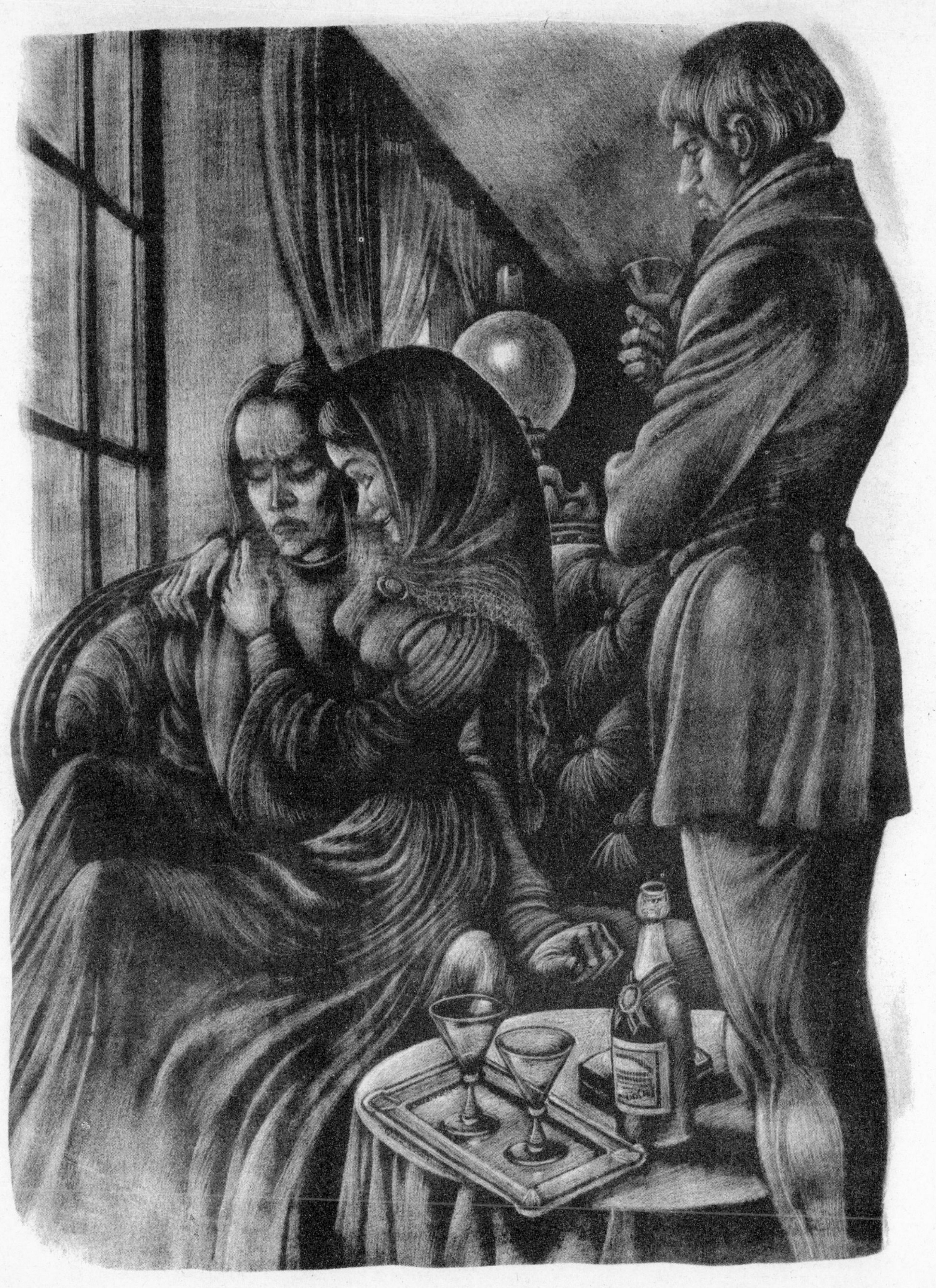

"DRINK TO THE GATES OF PARADISE"

what I am. And you hush, Rakitin, because you are telling lies. I had the low idea of trying to swallow him, but now you are lying, now it's all different. And don't let me hear anything more from you, Rakitin."

All this Grushenka said with extreme emotion.

"They are both crazy," said Rakitin, looking at them with amazement. "I feel as though I were in a madhouse. They're both weakening so that they'll begin crying in a minute."

"I shall begin to cry, I shall," repeated Grushenka. "He called me his sister and I shall never forget that. Only let me tell you, Rakitin, though I am bad, I did give away an onion."

"An onion? Hang it all, you really are crazy."

Rakitin wondered at their exaltation. He was aggrieved and annoyed, though he might have reflected that each of them was just passing through a spiritual crisis such as does not come often in a lifetime. But though Rakitin was very sensitive about everything that concerned himself, he was very obtuse as regards the feelings and sensations of others — partly because of his youth and inexperience, partly because of his intense egoism.

"You see, Alyosha," Grushenka turned to him with a nervous laugh, "I was boasting when I told Rakitin I had given away an onion, but it's not to boast I tell you about it. It's only a story, but it's a nice story. I heard it when I was a child from Matryona, my cook, who is still with me. It's like this. 'Once upon a time there was a peasant woman and a very wicked woman she was. And she died and did not leave a single good deed behind. The devils caught her and plunged her into a lake of fire. So her guardian angel stood and wondered what good deed of hers he could remember to tell to God; he did remember one and said to God: "She once pulled up an onion in her garden," said he, "and gave it to a beggar woman." And God answered: "You take that onion then, hold it out to her in the lake, and let her take hold of it. And if you can pull her out of the lake, let her come to Paradise, but if the onion breaks, then the woman must stay where she is." The angel ran to the woman and held out the onion to her. "Come," said he, "catch hold and I'll pull you out." And he began cautiously pulling her out. He had nearly pulled her out, when the other sinners in the lake, seeing how she was being drawn out, began catching hold of her so as to be pulled out with her. But she was a very wicked woman and she began kicking them. "I'm to be pulled out, not you. It's my onion, not yours." As soon as she said that, the onion broke. And the woman fell into the lake and she is burning there to this day. So the angel wept and went away.' So that's the story, Alyosha; I know it by heart, for I am that wicked woman myself. I boasted to Rakitin that I had given away an onion, but to you I'll say: 'I've done nothing but give away one onion all my life, that's the only good deed I've done.' So don't praise me, Alyosha, don't think me good, I am bad, I am a wicked woman and you make me ashamed if you praise me. Eh, I must confess everything. Listen, Alyosha. I was so anxious to get hold of you that I promised Rakitin twenty-five roubles if he would bring you to me. Stay, Rakitin, wait!" She went rapidly to the table, opened a drawer, pulled out a purse and took from it a twenty-five rouble note.

"What nonsense! What nonsense!" cried Rakitin, disconcerted.

"Take it, Rakitin, I owe it you, there's no fear of your refusing it, you asked for it yourself." And she threw the note to him.

"Likely I should refuse it," boomed Rakitin, obviously abashed, but carrying off his confusion with a swagger. "That will come in very handy; fools are made for wise men's profit."

"And now hold your tongue, Rakitin, what I am going to say now is not for your ears. Sit down in that corner and keep quiet. You don't like us, so hold your tongue."

"What should I like you for?" Rakitin snarled, not concealing his ill-humour. He put the twenty-five rouble note in his pocket and he felt ashamed at Alyosha's seeing it. He had reckoned on receiving his payment later, without Alyosha's knowing of it, and now, feeling ashamed, he lost his temper. Till that moment he had thought it discreet not to contradict Grushenka too flatly in spite of her snubbing, since he had something to get out of her. But now he, too, was angry:

"One loves people for some reason, but what have either of you done for me?"

"You should love people without a reason, as Alyosha does."

"How does he love you? How has he shown it, that you make such a fuss about it?"

Grushenka was standing in the middle of the room; she spoke with heat and there were hysterical notes in her voice.

"Hush, Rakitin, you know nothing about us! And don't dare to speak to me like that again. How dare you be so familiar! Sit in that corner and be quiet, as though you were my footman! And now, Alyosha, I'll tell you the whole truth, that you may see what a hussy I am! I am not talking to Rakitin, but to you. I wanted to ruin you, Alyosha, that's the holy truth; I quite meant to. I wanted to so much, that I bribed Rakitin to bring you. And why did I want to do such a thing? You knew nothing about it, Alyosha, you turned away from me, if you passed me, you dropped your eyes. And I've looked at you a hundred times before to-day, I began asking every one about you. Your face haunted my heart. 'He despises me,' I thought, 'he won't even look at me.' And I felt it so much at last that I wondered at myself for being so scared of a boy. I'll swallow him whole and laugh. I was full of spite and anger. Would you believe it, nobody here dares talk or think of coming to Agrafena Alexandrovna with any evil purpose. The old man is the only one I have anything to do with, I was bound and sold to him, Satan married us, but there has been no one else. But looking at you, I decided, I'll swallow him and laugh. You see what a spiteful cur I am, and you called me your sister! And now that man who wronged me has come; I sit here waiting for a message from him. And do you know what that man has been to me? Five years ago, when Kuzma brought me here, I used to shut myself up, that no one might have sight or sound of me. I was a silly slip of a girl; I used to sit here sobbing, I used to lie awake all night, thinking: 'Where is he now, the man who wronged me? He is laughing at me with another woman, most likely. If only I could see him, if I could meet him again, I'd pay him out, I'd pay him out!' At night I used to lie sobbing into my pillow in the dark, and I used to brood over it, I used to tear my heart on purpose and gloat over my anger. 'I'll pay him out, I'll pay him out!' That's what I used to cry out in the dark. And when I suddenly thought that I should really do nothing to him, and that he was laughing at me then, or perhaps had utterly forgotten me, I would fling myself on the floor, melt into helpless tears, and lie there shaking till dawn. In the morning I would get up more spiteful than a dog, ready to tear the whole world to pieces. And then what do you think? I began saving money, I became hard-hearted, grew plump — grew wiser, would you say? No, no one in the whole world sees it, no one knows it, but when night comes on, I sometimes lie as I did five years ago, when I was a silly girl, grinding my teeth and crying all night, thinking: 'I'll pay him out, I'll pay him out!' Do you hear? Well, then, now you understand me. A month ago a letter came to me — he was coming, he was a widower, he wanted to see me. It took my breath away, then I suddenly thought: 'If he comes and whistles to call me, I shall creep back to him like a beaten dog.' I couldn't believe myself. Am I so abject? Shall I run to him or not? And I've been in such a rage with myself all this month that I am worse than I was five years ago. Do you see now, Alyosha, what a violent, savage creature I am? I have shown you the whole truth! I played with Mitya to keep me from running to that other. Hush, Rakitin, it's not for you to judge me, I am not speaking to you. Before you came in, I was lying here waiting, brooding, deciding my whole future life, and you can never know what was in my heart. Yes, Alyosha, tell your young lady not to be angry with me for what happened the day before yesterday. . . . Nobody in the whole world knows what I am going through now, and no one ever can know. . . . For perhaps I shall take a knife with me to-day, I can't make up my mind . . ."

And at this "pathetic" phrase Grushenka broke down, hid her face in her hands, flung herself on the sofa pillows, and sobbed like a child. Alyosha got up and went to Rakitin.

"Misha," he said, "don't be angry. She wounded you, but don't be angry. You heard what she said just now? You mustn't ask too much of human endurance, one must be more merciful."

Alyosha said this at the instinctive prompting of his heart. He felt obliged to speak and he turned to Rakitin. If Rakitin had not been there, he would have spoken to the air. But Rakitin looked at him ironically and Alyosha stopped short.

"You were so primed up with your elder's teaching the other night that now you have to shoot it off at me, Alexey, man of God!" said Rakitin, with a smile of hatred.

"Don't laugh, Rakitin, don't grin, don't talk of the dead — he was better than any one on earth!" cried Alyosha, with tears in his voice. "I didn't get up to speak to you as a judge but as the lowest of the judged. What am I beside her? I came here seeking my ruin, and said to myself, 'What does it matter?' and that because of cowardice, but she, after five years in torment, as soon as any one says a word from the heart to her — she forgives everything, she forgets everything, and cries. The man who has wronged her has come back, he sends for her and she forgives him everything, and hastens joyfully to meet him and she won't take a knife with her. She won't! No, I am not like that. I don't know whether you are, Misha, but I am not like that. It's a lesson to me. . . . She loves better than we. . . . Have you heard her speak before of what she has just told us? No, you haven't; if you had, you'd have understood her long ago . . . and the person insulted the day before yesterday must forgive her, too! She will, when she knows . . . and she shall know. . . . This soul is not yet at peace with itself, one must spare it . . . there may be a treasure in that soul. . . ."

Alyosha stopped, because he was breathless. In spite of his ill-humour Rakitin looked at him with astonishment. He had never expected such a tirade from the gentle Alyosha.

"What an advocate she has found! Are you in love with her? Agrafena Alexandrovna, our monk's really in love with you, you've made a conquest!" he cried, with an insolent laugh.

Grushenka lifted her head from the pillow and looked at Alyosha with a tender smile shining on her face, which suddenly appeared swollen with tears.

"Let him alone, Alyosha, my cherub, you see the sort he is, he is not a person for you to speak to. Mihail Osipovich," she turned to Rakitin, "I meant to beg your pardon for being rude to you, but now I don't want to. Alyosha, come to me, sit down here." She beckoned to him with a happy smile. "That's right, sit here. Tell me," she took him by the hand and peeped into his face, smiling, "tell me, do I love that man or not? the man who wronged me, do I love him or not? Before you came, I lay here in the dark, asking my heart whether I loved him. Decide for me, Alyosha, the time has come, it shall be as you say. Am I to forgive him or not?"

"But you have forgiven him already," said Alyosha, smiling.

"Yes, I really have forgiven him," Grushenka murmured thoughtfully. "What a vile heart! To my vile heart!" She snatched up a glass from the table, emptied it at a gulp, lifted it in the air and flung it on the floor. The glass broke with a crash. A little cruel line came into her smile.

"Perhaps I haven't forgiven him, though," she said, with a sort of menace in her voice, and she dropped her eyes to the ground as though she were talking to herself. "Perhaps my heart is only getting ready to forgive. I shall yet struggle with my heart. You see, Alyosha, I've grown to love my tears awfully in these five years. . . . Perhaps I love only my resentment, not him. . . ."

"Well, I shouldn't care to be in his skin," hissed Rakitin.

"Well, you won't be, Rakitin, you'll never be in his skin. You shall black my shoes, Rakitin, that's the kind of work I'll make you do. You'll never get one like me . . . and he won't either, perhaps. . . ."

"Won't he? Then why are you dressed up like that?" said Rakitin, with a venomous sneer.

"Don't taunt me with dressing up, Rakitin, you don't know all that is in my heart! If I choose to tear off my finery, I'll tear it off at once, this minute," she cried in a resonant voice. "You don't know what that finery is for, Rakitin! Perhaps I shall come before him and say: 'Have you ever seen me look like this before?' He left me a thin, consumptive cry-baby of seventeen. I'll sit with him, fascinate him and work him up. 'Do you see what I am like now?' I'll say to him; 'well, and that's enough for you, my dear sir, there's many a slip twixt the cup and the lip!' That may be what the finery is for, Rakitin." Grushenka finished with a malicious laugh. "I'm violent and savage, Alyosha, I'll tear off my finery, I'll destroy my beauty, I'll scorch my face, slash it with a knife, and turn beggar. If I choose, I won't go anywhere now to see any one. If I choose, I'll send Kuzma back all he has ever given me, and all his money, to-morrow, and I'll go out charing for the rest of my life. You

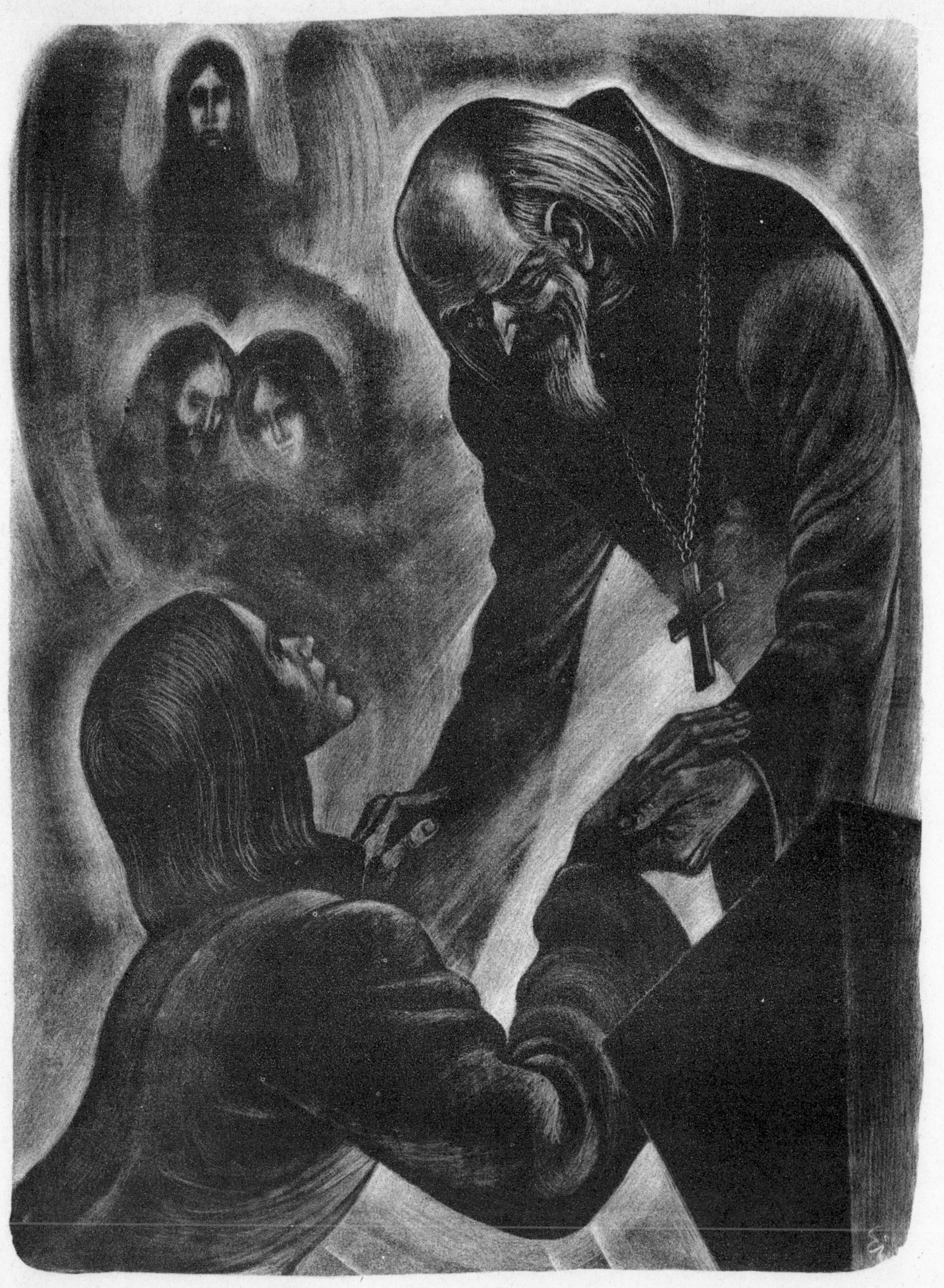

CANA OF GALILEE

think I wouldn't do it, Rakitin, that I would not dare to do it? I would, I would, I could do it directly, only don't exasperate me . . . and I'll send him about his business, I'll snap my fingers in his face, he shan't have me!"

She screamed the last words hysterically, but broke down again, hid her face in her hands, buried it in the pillow and shook with sobs.

Rakitin got up.

"It's time we were off," he said, "it's late, we shall be shut out of the monastery."

Grushenka leapt up from her place.

"Surely you don't want to go, Alyosha!" she cried, in mournful surprise. "What are you doing to me? You've shaken me, tortured me, and now you'll leave me to face this night alone!"

"He can hardly spend the night with you! Though if he wants to, let him! I'll go alone," Rakitin joked sneeringly.

"Hush, evil soul!" Grushenka cried savagely at him; "you never said such words to me as he has come to say."

"What has he said to you, after all?" muttered Rakitin irritably.

"I can't say, I don't know. I don't know what he said to me, it went straight to my heart; he has wrung my heart. . . . He is the first, the only one who has pitied me, that's what it is. Why did you not come before, you angel?" She fell on her knees before him as though in a sudden frenzy. "I've been waiting all my life for some one like you, I knew that some one like you would come and forgive me. I believed that, nasty as I am, some one would really love me, not only with a shameful love!"

"What have I done to you?" answered Alyosha, bending over her with a tender smile, and gently taking her by the hands; "I only gave you an onion, nothing but a tiny little onion, that was all!"

He was moved to tears himself as he said it. At that moment there was a sudden noise in the passage, some one came into the hall. Grushenka jumped up, seeming greatly alarmed. Fenya ran noisily into the room.

"Mistress, mistress darling, a messenger has galloped up," she cried, breathless and joyful. "A carriage from Mokroye for you, Timofey the driver, with a troika, they are just putting in fresh horses. . . . A letter, here's the letter, mistress."

A letter was in her hand and she waved it in the air all the while she talked. Grushenka snatched the letter from her and carried it to the candle. It was only a note, a few lines. She read it in one instant.

"He has sent for me," she cried, her face white and distorted, with a sickly smile; "he whistles! Crawl back, little dog!"

But only for one instant she stood as though hesitating; suddenly the blood rushed to her head and sent a glow to her cheeks.

"I'm going," she cried; "five years of my life! Good-bye! Good-bye, Alyosha, my fate is sealed. Go, go, leave me, all of you, don't let me see you again! Grushenka is flying to a new life. . . . Don't you remember evil against me either, Rakitin. I may be going to my death! Ugh! I feel as though I were drunk!"

She suddenly left them and ran into her bedroom.

"Well, she has no thoughts for us now!" grumbled Rakitin. "Let's go, or we may hear that female shriek again. I am sick of all these tears and screams."

Alyosha mechanically let himself be led

out. In the yard stood a covered carriage. Horses were being taken out of the shafts, men were running to and fro with a lantern. Three fresh horses were being led in at the open gate. But when Alyosha and Rakitin reached the bottom of the steps, Grushenka's bedroom window was suddenly opened and she called in a ringing voice after Alyosha:

"Alyosha, give my greetings to your brother Mitya and tell him not to remember evil against me, though I have brought him misery. And tell him, too, in my words: 'Grushenka has fallen to a scoundrel, and not to you, noble heart.' And add, too, that Grushenka loved him only one hour, only one short hour she loved him — so let him remember that hour all his life — say, 'Grushenka tells you to!' "

She ended in a voice full of sobs. The window was shut with a slam.

"H'm, h'm!" growled Rakitin, laughing, "she murders your brother Mitya and then tells him to remember it all his life! What carnality!"

Alyosha made no reply, he seemed not to have heard. He walked fast beside Rakitin as though in a terrible hurry. He was lost in thought and moved mechanically. Rakitin felt a sudden twinge as though he had been touched on an open wound. He had expected something quite different by bringing Grushenka and Alyosha together. Something very different from what he had hoped for had happened.

"He is a Pole, that officer of hers," he began again, restraining himself; "and indeed he is not an officer at all now. He served in the customs in Siberia, somewhere on the Chinese frontier, some puny little beggar of a Pole, I expect. Lost his job, they say. He's heard now that Grushenka's saved a little money, so he's turned up again — that's the explanation of the mystery."

Again Alyosha seemed not to hear. Rakitin could not control himself.

"Well, so you've converted the Magdalene?" he laughed spitefully. "You have turned the harlot into the path of virtue? Driven out the seven devils, eh? So that's where those long-expected miracles of ours have come to pass!"

"Hush, Rakitin," Alyosha answered, with an aching heart.

"So you despise me now for those twenty-five roubles? I've sold my friend, you think. But you are not Christ, you know, and I am not Judas."

"Oh, Rakitin, I assure you I'd forgotten about it," cried Alyosha, "you have reminded me of it yourself. . . ."

But this was the last straw for Rakitin.

"Damnation take you all and each of you!" he yelled suddenly; "why the devil did I have anything to do with you? I don't want to know you from now on. Take yourself off, there's your road!"

And he turned abruptly into another street, leaving Alyosha alone in the dark. Alyosha passed out of the town and walked across the fields to the monastery.

CHAPTER IV

CANA OF GALILEE

It was very late, according to monastery ideas, when Alyosha returned to the hermitage; the door-keeper let him in by a special entrance. It had struck nine o'clock — the hour of rest and repose after a day of such agitation for all. Alyosha timidly opened the door and went into the elder's cell where his coffin was now standing. There was no one in the cell but

Father Païssy, reading the Gospel in solitude over the coffin, and the young novice Porfiry, who, exhausted by the previous night's conversation and the exciting incidents of the day, was sleeping the sound sleep of youth on the floor of the other room. Though Father Païssy heard Alyosha come in, he did not even look in his direction. Alyosha turned from the door to the right-hand corner, fell on his knees and began to pray.

His soul was overflowing, but with mingled feelings; no single sensation stood out distinctly; on the contrary, one drove out another in a slow, continual rotation, as it were. But the moment was sweet to his heart and, strange to say, Alyosha was not surprised at it. Again he saw that coffin before him, the hidden dead figure so precious to him, but tearful, poignant grief no longer gnawed at his soul as it had in the morning. As soon as he came in, he fell down before the coffin as before a holy shrine, but joy, joy was glowing in his mind and in his heart. The one window of the cell was open, the air was fresh and cool. "So the smell must have become stronger, if they opened the window," thought Alyosha. But even this thought of the breath of corruption, which had seemed to him so dreadful and disgraceful a few hours before, no longer made him feel miserable or indignant. He began quietly praying, but he soon felt that he was praying almost mechanically. Fragments of thought floated through his soul, flashed like stars and went out again at once, to be succeeded by others. But yet there was reigning in his soul a sense of the wholeness of things — something steadfast and comforting — and he was aware of it himself. Sometimes he began praying ardently, he longed to pour out his thankfulness and love. . . .

But having begun to pray, he passed suddenly to something else, and sank into thought, forgetting both the prayer and what had interrupted it.

He began listening to what Father Païssy was reading, but in his great exhaustion he gradually began to doze.

"*And the third day there was a marriage in Cana of Galilee,*" read Father Païssy. "*And the mother of Jesus was there: And both Jesus was called, and his disciples, to the marriage.*"

"Marriage? What's that . . . marriage . . ." whirled through Alyosha's mind. "There is happiness for her, too. . . . She has gone to the feast. . . . No, she has not taken the knife. . . . That was only a pathetic phrase. . . . Well . . . pathetic phrases should be forgiven, they must be. Pathetic phrases comfort the heart. . . . Without them, sorrow would be too heavy for men to bear. Rakitin turned into the lane. As long as Rakitin broods over his wrongs, he will always turn into the lane. . . . But the high road . . . The high road is wide and straight and bright as crystal, and the sun is at the end of it. . . . Ah! . . . What's being read?" . . .

"*And when they wanted wine, the mother of Jesus saith unto him, They have no wine* . . ." Alyosha heard.

"Ah, yes, I had missed that, and I didn't want to miss it, I love that passage: it's Cana of Galilee, the first miracle. . . . Ah, that miracle! Ah, that sweet miracle! It was not men's grief, but their joy that Christ visited, He worked His first miracle to help men's gladness. . . . 'He who loves men loves their joy, too.' . . . The deceased was always repeating that, it was one of his leading ideas. . . . 'There's no living without joy,' Mitya says. . . . Yes, Mitya. . . . 'Everything that is true and good is always full of forgiveness,' *he* used to say that, too." . . .

"Jesus saith unto her, Woman, what have I to do with thee? Mine hour is not yet come."

"His mother saith unto the servants, Whatsoever he saith unto you, do it." . . .

"Do it. . . . Joy, the joy of some poor, very poor, people. . . . Of course they were poor, since they hadn't wine enough even at a wedding. . . . Historians write that, in those days, the people living about the Lake of Genesareth were the poorest that can possibly be imagined . . . and another great heart, that other great being, His mother, knew that He had come not only to make His great terrible sacrifice. She knew that His heart was open even to the simple, artless merry-making of some obscure, simple people, who had warmly bidden Him to their poor wedding. 'Mine hour is not yet to come,' He said, with a soft smile (He must have smiled gently to her). And indeed was it to make wine abundant at poor weddings He had come down to earth? And yet He went and did as she asked Him. . . . Ah, he is reading again." . . .

"Jesus saith unto them, Fill the waterpots with water. And they filled them up to the brim. And he saith unto them, Draw out now, and bear unto the governor of the feast. And they bare it.

When the ruler of the feast had tasted the water that was made wine, and knew not whence it was: (but the servants which drew the water knew;) the governor of the feast called the bridegroom,

And saith unto him, Every man at the beginning doth set forth good wine; and when men have well drunk, then that which is worse; but thou hast kept the good wine until now."

"But what's this, what's this? Why is the room growing wider? . . . Ah, yes. . . . It's the marriage, the wedding . . . yes, of course. Here are the guests, here are the young couple sitting, and the merry crowd and . . . Where is the wise governor of the feast? But who is this? Who? Again the walls are receding. . . . Who is getting up there from the great table? What! . . . He here, too? But he's in the coffin . . . but he's here, too. He has stood up, he sees me, he is coming here. . . . Lord! . . ."

Yes, he came up to him, to him, he, the little, thin old man, with tiny wrinkles on his face, joyful and laughing softly. There was no coffin now, and he was in the same dress as he had worn yesterday sitting with them, when the visitors had gathered about him. His face was open, his eyes were shining. How was this, then, he, too, had been called to the feast. He, too, at the marriage of Cana in Galilee. . . .

"Yes, my dear, I am called, too, called and bidden," he heard a soft voice saying over him. "Why have you hidden yourself here, out of sight? You come and join us, too."

It was his voice, the voice of Father Zosima. And it must be he, since he called him!

The elder raised Alyosha by the hand and he rose from his knees.

"We are making merry," the little, thin old man went on. "We are drinking the new wine, the wine of new, great joy; do you see how many guests there are? Here are the bride and bridegroom, here is the wise governor of the feast, he is tasting the new wine. Why do you wonder at me? I gave an onion to a beggar, so I, too, am here. And many here have given only an onion each — only one little onion. . . . What are all our deeds? And you, my gentle

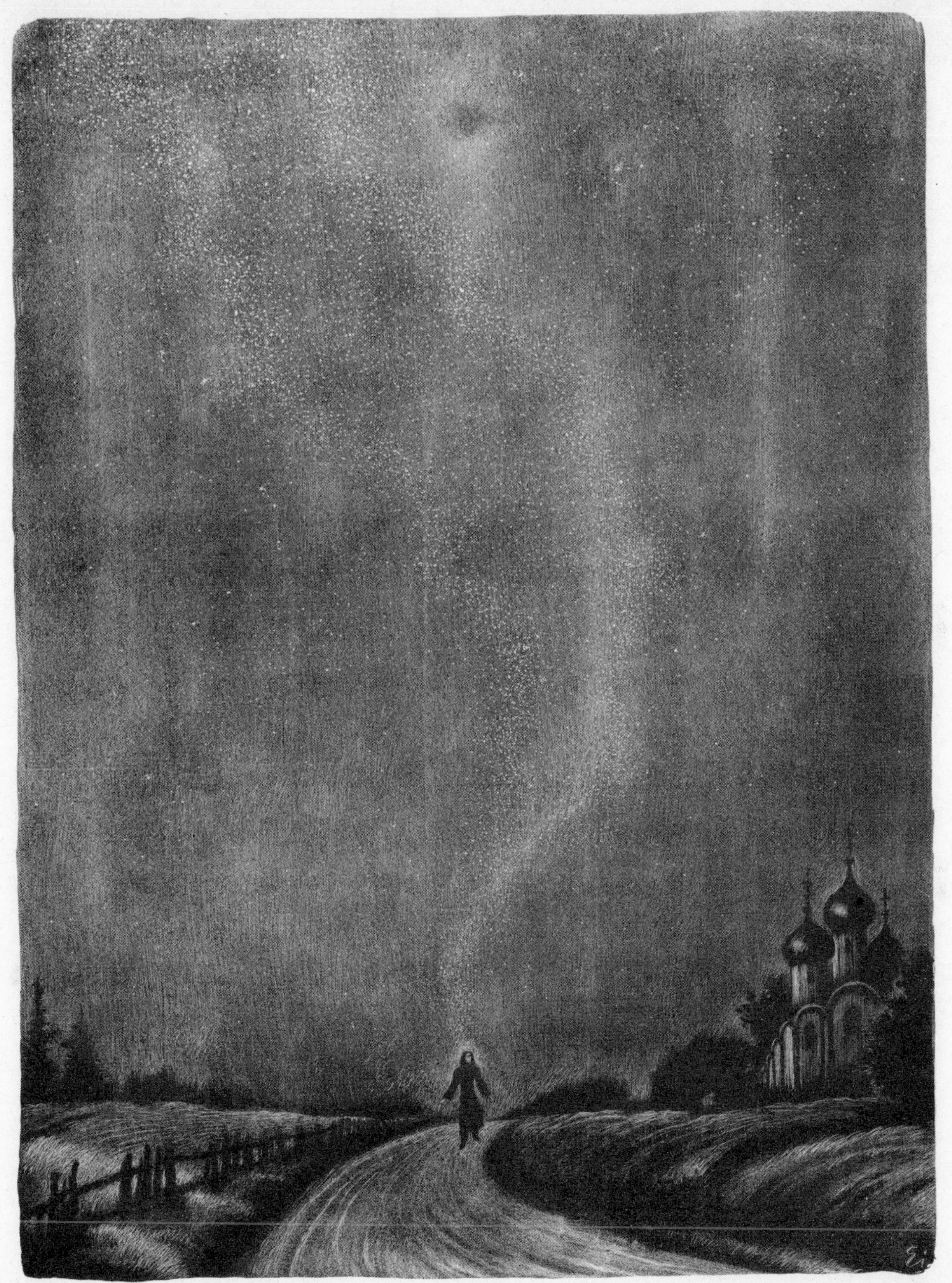

THE MYSTERY OF EARTH

one, you, my meek boy, you, too, have known how to give a famished woman an onion today. Begin your work, dear one, begin it, gentle one! . . . Do you see our Sun, do you see Him?"

"I am afraid . . . I dare not look," whispered Alyosha.

"Do not fear Him. He is terrible in His majesty, awful in His grandeur, but infinitely merciful. He has made Himself like unto us out of love and rejoices with us. He is changing the water into wine that the joy of the guests may not be cut short. He is expecting new guests, He is calling new ones unceasingly for ever and ever. . . . There they are bringing new wine. Do you see they are bringing the vessels . . ."

Something glowed in Alyosha's heart, something filled it till it ached, tears of rapture gushed from his soul. . . .

He stretched out his hands, uttered a cry and awoke.

Again the coffin, the open window, and the soft, solemn, distinct reading of the Gospel. But Alyosha no longer listened to the reading. Strange, he had fallen asleep on his knees, but now he was on his feet, and suddenly, as though flung forward, with three firm rapid steps he went right up to the coffin. His shoulder brushed against Father Païssy without his noticing it. Father Païssy raised his eyes for an instant from his book, but looked away again at once, seeing that something strange had happened to the boy. Alyosha gazed for half a minute at the coffin, at the covered, motionless dead man that lay in the coffin, with the ikon on his breast and the peaked cap with the Orthodox cross on his head. He had only just been hearing his voice, and that voice was still ringing in his ears. He was listening, still expecting other words, but suddenly he turned sharply and went out of the cell.

He did not stop on the steps either, but went quickly down; his soul, overflowing with rapture, yearned for freedom, space, breadth. The vault of heaven, full of soft, shining stars, stretched vast and limitless above him. The Milky Way ran in a pale double stream from the zenith to the horizon. The fresh, motionless, still night enfolded the earth. The white towers and golden domes of the cathedral gleamed out against the sapphire sky. The gorgeous autumn flowers, in the beds round the house, were slumbering till morning. The silence of earth seemed to melt into the silence of the heavens. The mystery of earth touched the mystery of the stars. . . .

Alyosha stood, gazed, and suddenly fell upon the earth as though mowed down. He did not know why he embraced it. He could not have told why he longed so irresistibly to kiss it, to kiss it all. But he kissed it weeping, sobbing, and watering it with his tears, and vowed passionately to love it, to love it for ever and ever. "Water the earth with the tears of your joy and love those tears," echoed in his soul. What was he weeping over?

Oh! in his rapture he was weeping even over those stars, which were shining to him from the abyss of space, and "he was not ashamed of that ecstasy." There seemed to be threads from all those innumerable worlds of God, linking his soul to them, and it was trembling all over "in contact with other worlds." He longed to forgive every one and for everything, and to beg forgiveness. Oh, not for himself, but for all men, for all and for everything. "And others are praying for me, too," echoed again in his soul. But with every instant he felt clearly and, as it were, tangibly, that something firm and unshakable as that vault of heaven had entered into his soul. It was as though some idea had seized the sovereignty of his mind — and it was for all his life and for ever and ever. He had fallen on the earth a weak boy, but he rose up a resolute fighter, and he knew and felt it suddenly at the very moment of his ecstasy. And never, never, all his life long, could Alyosha forget that minute.

"Some one visited my soul in that hour," he said afterwards, with firm faith in his words.

Three days later he left the monastery, which was in accordance, too, with the words of his elder, who had bidden him "sojourn in the world."

CHAPTER I

KUZMA SAMSONOV

As for Dmitri, to whom Grushenka, flying away to a new life, had left her last greetings, bidding him remember the hour of her love for ever, he knew nothing of what had happened to her, and was at that moment also in a condition of feverish agitation and activity. For the last two days he had been in such an inconceivable state of mind that he might easily have fallen ill with inflammation of the brain, as he said himself afterwards. Alyosha had not been able to find him the morning before, and Ivan had not succeeded in meeting him at the tavern on the same day. The people at his lodgings, by his orders, hid his traces.

He had spent those two days literally rushing in all directions, "struggling with his destiny and trying to save himself," as he expressed it himself afterwards, and for some hours he even made a dash out of the town on urgent business, terrible as it was to him to lose sight of Grushenka for a moment. All this became clear afterwards in detail, and was confirmed by documentary evidence; but for the present we will note only the most essential incidents of those two terrible days immediately preceding the awful catastrophe that broke so suddenly upon him.

Though Grushenka had, it is true, loved him for an hour, genuinely and sincerely, yet she tortured him sometimes cruelly and mercilessly. The worst of it was that he could never tell what she meant to do. To prevail upon her by force or kindness was also impossible: she would yield to nothing. She would only have become angry and turned away from him altogether, he knew that well already. He suspected, quite correctly, that she, too, was passing through an inward struggle, and was in a state of extraordinary indecision, that she was making up her mind to something, and was unable to determine upon it. And so, not without good reason, he divined, with a sinking heart, that at moments she must simply hate him and his passion. And so, perhaps, it was, but what was distressing Grushenka he did not understand. Properly speaking, for him, the whole tormenting question was expressed thus: "Either he, Mitya, or Fyodor Pavlovich."

Here, we must note, by the way, one established fact: he was firmly persuaded that Fyodor Pavlovich would offer, or perhaps had offered, Grushenka lawful wedlock, and did not for a moment believe that the old voluptuary hoped to get off by paying three thousand. Mitya had inferred this from his knowledge of Grushenka and her character. That was how it was that he could believe at times that all Grushenka's uneasiness rose from not knowing which of them to choose, which was most to her advantage.

Strange to say, during those days it never occurred to him to think of the approaching return of the "officer," that is, of the man who had been such a fatal influence in Grushenka's life, and whose arrival she was expecting with such emotion and dread. It is true that of late Grushenka had been very silent about it. Yet he was perfectly aware of a letter she had received a month ago from her former seducer, and had heard of it from her own lips. He partly knew, too, what the letter contained. In a moment of spite Grushenka had shown him that letter, but to her astonishment he attached hardly any consequence to it. It would be hard to say why this was so. Perhaps, weighed down by all the hideous horror of his struggle with his own father for this woman, he was incapable of imagining any danger more terrible, at any rate for the time. He simply did not believe in a suitor who suddenly turned up again after five years' absence, still less in his speedy arrival. Moreover, in the "officer's" first letter, which had been shown to Mitya, the possibility of his new rival's visit was very vaguely suggested. The letter was very vague, high-flown, and full of sentimentality. It must be noted that Grushenka had concealed from him the last lines of the letter, in which his return was spoken of more definitely. He had, besides, noticed at that moment, he remembered afterwards, a certain involuntary proud contempt for this missive from Siberia on Grushenka's face. Grushenka told him nothing of what had passed later between her and this rival; so that by degrees he had completely forgotten the officer's existence.

He felt that whatever might come later, whatever turn things might take, his final conflict with Fyodor Pavlovich was close upon him, and must be decided before anything else. With a sinking heart he was expecting every moment Grushenka's decision, always believing that it would come suddenly, on the impulse of the moment. All of a sudden she would say to him: "Take me, I'm yours for ever," and it would all be over. He would seize her and bear her away at once to the ends of the earth. Oh, then he would bear her away at once, as far, far away as possible; to the farthest end of Russia, if not of the earth, then he would marry her, and settle down with her incognito, so that no one would know anything about them, there, here, or anywhere. Then, oh, then, a new life would begin at once! Of this different, reformed, and "virtuous" life ("it must, it must be virtuous") he dreamed ecstatically and continually. He thirsted for this resurrection and renewal. The filthy morass, into which he had sunk of his own free will, was too revolting to him, and, like very many men in such cases, he put faith above all in change of place. If only it were not for these people, if only it were not for these circumstances, if only he could fly away from this accursed place — he would be altogether regenerated, would enter on a new path. That was what he believed in, and for that he was yearning.

But all this could only be in case of the first, the *happy* solution of the question. There was another possibility, a different and awful ending. Suddenly she might say to him: "Go away. I have just come to terms with Fyodor Pavlovich. I am going to marry him and don't want you" — and then . . . but then . . . But Mitya did not know what would happen then. Up to the last hour he didn't know. That must be said to his credit. He had no definite intentions, had planned no crime. He was simply watching and spying in agony, while he prepared himself for the first, happy issue. He drove away any other idea, in fact. But here began a quite different anxiety, a new, extraneous, but yet fatal and insoluble difficulty presented itself.

If she were to say to him: "I'm yours; take me away," how could he take her away? Where had he the means, the money to do it? It was just at this time that all sources of revenue from Fyodor Pavlovich, doles which had gone on without interruption for so many years, ceased. Grushenka had money, of course, but with regard to this Mitya suddenly evinced extraordinary pride; he wanted to carry her away and begin the new life with her himself, at his own expense, not at hers. He could not conceive of taking her money, and the very idea caused him a pang of intense repulsion. I won't enlarge on this fact or analyze it here, but confine myself to remarking that this was the bent of his mind at the moment. All this may have arisen indirectly and unconsciously from the secret stings of his conscience for the money of Katerina Ivanovna that he had dishonestly appropriated. "I've behaved like a scoundrel before one of them, and I shall behave like a scoundrel again before the other directly," was his feeling then, as he explained afterwards: "and if Grushenka found out, she herself wouldn't care for such a scoundrel."

Where then was he to get the means, where was he to get the fateful money? Without it, all would be lost and nothing could be done, "and only because I hadn't the money. Oh, the shame of it!"

To anticipate things: he did, perhaps, know where to get the money, knew, perhaps, where it lay at that moment. I will say no more of this here, as it will all be clear later. But his chief trouble, I must explain, however obscurely, lay in the fact that to have that sum he knew of, to *have the right* to take it, he must first restore Katerina Ivanovna's three thousand — if not, "I'm a common pick-pocket, I'm a scoundrel, and I don't want to begin a new life as a scoundrel," Mitya decided. And so he made up his mind to move heaven and earth to return that three thousand to Katerina Ivanovna, and that *first of all*. The final stage of this decision, so to say, had been reached only during the last hours, that is, after his last interview with Alyosha, two days before, on the high road, on the evening when Grushenka had insulted Katerina Ivanovna, and Mitya, after hearing Alyosha's account of it, had admitted that he was a scoundrel, and told him to tell Katerina Ivanovna so, if it could be any comfort to her. After parting from his brother on that night, he had felt in his frenzy that it would be better "to murder and rob some one than fail to pay my debt to Katya. I'd rather every one thought me a robber and a murderer, I'd rather go to Siberia than that Katya should have the right to say that I deceived her and stole her money, and used her money to run away with Grushenka and begin a virtuous life! That I can't do!" So Mitya spoke, grinding his teeth, and he might well fancy at times that he would end by having inflammation of the brain. But meanwhile he went on struggling. . . .

Strange to say, though one would have supposed there was nothing left for him but despair — for what chance had he, with nothing in the world, to raise such a sum? — yet to the very end he persisted in hoping that he would get that three thousand, that the money would somehow come to him, of itself, as though it might drop from heaven. That is just how it is with people who, like Dmitri, have never had anything to do with money, except to squander what has come to them by inheritance without any effort of their own, and have no notion how money is obtained. A whirl of the most fantastic notions took possession of his brain immediately after he had parted with Alyosha two days before, and threw his thoughts into a tangle of confusion. This is how it was he pitched first on a perfectly wild enterprise. And perhaps to men of that kind in such circumstances the most impossible, fantastic schemes occur first, and seem most practical.

He suddenly determined to go to Samsonov, the merchant who was Grushenka's protector, and to propose a "scheme" to him, whereby he would obtain from him at once the whole of the sum required. Of the commercial value of his scheme he had not the slightest doubt, and was only uncertain how Samsonov would look upon his vagary, supposing he were to consider it from any but the commercial point of view. Though Mitya knew the merchant by sight, he was not acquainted with him and had never spoken a word to him. But for some unknown reason he had long entertained the conviction that the old reprobate, who was lying at death's door, would perhaps not at all object now to Grushenka's securing a respectable position, and marrying a "dependable" man. And he believed not only that he would not object, but that this was what he desired, and, if opportunity arose, that he would be ready to further matters. From some rumour, or perhaps from some stray word of Grushenka's, he had gathered further that the old man would perhaps prefer him to Fyodor Pavlovich for Grushenka.

Possibly many of the readers of my novel will feel that in reckoning on such assistance, and being ready to take his bride, so to speak, from the hands of her protector, Dmitri showed great coarseness and want of delicacy. I will only observe that Mitya looked upon Grushenka's past as something completely done with. He looked on that past with infinite pity and resolved with all the fervour of his passion that when once Grushenka told him she loved him and would marry him, it would mean the beginning of a new Grushenka and a new Dmitri, free from every vice. They would forgive one another and would begin their lives afresh. As for Kuzma Samsonov, Dmitri looked upon him as a man who had exercised a fateful influence in that remote past of Grushenka's, though she had never loved him, and who was now himself a thing of the past, completely done with, and, so to say, non-existent. Besides, Mitya hardly looked upon him as a man at all, for it was known to every one in the town that he was only the ruin of one, whose relations with Grushenka had changed their character and were now simply fatherly, and that this had been so for a long time.

In any case there was much simplicity on Mitya's part in all this, for, in spite of all his vices, he was a very simple-hearted man. It was an instance of this simplicity that Mitya was seriously persuaded that, being on the eve of his departure for the next world, old Kuzma must sincerely repent of his past relations with Grushenka, and that she had no more devoted friend and protector in the world than this, now harmless, old man.

After his conversation with Alyosha, at the cross-roads, he hardly slept all night, and, at ten o'clock next morning, he was at the house of Samsonov and telling the servant to announce him. It was a very spacious and gloomy old house, of two storeys, with a wing and outhouses. In the lower storey lived Samsonov's two married sons with their families, his aged sister, and one unmarried daughter. In the wing lived two of his clerks, one of whom also had a large family. Both the wing and the lower storey were overcrowded, but the old man kept the upper floor to himself, and would not even let the daughter live there with him, though she waited upon him, and in spite of her asthma was obliged at certain fixed hours, and at any time he might call her, to run upstairs to him from below.

This upper floor contained a number of large rooms kept purely for show, furnished in the old-fashioned merchant style, with long, monotonous rows of clumsy mahogany chairs along the walls, with crystal chandeliers in covers, and gloomy mirrors on the walls. All these rooms were entirely empty and unused, for the old man kept to one room, a small, remote bedroom, where he was waited upon by an old servant with a kerchief on her head, and by a lad, who used to sit on the bench in the passage. Owing to his swollen legs, the old man could hardly walk at all, and was only rarely lifted from his leather armchair, when the old woman, supporting him, led him up and down the room once or twice. He was morose and taciturn even with this old woman.

When he was informed of the arrival of the "captain," he at once refused to see him. But Mitya persisted and sent his name up again. Samsonov questioned the lad minutely: What he looked like? Whether he was drunk?

Was he rowdy? The answer he received was: that he was sober, but wouldn't go away. The old man again refused to see him. Then Mitya, who had foreseen this, and purposely brought pencil and paper with him, wrote clearly on the piece of paper the words: "On most important business closely concerning Agrafena Alexandrovna," and sent it up to the old man.

After thinking a little Samsonov told the lad to take the visitor to the drawing-room, and sent the old woman downstairs with a summons to his younger son to come upstairs to him at once. This younger son, a man over six foot and of exceptional physical strength, who was closely shaven and dressed in the European style, though his father still wore a kaftan and a beard, came at once and without comment. All the family trembled before the father. The old man had sent for this giant, not because he was afraid of the "captain" (he was by no means of a timorous temper), but in order to have a witness in case of any emergency. Supported by his son and the servant-lad, he waddled at last into the drawing-room. It may be assumed that he felt considerable curiosity. The drawing-room in which Mitya was awaiting him was a vast, dreary room that crushed the heart with ennui. It had a double row of windows, a gallery, marbled walls, and three immense chandeliers with crystal lustres in covers.

Mitya was sitting on a little chair at the entrance, awaiting his fate with nervous impatience. When the old man appeared at the opposite door, seventy feet away, Mitya jumped up at once, and with his long, military stride walked to meet him. Mitya was decently dressed, in a frock-coat, buttoned up, with a round hat and black gloves in his hands, just as he had been three days before at the elder's, at the family meeting with his father and brothers. The old man waited for him, standing dignified and unbending, and Mitya felt at once that he had looked him through and through as he advanced. Mitya was greatly impressed, too, with Samsonov's immensely swollen face. His lower lip, which had always been thick, hung down now, looking like a bun. He bowed to his guest in dignified silence, motioned him to a low chair by the sofa, and, leaning on his son's arm, he began lowering himself on to the sofa opposite, groaning painfully, so that Mitya, seeing his painful exertions, immediately felt remorseful and sensitively conscious of his insignificance in the presence of the dignified person he had ventured to disturb.

"What is it you want of me, sir?" said the old man, deliberately, distinctly, severely, but courteously, when he was at last seated.

Mitya started, leapt up, but sat down again. Then he began at once speaking with loud, nervous haste, gesticulating, and in a positive frenzy. He was unmistakably a man driven into a corner, on the brink of ruin, catching at a straw, knowing that he was done for if this hope failed him.

Old Samsonov probably grasped all this in an instant, though his face remained cold and immovable as a statue's.

"Most honoured sir, Kuzma Kuzmich, you have no doubt heard, more than once, of my disputes with my father, Fyodor Pavlovich Karamazov, who robbed me of my inheritance from my mother . . . seeing the whole town is gossiping about it . . . for here every one's gossiping of what they shouldn't . . . and besides, it might have reached you through Grushenka . . . I beg your pardon, through Agrafena Alexandrovna . . . Agrafena Alexandrovna, the lady for whom I have the highest respect and esteem . . ."

So Mitya began, and broke down at the first sentence. We will not reproduce his speech word for word, but will only give a summary of it. Three months ago, he said, he had of express intention (Mitya purposely used these words instead of "intentionally") consulted a lawyer in the chief town of the province, "a distinguished lawyer, Kuzma Kuzmich, Pavel Pavlovich Korneplodov. You have perhaps heard of him? A man of vast intellect, the mind of a statesman . . . he knows you, too . . . spoke of you in the highest terms . . ." Mitya broke down again. But these breaks did not deter him. He leapt instantly over the gaps, and struggled on and on.

This Korneplodov, after questioning him minutely, and inspecting the documents he was able to bring him (Mitya alluded somewhat vaguely to these documents, and slurred over the subject with special haste) reported that they certainly might take proceedings concerning the village of Chermashnya, which ought, he said, to have come to him, Mitya, from his mother, and so checkmate the old villain, his father . . . "because every door was not closed and justice might still find a loophole." In fact, he might reckon on an additional sum of six or even seven thousand roubles from Fyodor Pavlovich, as Chermashnya was worth, at least, twenty-five thousand, he might say twenty-eight thousand, in fact, "thirty, thirty, Kuzma Kuzmich, and, would you believe it, I didn't get seventeen from that heartless man!" So he, Mitya, had thrown the business up, for the time, knowing nothing about the law, but on coming here was struck dumb by a cross-claim made upon him (here Mitya went adrift again, and again took a flying leap forward), "so will not you, excellent and honoured Kuzma Kuzmich, be willing to take up all my claims against that unnatural monster, and pay me a sum down of only three thousand? . . . You see, you cannot, in any case, lose on it. On my honour, my honour, I swear that. Quite the contrary, you may make six or seven thousand instead of three. . . ." Above all, he wanted this concluded that very day.

"I'll do the business with you at a notary's, or whatever it is . . . in fact, I'm ready to do anything. . . . I'll hand over all the deeds . . . whatever you want, sign anything . . . and we could draw up the agreement at once . . . and if it were possible, if it were only possible, this very morning. . . . You could pay me that three thousand, for there isn't a capitalist in this town to compare with you, and so you would save me from . . . would save my poor head, in fact . . . for a good, I might say an honourable, action. . . . For I cherish the most honourable feelings for a certain person, whom you know well, and care for as a father. I would not have come, indeed, if it had not been as a father. And, indeed, it's a struggle of three in this business, for it's fate — that's a fearful thing, Kuzma Kuzmich! Realism, Kuzma Kuzmich, realism! And as you've dropped out long ago, it's a tug-of-war between two. I'm expressing it awkwardly, perhaps, but I'm not a literary man. You see, I'm on the one side, and that monster on the other. So you must choose. It's either I or the monster. It all lies in your hands — the fate of three lives, and the happiness of two. . . . Excuse me, I'm making a mess of it, but you understand. I see from your esteemed eyes that you understand . . . and if you don't understand, I've got to drown myself . . . there!"

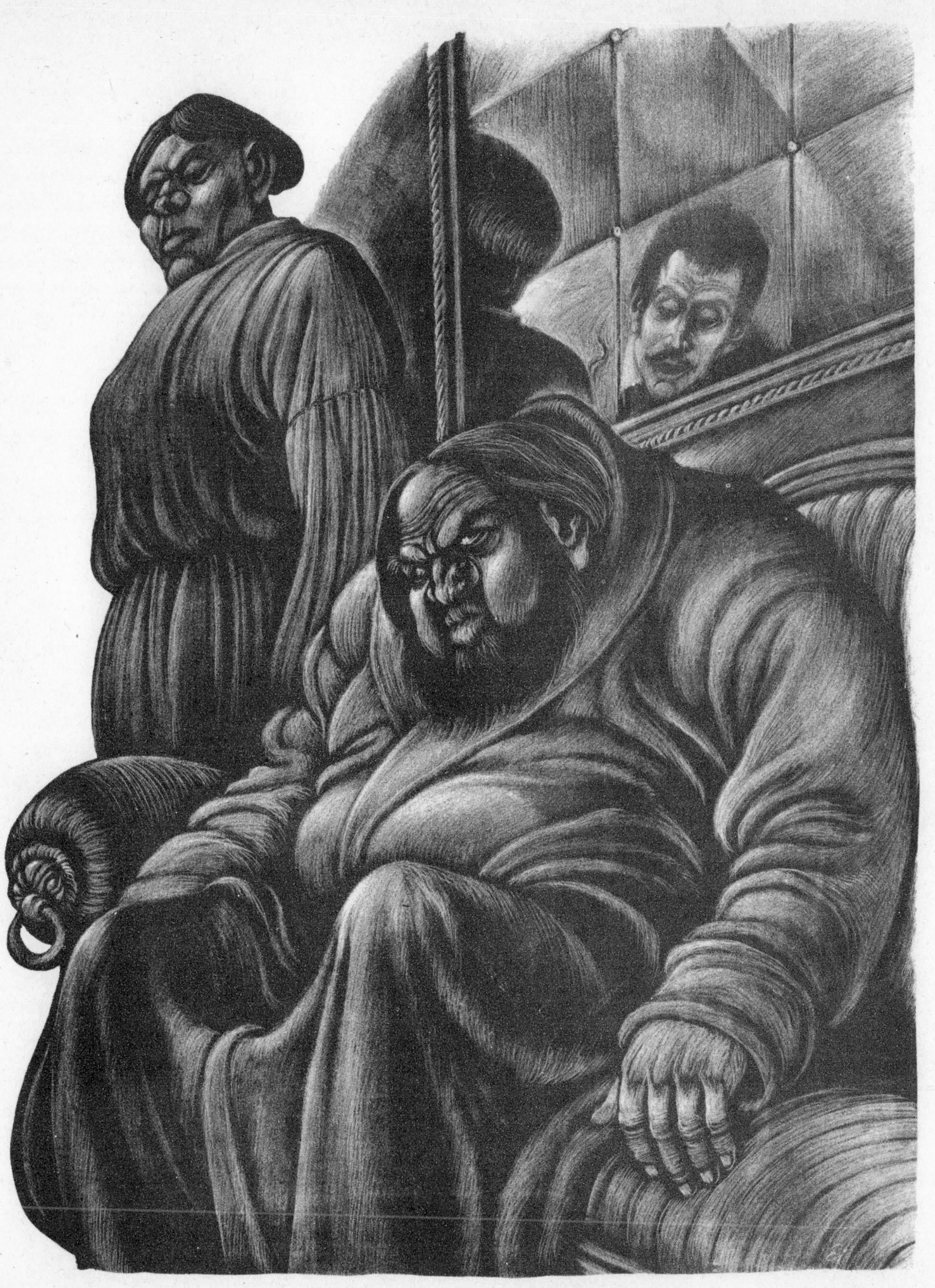

OLD SAMSONOV

Mitya broke off his absurd speech with that "there!" and, jumping up from his seat, awaited the answer to his foolish proposal. At the last phrase he had suddenly become hopelessly aware that it had all fallen flat, above all, that he had been talking utter nonsense.

"How strange it is! On the way here it seemed all right, and now it's nothing but nonsense." The idea suddenly dawned on his despairing mind. All the while he had been talking, the old man sat motionless, watching him with an icy expression in his eyes. After keeping him for a moment in suspense, Kuzma Kuzmich pronounced at last, in the most positive and chilling tone:

"Excuse me, we don't handle such business."

Mitya suddenly felt his legs growing weak under him.

"What am I to do now, Kuzma Kuzmich?" he muttered, with a pale smile. "I suppose it's all up with me — what do you think?"

"Excuse me . . ."

Mitya remained standing, staring motionless. He suddenly noticed a movement in the old man's face. He started.

"You see, sir, business of that sort's not in our line," said the old man slowly. "There's the court, and the lawyers — it's a wretched affair. But if you like, there is a man here you might apply to."

"Good heavens! Who is it? You're my salvation, Kuzma Kuzmich," faltered Mitya.

"He doesn't live here, and he's not here just now. He is a peasant, he does business in timber. His name is Lyagavy. He's been haggling with Fyodor Pavlovich for the last year, over your copse at Chermashnya. They can't agree on the price, maybe you've heard? Now he's come back again and is staying with the priest at Ilyinskoe, about twelve versts from the Volovya station. He wrote to me, too, about the business of the copse asking my advice. Fyodor Pavlovich means to go and see him, himself. So if you were to get ahead of Fyodor Pavlovich and to make Lyagavy the offer you've made me, he might possibly . . ."

"A stroke of genius!" Mitya interrupted ecstatically. "He's the very man, it would just suit him. He's haggling with him for it, being asked too much, and here he would have all the documents entitling him to the property itself. Ha-ha-ha!"

And Mitya suddenly went off into his short, wooden laugh, startling Samsonov.

"How can I thank you, Kuzma Kuzmich?" cried Mitya effusively.

"Don't mention it," said Samsonov, inclining his head.

"But you don't know, you've saved me. Oh, it was a true presentiment brought me to you. . . . So now to this priest!"

"No need of thanks."

"I'll make haste and fly there. I'm afraid I've overtaxed your strength. I shall never forget it. It's a Russian says that, Kuzma Kuzmich, a R-r-russian!"

"To be sure!"

Mitya seized his hand to press it, but there was a malicious gleam in the old man's eye. Mitya drew back his hand, but at once blamed himself for his mistrustfulness.

"It's because he's tired," he thought.

"For her sake! For her sake, Kuzma Kuzmich! You understand that it's for her," he cried, his voice ringing through the room. He bowed, turned sharply round, and with the same long stride walked to the door without looking back. He was trembling with ecstasy.

"Everything was on the verge of ruin and

my guardian angel saved me," was the thought in his mind. And if such a businessman as Samsonov (a most worthy old man, and what dignity!) had suggested this course, then . . . then success was assured. He would fly off immediately. "I will be back before night, I shall be back at night and the thing is done. Could the old man have been laughing at me?" exclaimed Mitya, as he strode towards his lodging. He could, of course, imagine nothing, but that the advice was practical "from such a businessman" with an understanding of business, with an understanding of this Lyagavy (curious surname!) Or — the old man was laughing at him.

Alas! the second alternative was the correct one. Much later, after the catastrophe had occurred, old Samsonov himself confessed, laughing, that he had made a fool of the "captain." He was a cold, spiteful, and sarcastic man, liable to morbid antipathies. Whether the old man was worked on by the "captain's" excited face, or by the foolish conviction of the "rake and spendthrift," that he, Samsonov, could be taken in by such a cock-and-bull story as his scheme, or by jealousy over Grushenka, in whose name this "scapegrace" had rushed in on him with such a tale to get money — I can't tell. But, at the instant when Mitya stood before him, feeling his legs grow weak under him, and frantically exclaiming that he was ruined, at that moment the old man looked at him with intense spite, and resolved to make a laughing-stock of him. When Mitya had gone, Kuzma Kuzmich, white with rage, turned to his son and bade him see to it that that beggar never be admitted again, and never be allowed even into the yard, or else he'd . . .

He did not utter his threat. But even his son, who often saw him enraged, trembled with fear. For a whole hour afterwards, the old man was shaking with anger, and by evening he was worse, and sent for the doctor.

CHAPTER II

LYAGAVY

So he must drive at full speed, and he had not the money for horses. He had forty copecks, and that was all, all that was left after so many years of prosperity! But he had at home an old silver watch which had long since ceased to go. He snatched it up and carried it to a Jewish watchmaker who had a shop in the market-place. The Jew gave him six roubles for it.

"And I didn't expect that," cried Mitya, ecstatically. (He was still in a state of ecstasy.) He seized his six roubles and ran home. At home he borrowed three roubles from the people of the house, who loved him so much that they were pleased to give it him, though it was all they had. Mitya in his excitement told them on the spot that his fate would be decided that day, and he described, in desperate haste, the whole scheme he had put before Samsonov, the latter's decision, his own hopes for the future, and so on. These people had been told many of their lodger's secrets before, and so looked upon him as a gentleman who was not at all proud, and almost one of themselves. Having thus collected nine roubles Mitya sent for posting-horses to take him to the Volovya station. This was how the fact came to be remembered and established that "at midday, on the day before the event, Mitya had not a farthing, and that he had sold his watch to get money and had borrowed three roubles from his landlord, all in the presence of witnesses."

I note this fact, later on it will be apparent why I do so.

Though he was radiant with the joyful anticipation that he would at last solve all his difficulties, yet, as he drew near Volovya station, he trembled at the thought of what Grushenka might be doing in his absence. What if she made up her mind to-day to go to Fyodor Pavlovich? This was why he had gone off without telling her and why he left orders with his landlady not to let out where he had gone, if any one came to inquire for him.

"I must, I must get back to-night," he repeated, as he was jolted along in the cart, "and I dare say I shall have to bring this Lyagavy back here . . . to draw up the deed." So mused Mitya, with a throbbing heart, but alas! his dreams were not fated to be carried out.

To begin with, he was late, taking a short cut from Volovya station which turned out to be eighteen versts instead of twelve. Secondly, he did not find the Ilyinskoe priest at home; he had gone off to a neighbouring village. While Mitya, setting off there with the same exhausted horses, was looking for him, it was almost dark.

The priest, a shy and amiable-looking little man, informed him at once that, though Lyagavy had been staying with him at first, he was now at Suhoy Posyolok, that he was staying the night in the forester's cottage, as he was buying timber there, too. At Mitya's urgent request that he would take him to Lyagavy at once, and by so doing "save him, so to speak," the priest agreed, after some demur, to conduct him to Suhoy Posyolok; his curiosity was obviously aroused. But, unluckily, he advised their going on foot, as it would not be "much over" a verst. Mitya, of course, agreed, and marched off with his yard-long strides, so that the poor priest almost ran after him. He was a very cautious man, though not old.

Mitya at once began talking to him, too, of his plans, nervously and excitedly asking advice in regard to Lyagavy, and talked all the way. The priest listened attentively, but gave little advice. He turned off Mitya's questions with: "I don't know. Ah, I can't say. How can I tell?" and so on. When Mitya began to speak of his quarrel with his father over his inheritance, the priest was positively alarmed, as he was in some way dependent on Fyodor Pavlovich. He inquired, however, with surprise, why he called the peasant-trader Gorstkin, Lyagavy, and obligingly explained to Mitya that, though the man's name really was Lyagavy, he was never called so, as he would be grievously offended at the name, and that he must be sure to call him Gorstkin, "or you'll do nothing with him; he won't even listen to you," said the priest in conclusion.

Mitya was somewhat surprised for a moment, and explained that that was what Samsonov had called him. On hearing this fact, the priest immediately dropped the subject, though he would have done well to have expressed to Dmitri Fyodorovich his conjecture: wasn't there something wrong about Samsonov having sent him to that peasant, and calling him Lyagavy, and wasn't Samsonov trying to put him into a ridiculous position? But Mitya had no time to pause over such trifles. He hurried, striding along, and only when he reached Suhoy Posyolok he realised that they had walked not one verst, nor one and a half, but at least three. This annoyed him, but he controlled himself.

They went into the hut. The forester, who was the priest's acquaintance, occupied one half of the hut, and Gorstkin was lodging in the other, the better half on the other side of the passage. They went into that room and lighted a tallow candle. The hut was extremely overheated. On the table there was a samovar that had gone out, a tray with cups, an empty rum bottle, a bottle of vodka partly full, and some half eaten crusts of wheaten bread. The occupant himself lay stretched at full length on the bench, with his coat crushed up under his head for a pillow, snoring heavily. Mitya stood in perplexity.

"Of course I must wake him. My business is too important. I've come in such haste. I'm in a hurry to get back today," he said in great agitation. But the priest and the forester stood in silence, not giving their opinion. Mitya went up and began trying to wake him himself; he tried vigorously, but the sleeper did not wake.

"He's drunk," Mitya decided. "Good Lord! What am I to do? What am I to do?" And, terribly impatient, he began pulling him by the arms, by the legs, shaking his head, lifting him up and making him sit on the bench. Yet, after prolonged exertions, he could only succeed in getting the drunken man to utter absurd grunts, and violent, but inarticulate oaths.

"No, you'd better wait a little," the priest pronounced at last, "for he's obviously not in a fit state."

"He's been drinking the whole day," the forester chimed in.

"Good heavens!" cried Mitya. "If only you knew how important it is to me and how desperate I am!"

"No, you'd better wait till morning," the priest repeated.

"Till morning? Mercy! that's impossible!"

And in his despair he was on the point of renewing his attempt to rouse the drunkard, but stopped short at once, realising the uselessness of his efforts. The priest said nothing, the sleepy forester looked gloomy.

"What terrible tragedies life contrives for people," said Mitya, in complete despair. The perspiration was streaming down his face. The priest seized the moment to put before him, very reasonably, that, even if he succeeded in wakening the man, he would still be drunk and incapable of conversation. "And your business is important," he said, "so you'd certainly better put it off till morning." With a gesture of despair Mitya agreed.

"Father, I will stay here with a light, and seize the favourable moment. As soon as he wakes I'll begin. I'll pay you for the light," he said to the forester, "for the night's lodging, too; you'll remember Dmitri Karamazov. Only, father, I don't know what we're to do with you. Where will you sleep?"

"No, I'm going home. I'll take his horse and get home," he said, indicating the forester. "And now I'll say good-bye. I wish you all success."

So it was settled. The priest rode off on the forester's horse, delighted to escape, though he shook his head uneasily, wondering whether he ought not, next day, inform his benefactor, Fyodor Pavlovich, of this curious incident, "or he may in an unlucky hour hear of it, be angry, and withdraw his favour."

The forester, scratching himself, went back to his room without a word, and Mitya sat on the bench to "seize the favourable moment," as he expressed it. Profound dejection clung to his soul like a heavy mist. A profound, intense dejection! He sat thinking, but could reach no conclusion. The candle burnt dimly, a cricket chirped; it became insufferably close in the overheated room. He suddenly pictured the garden, the path behind the garden, the door of his father's house mysteriously opening and Grushenka running in. He leapt up from the bench.

"It's a tragedy!" he said, grinding his teeth. Mechanically he went up to the sleeping man and looked in his face. He was a lean, middle-aged peasant, with a very long face, flaxen curls, and a long, thin, reddish beard, wearing a cotton shirt and a black waistcoat, from the pocket of which peeped the chain of a silver watch. Mitya looked at his face with intense hatred, and for some unknown reason his curly hair particularly irritated him.

What was insufferably humiliating was, that, after leaving things of such importance and making such sacrifices, he, Mitya, utterly worn out, should with business of such urgency be standing over this dolt on whom his whole fate depended, while he snored as though there were nothing the matter, as though he'd dropped from another planet.

"Oh, the irony of fate!" cried Mitya, and, quite losing his head, he fell again to rousing the tipsy peasant. He tried to rouse him with a sort of ferocity, pulled at him, pushed him, even beat him; but after five minutes of vain exertions, he returned to his bench in helpless despair, and sat down.

"Stupid! Stupid!" cried Mitya. "And how dishonourable it all is!" something made him add. His head began to ache horribly. "Should he fling it up and go away altogether?" he wondered. "No, wait till to-morrow now. I'll stay on purpose. What else did I come for? Besides, I've no means of going. How am I to get away from here now? Oh, the idiocy of it!"

But his head ached more and more. He sat without moving, dozed off and suddenly fell asleep as he sat. He seemed to have slept for two hours or more. He was waked up by his head aching so unbearably that he could have screamed. There was a hammering in his temples, and the top of his head ached. It was a long time before he could wake up fully and understand what had happened to him.

At last he realised that the room was full of charcoal fumes from the stove, and that he might die of suffocation. And the drunken peasant still lay snoring. The candle guttered and was about to go out. Mitya cried out, and ran staggering across the passage into the forester's room. The forester waked up at once, but hearing that the other room was full of fumes, to Mitya's surprise and annoyance, accepted the fact with strange unconcern, though he did go to see to it.

"But he's dead, he's dead! and . . . what shall I do then?" cried Mitya frantically.

They threw open the doors, opened a window and the chimney. Mitya brought a pail of water from the passage. First he wetted his own head, then, finding a rag of some sort, dipped it into the water, and put it on Lyagavy's head. The forester still treated the matter contemptuously, and when he opened the window said grumpily:

"It'll be all right, now."

He went back to sleep, leaving Mitya a lighted lantern. Mitya fussed about the drunken peasant for half an hour, wetting his head, and gravely resolved not to sleep all night. But he was so worn out that when he sat down for a moment to take breath, he closed his eyes, unconsciously stretched himself full length on the bench and slept like the dead.

It was dreadfully late when he waked. It

was somewhere about nine o'clock. The sun was shining brightly in the two little windows of the hut. The curly-headed peasant was sitting on the bench and had his coat on. He had another samovar and another bottle in front of him. Yesterday's bottle had already been finished, and the new one was more than half empty. Mitya jumped up and saw at once that the cursed peasant was drunk again, hopelessly and incurably. He stared at him for a moment with bulging eyes. The peasant was silently and slyly watching him, with insulting composure, and even a sort of contemptuous condescension, so Mitya fancied. He rushed up to him. "Excuse me, you see. . . . I . . . you've most likely heard from the forester here in the hut. I'm Lieutenant Dmitri Karamazov, the son of the old Karamazov whose copse you are buying."

"You're lying!" said the peasant, calmly and deliberately.

"I'm lying? You know Fyodor Pavlovich?"

"I don't know any of your Fyodor Pavloviches," said the peasant, speaking thickly.

"You're bargaining with him over the copse, the copse. Do wake up, and come to. Father Pavel of Ilyinskoe brought me here. You wrote to Samsonov, and he has sent me to you," Mitya gasped breathlessly.

"You're l — lying!" Lyagavy blurted out again. Mitya's legs went cold.

"For mercy's sake! It isn't a joke! You're drunk, perhaps. Yet you can speak and understand . . . or else . . . I understand nothing!"

"You're a house-painter!"

"For mercy's sake! I'm Karamazov, Dmitri Karamazov. I have an offer to make you, an advantageous offer . . . very advantageous offer, concerning the copse!"

The peasant stroked his beard importantly.

"No, you've contracted for the job and turned out a scamp. You're a scoundrel!"

"I assure you you're mistaken," cried Mitya, wringing his hands in despair. The peasant still stroked his beard, and suddenly screwed up his eyes cunningly.

"No, you show me this: you tell me the law that allows roguery. D'you hear? You're a scoundrel! Do you understand that?"

Mitya stepped back gloomily, and suddenly "something seemed to hit him on the head," as he said afterwards. In an instant a light seemed to dawn in his mind, "a light was kindled and I grasped it all." He stood, stupefied, wondering how he, after all a man of intelligence, could have yielded to such folly, have been led into such an adventure, and have kept it up for almost twenty-four hours, fussing round this Lyagavy, wetting his head.

"Why, the man's drunk, dead drunk, and he'll go on drinking now for a week; what's the use of waiting here? And what if Samsonov sent me here on purpose? What if she . . . ? Oh, God, what have I done?"

The peasant sat watching him and grinning. Another time Mitya might have killed the fool in a fury, but now he felt as weak as a child. He went quietly to the bench, took up his overcoat, put it on without a word, and went out of the hut. He did not find the forester in the next room; there was no one there. He took fifty copecks in small change out of his pocket and put them on the table for his night's lodging, the candle, and the trouble he had given. Coming out of the hut he saw nothing but forest all round. He walked at hazard, not knowing which way to turn out of the hut, to the right or to the left. Hurrying there the evening before with the priest, he had not noticed the road. He had no revengeful feeling in his heart for anybody, not even for Samsonov. He strode along a narrow forest path, aimless, dazed, without heeding where he was going. A child could have knocked him down, so weak was he in body and soul. He got out of the forest somehow, however, and a vista of fields, bare after the harvest, stretched as far as the eye could see.

"What despair! What death all round!" he repeated, striding on and on.

He was saved by meeting an old merchant who was being driven across country in a hired trap. When he overtook him, Mitya asked the way, and it turned out that the old merchant, too, was going to Volovya. After some discussion Mitya got into the trap. Three hours later they arrived. At Volovya, Mitya at once ordered posting-horses to drive to the town, and suddenly realised that he was appallingly hungry. While the horses were being harnessed, an omelette was prepared for him. He ate it all in an instant, ate a huge hunk of bread, ate a sausage, and swallowed three glasses of vodka. After eating, his spirits and his heart grew lighter. He flew towards the town, urged on the driver, and suddenly made a new and "unalterable" plan to procure that "accursed money" before evening. "And to think, only to think that a man's life should be ruined for the sake of that paltry three thousand!" he cried, contemptuously. "I'll settle it to-day." And if it had not been for the thought of Grushenka and of what might have happened to her, which never left him, he would perhaps have become quite cheerful again. . . . But the thought of her was stabbing him to the heart every moment, like a sharp knife. At last they arrived, and Mitya at once ran to Grushenka.

CHAPTER III

GOLD-MINES

This was the visit of Mitya of which Grushenka had spoken to Rakitin with such fear. She was just then expecting the "message," and was much relieved that Mitya had not been to see her that day or the day before. She hoped that, please God, he wouldn't come till she had gone, and he suddenly burst in on her. The rest we know already. To get him off her hands she suggested at once that he should walk with her to Samsonov's, where she said she absolutely must go "to count money," and when Mitya accompanied her at once, she said good-bye to him at the gate, making him promise to come at twelve o'clock to take her home again. Mitya, too, was delighted at this arrangement. If she was sitting at Samsonov's she could not be going to Fyodor Pavlovich's, "if only she's not lying," he added at once. But he thought she was not lying from what he saw.

He was that sort of jealous man who, in the absence of the beloved woman, at once invents all sorts of awful fancies of what may be happening to her, and how she may be betraying him, but, when shaken, heartbroken, convinced of her faithlessness, he runs back to her, at the first glance at her face, her gay, laughing, affectionate face, he revives at once, lays aside all suspicion and with joyful shame upbraids himself for his jealousy.

After leaving Grushenka at the gate he rushed home. Oh, he had so much still to do that night! But a load had been lifted from his heart, anyway.

"Now I must only make haste and find out from Smerdyakov whether anything happened there last night, whether, by any chance, she went to Fyodor Pavlovich; ough!" floated through his mind.

Before he had time to reach his lodging, jealousy had surged up again in his restless heart.

Jealousy! "Othello is not jealous, he is trustful," observed Pushkin. And that remark alone is enough to show the deep insight of our great poet. Othello's soul is shattered and his whole outlook clouded simply because *his ideal is destroyed*. But Othello will not hide, spy, peep. He is trustful. On the contrary, he has to be led up, pushed on, excited with great difficulty before he can entertain the idea of deceit. The truly jealous man is not like that. It is impossible to picture to oneself the shame and moral degradation to which the jealous man can descend without a qualm of conscience. And yet it's not as though the jealous were all vulgar and base souls. On the contrary, a man of lofty feelings, whose love is pure and full of self-sacrifice, may yet hide under tables, bribe the vilest people, and be familiar with the lowest ignominy of spying and eavesdropping.

Othello was incapable of reconciling himself to faithlessness — not incapable of forgiving it, but of reconciling himself to it — though his soul was as innocent and free from malice as a babe's. It is not so with the really jealous man. It is hard to imagine what some jealous men can get accustomed and reconciled to, and what they can forgive! The jealous are the readiest of all to forgive, and all women know it. The jealous man can forgive extraordinarily quickly (though, of course, after a violent scene), and he is able to forgive infidelity almost conclusively proved, the very kisses and embraces he has seen, if only he can somehow be convinced that it has all been "for the last time," and that his rival will vanish from that day forward, will depart to the ends of the earth, or that he himself will carry her away somewhere, where that dreaded rival will not get near her. Of course the reconciliation is only for an hour. For, even if the rival did disappear next day, he would invent another one and would be jealous of him. And one might wonder what there was in a love that had to be so watched over, what a love could be worth that needed such strenuous guarding. But that the jealous will never understand. And yet among them are men of noble hearts. It is remarkable, too, that those very men of noble hearts, standing hidden in some cupboard, listening and spying, never feel the stings of conscience at that moment, anyway, though they understand clearly enough with their "noble hearts" the shameful depths to which they have voluntarily sunk.

At the sight of Grushenka, Mitya's jealousy vanished, and for an instant he became trustful and generous, and positively despised himself for his evil feelings. But that only meant that, in his love for that woman, there was an element of something far higher than he himself imagined, that it was not only a sensual passion, not only the "curve of her body," of which he had talked to Alyosha. But, as soon as Grushenka vanished, Mitya began to suspect her of all the low cunning of faithlessness, and he felt no sting of conscience at it.

And so jealousy surged up in him again. He had, in any case, to make haste. The first thing to be done was to get hold of at least a small, temporary loan of money. The nine roubles had almost all gone on his expedition. And, as we all know, one can't take a step without money. But he had thought over in the carriage where he could get a loan. He had a brace of fine duelling pistols in a case, which he had not pawned till then because he prized them above all his possessions.

In the "Metropolis" tavern he had some time since made acquaintance with a young official and had learnt that this very opulent bachelor was passionately fond of weapons. He used to buy pistols, revolvers, daggers, hang them on his wall and show them to acquaintances. He prided himself on them, and was quite a specialist on the mechanism of the revolver. Mitya, without stopping to think, went straight to him, and offered to pawn his pistols to him for ten roubles. The official, delighted, began trying to persuade him to sell them outright. But Mitya would not consent, so the young man gave him ten roubles, protesting that nothing would induce him to take interest. They parted friends.

Mitya was in haste; he rushed towards Fyodor Pavlovich's by the back way, to his arbour, to get hold of Smerdyakov as soon as possible. In this way the fact was established that three or four hours before a certain event, of which I shall speak later on, Mitya had not a farthing, and pawned for ten roubles a possession he valued, though, three hours later, he was in possession of thousands. . . . But I am anticipating. From Marya Kondratyevna (the woman living near Fyodor Pavlovich's) he learnt the very disturbing fact of Smerdyakov's illness. He heard the story of his fall in the cellar, his fit, the doctor's visit, Fyodor Pavlovich's anxiety; he heard with interest, too, that his brother Ivan had set off that morning for Moscow.

"Then he must have driven through Volovya before me," thought Dmitri, but he was terribly distressed about Smerdyakov. "What will happen now? Who'll keep watch for me? Who'll bring me word?" he thought. He began greedily questioning the women whether they had seen anything the evening before. They quite understood what he was trying to find out, and completely reassured him. No one had been there. Ivan Fyodorovich had spent the night there; everything had been in perfect order. Mitya grew thoughtful. He would certainly have to keep watch to-night, but where? Here or at Samsonov's gate? He decided that he must be on the look-out both here and there, and meanwhile . . . meanwhile . . . The difficulty was that he had to carry out the new plan that he had made on the journey back. He was sure of its success, but he must not delay acting upon it. Mitya resolved to sacrifice an hour to it: "In an hour I shall know everything, I shall settle everything, and then, then, first of all to Samsonov's. I'll inquire whether Grushenka's there and instantly be back here again, stay till eleven, and then to Samsonov's again to bring her home." This was what he decided.

He flew home, washed, combed his hair, brushed his clothes, dressed, and went to Madame Hohlakov's. Alas! he had built his hopes on her. He had resolved to borrow three thousand from that lady. And what was more, he felt suddenly convinced that she would not refuse to lend it to him. It may be wondered why, if he felt so certain, he had not gone to her at first, one of his own sort, so to speak, instead of to Samsonov, a man he did not know, who was not of his own class, and to whom he hardly knew how to speak.

But the fact was that he had never known Madame Hohlakov well, and had seen nothing of her for the last month, and that he knew she could not endure him. She had detested him from the first because he was engaged to

Katerina Ivanovna, while she had, for some reason, suddenly conceived the desire that Katerina Ivanovna should throw him over, and marry the "charming, chivalrously refined Ivan, who had such excellent manners." Mitya's manners she detested. Mitya positively laughed at her, and had once said about her that she was just as lively and at her ease as she was uncultivated. But that morning in the carriage a brilliant idea had struck him: "If she is so anxious I should not marry Katerina Ivanovna" (and he knew she was positively hysterical upon the subject) "why should she refuse me now that three thousand, just to enable me to leave Katya and get away from her for ever. These spoilt fine ladies, if they set their hearts on anything, will spare no expense to satisfy their caprice. Besides, she's so rich," Mitya argued.

As for his "plan," it was just the same as before; it consisted of the offer of his rights to Chermashnya — but not with a commercial object, as it had been with Samsonov, not trying to allure the lady with the possibility of making a profit of six or seven thousand — but simply as a security for the debt. As he worked out this new idea, Mitya was enchanted with it, but so it always was with him in all his undertakings, in all his sudden decisions. He gave himself up to every new idea with passion. Yet, when he mounted the steps of Madame Hohlakov's house he felt a shiver of fear run down his spine. At that moment he saw fully, as a mathematical certainty, that this was his last hope, that if this broke down, nothing else was left him in the world but to "rob and murder some one for the three thousand." It was half-past seven when he rang the bell.

At first fortune seemed to smile upon him. As soon as he was announced he was received with extraordinary rapidity. "As though she were waiting for me," thought Mitya, and as soon as he had been led to the drawing-room, the lady of the house herself ran in, and declared at once that she was expecting him.

"I was expecting you! I was expecting you! Though I'd no reason to suppose you would come to see me, as you will admit yourself. Yet, I did expect you. You may marvel at my instinct, Dmitri Fyodorovich, but I was convinced all the morning that you would come."

"That is certainly wonderful, madam," observed Mitya, sitting down awkwardly, "but I have come to you on a matter of great importance. . . . On a matter of supreme importance for me that is, madam . . . for me alone . . . and I hasten . . ."

"I know you've come on most important business, Dmitri Fyodorovich; it's not a case of presentiment, no reactionary harking back to the miraculous (have you heard about Father Zosima?). This is a case of mathematics: you couldn't help coming, after all that has passed with Katerina Ivanovna; you couldn't, you couldn't, that's a mathematical certainty."

"The realism of actual life, madam, that's what it is. But allow me to explain . . ."

"Realism indeed, Dmitri Fyodorovich. I'm all for realism now. I've had a lesson as regards miracles. You've heard that Father Zosima is dead?"

"No, madam, it's the first time I've heard of it." Mitya was a little surprised. The image of Alyosha rose to his mind.

"Last night, and only imagine . . ."

"Madam," said Mitya, "I can imagine nothing except that I'm in a desperate position, and that if you don't help me, everything will go to the dogs, and I first of all. Excuse me for the triviality of the expression, but I'm in a fever . . ."

"I know, I know that you're in a fever. You could hardly fail to be, and whatever you may say to me, I know beforehand. I have long been thinking over your destiny, Dmitri Fyodorovich, I am watching over it and studying it. . . . Oh, believe me, I'm an experienced doctor of the soul, Dmitri Fyodorovich."

"Madam, if you are an experienced doctor, I'm certainly an experienced patient," said Mitya, with an effort to be polite, "and I feel that if you are watching over my destiny in this way, you will come to my help in my ruin, and so allow me at last to explain to you the plan with which I have ventured to come to you . . . and what I am hoping of you. . . . I have come, madam . . ."

"Don't explain it. It's of secondary importance. But as for help, you're not the first I have helped, Dmitri Fyodorovich. You have most likely heard of my cousin, Madame Belmesov. Her husband was perishing, was 'going to the dogs,' as you characteristically express it, Dmitri Fyodorovich. I recommended him to take to horse-breeding, and now he's flourishing. Have you any idea of horse-breeding, Dmitri Fyodorovich?"

"Not the faintest, madam; ah, madam, not the faintest!" cried Mitya, in nervous impatience, positively starting from his seat. "I simply implore you, madam, to listen to me. Only give me two minutes of free speech that I may just explain everything to you, the whole plan with which I have come. Besides I am short of time. I'm in a fearful hurry," Mitya cried hysterically, feeling that she was just going to begin talking again, and hoping to cut her short. "I have come in despair . . . in the last gasp of despair, to beg you to lend me the sum of three thousand, a loan, but on safe, most safe security, madam, with the surest guarantees! Only allow me to explain . . ."

"You must tell me all that afterwards, afterwards!" Madame Hohlakov in her turn motioned him to be silent, "and whatever you may tell me, I know it all beforehand; I've told you so already. You ask for a certain sum, you need three thousand, but I can give you more, immeasurably more, I will save you, Dmitri Fyodorovich, but you must listen to me."

Mitya started from his seat again.

"Madam, will you really be so good!" he cried, with strong feeling. "Good God, you've saved me! You have saved a man from a violent death, from a bullet. . . . My eternal gratitude . . ."

"I will give you more, infinitely more than three thousand!" cried Madame Hohlakov, looking with a radiant smile at Mitya's ecstasy.

"Infinitely? But I don't need so much. I only need that fatal three thousand, and on my part I can give security for that sum with infinite gratitude, and I propose a plan which . . ."

"Enough, Dmitri Fyodorovich, it's said and done." Madame Hohlakov cut him short, with the modest triumph of a benefactress: "I have promised to save you, and I will save you. I will save you as I did Belmesov. What do you think of gold-mines, Dmitri Fyodorovich?"

"Gold-mines, madam? I have never thought anything about them."

"But I have thought of them for you. Thought of them over and over again. I have been watching you for the last month. I've watched you a hundred times as you've walked past, saying to myself: that's a man of energy who ought to be at the gold-mines. I've studied your gait and come to the conclusion: that's a man who would find gold."

"From my gait, madam?" said Mitya, smiling.

"Yes, from your gait. You surely don't deny that character can be told from the gait, Dmitri Fyodorovich? The natural sciences support the idea. Oh, I'm a realist now. After all this business with Father Zosima, which has so upset me, from this very day I'm a perfect realist and I want to devote myself to practical activities. I'm cured. 'Enough!' as Turgenev says."

"But, madam, the three thousand you so generously promised to lend me . . ."

"It is yours, Dmitri Fyodorovich," Madame Hohlakov cut in at once. "The money is as good as in your pocket, not three thousand, but three million, Dmitri Fyodorovich, in less than no time. I'll make you a present of the idea: you shall find gold-mines, make millions, return and become a leading citizen, and wake us up and lead us to better things. Are we to leave it all to the Jews? You will erect buildings and start enterprises of all sorts. You will help the poor, and they will bless you. This is the age of railways, Dmitri Fyodorovich. You'll become famous and indispensable to the Department of Finance, which is so badly off at present. The depreciation of the rouble keeps me awake at night, Dmitri Fyodorovich; people don't know that side of me . . ."

"Madam, madam!" Dmitri interrupted with an uneasy presentiment. "I shall indeed, perhaps, follow your advice, your wise advice, madam. . . . I shall perhaps set off . . . to the gold-mines. . . . I'll come and see you again about it . . . many times, indeed . . . but now, that three thousand you so generously . . . oh, that would set me free, and if you could to-day . . . you see, I haven't a minute, a minute to lose to-day . . ."

"Enough, Dmitri Fyodorovich, enough!" Madame Hohlakov interrupted emphatically. "The question is, will you go to the gold-mines or not; have you quite made up your mind? Answer yes or no."

"I will go, madam, afterwards. . . . I'll go where you like . . . but now . . ."

"Wait!" cried Madame Hohlakov. And jumping up and running to a handsome bureau with numerous little drawers, she began pulling out one drawer after another, looking for something with desperate haste.

"The three thousand," thought Mitya, his heart almost stopping, "and at the instant . . . without any papers or formalities . . . that's doing things in gentlemanly style! She's a splendid woman, if only she didn't talk so much!"

"Here!" cried Madame Hohlakov, running back joyfully to Mitya, "here is what I was looking for!"

It was a tiny silver ikon on a cord, such as is sometimes worn next the skin with a cross.

"This is from Kiev, Dmitri Fyodorovich," she went on reverently, "from the relics of Varvara, the Great Martyr. Let me put it on your neck myself, and with it dedicate you to a new life, to a new career."

And she actually put the cord around his neck, and began arranging it. In extreme embarrassment, Mitya bent down and helped her, and at last he got it under his neck-tie and collar and next to his chest.

"Now you can set off," Madame Hohlakov pronounced, sitting down triumphantly in her place again.

"Madam, I am so touched. I don't know how to thank you, indeed . . . for such kindness, but . . . If only you knew how precious time is to me. . . . That sum of money, for which I shall be indebted to your generosity. . . . Oh, madam, since you are so kind, so touchingly generous to me," Mitya exclaimed impulsively, "then let me reveal to you . . . though, of course, you've known it a long time . . . that I love somebody here. . . . I have been false to Katya . . . Katerina Ivanovna I should say. . . . Oh, I've behaved inhumanly, dishonourably to her, but I fell in love here with another woman . . . a woman whom you, madam, perhaps, despise, for you know everything already, but whom I cannot leave on any account, and therefore that three thousand now . . ."

"Leave everything, Dmitri Fyodorovich," Madame Hohlakov interrupted in the most decisive tone. "Leave everything, especially women. Gold-mines are your goal, and there's no place for women there. Afterwards, when you come back rich and famous, you will find the companion of your heart in the highest society. That will be a modern girl, with education and without prejudices. By that time the budding woman question will have ripened, and the new woman will have appeared."

"Madam, that's not the point, not at all. . . ." Mitya clasped his hands in entreaty.

"Yes, it is, Dmitri Fyodorovich, just what you need; the very thing you're yearning for, though you don't realise it yourself. I am not at all opposed to the present woman's movement, Dmitri Fyodorovich. The development of woman, and even the political emancipation of woman in the near future — that's my ideal. I've a daughter myself, Dmitri Fyodorovich, people don't know that side of me. I wrote a letter to the author, Shchedrin, on that subject. He has taught me so much, so much about the vocation of woman. So last year I sent him an anonymous letter of two lines: 'I kiss and embrace you, my author, for the modern woman. Persevere.' And I signed myself, 'a Mother.' I thought of signing myself 'a contemporary Mother,' and hesitated, but I stuck to the simple 'Mother'; there's more moral beauty in that, Dmitri Fyodorovich. And the word 'contemporary' might have reminded him of 'The Contemporary' — a painful recollection owing to the censorship. . . . Good heavens, what is the matter with you?"

"Madam!" cried Mitya, jumping up at last, clasping his hands before her in helpless entreaty. "You will make me weep if you delay what you have so generously . . ."

"Oh, do weep, Dmitri Fyodorovich, do weep! That's a noble feeling . . . such a path lies open before you! Tears will ease your heart, and later on you will return rejoicing. You will hasten to me from Siberia on purpose to share your joy with me . . ."

"But allow me, too!" Mitya shouted suddenly. "For the last time I entreat you, tell me, can I have the sum you promised me today, if not, when may I come for it?"

"What sum, Dmitri Fyodorovich?"

"The three thousand you promised me . . . that you so generously . . ."

"Three thousand? Roubles? Oh, no, I haven't got three thousand," Madame Hohlakov announced with serene amazement. Mitya was stupefied.

"Why, you said just now . . . you said . . . you said it was as good as in my pocket."

"Oh, no, you misunderstood me, Dmitri Fyodorovich. In that case you misunderstood me. I was talking of the gold-mines. It's true I promised you more, infinitely more than three thousand, I remember it all now, but I was referring to the gold-mines."

"But the money? The three thousand?" Mitya exclaimed, awkwardly.

"Oh, if you meant money, I haven't any. I haven't a penny, now, Dmitri Fyodorovich. I'm in the midst of a fight with my steward, and I've just borrowed five hundred roubles from Miüsov, myself. No, no, I've no money. And, do you know, Dmitri Fyodorovich, if I had, I wouldn't give it to you. In the first place I never lend money. Lending money means losing friends. And I wouldn't give it to you particularly. I wouldn't give it you, because I like you and want to save you, for all you need is the gold-mines, the gold-mines, the gold-mines!"

"Oh, the devil!" roared Mitya, and with all his might brought his fist down on the table.

"Aie! Aie!" cried Madame Hohlakov, alarmed and she flew to the other end of the drawing-room.

Mitya spat, and strode rapidly out of the room, out of the house, into the street, into the darkness! He walked like one demented, beating himself on the breast, on the spot where he had struck himself two days previously, before Alyosha, the last time he saw him in the dark, on the road. What those blows upon his breast signified, *on that spot*, and what he meant by it — that was, for the time, a secret which was known to no one in the world, and had not been told even to Alyosha. But that secret meant for him more than disgrace; it meant ruin, suicide. So he had determined, if he did not get hold of the three thousand that would pay his debt to Katerina Ivanovna, and so remove from his breast, from *that spot on his breast*, the shame he carried upon it, that weighed on his conscience. All this will be fully explained to the reader later on, but now that his last hope had vanished, this man, so strong in appearance, burst out crying like a little child a few steps from the Hohlakovs' house. He walked on, and not knowing what he was doing, wiped away his tears with his fist. In this way he reached the square, and suddenly became aware that he had stumbled against something. He heard a piercing wail from an old woman whom he had almost knocked down.

"Good Lord, you've nearly killed me! Why don't you look where you're going, scapegrace?"

"Why, it's you!" cried Mitya, recognising the old woman in the dark. It was the old servant who waited on Samsonov, whom Mitya had particularly noticed the day before.

"And who are you, my good sir?" said the old woman in quite a different voice. "I don't know you in the dark."

"You live at Kuzma Kuzmich's. You're the servant there?"

"Just so, sir, I was only running out to Prohorich's . . . But I don't know you now."

"Tell me, my good woman, is Agrafena Alexandrovna there now?" said Mitya, beside himself with suspense. "I saw her to the house some time ago."

"She has been there, sir. She stayed a little while, and went off again."

"What? Went away?" cried Mitya. "When did she go?"

"Why, as soon as she came. She only stayed a minute. She only told Kuzma Kuzmich a tale that made him laugh, and then she ran away."

"You're lying, damn you!" roared Mitya.

"Aie! Aie!" shrieked the old woman, but Mitya had vanished.

He ran with all his might to the house where Grushenka lived. When he reached it, Grushenka had already left for Mokroye; she had not been gone for more than a quarter of an hour.

Fenya was sitting in the kitchen with her grandmother, the old cook, Matryona, when the "captain" ran in. Fenya uttered a piercing shriek on seeing him.

"You scream?" roared Mitya, "where is she?"

But without giving the terror-stricken Fenya time to utter a word, he fell all of a heap at her feet.

"Fenya, for the sake of our Lord Christ, tell me, where is she?"

"My sweet one, I don't know anything. Dmitri Fyodorovich, darling, I don't know anything. You may kill me but I don't know anything." Fenya swore and protested. "You went out with her yourself not long ago . . ."

"She came back!"

"Darling, she didn't. I swear by God she didn't come back."

"You're lying!" shouted Mitya. "From your fright I know where she is."

He dashed out. Fenya in her fright was glad she had got off so easily. But she knew very well that it was only that he was in such haste, or she might not have fared so well. But as he ran, he surprised both Fenya and old Matryona by an unexpected action. On the table stood a brass mortar, with a pestle in it, a small brass pestle, not much more than six inches long. Mitya had already opened the door with one hand when, with the other, he snatched up the pestle, thrust it in his side pocket, and was gone.

"Oh, Lord! He's going to murder some one!" cried Fenya, striking her hands together.

CHAPTER IV

IN THE DARK

WHERE was he running? "Where could she be except at Fyodor Pavlovich's? She must have run straight to him from Samsonov's, that was clear now. The whole intrigue, the whole deception was evident." . . . It all rushed whirling through his mind. He did not run to Marya Kondratyevna's. "There was no need to go there . . . not the slightest need . . . he must raise no alarm . . . they would run and tell directly. . . . Marya Kondratyevna was clearly in the plot, Smerdyakov, too, he, too, all had been bought over!"

He formed another plan of action: taking the long way, he ran round Fyodor Pavlovich's house, crossing the lane, running down Dmitrovsky Street, then over the little bridge, and so came straight to the deserted alley at the back, which was empty and uninhabited, with on one side the hurdle fence of a neighbour's kitchen-garden, on the other the strong high fence that ran all round Fyodor Pavlovich's garden. Here he chose a spot, apparently the very place where, according to the tradition he knew, Lizaveta had once climbed over the fence: "If she could climb over it," the thought, God knows why, occurred to him, "surely I can." He did in fact jump up, and instantly contrived to catch hold of the top of the fence. Then he vigorously pulled himself up and sat astride it. Close by, in the garden, stood the bath-house, but from the fence he could see the lighted windows of the house, too.

"Yes, the old man's bedroom is lighted up. She's there!" and he leapt from the fence into the garden. Though he knew Grigory was ill and very likely Smerdyakov, too, and that there was no one to hear him, he instinctively hid himself, stood still, and began to listen. But there was dead silence on all sides and, as though of design, complete stillness, not the slightest breath of wind.

"And only silence whispered there," the line for some reason rose to his mind. "If only no one heard me jump over the fence! I think not." Standing still for a minute, he walked softly across the grass in the garden, avoiding the trees and shrubs. He walked slowly, creeping stealthily at every step, listening to his own footsteps. It took him five minutes to reach the lighted window. He remembered that just under the window there were several thick and high bushes of elder and guelder-rose. The door from the house into the garden, on the left-hand side, was locked; he had carefully looked purposely to see, in passing. At last he reached the bushes and hid behind them. He held his breath. "I must wait now," he thought, "to reassure them, in case they heard my footsteps and are listening . . . if only I don't cough or sneeze."

He waited two minutes. His heart was beating violently, and, at moments, he was almost suffocated. "No, this throbbing of my heart won't stop," he thought. "I can't wait any longer." He was standing behind a bush in the shadow. The light of the window fell on the front part of the bush.

"How red the guelder-rose berries are!" he murmured, not knowing why. Softly and noiselessly, step by step, he approached the window, and raised himself on tiptoe. All Fyodor Pavlovich's bedroom lay open before him. It was not a large room, and was divided in two parts by a red screen, "Chinese," as Fyodor Pavlovich used to call it. The word "Chinese" flashed into Mitya's mind, "and behind the screen is Grushenka," thought Mitya. He began watching Fyodor Pavlovich, who was wearing his new striped-silk dressing-gown, which Mitya had never seen, and a silk cord with tassels round the waist. A clean, dandified shirt of fine linen with gold studs peeped out under the collar of the dressing-gown. On his head Fyodor Pavlovich had the same red bandage which Alyosha had seen.

"He has got himself up," thought Mitya.

His father was standing near the window, apparently lost in thought. Suddenly he jerked up his head, listened a moment, and, hearing nothing, went up to the table, poured out half a glass of brandy from a decanter, and drank it off. Then he breathed deeply, again stood still a moment, walked carelessly up to the looking-glass on the wall, with his right hand raised the red bandage on his forehead a little, and began examining his bruises and wounds, which had not yet disappeared.

"He's alone," thought Mitya, "in all probability he's alone."

Fyodor Pavlovich moved away from the looking-glass, turned suddenly to the window and looked out. Mitya instantly slipped away into the shadow.

"She may be there behind the screen. Perhaps she's asleep by now," he thought, with a pang at his heart. Fyodor Pavlovich moved away from the window. "He's looking for her out of the window, so she's not there. Why should he peer out into the dark? He's wild

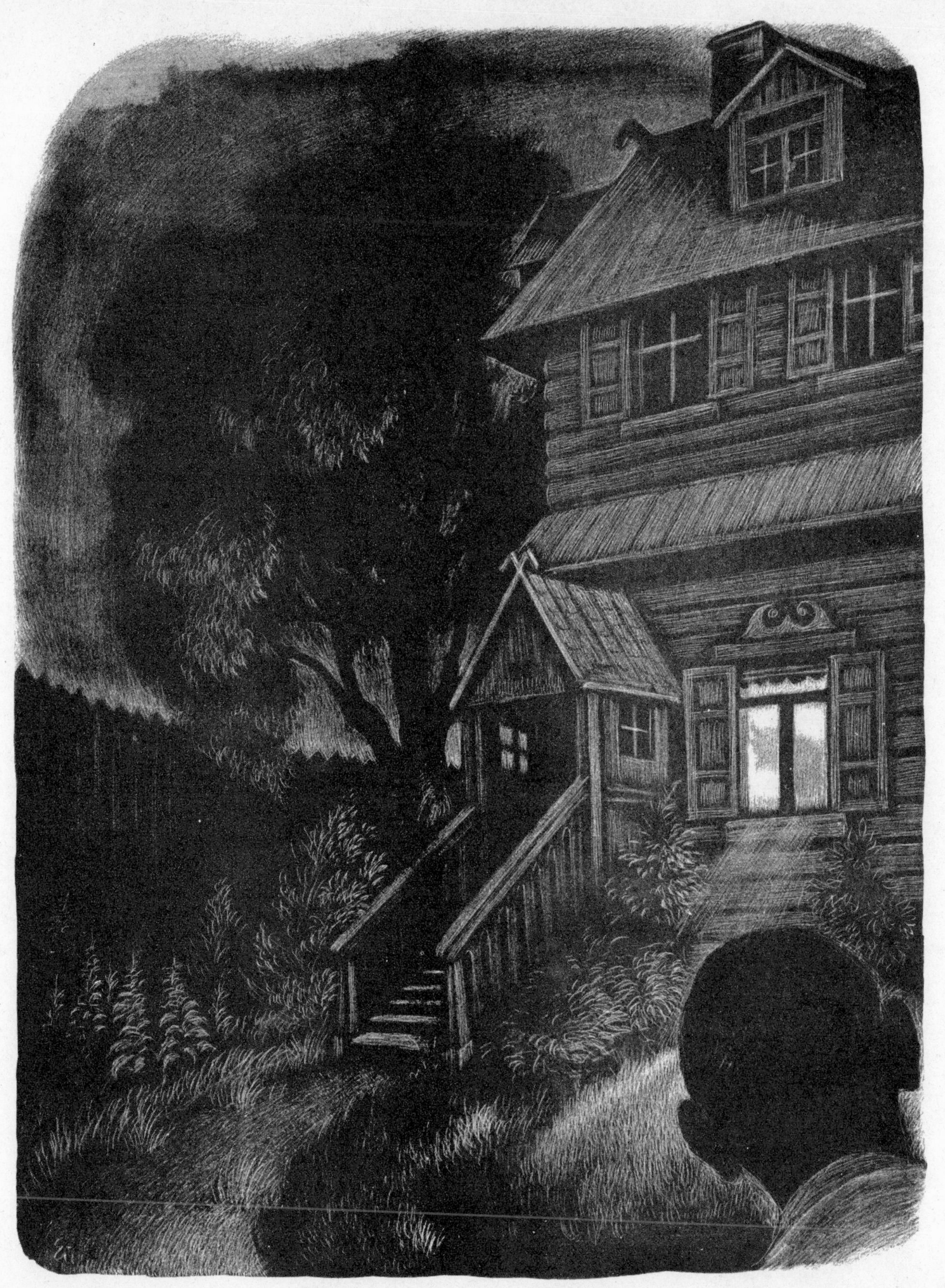

AN OCCURRENCE IN THE DARK

with impatience." . . . Mitya slipped back at once, and fell to gazing in at the window again. The old man was sitting down at the table, apparently disappointed. At last he put his elbow on the table, and laid his right cheek against his hand.

Mitya watched him eagerly.

"He's alone, he's alone!" he repeated again. "If she were here, his face would be different."

Strange to say, a queer, irrational vexation rose up in his heart that she was not here. "It's not that she's not here," he explained to himself, immediately, "but that I can't tell for certain whether she is or not." Mitya remembered afterwards that his mind was, at that moment, exceptionally clear, that he took in everything to the slightest detail, and missed no point. But a feeling of misery, the misery of uncertainty and indecision, was growing in his heart with every instant. "Is she here or not?" The angry doubt filled his heart, and suddenly, making up his mind, he put out his hand and softly knocked on the window frame. He knocked the signal the old man had agreed upon with Smerdyakov, twice slowly and then three times more quickly, the signal that meant "Grushenka has come!"

The old man started, jerked up his head, and, jumping up quickly, ran to the window. Mitya slipped away into the shadow. Fyodor Pavlovich opened the window and thrust his whole head out.

"Grushenka, is it you? Is it you?" he said, in a sort of trembling half-whisper. "Where are you, my angel, where are you?" He was fearfully agitated and breathless.

"He's alone," Mitya decided.

"Where are you?" cried the old man again; and he thrust his head out farther, thrust it out to the shoulders, gazing in all directions, right and left. "Come here, I've a little present for you. Come, I'll show you . . ."

"He means the package with the three thousand," thought Mitya.

"But where are you? Are you at the door? I'll open it directly."

And the old man almost climbed out of the window, peering out to the right, where there was a door into the garden, trying to see into the darkness. In another second he would certainly have run out to open the door without waiting for Grushenka's answer.

Mitya looked at him from the side without stirring. The old man's profile that he loathed so, his pendant Adam's apple, his hooked nose, his lips that smiled in greedy expectation, were all brightly lighted up by the slanting lamplight falling on the left from the room. A dreadful fury of hatred suddenly surged up in Mitya's heart. "There he was, his rival, the man who had tormented him, who had ruined his life!" It was a rush of that sudden, furious, vengeful anger of which he had spoken to Alyosha, as though foreseeing it, four days ago in the arbour, when, in answer to Alyosha's question, "How can you say you'll kill our father?" he had said, "I don't know, I don't know. Perhaps I shall not kill him, perhaps I shall. I'm afraid he'll suddenly be so loathsome to me at that moment. I hate his Adam's apple, his nose, his eyes, his shameless grin. I feel a personal loathing. That's what I'm afraid of, that's what may be too much for me." . . . This personal loathing was growing unendurable. Mitya was beside himself, he suddenly pulled the brass pestle out of his pocket. . . .

"God was watching over me then," Mitya himself said afterwards. At that very moment Grigory waked up on his bed of sickness. Earlier in the evening he had undergone the treatment which Smerdyakov had described to Ivan Fyodorovich. He had rubbed himself all over with vodka mixed with a secret very strong decoction, had drunk what was left of the mixture while his wife repeated a "certain prayer" over him, after which he had gone to bed. Marfa Ignatyevna had quaffed of the stuff, too, and, being unused to strong drink, slept like the dead beside her spouse.

But Grigory waked up in the night, quite suddenly, and, after a moment's reflection, though he immediately felt a sharp pain in his back, he sat up in bed. Then he deliberated again, got up and dressed hurriedly. Perhaps his conscience was uneasy at the thought of sleeping while the house was unguarded "in such perilous times." Smerdyakov, exhausted by his fit, lay motionless in the next room. Marfa Ignatyevna did not stir. "The stuff's been too much for the woman," Grigory thought, glancing at her, and, groaning, he went out on the steps. No doubt he only intended to look out from the steps, for he was hardly able to walk, the pain in his back and his right leg was intolerable. But he suddenly remembered that he had not locked the little gate into the garden that evening. He was the most punctual and precise of men, a man who adhered to an unchangeable routine, and habits that lasted for years. Limping and writhing with pain, he went down the steps and towards the garden. Yes, the gate stood wide open. Mechanically he stepped into the garden. Perhaps he fancied something, perhaps caught some sound, and, glancing to the left, he saw his master's window open. No one was looking out of it then.

"What's it open for? It's not summer now," thought Grigory, and suddenly, at that very instant, he caught a glimpse of something extraordinary before him in the garden. Forty paces in front of him a man seemed to be running in the dark, a shadow was moving very fast.

"Good Lord!" cried Grigory, beside himself, and forgetting the pain in his back, he hurried to intercept the running figure. He took a short cut, evidently he knew the garden better than the stranger; the flying figure went towards the bath-house, ran behind it, and rushed to the garden fence. Grigory followed, not losing sight of him, and ran, forgetting everything. He reached the fence at the very moment the man was climbing over it. Grigory cried out, beside himself, pounced on him, and clutched his leg in his two hands.

Yes, his foreboding had not deceived him. He recognised him, it was he, the "monster," the "parricide."

"Parricide!" the old man shouted so that the whole neighbourhood could hear, but he had not time to shout again, he fell at once, as though struck by lightning.

Mitya jumped back into the garden and bent over the fallen man. In Mitya's hands was a brass pestle, and he flung it mechanically into the grass. The pestle fell two paces from Grigory, not in the grass but on the path, in a most conspicuous place. For some seconds he examined the prostrate figure before him. The old man's head was all bloody. Mitya put out his hand and began feeling it. He remembered afterwards clearly that he had been awfully anxious to make sure whether he had broken the old man's skull, or simply stunned him with the pestle. But the blood was flowing horribly, and in a moment Mitya's trembling fingers were drenched with the hot stream. He remembered taking out of his pocket the clean white handkerchief with which he had provided himself for his visit to Madame Hohlakov, and putting it to the old man's head, senselessly trying to wipe the blood from his face and temples. But the handkerchief was instantly soaked with blood.

"Good heavens! what am I doing it for?" thought Mitya, suddenly pulling himself together. "If I have broken his skull, how can I find out now? And what difference does it make now?" he added, hopelessly. "If I've killed him, I've killed him . . . you've come to grief, old man, so there you must lie!" he said aloud. And suddenly, turning to the fence, he vaulted over it into the lane and fell to running — the handkerchief soaked with blood he held, crushed up, in his right fist, and, as he ran, he thrust it into the back pocket of his coat.

He ran headlong, and the few passers-by who met him in the dark, in the streets, remembered afterwards that they had met a man running that night. He flew back again to the widow Morozov's house.

Immediately after he had left it, that evening, Fenya had rushed to the chief porter, Nazar Ivanovich, and besought him, for Christ's sake, "not to let the captain in again to-day or to-morrow." Nazar Ivanovich promised, but went upstairs to his mistress who had suddenly sent for him, and meeting his nephew, a boy of twenty, who had recently come from the country, on the way up, told him to take his place, but forgot to mention the "captain." Mitya, running up to the gate, knocked. The lad instantly recognised him, for Mitya had more than once tipped him. Opening the gate at once, he let him in, and hastened to inform him with a good-humoured smile that "Agrafena Alexandrovna is not at home now, you know."

"Where is she then, Prohor?" asked Mitya, stopping short.

"She set off this evening, some two hours ago, with Timofey, to Mokroye."

"What for?" cried Mitya.

"That I can't say. To see some officer. Some one invited her and horses were sent to fetch her."

Mitya left him, and ran like a madman to Fenya.

CHAPTER V

A SUDDEN RESOLUTION

She was sitting in the kitchen with her grandmother; they were both just going to bed. Relying on Nazar Ivanovich, they had not locked themselves in. Mitya ran in, pounced on Fenya and seized her by the throat.

"Speak at once! Where is she? With whom is she now at Mokroye?" he roared, beside himself.

Both the women squealed.

"Aie! I'll tell you. Aie, Dmitri Fyodorovich, darling, I'll tell you everything directly, I won't hide anything," gabbled Fenya, frightened to death; "she's gone to Mokroye, to her officer."

"What officer?" roared Mitya.

"To her officer, the same one she used to know, the one who threw her over five years ago," cackled Fenya, as fast as she could speak.

Mitya withdrew the hands with which he was squeezing her throat. He stood facing her, pale as death, unable to utter a word, but his eyes showed that he realised it all, all, from the first word, and guessed the whole situation. Poor Fenya was not in a condition at that moment to observe whether he understood or not. She remained sitting on the trunk as she had been when he ran into the room, trembling all over, holding her hands out before her as though trying to defend herself. She seemed to have grown rigid in that position. Her wide-open, scared eyes were fixed immovably upon him. And to make matters worse, both his hands were smeared with blood. On the way, as he ran, he must have touched his forehead with them, wiping off the perspiration, so that on his forehead and his right cheek were red patches of smeared blood. Fenya was on the verge of hysterics. The old cook had jumped up and was staring at him like a mad-woman, almost unconscious with terror.

Mitya stood for a moment, then mechanically sank onto a chair next to Fenya. He was sitting, not so much sunk in thought as terror-stricken, so to speak, benumbed. Yet everything was clear as day: that officer, he knew about him, he knew everything perfectly, he had known it from Grushenka herself, had known that a letter had come from him a month before. So that for a month, for a whole month this had been going on in secret from him, till the very arrival of this new man, and he had never thought of him! But how could he, how could he not have thought of him? Why was it he had forgotten this officer, like that, forgotten him as soon as he heard of him? That was the question that faced him like some monstrous thing. And he looked at this monstrous thing with fear, growing cold with fear.

But suddenly, as gently and meekly as a gentle and affectionate child, he began speaking to Fenya as though he had utterly forgotten how he had scared and hurt her just now. He fell to questioning Fenya with an extreme preciseness, astonishing in his position, and though the girl looked wildly at his blood-stained hands, she, too, with wonderful readiness and haste, answered every question as though eager to put the whole truth and nothing but the truth before him. Little by little, even with a sort of enjoyment, she began explaining every detail, not wanting to torment him, but, as it were, eager to be of the utmost service to him. She described the whole of that day, in great detail, the visit of Rakitin and Alyosha, how she, Fenya, had been on the watch, how the mistress had set off, and how she had called out of the window to Alyosha to give him, Mitya, her greetings, and to tell him "to remember for ever how she had loved him for an hour."

Hearing of the message, Mitya suddenly smiled, and there was a flush of colour on his pale cheeks. At the same moment Fenya said to him, not a bit afraid now to be inquisitive:

"Look at your hands, Dmitri Fyodorovich. They're all over blood!"

"Yes," answered Mitya mechanically. He looked absent-mindedly at his hands and at once forgot them and Fenya's question.

He sank into silence again. Twenty minutes had passed since he had run in. His first horror was over, but evidently some new fixed determination had taken possession of him. He suddenly stood up, smiling dreamily.

"What has happened to you, sir?" said Fenya, pointing to his hands again. She spoke compassionately, as though she felt very near to him now in his grief. Mitya looked at his hands again.

"That's blood, Fenya," he said, looking at her with a strange expression. "That's human blood, and, my God! why was it shed? But . . . Fenya . . . there's a fence here" (he

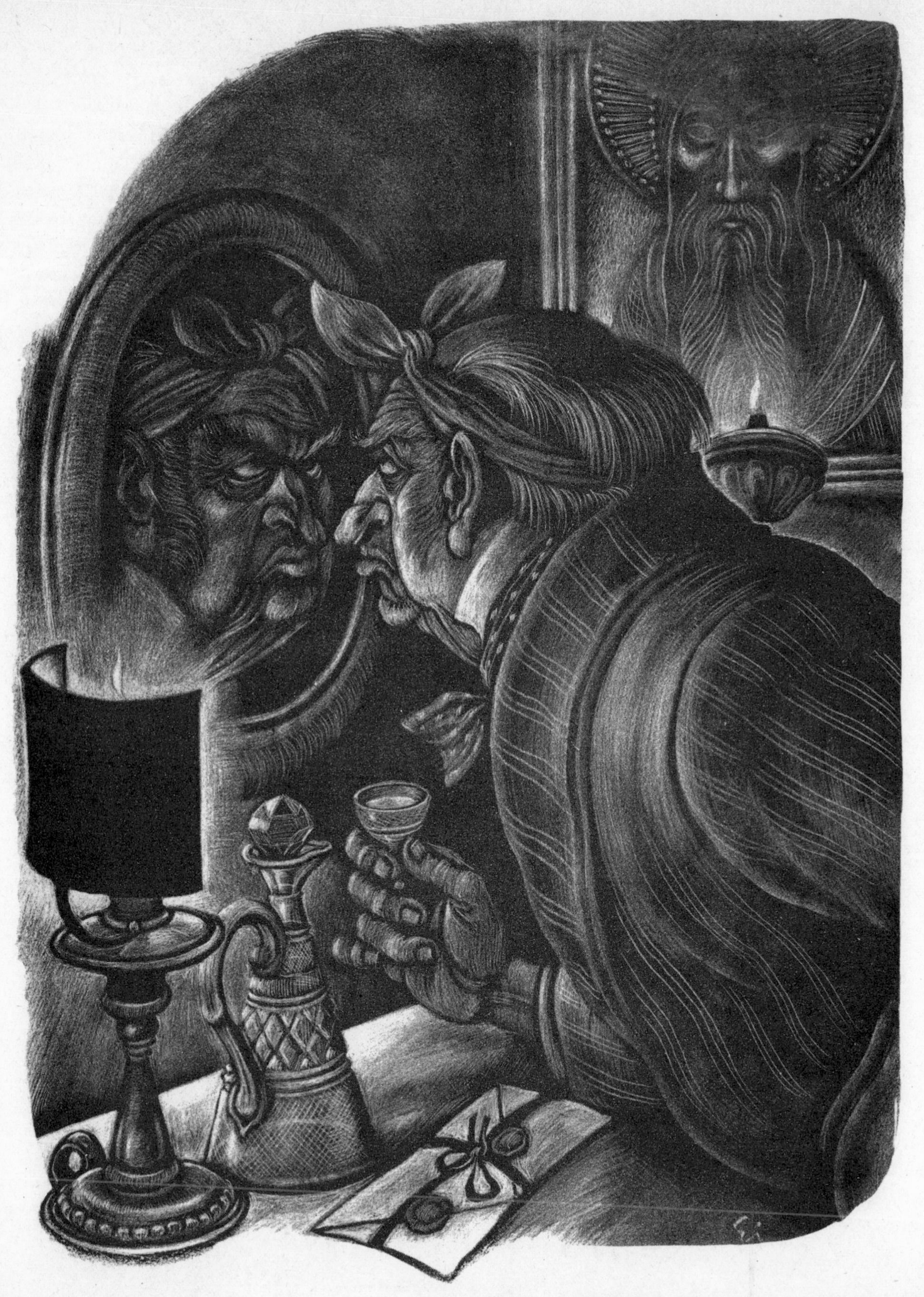

FYODOR PAVLOVICH EXAMINES HIS BRUISES

looked at her as though setting her a riddle), "a high fence, and terrible to look at. But, at dawn to-morrow, 'when the sun soars,' Mitya will leap over that fence. . . . You don't understand what fence, Fenya, and, never mind. . . . You'll hear to-morrow and understand everything . . . and now, good-bye. I won't stand in her way. I'll step aside, I know how to step aside. Live, my joy. . . . You loved me for an hour, so remember Mityenka Karamazov for ever. . . . She always used to call me Mityenka, do you remember?"

And with those words he walked suddenly out of the kitchen. Fenya was almost more frightened at this sudden departure than she had been when he ran in and attacked her.

Just ten minutes later Dmitri went in to Pyotr Ilyich Perhotin, the young official with whom he had pawned his pistols. It was by now half-past eight, and Pyotr Ilyich had finished his evening tea, and had just put his coat on again to go to the "Metropolis" to have a game of billiards. Mitya caught him coming out.

Seeing him with his face all smeared with blood, the young man uttered a cry of surprise.

"Good heavens! What is the matter?"

"I've come for my pistols," said Mitya, "and brought you the money. And thanks very much. I'm in a hurry, Pyotr Ilyich, please make haste."

Pyotr Ilyich's surprise increased; he suddenly caught sight of a bundle of bank-notes in Mitya's hand, and what was more, he had walked in holding the notes as no one walks in and no one carries money: he had them in his right hand, and held them outstretched as if to show them. Perhotin's servant, a young boy, who met Mitya in the passage, said afterwards that he walked into the passage in the same way, with the money in his outstretched hand, so he must have been carrying it like that even in the street. They were all rainbow-coloured hundred-rouble notes, and the fingers holding them were covered with blood.

When Pyotr Ilyich was questioned later on as to the sum of money, he said that it was difficult to judge at a glance, but that it might have been two thousand, or perhaps three, but it was a big "fat" bundle. "Dmitri Fyodorovich," so he testified afterwards, "seemed unlike himself, too; not drunk, but in a kind of ecstasy, as it were, absent-minded, but at the same time, as it were, absorbed, as though pondering and searching for something and unable to come to a decision. He was in great haste, answered abruptly and very strangely, and at moments seemed not at all dejected but quite cheerful."

"But what *is* the matter with you? What's wrong?" cried Pyotr Ilyich, looking wildly at his guest. "How is it that you're all covered with blood? Have you had a fall? Look at yourself!"

He took him by the elbow and led him to the glass.

Seeing his blood-stained face, Mitya started and scowled wrathfully.

"Damnation! That's the last straw," he muttered angrily, hurriedly changing the notes from his right hand to his left, and impulsively jerked the handkerchief out of his pocket. But the handkerchief turned out to be soaked with blood, too (it was the handkerchief he had used to wipe Grigory's head and face). There was scarcely a white spot on it, and it had not merely begun to dry, but had stiffened into a crumpled ball and could not be unfolded. Mitya threw it angrily on the floor. "Oh, damn it!" he said. "Haven't you a rag of some sort . . . to wipe my face?"

"So you're only stained, not wounded? You'd better wash," said Pyotr Ilyich. "Here's a wash-stand. I'll pour you out some water."

"A wash-stand? That's all right . . . but where am I to put this?"

With the strangest perplexity he indicated his bundle of hundred-rouble notes, looking inquiringly at Pyotr Ilyich as though it were for him to decide what he, Mitya, was to do with his own money.

"In your pocket, or on the table here. They won't be lost."

"In my pocket? Yes, in my pocket. All right. . . . But, I say, that's all nonsense," he cried, as though suddenly coming out of his absorption. "Look here, let's first settle that business of the pistols. Give them back to me. Here's your money . . . because I am in great need of them . . . and I haven't a minute, a minute to spare."

And taking the topmost note from the bundle, he held it out to Pyotr Ilyich.

"But I shan't have change enough. Haven't you less?"

"No," said Mitya, looking again at the bundle, and as though not trusting his own words he fingered two or three of the topmost ones.

"No, they're all alike," he added, and again he looked inquiringly at Pyotr Ilyich.

"How have you grown so rich?" the latter asked. "Wait, I'll send my boy to Plotnikovs', they close late — to see if they won't change it. Here, Misha!" he called into the passage.

"To Plotnikovs' shop — first rate!" cried Mitya, as though struck by an idea. "Misha," he turned to the boy as he came in, "look here, run to Plotnikovs' and tell them that Dmitri Fyodorovich sends his greetings, and will be there directly. . . . But listen, listen, tell them to have champagne, three dozen bottles ready before I come, and packed as it was to take to Mokroye. I took four dozen with me then," he added (suddenly addressing Pyotr Ilyich); "they know all about it, don't you trouble, Misha," he turned again to the boy. "Stay, listen; tell them to put in cheese, Strasburg pies, smoked fish, ham, caviare, and everything, everything they've got, up to a hundred roubles, or a hundred and twenty as before. . . . But wait: don't let them forget dessert, sweets, pears, watermelons, two or three or four — no, one melon's enough, and chocolate, candy, toffee, fondants; in fact, everything I took to Mokroye before, three hundred roubles' worth with champagne . . . let it be just the same again. And remember, Misha, if you are called Misha . . . His name is Misha, isn't it?" He turned to Pyotr Ilyich again.

"Wait a minute," Pyotr Ilyich intervened, listening and watching him uneasily, "you'd better go yourself and tell them. He'll muddle it."

"He will, I see he will! Eh, Misha! Why, I was going to kiss you for the commission. . . . If you don't make a mistake, there's ten roubles for you, run along, make haste. . . . Champagne's the chief thing, let them roll out champagne. And cognac, too, and red and white wine, and all I had then. . . . They know what I had then."

"But listen!" Pyotr Ilyich interrupted with some impatience. "I say, let him simply run and change the money and tell them not to close, and you go and tell them. . . . Give him your note. Be off, Misha! Shake a leg!"

Pyotr Ilyich seemed to hurry Misha off on

purpose, because the boy remained standing with his mouth and eyes wide open, apparently understanding little of Mitya's orders, gazing up with amazement and terror at his blood-stained face and the trembling blood-stained fingers that held the notes.

"Well, now come and wash," said Pyotr Ilyich sternly. "Put the money on the table or else in your pocket. . . . That's right, come along. But take off your coat."

And beginning to help him off with his coat, he cried out again:

"Look, your coat's covered with blood, too!"

"That . . . it's not the coat. It's only a little here on the sleeve. . . . And that's only here where the handkerchief lay. It must have soaked through. I must have sat on the handkerchief at Fenya's, and the blood's come through," Mitya explained at once with astonishing trustfulness. Pyotr Ilyich listened, frowning.

"Well, you must have been up to something; you must have had a fight with some one," he muttered.

They began to wash. Pyotr Ilyich held the jug and poured out the water. Mitya, in desperate haste, scarcely soaped his hands (they were trembling, and Pyotr Ilyich remembered it afterwards). But the young official insisted on his soaping them thoroughly and rubbing them more. He seemed to dominate Mitya, and more so as time passed. It may be noted in passing that he was a young man of far from timid character.

"Look, you haven't got your nails clean. Now rub your face; here, on your temples, by your ear. . . . Will you go in that shirt? Where are you going? Look, the whole cuff of your right sleeve is covered with blood."

"Yes, it's all bloody," observed Mitya, looking at the cuff of his shirt.

"Then change your shirt."

"I haven't time. You see I'll . . ." Mitya went on in the same confiding way, drying his face and hands on the towel, and putting on his coat. "I'll turn it up at the wrist. It won't be seen under the coat. . . . You see!"

"Tell me now, what game have you been up to? Have you been fighting with some one? In the tavern again, as before? Have you been beating that captain again?" Pyotr Ilyich asked him reproachfully. "Whom did you beat up now . . . or kill, perhaps?"

"Nonsense!" said Mitya.

"How 'nonsense'?"

"Don't worry," said Mitya, and he suddenly grinned. "I crushed an old woman in the market-place just now."

"Crushed? An old woman?"

"An old man!" cried Mitya, looking Pyotr Ilyich straight in the face, laughing, and shouting at him as though he were deaf.

"Confound it! An old woman, an old man. . . . Have you killed some one?"

"We made it up. We had a row — and made it up. In a place I know of. We parted friends. A fool. . . . He's forgiven me. . . . He's sure to have forgiven me by now . . . if he had got up, he wouldn't have forgiven me" — Mitya suddenly winked — "only, damn him, you know, I say, Pyotr Ilyich, damn him! Don't worry about him! I don't want to just now!" Mitya snapped out, resolutely.

"Whatever do you want to go picking quarrels with every one for? . . . Just as you did with that captain over some trifle. . . . You've been fighting and now you're rushing off on a spree — that's you all over! Three dozen champagne — what do you want all that for?"

"Bravo! Now give me the pistols. Upon my honour I've no time now. I should like to have a chat with you, my dear boy, but I haven't the time. And there's no need, it's too late for talking. Where's my money? Where have I put it?" he cried, thrusting his hands into his pockets.

"You put it on the table . . . yourself. . . . Here it is. Had you forgotten? Money's like dirt or water to you, it seems. Here are your pistols. It's an odd thing, at six o'clock you pledged them for ten roubles, and now you've got thousands. Two or three I should say."

"Three, you bet," laughed Mitya, stuffing the notes into the side pockets of his trousers.

"You'll lose it like that. Have you found a gold-mine?"

"The mines? The gold-mines?" Mitya shouted at the top of his voice and went off in a roar of laughter. "Would you like to go to the mines, Perhotin? There's a lady here who'll stump up three thousand for you, if only you'll go. She did it for me, she's so awfully fond of gold-mines. Do you know Madame Hohlakov?"

"I don't know her, but I've heard of her and seen her. Did she really give you three thousand? Did she really hand them over to you?" said Pyotr Ilyich, eyeing him dubiously.

"As soon as the sun soars to-morrow, as soon as Phœbus, ever young, soars upwards, praising and glorifying God, you go to her, this Madame Hohlakov, and ask her whether she did stump up that three thousand or not. Try and find out."

"I don't know on what terms you are . . . since you say it so positively, I suppose she did give it to you. You've got the money in your hand, but instead of going to Siberia you're spending it all. . . . Where are you really off to now, eh?"

"To Mokroye."

"To Mokroye? But it's night!"

"Once the lad had all, now the lad has naught," cried Mitya suddenly.

"How 'naught'? You say that with all those thousands!"

"I'm not talking about thousands. Damn thousands! I'm talking of the female character:

Credulous is woman's heart,
Mutable and full of vices;

I agree with Ulysses. That's what he says."

"I don't understand you!"

"Am I drunk?"

"Not drunk, but worse."

"I'm drunk in spirit, Pyotr Ilyich, drunk in spirit! But that's enough!"

"What are you doing, loading the pistol?"

"I'm loading the pistol."

Unfastening the pistol-case, Mitya actually opened the powder horn, and carefully placed and rammed in the charge. Then he took the bullet and, before inserting it, held it in two fingers in front of the candle.

"Why are you looking at the bullet?" asked Pyotr Ilyich, watching him with uneasy curiosity.

"Oh, a fancy. Why, if you meant to put that bullet in your brain, would you look at it when you charged the pistol, or not?"

"Why look at it?"

"It will go into my brain, so it's interesting to look and see what it's like. But that's foolishness, a moment's foolishness. Now that's done," he added, putting in the bullet and ramming it in with tow. "Pyotr Ilyich, my dear fellow, that's nonsense, all nonsense, and if only you knew what nonsense! Give me a little piece of paper now."

"Here's some paper."

"No, a smooth, clean piece, writing paper. That's right."

And taking a pen from the table, Mitya rapidly wrote two lines, folded the paper twice, and thrust it into his waistcoat pocket. He put the pistols in the case, locked it up, and took it in his hands. Then he looked at Pyotr Ilyich with a slow, thoughtful smile.

"Now, let's go," he said.

"Where are we going? No, wait a minute. . . . Are you thinking of putting that bullet in your brain, perhaps?" Pyotr Ilyich asked uneasily.

"The bullet is nonsense! I want to live. I love life! You may be sure of that. I love golden-haired Phœbus and his hot light. . . . Dear Pyotr Ilyich, do you know how to step aside?"

"What do you mean by 'stepping aside'?"

"Making way. Making way for a dear creature, and for one I hate. And to let the one I hate become dear — that's what making way means! And to say to them: God bless you, go your way, pass on, while I . . ."

"While you?"

"That's enough, let's go."

"Upon my word. I'll tell some one to prevent your going there," said Pyotr Ilyich, looking at him. "What are you going to Mokroye for, now?"

"There's a woman there, a woman. That's enough for you, Pyotr Ilyich. Finished."

"Listen, though you're such a savage I've always liked you. . . . I feel anxious."

"Thanks, old fellow. I'm a savage you say. Savages, savages! That's what I am always saying. Savages! Why, here's Misha! I was forgetting him."

Misha ran in, post haste, with a handful of notes in change, and reported that every one was in a bustle at the Plotnikovs'; "They're carrying down the bottles, and the fish, and the tea; it will all be ready directly." Mitya seized ten roubles and handed it to Pyotr Ilyich, then tossed another ten-rouble note to Misha.

"Don't dare to do such a thing!" cried Pyotr Ilyich. "I won't have it in my house, it's a bad, demoralising habit. Put your money away. Here, put it here, why waste it? It would come in handy to-morrow, and I dare say you'll be coming to me to borrow ten roubles again. Why do you keep putting the notes in your side pocket? Ah, you'll lose them!"

"I say, my dear fellow, let's go to Mokroye together."

"What should I go for?"

"I say, let's open a bottle at once, and drink to life! I want to drink, and especially to drink with you. I've never drunk with you, have I?"

"Very well, we can go to the 'Metropolis.' I was just going there."

"I haven't time for that. Let's drink at the Plotnikovs', in the back room. Shall I set you a riddle?"

"Go ahead."

Mitya took the piece of paper out of his waistcoat pocket, unfolded it and showed it. In a large, distinct hand was written:

"I punish myself for my whole life, my whole life I punish!"

"I certainly will speak to some one. I'll go at once," said Pyotr Ilyich, after reading.

"You won't have time, darling, come and have a drink. March!"

Plotnikovs' shop was at the corner of the street, next door but one to Pyotr Ilyich's. It was the largest grocery shop in our town, and by no means a bad one, owned by rich merchants. They kept everything that could be got in a Petersburg shop, delicacies of all sorts, wines "bottled by the brothers Eliseyev," fruits, cigars, tea, coffee, sugar, and so on. There were three shop-assistants and two errand boys always employed. Though our part of the country had grown poorer, the landowners had gone away, and trade had got worse, yet the grocery stores flourished as before, every year increasing in prosperity; there were plenty of purchasers for their goods.

They were awaiting Mitya with impatience in the shop. They had vivid recollections of how he had bought, three or four weeks ago, wine and provisions of all sorts to the value of several hundred roubles, paid for in cash (they would never have let him have anything on credit, of course). They remembered that then, as now, he had had a bundle of hundred-rouble notes in his hand, and had scattered them at random, without bargaining, without reflecting, or caring to reflect, what use so much wine and so many provisions would be to him. The story was told all over the town that, driving off then with Grushenka to Mokroye, he had "spent three thousand in one night and the following day, and had come back from the spree without a penny, in his birthday-suit." He had picked up a whole troop of gipsies (encamped in our neighbourhood at the time), who for two days got money without stint out of him while he was drunk, and drank no end of expensive wine. People used to tell, laughing at Mitya, how he had given champagne to grimy-handed peasants, and feasted the village women and girls on sweets and Strasburg pies. Though to laugh at Mitya to his face was rather a risky proceeding, there was much laughter behind his back, especially in the tavern, at his own ingenuous public avowal that all he had got out of Grushenka by this "escapade" was "permission to kiss her foot, and that was the utmost she had allowed him."

By the time Mitya and Pyotr Ilyich reached the shop, they found a carriage with three horses harnessed abreast with bells, and with Andrey, the driver, ready waiting for Mitya at the entrance. In the shop they had almost entirely finished packing one box of provisions, and were only waiting for Mitya's arrival to nail it down and put it in the troika. Pyotr Ilyich was astounded.

"Where did this troika come from in such a hurry?" he asked Mitya.

"I met Andrey as I ran to you, and told him to drive straight here to the shop. There's no time to lose. Last time I drove with Timofey, but Timofey now has gone on before me with an enchantress. Shall we be very late, Andrey?"

"They'll only get there an hour before us, at most, not even that maybe. I helped Timofey get ready. I know how he'll go. Their pace is nothing like ours, Dmitri Fyodorovich. How could it be? They won't get there an hour earlier!" Andrey, a lanky, red-haired, middle-aged driver, wearing a full-skirted coat, and with a kaftan on his arm, replied.

"A fifty roubles tip if we're only an hour behind them."

"I guarantee an hour, Dmitri Fyodorovich. Ech, they won't be half an hour ahead of us, let alone an hour."

Though Mitya bustled about seeing after

things, he gave his orders strangely, as it were disconnectedly, and inconsecutively. He began a sentence and forgot the end of it. Pyotr Ilyich found himself obliged to come to the rescue.

"Four hundred roubles' worth, not less than four hundred roubles' worth, just as it was then," commanded Mitya. "Four dozen champagne, not a bottle less."

"What do you want with so much? What's it for? Wait!" cried Pyotr Ilyich. "What's this box? What's in it? Surely there isn't four hundred roubles' worth here?"

The officious shopmen began explaining with oily politeness that the first box contained only half a dozen bottles of champagne, and only "the most indispensable articles" such as savouries, sweets, toffee, etc. But the main part of the provisions ordered would be packed and sent off, as on the previous occasion, in a special cart, also with three horses, travelling at full speed, so that it would arrive not more than an hour later than Dmitri Fyodorovich himself.

"Not more than an hour! Not more than an hour! And put in more toffee and fondants. The girls there are so fond of them," Mitya insisted hotly.

"The fondants are all right. But what do you want with four dozen of champagne? One would be enough," said Pyotr Ilyich, almost angry. He began bargaining, asking for an itemised bill, and refused to be satisfied. But he only succeeded in saving a hundred roubles. In the end it was agreed that only three hundred roubles' worth should be delivered.

"Well, you may go to the devil!" cried Pyotr Ilyich, on second thoughts. "What's it to do with me? Throw away your money, since it's cost you nothing."

"This way, my pinch-penny, this way, don't be angry." Mitya drew him into a room at the back of the shop. "They'll give us a bottle here directly. We'll taste it. Ech, Pyotr Ilyich, come along with me, for you're a nice fellow, the sort I like."

Mitya sat down on a wicker chair, before a little table, covered with the dirtiest napkin. Pyotr Ilyich sat down opposite, and the champagne soon appeared, and oysters were suggested to the gentlemen. "First-class oysters, the last lot in."

"Hang the oysters. I don't eat them. And we don't need anything," cried Pyotr Ilyich, almost angrily.

"There's no time for oysters," said Mitya. "And I have no appetite. Do you know, friend," he said suddenly, with feeling, "I never have liked all this disorder."

"Who does like it? Three dozen of champagne for peasants, upon my word, that's enough to make any one explode!"

"That's not what I mean. I'm talking of a higher order. There's no order in me, no higher order. But . . . that's all over. There's no need to grieve about it. It's too late, damn it! My whole life has been disorder, and one must set it in order. Is that a pun, eh?"

"You're raving, not making puns!"

"Glory be to God in heaven,
Glory be to God in me . . .

"That verse came from my heart once, it's not a verse, but a tear. . . . I made it up myself . . . not while I was pulling the captain's beard though. . . ."

"Why do you bring him in all of a sudden?"

"Why do I bring him in? Foolery! All things come to an end; all things are made equal. That's the long and the short of it."

"You know, I keep thinking of your pistols."

"That's all foolery, too! Drink, and don't be fanciful. I love life. I've loved life too much, shamefully much. Enough! To life, dear boy, let's drink to life, I propose a toast to life. Why am I pleased with myself? I'm a scoundrel, but I'm pleased with myself. And yet I'm tortured by the thought that I'm a scoundrel, but I'm pleased with myself. I bless creation. I'm ready right now to bless God and His creation, but . . . it is necessary to destroy one vile insect so that it should not crawl and spoil life for others. . . . Let us drink to life, dear brother. What can be more precious than life? Nothing! To life, and to a queen of queens!"

"Let's drink to life and to your queen, too, if you like."

They drank a glass each. Although Mitya was excited and expansive, yet he was melancholy, too. It was as though some heavy, overwhelming anxiety were weighing upon him.

"Misha . . . here's your Misha come! Misha, come here, my boy, drink this glass to Phœbus, the golden-haired, of to-morrow . . ."

"What are you giving it to him for?" cried Pyotr Ilyich irritably.

"Please let me! I want to!"

"E — ech!"

Misha emptied the glass, bowed, and ran out.

"He'll remember it longer," Mitya remarked. "Woman I love, woman! What is woman? The queen of the earth! My heart is sad, sad, Pyotr Ilyich. Do you remember Hamlet? 'I am sad, so sad, good Horatio! Alas, poor Yorick!' Perhaps that's me, Yorick? Yes, I'm Yorick now, and a skull afterwards."

Pyotr Ilyich listened in silence. Mitya, too, was silent for a while.

"What dog's that you've got here?" he suddenly asked the shopman, absent-mindedly, noticing a pretty little lap-dog with dark eyes, sitting in the corner.

"It belongs to Varvara Alexyevna, the mistress," answered the clerk. "She brought it and left it here. It must be taken back to her."

"I saw one like it . . . in the regiment . . ." murmured Mitya dreamily, "only that one had its hind leg broken. . . . By the way, Pyotr Ilyich, I wanted to ask you: have you ever stolen anything in your life?"

"What a question!"

"Oh, I didn't mean anything. From somebody's pocket, you know. I don't mean government money, every one steals that, and no doubt you do, too. . . ."

"You go to the devil."

"I'm talking of other people's money. Stealing straight out of a pocket? Out of a purse, eh?"

"I stole twenty copecks from my mother when I was nine years old. I took it off the table on the sly, and held it tight in my hand."

"Well, and what happened?"

"Oh, nothing. I kept it three days, then I felt ashamed, confessed, and gave it back."

"And what then?"

"Naturally I was whipped. But why do you ask? Have you stolen something?"

"I have," said Mitya, winking slyly.

"What have you stolen?" asked Pyotr Ilyich inquisitively.

"I stole twenty copecks from my mother when I was nine years old, and gave it back three days after."

As he said this Mitya suddenly got up.

"Dmitri Fyodorovich, won't you come now?" called Andrey from the door of the shop.

"Are you ready? We'll come!" Mitya started. " 'And now one final tale' and . . . A glass of vodka for Andrey before we start. And a glass of cognac, too. That box" (the one with the pistols) "put under my seat. Good-bye, Pyotr Ilyich, don't remember evil against me."

"But you're coming back to-morrow?"

"Of course."

"Will you settle the little bill now?" cried the clerk, springing forward.

"Oh, yes, the bill. Of course."

He pulled the bundle of notes out of his pocket again, picked out three hundred roubles, threw them on the counter, and ran hurriedly out of the shop. Every one followed him out, bowing and wishing him good luck. Andrey, clearing his throat after the brandy he had just swallowed, jumped up on the box. But Mitya was only just taking his seat when suddenly, to his surprise, he saw Fenya before him. She ran up panting, clasped her hands before him with a cry, and plumped down at his feet.

"Darling master, Dmitri Fyodorovich, don't harm my mistress. And it was I told you all about it. . . . And don't murder him, he came first, he's hers! He'll marry Agrafena Alexandrovna now. That's why he's come back from Siberia. Dmitri Fyodorovich, dear, don't take a fellow creature's life!"

"Tut-tut-tut! That's it, is it? So you're off there to make trouble!" muttered Pyotr Ilyich. "Now, it's all clear, as clear as daylight. Dmitri Fyodorovich, give me your pistols at once if you mean to behave like a man," he shouted aloud to Mitya. "Do you hear, Dmitri?"

"The pistols? Wait a bit, brother, I'll throw them into the pool on the road," answered Mitya. "Fenya, get up, don't lie there before me. Mitya won't do for any one, the silly fool won't do for any one again. But I say, Fenya," he shouted, after having taken his seat. "I insulted you just now, so forgive me and have pity on me, forgive the scoundrel. . . . But it doesn't matter if you don't. It's all the same now. Now then, Andrey, look alive, go full speed!"

Andrey whipped up the horses, and the bell tinkled.

"Farewell, Pyotr Ilyich! 'For you I shed my final tear!' . . ."

"He's not drunk, but he babbles like a lunatic," Pyotr Ilyich thought as he watched him go. He had half a mind to stay and see the cart packed with the remaining wines and provisions, knowing that Mitya would be deceived and defrauded. But, suddenly feeling vexed with himself, he turned away with a curse and went to the tavern to play billiards.

"He's a fool, though he's a good fellow," he muttered as he went. "I've heard of that officer, Grushenka's former flame. Well, if he has turned up . . . Ech, those pistols! Damn it all! I'm not his nurse! Let them do what they like! Besides, it'll all come to nothing. They're a set of brawlers, that's all. They'll drink and fight, fight and make friends again. They are not men who do anything real. What does he mean by 'I'm stepping aside, I'm punishing myself'? It'll come to nothing! He's shouted such stuff a thousand times, drunk, in the taverns. But now he's not drunk. 'Drunk in spirit' — they're fond of fine phrases, the scoundrels. Am I his nurse? He must have been fighting, his face was all over blood. With whom? I shall find out at the 'Metropolis.' And his handkerchief was soaked in blood. . . . It's still lying on my floor. . . . Hang it!"

He reached the tavern in a bad humour and at once got up a game. The game cheered him. He played a second game, and suddenly began telling one of his partners that Dmitri Karamazov had come in for some cash again — something like three thousand roubles, he had seen it himself, and had gone to Mokroye again to spend it with Grushenka. . . . This news roused singular interest in his listeners. They all spoke of it, not laughing, but with a strange gravity. They left off playing.

"Three thousand? But where can he have got three thousand?"

Questions were asked. The story of Madame Hohlakov's present was received skeptically.

"Hasn't he robbed his old father, that's the question?"

"Three thousand! There's something odd about it."

"He boasted aloud that he would kill his father; we all heard him, here. And it was three thousand he talked about . . ."

Pyotr Ilyich listened. All at once he became short and dry in his answers. He said not a word about the blood on Mitya's face and hands, though he had meant to speak of it at first.

They began a third game, and by degrees the talk about Mitya died away. But by the end of the third game, Pyotr Ilyich felt no more desire for billiards; he laid down the cue, and without having supper as he had intended, he walked out of the tavern. When he reached the market-place he stood still in perplexity, wondering at himself. He realised that what he wanted was to go to Fyodor Pavlovich's and find out if anything had happened there, "On account of some stupid nonsense — as it's sure to turn out — am I going to wake up the household and make a scandal? Faugh! damn it, is it my business to look after them?"

In a very bad humour he went straight home, and suddenly remembered Fenya. "Damn it all! I ought to have questioned her just now," he thought with vexation, "I should have heard everything." And the desire to speak to her, and so find out, became so pressing and importunate that when he was half-way home he turned abruptly and went towards the house where Grushenka lodged. Going up to the gate he knocked. The sound of the knock in the silence of the night suddenly sobered and annoyed him, as it were. And no one answered him; every one in the house was asleep.

"And I shall be making a scandal here, too!" he thought, with a feeling of positive distress. But instead of going away altogether, he fell to knocking again with all his might, filling the street with clamour. "No, but I will knock them up, I will!" he muttered at each knock, fuming at himself, but at the same time he redoubled his knocks on the gate.

CHAPTER VI

"I, MYSELF, AM COMING"

But Dmitri Fyodorovich was speeding along the road. It was a little more than twenty versts to Mokroye, but Andrey's three horses galloped at such a pace that the distance might be covered in an hour and a quarter. The swift motion suddenly refreshed Mitya, as it were. The air was fresh and cool, there were big stars shining in the sky. It was the very night, and perhaps the very hour, in which Alyosha fell on the earth, and rapturously swore to love it for ever and ever.

All was confusion, extreme confusion, in Mitya's soul, but although many things were harassing his soul, at that moment his whole being was straining irrepressibly towards her, his queen, to whom he was flying in order to look upon her for the last time. One thing I can say for certain; his heart was not angered for an instant. I shall perhaps not be believed when I say that this jealous lover felt not the slightest jealousy of this new man, this new rival, the "officer," who seemed to have sprung out of the earth. If any other had appeared on the scene, he would have been jealous at once, and would perhaps have stained his fierce hands with blood again. But as he flew through the night, he felt no jealous hate, no hostility even, towards the man who had been her first lover. . . . It is true he had not yet seen him. "There is no room for dispute here: it is her right and his; this was her first love whom, after five years, she has not forgotten; so all these five years she loved him only, and I, how do I come in? What rights have I? Step aside, Mitya, and make way! Why fret anyhow? Now everything is over even apart from the officer — even if he had not appeared, everything would be over. . . ."

These words would roughly have expressed his feelings, if he had been capable of reasoning. But he could no longer reason at that moment. His present determination had arisen without reasoning. At Fenya's first words, he had become aware of it, and adopted his plan in a flash, with all its consequences. And yet, in spite of his resolution, there was confusion in his soul, an agonising confusion: his resolution did not give him peace. There was so much behind that tortured him. And it seemed strange to him, at moments, to think that he had written his own sentence of death with pen and paper: "I punish myself," and the paper was lying there in his pocket, ready; the pistol was loaded; he had already resolved how, next morning, he would meet the first warm ray of "golden-haired Phœbus."

And yet he could not be quit of the past, of all that he had left behind and that tortured him. He felt that miserably, and the thought of it filled his heart with despair. There was one moment when he felt an impulse to stop Andrey, to jump out of the cart, to pull out his loaded pistol, and to make an end of everything without waiting for the dawn. But that moment flew by like a spark. The horses galloped on, "devouring space," and as he drew near his goal, again the thought of her, of her alone, took more and more complete possession of his spirit, chasing away the fearful images that had been haunting it. Oh, how he longed to look upon her, if only for a moment, if only from a distance!

"She's now with *him*," he thought, "now I shall see what she looks like with him, her first love, and that's all I want." Never had this woman, who was such a fateful influence in his life, aroused such love in his breast, such a novel and hitherto unexperienced feeling, surprising even to himself, a feeling tender to the point of adoration, of self-effacement before her! "And I will efface myself!" he said, in a rush of almost hysterical ecstasy.

They had been galloping nearly an hour. Mitya was silent, and though Andrey was, as a rule, a talkative peasant, he did not utter a word, either. He seemed afraid to talk, he only whipped up smartly his three lean, but mettlesome, bay horses. Suddenly Mitya cried out in horrible anxiety:

"Andrey! What if they're asleep?"

This thought fell upon him like a blow. It had not occurred to him before.

"It may well be that they've gone to bed, by now, Dmitri Fyodorovich."

Mitya frowned as though in pain. Yes, indeed . . . he was rushing there . . . with such feelings . . . while they were asleep . . . she was asleep, perhaps, there, too. . . . An evil feeling surged up in his heart.

"Drive on, Andrey! Whip them up! Look alive!" he cried, beside himself.

"But maybe they haven't gone to bed!" Andrey went on after a pause. "Timofey said there were a lot of them there . . ."

"At the station?"

"Not at the posting-station, but at Plastunov's, at the inn, where they furnish horses, too."

"I know. So you say there are a lot of them? How's that? Who are they?" cried Mitya, greatly dismayed at this unexpected news.

"Well, Timofey was saying they're all gentlefolk. Two from our town — who they are I can't say — and there are two others, strangers, maybe more besides. I didn't ask particularly. They've set to playing cards, so Timofey said."

"Cards?"

"So, maybe they're not in bed if they're at cards. It's most likely not more than eleven."

"Quicker, Andrey! Quicker!" Mitya cried again, nervously.

"May I ask you something, sir?" said Andrey, after a pause. "Only I'm afraid of angering you, sir."

"What is it?"

"Why, Fenya threw herself at your feet just now, and begged you not to harm her mistress, and some one else, too . . . so you see, sir . . . It's I am taking you there . . . forgive me, sir, it's my conscience . . . maybe it's stupid of me to speak of it . . ."

Mitya suddenly seized him by the shoulders from behind. "Are you a driver? A driver?" he asked frantically.

"Yes, sir . . ."

"Then you know that one has to make way. What would you say to a driver who wouldn't make way for any one, but would just drive on and crush people? No, a driver mustn't run over people. One can't run over a man. One can't spoil people's lives. And if you have spoilt a life — punish yourself. . . . If only you've spoilt, if only you've ruined any one's life — punish yourself and go away."

These phrases broke from Mitya almost hysterically. Though Andrey was surprised at him, he kept up the conversation.

"That's right, Dmitri Fyodorovich, you're quite right, one mustn't crush or torment a man, or any kind of creature, for every creature is created by God. Take a horse, for instance, some folks, even among us drivers, dash ahead, any which way. Nothing will restrain them, they just push ahead."

"To hell?" Mitya interrupted, and went off into his abrupt, short laugh. "Andrey, simple soul," he seized him by the shoulders again, "tell me, will Dmitri Fyodorovich Karamazov go to hell, or not?"

"I don't know, my dear, it depends on you, for you are . . . You see, sir, when the Son of God was nailed on the Cross and died, He went straight down to hell from the Cross, and set free all sinners that were in agony. And Hell groaned, because it looked as though no more sinners would get there. And God said to

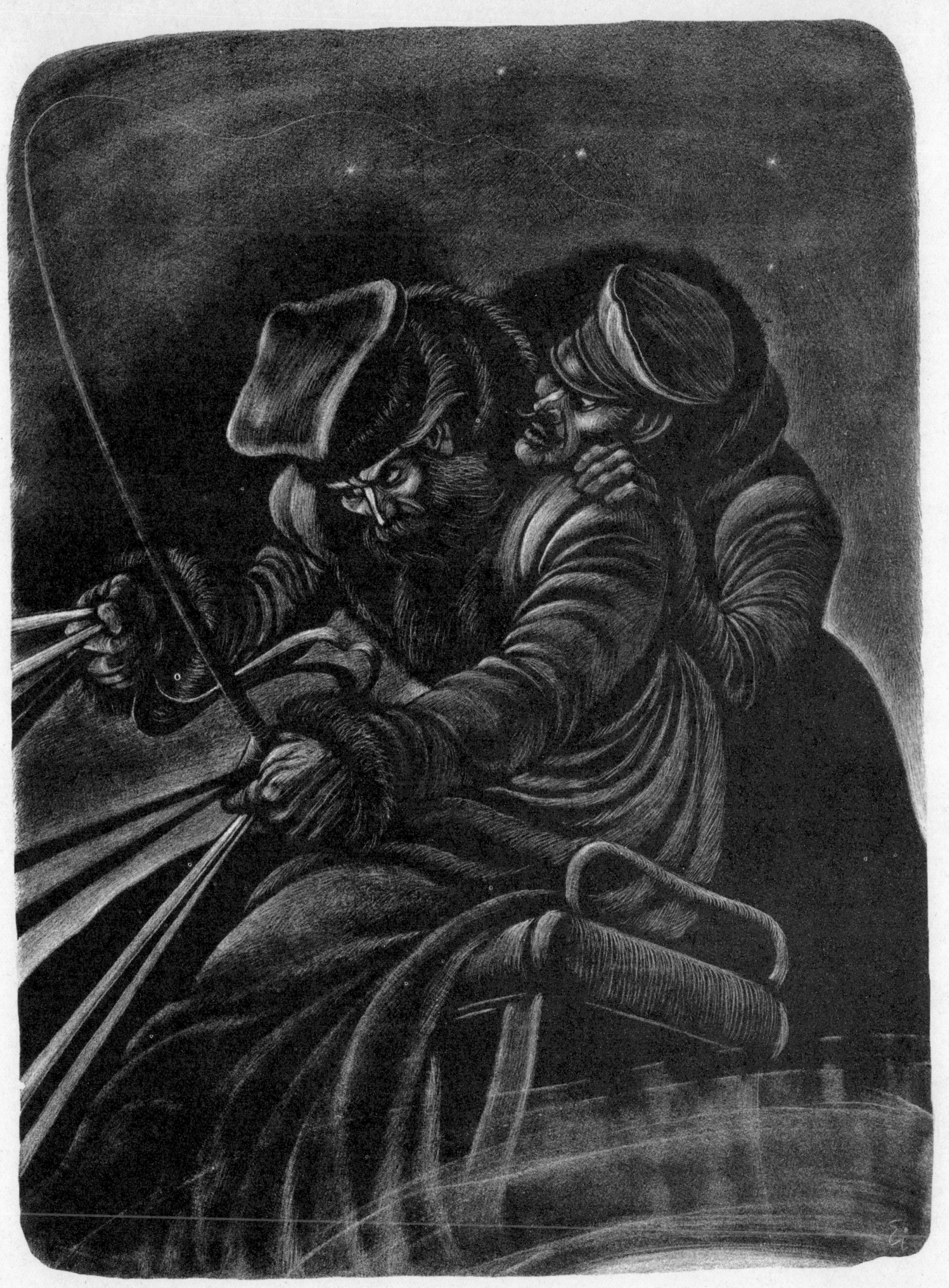

DMITRI ON THE ROAD

Hell, then, 'Don't groan, Hell, for you shall have all the mighty of the earth, the rulers, the chief judges, and the rich men, and shall be filled up as you have been in all the ages till I come again.' Those were His very words . . ."

"A folk legend! Capital! Whip up the left, Andrey!"

"So you see, sir, who it is hell's for," said Andrey, whipping up the left horse, "but you're like a little child . . . that's how we look on you . . . and though you're hasty-tempered, sir, yet God will forgive you for your kind heart."

"And you, do you forgive me, Andrey?"

"What should I forgive you for, sir? You've never done me any harm."

"No, for every one, for every one, you here alone, on the road, will you forgive me for every one? Speak, simple peasant heart!"

"Oh, sir! I feel afraid of driving you, your talk is so strange."

But Mitya did not hear. He was praying frantically and muttering fiercely to himself.

"Lord, receive me, in all my lawlessness, and do not judge me. Let me pass without Thy judgment . . . do not judge me, for I have condemned myself, do not judge me, for I love Thee, O Lord. I am vile, but I love Thee. If Thou sendest me to hell, I shall love Thee there, and from there I shall cry out that I love Thee for ever and ever. . . . But let me love to the end. . . . Here and now for just five hours . . . till the first burning beam of Thy day . . . for I love the queen of my soul . . . I love her and I cannot help loving her. Thou seest my whole heart. . . . I shall gallop up, I shall fall before her and say, 'You are right to pass on and leave me. Farewell, and forget your victim . . . never fret yourself about me!' "

"Mokroye!" cried Andrey, pointing ahead with his whip.

Through the pale darkness of the night loomed a solid black mass of buildings, scattered over a vast area. The village of Mokroye numbered two thousand inhabitants, but at that hour all were asleep, and only here and there a few lights still twinkled in the dark.

"Drive on, Andrey, I come!" Mitya exclaimed feverishly.

"They're not asleep," said Andrey again, pointing with his whip to the Plastunovs' inn, which was at the entrance to the village. The six windows, looking on the street, were all brightly lighted up.

"They're not asleep," Mitya repeated joyously. "Quicker, Andrey! Gallop! Drive up with a dash! Set the bells ringing! Let all know that I have come. I'm coming! I, myself, am coming!" Mitya exclaimed frantically.

Andrey lashed his exhausted team into a gallop, drove noisily and pulled up his steaming, panting horses at the high flight of steps.

Mitya jumped out of the cart just as the innkeeper, on his way to bed, peeped out from the steps, curious to see who had arrived.

"Trifon Borisovich, is that you?"

The innkeeper bent down, looked intently, ran down the steps, and rushed up to the guest with obsequious delight.

"Dmitri Fyodorovich, your honour! Is it you we're seeing again?"

Trifon Borisovich was a thick-set, robust peasant, of middle height, with a rather fat face. His expression was severe and uncompromising, especially with the peasants of Mokroye, but he had the power of assuming the most obsequious countenance when he had an inkling that it was to his interest. He dressed in Russian style, with a shirt buttoning down on one side, and a full-skirted coat. He had saved a good sum of money, but was for ever dreaming of bettering himself. More than half the peasants were in his clutches, every one in the neighbourhood was in debt to him. From the neighbouring landowners he bought and rented lands which were worked by the peasants, in payment of debts which they could never shake off. He was a widower, with four grown-up daughters. One of them was already a widow and lived in his house with her two children, his grandchildren, and worked for him like a charwoman. Another of his daughters was married to a petty official and in one of the rooms of the inn on the wall could be seen, among the family pictures, a miniature photograph of this official in uniform with epaulettes. The two younger daughters used to wear fashionable blue or green dresses, fitting tight at the back, and with trains a yard long, on Church holidays or when they went to pay visits. But the next morning they would get up at dawn, as usual, sweep out the rooms with a birch broom, empty the slops, and clean up after lodgers.

In spite of the thousands of roubles he had saved, Trifon Borisovich was very fond of emptying the pockets of a drunken guest, and, remembering that not a month ago he had, in twenty-four hours, made two if not three hundred roubles out of Dmitri, when he had come on his escapade with Grushenka, he met him now with eager welcome, scenting his prey by the very manner in which Mitya drove up to the steps.

"Dmitri Fyodorovich, dear sir, is it you we have with us again?"

"Hold on, Trifon Borisovich," began Mitya, "first and foremost, where is she?"

"Agrafena Alexandrovna?" The innkeeper understood at once, looking sharply into Mitya's face. "She, too, is here . . ."

"With whom? With whom?"

"Some strangers. One is an official, a Pole, to judge from his speech. He sent the horses for her from here; and there's another with him, a friend of his, or a fellow traveller, there's no telling. They're dressed like civilians."

"Well, are they on a spree? Have they money?"

"Spree, indeed! Small fry, Dmitri Fyodorovich."

"Small fry? And who are the others?"

"They're two gentlemen from the town. . . . They were returning from Cherny, and are putting up here. One's quite a young gentleman, a relative of Mr. Miüsov, he must be, but I've forgotten his name . . . and I expect you know the other, too, a gentleman called Maximov. He's been on a pilgrimage, so he says, to the monastery in the town. He's travelling with this young relation of Mr. Miüsov."

"Is that all?"

"Yes."

"Wait, listen, Trifon Borisovich. Tell me the chief thing: What of her? How is she?"

"Oh, she's only just come. She's sitting with them."

"Is she cheerful? Is she laughing?"

"No, I think she's not laughing much. She seems quite bored. She was combing the young gentleman's hair."

"The Pole's — the officer's?"

"He's not young, and he's not an officer, either. Not his hair, sir. It's the young gentleman that's Mr. Miüsov's relation . . . I forget his name."

"Kalganov?"

"That's it, Kalganov!"

"All right. I'll see for myself. Are they playing cards?"

"They have been playing, but they've left off. They've been drinking tea, the official called for liqueurs."

"Wait, Trifon Borisovich, wait, my good soul, I'll see for myself. Now answer one more question: are the gipsies here?"

"You can't have the gipsies now, Dmitri Fyodorovich. The authorities have chased them off. But we've Jews that play the cymbals and the fiddle in the village, so one might send for them. They'd come."

"Send for them. By all means send for them!" cried Mitya. "And you can get the girls together as you did then, Marya especially, Stepanida, too, and Arina. Two hundred roubles for a chorus!"

"Oh, for a sum like that I can rouse the whole village, though by now they're snoring. But are the peasants here worth such kindness, Dmitri Fyodorovich, or the girls either? To spend a sum like that on clodhoppers! What's the good of giving a peasant a cigarette to smoke, the stinking ruffian! And the girls are all lousy. Besides, I'll get my daughters up for nothing, let alone a sum like that. They've only just gone to bed, I'll kick them awake and set them singing for you. You gave the peasants champagne to drink the other day, e-ech!"

For all his pretended compassion for Mitya, Trifon Borisovich had hidden half a dozen bottles of champagne on the last occasion, and had picked up a hundred-rouble note under the table, and kept it in his fist. "Trifon Borisovich, I sent more than one thousand flying last time I was here. Do you remember?"

"You did send it flying. I remember very well. You must have left three thousand behind you."

"Well, I've come to do the same again, do you see?"

And he pulled out his roll of notes, and held them up before the innkeeper's nose.

"Now, listen and remember. In an hour's time the wine will arrive, savouries, pies, and sweets — bring them all up at once. That box Andrey has got is to be brought up at once, too. Open it, and serve champagne immediately. And the girls, we must have the girls, Marya especially."

He turned to the carriage and pulled the box of pistols out from under the seat.

"Here, Andrey, let's settle. Here's fifteen roubles for the drive, and fifty as a tip . . . for your readiness, for your love. . . . Remember Karamazov!"

"I'm afraid, sir," faltered Andrey. "Give me five roubles extra, but more I won't take. Trifon Borisovich, bear witness. Forgive my foolish words . . ."

"What are you afraid of?" asked Mitya, looking up and down. "Well, go to the devil, if that's it!" he cried, flinging him five roubles. "Now, Trifon Borisovich, take me up quietly and let me first get a look at them, so that they don't see me. Where are they? In the blue room?"

Trifon Borisovich looked apprehensively at Mitya, but at once obediently did his bidding. Leading him into the passage, he went himself into the first large room, adjoining that in which the visitors were sitting, and took the light away. Then he stealthily led Mitya in, and put him in a corner in the dark, whence he could freely watch the company without being seen. But Mitya did not look long, and, indeed, he could not see them, he saw her, his heart throbbed violently, and everything swam before his eyes.

She was sitting sideways at the table in an armchair, and beside her, on the sofa, was the pretty youth, Kalganov. She was holding his hand and seemed to be laughing, while he, seeming vexed and not looking at her, was saying something in a loud voice to Maximov, who sat on the other side of the table, facing Grushenka. Maximov was laughing violently at something. On the sofa sat *he*, and on a chair by the sofa there was another stranger. The one on the sofa was lolling backwards, smoking a pipe, and Mitya had an impression of a stoutish broad-faced short little man, who was apparently angry about something. His friend, the other stranger, struck Mitya as extraordinarily tall, but he could make out nothing more. He caught his breath. He could not bear it for a minute, he put the pistol-case on a chest, and with a throbbing heart, feeling cold all over, he walked straight into the blue room to face the company.

"Aie!" shrieked Grushenka, the first to notice him.

CHAPTER VII

THE FIRST AND RIGHTFUL LOVER

With his long, rapid strides, Mitya walked up close to the table.

"Gentlemen," he said in a loud voice, almost shouting, yet stammering over every word, "I . . . I'm all right! Don't be afraid!" he exclaimed, "I — there's nothing the matter," he turned suddenly to Grushenka, who had shrunk back in her chair in the direction of Kalganov, and clasped his hand tightly. "I . . . I'm travelling, too. I'm here till morning. Gentlemen, as a traveller . . . may I stay with you till morning? Only till morning, for the last time, in this same room?"

His last phrases were addressed to the fat little man, with the pipe, sitting on the sofa. The latter removed his pipe from his lips with dignity and observed severely:

"*Panie*, this is our private room. There are other rooms available."

"Why, it's you, Dmitri Fyodorovich! What do you mean?" answered Kalganov suddenly. "Sit down with us. How are you?"

"Delighted to see you, dear . . . and precious fellow, I always thought a lot of you," Mitya responded, joyfully and eagerly, at once holding out his hand across the table.

"Aie! How hard you squeeze! You've quite broken my fingers," laughed Kalganov.

"He always squeezes like that, always," Grushenka put in gaily, with a timid smile, seeming suddenly convinced by Mitya's expression that he was not going to make a scene. She was watching him with intense curiosity and still some uneasiness. She was impressed by something about him, and indeed the last thing she expected of him was that he would come in and speak like this at such a moment.

"Good evening," Maximov ventured blandly, on the left. Mitya rushed up to him, too.

"Good evening. You're here, too! How glad I am to find you here, too! Gentlemen, gentlemen, I . . ." (He addressed the Polish gentleman with the pipe again, evidently taking him for the most important person present.) "I flew here. . . . I wanted to spend my last day, my last hour in this room, in this very room . . . where I, too, adored . . . my queen. . . . Forgive me, *panie*," he cried wildly, "I flew here and made a vow. . . . Oh, don't be afraid, it's my last night! Let's drink to our good understanding. They'll serve the wine at once. . . . I brought this with me." (He suddenly pulled out his bundle of notes.) "Allow me, *panie!* I want music, noise, thunder, like last time. . . . But the worm, the useless worm, will crawl away, and there'll be no more of him! I will celebrate my day of joy on my last night!"

He nearly choked. There was so much, so much he wanted to say, but queer exclamations were all that came from his lips. The Pole gazed fixedly at him, at the bundle of notes in his hand; looked at Grushenka, and was obviously perplexed.

"If my queen will permit . . ." he began.

"What does he mean?" interrupted Grushenka. "I can't help laughing at you, the way you talk. Sit down, Mitya, what are you saying? Don't frighten us, please. You won't frighten us, will you? If you won't, I am glad to see you . . ."

"I, I frighten you?" cried Mitya, flinging up his hands. "Oh, pass me by, go your way, I won't hinder you! . . ."

And suddenly he surprised them all, and no doubt himself as well, by flinging himself on a chair and bursting into tears; he turned his head to the opposite wall, while his arms clasped the back of the chair tight, as though embracing it.

"Come, come, what a fellow you are!" cried Grushenka reproachfully. "That's just how he acted when he came to see me — he would begin talking, and I couldn't make out what he meant. He cried like that once before, and now he's crying again! For shame! Why are you crying? *As though you had anything to cry for!*" she added enigmatically, emphasising each word with a kind of irritability.

"I . . . I'm not crying. . . . Well, good evening!" He instantly turned round in his chair, and suddenly laughed, not his abrupt, wooden laugh, but a long, quivering, inaudible nervous laugh.

"Well, there you are again. . . . Come, cheer up, cheer up!" Grushenka said to him persuasively. "I'm very glad you've come, very glad, Mitya, do you hear, I'm very glad? I want him to stay here with us," she said peremptorily, addressing the whole company, though her words were obviously meant for the man sitting on the sofa. "I wish it, I wish it! And if he goes away I shall go, too!" she added with flashing eyes.

"What my queen commands is law!" pronounced the Pole, gallantly kissing Grushenka's hand. "I beg you, *panie*, to join our company," he added politely, addressing Mitya.

Mitya jumped up with the obvious intention of delivering another tirade, but the words did not come.

"Let's have a drink, *panie*," he blurted out instead of making a speech. Every one laughed.

"Good heavens! I thought he was going to make another speech!" Grushenka exclaimed nervously. "Do you hear, Mitya," she went on insistently, "don't jump up any more; and as for the champagne you've brought, that's fine. I want some myself, and I can't bear liqueurs. And best of all, you've come yourself. We were fearfully dull here. . . . You're on a spree again, I suppose? But put your money in your pocket. Where did you get such a lot?"

Mitya had been, all this time, holding in his hand the crumpled bundle of notes on which the eyes of all, especially the Poles, were fixed. In confusion he thrust them hurriedly into his pocket. He flushed. At that moment the innkeeper brought in an uncorked bottle of champagne, and glasses on a tray. Mitya snatched up the bottle, but he was so bewildered that he did not know what to do with it. Kalganov took it from him and poured out the champagne.

"Another! Another bottle!" Mitya cried to the innkeeper, and, forgetting to clink glasses with the Pole whom he had so solemnly invited to drink to their good understanding, he drank off his glass without waiting for any one else. His whole countenance suddenly changed. The solemn and tragic expression with which he had entered vanished completely, and a look of something childlike came into his face. He seemed to have become suddenly gentle and subdued. He looked shyly and happily at every one, with a continual nervous little laugh, and the grateful expression of a dog who has done wrong, been punished, and forgiven. He seemed to have forgotten everything, and was looking round at every one with a childlike smile of delight. He looked at Grushenka, laughing continually, and bringing his chair close up to hers. By degrees he had gained some idea of the two Poles, though he had formed no definite conception of them yet.

The Pole on the sofa struck him by his dignified demeanour and his Polish accent; and, above all, by his pipe. "Well, what of it? It's a good thing he's smoking a pipe," he reflected. The Pole's puffy face, the face of a man almost forty, with its tiny nose and two very thin, pointed, waxed, and saucy moustaches, had not so far roused any questions in Mitya's mind. He was not even particularly struck by the Pole's wretched little wig made in Siberia, with love-locks foolishly combed forward over the temples. "I suppose it's all right since he wears a wig," he went on, musing blissfully. The other, younger Pole, who was staring insolently and defiantly at the company and listening to the conversation with silent contempt, still only impressed Mitya by his great height, which was in striking contrast to that of the Pole on the sofa. "If he stood up he'd be six foot three." The thought flitted through Mitya's mind. It occurred to him, too, that this Pole must be the friend of the other, a "bodyguard," as it were, and no doubt the little Pole with the pipe was lording it over the big Pole. But this all seemed to Mitya perfectly right and unquestionable. In the little dog all feeling of rivalry had vanished.

Grushenka's mood and the enigmatic tone of some of her words he completely failed to grasp. All he understood, with thrilling heart, was that she was kind to him, that she had forgiven him, and made him sit by her. He was beside himself with delight, watching her sip her glass of champagne. The silence of the company seemed somehow to strike him, however, and he looked round at every one with expectant eyes.

"Why are we sitting here though, gentlemen? Why don't you begin doing something?" his smiling eyes seemed to ask.

"He keeps talking nonsense, and we were all laughing," Kalganov began suddenly, as though divining his thought, and pointing to Maximov. Mitya immediately stared at Kalganov and then at Maximov.

"He's talking nonsense?" — he laughed his short, wooden laugh, seeming suddenly delighted at something — "ha, ha!"

"Yes. Would you believe it, he will have it that all our cavalry officers in the twenties married Polish women. That's awful rot, isn't it?"

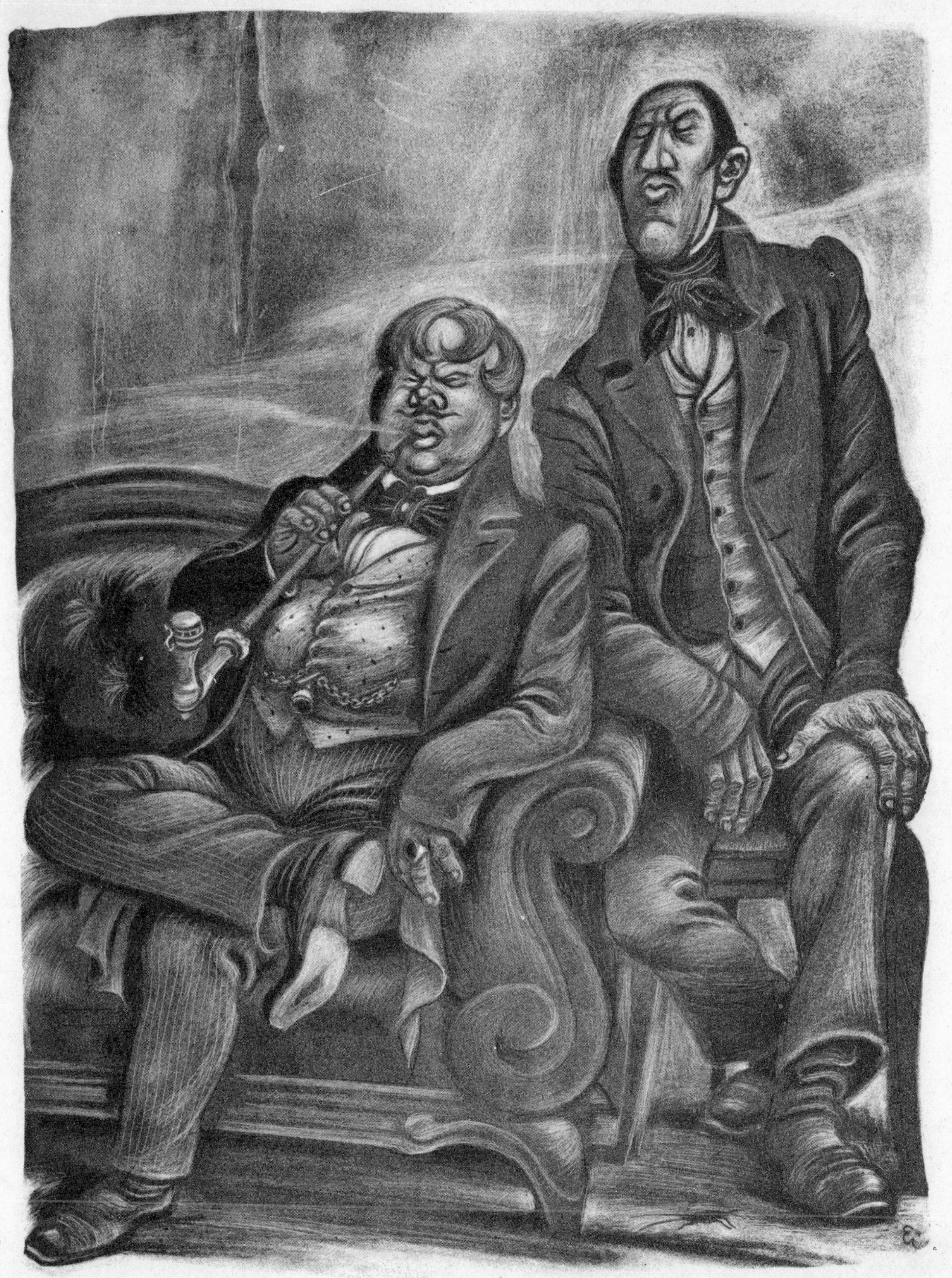

THE FIRST, THE RIGHTFUL LOVER

"Polish women?" repeated Mitya, perfectly ecstatic.

Kalganov was well aware of Mitya's attitude to Grushenka, and he guessed about the Pole, too, but that did not so much interest him, perhaps did not interest him at all; what he was interested in was Maximov. He had come here with Maximov by chance, and he met the Poles here at the inn for the first time in his life. Grushenka he had known before, and had once been with some one to see her; but she had not taken to him. But here she looked at him very affectionately: before Mitya's arrival, she had petted him, but he seemed somehow to be unmoved by it. He was a young man, not over twenty, dressed like a dandy, with a very charming fair-skinned face, and splendid thick, fair hair. From his fair face looked out beautiful pale blue eyes, with an intelligent and sometimes even deep expression, beyond his age indeed, although the young man sometimes looked and talked quite like a child, and was not at all embarrassed by it, even when he was aware of it himself. As a rule he was very wilful, even capricious, though always friendly. Sometimes there was something fixed and obstinate in his expression. He would look at you and listen, seeming all the while to be persistently dreaming about something else. Often he was listless and lazy, at other times he would grow excited, sometimes, apparently, over the most trivial matters.

"Only imagine, I've been taking him about with me for the last four days," he went on, indolently drawling his words, quite naturally though, without the slightest affectation. "Ever since your brother, do you remember, pushed him out of the carriage and sent him flying. That made me take an interest in him at the time, and I took him into the country, but he keeps talking such rot I'm ashamed to be with him. I'm taking him back."

"The gentleman has not seen Polish ladies, and says what is impossible," the Pole with the pipe observed to Maximov.

He spoke Russian fairly well, much better, anyway, than he pretended. If he used Russian words, he always distorted them in a Polish fashion.

"But I was married to a Polish lady myself," tittered Maximov.

"But did you serve in the cavalry? You were talking about the cavalry. Were you a cavalryman?" put in Kalganov at once.

"Was he a cavalryman indeed? Ha, ha!" cried Mitya, listening eagerly, and turning his inquiring eyes to each as he spoke, as though he expected to hear something wonderful from each.

"No, you see," Maximov turned to him, "what I mean is that those pretty Polish ladies . . . when they danced the mazurka with our Uhlans . . . when one of them dances a mazurka with an Uhlan she jumps on his knee like a kitten . . . a little white one . . . and the *pan*-father and *pan*-mother look on and allow it. . . . They allow it . . . and next day the Uhlan comes and offers her his hand. . . . That's how it is . . . offers her his hand, he—he!" Maximov ended, tittering.

"The gentleman is a *lajdak!*" The tall Pole on the chair growled suddenly and crossed one leg over the other. Mitya's eye was caught by his huge greased boot, with its thick, dirty sole. The dress of both the Poles looked rather greasy.

"Well, now it's *lajdak!* What's he scolding about?" said Grushenka, suddenly vexed.

"*Pani* Agrippina, what the gentleman saw

in Poland were peasant girls, and not ladies of good birth," the Pole with the pipe observed to Grushenka.

"You can reckon on that," the tall Pole snapped contemptuously.

"What next! Let him talk! People talk, why hinder them? It makes it cheerful," Grushenka said crossly.

"I'm not hindering them, *pani*," said the Pole in the wig, with a long look at Grushenka, and relapsing into dignified silence he sucked his pipe again.

"No, no. The Polish gentleman spoke the truth." Kalganov got excited again, as though it were a question of vast import. "He's never been in Poland, so how can he talk about it? I suppose you weren't married in Poland, were you?"

"No, in the Province of Smolensk. Only, an Uhlan had brought her to Russia before that, my future wife, with her mamma and her aunt, and another female relation with a grown-up son. He brought her straight from Poland and handed her over to me. He was a lieutenant in our regiment, a very nice young man. At first he meant to marry her himself. But he didn't marry her, because she turned out to be lame."

"So you married a lame woman?" cried Kalganov.

"Yes. They both deceived me a little bit at the time, and concealed it. I thought she was hopping; she kept hopping . . . I thought it was out of gaiety."

"So glad she was going to marry you!" yelled Kalganov, in a ringing, childish voice.

"Yes, so glad. But the reason turned out to be quite a different one. Afterwards, when we were married, after the wedding, that very evening, she confessed, and very touchingly asked forgiveness. 'I once jumped over a puddle when I was a child,' she said, 'and injured my leg.' He — he!"

Kalganov went off into the most childish laughter, almost falling on the sofa. Grushenka, too, laughed. Mitya was at the pinnacle of happiness.

"Do you know, that's the truth, he's not lying now," exclaimed Kalganov, turning to Mitya; "and do you know, he's been married twice; it's his first wife he's talking about. But his second wife, do you know, ran away, and is alive now."

"Is it possible?" said Mitya, turning quickly to Maximov with an expression of the utmost astonishment on his face.

"Yes. She did run away. I've had that unpleasant experience," Maximov modestly assented, "with a *monsieur*. And what was worse, she'd had all my little property transferred to her beforehand. 'You're an educated man,' she said to me. 'You can always earn your bread.' That's how she settled my business. A venerable bishop once said to me: 'One of your wives was lame, but the other was too light-footed.' He-he!"

"Listen, listen!" cried Kalganov, bubbling over, "if he's telling lies — and he often is — he's only doing it to amuse us all. That's not nasty, is it? You know, I sometimes like him. He's an awful scoundrel, but a natural scoundrel, eh? Don't you think so? Some people are scoundrels out of self-interest, but he's simply so by nature. Only fancy, he claims (he was arguing about it all the way yesterday) that in his 'Dead Souls' Gogol wrote about him. Do you remember, there's a landowner called Maximov in it, whom Nozdryov thrashed? He was tried, do you remember, 'for inflicting bodily injury with rods on the landowner Maximov in a drunken condition.' Would you believe it, he claims that he was that Maximov and that he was flogged! Now can it be so? Chitchikov made his journey, at the very latest, at the beginning of the twenties, so that the dates don't fit. He couldn't have been flogged then, he couldn't, could he?"

It was difficult to imagine what Kalganov was excited about, but his excitement was genuine.

Mitya fully shared his interest.

"Well, but if they did flog him!" he cried, laughing.

"It's not that they flogged me exactly, but what I mean is . . ." put in Maximov.

"What do you mean? Either they flogged you or they didn't."

"What o'clock is it, *panie?*" the Pole with the pipe asked his tall friend, with a bored expression. The other shrugged his shoulders in reply. Neither of them had a watch.

"Why not talk? Let the others talk, too. Must other people keep still because you're bored?" Grushenka flew at him with the evident intention of finding fault. Something seemed for the first time to flash through Mitya's mind. This time the Pole answered with unmistakable irritability.

"*Pani*, I didn't oppose it. I didn't say anything."

"All right then. Come, tell us your story," Grushenka cried to Maximov. "Why did you all stop talking?"

"There's nothing to tell, it's all so foolish," answered Maximov at once, with evident pleasure and some affectation. "Besides, all that's by way of allegory in Gogol, for he's made all the names have a meaning. Nozdryov was really called Nosov, and Kuvshinikov had quite a different name, he was called Shkvornev. Fenardi really was called Fenardi, only he wasn't an Italian but a Russian, Petrov, and Mamsel Fenardi was a pretty girl with her pretty little legs in tights, and she had a little short skirt with spangles, and she kept turning round and round, only not for four hours but for four minutes only, and she bewitched every one . . ."

"But what did they flog you for, what for?" cried Kalganov.

"For Piron, sir!" answered Maximov.

"What Piron?" cried Mitya.

"The famous French writer, Piron. We were all drinking then, a big party of us, in a tavern at that very fair. They'd invited me, and first of all I began reciting epigrams. 'Is that you, Boileau? What a funny get-up!' and Boileau answers that he's going to a masquerade, that is to the baths, he-he! And they took it personally, so I made haste to repeat another, very sarcastic, well known to all educated people:

You're Sappho, I'm Phaon, I see!
But one grief is weighing on me:
You don't know your way to the sea!

They were still more offended and began abusing me in the most unseemly way for it. And as ill-luck would have it, to set things right, I began telling a very cultivated anecdote about Piron, how he was not admitted to the French Academy, and to revenge himself wrote his own epitaph:

Ci-gît Piron qui ne fut rien
Pas même académicien.

They took and flogged me."

"But what for? What for?"

"For my education. People can flog a man

for anything," Maximov concluded, briefly and sententiously.

"Eh, that's enough! That's all nasty, I don't want to listen. I thought it would be amusing," Grushenka cut them short, suddenly.

Mitya started, and at once left off laughing. The tall Pole rose to his feet, and, with the haughty air of a man bored and out of his element, began pacing the room, from one end to the other, his hands behind his back.

"Ah, he can't sit still," said Grushenka, looking at him contemptuously. Mitya began to feel anxious. He noticed besides, that the Pole on the sofa was looking at him with an irritable expression.

"*Panie!*" cried Mitya, "let's drink! and the other *pan*, too! Let us drink."

In a flash he had pulled three glasses towards him, and filled them with champagne.

"To Poland, *panowie*, I drink to your Poland!" cried Mitya.

"I shall be delighted, *panie*," said the Pole on the sofa, with dignity and affable condescension, and he took his glass.

"And the other *pan*, what's his name? Drink, most illustrious, take your glass!" Mitya urged.

"*Pan* Wróblewski," put in the Pole on the sofa.

Pan Wróblewski came up to the table, swaying as he walked, and accepted the glass, standing.

"To Poland, *panowie!*" cried Mitya, raising his glass. "Hurrah!"

All three drank. Mitya seized the bottle and again poured out three glasses. "Now to Russia, *panowie*, and let us be brothers!"

"Pour out some for us," said Grushenka; "I'll drink to Russia, too!"

"So will I," said Kalganov.

"And I would, too . . . to Russia, the old grandmother!" tittered Maximov.

"All! All!" cried Mitya. "Trifon Borisovich, some more bottles!"

The other three bottles Mitya had brought with him were put on the table. Mitya filled the glasses.

"To Russia! Hurrah!" he shouted again. All drank the toast except the Poles, and Grushenka tossed off her whole glass at once. The Poles did not touch theirs.

"How's this, *panowie?*" cried Mitya, "won't you drink it?"

Pan Wróblewski took the glass, raised it, and said with a resonant voice:

"To Russia as she was before 1772."

"Come, that's better!" cried the other Pole, and they both emptied their glasses at once.

"You're fools, you *panowie*," broke suddenly from Mitya.

"*Panie!*" shouted both the Poles, menacingly, setting on Mitya like a couple of cocks. *Pan* Wróblewski was specially furious.

"Can one help loving one's own country?" he shouted.

"Be silent! Don't quarrel! I won't have any quarrelling!" cried Grushenka imperiously, and she stamped her foot on the floor. Her face glowed, her eyes were shining. The effects of the glass she had just drunk were apparent. Mitya was terribly alarmed.

"*Panowie*, forgive me! It was my fault, I'm sorry. Wróblewski, *panie* Wróblewski, I'm sorry."

"Hold your tongue, you, anyway! Sit down, you stupid!" Grushenka scolded with angry annoyance.

Every one sat down, all were silent, looking at one another.

"Gentlemen, I was the cause of it all," Mitya began again, unable to make anything of Grushenka's words. "Come, why are we sitting here? What shall we do . . . to amuse ourselves again?"

"Ach, it's certainly anything but amusing!" Kalganov mumbled lazily.

"Let's play faro again, as we did just now," Maximov tittered suddenly.

"Faro? Splendid!" cried Mitya. "If only the *panowie* . . ."

"It's late, *panowie*," the Pole on the sofa responded, as it were unwillingly.

"That's true," assented *Pan* Wróblewski.

"Late? What do you mean by 'late'?" asked Grushenka.

"Late, *pani!* 'a late hour' I mean," the Pole on the sofa explained.

"It's always late with them. They never let you do anything!" Grushenka almost shrieked in her anger. "They're dull themselves, so they want others to be dull. Before you came, Mitya, they sat there silently and kept turning up their noses at me."

"My goddess!" cried the Pole on the sofa. "As you say, so be it! I see you're not well-disposed towards me, that's why I'm gloomy. I'm ready, *panie*," added he, addressing Mitya.

"Begin, *panie*," Mitya assented, pulling his notes out of his pocket, and laying two hundred-rouble notes on the table. "I want to lose a lot to you. Take your cards. Make the bank."

"The cards must come from the innkeeper, *panie*," said the little Pole, gravely and emphatically.

"That's much the best way," chimed in *Pan* Wróblewski.

"From the innkeeper? Very good, I understand, let's get them from him. Cards!" Mitya shouted to the innkeeper.

The landlord brought in a new, unopened pack, and informed Mitya that the girls were getting ready, and that the Jews with the cymbals would most likely be there soon; but that the cart with the provisions had not yet arrived. Mitya jumped up from the table and ran into the next room to give orders, but only three girls had arrived, and Marya was not there yet. And he did not know himself what orders to give and why he had run out. He only told them to take out of the box the presents for the girls, the sweets, the toffee, and the fondants. "And vodka for Andrey, vodka for Andrey!" he cried in haste. "I was rude to Andrey!"

Suddenly Maximov, who had followed him out, touched him on the shoulder.

"Give me five roubles," he whispered to Mitya. "I'll stake something at faro, too, he-he!"

"Capital! Splendid! Take ten, here!"

Again he took all the notes out of his pocket and picked out a ten-rouble one. "And if you lose that, come again, come again."

"Very well, sir," Maximov whispered joyfully, and he ran back again. Mitya too, returned, apologising for having kept them waiting. The Poles had already sat down, and opened the pack. They looked much more amiable, almost cordial. The Pole on the sofa had lighted another pipe and was preparing to deal. He wore an air of solemnity.

"To your places, gentlemen," cried *Pan* Wróblewski.

"No, I'm not going to play any more," observed Kalganov, "I've lost fifty roubles to them just now."

"The gentleman had no luck, perhaps he'll

be lucky this time," the Pole on the sofa observed, glancing in his direction.

"How much in the bank? To correspond?" asked Mitya.

"Quite so, *panie*, maybe a hundred, maybe two hundred, as much as you will stake."

"A million!" Mitya guffawed.

"The *Pan* Captain has heard of *Pan* Podwysocki, perhaps?"

"Which Podwysocki?"

"In Warsaw, Podwysocki on one occasion comes to a gaming-house, sees a thousand gold-pieces, and stakes against the bank. The banker says, '*Panie* Podwysocki, are you laying down the gold, or must we trust to your honour?' 'To my honour, *panie*,' says Podwysocki. 'So much the better.' The banker deals out the cards. Podwysocki wins and takes a thousand gold-pieces. 'Wait, *panie*,' says the banker, and pulling out the drawer gives him a million. 'Take it, *panie*, this is your winnings.' There was a million in the bank. 'I didn't know that,' says Podwysocki. '*Panie* Podwysocki,' said the banker, 'you pledged your honour and we pledged ours.' Podwysocki took the million."

"That's not true," said Kalganov.

"*Panie* Kalganov, among gentlemen one doesn't say such things."

"As if a Polish gambler would give up a million, just like that!" cried Mitya, but checked himself at once. "Forgive me, *panie*, it's my fault again, he would, he would give away a million, for the sake of honour, Polish honour. You see how I talk Polish, ha-ha! Here, I stake ten roubles, the knave leads."

"And I put a rouble on the queen, the queen of hearts, the pretty little *panienochka*, he-he!" laughed Maximov, pulling out his queen, and, as though trying to conceal it from every one, he moved right up and crossed himself hurriedly under the table. Mitya won. The rouble won, too.

"A corner!" cried Mitya.

"I'll bet another rouble, a 'single' stake," Maximov muttered gleefully, hugely delighted at having won a rouble.

"Lost!" shouted Mitya. "A 'double' on the seven!"

The seven, too, was trumped.

"Stop!" cried Kalganov suddenly.

"Double! Double!" Mitya doubled his stakes, and each time he doubled the stake, the card he doubled was trumped by the Poles. The rouble stakes kept winning.

"On the double!" shouted Mitya, furiously.

"You've lost two hundred, *panie*. Will you stake another two hundred?" the Pole on the sofa inquired.

"What? Lost two hundred already? Then another two hundred! All doubles!"

And pulling his money out of his pocket, Mitya was about to fling two hundred roubles on the queen, but Kalganov covered it with his hand.

"That's enough!" he shouted in his ringing voice.

"What's the matter?" Mitya stared at him.

"That's enough! I don't want you to play any more. Don't!"

"Why?"

"Because I don't. Hang it, come away. That's why. I won't let you go on playing."

Mitya gazed at him in astonishment.

"Give it up, Mitya. He may be right. You've lost a lot as it is," said Grushenka, with a curious note in her voice. Both the Poles rose from their seats with a deeply offended air.

"Are you joking, *panie?*" said the short man, looking severely at Kalganov.

"How dare you!" *Pan* Wróblewski, too, growled at Kalganov.

"Don't dare to shout like that," cried Grushenka. "Ah, you turkey-cocks!"

Mitya looked at each of them in turn. But something in Grushenka's face suddenly struck him, and at the same instant something new flashed into his mind — a strange new thought!

"*Pani* Agrippina," the little Pole began, crimson with anger, when Mitya suddenly went up to him and slapped him on the shoulder.

"Most illustrious, two words with you."

"What do you want?"

"In the next room, I've two words to say to you, something pleasant, very pleasant. You'll be glad to hear it."

The little *pan* was taken aback and looked apprehensively at Mitya. He agreed at once, however, on condition that *Pan* Wróblewski went with them.

"The body-guard? Let him come, and I want him, too. I must have him!" cried Mitya. "March, *panowie!*"

"Where are you going?" asked Grushenka anxiously.

"We'll be back in one moment," answered Mitya.

There was a sort of boldness, a sudden confidence shining in his eyes. His face had looked very different when he entered the room an hour before.

He led the Poles, not into the large room where the chorus of girls was assembling and the table was being laid, but into the bedroom on the right, where the trunks and chests were kept, and there were two large beds, with pyramids of cotton pillows on each. There was a lighted candle on a small deal table in the corner. The small man and Mitya sat down at this table, facing each other, while the huge Wróblewski stood beside them, his hands behind his back. The Poles looked severe but were obviously curious.

"What can I do for you, *panie?*" lisped the little Pole.

"Well, look here, *panie*, I won't keep you long. Here's money for you," he pulled out his notes. "Would you like three thousand? Take it and go your way."

The Pole gazed open-eyed at Mitya, with a searching look.

"Three thousand, *panie?*" He exchanged glances with Wróblewski.

"Three, *panowie*, three! Listen, *panie*, I see you're a sensible man. Take three thousand and go to the devil, and take Wróblewski with you — d'you hear? But, at once, this very minute, and for ever. You understand that, *panie*, for ever. Here's the door, you go out of it. What have you got there, an overcoat, a fur coat? I'll bring it out to you. They'll get the horses out directly, and then — good-bye, *panie!* Eh?"

Mitya awaited an answer with assurance. He had no doubts. An expression of extraordinary resolution passed over the Pole's face.

"And the money, *panie?*"

"The money, *panie?* Five hundred roubles I'll give you this moment for the journey, and as a first instalment, and two thousand five hundred to-morrow, in town — I swear on my honour, I'll get it, I'll get it at any cost!" cried Mitya.

The Poles exchanged glances again. The short man's face looked more forbidding.

"Seven hundred, seven hundred, not five

hundred, at once, this minute, cash down!" Mitya added, feeling that something was wrong. "What's the matter, *panie?* Don't you trust me? I can't give you the whole three thousand straight off. If I give it, you may come back to her to-morrow. . . . Besides, I haven't the three thousand with me. I've got it at home in town," faltered Mitya, his spirit sinking at every word he uttered. "Upon my word, the money's there, hidden."

In an instant an extraordinary sense of personal dignity showed itself in the little man's face.

"What next?" he asked ironically. "For shame!" and he spat on the floor. *Pan* Wróblewski spat, too.

"You do that, *panie*," said Mitya, recognising with despair that all was over, "because you hope to make more out of Grushenka? You're a couple of capons, that's what you are!"

"This is a mortal insult!" The little Pole turned as red as a lobster, and he went out of the room, briskly, as though unwilling to hear another word. Wróblewski swung out after him, and Mitya followed, embarrassed and crestfallen. He was afraid of Grushenka, afraid that the *pan* would at once raise an outcry. And so indeed he did. The Pole walked into the room and threw himself in a theatrical attitude before Grushenka.

"*Pani* Agrippina, I have received a mortal insult!" he exclaimed. But Grushenka suddenly lost all patience, as though they had touched her in the tenderest spot.

"Speak Russian! Speak Russian!" she cried, "not another word of Polish! You used to talk Russian. You can't have forgotten it in five years."

She was red with anger.

"*Pani* Agrippina . . ."

"My name's Agrafena, Grushenka, speak Russian or I won't listen!"

The Pole gasped with offended dignity, and quickly and pompously delivered himself in broken Russian:

"*Pani* Agrafena, I came here to forget the past and forgive it, to forget all that has happened till to-day . . ."

"Forgive? Came here to forgive me?" Grushenka cut him short, jumping up from her seat.

"Just so, *pani*, I'm not small-minded, I'm magnanimous. But I was astounded when I saw your lovers. *Pan* Mitya offered me three thousand, in the other room, to depart. I spat in the *pan's* face."

"What? He offered you money for me?" cried Grushenka, hysterically. "Is it true, Mitya? How did you dare? Am I for sale?"

"*Panie, panie!*" shouted Mitya, "she's pure and shining, and I have never been her lover! That's a lie . . ."

"How dare you defend me before him?" shrieked Grushenka. "It wasn't virtue kept me pure, and it wasn't that I was afraid of Kuzma, but that I might hold up my head when I met him, and tell him he's a scoundrel. And did he actually refuse the money?"

"He took it! He took it!" cried Mitya; "only he wanted to get the whole three thousand at once, and I could only give him seven hundred straight off."

"I see: he heard I had money, and came here to marry me!"

"*Pani* Agrippina!" cried the little Pole. "I'm — a knight, I'm — a nobleman, and not a *lajdak*. I came here to make you my wife and I find you a different woman, wilful and shameless."

"Oh, go back where you came from! I'll tell them to turn you out and you'll be turned out," cried Grushenka, furious. "I've been a fool, a fool, to have tortured myself all these five years! And it wasn't for his sake, it was my anger made me miserable. And this isn't he at all! Was he like this? It might be his father! Where did you get your wig from? He was a falcon, but this is a gander. He used to laugh and sing to me. . . . And I've been crying for five years, damned fool that I was, low, shameless creature!"

She sank back in her armchair and hid her face in her hands.

At that instant the chorus of Mokroye girls began singing in the room on the left — a rollicking dance song.

"A regular Sodom!" Wróblewski roared suddenly. "Innkeeper, send the shameless hussies away!"

The innkeeper, who had been for some time past inquisitively peeping in at the door, hearing shouts and guessing that his guests were quarrelling, at once entered the room.

"What are you shouting for? D'you want to split your throat?" he said, addressing Wróblewski, with surprising rudeness.

"You beast!" bellowed *Pan* Wróblewski.

"Beast? And what sort of cards were you playing with just now? I gave you a pack and you hid it. You played with marked cards! I could send you to Siberia for playing with marked cards, d'you know that, for it's just the same as forged bank-notes . . ."

And going up to the sofa he thrust his fingers between the sofa-back and the cushion, and pulled out an unopened pack of cards.

"Here's my pack unopened!"

He held it up and showed it to all in the room. "From where I stood I saw him slip my pack away, and put his in place of it — you're a cheat and not a gentleman!"

"And I twice saw the *pan* change a card!" cried Kalganov.

"How shameful! How shameful!" exclaimed Grushenka, striking her hands together, and blushing for genuine shame. "Good Lord, he's come to that!"

"I thought so, too!" said Mitya. But before he had uttered the words, Wróblewski, abashed and infuriated, shook his fist at Grushenka, shouting:

"You common harlot!"

Mitya flew at him at once, seized him in both hands, lifted him in the air, and in one instant had carried him into the room on the right, from which they had just come.

"I've laid him on the floor, there," he announced, returning at once, gasping with excitement. "He's struggling, the scoundrel! But he won't come back, no fear of that! . . ."

He closed one half of the folding doors, and holding the other ajar called out to the little Pole:

"Most illustrious, will you be pleased to follow him? I beg you."

"My dear Dmitri Fyodorovich," said Trifon Borisovich, "make them give you back the money you lost. It's as good as stolen from you."

"I don't want my fifty roubles back," Kalganov declared suddenly.

"I don't want my two hundred, either," cried Mitya, "I wouldn't take it for anything! Let him keep it as a consolation."

"Bravo, Mitya! You're a trump, Mitya!" cried Grushenka, and there was a note of fierce anger in the exclamation.

The little *pan*, crimson with fury, but still mindful of his dignity, was making for the door, but he stopped short and said suddenly, addressing Grushenka:

"*Pani*, if you want to come with me, come. If not, good-bye."

And swelling with indignation and importance he went to the door. This was a man of character: he had so good an opinion of himself that after all that had passed, he still expected that she would go with him. Mitya slammed the door after him.

"Lock it," said Kalganov. But the key clicked on the other side, they had locked themselves in.

"That's capital!" exclaimed Grushenka angrily and ruthlessly. "That's capital! Serve them right!"

CHAPTER VIII

DELIRIUM

What followed was almost an orgy, a feast to which all were welcome. Grushenka was the first to call for wine.

"I want to drink. I want to be quite drunk, as we were before. Do you remember, Mitya, do you remember how we made friends here last time!"

Mitya himself was almost delirious, feeling that his happiness was at hand. But Grushenka was continually sending him away from her:

"Go and enjoy yourself. Tell them to dance, to make merry, 'let the stove and cottage dance'; as it was last time," she kept exclaiming. She was tremendously excited. And Mitya kept running out to give orders. The chorus had assembled in the next room. The room in which they had been sitting till that moment was too small, and was divided in two by cotton curtains, behind which was a huge bed with a puffy feather mattress and a pyramid of cotton pillows. In the four rooms for visitors there were beds. Grushenka settled herself just at the door. Mitya placed an easy-chair for her. She had sat in the same place to watch the dancing and singing "the time before," when they had made merry there the first time. The same girls had come again; the Jewish band with fiddles and zithers had come, too, and at last the long expected cart had arrived with the wines and provisions.

Mitya bustled about. Strangers, too, began coming into the room to look on, peasants and their women, who had been roused from sleep and attracted by the hopes of another marvellous entertainment such as they had enjoyed a month before. Mitya remembered their faces, greeting and embracing every one he knew. He uncorked bottles and poured out wine for every one who presented himself. Only the girls were very eager for the champagne. The men preferred rum, cognac, and, above all, hot punch. Mitya had chocolate made for all the girls, and ordered that three samovars should be kept boiling all night to provide tea and punch for all and sundry; every one could help himself.

In a word, disorder and absurdity reigned, but Mitya was in his native element, as it were, and the more absurd things grew, the higher his spirits rose. If a peasant had asked him for money at that moment, he would have pulled out his entire roll and proceeded to distribute the money right and left. This was probably why the innkeeper, Trifon Borisovich, kept hovering about Mitya to protect him. He seemed to have given up all idea of going to bed that night, though he drank little, only one glass of punch, and kept sharp watch over Mitya's interests after his own fashion. He intervened in the nick of time, tenderly and obsequiously persuading Mitya not to give "cigarettes and Rhine wine" and, God forbid, money, to the peasants as he had done before. He was very indignant, too, at the peasant girls drinking liqueur, and eating sweets.

"They're a lousy lot, Dmitri Fyodorovich," he said. "I'll give them a kick, every one of them, and I will order them to take it as an honour — that's all they're worth!"

Mitya remembered Andrey again, and ordered punch to be sent out to him. "I was rude to him just now," he repeated in a weak, melting voice. Kalganov did not want to drink, and at first did not care for the girls' singing; but after he had drunk a couple of glasses of champagne he became extraordinarily lively, strolling about the room, laughing and praising the music and the songs, admiring every one and everything. Maximov, blissfully drunk, never left his side. Grushenka, too, was beginning to get drunk. Pointing to Kalganov, she said to Mitya: "What a charming, what a wonderful boy he is!"

And Mitya, delighted, ran to kiss Kalganov and Maximov. Oh, he had high anticipations! She had said nothing yet, and seemed, indeed, purposely to refrain from speaking. But she looked at him from time to time with caressing and ardent eyes. At last she suddenly gripped his hand and drew him vigorously to her. She was sitting at the moment in the armchair by the door.

"How was it you came just now, eh? How you walked in! . . . I *was* frightened. So you wanted to give me up to him, did you? Did you really want to?"

"I didn't want to spoil your happiness!" Mitya faltered blissfully. But she did not need his answer.

"Well, go and enjoy yourself . . ." she sent him away once more. "Don't cry, I'll call you back again."

He would run away, and she listened to the singing and looked at the dancing, though her eyes followed him wherever he went. But in another quarter of an hour she would call him once more and again he would run back to her.

"Come, sit beside me, tell me, how did you hear about me, and my going off yesterday? From whom did you first hear it?"

And Mitya began telling her all about it, disconnectedly, incoherently, feverishly. He spoke strangely, often frowning, and stopping abruptly.

"What are you frowning at?" she asked.

"Nothing. . . . I left a sick man there. If only he got well, if only I knew that he was going to get well, I'd give ten years of my life for that right away!"

"Well, never mind him, if he's ill. So you meant to shoot yourself to-morrow! What a silly boy! What for? I like such reckless fellows as you," she lisped, with a rather halting tongue. "So you would go to any lengths for me, eh? Did you really mean to shoot yourself to-morrow, you stupid? No, wait a little. To-morrow I may have a little word to say to you. . . . I won't say it to-night, but to-morrow. You'd like it to be to-night? No, I don't want to to-night. Come, go along now, go and amuse yourself."

Once, however, she called him, as it were, puzzled and uneasy.

"Why are you sad? I see you're sad. . . . Yes, I see it," she added, looking intently into his eyes. "Though you keep kissing the peasants and shouting, I see something. No, be merry. I'm merry; you be merry, too. . . . I love somebody here. Guess who it is. Ah, look, my boy has fallen asleep, poor dear, he's drunk."

She meant Kalganov. He was, in fact, drunk, and had dropped asleep for a moment, sitting on the sofa. But he was not merely drowsy from drink; he felt suddenly dejected, or, as he said, "bored." He was intensely depressed by the girls' songs, which, as the drinking went on, gradually became coarse and more reckless. And the dances were as bad. Two girls dressed up as bears, and a lively girl, called Stepanida, with a stick in her hand, acted the part of showman, and began to "exhibit them."

"Look alive, Marya, or you'll get the stick!" she shouted.

The bears rolled on the ground at last in the most unseemly fashion, amid roars of laughter from the closely packed crowd of men and women.

"Well, let them! Let them!" said Grushenka sententiously, with a blissful expression on her face. "When they do get a day to enjoy themselves, why shouldn't folks be happy?"

Kalganov looked as though he had been besmirched with dirt.

"It's swinish, all this peasant foolery," he murmured, moving away; "these are spring games, they play them when they watch for the sun all through the summer night."

He particularly disliked one "new" song which they sang to a jaunty dance tune. It described how a gentleman came and tried his luck with the girls, to see whether they would love him:

The master came to ask the girls:
Would they love him, would they not?

But the girls could not love the master:

He would beat me cruelly:
I can't feel love for such as he.

Then a gipsy comes along and he, too, tries his luck:

The gipsy came and asked the girls:
Would they love him, would they not?

But they couldn't love the gipsy either:

The gipsy will be thieving,
And me, I will be grieving.

And many more men come to try their luck, among them a soldier:

The soldier came and asked the girls:
Would they love him, would they not?

But the soldier is rejected with contempt, in an unprintable couplet, which was sung with perfect frankness and produced a furore in the audience. The song ends with a merchant:

The merchant came and asked the girls:
Would they love him, would they not?

And it appears that he wins their love because:

The merchant will be trading,
And me, I'll be parading.

Kalganov was positively indignant:

"That song must have been made just yesterday," he said aloud. "Who writes such things for them? They might just as well have had a railway man or a Jew come to try his luck with the girls; they'd have carried all before them."

And, almost as though it were a personal affront, he declared, on the spot, that he was bored, sat down on the sofa and immediately

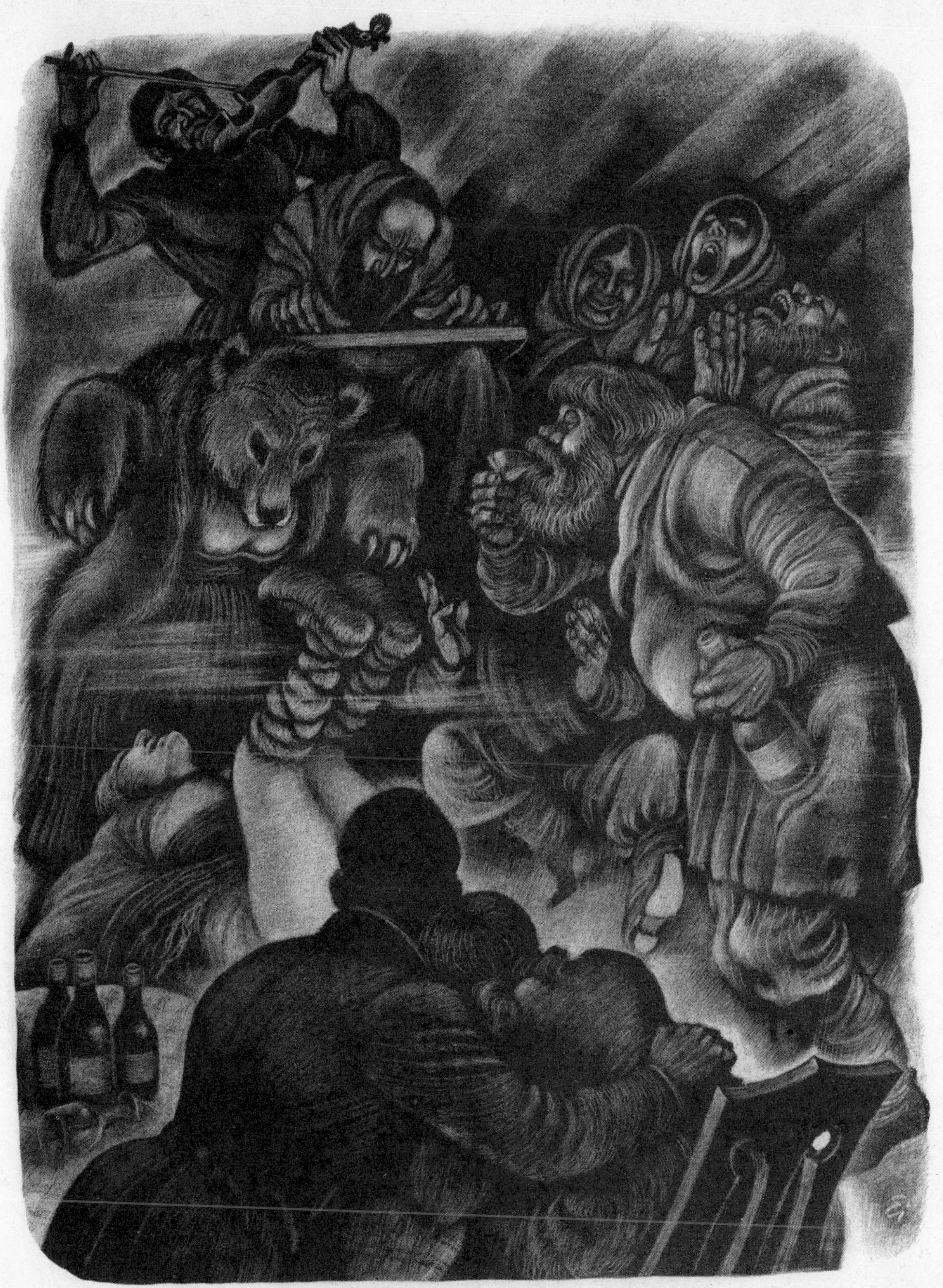

THE ORGY

fell asleep. His pretty little face grew rather pale, as it fell back on the sofa cushion.

"Look how pretty he is," said Grushenka, taking Mitya up to him. "I was combing his hair just now; his hair's like flax, and so thick . . ."

And, bending over him tenderly, she kissed his forehead. Kalganov instantly opened his eyes, looked at her, stood up, and with the most anxious air inquired where was Maximov?

"So that's who it is you want," Grushenka laughed. "Stay with me a minute. Mitya, run and find his Maximov."

Maximov, it appeared, could not tear himself away from the girls, only running away from time to time to pour himself out a glass of liqueur. He had drunk two cups of chocolate. His face was red, and his nose was crimson; his eyes were moist, and melting. He ran up and announced that he was going to dance the "*sabotière*."

"They taught me all those well-bred, aristocratic dances when I was little . . ."

"Go, go with him, Mitya, and I'll watch from here how he dances," said Grushenka.

"No, no, I'm coming to look on, too," exclaimed Kalganov, brushing aside in the most naïve way Grushenka's offer to sit with him. They all went to look on. Maximov actually danced his dance. But it roused no great admiration in any one but Mitya. It consisted of nothing but skipping and hopping, kicking up the heels, and at every skip Maximov slapped the upturned sole of his foot with his palm. Kalganov did not like it at all, but Mitya kissed the dancer.

"Well, thank you. You're tired perhaps? What are you looking for here? Would you like some sweets? A cigarette, perhaps?"

"A cigarette."

"Don't you want a drink?"

"I'll just have a liqueur. . . . Have you any chocolates?"

"Yes, there's a heap of them on the table there. Take one, you dear soul!"

"No, sir, I like one with vanilla . . . the old men's sort. He-he!"

"No, brother, we've none of that special sort."

"I say," the old man bent down to whisper in Mitya's ear. "That girl there, little Marya, he-he! How would it be if out of your kindness you were to help me make friends with her?"

"So that's what you're after! No, brother, that won't do!"

"I'd do no harm to any one," Maximov muttered disconsolately.

"Oh, all right, all right. They only come here to dance and sing, you know, brother. But damn it all, wait a bit! . . . Eat and drink and be merry, meanwhile. Don't you want money?"

"Later on perhaps," smiled Maximov.

"All right, all right. . . ."

Mitya's head was burning. He went outside to the wooden balcony which ran round the whole building on the inner side, overlooking the courtyard. The fresh air revived him. He stood alone in a dark corner, and suddenly clutched his head in both hands. His scattered thoughts suddenly came together; his sensations blended into a whole and threw a sudden light into his mind. A fearful and terrible light! "If I'm to shoot myself, when shall I, if not now?" passed through his mind. "Why not go for the pistols, bring them here, and here, in this dark, dirty corner, make an end?" Almost a minute he stood, undecided.

A few hours earlier, when he had been dashing here, he was pursued by disgrace, by the theft he had committed, and that blood, that blood! . . . But yet it was easier for him then. Then everything was over: he had lost her, given her up. She had perished as far as he was concerned; she had vanished — oh, then his death sentence had been easier for him; at least it had seemed necessary, inevitable, for what had he to stay on earth for?

But now? Was it the same as then? Now one phantom, one terror at least was at an end: that first, rightful lover, that fateful figure had vanished, leaving no trace. The terrible ghost had turned into something so small, so comic; it had been carried into the bedroom and locked in. It would never return. She was ashamed, and from her eyes he could see now whom she loved. Now to live, to live! . . . . But he could not go on living, he could not; oh, damnation! "Oh, God! restore to life the man I knocked down at the fence! Let this fearful cup pass from me! Lord, Thou hast wrought miracles for such sinners as me! But what, what if the old man's alive? Oh, then the shame of the other disgrace I would wipe away. I would restore the stolen money. I'd give it back; I'd get it somehow. . . . No trace of that shame will remain except in my heart for ever! But no, no; oh, impossible cowardly dreams! Oh, damnation!"

Yet there was a ray of light and hope in his darkness. He jumped up and ran back to the room — to her, to her, his queen for ever! Was not one moment of her love worth all the rest of life, even in the agonies of disgrace? This wild question clutched at his heart. "To her, to her alone, to see her, to hear her, to think of nothing, to forget everything, if only for that night, for an hour, for a moment!" Just as he turned from the balcony into the passage, he came upon the innkeeper, Trifon Borisovich. He thought he looked gloomy and worried, and fancied he was looking for him.

"What is it, Trifon Borisovich, are you looking for me?"

"No, sir." The innkeeper seemed disconcerted. "Why should I be looking for you? And you . . . where have you been?"

"Why do you look so glum? You're not angry, are you? Wait a bit, you shall soon get to bed. . . . What's the time?"

"It'll be three o'clock. Past three, it must be."

"We'll leave off soon. We'll leave off."

"Don't mention it; it doesn't matter. Keep it up as long as you like . . ."

"What's the matter with him?" Mitya wondered for an instant, and he ran back to the room where the girls were dancing. But she was not there. She was not in the blue room either; there was no one but Kalganov asleep on the sofa. Mitya peeped behind the curtain — she was there. She was sitting in the corner, on a trunk. Bent forward, with her head and arms on the bed close by, she was crying bitterly, doing her utmost to stifle her sobs that she might not be heard. Seeing Mitya, she beckoned him to her, and when he ran to her, she grasped his hand tightly.

"Mitya, Mitya, I loved him, you know," she began in a whisper. "How I have loved him these five years, all that time! Did I love him or only my own anger? No, him, him! It's a lie that it was my anger I loved and not him. Mitya, I was only seventeen then; he was so kind to me, so merry; he used to sing to me. . . . Or so it seemed to a silly girl like me. . . . And now, O Lord, it's not the same man. Even his face is not the same; he's different altogether. I shouldn't have known him. I drove here with Timofey, and all the way I was thinking how I should meet him, what I should say to him, how we should look at one another. My soul was faint, and all of a sudden it was just as though he had emptied a pail of dirty water over me. He talked to me like a schoolmaster, all so grave and learned; he met me so solemnly that I was struck dumb. I couldn't get a word in. At first I thought he was ashamed to talk before his great big Pole. I sat staring at him and wondering why I couldn't say a word to him now. It must have been his wife that spoiled him; you know he threw me over to get married. She must have changed him like that. Mitya, how shameful it is! Oh, Mitya, I'm ashamed, I'm ashamed of my whole life. Let those five years be cursed, cursed, cursed!"

And again she burst into tears, but clung tight to Mitya's hand and did not let it go.

"Mitya darling, stay, don't go away. I want to say one word to you," she whispered, and suddenly raised her face to him. "Listen, tell me who it is I love? I love one man here. Who is that man? That's what you must tell me."

A smile lighted up her face that was swollen with weeping, and her eyes shone in the half darkness.

"A falcon flew in, and my heart sank within me. 'Fool! that's the man you love!' That was what my heart whispered to me at once. You came in and everything grew bright. What's he afraid of? I wondered. For you were frightened; you couldn't speak. It's not them he's afraid of — could you be frightened of any one? It's me he's afraid of, I thought, only me. So Fenya told you, you little stupid, how I called to Alyosha out of the window that I'd loved Mityenka for one hour, and that I was going now to love . . . another. Mitya, Mitya, how could I be such a fool as to think I could love any one after you? Do you forgive me, Mitya? Do you forgive me or not? Do you love me? Do you love me?" She jumped up and held him with both hands on his shoulders. Mitya, dumb with rapture, gazed into her eyes, at her face, at her smile, and suddenly clasped her tightly in his arms and kissed her passionately.

"You will forgive me for having tormented you? It was through spite I tormented you all. It was for spite I drove the old man out of his mind. . . . Do you remember how you drank at my house one day and broke the wineglass? I remembered that and I broke a glass to-day and drank 'to my vile heart.' Mitya, my falcon, why don't you kiss me? He kissed me once, and now he draws back and looks and listens. Why listen to me? Kiss me, kiss me hard, that's right. If you love, well then love! I'll be your slave now, your slave for the rest of my life. It's sweet to be a slave. Kiss me! Beat me, torture me, injure me. . . . And I do deserve to suffer. Stay, wait, afterwards, I won't have that . . ." she suddenly thrust him away. "Go along, Mitya, I'll come and have some wine, I want to be drunk, I'm going to get drunk and dance; I must, I must!" She tore herself away from him and disappeared behind the curtain. Mitya followed like a drunken man.

"Yes, come what may — whatever may happen now, for one minute I'd give the whole world," he thought. Grushenka did, in fact, toss off a whole glass of champagne at one gulp, and became at once very tipsy. She sat down in the same chair as before, with a blissful smile on her face. Her cheeks were blazing, her lips were burning, her flashing eyes grew filmy; there was the lure of passion in her eyes. Even Kalganov's heart was stung and he went up to her.

"Did you feel how I kissed you when you were asleep just now?" she said thickly. "I'm drunk now, that's what it is. . . . And aren't you drunk? And why isn't Mitya drinking? Why don't you drink, Mitya? I drank, and you don't drink . . ."

"I am drunk! I'm drunk as it is . . . drunk with you . . . and now I'll be drunk with wine, too."

He drank off another glass, and — he thought it strange himself — that glass made him completely drunk. He was suddenly drunk, although till that moment he had been quite sober, he remembered that. From that moment everything whirled about him, as though he were delirious. He walked, laughed, talked to everybody, without knowing what he was doing. Only one persistent burning sensation made itself felt continually, "like a red-hot coal in his heart," he said afterwards. He went up to her, sat beside her, gazed at her, listened to her. . . . She became very talkative, kept calling every one to her, and beckoned to different girls out of the chorus. When the girl came up, she either kissed her or made the sign of the cross over her. In another minute she might have cried. She was greatly amused by the "little old man," as she called Maximov. He ran up every minute to kiss her hands, "each little finger," and finally he danced another dance to an old song, which he sang himself. He danced with special ardour to the refrain:

The little pig says — umph! umph! umph!
The little calf says — moo, moo, moo,
The little duck says — quack, quack, quack,
The little goose says — gabble, gabble, gabble.
The hen went strutting through the entry.
Cluck, cluck, cluck, cluck, cluck, she says,
Cluck, cluck, cluck, cluck, cluck, she says.

"Give him something, Mitya," said Grushenka. "Give him a present, he's poor, you know. Ah, the poor, the insulted. . . . Do you know, Mitya, I shall go into a nunnery. No, I really shall one day. Alyosha said something to me to-day that I shall remember all my life. . . . Yes. . . . But to-night let us dance. To-morrow to the nunnery, but to-night we'll dance. I want to play to-night, good people, and what of it? God will forgive us. If I were God, I'd forgive every one: 'My dear sinners, from this day forth I forgive you.' I'm going to beg forgiveness: 'Forgive me, good people, a silly woman.' I'm a beast, that's what I am. But I want to pray. I gave a little onion. Wicked as I've been, I want to pray. Mitya, let them dance, don't stop them. Every one in the world is good. Every one — even the worst of them. The world's a nice place. Though we're bad the world's all right. We're good and bad, good and bad. . . . Come tell me, I've something to ask you; come here every one, and I'll ask you: Why am I so good? You know I am good. I'm very good. . . . Come, why am I so good?"

So Grushenka babbled on, getting more and more drunk. At last she announced that she was going to dance, too. She got up from her chair, staggering. "Mitya, don't give me any more wine — if I ask you, don't give it to me. Wine gives me no peace. Everything's going round, the stove, and everything. I want to dance. Let every one see how I dance . . . let them see how beautifully I dance . . ."

She really meant it. She pulled a white cambric handkerchief out of her pocket, and took it by one corner in her right hand, to wave it in the dance. Mitya ran to and fro, the girls were quiet, and got ready to break into a dancing song at the first signal. Maximov, hearing that Grushenka wanted to dance, squealed with delight, and ran skipping about in front of her, humming:

"With legs so slim and sides so trim
And its little tail curled tight."

But Grushenka waved her handkerchief at him and drove him away.

"Sh-h! Mitya, why don't they come? Let every one come . . . to look on. Call them in, too, the ones that were locked in. . . . Why did you lock them in? Tell them I'm going to dance. Let them look on, too. . . ."

Mitya walked with a drunken swagger to the locked door, and began knocking at the door with his fist.

"Hi, you . . . Podwysockis! Come, she's going to dance. She wants you."

"*Lajdak!*" one of the Poles shouted in reply.

"You're a sub-*lajdak* yourself! You're a little scoundrel, that's what you are."

"Leave off laughing at Poland," said Kalganov sententiously. He, too, was drunk.

"Be quiet, boy! If I call him a scoundrel, it doesn't mean that I called all Poland so. One *lajdak* doesn't make a Poland. Be quiet, my pretty boy, eat a sweetmeat."

"Ach, what fellows! As though they were not human beings. Why won't they make friends?" said Grushenka, and went forward to dance. The chorus broke into "Ah, my entry, my new entry!" Grushenka flung back her head, half opened her lips, smiled, waved her handkerchief, and suddenly, with a violent lurch, stood still in the middle of the room, looking bewildered.

"I'm weak . . ." she said in an exhausted voice. "Forgive me. . . . I'm weak, I can't. . . . I'm sorry." She bowed to the chorus, and then began bowing in all directions.

"I'm sorry. . . . Forgive me. . . ."

"The lady's been drinking. The pretty lady has been drinking," voices were heard saying.

"The lady's drunk too much," Maximov explained to the girls, giggling.

"Mitya, lead me away . . . take me," said Grushenka helplessly. Mitya pounced on her, snatched her up in his arms, and carried the precious burden through the curtains.

"Well, now I'll go," thought Kalganov, and walking out of the blue room, he closed the two halves of the door after him. But the orgy in the larger room went on and grew louder and louder. Mitya laid Grushenka on the bed and kissed her on the lips.

"Don't touch me . . ." she faltered, in an imploring voice. "Don't touch me, till I'm yours. . . . I've told you I'm yours, but don't touch me . . . spare me. . . . With them here, with them close, you mustn't. He's here. It's nasty here . . ."

"I'll obey you! I won't think of it . . . I worship you!" muttered Mitya. "Yes, it's nasty here, it's despicable."

And still holding her in his arms, he sank on his knees by the bedside.

"I know, though you're a brute, you're noble-hearted," Grushenka articulated with difficulty. "It must be honourable . . . it shall be honourable in the future . . . and let us be honest, let us be good, not brutes, but good . . . take me away, take me far away, do you hear? I don't want it to be here, but far, far away. . . ."

"Oh, yes, yes, it must be!" said Mitya, pressing her in his arms. "I'll take you and we'll fly away. . . . Oh, I'd give my whole life for one year only to know about that blood!"

"What blood?" asked Grushenka, bewildered.

"Nothing," muttered Mitya, through his teeth. "Grusha, you wanted to be honest, but I'm a thief. But I've stolen money from Katya. . . . Disgrace, a disgrace!"

"From Katya, from that young lady? No, you didn't steal it. Give it her back, take it from me. . . . Why make a fuss? Now everything of mine is yours. What does money matter? We shall waste it anyway. . . . Folks like us are bound to run through money. But we'd better go and work the land. I want to dig the earth with my own hands. We must work, do you hear? Alyosha said so. I won't be your mistress, I'll be faithful to you, I'll be your slave, I'll work for you. We'll go to the young lady and bow down to her together, so that she may forgive us, and then we'll go away. And if she won't forgive us, we'll go, anyway. Take her her money and love me. . . . Don't love her. . . . Don't love her any more. If you love her, I will strangle her. . . . I'll put out both her eyes with a needle . . ."

"I love you. I love only you. I'll love you in Siberia . . ."

"Why Siberia? Never mind, Siberia if you like. I don't care . . . we'll work . . . there's snow in Siberia. . . . I love driving in the snow . . . and there must be bells. . . . Do you hear, there's a bell ringing? Where is that bell ringing? There are people coming. . . . Now it's stopped."

She closed her eyes, exhausted, and suddenly fell asleep for an instant. There had indeed been the sound of a bell in the distance, but the ringing had ceased. Mitya let his head sink on her breast. He did not notice that the bell had ceased ringing, nor did he notice that the songs had ceased, and that instead of singing and drunken clamour there was absolute stillness in the house. Grushenka opened her eyes.

"What's the matter? Was I asleep? Yes . . . a bell . . . I've been asleep and dreamt I was driving over the snow with bells, and I dozed. I was with some one I loved, with you. And far, far away. I was holding you and kissing you, nestling close to you. I was cold, and the snow glistened. . . . You know how the snow glistens at night when the moon shines. It was as though I was not on earth. I woke up, and my dear one is close to me. How sweet that is . . ."

"Close to you," murmured Mitya, kissing her dress, her bosom, her hands. And suddenly he had a strange fancy: it seemed to him that she was looking straight before her, not at him, not into his face, but over his head, with an intent, almost uncanny fixity. An expression of wonder, almost of alarm, came suddenly into her face.

"Mitya, who is that looking at us?" she whispered.

Mitya turned, and saw that some one had, in fact, parted the curtains and seemed to be watching them. And not one person alone, it seemed.

He jumped up and walked quickly to the intruder.

"Here, this way, kindly, come here," said a voice, speaking gently but firmly and peremptorily.

Mitya passed to the other side of the curtain and stood stock still. The room was filled

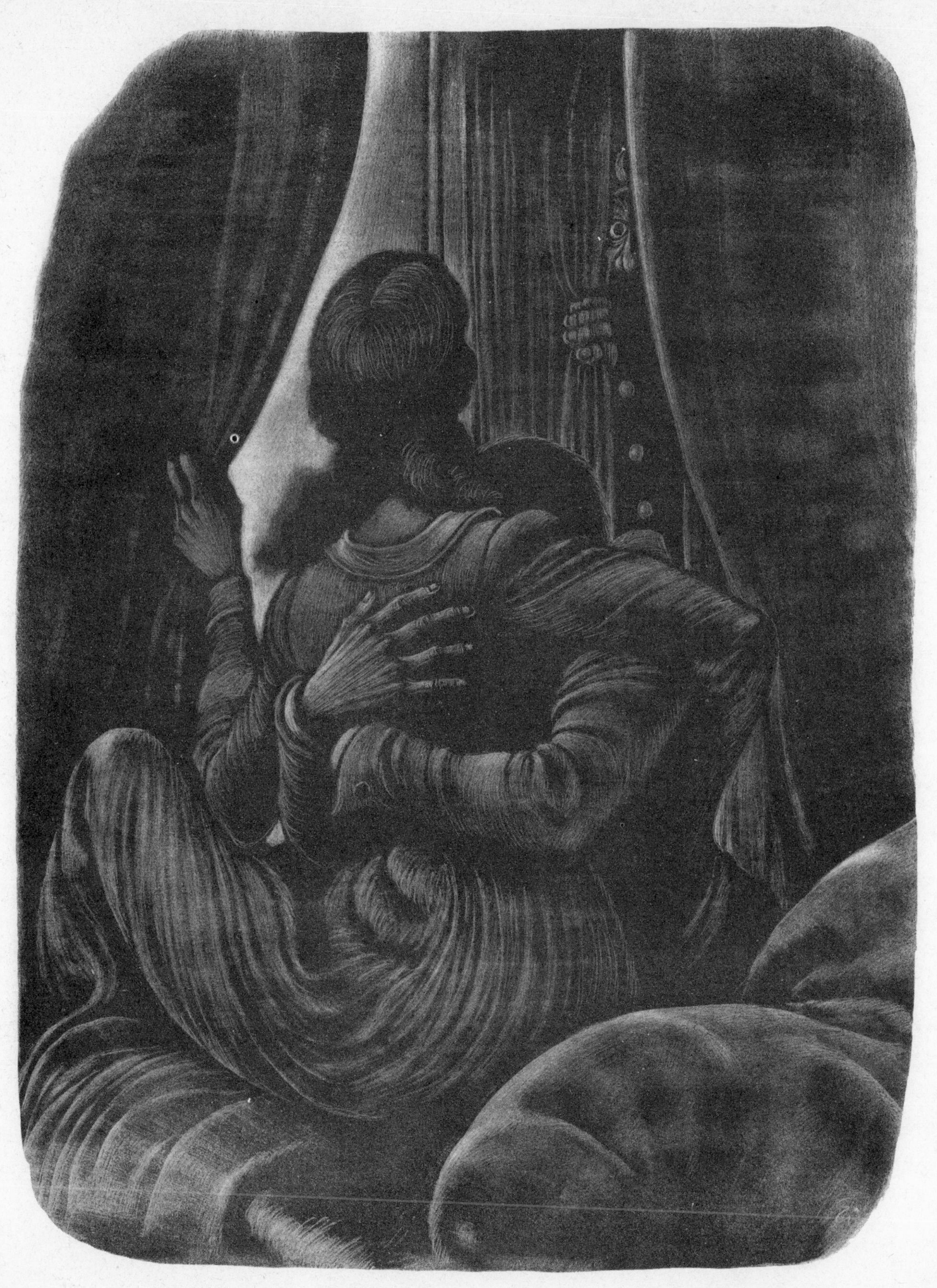

"I AM DRUNK WITH YOU"

with people, but not those who had been there before. An instantaneous shiver ran down his back, and he shuddered. He recognised all those people instantly. That tall, stout old man in the overcoat and the cap with a cockade — was the police captain, Mihail Makarovich. And that "consumptive-looking" trim dandy, "who always has such polished boots" — that was the assistant prosecutor. "He has a watch worth four hundred roubles; he showed it to me." And that small young man in spectacles . . . Mitya forgot his surname though he knew him, had seen him: he was the magistrate, the examining magistrate, from the "school of jurisprudence," who had only lately come to the town. And this man — the inspector of police, Mavriky Mavrikyevich, a man he knew well. And those fellows with the brass badges on, why are they here? And those other two . . . peasants. . . . And there at the door Kalganov with Trifon Borisovich. . . .

"Gentlemen! What's this for, gentlemen?" began Mitya, but suddenly, as though beside himself, not knowing what he was doing, he cried aloud, at the top of his voice:

"I un — der — stand!"

The young man in spectacles moved forward suddenly, and stepping up to Mitya, began with dignity, though hurriedly:

"We have to make . . . in brief, I beg you to come this way, this way to the sofa. . . . It is absolutely imperative for us to have a talk with you."

"The old man!" cried Mitya frantically. "The old man and his blood! . . . I understand." And he sank, almost fell, on a chair close by, as though he had been mown down by a scythe.

"You understand? He understands it! Monster and parricide! Your father's blood cries out against you!" the old captain of police roared suddenly, stepping up to Mitya.

He was beside himself, crimson in the face and quivering all over.

"This is impossible!" cried the small young man. "Mihail Makarovich, Mihail Makarovich, this won't do! It won't do, sir! . . . Allow me to be the one to speak. I should never have expected such behaviour from you . . ."

"This is delirium, gentlemen, raving delirium," cried the captain of police; "look at him: drunk, at this time of night, in the company of a disreputable woman, with the blood of his father upon him. . . . It's delirium!"

"I beg you most earnestly, dear Mihail Makarovich, to restrain your feelings," the prosecutor said in a rapid whisper to the old police captain, "or I shall be forced to resort to . . ."

But the little lawyer did not allow him to finish. He turned to Mitya, and delivered himself in a loud, firm, dignified voice:

"Ex-Lieutenant Karamazov, it is my duty to inform you that you are charged with the murder of your father, Fyodor Pavlovich Karamazov, perpetrated this night . . ."

He said something more, and the prosecutor, too, put in a word, but though Mitya heard them he did not understand them. He stared at them all with wild eyes.

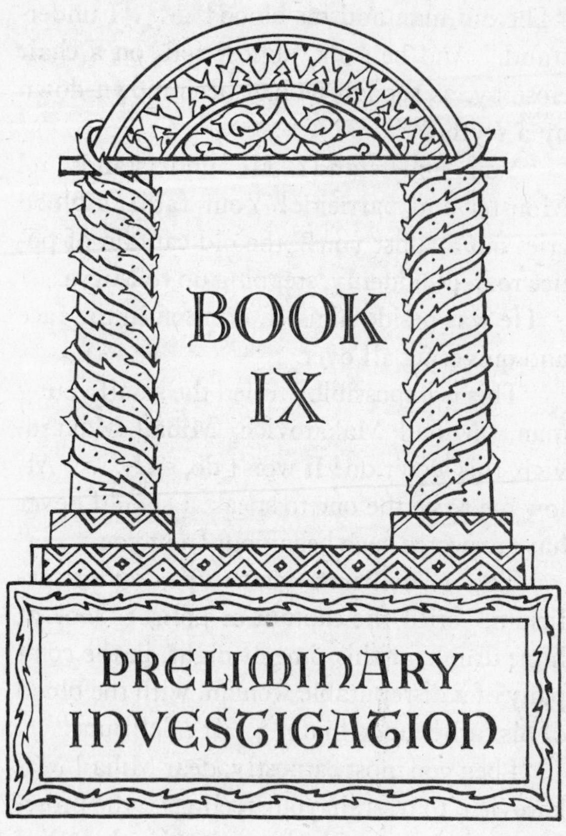

CHAPTER I

THE BEGINNING OF PERHOTIN'S OFFICIAL CAREER

Pyotr Ilyich Perhotin, whom we left knocking at the strong, locked gates of the widow Morozov's house, ended, of course, by making himself heard. Fenya, who was still excited by the fright she had had two hours before, and too much "upset" to go to bed, was almost frightened into hysterics on hearing the furious knocking at the gate. Though she had herself seen him drive away, she fancied that it must be Dmitri Fyodorovich knocking again, no one else could knock so rudely. She ran to the house-porter, who had already waked up and gone out to the gate, and began imploring him not to open it. But having questioned Pyotr Ilyich, and learnt that he wanted to see Fenya on very "important business," the man made up his mind at last to open. Pyotr Ilyich was admitted into Fenya's kitchen, but the girl begged him to allow the house-porter to be present, "because of her misgivings." He began questioning her and at once learnt the most vital fact, that is, that when Dmitri Fyodorovich had run out to look for Grushenka, he had snatched up a pestle from the mortar, and that when he returned, the pestle was not with him and his hands were bloody.

"And the blood was still dripping, dripping from them, dripping!" Fenya kept exclaiming. This horrible detail was simply the product of her disordered imagination. But Pyotr Ilyich had himself seen those hands stained with blood, although not "dripping," and had helped to wash them. Moreover, the question he had to decide was not how soon the blood had dried, but where Dmitri Fyodorovich had run with the pestle, or rather, whether it really was to Fyodor Pavlovich's, and how he could definitely deduce the fact. Pyotr Ilyich persisted in returning to this point, and though he found out nothing conclusive, yet he carried away a conviction that Dmitri Fyodorovich could have gone nowhere but to his father's house, and that therefore something must have happened there.

"And when he came back," Fenya added with excitement, "and I made a clean breast of it to him, then I began asking him: 'Why have you got blood on your hands, Dmitri Fyodorovich?' and he answered that that was human blood, and that he had just killed some one. He confessed it all to me, and suddenly ran off like a madman. I sat down and began thinking, where's he run off to now like a madman? He'll go to Mokroye, I thought, and kill my mistress there. I ran out to beg him not to kill her. I was running to his lodgings, but I looked at Plotnikov's shop, and saw him just setting off, and there was no blood on his hands then." (Fenya had noticed this and remembered it.) Fenya's old grandmother confirmed her evidence as far as she was able. After asking some further questions, Pyotr Ilyich left the house, even more upset and uneasy than he had been when he entered it.

It would seem that the most direct and the easiest thing for him to do would have been to go straight to Fyodor Pavlovich's, to find out whether anything had happened there, and if so, what; and only to go to the police captain, as Pyotr Ilyich firmly intended doing, when he had satisfied himself of the fact. But the night was dark, Fyodor Pavlovich's gates were strong, and he would have to knock again. His acquaintance with Fyodor Pavlovich was of the slightest, and what if, after he had aroused them, they opened to him, and nothing had happened, and Fyodor Pavlovich in his jeering way would go telling the story all over the town, how a stranger, Perhotin, the official, had broken in upon him at midnight to ask if any one had killed him. It would make a scandal. And scandal was what Pyotr Ilyich dreaded more than anything.

Yet the feeling that possessed him was so strong, that though he stamped his foot angrily and swore at himself, he set off again, not to Fyodor Pavlovich's, but to Madame Hohlakov's. He decided that if she denied having just given Dmitri Fyodorovich three thousand roubles, he would go straight to the police captain, but if she admitted having given him the money, he would go home and let the matter rest till next morning.

It is, of course, perfectly evident that there was even more likelihood of causing scandal by going at eleven o'clock at night to a fashionable lady, a complete stranger, and perhaps rousing her from her bed to ask her an amazing question, than by going to Fyodor Pavlovich. But that is just how it is, sometimes, especially in cases like the present one, with the decisions of the most precise and phlegmatic people. Pyotr Ilyich was by no means phlegmatic at that moment. He remembered all his life how an unconquerable uneasiness, which had gradually gained possession of him, had finally reached a point where it was actually painful and drove him on, against his will. Yet he kept cursing himself, of course, all the way for going to this lady, but "I will see it through, I will!" he repeated for the tenth time, grinding his teeth, and he carried out his intention.

It was exactly eleven o'clock when he entered Madame Hohlakov's house. He was admitted into the courtyard fairly quickly, but, in response to his inquiry whether the lady was resting or had not yet retired, the porter could give no answer, except that she was usually in bed by that time.

"Ask at the top of the stairs. If the lady wants to receive you, she'll receive you. If she won't, she won't."

Pyotr Ilyich went upstairs, but did not find things so easy here. The footman was unwilling to take in his name, but finally called a maid. Pyotr Ilyich politely but insistently begged her to inform her lady that a local official, called Perhotin, had called on particular business, and that, if it were not of the greatest importance, he would not have ventured to come. "Tell her in those words, in those words exactly," he asked the girl.

She went away. He remained waiting in the entry. Madame Hohlakov herself was already in her bedroom, though she had not yet retired. She had felt upset ever since Mitya's visit, and had a presentiment that she would not get through the night without the sick headache which always, with her, followed such excitement. She was surprised on hearing the announcement from the maid. She irritably declined to see him, however, though the unexpected visit at such an hour, of a "local official" who was a stranger, roused her feminine curiosity intensely. But this time Pyotr Ilyich was as obstinate as a mule. He begged the maid most earnestly to take another message in these very words:

"That he had come on business of the greatest importance, and that Madame Hohlakov might have cause to regret it later, if she refused to see him now."

"I plunged headlong," he described it afterwards.

The maid, gazing at him in amazement, went to take his message again. Madame Hohlakov was impressed. She thought a little, asked what he looked like, and learnt that he was "very well dressed, young, and so polite." We may note, parenthetically, that Pyotr Ilyich was a rather good-looking young man, and well aware of the fact. Madame Hohlakov made up her mind to see him. She was in her dressing-gown and slippers, but she flung a black shawl over her shoulders. The "official" was asked to walk into the drawing-room, the very room in which Mitya had been received shortly before. The lady came to meet her visitor, with a sternly inquiring countenance, and, without asking him to sit down, began at once with the question:

"What do you wish?"

"I have ventured to disturb you, madam, on a matter concerning our common acquaintance, Dmitri Fyodorovich Karamazov," Perhotin began.

But he had hardly uttered the name, when the lady's face showed signs of acute irritation. She almost shrieked, and interrupted him in a fury:

"How much longer am I to be tormented by that awful man?" she cried hysterically. "How dare you, sir, how could you venture to disturb a lady who is a stranger to you, in her own house at such an hour? . . . And to force yourself upon her to talk of a man who came here, to this very drawing-room, only three hours ago, to murder me, and went stamping out of the room, as no one would go out of a decent house. Let me tell you, sir, that I shall lodge a complaint against you, that I will not let it pass. Kindly leave me at once. . . . I am a mother. . . . I . . . I . . ."

"Murder! then he tried to murder you, too?"

"Why, has he killed somebody else?" Madame Hohlakov asked impulsively.

"If you would kindly listen, madam, for half a moment, I'll explain it all in a couple of words," answered Perhotin firmly. "At five o'clock this afternoon Dmitri Fyodorovich borrowed ten roubles from me, and I know for a fact that he had no money. Yet at nine o'clock, he came to see me with a bundle of hundred-rouble notes in his hand, about two or three thousand roubles in all. His hands and face were all covered with blood, and he looked like a madman. When I asked him where he had got so much money, he answered that he had just received it from you, that you had given him a sum of three thousand to go to the gold-mines . . ."

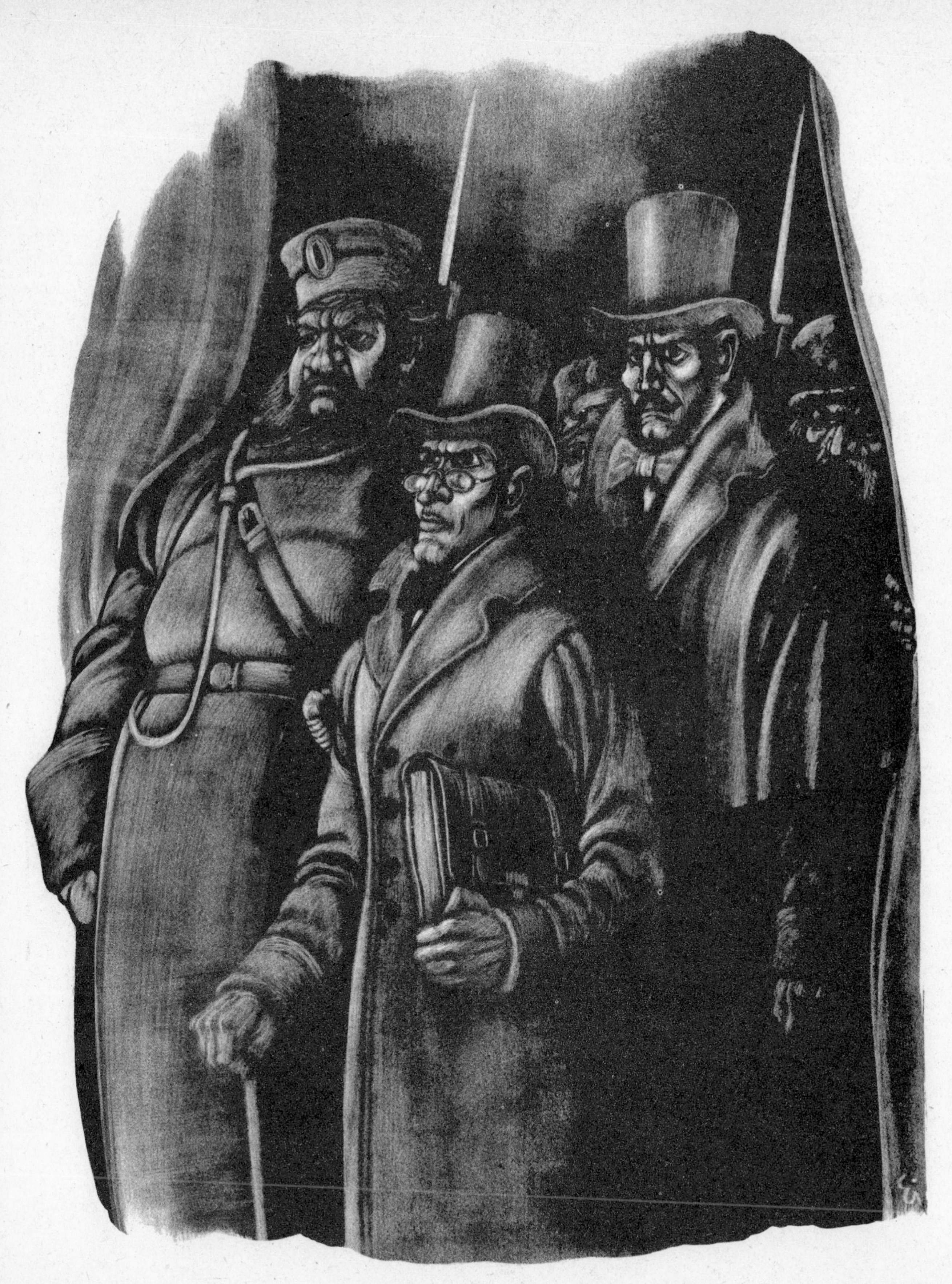

"YOU ARE CHARGED WITH THE MURDER OF YOUR FATHER"

Madame Hohlakov's face assumed an expression of intense and morbid excitement.

"Good God! He must have killed his old father!" she cried, striking her hands together. "I haven't given him any money at all, none whatsoever. Oh, run, run! . . . Don't say another word! Save the old man . . . run to his father . . . run!"

"Excuse me, madam, then you did not give him money? You remember distinctly that you did not give him any money?"

"No, I didn't, I didn't! I refused to give it him, for he could not appreciate it. He ran out in a fury, stamping. He rushed at me, but I slipped away. . . . And let me tell you, as I wish to hide nothing from you now, that he positively spat at me. Can you fancy that! But why are we standing? Ah, sit down. . . . Excuse me, I . . . or better run, run, you must run and save the poor old man from an awful death!"

"But if he has killed him already?"

"Ah, good heavens, yes! Then what are we to do now? What do you think we must do now?"

Meantime she had made Pyotr Ilyich sit down and sat down herself, facing him. Briefly, but rather clearly, Pyotr Ilyich told her the history of the affair, that part of it at least which he had himself witnessed. He described, too, his visit to Fenya, and told her about the pestle. All these details produced an overwhelming effect on the distracted lady, who kept uttering shrieks, and covering her face with her hands. . . .

"Would you believe it, I foresaw all this! I have that special faculty, whatever I imagine comes to pass. And how often I've looked at that awful man and always thought, that man will end by murdering me. And now it's happened . . . that is, if he hasn't murdered me, but only his own father, it's only because the finger of God preserved me, and what's more, he was ashamed to murder me because, on this very place, I put the holy ikon from the relics of the holy martyr, Saint Varvara, on his neck. . . . And to think how near I was to death at that minute, I went close up to him and he stretched out his neck to me! . . . Do you know, Pyotr Ilyich (I think you said your name was Pyotr Ilyich), I don't believe in miracles, but that ikon and this unmistakable miracle with me now — that shakes me, and I'm ready to believe in anything you like. Have you heard about Father Zosima? . . . But I don't know what I'm saying . . . and only fancy, with the ikon on his neck he spat at me. . . . He only spat, it's true, he didn't murder me and . . . he dashed away! But what shall we do, what must we do now? What do you think?"

Pyotr Ilyich got up, and announced that he was going straight to the police captain, to tell him all about it, and leave him to do what he thought fit.

"Oh, he's an excellent man, excellent! Mihail Makarovich, I know him. Of course, he's the person to go to. How practical you are, Pyotr Ilyich! How well it is that you've thought of everything! I should never have thought of it in your place!"

"Especially as I know the police captain very well, too," observed Pyotr Ilyich, who still continued to stand, and was obviously anxious to escape as quickly as possible from the impulsive lady, who would not let him say good-bye and go away.

"And be sure, be sure," she prattled on, "to come back and tell me what you see there, and what you find out . . . what comes to light

. . . how they'll try him . . . and what he's condemned to. . . . Tell me, we have no capital punishment, have we? But be sure to come, even if it's at three o'clock at night, at four, at half-past four. . . . Tell them to wake me, to wake me, to shake me, if I don't get up. . . . But, good heavens, I shan't sleep! But wait, hadn't I better come with you?"

"N-no. But if you would write three lines with your own hand, stating that you did not give Dmitri Fyodorovich money, it might, perhaps, be of use . . . in case it's needed. . . ."

"To be sure!" Madame Hohlakov skipped, delighted, to her bureau. "And you know I'm simply struck, amazed at your resourcefulness, your good sense in such affairs. Are you in the service here? I'm delighted to think that you're in the service here!"

And still speaking, she scribbled on half a sheet of note-paper the following lines:

"I've never in my life lent to that unhappy man, Dmitri Fyodorovich Karamazov (for, in spite of all, he is unhappy), three thousand roubles to-day. I've never given him money, never! That I swear by all that's holy!

"K. Hohlakov."

"Here's the note!" she turned quickly to Pyotr Ilyich. "Go, save him. It's a noble deed on your part!"

And she made the sign of the cross over him three times. She ran out to accompany him to the foyer.

"How grateful I am to you! You can't think how grateful I am to you for having come to me, first. How is it I haven't met you before? I shall feel flattered at seeing you at my house in the future. How delightful it is that you are in the service here! . . . Such precision! Such resourcefulness! . . . They must appreciate you, they must understand you. If there's anything I can do, believe me . . . oh, I love young people! I'm in love with young people! The younger generation are the one foundation of our suffering country. Her one hope. . . . Oh, go, go! . . ."

But Pyotr Ilyich had already run off or she would not have let him go so soon. Yet Madame Hohlakov had made a rather agreeable impression on him, which had somewhat softened his anxiety at being drawn into such an unpleasant affair. Tastes differ, as we all know. "She's by no means so elderly," he thought, feeling pleased, "on the contrary, I should have taken her for her daughter."

As for Madame Hohlakov, she was simply enchanted by the young man. "Such sense! such precision! in so young a man! in our day! and all that with such manners and appearance! They say the young people of to-day are no good for anything, but here's an example!" etc., etc. So she simply forgot this "dreadful affair," and it was only as she was getting into bed, that, suddenly recalling "how near death she had been," she exclaimed: "Ah, it is awful, awful!"

But she fell at once into a sound, sweet sleep.

I would not, however, have dwelt on such trivial and irrelevant details, if this eccentric meeting of the young official with the by no means elderly widow had not subsequently turned out to be the foundation of the whole career of that practical and precise young man. His story is remembered to this day with amazement in our town, and I shall perhaps have something to say about it, when I have finished my long tale of the Brothers Karamazov.

CHAPTER II

THE ALARM

Our police captain, Mihail Makarovich Makarov, a retired lieutenant-colonel, with the rank of court councillor, was a widower and an excellent man. He had come to us only three years previously, but had won general esteem, chiefly because he "knew how to bring people together." He was never without visitors, and it would seem that he could not have got on without them. Some one or other was always dining with him; he never sat down to table without guests. He gave regular dinners, too, on all sorts of occasions, sometimes most surprising ones. Though the fare was not *recherché*, it was abundant. The fish pies were excellent, and the wine made up in quantity for what it lacked in quality.

The first room his guests entered was a well-fitted billiard-room, with pictures of English race-horses, in black frames, on the walls, an essential decoration, as we all know, for a bachelor's billiard-room. There was card-playing every evening at his house, if only at one table. But at frequent intervals, all the best society of our town, with the mammas and young ladies, assembled at his house to dance. Though Mihail Makarovich was a widower, he did not live alone. His widowed daughter lived with him, with her two unmarried daughters, grown-up girls, who had finished their education. They were of agreeable appearance and lively character, and though every one knew they would have no dowry, they attracted all the young men of fashion to their grandfather's house.

Mihail Makarovich was by no means very efficient in his work, though he performed his duties no worse than many others. To speak plainly, he was a rather uneducated man. His understanding of the limits of his administrative power could not always be relied upon. It was not so much that he failed to grasp certain reforms enacted during the present reign, as that he made conspicuous blunders in his interpretation of them. This was not from any special lack of intelligence, but from carelessness, for he was always in too great a hurry to go into the subject.

"I have the heart of a soldier rather than a civilian," he used to say of himself. He had not even formed a definite idea of the fundamental principles of the reforms connected with the emancipation of the serfs, and he added to his knowledge of it, so to speak, from year to year, involuntarily increasing his understanding by practice. And yet he was himself a landowner. Pyotr Ilyich knew for certain that he would meet some of Mihail Makarovich's visitors there that evening, but he didn't know which. As it happened, at that moment there were sitting in his house, over a game of whist, the prosecutor, and Varvinsky, our district doctor, a young man, who had only just come to us from Petersburg after graduating with high honours from the Academy of Medicine. Ippolit Kirillovich, the prosecutor (he was really the assistant prosecutor, but we always called him the prosecutor), was a rather peculiar man, of about five and thirty, inclined to be consumptive, and married to a fat and childless woman. He was vain and irritable, though he had a good intellect, and even a kind heart. It seemed that all that was wrong with him was that he had a better opinion of himself than his ability warranted. And that made him seem constantly uneasy. He had, moreover, certain higher, even artistic, leanings, towards psychology, for instance, a special study of the human heart, a special knowledge of the criminal and his crime. He cherished a grievance on this score, considering that he had been passed over in the service, and being firmly persuaded that in higher spheres he had not been properly appreciated, and had enemies. In gloomy moments he even threatened to give up his post, and practise as a barrister in criminal cases. The unexpected Karamazov case involving parricide shook him to the depths: "It was a case that might well be talked about all over Russia." But I am anticipating.

Nikolay Parfenovich Nelyudov, the young examining magistrate, who had come from Petersburg only two months before, was sitting in the next room with the young ladies. People talked about it afterwards and wondered that all these gentlemen, as though intentionally, should have been gathered together at the house of the executive authority on the evening of "the crime." Yet it was perfectly simple and happened quite naturally.

Ippolit Kirillovich's wife had had toothache for the last two days, and, naturally, he had to run off somewhere to escape from her groans. The doctor, from the very nature of his being, could not spend an evening except at cards. As for Nikolay Parfenovich Nelyudov, he had been intending for three days past to drop in that evening at Mihail Makarovich's, so to speak casually, so as slyly to startle the eldest granddaughter, Olga Mihailovna, by showing that he knew her secret, that he knew it was her birthday, and that she was trying to conceal it on purpose, so as not to be obliged to give a dance. He anticipated a great deal of merriment, many playful jests about her age, and her being afraid to reveal it, about his knowing her secret and telling everybody, and so on. The charming young man was a great adept at such teasing; the ladies called him "naughty," and he seemed to be delighted at the nickname. He was extremely well bred, however, of good family, education, and feelings, and, though leading a life of pleasure, his sallies were always innocent and in good taste. He was short and delicate looking. On his white, slender little fingers he always wore a number of big, glittering rings. When he was engaged in his official duties, he always became extraordinarily grave, as though realising his position and the sanctity of the obligations laid upon him. He had a special gift for nonplussing murderers and other criminals from among the common people during interrogation, and if he did not win their respect, he certainly succeeded in arousing their wonder.

Pyotr Ilyich was simply dumbfounded when he went into the police captain's. He saw instantly that every one knew. They had positively thrown down their cards, all were standing up and talking. Even Nikolay Parfenovich had left the young ladies and run in, looking strenuous and ready for action. Pyotr Ilyich was met with the astounding news that old Fyodor Pavlovich really had been murdered that evening in his own house, murdered and robbed. The news had only just reached them in the following manner:

Marfa Ignatyevna, the wife of old Grigory, who had been knocked senseless near the fence, was sleeping soundly in her bed and might well have slept till morning after the draught she had taken. But all of a sudden she waked up, no doubt roused by a fearful epileptic scream from Smerdyakov, who was lying in the next room unconscious. That scream always preceded his fits, and always terrified and upset Marfa Ignatyevna. She could never get accustomed to it. She jumped up and ran half-awake to Smerdyakov's room. But it was dark there, and she could only hear the invalid beginning to gasp and struggle. Then Marfa Ignatyevna herself screamed out and was going to call her husband, but suddenly realised that when she had got up he was not beside her in bed. She ran back to the bedstead and began groping with her hands, but the bed was really empty. Then he must have gone out — where? She ran to the steps and timidly called him. She got no answer, of course, but she caught the sound of groans far away in the garden in the darkness. She listened. The groans were repeated, and it was evident they came from the garden.

"Good Lord! Just as it was with Lizaveta Smerdyashchaya!" she thought distractedly. She went timidly down the steps and saw that the gate into the garden was open.

"He must be out there, poor dear," she thought. She went up to the gate and all at once she distinctly heard Grigory calling her by name, "Marfa! Marfa!" in a weak, moaning, dreadful voice.

"Lord, preserve us from harm!" Marfa Ignatyevna murmured, and ran towards the voice, and that was how she found Grigory. But she found him not by the fence where he had been knocked down, but about twenty paces off. It appeared later that he had crawled away on coming to himself, and probably had been a long time getting so far, losing consciousness several times. She noticed at once that he was covered with blood, and screamed at the top of her voice. Grigory was muttering incoherently: "He has murdered . . . murdered his father . . . Why scream, silly . . . run . . . fetch some one . . ."

But Marfa continued screaming, and seeing that her master's window was open and that there was a candle alight in the window, she ran there and began calling Fyodor Pavlovich. But peeping in at the window, she saw a fearful sight. Her master was lying on his back, motionless, on the floor. His light-coloured dressing-gown and white shirt were soaked with blood. The candle on the table brightly lighted up the blood and the motionless dead face of Fyodor Pavlovich. Terror-stricken, Marfa rushed away from the window, ran out of the garden, drew the bolt of the big gate, and ran headlong by the back way to the neighbour, Marya Kondratyevna. Both mother and daughter were asleep, but they were waked up by Marfa's desperate and persistent screaming and knocking at the shutter. Marfa, shrieking and screaming incoherently, managed to tell them the main fact, and to beg for assistance. It happened that Foma had come back from his wanderings and was spending the night with them. They got him up immediately and all three ran to the scene of the crime. On the way, Marya Kondratyevna remembered that at about eight o'clock she had heard a dreadful and piercing scream from their garden, and this was no doubt Grigory's scream, "Parricide!" uttered when he caught hold of Mitya's leg with his hands, Mitya then being astride the fence.

"Some one screamed out and then was silent," Marya Kondratyevna explained as she ran. Running to the place where Grigory lay, the two women with the help of Foma carried him to the lodge. They lighted a candle and saw that Smerdyakov was no better, that he was writhing in convulsions, his eyes fixed in a squint, and that foam was flowing from his lips. They moistened Grigory's forehead with water mixed with vinegar, and the water revived him at once. He asked immediately:

"Is the master murdered?"

Then Foma and both the women ran to the house and saw this time that not only the window, but also the door into the garden was wide open, though Fyodor Pavlovich had for the last week locked himself in every night and did not allow even Grigory to come in on any pretext. Seeing that door open, they were afraid to go in to Fyodor Pavlovich "for fear anything should happen afterwards." And when they returned to Grigory, the old man told them to go straight to the police captain. Marya Kondratyevna ran there and gave the alarm to the whole party at the police captain's. She arrived only five minutes before Pyotr Ilyich, so that his story came, not as his own surmise and theory, but as the direct confirmation, by a witness, of the theory held by all, as to the identity of the criminal (a theory he had at the bottom of his heart refused to believe till that moment).

It was resolved to act energetically. The deputy police inspector of the town was immediately commissioned to take four witnesses, and they entered Fyodor Pavlovich's house and there opened an inquiry on the spot, according to the regular forms, which I will not go into here. The district doctor, a zealous man, new to his work, almost insisted on accompanying the police captain, the prosecutor, and the examining magistrate.

I will note briefly that Fyodor Pavlovich was found to be quite dead, with his head broken. But by what? Most likely with the same weapon with which Grigory had been attacked later. And immediately that weapon was found, Grigory, to whom all possible medical assistance was at once given, described in a weak and breaking voice how he had been knocked down. They began looking with a lantern by the fence and found the brass pestle dropped in a most conspicuous place on the garden path. There were no signs of disturbance in the room where Fyodor Pavlovich was lying. But by the bed, behind the screen, they picked up from the floor a big and thick envelope with the inscription: "A present of three thousand roubles for my angel Grushenka, if she will wish to come to me." And below had been added by Fyodor Pavlovich, "For my little chick." There were three big seals made with red sealing-wax on the envelope, but it had been torn open and was empty: the money had been removed. They found also on the floor a piece of narrow pink ribbon, with which the envelope had been tied up.

One piece of Pyotr Ilyich's evidence made a great impression on the prosecutor and the examining magistrate, namely, his idea that Dmitri Fyodorovich would shoot himself at daybreak, that he had resolved to do so, had spoken of it to Pyotr Ilyich, had taken the pistols, loaded them before him, written a note, put it in his pocket, etc., that when Pyotr Ilyich, though still unwilling to believe in it, had threatened to tell some one so as to prevent the suicide, Mitya had answered grinning: "You'll be too late." So they must make haste to Mokroye to catch the criminal, before he really did shoot himself.

"That's clear, that's clear!" repeated the prosecutor in great excitement. "That's just the way with mad fellows like that: 'I shall kill myself to-morrow, so I'll make merry before I die!' " The story of how he had bought the wine and provisions excited the prosecutor more than ever.

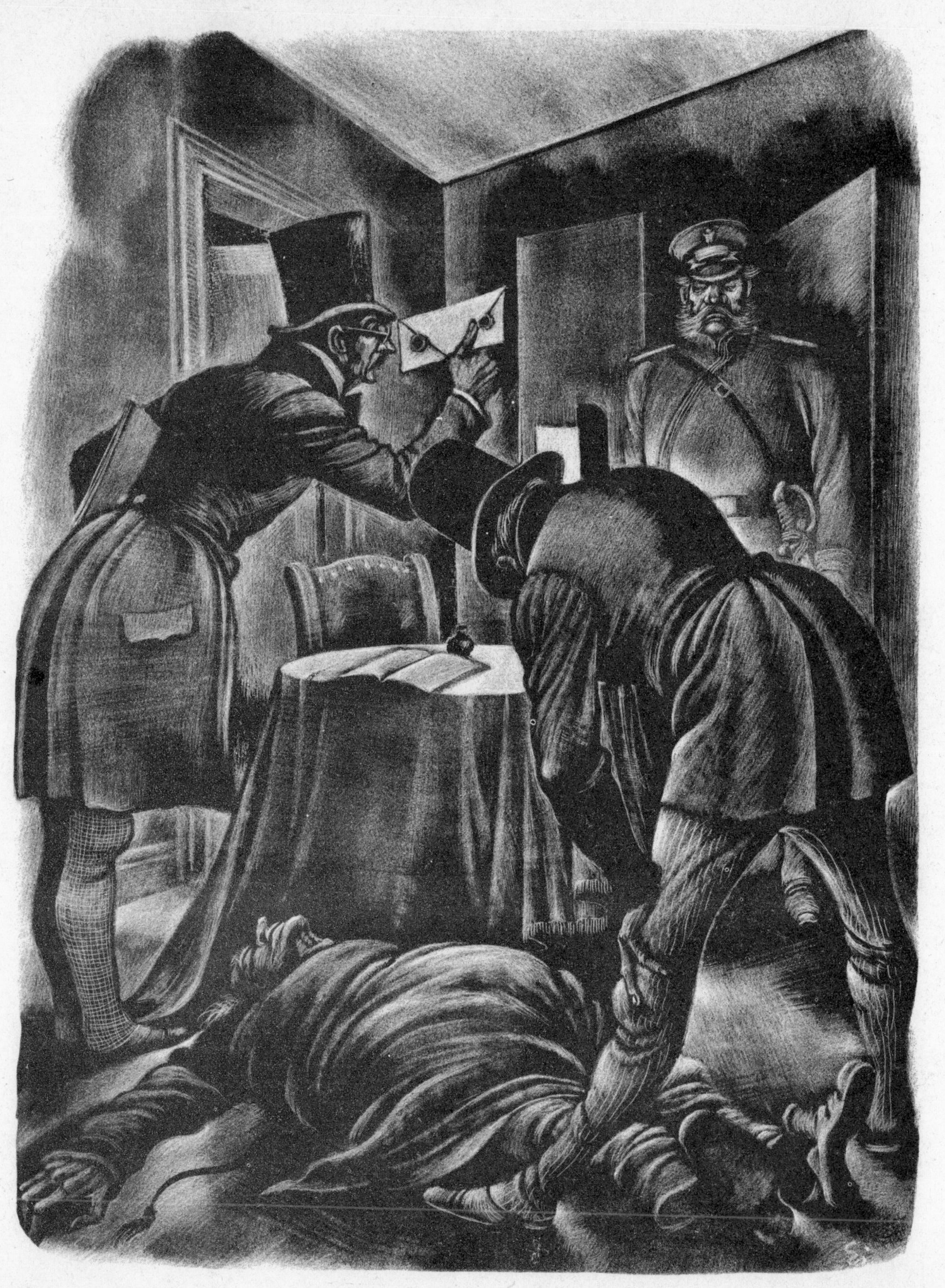

QUITE DEAD, WITH HIS HEAD BROKEN

"Do you remember the fellow that murdered a merchant called Olsufyev, gentlemen? He stole fifteen hundred, went at once to have his hair curled, and then, without even hiding the money, carrying it almost in his hand in the same way, he went off to the girls."

All were delayed, however, by the inquiry, the search, and the formalities, etc., in the house of Fyodor Pavlovich. It all took time and so, two hours before starting, they sent on ahead to Mokroye the officer of the rural police, Mavriky Mavrikyevich Shmertsov, who had arrived in the town the morning before to get his salary. He was instructed to avoid raising the alarm when he reached Mokroye, but to keep constant watch over the "criminal" till the arrival of the proper authorities, also to procure witnesses for the arrest, police constables, and so on. Mavriky Mavrikyevich did as he was told, preserving his incognito, and partly initiating only his old acquaintance, Trifon Borisovich, into the secret. He had spoken to him just before Mitya met the innkeeper on the balcony, looking for him in the dark, and noticed at once a change in Trifon Borisovich's face and voice. So neither Mitya nor any one else knew that he was being watched. The box with the pistols had been carried off by Trifon Borisovich and tucked away in a suitable place. Only after four o'clock, almost at sunrise, all the officials, the police captain, the prosecutor, the examining magistrate, drove up in two carriages, each drawn by three horses. The doctor remained at Fyodor Pavlovich's to make a post-mortem next day on the body. But he was particularly interested in the condition of the servant, Smerdyakov.

"Such violent and protracted epileptic fits, recurring continually for forty-eight hours, are rarely to be met with, and are of interest to science," he declared enthusiastically to his companions, and, as they left, they laughingly congratulated him on his find. The prosecutor and the examining magistrate distinctly remembered the doctor's saying that Smerdyakov could not outlive the night.

After these long, but, I think, necessary explanations, we return to that moment of our tale at which we broke off in the previous book.

CHAPTER III

THE SUFFERINGS OF A SOUL IN THE PLACE OF TORMENTS. THE FIRST ORDEAL

AND so Mitya sat looking wildly at the people round him, not understanding what was said to him. Suddenly he got up, flung up his hands and shouted aloud:

"I'm not guilty! I'm not guilty of that blood! I'm not guilty of my father's blood. . . . I meant to kill him. But I'm not guilty. Not I."

But he had hardly said this, before Grushenka rushed from behind the curtain and flung herself at the police captain's feet.

"It was my fault! Mine! My wickedness!" she cried, in a heart-rending voice, bathed in tears, stretching out her clasped hands towards them. "He did it through me. I tortured him and drove him to it. I tortured that poor old man that's dead, too, in my wickedness, and brought him to this! It's my fault, mine first, mine most, my fault!"

"Yes, you're the guilty one! You're the chief criminal! You're a fury! You're a loose woman! You're the most to blame!" shouted the police captain threatening her with his hand. But he was quickly and resolutely suppressed.

The prosecutor went so far as to restrain him with his arms.

"This is absolutely irregular, Mihail Makarovich!" he cried. "You are positively hindering the inquiry. . . . You're ruining the case . . ." he almost gasped.

"Take measures! Take measures!" cried Nikolay Parfenovich, fearfully excited, too, "otherwise it's absolutely impossible! . . ."

"Try us together!" Grushenka cried frantically, still kneeling. "Punish us together. I will go with him now, if it's to death!"

"Grusha, my life, my blood, my holy one!" Mitya fell on his knees beside her and held her tight in his arms. "Don't believe her," he cried, "she's not guilty of anything, of any blood, of anything!"

He remembered afterwards that he was forcibly dragged away from her by several men, and that she was led out, and that when he recovered himself he was sitting at the table. Beside him and behind him stood the men with metal badges. Facing him on the other side of the table sat Nikolay Parfenovich, the examining magistrate. He kept persuading him to drink a little water out of a glass that stood on the table.

"That will refresh you, that will calm you. Be calm, don't be frightened," he added, with extreme politeness. Mitya (he remembered it afterwards) became suddenly intensely interested in his big rings, one with an amethyst, and another with a transparent bright yellow stone, of great brilliance. And long afterwards he remembered with wonder how those rings had riveted his attention through all those terrible hours of interrogation, so that he was utterly unable to tear himself away from them and dismiss them, as things that had nothing to do with his position. On Mitya's left side, in the place where Maximov had been sitting at the beginning of the evening, the prosecutor was now seated, and on Mitya's right hand, where Grushenka had been, was a rosy-cheeked young man in a sort of shabby hunting jacket, with ink and paper before him. This was the secretary of the examining magistrate, who had brought him along. The police captain was now standing by the window at the other end of the room, beside Kalganov, who was sitting there.

"Have some water," said the examining magistrate softly, for the tenth time.

"I have had it, gentlemen, I have . . . but . . . come, gentlemen, crush me, punish me, decide my fate!" cried Mitya, staring with terribly fixed wide-open eyes at the investigating lawyer.

"So you positively declare that you are not guilty of the death of your father, Fyodor Pavlovich?" asked the examining magistrate softly but insistently.

"I am not guilty. I am guilty of the blood of another old man, but not of my father's. And I weep for it! I killed, I killed the old man and knocked him down. . . . But it's hard to have to answer for that murder with another, a terrible murder of which I am not guilty. . . . It's a terrible accusation, gentlemen, a knock-down blow. But who has killed my father, who has killed him? Who can have killed him if I didn't? It's miraculous, extraordinary, impossible."

"Yes, who can have killed him?" the examining magistrate was beginning, but Ippolit Kirillovich, the prosecutor, glancing at him, addressed Mitya.

"You need not worry yourself about the old servant, Grigory Vasilyevich. He is alive, he has recovered, and in spite of the terrible blows inflicted by you, according to his own and your statements, there seems no doubt that he will live, so the doctor says, at least."

"Alive? He's alive?" cried Mitya, striking his hands together. His face beamed. "Lord, I thank Thee for the miracle Thou hast wrought for me, a sinner and evil-doer. That's an answer to my prayer. I've been praying all night." And he crossed himself three times. He was almost choking.

"So from this Grigory we have received such important evidence concerning you, that . . ." The prosecutor would have continued, but Mitya suddenly jumped up from his chair.

"One minute, gentlemen, for God's sake, one minute; I will run to her ——"

"Excuse me, at this moment it's quite impossible," Nikolay Parfenovich almost shrieked. He, too, leapt to his feet. Mitya was seized by the men with the metal badges, but he sat down of his own accord. . . .

"Gentlemen, what a pity! I wanted to see her for one minute only; I wanted to tell her that it has been washed away, it has gone, that blood that was weighing on my heart all night, and that I am not a murderer now! Gentlemen, she is my betrothed!" he said ecstatically and reverently, looking round at them all. "Oh, thank you gentlemen! Oh, in one minute you have given me new life, new heart! . . . That old man used to carry me in his arms, gentlemen. He used to wash me in the tub when I was a baby three years old, abandoned by every one, he was like a father to me! . . ."

"And so you . . ." the examining magistrate began.

"Allow me, gentlemen, allow me one minute more," interposed Mitya, putting his elbows on the table and covering his face with his hands. "Let me have a moment to think, let me breathe, gentlemen. All this is horribly upsetting, horribly. A man is not a drum-head, gentlemen!"

"Take a little more water," murmured Nikolay Parfenovich.

Mitya took his hands from his face and laughed. His eyes were confident. He seemed completely transformed in a moment. His whole bearing was changed; he was once more the equal of these men, with all of whom he was acquainted, as though they had all met the day before, when nothing had happened, at some social gathering. We may note in passing that, on his first arrival, Mitya had been made very welcome at the police captain's, but later, during the last month especially, Mitya had hardly called at all, and when the police captain met him, in the street, for instance, Mitya noticed that he frowned and only bowed out of politeness. His acquaintance with the prosecutor was less intimate, though he sometimes paid his wife, a nervous and fanciful lady, visits of courtesy, without quite knowing why, and she always received him graciously and had, for some reason, taken an interest in him up to the last. He had not had time to get to know the examining magistrate, though he had met him and talked to him twice, each time about the fair sex.

"You're a most skilful examiner, I see, Nikolay Parfenovich," cried Mitya, laughing gaily, "but I can help you now. Oh, gentlemen, I feel like a new man, and don't be offended at my addressing you so simply and directly. I'm rather drunk, too, I'll tell you that frankly. I believe I've had the honour and pleasure of meeting you, Nikolay Parfenovich, at my kinsman Miusov's. Gentlemen, gentlemen, I don't pretend to be on equal terms with you. I understand, of course, in what character I am sitting before you. Oh, of course, there's a horrible suspicion . . . hanging over me . . . if Grigory has given evidence. . . . A horrible suspicion! It's awful, awful, I understand that! But to business, gentlemen, I am ready, and we will make an end of it in one moment; for, listen, listen, gentlemen! Since I know I'm innocent, we can put an end to it in a minute. Can't we? Can't we?"

Mitya spoke much and quickly, nervously and effusively, as though he positively took his listeners to be his best friends.

"So, for the present, we will write that you absolutely deny the charge brought against you," said Nikolay Parfenovich, impressively, and bending down to the secretary he dictated to him in an undertone what to write.

"Write it down? You want to write that down? Well, write it; I consent, I give my full consent, gentlemen, only . . . do you see . . . Stay, stay, write this. Of disorderly conduct he is guilty, of beating up a poor old man he is guilty. And there is something else at the bottom of my heart, of which I am guilty, too — but that you need not write down" (he turned suddenly to the secretary); "that's my personal life, gentlemen, that doesn't concern you, the bottom of my heart, that's to say. . . . But of the murder of my old father I'm not guilty. That's a wild idea. It's quite a wild idea! . . . I will prove it to you and you'll be convinced instantly. . . . You will laugh, gentlemen. You'll laugh yourself at your suspicion! . . ."

"Be calm, Dmitri Fyodorovich," said the examining magistrate, evidently trying to allay Mitya's excitement by his own composure. "Before we go on with our inquiry, I should like, if you will consent to answer, to hear you confirm the statement that you disliked your father, Fyodor Pavlovich, that you were involved in continual disputes with him. Here at least, a quarter of an hour ago, you exclaimed that you wanted to kill him: 'I didn't kill him,' you said, 'but I wanted to kill him'?"

"Did I say that? Ach, that may be so, gentlemen! Yes, unhappily, I did want to kill him . . . many times I wanted to . . . unhappily, unhappily!"

"You wanted to. Would you consent to explain what motives precisely led you to such a sentiment of hatred for the person of your parent?"

"What is there to explain, gentlemen?" Mitya shrugged his shoulders sullenly, looking down. "I have never concealed my feelings. All the town knows about it — every one knows in the tavern. Only lately I declared them in Father Zosima's cell at the monastery. . . . And the very same day, in the evening I beat my father. I nearly killed him, and I swore I'd come again and kill him, before witnesses. . . . Oh, a thousand witnesses! I've been shouting it aloud for the last month, any one can tell you that! . . . The fact stares you in the face, it speaks for itself, it cries aloud, but, feelings, gentlemen, feelings are another matter. You see, gentlemen" (Mitya frowned), "it seems to me that about feelings you've no right to question me. I know that you are invested with power, I quite understand that, but that's my affair, my private, intimate affair, yet . . . since I haven't concealed my feelings in the past . . . in the tavern, for instance, I've talked to every one, so . . . so I won't make a secret of it now. You see, I understand, gentlemen, that there is terrible evidence against me in this case. I told every one

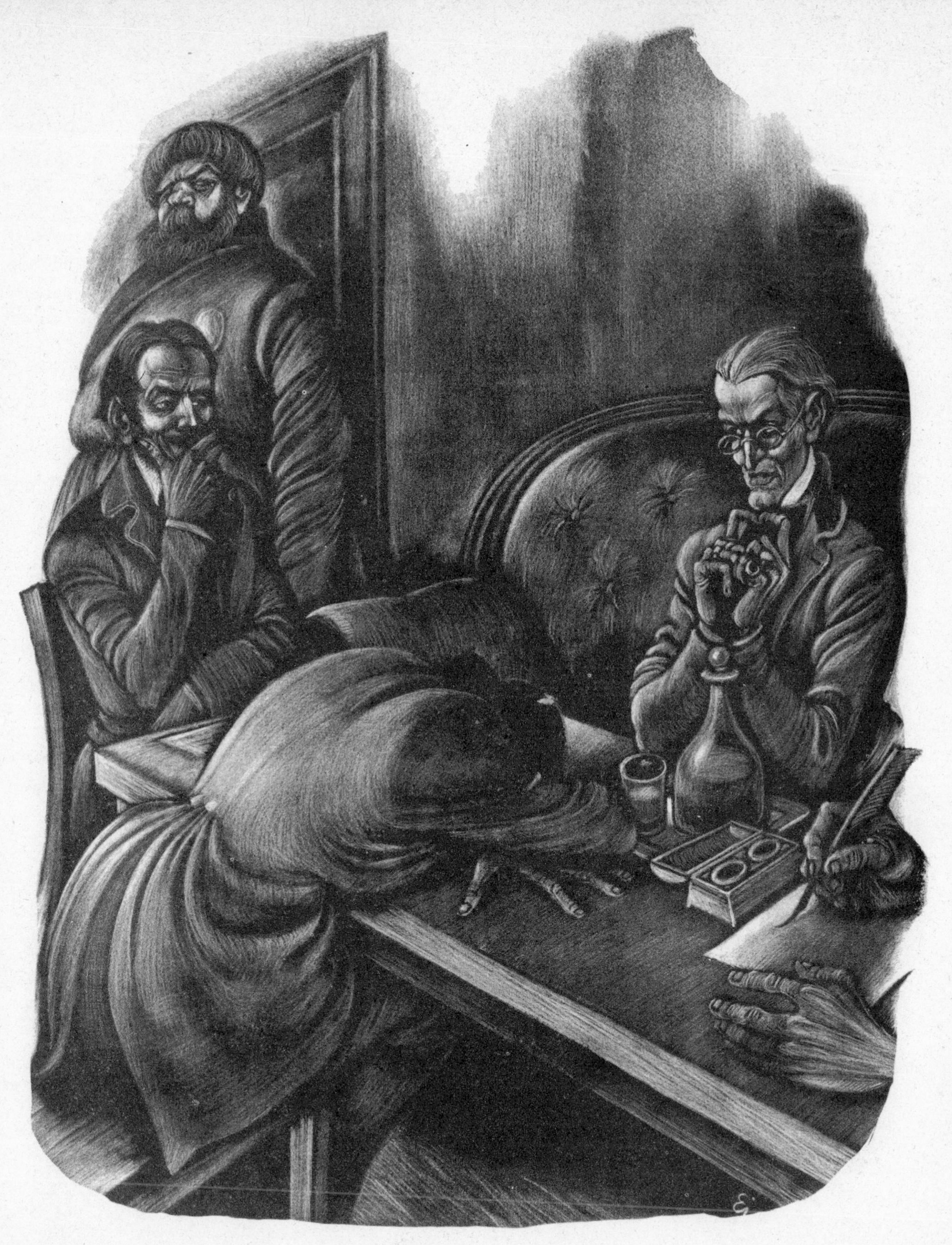

THE FIRST ORDEAL

that I'd kill him, and now, all of a sudden, he's been killed. So it must have been I! Ha, ha! I can make allowances for you, gentlemen, I can quite make allowances. I'm struck all of a heap myself, for who can have murdered him, if not I? That's what it comes to, isn't it? If not I, who can it be, who? Gentlemen, I want to know, I insist on knowing!" he exclaimed suddenly. "Where was he murdered? How was he murdered? How, and with what? Tell me," he asked quickly, looking at the two magistrates.

"We found him in his study, lying on his back on the floor, with his head broken," said the prosecutor.

"That's horrible, gentlemen!" Mitya shuddered and, putting his elbows on the table, hid his face in his right hand.

"We will continue," interposed Nikolay Parfenovich. "So what was it that impelled you to this sentiment of hatred? You have asserted in public, I believe, that it was based upon jealousy?"

"Well, yes, jealousy. And not only jealousy."

"Disputes about money?"

"Yes, about money, too."

"There was a dispute about three thousand roubles, I think, which you claimed as part of your inheritance?"

"Three thousand! More, more," cried Mitya hotly; "more than six thousand, more than ten, perhaps. I told every one so, shouted it at them. But I made up my mind to let it go at three thousand. I was desperately in need of that three thousand . . . so the bundle of notes for three thousand that I knew he kept under his pillow, ready for Grushenka, I considered as simply stolen from me. Yes, gentlemen, I looked upon it as mine, as my own property. . . ." The prosecutor looked significantly at the examining magistrate, and had time to wink at him on the sly.

"We will return to that subject later," said the examining magistrate promptly. "You will allow us to note that point and write it down; that you looked upon that money in the envelope as your own property?"

"Write it down, by all means. I know that's another fact that tells against me, but I'm not afraid of evidence and I give it against myself. Do you hear? Do you know, gentlemen, you take me for a different sort of man from what I am," he added, suddenly, gloomy and dejected. "You have to deal with a man of honour, a man of the highest honour; above all — don't lose sight of it — a man who's done a lot of nasty things, but has always been, and still is, honourable at bottom, in his inner being. I don't know how to express it. That's just what's made me wretched all my life, that I yearned to be honourable, that I was, so to say, a martyr to a sense of honour, seeking for it with a lantern, with the lantern of Diogenes, and yet all my life I've been doing filthy things like all of us, gentlemen . . . that is like me alone. That was a mistake, like me alone, me alone! . . . Gentlemen, my head aches. . . ." His brows contracted with pain. "You see, gentlemen, I couldn't bear the look of him, there was something in him ignoble, impudent, trampling on everything sacred, something sneering and irreverent, loathsome, loathsome. But now that he's dead, I feel differently."

"How do you mean?"

"I don't feel differently, but I wish I hadn't hated him so."

"You feel penitent?"

"No, not penitent, don't write that. I'm not much good myself, I'm not very beautiful, so I had no right to consider him repulsive. That's what I mean. Write that down, if you like."

Saying this Mitya became very mournful. He had grown more and more gloomy as the inquiry continued.

At that moment another unexpected scene followed. Though Grushenka had been removed, she had not been taken far away, only into the room next but one from the blue room, in which the examination was proceeding. It was a little room with one window, next beyond the large room in which they had danced and feasted so lavishly. She was sitting there with no one by her but Maximov, who was terribly bewildered, terribly scared, and clung to her side, as though for security. At their door stood one of the peasants with a metal badge on his breast. Grushenka was crying, and suddenly her grief was too much for her, she jumped up, flung up her arms, and with a loud wail of sorrow rushed out of the room to him, to her Mitya, and so unexpectedly that they had not time to stop her. Mitya, hearing her cry, trembled, jumped up, and with a yell rushed impetuously to meet her, not knowing what he was doing. But they were not allowed to come together, though they saw one another. He was seized by the arms. He struggled, and tried to tear himself away. It took three or four men to hold him. She was seized, too, and he saw her stretching out her arms to him, crying aloud as they carried her away. When the scene was over, he came to himself again, sitting in the same place as before, opposite the examining magistrate, and crying out to them:

"What do you want with her? Why do you torment her? She's innocent, innocent! . . ."

The magistrates tried to soothe him. About ten minutes passed like this. At last Mihail Makarovich, who had been absent, came hurriedly into the room, and said in a loud and excited voice to the prosecutor:

"She's been removed, she's downstairs. Will you allow me to say one word to this unhappy man, gentlemen? In your presence, gentlemen, in your presence."

"By all means, Mihail Makarovich," answered the examining magistrate. "In the present case we have nothing against it."

"Listen, Dmitri Fyodorovich, my dear fellow," began the police captain, and there was a look of warm, almost fatherly, compassion for the luckless man on his excited face. "I took your Agrafena Alexandrovna downstairs myself, and confided her to the care of the innkeeper's daughters, and that old fellow Maximov is with her all the time. And I soothed her, do you hear? I soothed and calmed her. I impressed on her that you have to clear yourself, so she mustn't hinder you, must not depress you, or you may lose your head and say the wrong thing in your evidence. In fact, I talked to her and she understood. She's a sensible girl, my boy, a good-hearted girl, she would have kissed my old hands, begging help for you. She sent me herself, to tell you not to worry about her. And I must go, my dear fellow, I must go and tell her that you are calm and comforted about her. And so you must be calm, do you understand? I was unfair to her; she is a Christian soul, gentlemen, yes, I tell you, she's a gentle soul, and not to blame for anything. So what am I to tell her, Dmitri Fyodorovich, will you sit quietly or not?"

The good-natured police captain said a great deal that was irregular, but Grushenka's suffering, a fellow creature's suffering, had touched his good-natured heart, and tears stood in his eyes. Mitya jumped up and rushed towards him.

"Forgive me, gentlemen, oh, allow me, allow me!" he cried. "You've the heart of an angel, an angel, Mihail Makarovich, I thank you for her. I will, I will be calm, cheerful, in fact. Tell her, in the measureless kindness of your heart, that I am cheerful, quite cheerful, that I shall be laughing in a minute, knowing that she has a guardian angel like you. I shall have done with all this directly, and as soon as I'm free, I'll be with her, she'll see, let her wait. Gentlemen," he said, turning to the two lawyers, "now I'll open my whole soul to you; I'll pour out everything. We'll finish this off directly, finish it off gaily. We shall laugh at it in the end, shan't we? But gentlemen, that woman is the queen of my heart. Oh, let me tell you that. That one thing I'll tell you now. . . . I see I'm with most honourable men. She is my light, she is my holy one, and if only you knew! Did you hear her cry, 'I'll go to death with you'? And what have I, a penniless beggar, done for her? Why such love for me? How can a clumsy, ugly brute like me, with my ugly face, deserve such love, that she is ready to go to exile with me? And how she fell down at your feet for my sake, just now! . . . and yet she's proud and has done nothing! How can I help adoring her, how can I help crying out and rushing to her as I did just now? Gentlemen, forgive me! But now, now I am comforted."

And he sank back in his chair and, covering his face with his hands, burst into tears. But they were happy tears. He recovered himself instantly. The old police captain seemed much pleased, and the lawyers also. They felt that the examination was passing into a new phase.

When the police captain went out, Mitya was positively gay.

"Now, gentlemen, I am at your disposal, entirely at your disposal. And if it were not for all these trivial details, we should understand one another in a minute. I'm at those details again. I'm at your disposal, gentlemen, but I declare that we must have mutual confidence, you in me and I in you, or there'll be no end to it. I speak in your interests. To business, gentlemen, to business, and don't rummage in my soul; don't vex it with trifles, but only ask me about facts and what matters, and I will satisfy you at once. And damn the details!" So spoke Mitya. The interrogation began again.

CHAPTER IV

THE SECOND ORDEAL

"You don't know how you encourage us, Dmitri Fyodorovich, by this readiness of yours," said Nikolay Parfenovich, with an animated air, and obvious satisfaction beaming in his very prominent, short-sighted, light grey eyes, from which he had removed his spectacles a moment before. "And you have made a very just remark about the mutual confidence, without which it is sometimes positively impossible to get on in cases of such importance, if the suspected party really hopes and desires to clear himself and is in a position to do so. We, on our side, will do everything in our power, and you can see for yourself how we are conducting the case. You approve, Ippolit Kirillovich?" He turned to the prosecutor.

"Oh, undoubtedly," replied the prosecutor. His tone was somewhat dry, compared with Nikolay Parfenovich's impulsiveness.

I will note once for all that Nikolay Parfenovich, who had but lately arrived among us, had from the first felt marked respect for Ippolit Kirillovich, our prosecutor, and had become almost his bosom friend. He was almost the only person who put implicit faith in the extraordinary talents as a psychologist and orator of our Ippolit Kirillovich, and who also fully believed that he had been slighted by his superiors. He had heard of him while he was still in Petersburg. On the other hand, young Nikolay Parfenovich was the only person in the whole world whom our "unappreciated" prosecutor genuinely liked. On their way to Mokroye they had time to come to an understanding about the present case. And now as they sat at the table, the sharp-witted junior caught and interpreted every indication on his senior colleague's face, every movement, half a word, a glance, a wink.

"Gentlemen, only let me tell my own story and don't interrupt me with trifles and I'll tell you everything in a jiffy," said Mitya excitedly.

"Excellent! Thank you. But before we proceed to listen to your communication, will you allow me to inquire as to another little fact of great interest to us. I mean the ten roubles you borrowed yesterday at about five o'clock on the security of your pistols, from your friend, Pyotr Ilyich Perhotin."

"I pawned them, gentlemen. I pawned them for ten roubles. What more? That's all about it. As soon as I got back to town I pawned them."

"You got back to town? Then had you been out of town?"

"Yes, I went a journey of forty versts into the country. Didn't you know?"

The prosecutor and Nikolay Parfenovich exchanged glances.

"Well, how would it be if you began your story with a systematic description of all you did yesterday, from the morning onwards? Allow us, for instance, to inquire why you were absent from the town, and just when you left and when you came back — all those facts."

"You should have asked me that from the beginning," cried Mitya, laughing aloud, "and, if you like, we won't begin from yesterday, but from the morning of the day before; then you'll understand how, why, and where I went. I went the day before yesterday, gentlemen, to a merchant of the town, called Samsonov, to borrow three thousand roubles from him on the best security. It was a pressing matter, gentlemen, it was a sudden necessity."

"Allow me to interrupt you," the prosecutor put in politely. "Why were you in such pressing need for just that sum, three thousand?"

"Oh, gentlemen, you needn't go into details, how, when, and why, and why just so much money, and not so much, and all that rigmarole. Why, it'll run to three volumes, and then you'll want an epilogue!"

Mitya said all this with the good-natured but impatient familiarity of a man who is anxious to tell the whole truth and is full of the best intentions.

"Gentlemen!" — he corrected himself hurriedly — "don't be vexed with me for my restiveness, I beg you again. Believe me once more, I feel the greatest respect for you and understand the true position of affairs. Don't think I'm drunk. I'm quite sober now. And, besides, even if I were drunk it would be no hindrance. It's with me, you know, like the saying: 'When he is sober, he is a fool; when he is drunk, he is a wise man.' Ha, ha! But I see, gentlemen, that for the time being it's not the proper thing for me to make jokes before you, till we've had our explanation, I mean. And I've my own dignity to keep up, too. I quite understand the difference for the moment. I come before you, after all, as a criminal, and so am far from being on an equal footing with you. And it's your business to watch me. I can't expect you to pat me on the head for what I did to Grigory, for one can't break old men's heads with impunity. I suppose you'll put me away on his account for six months, or a year perhaps, in a house of correction. I don't know what the punishment is — but it will be without loss of the rights of my rank, without loss of my rank, won't it, prosecutor? So you see, gentlemen, I understand the distinction between us. . . . But you must also admit that you could confuse God Himself with such questions. 'How did you step? Where did you step? When did you step? And on what did you step?' I shall get mixed up, if you go on like this, and you will put it all down against me, black on white. And what will that lead to? To nothing! And even if it's nonsense I'm talking now, let me finish, and you, gentlemen, being men of honour and education, forgive me! I'll finish by asking you, gentlemen, to drop that conventional method of questioning. I mean, beginning from some miserable trifle, how I got up, what I had for breakfast, how I spat, and where I spat, and so having distracted the attention of the criminal, suddenly stun him with an overwhelming question, 'Whom did you murder? Whom did you rob?' Ha, ha! That's your routine method, that's your rule, that's what all your cunning is based on. You can put peasants off their guard like that, but not me. I know the tricks. I've been in the service, too. Ha, ha, ha! You're not angry, gentlemen? You forgive my impertinence?" he cried, looking at them with a good-nature that was almost surprising. "It's only Mitya Karamazov, you know, so you can overlook it. It would be inexcusable in a sensible man; but you can forgive it in Mitya. Ha, ha!"

Nikolay Parfenovich listened, and laughed, too. Though the prosecutor did not laugh, he kept his eyes fixed keenly on Mitya, as though anxious not to miss the least syllable, the slightest movement, the smallest twitch of any feature of his face.

"That's how we have treated you from the beginning," said Nikolay Parfenovich, still laughing. "We haven't tried to put you out by asking how you got up in the morning and what you had for breakfast. We began, indeed, with questions of the greatest importance."

"I understand. I saw it and appreciated it, and I appreciate still more your present kindness to me, an unprecedented kindness, worthy of the noblest souls. We three here are gentlemen, and let everything be on the footing of mutual confidence such as obtains among educated, well-bred people, who have the common bond of noble birth and honour. In any case, allow me to look upon you as my best friends at this moment of my life, at this moment when my honour is humbled. That's no offence to you, gentlemen, is it?"

"On the contrary. You've expressed all that so admirably, Dmitri Fyodorovich," Nikolay Parfenovich answered with dignified approbation.

"And enough of those trivial questions, gentlemen, all those tricky questions!" cried Mitya enthusiastically. "Or there is simply no knowing where we shall get to! Is there?"

"I will follow your sensible advice entirely," the prosecutor interposed, addressing Mitya. "But I don't withdraw my question, however. It is now vitally important for us to know exactly why you needed that sum, I mean precisely three thousand."

"Why I needed it? . . . Oh, for one thing and another. . . . Well, it was to pay a debt."

"A debt to whom?"

"That I absolutely refuse to answer, gentlemen. Not because I couldn't, or because I daren't or because I am afraid, for it's all a paltry matter and absolutely trifling, but — I won't, because it's a matter of principle: that's my private life, and I won't allow any intrusion into my private life. That's my principle. Your question has no bearing on the case, and whatever has nothing to do with the case is my private affair. I wanted to pay a debt. I wanted to pay a debt of honour, but to whom I won't say."

"Allow me to make a note of that," said the prosecutor.

"By all means. Write down that I won't say, that I won't. Write that I should think it dishonourable to say. Ech! you can write it; you've nothing else to do with your time."

"Allow me to caution you, sir, and to remind you once more, if you are unaware of it," the prosecutor began, with a peculiar and stern impressiveness, "that you have a perfect right not to answer the questions put to you now, and we, on our side, have no right to extort an answer from you, if you decline to give it for one reason or another. That is entirely a matter for your personal decision. But it is our duty, on the other hand, in such cases as the present, to explain and set before you the degree of injury you will be doing yourself by refusing to give this or that piece of evidence. After which I will beg you to continue."

"Gentlemen, I'm not angry . . . I . . ." Mitya muttered in a rather disconcerted tone. "Well, gentlemen, you see, that Samsonov to whom I went then . . ."

We will, of course, not reproduce his account of what is known to the reader already. Mitya was impatiently anxious not to omit the slightest detail. At the same time he was in a hurry to get it over. But as he gave his evidence it was written down, and therefore they had continually to pull him up. Mitya disliked this, but submitted; got angry, though still good-humouredly. He did, it is true, exclaim, from time to time, "Gentlemen, this would enrage God Himself!" Or, "Gentlemen, do you know that you're only irritating me to no purpose!"

But even though he exclaimed, he still preserved for a time his genially expansive mood. So he told them how Samsonov had made a fool of him two days before. (He had completely realised by now that he had been fooled.) The sale of his watch for six roubles to obtain money for the journey was something new to the lawyers. They were at once greatly interested, and even, to Mitya's immeasurable indignation, thought it necessary to write the fact down as a secondary confirmation of the circumstance that he had hardly a farthing in his pocket at the time. Little by little Mitya began to grow surly. Then, after describing his journey to see Lyagavy, the night spent in the stifling hut, and so on, he came to his return to the town. Here he began, without being particularly urged, to give a minute account of the agonies of jealousy he endured on Grushenka's account.

He was heard with silent attention. They

inquired particularly into the circumstance of his having established a look-out in Marya Kondratyevna's house at the back of Fyodor Pavlovich's garden to keep watch on Grushenka, and of Smerdyakov's bringing him information. They laid particular stress on this, and noted it down. Of his jealousy he spoke hotly and at length, and though inwardly ashamed at exposing his most intimate feelings, so to speak, to "public ignominy," he evidently overcame his shame in order to tell the truth.

The impersonal severity, with which the examining magistrate, and still more the prosecutor, stared at him as he told his story, disconcerted him at last considerably.

"That boy, Nikolay Parfenovich, to whom I was talking nonsense about women only a few days ago, and that sickly prosecutor are not worth my telling this to," he reflected mournfully. "It's ignominious. 'Be patient, humble, do not speak.' " He wound up his reflections with that line. But he pulled himself together to go on again. When he came to telling of his visit to Madame Hohlakov, he regained his spirits and even wished to tell a little anecdote of that lady which had nothing to do with the case. But the investigating lawyer stopped him, and civilly suggested that he should pass on to "more essential matters." At last, when he described his despair and told them how, when he left Madame Hohlakov's he thought that he'd "get three thousand if he had to murder some one to do it," they stopped him again and noted down that he had "meant to murder some one." Mitya let them write it without protest. At last he reached the point in his story when he learned that Grushenka had deceived him and had returned from Samsonov's as soon as he left her there, though she had said that she would stay with the old man till midnight.

"If I didn't kill Fenya then, gentlemen, it was only because I hadn't time," broke from him suddenly at that point in his story. That, too, was carefully written down. Mitya waited gloomily, and was beginning to tell how he ran into his father's garden when the examining magistrate suddenly stopped him, and opening the big portfolio that lay on the sofa beside him he brought out the brass pestle.

"Do you recognise this object?" he asked, showing it to Mitya.

"Oh, yes." He grinned gloomily. "Of course I recognise it. Let me have a look at it. . . . Damn it, never mind!"

"You have forgotten to mention it," observed the examining magistrate.

"Hang it all, I didn't mean to conceal it from you. Do you suppose I could have told my story without it? It simply escaped my memory."

"Be so good as to tell us precisely how you came to arm yourself with it."

"Certainly I will be so good, gentlemen."

And Mitya described how he took the pestle and ran.

"But what object had you in view in arming yourself with such a weapon?"

"What object? No object. I just picked it up and ran off."

"What for, if you had no object?"

Mitya was boiling with anger. He looked intently at "the boy" and smiled gloomily and viciously. He was feeling more and more ashamed at having told "such people" the story of his jealousy so sincerely and spontaneously.

"Bother the pestle!" broke from him suddenly.

"But still . . ."

"Oh, to keep off dogs. . . . Oh, because it was dark. . . . In case anything turned up."

"But have you ever on previous occasions taken a weapon with you when you went out, since you're afraid of the dark?"

"Ugh! damn it all, gentlemen! There's positively no talking to you!" cried Mitya, exasperated beyond endurance, and turning to the secretary, crimson with anger, he said quickly, with a note of fury in his voice:

"Write down at once . . . at once . . . 'that I snatched up the pestle to go and kill my father . . . Fyodor Pavlovich . . . by hitting him on the head with it!' Well, now are you satisfied, gentlemen? Are your minds relieved?" he said, glaring defiantly at the magistrates.

"We quite understand that you made that statement just now through exasperation with us and the questions we put to you, which you consider trivial, though they are, in fact, essential," the prosecutor remarked drily in reply.

"Well, upon my word, gentlemen! Yes, I took the pestle . . . What does one pick things up for at such moments? I don't know what for. I snatched it up and ran — that's all. Faugh, gentlemen, *passons*, or I declare I'll stop talking."

He put his elbows on the table and rested his head on his hands. He sat sideways to them and gazed at the wall, struggling against an evil feeling. He had, in fact, an intense inclination to get up and declare that he wouldn't say another word, "not if you hang me for it."

"You see, gentlemen," he said at last, with difficulty controlling himself, "you see. I listen to you and am haunted by a dream. . . . It's a dream I have sometimes, you know. . . . I often dream it — it's always the same . . . that some one is chasing me, some one I'm awfully afraid of . . . that he's chasing me in the dark, in the night . . . tracking me, and I hide somewhere from him, behind a door or cupboard, hide in a degrading way, and the worst of it is, he always knows where I am, but he pretends not to know where I am on purpose, to prolong my agony, to enjoy my terror. . . . That's just what you're doing now. It's just like that!"

"Is that the sort of thing you dream about?" inquired the prosecutor.

"Yes, it is. Don't you want to write it down?" said Mitya, with a distorted smile.

"No; no need to write it down. But still you do have curious dreams."

"It's not a question of dreams now — this is realism, gentlemen, the realism of actual life! I'm a wolf and you're the hunters. Well, hunt him down!"

"You are wrong to make such comparisons . . ." began Nikolay Parfenovich, with extraordinary softness.

"No, I'm not wrong, gentlemen, not at all!" Mitya flared up again, though his outburst of wrath had obviously relieved his heart. He grew more good-humoured at every word. "You may not trust a criminal or a man on trial tortured by your questions, but an honourable man, the honourable impulses of the heart (I say that boldly!) — no! That you cannot disbelieve, you have no right indeed . . . but —

Be silent, heart,
Be patient, humble, do not speak.

Well, shall I go on?" he broke off gloomily.

"If you'll be so kind," answered Nikolay Parfenovich.

CHAPTER V

THE THIRD ORDEAL

THOUGH Mitya spoke sullenly, it was evident that he was trying more than ever not to forget or miss a single detail of his story. He told them how he had leapt over the fence into his father's garden; how he had gone up to the window; told them all that had passed at the window. Clearly, precisely, distinctly, he described the feelings that troubled him during those moments in the garden when he longed so terribly to know whether Grushenka was with his father or not. But, strange to say, both the lawyers listened now with a sort of awful reserve, looked coldly at him, asked few questions. Mitya could gather nothing from their faces.

"They're angry and offended," he thought. "Well, devil take them!"

When he told how he had made up his mind at last to make the "signal" to his father that Grushenka had come, so that he should open the window, the lawyers paid no attention to the word "signal," as though they entirely failed to grasp the meaning of the word in this connection: so much so, that Mitya noticed it. Coming at last to the moment when, seeing his father peering out of the window, his hatred flared up and he pulled the pestle out of his pocket, he suddenly, as though of design, stopped short. He sat gazing at the wall and was aware that their eyes were fixed upon him.

"Well?" said the examining magistrate. "You pulled out the weapon and . . . and what happened then?"

"Then? Why, then I murdered him . . . hit him on the head and cracked his skull. . . . I suppose that's your story. That's it!"

His eyes suddenly flashed. All his smothered wrath suddenly flamed up with extraordinary violence in his soul.

"Our story?" repeated Nikolay Parfenovich. "Well — and yours?"

Mitya dropped his eyes and was silent a long time.

"My story, gentlemen? Well, it was like this," he began softly. "Whether it was some one's tears, or my mother prayed to God, or a good angel kissed me at that instant, I don't know. But the devil was conquered. I rushed from the window and ran to the fence. My father was alarmed and then, for the first time, he saw me, cried out, and sprang back from the window. I remember that very well. I ran across the garden to the fence . . . and it was there that Grigory reached me, when I was sitting on the fence."

At that point he raised his eyes at last and looked at his listeners. They seemed to be staring at him with perfectly unruffled attention. A sort of paroxysm of indignation seized on Mitya's soul.

"Why, you're laughing at me at this moment, gentlemen!" he broke off suddenly.

"What makes you think that?" observed Nikolay Parfenovich.

"You don't believe one word — that's why! I understand, of course, that I have come to the vital point. The old man's lying there now with his skull broken, while I — after dramatically describing how I wanted to kill him, and how I snatched up the pestle — I suddenly run away from the window. An epic! In verse! As though one could take a fellow's word for it. Ha, ha! You are making game of me, gentlemen!" And he swung round on his chair so that it creaked.

"And did you notice," asked the prosecutor suddenly, as though not observing Mitya's excitement, "did you notice when you ran away from the window, whether the door into the garden, that is, the door at the other end of the wing, was open or not?"

"No, it was not open."

"It was not?"

"It was shut. And who could open it? Bah! the door. Wait a bit!" He seemed suddenly to bethink himself, and almost with a start:

"Why, did you find the door open?"

"Yes, it was open."

"Why, who could have opened it if you did not open it yourselves?" cried Mitya, tremendously astonished.

"The door stood open, and your father's murderer undoubtedly went in at that door, and, having accomplished the crime, went out again by the same door," the prosecutor pronounced deliberately, as though marking each word separately. "That is perfectly clear to us. The murder was apparently committed in the room and *not through the window;* that is absolutely certain from the examination that has been made, from the position of the body, and everything. There can be no doubt of that circumstance."

Mitya was absolutely dumbfounded.

"But that's utterly impossible!" he cried, completely at a loss. "I . . . I didn't go in. . . . I tell you positively, definitely, the door was shut the whole time I was in the garden, and when I ran out of the garden. I only stood at the window and saw him through the window. That's all, that's all. . . . I remember to the last minute. And if I didn't remember, it would be just the same. I know it, for no one knew the signals except Smerdyakov, and me, and the deceased. And he wouldn't have opened the door to any one in the world without the signals."

"Signals? What signals?" asked the prosecutor, with greedy, almost hysterical, curiosity. He instantly lost all trace of his reserve and dignity. He asked the question with a sort of cringing timidity. He scented an important fact of which he had known nothing, and was already filled with dread that Mitya might be unwilling to disclose it.

"So you didn't know!" Mitya winked at him with a malicious and mocking smile. "What if I won't tell you? From whom could you find out? No one knew about the signals except the deceased, myself, and Smerdyakov: that was all. Heaven knew, too, but it won't tell you. And the fact is a curious one. There's no knowing what you might build on it. Ha, ha! Take comfort, gentlemen, I'll reveal it. You've some foolish idea in your heads. You don't know the man you have to deal with! You have to do with a prisoner who gives evidence against himself, to his own damage! Yes, for I'm a man of honour and you — are not."

The prosecutor swallowed these pills without a murmur. He was trembling with impatience to learn the new fact. Fully and precisely, Mitya told them everything about the signals invented by Fyodor Pavlovich for Smerdyakov. He told them exactly what every tap on the window meant, tapped the signals on the table, and when Nikolay Parfenovich said that he supposed he, Mitya, had tapped the signal "Grushenka has come," when he tapped to his father, he answered precisely that he had tapped that signal, that "Grushenka had come."

"So now you can build up your tower," Mitya broke off, and again turned away from them contemptuously.

"So no one knew of the signals but your deceased parent, you, and the servant Smerdyakov? And no one else?" Nikolay Parfenovich inquired once more.

"Yes. The servant Smerdyakov, and heaven. Write down about heaven. That may be of use. Besides, you will need God yourselves."

And they had already, of course, begun writing it down. But while they wrote, the prosecutor said abruptly, as though suddenly stumbling on a new idea:

"But if Smerdyakov also knew of these signals and you absolutely deny the charge of having caused the death of your parent, was it not he, perhaps, who knocked the signal agreed upon, induced your father to open to him, and then . . . committed the crime?"

Mitya turned upon him a look of profound irony and intense hatred. His silent stare lasted so long that it made the prosecutor blink.

"You've caught the fox again," commented Mitya at last; "you've got the beast by the tail. Ha, ha! I see through you, Mr. Prosecutor. You thought, of course, that I should jump at that, catch at your prompting, and shout with all my might, 'Aie, it's Smerdyakov; he's the murderer.' Confess that's what you thought. Confess, and I'll go on."

But the prosecutor did not confess. He held his tongue and waited.

"You're mistaken. I'm not going to shout 'It's Smerdyakov,'" said Mitya.

"And you don't even suspect him?"

"Why, do you suspect him?"

"He was suspected, too."

Mitya fixed his eyes on the floor.

"Joking apart," he brought out gloomily. "Listen. From the very beginning, almost from the moment when I ran out to you from behind the curtain, I've had the thought of Smerdyakov in my mind. I've been sitting here, shouting that I'm innocent and thinking all the time 'Smerdyakov!' I can't get Smerdyakov out of my head. In fact, I, too, thought of Smerdyakov just now; but only for a second. Almost at once I thought, 'No, it's not Smerdyakov.' It's not his doing, gentlemen."

"In that case is there anybody else you suspect?" Nikolay Parfenovich inquired cautiously.

"I don't know any one it could be, whether it's the hand of heaven or of Satan, but . . . not Smerdyakov," Mitya snapped firmly.

"But what makes you affirm so confidently and emphatically that it's not he?"

"From my conviction — my impression. Because Smerdyakov is a man of the lowest sort and a coward. He's not a coward, he's the epitome of all the cowardice in the world walking on two legs. He was born of a chicken. When he talked to me, he was always trembling for fear I should kill him, though I never raised my hand against him. He fell at my feet and blubbered; he has kissed these very boots, literally, beseeching me 'not to frighten him.' Do you hear? 'Not to frighten him.' What a thing to say! Why, I gave him presents. He's a sickly chicken — epileptic, weak-minded — a boy of eight could thrash him. He has no character worth talking about. It's not Smerdyakov, gentlemen. Besides, he doesn't even care for money; he wouldn't take my presents. Besides, why should he murder the old man? Why, he's very likely his son, you know — his natural son. Do you know that?"

"We have heard that legend. But you are your father's son, too; yet you yourself told every one you wanted to murder him."

"That's a thrust! And a nasty, mean one, too! I'm not afraid! Oh, gentlemen, isn't it too base of you to say that to my face? It's base, because I told you that myself. I not only wanted to murder him, but I might have done it. And, what's more, I went out of my way to tell you of my own accord that I nearly murdered him. But, you see, I didn't murder him; you see, my guardian angel saved me — that's what you've not taken into account. And that's why it's so base of you. For I didn't kill him, I didn't kill him! Do you hear, Mr. Prosecutor, I did not kill."

He was almost choking. He had not been so agitated before during the whole interrogation.

"And what has he told you, gentlemen — Smerdyakov, I mean?" he added suddenly, after a pause. "May I ask that question?"

"You may ask any question," the prosecutor replied with frigid severity, "any question relating to the facts of the case, and we are, I repeat, bound to answer every inquiry you make. We found the servant Smerdyakov, concerning whom you inquire, lying unconscious in his bed, in an epileptic fit of extreme severity, that had recurred, possibly, ten times. The doctor who was with us told us, after seeing him, that he may possibly not outlive the night."

"Well, in that case, the devil must have killed father," broke suddenly from Mitya, as though until that moment he had been asking himself: "Was it Smerdyakov or not?"

"We will come back to this later," Nikolay Parfenovich decided. "Now, wouldn't you like to continue your statement?"

Mitya asked for a rest. His request was courteously granted. After resting, he went on with his story. But he was evidently depressed. He was exhausted, mortified, and morally shaken. To make things worse, the prosecutor began to irritate him continually, as though intentionally, by attaching himself to "details." Scarcely had Mitya described how, sitting on the wall, he had struck Grigory on the head with the pestle, while the old man had hold of his left leg, and how he had then jumped down to look at him, when the prosecutor stopped him to ask him to describe in greater detail how he was sitting on the wall. Mitya was astonished.

"Oh, I was sitting like this, astride, one leg on one side and one on the other."

"And the pestle?"

"The pestle was in my hands."

"Not in your pocket? Do you remember that precisely? Was it a hard blow you gave him?"

"It must have been a violent one. But why do you ask?"

"Would you mind sitting on the chair just as you sat on the fence then and showing us just how you swung your arm, and in what direction?"

"Are you making fun of me?" asked Mitya, looking haughtily at the speaker; but the latter did not flinch.

Mitya turned convulsively, sat astride on his chair, and swung his arm.

"This was how I struck him! That's how I knocked him down! What more do you want?"

"Thank you. May I trouble you now to explain why you jumped down, with what object, and what you had in view?"

"Oh, hang it! . . . I jumped down to look at the man I'd hurt . . . I don't know what for!"

"Though you were so excited and were running away?"

"Yes, though I was excited and running away."

"You wanted to help him?"

"Help! . . . Yes, perhaps I did want to help him. . . . I don't remember."

"You don't remember? Then you were in a kind of daze?"

"Oh, no, not at all. I remember everything — every detail. I jumped down to look at him, and wiped his face with my handkerchief."

"We have seen your handkerchief. Did you hope to restore him to consciousness?"

"I don't know whether I hoped it. I simply wanted to make sure whether he was alive or not."

"Ah! You wanted to be sure? Well, what then?"

"I'm not a doctor. I couldn't decide. I ran away thinking I'd killed him. And now he's recovered."

"Excellent," commented the prosecutor. "Thank you. That's all I wanted. Kindly proceed."

Alas! it never entered Mitya's head to tell them, though he remembered it, that he had jumped down out of pity, and standing over the prostrate figure had even uttered some words of regret: "You've come to grief, old man — there's no help for it. Well, there you must lie."

The prosecutor could draw only one conclusion: that the man had jumped down "at such a moment and in such excitement simply with the object of ascertaining whether the *only* witness of his crime were alive or not; and that therefore what must have been the man's strength, coolness, decision, and shrewdness even at such a moment . . ." and so on. The prosecutor was satisfied: "I've provoked the nervous fellow by 'details' and he has said more than he meant to." With painful effort Mitya went on. But this time he was pulled up immediately by Nikolay Parfenovich.

"How came you to run to the servant, Fedosya Markovna, with your hands so covered with blood, and, as it appears, your face, too?"

"Why, I didn't notice the blood at all at the time," answered Mitya.

"That's quite likely. That's how it happens." The prosecutor exchanged glances with Nikolay Parfenovich.

"I simply didn't notice. You're quite right there, prosecutor," Mitya assented suddenly.

Next came the account of Mitya's sudden determination to "step aside" and make way for their happiness. But he could not make up his mind to open up his heart to them as before, and tell them about "the queen of his soul." He disliked speaking of her before these chilly persons "who were nipping at him like bugs." And so in response to their reiterated questions he answered briefly and sharply:

"Well, I made up my mind to kill myself. What had I left to live for? That question stared me in the face. Her first, rightful lover had come back, the man who wronged her but who'd hurried back to offer his love, after five years, and atone for the wrong with marriage. . . . So I knew it was all over for me. . . . And behind me disgrace, and that blood — Grigory's. . . . What had I to live for? So I went to redeem the pistols I had pawned, in order to load them and put a bullet in my brain the next day."

"And a grand feast the night before?"

"Yes, a grand feast the night before. Damn it all, gentlemen! Hurry up and be done with it. I meant to shoot myself not far from here, beyond the village, and I'd planned to do it at five o'clock in the morning. And I had a note in my pocket already. I wrote it at Perhotin's when I loaded my pistols. Here's the note. Read it! It's not for you I tell it," he suddenly added with contempt. He took it from his waistcoat pocket and flung it on the table. The examiners read it with interest, and, as is usual, added it to the papers connected with the case.

"And you didn't even think of washing your hands at Perhotin's? You were not afraid then of arousing suspicion?"

"What suspicion? Suspicion or not, I should have galloped here just the same, and shot myself at five o'clock, and nothing could have been done. If it hadn't been for what's happened to my father, you would have known nothing about it, and wouldn't have come here. Oh, it's the devil's doing. It was the devil murdered father, it was through the devil that you found it out so soon. How did you manage to get here so quick? It's a marvel, a dream!"

"Mr. Perhotin informed us that when you came to him, you held in your hands . . . your blood-stained hands . . . your money . . . a great deal of money . . . a batch of hundred-rouble notes, and that his servant, a boy, saw it, too."

"That's true, gentlemen. I remember it was so."

"Now, there's one little point presents itself. Can you not inform us," Nikolay Parfenovich began, with extreme gentleness, "where you got so much money all of a sudden, when it appears from the facts, and by the reckoning of time, that you had not been home?" The prosecutor's brows contracted at the question being asked so plainly, but he did not interrupt Nikolay Parfenovich.

"No, I didn't go home," answered Mitya, apparently perfectly composed, but looking at the floor.

"Allow me then to repeat my question," Nikolay Parfenovich went on as though creeping along. "Where were you able to procure such a sum all at once, when, by your own confession, at five o'clock the same day you . . ."

"I was in want of ten roubles and pawned my pistols with Perhotin, and then went to Madame Hohlakov to borrow three thousand, which she wouldn't give me, and so on, and all the rest of it," Mitya interrupted sharply. "Yes, gentlemen, I was in want of it, and suddenly thousands turned up, eh? Do you know, gentlemen, you're both afraid now 'what if he won't tell us where he got it?' That's just what will happen. I'm not going to tell you, gentlemen. You've guessed right. You shall not know," Mitya suddenly pronounced, marking each word with extraordinary determination. The lawyers were silent for a moment.

"You must understand, Mr. Karamazov, that it is of vital importance for us to know," said Nikolay Parfenovich, softly and meekly.

"I understand; but still I won't tell you."

The prosecutor, too, intervened, and again reminded him that the prisoner was at liberty to refuse to answer questions, if he thought it to his interest, and so on. But in view of the damage he might do himself by his silence, especially in a case of such importance as . . .

"And so on, gentlemen, and so on. Enough! I've heard that rigmarole before," Mitya interrupted again. "I can see for myself how important it is, and that this is the vital point, and still I won't say."

"What is it to us? It's not our business, but it's yours. You are doing yourself harm," observed Nikolay Parfenovich very nervously.

"You see, gentlemen, joking apart" — Mitya lifted his eyes and looked firmly at them both — "I had an inkling from the first that we should come to loggerheads at this point. But at first when I began to give my evidence, it was all still far away and misty; it was all floating, and I was so simple that I began with the proposition of mutual confidence. Now I can see for myself that such confidence is out of the question, for in any case we were bound to come to this cursed stumbling-block. And now we've come to it! It's impossible and there's an end of it! But I don't blame you. You can't take my word for it. I understand that, of course."

He relapsed into gloomy silence.

"Couldn't you, without abandoning your resolution to be silent about the chief point, could you not, at the same time, give us some slight hint as to the nature of the motives which are strong enough to induce you to refuse to answer, at a point in the investigation which is so full of danger for you?"

Mitya smiled mournfully, almost dreamily.

"I'm much more good-natured than you think, gentlemen, and I'll tell you the reason why and give you that hint, though you don't deserve it. I refuse to speak, gentlemen, because the matter involves a disgrace for me. The answer to the question where I got the money involves me in a far greater disgrace than the murder and robbing of my father, if I had murdered and robbed him. That's why I can't speak. I can't because of the disgrace. What, gentlemen, are you going to write that down?"

"Yes, we'll write it down," lisped Nikolay Parfenovich.

"You ought not to write that down about 'disgrace.' I only told you that in the goodness of my heart. I needn't have told you. I made you a present of it, so to speak, and you pounce upon it at once. Oh, well, write — write what you like," he concluded, with scornful disgust. "I'm not afraid of you and I can still hold up my head before you."

"And can't you tell us the nature of that disgrace?" Nikolay Parfenovich hazarded.

The prosecutor frowned darkly.

"No, no, *c'est fini*, don't trouble yourselves. It's not worth while soiling one's hands. I have soiled myself enough through you as it is. You're not worth it — no one is . . . Enough, gentlemen. I'm not going on."

This was said too peremptorily. Nikolay Parfenovich did not insist further, but from Ippolit Kirillovich's eyes he saw that the latter had not given up hope.

"Can you not, at least, tell us what sum you had in your hands when you went into Mr. Perhotin's — that is, how many roubles exactly?"

"I can't tell you that, either."

"You spoke to Mr. Perhotin, I believe, of having received three thousand from Madame Hohlakov."

"Perhaps I did. Enough, gentlemen. I won't say how much I had."

"Will you be so good then as to tell us how you came here and what you have done since you arrived?"

"Oh! you might ask the people here about that. But I'll tell you if you like."

He proceeded to do so, but we will not repeat his story. He told it drily and rapidly. Of the raptures of his love he said nothing, but told them that he abandoned his determination to shoot himself, owing to "new factors in the case." He told the story without going into motives or details. And this time the lawyers did not worry him much. It was obvious that this was not of essential interest to them.

"We shall verify all that. We will come back to it during the examination of the witnesses, which will, of course, take place in your presence," said Nikolay Parfenovich in conclusion. "And now allow me to request you to lay on the table everything in your possession, especially all the money you still have about you."

"My money, gentlemen? Certainly. I understand that that is necessary. I'm surprised, indeed, that you haven't inquired about it before. It's true I couldn't get away anywhere. I'm sitting here where I can be seen. But here's my money — count it — take it. That's all, I think."

He took everything out of his pockets; even the small change — two twenty-copeck pieces — he pulled out of his waistcoat pocket. They counted the money, which amounted to eight hundred and thirty-six roubles, and forty copecks. "And is that all?" asked the examining magistrate.

"Yes."

"You stated just now in your evidence that you spent three hundred roubles at Plotnikovs'. You gave Perhotin ten, your driver twenty, here you lost two hundred at cards, then . . ."

Nikolay Parfenovich reckoned it all up. Mitya helped him readily. They recollected every farthing and included it in the reckoning. Nikolay Parfenovich hurriedly added up the total. "With this eight hundred you must have had about fifteen hundred at first?"

"I suppose so," snapped Mitya.

"How is it they all assert there was much more?"

"Let them assert it."

"But you asserted it yourself."

"Yes, I did, too."

"We will compare all this with the evidence of other persons not yet examined. Don't be anxious about your money. It will be properly taken care of and be at your disposal at the conclusion of . . . what is beginning . . . if it appears, or, so to speak, is proved that you have undisputed right to it. Well, and now . . ."

Nikolay Parfenovich, suddenly got up, and informed Mitya firmly that it was his duty and obligation to conduct a minute and thorough search "of your clothes and everything else . . ."

"By all means, gentlemen. I'll turn out all my pockets, if you like."

And he did, in fact, begin turning out his pockets.

"It will be necessary to take off your clothes, too."

"What! Strip? Ugh! Damn it! Won't you search me as I am? Can't you?"

"It's utterly impossible, Dmitri Fyodorovich. You must take off your clothes."

"As you like," Mitya submitted gloomily; "only, please, not here, but behind the curtains. Who will search them?"

"Behind the curtains, of course."

Nikolay Parfenovich bent his head in assent. His small face wore an expression of peculiar solemnity.

CHAPTER VI

THE PROSECUTOR CATCHES MITYA

SOMETHING utterly unexpected and amazing to Mitya followed. He could never, even a minute before, have conceived that any one could treat him, Mitya Karamazov, like that.

What was worst of all, there was something humiliating in it, and on their side something "supercilious and contemptuous." It was nothing to take off his coat, but he was asked to undress further, or rather not asked but "commanded," he quite understood that. From pride and contempt he submitted without a word. Several peasants accompanied the lawyers and remained on the same side of the curtain. "To be ready if force is required," thought Mitya, "and perhaps for some other reason, too."

"Well, must I take off my shirt, too?" he asked sharply, but Nikolay Parfenovich did not answer. He was busily engaged with the prosecutor in examining the coat, the trousers, the waistcoat, and the cap; and it was evident that they were both much interested in the scrutiny. "They make no bones about it," thought Mitya, "they don't show the most elementary politeness."

"I ask you for the second time — need I take off my shirt or not?" he said, still more sharply and irritably.

"Don't trouble yourself. We will tell you what to do," Nikolay Parfenovich said, and there was something dictatorial about his voice, or so it seemed to Mitya.

Meantime a consultation was going on in undertones between the examining magistrate and the prosecutor. There turned out to be on the coat, especially on the left side at the back, huge patches of blood, dry, and still stiff. There were bloodstains on the trousers, too. Nikolay Parfenovich, moreover, in the presence of the peasant witnesses, passed his fingers along the collar, the cuffs, and all the seams of the coat and trousers, obviously looking for something — money, of course. He didn't even hide from Mitya his suspicion that he was capable of sewing money up in his clothes.

"I am being treated not as an officer but as a thief," Mitya muttered to himself. They communicated their ideas to one another with amazing frankness. The secretary, for instance, who was also behind the curtain, fussing about and making himself useful, called Nikolay Parfenovich's attention to the cap, which they were also fingering.

"You remember Gridyenko, the copying-clerk," observed the secretary. "Last summer he received the wages of the whole office, and pretended to have lost the money when he was drunk. And where was it found? Why, in just such pipings in his cap. The hundred-rouble notes were screwed up in little rolls and sewed up in the piping."

Both the magistrates remembered Gridyenko's case perfectly, and so laid aside Mitya's cap, and decided that all his clothes must be more thoroughly examined later.

"Excuse me," cried Nikolay Parfenovich, suddenly, noticing that the right cuff of Mitya's shirt was turned in, and covered with blood, "excuse me, what's that, blood?"

"Yes," Mitya jerked out.

"That is, what blood . . . and why is the cuff turned in?"

Mitya told him how he had got the sleeve stained with blood looking after Grigory, and had turned it inside when he was washing his hands at Perhotin's.

"You must take off your shirt, too. That's very important as material evidence."

Mitya flushed red and flew into a rage.

"What, am I to stay naked?" he shouted.

"Don't disturb yourself. We will arrange something. And meanwhile take off your socks."

"You're not joking? Is that really necessary?" Mitya's eyes flashed.

"We are in no mood for joking," answered Nikolay Parfenovich sternly.

"Well, if I must . . ." muttered Mitya, and sitting down on the bed, he took off his socks. He felt unbearably awkward. All were clothed, while he was naked, and, strange to say, when he was undressed he felt somehow guilty in their presence, and was almost ready to believe himself that he was inferior to them, and that now they had a perfect right to despise him.

"When all are undressed, one is somehow not ashamed, but when one's the only one undressed and everybody is looking, it's disgraceful," he kept repeating to himself, again and again. "It's like a dream, I've sometimes dreamed of being in such degrading positions." It was a misery to him to take off his socks. They were very dirty, and so were his underclothes, and now everyone could see it. And what was worse, he disliked his feet. All his life he had thought both his big toes hideous. He particularly loathed the coarse, flat, crooked nail on the right one, and now they would all see it. Feeling intolerably ashamed made him, at once and intentionally, rougher. He pulled off his shirt, himself.

"Would you like to look anywhere else if you're not ashamed to?"

"No, there's no need to, at present."

"Well, am I to stay naked like this?" he added savagely.

"Yes, that can't be helped for the time. . . . Kindly sit down here for a while. You can wrap yourself in a quilt from the bed, and I . . . I'll see to all this."

All the things were shown to the witnesses. The report of the search was drawn up, and at last Nikolay Parfenovich went out, and the clothes were carried out after him. Ippolit Kirillovich went out, too. Mitya was left alone with the peasants, who stood in silence, never taking their eyes off him. Mitya wrapped himself up in the quilt. He felt cold. His bare feet stuck out, and he couldn't pull the quilt over so as to cover them. Nikolay Parfenovich seemed to be gone a long time, "an insufferable time." "He thinks of me as a puppy," thought Mitya, gnashing his teeth. "That rotten prosecutor has gone, too, contemptuous no doubt, it disgusts him to see me naked!"

Mitya imagined, however, that his clothes would be examined and returned to him. But what was his indignation when Nikolay Parfenovich came back with quite different clothes, brought in behind him by a peasant.

"Here are clothes for you," he observed airily, seeming well satisfied with the success of his mission. "Mr. Kalganov has kindly provided these for this unusual emergency, as well as a clean shirt. Luckily he had them all in his trunk. You can keep your own socks and underclothes." Mitya flew into a passion.

"I won't have other people's clothes!" he shouted menacingly, "give me my own!"

"It's impossible!"

"Give me my own. Damn Kalganov and his clothes, too!"

It was a long time before they could persuade him. But they succeeded somehow in quieting him down. They impressed upon him that his clothes, being stained with blood, must be "added to the other material evidence," and that they "had not even the right to let him have them now . . . taking into consideration the possible outcome of the case." Mitya at last understood this. He subsided into gloomy silence and hurriedly dressed himself. He merely observed, as he put them on, that the clothes were much better than his old ones, and that he disliked "gaining by the change." They were, besides, "shamefully narrow. Am I to be made to play the clown . . . for your amusement?"

They urged upon him again that he was exaggerating, that Kalganov was only a little taller, so that only the trousers might be a little too long. But the coat turned out to be really tight in the shoulders.

"Damn it all! I can hardly button it," Mitya grumbled. "Be so good as to tell Mr. Kalganov from me that I didn't ask for his clothes, and it's not my doing that they've dressed me up like a clown."

"He quite understands that, and is sorry . . . I mean, not sorry to lend you his clothes, but sorry about all this business," mumbled Nikolay Parfenovich.

"Confound his regrets! Well, where now, or am I to go on sitting here?"

He was asked to go back to the "other room." Mitya went in, scowling with anger, and trying to avoid looking at any one. Dressed in another man's clothes he felt himself disgraced, even in the eyes of the peasants, and of Trifon Borisovich, whose face appeared, for some reason, in the doorway, and vanished immediately. "He's come to look at me dressed up," thought Mitya. He sat down on the same chair as before. He had an absurd nightmarish feeling, as though he were out of his mind.

"Well, what now? Are you going to flog me? That's all that's left for you," he said, clenching his teeth and addressing the prosecutor. He would not turn to Nikolay Parfenovich, as though he disdained to speak to him.

"He looked too closely at my socks, and turned them inside out on purpose to show every one what dirty underclothes I wear — the scoundrel!"

"Well, now we must proceed to the examination of witnesses," observed Nikolay Parfenovich, as though in reply to Mitya's question.

"Yes," said the prosecutor thoughtfully, as though reflecting on something.

"We've done what we could in your interest, Dmitri Fyodorovich," Nikolay Parfenovich went on, "but having received from you such an uncompromising refusal to explain to us the source from which you obtained the money found upon you, we are, at the present moment . . ."

"What is the stone in your ring?" Mitya interrupted suddenly, as though awakening from a reverie. He pointed to one of the three rings adorning Nikolay Parfenovich's right hand.

"Ring?" repeated Nikolay Parfenovich with surprise.

"Yes, that one . . . on your middle finger, with the little veins in it, what stone is that?" Mitya persisted, like a peevish child.

"That's a smoky topaz," said Nikolay Parfenovich, smiling. "Would you like to look at it? I'll take it off . . ."

"No, no, don't take it off," cried Mitya furiously, suddenly waking up, and angry with himself. "Don't take it off . . . there's no need. . . . Damn it. . . . Gentlemen, you've sullied my soul! Can you suppose that I would conceal it from you, if I really had killed my father, that I would shuffle, lie, and hide myself? No, that's not like Dmitri Karamazov, that he couldn't bear, and if I were guilty, I swear I wouldn't have waited for your coming, or for the sunrise as I meant at first, but would have destroyed myself before this, without waiting for the dawn! I know that about myself now. I couldn't have learnt so much in twenty years as I've found out in this accursed night! . . . And should I have been like this on this night, and at this moment, sitting with you, could I have talked like this, could I have moved like this, could I have looked at you and at the world like this, if I had really been the murderer of my father, when the very thought of having accidentally killed Grigory gave me no peace all night — not from fear — oh, not simply from fear of your punishment! The digrace of it! And you want me to be open with such scoffers as you, who see nothing and believe in nothing, blind moles and scoffers, and to tell you another nasty thing I've done, another disgrace, even if that would save me from your accusation! No, better Siberia! The man who opened the door to my father and went in at that door, he killed him, he robbed him. Who was he — I'm racking my brains and can't think who. But I can tell you it was not Dmitri Karamazov, and that's all I can tell you, and that's enough, enough, leave me alone. . . . Exile me, execute me, but don't bother me any more. I'll say no more. Call your witnesses!"

Mitya uttered his sudden monologue as though he were determined to be absolutely silent for the future. The prosecutor watched him the whole time and only when he had ceased speaking, observed, as though it were the most ordinary thing, with the most frigid and composed air:

"Oh, about the open door of which you spoke just now, we may as well inform you, by the way, now, of a very interesting piece of evidence of the greatest importance both to you and to us, that has been given us by Grigory, the old man you wounded. On his recovery, he clearly and emphatically stated, in reply to our questions, that when, on coming out to the steps, and hearing a noise in the garden, he made up his mind to go into it through the little gate which stood open, before he noticed you running, as you have told us already, in the dark from the open window where you saw your father, he, Grigory, glanced to the left, and, while noticing the open window, observed at the same time, much nearer to him, the door, standing wide open — that door which you have stated to have been shut the whole time you were in the garden. I will not conceal from you that Grigory himself confidently affirms and bears witness that you must have run from that door, though, of course, he did not see you do so with his own eyes, since he only noticed you first some distance away in the garden, running towards the fence."

Mitya had leapt up from his chair half-way through this speech.

"Nonsense!" he yelled, in a sudden frenzy, "it's a bare-faced lie. He couldn't have seen the door open because it was shut. He's lying!"

"I consider it my duty to repeat that he is firm in his statement. He does not waver. He adheres to it. We've questioned him several times."

"Precisely. I have questioned him several times," Nikolay Parfenovich confirmed warmly.

"It's false, false! It's either slander, or the hallucination of a madman," Mitya still shouted. "He's simply raving, from loss of blood, from the wound. He must have fancied it when he came to. . . . He's raving."

"Yes, but he noticed the open door, not

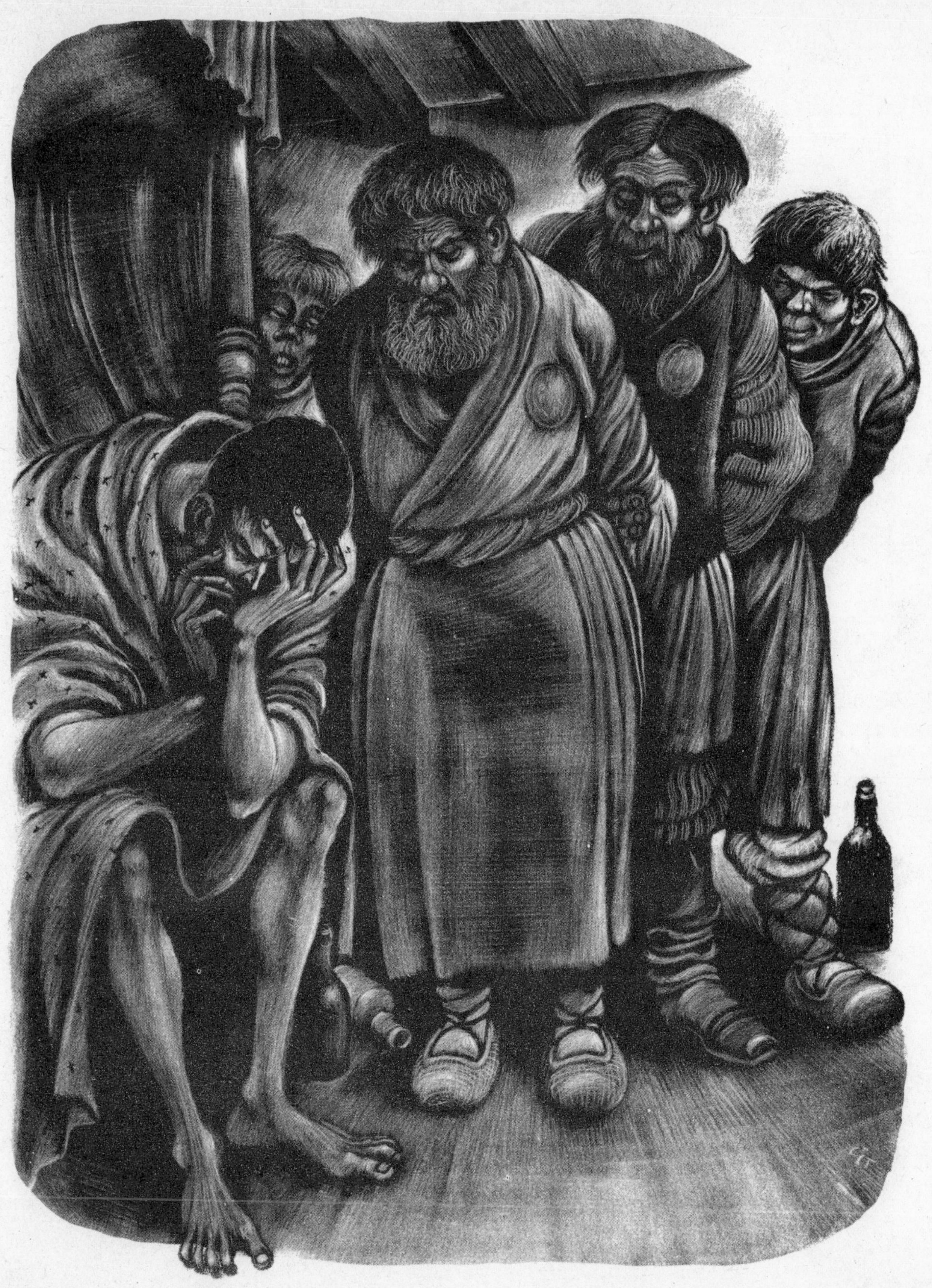

MITYA IS DISGRACED

when he came to after his injuries, but before that, as soon as he went into the garden from the lodge."

"But it's false, it's false! It can't be so! He's slandering me from spite. . . . He couldn't have seen it . . . I didn't run out of the door," gasped Mitya.

The prosecutor turned to Nikolay Parfenovich and said to him impressively:

"Confront him with it."

"Do you recognise this object?"

Nikolay Parfenovich laid upon the table a large and thick official envelope, on which three seals still remained intact. The envelope was empty, and slit open at one end. Mitya stared at it with open eyes.

"It . . . it must be that envelope of my father's, the envelope that contained the three thousand roubles . . . and if there's inscribed on it, allow me, 'for my little chick' . . . yes — three thousand!" he shouted, "do you see, three thousand, do you see?"

"Of course, we see. But we didn't find the money in it. It was empty, and lying on the floor by the bed, behind the screen."

For some seconds Mitya stood as though thunderstruck.

"Gentlemen, it's Smerdyakov!" he shouted suddenly, at the top of his voice. "It's he who's murdered him! He's robbed him! No one else knew where the old man hid the envelope. It's Smerdyakov, that's clear, now!"

"But you, too, knew of the envelope and that it was under the pillow."

"I never knew it. I've never seen it. This is the first time I've looked at it. I'd only heard of it from Smerdyakov. . . . He was the only one who knew where the old man kept it hidden, I didn't know . . ." Mitya was completely breathless.

"But you told us yourself that the envelope was under your deceased father's pillow. You especially stated that it was under the pillow, so you must have known it."

"We've got it written down," confirmed Nikolay Parfenovich.

"Nonsense! It's absurd! I'd no idea it was under the pillow. And perhaps it wasn't under the pillow at all. . . . It was just a chance guess that it was under the pillow. What does Smerdyakov say? Have you asked him where it was? What does Smerdyakov say? that's the chief point. . . . And I went out of my way to tell lies against myself. . . . I told you without thinking that it was under the pillow, and now you . . . . Oh, you know how one says the wrong thing, without meaning it. No one knew but Smerdyakov, only Smerdyakov, and no one else. . . . He didn't even tell me where it was! But it's his doing, his doing; there's no doubt about it, he murdered him, that's as clear as daylight now," Mitya exclaimed more and more frantically, repeating himself incoherently, and growing more and more exasperated and excited. "You must understand that, and arrest him at once. . . . He must have killed him while I was running away and while Grigory was unconscious, that's clear now. . . . He gave the signal and father opened to him . . . for no one but he knew the signal, and without the signal father would never have opened the door. . . ."

"But you're again forgetting the circumstance," the prosecutor observed, still speaking with the same restraint, though with a note of triumph, "that there was no need to give the signal if the door already stood open when you were there, while you were in the garden . . ."

"The door, the door," muttered Mitya, and

he stared speechless at the prosecutor. He sank back helpless in his chair. All were silent.

"Yes, the door! . . . It's a nightmare! God is against me!" he exclaimed, staring before him in complete stupefaction.

"Come, you see," the prosecutor went on with dignity, "and you can judge for yourself, Dmitri Fyodorovich. On the one hand we have the evidence of the open door from which you ran out, a fact which overwhelms you and us. On the other side your incomprehensible, persistent, and, so to speak, obdurate silence with regard to the source from which you obtained the money which was so suddenly seen in your hands, when only three hours earlier, on your own showing, you pledged your pistols for the sake of ten roubles! In view of all these facts, judge for yourself. What are we to believe, and what can we depend upon? And don't accuse us of being 'frigid, cynical, scoffing people,' who are incapable of believing in the generous impulses of your heart. . . . Try to enter into our position . . ."

Mitya was indescribably agitated. He turned pale.

"Very well!" he exclaimed suddenly, "I will tell you my secret. I'll tell you where I got the money! . . . I'll reveal my shame, that I may not have to blame myself or you hereafter."

"And believe me, Dmitri Fyodorovich," put in Nikolay Parfenovich, in a voice of almost pathetic delight, "that every sincere and complete confession on your part at this moment may, later on, immensely alleviate your lot, and may, indeed, moreover . . ."

But the prosecutor gave him a slight shove under the table, and he checked himself in time. Mitya, it is true, had not heard him.

CHAPTER VII

MITYA'S GREAT SECRET. RECEIVED WITH HISSES

"Gentlemen," he began, still in the same agitation, "I want to make a full confession: that money was *my own*."

The magistrates' faces lengthened. That was not at all what they expected.

"How do you mean?" faltered Nikolay Parfenovich, "when at five o'clock on the same day, by your own confession . . ."

"Damn five o'clock on the same day and my own confession. That's got nothing to do with it now! That money was my own, my own, that is, stolen by me . . . not mine, I mean, but stolen by me, and it was fifteen hundred roubles, and I had it on me all the time, all the time . . ."

"But where did you get it?"

"I took it off my neck, gentlemen, off this very neck . . . it was here, round my neck, sewn up in a rag, and I'd had it round my neck a long time, it's a month since I put it round my neck . . . to my shame and disgrace!"

"And from whom did you . . . obtain it?"

"You mean, 'steal it'? Speak out plainly now. Yes, I consider that I practically stole it, but, if you prefer, I 'appropriated it.' I consider I stole it. And last night I stole it for good."

"Last night? But you said that it's a month since you . . . obtained it? . . ."

"Yes. But not from my father. Not from my father, don't be uneasy. I didn't steal it from my father, but from her. Let me tell you without interruption. It's hard to do, you know. You see, a month ago, I was sent for by Katerina Ivanovna Verhovtzev, formerly my betrothed. Do you know her?"

"Yes, of course."

"I know you know her. She's a noble creature, noblest of the noble. But she has hated me ever so long, oh, ever so long . . . and hated me with good reason, good reason!"

"Katerina Ivanovna!" the examining magistrate exclaimed with amazement. The prosecutor, too, stared.

"Oh, don't take her name in vain! I'm a scoundrel to bring her into it. Yes, I've seen that she hated me . . . a long while. . . . From the very first, even that evening at my lodging . . . but enough, enough. You're unworthy even to know of that. No need of that at all. . . . I need only tell you that she sent for me a month ago, gave me three thousand roubles to send off to her sister and another relation in Moscow (as though she couldn't have sent it off herself!), and I . . . it was just at that fatal moment in my life when I . . . Well, in fact, when I'd just come to love another, *her*, the present one, the one who's sitting down below now, Grushenka. I carried her off here to Mokroye then, and squandered here in two days half that damned three thousand, but the other half I kept on me. Well, I've kept that other half, that fifteen hundred, like a locket round my neck, but yesterday I opened it, and spent it. What's left of it, eight hundred roubles, is in your hands now, Nikolay Parfenovich. That's the change out of the fifteen hundred I had yesterday."

"Excuse me. How's that? Why, when you were here a month ago you spent three thousand, not fifteen hundred, everybody knows that."

"Who knows it? Who counted the money? Did I let any one count it?"

"Why, you told every one yourself that you'd spent exactly three thousand."

"It's true, I did. I told the whole town so, and the whole town said so. And here, at Mokroye, too, every one reckoned it was three thousand. Yet I didn't spend three thousand, but fifteen hundred. And the other fifteen hundred I sewed into a little bag. That's how it was, gentlemen. That's where I got that money yesterday. . . ."

"This is almost miraculous," murmured Nikolay Parfenovich.

"Allow me to inquire," observed the prosecutor at last, "have you informed any one whatever of this circumstance before, I mean that you had fifteen hundred left about you a month ago?"

"I told no one."

"That's strange. Do you mean absolutely no one?"

"Absolutely no one. No one and nobody."

"What was your reason for this reticence? What was your motive for making such a secret of it? To be more precise: You have told us at last your secret, in your words, so 'disgraceful,' though in reality — that is, of course, comparatively speaking — this action, that is, the appropriation of three thousand roubles belonging to some one else, and, of course, only for a time, is, in my view at least, only an act of the greatest recklessness and not so disgraceful, when one takes into consideration your character. . . . Even admitting that it was an action in the highest degree discreditable, still, discreditable is not 'disgraceful.' . . . Many people have already guessed, during this last month, about the three thousand of Katerina Ivanovna's that you have spent, and I had heard the legend myself, apart from your confession. . . . Mihail Makarovich, for instance, had heard it, too, so that indeed, it was scarcely a legend, but the gossip of the whole town. There are indications, too, if I am not mistaken, that you confessed this yourself to some one, I mean that the money was Katerina Ivanovna's, and so, it's extremely surprising to me that hitherto, that is, up to the present moment, you have made such an extraordinary secret of the fifteen hundred you say you put by, apparently connecting a feeling of positive horror with that secret. . . . It's not easy to believe that it could cost you such distress to confess such a secret. . . . You cried out, just now, that Siberia would be better than confessing it. . . ."

The prosecutor ceased speaking. He was provoked. He did not conceal his vexation, which was almost anger, and gave vent to all his accumulated spleen, without choosing words, disconnectedly and incoherently.

"It's not the fifteen hundred that's the disgrace, but that I put it apart from the rest of the three thousand," said Mitya firmly.

"Why?" smiled the prosecutor irritably. "What is there disgraceful, to your thinking, in your having set aside half of the three thousand you had discreditably, if you prefer, 'disgracefully,' appropriated? Your taking the three thousand is more important than what you did with it. And by the way, why did you do that — why did you set apart that half, for what purpose, for what object did you do it? Can you explain that to us?"

"Oh, gentlemen, the purpose is the whole point!" cried Mitya. "I put it aside because I was vile, that is, because I was calculating, and to be calculating in such a case is vile . . . and that vileness has lasted a whole month."

"It's incomprehensible."

"I am surprised at you. But I'll make it clearer. Perhaps it really is incomprehensible. You see, attend to what I say. I appropriate three thousand entrusted to my honour, I spend it on a spree, say I spend it all, and next morning I appear before her and say, 'Katya, I've done wrong, I've squandered your three thousand,' well, is that right? No, it's not right — it's dishonest and mean, I'm a beast, with no more self-control than a beast, that's so, isn't it? But still I'm not a thief? Not a downright thief, you'll admit! I squandered it, but I didn't steal it. Now a second, rather more favourable alternative: follow me carefully, or I may get confused again — my head's going round — and so, for the second alternative: I squander here only fifteen hundred out of the three thousand, that is, only half. Next day I go and take that half to her: 'Katya, take this fifteen hundred from me, I'm a low beast, and an untrustworthy scoundrel, for I've squandered half the money, and I shall squander this, too, so keep me from temptation!' Well, what of that alternative? I should be a beast and a scoundrel, and whatever you like; but not a thief, not altogether a thief, for, if I were a thief, I should not have brought back what was left, but have kept that, too. She would see at once that since I brought back half, I should pay back what I'd squandered, that I should never give up trying to, that I should work to get it and pay it back. So in that case I should be a scoundrel, but not a thief, you may say what you like, not a thief!"

"I admit that there is a certain distinction," said the prosecutor, with a cold smile. "But it's strange that you see such a fateful difference."

"Yes, I see a fateful difference! Every man may be a scoundrel, and perhaps every man is a scoundrel, but not every one can be a thief, it takes an arch-scoundrel to be that. Oh, of course, I don't know how to make these fine distinctions . . . but a thief is lower than a scoundrel, that's my conviction. Listen, I carry the money about me a whole month, I may make up my mind to give it back to-morrow, and I'm a scoundrel no longer, but I cannot make up my mind, you see, though I'm making up my mind every day, and every day spurring myself on to do it, and yet for a whole month I can't bring myself to it, you see. Is that right to your thinking, is that right?"

"Certainly, that's not right, that I can quite understand, and that I don't dispute," answered the prosecutor with reserve. "And let us give up all discussions of these subtleties and distinctions, and, if you will be so kind, get back to the point. And the point is, that you have still not told us, although we've asked you, why, in the first place, you divided the money, squandering one half and hiding the other? For what purpose exactly did you hide it, what did you mean to do with that fifteen hundred? I insist upon that question, Dmitri Fyodorovich."

"Yes, of course!" cried Mitya, striking himself on the forehead; "forgive me, I'm tormenting you, and am not explaining the chief point, or you'd understand in a minute, for it's just the aim of it, the aim, that's the disgrace! You see, it all had to do with the old man, the deceased. He was always pestering Agrafena Alexandrovna, and I was jealous; I thought then that she was hesitating between me and him. So I kept thinking every day, suppose she were to make up her mind all of a sudden, suppose she were to leave off tormenting me, and were suddenly to say to me, 'I love you, not him; take me to the other end of the world.' And I'd only forty copecks; how could I take her away, what could I do? Why, I'd be lost. You see, I didn't know her then, I didn't understand her, I thought she wanted money, and that she wouldn't forgive my poverty. And so I fiendishly counted out the half of that three thousand, sewed it up cold-bloodedly, calculating on it, sewed it up before I went on a spree, and after I had sewn it up, I went off to get drunk on the rest. Yes, that was base. Do you understand now?"

Both the magistrates laughed aloud.

"I should have called it sensible and moral on your part not to have squandered it all," chuckled Nikolay Parfenovich, "for after all what does it amount to?"

"Why, that I stole it, that's what it amounts to! Oh, God, you horrify me by your lack of understanding! All the time that I carried that fifteen hundred sewn up round my neck, every day and every hour I said to myself, 'You're a thief! you're a thief!' Yes, that's why I've been so savage all this month, that's why I fought in the tavern, that's why I attacked my father, it was because I felt I was a thief. I couldn't make up my mind, I didn't dare even to tell Alyosha, my brother, about that fifteen hundred: I felt I was such a scoundrel and such a pickpocket. But, do you know, while I carried it I said to myself at the same time every hour: 'No, Dmitri Fyodorovich, perhaps you are not a thief yet.' Why? Because I might go next day and hand over that fifteen hundred to Katya. And only yesterday I made up my mind to tear my amulet off my neck, on my way from Fenya's to Perhotin. I hadn't been able till that moment to bring myself to it. And as soon as I tore it off, at that very moment I became a downright thief, a thief and a dishonest man for the rest of my life. Why?

Because with that I destroyed, too, my dream of going to Katya and saying, 'I'm a scoundrel, but not a thief!' Do you understand now? Do you understand?"

"What was it made you decide to do it yesterday?" Nikolay Parfenovich interrupted.

"Why? It's absurd to ask. Because I had condemned myself to die at five o'clock this morning, here, at dawn. I thought it made no difference whether I died a thief or a man of honour. But I see it's not so, it turns out that it does make a difference. Believe me, gentlemen, what has tortured me most during this night has not been the thought that I'd killed the old servant, and that I was in danger of Siberia just when my love was being rewarded, and heaven was open to me again. Oh, that did torture me, but not so much; not so much as the accursed consciousness that I had torn that damned money off my breast at last and spent it, and had become a downright thief! Oh, gentlemen, I tell you again, with a bleeding heart, I have learnt a great deal this night. I have learnt that it's not only impossible to live a scoundrel, but impossible to die a scoundrel. . . . No, gentlemen, one must die honest . . ." Mitya was pale. His face had a haggard and exhausted look, in spite of his being intensely excited.

"I am beginning to understand you, Dmitri Fyodorovich," the prosecutor said slowly, in a soft and almost compassionate tone. "But all this, if you'll excuse my saying so, is a matter of nerves, in my opinion . . . your overwrought nerves, that's what it is. And why, for instance, should you not have saved yourself such misery for almost a month, by going and returning that fifteen hundred to the lady who had entrusted it to you? And why could you not have explained things to her, and in view of your position, which you describe as being so awful, why could you not have had recourse to the plan which would so naturally have occurred to one's mind, that is, after honourably confessing your errors to her, why could you not have asked her to lend you the sum needed for your expenses, which, with her generous heart, she would certainly not have refused you in your distress, especially if it had been with some guarantee, or even on the security you offered to the merchant Samsonov, and to Madame Hohlakov. I suppose you still regard that security as of value?"

Mitya suddenly crimsoned.

"Surely you don't think me such an out and out scoundrel as that? You can't be speaking in earnest?" he said, with indignation, looking the prosecutor straight in the face, and seeming unable to believe his ears.

"I assure you I'm in earnest. . . . Why do you imagine I'm not serious?" It was the prosecutor's turn to be surprised.

"Oh, how base that would have been! Gentlemen, do you know, you are torturing me! Very well, I will tell you everything, if it must be so. I'll confess all my damnable vileness, but only in order to put you to shame, and you'll be surprised yourself at the depths of ignominy to which a medley of human passions can sink. You must know that I already had that plan myself, that plan you spoke of, just now, prosecutor! Yes, gentlemen, I, too, have had that thought in my mind all this accursed month, so that I was on the point of deciding to go to Katya — that's how mean I was. But to go to her, to tell her of my treachery, and for that very treachery, to carry out that treacherous act, for the expenses connected with it, to beg for money from her, Katya (to beg, do you hear, to beg), and straight from her to run away with the other, her rival, who hated her and had insulted her—to think of it! Why, you must have lost your mind, prosecutor!"

"I haven't lost my mind, but I did speak in haste, without thinking . . . of that feminine jealousy . . . if there could be jealousy in this case, as you assert . . . yes, perhaps there is something of the kind," said the prosecutor, smiling.

"But that would have been so infamous!" Mitya brought his fist down on the table fiercely. "That would have stunk beyond words! And do you know that she might have given me that money, yes, and she would have given it, too; she'd have been certain to give it, to be revenged on me, she'd have given it to satisfy her vengeance, to show her contempt for me, for hers is an infernal nature, too, and she's a woman of great wrath. I'd have taken the money, too, oh, I should have taken it; I should have taken it, and then, for the rest of my life . . . oh, God! Forgive me, gentlemen, I'm making such an outcry because I've had that thought in my mind so lately, only the day before yesterday, that night when I was having all that bother with Lyagavy, and afterwards yesterday, all day yesterday, I remember, till that happened . . ."

"Till what happened?" put in Nikolay Parfenovich inquisitively, but Mitya did not hear it.

"I have made you a dreadful confession," Mitya said gloomily in conclusion. "You must appreciate it, gentlemen, and what's more, you must feel it, for if not, if that leaves your souls untouched, then you've simply no respect for me, gentlemen, I tell you that, and I shall die of shame at having confessed it to men like you! Oh, I shall shoot myself! Yes, I see, I see already that you don't believe me. What, you want to write that down, too?" he cried in fear.

"And what you said just now," said Nikolay Parfenovich, looking at him in surprise, "that is, that up to the last hour you were still planning to go to Katerina Ivanovna to beg that sum from her. . . . I assure you, that's a very important piece of evidence for us, Dmitri Fyodorovich, I mean for the whole case . . . and particularly for you, particularly important for you."

"Have mercy, gentlemen!" Mitya flung up his hands. "Don't write that, anyway; have some shame. Here I've torn my heart in half before you, and you seize the opportunity and dig your fingers into the torn parts of both halves. . . . Oh, my God!"

In despair he hid his face in his hands.

"Don't worry yourself so, Dmitri Fyodorovich," observed the prosecutor, "everything that is written down will be read over to you afterwards, and what you don't agree to we'll alter as you like. But now I'll ask you one little question for the third time. Has no one, absolutely no one, heard from you of that money you sewed up in the bag? That, I must tell you, is almost impossible to believe."

"No one, no one, I told you so before, or you've not understood anything! Let me alone!"

"Very well, this matter is bound to be explained, and there's plenty of time for it, but meantime, consider; we have perhaps a dozen witnesses that you yourself spread it abroad, and even shouted almost everywhere, about the three thousand you'd spent here; three thousand, not fifteen hundred. And now, too, when you got hold of the money you had yesterday, you gave many people to understand that you had brought three thousand with you."

"You've got not dozens, but hundreds of witnesses, two hundred witnesses, two hundred have heard it, thousands have heard it!" cried Mitya.

"Well, you see, all bear witness to it. And the word *all* means something."

"It means nothing. I told a lie, and every one began repeating it."

"But what need had you to 'tell a lie,' as you put it?"

"The devil knows. Out of bravado perhaps . . . just so . . . to show I'd squandered so much money. . . . To try and forget that money I had sewn up, perhaps . . . yes, that was why . . . damn it . . . how often will you ask me that question? Well, I told a fib, and that was the end of it, once I'd said it I didn't care to correct it. What does a man tell lies for sometimes?"

"That's very difficult to decide, Dmitri Fyodorovich, what makes a man tell lies," observed the prosecutor impressively. "Tell me, though, was that 'amulet,' as you call it, on your neck, a big thing?"

"No, not big."

"How big, for instance?"

"If you fold a hundred-rouble note in half, that would be the size."

"You'd better show us the remains of it. You must have them somewhere."

"Damnation, what nonsense! I don't know where they are."

"But excuse me: where and when did you take it off your neck? According to your own evidence you didn't go home."

"When I was going from Fenya's to Perhotin's, on the way I tore it off my neck and took out the money."

"In the dark?"

"What should I want a light for? I did it with a finger in one minute."

"Without scissors, in the street?"

"On the square I think it was. Why scissors? It was an old rag. It ripped in a minute."

"What did you do with it afterwards?"

"I dropped it there."

"Where was it, exactly?"

"On the square, somewhere on the square! The devil knows just where. What do you want to know for?"

"That's extremely important, Dmitri Fyodorovich. It would be material evidence in your favour. How is it you don't understand that? Who helped you to sew it up a month ago?"

"No one helped me. I did it myself."

"Can you sew?"

"A soldier has to know how to sew. It doesn't take any skill."

"Where did you get the material, that is, the rag in which you sewed the money?"

"Are you laughing at me?"

"Not at all. And we are in no mood for laughing, Dmitri Fyodorovich."

"I don't know where I got the rag from — somewhere I suppose."

"I should have thought that you would remember it."

"Upon my word, I don't remember. I might have torn a bit off my linen."

"That's very interesting. We might find in your lodgings to-morrow the shirt or whatever it is from which you tore the rag. What sort of rag was it, cloth or linen?"

"Goodness only knows what it was. Wait a bit. . . . I believe I didn't tear it off anything. It was a bit of calico. . . . I believe I sewed it up in a cap of my landlady's."

"In your landlady's cap?"

"Yes. I took it from her."

"How did you get it?"

"You see, I remember once taking a cap for a rag, perhaps to wipe my pen on. I took it without asking, because it was a worthless rag. I tore it up, and I took the notes and sewed them up in it. I believe it was in that very rag I sewed it. An old piece of calico, washed a thousand times."

"And you remember that for certain now?"

"I don't know whether for certain. I think it was in the cap. But what does it matter?"

"In that case your landlady might at least remember that she had lost the thing."

"No, she won't, she didn't miss it. It was an old rag, I tell you, not worth a groat."

"And where did you get the needle and thread?"

"I'll stop now. I won't say any more. Enough of it!" said Mitya, losing his temper at last.

"It's strange that you should have so completely forgotten where you threw the pieces in the square."

"Give orders for the square to be swept tomorrow, and perhaps you'll find it," said Mitya, sneering. "Enough, gentlemen, enough!" he decided, in an exhausted voice. "I see clearly you don't believe me! Not for a moment! It's my fault, not yours. I ought not to have been so ready. Why, why did I degrade myself by confessing my secret to you? It's a joke to you. I see that from your eyes. You led me on to it, prosecutor! Sing a hymn of triumph if you can. . . . Damn you, you torturers!"

He bent his head, and hid his face in his hands. The magistrates were silent. A minute later he raised his head and looked at them almost vacantly. His face now expressed complete, hopeless despair, and he sat mute and passive as though hardly conscious of what was happening. In the meantime they had to finish what they were about. They had immediately to begin examining the witnesses. It was by now eight o'clock in the morning. The candles had been extinguished long ago. Mihail Makarovich and Kalganov, who had been continually in and out of the room all the while the interrogation had been going on, had now both gone out again. The magistrates, too, looked very tired. It was a wretched morning, the whole sky was overcast, and the rain streamed down in bucketfuls. Mitya gazed blankly out the window.

"May I look out the window?" he asked Nikolay Parfenovich suddenly. "Oh, as much as you like," the latter replied.

Mitya got up and went to the window. The rain lashed against the little greenish panes of the window. He could see the muddy road just below the window, and farther away, in the rainy mist, a row of poor, black, dismal huts, looking even blacker and poorer in the rain. Mitya thought of "Phœbus the golden-haired," and how he had meant to shoot himself at his first ray. "Perhaps it would be even better on a morning like this," he thought with a smile, and suddenly, dropping his hands, he turned to his "torturers."

"Gentlemen," he cried, "I see that I am lost! But she? Tell me about her. I beseech you. Surely she need not be ruined with me? She's innocent, you know, she was out of her mind when she cried last night 'It's all my fault!' She's done nothing, nothing! I've been grieving over her all night as I sat with you. . . . Can't you, won't you tell me what you are going to do with her now?"

"You can set your mind quite at rest on that score, Dmitri Fyodorovich," the prosecutor answered at once, with visible alacrity. "We have, so far, no grounds for troubling the person in whom you are so interested. I trust that it may be the same in the later development of the case. . . . On the contrary, we'll do everything that lies in our power in that matter. Set your mind completely at rest."

"Gentlemen, I thank you. I knew that you were honest, just people in spite of everything. You've taken a load off my heart. . . . Well, what are we to do now? I'm ready."

"Well, we ought to make haste. We must pass to examining the witnesses without delay. That must be done in your presence and therefore . . ."

"Shouldn't we have some tea first?" interposed Nikolay Parfenovich. "I think we've deserved it!"

They decided that if tea were ready downstairs (Mihail Makarovich had, no doubt, gone down to get some) they would have a glass and then "go on and on," putting off their proper breakfast until a more favourable opportunity. Tea really was ready below, and was soon brought up. Mitya at first refused the glass that Nikolay Parfenovich politely offered him, but afterwards he asked for it himself and drank it greedily. He looked surprisingly exhausted. It might have been supposed from his herculean strength that one night of carousing, even accompanied by the most violent emotions, could have had little effect on him. But he felt that he could hardly sit up, and from time to time all the objects about him seemed heaving and dancing before his eyes.

"A little more and I shall begin raving," he said to himself.

CHAPTER VIII

THE EVIDENCE OF THE WITNESSES. THE BABE

The examination of the witnesses began. But we will not continue our story in such detail as hitherto. And so we will omit to say how Nikolay Parfenovich impressed on every witness called that he must give his evidence in accordance with truth and conscience, and that he would afterwards have to repeat his evidence on oath, how every witness was called upon to sign his affidavit, and so on. We will only note that the point principally insisted upon in the examination was the question of the three thousand roubles, that is, was the sum spent here, at Mokroye, by Mitya on the first occasion, a month before, three thousand or fifteen hundred? And again had he spent three thousand or fifteen hundred the previous day? Alas, all the evidence, absolutely all, turned out to be against Mitya. There was not one deposition in his favour, and some witnesses introduced new, almost crushing facts, in contradiction of his, Mitya's, story.

The first witness examined was Trifon Borisovich. He was not in the least abashed as he stood before the magistrates. He had, on the contrary, an air of stern and severe indignation with the accused, which gave him an appearance of truthfulness and personal dignity. He spoke little, and with reserve, waited to be questioned, answered precisely and deliberately. Firmly and unhesitatingly he bore witness that the sum spent a month before could not have been less than three thousand, that all the peasants about here would testify that they had heard the sum of three thousand mentioned by Dmitri Fyodorovich himself. "What a lot of money he flung away on the gipsy girls alone. He wasted a thousand, I dare say, on them alone."

"I don't believe I gave them five hundred," was Mitya's gloomy comment on this. "It's a pity I didn't count the money at the time, but I was drunk . . ."

Mitya was sitting sideways with his back to the curtains. He listened gloomily, with a melancholy and exhausted air, as though he would say:

"Oh, say what you like. It makes no difference now."

"More than a thousand went to them, Dmitri Fyodorovich," retorted Trifon Borisovich firmly. "You flung it about at random and they picked it up. They were a rascally, thievish lot, horse-stealers, they've been driven away from here, or maybe they'd bear witness themselves how much they got from you. I saw the sum in your hands, myself — count it I didn't, you didn't let me, that's true enough — but by the look of it I should say it was far more than fifteen hundred . . . fifteen hundred, indeed! We've seen money, too. We can judge of amounts . . ."

As for the sum spent the day before, he asserted that Dmitri Fyodorovich had told him, as soon as he arrived, that he had brought three thousand with him.

"Come now, is that so, Trifon Borisovich?" replied Mitya. "Surely I didn't declare so positively that I'd brought three thousand?"

"You did say so, Dmitri Fyodorovich. You said it before Andrey. Andrey himself is still here. Send for him. And in the hall, when you were treating the chorus, you shouted straight out that you would leave your sixth thousand here — that is with what you spent before, we must understand. Stepan and Semyon heard it, and Pyotr Fomich Kalganov, too, was standing beside you at the time. Maybe he'd remember it. . . ."

The evidence as to the "sixth" thousand made an extraordinary impression on the two magistrates. They were delighted with this new mode of reckoning, three and three made six, three thousand then and three now made six, that was clear.

They questioned all the peasants mentioned by Trifon Borisovich, Stepan and Semyon, the driver Andrey, and Kalganov. The peasants and the driver unhesitatingly confirmed Trifon Borisovich's evidence. They noted down, with particular care, Andrey's account of the conversation he had had with Mitya on the road: " 'Where,' says he, 'am I, Dmitri Fyodorovich, going, to heaven or to hell, and shall I be forgiven in the next world or not?' "

The psychological Ippolit Kirillovich heard this with a subtle smile, and ended by recommending that these remarks as to where Dmitri Fyodorovich would go should be "included in the case."

Kalganov, when called, came in reluctantly, frowning and ill-humoured, and he spoke to the magistrates as though he had never met them before in his life, though they were acquaintances whom he had been meeting every day for a long time past. He began by saying that "he knew nothing about it and didn't want to." But it appeared that he had heard of the "sixth" thousand, and he admitted that he had been standing close by at the moment. So far as he could see he "didn't know" how much money Mitya had in his hands. He affirmed that the Poles had cheated at cards. In reply to reiterated questions he stated that, after the Poles had been turned out, Mitya's position with Agrafena Alexandrovna had certainly improved, and that she had said that she loved him. He spoke of Agrafena Alexandrovna with reserve and respect, as though she had been a lady of the best society, and did not once allow himself to call her Grushenka. In spite of the young man's obvious repugnance at giving evidence, Ippolit Kirillovich examined him at great length, and only from him learnt all the details of what made up Mitya's "love affair," so to say, on that night. Mitya did not once pull Kalganov up. At last they let the young man go, and he left the room with unconcealed indignation.

The Poles, too, were examined. Though they had gone to bed in their room, they had not slept all night, and on the arrival of the police officers they hastily dressed and got ready, realising that they would certainly be sent for. They gave their evidence with dignity, though not without some fear. The little Pole turned out to be a retired official of the twelfth class, who had served in Siberia as a veterinary surgeon. His name was Musialowicz. *Pan* Wróblewski turned out to be an unlicensed dentist. Although Nikolay Parfenovich asked them questions on their entering the room, they both addressed their answers to Mihail Makarovich, who was standing on one side, taking him in their ignorance for the most important person and in command, and addressed him at every word as "*Pan* Colonel." Only after several reproofs from Mihail Makarovich himself, they grasped that they had to address their answers only to Nikolay Parfenovich. It turned out that they could speak Russian quite correctly except for their pronunciation of some words. Of his relations with Grushenka, past and present, *Pan* Musialowicz spoke proudly and hotly, so that Mitya was roused at once and declared that he would not allow the "scoundrel" to speak like that in his presence! *Pan* Musialowicz at once called attention to the word "scoundrel," and begged that it should be entered in the record. Mitya fumed with rage.

"He's a scoundrel! A scoundrel! You can put that down. And put down, too, that in spite of the record I still declare that he's a scoundrel!" he cried.

Though Nikolay Parfenovich did insert this in the record, he showed the most praiseworthy tact and management. After sternly reprimanding Mitya, he cut short all further inquiry into the romantic aspect of the case, and hastened to pass to what was essential. One piece of evidence given by the Poles roused special interest in the magistrates: that was how, in that very room, Mitya had tried to buy off *Pan* Musialowicz, and had offered him three thousand roubles to resign his claims, seven hundred roubles down, and the remaining two thousand three hundred "to be paid next day in the town." He had sworn at the time that he had not the whole sum with him at Mokroye, but that his money was in the town. Mitya observed hotly that he had not said that he would be sure to pay him the remainder next day in the town. But *Pan* Wróblewski confirmed the statement, and Mitya, after thinking for a moment, admitted, frowning, that it must have been as the Poles stated, that he had been excited at the time, and might indeed have said so.

The prosecutor positively pounced on this piece of evidence. It seemed to establish for the prosecution (and they did, in fact, base this deduction on it) that half, or a part of, the three thousand that had come into Mitya's hands might really have been left somewhere hidden in the town, or even, perhaps, somewhere here, in Mokroye. This would explain the circumstance, so baffling for the prosecution, that only eight hundred roubles were to be found in Mitya's hands. This circumstance had been the one piece of evidence which, insignificant as it was, had hitherto told, to some extent, in Mitya's favour. Now this one piece of evidence in his favour had broken down. In answer to the prosecutor's inquiry, where he would have got the remaining two thousand three hundred roubles, since he himself had denied having more than fifteen hundred, Mitya confidently replied that he had meant to offer the "little chap," not money, but a formal deed of conveyance of his rights to the village of Chermashnya, those rights which he had already offered to Samsonov and Madame Hohlakov.

The prosecutor positively smiled at the "innocence of this subterfuge."

"And you imagine he would have accepted such a deed as a substitute for two thousand three hundred roubles in cash?"

"He certainly would have accepted it," Mitya declared hotly. "Why, look here, he might have grabbed not two thousand, but four or six, for it. He would have put his lawyers, Poles and Jews, on to the job, and might have got, not three thousand, but the whole property out of the old man."

The evidence of *Pan* Musialowicz was, of course, entered into the record in the fullest detail. Then they let the Poles go. The incident of the cheating at cards was hardly touched upon. Nikolay Parfenovich was too well pleased with them, as it was, and did not want to worry them with trifles; moreover, it was nothing but a foolish, drunken quarrel over cards. There had been drinking and disorder enough, that night. . . . So the two hundred roubles remained in the pockets of the Poles.

Then old Maximov was summoned. He came in timidly, approached with little steps, looking very dishevelled and sad. He had, all this time, taken refuge below with Grushenka, sitting silently beside her, and "now and then he'd begin blubbering over her and wiping his eyes with a blue-check handkerchief," as Mihail Makarovich described afterwards. So that she, herself, began trying to pacify and comfort him. The old man at once confessed that he had done wrong, that he had borrowed "ten roubles in my poverty," from Dmitri Fyodorovich, and that he was ready to refund it. To Nikolay Parfenovich's direct question, had he noticed how much money Dmitri Fyodorovich held in his hand, as he must have been able to see the sum better than any one when he took the note from him, Maximov, in the most positive manner, declared that there was twenty thousand.

"Have you ever seen as much as twenty thousand before, then?" inquired Nikolay Parfenovich, with a smile.

"To be sure I have, sir, not twenty, but seven, when my wife mortgaged my little property. She'd only let me look at it from a distance, boasting of it to me. It was a very thick bundle, sir, all rainbow-coloured notes. And Dmitri Fyodorovich's were all rainbow-coloured . . ."

He was soon dismissed. At last it was Grushenka's turn. The examiners were obviously apprehensive of the effect her appearance might have on Mitya, and Nikolay Parfenovich muttered a few words of admonition to him, but Mitya bowed his head in silence, giving him to understand "that he would not make a scene." Mihail Makarovich, himself, led Grushenka in. She entered with a stern and gloomy face, that looked almost composed, and sat down quietly on the chair offered her by Nikolay Parfenovich. She was very pale, she seemed to be cold, and wrapped herself closely in her magnificent black shawl. She was suffering from a slight feverish chill — the first symptom of the long illness which followed that night. Her grave air, her direct earnest look and quiet manner made a very favourable impression on every one. Nikolay Parfenovich was even somewhat "captivated." He admitted himself, when talking about it afterwards, that only then had he seen "how handsome the woman was," for, though he had seen her several times before, he had always looked upon her as something of a "provincial hetaira." "She has the manners of the best society," he said enthusiastically, gossiping about her in a circle of ladies. But this was received with positive indignation and he was immediately pronounced a "naughty man," to his great satisfaction.

As she entered the room, Grushenka only glanced for an instant at Mitya, who in his turn looked at her uneasily. But her appearance reassured him at once. After the first inevitable inquiries and admonitions, Nikolay Parfenovich asked her, hesitating a little, but preserving the most courteous manner, on what terms she was with the retired lieutenant, Dmitri Fyodorovich Karamazov. To this Grushenka firmly and quietly replied:

"He was an acquaintance. I have been receiving him this last month as an acquaintance." To further inquisitive questions she answered plainly and with complete frankness, that, though "at times" she had thought him attractive, she had not loved him, but that she had led him on, and his old father as well, "out of nasty spite," that she had seen that Mitya was very jealous of Fyodor Pavlovich and every one else; but that had only amused her. She had never meant to go to Fyodor Pavlovich, she had simply been laughing at him. "I had no thoughts for either of them all this last month. I was expecting another man, who had wronged me. But I think," she said in conclusion, "that there's no need for you to inquire about that, nor for me to answer you, for that's my own affair."

Nikolay Parfenovich immediately acted upon this hint. He again dismissed the "romantic" points in the case and passed to the serious one, that is, to the question of most importance, concerning the three thousand roubles. Grushenka confirmed the statement that three thousand roubles had certainly been spent on the first carousal at Mokroye, and, though she had not counted the money herself, she had heard that it was three thousand from Dmitri Fyodorovich himself.

"Did he tell you that alone, or before some one else, or did you only hear him speak of it to others in your presence?" the prosecutor inquired immediately.

To which Grushenka replied that she had heard him say so before other people, and had heard him say so when they were alone.

"Did he say it to you alone once, or several times?" inquired the prosecutor, and learned that he had told Grushenka several times.

Ippolit Kirillovich was very well satisfied with this piece of evidence. Further examination elicited that Grushenka knew, too, where that money had come from, and that Dmitri Fyodorovich had got it from Katerina Ivanovna.

"And did you never, once, hear that the money spent a month ago was not three thousand, but less, and that Dmitri Fyodorovich had saved half that sum for his own use?"

"No, I never heard that," answered Grushenka. It transpired further that Mitya had, on the contrary, often told her during that month that he hadn't a copeck.

"He was always expecting to get some from his father," said Grushenka in conclusion.

"Did he never say before you . . . casually, or in a moment of irritation," Nikolay Parfenovich put in suddenly, "that he intended to make an attempt on his father's life?"

"Oh, he did say so," sighed Grushenka.

"Once or several times?"

"He mentioned it several times, always in anger."

"And did you believe he would do it?"

"No, I never believed it," she answered firmly. "I had faith in his noble heart."

"Gentlemen, allow me," cried Mitya suddenly, "allow me to say one word to Agrafena Alexandrovna, in your presence."

"You may speak," Nikolay Parfenovich assented.

"Agrafena Alexandrovna!" Mitya got up from his chair, "have faith in God and in me. I am not guilty of the blood of my father who was murdered yesterday!"

Having uttered these words, Mitya sat down again on his chair. Grushenka stood up and crossed herself devoutly before the ikon.

"Glory to Thee, O Lord," she said, in a voice thrilling with ardent emotion, and, still standing, she turned to Nikolay Parfenovich and added:

"What he has just said, that you must believe! I know him. He'll say anything as a joke or out of obstinacy, but he'll never deceive you against his conscience. He will tell the whole truth, you may believe it."

"Thanks, Agrafena Alexandrovna, you've given my heart comfort," Mitya responded in a quivering voice.

As to the money spent the previous night, she declared that she did not know what the sum was, but had heard him tell several people that he had three thousand with him. And to the question where he got the money, she said that he had told her that he had "stolen" it from Katerina Ivanovna, and that she had replied to that that he hadn't stolen it, and that he must pay the money back next day. On the prosecutor's asking her emphatically whether the money he said he had stolen from Katerina Ivanovna was what he had spent the previous night, or what he had squandered here a month ago, she declared that he meant the money spent a month ago, and that that was how she understood him.

Grushenka was at last released, and Nikolay Parfenovich informed her impulsively that she might at once return to the town and that if he could assist her in any way, with horses for example, or if she would care for an escort he . . . would be . . .

"I thank you sincerely," said Grushenka, bowing to him, "I'm going with this old gentleman, I am driving him back to town with me, and meanwhile, if you'll allow me, I'll wait below to hear what you decide about Dmitri Fyodorovich."

She went out. Mitya was calm, and even looked more cheerful, but only for a moment. He felt more and more overcome by a strange physical weakness. His eyes were closing with fatigue. The examination of the witnesses was, at last, over. They proceeded to a final revision of the testimony. Mitya got up, moved from his chair to the corner by the curtain, lay down on a large chest covered with a rug, and instantly fell asleep. He had a strange dream, utterly out of keeping with the place and the time.

He was driving somewhere in the steppes, where he had been stationed long ago, and a peasant was driving him in a cart with a pair of horses, over a muddy road. He was cold, it was early in November, and the snow was falling in big wet flakes, melting as soon as it touched the earth. And the peasant drove him smartly; he had a fair, long beard. He was not an old man, somewhere about fifty, and he had on a grey peasant's smock. Not far off was a village, he could see the black huts, and half the huts were burnt down, there were only the charred beams sticking up. And as they drove in, there were peasant women drawn up along the road, a lot of women, a whole row, all thin and wan, with their faces a sort of brownish colour, especially one at the edge, a tall, bony woman, who looked forty, but might have been only twenty, with a long thin face. And in her arms was a little baby crying. And her breasts seemed so dried up that there was not a drop of milk in them. And the child cried and cried, and held out its little bare arms, with its little fists blue from cold.

"Why are they crying? Why are they crying?" Mitya asked, as they dashed gaily by.

"It's the babe," answered the driver, "the babe weeping."

And Mitya was struck by his saying, in his peasant way, "the babe," and he liked the peasant's calling it a "babe." There seemed more pity in it.

"But why is it weeping?" Mitya persisted stupidly, "why are its little arms bare? Why don't they wrap it up?"

"The babe's cold, its little clothes are frozen and don't warm it."

"But why is it? Why?" Mitya still persisted foolishly.

"Why, they're poor people, burnt out. They've no bread. They're begging because they've been burnt out."

"No, no." Mitya, as it were, still did not understand. "Tell me why it is those poor mothers stand there? Why are people poor? Why is the babe poor? Why is the steppe barren? Why don't they hug each other and kiss? Why don't they sing songs of joy? Why are they so black with black misery? Why don't they feed the babe?"

And he felt that, though his questions were unreasonable and senseless, yet he wanted to ask just that, and he had to ask it in just that way. And he felt that a passion of pity, such as he had never known before, was rising in his heart, that he wanted to cry, that he wanted to do something for them all, so that the babe should weep no more, so that the dark-faced, withered mother should not weep, that no one should shed tears again from that moment, and he wanted to do it at once, at once, regardless of all obstacles, with true Karamazov recklessness.

"And I'm coming with you. I won't leave you now for the rest of my life, I'm coming with you," he heard close beside him Grushenka's tender voice, thrilling with emotion. And his heart glowed, and he struggled forward towards the light, and he longed to live, to live, to go on and on, towards the new, beckoning light, and to hasten, hasten, now, at once!

"What! Where?" he exclaimed, opening his eyes, and sitting up on the chest, as though he had revived from a swoon, he smiled serenely. Nikolay Parfenovich was standing over him, suggesting that he should hear the

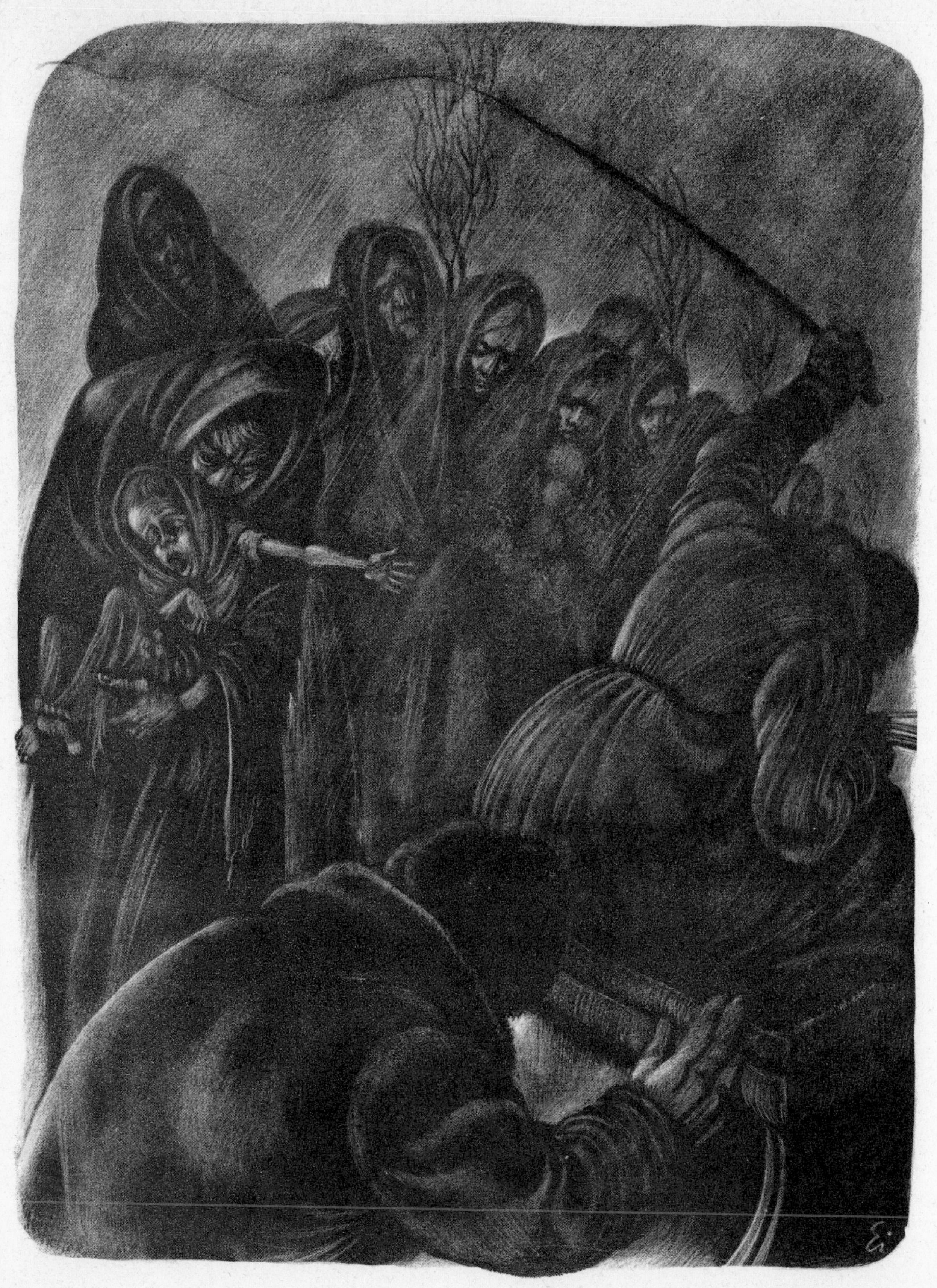

THE PEASANT CALLED IT A "BABE"

testimony read aloud and sign it. Mitya guessed that he had been asleep an hour or more, but he did not listen to Nikolay Parfenovich. He was suddenly struck by the fact that there was a pillow under his head, which hadn't been there when he had leant back, exhausted, on the chest.

"Who put that pillow under my head? Who was so kind?" he cried, with a sort of ecstatic gratitude, and tears in his voice, as though some great kindness had been shown him.

He never found out who this kind man was, perhaps one of the peasant witnesses, or Nikolay Parfenovich's little secretary had compassionately thought to put a pillow under his head, but his whole soul was quivering with tears. He went to the table and said that he would sign whatever they liked.

"I've had a good dream, gentlemen," he said in a strange voice, with a new face, radiant with joy.

CHAPTER IX

THEY CARRY MITYA AWAY

When the testimony had been signed, Nikolay Parfenovich turned solemnly to the prisoner and read him the "Commitment," setting forth that, in such a year, on such a day, in such a place, the examining magistrate of such-and-such a district court, having examined so-and-so (to wit, Mitya) accused of this and of that (all the charges were carefully itemized) and taking into consideration that the accused, pleading not guilty to the charges made against him, had brought forward nothing in his defence, while the witnesses, so-and-so and so-and-so, and the circumstances, such-and-such, testify against him, — the examining magistrate acting in accordance with such-and-such articles of the Penal Code, and so on, has ruled that, in order to preclude such-and-such (Mitya) from all means of evading examination and trial, the said person be detained in such-and-such a prison, of which circumstance he hereby notifies the accused, and further, the examining magistrate delivers a copy of this same "Commitment" to the deputy prosecutor, and so on, and so on.

In brief, Mitya was informed that he was, from that moment, a prisoner, and that he would be driven at once to the town, and there locked up in a very unpleasant place. Mitya listened attentively, and only shrugged his shoulders.

"Well, gentlemen, I don't blame you. I'm ready. . . . I understand that there's nothing else for you to do."

Nikolay Parfenovich informed him gently that he would be escorted at once by the rural police officer, Mavriky Mavrikyevich, who happened to be on the spot. . . .

"Wait," Mitya interrupted suddenly, and impelled by uncontrollable feeling he said, addressing all in the room:

"Gentlemen, we're all cruel, we're all monsters, we all make men weep, and mothers, and babes at the breast, but of all, let it be settled here, now, of all I am the lowest reptile! Every day of my life, beating my breast, I swore to reform, and every day I did the same filthy things. I understand now that such men as I need a blow, a blow of fate to catch them as with a noose, and bind them by an external force. Never, never should I have risen of myself! But the thunderbolt has fallen. I accept the torture of accusation, and my public shame, I want to suffer and by suffering I shall be purified. Perhaps I shall be purified, gentlemen, eh? But listen, for the last time, I am not guilty of my father's blood. I accept my punishment, not because I killed him, but because I meant to kill him, and perhaps I really might have killed him. Still I mean to fight it out with you, I warn you of that. I'll fight it out with you to the end, and then God will decide. Good-bye, gentlemen, don't be vexed with me for having shouted at you during the examination. Oh, I was still such a fool then. . . . In another minute I shall be a prisoner, but now, for the last time, as a free man, Dmitri Karamazov offers you his hand. Saying good-bye to you, I say it to all men."

His voice quivered and he stretched out his hand, but Nikolay Parfenovich, who happened to stand nearest to him, with a sudden, almost nervous movement, hid his hands behind his back. Mitya instantly noticed this, and started. He let his outstretched hand drop at once.

"The preliminary inquiry is not yet over," Nikolay Parfenovich faltered, somewhat embarrassed. "We will continue it in the town, and I, for my part, of course, am ready to wish you all success . . . in your defence. . . . As a matter of fact, Dmitri Fyodorovich, I've always been disposed to regard you as, so to speak, more unfortunate than guilty. All of us here, if I may make bold to speak for all, are ready to recognise that you are, at bottom, a young man of honour, but, alas, one who has been carried away by certain passions to a somewhat excessive degree. . . ."

Nikolay Parfenovich's little figure was positively majestic by the time he had finished speaking. It struck Mitya that in another minute this "boy" would take his arm, lead him to another corner, and renew their conversation about "women." But many quite irrelevant and inappropriate thoughts sometimes occur to a prisoner even when he is being led to execution.

"Gentlemen, you are good, you are humane, may I see *her* to say 'good-bye' for the last time?" asked Mitya.

"Certainly, but considering . . . in fact, now it's impossible except in the presence of . . ."

"Oh, well, if it must be so, it must!"

Grushenka was brought in, but the farewell was brief and laconic, and did not at all satisfy Nikolay Parfenovich. Grushenka made a deep bow to Mitya.

"I have told you I am yours, and I will be yours. I will follow you for ever, wherever they may send you. Farewell, you who have been your own undoing, though you are guiltless."

Her lips quivered, tears flowed from her eyes.

"Forgive me, Grusha, for my love, for undoing you, too, with my love."

Mitya would have said something more, but he broke off and went out. He was at once surrounded by men who kept a constant watch on him. At the bottom of the steps to which he had driven up with such a dash the night before with Andrey's three horses, two carts stood in readiness. Mavriky Mavrikyevich, a sturdy, thick-set man with a flabby face, was annoyed about something, some sudden irregularity. He was shouting angrily. He asked Mitya to get into the cart with somewhat excessive surliness.

"When I stood him drinks in the tavern, the man had quite a different face," thought Mitya, as he got in. At the gates there was a crowd of people, peasants, women and drivers. Trifon Borisovich came down the steps, too. All stared at Mitya.

"Forgive me at parting, God's people!" Mitya shouted suddenly from the cart.

"Forgive us, too!" he heard two or three voices.

"Farewell to you, too, Trifon Borisovich!"

But Trifon Borisovich did not even turn round. He was, perhaps, too busy. He, too, was shouting and fussing about something. It appeared that everything was not yet ready in the second cart, in which two constables were to accompany Mavriky Mavrikyevich. The peasant who had been ordered to drive the second cart was pulling on his smock, stoutly maintaining that it was not his turn to go, but Akim's. But Akim was not to be seen. They ran to fetch him. The peasant persisted and besought them to wait.

"You see what our people are, Mavriky Mavrikyevich. They've no shame!" exclaimed Trifon Borisovich. "Akim gave you twenty-five copecks the day before yesterday. You've drunk it all and now you cry out. I'm simply surprised at how kind you are to our louts, Mavriky Mavrikyevich, that's all I can say."

"But what do we want a second troika for?" Mitya put in. "Let's start with the one, Mavriky Mavrikyevich. I won't be unruly, I won't run away from you, old fellow. What do we want an escort for?"

"I'll trouble you, sir, to learn how to speak to me if you've never been taught. I'm not 'old fellow' to you, and you can keep your advice for another time!" Mavriky Mavrikyevich snapped out savagely, as though glad to vent his wrath.

Mitya was reduced to silence. He flushed all over. A moment later he felt suddenly very cold. The rain had ceased, but the dull sky was still overcast, and a keen wind was blowing straight in his face. "I've taken a chill," thought Mitya, twitching his shoulders.

At last Mavriky Mavrikyevich, too, got into the cart, sat down heavily, and, as though without noticing it, squeezed Mitya into the corner. It is true that he was out of humour and greatly disliked the task that had been laid upon him.

"Good-bye, Trifon Borisovich!" Mitya shouted again, and felt himself that he had not called out this time from good-nature, but involuntarily, from resentment.

But Trifon Borisovich stood proudly, with both hands behind his back, and staring straight at Mitya with a stern and angry face, he made no reply.

"Good-bye, Dmitri Fyodorovich, good-bye!" he heard all at once the voice of Kalganov, who had suddenly darted out. Running up to the cart, he held out his hand to Mitya. He had no cap on.

Mitya had time to seize and press his hand.

"Good-bye, dear fellow! I shan't forget your magnanimity," he cried warmly.

But the cart moved and their hands parted. The bell began ringing and Mitya was driven off.

Kalganov ran back, sat down in a corner, bent his head, hid his face in his hands, and burst out crying.

For a long while he sat like that, crying as though he were a little boy instead of a young man of twenty. Oh, he believed almost without doubt in Mitya's guilt.

"What are people like? What can men be after this?" he exclaimed incoherently, in bitter despondency, almost despair. At that moment he had no desire to live.

"Is it worth it? Is it worth it?" exclaimed the boy in his grief.

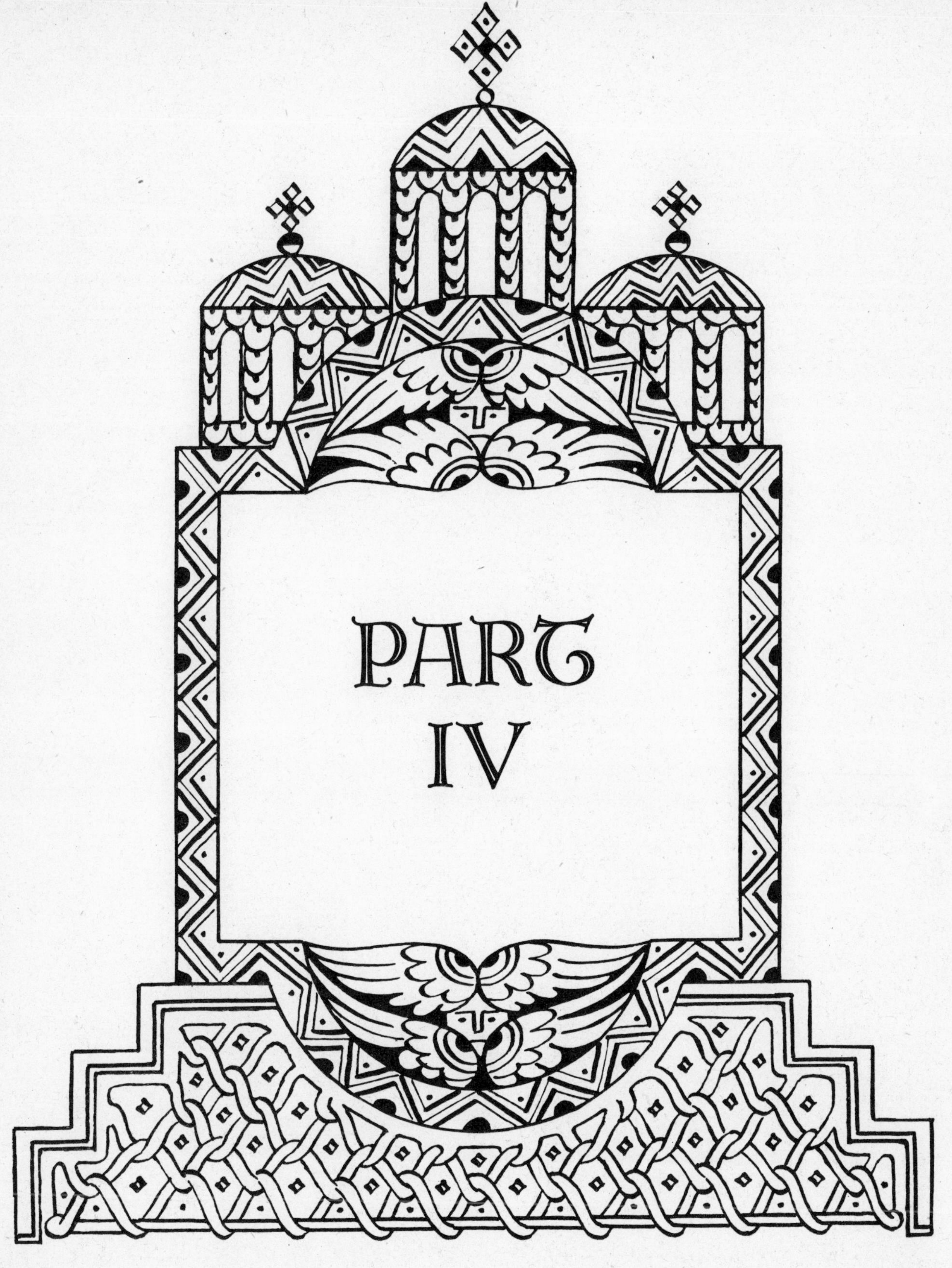
PART
IV

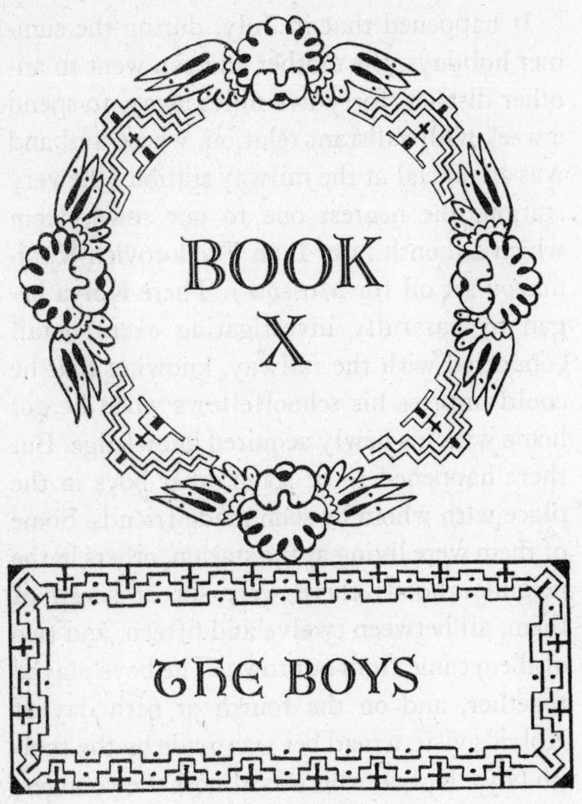

CHAPTER I

KOLYA KRASOTKIN

It was the beginning of November. There had been a hard frost, eleven degrees below zero, with ice under foot, and only a little dry snow had fallen on the frozen ground during the night. A keen dry wind was lifting and blowing it along the dreary streets of our town, especially about the market-place. It was a dull morning, but the snow had ceased.

Not far from the market-place, close to the Plotnikov shop, there stands a small house, very neat both without and within. It belongs to Madame Krasotkin, the widow of a former provincial secretary, who has been dead for fourteen years. His widow, still a good-looking woman and in her thirties, is living in her neat little house on her private income. She lives in respectable seclusion; she is of a soft but fairly cheerful disposition. She was about eighteen at the time of her husband's death; she had been married only a year and had just borne him a son. From the day of his death she devoted herself heart and soul to the bringing up of her darling boy Kolya. She loved him passionately all those fourteen years, though he had caused her far more suffering than happiness. She had been trembling and fainting with terror almost every day, afraid he would fall ill, would catch cold, do something naughty, climb on a chair and fall off it, and so on and so on. When Kolya began going to school, the mother devoted herself to studying all the subjects with him so as to help him, and go through his lessons with him. She hastened to make the acquaintance of the teachers and their wives, even made up to Kolya's schoolfellows, and fawned upon them in the hope of thus saving Kolya from being teased, laughed at, or beaten by them. She went so far that the boys actually began to mock at him on her account, and taunt him with being a "mamma's pet."

But the boy could stand up for himself. He was a daring boy, "tremendously strong," as was rumoured in his class, and soon proved to be the fact; he was agile, strong-willed, and of an audacious and enterprising temper. He was good at lessons, and there was a rumour in the school that he could beat the teacher, Dardanelov, himself at arithmetic and universal history. Though he looked down upon every one, and turned up his nose, he was a good comrade and not supercilious. He accepted his schoolfellows' respect as his due, but was friendly with them. Above all, he knew where to draw the line. He could restrain himself on occasion, and in his relations with the teachers he never overstepped that last forbidden limit beyond which a prank becomes an unpardonable breach of discipline. But he was as fond of mischief on every possible occasion as the smallest boy in the school, and not so much for the sake of mischief as for the sake of creating a sensation, inventing something, doing something effective and conspicuous. He was extremely vain. He knew how to make even his mother give in to him; he treated her almost despotically. She gave in to him, oh, she had begun giving in to him long ago. The one thought unendurable to her was that her boy did not love her enough. She was always fancying that Kolya was "unfeeling" towards her, and at times, dissolving into hysterical tears, she reproached him with coldness. The boy disliked this, and the more demonstrations of feeling were demanded of him the more he seemed intentionally to avoid them. Yet it was not intentional on his part but instinctive — it was his character. His mother was mistaken; he was very fond of her. He only disliked "sheepish sentimentality," as he expressed it in his schoolboy language.

There was a bookcase in the house containing a few books that had been his father's. Kolya was fond of reading, and had read several of them by himself. His mother did not mind that and only wondered sometimes at seeing the boy stand for hours by the bookcase poring over a book instead of going to play. And in that way Kolya read some things unsuitable for his age.

Though the boy, as a rule, knew where to draw the line in his mischief, he had of late begun to play pranks that caused his mother serious alarm. It is true there was nothing vicious, but a wild mad recklessness.

It happened that in July, during the summer holidays, the mother and son went to another district, forty-five miles away, to spend a week with a distant relation, whose husband was an official at the railway station (the very station, the nearest one to our town, from which a month later Ivan Fyodorovich Karamazov set off for Moscow). There Kolya began by carefully investigating every detail connected with the railway, knowing that he could impress his schoolfellows when he got home with his newly acquired knowledge. But there happened to be some other boys in the place with whom he soon made friends. Some of them were living at the station, others in the neighbourhood; there were six or seven of them, all between twelve and fifteen, and two of them came from our town. The boys played together, and on the fourth or fifth day of Kolya's visit, a mad bet was made by the foolish boys. Kolya, who was almost the youngest of the party and rather looked down upon by the others in consequence, was moved by vanity or by reckless bravado to bet them two roubles that he would lie down between the rails at night when the eleven o'clock train was due, and would lie there without moving while the train rolled over him at full speed. It is true they made a preliminary investigation, from which it appeared that it was possible to stretch out and lie so flat between the rails that the train could pass over without touching one, but to lie there was no joke! Kolya maintained stoutly that he would do it. At first they laughed at him, called him a little liar, a braggart, but that only egged him on. What piqued him most was that these boys of fifteen turned up their noses at him unbearably, and were at first disposed to treat him as "a small boy," not fit to associate with them, and that was an unendurable insult to him.

And so it was resolved to go in the evening to a point half a mile from the station, so that the train might have time to get up full speed after leaving the station. The boys assembled. It was a pitch-dark moonless night. At the appointed time, Kolya lay down between the rails. The five others who had taken the bet waited among the bushes below the embankment, their hearts beating with suspense, which was followed by alarm and remorse. At last they heard in the distance the rumble of the train leaving the station. Two red lights gleamed out of the darkness; the monster roared as it approached.

"Run, run off the tracks!" the boys cried to Kolya from the bushes, breathless with terror. But it was too late: the train dashed up and flew past. The boys rushed to Kolya. He lay without moving. They began pulling at him, lifting him up. He suddenly got up and walked off the embankment without a word. Then he explained that he had lain there as though he were unconscious to frighten them, but the fact was that he really had lost consciousness, as he confessed long after to his mother. In this way his reputation as "a desperate character," was established for ever. He returned home to the station as white as a sheet. Next day he had a slight attack of nervous fever, but he was in high spirits and well pleased with himself. The incident did not become known at once, but when they came back to the town it penetrated to the school and even reached the ears of the masters. But then Kolya's mother hastened to entreat the masters on her boy's behalf, and in the end Dardanelov, a respected and influential teacher, exerted himself in his favour, and the affair was hushed up.

Dardanelov was a middle-aged bachelor, who had been passionately in love with Madame Krasotkin for many years past, and had once already, about a year previously, ventured, faint with fear and the delicacy of his sentiments, to offer her most respectfully his hand in marriage. But she refused him pointblank, feeling that to accept him would be an act of treachery to her boy, though Dardanelov had reason for believing, to judge from certain mysterious symptoms, that he was not an object of aversion to the charming but too chaste and tender-hearted widow. Kolya's mad prank seemed to have broken the ice, and Dardanelov was rewarded for his intercession by an intimation of hope. The intimation, it is true, was a slight one, but then Dardanelov himself was such a paragon of purity and delicacy that it was enough for the time being to make him perfectly happy. He was fond of the boy, though he would have felt it beneath him to try and win him over, and was severe and strict with him in class. Kolya, too, kept him at a respectful distance. He learnt his lessons perfectly; he was second in his class, was reserved with Dardanelov, and the whole class firmly believed that Kolya was so good at universal history that he could "beat" even Dardanelov. Kolya did indeed ask him the question, "Who founded Troy?" to which Dardanelov had made a very vague reply, referring to the movements and migrations of races, to the remoteness of the period, to the mythical legends. But the question, "Who had founded Troy?" that is, what individuals, he could not answer, and even for some reason regarded the question as idle and frivolous. But the boys remained convinced that Dardanelov did not know who founded Troy. Kolya had read of the founders of Troy in

Smaragdov, whose history was among the books in his father's bookcase. In the end all the boys became interested in the question, who it was that had founded Troy, but Krasotkin would not tell his secret, and his reputation for knowledge remained unshaken.

After the incident on the railway a certain change came over Kolya's attitude to his mother. When Anna Fyodorovna (Madame Krasotkin) heard of her son's exploit, she almost went out of her mind with horror. She had such terrible attacks of hysterics, lasting with intervals for several days, that Kolya, seriously alarmed at last, promised on his honour that such pranks should never be repeated. He swore on his knees before the holy image, and swore by the memory of his father, at Madame Krasotkin's instance, and the "manly" Kolya burst into tears like a boy of six. And all that day the mother and son were constantly rushing into each other's arms sobbing. Next day Kolya woke up as "unfeeling" as before, but he had become more silent, more modest, sterner, and more thoughtful.

Six weeks later, it is true, he played another prank, which even brought his name to the ears of our justice of the peace, but it was a prank of quite another kind, amusing, foolish, and he did not, as it turned out, take the leading part in it, but was only implicated in it. But of this later. His mother still fretted and trembled, but the more uneasy she became, the greater were the hopes of Dardanelov. It must be noted that Kolya understood and divined what was in Dardanelov's heart and, of course, despised him profoundly for his "feelings"; he had in the past been so tactless as to show this contempt before his mother, hinting vaguely that he knew what Dardanelov was after. But from the time of the railway incident his behaviour in this respect also was changed; he did not allow himself the remotest allusion to the subject and began to speak more respectfully of Dardanelov before his mother, which the sensitive woman at once appreciated with boundless gratitude. But at the slightest mention of Dardanelov by a visitor in Kolya's presence, she would flush as pink as a rose. At such moments Kolya would either stare out the window scowling, or would investigate the state of his boots, or would shout angrily for "Perezvon," the big, shaggy, mangy dog, which he had picked up a month before, brought home, and kept for some reason secretly indoors, not showing him to any of his schoolfellows. He bullied him frightfully, teaching him all sorts of tricks, so that the poor dog howled for him whenever he was absent at school, and when he came in, whined with delight, rushed about as if he were crazy, begged, lay down on the ground and played dead, and so on; in fact, showed all the tricks he had taught him, not at the word of command, but simply from the zeal of his ecstatic and grateful heart.

I have forgotten, by the way, to mention that Kolya Krasotkin was the boy stabbed with a penknife by the boy already known to the reader as the son of Captain Snegiryov. Ilusha had been defending his father when the schoolboys jeered at him, shouting the nickname "bath-mop."

CHAPTER II

CHILDREN

And so on that frosty, windy day in November, Kolya Krasotkin was sitting at home. It was Sunday and there was no school. It had just struck eleven, and he particularly wanted to go out "on very urgent business," but he was left alone in charge of the house, for it so happened that all its elder occupants were absent owing to a sudden and singular event. Madame Krasotkin had let two little rooms, separated from the rest of the house by a passage, to a doctor's wife with her two small children. This lady was the same age as Anna Fyodorovna, and a great friend of hers. Her husband, the doctor, had taken his departure a year ago, going first to Orenburg and then to Tashkent, and for the last six months she had not heard a word from him. Had it not been for her friendship with Madame Krasotkin, which was some consolation to the forsaken lady, she would certainly have dissolved in tears completely. And now, to add to her misfortunes, Katerina, her only servant, was suddenly moved the evening before to announce, to her mistress's amazement, that she proposed to bring a child into the world by morning. How it was that no one had noticed the imminence of the event before seemed almost miraculous to every one. The astounded doctor's wife decided to move Katerina while there was still time to an establishment kept for such emergencies by a midwife in our town. As she set great store by her servant, she promptly carried out this plan, took her to the institution and remained there looking after her. Then, by morning, for some reason there arose the need of all the friendly sympathy and assistance of Madame Krasotkin herself. It was thought that on this occasion she might be able to appeal to some one and give aid and comfort.

So both the ladies were absent from home, while Madame Krasotkin's servant, Agafya, had gone to market, and Kolya was thus left for a time to protect and look after the "kids," that is, the son and daughter of the doctor's wife, who were left alone. Kolya was not afraid of taking care of the house, besides he had Perezvon, who had been ordered to lie flat, without moving, under the bench in the hall. Every time Kolya, walking to and fro through the rooms, came into the hall, the dog shook his head and gave two firm and wheedling taps on the floor with his tail, but alas! no summoning whistle was heard. Kolya looked sternly at the luckless dog, who relapsed again into obedient rigidity. The one thing that troubled Kolya was the "kids." He looked, of course, with the utmost scorn on Katerina's unexpected adventure, but he was very fond of the bereaved "kiddies," and had already taken them a picture book. Nastya, the elder, a girl of eight, could read, and Kostya, the boy, aged seven, was very fond of being read to by her. Krasotkin could, of course, have provided more diverting entertainment for them. He could have made them stand side by side and played soldiers with them, or sent them hiding all over the house. He had done so more than once before and was not above doing it, so much so that a report once spread at school that at home Krasotkin played horses with the little lodgers, prancing with his head on one side like a trace-horse. But Krasotkin haughtily parried this thrust, pointing out that to play horses with boys of one's own age, boys of thirteen, would certainly be disgraceful "at this date," but that he did it for the sake of the "kids" because he liked them, and no one had a right to call him to account for his feelings. The two "kids" adored him.

But on this occasion he was in no mood for games. He had very important business of his own before him, something almost mysterious.

Meanwhile time was passing and Agafya, with whom he could have left the children, would not come back from market. He had several times already crossed the passage, opened the door of the lodgers' apartment and looked anxiously at the "kids," who were sitting over the book, as he had bidden them. Every time he opened the door they grinned at him, hoping he would come in and would do something delightful and amusing. But Kolya was uneasy and did not go in.

At last it struck eleven and he made up his mind, once for all, that if that "damned" Agafya did not come back within ten minutes he would go out without waiting for her, making the "kids" "promise," of course, to be brave when he was away, not to be naughty, not to cry from fright. With this idea he put on his wadded winter overcoat with its sealskin collar, slung his satchel round his shoulder, and, regardless of his mother's constantly reiterated entreaties that he would always put on goloshes in such cold weather, he looked at them contemptuously as he crossed the hall and went out with only his boots on. Perezvon, seeing him in his outdoor clothes, began tapping vigorously on the floor with his tail. Nervously twitching all over, he even uttered a plaintive whine. But Kolya, seeing his dog's passionate excitement, decided that it was a breach of discipline, kept him for another minute under the bench, and only when he had opened the door into the passage he whistled for him. The dog leapt up like a mad creature and began bounding before him with rapture.

Having crossed the passage, Kolya opened the door to peep at the "kids." They were both sitting as before at the table, not reading but warmly disputing about something. The children often argued together about various exciting problems of life, and Nastya, being the elder, always got the best of it. If Kostya did not agree with her, he almost always appealed to Kolya Krasotkin, and his verdict was regarded as final by both of them. This time the "kids' " discussion rather interested Krasotkin, and he stood still in the passage to listen. The children saw he was listening and that made them argue with even greater heat.

"I shall never, never believe," Nastya prattled, "that midwives find babies among the cabbages in the kitchen garden. It's winter now and there are no cabbages, and so the midwife couldn't have taken Katerina a daughter."

"Phew!" Kolya whistled to himself.

"Or perhaps they do bring babies from somewhere, but only to those who are married."

Kostya stared at Nastya and listened, pondering profoundly.

"Nastya, how silly you are," he said at last, firmly and calmly. "How can Katerina have a baby when she isn't married?"

Nastya was exasperated.

"You know nothing about it," she snapped irritably. "Perhaps she has a husband, only he is in prison, so now she's got a baby."

"But is her husband in prison?" the matter-of-fact Kostya inquired gravely.

"Or, I tell you what," Nastya interrupted impulsively, completely rejecting and forgetting her first hypothesis. "She hasn't a husband, you are right there, but she wants to be married, and so she's been thinking of getting married, and thinking and thinking of it till now she's got it, that is, not a husband but a baby."

"Well, perhaps so," Kostya agreed, entirely vanquished. "But you didn't say so before. So how could I tell?"

"Well, young ones," said Kolya, stepping into the room. "You're a dangerous sort, I see."

"And Perezvon with you!" grinned Kostya, and began snapping his fingers and calling Perezvon.

"I am in trouble, kids," Krasotkin began solemnly, "and you must help me. Agafya must have broken a leg, since she has not turned up till now, that's certain. And I must go out. Will you let me go?"

The children looked anxiously at one another. Their smiling faces showed signs of uneasiness, but they did not yet fully grasp what was expected of them.

"You won't be naughty while I am gone? You won't climb on the cupboard and break your legs? You won't be frightened alone and cry?"

A look of profound despondency came into the children's faces.

"And I could show you something as a reward, a little copper cannon which can be fired with real gunpowder."

The children's faces instantly brightened. "Show us the cannon," said Kostya, beaming all over.

Krasotkin put his hand in his satchel, and pulling out a little brass cannon stood it on the table.

"Ah, you are bound to ask that! Look, it's on wheels." He rolled the toy along on the table. "And it can be fired off, too. It can be loaded with shot and fired off."

"And it could kill?"

"It would kill everybody; you've only got to aim it," and Krasotkin explained where the powder had to be put, where the shot should be rolled in, showed a tiny hole like a touch-hole, and told them that it kicked when it was fired.

The children listened with intense interest. What particularly struck their imagination was that the cannon kicked.

"And have you got any powder?" Nastya inquired.

"Yes."

"Show us the powder, too," she drawled with a smile of entreaty.

Krasotkin dived again into his satchel and pulled out a small flask containing a little real gunpowder. He had some shot, too, in a screw of paper. He even uncorked the flask and shook a little powder into the palm of his hand.

"One has to be careful there's no fire about, or it would blow up and kill us all," Krasotkin warned them to produce a sensation.

The children gazed at the powder with an awe-stricken fear that only intensified their enjoyment. But Kostya liked the shot better.

"And does the shot burn?" he inquired.

"No, it doesn't."

"Give me a little shot," he asked in an imploring voice.

"I'll give you a little shot; here, take it, but don't show it to your mother till I come back, or she'll be sure to think it's gunpowder, and will die of fright and give you a thrashing."

"Mother never does whip us," Nastya observed at once.

"I know, I only said it for the sake of the style. And don't you ever deceive your mother except just this once, until I come back. And so, kiddies, can I go out? You won't be frightened and cry when I'm gone?"

"We sha—all cry," drawled Kostya, on the verge of tears already.

"We shall cry, we shall be sure to cry," Nastya chimed in with timid haste.

"Oh, children, children, how fraught with peril are your years! There's no help for it, chicks, I shall have to stay with you. I don't know how long. And time is passing, time is passing, oogh!"

"Tell Perezvon to play dead!" Kostya begged.

"There's no help for it, we must have recourse to Perezvon. *Ici*, Perezvon." And Kolya began giving orders to the dog, who performed all his tricks.

He was a shaggy dog, of a very common size, with a coat of a sort of lilac-grey colour. He was blind in his right eye, and his left ear was torn. He whined and jumped, stood and walked on his hind legs, lay on his back with his paws in the air, and lay rigid as though he were dead. While this last performance was going on, the door opened and Agafya, Madame Krasotkin's servant, a stout pock-marked woman of forty, appeared on the threshold. She had come back from market and had a bag full of provisions in her hand. Holding up the bag of provisions in her left hand, she stood still to watch the dog. Though Kolya had been so anxious for her return, he did not cut short the performance, and after keeping Perezvon dead for the usual time, at last he whistled to him. The dog jumped up and began bounding about in his joy at having done his duty.

"Only think, a dog!" Agafya observed sententiously.

"Why are you late, female?" asked Krasotkin sternly.

"Female, indeed! Go on with you, you brat."

"Brat?"

"Yes, brat. What is it to you if I'm late; if I'm late, you may be sure I have good reason," muttered Agafya, busying herself about the stove, without a trace of anger or displeasure in her voice. She seemed quite pleased, in fact, to enjoy a chat with her merry young master.

"Listen, you frivolous old woman," Krasotkin began, getting up from the sofa, "can you swear by all you hold sacred in the world and something else besides, that you will watch vigilantly over the kids in my absence? I am going out."

"And what should I swear for?" laughed Agafya. "I shall look after them without that."

"No, you must swear on the salvation of your soul. Else I shan't go."

"Well, don't then. What does it matter to me? It's cold out; stay home."

"Kids," Kolya turned to the children, "this woman will stay with you till I come back or till your mother comes, for she ought to have been back long ago. She will give you some lunch, too. You'll give them something, Agafya, won't you?"

"That I can do."

"Good-bye, chicks, I go with my heart at rest. And you, granny," he added gravely, in an undertone, as he passed Agafya, "I hope you'll spare their tender years and not tell them any of your old woman's nonsense about Katerina. *Ici*, Perezvon!"

"Get along with you!" retorted Agafya, really angry this time. "Ridiculous boy! You want a whipping for saying such things, that's what you want!"

CHAPTER III

THE SCHOOLBOY

BUT Kolya did not hear her. At last he could go out. As he went out at the gate he looked round him, shrugged up his little shoulders, and saying "It is freezing," went straight along the street and turned off to the right towards the market-place. When he reached the last house but one before the market-place he stopped at the gate, pulled a whistle out of his pocket, and whistled with all his might as though giving a signal. He had not to wait more than a minute before a rosy-cheeked boy of about eleven, wearing a warm, neat, and even stylish coat, darted out to meet him. This was Smurov, a boy in the preparatory class (two classes below Kolya Krasotkin), son of a well-to-do official. Apparently he was forbidden by his parents to associate with Krasotkin, who was well known to be a desperately naughty boy, so Smurov was obviously slipping out on the sly. He was — if the reader has not forgotten — one of the group of boys who two months before had thrown stones across the ditch at Ilusha. He was the one who had told Alyosha Karamazov about Ilusha.

"I've been waiting for you for the last hour, Krasotkin," said Smurov stolidly, and the boys strode towards the market-place.

"I am late," answered Krasotkin. "I was detained by circumstances. You won't be thrashed for coming with me?"

"Come, I say, I'm never thrashed! And you've got Perezvon with you?"

"Yes."

"You're taking him, too?"

"Yes."

"Ah! if it were only Zhuchka!"

"That's impossible. Zhuchka doesn't exist. Zhuchka is lost in the mists of obscurity."

"Ah! couldn't we do this?" Smurov suddenly stood still. "You see Ilusha says that Zhuchka was a shaggy, greyish, smoky-looking dog like Perezvon. Couldn't you tell him this is Zhuchka, and maybe he'll believe it?"

"Boy, shun a lie, that's one thing; even a white lie — that's another. Above all, I hope you've not told them anything about my coming."

"Heaven forbid! I know what I am about. But you won't comfort him with Perezvon," said Smurov, with a sigh. "You know his father, the captain, the 'bath-mop,' told us that he was going to bring him a real mastiff pup, with a black nose, to-day. He thinks that would comfort Ilusha; but I doubt it."

"And how is Ilusha?"

"Ah, he is low, very low! I believe he's in consumption: he is quite conscious, but his breathing! He doesn't breathe well. The other day he asked them to lead him round the room. They put on his boots for him and he tried to walk, but he couldn't. 'Ah, I told you before, papa,' he said, 'that those boots were no good. I could never walk comfortably in them.' He fancied it was the boots that made him stagger, but it was simply weakness, really. He won't live another week. Herzenstube is looking after him. Now they are rich again — they've got heaps of money."

"They are rogues."

"Who are rogues?"

"Doctors and the whole medical crew collectively, and also, of course, individually. I'm against medicine. It's a useless institution. However, I mean to go into all that. But what's that sentimentality you've got up there? The whole class seems to be there every day?"

"Not the whole class: it's only ten of our fellows who go to see him every day. There's nothing in that."

"What surprises me in all this is the part that Alexey Karamazov is taking in it. His brother's going to be tried to-morrow or next day for such a crime, and yet he has so much time to spend on sentimentalities with boys."

"There's no sentimentality about it. Here you are going yourself now to make up with Ilusha."

"Make up? A ridiculous expression! Besides, I allow no one to analyse my actions."

"And how pleased Ilusha will be to see you! He has no idea that you are coming. Why was it, why was it you wouldn't come all this time?" Smurov cried with sudden heat.

"My dear boy, that's my business, not yours. I am going of my own accord because I choose to, but you've all been hauled there by Alexey Karamazov — there's a difference, you know. And how do you know? I may not be going to make up at all. A stupid expression."

"It's not Karamazov at all; it's not his doing. Our fellows began going there of themselves. Of course, they went with Karamazov at first. And there's been nothing of that sort — no silliness. First one went, and then another. His father was awfully pleased to see us. You know he will simply go out of his mind if Ilusha dies. He sees that Ilusha's dying. And he seems so glad we've made it up with Ilusha. Ilusha asked after you, that was all. He just asks and says no more. His father will go out of his mind or hang himself. He behaved like a madman before. You know he is a very decent man. We made a mistake then. It's all the fault of that murderer who thrashed him then."

"Karamazov's a riddle to me all the same. I might have made his acquaintance long ago, but I like to have a proper pride in some cases. Besides, I have a theory about him which I must work out and verify."

Kolya subsided into dignified silence. Smurov, too, was silent. Smurov, of course, worshipped Krasotkin and never dreamed of putting himself on a level with him. Now he was tremendously interested at Kolya's saying that he was "going of his own accord" to see Ilusha. He felt that there must be some mystery in Kolya's suddenly taking it into his head to go to him that day. They crossed the market-place, in which at that hour were many loaded wagons from the country and a great number of live fowls. The market women were selling pretzels, thread, etc., in their booths. These Sunday assemblies were naïvely called "fairs" in the town, and there were many such fairs in the year.

Perezvon ran about in the wildest spirits, sniffing about first on one side, then on the other. When he met other dogs he zealously sniffed them according to the rules of canine etiquette.

"I like to watch such realistic scenes, Smurov," said Kolya suddenly. "Have you noticed how dogs sniff at one another when they meet? It seems to be a law of their nature."

"Yes; it's a funny habit."

"No, it's not funny; you are wrong there. There's nothing funny in nature, however funny it may seem to man with his prejudices. If dogs could reason and criticise us they'd be sure to find just as much that would be funny to them, if not far more, in the social relations of men, their masters — far more, indeed. I repeat that, because I am convinced that there is far more foolishness among us. That's Rakitin's idea — a remarkable idea. I am a socialist, Smurov."

"And what is a socialist?" asked Smurov.

"That's when all are equal and all have property in common, there are no marriages, and every one has any religion and laws he likes best, and all the rest of it. You are not old enough to understand that yet. It's cold, though."

"Yes, twelve degrees below zero. Father looked at the thermometer just now."

"Have you noticed, Smurov, that in the middle of winter we don't feel so cold, even when there are fifteen or eighteen degrees below zero as we do now, in the beginning of winter, when there is a sudden frost of twelve degrees, especially when there is not much snow? It's because people are not used to it. Everything is habit with men, everything even in their social and political relations. Habit is the great motive-power. What a funny-looking peasant!"

Kolya pointed to a tall peasant, with a good-natured countenance, in a long sheepskin coat, who was standing by his wagon, clapping together his mittened hands to warm them. His long fair beard was all white with frost.

"That peasant's beard's frozen," Kolya cried in a loud provocative voice as he passed him.

"Lots of people's beards are frozen," the peasant replied, calmly and sententiously.

"Don't tease him," observed Smurov.

"It's all right; he won't be cross; he's a nice fellow. Good-bye, Matvey."

"Good-bye."

"Is your name Matvey?"

"Yes. Didn't you know?"

"No, I didn't. It was a guess."

"You don't say so! You are a schoolboy, I suppose?"

"Yes."

"You get whipped, I expect?"

"Nothing to speak of — sometimes."

"Does it hurt?"

"Well, yes, it does."

"Ech, what a life!" The peasant heaved a sigh from the bottom of his heart.

"Good-bye, Matvey."

"Good-bye. You are a nice chap, that you are."

The boys went on.

"That was a nice peasant," Kolya observed to Smurov. "I like talking to the peasants, and am always glad to do them justice."

"Why did you tell a lie, pretending we are thrashed?" asked Smurov.

"I had to say that to please him."

"How do you mean?"

"You know, Smurov, I don't like being asked the same thing twice. I like people to understand at the first word. Some things can't be explained. According to a peasant's notions, schoolboys are whipped, and must be whipped. What kind of a schoolboy would he be, if he were not whipped? And suddenly I tell him that they don't whip us, why, he'd be pained. But you don't understand that. One has to know how to talk to the peasants."

"Only don't tease them, please, or you'll get into another scrape as you did about that goose."

"So you're afraid?"

"Don't laugh, Kolya. Of course, I'm afraid. My father would be awfully cross. I am strictly forbidden to go out with you."

"Don't be uneasy, nothing will happen this time. Hullo, Natasha!" he shouted to a market woman in one of the booths.

"Call me Natasha! What next! My name is Marya," the middle-aged market woman shouted at him.

"I am so glad it's Marya. Good-bye!"

"Ah, you young rascal! A brat like you to carry on so!"

"I'm in a hurry. I can't stay now. You shall

tell me next Sunday." Kolya waved his hand at her, as though she had accosted him and not he her.

"I've nothing to tell you next Sunday. You set upon me, you impudent young monkey. I didn't say anything," bawled Marya. "You want a whipping, that's what you want, you saucy jackanapes!"

There was a roar of laughter among the other market women round her. Suddenly an angry man darted out from the arcade of shops close by. He was a young man, not a native of the town, with dark, curly hair and a long pale face, marked with smallpox. He wore a long blue coat and a visored cap, and looked like a merchant's clerk. He was in a state of stupid excitement and immediately started brandishing his fists at Kolya.

"I know you," he cried angrily, "I know you!"

Kolya stared at him. He could not recall when he could have had a row with the man. But he had been in so many rows in the street that he could hardly remember them all.

"Do you?" he asked ironically.

"I know you! I know you!" the man repeated idiotically.

"So much the better for you. Well, I haven't any time. Good-bye!"

"You are up to mischief again?" cried the man. "You are at it again? I know, you are at it again!"

"It's not your business, brother, if I am at it again," said Kolya, stopping and scanning him.

"Not my business?"

"No; it's not your business."

"Whose then? Whose then? Whose then?"

"It's Trifon Nikitich's business, not yours."

"What Trifon Nikitich?" asked the fellow, staring with loutish amazement at Kolya, but still as angry as ever.

Kolya looked him gravely up and down.

"Have you been to the Church of the Ascension?" he suddenly asked him, sternly and emphatically.

"What Church of Ascension? What for? No, I haven't," said the fellow, somewhat taken aback.

"Do you know Sabaneyev?" Kolya went on even more emphatically and severely.

"What Sabaneyev? No, I don't know him."

"Well, then you can go to the devil," said Kolya, cutting short the conversation, and turning sharply to the right he strode quickly on his way as though he disdained further conversation with a dolt who did not even know Sabaneyev.

"Stop, hey! What Sabaneyev?" The young man recovered from his momentary stupefaction and was as agitated as before. "What did he say?" He turned to the market women with a silly stare. The women laughed.

"He's a deep 'un, that boy," said one of them.

"What Sabaneyev did he mean?" the fellow repeated, still furious and brandishing his right arm.

"It must be the Sabaneyev who worked for the Kuzmichovs, that's who it must be," one of the women suggested.

The fellow stared at her wildly.

"For the Kuzmichovs?" repeated another woman. "But his name wasn't Trifon. His name's Kuzma, not Trifon; but the boy said Trifon Nikitich, so it can't be the same."

"His name is not Trifon and not Sabaneyev, it's Chizhov," suddenly put in a third woman, who had hitherto been silent, listening gravely.

"Alexey Ivanovich is his name. Chizhov, Alexey Ivanovich."

"Not a doubt about it, it's Chizhov," a fourth woman emphatically confirmed the statement.

The bewildered fellow looked from one to another.

"But what did he ask for, what did he ask for, good people?" he cried almost in desperation. " 'Do you know Sabaneyev?' says he. And who the devil's to know who Sabaneyev is?"

"You're a senseless fellow. I tell you it's not Sabaneyev, but Chizhov, Alexey Ivanovich Chizhov, that's who it is!" one of the women shouted at him impressively.

"What Chizhov? Who is he? Tell me, if you know."

"That tall, snivelling fellow who used to sit in the market in the summer."

"And what the devil's your Chizhov to do with me, good people, eh?"

"How can I tell what he's to do with you?" put in another. "You ought to know yourself what you want with him, if you make such a clamour about him. He spoke to you, he did not speak to us, you stupid. Don't you really know him?"

"Know whom?"

"Chizhov."

"The devil take Chizhov and you with him. I'll give him a hiding, that I will. He was laughing at me!"

"Give Chizhov a hiding! More likely he will give you one. You are a fool, that's what you are!"

"Not Chizhov, not Chizhov, you spiteful, mischievous woman. I'll give the boy a hiding. Catch him, catch him, he was laughing at me!"

The women guffawed. But Kolya was by now a good way off, marching along with a triumphant air. Smurov walked beside him, looking back at the shouting group far behind. He, too, was in high spirits, though he was still afraid of getting into some scrape in Kolya's company.

"What Sabaneyev did you mean?" he asked Kolya, foreseeing what his answer would be.

"How do I know? Now there'll be a hubbub among them all day. I like to stir up fools in every class of society. There's another blockhead, that peasant there. You know, they say 'there's no one stupider than a stupid Frenchman,' but a stupid Russian shows it in his face just as much. Can't you see it written all over his face that he is a fool, that peasant, eh?"

"Let him alone, Kolya. Let's go on."

"Not for anything, now I'm started. Hey, good-morning, peasant!"

A sturdy-looking peasant, with a round, simple face, and grizzled beard, who was walking by, and seemed already to have had a drop too much, raised his head and looked at the boy. "Good-morning, if you are not joking," he said deliberately in reply.

"And if I am?" laughed Kolya.

"Well, a joke's a joke. Laugh away. I don't mind. There's no harm in a joke."

"I apologise, brother, it was a joke."

"Well, God forgive you!"

"Do you forgive me, too?"

"I quite forgive you. Go along."

"I say, you seem a clever peasant."

"Cleverer than you," the peasant answered unexpectedly with the same gravity.

"I doubt it," said Kolya, somewhat taken aback.

"It's true though."

"Perhaps it is."

"It is, brother."

"Good-bye, peasant!"

"Good-bye!"

"There are all sorts of peasants," Kolya observed to Smurov, after a brief silence. "How could I tell I had hit on a clever one? I am always ready to recognise intelligence in the peasantry."

In the distance the cathedral clock struck half-past eleven. The boys made haste and they walked as far as Captain Snegiryov's lodging, a considerable distance, quickly and almost in silence. Twenty paces from the house Kolya stopped and told Smurov to go on ahead and ask Karamazov to come out to him.

"One must sniff round a bit first," he observed to Smurov.

"Why ask him to come out?" Smurov protested. "You go in; they will be awfully glad to see you. What's the sense of getting acquainted out here in the cold?"

"That's my business, why I want to see him out here in the cold," Kolya cut him short in the despotic tone he was fond of adopting with "small boys," and Smurov ran to do his bidding.

CHAPTER IV

THE LOST DOG

Kolya leaned against the fence with an air of importance, waiting for Alyosha to appear. Yes, he had long wanted to meet him. He had heard a great deal about him from the boys, but hitherto he had always maintained an appearance of disdainful indifference when he was mentioned, and he had even "criticised" Alyosha as he listened to what he was told about him. But secretly he had a great longing to make his acquaintance; there was something sympathetic and attractive in all he was told about Alyosha. So the present moment was important: to begin with, he had to show himself at his best, to show his independence. "Or he'll think of me as thirteen and take me for a boy like the rest of them. And what are these boys to him? I shall ask him when I get to know him. It's a pity I am so short, though. Tuzikov is younger than I am, yet he is half a head taller. But I have an intelligent face. I am not good-looking. I know I'm hideous, but I've an intelligent face. I mustn't talk too freely; if I throw myself into his arms all at once, he may think . . . Faugh! how horrible if he should think . . .!"

Kolya was thus agitated while he was doing his utmost to assume the most independent air. What distressed him most was his being so short; he did not mind his "hideous" face so much as being so short. At home on the wall in a corner he had the year before made a pencil mark to show his height, and every two months since, he had anxiously measured himself against it to see how much he had grown. But, alas! he was growing very slowly, and this sometimes reduced him almost to despair. His face was in reality by no means "hideous"; on the contrary, it was rather attractive, with a fair, pale skin, freckled. His small, lively grey eyes had a fearless look, and often glowed with feeling. He had rather high cheekbones; small lips, very red, but not very thick; his nose was small and unmistakably turned up. "I've a regular pug nose, a regular pug nose," Kolya used to mutter to himself when he looked in the mirror, and he always left it with indignation. "But perhaps I haven't got an intelligent face?" he sometimes thought, doubtful even of that. But it must not be supposed that his mind was wholly preoccupied with his face and his height. On the contrary, however bitter the moments before the looking-glass were to him, he quickly forgot them, and forgot them for a long time, "abandoning himself entirely to ideas and to real life," as he formulated it to himself.

Alyosha came out quickly and hurriedly went up to Kolya. Before he reached him, Kolya could see that he looked delighted. "Can he be so glad to see me?" Kolya wondered, feeling pleased. We may note here, in passing, that Alyosha's appearance had undergone a complete change since we saw him last. He had abandoned his cassock and was wearing now a well-cut coat, a soft, round hat, and his hair had been cropped short. All this was very becoming to him, and he looked quite handsome. His charming face always had a good-humoured expression; but there was a gentleness and serenity in his good-humour. To Kolya's surprise, Alyosha came out to him just as he was, without an overcoat. He had evidently come in haste. He held out his hand to Kolya at once.

"Here you are at last! How anxiously we've all been waiting for you!"

"There were reasons which you shall know directly. Anyway, I am glad to make your acquaintance. I've long been hoping for an opportunity, and have heard a great deal about you," Kolya muttered, a little breathless.

"We should have met anyway. I've heard a great deal about you, too; but you've been a long time coming here."

"Tell me, how are things going?"

"Ilusha is very ill. He will surely die."

"How awful! You must admit that medicine is a fraud, Karamazov," cried Kolya heatedly.

"Ilusha has mentioned you often, very often, even in his sleep, in delirium, you know. One can see that you used to be very, very dear to him . . . before the incident . . . with the knife. . . . Then there's another reason. . . . Tell me, is that your dog?"

"Mine. Perezvon."

"Not Zhuchka?" Alyosha looked at Kolya with eyes full of pity. "Is she lost for ever?"

"I know you would all like it to be Zhuchka. I've heard all about it." Kolya smiled mysteriously. "Listen, Karamazov, I'll tell you all about it. That's what I came for; that's what I asked you to come out here for, to explain the whole episode to you before we go in," he began with animation. "You see, Karamazov, Ilusha came into the preparatory class last spring. Well, you know what our preparatory class is — a lot of small boys. They began teasing Ilusha at once. I am two classes higher up, and, of course, I only look on at them from a distance. I saw the boy was weak and small, but he wouldn't give in to them; he fought with them. I saw he was proud, and his eyes were full of fire. I like them like that. And they teased him all the more. The worst of it was he was horribly dressed at the time, his breeches were too small for him, and there were holes in his boots. They teased him about that, too; they shamed him. No, that I don't like. I stood up for him at once, and gave it to them hot. I beat them, but they adore me, do you know, Karamazov?" Kolya bragged impulsively; "generally, I am fond of children. I've two chicks on my hands at home now — that's what detained me to-day. So they left off beating Ilusha and I took him under my protection. I saw the boy was proud. I tell you that, the boy was proud; but in the end he became slavishly devoted to me; he did my slightest bidding, obeyed me as though I were God, tried to copy me. In the intervals between classes he used to run to me at once, and we'd walk together. On Sundays, too. In our school they always laugh when an older boy makes friends with a younger one like that; but that's a prejudice. If it's my fancy, that's enough, isn't that so? I teach him, develop him. Why shouldn't I develop him if I like him? Here you, Karamazov, have taken up with all these young ones. I see you want to influence the younger generation — to develop them, to be of use to them, and I assure you this trait in your character, which I knew by hearsay, interests me more than anything. But let's get to the point, though. I noticed that there was a sort of softness and sentimentality coming over the boy, and you know I am a positive enemy of this sheepish sentimentality, and I have been since I was born. There were contradictions in him, too: he was proud, but he was slavishly devoted to me; he was slavishly devoted and yet all at once his eyes would flash and he'd refuse to agree with me; he'd argue, fly into a rage. I used sometimes to propound certain ideas; I could see that it was not so much that he disagreed with the ideas, but that he was simply rebelling against me, because I was cool in responding to his sentimentalities. And so, in order to harden him properly, the tenderer he was, the colder I became. I did it on purpose: that was my conviction. My object was to form his character, to lick him into shape, to make a man of him . . . and then . . . no doubt, you understand me without further words. Suddenly I noticed that for three days in succession he was downcast and dejected, not because of my coldness, but because of something else, something higher, more important. I wondered what the tragedy was. I pumped him and found out that he had somehow got to know Smerdyakov, the servant of your late father — it was before his death, of course — and he taught the little fool a silly trick — that is, a brutal, nasty trick. You take a piece of bread, stick a pin in it, and throw it to one of those curs who are so hungry that they swallow anything without chewing it, and then watch and see what happens. So they prepared a piece of bread like that and threw it to Zhuchka, that shaggy dog there's been such a fuss about. The people of the house it belonged to never fed it at all, though it barked all day. (Do you like that stupid barking, Karamazov? I can't stand it.) So it rushed at the bread, swallowed it, and began to squeal; it turned round and round and ran away, squealing as it ran out of sight. That was Ilusha's own account of it. He confessed it to me, and cried bitterly. He hugged me, shaking all over. He kept on repeating, 'He ran away squealing, he ran away squealing': the sight haunted him. Well, I see: remorse. I took it seriously. I had been wanting to give him a lesson for other things as well. So I must confess I wasn't quite straightforward, and pretended to be more indignant perhaps than I really was. 'You've done a nasty thing,' I said, 'you are a scoundrel. I won't tell of it, of course, but I shall have nothing more to do with you for a time. I'll think it over and let you know through Smurov (that's the boy who's just come with me and who has always been devoted to me) whether I will have anything to do with you in the future or whether I give you up for good as a scoundrel.' He was tremendously upset. I must own I felt I'd gone too far as I spoke, but there was no help for it. I did what I thought best at the time.

The day after, I sent Smurov to tell him that I would not speak to him again. That's what we call it when two schoolfellows refuse to have anything more to do with one another. Secretly I only meant to send him to Coventry for a few days and then, if I saw signs of repentance, to hold out my hand to him again. That was my firm intention. But what do you think happened? He heard Smurov's message, his eyes flashed. 'Tell Krasotkin from me,' he cried, 'that I will throw bread with pins in it to all the dogs — all — all of them!' 'So,' I thought, 'this is revolt. We must smoke it out of him.' And I began to treat him with complete contempt: whenever I met him I turned away or smiled ironically. And just then that affair with his father happened, the 'bath-mop,' you remember? You must realise that he was fearfully worked up by what had happened already. The boys, seeing I'd given him up, set on him and taunted him, shouting, 'Bath-mop, bath-mop!' It was then that those fights began, for which I am terribly sorry, because they seem to have given him one very bad beating. One day he flew at them, all in the court-yard as they were coming out of school. I stood ten paces off, looking on. And, I swear, I don't remember that I laughed then; it was quite the other way, I felt awfully sorry for him, in another minute I would have run up to take his part. But he suddenly met my eyes. I don't know what he fancied; but he pulled out a penknife, rushed at me, and struck at my thigh, here, my right leg. I didn't budge. I don't mind owning I am plucky sometimes, Karamazov. I simply looked at him contemptuously, as though to say, 'This is how you repay all my kindness! Do it again, if you like, I'm at your service.' But he didn't stab me again; he broke down, he was frightened at what he had done, he threw away the knife, burst out crying, and ran away. I did not sneak on him, of course, and I made them all keep quiet, so it shouldn't come to the ears of the masters. I didn't even tell my mother till it had healed up. And the wound was a mere scratch. And then I heard that the same day he'd been throwing stones and had bitten your finger — but you understand now what a state he was in! Well, it can't be helped: it was stupid of me not to come and forgive him — that is, to make it up with him — when he was taken ill. I am sorry for it now. But I had a special reason. So now I've told you all about it . . . but I'm afraid it was stupid of me."

"Oh, what a pity," exclaimed Alyosha, with feeling, "that I didn't know before what terms you were on with him, or I'd have come to you long ago to beg you to go to him with me. Would you believe it, when he was feverish he talked about you in his delirium. I didn't know how much you were to him! And you've really not succeeded in finding that dog? His father and the boys have been hunting all over the town for it. Would you believe it, since he's been ill, I've three times heard him repeat with tears, 'It's because I killed Zhuchka, father, that I am ill now. God is punishing me for it.' He can't get that idea out of his head. And if the dog were found and proved to be alive, one might almost fancy the joy would resurrect him. We have all rested our hopes on you."

"Tell me, what made you hope that I should be the one to find him?" Kolya asked, with great curiosity. "Why did you reckon on me rather than any one else?"

"There was a report that you were looking for the dog, and that you would bring it when you'd found it. Smurov said something of the sort. We've all been trying to persuade Ilusha that the dog is alive, that it's been seen. The boys brought him a live hare: he just looked at it, with a faint smile, and asked them to set it free in the fields. And so we did. His father has just this moment come back, bringing him a mastiff pup, hoping to comfort him with that; but I think it only made it worse."

"Tell me, Karamazov, what sort of man is the father? I know him, but what do you make of him — a mountebank, a buffoon?"

"Oh, no; there are people of deep feeling who have been somehow crushed. Buffoonery in them is a form of resentful irony against those to whom they daren't speak the truth, through having been for years humiliated and intimidated by them. Believe me, Krasotkin, that sort of buffoonery is sometimes tragic in the extreme. His whole life now is centred in Ilusha, and if Ilusha dies, he will either go mad with grief, or kill himself. I feel almost certain of that when I look at him now."

"I understand you, Karamazov. I see you understand human nature," Kolya added, with feeling.

"And as soon as I saw you with a dog, I thought it was Zhuchka you were bringing."

"Wait a bit, Karamazov, perhaps we shall find him yet; but this is Perezvon. I'll let him go in now and perhaps he will amuse Ilusha more than the mastiff pup. Wait a bit, Karamazov, you will learn something in a minute. But, good heavens, I am keeping you here!" Kolya cried suddenly. "You've no overcoat on in this bitter cold. You see what an egoist I am. Oh, we are all egoists, Karamazov!"

"Don't trouble; it is cold, but I don't often catch cold. Let us go in though, and, by the way, what is your name? I know you are called Kolya, but what else?"

"Nikolay — Nikolay Ivanovich Krasotkin, or, as they say in official documents, 'son of Krasotkin.'" Kolya laughed for some reason, but added suddenly, "Of course I hate my name Nikolay."

"Why so?"

"It's so trivial, so ordinary."

"You are thirteen?" asked Alyosha.

"No, fourteen — that is, I shall be fourteen very soon, in a fortnight. I'll confess one weakness of mine, Karamazov, just to you, since it's our first meeting, so that you may understand my character at once. I hate being asked my age, I more than hate it . . . and in fact . . . there's a libellous story going about me, that last week I played robbers with the 'preparatory' boys. It's a fact that I did play with them, but it's a perfect libel to say I did it for my own amusement. I have reasons for believing that you've heard the story; but I wasn't playing for my own amusement, it was for the sake of the children, because they couldn't think of anything to do by themselves. But they've always got some silly tale. This is an awful town for gossip, I can tell you."

"But what if you had been playing for your own amusement, what's the harm?"

"Come, I say, for my own amusement! You don't play horses, do you?"

"But you must look at it like this," said Alyosha, smiling. "Grown-up people go to the theatre and there the adventures of all sorts of heroes are represented — sometimes there are robbers, and battles, too — and isn't that just the same thing, in a different form, of course? And young people's games of soldiers or robbers in their play-time are also art in its first stage. You know, they spring from the growing artistic instincts of the young. And sometimes these games are much better than performances in the theatre; the only difference is that people go there to look at actors, while in these games the young people are the actors themselves. But that's only natural."

"You think so? Is that your conviction?" Kolya looked at him intently. "Oh, you know, that's rather an interesting notion. When I go home, I'll think it over. I'll admit I thought I might learn something from you. I've come to learn of you, Karamazov," Kolya concluded, in a voice full of spontaneous feeling.

"And I of you," said Alyosha, smiling and pressing his hand.

Kolya was much pleased with Alyosha. What struck him most was that he treated him exactly like an equal and that he talked to him just as if he were "quite grown up."

"I'll show you something directly, Karamazov; it's a theatrical performance, too," he said, laughing nervously. "That's why I've come."

"Let us go first to the landlord's, on the left. All the boys leave their coats in there, because the room is small and hot."

"Oh, I'm only coming in for a minute. I'll keep on my overcoat. Perezvon will stay here in the passage and play dead. *Ici*, Perezvon, lie down and play dead! You see he's dead. I'll go in first and reconnoitre, then I'll whistle to him when I think fit, and, you'll see, he'll dash in like mad. Only Smurov must not forget to open the door at the right moment. I'll arrange it all and you'll see a trick."

CHAPTER V

AT ILUSHA'S BEDSIDE

THE room inhabited by the family of the retired captain Snegiryov is already familiar to the reader. It was close and crowded at that moment with numerous visitors. Several boys were sitting with Ilusha and though all of them, like Smurov, were prepared to deny that it was Alyosha who had brought them and reconciled them with Ilusha, it was really so. All the art he had used had been to take them, one by one, to Ilusha, without "sheepish sentimentality," appearing to do so casually and without design. It was a great consolation to Ilusha in his suffering. He was greatly touched by seeing the almost tender affection and sympathy shown him by these boys, who had been his enemies. Krasotkin was the only one missing and his absence was a heavy load on Ilusha's heart. Perhaps the bitterest of all his bitter memories was his stabbing Krasotkin, who had been his one friend and protector. Clever little Smurov, who had been the first to make it up with Ilusha, thought it was so. But when Smurov hinted to Krasotkin that Alyosha wanted to come and see him about something, the latter cut him short, bidding Smurov tell "Karamazov" at once that he knew best what to do, that he wanted no one's advice, and that, if he went to see the patient, he would choose his own time for he had "his own reasons."

That was a fortnight before this Sunday. That was why Alyosha had not been to see him, as he had meant to. But though he waited, he sent Smurov to him again twice. Both times Krasotkin met him with a curt, impatient refusal, sending Alyosha a message not to bother him any more, adding that if he came himself, he, Krasotkin, would not go to Ilusha at all. Up to the very last day, Smurov did not know that Kolya meant to go to Ilusha that morning, and only the evening before, as he parted from Smurov, Kolya abruptly told him to wait at home for him next morning, for he would go with him to the Snegiryovs, but warned him on no account to say he was coming, as he wanted to drop in casually. Smurov obeyed. Smurov's fancy that Kolya would bring back the lost dog was based on the words Kolya had dropped that "they must be asses to be unable to find the dog, if it was alive." When Smurov, waiting for an opportunity, timidly hinted at his guess about the dog, Krasotkin flew into a violent rage. "I'm not such an ass as to go hunting about the town for other people's dogs when I've got a dog of my own! And how can you imagine a dog could be alive after swallowing a pin? Sheepish sentimentality, that's what it is!"

For the last fortnight Ilusha had not left his little bed under the ikons in the corner. He had not been to school since the day he met Alyosha and bit his finger. He was taken ill the same day, though for a month afterwards he was sometimes able to get up and walk about the room and the passage. But latterly he had become so weak that he could not move without help from his father. His father trembled over him. He even gave up drinking and was almost insane with terror that his boy would die. And often, especially after leading him round the room on his arm and putting him back to bed, he would run to a dark corner in the passage and, leaning his head against the wall, he would break into paroxysms of violent weeping, stifling his sobs that they might not be heard by Ilusha.

Returning to the room, he would usually begin doing something to amuse and comfort his precious boy: he would tell him stories, funny anecdotes, or would mimic comic people he had happened to meet, even imitate the funny howls and cries of animals. But Ilusha could not bear to see his father fooling and playing the buffoon. Though the boy tried not to show how he disliked it, he saw with an aching heart that his father was an object of contempt, and he was continually haunted by the memory of the "bath-mop" and that "terrible day."

Nina, Ilusha's gentle, crippled sister, did not like her father's buffoonery either (Varvara had been gone for some time past to Petersburg to study at the University). But the half-imbecile mother was greatly diverted and laughed heartily when her husband began capering about or performing. It was the only thing that amused her; all the rest of the time she was grumbling and complaining that now every one had forgotten her, that no one treated her with respect, that she was being slighted and so on. But during the last few days she had completely changed. She began looking constantly at Ilusha's bed in the corner and seemed lost in thought. She was more silent, quieter, and, if she cried, she cried quietly so as not to be heard. The captain noticed the change in her with bitter perplexity. The boys' visits at first only angered her, but later on their merry shouts and stories began to divert her, and at last she liked them so much that, if the boys had given up coming, she would have felt terribly dreary. When the children told some story or played a game, she laughed and clapped her hands. She called some of them to her and kissed them. She was particularly fond of Smurov.

As for the captain, the presence in his room of the children, who came to cheer up Ilusha, filled his heart from the first with ecstatic joy. He even hoped that Ilusha would now get over his depression, and that that would hasten his recovery. In spite of his alarm about Ilusha, he had not, till lately, felt one minute's doubt of his boy's ultimate recovery.

He met his little visitors with homage, waited upon them hand and foot, he was ready to be their horse and even began letting them ride on his back, but Ilusha did not like the game and it was given up. He began buying little things for them, gingerbread and nuts, gave them tea, and buttered sandwiches for them. It must be noted that all this time he had plenty of money. He had taken the two hundred roubles from Katerina Ivanovna just as Alyosha had predicted he would. And afterwards Katerina Ivanovna, learning more about their circumstances and Ilusha's illness, visited them herself, made the acquaintance of the family and succeeded in fascinating the half-imbecile mother. Since then she had been lavish in helping them, and the captain, terror-stricken at the thought that his boy might die, forgot his pride and humbly accepted her charity.

All this time Dr. Herzenstube, who was called in by Katerina Ivanovna, came punctually every other day, but little was gained by his visits and he dosed the invalid mercilessly. But on that Sunday morning a new doctor was expected, who had come from Moscow, where he had a great reputation. Katerina Ivanovna had sent for him from Moscow at great expense, not expressly for Ilusha, but for another purpose of which more will be said in its place hereafter. But, as he had come, she had asked him to see Ilusha as well, and the captain had been told to expect him. He hadn't the slightest idea that Kolya Krasotkin was coming, though he had long wished for a visit from the boy for whom Ilusha was yearning.

At the moment when Krasotkin opened the door and came into the room, the captain and all the boys were round Ilusha's bed, looking at a tiny mastiff pup, which had been born only the day before, though the captain had bespoken it a week ago to comfort and amuse Ilusha, who was still longing for the lost and probably dead Zhuchka. Ilusha, who had heard three days before that he was to be presented with a puppy, but not an ordinary puppy, but a real pedigree mastiff (an enormously important point, of course), tried from delicacy of feeling to pretend that he was pleased. But his father and the boys could not help seeing that the puppy only served to recall to his little heart the thought of the unhappy dog he had destroyed. The puppy lay beside him feebly moving and he, smiling morbidly, stroked it with his thin, pale, wasted hand. Clearly he liked the puppy, but . . . it wasn't Zhuchka; if he could have had Zhuchka and the puppy, too, then it would have been complete happiness.

"Krasotkin!" cried one of the boys suddenly. He was the first to see him come in.

Krasotkin's entrance made a general sensation, the boys moved away and stood on either side of the bed, so that he could get a full view of Ilusha. The captain ran eagerly to meet Kolya.

"Please, please, come in . . . you are most welcome!" he mumbled. "Ilusha, Mr. Krasotkin has come to see you!"

But Krasotkin, shaking hands with him hurriedly, instantly showed his complete knowledge of the manners of good society. He turned first to the captain's wife, who was sitting in her armchair, and who was very ill-humoured at the moment, grumbling that the boys stood between her and Ilusha's bed and did not let her see the new puppy. With the greatest courtesy he made her a bow, scraping his foot, and then turning to Nina, he made her, as the only other lady present, a similar bow.

This polite behaviour made an extremely favourable impression on the deranged lady.

"There, you can see at once he is a young man who has been well brought up," she commented aloud, throwing up her hands; "but as for our other visitors, they come in riding on each other's backs."

"How do you mean, mamma, riding on each other's backs, how is that?" muttered the captain affectionately, though a little anxious on her account.

"That's how they ride in. They get on each other's shoulders in the passage and prance in like that on a respectable family. Strange sort of visitors!"

"But who's come in like that, mamma?"

"Why, that boy came in riding on that one's back and this one on that one's."

Kolya was already at Ilusha's bedside. The sick boy turned visibly paler. He raised himself in the bed and looked intently at Kolya. Kolya had not seen his little friend for two months, and he was overwhelmed at the sight of him. He had never imagined that he would see such a wasted, yellow face, such enormous, feverishly glowing eyes, and such thin little hands. He noted, with grieved surprise, Ilusha's rapid, hard breathing and dry lips. He stepped close to him, held out his hand, and, almost overwhelmed, he said:

"Well, old man . . . how are you?" But his voice failed him, he couldn't achieve an appearance of ease; his face suddenly twitched and the corners of his mouth quivered. Ilusha smiled a pitiful little smile, still unable to utter a word. Something moved Kolya to raise his hand and pass it over Ilusha's hair.

"Never mind!" he murmured softly to him to cheer him up, or perhaps not knowing why he said it. For a minute they were silent again.

"Hullo, so you've got a new puppy?" Kolya said suddenly, in a most callous voice.

"Ye-es," answered Ilusha in a long whisper, gasping for breath.

"A black nose, that means he'll be fierce, a good watch-dog," Kolya observed gravely and stolidly, as if the only thing he cared about was the puppy and its black nose. But in reality he still had to do his utmost to control his feelings so as not to burst out crying like a little one, and do what he would he could not control them. "When it grows up, you'll have to keep it on the chain, I'm sure."

"He'll be a huge dog!" cried one of the boys.

"Of course he will," "a mastiff," "large," "like this," "as big as a calf," shouted several voices.

"As big as a calf, as a real calf," chimed in the captain. "I got one like that on purpose, one of the fiercest breed, and his parents are huge and very fierce, they stand as high as this from the floor. . . . Sit down here, on Ilusha's bed, or here on the bench. You are very welcome, dear visitor, we've been hoping to see you a long time. . . . You were so kind as to come with Alexey Fyodorovich?"

Krasotkin sat on the edge of the bed, at Ilusha's feet. Though he had perhaps prepared a free-and-easy opening for the conversation on his way, now he completely lost the thread of it.

"No . . . I came with Perezvon. I've got a dog now, called Perezvon. A Slavonic name. He's out there . . . if I whistle, he'll run in. I've brought a dog, too," he said, addressing Ilusha all at once. "Do you remember Zhuchka, old man?" He suddenly fired the question at him.

A spasm passed over Ilusha's little face. He looked with an agonised expression at Kolya. Alyosha, standing at the door, frowned and signed to Kolya not to speak of Zhuchka, but he did not or would not notice.

"Where . . . is Zhuchka?" Ilusha asked in a broken voice.

"Oh, well, my boy, your Zhuchka, whew! — he's lost and done for!"

Ilusha did not speak, but he fixed an intent gaze once more on Kolya. Alyosha, catching Kolya's eye, signed to him vigorously again, but again he turned away his eyes pretending not to have noticed.

"It must have run away somewhere and perished. It must have perished after a meal like that," Kolya rapped out pitilessly, though it seemed as though something had begun to choke him. "But I've got a dog, Perezvon . . . A Slavonic name. . . . I've brought him to show you."

"I don't want him!" said Ilusha suddenly.

"No, no, you really must see him . . . it will amuse you. I brought him on purpose. . . . He's the same sort of shaggy dog. . . . You allow me to call in my dog, madam?" He suddenly addressed Madame Snegiryov, with inexplicable and obvious excitement in his manner.

"I don't want him, I don't want him!" cried Ilusha, with a mournful break in his voice. There was a reproachful light in his eyes.

"You'd better . . ." the captain started up from the chest by the wall on which he had just sat down, "you'd better . . . another time," he muttered, but Kolya could not be restrained. He hurriedly shouted to Smurov, "Open the door," and as soon as it was open, he blew his whistle. Perezvon dashed headlong into the room.

"Jump, Perezvon, beg! Beg!" shouted Kolya, jumping up, and the dog stood erect on its hind legs by Ilusha's bedside. What followed was a surprise to every one: Ilusha started, lurched violently forward, bent towards Perezvon and gazed at him, faint with suspense.

"It's . . . Zhuchka!" he cried suddenly, in a voice breaking with joy and suffering.

"And who did you think it was?" Krasotkin shouted with all his might, in a ringing, happy voice, and bending down he seized the dog and lifted him up to Ilusha.

"Look, old man, you see, blind of one eye and the left ear is torn, just the marks you described to me. It was by those marks that I found him. I found him directly. He did not belong to anyone!" he explained, turning quickly to the captain, to his wife, to Alyosha, and then again to Ilusha. "He used to stay in the Fedotovs' back yard. Though he made his home there, they did not feed him. He was a stray dog that had run away from some farm . . . I found him. . . . You see, old man, he couldn't have swallowed what you gave him. If he had, he must have died, he must have! So he must have spat it out, since he is alive. You did not see him do it. But the pin pricked his tongue, that is why he squealed. He ran away squealing and you thought he'd swallowed it. He might well squeal, because the skin of dogs' mouths is so tender . . . tenderer than in men, much tenderer!" Kolya cried impetuously, his face glowing and radiant with delight. Ilusha could not speak. White as a sheet, he gazed open-mouthed at Kolya, with his great eyes almost starting out of his head. And if Krasotkin, who had no suspicion of it, had known what a disastrous and fatal effect such a moment might have on the sick child's health, nothing would have induced him to play such a trick on him. But Alyosha was perhaps the only person in the room who realised it. As for the captain he had himself turned, as it were, into a small boy.

"Zhuchka! So it's Zhuchka!" he cried in a blissful voice. "Ilusha, this is Zhuchka, your Zhuchka! Mamma, this is Zhuchka!" He was almost weeping.

"And I never guessed!" cried Smurov sorrowfully. "Bravo, Krasotkin, I said he'd find the dog and here he's found him."

"Here he's found him!" another boy repeated gleefully.

"Krasotkin's a brick!" cried a third voice.

"He's a brick, he's a brick!" cried the other boys, and they began clapping.

"Wait, wait," Krasotkin did his utmost to shout above them all. "I'll tell you how it happened, that's the whole point. I found him, I took him home and hid him at once. I kept him locked up at home and did not show him to any one till to-day. Only Smurov has known for the last fortnight, but I assured him this dog was called Perezvon and he did not guess. And meanwhile I taught the dog all sorts of tricks. You should only see all the things he can do! I trained him so as to bring you a well-trained dog, in fine fettle, old man, so as to be able to say to you, 'See, old man, what a fine dog your Zhuchka is now!' Haven't you a bit of meat? — he'll show you a trick that will make you die with laughing. A piece of meat, haven't you got any?"

The captain dashed across the passage to the landlady, where their cooking was done. Not to lose precious time, Kolya, in desperate haste, shouted to Perezvon, "Dead!" And the dog immediately turned round and lay on his back with its four paws in the air. The boys laughed, Ilusha looked on with the same suffering smile, but the person most delighted with the dog's performance was "mamma." She laughed at the dog and began snapping her fingers and calling it, "Perezvon, Perezvon!"

"Nothing will make him get up, nothing!" Kolya cried triumphantly, proud of his success. "He won't move for all the shouting in the world, but if I call to him, he'll jump up in a minute. *Ici*, Perezvon!" The dog leapt up and bounded about, squealing with delight. The captain ran in with a piece of cooked beef.

"Is it hot?" Kolya inquired hurriedly, with a businesslike air, taking the meat. "Dogs don't like hot things. No, it's all right. Look, everybody, look, Ilusha, look, old man; why aren't you looking? He does not look at him, now I've brought him."

The new trick consisted in making the dog stand motionless with his nose out and putting a tempting morsel of meat just on his nose. The luckless dog had to stand without moving, with the meat on his nose, as long as his master chose to keep him so, without a movement, perhaps for half an hour. But he kept Perezvon only for a brief moment.

"Take it!" cried Kolya, and the meat passed in a flash from the dog's nose to his mouth.

The audience, of course, expressed enthusiasm and surprise.

"Can you really have put off coming all this time simply to train the dog?" exclaimed Alyosha, with an involuntary note of reproach in his voice.

"Simply for that!" answered Kolya, with

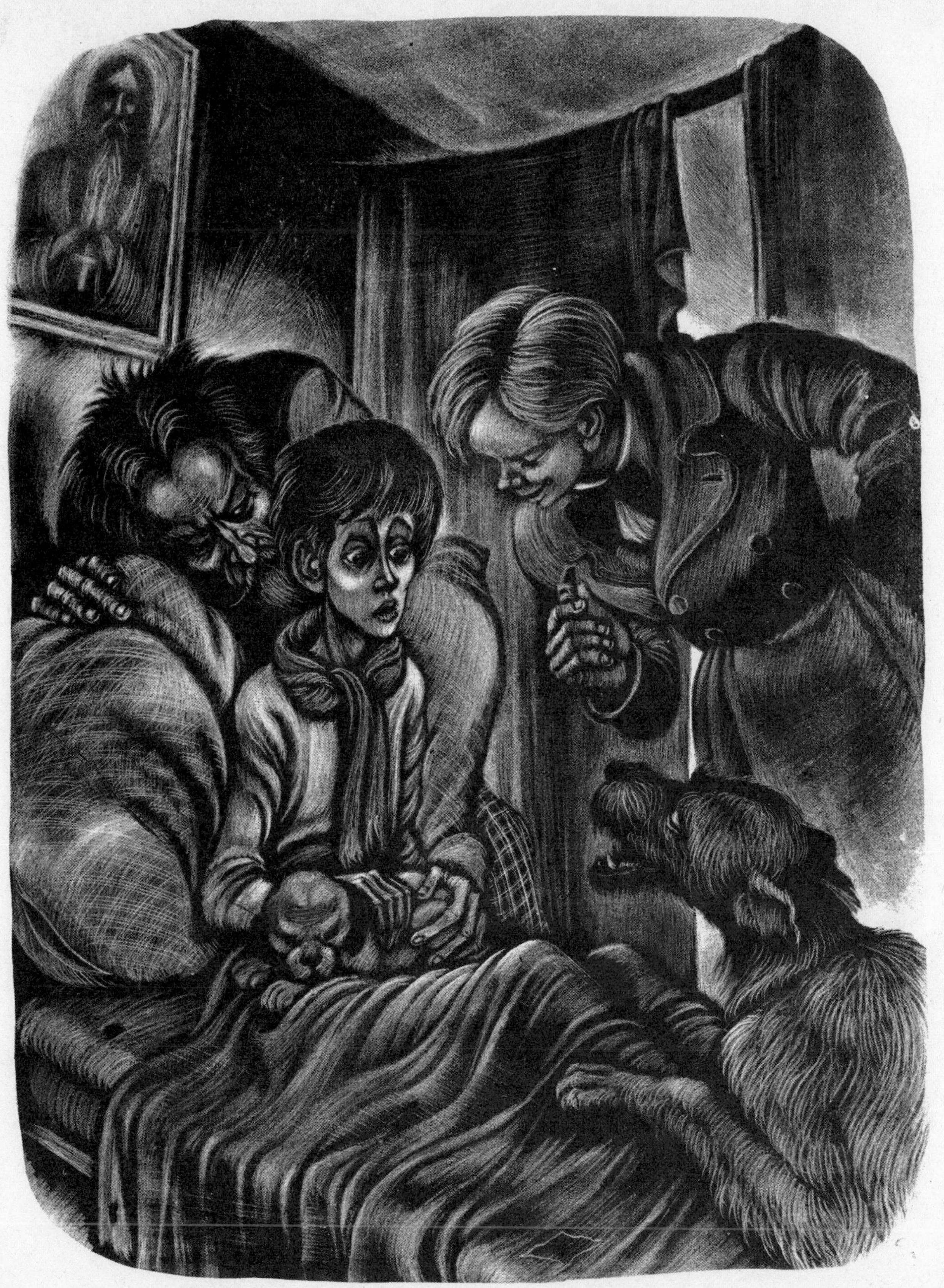

ILUSHA SICK

perfect simplicity. "I wanted to show him in all his glory."

"Perezvon! Perezvon," called Ilusha suddenly, snapping his thin fingers and beckoning to the dog.

"What is it? Let him jump up on the bed! *Ici*, Perezvon!" Kolya slapped the bed and Perezvon darted up to Ilusha. The boy threw both arms round his head and Perezvon instantly licked his cheek. Ilusha crept close to him, stretched himself out in bed and hid his face in the dog's shaggy coat.

"Dear, dear!" the captain kept exclaiming. Kolya sat down again on the edge of the bed.

"Ilusha, I can show you another trick. I've brought you a little cannon. You remember, I told you about it before and you said how much you'd like to see it. Well, here, I've brought it to you."

And Kolya hurriedly pulled out of his satchel the little brass cannon. He hurried, because he was happy himself. Another time he would have waited till the sensation made by Perezvon had passed off, now he hurried on regardless of all propriety. "You are all happy now," he felt, "so here's something to make you happier!" He was himself completely intoxicated.

"I've had my eye on this thing for a long while; for you, old man, for you. It belonged to Morozov, the official, it was no use to him, he had it from his brother. I swopped a book from father's bookcase for it, 'A Kinsman of Mahomet or Salutary Folly,' a scandalous book published in Moscow a hundred years ago, before they had any censorship. And Morozov has a taste for such things. He was grateful to me, too. . . ."

Kolya held the cannon in his hand so that all could see and enjoy it. Ilusha raised himself, and, with his right arm still round the dog, he gazed enchanted at the toy. The sensation was even greater when Kolya announced that he had gunpowder, too, and that it could be fired off at once "if it won't alarm the ladies." "Mamma" immediately asked to look closer at the toy and her request was granted. The little brass cannon on wheels delighted her immensely and she began rolling it to and fro on her lap. She readily gave permission for the cannon to be fired, without any idea of what she had been asked. Kolya showed the powder and the shot. The captain, as a former military man, undertook to load it, putting in a minute quantity of powder. He asked that the shot might be put off till another time. The cannon was placed on the floor, aiming at an empty part of the room, three grains of powder were thrust into the touch-hole and a match was put to it. A magnificent explosion followed. Mamma was startled, but at once laughed with delight. The boys gazed in speechless triumph. But the captain, looking at Ilusha, was more enchanted than any of them.

Kolya picked up the cannon and immediately presented it to Ilusha, together with the powder and the shot.

"I got it for you, for you! I've been keeping it for you for a long time," he repeated once more in his delight.

"Oh, give it to me! No, give the cannon to me!" Mamma began begging like a little child. Her face showed a piteous fear that she would not get it. Kolya was embarrassed. The captain fidgeted uneasily.

"Mamma, mamma," he ran to her, "the cannon's yours, of course, but let Ilusha have it, because it's a present to him, but it's just as good as yours. Ilusha will always let you play with it, it shall belong to both of you, both of you."

"No, I don't want it to belong to both of us, I want it to be mine altogether, not Ilusha's," persisted mamma, who was on the point of tears.

"Take it, mother, here, keep it!" Ilusha cried. "Krasotkin, may I give it to my mother?" He turned to Krasotkin with an expression of entreaty, as though he were afraid he might be offended at his giving his present to some one else.

"Of course, you may," Krasotkin assented heartily, and, taking the cannon from Ilusha, he handed it himself to mamma with a polite bow. She burst into tears with emotion.

"Ilusha, the darling, he's the one who loves his mamma!" she said tenderly, and at once began wheeling the cannon to and fro on her lap again.

"Mamma, let me kiss your hand." The captain darted up to her at once and did so.

"And I never saw such a charming fellow as this nice boy," said the grateful lady, pointing to Krasotkin.

"And I'll bring you as much powder as you like, Ilusha. We make the powder ourselves now. Borovikov found out how it's made — twenty-four parts of saltpetre, ten of sulphur and six of birchwood charcoal. It's all pounded together, mixed into a paste with water and rubbed through a skin — that's how it's done."

"Smurov told me about your powder, only father says it's not real gunpowder," responded Ilusha.

"Not real?" Kolya flushed. "It burns. I don't know, of course."

"No, I didn't mean that," put in the captain, with a guilty face. "I only said that real powder is not made like that, but that's nothing, it can be made so."

"I don't know, you know best. We lighted some in a pomatum pot, it burned splendidly, it all burned away leaving only a tiny ash. But that was only the paste, and if you rub it through a skin . . . but of course you know best, I don't know. . . . And Bulkin's father thrashed him on acount of our powder, did you hear?" He turned to Ilusha.

"Yes," answered Ilusha. He listened to Kolya with immense interest and enjoyment.

"We had prepared a whole bottle of it and he used to keep it under his bed. His father saw it. He said it might explode, and thrashed him on the spot. He was going to make a complaint against me to the masters. He is not allowed to go about with me now, no one is allowed to go about with me now. Smurov is not allowed to either, I've got a bad name with every one. They say I'm a 'desperate character.'" Kolya smiled scornfully. "It all began with what happened on the railway."

"Ah, we've heard of that exploit of yours, too," cried the captain. "How could you lie still there? Is it possible you weren't the least afraid, lying there under the train? Weren't you frightened?"

The captain was abject in his flattery of Kolya.

"N-not particularly," answered Kolya carelessly. "What's blasted my reputation more than anything here was that cursed goose," he said, turning again to Ilusha. But though he assumed an unconcerned air as he talked, he still could not control himself and was continually missing the note he tried to keep up.

"Ah! I heard about the goose!" Ilusha laughed, beaming all over. "They told me, but I didn't understand. Did they really take you to court?"

"The most stupid, trivial affair, they made a mountain of a mole-hill as they always do," Kolya began self-confidently. "I was walking through the market-place here one day, just when they'd driven in the geese. I stopped and looked at them. All at once a fellow, who is an errand boy at Plotnikovs', looked at me and said, 'What are you staring at the geese for?' I looked at him, he was a stupid, moon-faced fellow of twenty. I am always on the side of the people, you know. I like talking to peasants. . . . We've dropped behind the people — that's an axiom. I believe you are laughing, Karamazov?"

"No, heaven forbid, I am listening attentively," said Alyosha with a most good-natured air, and the sensitive Kolya was immediately reassured.

"My theory, Karamazov, is clear and simple," he hurried on again, looking pleased. "I believe in the people and am always glad to give them their due, but I am not for spoiling them, that is a *sine qua non*. . . . But I was telling you about the goose. So I turned to the fool and answered, 'I am wondering what the goose thinks about.' He looked at me quite stupidly. 'And what does the goose think about?' he asked. 'Do you see that cart full of oats?' I said. 'The oats are dropping out of the sack, and the goose has put its neck right under the wheel to gobble them up — do you see?' 'I see that quite well,' he said. 'Well,' said I, 'if that cart were to move on a little, would it break the goose's neck or not?' 'It'd be sure to break it,' and he grinned all over his face, highly delighted. 'Come on then,' said I, 'let's try.' 'Let's,' he said. And it did not take us long to arrange: he stood at the bridle without being noticed, and I stood on one side to direct the goose. And the owner wasn't looking, he was talking to some one, so I had nothing to do, the goose thrust its head in after the oats of itself, under the cart, just under the wheel. I winked at the lad, he tugged at the bridle, and crack! The goose's neck was broken in half. And, as luck would have it, all the peasants saw us at that moment and they kicked up a shindy at once. 'You did that on purpose!' 'No, not on purpose.' 'Yes, you did, on purpose!' Well, they shouted, 'Take him to the justice of the peace!' They took me, too. 'You were there, too,' they said, 'you helped, you're known all over the market!' And, for some reason, I really am known all over the market," Kolya added conceitedly. "We all went off to the justice's, they took the goose, too. The fellow was crying in a great funk, simply blubbering like a woman. And the farmer kept shouting that you could kill any number of geese like that. Well, of course, there were witnesses. The justice of the peace settled it in a minute, that the farmer was to be paid a rouble for the goose, and the fellow to have the goose. And he was warned not to play such pranks again. And the fellow kept blubbering like a woman. 'It wasn't me,' he said, 'it was he egged me on,' and he pointed to me. I answered with the utmost composure that I hadn't egged him on, that I simply expressed the fundamental thought, that I had spoken hypothetically. The justice of the peace smiled and was vexed with himself at once for having smiled. 'I'll complain to your masters of you, so that in the future you mayn't waste your time on such hypotheses, instead of sitting at your books and learning your lessons.' He didn't complain to the masters, that was a joke, but the matter was noised abroad and came to the ears of the authorities. Their ears are long, you know! The classical master, Kolbasnikov, was particularly aroused by it, but Dardanelov got me off again. But Kolbasnikov has a grudge against every one now like a green ass. Did you know, Ilusha, he just got married, got a dowry of a thousand roubles, and his bride's a regular fright of the first rank and the last degree? The third class fellows wrote an epigram on it.

Astounding news has reached the class:
Kolbasnikov has won a lass!

And so on, awfully funny, I'll bring it to you later on. I say nothing against Dardanelov, he is a man of learning, there's no doubt about it. I respect men like that and it's not because he stood up for me."

"But you took him down about the founders of Troy!" Smurov put in suddenly, unmistakably proud of Krasotkin at such a moment. He was particularly pleased with the story of the goose.

"Did you really take him down?" the captain inquired, in a flattering way. "On the question of who founded Troy? We heard of it, Ilusha told me about it at the time."

"He knows everything, father, he knows more than any of us!" put in Ilusha; "he only pretends to be like that, but really he is at the top in every subject . . ."

Ilusha looked at Kolya with infinite happiness.

"Oh, that's all nonsense about Troy, a trivial matter. I consider that an unimportant question," said Kolya with haughty humility. He had by now completely recovered his dignity, though he was still a little uneasy. He felt that he was greatly excited and that he had talked about the goose, for instance, with too little reserve, while Alyosha had looked serious and had not said a word all the time. And the vain boy began by degrees to have a rankling fear that Alyosha was silent because he despised him, and thought he was showing off before him. If he dared to think anything like that Kolya would . . .

"I regard the question as quite a trivial one," he rapped out again, proudly.

"And I know who founded Troy," a boy, who had not spoken before, said suddenly, to the surprise of every one. He was a taciturn, shy, handsome boy of about eleven, called Kartashov. He was sitting right near the door. Kolya looked at him with dignified amazement.

The fact was that the identity of the founders of Troy had become a mystery for the whole school, a mystery which could be penetrated only by reading Smaragdov, and no one had Smaragdov but Kolya. One day when Kolya's back was turned, Kartashov had hastily opened Smaragdov, which lay among Kolya's books, and had lighted directly on the passage relating to the founders of Troy. This had happened some time ago, but he felt uneasy and could not bring himself to announce publicly that he, too, knew who had founded Troy, afraid of what might happen and of Krasotkin's somehow putting him to shame over it.

But now he couldn't resist saying it. He had been longing to do it for ages.

"Well, who did found it?" asked Kolya, turning to him with haughty superciliousness. He saw from the boy's face that he really did know and, of course, at once prepared for the consequences. There was, so to speak, a discordant note in the general harmony.

"Troy was founded by Teucer, Dardanus,

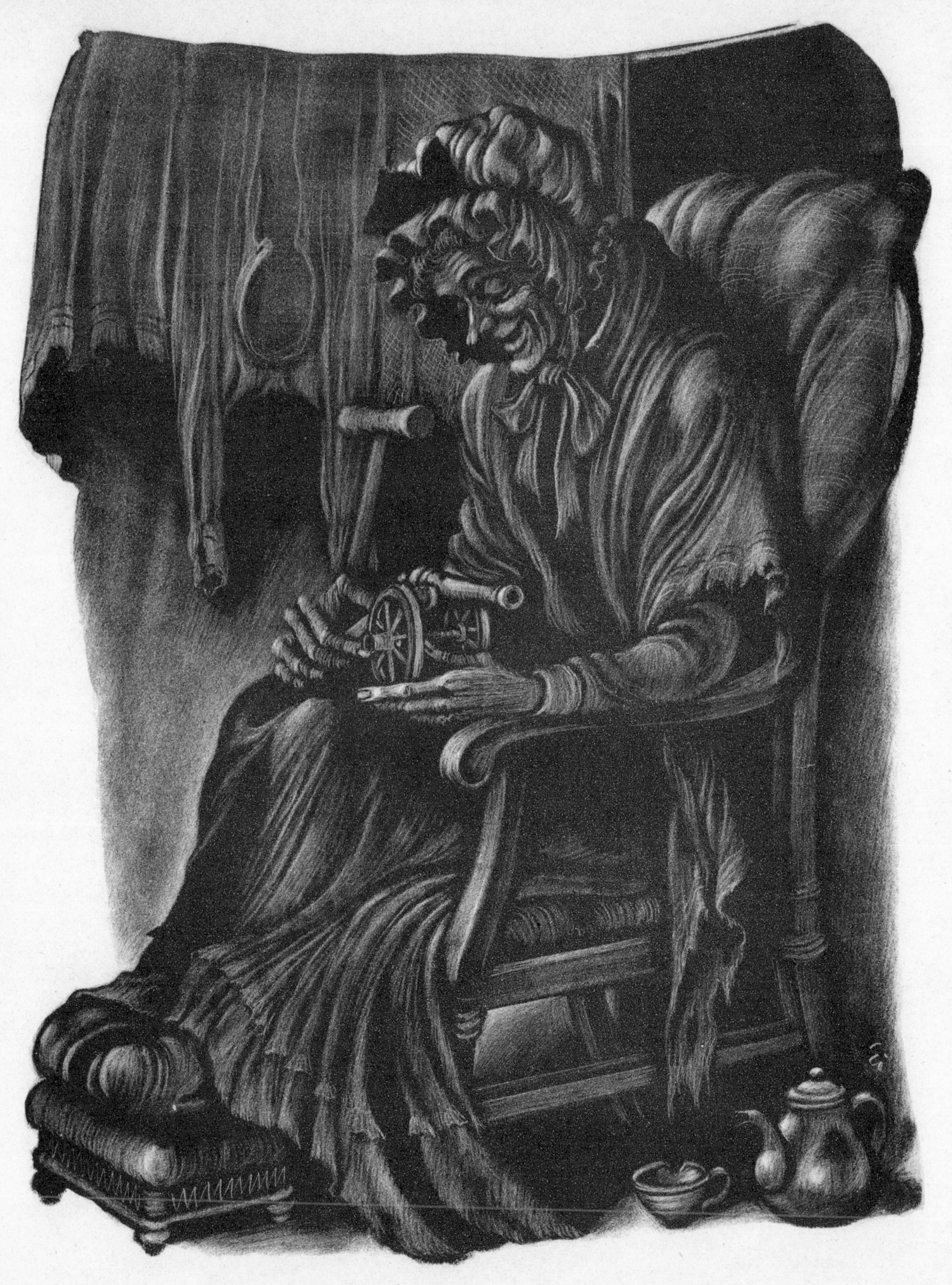

THE LITTLE BRONZE CANNON

Ilius, and Tros," the boy rapped out at once, and in the same instant he blushed, blushed so that it was pitiful to look at him. But the boys stared at him, stared at him for a whole minute, and then all the staring eyes turned at once and were fastened upon Kolya, who was still scanning the audacious boy with disdainful composure.

"In what sense did they found it?" he deigned to comment at last. "And what is meant by founding a city or a state? What did they do — did they go and each lay a brick, do you suppose?"

There was laughter. The offending boy turned from pink to crimson. He was silent and on the point of tears. Kolya held him so for a minute.

"Before you talk of a historical event like the foundation of a nationality, you must first understand what you mean by it," he admonished him in stern incisive tones. "But I attach no consequence to these old wives' tales and I don't think much of universal history in general," he added carelessly, addressing the company generally.

"Universal history?" the captain inquired, looking almost scared.

"Yes, universal history! It's the study of the successive follies of mankind and nothing more. The only subjects I respect are mathematics and natural science," said Kolya. He was showing off and he stole a glance at Alyosha, his was the only opinion he was afraid of there. But Alyosha was still silent and still serious as before. If Alyosha had said a word it would have stopped him, but Alyosha was silent and "it might be the silence of contempt" and that finally irritated Kolya.

"Again, take the classical languages . . . they are simply insanity, nothing more. You seem to disagree with me again, Karamazov?"

"I don't agree," said Alyosha, with a faint smile.

"The study of the classical languages, if you ask my opinion, is simply a police measure, that's the only reason why it has been introduced into our schools." By degrees Kolya began to get breathless again. "They were introduced because they are a bore and because they stupefy the intellect. It was dull before, so what could they do to make things duller? It was senseless enough before, so what could they do to make it more senseless? So they invented the classical languages. That's my opinion, I hope I shall never change it," Kolya finished abruptly. His cheeks were flushed.

"That's true," assented Smurov suddenly, in a ringing tone of conviction. He had listened attentively.

"And yet he is first in Latin himself," cried one of the group of boys suddenly.

"Yes, father, he says that and yet he is first in Latin," echoed Ilusha.

"What of it?" Kolya thought fit to defend himself, though the praise was very sweet to him. "I am fagging away at Latin, because I have to, because I promised my mother to pass my examination, and I think that whatever you do should be done well. But at heart I have a profound contempt for the classics and all that fraud. . . . You don't agree, Karamazov?"

"Why 'fraud'?" Alyosha smiled again.

"Well, all the classical authors have been translated into all languages, so it was not for the sake of studying the classics they introduced Latin, but solely as a police measure, and to stupefy the intelligence. So what can one call it but a fraud?"

"Why, who taught you all this?" cried Alyosha, surprised at last.

"In the first place, I am capable of thinking for myself without being taught. Besides, what I said just now about the classics being translated our teacher Kolbasnikov has said to the whole of the third class."

"The doctor has come!" cried Nina, who had been silent till then.

A carriage belonging to Madame Hohlakov drove up to the gate. The captain, who had been expecting the doctor all morning, rushed headlong out to meet him. "Mamma" pulled herself together and assumed a dignified air. Alyosha went up to Ilusha and began setting his pillows straight. Nina, from her invalid chair, anxiously watched him making the bed tidy. The boys hurriedly took leave. Some of them promised to come again in the evening. Kolya called Perezvon and the dog jumped off the bed.

"I won't go away, I won't go away," Kolya said hastily to Ilusha. "I'll wait in the passage and come back when the doctor's gone, I'll come back with Perezvon."

But by now the doctor had entered, an important-looking person with long, dark whiskers and a shiny, shaven chin, wearing a bearskin coat. As he crossed the threshold he stopped, taken aback; he probably fancied he had come to the wrong place. "How is this? Where am I?" he muttered, not removing his coat nor his peaked sealskin cap. The crowd, the poverty of the room, the washing hanging on a line in the corner, puzzled him. The captain, bent double, was bowing low before him.

"It's here, sir, here, sir," he muttered cringingly; "it's here, you've come to the right place, you were coming to us . . ."

"Sne-gi-ryov?" the doctor said loudly and pompously. "Mr. Snegiryov — is that you?"

"That's me, sir!"

"Ah!"

The doctor looked round the room with a squeamish air once more and threw off his coat, displaying to all eyes the grand decoration round his neck. The captain caught the fur coat in the air, and the doctor took off his cap.

"Where is the patient?" he asked loudly and emphatically.

CHAPTER VI

PRECOCITY

"WHAT do you think the doctor will say to him?" Kolya asked quickly. "What a repulsive mug though, hasn't he? I can't endure medicine!"

"Ilusha is dying. I think that's certain," answered Alyosha mournfully.

"They are rogues! Medicine's a fraud! I am glad to have made your acquaintance though, Karamazov. I have wanted to know you for a long time. I am only sorry we meet under such sad circumstances."

Kolya had a great inclination to say something even warmer and more demonstrative, but he felt ill at ease. Alyosha noticed this, smiled, and pressed his hand.

"I've long learnt to respect you as a rare person," Kolya muttered again, faltering and uncertain. "I have heard you are a mystic and have been in the monastery. I know you are a mystic but . . . that hasn't put me off. Contact with real life will cure you. . . . It's always so with characters like yours."

"What do you mean by mystic? Cure me of what?" Alyosha was rather astonished.

"Oh, God and all the rest of it."

"What, don't you believe in God?"

"On the contrary, I've nothing against God. Of course, God is only a hypothesis, but . . . I admit that He is needed . . . for order, for universal order and all that . . . and that if there were no God He would have to be invented," added Kolya, beginning to blush. He suddenly fancied that Alyosha might think he was trying to show off his knowledge and to prove that he was "grown up." "I haven't the slightest desire to show off my knowledge to him," Kolya thought indignantly. And all of a sudden he felt horribly annoyed.

"I must confess I can't endure entering on such discussions," he said with a final air. "It's possible for one who doesn't believe in God to love mankind, don't you think so? Voltaire didn't believe in God and loved mankind." ("I am at it again," he thought to himself.)

"Voltaire did believe in God, though not very much, I think, and I don't think he loved mankind very much either," said Alyosha quietly, gently, and quite naturally, as though he were talking to some one of his own age, or even older. Kolya was particularly struck by Alyosha's apparent diffidence about his opinion of Voltaire. He seemed to be leaving the question for him, little Kolya, to settle.

"Have you read Voltaire?" Alyosha finished.

"No, not to say read. . . . But I've read *Candide* in a Russian translation . . . in an absurd, grotesque, old translation." . . . ("At it again! again!")

"And did you understand it?"

"Oh, yes, everything. . . . That is . . . Why do you suppose I shouldn't understand it? There's a lot of salaciousness in it, of course. . . . Of course I can understand that it's a philosophical novel and written to advocate an idea. . . ." Kolya was getting confused by now. "I am a socialist, Karamazov, I am an incorrigible socialist," he announced suddenly, apropos of nothing.

"A socialist?" laughed Alyosha. "But when have you had time to become one? Why, I thought you are only thirteen?"

Kolya winced.

"In the first place, I am not thirteen, but fourteen, fourteen in a fortnight" — he flushed angrily — "and in the second place, I am at a complete loss to understand what my age has to do with it. The question is, what are my convictions, not what is my age, isn't it?"

"When you are older, you'll understand for yourself the influence of age on convictions. I fancied, too, that you were not using your own words," Alyosha answered serenely and modestly, but Kolya interrupted him hotly:

"Come, you want obedience and mysticism. You must admit that the Christian religion, for instance, has only been of use to the rich and the powerful to keep the lower classes in slavery, that's so, isn't it?"

"Ah, I know where you read that, and I am sure some one taught you this!" cried Alyosha.

"I say, what makes you think I read it? And certainly no one taught it to me. I can think for myself. . . . I am not opposed to Christ, if you like. He was an altogther humane person, and if He were alive to-day, He would be found in the ranks of the revolutionists, and would perhaps play a conspicuous part. . . . There's no doubt about that."

"Oh, where, where did you get that from? What fool have you made friends with?" exclaimed Alyosha.

"Come, the truth will out! Of course, it happens that I have often talked to Mr. Rakitin, but . . . old Belinsky said that, too, so they say."

"Belinsky? I don't remember. He hasn't written that anywhere."

"If he didn't write it, they say he said it. I heard that from a . . . but never mind."

"And have you read Belinsky?"

"Well, no . . . I haven't read all of him, but . . . I read the passage about Tatyana, asking why she didn't go off with Onyegin."

"Didn't go off with Onyegin? Surely you don't . . . understand that already?"

"Why, you seem to take me for little Smurov," said Kolya, with a grin of irritation. "But please don't suppose I am such a revolutionist. I often disagree with Mr. Rakitin. Though I mention Tatyana, I am not at all for the emancipation of women. I acknowledge that women are a subject race and must obey. *Les femmes tricottent*, as Napoleon said." Kolya, for some reason, smiled. "And on this subject at least I am quite of one mind with that pseudo-great man. I think, too, that to leave one's own country and escape to America is mean, worse than mean — stupid. Why go to America when one may be of great service to humanity here? Now especially. There's a perfect heap of fruitful activity open to us. That's what I answered."

"What do you mean? Answered whom? Has some one suggested your going to America already?"

"I must own, they've been at me to go, but I declined. That's between ourselves, of course, Karamazov; do you hear, not a word to any one. I say this only to you. I am not at all anxious to fall into the clutches of the secret police and take lessons at the Chain bridge,

Long will you remember
The house at the Chain bridge.

Do you remember? It's splendid. Why are you laughing? You don't suppose I am fibbing, do you?" ("What if he should find out that I've only that one number of *The Bell** in father's bookcase, and haven't read any more of it?" Kolya thought with a shudder.)

"Oh, no, I am not laughing and don't suppose for a moment that you are lying. No, indeed, I can't suppose so, for all this alas! is perfectly true. But tell me, have you read Pushkin, Onyegin, for instance? . . . You spoke just now of Tatyana."

"No, I haven't read it yet, but I want to read it. I have no prejudices; I want to hear both sides. What makes you ask?"

"Oh, nothing."

"Tell me, Karamazov, have you an awful contempt for me?" Kolya rapped out suddenly and drew himself up before Alyosha, as though he were on drill. "Be so kind as to tell me, without beating about the bush."

"I have a contempt for you?" Alyosha looked at him wonderingly. "What for? I am only sad that a charming nature such as yours should be perverted by all this crude nonsense before you have begun life."

"Don't be anxious about my nature," Kolya interrupted, not without complacency. "But it's true that I am stupidly sensitive, crudely sensitive. You smiled just now, and I fancied you seemed to . . . "

"Oh, my smile meant something quite different. I'll tell you why I smiled. Not long ago I read the opinion of a German who had lived in Russia, about our present-day student-body. 'Show a Russian schoolboy,' he writes, 'a map of the stars, which he knows nothing about, and he will give you back the map next day with corrections on it.' No knowledge

* A review published abroad under Herzen's editorship, and smuggled into Russia. *Editor's note.*

and unbounded conceit — that's what the German meant to say about the Russian schoolboy."

"Yes, that's perfectly right," Kolya laughed suddenly, "exactly so! Bravo, German! But the numbskull did not see the good side, what do you think? Conceit — maybe, that comes from youth, that will be corrected if need be, but, on the other hand, there is an independent spirit almost from childhood, boldness of thought and conviction, and not the spirit of these sausage-makers, grovelling before authority. . . . But the German was right all the same. Bravo, German! But Germans want strangling all the same. Though they are so good at science and learning, they must be strangled."

"Strangled, what for?" smiled Alyosha.

"Well, perhaps I am talking nonsense, I agree. I am awfully childish sometimes, and when I am pleased about anything I can't restrain myself and am ready to talk stuff. But, I say, we are chattering away here about trifles, and that doctor has been in there a long time. But perhaps he's examining 'mamma' and that poor crippled Nina. I liked that Nina, you know. She whispered to me suddenly as I was coming away, 'Why didn't you come before?' And in such a voice, so reproachfully! I think she is awfully kind and pitiful."

"Yes, yes! Well, you'll be coming often, you will see what she is like. It would do you a great deal of good to know people like that, to learn to value a great deal which you will find out from knowing these people," Alyosha observed warmly. "That would have more effect on you than any thing."

"Oh, how I regret and how I blame myself for not having come sooner!" Kolya exclaimed, with bitter feeling.

"Yes, it's a great pity. You saw for yourself how delighted the poor child was to see you. And how he was fretting, waiting for you to come!"

"Don't tell me! You make it worse! But it serves me right. What kept me from coming was my conceit, my egoistic vanity, and the beastly wilfulness, which I never can get rid of, though I've been struggling with it all my life. I see that now. I am a beast in lots of ways, Karamazov!"

"No, you have a charming nature, though it's been distorted, and I quite understand why you have had such an influence on this generous, morbidly sensitive boy," Alyosha answered warmly.

"And you say that to me!" cried Kolya; "and would you believe it, I thought — I've thought several times since I've been here — that you despised me! If only you knew how I prize your opinion!"

"But are you really so sensitive? At your age! Would you believe it, just now, when you were telling your story, I thought, as I watched you, that you must be very sensitive!"

"You thought so? What an eye you've got, I say! I bet that was when I was talking about the goose. That was just when I was fancying you had a great contempt for me for being in such a hurry to show off, and for a moment I quite hated you for it, and began talking like a fool. Then I fancied — here, just now — when I said that if there were no God He would have to be invented, that I was in too great a hurry to display my information, especially as I got that phrase out of a book. But I swear I wasn't showing off out of vanity, but just so, I really don't know why, because I was so overjoyed, yes, I believe it was because I was so overjoyed . . . though it's perfectly disgraceful for any one to be gushing directly they are pleased, I know that. But I am convinced now that you don't despise me; it was all my imagination. Oh, Karamazov, I am profoundly unhappy. I sometimes fancy all sorts of things, that every one is laughing at me, the whole world, and then I feel ready to destroy the whole order of things."

"And you torment every one about you," smiled Alyosha.

"Yes, I torment every one about me, especially my mother. Karamazov, tell me, am I very ridiculous now?"

"Don't think about that, don't think of it at all!" cried Alyosha. "And what does ridiculous mean? Isn't every one constantly being or seeming ridiculous? Besides, nearly all clever people now are fearfully afraid of being ridiculous, and that makes them unhappy. All I am surprised at is that you should be feeling that so early, though I've observed it for some time past, and not only in you. Nowadays the very children have begun to suffer from it. It's almost a sort of insanity. The devil has taken the form of that vanity and entered into the whole generation; it's simply the devil," added Alyosha, without a trace of the smile that Kolya, staring at him, expected to see. "You are like every one else," said Alyosha, in conclusion, "that is, like very many others. Only you must not be like everybody else, that's all."

"Even if every one is like that?"

"Yes, even if every one is like that. You be the only one not like it. You really are not like every one else, here you are not ashamed to confess to something bad and even ridiculous. And who will admit so much in these days? No one. And people have even ceased to feel the impulse to self-criticism. Don't be like every one else, even if you were the only one."

"Splendid! I was not mistaken in you. You know how to console one. Oh, how I have longed to know you, Karamazov. I've long been eager for this meeting. Can you really have thought about me, too? You said just now that you thought of me, too?"

"Yes, I'd heard of you and had thought of you, too . . . and if it's partly vanity that makes you ask, it doesn't matter."

"Do you know, Karamazov, our talk has been like a declaration of love," said Kolya, in a bashful and melting voice. "That's not ridiculous, is it?"

"Not at all ridiculous, and if it were, it wouldn't matter, because it's been a good thing." Alyosha smiled serenely.

"But do you know, Karamazov, you must admit that you are a little ashamed yourself, now. . . . I see it by your eyes." Kolya smiled slyly but with a kind of happiness.

"Why ashamed?"

"Well, why are you blushing?"

"It was you made me blush," laughed Alyosha, and he really did blush. "Oh, well, I am a little, goodness knows why, I don't know . . ." he muttered, almost embarrassed.

"Oh, how I love you and value you at this moment just because you, too, are rather ashamed! Because you are just like me," cried Kolya, in positive ecstasy. His cheeks glowed, his eyes beamed.

"You know, Kolya, you will be very unhappy in your life," something made Alyosha say suddenly.

"I know, I know. How you know it all beforehand!" Kolya agreed at once.

"But you will bless life on the whole, all the same."

"Just so, hurrah! You are a prophet. Oh, we shall be friends, Karamazov! Do you know, what delights me most, is that you treat me quite like an equal. But we are not equals, no, we are not, you are better! But we shall be friends. Do you know, all this last month I've been saying to myself, 'either we shall be friends at once, for ever, or we shall part enemies to the grave!'"

"And saying that, of course, you loved me." Alyosha laughed gaily.

"I did. I loved you awfully. I've been loving you and dreaming of you. And how do you know it all beforehand? Ah, here's the doctor. Goodness! What will he tell us? Look at his face!"

CHAPTER VII

ILUSHA

THE doctor came out of the room again, muffled in his fur coat and with his cap on his head. His face looked almost angry and disgusted, as though all the time he were afraid of being soiled. He cast a cursory glance round the passage, and looked sternly at Alyosha and Kolya as he did so. Alyosha waved from the door to the coachman, and the carriage that had brought the doctor drove up. The captain darted out after the doctor, and, bent over, almost wriggling before him, stopped him to get the last word. The poor fellow looked utterly crushed; there was a scared look in his eyes.

"Your Excellency, your Excellency . . . is it possible?" he began, but could not go on and struck his hands together in despair. Yet he still gazed imploringly at the doctor, as though a word from him might still change the verdict concerning the poor boy.

"What can I do! I am not God!" the doctor answered offhand, though with the customary impressiveness.

"Doctor . . . your Excellency . . . and will it be soon, soon?"

"You must be prepared for anything," said the doctor in emphatic and incisive tones, and, dropping his eyes, he was about to cross the threshold and step into the coach.

"Your Excellency, for Christ's sake," the terror-stricken captain stopped him again. "Your Excellency! but can nothing, absolutely nothing save him now?"

"It's not in my hands now," said the doctor impatiently, "but h'm . . ." He stopped suddenly. "If you could, for instance . . . send . . . your patient . . . at once, without delay" (the words "at once, without delay" the doctor uttered with an almost wrathful sternness that made the captain start), "to Syracuse, the change to the new be-ne-ficial climatic conditions might possibly affect . . ."

"To Syracuse!" cried the captain, unable to grasp what was said.

"Syracuse is in Sicily," Kolya jerked out suddenly in explanation. The doctor looked at him.

"Sicily! your Excellency," faltered the captain, "but you've seen"—he spread out his hands, indicating his surroundings—"and what about mamma and the family?"

"N-no, Sicily is not the place for the family, the family should go to the Caucasus in the early spring . . . your daughter must go to the Caucasus, and your spouse . . . after a course of the waters in the Caucasus for her rheumatism . . . must be sent straight to Paris to the mental specialist Lepelletier; I could give you a note to him, and then . . . there might be a change . . ."

"Doctor, doctor! But you see!" The captain flung wide his hands again despairingly, indicating the bare wooden walls of the passage.

"Well, that's not my business," grinned the doctor. "I have only told you the answer of medical science to your question as to possible treatment. As for the rest, to my regret . . ."

"Don't be afraid, apothecary, my dog won't bite you," Kolya rapped out loudly, noticing the doctor's rather uneasy glance at Perezvon, who was standing in the doorway. There was a wrathful note in Kolya's voice. He used the word apothecary instead of doctor on purpose, and, as he explained afterwards, "I used it to insult him."

"What's that?" The doctor flung up his head, staring with surprise at Kolya. "Who's this?" He addressed Alyosha, as though demanding an accounting from him.

"It's Perezvon's master, don't worry about my person, apothecary," Kolya said incisively again.

"Perezvon,"* repeated the doctor, perplexed.

"He hears the bell, but where it is he cannot tell. Good-bye, apothecary, we shall meet in Syracuse."

"Who's this? Who's this?" The doctor flew into a terrible rage.

"He is a schoolboy, doctor, he is a mischievous boy; take no notice of him," said Alyosha, frowning and speaking quickly. "Kolya, hold your tongue!" he cried to Krasotkin. "Take no notice of him, doctor," he repeated, rather impatiently.

"He wants a thrashing, a good thrashing!" The doctor stamped in a perfect fury.

"And you know, apothecary, my Perezvon might bite!" said Kolya, turning pale, with quivering voice and flashing eyes. "*Ici*, Perezvon!"

"Kolya, if you say another word, I'll break with you for ever," Alyosha cried peremptorily.

"Apothecary, there is only one man in the world who can command Nikolay Krasotkin—this is the man" (Kolya pointed to Alyosha). "I obey him, good-bye!"

He dashed from the spot and, opening the door, quickly went into the room. Perezvon flew after him. The doctor stood still for five seconds in amazement, looking at Alyosha; then he suddenly spat and went out quickly to the carriage, repeating aloud, "This is . . . this is . . . I don't know what it is!" The captain darted forward to help him into the carriage. Alyosha followed Kolya into the room. He was already at Ilusha's bedside. The sick boy was holding his hand and calling for his father. A minute later the captain, too, came back.

"Father, father, come . . . we . . ." Ilusha faltered in violent excitement but, apparently unable to go on, he flung his wasted arms round his father and Kolya, uniting them in one embrace, and hugging them as tightly as he could. The captain suddenly began to shake with dumb sobs, and Kolya's lips and chin twitched.

"Father, father! How sorry I am for you!" Ilusha moaned bitterly.

"Ilusha . . . darling . . . the doctor said . . . you would be all right . . . we shall be happy . . . the doctor . . ." the captain began.

"Ah, father! I know what the new doctor said to you about me . . . didn't I see!" cried Ilusha, and again he hugged them both with all his strength, hiding his face on his father's shoulder.

* *i.e.*, a chime of bells.

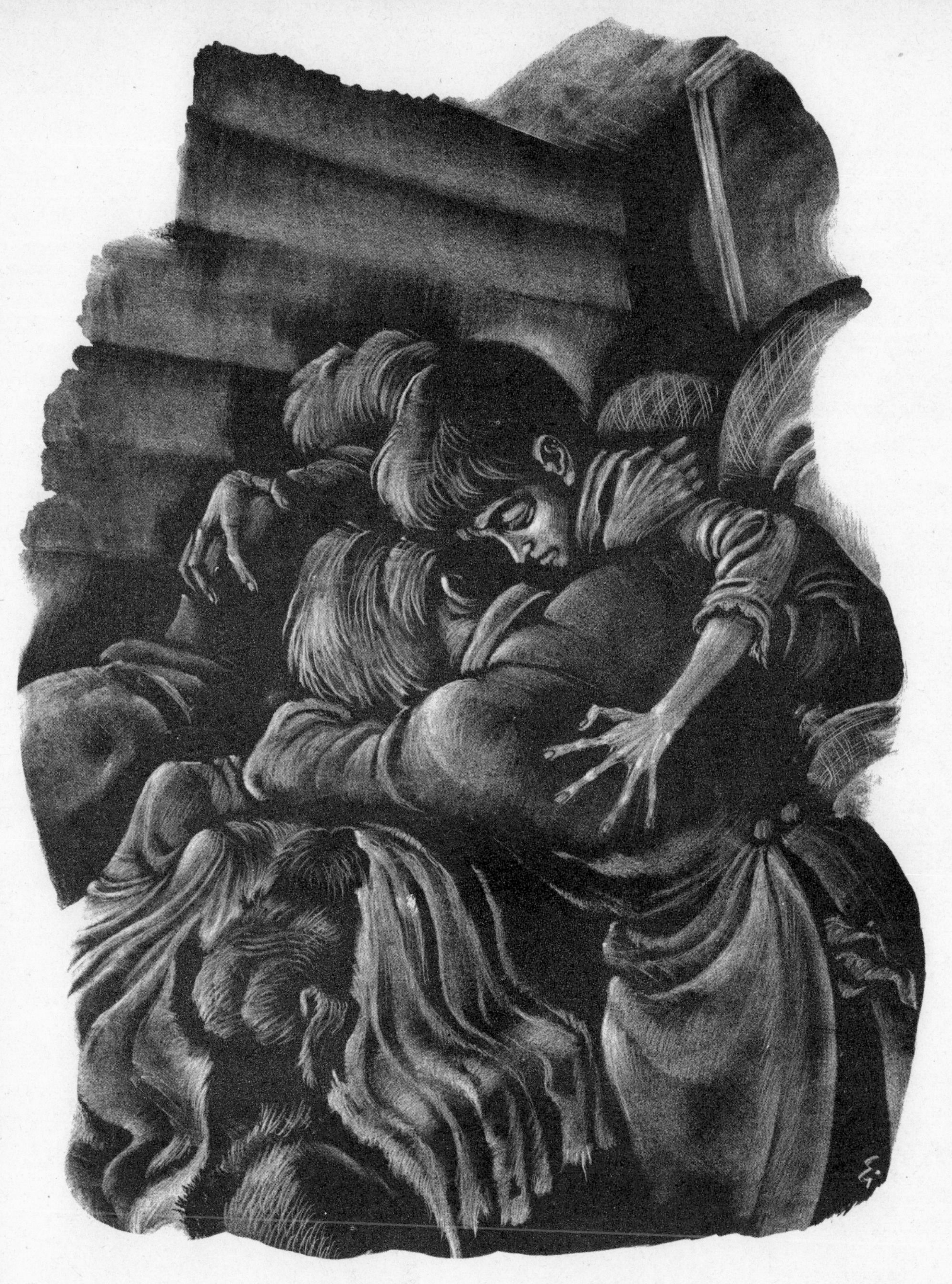

KRASOTKIN AND HIS SON

"Father, don't cry, and when I die get a good boy, another one . . . choose one of them all, a good one, call him Ilusha and love him instead of me . . ."

"Hush, old man, you'll get well," Krasotkin cried suddenly, as though getting angry.

"But don't ever forget me, father," Ilusha went on, "come to my grave . . . and, father, bury me by our big stone, where we used to go for our walk, and come to me there with Krasotkin in the evening . . . and Perezvon . . . I shall expect you. . . . Father, father!"

His voice broke. They were all three silent, still embracing.

Nina was crying quietly in her chair, and at last, seeing them all crying, "mamma," too, burst into tears.

"Ilusha! Ilusha!" she exclaimed.

Krasotkin suddenly released himself from Ilusha's embrace.

"Good-bye, old man, mother expects me back to dinner," he said quickly. "What a pity I did not tell her! She will be dreadfully anxious. . . . But after dinner I'll come back to you for the whole day, for the whole evening, and I'll tell you all sorts of things, all sorts of things. And I'll bring Perezvon, but now I will take him with me, because he will begin to howl when I am away and bother you. Good-bye!"

And he ran out into the passage. He didn't want to cry, but in the passage he burst into tears. Alyosha found him crying.

"Kolya, you must be sure to keep your word and come, or he will be in agony," Alyosha said emphatically.

"I will! Oh, how I curse myself for not having come before," muttered Kolya, crying, and no longer ashamed of it.

At that moment the captain flew out of the room, and at once closed the door behind him. His face looked frenzied, his lips were trembling. He stood before the two lads and flung up his arms.

"I don't want a good boy! I don't want another boy!" he muttered in a wild whisper, clenching his teeth. "If I forget thee, Jerusalem, may my tongue . . ." He broke off with a sob and sank on his knees before the wooden bench. Pressing his fists against his head, he began sobbing with absurd whimpering cries, doing his utmost that his cries should not be heard in the room.

Kolya ran out into the street.

"Good-bye, Karamazov! Will you come yourself?" he cried sharply and angrily to Alyosha.

"I will certainly come in the evening."

"What was that he said about Jerusalem? . . . What did he mean by that?"

"It's from the Bible. 'If I forget thee, Jerusalem,' that is, if I forget all that is most precious to me, if I let anything take its place, then may . . ."

"I understand, that's enough! Mind you come! *Ici*, Perezvon!" he cried with positive ferocity to the dog, and with rapid strides he went home.

CHAPTER I

AT GRUSHENKA'S

ALYOSHA went towards the cathedral square to the widow Morozov's house to see Grushenka, who had sent Fenya to him early in the morning with an urgent message begging him to come. On questioning Fenya, Alyosha learnt that her mistress had been particularly distressed since the previous day. During the two months that had passed since Mitya's arrest, Alyosha had called frequently at the widow Morozov's house, both because of his own inclination and in order to take messages for Mitya. Three days after Mitya's arrest, Grushenka was taken very sick and was ill for nearly five weeks. For one whole week she was unconscious. She was very much changed — thinner and a little sallow, though she had for the past fortnight been well enough to go out. But to Alyosha her face was even more attractive than before, and he liked to meet her eyes when he went in to her. A look of firmness and intelligent purpose had developed in her face. There were signs of a spiritual transformation in her, and a steadfast, fine, and humble determination that nothing could shake could be discerned in her. There was a small vertical wrinkle between her brows which gave her charming face a look of concentrated thought, almost austere at the first glance. There was scarcely a trace of her former frivolity.

It seemed strange to Alyosha, too, that in spite of the calamity that had overtaken the poor woman, betrothed to a man who had been arrested for a terrible crime, almost at the instant of their betrothal, in spite of her illness and the almost inevitable sentence hanging over Mitya, Grushenka had yet not lost her youthful cheerfulness. There was a soft light in the once proud eyes, though at times they gleamed with the old sinister fire when she was visited by one worry which had become stronger than ever in her heart. The object of that uneasiness was the same as ever — Katerina Ivanovna, of whom Grushenka had even raved when she lay in delirium. Alyosha knew that she was fearfully jealous of her, in spite of the fact that Katerina Ivanovna had not once visited Mitya in prison, though she might have done it whenever she liked. All this made a difficult problem for Alyosha, for he was the only person to whom Grushenka opened her heart and from whom she was continually asking advice. Sometimes he was unable to say anything.

Full of anxiety he entered her lodging. She was at home. She had returned from seeing Mitya half an hour before, and from the rapid movement with which she leapt up from her chair to meet him he saw that she had been waiting for him with great impatience. A pack of cards dealt for a game of "fools" lay on the table. A bed had been made up on the leather sofa on the other side of the table and Maximov lay, half reclining, on it. He wore a dressing-gown and a cotton nightcap, and was evidently ill and weak, though he was smiling blissfully. When the homeless old man had returned with Grushenka from Mokroye two months before, he had simply stayed on and was still staying with her. Having come with her through rain and mud, he had sat down on the sofa, drenched and scared, and gazed mutely at her with a timid, appealing smile. Grushenka, who was in terrible grief and in the first stage of fever, almost forgot his existence in all she had to do the first half-hour after her arrival. Suddenly she looked at him closely: he gave a pitiful, helpless little titter. She called Fenya and told her to give him something to eat. All that day he sat in the same place, almost without stirring. When it got dark and the shutters were closed, Fenya asked her mistress:

"Is the gentleman going to stay the night, mistress?"

"Yes; make him a bed on the sofa," answered Grushenka.

Questioning him in more detail, Grushenka learnt from him that he had literally nowhere to go, and that "Mr. Kalganov, my benefactor, told me straight that he wouldn't receive me again and gave me five roubles."

"Well, God bless you, you'd better stay then," Grushenka decided in her anguish, smiling compassionately at him. Her smile wrung the old man's heart and his lips twitched with grateful weeping. And so the wandering pensioner had stayed with her ever since. He did not leave the house even when she was ill. Fenya and her grandmother, the cook, did not turn him out, but went on serving him meals and making up his bed on the sofa. Grushenka had grown used to him, and coming back from seeing Mitya (whom she had begun to visit in prison before she was really well), she would sit down and begin talking to "Maximushka" about trifling matters, to keep her from thinking of her sorrow. The old man turned out to be a good story-teller on occasion, so that at last he became necessary to her. Grushenka saw scarcely any one else besides Alyosha, who did not come every day and never stayed long. Her old merchant lay seriously ill at this time, "at his last gasp," as they said in the town, and he did, in fact, die a week after Mitya's trial. Three weeks before his death, feeling the end approaching, he made his sons, their wives and children, come upstairs to him at last and bade them not leave him again. From that moment he gave strict orders to his servants not to admit Grushenka and to tell her if she came, "The master wishes you long life and happiness and tells you to forget him." But Grushenka sent almost every day to inquire after him.

"You've come at last!" she cried, flinging down the cards and joyfully greeting Alyosha, "and Maximushka's been scaring me that perhaps you wouldn't come. Ah, how I need you! Sit down at the table. What will you have — coffee?"

"Yes, please," said Alyosha, sitting down at the table. "I am very hungry."

"That's right. Fenya, Fenya, coffee," cried Grushenka. "It's been boiling a long time, it's waiting for you. And bring some little pies, and mind they are hot. Do you know, we've had a storm over those pies to-day. I took them to the prison for him, and, would you believe it, he threw them back at me: he would not eat them. He flung one of them on the floor and stamped on it. So I said to him: 'I shall leave them with the warden; if you don't eat them before evening, it will mean that you feed on your venomous spite!' With that I went away. We quarrelled again, would you believe it? Whenever I go we quarrel."

Grushenka said all this in one breath in her agitation. Maximov, suddenly grown timid, smiled with downcast eyes.

"What did you quarrel about this time?" asked Alyosha.

"I didn't expect it in the least. Only fancy, he is jealous of the Pole. 'Why are you keeping him?' he said. 'So you've begun keeping him.' He is jealous, jealous of me all the time, jealous eating and sleeping! He even took it into his head to be jealous of Kuzma last week."

"But he knew about the Pole before?"

"Yes, but there it is. He has known about him from the very beginning, but to-day he suddenly got up and began scolding about him. I am ashamed to repeat what he said. Fool! Rakitin went in as I came out. Perhaps Rakitin is egging him on. What do you think?" she added absent-mindedly, as it were.

"He loves you, that's what it is; he loves you so much. And now he is particularly irritable."

"I should think he might be, with the trial to-morrow. And I went to him to say something about to-morrow, for I dread to think what's going to happen then. You say that he is irritable, but how irritable I am! And he talks about the Pole! What a fool! He is not jealous of Maximushka yet, anyway."

"My wife was dreadfully jealous of me, too," Maximov put in his word.

"Jealous of you?" Grushenka laughed in spite of herself. "Of whom could she have been jealous?"

"Of the servant girls."

"Hold your tongue, Maximushka, I am in no laughing mood now, I feel angry. Don't ogle the pies. I shan't give you any; they are not good for you, and I won't give you any vodka either. I have to look after him, too, just as though I kept an alms-house," she laughed.

"I don't deserve your kindness. I am a worthless creature," said Maximov, with tears in his voice. "You would do better to spend your kindness on people of more use than me."

"Ah, every one is of use, Maximushka, and how can we tell who's of most use. If only that Pole weren't there at all, Alyosha. He's taken it into his head to fall ill, too, to-day. I've been to see him also. And I shall send him some pies, too, on purpose. I hadn't sent him any, but Mitya accused me of it, so now I shall send some on purpose! Ah, here's Fenya with a letter! Yes, it's from the Poles — begging again!"

Pan Musialowicz had indeed sent an extremely long and, as usual, high-flown letter in which he begged her to lend him three roubles. In the letter was enclosed a receipt for the sum, with a promise to repay it within three months, signed by *Pan* Wróblewski as well. Grushenka had received many such letters, accompanied by such receipts, from her former lover during the fortnight of her convalescence. But she knew that the two Poles had been to ask after her health during her illness. The first letter Grushenka got from them was a long one, written on large note-paper and with a big family crest on the seal. It was so obscure and rhetorical that Grushenka put it down before she had read half, unable to make head or tail of it. She could not attend to letters then. The first letter was followed next day by another in which *Pan* Musialowicz begged her for a loan of two thousand roubles for a very short period. Grushenka left that letter, too, unanswered. A whole series of letters had followed — one every day — all as pompous and rhetorical, but the loan asked for, gradually diminishing, dropped to a hundred roubles, then to twenty-five, to ten, and finally Grushenka received a letter in which both the Poles begged her for only one rouble and included a receipt signed by both.

Then Grushenka suddenly felt sorry for them, and at dusk she went round herself to their lodging. She found the two Poles in great poverty, almost destitution, without food or fuel, without cigarettes, in debt to their landlady. The two hundred roubles they had carried off from Mitya at Mokroye had soon disappeared. But Grushenka was surprised at their meeting her with arrogant dignity and self-assertion, with the greatest formality and pompous speeches. Grushenka simply laughed, and gave her former admirer ten roubles. Then, laughing, she told Mitya of it and he was not in the least jealous. But ever since, the Poles had attached themselves to Grushenka and bombarded her daily with requests for money and she had always sent them small sums. And now that day Mitya had taken it into his head to be fearfully jealous.

"Like a fool, I went round to him just for a minute, on the way to see Mitya, for he is ill, too, my Pole," Grushenka began again with nervous haste. "I was laughing, telling Mitya about it. 'Fancy,' I said, 'my Pole had the happy thought of singing his old songs to me to the guitar. He thought I would be touched and marry him!' Mitya leapt up swearing. . . . So, there, I'll send them the pies! Fenya, is it that little girl they've sent? Here, give her three roubles and wrap a dozen pies up in a paper and tell her to take them. And you, Alyosha, be sure to tell Mitya that I did send them the pies."

"I wouldn't tell him for anything," said Alyosha, smiling.

"Oh! You think he is unhappy about it. Why, he's jealous on purpose. He doesn't care," said Grushenka bitterly.

"On purpose?" queried Alyosha.

"I tell you you are silly, Alyosha. You understand nothing about it, with all your cleverness. I am not offended because he is jealous of a girl like me. I would be offended if he were not jealous. I am like that. I am not offended by jealousy. I have a fierce heart, too. I can be jealous myself. Only what offends me is that he doesn't love me at all. I tell you he is jealous now *on purpose*. Am I blind? Don't I see? He began talking to me just now of that woman, of Katerina, saying she was this and that, how she had called in a doctor from Moscow for the trial, to try and save him; how she had sent for the best counsel, the most learned one, too. So he loves her, if he'll praise her to my face, more shame to him! He's guilty before me himself, so he attacked me, to make out I was in fault first and to put it all on me. 'You were with your Pole before I came, so I can't be blamed for Katerina,' that's what it amounts to. He wants to put the whole blame on me. He attacked me on purpose, on purpose, I tell you, but I'll . . ."

Grushenka did not finish saying what she would do. She hid her eyes in her handkerchief and broke into violent sobs.

"He doesn't love Katerina Ivanovna," said Alyosha firmly.

"Well, whether he loves her or not I'll soon find out for myself," said Grushenka, with a menacing note in her voice, taking the handkerchief from her eyes. Her face was distorted. Alyosha saw sorrowfully that from being mild and serene it had become sullen and spiteful.

"Enough of this foolishness," she said suddenly; "it's not for that I sent for you. Alyosha, darling, to-morrow — what will happen to-morrow? That's what worries me! And it's only me it worries! I look at every one and no one is thinking of it. No one cares about it. Are you thinking about it even? To-morrow he'll be tried, you know. Tell me, how will he be tried? You know it's the valet, the valet killed him! Good heavens! Can they condemn him in place of the valet and will no one stand up for him? They haven't troubled the valet at all, have they?"

"He's been severely cross-examined," observed Alyosha thoughtfully; "but every one came to the conclusion it was not he. Now he is lying very ill. He has been ill ever since that attack. Really ill," added Alyosha.

"Oh, dear! Couldn't you go to that counsel yourself and tell him the whole thing in private? He's been brought from Petersburg for three thousand roubles, they say."

"We gave these three thousand together — Ivan, Katerina Ivanovna, and I — but she paid two thousand for the doctor from Moscow herself. The counsel Fetyukovich would have charged more, but the case has become known all over Russia; it's in all the newspapers and reviews. Fetyukovich agreed to come more for the glory, because the case has become so notorious. I saw him yesterday."

"Well? Did you talk to him?" Grushenka put in eagerly.

"He listened and said nothing. He told me that he had already formed his opinion. But he promised to give my words consideration."

"Consideration! Ah, they are swindlers! They'll ruin him. And why did she send for the doctor?"

"As an expert. They want to prove that Mitya's mad and committed the murder when he didn't know what he was doing"; Alyosha smiled gently; "but Mitya won't agree to that."

"Yes; but that would be the truth if he had killed him!" cried Grushenka. "He was mad then, perfectly mad, and that was my fault, wretch that I am! But, of course, he didn't do it, he didn't do it! And they are all against him, saying he is the murderer, the whole town. Even Fenya's evidence went to prove he had done it. And the people at the shop, and that official, and at the tavern, too, before, people had heard him say so! They are all, all against him, all crying out against him."

"Yes, there's a fearful accumulation of evidence," Alyosha observed grimly.

"And Grigory — Grigory Vasilyevich — sticks to his story that the door was open, insists that he saw it — there's no shaking him. I went and talked to him myself. He's rude about it, too."

"Yes, that's perhaps the strongest evidence against him," said Alyosha.

"And as for Mitya's being mad, he certainly seems like it now," Grushenka began with a peculiarly anxious and mysterious air. "Do you know, Alyosha, I've been wanting to talk to you about it for a long time. I go to him every day and simply wonder at him. Tell me, now, what do you suppose he's always talking about? He talks and talks and I can make nothing of it. I fancied he was talking of something intellectual that I couldn't understand in my foolishness. Only he suddenly began talking to me about a babe — that is, about some child. 'Why is the babe poor?' he said. 'It's for that babe I am going to Siberia now. I did not kill, but I must go to Siberia!' What that meant, what babe, I couldn't tell for the life of me. Only I cried when he said it, because it was so fine the way he said it. He cried himself, and I cried, too. He suddenly kissed me and made the sign of the cross over me. What did it mean, Alyosha, tell me? What is this babe?"

"It must be Rakitin, who's been going to see him lately," smiled Alyosha, "though . . . that's not Rakitin's doing. I didn't see Mitya yesterday. I'll see him to-day."

"No, it's not Rakitin; it's his brother Ivan Fyodorovich upsetting him. It's his going to see him, that's what it is," Grushenka began, and suddenly broke off.

Alyosha gazed at her in amazement. "Ivan's going? Has he been to see him? Mitya told me himself that Ivan hasn't been once."

"There . . . there! What a girl I am! Blurting things out!" exclaimed Grushenka, confused and suddenly blushing. "Wait, Alyosha, hush! Since I've said so much I'll tell the whole truth — he's been to see him twice, the first time directly he arrived. He galloped here from Moscow at once, of course, before I was taken ill; and the second time was a week ago. He told Mitya not to tell you about it, under any circumstances; and not to tell any one, in fact. He came secretly."

Alyosha sat plunged in thought, considering. The news evidently astonished him.

"Ivan doesn't talk to me of Mitya's case," he said slowly. "He's said very little to me these last two months. And whenever I go to see him, he seems vexed at my coming, so I've not been to him for the last three weeks. H'm! . . . if he was there a week ago . . . there certainly has been a change in Mitya this week."

"There has been a change," Grushenka assented quickly. "They have a secret, they had a secret! Mitya told me himself there was a secret, and such a secret that Mitya can't rest. Before then, he was cheerful — and, indeed, he is cheerful now — but when he begins shaking his head like that, you know, and strides about the room and keeps pulling at the hair on his right temple with his right hand, I know there is something on his mind worrying him. . . . I know! He was cheerful before, though, indeed, he is cheerful to-day."

"But you said he was irritable."

"Yes, he is irritable and yet cheerful. He keeps on being irritable for a minute and then cheerful and then irritable again. And you know, Alyosha, I am constantly wondering at him — with this awful thing hanging over him, he sometimes laughs at such trifles as though he were a baby himself."

"And did he really tell you not to tell me about Ivan? Did he say 'don't tell him'?"

"Yes, he told me 'don't tell him.' It's you that Mitya's most afraid of. Because it's a secret: he said himself it was a secret. Alyosha, darling, go to him and find out what their secret is and come and tell me," Grushenka besought him with sudden eagerness. "Set my mind at rest that I may know the worst that's in store for me. That's why I sent for you."

"You think it's something to do with you? If it were, he wouldn't have told you there was a secret."

"I don't know. Perhaps he wants to tell me, but doesn't dare to. He warns me. There is a secret, he tells me, but he won't tell me what it is."

"What do you think yourself?"

"What do I think? It's the end of me, that's what I think. They all three have been plotting my end, for Katerina's in it. It's all Katerina, it all comes from her. She is this and that, which means I am not this and that. He tells me that beforehand — warns me. He is planning to throw me over, that's the whole secret. They've planned it together, the three of them — Mitya, Katerina, and Ivan Fyodorovich. Alyosha, I've been wanting to ask you a long time. A week ago he suddenly told me that Ivan was in love with Katerina, because he often goes to see her. Did he tell me the truth or not? Tell me, on your conscience, knife me."

"I won't tell you a lie. Ivan is not in love with Katerina Ivanovna, I think."

"Oh, that's what I thought! He is lying to me, shameless deceiver, that's what it is! And he was jealous of me just now, so as to put the blame on me afterwards. He is stupid, he can't cover his traces; he is so open, you know. . . . But I'll give it to him, I'll give it to him! 'You believe I killed,' he said. He said that to me, to me. He reproached me with that! God forgive him! You wait, I'll make it hot for Katerina at the trial! I'll just say a word then . . . I'll tell everything then!"

And again she cried bitterly.

"This I can tell you for certain, Grushenka," Alyosha said, getting up. "First, that he loves you, loves you more than any one in the world, and you only, believe me. I know. I do know. The second thing is that I don't want to worm his secret out of him, but if he'll tell me of himself to-day, I shall tell him straight out that I have promised to tell you. Then I'll come to you to-day and tell you. Only . . . I fancy . . . Katerina Ivanovna has nothing to do with it, and that the secret is about something else. That's certain. It isn't likely it's about Katerina Ivanova, it seems to me. Good-bye for the present."

Alyosha shook hands with her. Grushenka was still crying. He saw that she put little faith in his consolation, but she was better for having poured her sorrow out, for having spoken of it. He was sorry to leave her in such a state of mind, but he was in haste. He had a great many things to do.

CHAPTER II

THE INJURED FOOT

The first of these things was at the house of Madame Hohlakov, and he hurried there to get it over as quickly as possible and not be too late for Mitya. Madame Hohlakov had been slightly ailing for the last three weeks: her foot had for some reason swollen up, and though she was not in bed, she lay all day half reclining on the couch in her boudoir, in fascinating but decorous *déshabillé*. Alyosha had once noted with innocent amusement that, in spite of her illness, Madame Hohlakov had begun to be rather dressy — little caps, ribbons, *négligés*, had made their appearance, and he had an inkling of the reason, though he dismissed such ideas from his mind as idle. During the last two months the young official, Perhotin, had become a regular visitor at the house.

Alyosha had not called for four days and he was in haste to go straight to Lise, as it was with her he had to speak, for Lise had sent a maid to him the previous day, specially asking him to come to her "about something very important," a request which, for certain reasons, interested Alyosha. But while the maid went to take his name in to Lise, Madame Hohlakov heard of his arrival from some one, and immediately sent to beg him to come to her "just for one minute." Alyosha reflected that it was better to accede to the mamma's request, or else she would be sending down to Lise's room every minute that he was there. Madame Hohlakov was lying on a couch. She was dressed very festively and was evidently in a state of extreme nervous excitement. She greeted Alyosha with cries of rapture.

"It's ages, ages, perfect ages since I've seen you! It's a whole week — only think of it! Ah, but you were here only four days ago, on Wednesday. You have come to see Lise. I'm sure you meant to slip into her room on tiptoe, without my hearing you. My dear, dear Alexey Fyodorovich, if you only knew how worried I am about her! But of that later, though that's the most important thing, of that later. Dear Alexey Fyodorovich, I trust you implicitly with my Lise. Since the death of Father Zosima — God rest his soul!" (she crossed herself) — "I look upon you as a monk, though you look charming in your new suit. Where did you find such a tailor in these parts? No, no, that's not the chief thing — of that later. Forgive me for sometimes calling you Alyosha; an old woman like me may take liberties," she smiled coquettishly; "but that will do later, too. The important thing is that I shouldn't forget what is important. Please remind me of it yourself. As soon as my tongue runs away with me, you just say, 'The important thing?' Ah! how do I know now what is of most importance? Ever since Lise took back her promise — her childish promise, Alexey Fyodorovich — to marry you, you've realised, of course, that it was only the playful fancy of a sick child who had been so long confined to her chair — thank God, she can walk now! . . . that new doctor Katya sent for from Moscow for your unhappy brother, who will to-morrow . . . But why speak of to-morrow? I am dying at the very thought of to-morrow. Dying of curiosity. . . . In a word, that doctor was here yesterday and saw Lise. . . . I paid him fifty roubles for the visit. But that's not the point, that's not the point again. You see, I'm mixing everything up. I am in such a hurry. Why am I in a hurry? I don't understand. It's awful how I seem growing unable to understand anything. Everything seems mixed up in a sort of tangle. I am afraid you are so bored you will jump up and run away, and that will be all I shall see of you. Goodness! Why are we sitting here and no coffee? Yulia, Glafira, coffee!"

Alyosha made haste to thank her, and said that he had only just had coffee.

"Where?"

"At Agrafena Alexandrovna's."

"At . . . at that woman's? Ah, it's she has brought ruin on every one. I know nothing about it though. They say she has become a saint, though it's rather late in the day. She had better have done it before. What use is it now? Hush, hush, Alexey Fyodorovich, for I have so much to say to you that I am afraid I shall tell you nothing. This awful trial . . . I shall certainly go, I am making arrangements. I shall be carried there in my chair; besides I can sit up. I shall have people with me. And, you know, I am a witness. How shall I speak, how shall I speak? I don't know what I shall say. One has to take an oath, hasn't one?"

"Yes; but I don't think you will be able to go."

"I can sit up. Ah, you put me out! Ah! this trial, this savage act, and then they are all going to Siberia, others get married, and all this so quickly, so quickly, everything's changing, and at last — nothing. All grow old and have death to look forward to. Well, so be it! I am tired. This Katya, *cette charmante personne*, has blasted all my hopes. Now she is going to follow one of your brothers to Siberia, and your other brother is going to follow her, and will live in the nearest town, and they will all torment one another. It drives me out of my mind. Worst of all — the publicity. The story has been told a million times over in all the papers in Moscow and Petersburg. Ah! yes, would you believe it, they've written about me, too, that I was 'a dear friend' of your brother's ——, I can't repeat the horrid word. Just fancy, just fancy!"

"Impossible! Where did it appear? What did it say?"

"I'll show you directly. I got the paper and read it yesterday. Here, in the Petersburg paper *Rumour*. The paper began coming out this year. I am awfully fond of gossip, and I take it in, and now it pays me out — this is what gossip comes to! Here it is, here, this passage. Read it."

And she handed Alyosha a sheet of newspaper which had been under her pillow.

It was not exactly that she was upset, she seemed overwhelmed, and perhaps everything really was mixed up in a tangle in her head. The newspaper notice was very typical, and must have been an annoyance to her, but, fortunately perhaps, she was unable to keep her mind fixed on any one subject at that moment, and so might race off in a minute to something else and quite forget the newspaper.

Alyosha was well aware that the story of the terrible case had spread all over Russia. And, good heavens! what wild rumours about his brother, about the Karamazovs, and about himself he had read in the course of those two months, among other equally credible items. One paper had even stated that he had gone into a monastery and become a monk, in horror at his brother's crime. Another contradicted this, and stated that he and his elder, Father Zosima, had broken into the monastery chest and "made tracks from the monastery." The present paragraph in the paper *Rumour* was under the heading, "The Karamazov Case at Skotoprigonyevsk."* (That, alas! was the name of our little town. I had hitherto kept it concealed.) It was brief, and Madame Hohlakov was not directly mentioned in it. No names appeared, in fact. It was merely stated that the criminal, whose approaching trial was making such a sensation — retired army captain, a swagger, an idler, and a retrograde bully — was continually involved in amorous intrigues, and particularly popular with certain ladies "who were bored with solitude." One such lady, a bored widow, who tried to seem young though she had a grown-up daughter, was so fascinated by him that only two hours before the crime she had offered him three thousand roubles, on condition that he would elope with her to the gold-mines. But the criminal, counting on escaping punishment, had preferred to murder his father to get the three thousand, rather than go off to Siberia with the middle-aged charms of his bored lady. This playful notice wound up, of course, with an outburst of high-minded in-

* The name suggests a cattle-pen, or something of the sort. *Editor's note.*

dignation at the wickedness of parricide and of the lately abolished institution of serfdom. Having read it with curiosity, Alyosha folded up the paper and handed it back to Madame Hohlakov.

"Well, that must be me," she hurried on again. "Of course I am meant. Scarcely more than an hour before, I suggested gold-mines to him, and here they talk of 'middle-aged charms' as though that were my motive! He writes that out of spite! God Almighty forgive him for the middle-aged charms, as I forgive him! You know it's . . . Do you know who it is? It's your friend Rakitin."

"Perhaps," said Alyosha, "though I've heard nothing about it."

"It's he, it's he! No 'perhaps' about it. You know I turned him out of the house. . . . You know that whole story, don't you?"

"I know that you asked him not to visit you in future, but why it was I hadn't heard . . . from you, at least."

"Ah, then you've heard it from him! He abuses me, I suppose, abuses me dreadfully?"

"Yes, he does; but then he abuses every one. But why you've closed your doors to him I haven't heard from him either. I meet him very seldom now, indeed. We are not friends."

"Well, then, I'll tell you all about it. There's no help for it, I'll confess, for there is one point in which I was perhaps to blame. Only a little, little point, so little that perhaps it doesn't count. You see, my dear boy" — Madame Hohlakov suddenly looked arch and a charming, though enigmatic, smile played about her lips — "you see, I suspect . . . You must forgive me, Alyosha. I am like a mother to you. . . . No, no; quite the contrary. I speak to you now as though you were my father — mother's quite out of place. Well, it's as though I were confessing to Father Zosima, that's just it. I called you a monk just now. Well, that poor young man, your friend, Rakitin (Mercy on us! I can't be angry with him. I feel cross, but not very), in a word, that frivolous young man, would you believe it, seems to have taken it into his head to fall in love with me. I only noticed it later, later. At first — that is, a month ago — he began to come oftener to see me, almost every day; though, of course, we were acquainted before. I knew nothing about it . . . and suddenly it dawned upon me, and I began to notice things with surprise. You know, two months ago, that modest, charming, excellent young man, Pyotr Ilyich Perhotin, who's in the service here, began to be a regular visitor at the house. You've met him here ever so many times yourself. And he is a worthy, earnest young man, isn't he? He comes once every three days, not every day (though I should be glad to see him every day), and always so well dressed. Altogether, I love young people, Alyosha, talented, modest, like you, and he has almost the mind of a statesman, he talks so charmingly, and I shall certainly, certainly try and get promotion for him. He is a future diplomat. On that awful day he almost saved me from death by coming in the night. And your friend Rakitin comes in such boots, and always stretches them out on the carpet. . . . In a word, he began hinting at his feelings, in fact, and one day, as he was going, he squeezed my hand terribly hard. My foot began to swell directly after he pressed my hand like that. He had met Pyotr Ilyich here before, and, would you believe it, he is always gibing at him, growling at him, for some reason. I simply looked at the way they went on together and laughed inwardly. So I was sitting here alone

— no, I was laid up then. Well, I was lying here alone and suddenly Rakitin comes in, and only fancy! brought me some verses of his own composition — a short poem, on my bad foot: that is, he described my foot in a poem. Wait a minute — how did it go?

This little foot, for heaven's sake!
Has suddenly commenced to ache.

It began somehow like that. I can never remember poetry. I've got it here. I'll show it to you later. But it's a charming thing — charming; and, you know, it's not only about the foot, it had a good moral, too, a charming idea, only I've forgotten it; in fact, it was just the thing for an album. So, of course, I thanked him, and he was obviously flattered. I'd hardly had time to thank him when in comes Pyotr Ilyich, and Rakitin suddenly looked as black as night. I could see that Pyotr Ilyich was in the way, for Rakitin certainly wanted to say something after giving me the verses. I had a presentiment of it; but Pyotr Ilyich came in. I showed Pyotr Ilyich the verses and didn't say who was the author. But I am convinced that he guessed, though he won't own it to this day, and declares he had no idea. But he says that on purpose. Pyotr Ilyich began to laugh at once, and fell to criticising it. 'Wretched doggerel,' he said it was, 'some divinity student must have written it,' and with such vehemence, such vehemence! Then, instead of laughing, your friend flew into a rage. 'Good gracious!' I thought, 'they'll fly at each other.' 'It was I who wrote it,' said he. 'I wrote it as a joke,' he said, 'for I think it degrading to write verses. . . . But they are good poetry. They want to put a monument to your Pushkin for writing about women's feet, while I wrote with a moral purpose, and you,' said he, 'are an advocate of serfdom. You've no humane ideas,' said he. 'You have no modern, enlightened feelings, you are uninfluenced by progress, you are a mere official,' he said, 'and you take bribes.' Then I began screaming and imploring them. And, you know, Pyotr Ilyich is anything but a coward. He at once took up the most gentlemanly tone, looked at him sarcastically, listened, and apologised. 'I'd no idea,' said he. 'I shouldn't have said it, if I had known. I should have praised it. Poets are all so irritable,' he said. In short, he laughed at him under cover of the most gentlemanly tone. He explained to me afterwards that it was all sarcastic. I thought he was in earnest. Only as I lay there, just as before you now, I thought, would it, or would it not, be the proper thing for me to turn Rakitin out for shouting so rudely at a visitor in my house? And, would you believe it, I lay here, shut my eyes, and wondered, would it be the proper thing or not, and I couldn't decide, and I kept worrying and worrying, and my heart began to beat, and I couldn't make up my mind whether to make an outcry or not. One voice seemed to be telling me, 'Cry out,' and the other, 'No, don't cry out.' And no sooner had the second voice said that than I cried out, and fainted. Of course, there was a fuss. I got up suddenly and said to Rakitin, 'It's painful for me to say it, but I don't wish to see you in my house again.' So I turned him out. Ah! Alexey Fyodorovich, I know myself I did wrong. I was putting it on. I wasn't angry with him at all really; but I suddenly fancied — that was what did it — that it would be such a fine scene. . . . And yet, believe me, it was quite natural, for I really shed tears and cried for several days afterwards, and then suddenly, one afternoon,

I forgot all about it. So it's a fortnight since he's stopped coming, and I kept wondering whether he would come again. I wondered even yesterday, then suddenly last night came this issue of *Rumour*. I read it and gasped. Who could have written it? He must have written it. He went home, sat down, wrote it on the spot, sent it, and they printed it. It was a fortnight ago, you see. But, Alyosha, it's awful how I keep talking and don't say what I want to say. Ah! the words come of themselves!"

"It's very important for me to be in time to see my brother to-day," Alyosha faltered.

"To be sure, to be sure! You bring it all back to me. Listen, what is an aberration?"

"What aberration?" asked Alyosha, wondering.

"In the legal sense. An aberration in which everything is pardonable. Whatever you do, you will be acquitted at once."

"What do you mean?"

"I'll tell you. This Katya . . . Ah! she is a charming, charming creature, only I never can make out who it is she is in love with. She was with me some time ago and I couldn't get anything out of her. Especially as she won't talk to me except superficially now. She is always talking about my health and nothing else, and she takes such a tone with me, too. I simply said to myself, 'Well, so be it. I don't care.' . . . Oh, yes. I was talking of aberration. This doctor has come. You know a doctor has come? Of course you know it — the one who discovers madmen. You sent for him. No, it wasn't you, but Katya. It's all Katya's doing. Well, you see, a man may be sitting there perfectly sane and suddenly have an aberration. He may be conscious and know what he is doing and yet be in a state of aberration. And there's no doubt that Dmitri Fyodorovich had an aberration. They found out about aberration as soon as the law courts were reformed. It's all the good effect of the reformed law courts. The doctor has been here and questioned me about that evening, about the gold-mines. 'How did he seem then?' he asked me. He must have been in a state of aberration. He came in shouting, 'Money, money, three thousand! Give me three thousand!' and then went away and immediately committed the murder. 'I don't want to kill,' he said, 'I don't want to,' and he suddenly went and killed. That's why they'll acquit him, because he resisted the impulse and yet killed."

"But he didn't kill," Alyosha interrupted rather sharply. He was increasingly overcome by anxiety and impatience.

"I know, it was that old man Grigory committed the murder."

"Grigory?" cried Alyosha.

"Yes, yes; it was Grigory. He lay where Dmitri Fyodorovich struck him down, and then got up, saw the door open, went in and killed Fyodor Pavlovich."

"But why, why?"

"Got an aberration. When he recovered from the blow Dmitri Fyodorovich gave him on the head, he got an aberration: then he went and killed. As for his saying he didn't, he very likely doesn't remember. Only, you know, it'll be better, ever so much better, if Dmitri Fyodorovich committed the murder. And that's how it must have been, though I say it was Grigory. It certainly was Dmitri Fyodorovich, and that's better, ever so much better! Oh! not better that a son should have killed his father, I don't admire that. On the contrary, children ought to honour their parents, and yet it would be better if it were he, as you'd have nothing to cry over then, for he did it when he was unconscious or rather when he was conscious, but did not know what he was doing. Let them acquit him — that's so humane, and would show what a blessing reformed law courts are. I knew nothing about it, but they say they have been so a long time. And when I heard it yesterday, I was so struck by it that I wanted to send for you at once. And if he is acquitted, make him come straight from the law courts to dinner with me, and I'll have a party of friends, and we'll drink to the reformed law courts. I don't believe he'd be dangerous; besides, I'll invite a great many friends, so that he could always be led out if he did anything. And then he might be made a justice of the peace or something in another town, for those who have been in trouble themselves make the best judges. And, besides, who isn't suffering from aberration nowadays? — you, I, all of us are in a state of aberration, and there are ever so many examples of it: a man sits singing a song, suddenly something annoys him, he takes a pistol and shoots the first person he comes across, and no one blames him for it. I read that lately, and all the doctors confirm it. Nowadays doctors are always confirming; they confirm anything. Why, my Lise is in a state of aberration. She made me cry again yesterday, and the day before, too, and to-day I suddenly realised that it's all due to aberration. Oh, Lise grieves me so! I believe she's quite mad. Why did she send for you? Did she send for you or did you come of yourself?"

"Yes, she sent for me, and I am going to her directly." Alyosha got up resolutely.

"Oh, my dear, dear Alexey Fyodorovich, perhaps that's what's most important," Madame Hohlakov cried, suddenly bursting into tears. "God knows I trust Lise to you with all my heart, and it's no matter her sending for you on the sly, without telling her mother. But forgive me, I can't trust my daughter so easily to your brother Ivan Fyodorovich, though I still consider him the most chivalrous young man. But only fancy, he's been to see Lise and I knew nothing about it!"

"How? What? When?" Alyosha was terribly surprised. He had not sat down again and listened standing.

"I will tell you, that's perhaps why I asked you to come, for I don't know now why I did ask you to come. Well, Ivan Fyodorovich has been to see me twice, since he came back from Moscow. First time he came as a friend to call on me, and the second time Katya was here and he came because he heard she was here. I didn't, of course, expect him to come often, knowing what a lot he has to do as it is, *vous comprenez, cette affaire et la mort terrible de votre papa*. But I suddenly heard he'd been here again, not to see me but to see Lise. That's six days ago now. He came, stayed five minutes, and went away. And I didn't hear of it till three days afterwards, from Glafira, so it was a great shock to me. I sent for Lise directly. She laughed. 'He thought you were asleep,' she said, 'and came in to me to ask after your health.' Of course, that's how it happened. But Lise, Lise, mercy on us, how she distresses me! Would you believe it, one night, four days ago, just after you saw her last, and had gone away, she suddenly had a fit, screaming, shrieking hysterics! Why is it I never have hysterics? Then next day another fit and the same thing on the third, and yesterday, too, and then yesterday that aberration. She suddenly screamed out, 'I hate Ivan Fyodorovich. I demand that you do not receive him, that you refuse him the house.' I was struck dumb at these amazing words, and answered, 'On what grounds could I refuse to see such an excellent young man, a young man of such learning, too, and so unfortunate,' for all this business is a misfortune, isn't it? She suddenly burst out laughing at my words, and so rudely, you know. Well, I was pleased, I thought I had amused her and the fits would pass off, especially as I wanted to refuse to see Ivan Fyodorovich anyway on account of his strange visits without my consent, and meant to ask him for an explanation. But early this morning Lise waked up and flew into a passion with Yulia and, would you believe it, slapped her in the face. That's monstrous, I am always polite to my servants. And an hour later she was hugging and kissing Yulia's feet. She sent a message to me, that she wasn't coming to me at all, and would never come and see me again, and when I dragged myself down to her, she rushed to kiss me, crying, and, as she kissed me, she pushed me out of the room without saying a word, so I couldn't find out what was the matter. Now, dear Alexey Fyodorovich, I rest all my hopes on you, and, of course, my whole life is in your hands. I simply beg you to go to Lise and find out everything from her, as you alone can, and come back and tell me — me, her mother, for you understand it will be the death of me, simply the death of me, if this goes on, or else I shall run away from the house. I can stand no more. I have patience; but I may lose it, and then . . . then something awful will happen. Ah, dear me! At last, Pyotr Ilyich!" cried Madame Hohlakov, beaming all over as she saw Perhotin enter the room. "You are late, you are late! Well, sit down, speak, put us out of suspense. What does the counsel say? Where are you off to, Alexey Fyodorovich?"

"To Lise."

"Oh, yes. You won't forget, you won't forget what I asked you? It's a question of life and death!"

"Of course, I won't forget, if I can . . . but I am so late," muttered Alyosha, beating a hasty retreat.

"No, be sure, be sure to come in; don't say 'if you can.' I shall die if you don't," Madame Hohlakov called after him, but Alyosha had already left the room.

CHAPTER III

THE IMP

Going in to Lise, he found her half reclining in the invalid chair, in which she had been wheeled when she was unable to walk. She did not move to meet him, but her sharp keen eyes simply bored into his face. There was a feverish look in her eyes, her face was pale and yellow. Alyosha was amazed at the change that had taken place in her in three days. She was positively thinner. She did not hold out her hand to him. He touched the thin, long fingers which lay motionless on her dress, then he sat down facing her, without a word.

"I know you are in a hurry to get to the prison," Lise said curtly, "and mamma's kept you there for hours, she's just been telling you about me and Yulia."

"How do you know?" asked Alyosha.

"I've been eavesdropping. Why do you stare at me? I want to eavesdrop and I do eavesdrop, there's nothing bad about that. I don't apologise."

"You are upset about something?"

"On the contrary, I am very happy. I've only just been reflecting for the thirtieth time what a good thing it is I refused you and shall not be your wife. You are not fit to be a husband. If I were to marry you and give you a note to take to the man I loved after you, you'd take it and be sure to give it to him and bring an answer back, too. If you were forty, you would still go on carrying my love-letters for me."

She suddenly laughed.

"There is something spiteful and yet open-hearted about you." Alyosha smiled at her.

"The open-heartedness consists in my not being ashamed before you. What's more, I don't want to feel ashamed before you, just before you. Alyosha, why is it I don't respect you? I am very fond of you, but I don't respect you. If I respected you, I shouldn't talk to you without shame, should I?"

"No."

"But do you believe that I am not ashamed before you?"

"No, I don't believe it."

Lise laughed nervously again; she spoke rapidly.

"I sent some sweets to your brother, Dmitri Fyodorovich, in prison. Alyosha, you know, you are very handsome! I shall love you awfully for having so quickly allowed me not to love you."

"Why did you send for me to-day, Lise?"

"I wanted to tell you of a desire I have. I should like some one to torture me, marry me and then torture me, deceive me and go away. I don't want to be happy."

"You are in love with disorder?"

"Yes, I want disorder. I keep wanting to set fire to the house. I keep imagining how I'll creep up and set fire to the house on the sly, it must be on the sly. They'll try to put it out, but it'll go on burning. And I shall know and say nothing. Ah, what silliness! And how bored I am!"

She waved her hand with a look of repulsion.

"It's your luxurious life," said Alyosha softly.

"Is it better then to be poor?"

"Yes, it is better."

"That's what your deceased monk taught you. That's not true. Let me be rich and all the rest poor. I'll eat sweets and drink cream and not give any to any one else. Ah, don't speak, don't say anything," she shook her hand at him, though Alyosha had not opened his mouth. "You've told me all that before, I know it all by heart. It bores me. If I am ever poor, I shall murder somebody, and even if I am rich, I may murder some one, perhaps—why do nothing? But do you know, I should like to reap, reap rye? I'll marry you, and you shall become a peasant, a real peasant; we'll keep a colt, shall we? Do you know Kalganov?"

"Yes."

"He is always wandering about, dreaming. He says, why endure real life, it's better to dream. One can dream the jolliest things, but real life is a bore. But he'll be married soon for all that, he's been making love to me already. Can you spin tops?"

"Yes."

"Well, he's just like a top: he wants to be wound up and set spinning and then to be lashed, lashed, lashed with a whip. If I marry him, I'll keep him spinning all his life. You are not ashamed to be with me?"

"No."

"You are awfully cross, because I don't talk about holy things. I don't want to be holy. What will they do to one in the next world for the greatest sin? You must know all about that."

"God will condemn you." Alyosha was watching her steadily.

"That's just what I should like. I would go up and they would condemn me and I would burst out laughing in their faces. I should dreadfully like to set fire to the house, Alyosha, to our house, you still don't believe me?"

"Why not? There are children twelve years old who have a longing to set fire to something and they do set things on fire, too. It's a sort of disease."

"That's not true, that's not true, there may be children like that, but that's not what I mean."

"You mistake evil for good; it's a passing crisis, it's the result of your illness, perhaps."

"You do despise me though! It's simply that I don't want to do good, I want to do evil, and it has nothing to do with illness."

"Why do evil?"

"So that nothing may be left anywhere. Ah, how nice it would be if nothing were left anywhere! You know, Alyosha, I sometimes think of doing a fearful lot of harm and everything bad, and I should do it for a long while on the sly and suddenly every one would find it out. All would stand round and point their fingers at me and I would look at them all. That would be very pleasant. Why would it be so pleasant, Alyosha?"

"Just so. It's a craving to destroy something good or, as you say, to set fire to something. It happens sometimes."

"I not only say it, I shall do it."

"I believe you."

"Ah, how I love you for saying you believe me. And you are not lying one little bit. But perhaps you think that I am saying all this on purpose to tease you?"

"No, I don't think that . . . though perhaps there is a little desire to do that in it, too."

"There is a little. I never can tell lies to you," she declared, with a strange fire in her eyes.

What struck Alyosha above everything was her earnestness. There was not a trace of humour or jesting in her face now, though, formerly, fun and gaiety had never deserted her even at her most "earnest" moments.

"There are moments when people love crime," said Alyosha thoughtfully.

"Yes, yes! You have uttered my thought, they love crime, every one loves crime, they love it always, not at some 'moments.' You know, it's as though people long ago made an agreement to lie about it and have lied about it ever since. They all say that they hate evil, but secretly they all love it."

"And are you still reading nasty books?"

"Yes, I am. Mamma reads them and hides them under her pillow and I steal them."

"Aren't you ashamed to destroy yourself?"

"I want to destroy myself. There's a boy here who lay down between the rails when the train was passing. Lucky fellow! Listen, your brother is being tried now for murdering his father and every one loves his having killed his father."

"Loves his having killed his father?"

"Yes, loves it, every one loves it! Everybody says it's awful, but secretly they simply love it. I for one love it."

"There is some truth in what you say about every one," said Alyosha softly.

"Oh, what ideas you have!" Lise shrieked with delight. "And you a monk, too! You wouldn't believe how I respect you, Alyosha, for never telling lies. Oh, I must tell you a funny dream of mine. I sometimes dream of devils. It's night, I am in my room with a candle and suddenly there are devils all over the place, in all the corners, under the table, and they open the doors, there's a crowd of them behind the doors and they want to come and seize me. And they are just coming, just seizing me. But I suddenly cross myself and they all draw back, afraid, though they don't go away altogether, they stand at the doors and in the corners, waiting. And suddenly I have a frightful longing to revile God aloud, and so I begin, and then they come crowding back to me, delighted, and seize me again and I cross myself again and they all draw back. It's awful fun, it takes one's breath away."

"I've had the same dream, too," said Alyosha suddenly.

"Really?" cried Lise, surprised. "I say, Alyosha, don't laugh, that's awfully important. Could two different people have the same dream?"

"It seems they can."

"Alyosha, I tell you, it's awfully important," Lise went on, with really excessive amazement. "It's not the dream that's important, but your having the same dream as I. You never lie to me, don't lie now: is it true? You are not laughing?"

"It's true."

Lise seemed extraordinarily impressed and for half a minute she was silent.

"Alyosha, come and see me, come and see me more often," she said suddenly, in a supplicating voice.

"I'll always come to see you, all my life," answered Alyosha firmly.

"You are the only person I can talk to, you know," Lise began again. "I talk to no one but myself and you. Only you in the whole world. And to you more readily than to myself. And I am not a bit ashamed before you, not a bit. Alyosha, why am I not ashamed before you, not a bit? Alyosha, is it true that at Easter the Jews steal children and slaughter them?"

"I don't know."

"There's a book here in which I read about the trial of a Jew, who took a four-year-old boy and cut off the fingers from both hands, and then crucified him on the wall, hammered nails into him and crucified him, and afterwards, when he was tried, he said that the child died soon, within four hours. That was 'soon'! He said the child moaned, kept on moaning, and he stood gloating over it. That's good!"

"Good?"

"Good. I sometimes imagine that it was I who did the crucifying. He would hang there moaning and I would sit opposite him eating pineapple compote. I am awfully fond of pineapple compote. Do you like it?"

Alyosha looked at her in silence. Her pale, sallow face was suddenly contorted, her eyes burned.

"You know, after I read about that Jew I shook with sobs all night. I kept fancying how the little thing cried and moaned (a child four years old understands, you know) and all the while the thought of pineapple compote haunted me. In the morning I wrote a letter to a certain person, begging him to come and see me *without fail*. He came and I suddenly told him all about the boy and the pineapple compote. *All* about it, *all*, and said that it was good. He laughed and said it really was good. Then he got up and went away. He was here only five minutes. Did he despise me? Did he? Tell me, tell me, Alyosha, did he despise me or not?" She sat up on the couch, with flashing eyes.

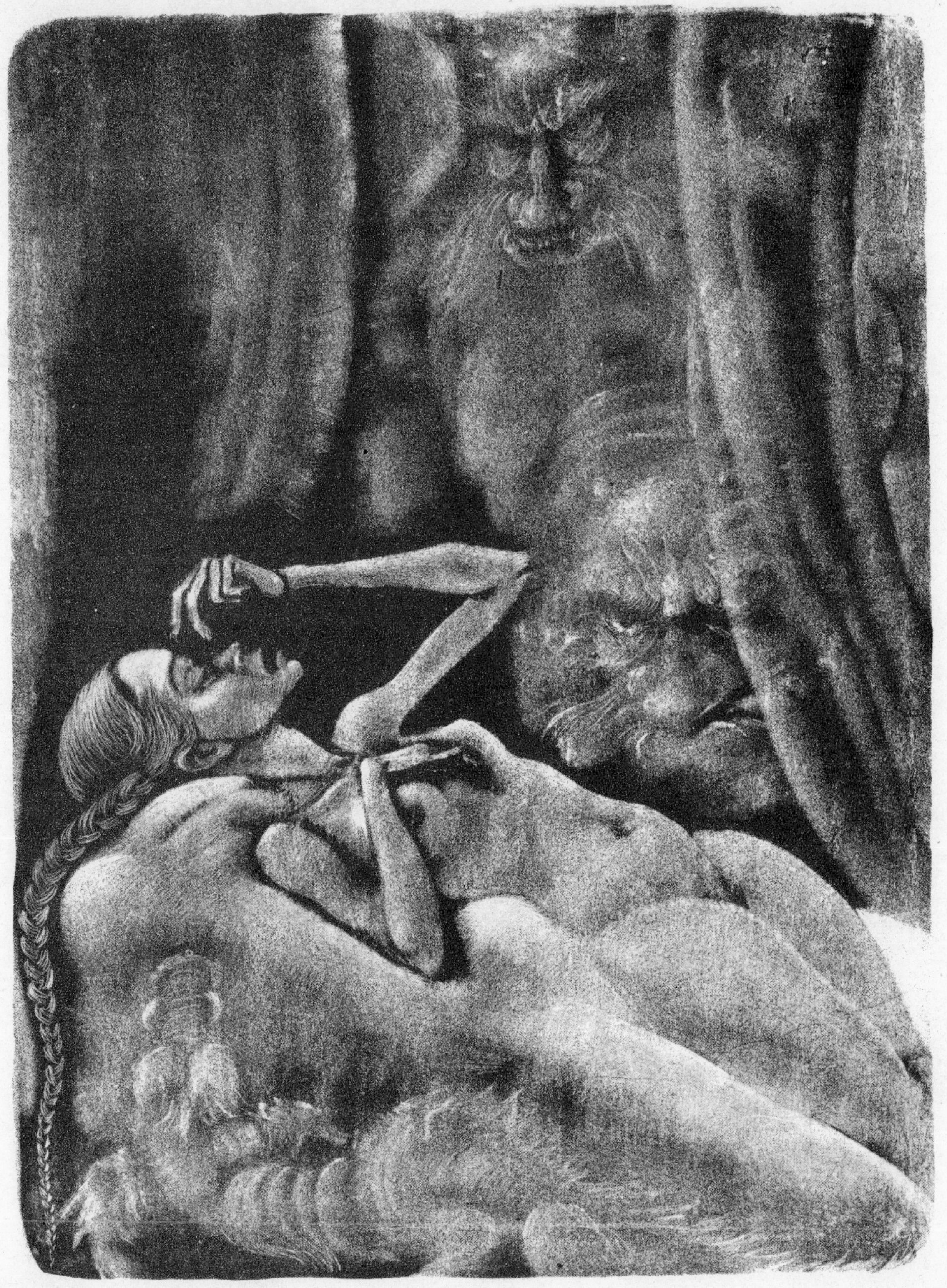

THE IMP

"Tell me," Alyosha asked anxiously, "did you send for that person yourself?"

"Myself."

"Did you send him a letter?"

"Yes."

"Simply to ask about that, about that child?"

"No, not about that at all. But when he came, I asked him about that at once. He answered, laughed, got up and went away."

"That person behaved honourably," Alyosha murmured.

"And did he despise me? Did he laugh at me?"

"No, for perhaps he believes in the pineapple compote himself. He is very ill now, too, Lise."

"Yes, he does believe in it," said Lise, with flashing eyes.

"He doesn't despise any one," Alyosha went on. "Only he does not believe any one. If he doesn't believe in people, of course, he does despise them."

"Then he despises me, me?"

"You, too."

"That's good." Lise seemed to grind her teeth. "When he went out laughing, I felt that it was good to be despised. The boy with his fingers cut off is good and to be despised is good. . . ."

And she laughed in Alyosha's face, a feverish, malicious laugh.

"Do you know, Alyosha, do you know, I should like . . . Alyosha save me!" She suddenly jumped from the couch, rushed to him and seized him with both hands. "Save me!" she almost groaned. "Is there any one in the world I could tell what I've told you? I've told you the truth, the truth. I shall kill myself, because I loathe everything! I don't want to live, because I loathe everything! I loathe everything, everything. Alyosha, why don't you love me in the least?" she finished in a frenzy.

"But I do love you!" answered Alyosha hotly.

"And will you weep over me, will you?"

"Yes."

"Not because I won't be your wife, but simply weep for me?"

"Yes."

"Thank you! It's only your tears I want. Every one else may punish me and trample me under foot, every one, every one, not excepting *any one*. For I don't love any one. Do you hear, not any one! On the contrary, I hate them! Go, Alyosha, it's time you went to your brother." She tore herself away from him suddenly.

"How can I leave you like this?" said Alyosha, almost in alarm.

"Go to your brother, the prison will be shut, go, here's your hat. Kiss Mitya, go, go!"

And she almost forcibly pushed Alyosha out the door. He looked at her with pained surprise, when he was suddenly aware of a letter in his right hand, a tiny letter folded up tight and sealed. He glanced at it and instantly read the address "To Ivan Fyodorovich Karamazov." He looked quickly at Lise. Her face had become almost menacing.

"Give it to him, give it to him without fail!" she ordered him, trembling and beside herself. "To-day, at once, or I'll poison myself! That's why I sent for you."

And she slammed the door quickly. The bolt clicked. Alyosha put the note in his pocket and went straight downstairs, without going back to Madame Hohlakov, forgetting her, in fact. As soon as Alyosha had gone, Lise unbolted the door, opened it a little, put her finger in the crack and slammed the door with all her might, pinching her finger. Ten seconds after, releasing her hand, she walked softly, slowly to her chair, sat up straight in it and looked intently at her blackened finger and at the blood that oozed from under the nail. Her lips were quivering and she kept whispering rapidly to herself:

"I am vile, vile, vile, vile!"

CHAPTER IV
A HYMN AND A SECRET

It was quite late (days are short in November) when Alyosha rang at the prison gate. Already dusk was falling. But Alyosha knew that he would be admitted without difficulty. Things were managed in our little town, as everywhere else. At first, of course, on the conclusion of the preliminary inquiry, relatives and a few other persons could obtain interviews with Mitya only by going through certain inevitable formalities. But later, though the formalities were not relaxed, exceptions were made for some, at least, of Mitya's visitors. So much so, that sometimes the interviews with the prisoner in the room set aside for the purpose were practically *tête-à-tête*.

Exceptions, however, were made for only a few, namely, Grushenka, Alyosha, and Rakitin. But the captain of the police, Mihail Mihailovich, was very favourably disposed towards Grushenka. His abuse of her at Mokroye weighed on the old man's conscience, and when he learned the whole story, he completely changed his view of her. And, strange to say, though he was firmly persuaded of Mitya's guilt, yet, after the latter was once in prison, the old man came to take a more and more lenient view of him. "He was a man of good heart, perhaps," he thought, "who had come to grief through drinking and dissipation." His first horror had been succeeded by pity. As for Alyosha, the police captain was very fond of him and had known him for a long time. Rakitin, who had of late taken to coming very often to see the prisoner, was one of the most intimate acquaintances of the "police captain's young ladies," as he called them, and was always hanging about their house. Also, he gave lessons in the house of the prison superintendent, who, though scrupulous in the performance of his duties, was a kind-hearted old man. Again, Alyosha had an intimate acquaintance of long standing with the superintendent, who was fond of talking to him, generally on edifying subjects. He respected Ivan Fyodorovich, and, indeed, stood in awe of his opinions, though he was a great philosopher himself; a "homespun" one, of course. But Alyosha had an irresistible attraction for him. During the last year the old man had taken to studying the Apocryphal Gospels, and constantly talked over his impressions with his young friend. He used to come to see him in the monastery and argued for hours together with him and with the monks. So even if Alyosha was late at the prison, he had only to go to the superintendent and everything was made easy. Besides, every one in the prison, down to the humblest watchman, had grown used to Alyosha. The sentry, of course, did not trouble him so long as the authorities were satisfied.

When Mitya was summoned from his cell, he always went downstairs, to the place set aside for interviews. As Alyosha entered the room he came upon Rakitin, who was just taking leave of Mitya. They were both talking loudly. Mitya was laughing heartily as he saw him out, while Rakitin seemed grumbling. Rakitin did not like meeting Alyosha, especially of late. He scarcely spoke to him, and bowed to him stiffly. Seeing Alyosha enter now, he frowned more than usual and looked away, as though he were entirely absorbed in buttoning his big, warm, fur-trimmed overcoat. Then he began looking at once for his umbrella.

"I must mind not to forget my belongings," he muttered, simply to say something.

"Mind you don't forget other people's belongings," said Mitya, as a joke, and laughed at once at his own wit. Rakitin fired up instantly.

"You'd better give that advice to your own family, who've always been a serf-owning lot, and not to Rakitin," he cried, suddenly trembling with anger.

"What's the matter? I was joking," cried Mitya. "Damn it all! They are all like that," he turned to Alyosha, nodding towards Rakitin's hurriedly retreating figure. "He was sitting here, laughing and cheerful, and all at once he boils up like that. He didn't even nod to you. Have you broken with him completely? Why are you so late? I've not been simply waiting, but thirsting for you the whole morning. But never mind. We'll make up for it now."

"Why does he come here so often? Surely you are not such great friends?" asked Alyosha. He, too, nodded at the door through which Rakitin had disappeared.

"Great friends with Rakitin? No, not as much as that. Is it likely — a pig like that? He considers I am . . . a blackguard. They can't understand a joke either, that's the worst of such people. They never understand a joke, and their souls are dry, dry and flat; they remind me of prison walls when I was first brought here. But he is a clever fellow, very clever. Well, Alexey, it's all over with me now."

He sat down on the bench and made Alyosha sit down beside him.

"Yes, the trial's to-morrow. Are you so hopeless, brother?" Alyosha said, with an apprehensive feeling.

"What are you talking about?" said Mitya, looking at him rather uncertainly. "Oh, you mean the trial! Damn it all! Till now we've been talking of things that don't matter, about this trial, but I haven't said a word to you about the chief thing. Yes, the trial is to-morrow; but it wasn't the trial I meant, when I said it was all over with me. Why do you look at me so critically?"

"What do you mean, Mitya?"

"Ideas, ideas, that's all! Ethics! What is ethics?"

"Ethics?" asked Alyosha, wondering.

"Yes; is it a science?"

"Yes, there is such a science . . . but . . . I confess I can't explain to you what sort of science it is."

"Rakitin knows. Rakitin knows a lot, damn him! He's not going to be a monk. He means to go to Petersburg. There he'll go in for criticism of an elevating tendency. Who knows, he may be of use and make his own career, too. Ugh! they are first-rate, these people, at making a career! Damn ethics. I am done for, Alexey, I am, you man of God! I love you more than any one. It makes my heart quake to look at you. Who was Karl Bernard?"

"Karl Bernard?" Alyosha was surprised again.

"No, not Karl. Wait, I made a mistake.

Claude Bernard. What was he? Chemist or what?"

"He must be a savant," answered Alyosha; "but I confess I can't tell you much about him, either. I've heard of him as a savant, but what sort I don't know."

"Well, damn him, then! I don't know either," Mitya cursed. "A scoundrel of some sort, most likely. They are all scoundrels. And Rakitin will make his way. Rakitin will get on anywhere; he is another Bernard. Ugh, these Bernards! They are all over the place."

"But what is the matter?" Alyosha asked insistently.

"He wants to write an article about me, about my case, and so begin his literary career. That's what he comes for; he said so himself. He wants to prove some theory. He wants to say 'he couldn't help murdering his father, he was corrupted by his environment,' and so on. He explained it all to me. He is going to put in a tinge of socialism, he says. But there, damn the fellow, he can put in a tinge, if he likes, I don't care. He can't bear Ivan, he hates him. He's not fond of you, either. But I don't turn him out, for he is a clever fellow. Awfully conceited though. I said to him just now, 'The Karamazovs are not blackguards, but philosophers; for all true Russians are philosophers, and though you've studied, you are not a philosopher — you are a churl.' He laughed, so maliciously. And I said to him, *de thoughtibus non est disputandum*.' Isn't that rather good? I, too, can set up for being a classical scholar, you see!" Mitya laughed suddenly.

"Why is it all over with you? You said so just now," Alyosha interposed.

"Why is it all over with me? H'm! . . . The fact of it is . . . if you take it as a whole, I am sorry to lose God — that's what it is."

"What do you mean by 'sorry to lose God'?"

"Imagine: inside, in the nerves, in the head — that is, these nerves are there in the brain . . . (damn them!) — there are sort of little tails, the little tails of those nerves, and as soon as they begin quivering . . . that is, you see, I look at something with my eyes and then they begin quivering, those little tails . . . and when they quiver, then an image appears . . . it doesn't appear at once, but an instant, a second, passes . . . and then something like a moment appears; that is, not a moment — devil take the moment! — but an image; that is, an object, or a happening, damn it! That's why I see and then think, because of those tails, not at all because I've got a soul, and that I am some sort of image and likeness. All that is nonsense! Rakitin explained it all to me yesterday, brother, and it simply bowled me over. It's magnificent, Alyosha, this science! A new man's arising — that I understand. . . . And yet I am sorry to lose God!"

"Well, that's a good thing, anyway," said Alyosha.

"That I am sorry to lose God? It's chemistry, brother, chemistry! There's no help for it, your reverence, you must make way for chemistry. And Rakitin does dislike God. Ugh! doesn't he dislike Him! That's the sore point with all of them. But they conceal it. They tell lies. They pretend. 'Will you preach this in your reviews?' I asked him. 'Oh, well, if I did it openly, they wouldn't let it through,' he said. He laughed. 'But what will become of men then?' I asked him, 'without God and the hereafter? In that case everything is lawful now, one can do everything?' 'Didn't you know it?' he said, laughing, 'a clever man can do what he likes,' he said. 'A clever man knows his way about, but you committed a murder and got in bad, and now you are rotting in prison.' He says that to my face! A regular swine! I used to kick such people out, but now I listen to them. He talks a lot of sense, too. And he writes cleverly. He began reading me an article last week. I copied out three lines of it. Wait a minute. Here it is."

Mitya hurriedly pulled out a piece of paper from his vest-pocket and read:

" 'In order to settle this question, it is above all essential to place one's personality counter to one's reality.' Do you understand that?"

"No, I don't," said Alyosha. He looked at Mitya and listened to him with curiosity.

"I don't understand either. It's dark and obscure, but intellectual. 'Every one writes like that now,' he says, 'it's the effect of their environment.' They are afraid of the environment. He writes poetry, too, the rascal. He's celebrated Madame Hohlakov's foot. Ha, ha, ha!"

"I've heard about it," said Alyosha.

"And have you heard the poem?"

"No."

"I've got it. Here it is. I'll read it to you. You don't know — I haven't told you — there's quite a story about it. The rogue! Three weeks ago he began to tease me. 'You've got yourself into a mess, like a fool, for the sake of three thousand, but I'm going to collar a hundred and fifty thousand. I am going to marry a widow and buy a stone house in Petersburg.' And he told me he was courting Madame Hohlakov. She hadn't much brains in her youth, and now at forty she had lost what she had. 'But she's awfully sentimental,' he says; 'that's how I shall get hold of her. When I marry her, I shall take her to Petersburg and there I shall start a newspaper.' And his mouth was simply watering, the beast, not for the widow, but for the hundred and fifty thousand. And he made me believe it. He came to see me every day. 'She is coming round,' he declared. He was beaming with delight. And then, all of a sudden, he was turned out of the house. Perhotin's carrying everything before him, bravo! I could kiss the silly old noodle for turning him out of the house. And he had written this doggerel. 'It's the first time I've soiled my hands with writing poetry,' he said. 'It's for the sake of seduction, so it's in a useful cause. When I get hold of the silly woman's fortune, I can be a great civic utility.' They have this civic justification for every nasty thing they do! 'Anyway it's better than your Pushkin's poetry,' he said, 'for I've managed to inject civic feeling even in that.' I understand what he means about Pushkin, I quite see that, if he really was a man of talent and yet wrote only about women's feet. But wasn't Rakitin stuck up about his doggerel! The vanity of these fellows! 'Lines on the recovery of the swollen foot of the object of my affections' — he thought of that for a title. The wag!

A captivating little foot,
Though swollen, red and tender!
The doctors come and plasters put,
But still they cannot mend her.

Yet 'tis not for her feet I pine —
A theme for Pushkin, not for me —
I fear to note the sad decline
Of intellectuality!

For as her foot swells, strange to say,
Her intellect is on the wane —
Oh, for some remedy I pray
That may restore both foot and brain!

He is a swine, a regular swine, but he's very arch, the rascal! And he really has put in a civic idea. And wasn't he angry when she kicked him out! He was gnashing his teeth!"

"He's taken his revenge already," said Alyosha. "He's gotten a notice published about Madame Hohlakov."

And Alyosha told him briefly about the notice in *Rumour*.

"That's his doing, that's his doing!" Mitya assented, frowning. "That's him! These notices . . . I know . . . the nasty things that have been written about Grushenka, for instance. . . . And about the other one, about Katya, too. . . . H'm!"

He walked across the room with a harassed air.

"Brother, I cannot stay long," Alyosha said, after a pause. "To-morrow will be a great and awful day for you, the judgment of God will be accomplished . . . I am amazed at you, you walk about here, talking of I don't know what . . ."

"No, don't be amazed at me," Mitya broke in hotly. "Am I to talk of that stinking dog? Of the murderer? We've talked enough of him. I don't want to say more of the stinking son of Stinking Lizaveta! God will kill him, you will see. Hush!"

He went up to Alyosha excitedly and kissed him. His eyes glowed.

"Rakitin wouldn't understand it," he began in a sort of exaltation; "but you, you'll understand it all. That's why I was thirsting for you. You see, there's so much I've been wanting to tell you for ever so long, here, within these peeling walls, but I haven't said a word about what matters most; it was as though the time hadn't come. Now I need wait no longer. I must pour out my heart to you. Brother, these last two months I've felt a new man within me. A new man has risen up in me. He was hidden in me, but would never have come to the surface, if it hadn't been for this blow from heaven. It's fearful! And what do I care if I spend twenty years in the mines, hammering out the ore? I am not a bit afraid of that — it's something else I am afraid of now: that that new man may leave me. Even there, in the mines, underground, I may find a human heart in another convict and murderer by my side, and I may make friends with him, for even there one may live and love and suffer. One may arouse and revive in that convict a lifeless heart, one may wait upon him for years, and at last bring up from the dark depths a lofty soul, a feeling, suffering creature; one may revive an angel, raise up a hero! There are so many of them, hundreds of them, and we are all to blame for them. Why was it I dreamed that 'babe' at such a moment? 'Why is the babe so poor?' That was a prophecy to me at that moment. It's for the babe I will go. Because we are all responsible for all. For all the 'babes,' for there are big children as well as little children. All are 'babes.' I go for all, because some one must go for all. I didn't kill father, but I've got to go. I accept it. It's all come to me here, here, within these peeling walls. There are numbers of them there, hundreds of them underground, with hammers in their hands. Oh, yes, we shall be in chains and there will be no freedom, but then, in our great sorrow, we shall rise again to joy, without which man cannot live nor God exist, for God gives joy: it's His privilege — a great one. Lord, let man be dissolved in prayer! How shall I exist there underground without God? Rakitin's lying! If they drive God from the earth, we shall shelter

Him underground. A convict cannot exist without God; it's even more impossible for him than for those who are not convicts. And then we men underground will raise from the bowels of the earth a tragic hymn to God, with Whom is joy. Hail to God and His joy! I love Him!"

Mitya was almost gasping for breath as he uttered his wild speech. He turned pale, his lips quivered, and tears rolled down his cheeks.

"No, life is full, there is life even underground," he began again. "You wouldn't believe, Alexey, how I want to live now, what a thirst for existence and consciousness has sprung up in me within these peeling walls. Rakitin doesn't understand that; all he cares about is building a house and letting flats. But I've been longing for you. And what is suffering? I am not afraid of it, even if it were beyond reckoning. I am not afraid of it now. I was afraid of it before. Do you know, perhaps I won't answer at the trial at all. . . . And I seem to have such strength in me now, that I think I could stand anything, any suffering, only to be able to say and to repeat to myself every moment, 'I am.' In thousands of agonies — I am. I'm tormented on the rack — but I am! Though I sit alone in a dungeon — I am! I see the sun, and if I don't see the sun, I know it's there. And to know that the sun is there, why, that's all of life. Alyosha, my angel, all these philosophies are the death of me. Damn them! Brother Ivan . . ."

"What of brother Ivan?" interrupted Alyosha, but Mitya did not hear.

"You see, I never had any of these doubts before, but it was all hidden away in me. It was perhaps just because unrealised ideas were raging up in me, that I used to drink and fight and carry on. It was to quench them in myself, to still them, to smother them. Ivan is not a Rakitin, there is an idea in him. Ivan is a sphinx and is silent; he is always silent. And as for me, God torments me. That's the only thing that's tormenting me. What if He doesn't exist? What if Rakitin's right — that it's an artificial idea produced by mankind? Then, if He doesn't exist, man is the ruler of the earth, of the universe. Magnificent! Only how is he going to be virtuous without God? That's the question. I always come back to that. For, whom is man going to love then? To whom will he be thankful? To whom will he sing the hymn? Rakitin laughs. Rakitin says that one can love humanity without God. Well, only a snivelling idiot can maintain that. I can't understand it. Life's easy for Rakitin. 'You'd better think about the extension of civic rights,' he says to me to-day, 'or even of keeping down the price of meat. You will show your love for humanity more simply and directly by that, than by philosophy.' I answered him, 'Well, but you, without a God, are more likely to raise the price of meat, if it suits you, and make a rouble on every copeck.' He lost his temper. But after all, what is virtue? Answer me that, Alexey. Virtue is one thing with me and another with a Chinaman, so it's a relative thing. Or isn't it? Is it not relative? A treacherous question! You won't laugh if I tell you it's kept me awake two nights. I only wonder now how people can live and think nothing about it. Vanity! Ivan has no God. He has an idea. It's beyond me. But he is silent. I believe he is a freemason. I asked him, but he is silent. I wanted to drink from his spring — he was silent. But once he did drop a word."

"What did he say?" Alyosha took it up quickly.

"I said to him, 'Then everything is lawful, if it is so?' He frowned. 'Fyodor Pavlovich, our papa,' he said, 'was a pig, but he reasoned correctly enough.' That was what he dropped. That was all he said. That was going one better than Rakitin."

"Yes," Alyosha assented bitterly. "When did he come to see you?"

"Of that later, now I must speak of something else. I have said nothing about Ivan to you before. I put it off to the last. When my business here is over and the verdict has been pronounced, then I'll tell you something. I'll tell you everything. We've something terrible on hand. . . . And you shall be my judge in this matter. But don't begin about that now; mum's the word. You talk of to-morrow, of the trial; but, would you believe it, I know nothing about it."

"Have you talked to the counsel?"

"What's the use of the counsel? I told him all about it. He's a soft, city-bred rogue — a Bernard! But he doesn't believe me — not a bit of it. Only imagine, he believes that I killed. I see it. 'In that case,' I asked him, 'why have you come to defend me?' Hang them all! They've got a doctor down, too, want to prove I'm mad. I won't have that! Katerina Ivanovna wants to do her 'duty' to the end, whatever the strain!" Mitya smiled bitterly. "The cat! Hard-hearted creature! She knows that I said of her at Mokroye that she was a woman of 'great wrath.' They repeated it to her. Yes, the facts against me have grown numerous as the sands of the sea. Grigory sticks to his point. Grigory's honest, but a fool. Many people are honest because they are fools: that's Rakitin's idea. Grigory's my enemy. And there are some people whom it's better to have as foes than as friends. I mean Katerina Ivanovna. I am afraid, oh, I am afraid she will tell how she bowed to the ground after that four thousand five hundred. She'll pay it back to the last farthing. I don't want her sacrifice; they'll put me to shame at the trial. I wonder how I can stand it. Go to her, Alyosha, ask her not to speak of that in court, can't you? But damn it all, it doesn't matter! I shall get through somehow. I don't pity her. It's her own doing. It serves her right. I shall have my own story to tell, Alexey." He smiled bitterly again. "Only . . . only Grusha, Grusha! Good Lord! Why should she have such suffering to bear?" he exclaimed suddenly, with tears. "Grusha's killing me; the thought of her's killing me, killing me. She was here just now . . ."

"She told me she was very much grieved by you to-day."

"I know. Confound my temper! It was jealousy. As she was leaving, I repented, I kissed her. I didn't ask her forgiveness."

"Why didn't you?" exclaimed Alyosha.

Suddenly Mitya laughed almost mirthfully.

"God preserve you, my dear boy, from ever asking forgiveness for a fault from a woman you love. From one you love especially, however greatly you may have been in fault. For a woman — devil only knows what a woman is! I know something about them, anyway. But try acknowledging you are in fault to a woman. Say, 'I am sorry, forgive me,' and a shower of reproaches will follow! Nothing will make her forgive you simply and directly, she'll humble you to the dust, bring forward things that have never happened, recall everything, forget nothing, add something of her own, and only then forgive you. And even the best, the best of them do it. She'll scrape up all the scrapings and load them on your head. They are ready to flay you alive, I tell you, every one of them, all these angels without whom we cannot live! I tell you plainly and openly, dear boy, every decent man ought to be under some woman's thumb. That's my conviction — not conviction, but feeling. A man ought to be magnanimous, and it's no disgrace to a man! No disgrace to a hero, not even a Cæsar! But don't ever beg her pardon all the same for anything. Remember that rule given you by your brother Mitya, who's come to ruin through women. No, I'd better make it up to Grusha somehow, without begging pardon. I worship her, Alexey, worship her. Only she doesn't see it. No, she still thinks I don't love her enough. And she tortures me, tortures me with her love. The past was nothing! In the past it was only those infernal curves of hers that tortured me, but now I've taken all her soul into my soul and through her I've become a man myself. Will they marry us? If they don't, I shall die of jealousy. I imagine something every day. . . . What did she say to you about me?"

Alyosha repeated all Grushenka had said to him that day. Mitya listened, made him repeat things, and seemed pleased.

"Then she is not angry at my being jealous?" he exclaimed. "She is a regular woman! 'I've a fierce heart myself!' Ah, I love such fierce hearts, though I can't bear any one's being jealous of me. I can't endure it. We shall fight. But I shall love her, I shall love her infinitely. Will they marry us? Do they let convicts marry? That's the question. And without her I can't exist . . ."

Mitya walked frowning across the room. It was almost dark. He suddenly seemed terribly worried.

"So there's a secret, she says, a secret? We have got up a plot against her, and Katya is mixed up in it, she thinks. No, my good Grushenka, that's not it. You are very wide of the mark, in your foolish feminine way. Alyosha, darling, well, here goes! I'll tell you our secret!"

He looked round, quickly went close up to Alyosha, who was standing before him, and whispered to him with an air of mystery, though in reality no one could hear them: the old watchman was dozing in the corner, and not a word could reach the ears of the soldiers on guard.

"I will tell you our whole secret," Mitya whispered hurriedly. "I meant to tell you later, for how could I decide on anything without you? You are everything to me. Though I say that Ivan is superior to us, you are my angel. It's your word will decide it. Perhaps it's you who are superior and not Ivan. You see, it's a question of conscience, a question of the higher conscience — the secret is so important that I can't deal with it alone, and I've put it off till I could speak to you. But anyway it's too early to decide now, for we must wait for the verdict. As soon as the verdict is pronounced, you shall decide my fate. Don't decide it now. I'll tell you now. You listen, but don't decide. Stand there and keep quiet. I won't tell you everything. I'll only tell you the idea, without details, and you keep quiet. Not a question, not a movement. You agree? But, Lord, what shall I do with your eyes? I'm afraid your eyes will tell me your decision, even if you don't speak. Oo! I'm afraid! Alyosha, listen! Ivan suggests my *escaping*. I won't tell you the details: it's all been thought out: it can all be arranged. Hush, don't decide. I should go to America with Grusha. You know I can't live without

Grusha! What if they won't let her follow me to Siberia? Do they let convicts get married? Ivan thinks not. And without Grusha what should I do there underground with a hammer? I should only smash my head with the hammer! But, on the other hand, my conscience? I should have run away from suffering. A sign was granted, I rejected the sign. There was a way of salvation and I turned my back on it. Ivan says that in America, 'with good inclinations,' one can be of more use than underground. But where then will our underground hymn be? What's America? America is vanity again! And there's a lot of swindling in America, too, I expect. I should have run away from crucifixion! I tell you this, you know, Alexey, because you are the only person who can understand this. There's no one else. To others, it's folly, madness, all I've told you of the hymn. They'll say I'm out of my mind or a fool. I am not out of my mind and I am not a fool. Ivan understands about the hymn, too. He understands, only he doesn't answer — he doesn't speak. He doesn't believe in the hymn. Don't speak, don't speak. I see how you look! You have already decided. Don't decide, spare me! I can't live without Grusha. Wait till after the trial!"

Mitya was beside himself as he finished. He held Alyosha by his shoulders, and his yearning, feverish eyes were fixed on his brother's.

"They don't let convicts marry, do they?" he repeated for the third time in a supplicating voice.

Alyosha listened with extreme surprise and was deeply shaken.

"Tell me one thing," he said, "does Ivan insist on it, and whose idea was it?"

"His, his, and he insists on it. He didn't come to see me at first, then he suddenly came a week ago and he broached the subject straight away. He is awfully keen on it. He doesn't ask me, but orders me to escape. He doesn't doubt of my obeying him, though I turned my heart inside out before him as I have before you, and told him about the hymn, too. He told me he'd arrange it; he's found out about everything. But of that later. He's simply set on it. It's all a matter of money: here, he says, is ten thousand for your escape and twenty thousand for America. And he says we can arrange a magnificent escape for ten thousand."

"And he told you on no account to tell me?" Alyosha asked again.

"To tell no one, and especially not you; on no account to tell you. He is afraid, no doubt, that you'll stand before me as my conscience. Don't tell him I told you. Don't tell him, for anything."

"You are right," Alyosha pronounced; "it's impossible to decide anything before the verdict. After the trial you'll decide for yourself. Then you'll find that new man in yourself and he will decide."

"A new man, or a Bernard who'll decide *à la* Bernard, for I believe I'm a contemptible Bernard myself," said Mitya, with a bitter grin.

"But, brother, have you no hope then of being acquitted?"

Mitya shrugged his shoulders nervously and shook his head.

"Alyosha, darling, it's time you were going," he said, with sudden haste. "There's the superintendent shouting in the yard. He'll be here directly. We are late; it's irregular. Embrace me quickly. Kiss me! Make the sign of the cross over me, darling, for the cross I have to bear to-morrow."

They embraced and kissed.

"Ivan," said Mitya suddenly, "suggests my escaping; but, of course, he believes that I killed."

A mournful smile came to his lips.

"Have you asked him whether he believes it?" asked Alyosha.

"No, I haven't. I wanted to, but I couldn't. I hadn't the courage. But I saw it from his eyes. Well, good-bye!"

Once more they kissed hurriedly, and Alyosha was just going out, when Mitya suddenly called him back.

"Stand facing me! That's right!" And again he seized Alyosha, putting both hands on his shoulders. His face became suddenly quite pale, so that it was dreadfully apparent, even through the gathering darkness. His lips twitched, his eyes fastened upon Alyosha.

"Alyosha, tell me the whole truth, as you would before the Lord God. Do you believe that I killed, or don't you believe it? Do you, do you yourself, believe it or not? The whole truth, don't lie!" he cried frantically.

Everything seemed heaving before Alyosha, and he felt something like a stab at his heart.

"Hush! What do you mean?" he faltered helplessly.

"The whole truth, the whole, don't lie!" repeated Mitya.

"I've never for one instant believed that you were the murderer!" broke suddenly in a shaking voice from Alyosha, and he raised his right hand, as though calling God to witness his words.

Mitya's whole face was lighted up with bliss.

"Thank you!" he articulated slowly, as though sighing after a swoon. "Now you have given me new life. Would you believe it, till this moment I've been afraid to ask you, you, even you. Well, go! You've given me strength for to-morrow. God bless you! Come, go along! Love Ivan!" was Mitya's last word.

Alyosha went out in tears. Such distrustfulness in Mitya, such lack of confidence even in him, in Alyosha — all this suddenly opened before Alyosha an unsuspected abyss of hopeless grief and despair in the soul of his unhappy brother. Intense, infinite compassion overwhelmed him instantly and tortured him. There was a poignant ache in his torn heart. "Love Ivan" — he suddenly recalled Mitya's words. And he was going to Ivan. He had wanted to see Ivan badly since morning. He was as much worried about Ivan as about Mitya, and more than ever now.

CHAPTER V

NOT YOU, NOT YOU!

On the way to Ivan he had to pass the house where Katerina Ivanovna was living. There was light in the windows. He suddenly stopped and resolved to go in. He had not seen Katerina Ivanovna for more than a week. But now it struck him that Ivan might be with her, especially on the eve of the terrible day. Having rung the bell and mounted the staircase, which was dimly lighted by a Chinese lantern, he saw a man coming down, and as they met he recognised his brother. So he was just coming from Katerina Ivanovna.

"Ah, it's only you," said Ivan drily. "Well, good-bye! You are going to her?"

"Yes."

"I don't advise you to; she's upset and you'll upset her more."

A door was instantly flung open above, and a voice cried suddenly:

"No, no! Alexey Fyodorovich, have you come from him?"

"Yes, I have been with him."

"Has he sent me any message? Come up, Alyosha, and you, Ivan Fyodorovich, you must come back, you must. Do you hear?"

There was such a peremptory note in Katya's voice that Ivan, after a moment's hesitation, made up his mind to go upstairs again with Alyosha.

"She was eavesdropping," he murmured angrily to himself, but Alyosha heard it.

"Excuse my keeping my greatcoat on," said Ivan, going into the drawing-room. "I won't sit down. I won't stay more than a minute."

"Sit down, Alexey Fyodorovich," said Katerina Ivanovna, though she remained standing. She had changed very little during this time, but there was an ominous gleam in her dark eyes. Alyosha remembered afterwards that she had struck him as particularly beautiful at that moment.

"What did he ask you to tell me?"

"Only one thing," said Alyosha, looking her straight in the face, "that you would spare yourself and say nothing at the trial of what" (he hesitated a little) ". . . passed between you . . . at the time of your first acquaintance . . . in that town."

"Ah! that I bowed down to the ground for that money!" She broke into a bitter laugh. "Why, is he afraid for me or for himself? He asks me to spare — whom? Him or myself? Tell me, Alexey Fyodorovich!"

Alyosha watched her intently, trying to understand her. "Both yourself and him," he answered softly.

"I am glad to hear it," she snapped out maliciously, and she suddenly blushed.

"You don't know me yet, Alexey Fyodorovich," she said menacingly. "And I don't know myself yet. Perhaps you'll want to trample me under foot after my testimony to-morrow."

"You will give your evidence honestly," said Alyosha; "that's all that's wanted."

"Women are often dishonest," she said, grinding her teeth. "Only an hour ago I was thinking I was horrified at the thought of touching that monster . . . as though he were a reptile . . . but no, he is still a human being to me! But did he kill? Is he the murderer?" she cried, all of a sudden, hysterically, turning quickly to Ivan. Alyosha saw at once that she had asked Ivan that question before, perhaps only a moment before he came in, and not for the first time, but for the hundredth, and that they had ended by quarrelling.

"I've been to see Smerdyakov. . . . It was you, you who persuaded me that he murdered his father. It's only you I believed!" she continued, still addressing Ivan. He gave her a sort of strained smile. Alyosha was startled to note that she addressed him familiarly. He had not suspected such intimacy between them.

"Well, that's enough, anyway," Ivan cut short the conversation. "I am going. I'll come to-morrow." And turning at once, he walked out of the room and went straight downstairs.

With an imperious gesture, Katerina Ivanovna seized Alyosha by both hands.

"Follow him! Overtake him! Don't leave him alone for a minute!" she said, in a hurried whisper. "He's mad! Don't you know that he's mad? He is in a fever, nervous fever. The doctor told me so. Go, run after him. . . ."

Alyosha jumped up and ran after Ivan, who was not fifty paces ahead of him.

"What do you want?" He turned quickly on Alyosha, seeing that he was running after him. "She told you to run after me, because I'm mad. I know it all by heart," he added irritably.

"She is mistaken, of course; but she is right that you are ill," said Alyosha. "I was looking at your face just now. You look very ill, Ivan." Ivan walked on without stopping. Alyosha followed him.

"And do you know, Alexey Fyodorovich, how people go out of their mind?" Ivan asked, his voice suddenly quiet, without a trace of irritation, in a tone of the simplest curiosity.

"No, I don't. I suppose there are all kinds of insanity."

"And can one observe that one's going mad oneself?"

"I imagine one can't see oneself clearly in such circumstances," Alyosha answered with surprise.

Ivan paused for half a minute.

"If you want to talk to me, please change the subject," he said suddenly.

"Oh, while I think of it, I have a letter for you," said Alyosha timidly, and he took Lise's note from his pocket and held it out to Ivan. They had just come up to a lamp-post. Ivan recognised the handwriting at once.

"Ah, from that imp!" he laughed maliciously, and, without opening the envelope, he tore it into bits and threw it to the wind. The bits were scattered.

"She's not sixteen yet, I believe, and already offering herself," he said contemptuously, striding along the street again.

"How do you mean, offering herself?" exclaimed Alyosha.

"As loose women offer themselves, to be sure."

"How can you, Ivan, how can you?" Alyosha cried hotly and sorrowfully. "She is a child; you are insulting a child! She is ill; she is very ill, too. She is on the verge of insanity, too, perhaps . . . I couldn't help handing her letter to you . . . I had hoped to hear something from you . . . that would save her."

"You'll hear nothing from me. If she is a child I am no nurse for her. Be quiet, Alexey. Don't go on about her. I am not even thinking about it."

They were silent again for a moment.

"She will be praying all night now to the Mother of God to show her how to act to-morrow at the trial," he said sharply and angrily again.

"You . . . you mean Katerina Ivanovna?"

"Yes. Whether she's to save Mitya or ruin him. She'll pray for light from above. She can't make up her mind for herself, you see. She has not had time to prepare herself yet. She takes me for her nurse, too. She wants me to sing lullabies to her."

"Katerina Ivanovna loves you, brother," said Alyosha sadly.

"Perhaps; but I am not very keen on her."

"She is suffering. Why do you . . . sometimes say things to her that give her hope?" Alyosha went on, with timid reproach. "I know that you've given her hope. Forgive me for speaking to you like this," he added.

"I can't behave to her as I ought—break off altogether and tell her so straight out," said Ivan irritably. "I must wait till sentence is passed on the murderer. If I break off with her now, she will avenge herself on me by ruining that scoundrel to-morrow at the trial, for she hates him and knows she hates him.

It's all a lie — lie upon lie! As long as I don't break off with her, she goes on hoping, and she won't ruin that monster, knowing how I want to get him out of trouble. If only that damned verdict would come!"

The words "murderer" and "monster" echoed painfully in Alyosha's heart.

"But how can she ruin Mitya?" he asked, pondering on Ivan's words. "What evidence can she give that would ruin Mitya?"

"You don't know that yet. She's got a document in her hands, in Mitya's own writing, that proves conclusively that he did murder Fyodor Pavlovich."

"That's impossible!" cried Alyosha.

"Why is it impossible? I've read it myself."

"There can't be such a document!" Alyosha repeated hotly. "There can't be, because he's not the murderer. It's not he murdered father, not he!"

Ivan suddenly stopped.

"Who is the murderer then, according to you?" he asked, with apparent coldness. There was even a supercilious note in his voice.

"You know who," Alyosha pronounced in a low, inward voice.

"Who? You mean the story about the crazy idiot, the epileptic, Smerdyakov?"

Alyosha suddenly felt himself trembling all over. "You know who," broke helplessly from him. He could scarcely breathe.

"Who? Who?" Ivan cried almost fiercely. All his restraint suddenly vanished.

"I know only one thing," Alyosha went on, still almost in a whisper, "*it wasn't you* killed father."

"Not you! What do you mean by 'not you'?" Ivan was thunderstruck.

"It was not you killed father, not you!" Alyosha repeated firmly.

The silence lasted for half a minute.

"I know I didn't. Are you raving?" said Ivan, with a pale, distorted smile. His eyes were riveted on Alyosha. They were standing again beside a lamp-post.

"No, Ivan. You've told yourself several times that you are the murderer."

"When did I say so? I was in Moscow. . . . When have I said so?" Ivan faltered helplessly.

"You've said so to yourself many times, when you've been alone during these two dreadful months," Alyosha went on softly and distinctly as before. Yet he was speaking now, as it were, not of himself, not of his own will, but obeying some irresistible command. "You have accused yourself and have confessed to yourself that you are the murderer and no one else. But you didn't do it: you are mistaken: you are not the murderer. Do you hear? It was not you! God has sent me to tell you so."

They were both silent. The silence lasted a whole long minute. They were both standing still, gazing into each other's eyes. They were both pale. Suddenly Ivan began trembling all over, and clutched Alyosha's shoulder.

"You've been in my room!" he whispered hoarsely. "You've been there at night, when he came. . . . Confess . . . have you seen him, have you seen him?"

"Whom do you mean — Mitya?" Alyosha asked bewildered.

"Not him, damn the monster!" Ivan shouted, in a frenzy. "Do you know that he visits me? How did you find out? Speak!"

"Who is *he?* I don't know whom you are talking about," Alyosha faltered, beginning to be alarmed.

"Yes, you do know . . . or how could you . . . ? It's impossible that you shouldn't know." Suddenly he seemed to check himself. He stood still and seemed to reflect. A strange grin contorted his lips.

"Brother," Alyosha began again, in a shaking voice, "I have said this to you because you'll believe my word, I know that. I tell you once and for all, it's not you. You hear, once for all! God has put it into my heart to say this to you, even though it may make you hate me from this hour."

But by now Ivan had apparently regained his self-control.

"Alexey Fyodorovich," he said, with a cold smile, "I can't endure prophets and epileptics — God's messengers especially — and you know that only too well. I break off all relations with you from this moment and probably for ever. I beg you to leave me at this turning. It's the way to your lodgings, too. You'd better be particularly careful not to come to me to-night! Do you hear?"

He turned and walked on with a firm step, not looking back.

"Brother," Alyosha called after him, "if anything happens to you to-night, turn to me before any one!"

But Ivan made no reply. Alyosha stood beside the lamp-post at the cross-roads, till Ivan had vanished into the darkness. Then he turned and walked slowly homewards. Both Alyosha and Ivan were living in lodgings; neither of them was willing to live in Fyodor Pavlovich's empty house. Alyosha had a furnished room in the house of some simple people. Ivan lived quite a distance from him. He had taken roomy and fairly comfortable quarters in the wing of a fine house that belonged to a well-to-do lady, the widow of an official. But his only attendant was a deaf and rheumatic old crone who went to bed at six o'clock every evening and got up at six in the morning. Ivan had become remarkably indifferent to his comforts of late, and very fond of being alone. He did everything for himself in the one room he lived in, and rarely entered any of the other rooms in his lodging.

He reached the gate of the house and had his hand on the bell, when he suddenly stopped. He felt that he was trembling all over with anger. Suddenly he let go of the bell, spat, turned back, and walked with rapid steps in the opposite direction. He walked a mile and a half to a tiny, crooked, wooden house, almost a peasant hut, where Marya Kondratyevna, the neighbour who used to come to Fyodor Pavlovich's kitchen for soup and to whom Smerdyakov had once sung his songs and played on the guitar, was now lodging. She had sold their little house, and was now living here with her mother. Smerdyakov, who was ill — almost dying — had been with them ever since Fyodor Pavlovich's death. It was to him Ivan was now going, moved by a sudden and irresistible prompting.

CHAPTER VI

THE FIRST INTERVIEW WITH SMERDYAKOV

This was the third time that Ivan had been to see Smerdyakov since his return from Moscow. The first time he had seen him and talked to him after the catastrophe was on the first day of his arrival, then he had visited him once more, a fortnight later. But his visits had ended with that second one, so that it was now over a month since he had seen him. And he had scarcely heard anything of him.

Ivan had only returned five days after his father's death, so that he had not been present at the funeral, which took place the day before he came back. The cause of his delay was that

Alyosha, not knowing his Moscow address, had to apply to Katerina Ivanovna to telegraph to him, and she, not knowing his correct address either, had telegraphed to her sister and aunt, reckoning on Ivan's going to see them as soon as he arrived in Moscow. But he had not gone to them till four days after his arrival. When he got the telegram, he had of course, set off post-haste for our town. The first to meet him was Alyosha, and Ivan was greatly surprised to find that, in opposition to the general opinion of the town, he refused to entertain a suspicion against Mitya, and pointed unhesitatingly to Smerdyakov as the murderer. Later on, after seeing the police captain and the prosecutor, and hearing the details of the charge and the arrest, he was still more surprised at Alyosha, and ascribed his opinion only to his exaggerated brotherly feeling and sympathy with Mitya, of whom Alyosha, as Ivan knew, was very fond.

By the way, let us say a word or two of Ivan's feeling towards his brother Dmitri. He positively disliked him, at most, felt pity for him sometimes, and even that was mixed with great contempt, almost repugnance. Mitya's whole personality, even his appearance, was extremely unattractive to him. On Katerina Ivanovna's love for his brother Ivan looked with indignation. Yet he went to see Mitya on the first day of his arrival, and that interview, far from shaking Ivan's belief in his guilt, positively strengthened it. He found his brother agitated, morbidly excited. Mitya was talkative, but very absent-minded and incoherent. He used violent language, accused Smerdyakov, and was fearfully muddled. He talked principally about the three thousand roubles, which he said had been "stolen" from him by his father.

"The money was mine, it was my money," Mitya kept repeating. "Even if I had stolen it, I should have had the right."

He hardly contested the evidence against him, and if he tried to turn a fact to his advantage, it was in an absurd and incoherent way. He hardly seemed to wish to defend himself before Ivan or any one else. Quite the contrary, he was angry and proudly scornful of the charges against him; he was abusing every one and was in a continual rage. He only laughed contemptuously at Grigory's evidence about the open door, and declared that it was "the devil that opened it." But he could not bring forward any coherent explanation of the fact. He even succeeded in insulting Ivan during their first interview, telling him sharply that it was not for people who declared that "everything was lawful" to suspect and question him. Altogether he was anything but friendly with Ivan on that occasion. Immediately after that interview with Mitya, Ivan had gone for the first time to see Smerdyakov.

In the railway train on his way from Moscow, he kept thinking of Smerdyakov and of his last conversation with him on the evening before he went away. Many things seemed to him puzzling and suspicious. But when he gave his evidence to the examining magistrate Ivan said nothing, for the time, of that conversation. He put that off till he had seen Smerdyakov, who was at that time in the hospital.

Dr. Herzenstube and Varvinsky, the doctor he met in the hospital, confidently asserted, in reply to Ivan's persistent questions, that Smerdyakov's epilepsy was unmistakably genuine, and were surprised indeed at Ivan's asking whether he might not have been shamming on the day of the catastrophe. They gave him to

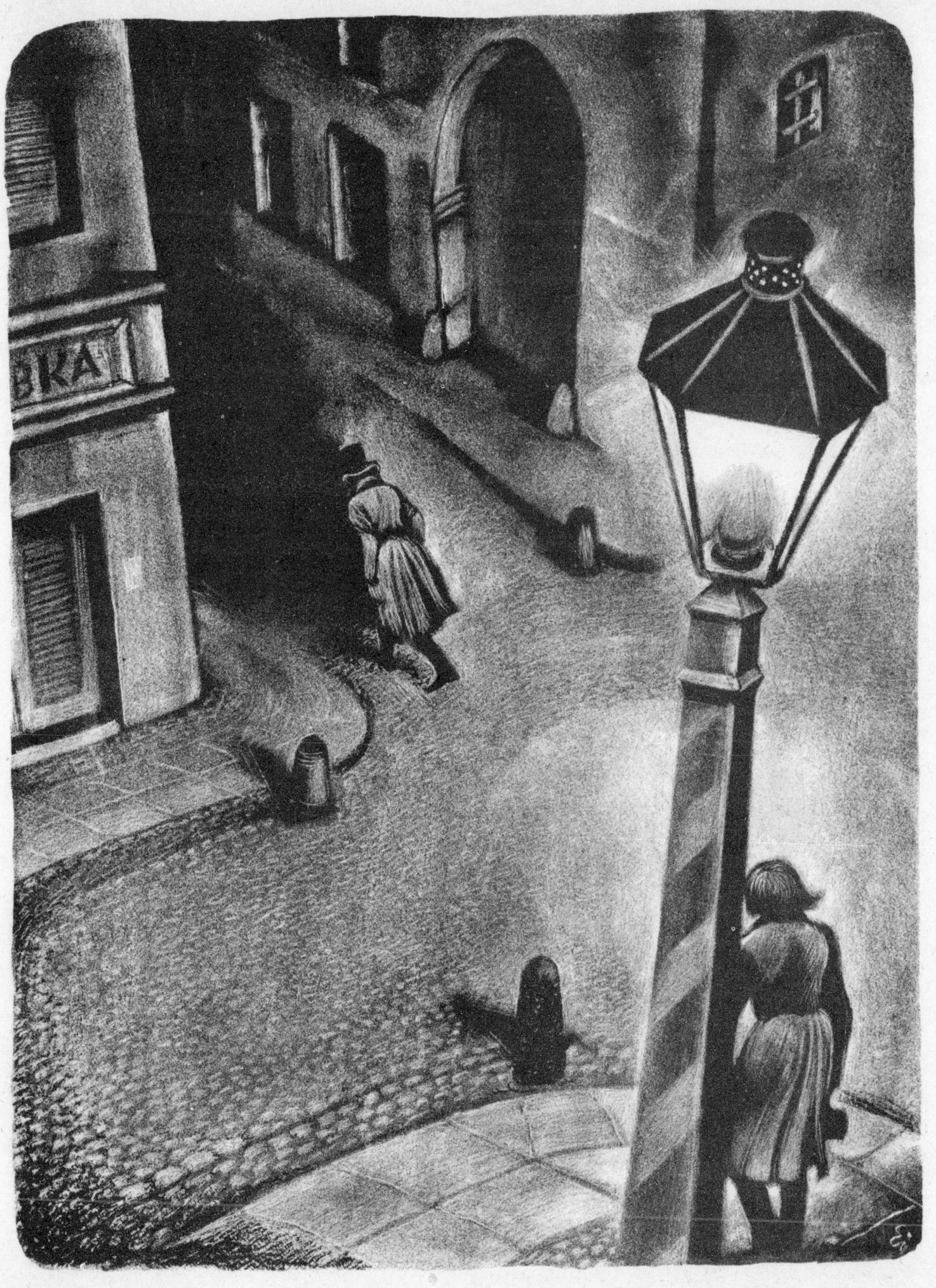

"BROTHER, TURN TO ME!"

understand that the attack was an exceptional one, the fits persisting and recurring several times, so that the patient's life was positively in danger, and it was only now, after they had taken measures, that they could assert with confidence that the patient would survive. "Though it might well be," added Dr. Herzenstube, "that his reason would be impaired for a considerable period, if not permanently." On Ivan's asking impatiently whether that meant that he was now mad, they told him that this was not yet the case, in the full sense of the word, but that certain abnormalities were perceptible. Ivan decided to find out for himself what those abnormalities were.

At the hospital he was at once allowed to see the patient. Smerdyakov was lying on a cot in a separate ward. There was only one other bed in the room, occupied by a tradesman of the town, swollen with dropsy, who was obviously going to die the following day or the day after that; he could be no hindrance to their conversation. Smerdyakov grinned distrustfully on seeing Ivan, and for the first instant seemed to be taken aback, as it were. So at least Ivan fancied. But that was only momentary. For the rest of the time he was struck, on the contrary, by Smerdyakov's composure. From the first glance Ivan had no doubt that he was very ill. He was very weak; he spoke slowly, seeming to move his tongue with difficulty; he had grown thin and sallow. Throughout the interview, which lasted twenty minutes, he kept complaining of a headache and of aches in all his limbs. His thin eunuch's face seemed to have become so tiny; the hair on his temples was ruffled, and his crest of curls in front stood up in a thin tuft. But the left eye, which was screwed up and seemed to be insinuating something, betrayed the old Smerdyakov. "A clever man is worth talking to." Ivan was reminded of that at once. He sat down on the stool at his feet. Smerdyakov, with a painful effort, shifted his position in bed, but he was not the first to speak. He remained silent, and did not even look much interested.

"Can you talk to me?" asked Ivan. "I won't tire you much."

"Certainly I can," mumbled Smerdyakov, in a faint voice. "Have you been back long, sir?" he added condescendingly, as though encouraging an embarrassed visitor.

"I arrived only to-day. . . . To clear up the mess you are in here."

Smerdyakov sighed.

"Why do you sigh? You knew of it all along," Ivan blurted out.

Smerdyakov was stolidly silent for a while.

"How could I help knowing, sir? It was clear beforehand. But how could I tell it would turn out like that?"

"What would turn out? Don't try to wriggle out! You foretold, didn't you, that you'd have a fit, on the way down to the cellar, you know. You mentioned the very spot."

"Have you said so at the examination yet?" Smerdyakov queried with composure.

Ivan felt suddenly angry.

"No, I haven't yet, but I will, without fail. You must explain a great deal to me, my man, and let me tell you, I am not going to let you play with me!"

"Why should I play with you, sir, when I put my whole trust in you, as in God Almighty?" said Smerdyakov, with the same composure, only for a moment closing his little eyes.

"In the first place," began Ivan, "I know that epileptic fits can't be foretold beforehand.

I've inquired, don't try to wriggle out of it. You can't foretell the day and the hour. How was it you told me the day and the hour beforehand, and about the cellar, too? How could you tell that you would fall down the cellar stairs in a fit, if you didn't sham a fit on purpose?"

"I had to go to the cellar, sir, anyway, several times a day, sir, indeed," Smerdyakov drawled deliberately. "I fell from the garret just in the same way a year ago. It's quite true you can't foretell the day and hour of a fit beforehand, but you can always have a presentiment of it."

"But you did foretell the day and the hour!"

"In regard to my epilepsy, sir, you had much better inquire of the doctors here. You can ask them whether it was a real fit or a sham; it's no use my saying any more about it."

"And the cellar? How could you know beforehand about the cellar?"

"You don't seem able to get over that cellar! As I was going down to the cellar, I was in terrible dread and doubt. What frightened me most was losing you and being left without protection in the whole world. So I went down into the cellar thinking, 'Here, it'll come on directly, it'll strike me down directly, shall I fall or not?' And it was through this fear that I suddenly felt the spasm in my throat that always comes . . . and so I went flying. All that and all my previous conversation with you at the gate the evening before when I told you how frightened I was and spoke of the cellar, I told all that to Dr. Herzenstube and Nikolay Parfenovich, the examining magistrate, and it's all in the record. And the doctor here, Mr. Varvinsky, maintained to all of them that it was just the thought of it brought it on, the apprehension that I might fall. It was just then that the fit seized me. And so they've written it down, that that's just how it must have happened, simply because of my fear."

As he finished, Smerdyakov drew a deep breath, as though exhausted.

"Then you have said all that in your evidence?" said Ivan, somewhat taken aback. He had meant to frighten him with the threat of repeating their conversation, and it appeared that Smerdyakov had already reported it all himself.

"What have I to be afraid of? Let them write down the whole truth," Smerdyakov pronounced firmly.

"And have you told them every word of our conversation at the gate?"

"No, not exactly every word."

"And did you tell them that you can sham fits, as you boasted then?"

"No, I didn't tell them that either."

"Tell me now, why did you send me to Chermashnya that time?"

"I was afraid you'd go away to Moscow, Chermashnya is nearer, anyway."

"You are lying, you suggested my going away yourself; you told me to get out of the way of trouble."

"That was simply out of affection and my sincere devotion to you, sir, foreseeing trouble in the house, to spare you, sir. Only I wanted to spare myself even more. That's why I told you to get out of harm's way, sir, that you might understand that there would be trouble in the house, and would remain at home to protect your father."

"You might have said it more directly, you blockhead!" Ivan suddenly fired up.

"How could I have said it more directly then? It was simply my fear that made me speak, sir; and besides, you might have gotten angry, too. I might well have been apprehensive that Dmitri Fyodorovich would make a scandal and carry away that money, for he considered it as good as his own, but who could tell that it would end in a murder like this? I thought that he would only carry off the three thousand that lay under the master's mattress in the envelope, and you see, he's murdered him. How could you guess it either, sir?"

"But if you say yourself that it couldn't be guessed, how could I have guessed and stayed at home? You contradict yourself!" said Ivan, pondering.

"You might have guessed from my sending you to Chermashnya and not to Moscow."

"How could I guess it from that?"

Smerdyakov seemed much exhausted, and again he was silent for a minute.

"You might have guessed from the fact of my asking you not to go to Moscow, but to Chermashnya, sir, that I wanted to have you nearer, for Moscow's a long way off, and Dmitri Fyodorovich, knowing you are not far off, would not be so bold. And if anything had happened, you might have come to protect me, too, for I warned you of Grigory Vasilyevich's illness, and that I was afraid of having a fit. And when I explained those knocks to you, by means of which one could go in to the deceased, and that Dmitri Fyodorovich knew them all through me, I thought that you would guess yourself that he would be sure to do something, and so you wouldn't go to Chermashnya even, but would stay."

"He talks very coherently," thought Ivan, "though he does mumble; what's the derangement of his faculties that Herzenstube talked of?"

"You are playing a double game with me, damn you," he exclaimed, getting angry.

"But I thought at the time that you quite guessed," Smerdyakov parried with the most naïve air.

"If I'd guessed, I should have stayed," cried Ivan.

"Why, I thought that it was because you guessed that you went away in such a hurry, sir, only to get out of trouble, only to run away and save yourself in your fright."

"You thought that every one was as great a coward as yourself?"

"Forgive me, sir, I thought you were like me."

"Of course, I ought to have guessed," Ivan said in agitation, "and I did guess there was some mischief brewing on your part . . . only you are lying, you are lying again," he cried, suddenly recollecting. "Do you remember how you went up to the carriage and said to me, 'A clever man is worth talking to'? So you were glad I went away, since you praised me?"

Smerdyakov sighed again and again. A trace of colour came into his face.

"If I was pleased," he articulated rather breathlessly, "it was simply beeause you agreed not to go to Moscow, but to Chermashnya. For it was nearer, anyway. Only when I said those words to you, it was not by way of praise, but of reproach, sir. You didn't understand it, sir."

"What reproach?"

"Why, that foreseeing such a calamity you deserted your own parent, and would not protect us, for I might have been taken up any time on the charge of having stolen that three thousand."

"Damn you!" Ivan swore again. "Wait, did you tell the prosecutor and the examining magistrate about those knocks?"

"I told them everything just as it was."

Ivan wondered inwardly again.

"If I thought of anything then," he began again, "it was solely of some dirty trick on your part. Dmitri might kill, but that he would steal — I did not believe that then. . . . But I was prepared for any dirty trick from you. You told me yourself you could sham a fit. What did you say that for?"

"It was just through my simplicity, and I never have shammed a fit on purpose in my life. And I only said so then to boast to you. It was just foolishness, sir. I liked you so much then, and was open-hearted with you."

"My brother plainly accuses you of having killed and stolen."

"What else is left for him to do?" said Smerdyakov, with a bitter grin. "And who will believe him with all the evidence against him? Grigory Vasilyevich saw the door open. What can he say after that, sir? But, well, God help him! He is trembling for his own skin."

He was quiet for a while, and suddenly, as though on reflection, added:

"And look here again, sir: he wants to lay the blame on me and make out that it is the work of my hands — I've heard that already, sir. But as to my being clever at shamming a fit: should I have told you beforehand that I could sham one, if I really had had such a design against your father? If I had been planning such a murder could I have been such a fool as to give such evidence against myself beforehand? And to his own son, too! Upon my word! Is that likely? As if that could be, such a thing has never happened. No one hears this talk of ours now, except Providence itself, and if you were to tell of it to the prosecutor and Nikolay Parfenovich you might defend me completely by doing so, for who would be likely to be such a criminal, if he is so open-hearted beforehand? Any one can see that."

"Well," and Ivan got up to cut short the conversation, struck by Smerdyakov's last argument, "I don't suspect you at all, and indeed I think it's absurd to accuse you. On the contrary, I am grateful to you for setting my mind at rest. Now I am going, but I'll come again. Meanwhile, good-bye. Get well. Is there anything you want?"

"I am very thankful for everything, sir. Marfa Ignatyevna does not forget me, and provides me with whatever I want, in her kindness. Good people visit me every day."

"Good-bye. But I shan't say anything of your being able to sham a fit, and I don't advise you to, either," something made Ivan say suddenly.

"I quite understand. And if you don't speak of that, I shall say nothing of our whole conversation at the gate."

Then it happened that Ivan went out, and only when he had gone a dozen steps along the corridor, he suddenly felt that there was an insulting significance in Smerdyakov's last words. He was almost on the point of turning back, but it was only a passing impulse, and muttering, "Nonsense!" he went out of the hospital.

His chief feeling was one of relief at the fact that it was not Smerdyakov, but Mitya, who had committed the murder, though he might have been expected to feel the opposite. He did not want to analyse the reason for this feeling, and even felt a positive repugnance at prying into his sensations. He felt as though he wanted to make haste to forget something. In the following days he became convinced of Mitya's guilt, as he acquainted himself with all the evidence against him. There was the evidence of people of no importance, Fenya and her mother, for instance, but the weight of it was almost overpowering, let alone the testimony of Perhotin, the people at the tavern, and at Plotnikovs' shop, as well as that of the witnesses at Mokroye. It was the details that were so damning. The secret knocks impressed the lawyers almost as much as Grigory's evidence as to the open door. Grigory's wife, Marfa, in answer to Ivan's questions, declared that Smerdyakov had been lying all night the other side of the partition, "He was not three paces from our bed," and that although she was a sound sleeper she waked several times and heard him moaning, "He was moaning the whole time, moaning continually."

Talking to Herzenstube, and giving it as his opinion that Smerdyakov was not mad, but only rather weak, Ivan only evoked from the old man a subtle smile.

"Do you know how he spends his time now?" he asked, "learning lists of French words by heart. He has an exercise-book under his pillow with the French words written out in Russian letters for him by some one, he, he, he!"

Ivan ended by dismissing all doubts. He could not think of Dmitri without repulsion. Only one thing was strange, however. Alyosha persisted that Dmitri was not the murderer, and that "in all probability" Smerdyakov was. Ivan always felt that Alyosha's opinion meant a great deal to him, and so he was disturbed by it now. Another thing that was strange was that Alyosha did not make any attempt to talk about Mitya with Ivan, that he never began on the subject and only answered his questions. This, too, struck Ivan particularly.

But he was very much preoccupied at this time with something quite apart from that. On his return from Moscow, he had abandoned himself hopelessly to his mad and consuming passion for Katerina Ivanovna. This is not the place to begin to speak of this new passion of Ivan's, which left its mark on the rest of his life: this would furnish the subject for another story, another novel, which I may perhaps never undertake. But I cannot omit to mention here that when Ivan, on leaving Katerina Ivanovna with Alyosha, as I've related already, told him, "I am not keen on her," it was an absolute lie: he loved her madly, though at times he hated her so that he could have murdered her. Many causes helped to bring about this feeling. Shattered by what had happened to Mitya, on Ivan's return she rushed to meet him as her one salvation. She was hurt, insulted, humiliated. And here the man had come back to her, who had loved her so ardently before (oh, she knew that very well), and whose heart and intellect she considered so superior to her own. But the stern girl did not abandon herself altogether to the man, in spite of the Karamazov violence of his passions and the great fascination he had for her. She was continually tormented at the same time by remorse for having deserted Mitya, and in moments of discord and violent anger (and they were numerous) she told Ivan so plainly. This was what he had called to Alyosha "lies upon lies." There was, of course, much that was false in it, and that angered Ivan more than anything. . . .

But of all this later.

In a word, for a time he almost forgot Smerdyakov's existence, and yet, a fortnight after his first visit to him, he began to be tormented by the same strange thoughts as before. It's enough to say that he was continually asking himself why it was that on that last night in Fyodor Pavlovich's house he had crept out on to the stairs like a thief and listened to hear what his father was doing below. Why had he recalled that afterwards with repulsion; why, next morning, had he been suddenly so depressed on the journey; why, as he reached Moscow, had he said to himself, "I am a scoundrel"? And now he almost fancied that these tormenting thoughts would make him even forget Katerina Ivanovna, so completely did they take possession of him again. It was just after fancying this that he met Alyosha in the street. He stopped him at once, and put a question to him:

"Do you remember when Dmitri burst in after dinner and gave father a beating, and afterwards I told you in the yard that I reserved for myself 'the right to desire' . . . tell me, did you think then that I desired father's death or not?"

"I did think so," answered Alyosha softly.

"It was so, too; it was not a matter of guessing. But didn't you fancy then that what I wished was just that 'one reptile should devour another'; that is, just that Dmitri should kill father, and as soon as possible . . . and that I myself was even prepared to help to bring that about?"

Alyosha turned rather pale, and looked silently into his brother's eyes.

"Speak!" cried Ivan. "I want above everything to know what you thought then. I want the truth, the truth!"

He drew a deep breath, looking angrily at Alyosha in anticipation of his answer.

"Forgive me, I did think that, too, at the time," whispered Alyosha, and ceased, without mentioning a single mitigating circumstance.

"Thanks," snapped Ivan, and, leaving Alyosha, he went quickly on his way. From that time on Alyosha noticed that Ivan obviously began to avoid him and seemed even to have taken a dislike to him, so much so that Alyosha gave up going to see him. Immediately after that meeting with him, Ivan, instead of going home, went straight to Smerdyakov again.

CHAPTER VII

THE SECOND VISIT TO SMERDYAKOV

By that time Smerdyakov had been discharged from the hospital. Ivan knew his new lodging, the dilapidated little wooden house, divided in two by a passage, on one side of which lived Marya Kondratyevna and her mother, and on the other, Smerdyakov. No one knew on what terms he lived with them, whether as a friend or as a lodger. It was supposed afterwards that he had come to stay with them as Marya Kondratyevna's betrothed, and was living there for a time without paying for board or lodging. Both mother and daughter had the greatest respect for him and looked upon him as greatly superior to themselves.

Ivan knocked, and, on the door's being opened, went into the passage. By Marya Kondratyevna's directions he went straight to the better room on the left, occupied by Smerdyakov. There was a tiled stove in the room and it was extremely hot. The walls were gay with blue paper, which was a good deal worn, however, and in the cracks under it cockroaches swarmed in amazing numbers, so that they made a continual rustling. The furniture was very scanty: two benches along the walls and two chairs by the table. The table of plain wood was covered with a cloth with a pink pattern. There was a pot of geranium at each of the two little windows. In the corner there was an ikon-case. On the table stood a little copper samovar with many dents in it, and a tray with two cups. But Smerdyakov had finished tea and the samovar was out. He was sitting at the table on a bench. He was looking at an exercise book and drawing lines with a pen. There was an inkwell by him and a short iron candlestick, but with a stearin candle. Ivan saw at once from Smerdyakov's face that he had completely recovered from his illness. His face was fresher, fuller, his hair stood up jauntily in front and was plastered down on his temples. He was sitting in a parti-coloured, wadded dressing-gown, rather dirty and frayed, however. He had spectacles on his nose, which Ivan had never seen him wear before. This trifling circumstance suddenly redoubled Ivan's irritation: "A creature like that and wearing spectacles!"

Smerdyakov slowly raised his head and looked intently at his visitor through his spectacles; then he slowly took them off and rose from the bench, but by no means respectfully, almost lazily, solely to preserve the most elementary civility. All this struck Ivan instantly, he took it all in and noted it at once — most of all the look in Smerdyakov's eyes, positively malicious, churlish, and even haughty. "Why are you barging in here?" it seemed to say; "we settled everything then, why have you come again?" Ivan could scarcely control himself.

"It's hot here," he said, still standing, and unbuttoned his overcoat. "Take off your coat," Smerdyakov conceded.

Ivan took off his coat and threw it on a bench. With trembling hands he took a chair, moved it quickly to the table and sat down. Smerdyakov managed to sit down on his bench before him.

"To begin with, are we alone?" Ivan asked sternly and impulsively. "Can they overhear us in there?"

"No one can hear anything. You've seen for yourself: there's a passage."

"Listen, my good fellow, what was that you babbled, as I was leaving the hospital, that if I said nothing about your being a past master at shamming fits, you wouldn't tell the examining magistrate our whole conversation at the gate? What do you mean by the *whole* conversation? What could you mean by it? Were you threatening me? Have I entered into some sort of compact with you? Do you suppose I am afraid of you?"

Ivan said this in a perfect fury, giving him to understand with obvious intention that he scorned any subterfuge or indirectness and meant to show his cards. Smerdyakov's eyes gleamed resentfully, his left eye winked, and he at once gave his answer, with his habitual composure and deliberation: "You want to have everything above-board, very well, you shall have it," he seemed to say.

"This is what I meant then, and this is why I said what I did: I meant that you, knowing beforehand of this murder of your own parent, left him to his fate, and that people might afterwards think evil of your feelings and perhaps of something else, too — that's what I promised then not to tell the authorities."

Though Smerdyakov spoke without haste and was obviously controlling himself, yet there was in his voice something determined and emphatic, resentful and insolently defiant. He stared impudently at Ivan. A mist passed before Ivan's eyes for the first moment.

"How? What? Are you out of your mind?"

"I'm in perfect possession of all my faculties."

"Do you suppose I *knew* of the murder?" Ivan cried at last, and he brought his fist down violently on the table. "What do you mean by 'something else, too'? Speak, scoundrel!"

Smerdyakov was silent and still scanned Ivan with the same insolent stare.

"Speak, you stinking rogue, what is that 'something else, too'?" he shouted.

"The 'something else' I meant was that you probably, too, were very desirous of your parent's death."

Ivan jumped up and struck him with all his might on the shoulder, so that he fell back against the wall. In an instant his face was bathed in tears, and saying, "It's a shame, sir, to strike a sick man," he suddenly covered his eyes with his very dirty blue-check cotton handkerchief and sank into quiet weeping. A minute passed.

"That's enough! Leave off," Ivan said peremptorily, sitting down again. "Don't put me out of all patience."

Smerdyakov took the rag from his eyes. Every line of his puckered face reflected the insult he had just received.

"So you thought then, you scoundrel, that together with Dmitri I meant to kill my father?"

"I didn't know what thoughts were in your mind then," said Smerdyakov in an injured tone; "and so I stopped you then at the gate to sound you on that very point."

"To sound me, how?"

"Why, as to that very circumstance, whether or not you wanted your father to be murdered?"

What infuriated Ivan more than anything was the aggressive, insolent tone which Smerdyakov persisted in using.

"You murdered him!" he cried suddenly.

Smerdyakov smiled contemptuously.

"That it wasn't I who murdered him you know for a fact, yourself. And I should have thought that there was no need for a sensible man to speak of it again."

"But why, why had you such a suspicion about me at the time?"

"As you know already, it was simply from fear. For I was in such a position, that, shaking with fear, I suspected everyone. I resolved to sound you, too, for I thought if you wanted the same thing that your brother did, then the business was as good as settled and I should be crushed like a fly, too."

"Look here, you didn't say that a fortnight ago."

"I meant that when I talked to you in the hospital, only I thought you'd understand without wasting words, and that being such a sensible man you didn't care to talk of it openly."

"What next! Come, answer, answer, I insist: what was it . . . what could I have done to put into your vile soul a suspicion so degrading to me?"

"As for the murder, you couldn't have done that and didn't want to, but as for wanting some one else to do it, that was just what you did want."

"And how coolly, how coolly he speaks! But why should I have wanted it, what grounds had I for wanting it?"

"What grounds had you? What about the

inheritance?" said Smerdyakov sarcastically, and as it were vindictively. "Why, after your parent's death, sir, there was at least forty thousand to come to each of you, and very likely more, but if Fyodor Pavlovich had got married then to that lady, Agrafena Alexandrovna, she would have had all his capital made over to her directly after the wedding, for she's plenty of sense, sir, so that your parent would not have left you two roubles among the three of you. And were they far from a wedding, either? Not a hair's-breadth: that lady had only to lift her little finger, sir, and he would have run after her to church, with his tongue out."

Ivan restrained himself with effort.

"Very good," he commented at last, "you see, I haven't jumped up, I haven't knocked you down, I haven't killed you. Speak on. So, according to you, I had fixed on Dmitri to do it, I was reckoning on him?"

"How could you help reckoning on him, sir? If he killed him, then he would lose all the rights of a nobleman, his rank and property, and would go off to exile, so his share of the inheritance would come to you, sir, and your brother Alexey Fyodorovich, in equal parts, so you'd each have not forty, but sixty thousand. There's not a doubt, sir, you did reckon on Dmitri Fyodorovich."

"What I put up with from you! Listen, scoundrel, if I had reckoned on any one then, it would have been on you, not on Dmitri, and I swear I did expect some dirty trick from you . . . at the time . . . I remember my impression!"

"I thought, too, for a minute, at the time, that you were reckoning on me as well," said Smerdyakov, with a sarcastic grin. "So that it was just by that more than anything else that you gave yourself away. For if you had a foreboding about me and yet went away, you as good as said to me, 'You can murder my parent, I won't hinder you!' "

"You scoundrel! So that's how you understood it!"

"It was all that going to Chermashnya. Why! You were meaning to go to Moscow, sir, and refused all your father's entreaties to go to Chermashnya — and simply at a foolish word from me, sir, you consented at once! What reason had you to consent to go to Chermashnya? Since you went to Chermashnya with no reason, simply at my word, it shows that you must have expected something from me, sir."

"No, I swear I didn't!" shouted Ivan, grinding his teeth.

"You didn't? Then you ought, as your father's son, to have had me taken to the lock-up, sir, and thrashed at once for my words then . . . or at least to have given me a punch in the face on the spot, but you were not a bit angry, if you please, and at once in a friendly way acted on my foolish word and went away, which was utterly absurd, sir, for you ought to have stayed to save your parent's life. How could I help drawing my conclusions?"

Ivan sat scowling, both his fists convulsively pressed on his knees.

"Yes, I am sorry I didn't punch you in the face," he said with a bitter smile. "I couldn't have taken you to the lock-up just then. Who would have believed me and what charge could I bring against you? But the punch in the face . . . oh, I'm sorry I didn't think of it. Though blows are forbidden, I should have pounded your ugly phiz to a jelly."

Smerdyakov looked at him almost with delight.

"On ordinary occasions, sir," he said in the same complacent and sententious tone in which he had taunted Grigory and argued with him about religion at Fyodor Pavlovich's table, "on ordinary occasions, blows on the face are forbidden nowadays by law and people have given them up, but on exceptional occasions people still resort to blows, sir, not only among us but all over the world, be it even the fullest Republic of France, just as in the time of Adam and Eve, and they never will leave off, but you, sir, even in an exceptional case, did not dare."

"What are you learning French words for?"

Ivan nodded towards the exercise book lying on the table.

"Why shouldn't I learn them, sir, and so improve my education, supposing that I may myself chance to go some day to those happy parts of Europe?"

"Listen, monster." Ivan's eyes flashed and he trembled all over. "I am not afraid of your accusations, you can say what you like about me on the witness stand, and if I don't beat the life out of you, it's simply because I suspect you of that crime and I'll drag you to justice. I'll unmask you."

"To my thinking, you'd better keep quiet, sir, for what can you say against me, considering my absolute innocence; and who would believe you? Only if you begin, I shall tell everything, too, sir, for I must defend myself."

"Do you think I am afraid of you now?"

"If the court doesn't believe all I've said to you just now, sir, the public will, and you will be put to shame, sir."

"That's as much as to say 'A clever man is worth talking to,' eh?" snarled Ivan.

"You hit the mark, indeed, sir. And you'd better be sensible, sir."

Ivan got up, shaking all over with indignation, put on his coat, and without replying further to Smerdyakov, without even looking at him, walked quickly out of the cottage. The cool evening air refreshed him. There was a bright moon in the sky. A nightmare of ideas and sensations filled his soul. "Shall I go at once and give information against Smerdyakov? But what information can I give? He is not guilty, anyway. On the contrary, he'll accuse me. And as a matter of fact, why did I set off for Chermashnya then? What for? What for?" Ivan asked himself. "Yes, of course, I was expecting something and he is right . . ." And he remembered for the hundredth time how, on that last night in his father's house, he had listened on the stairs. But he remembered it now with such anguish that he stood still on the spot as though he had been stabbed. "Yes, I expected it then, that's true! I wanted the murder, I did want the murder! Did I want the murder? Did I want it? I must kill Smerdyakov! If I don't dare kill Smerdyakov now, life is not worth living!"

Ivan did not go home, but went straight to Katerina Ivanovna, alarming her by his appearance. He was like a madman. He repeated his whole conversation with Smerdyakov, every syllable of it. He couldn't be calmed, however much she tried to soothe him: he kept pacing the room, speaking strangely, disconnectedly. At last he sat down, put his elbows on the table, leaned his head on his hands and pronounced this strange aphorism: "If it's not Dmitri, but Smerdyakov who's the murderer, I share his guilt, for I put him up to it. Whether I really did, I don't know yet. But if he is the murderer, and not Dmitri, then, of course, I am the murderer, too."

When Katerina Ivanovna heard that, she got up from her seat without a word, went to her writing-table, opened a box standing on it, took out a sheet of paper and laid it before Ivan. This was the document of which Ivan spoke to Alyosha later on as a "mathematical proof" that Dmitri had killed their father. This was the letter written by Mitya to Katerina Ivanovna when he was drunk, on the very evening he met Alyosha at the cross-roads on the way to the monastery, after the scene at Katerina Ivanovna's, when Grushenka had insulted her. Then, parting from Alyosha, Mitya had rushed to Grushenka. It is not known whether he saw her, but in the evening he was at the "Metropolis," where he got thoroughly drunk. Then he asked for pen and paper and wrote a document of weighty consequences to himself. It was a wordy, disconnected, frantic letter, a drunken letter in fact. It was like the talk of a drunken man, who, on his return home, begins with extraordinary heat telling his wife or one of his household how he has just been insulted, what a rascal has just insulted him, what a fine fellow he is, on the other hand, and how he will pay that scoundrel out; and all that at great length, incoherently and excitedly, with drunken tears and blows on the table. The letter was written on a dirty piece of ordinary paper of the cheapest kind. It had been provided by the tavern and there were figures scrawled on the back of it.

There was evidently not space enough for his drunken verbosity and Mitya had not only filled the margins but had written the last lines right across the rest. The letter ran as follows:

"FATAL KATYA! To-morrow I will get the money and repay your three thousand, and farewell, woman of great wrath, but farewell, too, my love! Let us make an end! To-morrow I shall try and get it from every one, and if I can't get it, I give you my word of honour I shall go to my father and break his head and take the money from under the pillow, if only Ivan has gone. If I have to go to Siberia for it, I'll give you back your three thousand. And farewell. I bow down to the ground before you, for I've been a scoundrel to you. Forgive me! No, better not forgive me, you'll be happier and so shall I! Better Siberia than your love, for I love another woman and you got to know her too well to-day, so how can you forgive? I will murder the man who's robbed me! I'll leave you all and go to the East so as to know no one. Not *her* either, for you are not my only tormentor, she is, too. Farewell!"

"P.S. — I write my curse, but I adore you! I hear it in my heart. One string is left, and it vibrates. Better tear my heart in two! I shall kill myself, but first of all the cur. I shall tear three thousand from him and fling it to you. Though I've been a scoundrel to you, I am not a thief! You can expect three thousand. The cur keeps it under his mattress, in pink ribbon. I am not a thief, but I'll murder my thief. Katya, don't look disdainful. Dmitri is not a thief; but a murderer! He has murdered his father and ruined himself to hold his ground, rather than endure your pride. And he doesn't love you.

"P.P.S. — I kiss your feet, farewell! P.P.P.S. — Katya, pray to God that some one'll give me the money. Then there will be no blood on me, and if no one does — there will! Kill me! Slave and enemy,

D. KARAMAZOV."

Having read this "document," Ivan rose convinced. So then it was his brother who killed, not Smerdyakov. And if not Smerdyakov, then not he, Ivan. This letter at once assumed in his eyes the aspect of a mathematical proof. There could be no longer the slightest doubt of Mitya's guilt. The suspicion never occurred to Ivan, by the way, that Mitya might have committed the murder with Smerdyakov as an accomplice, and indeed such a theory did not fit in with the facts. Ivan was completely reassured. The next morning he thought of Smerdyakov and his gibes only with contempt. A few days later he positively wondered how he could have been so horribly distressed at his suspicions. He resolved to dismiss him with contempt and forget him. So passed a month. He made no further inquiry about Smerdyakov, but twice he happened to hear that he was very ill and out of his mind.

"He'll end in madness," the young doctor, Varvinsky, observed about him and Ivan remembered this. During the last week of that month Ivan himself began to feel very ill. He went to consult the Moscow doctor who had been sent for by Katerina Ivanovna just before the trial. And just at that time his relations with Katerina Ivanovna became acutely strained. They were like two enemies in love with each other. Katerina Ivanovna's "returns" to Mitya, that is, her brief but violent revulsions of feeling in his favour, drove Ivan to perfect frenzy. Strange to say, until that last scene described above, when Alyosha came from Mitya to Katerina Ivanovna, Ivan had never once, during that month, heard her express a doubt of Mitya's guilt, in spite of those "returns" that were so hateful to him. It is remarkable, too, that while he felt that he hated Mitya more and more every day, he realised that it was not on account of Katya's "returns" that he hated him, but just *because he was the murderer of his father*. He was conscious of this and fully recognised it.

Nevertheless, he went to see Mitya ten days before the trial and proposed to him a plan of escape — a plan he had obviously conceived a long time ago. He was partly impelled to do this by a sore place still left in his heart by a phrase of Smerdyakov's, that it was to his, Ivan's, advantage that his brother should be convicted, as that would increase his inheritance and Alyosha's from forty to sixty thousand roubles. He determined to sacrifice thirty thousand on arranging Mitya's escape. On his return from seeing him, he was very mournful and dispirited; he suddenly began to feel that he was anxious for Mitya's escape, not only to heal that sore place by sacrificing thirty thousand, but for another reason. "Is it because I am as much a murderer at heart?" he asked himself. Something very deep down seemed burning and rankling in his soul. His pride above all suffered cruelly all that month. But of that later. . . .

When, after his conversation with Alyosha, Ivan suddenly decided with his hand on the bell of his lodging to go to Smerdyakov, he obeyed a sudden and peculiar impulse of indignation. He suddenly remembered how Katerina Ivanovna had only just cried out to him in Alyosha's presence: "It was you, you alone, persuaded me of his" (that is, Mitya's) "guilt!" Ivan was thunderstruck when he recalled it. He had never once tried to persuade her that Mitya was the murderer; on the contrary, he had suspected himself in her presence, that time when he came back from Smerdyakov. It was *she*, she, who had produced that "document" and proved his brother's guilt. And now she suddenly exclaimed: "I've been at Smerdyakov's myself!" When had she been there? Ivan had known nothing of it. So she was not at all so sure of Mitya's guilt! And what could Smerdyakov have told her? What, what, had he said to her? His heart burned with violent anger. He could not understand how he could, half an hour before, have let those words pass and not have cried out at the moment. He let go of the bell and rushed off to Smerdyakov. "I shall kill him perhaps this time," he thought on the way.

CHAPTER VIII

THE THIRD AND LAST INTERVIEW WITH SMERDYAKOV

When he had gone half-way, the keen dry wind that had been blowing early that morning rose again, and a fine dry snow began falling thickly. It did not stay on the ground, but was whirled about by the wind, and soon there was a regular snowstorm. There were scarcely any street-lamps in the part of the town where Smerdyakov lived. Ivan strode through the darkness, unconscious of the storm, instinctively picking his way. His head ached and there was a painful throbbing in his temples. He felt that his hands were twitching convulsively. Not far from Marya Kondratyevna's cottage, Ivan suddenly came upon a solitary drunken little peasant. He was wearing a coarse and patched coat, and was walking in zigzags, grumbling and swearing to himself. Then suddenly he would begin singing in a husky drunken voice:

"Ah, Vanka's gone to Petersburg
I won't wait till he comes back."

But he broke off every time at the second line and began swearing again; then he would begin the same song again. Ivan felt an intense hatred for him without even thinking about him at all. Suddenly he realised his presence and felt an irresistible impulse to knock him down. At that moment they met, and the peasant with a violent lurch fell full tilt against Ivan, who pushed him back furiously. The peasant went flying backwards and fell like a log on the frozen ground. He uttered one plaintive "O-oh!" and then was silent. Ivan stepped up to him. He was lying on his back, without movement or consciousness. "He will freeze to death," thought Ivan, and he went on his way to Smerdyakov's.

In the passage, Marya Kondratyevna, who ran out to open the door with a candle in her hand, whispered that Smerdyakov was very ill; "it's not that he's laid up, but it's as though he has gone out of his mind, and he even told us to take the tea away; he wouldn't have any."

"Why, has he been making a row?" asked Ivan coarsely.

"Oh, dear, no, quite the contrary, he's very quiet. Only please don't talk to him too long," Marya Kondratyevna begged him. Ivan opened the door and stepped into the room.

It was overheated as before, but there were changes in the room. One of the benches at the side had been removed, and in its place had been put a large old mahogany sofa, upholstered in leather, on which a bed had been made up, with fairly clean white pillows. Smerdyakov was sitting on the sofa, wearing the same dressing-gown. The table had been brought out in front of the sofa, so that there was hardly room to move. On the table lay a thick book in a yellow cover, but Smerdyakov was not reading it. He seemed to be sitting doing nothing. He met Ivan with a slow silent look, and was apparently not at all surprised at his coming. There was a great change in his face; he was much thinner and sallower. His eyes were sunken and his lower lids were blue.

"So you are really ill, eh!" Ivan stopped short. "I won't keep you long, I won't even take off my coat. Where can one sit down?"

He went to the other end of the table, moved up a chair and sat down on it.

"Why do you look at me without speaking? I've only come with one question, and I swear I won't go without an answer. Has the young lady, Katerina Ivanovna, been to see you?"

Smerdyakov still remained silent, looking quietly at Ivan as before. Suddenly, with a motion of his hand, he turned his face away.

"What's the matter with you?" cried Ivan.

"Nothing."

"What do you mean by 'nothing'?"

"Well, she has. It doesn't matter to you. Let me alone."

"No, I won't let you alone. Tell me, when was she here?"

"Why, I'd quite forgotten about her," said Smerdyakov, with a scornful smile, and, turning his face to Ivan again, he stared at him with a look of frenzied hatred, the same look that he had fixed on him at their last interview, a month before.

"You seem very ill yourself, your face is pinched; you don't look like yourself," he said to Ivan.

"Never mind my health, answer my question."

"But why are your eyes so yellow? The whites are quite yellow. Are you so tormented?" He smiled contemptuously and suddenly laughed outright.

"Listen, I've told you I won't go away without an answer!" Ivan cried.

"Why do you keep pestering me? Why do you torment me?" said Smerdyakov, with a look of suffering.

"Damn it! I've nothing to do with you. Just answer my question and I'll go away."

"I've no answer to give you," said Smerdyakov, looking down again.

"You may be sure I'll make you answer!"

"Why are you so uneasy?" Smerdyakov stared at him, not simply with contempt, but almost with a kind of repulsion. "Is this because the trial begins to-morrow? Nothing will happen to you, can't you believe that at last? Go home, go to bed and sleep in peace, don't be afraid of anything."

"I don't understand you. . . . What have I to be afraid of to-morrow?" Ivan articulated in astonishment, and suddenly a chill breath of fear did in fact pass over his soul. Smerdyakov measured him with his eyes.

"You don't understand?" he drawled reproachfully. "It's a strange thing a clever man should care to play such a farce!"

Ivan looked at him, speechless. The startling, incredibly supercilious tone of this man, who had once been his valet, was extraordinary in itself. He had not taken such a tone even at their last interview.

"I tell you, you've nothing to fear. I won't say anything about you, there's no evidence against you. I say, how your hands are trembling. Why are your fingers twitching like that? Go home, *you* did not kill."

Ivan started. He remembered Alyosha.

"I know it was not I," he faltered.

"Do you?" Smerdyakov caught him up again.

Ivan jumped up and seized him by the shoulder. "Say everything, you reptile! Say everything!"

Smerdyakov was not in the least scared. He only riveted his eyes on Ivan with insane hatred.

"Well, it was you who murdered him, if that's the case," he whispered furiously.

Ivan sank back in his chair, as though pondering something. He grinned angrily.

"You mean my going away. What you talked about last time?"

"You stood before me last time and understood it all, and you understand it now, too."

"All I understand is that you are mad."

"Aren't you tired of it? Here we are face to face; what's the use of fooling each other and keeping up a farce? Are you still trying to put it all on me, to my face? *You* killed; you are the real murderer, I was only your accomplice, your faithful servant, and it was at your word I did it."

"*Did* it? Why, did you kill?" Ivan turned cold.

Something seemed to give way in his brain, and he shuddered all over with a cold shiver. Then Smerdyakov himself looked at him wonderingly; probably the genuineness of Ivan's horror struck him.

"You don't mean to say you really did not know?" he faltered mistrustfully, looking with a crooked smile into his eyes. Ivan still stared at him, and seemed unable to speak.

Ah, Vanka's gone to Petersburg
I won't wait till he comes back,

suddenly echoed in his head.

"Do you know, I am afraid that you are a dream, a ghost sitting before me," he muttered.

"There's no ghost here, sir, but only us two and one other. No doubt he is here, that third, between us."

"Who is he? Who is here? What third person?" Ivan cried in alarm, looking about him, his eyes hastily searching every corner.

"That third is God Himself, sir, Providence. He is the third beside us now. Only don't look for him, sir, you won't find him."

"It's a lie that you killed him!" Ivan cried madly. "You are mad, or teasing me as you did last time!"

Smerdyakov, as before, watched him curiously, with no sign of fear. He could still scarcely get over his incredulity; he still fancied that Ivan knew everything and was merely pretending in order to "put it all on him to his face."

"Wait a minute, sir," he said at last in a weak voice, and suddenly bringing up his left leg from under the table, he began tucking up his trouser leg. He was wearing long white stockings and slippers. Without haste Smerdyakov took off his garter and thrust his fingers down into his stocking. Ivan stared at him, and suddenly shuddered in a paroxysm of terror.

"He's mad!" he cried, and, rapidly jumping up, he drew back, so that he knocked his back against the wall and stood up against it, stiff and straight. He looked with insane terror at Smerdyakov, who, entirely unaffected by his terror, continued fumbling in his stocking, as though he were making an effort to get hold of something with his fingers and pull it out. At last he got hold of it and began pulling it out. Ivan saw that it was a piece of paper, or perhaps a roll of papers. Smerdyakov pulled it out and laid it on the table.

"Here, sir," he said quietly.

"What is it?" responded Ivan, trembling.

"Kindly look at it, sir," Smerdyakov answered, still in the same low tone.

Ivan stepped up to the table, took up the

roll of paper and began unfolding it, but suddenly he drew back his fingers, as though from contact with a loathsome, fearful reptile.

"Your hands keep twitching, sir," observed Smerdyakov, and he deliberately unfolded the bundle himself. In the wrapper were three packets of hundred-rouble notes.

"They are all here, sir, all the three thousand roubles; you need not count them. Take them, sir," Smerdyakov suggested to Ivan, nodding at the notes. Ivan sank back in his chair. He was as white as a handkerchief.

"You frightened me . . . with your stocking," he said, with a strange grin.

"Can you really not have known till now?" Smerdyakov asked once more.

"No, I did not know. I kept thinking of Dmitri. Brother, brother! Ah!" He suddenly clutched his head in both hands. "Listen. Did you kill him alone? With my brother's help or without?"

"It was only with you, sir, together with you, I killed him, and Dmitri Fyodorovich is quite innocent."

"All right, all right. Talk about me later. Why do I keep on trembling? I can't speak properly."

"You were bold enough then, sir. You said 'everything is permitted,' and how frightened you are now," Smerdyakov muttered in surprise. "Won't you have some lemonade? I'll order some at once. It's very refreshing. Only I must hide this first."

And again he motioned towards the notes. He was just going to get up and call at the door to Marya Kondratyevna to make some lemonade and serve it, but, looking for something to cover up the notes that she might not see them, he first took out his handkerchief, and, as it turned out to be very dirty, took up the big yellow book that Ivan had noticed at first lying on the table, and put it over the notes. The book was "The Sayings of our Holy Father Isaac the Syrian." Ivan read the title mechanically.

"I won't have any lemonade," he said. "Of me later. Sit down and tell me how you did it. Tell me all about it."

"You'd better take off your greatcoat, sir, or you'll be too hot." Ivan, as though he'd only just thought of it, tore off his coat, and, without getting up from his chair, threw it on the bench. "Speak, please, speak."

He seemed calmer. He waited, feeling sure that Smerdyakov would tell him *all* now.

"How it was done?" sighed Smerdyakov. "It was done in a most natural way, sir, in accordance with your very words."

"Of my words later," Ivan broke in again, apparently with complete self-possession, speaking firmly, and not shouting as before. "Only tell me in detail how you did it. Everything, as it happened. Don't forget anything. The details, above everything, the details, I beg you."

"You'd gone away, sir, then I fell into the cellar."

"In a fit or did you sham?"

"I shammed, naturally. I shammed it all. I went quietly down the steps to the very bottom and lay down quietly, and as I lay down I gave a scream, and struggled, till they carried me out."

"Wait! And were you shamming all along, afterwards, and in the hospital?"

"No, not at all. Next day, in the morning, before they took me to the hospital, I had a real attack, and a more violent one than I've had for years. For two days I was quite unconscious."

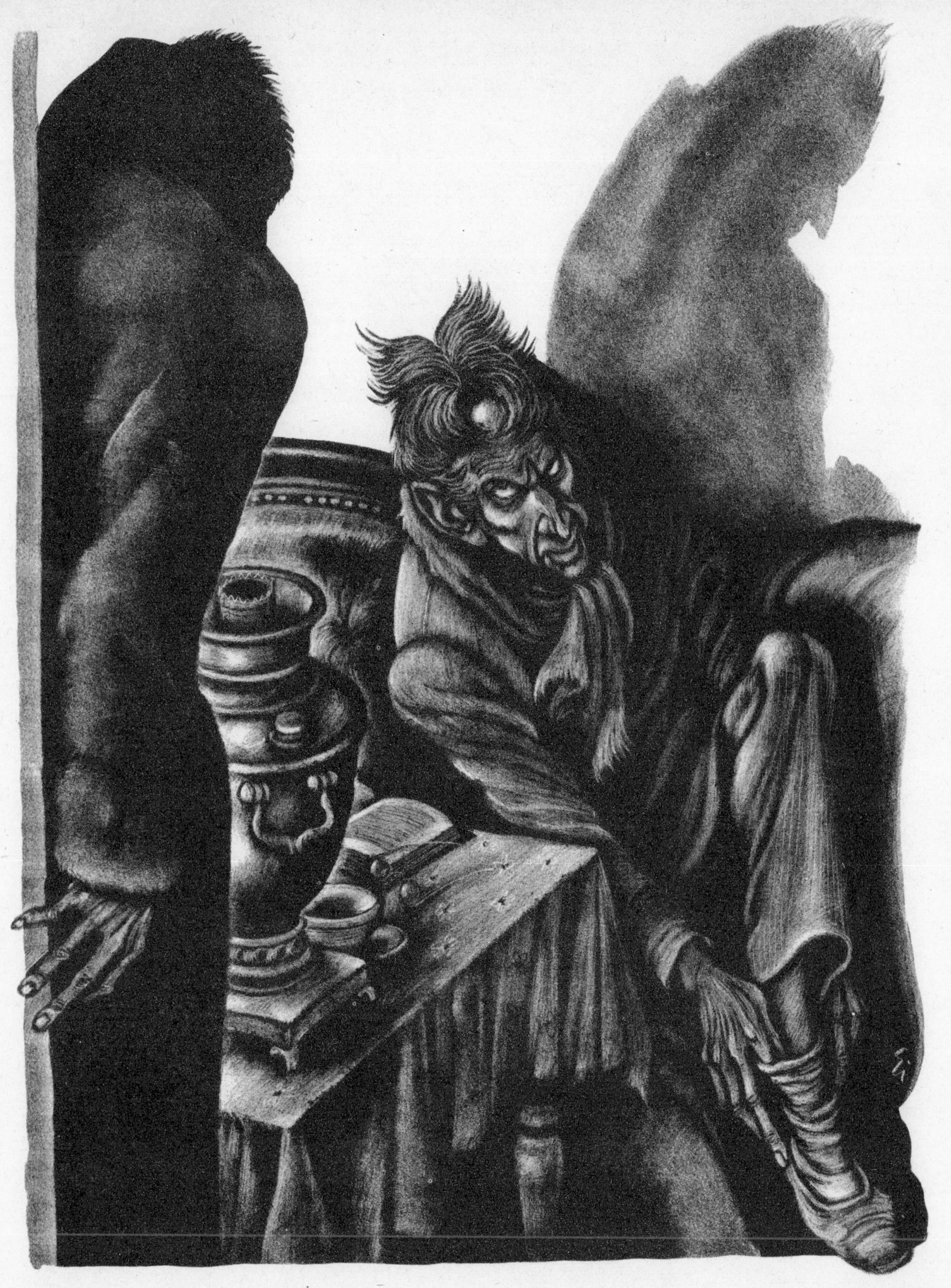

LAST INTERVIEW WITH SMERDYAKOV

"All right, all right. Go on."

"They laid me on this cot. I knew I'd be the other side of the partition, for whenever I was ill Marfa Ignatyevna used to put me there, near them. She's always been very kind to me from my birth up. At night I moaned, but quietly. I kept expecting Dmitri Fyodorovich to come."

"Expecting him? To come to you?"

"Not to me. I expected him to come into the house, for I'd no doubt that he'd come that night, for being without me and getting no news, he'd be sure to come and climb over the fence, as he used to and do something or other."

"And if he hadn't come?"

"Then nothing would have happened, sir. I should never have brought myself to it without him."

"All right, all right . . . speak more intelligibly, don't hurry; above all, don't leave anything out!"

"I expected him to kill Fyodor Pavlovich. I thought that was certain, for I had prepared him for it . . . during the last few days. . . . He knew about the knocks, that was the chief thing. With his suspiciousness and the fury which had been growing in him all those days, he was bound to get into the house by means of those taps. That was inevitable, so I was expecting him, sir."

"Wait," Ivan interrupted, "if he had killed him, he would have taken the money and carried it away; that's how you must have reasoned. What would you have got by it afterwards? I don't see."

"But he would never have found the money. That was only what I told him, that the money was under the mattress. But that wasn't true, sir. At first it was lying in a drawer, that's how it was. And afterwards I suggested to Fyodor Pavlovich, as I was the only person he trusted, to hide the envelope with the notes in the corner behind the ikons, for no one would have guessed that place, especially if he came in a hurry. So that's where the envelope lay, in the corner behind the ikons, sir. It would have been absurd to keep it under the mattress, the drawer, anyway, could be locked. But everybody here believes it was under the mattress. A stupid idea. So if Dmitri Fyodorovich had committed the murder, finding nothing, he would either have run away in a hurry, afraid of every sound, as always happens with murderers, or he would have been arrested. So I could always have clambered up to the ikons and have taken away the money next morning or even that night, and it would have all been blamed on Dmitri Fyodorovich. I could reckon. upon that."

"But what if he would not have killed him, but only stunned him?"

"If he would not have killed him, of course, I would not have dared to take the money, and nothing would have happened. But I calculated that he would beat him senseless, and I should have time to take it then, and then I'd make out to Fyodor Pavlovich that it was no one but Dmitri Fyodorovich who had taken the money after giving him a thrashing."

"Stop . . . I am getting mixed. Then it was Dmitri after all who killed him, you only took the money?"

"No, he didn't kill him, sir. Of course, I could tell you even now that he is the murderer. . . . But I don't want to lie to you now, because . . . because if you really haven't understood till now, as I see for myself, and have not been pretending, so as to put your guilt on me to my very face, you are still responsible for it all, sir, since you knew of the murder and charged me to do it, and went away knowing all about it. And so I want to prove to your face this evening that you are the chief murderer in the whole affair, and I am the merest accomplice, although it was I who did the killing. It is you who are the rightful murderer."

"Why, why, am I the murderer? Oh, God!" Ivan cried, unable to restrain himself at last, and forgetting that he had put off discussing himself till the end of the conversation. "You still mean that Chermashnya business? Wait, tell me, why did you want my consent, if you really took Chermashnya for consent? How will you explain that now?"

"Assured of your consent, I should have known that you wouldn't have made an outcry over those three thousand being lost, even if the authorities had suspected me, instead of Dmitri Fyodorovich, or as his accomplice; on the contrary, you would have protected me from others. . . . And when you got your inheritance you could have rewarded me now and again, all the rest of your life. For you'd have received your inheritance through me, seeing that if he had married Agrafena Alexandrovna, you'd have gotten nothing."

"Ah! Then you intended to pester me all my life afterwards," snarled Ivan. "And what if I hadn't gone away then, but had informed against you?"

"What could you have said? That I persuaded you to go to Chermashnya? That's all nonsense. Besides, after our conversation you would either have gone away or have stayed. If you had stayed, nothing would have happened. I should have known that you didn't want it done, and should have attempted nothing. As you went away, it meant you assured me that you wouldn't dare to inform against me at the trial, and that you'd overlook my having the three thousand. And, indeed, you couldn't have prosecuted me afterwards, because then I should have told it all in the court; that is, not that I had stolen the money or killed him — I shouldn't have said that — but that you'd put me up to the theft and the murder, though I didn't consent to it. That's why I needed your consent, so that you couldn't have cornered me afterwards, for what proof could you have had? I could always have cornered you, revealing your eagerness for your father's death, and I give you my word the public would all have believed it, and you would have been ashamed for the rest of your life."

"Was I so eager then, was I?" Ivan said again, gnashing his teeth.

"To be sure you were, and by your consent, sir, you silently permitted me to do the deed." Smerdyakov looked resolutely at Ivan. He was very weak and spoke softly and wearily, but some hidden inner force urged him on. He evidently had some design. Ivan felt that.

"Go on," he said. "Go on telling me what happened that night."

"What more is there to tell! I lay there and I thought I heard the master shout. And before that Grigory Vasilyevich had suddenly got up and came out, and he suddenly gave a scream, and then all was silence and darkness. I lay there waiting, my heart beating; I couldn't bear it. I got up at last, went out. I saw the window open on the left into the garden, and I stepped to the left to listen and find out whether he was alive there, and I heard the master moving about, sighing, so I knew he was alive. Well! I thought. I went to the window and shouted to the master, 'It's I.' And he shouted to me, 'He's been, he's been; he's run away.' He meant Dmitri Fyodorovich had been there. 'He's killed Grigory!' 'Where?' I whispered. 'There, in the corner,' he pointed. He was whispering, too. 'Wait a bit,' I said. I went to the corner of the garden to look, and there I came upon Grigory Vasilyevich lying by the wall, covered with blood, senseless. So it's true that Dmitri Fyodorovich has been here, was the thought that came into my head, and I determined on the spot to make an end of it, as Grigory Vasilyevich, even if he were alive, would see nothing of it, as he lay there senseless. The only risk was that Marfa Ignatyevna might wake up. I felt that at the moment, but this desire seized me, till I could scarcely breathe. I went back to the window to the master and said, 'She's here, she's come; Agrafena Alexandrovna has come, wants to be let in.' He started like a baby. 'Where is she, where?' he fairly gasped, but couldn't believe it. 'She's standing there,' said I, 'open.' He looked at me through the window, half believing and half distrustful, but afraid to open. 'Why, it's me he is afraid of now,' I thought. And here is a funny thing: I had the idea of tapping on the window frame before his eyes, the taps that meant, as we'd agreed, that Grushenka had come. He didn't seem to believe my words, but as soon as he heard the taps, he ran at once to open the door. He opened it. I would have gone in, but he stood in the way to prevent me passing. 'Where is she? Where is she?' He looked at me, all of a tremble. Well, thought I, if he's so frightened of me as all that, it's a bad look-out! And my legs went weak with the fear that he wouldn't let me in or would call out, or Marfa Ignatyevna would run up, or something else might happen. I don't remember now, but I must have stood pale, facing him. I whispered to him, 'Why, she's there, there, under the window, how is it you don't see her?' I said. 'Bring her then, bring her.' 'She's afraid,' said I, 'she was frightened at the noise, she's hidden in the bushes; go and call to her yourself from the study.' He ran to the window, put the candle in the window. 'Grushenka,' he cried, 'Grushenka, are you there?' Though he cried that, he didn't want to lean out of the window, he didn't want to move away from me, for he was panic-stricken; he was so afraid of me that he didn't dare to move away from me. 'Why, here she is,' said I. I went up to the window and leaned right out of it. 'Here she is, she's in the bushes, smiling at you, don't you see her?' He suddenly believed it; he was all of a shake — he was so madly in love with her — and he leaned right out of the window. I snatched up that iron paper weight from his table — do you remember it, sir? — weighing about three pounds. I swung it and hit him on the pate with the corner of it. He didn't even cry out. He only sank down suddenly, and I hit him again and a third time. And the third time I knew I'd broken his skull. He suddenly rolled on his back, face upwards, covered with blood. I looked round. There was no blood on me, not a spot. I wiped the paper weight, put it back, went up to the ikons, took the money out of the envelope, and flung the envelope on the floor and the pink ribbon beside it. I went out into the garden all of a tremble, straight to the apple tree with a hollow in it — you know that hollow. I'd marked it long before and had a rag and a piece of paper ready in it. I wrapped all the notes in the paper and then in the rag and stuffed it deep down into the hole. And there it stayed for over a fortnight. I took it out later, when I came out of the hospital. I went back to my bed, lay down and thought in fear, 'If Grigory Vasilyevich has been killed outright, it may be a bad job for me, but if he is not killed and recovers, it will be first rate, for then he'll bear witness that Dmitri Fyodorovich has been here, and so he must have killed him and taken the money.' Then I began groaning with suspense and impatience, so as to wake Marfa Ignatyevna as soon as possible. At last she got up, and she rushed to me, but when she saw Grigory Vasilyevich was not there, she ran out, and I heard her scream in the garden. And that set it all going and put my mind at rest."

He stopped. Ivan had listened all the time in dead silence without stirring or taking his eyes off him. As he told his story Smerdyakov glanced at him from time to time, but for the most part kept his eyes averted. When he had finished he was evidently agitated and was breathing hard. The perspiration stood out on his face. But it was impossible to tell whether it was remorse he was feeling, or what.

"Wait," cried Ivan, pondering. "What about the door? If he only opened the door to you, how could Grigory have seen it open before? For Grigory saw it before you went."

It was remarkable that Ivan spoke quite amicably, in a different tone, not angry as before, so if any one had opened the door at that moment and peeped in at them, he would certainly have concluded that they were talking peaceably about some ordinary, though interesting, subject.

"As for that door and Grigory Vasilyevich's having seen it open, that's only his fancy," said Smerdyakov, with a wry smile. "He is not a man, I assure you, but an obstinate nag. He didn't see it, but fancied he had seen it, and there's no shaking him. It's just your luck and mine that he took that notion into his head, for they can't fail to convict Dmitri Fyodorovich after that."

"Listen . . ." said Ivan, beginning to seem bewildered again and making an effort to grasp something. "Listen. There are a lot of questions I want to ask you, but I forget them . . . I keep forgetting and getting mixed up. Yes. Tell me this at least, why did you open the envelope and leave it there on the floor? Why didn't you simply carry off the envelope? . . . When you were telling me, I thought you spoke about it as though it were the right thing to do . . . but why, I can't understand . . ."

"I did that for a good reason, sir. For if a man had known all about it, as I did for instance, if he'd seen those notes before, and perhaps had put them in that envelope himself, and had seen the envelope sealed up and addressed, with his own eyes, if such a man had done the murder, what should have made him tear open the envelope afterwards, especially in such desperate haste, since he'd know for certain the notes must be in the envelope? No, if the robber had been some one like me, he'd simply have put the envelope straight in his pocket without opening it and got away with it as fast as he could. But it'd be quite different with Dmitri Fyodorovich. He only knew about the envelope by hearsay; he had not seen it, and if he'd found it, for instance, under the mattress, he'd have torn it open as quickly as possible to make sure the notes were in it. And he'd have thrown the envelope down, without having time to think that it would be evidence against him. Because he was not an habitual thief and had never directly stolen anything before, for he is a gentleman born, and if he did bring himself to steal, it would not be regular stealing, but simply taking what was his own, for he'd told the whole town he meant to before, and had even bragged aloud before every one that he'd go and take his property from Fyodor Pavlovich. I didn't say that openly to the prosecutor when I was being examined, but quite the contrary, I brought him to it by a hint, as though I didn't see it myself, and as though he'd thought of it himself and I hadn't prompted him; so that Mr. Prosecutor's mouth positively watered at my suggestion."

"But can you possibly have thought of all that on the spot?" cried Ivan, overcome with astonishment. He looked at Smerdyakov again with alarm.

"Mercy on us! Could any one think of it all in such a desperate hurry? It was all thought out beforehand."

"Well . . . well, it was the devil helped you!" Ivan cried again. "No, you are not a fool, you are far cleverer than I thought . . ."

He got up, obviously intending to walk across the room. He was in terrible distress. But as the table blocked his way, and there was hardly room to pass between the table and the wall, he only turned round where he stood and sat down again. Perhaps the impossibility of moving irritated him, as he suddenly cried out almost as furiously as before.

"Listen, you miserable, contemptible man! Don't you understand that if I haven't killed you, it's simply because I am keeping you to answer to-morrow at the trial? God sees," Ivan raised his hand, "perhaps I, too, was guilty; perhaps I really had a secret desire for my father's . . . death, but I swear I was not as guilty as you think, and perhaps I didn't urge you on at all. No, no, I didn't urge you on! But no matter, I will give evidence against myself to-morrow, at the trial. I'm determined to! I shall tell everything, everything. But we'll make our appearance together. And whatever you may say against me at the trial, whatever evidence you give, I'll face it, I am not afraid of you. I'll confirm it all myself! But you must confess, too! You must, you must, we'll go together. That's how it shall be!"

Ivan said this solemnly and forcefully, and from his flashing eyes alone it could be seen that it would be so.

"You are ill, sir, I see, you are quite ill. Your eyes are yellow, sir," Smerdyakov commented, without the least irony, with apparent sympathy in fact.

"We'll go together," Ivan repeated. "And if you won't go, no matter, I'll confess alone."

Smerdyakov paused as though pondering.

"There'll be nothing of the sort, and you won't go, sir," he concluded at last with finality.

"You don't understand me," Ivan exclaimed reproachfully.

"You'll be too much ashamed, if you confess it all. And, what's more, it will be no use at all, for I shall say straight out that I never said anything of the sort to you, and that you are either ill (and it looks like it, too), or that you're so sorry for your brother that you are sacrificing yourself to save him and have invented it all against me, for you've always thought no more of me than if I'd been a fly and not a human being. And who will believe you, and what single proof have you got?"

"Listen, you showed me those notes just now to convince me."

Smerdyakov lifted the book off the notes and laid it on one side.

"Take that money away with you," Smerdyakov sighed.

"Of course I shall take it. But why do you give it to me, if you committed the murder for the sake of it?" Ivan looked at him with great surprise.

"I don't want it," Smerdyakov articulated in a shaking voice, with a gesture of refusal. "I did have an idea of beginning a new life with that money in Moscow or, better still, abroad. I did dream of it, chiefly because 'everything is permitted.' That was quite right what you taught me, sir, for you talked a lot to me about that. For if there's no infinite God, there's no such thing as virtue, and there's no need of it. You were right there. So that's how I looked at it."

"Did you reach that conclusion by yourself?" asked Ivan, with a wry smile.

"With your guidance, sir."

"And now, I suppose, you believe in God, since you are giving back the money?"

"No, I don't believe," whispered Smerdyakov.

"Then why are you giving it back?"

"Leave off . . . that's enough!" Smerdyakov waved his hand again. "You used to say yourself that everything was lawful, so now why are you so upset, too? You even want to go and give evidence against yourself. . . . Only there'll be nothing of the sort! You won't go to give evidence," Smerdyakov decided with conviction.

"You'll see," said Ivan.

"It isn't possible. You are very clever. You are fond of money, I know that. You like to be respected, too, for you're very proud; you are far too fond of female charms, too, and you care most of all about living in undisturbed comfort, without having to depend on any one — that's what you care most about. You won't want to spoil your life for ever by taking such a disgrace on yourself. You are like Fyodor Pavlovich, you are more like him than any of his children; you've the same soul as he had."

"You are not a fool," said Ivan, as though struck. The blood rushed to his face. "I used to think you were a fool. You are serious now!" he observed, looking suddenly at Smerdyakov with a different expression.

"It was your pride made you think I was a fool. Take the money."

Ivan took the three rolls of notes and put them in his pocket without wrapping them in anything.

"I shall show them at court to-morrow," he said.

"Nobody will believe you, as you've plenty of money of your own; you may simply have taken it out of your cash-box and brought it to court."

Ivan rose from his seat.

"I repeat," he said, "the only reason I haven't killed you is that I need you for to-morrow, remember that, don't forget it!"

"Well, kill me. Kill me now," Smerdyakov said, all at once looking strangely at Ivan. "You won't dare do that even!" he added, with a bitter smile. "You won't dare to do anything, you, who used to be so bold!"

"Till to-morrow," cried Ivan, and moved to go out.

"Wait a moment. . . . Show me those notes again."

Ivan took out the notes and showed them to him. Smerdyakov looked at them for ten seconds. "Well, you can go," he said, with a wave of his hand. "Ivan Fyodorovich!" he called after him again.

"What do you want?" Ivan turned without stopping.

"Farewell!" "Till to-morrow!" Ivan cried again, and he walked out of the cottage.

The snowstorm was still raging. He walked the first few steps boldly, but suddenly began staggering, as it were. "It's something physical," he thought, with a grin. Something like joy was springing up in his heart. He was conscious of unbounded resolution; he would make an end of the wavering that had so tortured him of late. His determination was taken, "and now it will not be changed," he thought with happiness. At that moment he stumbled against something and almost fell down. Stopping short, he made out at his feet the peasant he had knocked down, still lying senseless and motionless. The snow had covered his face. Ivan seized him and lifted him in his arms. Seeing a light in the little house to the right he went up, knocked at the shutters, and asked the man to whom the house belonged to help him carry the peasant to the police-station, promising him three roubles. The man got ready and came out. I won't describe in detail how Ivan succeeded in his object, bringing the peasant to the police-station and arranging for a doctor to see him at once, providing with a liberal hand for the expenses. I will only say that this business took a whole hour, but Ivan was well content with it. His mind wandered and worked incessantly.

"If I had not taken my decision so firmly about to-morrow," he reflected with delight, "I should not have stayed a whole hour to look after the peasant, but should have passed by, without caring about his being frozen. I am quite capable of watching myself, by the way," he thought at the same instant, with still greater delight, "although they have decided that I am going out of my mind!"

Just as he reached his own house he stopped short, asking himself suddenly hadn't he better go at once now to the prosecutor and tell him everything. He decided the question by turning back to the house. "Everything together to-morrow!" he whispered to himself, and, strange to say, almost all his gladness and self-satisfaction passed in one instant.

As he entered his own room he felt something like a touch of ice on his heart, like a recollection or, more exactly, a reminder, of something agonising and revolting that was in that room now, at that moment, and had been there before. He sank wearily on his sofa. The old woman brought him a samovar; he made tea, but did not touch it. He sent the old woman away for the night. He sat on the sofa and felt giddy. He felt that he was ill and helpless. He was beginning to drop asleep, but got up uneasily and walked across the room to shake off his drowsiness. At moments he fancied he was delirious, but it was not illness that he thought of most. Sitting down again, he began looking round, as though searching for something. This happened several times. At last his eyes were fastened intently on one point. Ivan smiled, but an angry flush suffused his face. He sat a long time in his place, his head propped on both arms, though he looked sideways at the same point, at the sofa that stood against the opposite wall. There was evidently something, some object, that irritated him there, worried him and tormented him.

CHAPTER IX

THE DEVIL. IVAN'S NIGHTMARE

I AM not a doctor, and yet I feel that the moment has come when I positively must give the reader some account of the nature of Ivan

Fyodorovich's illness. Anticipating events, I shall say at least one thing: he was at that moment on the very eve of an attack of brain fever. Though his health had long been affected, it had offered a stubborn resistance to the fever which in the end gained complete mastery over it. Though I know nothing of medicine, I venture to hazard the suggestion that he really had perhaps, by a terrible effort of will, succeeded in delaying the attack for a time, hoping, of course, to check it completely. He knew that he was unwell, but he loathed the thought of being ill at that fatal time, at the approaching crisis in his life, when he needed to have all his presence of mind, to say what he had to say boldly and resolutely and "to justify himself to himself."

He had, however, consulted the new doctor, who had been brought from Moscow thanks to a fantastic notion of Katerina Ivanovna's, to which I have referred already. After listening to him and examining him the doctor came to the conclusion that he was actually suffering from some disorder of the brain, and was not at all surprised by an admission which Ivan had reluctantly made him. "Hallucinations are quite likely in your condition," the doctor opined, "though it would be better to verify them . . . you must have yourself treated seriously at once, without a moment's delay, or things will go badly with you." But Ivan did not follow this judicious advice and did not take to his bed to be nursed. "I am still on my feet, I am still strong enough; if I drop, it'll be different then, any one may treat me who likes," he decided, dismissing the subject with a wave of the hand.

And so he was sitting almost conscious himself of his delirium and, as I have said already, looking persistently at some object on the sofa against the opposite wall. Suddenly some one proved to be sitting there, though goodness knows how he had come in, for he had not been in the room when Ivan came into it, on his return from Smerdyakov. This was a man or, more accurately speaking, a Russian gentleman of a certain kind, no longer young, *qui frisait la cinquantaine*, as the French say, with rather long, still thick, dark hair, slightly streaked with grey, and a small pointed beard. He was wearing a brownish jacket, evidently made by a good tailor though already shabby, made perhaps three years ago and quite out of fashion, so that smart and well-to-do people had not been wearing this style for the last two years. His linen and his long neck-tie in the form of a scarf were all such as are worn by gentlemen who aim at being stylish, but on closer inspection his linen was not over-clean and his wide scarf was very threadbare. The visitor's check trousers fitted admirably, but were too light in colour and too tight for the present fashion. His soft fluffy white hat was out of keeping with the season.

In brief, there was every appearance of gentility on straitened means. It looked as though the gentleman belonged to that class of lily-handed landowners who used to flourish in the days of serfdom. He had unmistakably been, at some time, in fashionable society, had once had good connections, had possibly preserved them indeed, but, after a gay youth, becoming gradually impoverished on the abolition of serfdom, he had sunk into the position of a hanger-on of the better class, wandering from one good old friend to another and received by them for his companionable and accommodating disposition and as being, after all, a gentleman who could be asked to sit down with any one, though, of course, not in

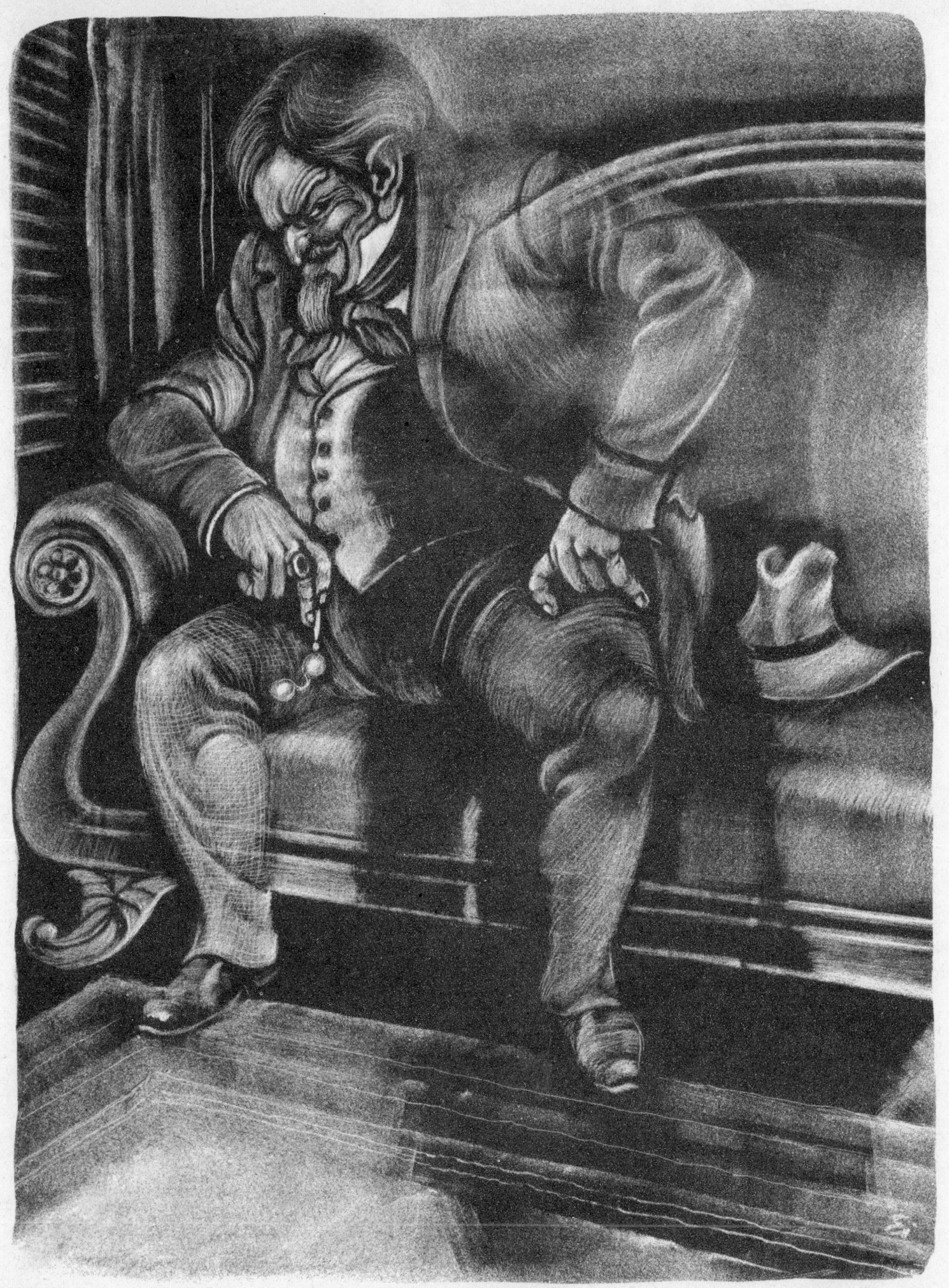

IVAN AND THE DEVIL

a place of honour. Such hangers-on, gentlemen of accommodating temper, who can tell a story, take a hand at cards, and who have a distinct aversion for any commissions if they are forced upon them, are usually solitary creatures, either bachelors or widowers. Sometimes they have children, but, if so, the children are always being brought up at a distance, at some aunt's, to whom these gentlemen never allude in good society, as though somewhat ashamed of the relationship. They gradually lose sight of their children altogether, though at intervals they receive a birthday or Christmas letter from them and sometimes even answer it.

The countenance of the unexpected visitor was not so much good-natured as accommodating and ready to assume any amiable expression as occasion might arise. He had no watch, but he had a tortoise-shell lorgnette on a black ribbon. On the middle finger of his right hand was a massive gold ring with a cheap opal stone in it.

Ivan was angrily silent and would not begin the conversation. The visitor waited and sat exactly like a dependant who had come down from his room to keep his host company at tea, and was discreetly silent, seeing that his host was frowning and preoccupied. But he was ready for any affable conversation as soon as his host should begin it. All at once his face expressed a sudden solicitude.

"I say," he began to Ivan, "excuse me, I only mention it to remind you. You went to Smerdyakov's to find out about Katerina Ivanovna, but you came away without having found out anything about her, you probably forgot . . ."

"Ah, yes," broke from Ivan and his face grew gloomy with care. "Yes, I'd forgotten . . . but it doesn't matter now, never mind, let it all wait till to-morrow," he muttered to himself; "and you," he added, addressing his visitor, "I should have remembered that myself in a minute, for that was just what was tormenting me! Why did you pop up, do you think I'm going to believe that you prompted me, and that I didn't remember it of myself?"

"Don't believe it then," said the gentleman, smiling affably, "what's the good of forcing yourself to believe? Besides, proofs do not help one to believe, especially material proofs. Thomas believed, not because he saw Christ risen, but because he wanted to believe, before he saw. Look at the spiritists, for instance. . . . I am very fond of them . . . only fancy, they imagine that they are serving the cause of religion, because the devils show them their horns from the other world. That, they say, is a material proof, so to speak, of the existence of the hereafter. The hereafter and material proofs, tra-la-la! And if you come to that, does proving there's a devil prove that there's a God? I want to join a society of idealists, I'll lead the opposition in it, I'll say I am a realist, and not a materialist, he-he!"

"Listen." Ivan suddenly got up from the table. "I seem to be delirious . . . I am delirious, in fact, talk any nonsense you like, I don't care! You won't drive me to fury, as you did last time. But I feel somehow ashamed . . . I want to walk about the room . . . I sometimes don't see you and don't even hear your voice as I did last time, but I always guess what you are gabbling, for it's I, *I myself speaking, not you*. Only I don't know whether I was dreaming last time or whether I really saw you. I'll wet a towel and put it on my head and perhaps you'll vanish into thin air."

Ivan went into the corner, took a towel, and

did as he said, and with a wet towel on his head began walking up and down the room.

"I am so glad that from the first we have been on terms of familiarity," the visitor began.

"Fool," laughed Ivan, "do you suppose I should stand on ceremony with you? I am in good spirits now, though I've a pain in my temple . . . and in the top of my head . . . only please don't talk philosophy, as you did last time. If you can't take yourself off, talk of something amusing. Give me some gossip, you are a hanger-on, you ought to gossip. What a nightmare to have! But I am not afraid of you. I'll get the better of you. I won't be taken to a mad-house!"

"*C'est charmant*, hanger-on. Yes, I am in my natural shape. For what am I on earth but a hanger-on? By the way, I am listening to you and am rather surprised to find you are actually beginning to take me for something real, not simply your fancy, as you persisted in declaring last time . . ."

"Never for one minute have I taken you for reality," Ivan cried with a sort of fury. "You are a lie, you are my illness, you are a phantom. It's only that I don't know how to destroy you and I see I must suffer for a time. You are my hallucination. You are the incarnation of myself, but only of one side of me . . . of my thoughts and feelings, but only the nastiest and stupidest of them. From that point of view you might be of interest to me, if only I had time to be bothered with you . . ."

"Excuse me, excuse me, I'll show you up. When you flew out at Alyosha at the lamppost this evening and shouted to him, 'You learnt it from *him!* How do you know that *he* visits me?' you were thinking of me then. So for one brief moment you did believe that I really exist." The gentleman laughed blandly.

"Yes, that was a moment of weakness . . . but I couldn't believe in you. I don't know whether I was asleep or awake last time. Perhaps I was only dreaming then and didn't see you really at all . . ."

"And why were you so harsh with Alyosha just now? He is a dear; I've wronged him over Father Zosima."

"Don't talk of Alyosha! How dare you, you flunkey!" Ivan laughed again.

"You scold me, but you laugh — that's a good sign. But to-night you are ever so much more polite to me than you were last time and I know why: that great resolution of yours."

"Don't speak of my resolution," cried Ivan savagely.

"I understand, I understand, *c'est noble, c'est charmant*, you are going to defend your brother to-morrow and to sacrifice yourself . . . *C'est chevaleresque*."

"Hold your tongue, I'll kick you!"

"I shan't be altogether sorry, for then my object will be attained. If you kick me, you must believe in my reality, for people don't kick ghosts. Joking apart, it doesn't matter to me, scold if you like, though it's better to be a trifle more polite even to me. 'Fool, flunkey!' what words!"

"Scolding you, I scold myself," Ivan laughed again, "you are myself, myself, only with a different mug. You just say what I am thinking . . . and are incapable of saying anything new!"

"If my way of thinking agrees with you, it's all to my credit," the gentleman declared, with delicacy and dignity.

"You pick out only my worst thoughts, and what's more, the stupid ones. You are stupid and vulgar. You are awfully stupid. No, I can't bear you! What am I to do, what am I to do!" Ivan said through his clenched teeth.

"My friend, above all things I want to be a gentleman and to be recognised as such," the visitor began in an access of the good-humoured and conciliatory pride typical of a dependant. "I am poor, but . . . I won't say very honest, but . . . it's an axiom generally accepted in society that I am a fallen angel. By God! I can't conceive how I can ever have been an angel. If I was, it must have been so long ago that there's no sin in forgetting it. Now I prize only my reputation as a well-bred person and live as I can, trying to make myself agreeable. I love men genuinely, I've been much maligned! When from time to time I settle here among you, my life gains a kind of reality and that's what I like most of all. You see, like you, the fantastic makes me suffer, and so I love your earthly realism. Here, with you, everything is circumscribed, here everything is formula, geometry, while with us it's all indeterminate equations! I wander about here dreaming. I love dreaming. Besides, on earth I become superstitious. Please don't laugh, that's just what I like, to become superstitious. I adopt all your habits here: I've grown fond of going to the public baths, would you believe it, and I enjoy steaming myself with merchants and priests. My dream is to become incarnate once for all and irrevocably in the form of some merchant's wife weighing two hundred and fifty pounds, and to believe all she believes. My ideal is to go to church and offer a candle in simple-hearted faith, I swear by God it is. Then there would be an end to my sufferings. I like being doctored, too; in the spring there was an outbreak of smallpox and I went and was vaccinated in a foundling hospital — if only you knew how I enjoyed myself that day. I subscribed ten roubles to the cause of the Slavs! . . . But you are not listening. Do you know, you are not yourself to-night," the gentleman said, after a pause. "I know you went yesterday to that doctor . . . well, what about your health? What did the doctor say?"

"Fool!" Ivan snapped out.

"But you're a clever one. You are scolding again? I didn't ask out of sympathy, but just like that. You needn't answer. Now rheumatism has come in again . . ."

"Fool!" repeated Ivan.

"You keep saying the same thing; but I had such an attack of rheumatism last year that I still remember it."

"The devil has rheumatism?"

"Why not, if I sometimes become incarnate? I become incarnate and I take the consequences. Satan *sum et nihil humanum a me alienum puto*."

"What, what? Satan *sum et nihil humanum* . . . that's not bad for the devil!"

"I am glad I've pleased you at last."

"But you didn't get that from me." Ivan stopped suddenly, seeming struck. "That never entered my head, that's strange."

"*C'est du nouveau, n'est ce pas?* This time I'll act honestly and explain it to you. Listen, in dreams and especially in nightmares, from indigestion or whatever it may be, a man sometimes has such artistic dreams, so complex and realistic, so full of events, even a whole world of events, woven into such a plot, with such unexpected details from the most exalted matters to the last button on a cuff, as I swear Leo Tolstoy will never invent. Yet such dreams are sometimes dreamed not by novelists, but by the most ordinary people, officials, journalists, priests. . . . The subject is a complete enigma. A statesman confessed to me, indeed, that all his best ideas came to him when he was asleep. Well, that's how it is now, too, though I am your hallucination, yet, just as in a nightmare, I say original things which had not entered your head before. So I don't repeat your ideas, yet I am only your nightmare, nothing more."

"You are lying, your aim is to convince me you have an existence of your own, and are not my nightmare, and now you are asserting you are a dream."

"My dear fellow, I've adopted a peculiar method to-day, I'll explain it to you afterwards. Wait, where did I break off? Oh, yes! I caught cold then, only not here but yonder."

"Where is yonder? Tell me, will you be here long? Can't you go away?" Ivan exclaimed almost in despair. He ceased walking to and fro, sat down on the sofa, leaned his elbows on the table again and held his head tight in both hands. He pulled the wet towel off and flung it away in vexation. It was evidently of no use.

"Your nerves are out of order," observed the gentleman, with a carelessly easy, though perfectly friendly, air. "You are angry with me even for being able to catch cold, though it happened in a most natural way. I was hurrying to a diplomatic *soirée* at the house of a lady of high rank in Petersburg, who was aiming at influence in the Ministry. Well, evening dress, white tie, gloves, though I was God knows where and had to fly through space to reach your earth. . . . Of course, it took only an instant, but you know a ray of light from the sun takes a full eight minutes, and fancy in evening dress and open waistcoat. Spirits don't freeze, but when one is incarnate, well . . . in brief, I acted rashly, and set off, and you know in those ethereal spaces, in the waters that were above the firmament, there's such a frost . . . at least one can't call it frost, you can fancy, 150° below zero! You know the game the village girls play — they invite the unwary to lick an axe when it's 30° below, the tongue instantly freezes to it and the dupe tears the skin off, so it bleeds. But that's only when it's 30°, when it's 150° I imagine it would be enough to put your finger on the axe and it would be the end of it . . . if only there could be an axe there."

"And can there be an axe there?" Ivan interrupted, absent-mindedly and squeamishly. He was exerting himself to the utmost not to believe in the delusion and not to sink into complete insanity.

"An axe?" the guest interrupted in surprise.

"Yes, what would become of an axe there?" Ivan cried suddenly, with a sort of savage and insistent obstinacy.

"What would become of an axe in space? *Quelle idée!* If it were far enough away, it would begin, I think, to revolve round the earth without knowing why, like a satellite. The astronomers would calculate the rising and the setting of the axe, Gatzuk would put it in his almanac, that's all."

"You are stupid, awfully stupid," said Ivan peevishly. "Lie more cleverly or I won't listen. You want to get the better of me by realism, to convince me that you exist, but I don't want to believe you exist! I won't believe it!"

"But I am not lying, it's all the truth; the truth is unhappily hardly ever amusing. I see you persist in expecting something big of me, and perhaps something fine. That's a great pity, for I only give what I can . . ."

"Don't talk philosophy, you ass!"

"Philosophy, indeed, when all my right side is numb and I am moaning and groaning. I've tried the whole medical faculty: they can diagnose beautifully, they have the whole of your disease at their finger-tips, but they've no idea how to cure you. There was an enthusiastic little student here, 'Even if you die,' said he, 'you'll know perfectly well what disease you died of!' And then this way they have of sending you to specialists. 'We only diagnose,' they say, 'but go to such-and-such a specialist, he'll cure you.' The old doctor who used to cure all sorts of diseases has completely disappeared, I assure you, now there are only specialists and they all advertise in the newspapers. If anything is wrong with your nose, they send you to Paris: there, they say, is a European specialist who cures noses. If you go to Paris, he'll look at your nose; I can cure only your right nostril, he'll tell you, for I don't cure the left nostril, that's not my specialty, but go to Vienna, there there's a specialist who will cure your left nostril. What are you to do? I fell back on popular remedies, a German doctor advised me to rub myself with honey and salt in the bath-house. Solely to get an extra bath I went, smeared myself all over, and it did me no good at all. In despair I wrote to Count Mattei in Milan. He sent me a book and some drops, bless him, and, only fancy, Hoff's malt extract cured me! I bought it by accident, drank a bottle and a half of it, and I was ready to dance, it took it away completely. I made up my mind to write to the papers to thank him, I was prompted by a feeling of gratitude, and, only fancy, it led to no end of bother: not a single paper would take my letter. 'It would be very reactionary,' they said, 'no one will believe it. *Le diable n'existe point*. You'd better print it anonymously,' they advised me. What use is a letter of thanks if it's anonymous? I laughed with the men at the newspaper office. 'It's reactionary to believe in God in our days,' I said, 'but I am the devil, so I may be believed in.' 'We quite understand that,' they said. 'Who doesn't believe in the devil? Yet it won't do, it might injure our reputation. Perhaps as a joke, if you like.' But I thought as a joke it wouldn't be very witty. So it wasn't printed. And do you know, I have felt sore about it to this day. My best feelings, gratitude, for instance, are literally denied me simply because of my social position."

"Philosophical reflections again?" Ivan snarled with hatred.

"God forbid, but one can't help complaining sometimes. I am a slandered man. You upbraid me every moment with being stupid. One can see you are young. My dear fellow, intelligence isn't the only thing! I have naturally a kind and merry heart. 'I also write vaudevilles of all sorts.' You seem to take me for Hlestakov* grown old, but my fate is a far more serious one. Before time was, by some decree which I could never make out, I was predestined 'to deny' and yet I am genuinely good-hearted and not at all inclined to negation. 'No, you must go and deny, without denial there's no criticism and what would a journal be without a department of criticism?' Without criticism it would be nothing but one 'hosannah.' But nothing but hosannah is not enough for life, the hosannah must be tried in the crucible of doubt and so on, in the same style. But I don't meddle in that, I am not the creator, I am not answerable. Well, they've

* The hero of Gogol's "Inspector-General." *Editor's note.*

chosen their scapegoat, they've made me head the department of criticism and so life was made possible. We understand that comedy; I, for instance, simply ask for annihilation. No, live, I am told, for there'd be nothing without you. If everything on earth were sensible, nothing would happen. There would be no events without you, and there must be events. So against the grain I serve so that there may be events, and do what's unreasonable because I am commanded to. For all their indisputable intelligence, men take this farce as something serious, and that is their tragedy. They suffer, of course . . . but then they live, they live a real life, not a fantastic one, for it is suffering that is life. Without suffering what would be the pleasure of it? It would be transformed into an endless church service; it would be holy, but tedious. But what about me? I suffer, but still, I don't live. I am *x* in an indeterminate equation. I am a sort of phantom in life who has lost all beginnings and ends, and who has even forgotten his own name. You are laughing — no, you are not laughing, you are angry again. You are for ever angry, all you care about is intelligence, but I repeat again that I would give away all this super-stellar life, all the ranks and honours, simply to be transformed into the soul of a merchant's wife weighing two hundred and fifty and set candles before God's shrine."

"Then even you don't believe in God?" said Ivan, with a smile of hatred.

"That is, — how shall I put it? — if only you are in earnest . . ."

"Is there a God or not?" Ivan cried with the same savage persistence.

"Ah, then you are in earnest! My dear fellow, upon my word I don't know. There! I've said it now!"

"You don't know, but you see God? No, you are not some one apart, you are myself, you are I and nothing more! You are rubbish, you are my fancy!"

"Well, if you like, we have the same philosophy, that would be true. *Je pense, donc je suis,* I know that for a fact, all the rest, all these worlds, God and even Satan — all that is not proved, to my mind. Does all that exist of itself, or is it only an emanation of myself, a logical development of my ego which alone has existed for ever: but I make haste to stop, for I believe you will be jumping up to beat me directly."

"You'd better tell me some anecdote!" said Ivan miserably.

"There is an anecdote precisely on our subject, or rather a legend, not an anecdote. You reproach me with unbelief, you say that I see, yet don't believe. But, my dear fellow, I am not the only one like that. We are all in a muddle over there now and all through your science. As long as there were atoms, five senses, four elements, everything hung together somehow. There were atoms in the ancient world even, but since we've learnt that you've discovered the chemical molecule and protoplasm and the devil knows what, we put our tails between our legs. It was just chaos, and, above all, superstition, scandal; there's as much scandal among us as among you, you know; a little more in fact, and indeed, we have informers, for we, too, have a place where certain 'information' is welcome. Well, this wild legend belongs to our middle ages — not yours, but ours — and no one believes it even among us, except the merchants' wives weighing two hundred and fifty pounds, not your merchants' wives I mean, but ours. Everything you have, we have, too, I am revealing one of our secrets out of friendship for you; though it's forbidden. This legend is about Paradise. There was, they say, here on earth a thinker and philosopher. He rejected everything, 'laws, conscience, faith,' and, above all, the future life. He died; he expected nothing but darkness and death and he found a future life before him. He was astounded and indignant. 'This is against my principles!' he said. And he was punished for that . . . that is, you must excuse me, I am just repeating what I heard myself, it's only a legend . . . he was sentenced to walk a quadrillion kilometres in the dark (we've adopted the metric system, you know) and when he had finished that quadrillion, the gates of heaven would be opened to him and he would be forgiven . . ."

"And what tortures have you in the other world besides the quadrillion kilometres?" asked Ivan, with a strange eagerness.

"What tortures? Ah, don't ask. In the old days we had all sorts, but now they have taken chiefly to moral punishments — 'remorse' and all that nonsense. We got that, too, from you, from the softening of your manners. And who's the better for it? Only those who have got no conscience, for how can they be tortured by remorse when they have no conscience? But decent people who have a conscience and a sense of honour suffer for it. Reforms, when the ground has not been prepared for them, especially if they are institutions copied from abroad, do nothing but mischief! The ancient hell-fire was better. Well, this man, who was condemned to the quadrillion kilometres, stood still, looked round, and lay down across the road. 'I won't go, I refuse on principle!' Take the soul of an enlightened Russian atheist and mix it with the soul of the prophet Jonah, who sulked for three days and nights in the belly of the whale, and you get the character of that thinker who lay across the road."

"What did he lie on there?"

"Well, I suppose there was something to lie on. You are not laughing?"

"Bravo!" cried Ivan, still with the same strange eagerness. Now he was listening with an unexpected curiosity. "Well, is he lying there now?"

"That's the point, that he isn't. He lay there almost a thousand years and then he got up and went on."

"What an ass!" cried Ivan, laughing nervously and still seeming to be pondering something intently. "Does it make any difference whether he lies there for ever or walks the quadrillion kilometres? It would take a billion years to walk it?"

"Much more than that. I haven't got a pencil and paper or I could work it out. But he got there long ago and that's where the story begins."

"What, he got there? But how did he get the billion years to do it?"

"Why, you keep thinking of our present earth! But our present earth may have been repeated a billion times. Why, it became extinct, froze, cracked, broke to bits, disintegrated into its elements, again 'the waters above the firmament,' then again a comet, again a sun, again an earth from the sun — and the same sequence may have been repeated endlessly and exactly the same to every detail. How disgustingly boring . . ."

"Well, well, what happened when he arrived?"

"Why, the moment the gates of Paradise were open and he walked in, before he had been there two seconds, by his watch (though to my thinking his watch must have long dissolved into its elements in his pocket on the way), he cried out that those two seconds were worth walking not a quadrillion kilometres but a quadrillion of quadrillions, raised to the quadrillionth power! In fact, he sang 'hosannah' and overdid it so that some persons there of a nobler way of thinking wouldn't shake hands with him at first — he'd become too rapidly reactionary, they said. The Russian temperament. I repeat, it's a legend. I offer it for what it's worth. So that's the sort of ideas we have on such subjects even now."

"I've caught you!" Ivan cried, with an almost childish delight, as though he had succeeded in remembering something at last. "That anecdote about the quadrillion years, I made up myself! I was seventeen then, I was at high school. I made up that anecdote and told it to a schoolfellow called Korovkin, it was in Moscow. . . . The anecdote is so characteristic that I couldn't have taken it from anywhere. I thought I'd forgotten it . . . but I've unconsciously recalled it — I recalled it myself — it was not you telling it! Thousands of things are unconsciously remembered like that even when people are being taken to execution . . . it's come back to me in a dream. You are that dream! You are a dream, you don't exist!"

"From the vehemence with which you deny my existence," laughed the gentleman, "I am convinced that you believe in me."

"Not in the slightest! I haven't a hundredth part of a grain of faith in you!"

"But you have the thousandth of a grain. Homeopathic doses perhaps are the strongest. Confess that you have faith even to the ten-thousandth of a grain."

"Not for one minute," cried Ivan furiously. "But I should like to believe in you," he added strangely.

"Aha! There's an admission! But I am good-natured. I'll come to your assistance again. Listen, it was I caught you, not you me. I told you your anecdote you'd forgotten, on purpose, so as to destroy your faith in me completely."

"You are lying. The object of your visit is to convince me of your existence!"

"Just so. But hesitation, suspense, conflict between belief and disbelief — is sometimes such torture to a conscientious man, such as you are, that it's better to hang oneself. Knowing that you are inclined to believe in me, I administered some disbelief by telling you that anecdote. I lead you to belief and disbelief in turn, and in doing it I have a purpose of my own. It's the new method. As soon as you disbelieve in me completely, you'll begin assuring me to my face that I am not a dream but a reality. I know you. Then I shall have attained my object, which is an honourable one. I shall sow in you only a tiny grain of faith and it will grow into an oak-tree — and such an oak-tree that, sitting on it, you will long to enter the ranks of 'the hermits in the wilderness and the saintly women,' for that is what you are secretly longing for. You'll dine on locusts, you'll drag yourself into the wilderness to save your soul!"

"Then it's for the salvation of my soul you are working, is it, you scoundrel?"

"One must do a good deed sometimes. You are ill-humoured, I see."

"Clown! Did you ever tempt those holy men who ate locusts and prayed seventeen years in the wilderness till they were overgrown with moss?"

"My dear fellow, I've done nothing else.

One forgets the whole world and all the worlds, and sticks to one such saint, because he is a very precious diamond. One such soul, you know, is sometimes worth a whole constellation. We have our own arithmetic, you know. The conquest is priceless! And some of them, on my word, are not inferior to you in culture, though you won't believe it. They can contemplate such depths of belief and disbelief at the same moment that sometimes it really seems that they are within a hair's-breadth of being 'turned upside down,' as the actor Gorbunov says."

"Well, did you get your nose pulled?"*

"My dear fellow," observed the visitor sententiously, "it's better to get off with your nose pulled than without a nose at all. As an afflicted marquis observed not long ago (he must have been treated by a specialist) in confessing to his spiritual father — a Jesuit. I was present, it was simply charming. 'Give me back my nose!' he said, and he beat his breast. 'My son,' said the priest evasively, 'all things are accomplished in accordance with the inscrutable decrees of Providence, and what seems a misfortune sometimes leads to extraordinary, though unapparent, benefits. If stern destiny has deprived you of your nose, it's to your advantage that as long as you live no one will dare say that he will pull your nose for you.' 'Holy father, that's no comfort,' cried the despairing marquis. 'I'd be delighted to have my nose pulled every day of my life, if it were only in its proper place.' 'My son,' sighed the priest, 'you can't ask for all the blessings at once. That would be murmuring against Providence, who even in this has not forgotten you, for if you cry out as you cried out just now, declaring you'd be glad to have your nose pulled for the rest of your life, your desire has already been fulfilled indirectly, for when you lost your nose, you were led by the nose.' "

"Faugh, how stupid!" cried Ivan.

"My dear friend, I only wanted to amuse you. But I swear that's the genuine Jesuit casuistry and I swear that it all happened word for word as I've told you. It happened lately and gave me a great deal of trouble. The unhappy young man shot himself that very night when he got home. I was by his side till the very last moment. As for those Jesuit confessionals, they are really my most delightful diversion at melancholy moments. Here's another incident that happened only the other day. A little blonde Norman girl of twenty — a buxom, unsophisticated beauty who would make your mouth water — comes to an old priest. She bends down and whispers her sin through the grating. 'Why, my daughter, have you fallen again already?' cries the priest. 'O Sancta Maria, what do I hear! Not the same man this time, how long will this go on? Aren't you ashamed!' *'Ah, mon père,'* answers the sinner with tears of penitence, *'ça lui fait tant de plaisir, et à moi si peu de peine!'* Fancy, such an answer! I drew back. It was the cry of nature, better than innocence itself, if you like. I absolved her sin on the spot and was turning to go, but I was forced to return. I heard the priest at the grating making an appointment with her for the evening — though he was an old man hard as flint, he fell in an instant! It was nature, the truth of nature asserted its rights! What, you are turning up your nose again? Angry again? I don't know how to please you . . ."

"Leave me alone, you are throbbing in my

* Literally: "Did you get off with a nose?" — meaning, "Did you fail?" *Editor's note.*

brain like a haunting nightmare," Ivan moaned miserably, helpless before his apparition. "I am bored with you, agonisingly and insufferably. I would give anything to be able to shake you off!"

"I repeat, moderate your expectations, don't demand of me 'everything great and noble' and you'll see how well we shall get on," said the gentleman impressively. "You are really angry with me for not having appeared to you in a red glow, with thunder and lightning, with scorched wings, and for showing myself in such a modest guise. You are wounded, in the first place, in your æsthetic feelings, and, secondly, in your pride. How could such a vulgar devil visit such a great man as you! Yes, there is that romantic strain in you, that was so derided by Belinsky. I can't help it, young man, as I got ready to come to you I did think of appearing as a joke in the form of a retired general who had served in the Caucasus, with a star of the Lion and the Sun on my coat. But I was positively afraid to do it, for you'd have thrashed me for daring to pin the Lion and the Sun on my coat, instead of, at least, the Polar Star or the Sirius. And you keep on saying I am stupid, but, mercy on us! I make no claim to be equal to you in intelligence. Mephistopheles declared to Faust that he desired evil, but did only good. Well, he can say what he likes, it's quite the opposite with me. I am perhaps the one man in all creation who loves the truth and genuinely desires good. I was there when the Word, Who died on the Cross, rose up into heaven bearing on His bosom the soul of the penitent thief. I heard the glad shrieks of the cherubim singing and shouting hosannah and the seraphim's thunderous shout of rapture which shook heaven and all creation, and I swear to you by all that's sacred I longed to join the chorus and shout hosannah with them all. The word had almost escaped me, had almost broken from my lips . . . . you know how susceptible and æsthetically impressionable I am. But common sense — oh, a most unhappy trait in my character — kept me in due bounds and I let the moment pass! For what would have happened, I reflected, what would have happened after my hosannah? Everything on earth would have been extinguished at once and no events could have occurred. And so, solely from a sense of duty and because of my social position, I was forced to suppress the good impulse and to stick to my nasty task. Somebody takes all the credit for goodness to himself, and nothing but nastiness is left for me. But I don't covet the honour of leading a cheat's life, I am not ambitious. Why am I, of all creatures in the world, doomed to be cursed by all decent people and even to be kicked, for if I put on mortal form I am bound to take such consequences sometimes. I know, of course, there's a secret in it, but they won't tell me the secret for anything, for then perhaps, seeing the meaning of it, I might bawl hosannah, and the indispensable minus would disappear at once and good sense would reign supreme throughout the whole world. And that, of course, would mean the end of everything, even of magazines and newspapers, for who would take them in? I know that at the end of all things I shall be reconciled. I, too, shall walk my quadrillion and learn the secret. But till that happens I shall sulk and fulfil my destiny though it's against the grain — that is, ruin thousands for the sake of saving one. How many souls have had to be ruined and how many honourable reputations destroyed for the sake of that one righteous man,

Job, over whom they made such a fool of me in the old days. Yes, till the secret is revealed, there are two sorts of truths for me — one, their truth, yonder, which I know nothing about so far, and the other my own. And there's no knowing which will turn out the better. . . . Are you asleep?"

"I might well be," Ivan groaned angrily. "All my stupid ideas — outgrown, thrashed out long ago, and flung aside like a dead carcass — you present to me as something new!"

"There's no pleasing you! And I thought I should fascinate you by my literary style. That hosannah in the skies really wasn't bad, was it? And then that ironical tone *à la* Heine, eh?"

"No, I was never such a flunkey! How then could my soul beget a flunkey like you?"

"My dear fellow, I know a most charming and attractive young Russian gentleman, a young thinker and a great lover of literature and art, the author of a promising poem entitled 'The Grand Inquisitor.' I was only thinking of him!"

"I forbid you to speak of 'The Grand Inquisitor,' " cried Ivan, crimson with shame.

"And the 'Geological Cataclysm.' Do you remember? That was a poem, now!"

"Hold your tongue, or I'll kill you!"

"You'll kill me? No, excuse me, I will speak. I came to treat myself to that pleasure. Oh, I love the dreams of my ardent young friends, quivering with eagerness for life! 'New men are there,' you decided last spring, when you were meaning to come here, 'they propose to destroy everything and begin with cannibalism. Stupid fellows! they didn't ask my advice! I maintain that nothing need be destroyed, that we need to destroy only the idea of God in mankind; that's how we have set to work. That's what one should begin with. That's what, that's what one should begin with. Oh, blind race of men who have no understanding! As soon as men have all of them denied God — and I believe that period, analogous with geological periods, will come to pass — the old conception of the universe will fall of itself without cannibalism and, what's more, the old morality, and everything will begin anew. Men will unite to take from life all it can give, but only for joy and happiness in the present world. Man will be lifted up with a spirit of divine Titanic pride and the man-god will appear. From hour to hour extending his conquest of nature infinitely by his will and his science, man will feel such lofty joy from hour to hour in doing it that it will make up for all his old hopes of attaining the joys of heaven. Every one will know that he is wholly mortal, that there is no resurrection, and will accept death proudly and serenely like a god. His pride will teach him that it's useless for him to murmur because life is but a moment, and he will love his brother without need of reward. Love will be sufficient unto the moment of life, but the very consciousness of its momentariness will intensify its fire, which now is dissipated in dreams of eternal love beyond the grave' . . . and so on and so on in the same style. Very charming!"

Ivan sat with his eyes on the floor and his hands pressed to his ears, but he began trembling all over. The voice continued.

"The question now is, my young thinker reflected, is it possible that such a period will ever come? If it does, everything is determined and humanity is settled for ever. But as, owing to man's inveterate stupidity, this cannot come about for at least a thousand years, every one who recognises the truth even now may legitimately order his life as he pleases, on the new principles. In that sense, 'everything is permitted' for him. What's more, even if this period never comes to pass, since there is anyway no God and no immortality, the new man may well become the man-god, even if he is the only one in the whole world, and, promoted to his new rank, he may lightheartedly overstep all the barriers of the morality of the old slave-man, if necessary. There is no law for God. Where God stands, the place is holy. Where I stand will be at once the foremost place . . . 'everything is permitted' and that's the end of it! That's all very charming; but if you want to swindle, why do you want a moral sanction for doing it? But that's our modern Russian all over. He can't bring himself to swindle without a moral sanction. He is so in love with truth . . ."

The visitor talked, obviously carried away by his own eloquence, speaking louder and louder and looking ironically at his host. But he did not succeed in finishing; Ivan suddenly snatched a glass from the table and flung it at the orator.

"*Ah, mais c'est bête enfin,*" cried the latter, jumping up from the sofa and shaking the drops of tea off himself. "He has remembered Luther's inkstand! He takes me for a dream and throws glasses at a dream! It's like a woman! I suspected you were only pretending to stop up your ears, but you were listening to me."

A loud, persistent knocking was suddenly heard at the window. Ivan jumped up from the sofa. "Do you hear? You'd better open," cried the visitor; "it's your brother Alyosha with the most interesting and surprising news, I'll be bound!"

"Be silent, deceiver, I knew it was Alyosha, I felt he was coming, and of course he has not come for nothing; of course he brings 'news,' " Ivan exclaimed frantically.

"Open, open to him. There's a snowstorm and he is your brother. *Monsieur sait-il le temps qu'il fait? C'est à ne pas mettre un chien dehors.*"

The knocking continued. Ivan wanted to rush to the window, but something seemed to fetter his arms and legs. He strained every nerve to break his chains, but in vain. The knocking at the window grew louder and louder. At last the chains were broken and Ivan leapt up from the sofa. He looked round him wildly. Both candles had almost burnt out, the glass he had just thrown at his visitor stood before him on the table, and there was no one on the sofa opposite. The knocking on the window frame went on persistently, but it was by no means so loud as it had seemed in his dream; on the contrary, it was quite subdued. "It was not a dream! No, I swear it was not a dream, it all happened just now!" cried Ivan. He rushed to the window and opened the movable pane.

"Alyosha, I told you not to come," he cried fiercely to his brother. "In two words, what do you want? In two words, do you hear?"

"An hour ago Smerdyakov hanged himself," Alyosha answered from the yard.

"Come round to the steps, I'll open at once," said Ivan, and went to open the door to Alyosha.

CHAPTER X

"IT WAS HE WHO SAID THAT"

ALYOSHA, coming in, told Ivan that a little over an hour ago Marya Kondratyevna had come to his rooms and informed him that

Smerdyakov had taken his own life. "I go in to clear away the samovar and I see he is hanging on a nail in the wall." On Alyosha's inquiring whether she had informed the police, she answered that she had told no one, "but I flew straight to you, I've run all the way." She was like one crazed, Alyosha reported, and was shaking like a leaf. When Alyosha ran with her to the cottage, he found Smerdyakov still hanging. On the table lay a note: "I destroy my life of my own will and desire, so as to put no blame on any one." Alyosha left the note on the table and went straight to the police captain and told him all about it. "And from him I've come straight to you," said Alyosha, in conclusion, looking intently into Ivan's face. He had not taken his eyes off him while he told his story, as though struck by something in his expression.

"Brother," he cried suddenly, "you must be terribly ill. You stare and don't seem to understand what I tell you."

"It's a good thing you came," said Ivan, as though brooding, and not hearing Alyosha's exclamation. "I knew he had hanged himself."

"From whom?"

"I don't know. But I knew. Did I know? Yes, he told me. He told me so just now."

Ivan stood in the middle of the room, and still spoke in the same brooding tone, looking at the ground.

"Who is *he?*" asked Alyosha, involuntarily looking round.

"He's slipped away."

Ivan raised his head and smiled softly.

"He was scared of you, of you, the dove. You are a 'pure cherub.' Dmitri calls you a cherub. Cherub! . . . the seraphim's thunderous shout of rapture. What are seraphim? Perhaps a whole constellation. But perhaps that constellation is only a chemical molecule. Is there a constellation of the Lion and the Sun? Do you know?"

"Brother, sit down," said Alyosha in alarm. "For goodness' sake, sit down on the sofa! You are delirious; put your head on the pillow, that's right. Would you like a wet towel on your head? Perhaps it will do you good."

"Give me the towel: it's here on the chair. I just threw it down there."

"It's not here. Don't worry yourself. I know where it is — here," said Alyosha, finding a clean towel, folded up and unused, by Ivan's dressing-table in the other corner of the room. Ivan looked strangely at the towel: recollection seemed to come back to him for an instant.

"Wait" — he got up from the sofa — "an hour ago I took that new towel from there and wetted it. I wrapped it round my head and threw it down here . . . How is it it's dry? There was no other."

"You put that towel on your head?" asked Alyosha.

"Yes, and walked up and down the room an hour ago . . . Why have the candles burnt down so? What's the time?"

"Nearly twelve."

"No, no, no!" Ivan cried suddenly. "It was not a dream. He was here; he was sitting here, on that sofa. When you knocked at the window, I threw a glass at him . . . this one. Wait a minute. I was asleep last time, but this dream was not a dream. It has happened before. I have dreams now, Alyosha . . . yet they are not dreams, but reality. I walk about, talk, and see . . . though I am asleep. But he was sitting here, on that sofa there. . . . He is frightfully stupid, Alyosha, frightfully stupid." Ivan laughed suddenly and began pacing about the room.

"Who is stupid? Of whom are you talking, brother?" Alyosha asked anxiously again.

"The devil! He's taken to visiting me. He's been here twice, almost three times. He taunted me with being angry at his being a simple devil and not Satan, with scorched wings, in thunder and lightning. But he is not Satan: that's a lie. He is an impostor. He is simply a devil — a paltry, trivial devil. He goes to the baths. If you undressed him, you'd be sure to find he had a tail, long and smooth like a Danish dog's, a yard long, dun colour. . . . Alyosha, you are cold. You've been out in the snow. Would you like some tea? What? Is it cold? Shall I tell her to bring some? *C'est à ne pas mettre un chien dehors* . . . ."

Alyosha ran to the wash-stand, wetted the towel, persuaded Ivan to sit down again, and put the wet towel round his head.

"What were you telling me just now about Lise?" Ivan began again. (He was becoming very talkative.) "I like Lise. I said something nasty about her. It was a lie. I like her . . . I am afraid for Katya to-morrow. I am afraid for her most of all. On account of the future. She will cast me off to-morrow and trample me under foot. She thinks that I am ruining Mitya from jealousy on her account! Yes, she thinks that! But it's not so. To-morrow the cross, but not the gallows. No, I shan't hang myself. Do you know, I can never commit suicide, Alyosha. Is it because I am base? I am not a coward. Is it because of the thirst for life? How did I know that Smerdyakov had hanged himself? Yes, it was *he* told me so."

"And you are quite convinced that there has been some one here?" asked Alyosha.

"Yes, on that sofa in the corner. You would have driven him away. You did drive him away: he disappeared when you arrived. I love your face, Alyosha. Did you know that I love your face? And *he* is myself, Alyosha. All that's base in me, all that's mean and contemptible. Yes, I am a romantic. He noticed it . . . though it's a libel. He is frightfully stupid; but that's his advantage. He has cunning, animal cunning — he knew how to infuriate me. He kept taunting me with believing in him, and that was how he made me listen to him. He fooled me like a boy. He told me a great deal that was true about myself, though. I should never have owned it to myself. Do you know, Alyosha," Ivan added in an intensely earnest and confidential tone, "I should be awfully glad to think it was *he* and not I."

"He has worn you out," said Alyosha looking compassionately at his brother.

"He's been teasing me. And you know he does it so cleverly, so cleverly. 'Conscience! What is conscience? I make it up myself. Why am I tormented by it? Out of habit. Out of the seven-thousand-year-old universal human habit. So let us give it up, and we shall be as gods.' It was he said that, it was he said that!"

"And not you, not you?" Alyosha could not help crying, looking frankly at his brother. "Never mind him, anyway; have done with him and forget him. And let him take with him all that you curse now, and never come back!"

"Yes, but he is spiteful. He laughed at me. He was insolent, Alyosha," Ivan said, with a shudder of offense. "But he slandered me, slandered me in many ways. He told lies about me to my face. 'Oh, you are going to perform an act of heroic virtue: to confess you murdered your father, that the valet murdered him at your instigation.' "

"Brother," Alyosha interposed, "restrain yourself. It was not you who murdered him. It's not true!"

"That's what he says, he, and he knows it. 'You are going to perform an act of heroic virtue, and you don't believe in virtue; that's what tortures you and makes you angry, that's why you are so vindictive.' He said that to me about myself and he knows whereof he speaks."

"It's you say that, not he," exclaimed Alyosha mournfully, "and you say it because you are ill and delirious, tormenting yourself."

"No, he knows whereof he speaks. 'You are going out of pride,' he says. 'You'll stand up and say it was I who killed, and why do you writhe with horror? You are lying! I despise your opinion, I despise your horror!' He said that about me. 'And do you know you are longing for their praise — "He is a criminal, a murderer, but what a generous soul; he wanted to save his brother and he confessed." ' That's a lie, Alyosha!" Ivan cried suddenly, with flashing eyes. "I don't want the low rabble to praise me, I swear I don't! That's a lie! That's why I threw the glass at him and it broke against his ugly face."

"Brother, calm yourself, stop!" Alyosha entreated him.

"Yes, he knows how to torment one. He's cruel," Ivan went on, unheeding. "I had an inkling from the first as to what he came for. 'Granting that you go out of pride, still you had a hope that Smerdyakov might be convicted and sent to Siberia, and Mitya would be acquitted, while you would only be condemned *morally*' (Do you hear? he laughed then) — 'and some people will praise you. But now Smerdyakov's dead, he has hanged himself, and who'll believe you alone? But yet you are going, you are going, you'll go all the same, you've decided to go. What are you going for now?' That's awful, Alyosha. I can't endure such questions. Who dares ask me such questions?"

"Brother," interposed Alyosha — his heart sank with terror, but he still seemed to hope to bring Ivan to reason — "how could he have told you of Smerdyakov's death before I came, when no one knew of it and there was no time for any one to know of it?"

"He told me," said Ivan firmly, refusing to admit a doubt. "It was all he did talk about, if you come to that. 'And it would be all right if you believed in virtue,' he said. ' "No matter if they disbelieve me, I am going for the sake of a principle." But you are a little pig like Fyodor Pavlovich and what is virtue to you? Why do you want to go meddling if your sacrifice is of no use to any one? Because you don't know yourself why you go! Oh, you'd give a great deal to know yourself why you go! And can you have made up your mind? You've not made up your mind. You'll sit all night deliberating whether to go or not. But you will go; you know you'll go. You know that whichever way you decide, the decision does not depend on you. You'll go because you won't dare not to go. Why won't you dare? You must guess that for yourself. That's a riddle for you!' He got up and went away. You came and he went. He called me a coward, Alyosha! *Le mot de l'énigme* is that I am a coward. 'It is not for such eagles to soar above the earth.' It was he added that — he! And Smerdyakov said the same. He must be killed! Katya despises me. I've seen that for a month past. Even Lise will begin to despise me! 'You are going in order to be praised.' That's a brutal lie! And you despise me, too, Alyosha. Now I am going to hate you again! And I hate the monster, too! I hate the monster! I don't want to save the monster. Let him rot in Siberia! He's begun singing a hymn! Oh, to-morrow I'll go, stand before them, and spit in their eyes!"

He jumped up in a frenzy, flung off the towel, and fell to pacing the room again. Alyosha recalled what he had just said. "I seem to be sleeping awake. . . . I walk, I speak, I see, but I am asleep." It seemed to be just like that now. Alyosha did not leave him. The thought passed through his mind to run for a doctor, but he was afraid to leave his brother alone: there was no one to whom he could leave him. By degrees Ivan lost consciousness completely at last. He still went on talking, talking incessantly, but quite incoherently, and even articulated his words with difficulty. Suddenly he staggered violently; but Alyosha was in time to support him. Ivan let him lead him to his bed. Alyosha undressed him somehow and put him to bed. He sat watching over him for another two hours. The sick man slept soundly, without stirring, breathing softly and evenly. Alyosha took a pillow and lay down on the sofa, without undressing.

As he fell asleep he prayed for Mitya and Ivan. He began to understand Ivan's illness. "The anguish of a proud determination. An earnest conscience!" God, in Whom he disbelieved, and His truth were gaining mastery over his heart, which still refused to submit. "Yes," the thought floated through Alyosha's head as it lay on the pillow, "yes, if Smerdyakov is dead, no one will believe Ivan's evidence; but he will go and give it." Alyosha smiled softly. "God will conquer!" he thought. "He will either rise up in the light of truth, or . . . he'll perish in hate, revenging on himself and on every one his having served the cause he does not believe in," Alyosha added bitterly, and again he prayed for Ivan.

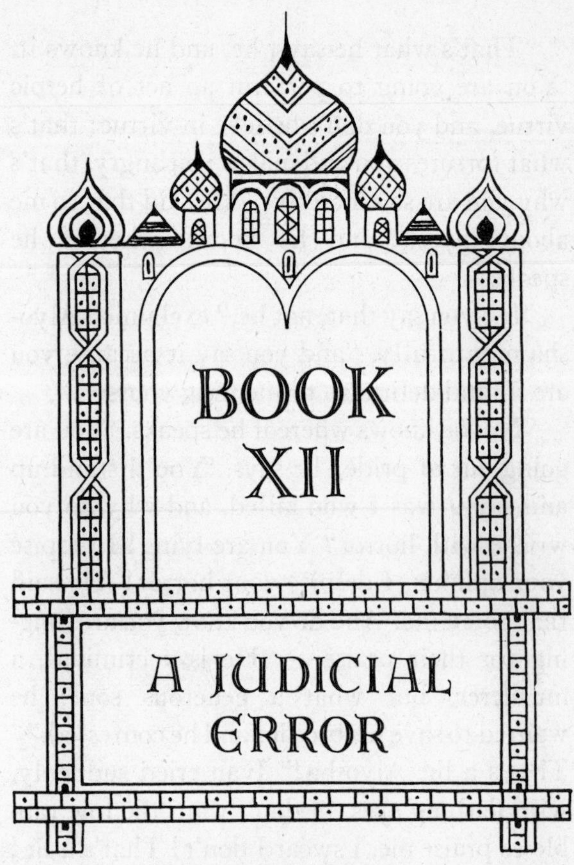

CHAPTER I

THE FATAL DAY

At ten o'clock in the morning of the day following the events I have described, the trial of Dmitri Karamazov began in our district court.

I hasten to emphasize the fact that I am far from esteeming myself capable of reporting all that took place at the trial in full detail, or even in proper order. I imagine that to recall everything, and to explain it all duly, would fill a whole volume, even a very large one. And so I trust I may not be reproached for confining myself to what struck me personally, and what I specially remembered. I may have mistaken what was of secondary importance for the main thing, and may have omitted the most prominent and essential features. But I see I shall do better not to apologise. I will do my best and the reader will see for himself that I have done all I can.

And, to begin with, before we enter the court-room, I will mention what surprised me most on that day. Indeed, as it appeared later, every one was surprised at it, too. We all knew that the affair had aroused great interest, that every one was burning with impatience for the trial to begin, that it had been a subject of talk, conjecture, exclamation, and surmise for the last two months in local society. Every one knew, too, that the case had become known throughout Russia, and yet we had not imagined that it had aroused such burning, such intense, interest in all and sundry, not only among ourselves, but everywhere. This became evident at the trial that day.

Visitors had arrived not only from the chief town of our province, but from several other Russian cities, as well as from Moscow and Petersburg. There came lawyers, several distinguished personages, and also some ladies. Every ticket of admission had been snatched up. A special place behind the table at which the court sat was set apart for the most distinguished and important of the male visitors; a row of armchairs had been placed there — something which had never been allowed before. A large proportion — not less than half of the public — were ladies. So many lawyers had arrived that they did not know where to seat them, for all the tickets had long since been distributed, or obtained by pleading and entreaty. I saw at the end of the room, behind the platform, a special partition hurriedly put up, behind which all these lawyers were admitted, and they thought themselves lucky to have standing room there, for all chairs had been removed to gain space, and the crowd behind the partition stood throughout the case closely packed, shoulder to shoulder.

Some of the ladies, especially those who came from a distance, made their appearance in the gallery very smartly dressed, but the majority of the ladies were oblivious even to dress. Their faces betrayed hysterical, eager, almost morbid, curiosity. A peculiar fact — established afterwards by many observations — that almost all the ladies, or, at least the vast majority of them, were on Mitya's side and in favour of his being acquitted. This was perhaps chiefly owing to his reputation as a heart-breaker. It was known that two women who were rivals were to appear in the case. One of them — Katerina Ivanovna — was an object of particular interest. All sorts of extraordinary tales were told about her, amazing anecdotes of her passion for Mitya, in spite of his crime. Her pride and "aristocratic connections" were particularly insisted upon (she had called upon scarcely any one in the town). People said she intended to petition the Government for leave to accompany the criminal to Siberia and to be married to him somewhere in the mines, underground. The appearance of Grushenka in court, as Katerina Ivanovna's rival, was awaited with no less agitation. The public was looking forward with anxious curiosity to the meeting of the two rivals — the proud aristocratic girl and "the hetaira." But Grushenka was a more familiar figure to the ladies of the district than Katerina Ivanovna. They had already seen "the woman who had ruined Fyodor Pavlovich and his unhappy son," and all, almost without exception, wondered how father and son could be so in love with "such a very common, ordinary Russian girl, who was not even pretty."

In brief, there was a great deal of talk. I know for a fact that there were several serious family quarrels on Mitya's account in our town. Many ladies quarrelled violently with their husbands because of differences of opinion about the dreadful case, and it was only natural that the husbands of these ladies should enter the court-room not only unfavourably disposed towards the accused, but actually full of bitter hostility towards him. In fact, one may say positively that the masculine, as distinguished from the feminine, part of the audience was biased against the accused. There were numbers of severe, frowning, even vindictive, faces. Mitya, indeed, had managed to offend many people during his stay in the town. Some of the visitors were, of course, in excellent spirits and quite unconcerned as to the fate of Mitya personally. But all were interested in the trial, and the majority of the men were certainly hoping for the conviction of the criminal, except perhaps the lawyers, who were interested in the legal, so to speak, rather than the moral aspect of the case.

Everybody was excited by the presence of the celebrated Fetyukovich. His talent was known everywhere, and this was not the first time he had appeared for the defence in notorious criminal cases in the provinces. And when he did, such cases became celebrated and long remembered all over Russia. There were stories, too, about our prosecutor and about the presiding judge. It was said that our prosecutor was trembling at the thought of meeting Fetyukovich, and that they had been inveterate enemies from the beginning of their careers in Petersburg, that our touchy Ippolit Kirillovich, who always considered that he had been offended by some one in Petersburg because his talents had not been properly appreciated, was keenly excited over the Karamazov case, and was even dreaming of rebuilding his flagging fortunes by means of it, but that Fetyukovich was his one anxiety. But these rumours were not quite justified. Our prosecutor was not one of those men who lose heart in the face of danger. On the contrary, his self-confidence increased with the increase of danger. It must be noted that our prosecutor was in general too hasty and morbidly impressionable. He would put his whole soul into some case and work at it as though his whole fate and his whole fortune depended on its result. This was the subject of some ridicule in the legal world, for just by this characteristic our prosecutor had gained a wider notoriety than could have been expected from his modest position. People laughed particularly at his passion for psychology. In my opinion, they were wrong, and our prosecutor was, I believe, a character of greater earnestness than was generally supposed. But because of his morbidity he had failed to impress himself on people at the outset of his career or at any time later.

As for the presiding judge, I can only say that he was a humane and cultured man, who had a practical knowledge of his work and the most advanced views. He was rather ambitious, but did not concern himself greatly about his career. The great aim of his life was to be a progressive. He had, too, connections with wealth. He felt, as we learnt afterwards, rather strongly about the Karamazov case, but not in any personal way. He was interested in it as a social phenomenon, in its classification and its character as a product of our social conditions, as typical of the national character, and so on, and so on. His attitude to the personal aspect of the case, to its tragic significance and the persons involved in it, including the prisoner, was rather indifferent and abstract, as was perhaps fitting, indeed.

The court-room was packed to overflowing long before the judges made their appearance. Our court-room is the best hall in the town — spacious, lofty, and with good acoustics. On the right of the judges, who were on a raised platform, a table and two rows of chairs had been placed for the jury. On the left was the place for the defendant and his counsel. In the middle of the court, near the judges, was a table with the "material evidence." On it lay Fyodor Pavlovich's white silk dressing-gown, stained with blood; the fatal brass pestle with which the supposed murder had been committed; Mitya's shirt, with a bloodstained sleeve; his coat, stained with blood in patches over the pocket in which he had put his handkerchief; the handkerchief itself, stiff with blood and by now quite yellow; the pistol loaded by Mitya at Perhotin's with a view to suicide, and taken from him on the sly at Mokroye by Trifon Borisovich; the envelope in which the three thousand roubles had been kept ready for Grushenka, the narrow pink ribbon with which it had been tied, and many other articles which I don't remember. Some distance farther back in the room were the seats for the public. But in front of the balustrade a few chairs had been placed for witnesses who were to be retained in court after giving their evidence.

At ten o'clock the three judges arrived — the presiding judge, one honorary justice of the peace, and one other. The prosecutor, of course, entered immediately after. The presiding judge was a short, stout, thick-set man of fifty, with a dyspeptic complexion, dark hair turning grey and cut short, and a red ribbon, of what Order I don't remember. The prosecutor struck me and the others, too, as looking particularly pale, almost green. His face seemed to have grown suddenly thinner, perhaps in a single night, for I had seen him looking as usual only two days before. The presiding judge began by asking the court attendant whether all the jurymen were present.

But I see I can't go on like this, partly because many things I did not hear, others I did not grasp, and others I have forgotten, but most of all because, as I have said before, I have literally no time or space to mention everything that was said and done. I only know that neither side objected to many of the jurymen. I remember the twelve jurymen — four were petty officials of the town, two were merchants, and six peasants and local townspeople. I remember, long before the trial, questions were continually asked with some surprise, especially by ladies, "Can such a delicate, complex and psychological case be submitted for decision to petty officials and even peasants?" and "What can an official, still more a peasant, understand in such an affair?" All the four officials on the jury were, in fact, men of no consequence and of low rank. Except for one who was rather younger, they were grey-headed men, little known in society, who had vegetated on a pitiful salary, and who probably had elderly, unpresentable wives and crowds of children, perhaps even without shoes and stockings. At best, they spent their leisure over cards and, of course, had never read a single book. The two merchants looked respectable, but were strangely silent and stolid. One of them had shaved his beard, and was dressed in European style; the other had a small, grey beard, and wore a red ribbon with some sort of medal upon it on his neck. There is no need to speak of the townspeople and the peasants. Our townspeople are almost peasants, and even work on the land. Two of them also wore European dress, and, perhaps for that reason, were dirtier and more uninviting-looking than the others. So that one might well wonder, as I did as soon as I had looked at them, "what men like that could possibly make of such a case?" Yet their faces wore a strangely imposing, almost menacing, expression; they were stern and frowning.

At last the presiding judge opened the case of the murder of Fyodor Pavlovich Karamazov, retired titular councillor. I don't quite remember how he expressed himself. The court attendant was told to bring in the prisoner, and Mitya made his appearance. There was a hush in the court. One could have heard a fly. I don't know how it was with others, but Mitya made a most unfavourable impression on me. He looked an awful dandy in a brand-new frock-coat. I heard afterwards that he had ordered it in Moscow expressly for the occasion from his own tailor, who had his measure. He wore immaculate black kid gloves and elegant linen. He walked in with his yard-long strides, looking stiffly straight in front of him, and sat down in his place with a most unperturbed air.

At the same moment the counsel for the defence, the celebrated Fetyukovich, entered, and a sort of subdued hum passed through the court. He was a tall, spare man, with long thin legs, with extremely long, thin, pale fingers, clean-shaven face, rather short hair, demurely brushed, and thin lips that were at times curved into something between a sneer and a smile. He looked about forty. His face would have been pleasant, if it had not been for his eyes, which, in themselves small and inexpressive, were set remarkably close together, with only the thin, long nose as a dividing line between them. In fact, there was something strikingly birdlike about his face. He wore a frock-coat and white tie.

I remember the presiding judge's first question to Mitya, about his name, his status, and so on. Mitya answered sharply, and his voice was so unexpectedly loud that it made the judge start and look at the prisoner almost with surprise. Then followed the reading of a list of persons who had been summoned to take part in the trial — that is, as witnesses and experts. It was a long list. Four of the witnesses did not appear — Miüsov, who had testified at the preliminary inquiry, but was now in Paris; Madame Hohlakov and Maximov, who were absent through illness; and Smerdyakov, through his sudden death, a police certificate of which was presented. The news of Smerdyakov's death produced a sudden stir and whisper in the court. Many in the audience, of course, had not heard of the sudden suicide. What struck people most was Mitya's sudden outburst. As soon as the statement of Smerdyakov's death was made, he cried out aloud from his place:

"The dog died like a dog!"

I remember how his counsel rushed to him, and how the presiding judge addressed him, threatening to take stern measures if such irregular behaviour repeated itself. Mitya nodded and in a subdued voice repeated several times abruptly to his counsel, with no show of regret:

"I won't again, I won't. It escaped me. I won't do it again."

And, of course, this brief episode did him no good with the jury or the public. His character was displayed, and it spoke for itself. It

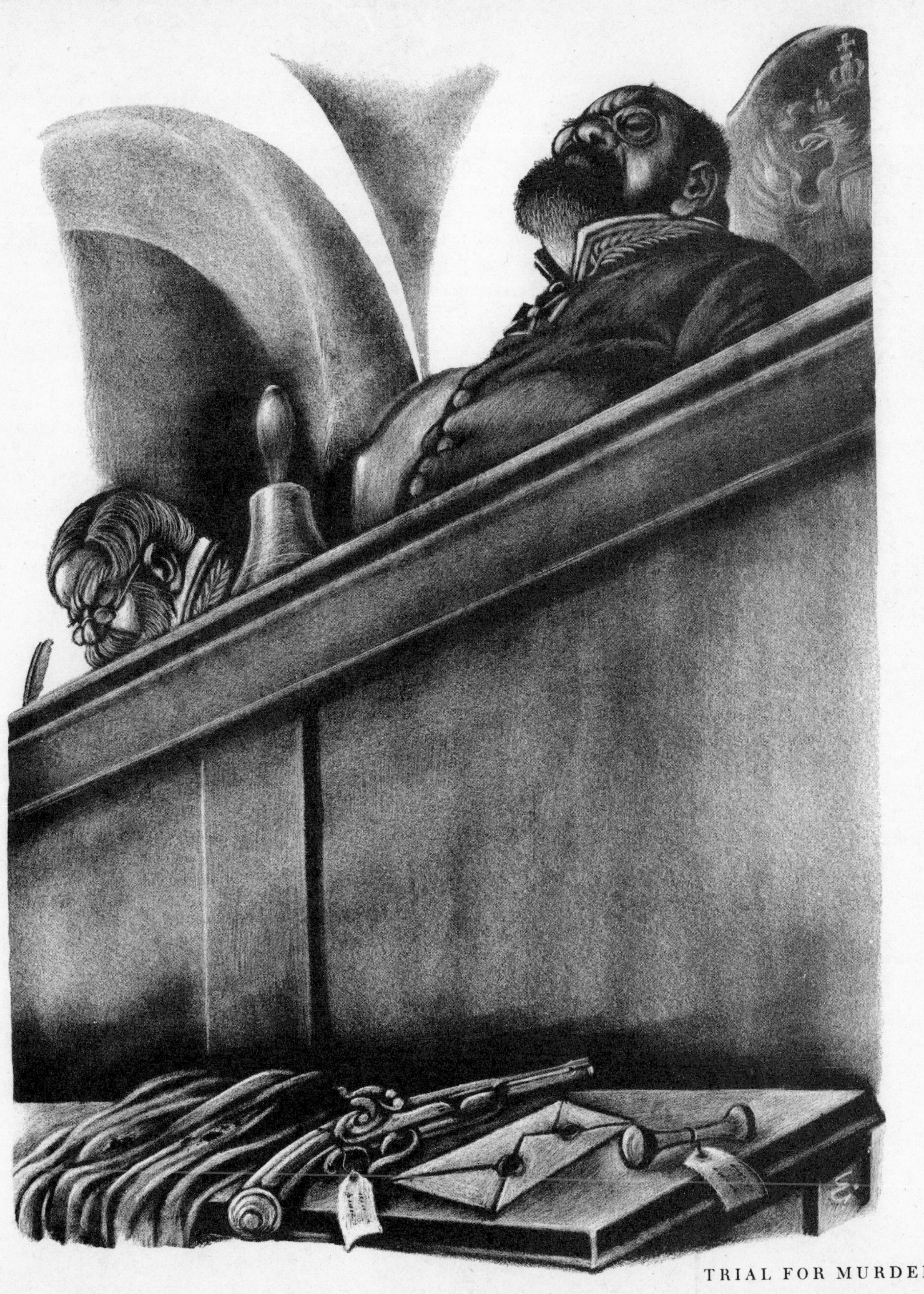

TRIAL FOR MURDER

was under the influence of this incident that the court clerk read the bill of indictment. It was rather short, but circumstantial. It contained only the chief reasons why so-and-so had been arrested, why he must be tried, and so on. Yet it made a great impression on me. The clerk read it loudly and distinctly. The whole tragedy was suddenly unfolded before us, in concentrated form, in bold relief, in a fatal and pitiless light. I remember how, immediately after it had been read, the presiding judge asked Mitya in a loud, impressive voice:

"Prisoner, do you plead guilty?"

Mitya suddenly rose from his seat.

"I plead guilty to drunkenness and dissipation," he exclaimed, again in a startling, almost frenzied, voice, "to idleness and debauchery. I meant to become an honest man for good, just at the moment when I was cut down by fate. But of the death of the old man, my enemy and my father, I am not guilty. But of robbing him, no, no, I am not guilty! I could not be. Dmitri Karamazov is a scoundrel, but not a thief."

Having shouted thus, he sat down, visibly trembling all over. The presiding judge again briefly, but impressively, admonished him to answer to the point, and not to go off into irrelevant exclamations. Then he ordered the case to proceed. All the witnesses were led up to take the oath. Here I saw them all together. The brothers of the accused were, however, allowed to give evidence without taking the oath.

After an exhortation from the priest and the presiding judge, the witnesses were led away and were seated as far apart from one another as possible. Then they began calling them up one by one.

CHAPTER II

DANGEROUS WITNESSES

I do not know whether the witnesses for the defence and for the prosecution were separated into groups by the presiding judge, and in what order they were to be called. But no doubt some arrangement existed. I only know that the witnesses for the prosecution were called first. I repeat I don't intend to describe all the questioning step by step. Besides, my account would be to some extent superfluous, because in the speeches of the prosecutor and the counsel for the defence all the testimony presented was brought together and set in a strong and significant light, and I took down parts of those two remarkable speeches in full, and will quote them in due time, and I shall also describe one extraordinary and quite unexpected episode, which occurred before the final speeches, and undoubtedly influenced the sinister and fatal outcome of the trial.

I will only observe that from the first moments of the trial one peculiar characteristic of the case was conspicuous and observed by all, that is, the overwhelming strength of the prosecution as compared with the arguments and means at the disposal of the defence. Every one realised it from the first moment when in this stern court-room the facts began to accumulate round a single point, and the whole horrible and bloody crime was gradually revealed. Every one, perhaps, felt from the first that the case was beyond dispute, that there was no doubt about it, that there could be really no discussion, and that the arguing would be only a matter of form, and that the criminal was guilty, obviously and conclusively guilty. I imagine that even the ladies, who were so impatiently longing for the acquittal of the interesting prisoner, were at the same time, without exception, convinced of his guilt. What's more, I believe they would have been mortified if his guilt had not been so firmly established, as that would have lessened the effect of the closing scene of the criminal's acquittal. That he would be acquitted all the ladies, strange to say, were firmly persuaded up to the very last moment. "He is guilty, but he will be acquitted, from motives of humanity, because of the new ideas, the new sentiments that have come into fashion," and so on, and so on. And that was why they had crowded into the court so impatiently. The men were more interested in the contest between the prosecutor and the famous Fetyukovich.

All were wondering and asking themselves what could even a talent like Fetyukovich's make of such a lost cause; and so they followed his achievements, step by step, with concentrated attention.

But Fetyukovich remained an enigma to all up to the very end, up to his speech. Persons of experience suspected that he had a system, that he had some design, that he was working towards some object, but it was almost impossible to guess what it was. His confidence and self-reliance were unmistakable, however. Every one noticed with pleasure, moreover, that, after so short a stay, not more than three days, perhaps, among us, he had so wonderfully succeeded in mastering the case and "had studied it to a nicety." People described with relish, afterwards, how cleverly he had "taken down" all the witnesses for the prosecution, and as far as possible perplexed them and, what's more, had aspersed their reputation and so depreciated the value of their evidence. But it was supposed that he did this rather by way of sport, so to speak, for professional glory, to show nothing had been omitted of the accepted methods, for all were convinced that he could do no real good by such disparagement of the witnesses, and that he probably was more aware of this than any one, having some idea of his own in the background, some concealed weapon of defence, which he would suddenly reveal when the time came. But meanwhile, conscious of his strength, he seemed to be playing and gambolling.

So, for instance, when Grigory, Fyodor Pavlovich's old servant, who had given the most damning piece of evidence about the open door, was examined, the counsel for the defence positively pounced upon him when his turn came to question him. It must be noted that Grigory entered the hall with a composed and almost stately air, not the least disconcerted by the majesty of the court or the vast audience listening to him. He testified with as much confidence as though he had been talking with his Marfa, only perhaps more respectfully. It was impossible to confuse him. The prosecutor questioned him first in detail about the family life of the Karamazovs. The family picture stood out in lurid colours. It was plain to ear and eye that the witness was guileless and impartial. In spite of his profound reverence for the memory of his deceased master, he yet bore witness that he had been unjust to Mitya and "hadn't brought up his children as he should. He'd have been devoured by lice when he was little, if it hadn't been for me," he added, describing Mitya's early childhood. "It wasn't fair either of the father to wrong his son over his mother's property, which was by right his."

In reply to the prosecutor's question what

grounds he had for asserting that Fyodor Pavlovich had wronged his son in their money relations, Grigory, to the surprise of every one, had no proof at all to bring forward, but he still persisted that the arrangement with the son was "unfair," and that he ought "to have paid him several thousand roubles more." I must note, by the way, that the prosecutor asked this question whether Fyodor Pavlovich had really kept back part of Mitya's inheritance with marked persistence of all the witnesses who could be asked it, not excepting Alyosha and Ivan, but he obtained no exact information from any one; all alleged that it was so, but were unable to bring forward any clear proof. Grigory's description of the scene at the dinner-table, when Dmitri had burst in and given his father a beating, threatening to come back to kill him, made a sinister impression on the court, especially as the old servant told his story quietly, without more words than necessary, and using a peculiar phraseology, so that it was all very eloquent. He observed that he was not angry with Mitya for having knocked him down and struck him on the face; he had forgiven him long ago, he said. Of the deceased Smerdyakov he observed, crossing himself, that he was a lad of ability, but stupid and afflicted with disease, and, worse still, an unbeliever, and that it was Fyodor Pavlovich and his elder son who had taught him atheism. But he defended Smerdyakov's honesty almost with warmth, and related how Smerdyakov had once found the master's money in the yard, and, instead of concealing it, had taken it to his master, who had rewarded him with a "gold-piece" for it, and trusted him implicitly from that time forward. He maintained obstinately that the door into the garden had been open. But he was asked so many questions that I can't recall them all.

At last the counsel for the defence began to cross-examine him, and the first question he asked was about the envelope in which Fyodor Pavlovich was supposed to have put three thousand roubles for "a certain person." "Have you ever seen it, you, who were for so many years in close attendance on your master?" Grigory answered that he had not seen it and had never heard of the money from any one "till everybody was talking about it." This question about the envelope Fetyukovich put to every one who could conceivably have known of it, as persistently as the prosecutor asked his question about Dmitri's inheritance, and got the same answer from all, that no one had seen the envelope, though many had heard of it. From the beginning every one noticed Fetyukovich's insistence on this subject.

"Now, with your permission I'll ask you a question," Fetyukovich said, suddenly and unexpectedly. "Of what was that balsam, or, rather, decoction, made, which, as we learn from the preliminary inquiry, you used on that evening to rub your lame back, in the hope of curing it?"

Grigory looked blankly at the questioner, and after a brief silence muttered "there was saffron in it."

"Nothing but saffron? Don't you remember any other ingredient?"

"There was plantain in it, too."

"And pepper perhaps?" Fetyukovich queried.

"Yes, there was pepper, too."

"And so on. And all soaked in vodka?"

"In spirits."

There was a faint sound of laughter in the court.

"You see, in spirits. After rubbing your back, I believe, you drank what was left in the bottle with a certain pious prayer, known only to your spouse, didn't you?"

"I did."

"Did you drink much? Roughly speaking, a wine-glass or two?"

"It might have been a tumblerful."

"A tumblerful, even. Perhaps a tumbler and a half?" Grigory did not answer. He seemed to see what was meant.

"A glass and a half of neat spirits — is not at all bad, don't you think? You might see the gates of heaven open, not only the door into the garden?"

Grigory remained silent. There was another laugh in the court. The presiding judge stirred.

"Do you know for a fact," Fetyukovich persisted, "whether you were awake or not when you saw the open door?"

"I was on my legs."

"That's not a proof that you were awake." (There was again laughter in the court.) "Could you have answered at that moment, if any one had asked you a question — for instance, what year it is?"

"That I don't know."

"And what year is it, what year of our era, Anno Domini, do you know?"

Grigory stood with a perplexed face, looking straight at his tormentor. Strange to say, it appeared he really did not know what year it was.

"But perhaps you can tell me how many fingers you have on your hand?"

"I am a servant," Grigory said suddenly, in a loud and distinct voice. "If the authorities think fit to make game of me, it is my duty to suffer it."

Fetyukovich was a little taken aback, and the presiding judge intervened, reminding him that he must ask more relevant questions. Fetyukovich bowed with dignity and said that he had no more questions to ask of the witness. The public and the jury, of course, were left with a grain of doubt in their minds as to the evidence of a man who might, while undergoing a certain cure, have seen "the gates of heaven," and who did not even know what year he was living in, so that the lawyer to some extent achieved his purpose. But before Grigory left the box another episode occurred. The presiding judge, turning to the accused, asked him whether he had any comment to make on the evidence of the last witness.

"Except about the door, all he has said is true," cried Mitya, in a loud voice. "For combing the lice off me, I thank him; for forgiving my blows, I thank him. The old man has been honest all his life and as faithful to my father as seven hundred poodles."

"Prisoner, choose your words," the judge admonished him.

"I am not a poodle," Grigory muttered.

"All right, it's I am a poodle myself," cried Mitya. "If it's an insult, I take it on myself and I beg his pardon. I was a beast and cruel to him. I was cruel to Æsop, too."

"What Æsop?" the judge asked sternly again.

"Oh, Pierrot . . . my father, Fyodor Pavlovich."

The judge again and again warned Mitya impressively and very sternly to be more careful in his language.

"You are injuring yourself in the opinion of your judges."

The counsel for the defence was equally clever in dealing with the evidence of Rakitin.

I may remark that Rakitin was one of the leading witnesses and one to whom the prosecutor attached great significance. It appeared that he knew everything; his knowledge was amazing, he had been everywhere, seen everything, talked to everybody, knew every detail of the biography of Fyodor Pavlovich and all the Karamazovs. Of the envelope, it is true, he had only heard from Mitya himself. But he described minutely Mitya's exploits at the "Metropolis," all his compromising doings and sayings, and told the story of Captain Snegiryov's "bath-mop." But even Rakitin could say nothing positive about Mitya's inheritance, and confined himself to contemptuous generalities.

"Who could tell which of them was to blame, and which was in debt to the other, with their crazy Karamazov way of muddling things so that no one could make head or tail of it." The tragedy of the crime he presented as the product of the ancient way of living based on serfdom and the disorderly state of Russia, due to the lack of proper institutions. He was, in fact, allowed some latitude of speech. This was the first occasion on which Rakitin showed what he could do, and attracted notice. The prosecutor knew that the witness was preparing a magazine article on the case, and afterwards in his speech, as we shall see later, quoted some ideas from the article, showing that he had seen it already. The picture drawn by the witness was a gloomy and sinister one, and greatly strengthened the case for the prosecution. Altogether, Rakitin's discourse fascinated the public by its independence and the extraordinary nobility of its ideas. There were even two or three outbreaks of applause when he spoke of serfdom and the disorderly state of Russia.

But Rakitin, in his youthful ardour, made a slight blunder, of which the counsel for the defence at once adroitly took advantage. Answering certain questions about Grushenka, and carried away by the loftiness of his own sentiments and his success, of which he was, of course, conscious, he went so far as to speak somewhat contemptuously of Agrafena Alexandrovna as "Samsonov's kept woman." He would have given a good deal to take back his words afterwards, for Fetyukovich caught him out over it at once. And it was all because Rakitin had not reckoned on the lawyer's having been able to become so intimately acquainted with every detail in so short a time.

"Allow me to ask," began the counsel for the defence, with the most affable and even respectful smile, "you are, of course, the same Mr. Rakitin whose pamphlet, 'The Life of Father Zosima, the Elder, Deceased in the Lord,' published by the diocesan authorities, full of profound and religious reflections and preceded by an excellent and devout dedication to the Bishop, I have just read with such pleasure?"

"I did not write it for publication . . . it was published afterwards," muttered Rakitin, for some reason fearfully disconcerted and almost ashamed.

"Oh, that's excellent! A thinker like you can, and indeed ought to, take the broadest view of every social phenomenon. Your most instructive pamphlet has been widely circulated through the patronage of the Bishop, and has been of appreciable service. . . . But this is the chief thing I should like to learn from you. You stated just now that you were very intimately acquainted with Madame Svyetlov."

(It must be noted that Grushenka's surname was Svyetlov. I heard it for the first time that day, during the trial.)

"I cannot answer for all my acquaintances. . . . I am a young man . . . and who can be responsible for every one he meets?" cried Rakitin, flushing all over.

"I understand, I quite understand," cried Fetyukovich, as though he, too, were embarrassed and in haste to excuse himself. "You, like any other, might well be interested in an acquaintance with a young and beautiful woman who would readily entertain the *élite* of the youth of the neighbourhood, but . . . I only wanted to know . . . it has come to my knowledge that Madame Svyetlov was particularly anxious a couple of months ago to make the acquaintance of the younger Karamazov, Alexey Fyodorovich, and promised you twenty-five roubles if you would bring him to her in his monastic dress. And that actually took place on the evening of the day on which the terrible crime, which is the subject of the present investigation, was committed. You brought Alexey Karamazov to Madame Svyetlov, and did you receive the twenty-five roubles from Madame Svyetlov as a reward, that's what I wanted to hear from you?"

"It was a joke. . . . I don't see of what interest that can be to you. . . . I took it for a joke . . . meaning to give it back later . . ."

"Then you did take . . . But you have not given it back yet . . . or have you?"

"That's of no consequence," muttered Rakitin, "I refuse to answer such questions. . . . Of course I shall give it back."

The judge intervened, but Fetyukovich declared he had no more questions to ask of the witness. Mr. Rakitin left the witness-box not absolutely without a stain upon his character. The effect left by the lofty idealism of his speech was somewhat marred, and Fetyukovich's expression, as he watched him walk away, seemed to suggest to the public, "this is a specimen of the lofty-minded persons who accuse him." I remember that this incident, too, did not pass off without an outbreak from Mitya. Enraged by the tone in which Rakitin had referred to Grushenka, he suddenly shouted, "Bernard!" When, after Rakitin's cross-examination, the judge asked the prisoner if he had anything to say, Mitya cried loudly:

"Since I've been arrested, he has borrowed money from me! He is a contemptible Bernard and careerist, and he doesn't believe in God; he cheated the Bishop!"

Mitya, of course, was pulled up again for the intemperance of his language, but Rakitin was done for. Captain Snegiryov's testimony was a failure, too, but for quite a different reason. He appeared in ragged and dirty clothes, muddy boots, and in spite of the vigilance exercised and preliminary examination by an expert, he turned out to be hopelessly drunk. On being asked about Mitya's attack upon him, he refused to answer.

"God bless him. Ilusha told me not to. God will make it up to me yonder."

"Who told you not to tell? Of whom are you talking?"

"Ilusha, my little son. 'Father, father, how he insulted you!' He said that at the stone. Now he is dying . . ."

The captain suddenly began sobbing, and plumped down on his knees before the judge. He was hurriedly led away amidst the laughter of the public. The effect prepared by the prosecutor did not come off at all.

Fetyukovich went on making the most of every opportunity, and amazed people more and more by his minute knowledge of the case. Thus, for example, Trifon Borisovich made a great impression, of course, very prejudicial to Mitya. He calculated almost on his fingers that on his first visit to Mokroye, Mitya must have spent three thousand roubles, "or very little less. Just think what he squandered on those gipsy girls alone! And as for our lousy peasants, it wasn't a case of flinging half a rouble in the street, he made them presents of twenty-five roubles each, he didn't give them less. And what a lot of money was simply stolen from him! And if any one did steal, he did not leave a receipt. How could one catch the thief when he was flinging his money away all the time? Our peasants are robbers, you know; they have no care for their souls. And the way he went on with the girls, our village girls! They're completely set up since then, I tell you, they used to be poor." He recalled, in fact, every item of expense and added it all up. So the theory that only fifteen hundred had been spent and the rest had been put aside in a little bag seemed inconceivable.

"I saw three thousand as clear as a penny in his hands, I saw it with my own eyes; I should think I ought to know how to reckon money," cried Trifon Borisovich, doing his best to please "the authorities."

When it was Fetyukovich's turn to cross-examine him, he scarcely tried to refute his evidence, but began asking him about an incident at the first carousal at Mokroye, a month before the arrest, when Timofey and another peasant called Akim had picked up on the floor in the passage a hundred roubles dropped by Mitya when he was drunk, and had given them to Trifon Borisovich, and received a rouble each from him for doing so. "Well," asked the lawyer, "did you give that hundred roubles back to Mr. Karamazov?" Trifon Borisovich shuffled in vain. . . . He was obliged, after the peasants had been examined, to admit the finding of the hundred roubles, only adding that he had religiously returned it all to Dmitri Fyodorovich "in perfect honesty, and it's only because his honour was in liquor at the time, he wouldn't remember it." But, as he had denied the incident of the hundred roubles till the peasants had been called to prove it, his evidence as to returning the money to Mitya was naturally regarded with great suspicion. So one of the most dangerous witnesses brought forward by the prosecution was again discredited.

The same thing happened with the Poles. They assumed an attitude of pride and independence; they asserted loudly that they had both been in the service of the Crown, and that "*Pan* Mitya" had offered them three thousand "to buy their honour," and that they had seen a large sum of money in his hands. *Pan* Musialowicz introduced a terrible number of Polish words into his sentences, and seeing that this only raised him in the eyes of the judge and the prosecutor, grew more and more pompous, and ended by talking in Polish altogether. But Fetyukovich caught them, too, in his snares. Trifon Borisovich, recalled, was forced, in spite of his evasions, to admit that *Pan* Wróblewski had substituted another pack of cards for the one he had provided, and that *Pan* Musialowicz had cheated during the game. Kalganov confirmed this, and both the Poles left the witness-box with damaged reputations, amidst laughter from the public.

Then exactly the same thing happened with almost all the most dangerous witnesses. Fetyukovich succeeded in casting a slur on all of them, and dismissing them with a certain derision. Both the amateurs and the professional lawyers were lost in admiration, and were only puzzled as to what good purpose could be served by it, for all, I repeat, felt that the case for the prosecution could not be refuted, but was growing more and more tragically overwhelming. But from the confidence of the "great magician" they saw that he was serene. They waited, feeling that "such a man" had not come from Petersburg for nothing, and that he was not a man to return unsuccessful.

CHAPTER III

THE MEDICAL EXPERTS AND A POUND OF NUTS

THE evidence of the medical experts, too, was of little use to the accused. And it appeared later that Fetyukovich had not reckoned much upon it. The medical line of defence had only been taken up through the insistence of Katerina Ivanovna, who had sent for a celebrated doctor from Moscow on purpose. The case for the defence could, of course, lose nothing by it and might, with luck, gain something from it. There was, however, an element of comedy about it, owing to the difference of opinion among the doctors. The medical experts were the famous doctor from Moscow, our doctor, Herzenstube, and the young doctor, Varvinsky. The two latter appeared also as witnesses for the prosecution.

The first to be called in the capacity of expert was Dr. Herzenstube. He was a grey and bald old man of seventy, of middle height and sturdy build. He was much esteemed and respected by every one in the town. He was a conscientious doctor and an excellent and pious man, a Herrnhuter or Moravian brother, I am not quite sure which. He had been living amongst us for many years and behaved with extraordinary dignity. He was a kind-hearted and humane man. He treated the sick poor and peasants for nothing, visited them in their slums and huts, and left money for medicine, but he was as obstinate as a mule. If once he had taken an idea into his head, there was no shaking him. Almost every one in the town was aware, by the way, that the famous doctor had, within the first two or three days of his presence among us, made some extremely offensive remarks as to Dr. Herzenstube's qualifications. Though the Moscow doctor asked twenty-five roubles for a visit, several people in the town were glad to take advantage of his arrival, and rushed to consult him regardless of expense. All these had, of course, previously been patients of Dr. Herzenstube's, and the celebrated doctor had criticised his treatment with extreme harshness. Finally, he had asked the patients as soon as he saw them, "Well, who has been cramming you with nostrums? Herzenstube? He, he!" Dr. Herzenstube, of course, heard all this, and now all the three doctors made their appearance, one after another, to be examined.

Dr. Herzenstube roundly declared that the abnormality of the prisoner's mental faculties was self-evident. Then giving his grounds for this opinion, which I omit here, he added that the abnormality was not only evident in many of the prisoner's actions in the past, but was apparent even now at this very moment. When he was asked to explain how it was apparent now at this moment, the old doctor, with simple-hearted directness, pointed out that the prisoner on entering the court had "an extraordinary air, remarkable under the circumstances"; that he had "marched in like a soldier, looking straight before him, though it would have been more natural for him to look to the left where, among the public, the ladies were sitting, seeing that he is a great admirer of the fair sex and must be thinking much of what the ladies are saying of him now," the old man concluded in his peculiar language.

I must add that he spoke Russian readily, but somehow every sentence was formed in the German manner, which did not, however, trouble him, for it had always been a weakness of his to believe that he spoke Russian perfectly, better indeed than Russians. And he was very fond of using Russian proverbs, always declaring that the Russian proverbs were the best and most expressive sayings in the whole world. I may remark, too, that in conversation, through absent-mindedness, he often forgot the most ordinary words, which sometimes went out of his head, though he knew them perfectly. The same thing happened, though, when he spoke German, and at such times he always waved his hand before his face as though trying to catch the lost word, and no one could induce him to go on speaking till he had found the missing word. His remark that the accused ought to have looked at the ladies on entering roused a whisper of amusement in the audience. All our ladies were very fond of our old doctor; they knew, too, that, having been a bachelor all his life and a chaste, religious man, he looked upon women as superior and ideal creatures. And so his unexpected observation struck every one as very queer.

The Moscow doctor, being questioned in his turn, definitely and emphatically affirmed that he considered the prisoner's mental condition abnormal in the highest degree. He talked at length and with erudition of "aberration" and "mania," and argued that, from all the facts collected, the prisoner had undoubtedly been in a condition of aberration for several days before his arrest, and, if the crime had been committed by him, it must, even if he were conscious of it, have been almost involuntary, as he had not the power to control the morbid impulse that possessed him.

But apart from temporary aberration, the doctor diagnosed mania, which promised, in his words, to lead to complete insanity in the future. (It must be noted that I report this in my own words, the doctor made use of very learned and technical language.) "All his actions are in contravention of common sense and logic," he continued. "Not to refer to what I have not seen, that is, the crime itself and the whole catastrophe, the day before yesterday, while he was talking to me, he had an unaccountably fixed look in his eye. He laughed unexpectedly when there was nothing to laugh at. He showed continual and inexplicable irritability, using strange words, 'Bernard!' 'Ethics!' and others equally inappropriate." But the doctor detected mania, above all, in the fact that the accused could not even speak of the three thousand roubles, of which he considered himself to have been cheated, without extraordinary irritation, though he could speak comparatively lightly of other misfortunes and grievances. According to all accounts, he had even in the past, whenever the subject of the three thousand roubles was touched on, flown into a perfect frenzy, and yet he was reported to be a disinterested and not grasping man.

"As to the opinion of my learned colleague," the Moscow doctor added ironically in conclusion, "that on entering the court, the accused would have naturally looked at the ladies and not straight before him, I will only say that, apart from the playfulness of this theory, it is radically unsound. For though I fully agree that the accused, on entering the court where his fate will be decided, would not naturally look straight before him in that fixed way, and that that may really be a sign of his abnormal mental condition, at the same time I maintain that he would naturally not look to the left at the ladies, but, on the contrary, to the right to find his legal adviser, on whose help all his hopes rest and on whose defence his fate depends." The doctor expressed his opinion resolutely and emphatically.

But the unexpected pronouncement of Dr. Varvinsky gave the last touch of comedy to the difference of opinion between the experts. In his opinion the accused was now, and had been all along, in a perfectly normal condition, and, although he certainly must have been in a nervous and exceedingly excited state before his arrest, this might have been due to several perfectly obvious causes, jealousy, anger, continual drunkenness, and so on. But this nervous condition would not involve the mental aberration of which mention had just been made. As to the question whether the accused should have looked to the left or to the right on entering the court, "in his modest opinion," the accused would naturally look straight before him on entering the court, as he had in fact done, as that was where the judges, on whom his fate depended, were sitting. So that it was just by looking straight before him that he showed his perfectly normal state of mind at present. The young doctor concluded his "modest" testimony with some heat.

"Bravo, doctor!" cried Mitya, from his seat, "just so!"

Mitya, of course, was checked, but the young doctor's opinion had a decisive influence on the judges and on the public, and, as appeared afterwards, every one agreed with him. But Dr. Herzenstube, when called as a witness, was quite unexpectedly of use to Mitya. As an old resident in the town who had known the Karamazov family for years, he furnished some facts of great value for the prosecution, and suddenly, as though recalling something, he added: "But the poor young man might have had a very different life, for he had a good heart both in childhood and after childhood, that I know. But the Russian proverb says, 'If a man has one head, it's good, but if another clever man comes to visit him, it would be better still, for then there will be two heads and not only one.' "

"One head is good, but two are better," the prosecutor put in impatiently. He knew the old man's habit of talking slowly and deliberately, regardless of the impression he was making and of the delay he was causing, and highly prizing his flat, dull, and always gleefully complacent German wit. The old man was fond of making jokes.

"Oh, yes, that's what I say," he went on stubbornly. "One head is good, but two are much better, but he did not meet another head with wits, and his wits went. Where did they go? I've forgotten the word." He went on, passing his hand before his eyes, "Oh, yes, *spazieren*."

"Wandering?".

"Oh, yes, wandering, that's what I say. Well, his wits went wandering and fell in such a deep hole that he lost himself. And yet he was a grateful and sensitive boy. Oh, I remember him very well, a little chap so high, left neglected by his father in the back yard, when he ran about without boots on his feet, and his little breeches hanging by one button."

A note of feeling and tenderness suddenly

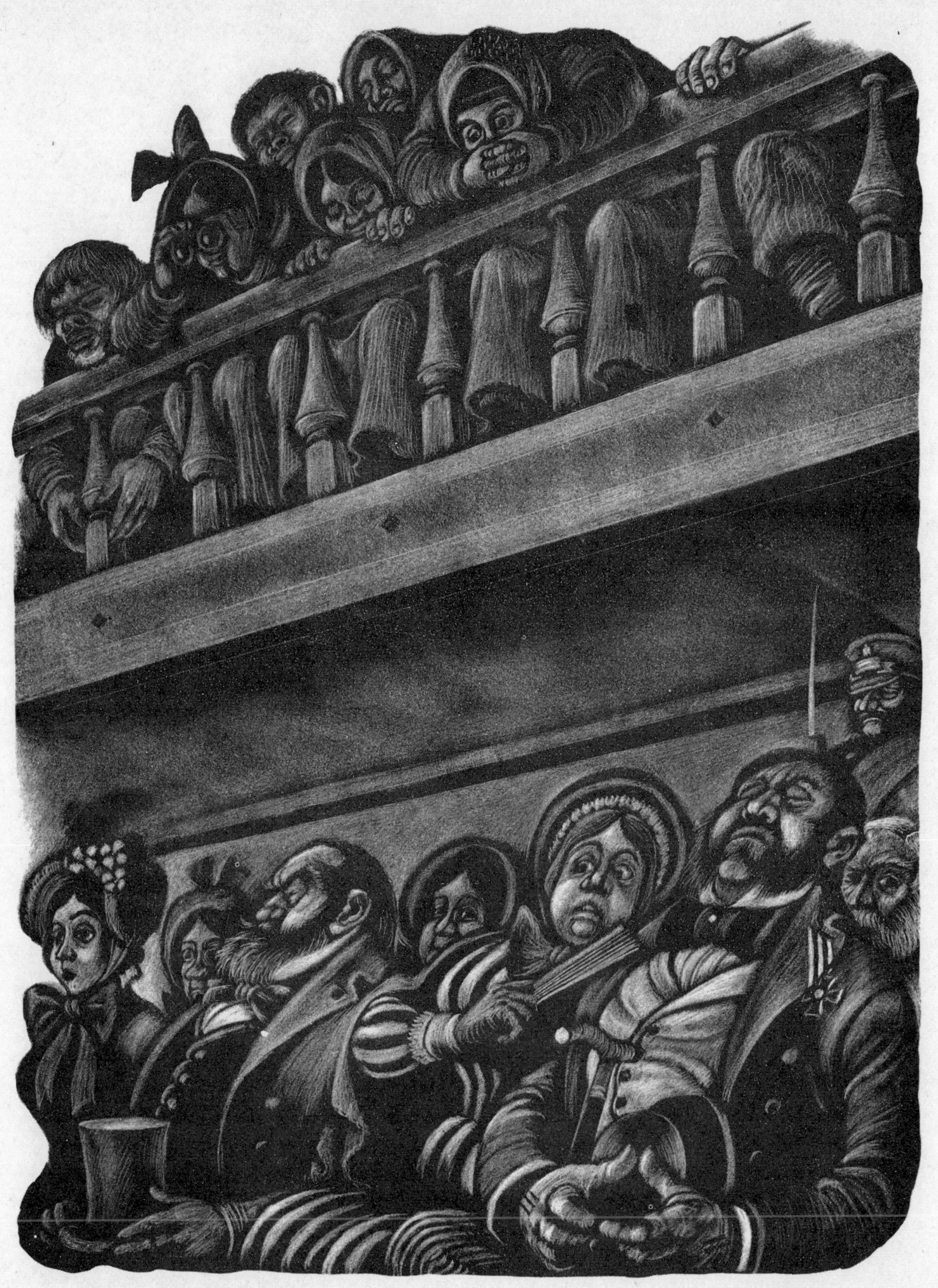

HE SAT RIGID IN HIS PLACE

came into the honest old man's voice. Fetyukovich positively started, as though scenting something and caught at it instantly.

"Oh, yes, I was a young man then. . . . I was . . . well, I was forty-five then, and had only just come here. And I was so sorry for the boy then; I asked myself why shouldn't I buy him a pound of . . . . a pound of what? I've forgotten what it's called. A pound of what children are very fond of, what is it, what is it?" The doctor began waving his hands again. "It grows on a tree and is gathered and given to every one . . ."

"Apples?"

"Oh, no, no. You have a dozen of apples, not a pound. . . . No, there are a lot of them, and all little. You put them in the mouth and crack."

"Nuts?"

"Quite so, nuts, I say so," the doctor repeated in the calmest way as though he had been at no loss for a word. "And I bought him a pound of nuts, for no one had ever bought the boy a pound of nuts before. And I lifted my finger and said to him, 'Boy, *Gott der Vater*.' He laughed and said, '*Gott der Vater*.' . . . '*Gott der Sohn*.' He laughed again and lisped, '*Gott der Sohn*.' '*Gott der heilige Geist*.' Then he laughed and said as best he could, '*Gott der heilige Geist*.' I went away, and two days after I happened to be passing, and he shouted to me of himself, 'Uncle, *Gott der Vater*, *Gott der Sohn*,' and he had only forgotten '*Gott der heilige Geist*.' But I reminded him of it and I felt very sorry for him again. But he was taken away, and I did not see him again. Twenty-three years passed. I am sitting one morning in my study, a white-haired old man, when there walks into the room a blooming young man, whom I should never have recognised, but he held up his finger and said, laughing, '*Gott der Vater*, *Gott der Sohn*, and *Gott der heilige Geist*. I have just arrived and have come to thank you for that pound of nuts, for no one else ever bought me a pound of nuts; you are the only one that ever did.' And then I remembered my happy youth and the poor child in the yard, without boots on his feet, and my heart was touched and I said, 'You are a grateful young man, for you have remembered all your life the pound of nuts I bought you in your childhood.' And I embraced him and blessed him. And I wept. He laughed, but he wept, too . . . for the Russian often laughs when he ought to be weeping. But he did weep; I saw it. And now, alas!"

"And I am weeping now, German, I am weeping now, too, you saintly man," Mitya cried suddenly.

In any case the anecdote made a certain favourable impression on the public. But the chief sensation in Mitya's favour was created by the evidence of Katerina Ivanovna, which I will describe directly. Indeed, when the witnesses *à décharge*, that is, called by the defence, began giving evidence, fortune seemed all at once markedly more favourable to Mitya, and, what was particularly striking, this was a surprise even to the counsel for the defence. But before Katerina Ivanovna was called, Alyosha was examined, and he recalled a fact which seemed to furnish positive evidence against one important point made by the prosecution.

CHAPTER IV

FORTUNE SMILES ON MITYA

It came quite as a surprise even to Alyosha himself. He was not required to take the oath, and I remember that both sides addressed him very gently and sympathetically. It was evident that his good reputation had preceded him. Alyosha gave his evidence modestly and with restraint, but his warm sympathy for his unhappy brother was unmistakable. In answer to one question, he sketched his brother's character as that of a man, violent-tempered perhaps and carried away by his passions, but at the same time honourable, proud, and generous, capable of self-sacrifice, if necessary. He admitted, however, that, through his passion for Grushenka and his rivalry with his father, his brother had been of late in an intolerable position. But he repelled with indignation the suggestion that his brother might have committed a murder with intent to rob, though he recognised that the three thousand roubles had become almost an obsession with Mitya; that he had looked upon them as part of the inheritance he had been cheated of by his father, and that, indifferent as he was to money as a rule, he could not even speak of that three thousand without fury. With regard to the rivalry of the two "ladies," as the prosecutor expressed it — that is, of Grushenka and Katya — he spoke evasively and was even unwilling to answer one or two questions altogether.

"Did your brother tell you, anyway, that he intended to kill your father?" asked the prosecutor. "You can refuse to answer if you think necessary," he added.

"He did not tell me so directly," answered Alyosha.

"How so? Did he indirectly?"

"He spoke to me once of his hatred for our father and of his fear that in an extreme moment . . . in a moment of disgust, he might perhaps murder him."

"And you believed him?"

"I am afraid to say that I did. But I never doubted that some higher feeling would always save him at the fatal moment, as it has indeed saved him, for *it was not he* killed my father," Alyosha said firmly, in a loud voice that was heard throughout the court.

The prosecutor started like a warhorse at the sound of a trumpet.

"Let me assure you that I fully believe in the complete sincerity of your conviction and do not explain it by or identify it with your affection for your unhappy brother. Your peculiar view of the whole tragic episode is known to us already from the preliminary investigation. I won't attempt to conceal from you that it is highly subjective and contradicts all the other evidence collected by the prosecution. And so I think it essential to press you to tell me what facts have led you to this conviction of your brother's innocence and of the guilt of another person whom you clearly indicated at the preliminary inquiry?"

"At the preliminary inquiry I only answered the questions which I was asked," replied Alyosha, slowly and calmly. "For my own part, I made no accusation against Smerdyakov."

"Yet you pointed to him?"

"I was led to do so by my brother Dmitri's words. Already before the inquiry I was told what took place at his arrest and how he had then pointed to Smerdyakov. I believe absolutely that my brother is innocent, and if he didn't commit the murder, then . . ."

"Then Smerdyakov? Why Smerdyakov? And why are you so completely persuaded of your brother's innocence?"

"I cannot help believing my brother. I know he wouldn't lie to me. I saw from his face he wasn't lying."

"Only from his face? Is that all the proof you have?"

"I have no other proof."

"And of Smerdyakov's guilt have you no proof whatever but your brother's word and the expression of his face?"

"No, I have no other proof."

The prosecutor dropped the examination at this point. The impression left by Alyosha's evidence on the public was most disappointing. There had been talk about Smerdyakov before the trial; some one had heard something, some one had pointed out something else, it was said that Alyosha had gathered together some extraordinary proofs of his brother's innocence and Smerdyakov's guilt, and after all there was nothing, no evidence except certain moral convictions so natural in a brother.

But Fetyukovich began his cross-examination. On his asking Alyosha when it was that the accused had told him of his hatred for his father and that he might kill him, and whether he had heard it, for instance, at their last meeting before the catastrophe, Alyosha started as he answered, as though only just recollecting and grasping something.

"I remember one circumstance now which I'd quite forgotten myself. It wasn't clear to me at the time, but now . . ."

And, obviously only now for the first time struck by an idea, he recounted eagerly how, at his last interview with Mitya that evening under the tree, on the road to the monastery, Mitya had struck himself on the breast, "the upper part of the breast," and had repeated several times that he had a means of restoring his honour, that that means was here, here on his breast. "I thought, when he struck himself on the breast, he meant that it was in his heart," Alyosha continued, "that he might find in his heart strength to save himself from some awful disgrace which was awaiting him and which he did not dare confess even to me. I must own I did think at the time that he was speaking of our father, and that the disgrace he was shuddering at was the thought of going to our father and doing some violence to him. Yet it was just then that he pointed to something on his breast, so that I remember the idea struck me at the time that the heart is not in that part of the breast, but below, and that he struck himself much too high, just below the neck, and kept pointing to that place. My idea seemed silly to me at the time, but he was perhaps pointing then to that little bag in which there were sewn up these fifteen hundred roubles!"

"Just so," Mitya cried from his place. "That's right, Alyosha, it was the little bag I struck with my fist."

Fetyukovich flew to him in hot haste entreating him to keep quiet, and at the same instant pounced on Alyosha. Alyosha, carried away himself by his recollection, warmly expressed his theory that this disgrace was probably just that fifteen hundred roubles on him, which he might have returned to Katerina Ivanovna as half of what he owed her, but which he had yet determined not to repay her and to use for another purpose: to enable him to elope with Grushenka, if she consented.

"It is so, it must be so," exclaimed Alyosha, in sudden excitement. "My brother cried several times that half of the disgrace, half of it (he said *half* several times) he could free himself from at once, but that his character was unhappily so weak that he wouldn't do it . . . that he knew beforehand he was incapable of doing it!"

"And you clearly, confidently remember that he struck himself just on this part of the breast?" Fetyukovich asked eagerly.

"Clearly and confidently, for I thought at the time, 'Why does he strike himself up there when the heart is lower down?' and the thought seemed foolish to me at the time . . . I remember its seeming foolish . . . it flashed through my mind. That's what brought it back to me just now. How could I have forgotten it till now! It was that little bag he meant when he said he had the means but wouldn't give back that fifteen hundred. And when he was arrested at Mokroye he cried out — I know, I was told it — that he considered it the most disgraceful act of his life that when he had the means of repaying Katerina Ivanovna half (half, note!) of what he owed her, he yet could not bring himself to repay the money and preferred to remain a thief in her eyes rather than part with it. And what torture, what torture that debt has been to him!" Alyosha exclaimed in conclusion.

The prosecutor, of course, intervened. He asked Alyosha to describe once more how it had all happened, and several times insisted on the question, had the prisoner seemed to point to anything. Perhaps he had simply struck himself with his fist on the breast?

"But it was not with his fist," cried Alyosha; "he pointed with his fingers and pointed here, very high up. . . . How could I have so completely forgotten it till this moment!"

The judge asked Mitya what he had to say about this evidence. Mitya confirmed it, saying that he had been pointing to the fifteen hundred roubles which were on his breast, just below the neck, and that that was, of course, the disgrace. "A disgrace I cannot deny, the most shameful act of my whole life," cried Mitya. "I might have repaid it and didn't repay it. I preferred to remain a thief in her eyes rather than give it back. And the most shameful part of it was that I knew beforehand I shouldn't give it back! You are right, Alyosha! Thanks, Alyosha!"

So Alyosha's cross-examination ended. What was important and striking about it was that one fact at least had been found, and even though this were only one tiny bit of evidence, a mere hint at evidence, it did go some little way towards proving that the bag had existed and had contained fifteen hundred roubles and that the prisoner had not been lying at the preliminary inquiry when he alleged at Mokroye that those fifteen hundred roubles were "his own." Alyosha was glad. With a flushed face he moved away to the seat assigned to him. He kept repeating to himself: "How was it I forgot! How could I have forgotten it! And what made it come back to me now?"

The examination of Katerina Ivanovna began. As she appeared there was a great commotion in the court-room. The ladies clutched their lorgnettes and opera-glasses. There was a stir among the men: some stood up to get a better view. Everybody alleged afterwards that Mitya had turned "white as a sheet" on her entrance. All in black, she advanced modestly, almost timidly. It was impossible to tell from her face that she was agitated; but there was a resolute gleam in her dark and gloomy eyes. I may remark that many people mentioned that she looked particularly handsome at that moment. She spoke softly but clearly, so that she was heard all over the court. She expressed herself with composure, or at least tried to appear composed. The presiding judge began his examination discreetly and respectfully, as though afraid to touch "certain chords," and showing consideration for her great misfortune. But in answer to one of the first questions Katerina Ivanovna replied firmly that she had been betrothed to the accused "until he left me of his own accord . . ." she added quietly. When they asked her about the three thousand she had entrusted to Mitya to post to her relations, she said firmly, "I didn't give him the money simply to send it off. I felt at the time that he was in great need of money. . . . I gave him the three thousand with the understanding that he should post it within the month if he cared to. There was no need for him to worry himself about that debt afterwards."

I am not repeating all the questions asked her and all her answers word for word. I am only giving the substance of her testimony.

"I was firmly convinced that he would send off that sum as soon as he got money from his father," she went on. "I have never doubted his disinterestedness and his honesty . . . his scrupulous honesty . . . in money matters. He felt quite certain that he would receive three thousand roubles from his father, and spoke to me several times about it. I knew he had a feud with his father and have always believed that he had been unfairly treated by his father. I don't remember any threat uttered by him against his father. He certainly never uttered any such threat in my presence. If he had come to me at that time, I should have at once relieved his anxiety about that wretched three thousand, but he had given up coming to see me . . . and I myself was put in such a position . . . that I could not invite him. . . . And I had no right, indeed, to be exacting about that money," she added suddenly, and there was a ring of resolution in her voice. "I once received a loan from him of more than three thousand, and I accepted it, although I could not at that time foresee that I should ever be in a position to repay my debt."

There was a note of defiance in her voice. It was then Fetyukovich began his cross-examination.

"Did that take place not here, but at the beginning of your acquaintance?" Fetyukovich suggested cautiously, feeling his way, instantly scenting something favourable. I must mention in parenthesis that, though Fetyukovich had been brought from Petersburg partly at the instance of Katerina Ivanovna herself, he knew nothing about the episode of the five thousand roubles given her by Mitya, and of her "bowing to the ground to him." She concealed this from him and said nothing about it, and that was strange. It may be pretty certainly assumed that she herself did not know till the very last minute whether she would speak of that episode in court, and waited for the inspiration of the moment.

No, I can never forget those moments. She began telling her story. She told everything, the whole episode that Mitya had told Alyosha, and her bowing to the ground, and her reason. She told about her father and her going to Mitya, and did not in one word, in a single hint, suggest that Mitya had himself, through her sister, proposed they should "send him Katerina Ivanovna" to fetch the money. She generously concealed that and was not ashamed to make it appear as though she had of her own impulse run to the young officer, hoping for something . . . to beg him for the money. It was something tremendous! I turned cold and trembled as I listened. The court was hushed, trying to catch every word. It was something unexampled. Even from such a self-willed and contemptuously proud girl as she was, such an extremely frank avowal, such sacrifice, such self-immolation, seemed incredible. And for what, for whom? To save the man who had deceived and insulted her and in however small a degree to help save him, by creating a strong impression in his favour. And, indeed, the figure of the young officer who, with a respectful bow to the innocent girl, handed her his last five thousand roubles — all he had in the world — was thrown into a very sympathetic and attractive light, but . . . my heart contracted painfully! I felt that calumny might come of it later (and it did, in fact, it did). It was repeated all over the town afterwards with spiteful laughter that the story was perhaps not quite exact — that is, in the statement that the officer had let the young lady depart "with nothing but a respectful bow." It was hinted that something was omitted here.

"And even if nothing had been omitted, if this were the whole truth," the most highly respected of our ladies maintained, "even then it's very doubtful whether it was creditable for a young girl to behave in that way, even for the sake of saving her father."

And can Katerina Ivanovna, with her intelligence, her morbid sensitiveness, have failed to understand that people would talk like that? She must have understood it, yet she made up her mind to tell everything. Of course, all these nasty little suspicions as to the truth of her story arose only afterwards and at the first moment all were deeply impressed by it. As for the judges and the lawyers, they listened in reverent, almost shamefaced silence to Katerina Ivanovna. The prosecutor did not venture upon even one question on the subject. Fetyukovich made a low bow to her. Oh, he was almost triumphant! Much ground had been gained. For a man to give his last five thousand on a generous impulse and then for the same man to murder his father at night for the sake of robbing him of three thousand — the idea seemed too incongruous. Fetyukovich felt that now the charge of theft, at least, was as good as disproved. "The case" was thrown into quite a different light. There was a wave of sympathy for Mitya. As for him . . . I was told that once or twice, while Katerina Ivanovna was giving her evidence, he jumped up from his seat, sank back again, and hid his face in his hands. But when she had finished, he suddenly cried in a sobbing voice:

"Katya, why have you ruined me?" and his sobs were audible all over the court. But he instantly restrained himself, and cried again:

"Now I am condemned!"

Then he sat rigid in his place, with his teeth clenched and his arms across his chest. Katerina Ivanovna remained in court and sat down in her place. She was pale and sat with her eyes cast down. Those who were sitting near her declared that for a long time she shivered all over as though in a fever. Grushenka was called.

I am approaching the sudden catastrophe which was perhaps the final cause of Mitya's ruin. For I am convinced, so is every one — all the lawyers said the same afterwards — that if the episode had not occurred, the accused would at least have received a light sentence. But of that later. A couple of words first about Grushenka.

She, too, was dressed entirely in black, with her magnificent black shawl on her shoulders. She walked to the witness-box with her smooth, noiseless tread, with the slightly swaying gait common in women of full figure. She looked steadily at the presiding judge, turning her eyes neither to the right nor to the left. To my thinking she looked very handsome at that moment, and not at all pale, as the ladies alleged afterwards. They declared, too, that she had a concentrated and spiteful expression. I believe that she was simply irritated and painfully conscious of the contemptuous and inquisitive eyes of our scandal-loving public. She was proud and could not stand contempt. She was one of those people who flare up, angry and eager to retaliate, at the mere suggestion of contempt. There was an element of timidity, too, of course, and inward shame at her own timidity, so it was not strange that her tone kept changing. At one moment it was angry, contemptuous, and rude, and at another there was a sincere note of self-condemnation. Sometimes she spoke as though she were taking a desperate plunge; as though she felt, "I don't care what happens, I'll say it. . . ." Apropos of her acquaintance with Fyodor Pavlovich, she remarked curtly, "That's all nonsense, and was it my fault that he would pester me?" But a minute later she added, "It was all my fault. I was laughing at them both — at the old man and at him, too — and I brought both of them to this. It was all on account of me it happened."

Samsonov's name came up somehow. "That's nobody's business," she snapped at once, with a sort of insolent defiance. "He was my benefactor; he took me when I went barefoot, when my family had turned me out." The presiding judge reminded her, though very politely, that she must answer the questions directly, without going off into irrelevant details. Grushenka crimsoned and her eyes flashed.

The envelope with the notes in it she had not seen, but had only heard from "that wicked wretch" that Fyodor Pavlovich had an envelope with three thousand in it. "But that was all foolishness. I was only joking. I wouldn't have gone there for anything."

"To whom are you referring as 'that wicked wretch'?" inquired the prosecutor.

"The lackey, Smerdyakov, who murdered his master and hanged himself last night."

She was, of course, at once asked what grounds she had for such a definite accusation; but it appeared that she, too, had no grounds for it.

"Dmitri Fyodorovich told me so himself; you can believe him. The woman who came between us has ruined him; she is the cause of it all, let me tell you," Grushenka added. She seemed to be quivering with hatred, and there was a vindictive note in her voice.

She was again asked to whom she was referring.

"The young lady, Katerina Ivanovna there. She sent for me, offered me chocolate, tried to fascinate me. There's not much true shame about her, I can tell you that . . ."

At this point the presiding judge checked her sternly, begging her to moderate her language. But the jealous woman's heart was burning, and she did not care what she did.

"When the prisoner was arrested at Mokroye," the prosecutor asked, "every one saw and heard you run out of the next room and cry out: 'It's all my fault. We'll go to Siberia together!' So you already believed him to have murdered his father?"

"I don't remember what I felt at the time," answered Grushenka. "Every one was crying out that he had killed his father, and I felt that it was my fault, that it was on my account he had murdered him. But when he said he wasn't guilty, I believed him at once, and I believe him now and always shall believe him. He is not the man to tell a lie."

Fetyukovich began his cross-examination. I remember that among other things he asked about Rakitin and the twenty-five roubles "you paid him for bringing Alexey Fyodorovich Karamazov to see you."

"There was nothing strange about his taking the money," sneered Grushenka, with angry contempt. "He was always coming to me for money: he used to get thirty roubles a month at least out of me, chiefly for luxuries: he had enough to keep him without my help."

"What led you to be so liberal to Mr. Rakitin?" Fetyukovich asked, in spite of an uneasy movement on the part of the presiding judge.

"Why, he is my cousin. His mother was my mother's sister. But he's always begged me not to tell any one here of it, he is so dreadfully ashamed of me."

This fact was a complete surprise to every one; no one in the town nor in the monastery, not even Mitya, knew of it. I was told that Rakitin turned purple with shame where he sat. Grushenka had somehow heard before she came into court that he had given evidence against Mitya, and so she was angry. The whole effect on the public, of Rakitin's speech, of his noble sentiments, of his attacks upon serfdom and the political disorder of Russia, was this time finally ruined. Fetyukovich was satisfied: it was another godsend. Grushenka's cross-examination did not last long and, of course, there could be nothing particularly new in her testimony. She left a very disagreeable impression on the public; hundreds of contemptuous eyes were fixed upon her, as she finished giving her evidence and sat down again in the court-room, at a good distance from Katerina Ivanovna. Mitya was silent throughout her testimony. He sat as though turned to stone, with his eyes fixed on the ground.

Ivan was called to give evidence.

CHAPTER V

A SUDDEN CATASTROPHE

I MAY note that he had been called before Alyosha. But the court attendant announced to the presiding judge that, owing to an attack of illness or some sort of fit, the witness could not appear at the moment, but was ready to give his evidence as soon as he recovered. But no one seemed to have heard it and it only came out later.

His entrance was at first almost unnoticed. The principal witnesses, especially the two rival women, had already been questioned. Curiosity was satisfied for the time; the public was feeling almost fatigued. Several more witnesses were still to be heard, who probably had little information to give after all that had been given. Time was passing. Ivan walked up with extraordinary slowness, looking at no one, and with his head bowed, as though plunged in gloomy thought. He was irreproachably dressed, but his face made a painful impression, on me at least: there was an earthy look in it, a look like a dying man's. His eyes were lusterless; he raised them and looked slowly round the court. Alyosha jumped up from his seat and moaned "Ah!" I remember that, but it was hardly noticed.

The presiding judge began by informing him that he was a witness not on oath, that he might answer or refuse to answer, but that, of course, he must bear witness according to his conscience, and so on and so on. Ivan listened and looked at him blankly, but his face gradually relaxed into a smile, and just as the judge, looking at him in astonishment, finished, he suddenly laughed outright.

"Well, and what else?" he asked in a loud voice.

There was a hush in the court; there was a feeling of something strange. The judge showed signs of uneasiness.

"You . . . are perhaps still unwell?" he began, seeking the attendant with his eyes.

"Don't trouble yourself, your Excellency, I am well enough and can tell you something interesting," Ivan answered with sudden calmness and respectfulness.

"You have some special communication to make?" the judge went on, still mistrustfully.

Ivan looked down, waited a few seconds, and, raising his head, answered, almost stammering:

"No . . . I haven't. I have nothing particular to say."

They began asking him questions. He answered, as it were, reluctantly, with extreme brevity, with a sort of disgust which grew more and more marked, though he answered rationally. To many questions he answered that he did not know. He knew nothing of his father's money relations with Dmitri. "I wasn't interested in the subject," he added. Threats to murder his father he had heard from the accused. Of the money in the envelope he had heard from Smerdyakov.

"It's all the same thing over and over again," he interrupted suddenly, with a look of weariness. "I have nothing particular to tell the court."

"I see you are unwell and understand your feelings," the judge began.

He turned to the prosecutor and the counsel for the defence to invite them to examine the witness, if necessary, when Ivan suddenly asked in an exhausted voice:

"Let me go, your Excellency, I feel very ill."

And with these words, without waiting for permission, he turned to walk out of the court. But after taking four steps he stood still, as though he had reached a decision, smiled slowly, and went back.

"I am like that peasant girl, your Excellency . . . you know. How does it go? 'I'll stand up if I like, and I won't if I don't.' They were trying to put on her sarafan to take her to church to be married, and she said, 'I'll stand up if I like, and I won't if I don't.' . . . It's in some book about the peasantry."

"What do you mean by that?" the judge asked severely.

"Why, this," Ivan suddenly pulled out a roll of notes. "Here's the money . . . the notes that lay in that envelope" (he nodded towards the table on which lay the material evidence) "for the sake of which our father was murdered. Where shall I put them? Here, officer, take them."

The court attendant took the whole roll and handed it to the judge.

"How could this money have come into your possession if it is the same money?" the judge asked wonderingly.

"I got it from Smerdyakov, from the murderer, yesterday. . . . I was with him just before he hanged himself. It was he, not my brother, killed our father. He did the killing, and I instructed him to do it. . . . Who doesn't desire his father's death?"

"Are you in your right mind?" broke involuntarily from the judge.

"I should think I am in my right mind . . . in the same nasty mind as all of you . . . as all these . . . ugly faces." He turned suddenly to the audience. "My father has been murdered and they pretend they are horrified," he snarled, with furious contempt. "They keep up the sham before one another. Liars! They all desire the death of their fathers. One reptile devours another. . . . If there hadn't been parricide, they'd have been angry and gone home ill-humoured. It's circuses they want! Bread and circuses! Though I am one to talk! Have you any water? Give me a drink for Christ's sake!" He suddenly clutched his head.

The attendant at once approached him. Alyosha jumped up and cried, "He is ill. Don't believe him: he has brain fever." Katerina Ivanovna rose impulsively from her seat and, rigid with horror, gazed at Ivan. Mitya stood up and greedily looked at his brother and listened to him with a wild, strange smile.

"Don't disturb yourselves. I am not mad, I am only a murderer," Ivan began again. "You can't expect eloquence from a murderer," he added suddenly for some reason and laughed crookedly.

The prosecutor leaned over to the presiding judge in obvious dismay. The two other judges whispered to each other in agitation. Fetyukovich pricked up his ears as he listened: the hall was hushed in expectation. The presiding judge seemed suddenly to recollect himself.

"Witness, your words are incomprehensible and impossible here. Calm yourself, if you can, and tell your story . . . if you really have something to tell. How can you confirm your statement . . . if indeed you are not delirious?"

"That's just it. I have no proof. That cur Smerdyakov won't send you proofs from the other world . . . in an envelope. You think of nothing but envelopes — one is enough. I've no witnesses . . . except one, perhaps," he smiled thoughtfully.

"Who is your witness?"

"He has a tail, your excellency, and that would be irregular! *Le diable n'existe point!* Don't pay attention: he is a paltry, pitiful devil," he added suddenly. He ceased laughing and spoke, as it were, confidentially. "He is here somewhere, no doubt — under that table with the material evidence on it, perhaps. Where should he sit if not there? You see, listen to me. I told him I didn't want to keep quiet, and he talked about the geological cataclysm . . . idiocy! Come, release the monster . . . he's been singing a hymn. That's because his heart is light! It's like a drunken man in the street bawling how 'Vanka went to Petersburg,' and I would give a quadrillion quadrillions for two seconds of joy. You don't know me! Oh, how stupid all this business is! Come, take me instead of him! I didn't come for nothing. . . . Why, why is everything so stupid? . . ."

And he began slowly, and as it were reflectively, looking round him again. But the court was all excitement by now. Alyosha rushed towards him, but the court attendant had already seized Ivan by the arm.

"What are you about?" he cried, staring into the man's face, and, suddenly seizing him by the shoulders, he flung him violently to the floor. But the police were on the spot and he was seized. He screamed furiously. And all the time he was being removed, he yelled and screamed something incoherent.

The whole court was thrown into confusion. I don't remember everything just as it happened. I was excited myself and could not follow. I only know that afterwards, when everything was quiet again and every one understood what had happened, the court attendant came in for a reprimand, though he very reasonably explained that the witness had been quite well, that the doctor had seen him an hour ago, when he had a slight attack of giddiness, but that, until he had come into court, he had talked quite sensibly, so that nothing could have been foreseen — that he had, in fact, insisted on giving evidence. But before all had completely regained their composure and recovered from this scene, it was followed by another. Katerina Ivanovna had an attack of hysterics. She sobbed, shrieking loudly, but refused to leave the court-room, struggled, and besought them not to remove her. Suddenly she cried to the presiding judge:

"There is more evidence I must give at once . . . at once! Here is a document, a letter . . . take it, read it quickly, quickly! It's a letter from that monster . . . that man there, there!" she pointed to Mitya. "It was he killed his father, you will see that directly. He wrote to me how he would kill his father! But the other one is ill, he is ill, he is delirious! For the past three days I've seen that he was delirious!" she kept crying out, beside herself.

The court attendant took the document she held out to the judge, and she, dropping into her chair, hiding her face in her hands, began convulsively and noiselessly sobbing, shaking all over, and stifling every sound for fear she should be ejected from the court-room. The document she had handed up was that letter Mitya had written at the "Metropolis" tavern, which Ivan had spoken of as a "mathematical proof." Alas! its mathematical conclusiveness was recognised, and had it not been for that letter, Mitya might have escaped his doom or, at least, that doom would have been less terrible. It was, I repeat, difficult to follow the details. What ensued is still confused to my mind. The presiding judge must, I suppose, have at once passed on the document to the judges, the jury, and the lawyers on both sides. I only remember how they began examining the witness. On being gently asked by the presiding judge whether she had recovered sufficiently, Katerina Ivanovna exclaimed impetuously:

"I am ready, I am ready! I am quite able to answer you," she added, evidently still afraid that for some reason she would not be listened to. She was asked to explain in detail what this letter was and under what circumstances she had received it.

"I received it the day before the crime was committed, but he wrote it the day before that, at the tavern — that is, two days before he committed the crime. Look, it is written on some sort of bill!" she cried breathlessly. "He hated me at that time, because he had behaved contemptibly and had run after that creature . . . and because he owed me that three thousand. . . . Oh! he was humiliated by that three thousand on account of his own meanness! This is how it happened with that three thousand. I beg you, I beseech you, to hear me out! One morning, three weeks before he murdered his father, he came to me. I knew he was in want of money, and what he wanted it for. Yes, yes — to seduce that creature and carry her off. I knew then that he had been false to me and meant to abandon me, and it was I, I, who gave him that money, who offered it to him on the pretext of his sending it to my sister in Moscow. And as I gave it him, I looked him in the face and said that he could send it when he liked, 'in a month's time would do.' How, how could he have failed to understand that I was practically telling him to his face, 'You want money to be false to me with your creature, so here's the money for you. I give it to you myself. Take it, if you have so little honour as to take it!' I wanted to show him in his true colours, and what happened? He took it, he took it, and carried it off, and squandered it with that creature in one night. . . . But he understood, he understood that I knew it all. I assure you he understood, too, that I gave him that money to test him, to see whether he was so dishonourable as to take it from me. I looked into his eyes and he looked into mine, and he understood it all and he took it — he carried off my money!"

"That's true, Katya," Mitya roared suddenly, "I looked into your eyes and I knew that you were dishonouring me, and yet I took your money. Despise me as a scoundrel, despise me, all of you! I've deserved it!"

"Prisoner," cried the presiding judge, "another word and I will order you to be removed."

"That money was a torment to him," Katya went on with impulsive haste. "He wanted to repay it. He wanted to, that's true; but he needed money for that creature, too. So he murdered his father, but he didn't repay me, and went off with her to that village where he was arrested. There, again, he squandered the money he had stolen from his father, whom he had murdered. And a day before the murder he wrote me this letter. He was drunk when he wrote it. I saw it at once, at the time. He wrote it from spite, and feeling certain, positively certain, that I should never show it to any one, even if he did kill him. Or else he wouldn't have written it. For he knew I shouldn't want to revenge myself and ruin him! But read it, read it carefully — more carefully, please — and you will see that he had described it all in his letter, all beforehand, how he would kill his father and where the old man's money lay. Look, please, don't overlook that, there's one phrase there, 'I shall kill him as soon as Ivan has gone away.' So he thought it all out beforehand how he would kill him," Katerina Ivanovna prompted the court venomously and malignantly. Oh! it was clear she had read the fatal letter with the closest attention and had studied every line of it. "If he hadn't been drunk, he wouldn't have written to me; but, look, everything is described there in advance, point by point, just as he committed the murder afterwards, the whole programme!"

She exclaimed thus, frantically, reckless now of all consequences to herself, though, no doubt, she had foreseen them even a month ago, for even then, perhaps, shaking with anger, she had pondered whether to show the letter at the trial or not. Now she had taken the fatal plunge.

I remember that the letter was read aloud by the clerk, directly afterwards, I believe. It made an overwhelming impression. They asked Mitya whether he admitted having written the letter.

"It's mine, mine!" cried Mitya. "I wouldn't have written it, if I hadn't been drunk! . . . We've hated each other for many things, Katya, but I swear, I swear I loved you even while I hated you, and you didn't love me!"

He sank back on his seat, wringing his hands in despair. The prosecutor and the counsel for the defence began cross-examining her, chiefly to ascertain what had induced her to conceal such a document and to give her evidence in quite a different tone and spirit just before.

"Yes, yes. I was telling lies just now. I was lying against my honour and my conscience, but I wanted to save him, for he has hated and despised me so!" Katya cried like a madwoman. "Oh, he has despised me horribly, he has always despised me, and do you know, he despised me from the very moment that I bowed down to him for that money. I saw that. . . . I felt it at once at the time, but for a long time I wouldn't believe it. How often I have read in his eyes, 'you came of yourself, though.' Oh, he didn't understand, he had no idea why I ran to him, he can suspect nothing but baseness, he judged me by himself, he thought every one was like himself!" Katya hissed furiously, in a perfect frenzy. "And he only wanted to marry me because I'd inherited a fortune, because of that, because of that! I always suspected it was because of that! Oh, he is a beast! He was always convinced that I should be trembling with shame all my life before him, because I went to him then, and that he had a right to despise me for ever for it, and so to be superior to me — that's why he wanted to marry me! That's so, that's all so! I tried to conquer him by my love — a love that knew no bounds. I even tried to forgive his faithlessness; but he understood nothing, nothing! How could he understand indeed? He is a monster! I received that letter only the next evening: it was brought me from the tavern — and only that morning, only that morning I wanted to forgive him everything, everything — even his treachery!"

The presiding judge and the prosecutor, of course, tried to calm her. I can't help thinking that they felt ashamed of taking advantage of her hysteria and of listening to such avowals. I remember hearing them say to her, "We understand how hard it is for you; be sure we are able to feel for you," and so on, and so on. And yet they dragged the evidence out of the raving, hysterical woman. She described at last with extraordinary clearness, which is so often manifested, though only for a moment, even in such overwrought states, how Ivan had been driven nearly out of his mind during the last two months trying to save "the monster and murderer," his brother.

"He tortured himself," she exclaimed, "he was always trying to minimise his brother's guilt and confessing to me that he, too, had never loved his father, and perhaps desired his death himself. Oh, he has a deep, deep conscience! His conscience simply ravaged him! He told me everything, everything! He came every day and talked to me as his only friend. I have the honour to be his only friend!" she cried suddenly with a sort of defiance, and her eyes flashed. "He had been twice to see Smerdyakov. One day he came to me and said, 'If it was not my brother, but Smerdyakov who committed the murder (for the legend was circulating everywhere that Smerdyakov had done it), perhaps I, too, am guilty, for Smerdyakov knew I didn't like my father and perhaps believed that I desired my father's death.' Then I brought out that letter and showed it him. He was entirely convinced that his brother had done it, and he was overwhelmed by it. He couldn't endure the thought that his own brother was a parricide! Only a week ago I saw that it was making him ill. During the last few days he has talked incoherently in my presence. I saw his mind was giving way. He walked about, raving; he was seen muttering in the streets. The doctor from Moscow, at my request, examined him the day before yesterday and told me that he was on the eve of brain fever — and all on his account, on account of this monster! And last night he learnt that Smerdyakov was dead! It was such a shock that it drove him out of his mind . . . and all through this monster, all for the sake of saving the monster!"

Oh, of course, such an outpouring, such an avowal is possible only once in a lifetime — at the hour of death, for instance, on the way to the scaffold! But it was in Katya's character, and it was such a moment in her life. It was the same impetuous Katya who had thrown herself on the mercy of a young profligate to save her father; the same Katya who had just before, in her pride and chastity, sacrificed herself and her maidenly modesty before all these people, telling of Mitya's generous act, in the hope of softening his fate a little. And now, again, she sacrificed herself; but this time it was for another, and perhaps only now — perhaps only at this moment — she felt and knew how dear that other was to her! She had sacrificed herself in terror for him, conceiving all of a sudden that he had ruined himself by his confession that it was he who had committed the murder, not his brother, she had sacrificed herself to save him, to save his good name, his reputation!

And yet one terrible doubt occurred to the audience — was she lying in her description of her former relations with Mitya? — that was the question. No, she had not intentionally slandered him when she cried that Mitya despised her for her bowing down to him! She believed it herself. She had been firmly convinced, perhaps ever since that bow, that the simple-hearted Mitya, who then still adored her, was laughing at her and despising her. She had conceived for him an hysterical, "lacerated" love only because of pride, wounded pride, and that love was not like love, but more like revenge. Oh! perhaps that lacerated love would have grown into real love, perhaps Katya longed for nothing more than that, but Mitya's faithlessness had wounded her to the bottom of her heart, and her heart could not forgive him. The moment of revenge had come upon her suddenly, and all that had been accumulating so long and so painfully in the offended woman's breast burst out all at once and unexpectedly. She betrayed Mitya, but she betrayed herself, too. And no sooner had she given full expression to her feelings than the tension, of course, was over and she was overwhelmed with shame. Hysterics began again: she fell on the floor, sobbing and screaming. She was carried out. At that moment Grushenka, with a wail, rushed towards Mitya before they had time to prevent her.

"Mitya," she wailed, "your serpent has destroyed you! There, she has shown you what she is!" she shouted to the judges, shaking with anger. At a signal from the presiding judge they seized her and tried to remove her from the court-room. She wouldn't allow it. She fought and struggled to get back to Mitya. Mitya uttered a cry and struggled to get to her. He was overpowered.

Yes, I think the ladies who came to see the spectacle must have been satisfied — the show had been a rich one. Then I remember the Moscow doctor appeared on the scene. I believe the presiding judge had previously sent the court attendant to arrange for medical aid for Ivan. The doctor announced to the court that the patient was suffering from a dangerous attack of brain fever and that he must be at once removed. In answer to questions from the prosecutor and the counsel for the defence he said that the patient had come to him of his own accord the day before yesterday and that he had warned him that he had such an attack coming on, but he had not consented to be looked after. "He was certainly not in a normal state of mind: he told me himself that he saw visions when he was awake, that he met several persons in the street, who were dead, and that Satan visited him every evening," said the doctor, in conclusion. Having given his evidence, the celebrated doctor withdrew. The letter produced by Katerina Ivanovna was added to the material evidence. After some deliberation, the judges decided to proceed with the trial and to enter both the unexpected pieces of evidence (given by Ivan and Katerina Ivanovna) into the record.

But I will not detail the evidence of the other witnesses, who only repeated and confirmed what had been said before, though all with their characteristic peculiarities. I repeat, all was brought together in the prosecutor's speech, to which I shall pass directly. Every one was excited, every one was electrified by the last incident, and with burning impatience all were awaiting the dénouement, that is, the speeches of the prosecutor and the counsel for the defence, and the verdict. Fetyukovich was obviously shaken by Katerina Ivanovna's evidence. But the prosecutor was triumphant. When all the evidence had been taken, the court was adjourned for almost an hour. Finally the presiding judge resumed the trial. I believe it was just eight o'clock when our prosecutor, Ippolit Kirillovich began his speech.

CHAPTER VI

THE PROSECUTOR'S SPEECH. CHARACTERIZATION

IPPOLIT KIRILLOVICH began his speech trembling with nervousness, with cold sweat on his forehead and temples, feeling chills and fever all over by turns. He described this himself afterwards. He regarded this speech as his *chef d'œuvre*, the *chef d'œuvre* of his whole life, his swan-song. He died, it is true, nine months later of consumption, so that he would have had the right, had he had a presentiment of his end, to compare himself to a swan singing his last song. He had put his whole heart and all the brain he had into that speech. And he unexpectedly revealed that civic sentiment and a feeling for "the accursed questions" lay concealed in him, at least to the degree possible to our poor Ippolit Kirillovich. Where his speech really excelled was in its sincerity. He genuinely believed in the prisoner's guilt; he was accusing him not only as a matter of form and of official duty, and in calling for vengeance he quivered with a genuine desire to "save society." Even the ladies in the audience, though they remained hostile to Ippolit Kirillovich, admitted that he made an extraordinary impression on them. He began in a cracked, broken voice, but it soon gained strength and filled the court to the end of his speech. But as soon as he had finished, he almost fainted.

"Gentlemen of the jury," began the prosecutor, "this case has made a stir throughout Russia. But what is there to wonder at, what is there so peculiarly horrifying in it for us? We are people accustomed to all this! That's what's so horrible, that such dark deeds have ceased to horrify us. What ought to horrify us is that we are so accustomed to it, and not this or that isolated crime. What are the causes of our indifference, our lukewarm attitude to such deeds, to such signs of the times, auguring an unenviable future? Is it our cynicism, is it the premature exhaustion of intellect and imagination in a society that is sinking into decay, in spite of its youth? Is it that our moral principles are shattered to their foundations, or is it, perhaps, a complete lack of such principles among us? I cannot answer such questions; nevertheless they are disturbing, and every citizen not only must, but ought to be harassed by them. Our young and still timid press has done good service to the public already, for without it we should never have heard of the horrors of unbridled violence and moral degradation which are continually made known by the press, not merely to those who attend the new public courts vouchsafed to us in the present reign, but to every one. And what do we read almost daily? Of things beside which the present case grows pale, and seems almost commonplace. But what is most important is that the majority of our national crimes of violence bear witness to a widespread evil that has struck such deep root among us that it is difficult to contend against it.

"One day we see a brilliant young officer of high society, at the very outset of his career, in a cowardly underhand way, without a pang of conscience, murdering an official who had once been his benefactor, and the servant girl, to steal his own IOU and what ready money he could find on him; 'it will come in handy for my pleasures in the fashionable world and for my career in the future.' After knifing them, he puts a pillow under the head of each of his victims, and goes away. Next, a young hero 'decorated for bravery' kills the mother of his chief and benefactor, like a highwayman, and to urge his companions to join him he asserts that 'she loves him like a son, and so will follow all his directions and take no precautions.' Granted that he is a monster, yet I dare not say in these days that he is unique. Another man will not kill, but will feel and think like him: his soul is equally dishonourable. In silence, alone with his conscience, he asks himself perhaps, 'What is honour, and isn't the condemnation of bloodshed a prejudice?'

"Perhaps people will cry out against me that I am morbid, hysterical, that it is a monstrous slander, that I am raving, exaggerating. Let them say so — and heavens! I should be the first to rejoice if it were so! Oh, don't believe me, think of me as morbid, but remember my words; if only a tenth, if only a twentieth part of what I say is true — even so it's horrible! Look how our young people commit suicide: they do not ask themselves the Hamletic question, 'What is there beyond?' — there is no sign of such a question, as though the whole matter of our soul and what awaits us beyond the grave had long since been erased from their nature and buried under the sands. Look at our dissoluteness, at our sensualists. Fyodor Pavlovich, the luckless victim in the present case, is almost an innocent babe compared with many of them. And yet we all knew him, 'he lived among us!' . . .

"Yes, one day perhaps the leading intellects of Russia and of Europe will study the psychology of Russian crime, for the subject is worth it. But this study will come later, at leisure, when all the tragic topsy-turvydom of to-day is farther behind us, so that it's possible to examine it with more insight and more impartiality than such men as I have. Now we are either horrified or pretend to be horrified, though we really gloat over the spectacle, and love strong and eccentric sensations which tickle our cynical, pampered idleness. Or, like little children, we brush the dreadful ghosts away and hide our heads in the pillow so as to return to our sports and merriment as soon as the terrible spectre has vanished. But we must one day begin life in sober earnest, we, too, must look upon ourselves as a society; it's time we tried to grasp something of our interests as a group, or at least to make a beginning in that direction.

"A great writer* of the last epoch, comparing Russia to a swift troika galloping towards an unknown goal, exclaims at the close of his greatest work, 'Oh, troika, birdlike troika, who invented thee!' and adds, in proud ecstasy, that all the peoples of the world stand aside respectfully to make way for the recklessly galloping troika. That may be, they may stand aside, respectfully or no, but in my poor opinion the great writer ended his book in this way either in an access of childish and naïve optimism, or simply in fear of the censorship of the day. For if the troika were drawn by his heroes, Sobakevich, Nozdryov, Chichikov, it could reach no rational goal, whoever might be driving it. And those were the steeds of old, ours are worse specimens still . . ."

At this point Ippolit Kirillovich's speech was interrupted by applause. The Liberal significance of the reference to the Russian troika was appreciated. The applause was, it's true, of brief duration, so that the judge did not think it necessary to caution the public, and only looked severely in the direction of the offenders. But Ippolit Kirillovich was encouraged; he had never been applauded before! He had been all his life unable to get a hearing, and now he suddenly had an opportunity of securing the ear of all Russia.

"What, after all, is this Karamazov family, which has gained such sad notoriety throughout Russia?" he continued. "Perhaps I am exaggerating, but it seems to me that certain general fundamental features of the educated class of to-day flash upon the eye, as it were, in the picture of this family, — oh, not all and only, of course, in miniature, reflected 'like the sun in a small drop of water.' Nevertheless, they are reflected, they do show themselves. Think of that unhappy, dissolute, unbridled old man, this head of a family, who has met with such a melancholy end! Born into the nobility, but from the first a poverty-stricken dependent, he comes into a small fortune, through an unexpected marriage. A petty knave, a toady and buffoon, of fairly good, though undeveloped, intelligence, he is, above all, a usurer. As the years pass, and his little capital increases, he grows bolder. His abjectness and servility disappear, there remains only a sarcastic and malicious cynic and sensualist. The spiritual side is entirely obliterated, but his thirst for life is excessive. He sees nothing in life but sensual pleasure, and he brings his children up to do likewise. He has no sense of his spiritual duties as a father. He ridicules those duties. He leaves his little children to the servants, and is glad to be rid of them, forgets about them completely. The old man's maxim is *après moi le déluge*. He embodies the very opposite of what is meant by a citizen, he represents the most complete divorce from, and, indeed, hostility to, society. 'The world may burn for aught I care, so long as I am at my ease,' and he is at his ease; he is content, he is eager to go on living

* Gogol is meant. *Translator's note.*

in the same way for another twenty or thirty years. He swindles his own son and with that money which he withholds from him, his maternal inheritance, tries to get his mistress away from him, from his own son. No, I don't intend to leave the prisoner's defence altogether to my talented colleague from Petersburg. I will speak the truth myself, I can well understand what resentment he had heaped up in his son's heart against him.

"But enough, enough of that unhappy old man; he has paid the penalty. Let us remember, however, that he was a father, and one of the typical fathers of to-day. Am I unjust, indeed, in saying that he is typical of many modern fathers? Alas! many of them differ only in not openly professing such cynicism, for they are better educated, more cultured, but their philosophy is essentially the same as his. Perhaps I am a pessimist, but you have agreed to forgive me. Let us agree beforehand, you need not believe me, but let me speak. Let me say what I have to say, and remember something of my words.

"Now for the children of this father, this head of a family. One of them is the prisoner before us, all the rest of my speech will deal with him. Of the other two I will speak only in passing.

"The elder is one of those modern young men of brilliant education and vigorous intellect, who has lost all faith in everything. He has denied and rejected much already, like his father. We have all heard him, he was a welcome guest in local society. He never concealed his opinions, quite the contrary in fact, which justifies me in speaking rather openly of him now, of course, not as a private person, but as a member of the Karamazov family. Another person closely connected with the case died here by his own hand last night. I mean a sickly idiot, a former servant, and possibly the illegitimate son of Fyodor Pavlovich — Smerdyakov. At the preliminary inquiry, he told me with hysterical tears how the young Ivan Karamazov had horrified him by his spiritual unrestraint. 'Everything in the world is permitted according to him, and nothing must be forbidden in the future — that is what he always taught me.' I believe that idiot was driven out of his mind by this thesis which he had been taught, though, of course, the epileptic attacks from which he suffered, and this terrible catastrophe, have helped to unhinge his mind. But he dropped one very interesting observation, which would have done credit to a more intelligent observer, and that is, indeed, why I've mentioned it, 'If there is one of the sons that is like Fyodor Pavlovich in character, it is Ivan Fyodorovich.'

"With that remark I conclude my sketch of his character, feeling it indelicate to continue further. Oh, I don't want to draw any further conclusions and croak like a raven over the young man's future. We've seen to-day in this court that there are still good impulses in his young heart, that family feeling has not been destroyed in him by lack of faith and moral cynicism, which has come to him rather by inheritance than by the exercise of independent thought.

"Then the third son. Oh, he is a devout and modest youth, who does not share his elder brother's gloomy and destructive theory of life. He has sought to cling to the 'folk ideals,' or to what goes by that name in some circles of our intellectual class. He clung to the monastery, and was within an ace of becoming a monk. He seems to me to have betrayed unconsciously, and so early, that timid despair which leads so many in our unhappy society, who dread cynicism and its corrupting influences, and mistakenly attribute all the mischief to European enlightenment, to cast themselves upon their 'native soil,' as they say, into the motherly embraces of their native land, like children frightened by ghosts, yearning to fall asleep on the withered bosom of their decrepit mother, and to sleep there for ever, only to escape the horrors that terrify them.

"For my part I wish the excellent and gifted young man every success; I trust that his youthful idealism and his striving towards the ideals of the people may never degenerate, as often happens, on the moral side into gloomy mysticism, and on the civic side into obtuse chauvinism — two evils which are even a greater menace to Russia than the premature decay, due to misunderstanding and to the gratuitous adoption of European enlightenment, from which his elder brother is suffering."

Two or three people clapped their hands at the mention of chauvinism and mysticism. Ippolit Kirillovich had, indeed, been carried away by his own eloquence. All this had little to do with the case in hand, to say nothing of the fact of its being somewhat vague, but the sickly and consumptive man was overcome by the desire to express himself once in his life. People said afterwards that he was actuated by unworthy motives in his criticism of Ivan, because the latter had on one or two occasions got the better of him in argument, and Ippolit Kirillovich, remembering it, tried now to take his revenge. But I don't know whether it was true.

All this was only introductory, however, and the speech passed to more direct consideration of the case.

"But to return to the eldest son," Ippolit Kirillovich went on. "He is in the dock before us. We have his life and his actions, too, before us; the fatal day has come and all has come out into the open. While his brothers seem to stand for 'Europeanism' and 'the principles of the people,' he seems to represent Russia in its spontaneity. Oh, not all Russia, not all! God preserve us, if it were! Yet, here we have her, our mother Russia, the very scent and sound of her. Oh, we are spontaneous, we are a marvellous mingling of good and evil, we are a lover of culture and Schiller, yet we brawl in taverns and pluck out the beards of our boon companions. Oh, we, too, can be good and noble, but only when all goes well with us. What is more, we can be carried off our feet, positively carried off our feet by noble ideals, but only if they come of themselves, if they fall down to us from heaven, if they are gratuitous, gratuitous, if they need not be paid for. We hate paying for anything, but are very fond of receiving, and that's so with us in everything. Oh, give us every possible good that life can offer (we couldn't be content with less), and put no obstacle in our way, and we will show that we, too, can be noble. We are not greedy, no, but we must have money, a great deal of money, and you will see how generously, with what scorn of filthy lucre, we will fling it all away in the reckless dissipation of one night. But if the money is not handed to us, we will show what we can do to get it when we want it badly. But of this later, let us take events in their chronological order.

"First, we have before us a poor abandoned child, running about the back yard, 'without boots to his feet,' as our worthy and esteemed fellow citizen, of foreign origin, alas! expressed it just now. I repeat it again, I yield to no one the defence of the criminal. I am here to accuse him, but to defend him also. Yes, I, too, am human; I, too, can weigh the influence of home and childhood on the character. But the boy grows up and becomes an officer; on account of a duel and other reckless conduct he is exiled to one of the remote frontier towns of our prosperous Russia. There he leads a wild life as an officer. And, of course, a big ship must travel far. We need money, money before all things, and so after prolonged wrangling he comes to a settlement with his father, and the last six thousand is sent him. A letter is in existence in which he practically gives up his claim to the rest and settles his dispute with his father over the inheritance on the payment of this six thousand.

"Then comes his meeting with a young girl of lofty character and brilliant education. Oh, I do not venture to repeat the details; you have only just heard them. Honour, self-sacrifice were displayed there, and I am silent. The figure of the young officer, frivolous and dissolute, but bowing before true nobility and a lofty ideal, was shown in a very sympathetic light before us. But the other side of the medal was unexpectedly turned to us immediately after in this very court. Again I will not venture to conjecture why it happened so, but there were causes. The same lady, bathed in tears of long-concealed indignation, has declared to us that he, he of all men, was the first to despise her for her impulse, which, though incautious, reckless perhaps, was still dictated by lofty and generous motives. He, he, the girl's betrothed, looked at her with that smile of mockery, which was more insufferable from him than from any one. And knowing that he had already deceived her (he had deceived her, believing that she was bound to endure everything from him, even treachery), she intentionally offers him three thousand roubles, and clearly, too clearly, lets him understand that she is offering him money with which to betray her. 'Well, will you take it or not, are you so lost to shame?' is the dumb question in her scrutinising eyes. He looks at her, sees clearly what is in her mind (he's admitted here before you that he understood it all), appropriates that three thousand unconditionally, and squanders it in two days with the new object of his affections.

"What are we to believe then? The first legend of the young officer sacrificing his last farthing in a noble impulse of generosity and doing reverence to virtue, or this other revolting picture? As a rule, between two extremes one has to find the mean, but in the present case this is not true. The probability is that in the first case he was genuinely noble, and in the second as genuinely base. And why? Precisely because we have the broad Karamazov nature — that's just what I am leading up to — capable of combining the most incongruous contradictions, and capable of contemplating at once the two abysses: the abyss above us, the abyss of the highest ideals, and the abyss below us, the abyss of the lowest and foulest degradation. Remember the brilliant remark made by a young observer who has seen the Karamazov family at close quarters — Mr. Rakitin: 'The sense of their own degradation is as essential to these reckless, unbridled natures as the sense of the highest nobility.' And that's true, they need continually this unnatural mixture. Two abysses, gentlemen, two abysses at the same moment, or we are miserable and dissatisfied and our existence is incomplete. We are wide, wide as mother Russia; we include everything and put up with everything.

"By the way, gentlemen of the jury, we've just touched upon that three thousand roubles, and I will venture to anticipate a little. Can you conceive that a man like that, on receiving that sum and in such a way, at the price of such shame, such disgrace, such utter degradation, could have been capable that very day of setting apart half that sum, that very day, and sewing it up in a little bag, and would have had the firmness of character to carry it about with him for a whole month afterwards, in spite of every temptation and his extreme need of it! Neither in drunken debauchery in taverns, nor when he was flying into the country, trying to get from God knows whom the money so essential to him to remove the object of his affections from being tempted by his father, did he bring himself to touch that little bag! Why, if only to avoid exposing his mistress to being tempted by the old man of whom he was so jealous, he would have been certain to have opened that bag and to have stayed at home to keep watch over her, awaiting the moment when she would say to him at last, 'I am yours,' so as to fly with her far from their fatal surroundings.

"But no, he does not touch his talisman, and what is the reason he gives for it? The primary reason, as I have just said, was that when she would say, 'I am yours, take me where you will,' he might have the wherewithal to take her. But that first reason, in the prisoner's own words, paled beside the second. While I have that money on me, he said, I am a scoundrel, not a thief, for I can always go to my insulted betrothed, and, laying down half the sum I have fraudulently appropriated, I can always say to her, 'You see I've squandered half your money, and shown I am a weak and immoral man, and, if you like, a scoundrel' (I use the prisoner's own expressions), 'but though I am a scoundrel, I am not a thief, for if I had been a thief, I shouldn't have brought you back this half of the money, but should have appropriated it as I did the other half!' A surprising explanation! This frantic, but weak man, who could not resist the temptation of accepting the three thousand roubles at the price of such disgrace, this very man suddenly develops the most stoical firmness, and carries about thousands of roubles without daring to touch them. Does that fit in at all with the character we have analysed? No, and I venture to tell you how the real Dmitri Karamazov would have behaved in such circumstances, if he really had brought himself to sew up the money in a little bag.

"At the first temptation — for instance, to entertain the woman with whom he had already squandered half the money — he would have ripped open his little bag and have taken out some hundred roubles, for why should he have taken back precisely half the money, that is, fifteen hundred roubles; why not fourteen hundred? He could just as well have said then that he was not a thief, because he brought back fourteen hundred roubles. Then a little later he would have ripped it open again and taken out another hundred, and then a third, and then a fourth, and before the end of the month he would have taken the last note but one, feeling that if he took back only a hundred it would answer the purpose, for a thief would have stolen it all. And then he would have looked at this last note, and have said to himself, 'It's really not worth while to give back one hundred; let's spend that, too!' That's how the real Dmitri Karamazov, as we know him, would have behaved. One cannot imagine anything more incongruous with the actual facts than this legend of the little bag. Nothing could be more inconceivable. But we shall return to that later."

After touching upon what had come out in the proceedings concerning the financial relations of father and son, and arguing again and again that it was utterly impossible, from the facts known, to determine which was in the wrong, Ippolit Kirillovich passed to the evidence of the medical experts in reference to Mitya's fixed idea about the three thousand owing him.

CHAPTER VII

AN HISTORICAL SURVEY

"The medical experts have striven to convince us that the prisoner is out of his mind and, in fact, a maniac. I maintain that he is in his right mind, but it's just this that's worst of all: if he had not been, he would have behaved more cleverly. As for his being a maniac, that I would agree to, but only as regards one point, that is, his fixed idea about the three thousand that his father had failed to pay up. Yet I think one might find a much more plausible explanation of his frenzy over the money than his tendency to insanity. For my part I agree thoroughly with the young doctor who maintained that the prisoner's mental faculties have always been normal, and that he has only been irritable and exasperated. The reason for the prisoner's continual and violent anger was not the sum itself; there was a special motive at the bottom of it. That motive is jealousy!"

Here Ippolit Kirillovich described at length the prisoner's fatal passion for Grushenka. He began from the moment when the prisoner went to the "young person's" lodgings "to give her a beating" — "I use his own expression," the prosecutor explained — "but instead of beating her, he remained at her feet. That was the beginning of this passion. At the same time the old man, the father of the accused, casts his eye upon the same person — a strange and fatal coincidence, for they both lost their hearts to her simultaneously, though both had known her before. And she inspired in both of them the most violent, characteristically Karamazov passion. We have her own confession: 'I was laughing at both of them.' Yes, the sudden desire to make mock of them came over her, formerly she had not wished this, but now suddenly the notion came into her head — it ended by both of them being conquered by her. The old man, who worshipped money as though it were God, at once set aside three thousand roubles as a reward for one visit from her, but soon after that, he would have been happy to lay his property and his name at her feet, if only she would become his lawful wife. We have good evidence of this. As for the prisoner, his tragedy is plain; it is before us. But such was the young person's 'game.' The enchantress gave the unhappy young man no hope until the last moment, when he knelt before her, stretching out hands that were already stained with the blood of his father and rival. It was in that position that he was arrested. 'Send me to Siberia with him, I have brought him to this, I am most to blame,' the woman herself cried, in genuine remorse, at the moment of his arrest.

"The talented young man, who took it upon himself to describe the present case, Mr.

Rakitin, to whom I have referred already, characterised this heroine in a few brief and graphic terms: 'Early disillusionment, early betrayal and fall, abandonment by her betrothed, who had seduced her; then poverty, repudiation by her respectable family, and finally, the protection of a wealthy old man, whom she still, however, considers as her benefactor. There was perhaps much that was good in her young heart, but it was embittered too early. She became prudent and saved money. She grew sarcastic and revengeful towards society.' After this sketch of her character it may well be understood that she might laugh at both of them simply from mischief, from malice.

"During this month of hopeless love and moral degradation, when he betrayed his betrothed and appropriated money entrusted to his honour, the prisoner was driven almost to frenzy, almost to madness by continual jealousy — and of whom? His father! And the worst of it was that the crazy old man was trying to seduce and entice the object of his passion by means of that very three thousand roubles which the son looked upon as his own property, part of his inheritance from his mother, of which his father was cheating him. Yes, I admit it was hard to bear! It might well drive a man to madness. It was not the money, but the fact that this money was used with such revolting cynicism to ruin his happiness!"

Then the prosecutor went on to describe how the idea of murdering his father had entered the prisoner's head, and traced it by means of the evidence.

"At first we only shout about it in taverns — we shout about it all that month. Ah, we like being always surrounded with company, and we like to tell our companions everything, even our most diabolical and dangerous ideas; we like to share every thought with others, and expect, for some reason, that those we confide in will respond to us with perfect sympathy, enter into all our troubles and anxieties, agree with us and not oppose us in anything. If not, we fly into a rage and smash up everything in the tavern." (Then followed the anecdote about Captain Snegiryov.) "Those who saw and heard the prisoner during that month began to think at last that he might mean more than threats, and that such a frenzy might turn threats into actions."

Here the prosecutor described the meeting of the family at the monastery, the conversations with Alyosha, and the abominable scene of violence when the prisoner rushed into his father's house just after dinner.

"I cannot positively assert," the prosecutor continued, "that the prisoner actually intended to murder his father before that incident. Yet the idea had several times presented itself to him, and he had deliberated on it — as regards that we have facts, the testimony of witnesses, and his own admission. I confess, gentlemen of the jury," he added, "that till to-day I have been uncertain whether to attribute to the prisoner conscious premeditation in the matter of the murder. I was firmly convinced that he had pictured the fatal moment beforehand, but had only pictured it, contemplating it as a possibility. He had not definitely considered when and how he might commit the crime.

"But I was uncertain only till to-day, till that fatal document was presented to the court just now. You yourselves heard that young lady's exclamation, 'It is the plan, the programme of the murder!' That is how she defined that miserable, drunken letter of the unhappy prisoner. And, in fact, that letter indicates a programme and a premeditated plan. It was written two days before the crime and so we know now for a fact that, forty-eight hours before the perpetration of his terrible design, the accused swore that, if he could not get money next day, he would kill his father in order to take money contained in the envelope with the pink ribbon from under his pillow, 'as soon as Ivan had left.' You hear that — 'as soon as Ivan had gone away'; so everything had been thought out, the circumstances had been weighed; and he carried it all out just as he had written it. The proof of premeditation is conclusive; the crime must have been committed for the sake of the money, that is stated clearly, that is written and signed. The accused does not deny his signature.

"I shall be told he was drunk when he wrote it. But that does not diminish the value of the letter, quite the contrary; he wrote when drunk what he had planned when sober. Had he not planned it when sober, he would not have written it when drunk. I shall be asked: Then why did he shout about his plan in the taverns? A man who premeditates such a crime holds his peace and keeps it to himself. Yes, but he talked about it before he had formed a plan, when he had only the desire, only the impulse to do it. Afterwards he talked less about it. On the evening he wrote that letter at the 'Metropolis' tavern, contrary to his custom he was silent, though he had been drinking. He did not play billiards, he sat in a corner, talked to no one. He did indeed turn a shopman out of his seat, but that was done almost unconsciously, because he could never enter a tavern without making a disturbance. It is true that after he had taken the final decision, he must have felt apprehensive that he had talked too much about his design beforehand, and that this might lead to his arrest and prosecution afterwards. But there was nothing for it; he could not take his words back, but his luck had served him before, it would serve him again. We believed in our star, gentlemen! I must confess, too, that he did a great deal to elude the fatal moment, that he made many efforts to avoid the bloody conclusion. 'To-morrow I will try and borrow the money from every one,' as he writes in his peculiar style, 'and if they won't give it to me, there will be bloodshed.' Again, what is written when drunk is carried out when sober."

Here Ippolit Kirillovich passed to a detailed description of all Mitya's efforts to borrow the money in order to avoid the crime. He described his adventure with Samsonov, his journey to Lyagavy, everything on the basis of documentary evidence. "Harassed, jeered at, hungry, after selling his watch to pay for the journey (though he tells us he had fifteen hundred roubles on him — a likely story), tortured by jealousy at having left the object of his passion in the town, suspecting that she would go to Fyodor Pavlovich in his absence, he returns at last to the town, to find, to his joy, that she has not been near his father. He accompanies her himself to her protector, Samsonov. (Strange to say, we are not jealous of Samsonov, which is psychologically interesting.) Then he hastens back to his ambush in the back yard, and there learns that Smerdyakov is in a fit, that the other servant is ill — the coast is clear and he knows the 'signals' — what a temptation! Nevertheless he resists it; he goes off to a lady who has for some time been residing in the town, and who is highly esteemed among us, Madame Hohlakov. That lady, who had long watched his career with compassion, gave him the most judicious advice, to give up his dissipated life, his unseemly love-affair, his frequenting of taverns, the waste of his youth and vigour, and to set off to Siberia to the gold-mines: 'that would be an outlet for your turbulent energies, your romantic character, your thirst for adventure.' "

After describing the result of this conversation and the moment when the prisoner learnt that Grushenka had not remained at Samsonov's, the sudden frenzy of the luckless man, worn out with jealousy and nervous exhaustion, at the thought that she had deceived him and was now with his father, Ippolit Kirillovich concluded by dwelling upon the fatal influence of chance. "Had the maid told him that her mistress was at Mokroye with her former lover, nothing would have happened. But she lost her head, she could only swear and protest her ignorance, and if the accused did not kill her on the spot, it was only because he flew in pursuit of his false mistress.

"But note, frantic as he was, he took with him a brass pestle. Why that? Why not some other weapon? But since we had been contemplating our plan and preparing ourself for it for a whole month, we would snatch up anything like a weapon that caught our eye. We had realised for a month past that any object of the kind would serve as a weapon, so we instantly, without hesitation, recognised that it would serve our purpose. So it was by no means unconsciously, by no means involuntarily, that he snatched up that fatal pestle. And then we find him in his father's garden — the coast is clear, there are no witnesses, it's a dark night, jealousy rages. The suspicion that she is there, with him, with his rival, in his arms, and perhaps laughing at him at that moment — takes his breath away. And it was not mere suspicion, the deception was open, obvious. She must be there, in that lighted room, she must be behind the screen; and the unhappy man would have us believe that he stole up to the window, peeped respectfully in, resigned himself decently, and discreetly withdrew, for fear something dangerous and immoral should happen. And he tries to persuade us of that, us, who know his character, who understand his state of mind at the moment, and who are aware that he knew the signals by which he could at once enter the house."

At this point Ippolit Kirillovich broke off to discuss exhaustively the suspected connection of Smerdyakov with the murder, in order to dispose of that theory once for all. He did this very circumstantially, and every one realised that, although he professed to despise that suspicion, he thought the subject of great importance.

CHAPTER VIII

A TREATISE ON SMERDYAKOV

"To begin with, how did this suspicion arise?" Ippolit Kirillovich began. "The first person to cry out that Smerdyakov had committed the murder was the accused himself at the moment of his arrest, yet from that time to this he has not brought forward a single fact to confirm the charge, nor the faintest suggestion of a fact. The charge is confirmed by three persons only — the two brothers of the accused and Madame Svyetlov. The elder of these brothers expressed his suspicions only to-day, when he was undoubtedly suffering from brain fever. But we know that for the last two months he has completely shared our conviction of his brother's guilt and did not attempt to combat that idea. But of that later. The younger brother has admitted that he has not the slightest fact to support his notion of Smerdyakov's guilt, and has been led to that conclusion only from the prisoner's own words and the expression of his face. Yes, that astounding piece of evidence has been brought forward twice to-day by him. Madame Svyetlov was even more astounding. 'What the accused tells you, you must believe; he is not a man to tell a lie.' That is all the evidence against Smerdyakov produced by these three persons, who are all deeply concerned in the prisoner's fate. And yet the theory of Smerdyakov's guilt has been noised about, has been and is still maintained. Is it credible? Is it conceivable?"

Here Ippolit Kirillovich found it necessary to describe the personality of Smerdyakov, "who had cut short his life in a fit of morbid derangement." He depicted him as a man of weak intellect, with a smattering of education, who had been thrown off his balance by philosophical ideas beyond his grasp and frightened by certain modern theories of duty and obligation which he learnt in practice from the reckless life of his master, who was also perhaps his father — Fyodor Pavlovich; and, theoretically, from various strange philosophical conversations with his master's elder son, Ivan Fyodorovich, who readily indulged in this diversion, probably out of boredom or wishing to amuse himself at the valet's expense. He spoke to me himself of his psychological condition during the last few days at his father's house," Ippolit Kirillovich explained; "but others, too, have borne witness to it — the accused himself, his brother, and the servant Grigory — that is, all who knew him well.

"Moreover, Smerdyakov, depressed by his attacks of epilepsy, was as cowardly as a chicken. 'He fell at my feet and kissed them,' the accused himself has told us, before he realised how damaging such a statement was to himself. 'He is an epileptic chicken,' he declared about him in his characteristic language. And it was he whom the accused chose for his confidant (we have his own word for it) and he frightened him into consenting at last to act as his spy and informer. In that capacity he deceived his master, revealing to the accused the existence of the envelope with the notes in it and the signals by means of which he could get into the house. How could he help telling him, indeed? 'He would have killed me, I could see that he would have killed me,' he said at the inquiry, trembling and shaking even before us, though the tormentor who had scared him so was by that time under arrest and could do him no harm. 'He suspected me every minute. In fear and trembling I hastened to tell him every secret to pacify him, that he might see that I had not deceived him and let me off alive.' Those are his own words. I wrote them down and I remember them. 'When he began shouting at me, I would fall on my knees.'

"He was by nature a very honest young man and enjoyed the complete confidence of his master, ever since he had restored him some money he had lost. So it may be supposed that the poor fellow suffered pangs of remorse at having deceived his master, whom he loved as his benefactor. Persons severely afflicted with epilepsy are, so the most skilful doctors testify, always prone to continual and morbid self-reproach. They are tormented by a sense of being 'guilty' of something and before somebody, they are tormented by pangs of conscience, often entirely without cause; they exaggerate and often invent all sorts of faults and crimes. And here we have a man of that type who had really been driven to wrongdoing by terror and intimidation.

"He had, besides, a strong presentiment that something bad would be the outcome of the situation that was developing before his eyes. When Ivan Fyodorovich was leaving for Moscow, just before the catastrophe, Smerdyakov besought him to remain, though he was too timid to tell him clearly and categorically what he feared. He confined himself to hints, but his hints were not understood.

"It must be observed that he looked on Ivan Fyodorovich as a protector, whose presence in the house was a guarantee that no harm would come to pass. Remember the phrase in Dmitri Karamazov's drunken letter, 'I will kill the old man, if only Ivan goes away.' So Ivan Fyodorovich's presence seemed to every one a guarantee of peace and order in the house.

"But he went away, and within an hour of his young master's departure Smerdyakov was taken with an epileptic fit. But that's perfectly intelligible. Here I must mention that Smerdyakov, oppressed by fears and a sort of despair, had felt during those last few days the possibility of an approaching epileptic attack, of the kind from which he had suffered before at moments of moral stress and strain. The day and hour of such an attack cannot, of course, be foreseen, but every epileptic can feel beforehand that he is likely to have one. So the doctors tell us. And so, as soon as Ivan Fyodorovich has left the house, Smerdyakov, depressed by his lonely and unprotected position, goes on an errand to the cellar. He walks down the stairs wondering if he will have a fit or not, and what if it is to come upon him at once. And just because of this very mood, this very apprehension, these very questions, he is seized by the spasm in his throat that always precedes such attacks, and he falls unconscious onto the floor of the cellar. And in this perfectly natural occurrence people try to detect a suspicion, a hint that he was shamming an attack *on purpose*. But, if it were on purpose, the question arises at once, what was his motive? What was he reckoning on? What was he aiming at? I say nothing about medicine: science, I am told, may lie, science may go astray: the doctors were not able to discriminate between the counterfeit and the real. That may be so, but answer me one question: what motive had he for shamming? Is it that, having plotted the murder, he desired to attract the attention of the household by having a fit just before the crime?

"You see, gentlemen of the jury, on the night of the murder, there were five persons in Fyodor Pavlovich's house — Fyodor Pavlovich himself (but he did not kill himself, that's evident); then his servant, Grigory, but he was almost killed himself; the third person was Grigory's wife, Marfa Ignatyevna, but it would be simply shameful to imagine her murdering her master. Two persons are left — the accused and Smerdyakov. But, if we are to believe the statement of the accused that he did not do the killing, then Smerdyakov must have done it, for there is no other alternative, no one else can be found. Thus arose this 'shrewd,' colossal accusation against the unhappy idiot who committed suicide yesterday. It came about for the sole reason that no other suspect could be found. Had a shadow of suspicion rested on any one else, had there been any sixth person, I am persuaded that even the prisoner would have been ashamed to accuse

Smerdyakov, and would have accused that sixth person, for to charge Smerdyakov with that murder is perfectly absurd.

"Gentlemen, let us lay aside psychology, let us lay aside medicine, let us even lay aside logic, let us turn only to the facts and see what the facts tell us. If Smerdyakov killed, how did he do it? Alone or in collusion with the accused? Let us consider the first alternative — that he did it alone. If he had killed him it must have been with some object, for some advantage to himself. But not having a shadow of the motive that the accused had for the murder — hatred, jealousy, and so on — Smerdyakov could have murdered him only for the sake of gain, in order to appropriate the three thousand roubles he had seen his master put in the envelope. And yet he tells another person — and a person most closely interested, that is, the accused — everything about the money and the signals, where the envelope lay, what was written on it, what it was tied up with, and, above all, told him of those signals by which he could enter the house. Did he do this simply to betray himself, or in order to find a rival who would be anxious to get that envelope for himself? 'Yes,' I shall be told, 'but he spoke out of fear.' But how do you explain this? A man who could conceive such an audacious, savage act, and afterwards carry it out, tells facts which are known to no one else in the world, and which, if he held his tongue, no one in the whole world would ever have guessed!

"No, however cowardly he might be, if he had plotted such a crime, nothing would have induced him to tell any one about the envelope and the signals, for that was as good as betraying himself beforehand. He would have invented something, he would have told some lie if he had been forced to give information, but he would have been silent about that. On the contrary, I repeat, if he had said nothing about the money but had committed the murder and stolen the money, no one in the world could have charged him with murder for the sake of robbery, since no one but he had seen the money, no one but he knew of its existence in the house. Even if he had been accused of the murder, it could only have been thought that he had committed it from some other motive. But since no one had observed any such motive in him beforehand, and every one saw, on the contrary, that his master was fond of him and honoured him with his confidence, he would, of course, have been the last to be suspected. People would have suspected first the man who had a motive, a man who had himself declared he had such motives, who had made no secret of it; they would, in fact, have suspected the son of the murdered man, Dmitri Fyodorovich. Had Smerdyakov killed and robbed him, and the son been accused of it, that would, of course, have suited Smerdyakov. Yet are we to believe that, though plotting the murder, he told that son, Dmitri, about the money, the envelope, and the signals? How logical! How clear!

"The day comes for the murder planned by Smerdyakov, and we have him falling downstairs in a *feigned* fit of epilepsy — with what object? In the first place that Grigory, who had been intending to take his medicine, might put it off and remain on guard, seeing there was no one to look after the house, and, in the second place, I suppose, that his master, seeing that there was no one to guard him, and in terror of a visit from his son, might redouble his vigilance and precaution. And, most of all, I suppose that he, Smerdyakov, disabled by the fit, might be carried from the kitchen, where he always slept, apart from all the rest, and where he could go in and out as he liked, to Grigory's room at the other end of the lodge, where he was always put, shut off by a screen three paces from their own bed. This was the immemorial custom established by his master and the kind-hearted Marfa Ignatyevna, whenever he had a fit. There, lying behind the screen, he would most likely, to keep up the sham, have begun groaning, and so keeping them awake all night (as Grigory and his wife testified). And all this, we are to believe, that he might more conveniently get up and murder his master!

"But I shall be told that he shammed illness on purpose that he might not be suspected and that he told the accused of the money and the signals to tempt him to commit the murder, and when he had murdered him and had gone away with the money, making a noise, most likely, and waking people, Smerdyakov got up, am I to believe, and went in — what for? To murder his master a second time and carry off the money that had already been stolen? Gentlemen, are you laughing? I am ashamed to put forward such suggestions, but, incredible as it seems, that's just what the accused alleges. When he had left the house, had knocked Grigory down and raised an alarm, he tells us Smerdyakov got up, went in and murdered his master and stole the money! I won't press the point that Smerdyakov could hardly have reckoned on this beforehand, and have foreseen that the furious and exasperated son would simply come to peep in respectfully, though he knew the signals, and beat a retreat, leaving Smerdyakov his booty. Gentlemen of the jury, I put this question to you in earnest; when was the moment when Smerdyakov could have committed his crime? Name that moment, for without that it's impossible to accuse him.

"But, perhaps, the epileptic fit was a real one, the sick man suddenly came to himself, heard a shout, and went out. Well — what then? He looked about him and said to himself, 'Let me go and kill the master'? And how did he know what had happened, since he had been lying unconscious till that moment? But there's a limit, gentlemen, to these flights of fancy.

" 'Quite so,' some astute people will tell me, 'but what if they were in collusion? What if they murdered him together and shared the money — what then?' A weighty suspicion, truly! And the evidence confirming it is astounding: one man commits the murder and takes all the trouble while his accomplice lies on his side shamming a fit, precisely to arouse suspicion in every one, alarm in his master and alarm in Grigory. It would be curious to know what motives could have induced the two accomplices to form such an insane plan.

"But perhaps it was not a case of active complicity on Smerdyakov's part, but only of passive acquiescence; perhaps Smerdyakov was intimidated and agreed not to prevent the murder, and, foreseeing that he would be blamed for letting his master be murdered, without screaming for help or resisting, he may have obtained permission from Dmitri Karamazov to get out of the way by shamming a fit — 'you may murder him as you like; it's nothing to me.' But as this attack of Smerdyakov's was bound to throw the household into confusion, Dmitri Karamazov could never have agreed to such a plan. I will waive that point, however. Supposing that he did agree, it would still follow that Dmitri Karamazov is the murderer, the actual murderer and the instigator, and Smerdyakov is only a passive accomplice, and not even an accomplice, but merely acquiesced against his will out of terror.

"But what do we see? As soon as he is arrested the prisoner instantly throws all the blame on Smerdyakov, not accusing him of being his accomplice, but of being himself the murderer. He did it alone, he says. He did the murdering and robbing, it was the work of his hands. Strange sort of accomplices who begin to accuse one another at once — that never happens. And think of the risk for Karamazov: he is the chief murderer, Smerdyakov is not the chief murderer, he is only the abettor, and all the time he was lying in bed behind the partition, and it is on this man that Karamazov puts the blame. But he, the man who lay in bed, might well have resented it and in self-preservation, if nothing else, might well have confessed the truth: 'We both had a hand in it, but I didn't kill, but only permitted and abetted the murder out of fear.' For he might well have seen that the court would at once estimate the degree of his guilt, and so he might well have reckoned that even if he were punished, it would be a far less severe punishment than the one meted out to the chief murderer, who wished to throw all the blame on him. But in that case he would have been certain to make a confession, yet he has not done so. Smerdyakov never hinted at their complicity, though the actual murderer persisted in accusing him and declaring that he had committed the crime alone.

"What's more, Smerdyakov at the inquiry volunteered the statement that it was *he* who had told the accused of the envelope with the money and of the signals, and that, but for him, Karamazov would have known nothing about them. If he had really been a guilty accomplice, would he so readily have stated at the inquiry that he had himself told everything to the accused? On the contrary, he would have tried to conceal it, to distort the facts or minimise them. But he neither distorted nor minimised them. No one but an innocent man, who had no fear of being charged with complicity, could have acted as he did. And in a fit of morbid melancholy arising from his disease and this catastrophe he hanged himself yesterday. He left a note written in his peculiar style, 'I destroy myself of my own will and inclination so as to throw no blame on any one.' What would it have cost him to add: 'I am the murderer, not Karamazov'? But that he did not add. Did his conscience lead him to suicide and not to avowing his guilt?

"And what followed? Notes for three thousand roubles were brought into the court just now, and we were told that they were the same that lay in the envelope now on the table before us, and that the witness had received them from Smerdyakov the day before. But you, gentlemen of the jury, yourselves recall the painful scene which took place here. I shall not recall the details, I shall only allow myself to make comments on two or three points, selecting such trivial ones as might not be obvious at first sight to every one, and so may be overlooked. In the first place, Smerdyakov must have given back the money and hanged himself yesterday from remorse (for without remorse he would not have returned the money). And it was, of course, only last night that he confessed his guilt to Ivan Karamazov, for the first time, as the latter informs us. If it were not so, indeed, why should Ivan Fyodorovich have kept silence till now? And so he confessed, but why, I ask again, did he not avow the whole truth in the last letter he left behind, knowing that the innocent prisoner had to face this terrible ordeal the next day?

"The money alone is no proof. A week ago, quite by chance, the fact came to the knowledge of myself and two other persons in this court that Ivan Fyodorovich had sent two five per cent notes of five thousand each — that is, ten thousand in all — to the chief town of the province to be changed. I only mention this to point out that any one may have money on a given date, and that it can't be proved that these notes are the same as were in Fyodor Pavlovich's envelope.

"Ivan Karamazov, after receiving yesterday a communication of such importance from the real murderer, did not stir. Why didn't he report it at once? Why did he put it all off till morning? I think I have a right to conjecture why.

"His health had been giving way for a week past: he had admitted to a doctor and to his most intimate friends that he was seeing visions and encountering phantoms of the dead: he was on the eve of the attack of brain fever by which he has been stricken to-day. In this condition he suddenly heard of Smerdyakov's death, and at once reflected, 'The man is dead, I can throw the blame on him and save my brother. I have money. I will take a roll of notes and say that Smerdyakov gave them to me before his death.' You will say that was dishonourable: it's dishonourable to slander even the dead, even to save a brother. True, but what if he lied unconsciously? What if, finally unhinged by the sudden news of the valet's death, he imagined it really was so? You saw the recent scene: you have seen the witness's condition. He was standing up and was speaking, but where was his mind?

"Then followed the document, the prisoner's letter addressed to Madame Verhovtzev written two days before the crime and containing a complete programme of the murder. Why, then, are we looking for a programme and its authors? The crime was committed precisely according to this programme, and by no other than the writer of it. Yes, gentlemen of the jury, it went off without a hitch! No, we didn't, we didn't run respectfully and timidly away from our father's window, being besides firmly convinced that the object of our affections was with him. No, that is absurd and incredible! He went in and did the deed. Most likely he killed him in anger, burning with resentment, as soon as he looked on his hated rival. But having killed him, probably with one blow of the brass pestle, and having convinced himself, after careful search, that she was not there, he did not, however, forget to put his hand under the pillow and take out the envelope with the money, the torn envelope which lies now on the table before us.

"I mention this fact that you may note one, to my thinking, very characteristic circumstance. Had he been an experienced murderer and had he committed the murder for the sake of robbing only, would he have left the torn envelope on the floor as it was found, beside the corpse? Had it been Smerdyakov, for instance, murdering his master to rob him, he would have simply carried away the envelope with him, without troubling himself to open it over his victim's corpse, for he would have known for certain that the notes were in the envelope — they had been put in and sealed up in his presence — and had he taken the envelope with him, no one would ever have known of the robbery. I ask you, gentlemen of the jury, would Smerdyakov have behaved in that way? Would he have left the envelope on the floor?

"No, this was precisely the action of a frantic murderer, a murderer whose reason was already clouded, who was not a thief and had never stolen before that day, who snatched the notes from under the pillow, not like a thief stealing them, but as though seizing his own property from the thief who had stolen it. For that was the idea which had become almost an insane obsession with Dmitri Karamazov in regard to that money. And pouncing upon the envelope, which he had never seen before, he tore it open to make sure that the money was in it, and ran away with the money in his pocket, even forgetting to consider that he had left an astounding piece of evidence against himself in that torn envelope on the floor. All because it was Karamazov, not Smerdyakov, he doesn't think, he doesn't reflect, and how should he? He runs away; he hears behind him the servant cry out; the old man catches him, stops him, and is felled to the ground by the brass pestle.

"The accused, moved by pity, leaps down to look at him. Would you believe it, he tells us that he leapt down out of pity, out of compassion, to see whether he could do anything for him. Was that a moment to show compassion? No; he jumped down simply to make certain whether the only witness of his crime was dead or alive. Any other feeling, any other motive would be unnatural. Note that he took trouble over Grigory, wiped his head with his handkerchief, and, convincing himself he was dead, he ran like one lost to the house of his mistress, covered with blood. How was it he never thought that he was covered with blood and would be at once detected? But the accused himself assures us that he paid no attention to the fact that he was covered with blood. That may be believed, that is very possible, that always happens at such moments with criminals. On one point they will show diabolical cunning, while another will escape them altogether. But he was thinking at that moment of one thing only — where was *she?* He had to find out at once where she was, so he ran to her lodging and learnt an unexpected and astounding piece of news — she had gone off to Mokroye to meet her former lover."

CHAPTER IX

PSYCHOLOGY AT FULL STEAM. THE GALLOPING TROIKA. THE END OF THE PROSECUTOR'S SPEECH

HAVING reached this moment in his speech, Ippolit Kirillovich, who had chosen the historical method of exposition, beloved by all nervous orators, since they find in its limitations a check on their own eager rhetoric, went off into a dissertation on Grushenka's "former and indubitable lover," and brought forward several interesting thoughts on this subject.

"Karamazov, who had been frantically jealous of every one, collapsed, so to speak, and effaced himself at once before this former lover. What makes it all the more strange is that he seems to have paid practically no attention to the new danger that assailed him in the person of this unexpected rival. But he had looked upon him as a remote danger, and Karamazov always lives in the present. Possibly he regarded him as a fiction. But his wounded heart grasped instantly that perhaps the woman had been concealing this new rival and deceiving him, because this newcomer was anything but a fiction and a fantasy to her, but was the one, the one hope of her life. Grasping this instantly, he resigned himself.

"Gentlemen of the jury, I cannot pass over in silence this unexpected trait in the character of the accused. He suddenly evinces an irresistible desire for justice, a respect for woman and a recognition of the rights of her heart. And all this at the very moment when he had stained his hands with his father's blood for her sake! It is true that the blood he had shed was already crying out for vengeance, for, after having ruined his soul and his earthly destiny, he was involuntarily forced to ask himself at that same instant what he meant and what he could mean *now* to her, to that being, dearer to him than his own soul, in comparison with that former and indubitable lover who had returned to the woman he had once betrayed, penitent, with new love, with honourable offers, with the promise of a reformed and happy life. And he, luckless man, what could he give her now, what could he offer her?

"Karamazov understood all this, he understood that all ways were barred to him by his crime and that he was a criminal under sentence, and not a man with life before him! This thought crushed and annihilated him. And so he instantly seizes upon one frantic plan, which, given Karamazov's character, could not but appear to him as the sole and fatal way out of his terrible position. That way out was suicide. He runs for the pistols he had left in pledge with Perhotin and on the way, as he runs, he pulls out of his pocket the money, for the sake of which he had stained his hands with his father's blood. Oh, now he needs money more than ever. Karamazov dies, Karamazov shoots himself and it will be remembered! It is not for nothing that we are a poet and it is not for nothing that we burnt the candle at both ends. 'To her, to her! and there, oh, there I will give a feast to the whole world, such as never was before, that will be remembered and talked of long after! In the midst of shouts of wild merriment, reckless gipsy songs and dances we shall raise the glass and drink to the woman we adore and her new-found happiness! And then, on the spot, at her feet, we shall dash out our brains before her and destroy our life! She will remember Mitya Karamazov sometimes, she will see how Mitya loved her, she will pity Mitya!'

"There is much here that is love of effect, romantic frenzy and sentimentality, the wild recklessness of the Karamazovs. Yes, but there is something else, gentlemen of the jury, something that cries out in the soul, throbs incessantly in the mind, and poisons the heart unto death — that *something* is conscience, gentlemen of the jury, its judgment, its terrible torments! But the pistol will settle everything, the pistol is the only way out! But *beyond* — I don't know whether Karamazov wondered at that moment, 'What lies beyond?' and whether Karamazov could, like Hamlet, wonder what lies beyond. No, gentlemen of the jury, they have Hamlets, but we still have Karamazovs!"

Here Ippolit Kirillovich drew a minute picture of Mitya's preparations, the scene at Perhotin's, at the shop, with the drivers. He cited numerous words, remarks, gestures, all confirmed by witnesses, and the picture made a terrible impression on the audience. What chiefly impressed people were the facts taken as a whole. The guilt of this man, frenzied and already careless of any precautions, stood out clear and incontrovertible.

"What need had he of precautions? Two or three times he almost confessed fully, hinted at it, all but spoke out." (Then followed the evidence given by witnesses.) "He even cried out to the peasant who drove him, 'Do you know, you are driving a murderer!' But it was impossible for him to speak out, he had to get to Mokroye and there to finish his romance. But what was awaiting the luckless man? Almost from the first minute at Mokroye he saw that his indubitable rival was perhaps by no means so indubitable, that the toast to their new-found happiness was not desired and would not be acceptable. But you know the facts, gentlemen of the jury, from the preliminary inquiry. Karamazov's triumph over his rival was complete and his soul passed into quite a new phase, perhaps the most terrible phase through which his soul has passed or will pass.

"One may say with certainty, gentlemen of the jury," the prosecutor exclaimed, "that outraged nature and the criminal heart bring their own vengeance more completely than any earthly justice. What's more, justice and punishment on earth positively alleviate the punishment of nature and are, indeed, necessary to the soul of the criminal at such moments, as its salvation from despair. For I cannot imagine the horror and moral suffering of Karamazov when he learnt that she loved him, that for his sake she had rejected her first lover, that she was summoning him, Mitya, to a new life, that she was promising him happiness — and when? When everything was over for him and nothing was possible!

"By the way, I will note in parenthesis a point of importance for the light it throws on the prisoner's position at the moment. This woman, this love of his, had been till the last moment, till the very instant of his arrest, a being unattainable, passionately desired by him but unattainable. Yet why did he not shoot himself then, why did he relinquish his design and even forget where his pistol was? It was just that passionate desire for love and the hope of satisfying it that restrained him. In the dizzy atmosphere of their revels he kept close to his adored mistress, who was feasting with him and was more charming and fascinating to him than ever — he did not leave her side, he filled his eyes with her, he melted before her.

"His passion might well, for a moment, stifle not only the fear of arrest, but even the torments of conscience. For a moment, oh, only for a moment. I can picture the state of mind of the criminal hopelessly enslaved by these influences — first, the influence of drink, of noise and excitement, of the thud of the dance and the scream of the songs, and of her, flushed with wine, singing and dancing and laughing to him in her drunken state! Secondly, the hope in the background that the fatal end might still be far off, that not till next morning, at least, would they come and take him. So he had a few hours and that's much, very much! In a few hours one can think up many things. I imagine that he felt something like what criminals feel when they are being taken to the gallows. They have another long, long street to ride down and at walking pace, past thousands of people. Then there will be a turning into another street and only at the end of that street the dread square! I fancy that at the beginning of the journey the condemned man, sitting on his shameful cart, must feel that he has infinite life still before him. But the houses recede, the cart moves on — oh, that's nothing, it's still far to the turning into the second street and he still looks boldly right and left at those thousands of callously curious people with their eyes fixed on him, and he still fancies that he is just such a man as they. But now comes the turning into the next street. Oh, that's nothing, nothing, there's still a whole street before him, and however many houses have been passed, he will still think there are many left. And so to the very end, to the very square.

"This I imagine is how it was with Karamazov then. 'They've not had time yet,' he must have thought, 'I may still find some way out, or, there's still time to make some plan of defence, and now, now — she is so fascinating!'

"His soul was full of confusion and dread, but he managed, however, to put aside half his money and hide it somewhere — I cannot otherwise explain the disappearance of quite half of the three thousand he had just taken from his father's pillow. He had been in Mokroye more than once before, he had caroused there for two days together already, he knew the old big house with all its passages and outbuildings. I imagine that part of the money was hidden in that house, not long before the arrest, in some crevice, under some floor, in some corner, under the roof. With what object? I shall be asked. Why, the catastrophe may take place at once, of course; he hadn't yet considered how to meet it, he hadn't the time, his head was throbbing and his heart was with *her*, but money — money was indispensable in any case! With money a man is everywhere a man. Perhaps such prudence at such a moment may strike you as unnatural? But he assures us himself that a month before, at a most exciting and fateful moment, he had withdrawn half of three thousand and sewn it up in a little bag. And though that was not true, as we shall prove directly, it shows the idea was a familiar one to Karamazov, he had contemplated it. What's more, when he declared at the inquiry that he had put fifteen hundred roubles in a bag (which never existed) he may have invented that little bag on the inspiration of the moment, because two hours before he had removed his money and hidden it at Mokroye till morning, in case of emergency, simply not to have it on his person. Two abysses, gentlemen of the jury, remember that Karamazov can contemplate two abysses and both at once.

"We have searched the house, but we haven't found the money. It may still be there or it may have disappeared next day and be in the prisoner's hands now. In any case, he was arrested at her side, on his knees before her, she was lying on the bed, he had his hands stretched out to her and he had so entirely forgotten everything that he did not even hear the men coming to arrest him. He hadn't time to prepare any line of defence in his mind. Both he and his mind were caught unawares.

"And here he is, before his judges, the arbiters of his destiny. Gentlemen of the jury, there are moments in the execution of our duties when it is terrible for us to face a man, terrible on his account, too! Those are the moments of contemplating that animal fear, when the criminal sees that all is lost, but still struggles, still intends to offer resistance. Those are the moments when every instinct of self-preservation rises up in him at once and he, to save himself, looks at you with penetrating, questioning, and suffering eyes, studies you, your face, your thoughts, uncertain on which side you will strike, and his distracted mind frames thousands of plans in an instant, but he is still afraid to speak, afraid of giving himself away! This journey through the purgatory of the spirit, this animal thirst for self-preservation, these humiliating moments of the human soul, are awful, and sometimes arouse horror and compassion for the criminal even in the examining magistrate. And this was what we all witnessed then.

"At first he was thunderstruck and in his terror dropped some very compromising words. 'Blood! I've deserved it!' But he quickly restrained himself. He had not prepared what he was to say, what answer he was to make, he had nothing but a bare denial ready. 'I am not guilty of my father's death.' That was his fence for the moment and behind it he hoped to throw up a barricade of some sort. His first compromising exclamations he hastened to explain by declaring that he was responsible for the death of the servant Grigory only. 'Of that bloodshed I am guilty, but who has killed my father, gentlemen, who has killed him? Who can have killed him, *if not I?*' Do you hear, he asked us that, us, who had come to ask him that question! Do you hear that phrase uttered with such premature haste — 'if not I' — the animal cunning, the naïveté, the Karamazov impatience of it? 'I didn't kill him and you mustn't think I did! I wanted to kill him, gentlemen, I wanted to kill him,' he hastens to admit (he was in a hurry, in a terrible hurry), 'but still I am not guilty, it is not I murdered him.' He concedes to us that he wanted to murder him, as though to say, you can see for yourselves how sincere I am, so you'll believe all the sooner that I didn't murder him. Oh, in such cases the criminal is often amazingly frivolous and credulous.

"At that point one of the lawyers asked him, as it were casually, the simplest question, 'Wasn't it Smerdyakov killed him?' What followed, we expected: he was horribly angry at our having anticipated him and caught him unawares, before he had time to pave the way to choose and snatch the most suitable moment for bringing in Smerdyakov's name. In keeping with his character, he rushed at once to the other extreme, and began to assure us that Smerdyakov could not have killed him, was not capable of it. But don't believe him, that was only his cunning; he didn't really give up the idea of Smerdyakov; on the contrary, he would yet bring him forward again; for, indeed, he had no one else to bring forward, but he would do that later, because for the moment that line was spoiled for him. He would bring him forward perhaps next day, or even a few days later, choosing an opportunity to cry out to us, 'You see, I myself was more sceptical about Smerdyakov than you, you remember that yourselves, but now I am convinced. He killed, who but he!' And for the present he falls back upon a gloomy and irritable denial. Impatience and anger prompt him, however, to the most inept and incredible explanation of how he looked into his father's window and how he respectfully withdrew. Above all, he does not yet know the circumstances, the evidence given by Grigory.

"We proceed to search him. The search angers, but encourages him, the whole three thousand have not been found on him, only half of it. And no doubt only at that moment of angry silence and denial the notion of the little bag first enters his head. No doubt he is conscious himself of the improbability of the invention and strives painfully to make it sound more likely, to weave it into a romance that will sound plausible. In such cases the first duty, the chief task of the examining magistrates, is to prevent the criminal from preparing himself, to pounce upon him unexpectedly so that he may blurt out his cherished ideas in all their simplicity, improbability, and inconsistency. The criminal can be made to speak only by the sudden and apparently incidental communication of some new fact, of some circumstance of great importance in the case, of which he had no previous idea and could not have foreseen. We had such a fact in readiness — that was Grigory's evidence about the open door through which the prisoner had run out. He had completely forgotten about that door and had not even suspected that Grigory could have seen it.

"The effect of it was amazing. He leapt up and shouted to us, 'It was Smerdyakov murdered him, Smerdyakov!' and so betrayed his most cherished, basic idea in its most improbable shape, for Smerdyakov could have committed the murder only after he had knocked Grigory down and run away. When we told him that Grigory saw the door was open before he fell down, and had heard Smerdyakov groan behind the partition as he came out of his bedroom — Karamazov was positively crushed. My esteemed and witty colleague, Nikolay Parfenovich, told me afterwards that he was almost moved to tears at the sight of him. And to improve matters, the prisoner hastened to tell us about the famous little bag — so be it, you shall hear this tale!

"Gentlemen of the jury, I have told you already, why I consider this invention not only an absurdity, but the most improbable fiction that could have been brought forward under the circumstances. If one tried on a bet to invent the most unlikely story, one could hardly find anything more incredible. The worst of such stories is that the triumphant romancers can always be put to confusion and crushed by the very details in which real life is so rich and which these unhappy and involuntary story-tellers neglect as insignificant trifles. Oh, they have no thought to spare for such details, their minds are concentrated on their grand invention as a whole, and fancy any one daring to pull them up for a trifle! But that's how they are caught. The accused is asked the question, 'Where did you get the stuff for your little bag and who made it for you?' 'I made it myself.' 'And where did you get the linen?' The accused is already offended, he considers it almost insulting to ask him such a trivial question, and, would you believe it, his resentment is genuine! But they are all like that. 'I tore it off my shirt.' 'Very well, then we shall find that shirt among your linen to-morrow, with a piece torn off.' And only fancy, gentlemen of the jury, if we really had found that torn shirt (and how could we have failed to find it in his chest of drawers or trunk if such a shirt really existed?) that would have been a fact, a material fact in support of his statement! But he was incapable of that reflection. 'I don't remember, it may not have been off my shirt, I sewed it up in my landlady's cap.' 'What sort of cap?' 'It was an old cotton rag of hers lying about.' 'And do you remember that clearly?' 'No, I don't.' And he is angry, very angry, and yet imagine not remembering it! At the most terrible moments of a man's life, for instance when he is being led to execution, he remembers just such trifles. He will forget anything but some green roof that has flashed past him on the road, or a jackdaw on a cross — that he will remember. Obviously, when he was making that little bag he was hiding from the people in the house and he must have remembered his humiliating fear that some one might come in and find him needle in hand, how at the slightest noise he jumped up and slipped behind the partition (there is a partition in his lodgings).

"But, gentlemen of the jury, why do I tell you all this, all these details, trifles?" cried Ippolit Kirillovich suddenly. "Just because the accused still persists in these absurdities to this moment. He has not explained anything since that fatal night two months ago, he has not added one actual illuminating fact to his former fantastic statements. 'Those are all trivialities. You must believe me on my honour.' Oh, we are glad to believe it, we are eager to believe it, even if only on his word of honour! Are we jackals thirsting for human blood? Give us, show us a single fact in the prisoner's favour and we shall rejoice; but let it be a substantial, real fact, and not a conclusion drawn from the prisoner's facial expression by his own brother, or that when he beat himself on the breast he must have meant to point to the little bag, and that in the darkness, too. We shall rejoice at the new fact, we shall be the first to repudiate our charge, we shall hasten to repudiate it. But now justice cries out and we persist, we cannot repudiate anything."

Ippolit Kirillovich passed to his final peroration. He looked as though he was in a fever, he spoke of the blood that cried for vengeance, the blood of the father murdered by his son, with the base motive of robbery! He pointed to the tragic and blaring totality of the facts.

"And whatever you may hear from the talented and celebrated counsel for the defence," Ippolit Kirillovich could not resist adding, "whatever eloquent and touching appeals may be made to your sensibilities, remember that at this moment you are in a temple of justice. Remember that you are the champions of our justice, the champions of our holy Russia, of her foundations, her family, everything that she holds sacred! Yes, you represent Russia here at this moment, and your verdict not only will be heard in this hall but will reecho throughout the whole of Russia, and all Russia will hear you, as her champions and her judges, and she will be encouraged or disheartened by your verdict. Do not disappoint Russia and her expectations. Our fatal troika dashes on in her headlong flight perhaps to destruction, and for a long time throughout Russia men have stretched out imploring hands and called a halt to its furious reckless course. And if other nations stand aside from that troika that may be, not out of respect to her, as the poet would fain believe, but simply out of horror. Out of horror, perhaps out of disgust. And well it is that they stand aside, but maybe they will cease one day to do so and will form a firm wall confronting the hurrying apparition and will check the frenzied rush of our lawlessness, for the sake of saving themselves, enlightenment, and civilisation! Already we have heard voices of alarm from Europe, they already begin to sound. Do not tempt them! Do not heap up their growing hatred by a sentence justifying the murder of a father by his own son!"

In a word, though Ippolit Kirillovich was genuinely moved, he wound up his speech with this rhetorical appeal — and indeed, the effect produced by him was extraordinary. When he had finished his speech, he went out hurriedly and, as I have mentioned before, almost fainted in the adjoining room. There was no applause in the court, but serious people were pleased. The ladies were not so well satisfied, though even they were pleased with his eloquence, especially as they had no apprehensions as to the outcome of the trial and had full trust in Fetyukovich. "He will speak at last and of course carry all before him."

Every one looked at Mitya; he sat silent through the whole of the prosecutor's speech, with his hands clasped, his teeth clenched, and his head bowed. Only from time to time he raised his head and listened, especially when Grushenka was spoken of. When the prosecutor mentioned Rakitin's opinion of her, a smile of contempt and anger passed over his face and he murmured rather audibly, "The Bernards!" When Ippolit Kirillovich described how he questioned and tortured him at Mokroye, Mitya raised his head and listened with intense curiosity. At one point he seemed about to jump up and cry out, but controlled himself and only shrugged his shoulders disdainfully. People talked afterwards of the end of the speech, of the prosecutor's feat in examining the prisoner at Mokroye, and jeered at Ippolit Kirillovich. "The man could not resist boasting of his cleverness," they said.

The court was adjourned, but only for a short interval, a quarter of an hour or twenty minutes at most. There was a hum of conversation and exclamations in the audience. I remember some of them.

"A serious speech," a gentleman in one group observed frowningly.

"He unreeled too much psychology," said another voice.

"But it was all true, the absolute truth!"

"Yes, he is first rate at it."

"He summed it all up."

"Yes, he summed us up, too," chimed in another voice. "Do you remember, at the beginning of his speech, making out we were all like Fyodor Pavlovich?"

"And at the end, too. But that was all rot."

"And obscure, too."

"He was a little too much carried away."

"It's unjust, sir, it's unjust."

"No, it was smartly done, anyway. He's had long to wait, but he's had his say, ha-ha!"

"What will the counsel for the defence say?"

In another group I heard:

"He had no business to make a thrust at the Petersburg man like that: 'appealing to your sensibilities' — do you remember?"

"Yes, that was awkward of him."

"He was in too great a hurry."

"A nervous fellow."

"We laugh, but what must the accused be feeling?"

"Yes, what must it be for Mitya?"

"What will counsel for the defence say?"

In a third group:

"Who is that lady, the fat one, with the lorgnette, sitting at the end?"

"She is a general's wife, divorced, I know her."

"That's why she has the lorgnette."

"She is not good for much."

"Oh, no, she is a piquant little woman."

"Two places beyond her there is a little blonde, she is prettier."

"Clever work at Mokroye, wasn't it, eh?"

"Oh, it was clever enough. We've heard it before, how often he has told the story at people's houses!"

"And he couldn't resist doing it now. That's vanity."

"He is a man with a chip on his shoulder, he-he!"

"Yes, and quick to take offence. And there was too much rhetoric, such long sentences."

"Notice, he scares us, he kept trying to scare us. Do you remember about the troika? 'They have Hamlets, but we have, so far, only Karamazovs!' That was clever!"

"That was to get in well with the Liberals. He is afraid of them."

"Yes, and he is afraid of the lawyer, too."

"Yes, what will Fetyukovich say?"

"Whatever he says, he won't get round our peasants."

"Don't you think so?"

A fourth group:

"What he said about the troika was good, that bit about the other nations."

"And that was true what he said about other nations not standing for it."

"What do you mean?"

"Why, in the English Parliament a Member got up last week and speaking about the Nihilists asked the Ministry whether it was not high time to intervene, to educate this barbarous nation. Ippolit was thinking of him, I know he was. He was talking about that last week."

"Not an easy job."

"Not an easy job? Why not?"

"Why, we'd shut up Kronstadt and not let them have any corn. Where would they get it?"

"In America. They get it from America now."

"Nonsense!"

But the bell rang, all rushed to their places. Fetyukovich mounted the tribune.

CHAPTER X

THE SPEECH FOR THE DEFENCE. A TWO-EDGED WEAPON

ALL was hushed as the first words of the famous orator rang out. The eyes of the audience were fastened upon him. He began very simply and directly, with an air of conviction, but not the slightest trace of conceit. He did not make the slightest attempt at eloquence, at rhetoric, or at phrases ringing with emotion. He was like a man speaking in an intimate circle of sympathetic friends. He had a beautiful voice, sonorous and appealing, and there was something genuine and simple in the very sound of it. But every one realised at once that the speaker might suddenly rise to true pathos and "pierce the heart with wondrous power." His language was perhaps more irregular than Ippolit Kirillovich's, but he spoke without long phrases, and, indeed, with more precision. One thing did not please the ladies: he kept bending forward, especially at the beginning of his speech, not exactly bowing, but as though he were straining towards and darting at his listeners, bending his long narrow back in the middle, as though there were a hinge there that enabled him to bend almost at a right angle.

At the beginning of his speech he spoke rather disconnectedly, without system, one may say, dealing with facts separately, but in the end these facts formed a whole. His speech might be divided into two halves, the first consisting of criticism in refutation of the charge, sometimes malicious and sarcastic. But in the second half he suddenly changed his tone, and even his manner, and at once rose to pathos. The audience seemed on the look-out for it, and quivered with delight.

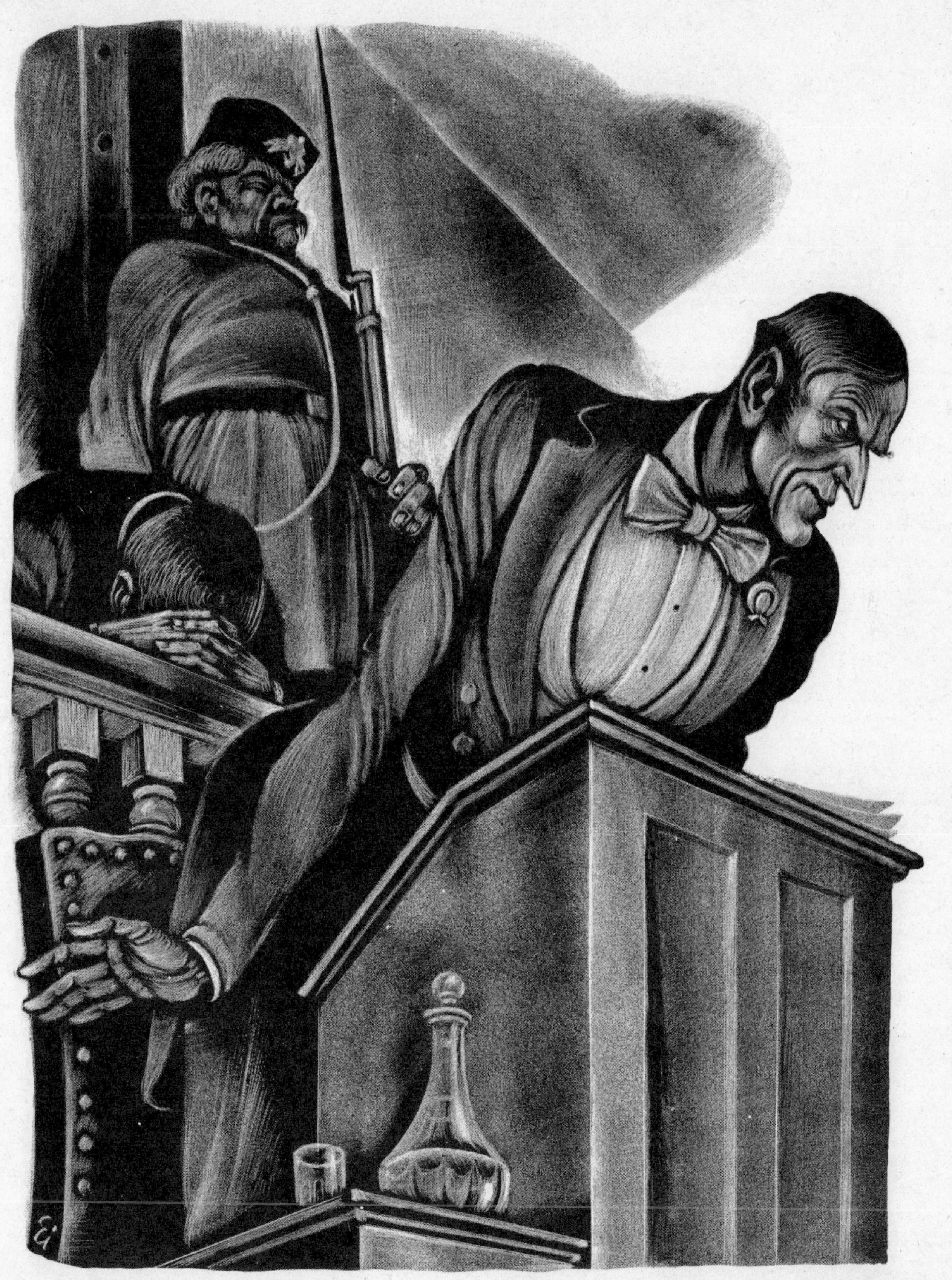

SPEECH FOR THE DEFENCE

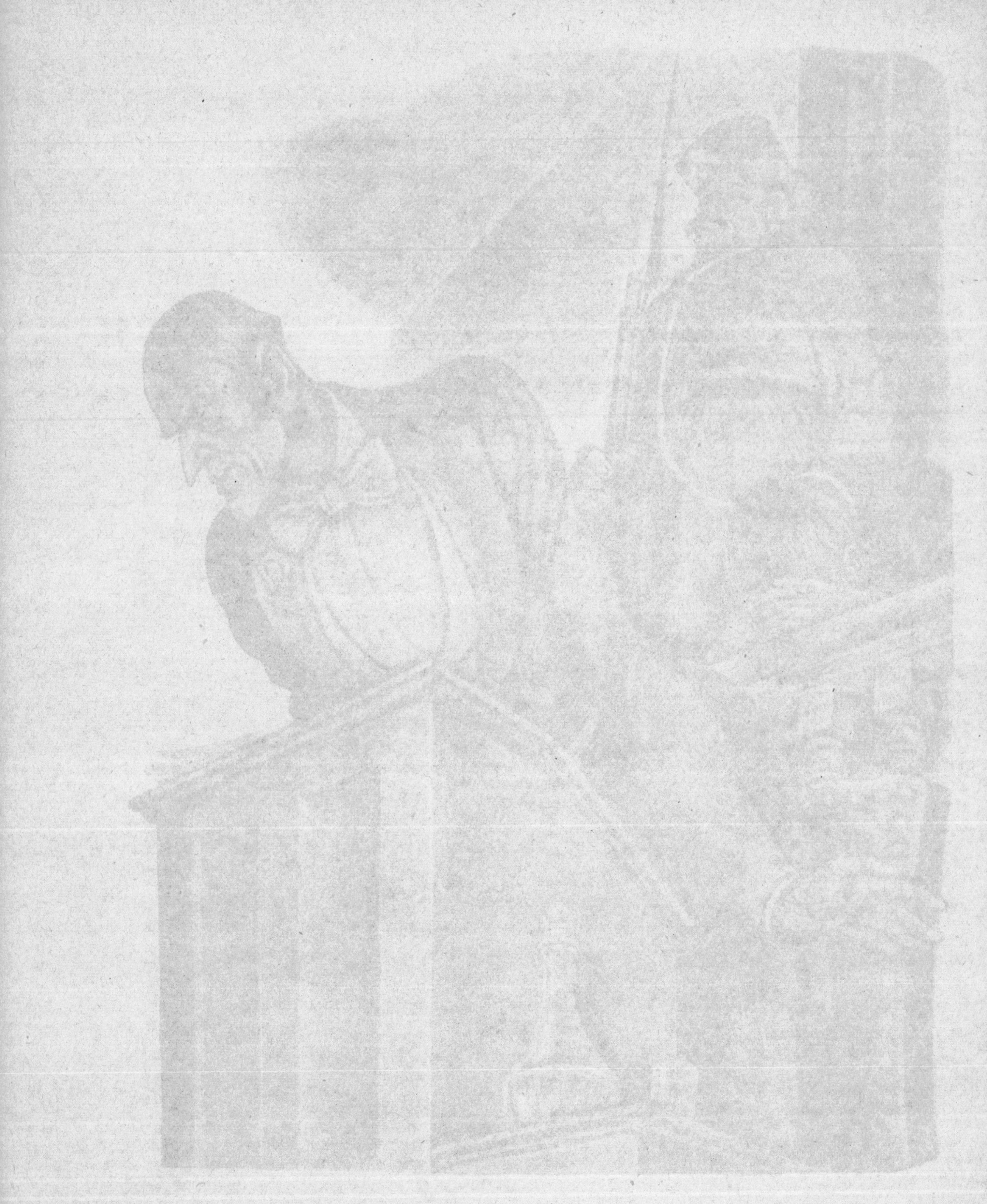

He went straight to the point, and began by saying that although he practised in Petersburg, he had more than once visited provincial towns to defend those whom he believed to be innocent or concerning whose innocence he had a kind of presentiment. "That is what has happened to me in the present case," he explained. "From the very first accounts in the newspapers I was struck by something which strongly prepossessed me in the prisoner's favour. In a word, what interested me most was a fact which often occurs in legal practice, but rarely, I think, in such an extreme and peculiar form as in the present case. I ought to formulate that peculiarity only at the end of my speech, but I will do so at the very beginning, for it is my weakness to come to the point directly, not keeping my effects in reserve and economising impressions. That may be imprudent on my part, but then it's sincere. What I have in my mind is this: there is an overwhelming accumulation of evidence against the accused, and at the same time not one fact that will stand criticism, if it is examined separately, by itself. As I followed the case more closely in the papers and through rumours, I was more and more confirmed in my idea, and I suddenly received from the relatives of the accused a request to undertake his defence. I at once hurried here, and here I became completely convinced. It was to break down this terrible chain of facts, and to show that each piece of evidence taken separately was unproved and fantastic, that I undertook the case."

So Fetyukovich began.

"Gentlemen of the jury," he suddenly protested, "I am new to this district. I have no preconceived ideas. The accused, a man of turbulent and unbridled temper, has not insulted me, as he has insulted perhaps hundreds of persons in this town, and so prejudiced many people against him beforehand. Of course I recognise that the moral sentiment of local society is justly excited against him. The accused is of turbulent and violent temper. Yet he was received in society here; he was even welcome in the family of my talented friend, the prosecutor."

(N.B. At these words there were two or three laughs in the audience, quickly suppressed, but noticed by all. All of us knew that the prosecutor received Mitya against his will, solely because he had somehow found favour with the prosecutor's wife — a lady most virtuous and highly respected, but fanciful, capricious, and fond of opposing her husband, especially in trifles. Mitya's visits, however, had not been frequent.)

"Nevertheless I venture to suggest," Fetyukovich continued, "that in spite of his independent mind and just character, my opponent may have formed a mistaken prejudice against my unfortunate client. Oh, that is so natural; the unfortunate man has only too well deserved to be regarded with such prejudice. Outraged morality, and still more outraged taste, is often inexorable. Of course, we have, in the prosecutor's excellent speech, heard a stern analysis of the prisoner's character and conduct, and his severe critical attitude towards the case was evident. And, what's more, he went into psychological subtleties to explain the esssence of the matter, subtleties into which he could not have entered, if he had the least conscious and malicious prejudice against the personality of the accused. But there are things which are even worse, even more fatal in such cases, than the most malicious and consciously unfair attitude. It is worse if we are carried away by the artistic instinct, by the desire to create, so to speak, a romance, especially if God has endowed us with psychological insight. Before I started on my way here, I was warned in Petersburg, and was myself aware, that I should find here a talented opponent whose psychological insight and subtlety had gained him peculiar renown in our legal world, which is still young. But profound as psychology is, gentlemen, it's a two-edged weapon." (Laughter among the public.) "You will, of course, forgive me my trivial comparison; I can't boast of eloquence. But I will take as an example any point in the prosecutor's speech.

"The accused, running away in the garden at night, climbs over the fence, and knocks down with a brass pestle the servant who has grabbed his leg. Then he jumps back into the garden and spends five minutes over the man, trying to discover whether he has killed him or not. Now the prosecutor refuses to believe the accused's statement that he ran to old Grigory out of pity. 'No,' he says, 'such sensibility is impossible at such a moment, that's unnatural; he ran to find out whether the only witness of his crime was dead or alive, and so showed that he had committed the murder, since he would not have run back for any other reason.'

"Here you have psychology; but let us take the same method and apply it to the case the other way round, and our result will be no less probable. The murderer, we are told, leapt down to find out, out of prudence, whether the witness was alive or not, yet he had just left in his murdered father's study, as the prosecutor himself argues, an amazing piece of evidence in the shape of a torn envelope, with an inscription that there had been three thousand roubles in it. 'If he had carried that envelope away with him, no one in the world would have known of the existence of that envelope and of the notes in it, and that the money had been stolen by the accused.' Those are the prosecutor's own words. So on one side you see a complete absence of precaution, a man who has lost his head and run away in a fright, leaving that clue on the floor, and two minutes later, when he has struck another man, we are asked to assume the most heartless and calculating prudence in him. But even admitting this was so, it is psychological subtlety, I suppose, that discerns that under certain circumstances I become as bloodthirsty and keen-sighted as a Caucasian eagle, while at the next I am as timid and blind as a mole. But if I am so bloodthirsty and cruelly calculating that when I kill a man I run back only to find out whether he is alive to bear witness against me, why should I spend five minutes looking after my victim at the risk of encountering other witnesses? Why soak my handkerchief, wiping the blood off his head so that it may be evidence against me later? If we are so cold-hearted and calculating, why not hit the servant on the head again and again with the same pestle so as to kill him outright and relieve ourself of all anxiety about the witness?

"And finally I jump down to see whether the witness is alive or not, and right there on the path I leave another witness, namely, that brass pestle which I took from the two women, and which they could always recognise afterwards as theirs, and testify that I had taken it from them. And it is not as though we had forgotten it on the path, dropped it through carelessness or haste, no, we flung away our weapon, for it was found fifteen paces from where Grigory lay. Why did we do so? Just because we were grieved at having killed a man, an old servant; and we flung away the pestle with a curse, as a murderous weapon. That's how it must have been, what other reason could we have had for throwing it so far? And if we were capable of feeling grief and pity at having killed a man, it was of course because we did not kill our father. Had we murdered him, we would never have run to another victim out of pity; then we would have felt differently; our thoughts would have been centred on self-preservation. We would have had none to spare for pity, that is beyond doubt. On the contrary, I repeat, we would have broken his skull instead of spending five minutes looking after him. There was room for pity and good-feeling just because our conscience had been clear till then. Here we have a different psychology. I have purposely resorted to this method, gentlemen of the jury, to show that you can prove anything by it. It all depends on who makes use of it. Psychology lures even most serious people into romancing, and quite unconsciously.

"I am speaking of excessive psychology, gentlemen of the jury, of the abuse of psychology, as it were."

Sounds of approval and laughter, at the expense of the prosecutor, were again audible in the court. I will not repeat the speech in detail; I will only quote some passages from it, some leading points.

CHAPTER XI

THERE WAS NO MONEY. THERE WAS NO ROBBERY

THERE was one point that struck every one in Fetyukovich's speech. He flatly denied the existence of the fatal three thousand roubles, and consequently the possibility of their having been stolen.

"Gentlemen of the jury," he began. "Every new and unprejudiced observer must be struck by a characteristic peculiarity in the present case, namely, the charge of robbery, and the complete impossibility of determining precisely what was stolen. We are told that money was stolen — three thousand roubles — but whether those roubles ever existed, nobody knows. Consider, how did we learn of that sum, and who has seen the notes? The only person who saw them, and stated that they had been put in the envelope with an inscription, was the servant, Smerdyakov. It was he also who had spoken of it to the accused and his brother, Ivan Fyodorovich, before the catastrophe. Madame Svyetlov, too, had been told of it. But not one of these three persons had actually seen the notes, no one but Smerdyakov had seen them.

"Here the question arises, if it's true that they did exist, and that Smerdyakov had seen them, when did he see them for the last time? What if his master had taken the notes from under his bed and put them back in his cashbox without telling him? Note, that according to Smerdyakov's story the notes were kept under the mattress; the accused must have pulled them out, and yet the bed was absolutely unrumpled; that is carefully set down in the record. How could the accused have found the notes without disturbing the bed? How could he have helped soiling with his bloodstained hands the fine and spotless linen with which the bed had purposely been made?

"But I shall be asked: what about the envelope on the floor? Yes, it's worth saying a word or two about that envelope. I was somewhat surprised just now to hear the highly talented prosecutor declare of himself — of himself, observe — that but for that envelope, but for its being left on the floor as a clue, but for the robber's not having taken it with him, no one in the world would have known of the existence of that envelope and the notes in it, and therefore of the accused's having stolen it. And so that torn scrap of paper is, by the prosecutor's own admission, the sole proof on which the charge of robbery rests, 'otherwise no one would have known of the robbery, nor perhaps even of the money.' But is the mere fact that that scrap of paper was lying on the floor a proof that there was money in it, and that that money had been stolen? Yet, it will be objected, Smerdyakov had seen the money in the envelope. But when, when had he seen it for the last time? I ask you that. I talked to Smerdyakov, and he told me that he had seen the notes two days before the catastrophe. Then why may I not suppose, for instance, that old Fyodor Pavlovich, locked up alone in impatient and hysterical expectation of the object of his adoration, may have whiled away the time by breaking open the envelope and taking out the notes. 'What's the use of the envelope,' he may have asked himself, 'she won't believe the notes are there, but when I show her the thirty rainbow-coloured notes in one roll, it will make more impression, you may be sure, it will make her mouth water.' And so he tears open the envelope, takes out the money, and flings the envelope on the floor, conscious of being the owner and untroubled by any fears of leaving evidence.

"Listen, gentlemen, could anything be more likely than such a supposition and such an action? Why is it impossible? But if anything of the sort could have taken place, the charge of robbery falls to the ground; there was no money, and therefore no robbery. If the envelope on the floor may be taken as evidence that there had been money in it, why may I not maintain the opposite, namely, that the envelope was on the floor because the money had previously been taken out of it by its owner?

"But I shall be asked, what became of the money if Fyodor Pavlovich took it out of the envelope, since it was not found when the police searched the house? In the first place, part of the money was found in a drawer, and secondly, he might have taken it out that morning or the evening before to make some other use of it, to give or send it away; he may have changed his idea, his plan of action completely, without thinking it necessary to announce the fact to Smerdyakov beforehand. And if there is the barest possibility of such an explanation, how can the prisoner be so positively accused of having committed murder for the sake of robbery, and of having actually carried out that robbery? This is encroaching on the domain of romance. If it is maintained that something has been stolen, the thing must be produced, or at least its existence must be proved beyond doubt. Yet no one had ever seen these notes.

"Not long ago in Petersburg a young man of eighteen, hardly more than a boy, who carried on a small business as a costermonger, went in broad daylight into a money-changer's shop with an axe, and with extraordinary, typical audacity killed the master of the shop and carried off fifteen hundred roubles. Five hours later he was arrested, and, except for fifteen roubles he had already managed to spend, the whole sum was found on him. Moreover, the shopman, on his return to the shop after the murder, informed the police not only of the exact sum stolen, but even of the notes and gold coins of which that sum was made up, and those very notes and coins were found on the criminal. This was followed by a full and genuine confession on the part of the murderer. That's what I call evidence, gentlemen of the jury! In that case I know, I see, I touch the money, and cannot deny its existence. Is it the same in the present case? And yet it is a question of life and death, of a man's fate.

"Yes, I shall be told, but he was carousing that night, squandering money; he was shown to have had fifteen hundred roubles — where did he get the money? But the very fact that only fifteen hundred could be found, and the other half of the sum could nowhere be discovered, shows that that money was not the same, and had never been in any envelope. By strict calculation of time it was proved at the preliminary inquiry that the accused ran straight from those women servants to Perhotin's without going home, and that he had been nowhere. So he had been all the time in company and therefore could not have divided the three thousand in half and hidden half in the town. It's just this consideration that has led the prosecutor to assume that the money is hidden in some crevice at Mokroye. Why not in the dungeons of the castle of Udolpho, gentlemen? Isn't this supposition really too fantastic and too romantic? And observe, if that supposition breaks down, the whole charge of robbery is scattered to the winds, for in that case what could have become of the other fifteen hundred roubles? By what miracle could they have disappeared, since it's proved that the accused went nowhere? And we are ready to ruin a man's life with such tales!

"I shall be told that he could not explain where he got the fifteen hundred that he had, and every one knew that he was without money before that night. Who knew it, pray? The accused has made a clear and unflinching statement of the source of that money, and if you will have it so, gentlemen of the jury, nothing can be more probable than that statement, and more consistent with the temper and spirit of the accused. The prosecutor is charmed with his own romance. A man of weak will, who had brought himself to take the three thousand so insultingly offered by his betrothed, could not, we are told, have set aside half and sewn it up, but would, even if he had done so, have opened it every two days and taken out a hundred, and so would have spent it all in a month. All this, you will remember, was put forward in a tone that brooked no contradiction. But what if the thing happened quite differently? What if you've been weaving a romance, and about quite a different kind of man? That's just it, you have invented quite a different person!

"I shall be told, perhaps, that there are witnesses that he spent on one day that whole three thousand given him by his betrothed a month before the catastrophe, so he could not have divided the sum in half. But who are these witnesses? The value of their testimony has been shown in court already. Besides, in another man's hand a crust always seems larger, and no one of these witnesses counted that money; they all judged simply at sight. And didn't the witness Maximov testify that the accused had twenty thousand in his hand? You see, gentlemen of the jury, psychology is a two-edged weapon. Let me use the other edge now and see what comes of it.

"A month before the catastrophe the accused was entrusted by Katerina Ivanovna with three thousand roubles to send off by mail. But the question is: is it true that they were entrusted to him in such an insulting and degrading way as was proclaimed just now? The first statement made by the young lady on the subject was different, absolutely different. In the second statement we heard only cries of resentment and revenge, cries of long-concealed hatred. And the very fact that the witness gave her first testimony incorrectly, gives us a right to conclude that her second piece of evidence may have been incorrect also. The prosecutor will not, dare not (his own words) touch on that story. So be it. I will not touch on it either, but will only venture to observe that if a lofty and high-principled person, such as that highly respected young lady unquestionably is, if such a person, I say, allows herself suddenly in court to contradict her first statement, with the obvious motive of ruining the accused, it is clear that this testimony has been given not dispassionately, not coolly. Have not we the right to assume that a revengeful woman might have exaggerated much? Yes, she may well have exaggerated, in particular, the insult and humiliation of her offering him the money. On the contrary, it was offered in such a way that it was possible to take it, especially for a man so easy-going as the accused; above all, as he expected to receive shortly from his father the three thousand roubles that he reckoned was owing to him. It was unreflecting of him, but it was just his irresponsible want of reflection that made him so confident that his father would give him the money, that he would get it, and so could always despatch the money entrusted to him and settle the debt.

"But the prosecutor refuses to allow that he could the same day have set aside half the money and sewn it up in a little bag. That's not his character, he tells us, he couldn't have had such feelings. But yet you cried out yourself that the Karamazov nature was broad; you cried out about the two abysses which a Karamazov can contemplate at once. Karamazov is just such a two-sided nature, fluctuating between two abysses, so that even when moved by the most violent craving for riotous gaiety, he can pull himself up, if something strikes him from another quarter. And in the other quarter is love — that new love which had flamed up in his heart, and for that love he needed money; oh, far more than for carousing with his mistress. If she were to say to him, 'I am yours, I won't have Fyodor Pavlovich,' then he must have money to seize her and carry her off. That was more important than carousing. Could a Karamazov fail to understand it? That anxiety was just what he was suffering from — what is there improbable in his laying aside that money and concealing it in case of emergency?

"But time passes, and Fyodor Pavlovich does not give the accused the expected three thousand; on the contrary, the latter hears that he means to use this sum to seduce the woman he, the accused, loves. 'If Fyodor Pavlovich doesn't hand over the money to me,' he thinks, 'I shall be put in the position of a thief before Katerina Ivanovna.' And then the idea presents itself to him that he will go to Katerina Ivanovna, lay before her the fifteen hundred roubles he still carries round his neck, and say, 'I am a scoundrel, but not a thief.' So here we have already a twofold reason why he should guard that sum of money as the apple of his eye, why he shouldn't open the little bag and spend it a hundred at a time. Why should you deny the accused a sense of honour? Yes, he has a sense of honour, granted that it's misdirected, granted it's often mistaken, yet it exists and amounts to a passion, and he has proved that.

"But now the affair becomes even more complex; his jealous torments reach a climax, and those same two questions torture his fevered brain more and more: 'If I repay Katerina Ivanovna, where can I find the means to carry Grushenka off?' If he behaved wildly, drank, and made disturbances in the taverns in the course of that month, it was perhaps because he was wretched and strained beyond his powers of endurance. These two questions became so acute that they drove him at last to despair. He sent his younger brother to beg for the last time for the three thousand roubles, but, without waiting for a reply, burst in himself and ended by beating up the old man in the presence of witnesses. After that he had no prospect of getting it from any one; his father would not give it him after that beating.

"The same evening he strikes himself on the breast, just on the upper part of the breast where the little bag is, and swears to his brother that he has the means to prevent his being a scoundrel, but that still he will remain a scoundrel, for he foresees that he will not use that means, that he won't have the character, that he won't have the will-power to do it. Why, why does the prosecutor refuse to believe the testimony of Alexey Karamazov, given so genuinely and sincerely, so spontaneously and convincingly? And why, on the contrary, does he force me to believe in money hidden in a crevice, in the dungeons of the castle of Udolpho?

"The same evening, after his talk with his brother, the accused writes that fatal letter, and that letter is the chief, the most stupendous proof of the accused's having committed robbery! 'I will beg from every one, and if I don't get it I will murder my father and will take the envelope with the pink ribbon on it from under his mattress as soon as Ivan has gone.' A full programme of the murder, we are told, so it must have been he. 'It has all been done as he wrote,' cries the prosecutor.

"But in the first place, it's the letter of a drunken man and written in great irritation; secondly, he writes of the envelope what he has heard from Smerdyakov again, for he has not seen the envelope himself; and thirdly, he wrote it indeed, but how can you prove that he did it? Did the accused take the envelope from under the pillow, did he find the money, did that money exist indeed? And was it to get money that the accused ran off, if you remember? He ran off post-haste not to rob, but to find out where she was, the woman who had crushed him. He was not running to carry out a programme, to carry out what he had written, that is, not for an act of premeditated robbery, but he ran suddenly, spontaneously, in a jealous fury. Yes! I shall be told, but when he got there and murdered him he seized the money, too. But did he murder him after all? The charge of robbery I repudiate with indignation. A man cannot be accused of robbery, if it's impossible to state accurately what he has stolen; that's an axiom. But did he murder him without robbery, did he murder him at all? Is that proved? Isn't that, too, a fiction?"

CHAPTER XII

AND THERE WAS NO MURDER EITHER

"Allow me, gentlemen of the jury, to remind you that a man's life is at stake and that you must be more careful. We have heard the prosecutor himself admit that until to-day he hesitated to accuse the prisoner of a full and conscious premeditation of the crime; he hesitated till he saw that fatal drunken letter which was produced in court to-day. 'All was done as written.' But, I repeat again, he was running to her, to seek her, solely to find out where she was. That's a fact that can't be disputed. Had she been at home, he would not have run away, but would have remained at her side, and so would not have done what he promised in the letter. He ran suddenly and accidentally, and by that time very likely he did not even remember his drunken letter. 'He snatched up the pestle,' they say, and you will remember how a whole edifice of psychology was built on that pestle — why he was bound to look at that pestle as a weapon, to snatch it up as a weapon, and so on, and so on. A very commonplace idea occurs to me at this point: What if that pestle had not been in sight, had not been lying on the shelf from which it was snatched by the accused, but had been put away in a cupboard? It would not have caught the prisoner's eye, and he would have run away without a weapon, with empty hands, and then he would certainly not have killed any one. How then can I look upon the pestle as a proof of arming and of premeditation?

"Yes, but he talked in the taverns of murdering his father, and two days before, on the evening when he wrote his drunken letter, he was quiet and only quarrelled with a shopman in the tavern, because a Karamazov could not help quarrelling, forsooth! But my answer to that is, that, if he was planning such a murder in accordance with his letter, he certainly would not have quarrelled even with a shopman, and probably would not have gone into the tavern at all, because a person plotting such a crime seeks quiet and retirement, seeks to efface himself, to avoid being seen and heard, and that not from calculation, but from instinct. Gentlemen of the jury, the psychological method is a two-edged weapon, and we, too, can use it. As for all this shouting in taverns throughout the month, don't we often hear children, or drunkards coming out of taverns shout, 'I'll kill you'? but they don't murder any one. And that fatal letter — isn't that simply drunken irritability, too? Isn't that simply the shout of the brawler outside the tavern, 'I'll kill you! I'll kill the lot of you!' Why not, why could it not be that? What reason have we to call that letter 'fatal' rather than ridiculous? Because his father has been found murdered, because a witness saw the accused running out of the garden with a weapon in his hand, and was knocked down by him: therefore, we are told, everything was done as he had planned in writing, and the letter was not 'ridiculous,' but 'fatal.'

"Now, thank God! we've come to the real point: 'since he was in the garden, he must have murdered him.' In those few words, 'since he *was*, then he *must*,' lies the whole case for the prosecution. He was there, so he must have. And what if there is no *must* about it, even if he was there? Oh, I admit that the chain of evidence — the coincidences — are really quite eloquent. But examine all these facts separately, regardless of the way they hang together. Why, for instance, does the prosecution refuse to admit the truth of the prisoner's statement that he ran away from his father's window? Remember the sarcasms in which the prosecutor indulged at the expense of the respectful and 'pious' sentiments which suddenly came over the murderer. But what if there was something of the sort, a feeling of religious awe, if not of filial respect? 'My mother must have been praying for me at that moment,' were the accused's words at the preliminary inquiry, and so he ran away as soon as he convinced himself that Madame Svyetlov was not in his father's house. 'But he could not convince himself by looking through the window,' the prosecutor objects. But why couldn't he? Why? The window opened at the signals given by the accused. Some word might have been uttered by Fyodor Pavlovich, some exclamation which showed the accused that she was not there. Why should we assume everything as we imagine it, as we make up our minds to imagine it? A thousand things may happen in reality which elude the imagination of the subtlest romancer.

" 'Yes, but Grigory saw the door open and so the prisoner certainly was in the house, therefore he killed him.' Now about that door, gentlemen of the jury. . . . Observe that we have only the statement of one witness as to that door, and he was at the time in such a condition, that . . . But supposing the door was open; supposing the accused has lied in denying it, from an instinct of self-defence, natural in his position; supposing he did go into the house — well, what then? How does it follow that because he was there he committed the murder? He might have dashed in, run through the rooms; might have pushed his father away; might have struck him; but as soon as he had made sure Madame Svyetlov was not there, he may have run away rejoicing that she was not there and that he had not killed his father. And it was perhaps just because he had escaped from the temptation to kill his father, because he had a clear conscience and was rejoicing at not having killed him, that he was capable of a pure feeling, the feeling of pity and compassion, and leapt off the fence a minute later to the assistance of Grigory after he had, in his excitement, knocked him down.

"With terrible eloquence the prosecutor has described to us the dreadful state of the prisoner's mind at Mokroye when love again lay before him calling him to new life, while love was impossible for him because he had his father's blood-stained corpse behind him and beyond that corpse — retribution. And yet the prosecutor nevertheless did allow him love, which he explained in his own way: 'a drunken condition, a criminal taken to the gallows, the end still far off,' and so on and so on. But again I ask, Mr. Prosecutor, have you not invented a new personality? Is the accused so coarse and heartless as to be able to think at that moment of love and of dodges to escape punishment, if his father's blood was really upon him? No, no, and no! As soon as it was made plain to him that she loved him and called him to her side, promising him new happiness, oh! then, I protest he must have felt the impulse to suicide doubled, trebled, and would have killed himself without fail, if he had his father's murder on his conscience. Oh, no! he would not have forgotten where his pistols lay! I know the accused: the savage, stony heartlessness ascribed to him by the prosecutor is inconsistent with his character. He would have killed himself, that's certain. He did not kill himself just because 'his mother's prayers had saved him,' and he was innocent of his father's blood. He was troubled, he was grieving that night at Mokroye only about old Grigory and praying to God that the old man would recover, that his blow had not been fatal, and that he would not have to suffer for it. Why not accept such an interpretation of the facts? What trustworthy proof have we that the accused is lying?

"But we shall be told at once again, 'There is his father's corpse! If he ran away without murdering him, who did murder him?' Here, I repeat, you have the whole logic of the prosecution. Who murdered him, if not he? There's no one to put in his place.

"Gentlemen of the jury, is that really so? Is it positively, actually true that there is no one else at all? We've heard the prosecutor count on his fingers all the persons who were in that house that night. They were five in number; three of them, I agree, could not have been responsible — the murdered man himself, old Grigory, and his wife. There are left then the accused and Smerdyakov, and the prosecutor dramatically exclaims that the accused pointed to Smerdyakov because he had no one else to fix on, that had there been a sixth person, even a phantom of a sixth person, he would have abandoned the charge against Smerdyakov at once in shame and have accused that other. But, gentlemen of the jury, why may I not draw the very opposite conclusion? There are two persons — the accused and Smerdyakov. Why can I not say that you accuse my client simply because you have no one else to accuse? And you have no one else only because you have determined to exclude Smerdyakov from all suspicion.

"It's true, indeed, Smerdyakov is accused only by the prisoner, his two brothers, and Madame Svyetlov. But there are others who point to him: there are vague rumours of a question, of a suspicion, an obscure report, a feeling of expectation. Finally, we have the evidence of a combination of facts very suggestive, though, I admit, inconclusive. In the first place, we have precisely on the day of the catastrophe that fit, the genuineness of which the prosecutor, for some reason, has felt obliged so carefully to uphold and defend. Then Smerdyakov's sudden suicide on the eve of the trial. Then the equally startling evidence given in court to-day by the elder of the accused's brothers, who until now had believed in his guilt, but who has to-day produced the money and proclaimed Smerdyakov as the murderer. Oh, I fully share the court's and the prosecutor's conviction that Ivan Karamazov is suffering from brain fever, that his statement may really be a desperate effort, planned in delirium, to save his brother by throwing the guilt on the dead man. But again Smerdyakov's name is pronounced, again there is a suggestion of mystery. There is something half-expressed here, as it were, something incomplete, gentlemen of the jury. And perhaps it may one day be stated in full. But we won't go into that now. Of that later.

"The court has resolved to go on with the trial, but, meantime, I might make a few remarks about the character sketch of Smerdyakov drawn with such subtlety and talent by the prosecutor. But while I admire his talent I cannot agree with the substance of his characterisation. I have visited Smerdyakov, I have seen him and talked to him, and he made a very different impression on me. He was weak in health, it is true; but in character, in spirit, oh, no, he was by no means the weak man the prosecutor has made him out to be. Especially, I found in him no trace of the timidity on which the prosecutor so insisted. There was no simplicity about him, either. I found in him, on the contrary, an extreme mistrustfulness concealed under a mask of naïveté, and an intelligence of considerable range. The prosecutor was too simple in taking him for weak-minded. He made a very definite impression on me: I left him with the conviction that he was a distinctly spiteful creature, excessively ambitious, vindictive, and intensely envious. I made some inquiries: he hated his origin, was ashamed of it, and would clench his teeth when he remembered that he was the son of 'Stinking Lizaveta.' He was disrespectful to the servant Grigory and his wife, who had cared for him in his childhood. He cursed and jeered at Russia. He dreamed of going to France and becoming a Frenchman. He used often to say that he hadn't the means to do so. I fancy he loved no one but himself and had a strangely high opinion of himself. His conception of culture was limited to good clothes, clean shirt fronts, and polished boots. Believing himself to be the illegitimate son of Fyodor Pavlovich (there is evidence of this), he might well have resented his position, compared with that of his master's legitimate sons. They had everything, he nothing. They had all the rights, they had the inheritance, while he was only the cook. He told me himself that he had helped Fyodor Pavlovich to put the money in the envelope. The destination of that sum — a sum which would have made his career — was, of course, hateful to him. Moreover, he saw three thousand roubles in new rainbow-coloured notes. (I asked him about that on purpose.) Oh, beware of showing an ambitious and envious man a large sum of money at once! And it was the first time he had seen so much money all at once. The sight of the rainbow-coloured notes may have made a morbid impression on his imagination, but with no immediate results.

"The talented prosecutor, with extraordinary subtlety, sketched for us all the arguments for and against the hypothesis of Smerdyakov's guilt, and asked us in particular what motive he had in feigning a fit. But he may not have been feigning at all, the fit may have happened quite naturally, but it may have passed off quite naturally, and the sick man may have recovered, not completely perhaps, but still regaining consciousness, as happens with epileptics.

"The prosecutor asks at what moment Smerdyakov could have committed the murder. But it is very easy to point out that moment. He might have waked up from deep sleep (for he was only asleep — an epileptic fit is always followed by a deep sleep) at that moment when the old man, Grigory, having grabbed the leg of the accused, who was then astride the fence, shouted at the top of his voice, 'Parricide!' That strange shout resounding in the stillness of the night may have waked Smerdyakov, whose sleep was perhaps less sound at the moment: he might naturally have begun to come out of his stupor an hour before.

"Getting out of bed, he goes almost unconsciously and with no definite motive towards the sound to see what's the matter. His head is still clouded by his attack, his mind is half asleep; but, once in the garden, he walks to the lighted windows and he hears the terrible news from his master, who would, of course, be glad to see him. His head clears up at once. He learns all the details from his frightened master, and gradually in his sick and disordered brain an idea shapes itself — terrible, but seductive and irresistibly logical: to kill the old man, take the three thousand, and throw all the blame on his young master. Who will be suspected if not the young master? Who will be accused if not the young master?

There is all this evidence; he was here. A terrible lust for money, for booty, might seize upon him together with the thought that he could act with impunity. Oh! these sudden and irresistible impulses come so often when there is a favourable opportunity, and especially with murderers who a moment earlier have had no idea of committing a murder. And Smerdyakov may have gone in and carried out his plan. With what weapon? Why, with any stone picked up in the garden. But what for, with what object? Why, the three thousand which means a career for him. Oh, I am not contradicting myself — the money may have existed. And perhaps Smerdyakov alone knew where to find it, where his master kept it. And the wrapper — the torn envelope on the floor? Just now, when the prosecutor was explaining his subtle theory that only an inexperienced thief like Karamazov would have left the envelope on the floor, and not one like Smerdyakov, who would have avoided leaving a piece of evidence against himself, I thought as I listened that I was hearing something very familiar, and, would you believe it, I have heard that very argument, that very conjecture, of how Karamazov would have behaved, precisely two days before, from Smerdyakov himself. What's more, it struck me at the time. I fancied that there was an artificial simplicity about him; that he was in a hurry to suggest this idea to me that I might fancy it was my own. He prompted me, as it were. Did he not insinuate the same idea at the inquiry and suggest it to the talented prosecutor?

"I shall be asked, 'What about the old woman, Grigory's wife? She heard the sick man moaning close by, all night.' Yes, she heard it, but that evidence is extremely unreliable. I knew a lady who complained bitterly that she had been kept awake all night by a dog in the yard. Yet the poor beast, it appeared, had yelped only once or twice in the night. And that's natural. A person is asleep and hears a groan — he wakes up, annoyed at being waked, but instantly falls asleep again. Two hours later, again a groan, he wakes up and falls asleep again; and the same thing again two hours later — three times altogether during the night. Next morning the sleeper wakes up and complains that some one has been groaning and keeping him awake all night. And it is bound to seem so to him: the intervals of two hours of sleep he does not remember, he remembers only the moments of waking, so he feels he has been kept awake all night.

"But why, why, asks the prosecutor, did not Smerdyakov confess in his last letter? Why did his conscience prompt him to one step and not to the other? But, allow me, conscience implies penitence, and the suicide may not have felt penitence, but only despair. Despair and penitence are two very different things. Despair may be vindictive and irreconcilable, and the suicide, laying hands on himself, may well have felt redoubled hatred for those whom he had envied all his life.

"Gentlemen of the jury, beware of a miscarriage of justice! What is there unlikely in all I have put before you just now? Find the error in my reasoning; find the impossibility, the absurdity. And if there is but a shade of possibility, but a shade of probability in my propositions, do not condemn him. And is there only a shade? I swear by all that is sacred, I fully believe in the explanation of the murder I have just put forward. What troubles me and makes me indignant is that of all the mass of facts heaped up by the prosecution against the accused, there is not a single one certain and irrefutable. And yet the unhappy man is to be ruined by the accumulation of these facts. Yes, the accumulated effect is awful: the blood, the blood dripping from his fingers, the bloodstained shirt, the dark night resounding with the shout 'Parricide!' and the old man falling with a broken head. And then this mass of utterances, statements, gestures, shouts! Oh! this has so much influence, it can so bias the mind; but, gentlemen of the jury, can it bias your minds? Remember, you have been given absolute power to bind and to loose, but the greater the power, the more terrible its responsibility.

"I do not draw back one iota from what I have said just now, but suppose for one moment I agreed with the prosecution that my luckless client had stained his hands with his father's blood. This is only a conjecture, I repeat; I never for one instant doubt his innocence. But, let me assume that my client is guilty of parricide. Even so, hear what I have to say. I have it in my heart to say something more to you, for I feel that there must be a great conflict in your hearts and minds. . . . Forgive my referring to your hearts and minds, gentlemen of the jury, but I want to be truthful and sincere to the end. Let us all be sincere!"

At this point the speech was interrupted by rather loud applause. The last words, indeed, were pronounced with a note of such sincerity that every one felt that he really might have something to say. But the presiding judge, hearing the applause, threatened to clear the court if such an incident were repeated. Every sound was hushed and Fetyukovich began in a voice full of feeling quite unlike the tone he had used hitherto.

CHAPTER XIII

A CORRUPTER OF THOUGHT

"It's not only the accumulation of facts that threatens my client with ruin, gentlemen of the jury," he began, "what threatens my client with ruin is really one fact — the dead body of his old father. Had it been an ordinary case of murder you would have rejected the charge in view of the triviality, the incompleteness, and the fantastic character of the evidence, if you examine each part of it separately; or, at least, you would have hesitated to ruin a man's life simply from the prejudice against him which he has, alas! only too well deserved. But it's not an ordinary case of murder, it's a case of parricide. That impresses men's minds, and to such a degree that the very triviality and incompleteness of the evidence becomes less trivial and less incomplete even to an unprejudiced mind. How can such a prisoner be acquitted? What if he committed the murder and gets off unpunished? That is what every one, almost involuntarily, instinctively, feels at heart.

"Yes, it's a fearful thing to shed a father's blood — the father who has begotten me, loved me, not spared his life for me, grieved over my illnesses from childhood up, suffered all his life for my happiness, and has lived in my joys, in my successes. To murder such a father — that's inconceivable. Gentlemen of the jury, what is a father — a real father? What is the meaning of that great word? What is the great idea in that name? We have just indicated in part what a true father is and what he ought to be. In the case with which we are now so deeply occupied and over which our hearts are aching — in the present case, the father, the late Fyodor Pavlovich

Karamazov, did not correspond to that conception of a father to which we have just referred. That's the misfortune. And indeed some fathers are a misfortune. Let us examine this misfortune rather more closely: we must shrink from nothing, gentlemen of the jury, considering the importance of the decision you have to make. It's our particular duty not to shrink from any idea, like children or frightened women, as the talented prosecutor happily expresses it.

"But in the course of his heated speech my esteemed opponent (and he was my opponent before I opened my lips) exclaimed several times, 'Oh, I will not yield the defence of the accused to the lawyer who has come down from Petersburg. I accuse, but I defend also!' He exclaimed that several times, but forgot to mention that if this terrible accused was for twenty-three years so grateful for a mere pound of nuts given him by the only man who had been kind to him, as a child in his father's house, might not such a man well have remembered for twenty-three years how he ran in his father's back yard, 'without boots to his feet and with his little trousers hanging by one button' — to use the expression of the kind-hearted doctor, Herzenstube?

"Oh, gentlemen of the jury, why need we look more closely at this misfortune, why repeat what we all know already? What did my client meet with when he arrived here, at his father's house, and why depict my client as a heartless egoist and monster? He is uncontrolled, he is wild and unruly — we are trying him now for that — but who is responsible for his fate? Whose guilt is it that in spite of his excellent disposition and his grateful and sensitive heart he received such an absurd upbringing? Did any one instruct him in the way he should go? Was he schooled in the sciences? Did any one love him ever so little in his childhood? My client was left to the care of Providence like a beast of the field. He thirsted perhaps to see his father after long years of separation. A thousand times perhaps he may, recalling his childhood, have driven away the loathsome phantoms that haunted his childish dreams and with all his heart he may have longed to embrace and to forgive his father! And what awaited him? He was met by cynical taunts, suspicions, and wrangling about money. He heard nothing but revolting talk and vicious precepts uttered daily over the cognac, and at last he saw his father trying to take his mistress away from him with his own money. Oh, gentlemen of the jury, that was cruel and revolting! And that old man was always complaining of the disrespect and cruelty of his son. He slandered him in society, injured him, calumniated him, bought up his unpaid debts to get him thrown into prison.

"Gentlemen of the jury, people like my client, who are fierce, unruly, and uncontrolled on the surface, are sometimes, most frequently indeed, exceedingly tender-hearted, only they don't show it. Don't laugh, don't laugh at my idea! The talented prosecutor laughed mercilessly just now at my client for loving Schiller — loving the beautiful and the sublime! I should not have laughed at that if I were he. Yes, such natures — oh, let me speak in defence of such natures, so often and so unjustly misunderstood — these natures often thirst for tenderness, goodness, and justice, in contrast to themselves, as it were, their unruliness, their ferocity — they thirst for it unconsciously, truly thirst. Passionate and cruel on the surface, they are painfully capable of falling in love with a woman, for instance, and loving her with a spiritual and elevated love. Again do not laugh at me, this is very often the case with such natures. But they cannot hide their passions — sometimes very coarse — and that is conspicuous and is noticed, but the inner man is unseen. All their passions are quickly satisfied; but, by the side of a noble and lofty creature that seemingly coarse and rough man seeks a new life, seeks the possibility of reforming himself, of becoming better, of becoming noble and honourable, 'sublime and beautiful,' however much the expression has been ridiculed.

"I said just now that I would not venture to touch upon my client's affair with Madame Verhovtzev. But I may say half a word. What we heard just now was not evidence, but only the outcry of a frenzied and revengeful woman, and it was not for her — oh, not for her! — to reproach him with treachery, for she has betrayed him herself! If she had had but a little time for reflection she would not have given such evidence. Oh, do not believe her! No, my client is not a monster, as she called him!

"The Lover of Mankind on the eve of His Crucifixion said: 'I am the Good Shepherd. The good shepherd lays down his life for his sheep, so that not one of them might perish.' Let not a man's soul perish through us!

"I asked just now what does 'father' mean, and exclaimed that it is a great word, a precious name. But one must use words honestly, gentlemen, and I venture to call things by their right names: such a father as old Karamazov cannot be called a father and does not deserve to be. Filial love for an unworthy father is an absurdity, an impossibility. Love cannot be created out of nothing: for only God can create something out of nothing.

" 'Fathers, provoke not your children to wrath,' the apostle writes, from a heart glowing with love. It's not for the sake of my client that I quote these sacred words, I mention them for the sake of all fathers. Who has authorised me to preach to fathers? No one. But as a man and a citizen I appeal — *vivos voco!* We are not long on earth, we do many evil deeds and say many evil words. So let us all catch a favourable moment when we are all together to say a good word to each other. That's what I am doing: while I am in this place I take advantage of my opportunity. Not for nothing is this tribune given us by the highest authority — all Russia hears us! I am not speaking only for the fathers here present, I cry aloud to all fathers: 'Fathers, provoke not your children to wrath.' Yes, let us first fulfil Christ's injunction ourselves and only then venture to expect it of our children. Otherwise we are not fathers, but enemies of our children, and they are not our children, but our enemies, and we have made them our enemies ourselves. 'What measure ye mete it shall be measured unto you again' — it's not I who say that, it's the Gospel precept, measure to others according as they measure to you. How can we blame children if they measure to us according to our measure?

"Not long ago a servant girl in Finland was suspected of having secretly given birth to a child. She was watched, and a chest of which no one knew anything was found in the corner of the loft, behind some bricks. It was opened and inside was found the body of a new-born child which she had killed. In the same chest were found the skeletons of two other babies which, according to her own confession, she had killed at the moment of their birth.

"Gentlemen of the jury, was she a mother to her children? She gave birth to them, indeed; but was she a mother to them? Would any one venture to give her the sacred name of mother? Let us be bold, gentlemen of the jury, let us be audacious even: it's our duty to be so at this moment and not to be afraid of certain words and ideas like the merchants' wives of Moscow in Ostrovsky's play, who are scared by the sound of certain words. No, let us prove that the progress of the last few years has touched us, too, and let us say plainly, the father is not merely he who begets the child, but he who begets it and does his duty by it.

"Oh, of course, there is the other meaning, there is the other interpretation of the word 'father,' which demands that my father, even though he be a monster, even though he be the enemy of his children, still remains my father simply because he begot me. But this is, so to say, the mystical meaning which I cannot comprehend with my mind, but can only accept by faith, or, better to say, *on faith*, like many other things which I do not understand, but which religion bids me believe. But in that case let it be kept outside the sphere of actual life. In the sphere of actual life, which has, indeed, its own rights, but also lays upon us great obligations, in that sphere, if we want to be humane — Christian, in fact — we must, or ought to, act only upon convictions justified by reason and experience, which have been passed through the crucible of analysis; in a word, we must act rationally, and not senselessly as though in a dream or in delirium, that we may not do harm, that we may not torment and ruin a man. Then it will be real Christian work, not only mystic, but rational and truly a work of loving-kindness. . . ."

At this juncture there was violent applause from many parts of the court, but Fetyukovich waved his hands as though imploring them to let him finish without interruption. The court relapsed into silence. The orator went on.

"Do you suppose, gentlemen of the jury, that our children as they grow up and begin to reason can avoid such questions? No, they cannot, and we will not impose on them an impossible restriction. The sight of an unworthy father involuntarily suggests tormenting questions to a youth, especially when he compares him with the excellent fathers of his companions. The conventional answer to this question is: 'He begot you, and you are his flesh and blood, and therefore you are bound to love him.' The youth involuntarily reflects: 'But did he love me when he begot me?' he asks, wondering more and more. 'Was it for my sake he begot me? He did not know me, not even my sex, at that moment, at the moment of passion, perhaps inflamed by wine, and he has only transmitted to me a propensity to drunkenness — that's the sum of his benefactions to me. . . . Why am I bound to love him, simply for begetting me when he has cared nothing for me all my life after?'

"Oh, perhaps these questions strike you as coarse and cruel, but do not expect an impossible restraint from a young mind. 'Drive nature out of the door and it will fly in at the window,' and, above all, let us not be afraid of words, but decide the question according to the dictates of reason and humanity and not of mystic ideas. How shall it be decided? Why, like this. Let the son stand before his father and ask him, 'Father, tell me, why must I love you? Father, show me that I must love you,' and if that father is able to answer him and show him good reason, we have a real, normal family, resting not on mystical prejudice, but on rational, responsible, and strictly humane foundations. But if he does not, there's an end to the family tie. He is not a father to him, and the son has a right to look upon him as a stranger, and even an enemy. Our tribune, gentlemen of the jury, ought to be a school of true and sane ideas."

Here the orator was interrupted by irrepressible and almost frantic applause. Of course, it was not the whole audience, but a good half of it applauded. Fathers applauded, and mothers. Shrieks and exclamations were heard from the gallery, where the ladies were sitting. Handkerchiefs were waved. The presiding judge began ringing his bell with all his might. He was obviously irritated by the behaviour of the audience, but did not venture to clear the court as he had threatened before. Even persons of high position, old men with stars on their frock-coats, sitting on specially reserved seats behind the judges, applauded the orator and waved their handkerchiefs. So that when the noise died down, the presiding judge confined himself to repeating his stern threat to clear the court, and Fetyukovich, excited and triumphant, continued his speech.

"Gentlemen of the jury, you remember that awful night of which so much has been said to-day, when the son jumped over the fence, entered his father's house, and stood face to face with the enemy and persecutor who had begotten him. I insist most emphatically it was not for money he ran to his father's house: the charge of robbery is an absurdity, as I proved before. And it was not to murder him he broke into the house, oh, no! If he had had that design he would, at least, have taken the precaution of arming himself beforehand. The brass pestle he caught up instinctively without knowing why he did it. Granted that he deceived his father by tapping at the window, granted that he made his way in — I've said already that I do not for a moment believe that legend, but let it be so, let us suppose it for a moment. Gentlemen, I swear to you by all that's holy, if it had not been his father, but an ordinary enemy, he would, after running through the rooms and satisfying himself that the woman was not there, have made off, post-haste, without doing any harm to his rival. He would have struck him, pushed him away perhaps, nothing more, for he had no thought and no time to spare for that. What he wanted to know was where she was. But his father, his father! The mere sight of the father who had hated him from his childhood, who had been his enemy, his persecutor, and now his unnatural rival, was enough! A feeling of hatred came over him involuntarily, irresistibly, clouding his reason. It all surged up in one moment! It was an impulse of madness and insanity, but also an impulse of nature, irresistibly and unconsciously (like everything in nature) avenging the violation of eternal laws.

"But the accused even then did not murder him — I maintain that, I cry it aloud! — no, he only brandished the pestle in a burst of indignant disgust, not meaning to kill him, not knowing that he would kill him. Had he not had this fatal pestle in his hand, he would have only knocked his father down perhaps, but would not have killed him. As he ran away, he did not know whether he had killed the old man. Such a murder is not a murder. Such a murder is not a parricide. No, the murder of such a father cannot be called parricide. Such a murder can be reckoned parricide only out of prejudice.

"But I appeal to you again and again from the depths of my soul: did this murder actually take place? Gentlemen of the jury, if we convict and punish him, he will say to himself: 'These people have done nothing for my bringing up, for my education, nothing to improve my lot, nothing to make me better, nothing to make me a man. These people have not given me to eat and to drink, have not visited me in prison and nakedness, and here they have sentenced me to penal servitude. I am quits, I owe them nothing now, and owe no one anything for ever. They are vicious and I will be vicious. They are cruel and I will be cruel.' That is what he will say, gentlemen of the jury. And I swear, by finding him guilty you will only make it easier for him: you will ease his conscience, he will curse the blood he has shed and will not regret it. At the same time you will destroy in him the possibility of becoming a new man, for he will remain in his wickedness and blindness all his life.

"But do you want to punish him fearfully, terribly, with the most awful punishment that could be imagined, and at the same time to save him and regenerate his soul? If so, overwhelm him with your mercy! You will see, you will hear how he will tremble and be horror-struck: 'How can I endure this mercy? How can I endure so much love? Am I worthy of it?' That's what he will exclaim.

"Oh, I know, I know that heart, that wild but noble heart, gentlemen of the jury! It will bow before your mercy; it thirsts for a great act of love, it will flame up and be for ever resurrected. There are souls which, in their limitation, blame the whole world. But subdue such a soul with mercy, show it love, and it will curse its deed, for there are many good impulses in it. Such a heart will expand and see that God is merciful and that men are good and just. He will be horror-stricken; he will be crushed by remorse and the vast obligation laid upon him henceforth. And he will not say then, 'I am quits,' but will say, 'I am guilty in the sight of all men and am more unworthy than all.' With tears of penitence and burning, anguished emotion, he will exclaim: 'People are better than I, they wanted to save me, not to ruin me!' Oh, this act of mercy is so easy for you, for in the absence of anything like real evidence it will be too awful for you to pronounce: 'Yes, he is guilty.'

"Better acquit ten guilty men than punish one innocent man!* Do you hear, do you hear that majestic voice from the past century of our glorious history? It is not for an insignificant person like me to remind you that Russian justice does not exist for the punishment only, but also for the salvation of the criminal!

"Let other nations cling to punishment and the letter of the law, we will cling to the spirit and the meaning — the salvation and the reformation of the lost. If this is true, if Russia and her justice are such, then forward, Russia! And do not scare us, oh, do not scare us with your frenzied troikas from which all the nations stand aside in disgust. Not a runaway troika, but the stately chariot of Russia will move calmly and majestically to its goal. In your hands is the fate of my client, in your hands is the fate of Russian justice. You will defend it, you will save it, you will prove that there are men to watch over it, that it is in good hands!"

* An aphorism attributed to Peter the Great. *Editor's note.*

CHAPTER XIV

THE PEASANTS STAND THEIR GROUND

THIS was how Fetyukovich concluded his speech, and the enthusiasm of the audience burst like an irresistible storm. It was out of the question to stop it: the women wept, many of the men wept, too, even two important personages shed tears. The presiding judge submitted, and even postponed ringing his bell. "To suppress such an enthusiasm would have been an attempt on something sacred," the ladies cried afterwards. The orator himself was genuinely touched.

And it was at this moment that Ippolit Kirillovich got up to make objections. People looked at him with hatred. "What? What's the meaning of it? He positively dares to make objections," the ladies babbled. But if the whole world of ladies, including his wife, had protested, he could not have been stopped at that moment. He was pale, he was shaking with emotion, his first phrases were even unintelligible, he gasped for breath, could hardly speak clearly, lost the thread. But he soon recovered himself. But of this new speech of his I shall quote only a few phrases.

". . . We are reproached with having woven romances. But what has the counsel for the defence done, if not pile one romance on top of another? All that was lacking was verse. Fyodor Pavlovich, while waiting for his mistress, tears open the envelope and throws it on the floor. We are even told what he said while engaged on this amazing occasion. Is not this a poetic fantasy? And what proof have we that he had taken out the money? Who heard what he said? The weak-minded idiot, Smerdyakov, transformed into a Byronic hero, revenging himself on society for his illegitimate birth — isn't this a poem in the Byronic manner? And the son who breaks into his father's house and murders him without murdering him is not even a romance, not a poem — it is a sphinx setting us a riddle which he cannot solve himself. If he killed, then he killed, and what's the meaning of his killing without having killed — who can make head or tail of this?

"Then we are informed that our tribune is a tribune of true and sane ideas and from this tribune of 'sane ideas' is heard a solemn declaration that to call the murder of a father 'parricide' is nothing but a prejudice! But if parricide is a prejudice, and if every child is to ask his father: 'Father, why should I love you?' what will become of us? What will become of the foundations of society? What will become of the family? Parricide, it appears, is only a bogey with which to scare a Moscow merchant's wife. The most precious, the most sacred foundations of the destiny and future of Russian justice are presented to us in a perverted and frivolous form, simply to attain an object — to obtain the justification of something which cannot be justified. 'Oh, crush him by mercy,' cries the counsel for the defence; but that's all the criminal wants, and to-morrow it will be seen how much he is crushed. And is not the counsel for the defence too modest in asking for only the acquittal of the prisoner? Why not demand the establishment of a Fund in honour of the parricide to immortalise his exploit both for the younger generation and for posterity? Religion and the Gospel are corrected — that's all mysticism, we are told, and ours is the only true Christianity which has been subjected to the analysis of reason and sane ideas. And so a false image of Christ is set up before us!

'What measure ye mete so it shall be meted unto you again,' cries the counsel for the defence, and instantly deduces that Christ teaches us to measure as it is measured to us — and this from the tribune of truth and sane ideas! We peep into the Gospel only on the eve of making speeches, in order to dazzle the audience by our acquaintance with what is, anyway, a rather original composition, which may be of use to produce a certain effect — should the need arise! But what Christ commands us is something very different: He bids us beware of doing this, because the wicked world does this, but we ought to forgive and to turn the other cheek, and not to measure to those who trespass against us as they measure to us. This is what our God has taught us and not that to forbid children to murder their fathers is a prejudice. And we will not from the tribune of truth and sane ideas correct the Gospel of our Lord, Whom the counsel for the defence deigns to call only 'the crucified lover of humanity,' in opposition to all orthodox Russia, which cries to Him, 'For Thou art our God!' "

At this point the presiding judge intervened and checked the over-zealous speaker, begging him not to exaggerate, not to overstep the bounds, and so on, as presiding judges always do in such cases. The audience, too, was uneasy. The public was restless: there were even exclamations of indignation. Fetyukovich did not so much as make a formal rebuttal; he only mounted the tribune to lay his hand on his heart and, in an offended voice, utter a few words full of dignity. He only touched again, lightly and ironically, on "romancing" and "psychology," and in an appropriate place quoted, "Jupiter, you are angry, therefore you are wrong," which provoked a burst of approving laughter in the audience, for Ippolit Kirillovich by no means resembled Jupiter. Then, apropos of the accusation that he allowed the young generation to murder their fathers, Fetyukovich observed, with great dignity, that he would not even answer. As for the "false image of Christ" and the prosecutor's charge that he did not deign to call Christ God, but called Him "the crucified lover of humanity," which is "contrary to orthodoxy and could not be uttered from the tribune of truth and sane ideas," Fetyukovich hinted that it was a personal insinuation and that he had expected in this court to be secure from accusations "damaging to my reputation as a citizen and a loyal subject." . . . But at these words the presiding judge pulled him up, too, and Fetyukovich concluded his remarks with a bow, amid a hum of universal approbation in the court. And Ippolit Kirillovich was, in the opinion of our ladies, "crushed for good."

Then the accused was allowed to speak. Mitya stood up, but said very little. He was fearfully exhausted, physically and spiritually. The look of strength and independence with which he had entered in the morning had almost disappeared. It seemed as though he had passed through an experience that day which had taught him for the rest of his life something very important he had not understood till then. His voice had grown weak, he did not shout as before. In his words there was a new note of humility, defeat, and submission.

"What am I to say, gentlemen of the jury? The hour of judgment has come for me, I feel the hand of God upon me! The end has come for a profligate! But, before God, I repeat to you, 'No, I am not guilty of my father's blood!' For the last time I repeat, it wasn't I

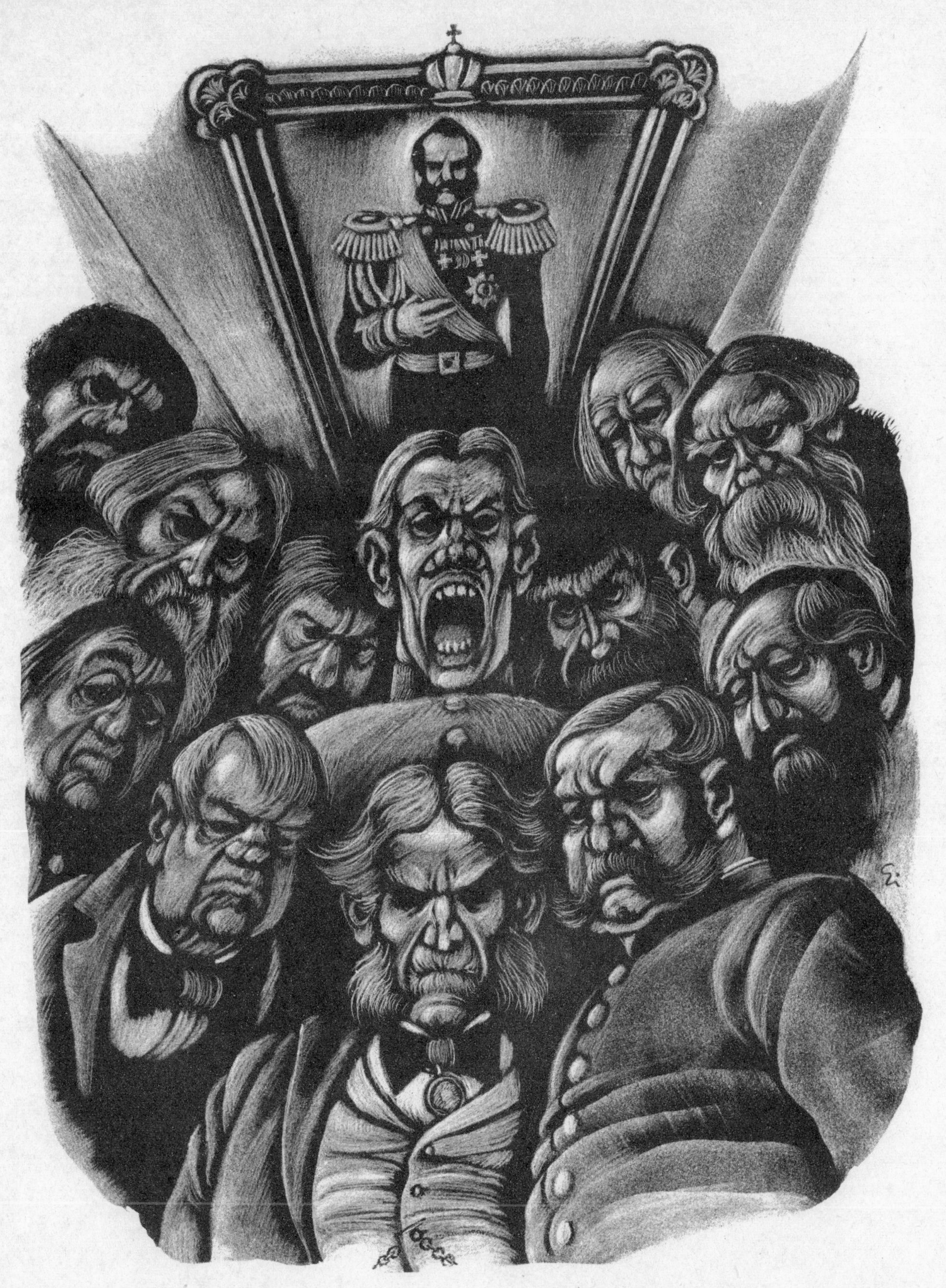

"GENTLEMEN OF THE JURY"

who killed him! I was a waster, but I loved goodness. Every instant I strove to reform, but I lived like a wild beast. I thank the prosecutor, he told me many things about myself that I did not know; but it's not true that I killed my father, the prosecutor is mistaken. I thank my counsel, too. I cried listening to him; but it's not true that I killed my father, and he needn't have supposed it. And don't believe the doctors. I am perfectly sane, only my heart is heavy. If you spare me, if you let me go, I will pray for you. I will be a better man. I give you my word, before God I will! And if you condemn me, I'll break my sword over my head myself and kiss the pieces. But spare me, do not deprive me of my God! I know myself, I shall cry out in rebellion! My heart is heavy, gentlemen . . . spare me!"

He almost fell back in his place: his voice broke: he could hardly articulate the last phrase. Then the judges proceeded to put the questions and began to ask both sides to formulate their conclusions. But I shall not describe the details. At last the jury rose to retire for consultation. The presiding judge was very tired, and so his last charge to the jury was rather feeble. "Be impartial, don't be influenced by the eloquence of the defence, but yet weigh the arguments. Remember that there is a great responsibility laid upon you," and so on and so on.

The jury withdrew and the court adjourned. People could get up, move about, exchange their accumulated impressions, refresh themselves at the buffet. It was very late, almost an hour past midnight, but nobody went away: all were so excited that they could not think of rest. All waited with sinking hearts; though that is, perhaps, too much to say, for the ladies were only in a state of hysterical impatience and their hearts were untroubled. An acquittal, they thought, was inevitable. They all prepared themselves for a dramatic moment of general enthusiasm. I must own there were many among the men, too, who were convinced that an acquittal was inevitable. Some were pleased, others frowned, while some were simply dejected, not wanting him to be acquitted. Fetyukovich himself was confident of his success. He was surrounded by people congratulating him and fawning upon him.

"There are," he said to one group, as I was told afterwards, "there are invisible threads binding the counsel for the defence to the jury. While one is speaking one has a presentiment as to whether or not they are being woven. I was aware of them. They exist. Our cause is won. Set your mind at rest."

"Well, I wonder what our peasants will say now?" said one stout, cross-looking, pockmarked gentlemen, a landowner of the neighbourhood, approaching a group of gentlemen engaged in conversation.

"But they are not all peasants. There are four government clerks among them."

"Yes, there are clerks," said a member of the district council, joining the group.

"And do you know that Nazaryev, the merchant with the medal, a juryman?"

"What of him?"

"He is a man with brains."

"But he never speaks."

"He is no great talker, but so much the better. There's no need for the Petersburg man to teach him: he could teach all Petersburg himself. He's the father of twelve children. Think of that!"

"Upon my word, you don't suppose they won't acquit him?" one of our young officials exclaimed in another group.

"They'll acquit him for certain," said a resolute voice.

"It would be shameful, disgraceful, not to acquit him!" cried the official. "Suppose he did murder him — there are fathers and fathers! And, besides, he was in such a frenzy. . . . He really may have done nothing but swing the pestle in the air, and so knocked the old man down. But it was a pity they dragged the valet in. That was simply a ridiculous episode! If I'd been in Fetyukovich's place, I should simply have said straight out: 'He murdered him; but he is not guilty, hang it all!' "

"That's what he did, only without saying, 'Hang it all!' "

"No, Mihail Semyonovich, he almost said that, too," put in a third voice.

"Why, gentlemen, last year during Lent an actress was acquitted in our town who had cut the throat of her lover's lawful wife."

"Oh, but she did not finish cutting it."

"That makes no difference. She began cutting it."

"What did you think of what he said about children? Splendid, wasn't it?"

"Splendid!"

"And about mysticism, too!"

"Oh, drop mysticism, do!" cried some one else; "think of Ippolit and his fate from this day forth. His wife will scratch his eyes out to-morrow on account of Mitya."

"Is she here?"

"What an idea! If she'd been here she'd have scratched them out in court. She is at home with toothache. He, he, he!"

"He, he, he!"

In a third group:

"I dare say they will acquit Mitenka, after all."

"I should not be surprised if he turns the 'Metropolis' upside down to-morrow. He will be drinking for ten days!"

"Oh, the devil!"

"The devil's bound to have a hand in it. Where should he be if not here?"

"Well, gentlemen, I admit it was eloquent. But still it's not the thing to break your father's head with a steelyard! Or what are we coming to?"

"The chariot! Do you remember the chariot?"

"Yes; he turned a cart into a chariot!"

"And to-morrow he will turn a chariot into a cart, should the need arise."

"What shrewd chaps there are nowadays. Is there any justice among us in Russia, gentlemen, or not?"

But the bell rang. The jury deliberated for exactly an hour, neither more nor less. A profound silence reigned in the court as soon as the public had taken their seats. I remember how the jurymen walked into the court. At last! I won't repeat the questions in order, and, indeed, I have forgotten them. I remember only the answer to the first and chief question of the presiding judge: "Did the accused commit the murder for the sake of robbery and with premeditation?" (I don't remember the exact words.) There was a complete hush. The foreman of the jury, the youngest of the clerks, pronounced, in a clear, loud voice, amidst the deathlike stillness of the court:

"Yes, guilty!"

And the same answer was repeated to every question: "Yes, guilty!" and without the least word of extenuation. This no one had expected; almost every one had reckoned upon a recommendation to mercy, at least. The deathlike silence in the court was not broken

— all seemed petrified: those who had desired his conviction as well as those who had been eager for his acquittal. But that was only for the first instant, and it was followed by fearful confusion. Many of the men in the audience were pleased. Some were rubbing their hands with no attempt to conceal their joy. Those who disagreed with the verdict seemed crushed, shrugged their shoulders, whispered, but still seemed unable to realise it. But good Lord! how shall I describe the state the ladies were in? I thought they would start a mutiny. At first they could scarcely believe their ears. Then suddenly the whole court rang with exclamations: "What's the meaning of it? What next?" They leapt up from their places. They seemed to fancy that the verdict might be at once reconsidered and reversed. At that instant Mitya suddenly stood up and cried in a heart-rending voice, stretching his hands out before him:

"I swear by God and the dreadful Day of Judgment I am not guilty of my father's blood! Katya, I forgive you! Brothers, friends, have pity on the other woman!"

He could not go on, and broke into a terrible sobbing wail that was heard all over the court in a strange, unnatural voice unlike his own. From the farthest corner at the back of the gallery came a piercing shriek — it was Grushenka. She had succeeded in begging admittance to the court again before the beginning of the lawyers' speeches. Mitya was taken away. The pronouncement of the sentence was deferred till next day. The whole court was in hubbub but I did not wait to hear anything further. I only remember a few exclamations I heard on the steps as I went out.

"He'll have a twenty years' spell at the mines!"

"Not less."

"Well, our peasants have stood their ground."

"And have done for our Mitya."

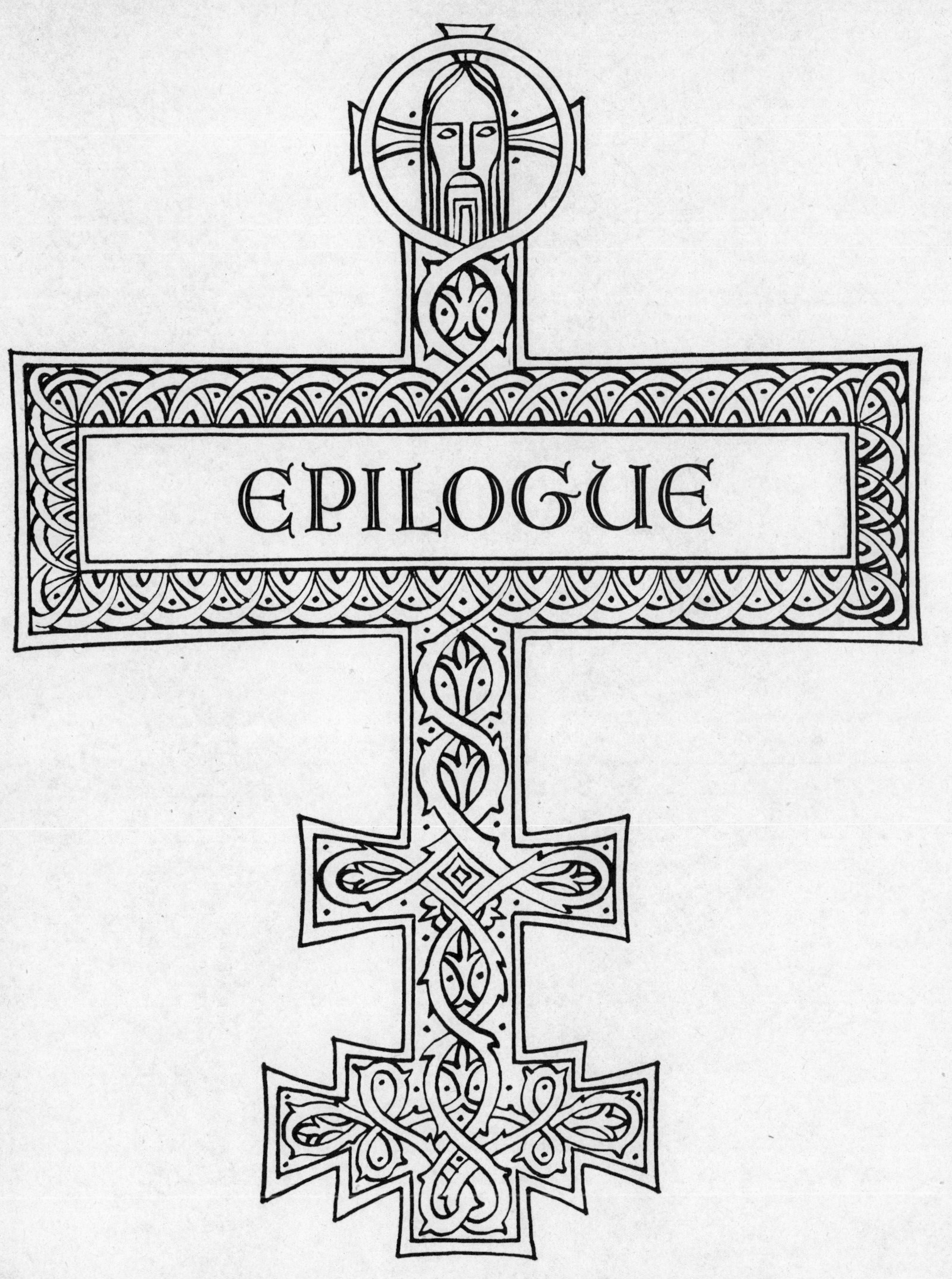
EPILOGUE

CHAPTER I

PLANS FOR SAVING MITYA

VERY early, at nine o'clock in the morning, five days after the trial, Alyosha came to Katerina Ivanovna's to talk over a matter of great importance to both of them, and to give her a message. She sat and talked to him in the very room in which she had once received Grushenka. In the next room Ivan Fyodorovich lay unconscious in a high fever. Immediately after the scene at the trial Katerina Ivanovna had ordered the sick and unconscious man to be carried to her house, disregarding the inevitable gossip and general disapproval of the public. One of the two relations who lived with her had departed to Moscow immediately after the scene at court, the other remained. But if both had gone away, Katerina Ivanovna would have adhered to her resolution, and would have gone on nursing the sick man and sitting by him day and night. Varvinsky and Herzenstube were attending him. The famous doctor had gone back to Moscow, refusing to give an opinion as to the probable outcome of the illness. Though the doctors encouraged Katerina Ivanovna and Alyosha, it was evident that they could not yet give them positive hopes of recovery.

Alyosha came to see his sick brother twice a day. But this time he had specially urgent business, and he foresaw how difficult it would be to approach the subject, yet he was in great haste. He had other and urgent business for that same morning, and there was need of haste.

They had been talking for a quarter of an hour. Katerina Ivanovna was pale and terribly fatigued, yet at the same time in a state of morbid excitement. She had a presentiment of the reason why Alyosha had come to her.

"Don't worry about his decision," she said, with confident emphasis to Alyosha. "One way or another, he is bound to accept this way out. He must escape. This unhappy man, this hero, all honour and conscience — not that one, not Dmitri Fyodorovich, but the man lying the other side of that door, who has sacrificed himself for his brother," Katya added, with flashing eyes, "told me the whole plan of escape long ago. You know he has already entered into negotiations. . . . I've told you something already. . . . You see, it will probably come off at the third halting-place, when the party of convicts is being taken to Siberia. Oh, it will take a long time yet. Ivan Fyodorovich has already visited the official in charge of the third station. But we don't know yet who will be in charge of the party, and it's impossible to find that out so long beforehand. To-morrow perhaps I will show you in detail the whole plan which Ivan Fyodorovich left me on the eve of the trial in case of need. . . . That was when — do you remember? — you found us quarrelling. He had just gone downstairs, but seeing you I made him come back; do you remember? Do you know what we were quarrelling about then?"

"No, I don't," said Alyosha.

"Of course he did not tell you. It was about that plan of escape. He had disclosed the main idea to me three days before, and we began quarrelling about it at once and quarrelled for three days. We quarrelled because when he told me that, if Dmitri Fyodorovich were convicted, he would escape abroad with that creature, I felt furious at once — I can't tell you why, I don't know myself why. . . . Oh, of course, I was furious then because of that creature, and that she, too, should go abroad with Dmitri!" Katerina Ivanovna exclaimed suddenly, her lips quivering with anger. "As soon as Ivan Fyodorovich saw that I was furious because of that woman, he instantly imagined I was jealous of Dmitri, and that I still loved Dmitri. That is how our first quarrel began. I would not give an explanation, I could not ask forgiveness. I could not bear to think that such a man could suspect me of still loving that . . . and when I myself had told him long before that I did not love Dmitri, that I loved no one but him! It was only resentment against that creature that made me angry with him. Three days later, on the evening you came, he brought me a sealed envelope, which I was to open at once, if anything happened to him. Oh, he foresaw his illness! He told me that the envelope contained the details of the escape, and that if he died or was taken dangerously ill, I was to save Mitya alone. Then he left me money, nearly ten thousand — those notes to which the prosecutor referred in his speech, having learnt from some one that he had sent them to be changed. I was tremendously impressed to find that Ivan Fyodorovich had not given up his idea of saving his brother, and was confiding this plan of escape to me, though he was still jealous of me and still convinced that I loved Mitya. Oh, that was a sacrifice! No, you cannot understand the greatness of such self-sacrifice, Alexey Fyodorovich. I wanted to fall at his feet in reverence, but I thought at once that he would take it only for my joy at the thought of Mitya's being saved (and he certainly would have imagined that!), and I was so exasperated at the mere possibility of such an unjust thought on his part that I lost my temper again, and, instead of kissing his feet, made him a scene again! Oh, I am unhappy! It's my character, my awful, unhappy character! Oh, you will see, I shall end by driving him, too, to abandon me for another with whom he can get on better, as Dmitri did. But . . . no, I could not bear it, I should kill myself. And when you came in then, and when I called to you and told him to come back, I was so enraged by the look of contempt and hatred he turned on me that — do you remember? — I cried out to you that it was he, he alone who had persuaded me that his brother Dmitri was a murderer! I told that lie on purpose to wound him again. He had never, never tried to persuade me that his brother was a murderer. On the contrary, it was I who persuaded him! Oh, my vile temper was the cause of everything! I paved the way to that accursed scene at the trial. He wanted to show me that he was an honourable man, and that, even if I loved his brother, he would not ruin him out of revenge or jealousy. So he spoke out in court . . . I am the cause of it all, I alone am to blame!"

Katya never had made such confessions to Alyosha before, and he felt that she was now at that stage of unbearable suffering when even the proudest heart painfully crushes its pride and falls vanquished by grief. Oh, Alyosha knew another terrible reason for her present misery, though she had carefully concealed it from him during those days since the trial; but it would have been for some reason too painful to him if she had been brought so low as to speak to him now about that. She was suffering for her "treachery" at the trial, and Alyosha felt that her conscience was impelling her to confess it to him, to him, Alyosha, with tears and shrieks and hysterical writhings on the floor. But he dreaded that moment and longed to spare her. It made the commission on which he had come even more difficult. He spoke of Mitya again.

"It's all right, it's all right, don't be anxious about him!" she began again, sharply and stubbornly. "All that is only a passing thing with him, I know him, I know his heart only too well. You may be sure he will consent to escape. It's not as though it would be immediately; he will have time to make up his mind to it. Ivan Fyodorovich will be well by that time and will manage it all himself, so that I shall have nothing to do with it. Don't be anxious; he will consent to run away. He has agreed already: do you suppose he would give up that creature? And they won't let her go to Siberia, so he is bound to escape. It's you he's most afraid of, he is afraid you won't approve of his escape on moral grounds. But you must generously *allow* it, if your sanction is so necessary," Katya added viciously. She paused and smiled.

"He talks about some hymn," she went on again, "some cross he has to bear, some duty; I remember Ivan Fyodorovich told me a great deal about it, and if you knew how he talked!" Katya cried suddenly, with irrepressible emotion, "if you knew how he loved that wretched man at the moment he told me, and how he hated him, perhaps, at the same moment. And I, oh, I heard his story and his tears with sneering disdain. Brute! Yes, I am a brute. It is I who gave him that fever. But that man, the convict, is he capable of suffering?" Katya concluded irritably. "Can such a man suffer? Men like him never suffer!"

There was a note of hatred and squeamish contempt in her words. And yet it was she who had betrayed him. "Perhaps because she feels how she's wronged him she hates him at moments," Alyosha thought to himself. He hoped that it was only "at moments." In Katya's last words he detected a challenging note, but he did not take it up.

"I sent for you this morning to make you promise to persuade him yourself. Or do you, too, consider that to escape would be dishonourable, cowardly, or something . . . unchristian, perhaps?" Katya added, even more defiantly.

"Oh, no. I'll tell him everything," muttered Alyosha. "He asks you to come and see him to-day," he blurted out suddenly, looking her steadily in the face. She started, and drew back a little from him on the sofa.

"Me? Can that be?" she faltered, turning pale.

"It can and ought to be!" Alyosha began emphatically, growing more animated. "He needs you particularly just now. I would not have broached the subject and worried you, if it were not necessary. He is ill, he is beside himself, he keeps asking for you. It is not to be reconciled with you that he wants you, but only that you should come and show yourself on his threshold. So much has happened to him since that day. He realises that he is guilty before you beyond all reckoning. He does not ask your forgiveness; 'it's impossible to forgive me,' he says himself, but only that you should show yourself in his doorway."

"It's so sudden . . ." faltered Katya. "I had a presentiment all these days that you would come with that message. I knew he would call me. It's impossible!"

"Let it be impossible, but do it. Only think, he realises for the first time how he has wounded you, the first time in his life; he had never grasped it so fully before. He said, 'If she refuses to come I shall be unhappy all my life.' Do you hear? Though he is condemned to penal servitude for twenty years, he is still planning to be happy — is not that piteous? Think — you shall visit a man who is ruined through no guilt of his own," broke like a challenge from Alyosha. "His hands are clean, there is no blood on them! For the sake of his infinite future suffering, visit him now. Go, see him off on his way into the darkness — stand at his door, that is all. . . . You must do it, you must!" Alyosha concluded, laying immense stress on the word "must."

"I must . . . but I cannot . . ." Katya moaned. "He will look at me. . . . I can't."

"Your eyes ought to meet. How will you live all your life, if you don't make up your mind to do it now?"

"Better suffer all my life."

"You must go, you must go," Alyosha repeated with merciless emphasis.

"But why to-day, why at once? . . . I can't leave the patient . . ."

"You can for a moment. It will be only a moment. If you don't come, he will be delirious by to-night. I would not tell you a lie; have pity on him!"

"Have pity on *me!*" Katya said, with bitter reproach, and she burst into tears.

"Then you will come," said Alyosha firmly, seeing her tears. "I'll go and tell him you will come directly."

"No, don't tell him so on any account," cried Katya in alarm. "I will come, but don't tell him beforehand, for perhaps I may come, but not go in . . . I don't know yet . . ."

Her voice failed her. She gasped for breath. Alyosha got up to go.

"And what if I meet any one?" she said suddenly, in a low voice, turning white again.

"That's just why you must go now, to avoid meeting any one. There will be no one there, I can tell you that for certain. We shall expect you," he concluded emphatically, and went out of the room.

CHAPTER II

FOR A MOMENT THE LIE BECOMES TRUTH

He hurried to the hospital where Mitya was lying now. The day after his sentence was pronounced, Mitya had fallen ill with nervous fever, and was sent to the prison division of the town hospital. But at the request of Alyosha and many other people (Madame Hohlakov, Lise, etc.), Dr. Varvinsky had not put Mitya with other prisoners, but in a separate little room, the one where Smerdyakov had lain. It is true that there was a sentinel at the end of the corridor, and there was a grating over the window, so that Varvinsky could be at ease about the indulgence he had shown, which was not quite legal, indeed; but he was a kind-hearted and compassionate young man. He knew how hard it would be for a man like Mitya to pass at once so suddenly into the society of robbers and murderers, and that he must get used to it by degrees. The visits of relations and friends were informally sanctioned by the doctor and superintendent, and even by the police captain. But only Alyosha and Grushenka had visited Mitya. Rakitin had tried to force his way in twice, but Mitya persistently begged Varvinsky not to admit him.

Alyosha found him sitting on his bed in a hospital dressing-gown, rather feverish, with a towel, soaked in vinegar and water, round his head. He looked at Alyosha as he came in with an undefined expression, but there was a shade of something like dread discernible in it. He had become terribly thoughtful since the trial; sometimes he would be silent for half an hour together, and seemed to be pondering something heavily and painfully, oblivious to everything about him. If he roused himself from his brooding and began to talk, he always spoke with a kind of abruptness and never of what he really wanted to say. He looked sometimes with a face of suffering at his brother. He seemed to be more at ease with Grushenka than with Alyosha. It is true, he scarcely spoke to her at all, but as soon as she came in, his whole face lighted up with joy.

Alyosha sat down beside him on the bed in silence. This time Mitya was waiting for Alyosha in suspense, but he did not dare ask him a question. He felt it almost unthinkable that Katya would consent to come, and at the same time he felt that if she did not come, something utterly impossible would happen. Alyosha understood his feelings.

"Trifon Borisovich," Mitya began nervously, "has pulled his whole inn to pieces, I am told. He's taken up the flooring, pulled apart the planks, split up the whole gallery, I am told. He is seeking the treasure — the fifteen hundred roubles which the prosecutor said I'd hidden there. He began playing these tricks, they say, as soon as he got home. Serve him right, the swindler! The guard here told me yesterday; he comes from there."

"Listen," began Alyosha. "She will come, but I don't know when. Perhaps to-day, perhaps in a few days, that I can't tell. But she will come, she will, that's certain."

Mitya started, would have said something, but was silent. The news had a tremendous effect on him. It was evident that he would have liked terribly to know in detail what had been said, but he was again afraid to ask. Something cruel and contemptuous from Katya would have cut him like a knife.

"This was what she said among other things; that I must be sure to set your conscience at rest about escaping. If Ivan is not well by then she will see to it all herself."

"You've spoken of that already," Mitya observed musingly.

"And you have repeated it to Grusha," observed Alyosha.

"Yes," Mitya admitted. "She won't come this morning." He looked timidly at his brother. "She won't come till the evening. When I told her yesterday that Katya was taking measures, she was silent, but her lips twitched. She only whispered, 'Let her!' She understood that it was important. I did not dare to try her further. She understands now, I think, that Katya no longer cares for me, but loves Ivan."

"Does she?" broke from Alyosha.

"Perhaps she does not. Only she is not coming this morning," Mitya hastened to explain again; "I asked her to do something for me. You know, brother Ivan will outstrip all. He ought to live, not we. He will recover."

"Would you believe it, though Katya trembles for him, she scarcely doubts of his recovery," said Alyosha.

"That means that she is convinced he will die. It's because she is frightened she's so sure he will get well."

"Ivan has a strong constitution, and I, too, believe there's every hope that he will get well," Alyosha observed with alarm.

"Yes, he will get well. But she is convinced that he will die. She has a great deal of sorrow to bear. . ."

A silence followed. A grave anxiety was fretting Mitya.

"Alyosha, I love Grusha terribly," he said suddenly in a shaking voice, full of tears.

"They won't let her go out there to you," Alyosha put in at once.

"And there is something else I wanted to tell you," Mitya went on, with a sudden ring in his voice. "If they start beating me on the way or out there, I won't submit to it. I shall kill some one, and shall be shot for it. And this will be going on for twenty years! They begin to speak rudely to me as it is. The guards do it. I've been lying here all night, passing judgment on myself. I am not ready! I haven't the strength to accept my fate. I wanted to sing a 'hymn'; but if a guard speaks rudely to me, I have not the strength to bear it. For Grusha I would bear anything . . . anything except blows. . . . But they won't let her come *there*."

Alyosha smiled gently.

"Listen, brother, once for all," he said. This is what I think about it. And you know that I would not tell you a lie. Listen: you are not ready, and such a cross is not for you. What's more, you don't need such a martyr's cross when you are not ready for it. If you had murdered our father, it would grieve me that you should reject your punishment. But you are innocent, and such a cross is too much for you. You wanted to make yourself another man by suffering. I say, only remember that other man always, all your life and wherever you may escape to; and that will be enough for you. Your refusal of that great cross will only serve to make you feel all your life an even greater duty, and that constant feeling will do more to make you a new man, perhaps, than if you went *there*. For there you would not endure it and would rebel, and perhaps at last would say: 'I am quits.' The lawyer was right about that. Such heavy burdens are not for all men. For some they are impossible. These are my thoughts about it, if you want them so much. If other men would have to answer for your escape, officers or soldiers, then I would not have 'allowed' you," smiled Alyosha. "But they declare — the superintendent of that station told Ivan himself — that if it's well managed there will be no great inquiry, and that they can get off easily. Of course, bribing is dishonest even in such a case, but I can't undertake to judge about it, because if Ivan and Katya commissioned me to act for you, I know I should go and give bribes. I must tell you the truth. And so I can't judge of your own action. But let me assure you that I shall never condemn you. And it would be a strange thing if I could judge you in this. Now I think I've gone into everything."

"But I shall condemn myself!" cried Mitya. "I shall escape, that was settled apart from you; could Mitya Karamazov do anything but run away? But I shall condemn myself, and I will pray for my sin for ever. That's how the Jesuits talk, isn't it? Just as we are doing?"

"Yes." Alyosha smiled gently.

"I love you for always telling the whole truth and never hiding anything," cried Mitya, with a joyful laugh. "So I've caught my Alyosha being Jesuitical. I must kiss you for that. Now listen to the rest; I'll open the other side of my heart to you. This is what I planned and decided. If I run away, even with money and a passport, and even to America, I should be cheered up by the thought that I am not running away for pleasure, not for happiness, but to another form of forced labor as bad, perhaps, as Siberia. It is as bad, Alyosha, it is! I hate that America, damn it, already. Even though Grusha will be with me. Just look at her; is she an American? She is Russian, Russian to the bone; she will be homesick for her own country, and I shall see every hour that she is suffering for my sake, that she has taken up that cross for me. And what harm has she done? And how shall I, too, put up with the rabble out there, though they may be better than I, every one of them. I hate that America already! And though they may be wonderful at machinery, every one of them, damn them, they are not my kind, they are strangers to my soul. I love Russia, Alyosha, I love the Russian God, though I am a scoundrel myself. I shall croak there!" he exclaimed, his eyes suddenly flashing. His voice was trembling with tears. "So this is what I've decided, Alyosha, listen," he began again, mastering his emotion. "As soon as I arrive there with Grusha, we will set to work at once on the land, in solitude, in some remote place, with wild bears. There must be some remote parts even there. I am told there are still redskins there, somewhere, on the edge of the horizon. So off to that country, to the 'Last of the Mohicans,' and there we'll tackle the grammar at once, Grusha and I. Work and grammar — that's how we'll spend three years. And by that time we shall speak English like any Englishman. And as soon as we've learnt it — good-bye to America! We'll flee here, to Russia, as American citizens. Don't be uneasy — we would not come to this little town. We'd hide somewhere, a long way off, in the north or in the south. I shall be changed by that time, and she will, too, in America. A doctor will make me some sort of wart on my face — it's not for nothing that they're such mechanics! — or else I'll put out one eye, let my beard grow a yard, and I shall turn grey, fretting for Russia. I dare say they won't recognise us. And if they do, let them send us to Siberia — I don't care. It will show it's our fate. We'll work on the land here, too, somewhere in the wilds, and I'll pretend to be an American all my life. But we shall die on our native soil. That's my plan, and it shan't be altered. Do you approve?"

"Yes," said Alyosha, not wanting to contradict him. Mitya paused for a minute and said suddenly: "And how they worked it up at the trial! Didn't they work it up!"

"If they had not, you would have been convicted just the same," said Alyosha, with a sigh.

"Yes, people are sick of me here! God bless them, but it's hard," Mitya moaned miserably. Again there was silence for a minute.

"Alyosha, knife me at once!" he exclaimed suddenly. "Tell me, is she coming now, or not? Tell me? What did she say? How did she say it?"

"She said she would come, but I don't know whether she will come to-day. It's hard for her, you know." Alyosha looked timidly at his brother.

"I should think it is hard for her! Alyosha, it will drive me out of my mind. Grusha keeps looking at me. She understands. My God, calm my heart: what is it I want? I want Katya! Do I understand what I want? It's the headstrong, evil Karamazov spirit! No, I am not fit for suffering. I am a scoundrel, that's all one can say."

"Here she is!" cried Alyosha.

At that instant Katya appeared in the doorway. For a moment she stood still, gazing at Mitya with a lost look, as it were. He leapt impulsively to his feet, and a scared look came into his face. He turned pale, but a timid, pleading smile appeared on his lips at once, and with an irresistible impulse he held out both hands to Katya. Seeing it, she flew impetuously to him. She seized him by the hands, and almost by force made him sit down on the bed. She sat down beside him, and still keeping his hands pressed them violently, convulsively. Several times they both strove to speak, but stopped short and again gazed speechless with a strange smile, their eyes fastened on each other. So passed two minutes.

"Have you forgiven me?" Mitya faltered at last, and at the same moment turning to Alyosha, his face working with joy, he cried, "Do you hear what I am asking, do you hear?"

"That's what I loved you for, that you are generous at heart!" broke from Katya. "My forgiveness is no good to you, nor yours to me; whether you forgive me or not, you will always be a wound in my heart, and I in yours — and so it ought to be. . . ." She stopped to take breath. "What have I come for?" she began again frantically and hastily: "to embrace your feet, to press your hands like this, till it hurts — you remember how in Moscow I used to squeeze them — to tell you again that you are my god, my joy, to tell you that I love you madly," she moaned in anguish, and suddenly pressed her lips greedily to his hand. Tears streamed from her eyes. Alyosha stood speechless and confounded; he had never expected what he was seeing.

"Love is over, Mitya!" Katya began again, "but the past is painfully dear to me. Know that will always be so. But now let what might have been come true for one minute," she faltered, with a crooked smile, looking into his face joyfully again. "You love another woman now, and I love another man, and yet I shall love you for ever, and you will love me; do you know that? Do you hear? Love me, love me all your life!" she cried, with a quiver, almost of menace, in her voice.

"I shall love you, and . . . do you know, Katya," Mitya began, drawing a deep breath at each word, "do you know, five days ago, that same evening, I loved you. . . . When you fell down and were carried out . . . All my life! So it will be, so it will always be."

So they murmured to each other words almost meaningless, and frantic, perhaps not even true, but at that moment it was all true, and they both believed implicitly what they said.

"Katya," cried Mitya suddenly, "do you believe I killed? I know you don't believe it now, but then . . . when you testified. . . . Could you, could you have believed it?"

"I did not believe it even then. I've never believed it. I hated you, and for a moment I persuaded myself. While I was testifying I persuaded myself and believed it, but when I'd finished speaking I left off believing it at once. Don't doubt that! I have forgotten that I came here to punish myself," she said, with a new expression in her voice, quite unlike the loverly tones of a moment before.

"Woman, yours is a heavy burden," broke, as it were, involuntarily from Mitya.

"Let me go," she whispered. "I'll come again. It's more than I can bear now."

She was getting up from her place, but suddenly uttered a loud scream and staggered back. Grushenka walked suddenly and noiselessly into the room. No one had expected her. Katya moved swiftly to the door, but when she reached Grushenka, she stopped suddenly, turned as white as chalk, and moaned softly, almost in a whisper:

"Forgive me!"

Grushenka stared at her and, pausing for an instant, in a vindictive, venomous voice, answered:

"We are full of hatred, my girl, you and I! We are both full of hatred! As though we could forgive each other! Save him, and I'll worship you all my life."

"You won't forgive her!" cried Mitya, with frantic reproach.

"Don't be anxious, I'll save him for you!" Katya whispered rapidly, and ran out of the room.

"And you could refuse to forgive her when she begged your forgiveness herself?" Mitya exclaimed bitterly again.

"Mitya, don't dare to reproach her; you have no right to!" Alyosha cried hotly.

"Her proud lips spoke, not her heart," Grushenka brought out in a tone of disgust. "If she saves you I'll forgive her everything . . ."

She stopped speaking, as though suppressing something. She could not yet recover herself. She had come in, as appeared afterwards, accidentally, with no suspicion, no expectation of what she would meet.

"Alyosha, run after her!" Mitya cried to his brother; "tell her . . . I don't know . . . don't let her go away like this!"

"I'll come to you again at nightfall," said Alyosha, and he ran after Katya. He overtook her outside the hospital grounds. She was walking fast, but as soon as Alyosha caught up with her she said quickly:

"No, before that woman I can't punish myself! I asked her forgiveness because I wanted to punish myself to the bitter end. She would not forgive me. . . . I love her for that!" she added, in an unnatural voice, and her eyes flashed with fierce resentment.

"My brother did not expect this in the least," muttered Alyosha. "He was sure she would not come . . ."

"No doubt. Let us leave that," she snapped. "Listen: I can't go with you to the funeral now. I've sent them flowers. I think they still have money. If necessary, tell them I'll never abandon them. . . . Now leave me, leave me, please. You are late as it is — the bells are ringing for the service. . . . Leave me, please!"

CHAPTER III

ILUSHA'S FUNERAL. THE SPEECH AT THE STONE

He really was late. They had waited for him and had already decided to bear the pretty flower-decked little coffin to the church without him. It was the coffin of poor little Ilusha. He had died two days after Mitya was sentenced. At the gate of the house Alyosha was met by the shouts of the boys, Ilusha's schoolfellows. They had all been impatiently expecting him and were glad that he had come at last. There were about twelve of them, they all had their school-bags or satchels on their shoulders. "Papa will cry, be with papa," Ilusha had told them as he lay dying, and the boys remembered it. Kolya Krasotkin was at the head of them.

"How glad I am you've come, Karamazov!" he cried, holding out his hand to Alyosha. "It's awful here. It's really painful to see it. Snegiryov is not drunk, we know for a fact he's had nothing to drink to-day, but he behaves as if he were drunk. . . . I always have a grip on myself, but this is awful. Karamazov, if I am not keeping you, one question before you go in?"

"What is it, Kolya?" said Alyosha.

"Is your brother innocent or guilty? Was it he killed your father or was it the valet? As you say, so it will be. I haven't slept for the last four nights thinking of it."

"The valet killed him, my brother is innocent," answered Alyosha.

"That's what I said," cried Smurov.

"So he will perish for the truth, an innocent victim!" exclaimed Kolya; "though he is ruined he is happy! I am ready to envy him!"

"What do you mean? How can you? And what for?" cried Alyosha, surprised.

"Oh, if I, too, could sacrifice myself some day for truth!" said Kolya with enthusiasm.

"But not in such a cause, not with such disgrace and such horror!" said Alyosha.

"Of course . . . I should like to die for all humanity, and as for disgrace, I don't care about that — let our names perish. I respect your brother!"

"And so do I!" the boy who had once declared that he knew who had founded Troy cried suddenly and unexpectedly and he blushed up to his ears like a peony as he had done on that occasion.

Alyosha went into the room. Ilusha lay with his hands folded and his eyes closed, in a blue coffin with a white frill round it. The features of his emaciated face were hardly altered at all, and, strange to say, there was no smell of decay from the corpse. The expression of his face was serious and, as it were, thoughtful. His hands, crossed over his breast, looked particularly beautiful, as though chiselled in marble. There were flowers in his hands and the coffin, inside and out, was decked with flowers, which had been sent early in the morning by Lise Hohlakov. But there were flowers, too, from Katerina Ivanovna, and when Alyosha opened the door, the captain had a bunch in his trembling hands and was strewing them again over his dear boy. He scarcely glanced at Alyosha when he came in, and he would not look at any one, even at his crazy weeping wife, "mamma," who kept trying to stand on her crippled legs to get a closer look at her dead boy. As for Nina, the boys had pushed her in her chair close up to the coffin. She sat with her head pressed against it and she, too, was no doubt quietly weeping. Snegiryov's face looked eager, yet bewildered and exasperated. There was something witless about his gestures and the words that broke from him. "Old man, dear old man!" he exclaimed every minute, gazing at Ilusha. It had been his habit to call Ilusha "old man" as a term of affection when he was alive.

"Father, give me a flower, too; take that white one out of his hand and give it me," the crazy mother begged, whimpering. Either because the little white rose in Ilusha's hand had caught her fancy or because she wanted one from his hand to keep in memory of him, she shifted restlessly, stretching out her hands for the flower.

"I won't give it to any one, I won't give you anything," Snegiryov cried callously. "They are his flowers, not yours! Everything is his, nothing is yours!"

"Father, give mother a flower!" said Nina, lifting her face wet with tears.

"I won't give away anything and to her less than any one! She didn't love Ilusha. She took away his little cannon and he gave it to her." The captain broke into loud sobs at the thought of how Ilusha had given up his cannon to his mother. The poor crazy creature was bathed in noiseless tears, hiding her face in her hands.

The boys, seeing that the father would not leave the coffin and that it was time to carry it out, stood round it in a close circle and began to lift it up.

"I don't want him to be buried in the

churchyard," Snegiryov wailed suddenly; "I'll bury him by the stone, by our stone! Ilusha told me to. I won't let him be carried out!"

He had been saying for the last three days that he would bury him by the stone, but Alyosha, Krasotkin, the landlady, her sister, and all the boys interfered.

"What an idea, bury him by an unholy stone, as though he had hanged himself," the old landlady said sternly. "There in the churchyard the ground is consecrated. He'll be prayed for there. One can hear the singing in church and the deacon reads so clearly and distinctly that it will reach him every time just as though it were read over his grave."

At last the captain made a gesture of despair, as though to say, "Take him where you will." The boys raised the coffin, but as they passed the mother they stopped for a moment and lowered it that she might say good-bye to Ilusha. But on seeing that precious little face, which for the last three days she had only looked at from a distance, she trembled all over and her grey head began twitching spasmodically over the coffin.

"Mother, make the sign of the cross over him, give him your blessing, kiss him," Nina cried to her. But her head still twitched like that of an automaton and with a face contorted with bitter grief she began, without a word, beating her breast with her fist. They carried the coffin past her. Nina pressed her lips to her brother's for the last time as they bore the coffin by her. As Alyosha went out of the house he begged the landlady to look after those who were left behind, but she interrupted him before he had finished. "To be sure, I'll stay with them, we are Christians, too." The old woman wept as she said it.

They had not far to carry the coffin to the church, not more than three hundred paces. It was a still clear day, with a slight frost. The church bells were still ringing. Snegiryov, distraught and forlorn, ran after the coffin, in his short old overcoat, almost as thin as a summer one, with his head bare and his soft, old, wide-brimmed hat in his hand. He seemed endlessly fretted. At one minute he stretched out his hand to support the head of the coffin and only hindered the bearers, at another he ran alongside and tried to find a place for himself there. A flower fell on the snow and he rushed to pick it up as though everything in the world depended on the loss of that flower.

"And the crust of bread, we've forgotten the crust!" he cried suddenly in terrible dismay. But the boys reminded him at once that he had taken the crust of bread already and that it was in his pocket. He instantly pulled it out and was reassured.

"Ilusha told me to, Ilusha," he explained at once to Alyosha. "I was sitting by him one night and he suddenly told me: 'Papa, when my grave is filled up crumble a piece of bread on it so that the sparrows may fly down, I shall hear and it will cheer me up not to be lying alone.' "

"That's a good thing," said Alyosha, "we must often take some."

"Every day, every day!" said the captain quickly, growing animated, as it were.

They reached the church at last and set the coffin in the middle of it. The boys surrounded it and remained reverently standing so, all through the service. It was an ancient and rather poor church. Many of the ikons were without settings but such churches are the best for praying in. During the mass Snegiryov became somewhat calmer, though at times he had outbursts of the same unconscious and, as it were, incoherent anxiety. At one moment he went up to the coffin to set straight the pall or the chaplet, when a candle fell out of the candlestick he rushed to replace it and was a fearful time fumbling over it, then he subsided and stood quietly by the coffin with a look of blank uneasiness and perplexity. After the passage from the Epistle he suddenly whispered to Alyosha, who was standing beside him, that it had not been read properly but did not explain what he meant. During the prayer, "Like the Cherubim," he joined in the singing but he did not go on to the end. Falling on his knees, he pressed his forehead to the stone floor and lay so for a long while.

At last came the funeral service itself and candles were distributed. The crazed father began fussing about again, but the touching and impressive funeral prayers moved and shook his soul. He seemed suddenly to shrink together and broke into rapid, short sobs, which he tried at first to smother, but at last he sobbed aloud. When they began taking leave of the dead and closing the coffin, he flung his arms about, as though he would not allow them to cover Ilusha, and began greedily and persistently kissing his dead boy on the lips. At last they succeeded in persuading him to come away from the step, but suddenly he impulsively stretched out his hand and snatched a few flowers from the coffin. He looked at them and a new idea seemed to dawn upon him, so that he apparently forgot his grief for a minute. Gradually he seemed to sink into brooding and did not resist when the coffin was lifted up and carried to the grave. It was an expensive one in the churchyard close to the church, Katerina Ivanovna had paid for it. After the customary rites the grave-diggers lowered the coffin. Snegiryov with his flowers in his hands bent down so low over the open grave that the boys caught hold of his coat in alarm and pulled him back. But he did not seem to understand fully what was happening. When they began filling up the grave, he suddenly pointed anxiously at the falling earth and began trying to say something, but no one could make out what he meant, and he grew quiet suddenly. Then he was reminded that he must crumble the bread and he was awfully excited, snatched up the bread and began pulling it to pieces and flinging the morsels on the grave.

"Come, fly down, birds, fly down, sparrows!" he muttered anxiously.

One of the boys observed that it was awkward for him to crumble the bread with the flowers in his hands and suggested he should give them to some one to hold for a time. But he would not do this and seemed indeed suddenly alarmed for his flowers, as though they wanted to take them from him altogether. And after looking at the grave and, as it were, satisfying himself that everything had been done and the bread had been crumbled, he suddenly, to the surprise of every one, turned, quite composedly even, and made his way homewards. But his steps became more and more hurried, he almost ran. The boys and Alyosha kept up with him.

"The flowers are for mamma, the flowers are for mamma! We were unkind to mamma," he began exclaiming suddenly.

Some one called to him to put on his hat as it was cold. But he flung the hat in the snow as though he were angry and kept repeating, "I don't want the hat, I don't want the hat." Smurov picked it up and carried it after him. All the boys were crying, and Kolya and the boy who had discovered Troy most of all. Though Smurov with the captain's hat in his hand, was crying bitterly, too, he managed, as he ran, to snatch up a piece of red brick that lay on the snow of the path, to fling it at the flock of sparrows that was flying by. He missed them, of course, and went on crying as he ran. Half way, Snegiryov suddenly stopped, stood still for a half a minute, as though struck by something, and, suddenly turning back to the church, ran towards the deserted grave. But the boys instantly overtook him and, surrounding him, caught hold of him. Then he fell helpless on the snow as though he had been knocked down, and struggling, sobbing, and wailing, he began crying out, "Ilusha, old man, dear old man!" Alyosha and Kolya tried to lift him up, soothing and persuading him.

"Captain, give over, a brave man must bear up," muttered Kolya.

"You'll spoil the flowers," said Alyosha, "and mamma is expecting them, she is sitting crying because you would not give her any before. Ilusha's little bed is still there . . ."

"Yes, yes, mamma!" Snegiryov suddenly recollected; "they'll take away the bed, they'll take it away," he added as though afraid that they really would. He jumped up and ran homewards again. But it was not far off and they all arrived together. Snegiryov opened the door hurriedly and called to his wife, with whom he had so cruelly quarrelled just before:

"Mamma, darling, oh, your poor legs, Ilusha has sent you these flowers!" he cried, holding out to her a little bunch of flowers that had been frozen and broken while he was struggling in the snow. But at that instant he saw in the corner, by the little bed, Ilusha's little boots, which the landlady had put tidily side by side. Seeing the old, patched, rusty-looking, stiff boots he flung up his hands and rushed to them, fell on his knees, snatched up one boot and, pressing his lips to it, began kissing it greedily, crying, "Ilusha, old man, dear old man, where are your little feet?"

"Where have you taken him to? Where have you taken him?" the lunatic cried in a heart-rending voice. Nina, too, broke into sobs. Kolya ran out of the room, the boys followed him. At last Alyosha, too, went out.

"Let them weep," he said to Kolya, "it's no use trying to comfort them just now. Let us wait a minute and then go back."

"No, it's no use, it's awful," Kolya assented. "Do you know, Karamazov," he dropped his voice so that no one could hear them, "I feel dreadfully sad, and if it were only possible to raise him from the dead, I'd give anything in the world to do it."

"Ah, so would I," said Alyosha.

"What do you think, Karamazov, had we better come back here to-night? He'll be drunk, you know."

"Perhaps he will. Let us come together, you and I, that will be enough, to spend an hour with them, with the mother and Nina. If we all come together we shall remind them of everything again," Alyosha suggested.

"The landlady is laying the table for them now — there'll be a funeral feast or something, the priest is coming; shall we go back to it, Karamazov?"

"Of course," said Alyosha.

"It's all so strange, Karamazov, such sorrow and suddenly pancakes, it all seems so unnatural the way we do it, according to our religion."

"They are going to have salmon, too," the boy who had discovered Troy observed in a loud voice.

"I beg you most earnestly, Kartashov, not to interrupt again with your idiotic remarks, especially when one is not talking to you and doesn't care to know whether you exist or not!" Kolya snapped out irritably. The boy flushed crimson but did not dare to make any reply.

Meantime they were strolling slowly along the path and suddenly Smurov exclaimed:

"There's Ilusha's stone, under which they wanted to bury him."

They all stood still by the big stone. Alyosha looked and the whole picture of what Snegiryov had described to him that day, how Ilusha, weeping and hugging his father, had cried, "Papa, papa, how he insulted you," rose at once before his imagination. Something suddenly shook his soul, as it were. With a serious and grave expression he looked from one to another of the dear, bright faces of Ilusha's school-fellows, and suddenly said to them:

"Boys, I should like to say one word to you, here on this spot."

The boys stood round him and at once bent attentive and expectant eyes upon him.

"Boys, we shall soon part. I shall be for some time with my two brothers, of whom one is going to Siberia and the other is lying at death's door. But soon I shall leave this town, perhaps for a long time, so we shall part. Let us make a compact, here, at Ilusha's stone, that we will never forget first, Ilusha, and, second, each other. And whatever happens to us later in life, even if we don't meet for twenty years, let us always remember how we buried the poor boy at whom we once threw stones — do you remember, by the bridge? — and afterwards we all grew so fond of him. He was a fine boy, a kind-hearted, brave boy, he felt for his father's honour and resented the cruel insult to him and stood up for him. And so, in the first place, we will remember him, boys, all our lives. And even if we are occupied with most important things, if we attain to honour or meet with great misfortune — still let us remember how good it was once here, when we were all together, united by a good and kind feeling which made us, for the time we were loving that poor boy, better perhaps than we are in reality. My little doves — let me call you so, for you are very like them, those pretty blue birds, at this minute as I look at your good dear faces. My dear children, perhaps you won't understand what I am saying to you, because I often speak very unintelligibly, but you'll remember it all the same and will agree with my words some day. You must know that there is nothing higher and stronger and more wholesome and useful for life in after years than some good memory, especially a memory connected with childhood, with home. People talk to you a great deal about your education, but some fine, sacred memory, preserved from childhood, is perhaps the best education. If a man carries many such memories with him into life, he is safe to the end of his days, and if we have only one good memory left in our hearts, even that may sometime be the means of saving us. Perhaps we may even grow wicked later on, may be unable to refrain from a bad action, may laugh at men's tears and at those people who say as Kolya did just now, 'I want to suffer for all men,' and may even jeer spitefully at such people. But however bad we may become — which God forbid — yet, when we recall how we buried Ilusha, how we loved him in his last days, and how we have been talking like friends all together, at this stone, then the cruellest and most mock-

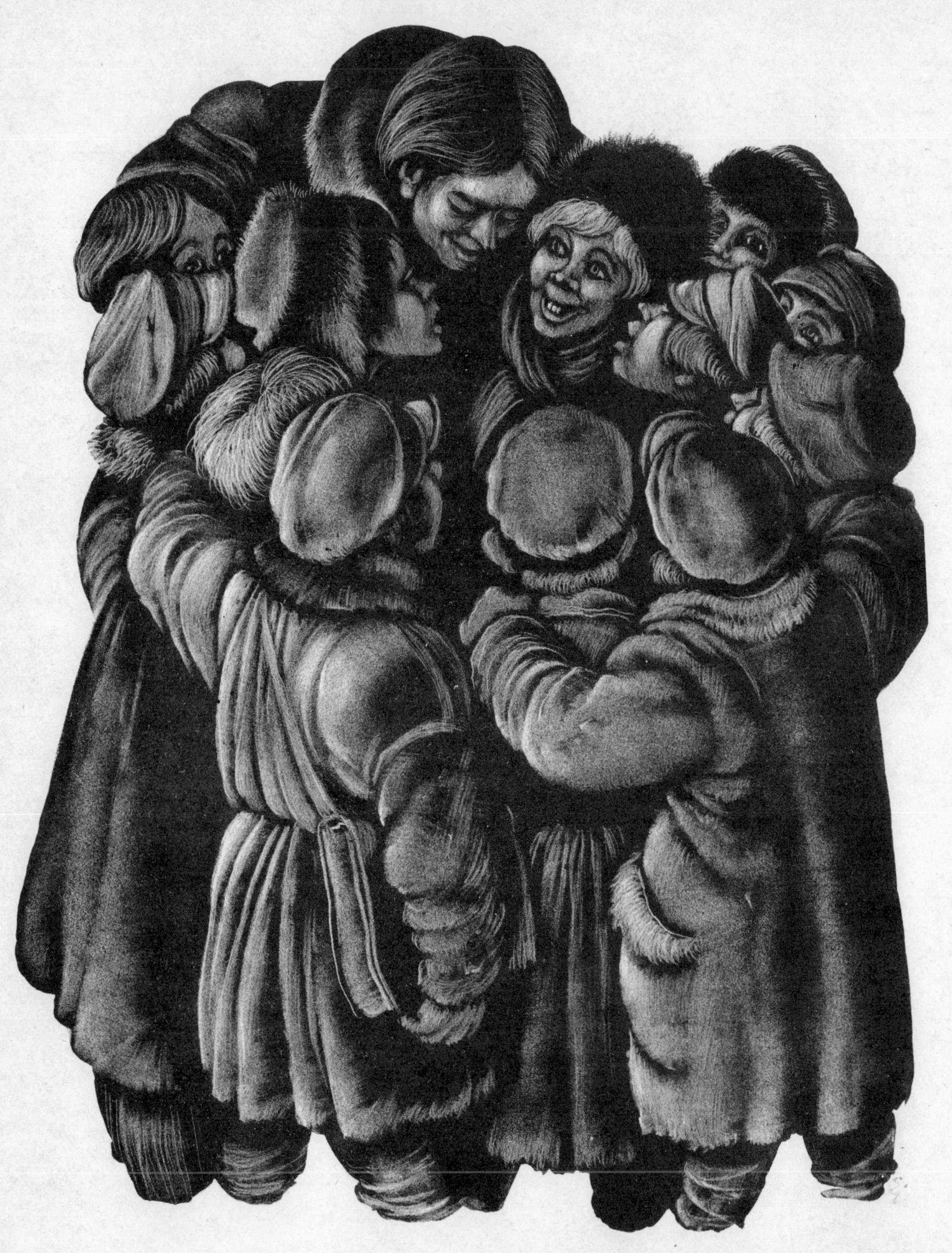

"HURRAH FOR KARAMAZOV!"

ing of us — if we do become so — will not dare to laugh inwardly at having been kind and good at this moment! What's more, perhaps, that one memory may keep him from great evil and he will reflect and say, 'Yes, I was good and brave and honest then!' Let him laugh to himself, that's no matter, a man often laughs at what's good and kind. That's only out of frivolity. But I assure you, boys, that as he laughs he will say at once in his heart, 'No, I do wrong to laugh, for that's not a thing to laugh at.' "

"That will be so, I understand you, Karamazov!" cried Kolya, with flashing eyes.

The boys were excited and they, too, wanted to say something, but they restrained themselves, looking with intentness and emotion at the speaker.

"I say this in case we become bad," Alyosha went on, "but there's no reason why we should become bad, is there, boys? Let us be, first and above all, kind, then honest, and then let us never forget each other! I say that again. I give you my word for my part that I'll never forget one of you. Every face looking at me now I shall remember even for thirty years. Just now Kolya said to Kartashov that we did not care to know whether he exists or not. But I cannot forget that Kartashov exists and that he is not blushing now as he did when he discovered Troy, but is looking at me with his jolly, kind, dear little eyes. Boys, my dear boys, let us all be generous and brave like Ilusha, intelligent, brave, and generous like Kolya (though he will be ever so much more intelligent when he is grown up), and let us all be as modest, as clever and sweet as Kartashov. But why am I talking about those two! You are all dear to me, boys, from this day forth, I shall shut you all in my heart, and I beg you to shut me within your hearts! Well, and who has united us in this kind, good feeling which we shall remember and intend to remember all our lives? Who, if not Ilusha, the good boy, the dear boy, precious to us for ever! Let us never forget him. May his memory live for ever in our hearts from this time forth and for evermore!"

"Yes, yes, for ever, for ever!" the boys cried in their ringing voices, with softened faces.

"Let us remember his face and his clothes and his poor little boots, his coffin and his unhappy, sinful father, and how boldly he stood up for him alone against the whole school."

"We will remember, we will remember," cried the boys. "He was brave, he was good!"

"Ah, how I loved him!" exclaimed Kolya.

"Ah, children, ah, dear friends, don't be afraid of life! How good life is when one does something good and true!"

"Yes, yes," the boys repeated enthusiastically.

"Karamazov, we love you!" a voice, probably Kartashov's, cried impulsively.

"We love you, we love you!" they all caught it up. There were tears in the eyes of many of them.

"Hurrah for Karamazov!" Kolya shouted ecstatically.

"And may the dead boy's memory live for ever!" Alyosha added again with feeling.

"For ever!" the boys chimed in again.

"Karamazov," cried Kolya, "can it be true what's taught us in religion, that we shall all rise again from the dead and shall live and see each other again, all, Ilusha, too?"

"Certainly we shall all rise again, certainly we shall see each other and shall tell each other with joy and gladness all that has happened!"

Alyosha answered, half laughing, half enthusiastic.

"Ah, how splendid it will be!" broke from Kolya.

"Well, now we will finish talking and go to his funeral feast. Don't be put out at our eating pancakes — it's an old, old custom and there's something good in that!" laughed Alyosha. "Well, let us go! And now we go hand in hand."

"And always so, all our lives hand in hand! Hurrah for Karamazov!" Kolya cried once more rapturously, and once more the boys took up his exclamation.